Movement Disorders

Notice

Movement Disorders

Third Edition

Editors

Ray L. Watts, MD
John N. Whitaker Professor and Chairman of Neurology
Director of Clinical Research
Parkinson's Disease and Movement Disorder Research Program
University of Alabama at Birmingham

David G. Standaertt, MD, PhD
John and Juanelle Strain Professor of Neurology
Director, Program for Neurodegeneration and Experimental Therapeutics
Director, Movement Disorders Program
Vice-Chair of Neurology
University of Alabama at Birmingham

Jose A. Obeso, MD
Consultant and Professor of Neurology
Clinica Universitaria and Medical School
Senior Researcher, Neuroscience, CIMA
University of Navarra
Pamplona, Spain

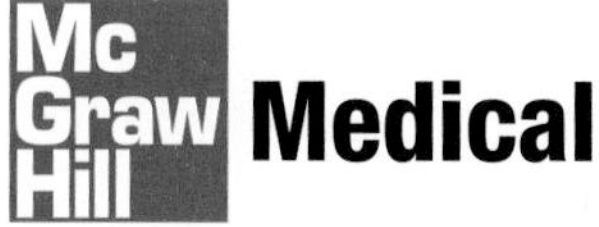

New York Chicago San Francisco Lisbon London Madrid Mexico City Milan
New Delhi San Juan Seoul Singapore Sydney Toronto

The McGraw-Hill Companies

Movement Disorders, Third Edition

1 2 3 4 5 6 7 8 9 0 CTP/CTP 15 14 13 12 11

Set ISBN 978-0-07-161310-1
Set MHID 0-07-161310-2

Book ISBN 978-0-07-161312-5
Book MHID 0-07-161312-9

DVD ISBN 978-0-07-161313-2
DVD MHID 0-07-161313-7

This book was set in ITC Garamond by Thomson Digital.
The editors were Anne M. Sydor and Christie Naglieri.
The production supervisor was Sherri Souffrance.
Project management was provided by Aakriti Kathuria, Thomson Digital.
The index was prepared by Thomson Digital.
China Translation & Printing, Ltd. was printer and binder.

This book is printed on acid-free paper.

Library of Congress Cataloging-in-Publication Data

Movement disorders / editors, Ray L. Watts, David G. Standaertt,
Jose A. Obeso. — 3rd ed.
p. ; cm.
Includes bibliographical references and index.
ISBN-13: 978-0-07-161310-1 (set)
ISBN-13: 978-0-07-161312-5 (hardcover : alk. paper)
ISBN-10: 0-07-161312-9 (hardcover : alk. paper)
ISBN-13: 978-0-07-161313-2 (dvd)
[etc.]
1. Movement disorders. I. Watts, Ray L. (Ray Lannom), 1953- II.
Standaertt, David G. III. Obeso, J. A.
[DNLM: 1. Movement Disorders. WL 390]
RC376.5.M69 2011
616.8'3—dc22

2010027858

CONTENTS

SECTION III CLINICAL DISORDERS

I. PARKINSONIAN STATES: PARKINSON'S DISEASE

OTHER PARKINSONIAN SYNDROMES

II. PARKINSONIAN STATES: AKINETIC-RIGID SYNDROMES

CONTRIBUTORS

Octavian R. Adam, MD
LCDR, MC, USN
Division of Neurology
Naval Medical Center Portsmouth
Portsmouth, Virginia

Amy W. Amara, MD, PhD
Francis and Ingeborg Heide Schumann Fellow in Parkinson Disease Research
Department of Neurology
University of Alabama at Birmingham
Birmingham, Alabama

Urmas Arumäe, PhD
Docent, Group Leader
Centre of Excellence for Molecular and Integrated Neuroscience Research, Institute of Biotechnology
University of Helsinki
Helsinki, Finland

Erika F. Augustine, MD
Senior Instructor
Department of Neurology and Department of Pediatrics
University of Rochester Medical Center
Rochester, New York

Donald L. Bliwise, PhD
Professor
Department of Neurology
Emory University School of Medicine
Atlanta, Georgia

Susan B Bressman, MD
Alan and Joan Mirken Chair and Professor
Departments of Neurology
Beth Israel Medical Center and Albert Einstein College of Medicine
New York, New York and Bronx, New York

David J. Brooks, MD, DSc, FRCP, FMedSci
Hartnett Professor of Neurology and Head of Neuroscience
Department of Medicine
Imperial College
London, UK

David J. Burn, FRCP, MD
Professor of Movement Disorders Neurology
Institute for Ageing and Health
Newcastle University
Newcastle upon Tyne, UK

Donald B. Calne, MD
Professor Emeritus
University of British Columbia
Pacific Parkinson's Research Centre
Vancouver, British Columbia

Susana Cantarero, MD
Médico Especialista en Neurología
Department of Neurology
Hospital de Móstoles,
Mostoles, Madrid, Spain

Maria Graciela Cersosimo, MD
Program of Movement Disorders and Parkinson's Disease
University of Buenos Aires
Buenos Aires, Argentina

Jang-Ho Cha, MD
Associate Professor of Neurology
Massachusetts General Hospital
Boston, Massachusetts

Amy Colcher, MD
Clinical Associate Professor
Department of Neurology
University of Pennsylvania
Philadelphia, Pennsylvania

Candan Depboylu, MD
Department of Neurology
Philipps University Marburg
Marburg, Germany

Dennis W. Dickson, MD
Robert E. Jacoby Professor of Alzheimer's Research
Mayo Clinic
Jacksonville, Florida

Milind Deogaonkar, MD
Staff Neurosurgery, Neurosciences and Gamma Knife
Center for Neurological Restoration
Department of Neurosurgery
Cleveland Clinic Foundation
Cleveland, Ohio

Justo Garcia de Yébenes, MD, PhD
Head, Unit of Neurodegenerative Diseases
Department of Neurology
Hospital Ramon y Cajal, Universidad de Alcalá de Henares
School of Medicine
Madrid, Madrid, Spain

John E. Duda, MD
Director, Parkinson's Disease Research, Education and Clinical Center
Philadelphia VA Medical Center
Assistant Professor of Neurology
University of Pennsylvania School of Medicine
Philadelphia, Pennsylvania

Leon S. Dure, IV, MD
Bew White Professor of Pediatrics and Neurology
Departments of Pediatrics and Neurology
University of Alabama at Birmingham

Rodger J. Elble, MD, PhD
Professor and Chair of Neurology
Department of Neurology
Southern Illinois University School of Medicine
Springfield, Illinois

Murat Emre, MD
Professor of Neurology
Department of Neurology, Behavioral Neurology and Movement Disorders Unit
İstanbul University, İstanbul Faculty of Medicine
İstanbul, Turkey

Robert J. Ferrante, PhD, MSc
Director, Experimental Neuropathology and Translational Therapeutics Laboratory and
Professor, Neurology, Laboratory Medicine and Pathology, and Psychiatry
Geriatric Research Education Clinical Center
New England Veterans Administration VISN 1
Bedford, Massachusetts
Neurology, Laboratory Medicine and Pathology, and Psychiatry Departments
Boston University School of Medicine
Boston, Massachusetts

Nestor Galvez-Jimenez, MD, MSc, MHSA, FACP
Chairman and Associate Clinical Professor of Neurology
The Herbert Wertheim College of Medicine-Florida Atlantic University
Department of Neurology
Cleveland Clinic in Florida
Weston (Fort Lauderdale), Florida

Oscar S. Gershanik, MD
Professor and Scientific Director
Institute for Neuroscience
Favaloro Foundation University Hospital
Buenos Aires, Argentina

Christopher G. Goetz, MD
Professor of Neurological Sciences
Professor of Pharmacology
Rush University Medical Center
Chicago, Illinois

Lawrence I. Golbe, MD
Professor
Department of Neurology
University of Medicine and Dentistry of New Jersey - Robert Wood Johnson Medical School
New Brunswick, New Jersey

Asier Gómez, MD
Department of Neurology and Neurosurgery
Clínica Universidad de Navarra,
Pamplona, Spain

Rafael González-Redondo, MD
Department of Neurosciences
Movement Disorders Group
Center for Applied Medical Research
University of Navarra
Pamplona, Spain
and
Centro de Investigación Biomédica en Red sobre Enfermedades Neurodegenerativas
Instituto Carlos III
Ministerio de Investigacion y Ciencias, Spain
and
Department of Neurology and Neurosurgery
Clínica Universidad de Navarra,
Pamplona, Spain

James F. Gusella, PhD
Bullard Professor of Neurogenetics in the Department of Genetics, Harvard Medical School and Director, Center for Human
Genetic Research, Massachusetts General Hospital
Boston, Massachusetts

Mark Hallett, MD
Chief, Human Motor Control Section
Medical Neurology Branch
National Institute of Neurological Disorders and Stroke
National Institutes of Health
Bethesda, Maryland

Haşmet Hanağası, MD
Associate Professor of Neurology
Department of Neurology, Behavioral Neurology and Movement Disorders Unit
İstanbul University, İstanbul Faculty of Medicine
İstanbul, Turkey

Nobutaka Hattori, MD
Professor and Chairman
Department of Neurology
Juntendo University School of Medicine
Bunkyo, Tokyo

Steven M. Hersch, MD, PhD
Professor of Neurology
MassGeneral Institute for Neurodegenerative Disease
Massachusetts General Hospital, Harvard Medical School
Charlestown, Massachusetts

Stacy Horn, DO
Assistant Clinical Professor
Department of Neurological Sciences
University of Pennsylvania
Philadelphia, Pennsylvania

Howard I. Hurtig, MD
Frank and Gladys Elliott Professor of Neurology
Department of Neurology
University of Pennsylvania
Philadelphia, Pennsylvania

Joseph Jankovic, MD
Professor of Neurology
Distinguished Chair in Movement Disorders
Director, Parkinson's Disease Center
and Movement Disorders Clinic
Baylor College of Medicine
Department of Neurology
Houston, Texas

Jorge L. Juncos, MD
Associate Professor of Neurology
Movement Disorders Program
Emory University School of Medicine
Atlanta, Georgia

Anthony E. Lang, MD, FRCPC, FAAN
Jack Clark Chair for Parkinson's Disease Research and Director of Division of Neurology
Department of Medicine
University of Toronto
Toronto, Ontario, Canada

Päivi Lindholm, PhD
Postdoctoral Fellow
Centre of Excellence for Molecular and Integrated Neuroscience Research, Institute of Biotechnology
University of Helsinki
Helsinki, Finland

Olle Lindvall, MD, PhD
Professor and Chairman
Division of Neurology, Department of Clinical Sciences
University of Lund
Lund, Sweden

Kelly E. Lyons, PhD
Research Associate Professor
Department of Neurology
University of Kansas
School of Medicine
Kansas City, Kansas

Andre Machado, MD, PhD
Director
Center for Neurological Restoration
Neurological Institute
Cleveland Clinic
Cleveland, Ohio

Philipp Mahlknecht, MD
Department of Neurology
Innsbruck Medical University
Anichstrasse 35, A-6020 Innsbruck
Innsbruck, Austria

Marcy E. MacDonald, PhD
Professor of Neurology, Harvard Medical School and Molecular Neurogenetics Unit, Center for Human Genetic Research,
Massachusetts General Hospital

Margery H. Mark, MD
Associate Professor of Neurology and Psychiatry
UMDNJ-Robert Wood Johnson Medical School
New Brunswick, New Jersey

Bala V. Manyam, MD
Professor and Director
Plummer Movement Disorders Center
Department of Neurology
Scott & White Clinic and Memorial Hospital
The Texas A&M University System Health Science Center College of Medicine
Temple, Texas

Connie Marras, MD, PhD
Assistant Professor, Department of Medicine (Neurology)
University of Toronto
Toronto, Ontario, Canada

MJ Marti, MD
Neurology Service
Hospital Clinic Universitari
University of Barcelona
Barcelona, Spain

Shyamal H. Mehta, MD, PhD
Assistant Professor of Neurology
Movement Disorders Program
Medical College of Georgia
Augusta, Georgia

Federico Micheli, MD, PhD
Professor of Neurology
Director of the Program of Movement Disorders and Parkinson's Disease
Institute of Applied Sciences
Hospital de Clinicas
University of El Salvador and University of Buenos Aires
Buenos Aires, Argentina

Jonathan W. Mink, MD, PhD
Professor and Chief of Child Neurology
Departments of Neurology, Neurobiology & Anatomy, and Pediatrics
University of Rochester School of Medicine and Dentistry
Rochester, New York

Yoshikuni Mizuno, MD
Director of Juntendo Koshigaya Hospital
Director of Juntendo Koshigaya Hospital
Juntendo University School of Medicine
Koshigaya, Saitama

Hideki Mochizuki, MD
Professor and Chairman
Department of Neurology
Kitasato University School of Medicine
Sagamihara, Kanagawa

Jens Carsten Möller, MD
Consultant
Neurocenter of Southern Switzerland
Ospedale Regionale di Lugano
Lugano, Switzerland

Anthony Nicholas, MD
Associate Professor
Department of Neurology
University of Alabama at Birmingham
School of Medicine
Birmingham, Alabama

José A. Obeso, MD
Professor and Consultant, Neurology, Univ. of Navarra
Pamplona, Spain

Wolfgang H. Oertel, MD
Director
Department of Neurology
Center of Nervous Disease
Philipps-University of Marburg
Marburg, Germany

Rajesh Pahwa, MD
Laverne & Joyce Rider Professor
Department of Neurology
University of Kansas
School of Medicine
Kansas City, Kansas

Henry L. Paulson, MD, PhD
Lucile Groff Professor
Department of Neurology
University of Michigan Health System
Ann Arbor, Michigan

Nicola Pavese, MD
Senior Lecturer in Neurology
Department of Medicine
Imperial College
London, UK

Ronald F. Pfeiffer, MD
Professor and Vice Chair
Department of Neurology
University of Tennessee Health Science Center
Memphis, Tennessee

Werner Poewe, MD
Professor and Chairman
Department of Neurology
Innsbruck Medical University
Anichstrasse 35, A-6020 Innsbruck
Innsbruck, Austria

Seth L. Pullman, MD
Professor of Clinical Neurology
Department of Neurology
Clinical Motor Physiology Laboratory
Columbia University Medical Center
New York, New York

Bradley J. Robottom, MD
Assistant Professor
Department of Neurology
University of Maryland School of Medicine
Baltimore, Maryland

Manuel Rodríguez, MD, PhD
Department of Physiology
Medical School
University of La Laguna
Tenerife, Spain

María C. Rodríguez-Oroz, MD, PhD
Department of Neurosciences
Movement Disorders Group
CIMA, University of Navarra
Pamplona, Spain
and
Department of Neurology and Neurosurgery
Clínica Universidad de Navarra and Medical School,
Pamplona, Spain

H. Diana Rosas, MD, MSc
Director, Center for Neuroimaging of Aging and Neurodegenerative Diseases; Co-Director, HDSA New England Center of Excellence
Department of Neurology
Massachusetts General Hospital, Harvard Medical School
Charlestown, Massachusetts

David B. Rye, MD, PhD
Professor
Department of Neurology
Emory University School of Medicine
Atlanta, GA

Daniel S. Sa, MD
Director, Movement Disorders Center
Marshfield Clinic Neurosciences
Marshfield, Wisconsin

Mart Saarma, PhD
Academy Professor and Director
Centre of Excellence for Molecular and Integrated Neuroscience Research, Institute of Biotechnology
University of Helsinki
Helsinki, Finland

Rachel Saunders-Pullman, MD, MPH
Associate Professor of Neurology
Department of Neurology
Albert Einstein School of Medicine
Beth Israel Medical Center
New York, New York

Jose Lopez Sendon, MD
Médico Especialista en Neurología
Department of Neurology
Hospital Ramon y Cajal, Universidad de Alcalá de Henares
School of Medicine
Madrid, Madrid, Spain

Kapil D. Sethi, MD, FRCP
Professor of Neurology
Director Movement Disorders Program
Georgia Health Sciences University
Augusta, Georgia

Lisa M. Shulman, MD
Eugenia Brin Professor of Parkinson's Disease and Movement Disorders
Department of Neurology
University of Maryland School of Medicine
Baltimore, Maryland

Yoland Smith, PhD
Professor
Yerkes National Primate Research Center and Department of Neurology
Emory University
School of Medicine
Atlanta, Georgia

David G. Standaert, MD, PhD
John and Juanelle Strain Professor and Vice Chairman
Director, Center for Neurodegeneration and Experimental Therapeutics
Department of Neurology
University of Alabama at Birmingham
Birmingham, Alabama

Matthew B. Stern, MD
Parker Family Professor of Neurology
Director, Parkinson's Disease and Movement Disorders Center
University of Pennsylvania
Co-Director, Parkinson's Disease Research, Education and Clinical Center
Philadelphia VA Medical Center
Philadelphia, Pennsylvania

Natividad P. Stover, MD
Assistant Professor
Department of Neurology
University of Alabama at Birmingham
Birmingham, Alabama

S. H. Subramony, MD
Professor
Department of Neurology,
McKnight Brain Institute at University of Florida
Gainesville, Florida

Lewis Sudarsky, MD
Director of Movement Disorders
Brigham and Women's Hospital, Boston
Associate Professor of Neurology
Harvard Medical School, Boston

Cesar Tabernero, MD
Médico Especialista en Neurología
Department of Neurology
Hospital de Segovia,
Segovia, Segovia, Spain

Caroline M Tanner, MD, PhD, FAAN
Director, Clinical Research
Parkinson's Institute
Sunnyvale, California

W. Thomas Thach, Jr., MD
Professor of Neurobiology
Department of Anatomy and Neurobiology
Washington University
School of Medicine
St. Louis, Missouri

Eduardo Tolosa, MD
Professor of Neurology
Neurology Service
Hospital Clinic Universitari
University of Barcelona
Barcelona, Spain

Camilo Toro, MD
Staff Clinician
National Human Genome Research Institute
National Institutes of Health
Bethesda, Maryland

Lynn Marie Trotti, MD
Assistant Professor
Department of Neurology
Emory University School of Medicine
Atlanta, Georgia

Jerrold L. Vitek, MD, PhD
Professor and Chair
Department of Neurology
University of Minnesota
Minneapolis, Minnesota

Ana Victoria Vazquez, MD
Médico Especialista en Neurología
Department of Neurology
Hospital de Leganés,
Leganes, Madrid, Spain

Sarah Wahlster, MD
Departments of Neurology
Massachusetts General Hospital and Brigham and Women's Hospital
Boston, Massachusetts

Ray L. Watts, MD
John N. Whitaker Professor of Neurology
Senior Vice President and Dean of the School of Medicine at UAB
University of Alabama at Birmingham
Birmingham, Alabama

William J. Weiner, MD
Professor and Chairman
Department of Neurology
University of Maryland School of Medicine
Baltimore, Maryland

Daniel Weintraub, MD
Associate Professor of Psychiatry
University of Pennsylvania School of Medicine
Parkinson's Disease and Mental Illness Research, Education and Clinical Centers
Philadelphia Veterans Affairs Medical Center
Philadelphia, Pennsylvania

Andrew West, PhD
Assistant Professor
Department of Neurology
University of Alabama at Birmingham
School of Medicine
Birmingham, Alabama

Vanessa C. Wheeler, PhD
Assistant Professor of Neurology, Harvard Medical School and Molecular Neurogenetics Unit, Center for Human Genetic Research,
Massachusetts General Hospital
Boston, Massachusetts

Jayne R. Wilkinson, MD
Assistant Professor of Clinical Neurology
Department of Neurology
University of Pennsylvania School of Medicine
Associate Clinical Director
Parkinson's Disease, Research, Education and Clinical Center
Philadelphia Veterans Affairs Medical Center
Philadelphia, Pennsylvania

George R. Wilmot, MD, PhD
Assistant Professor
Department of Neurology
Emory University School of Medicine
Atlanta, Georgia

G. Frederick Wooten, MD
Mary Anderson Harrison Professor
Department of Neurology
University of Virginia
Charlottesville, Virginia

Zbigniew K. Wszolek, MD
Consultant and Professor of Neurology
Department of Neurology
Mayo Clinic Florida
Jacksonville, Florida

Talene A. Yacoubian, MD, PhD
Assistant Professor
Center for Neurodegeneration and Experimental Therapeutics
Department of Neurology
University of Alabama at Birmingham School of Medicine
Birmingham, Alabama

PREFACE

Since the publication of the second edition of *Movement Disorders: Neurologic Principles and Practice* there have been major advances in understanding the molecular basis and range of clinical expression of many of the diseases that make up this spectrum of neurological disorders, hence the need for this third edition. In this new volume we have retained an organization of sections that is based principally on clinical patterns of disease expression the same (phenotypic approach), but we have placed greater emphasis on the molecular etiologies, where known (molecular genetic approach). Future editions will likely emphasize this mechanistic approach even more strongly as our knowledge of underlying causes continues to advance.

As in the first two editions, we have sought to present the material in a logical fashion beginning with Part I: Introduction to Movement Disorders (Chapters 1–3), followed by Part II: Neuroscientific Foundations (Chapters 4–8), and concluding with Part III: Clinical Disorders (Chapters 9-49, further segregated to address the major categories of movement disorders). We have added a new chapter on "Assessing Disability in Movement Disorders: Quantitative Techniques and Rating Scales" (Chapter 2), a new chapter on "Neuroprotective Therapies for Parkinson's Disease" (Chapter 14), and a new chapter on "Restless Legs Syndrome and Periodic Leg Movements of Sleep" (Chapter 47). We consolidated some smaller chapters where warranted. A large number of tables and figures are included that help present data more succinctly and are useful teaching aids; unique to this third edition is a new DVD with videos of representative patients with various movement disorders.

We are deeply appreciative for the support of our families and professional colleagues throughout the preparation of this second edition, and we are grateful for the assistance of the editorial and publishing staff of McGraw-Hill (especially Anne Sydor and Christine Naglieri). Particular appreciation is extended to Katherine (Kate) Tully of the University of Alabama at Birmingham (UAB) for her assistance with many aspects of the organizational, editorial, and publication processes that brought this third edition to fruition, and to Amy Amara, MD, PhD, a Movement Disorders Fellow at UAB, who was very helpful with the creation of the DVD with patient videos.

We dedicate this third edition to the work and memory of our dear colleague, William C. Koller, MD, PhD, who was a co-editor of the first two editions.

It is our hope that readers will find this third edition of even greater usefulness than the first two.

Ray L. Watts, MD
David G. Standaertt, MD, PhD
Jose A. Obeso, MD

SECTION I

INTRODUCTION TO MOVEMENT DISORDERS

CHAPTER 1

Overview of Movement Disorders and Approach to the Patient

Zbigniew K. Wszolek and Donald B. Calne

▶ INTRODUCTION

The term "movement disorders" has been coined for diseases characterized by abnormal or excessive movements occurring in conscious patients. "Extrapyramidal disorder" is an older classification of central motor disturbances not involving the corticospinal pathway. Involuntary movement can occur in a setting where there is also difficulty in initiating or executing voluntary movement. The commonest example of combined hyperkinetic and hypokinetic features is Parkinsonism, where tremor is frequently associated with bradykinesia and rigidity.

"Movement disorders" is used in two ways: (1) to describe a symptom or physical sign of involuntary movement; (2) to describe a syndrome in which abnormal movements occur. Abnormal movements may be the only manifestation of a disease [e.g., essential tremor (ET), hemifacial spasm (HS)], or they can be part of a constellation of deficits [e.g., Parkinson's disease (PD), Huntington's disease (HD), progressive supranuclear palsy (PSP), Creutzfeldt–Jakob disease (CJD)]. Frequently, there may be more than one type of movement disorder associated with a disease [e.g., chorea, dystonia, and tremor in HD and Wilson's disease (WD)] (see Table 1–1).

The first step when assessing a patient with a movement disorder is to designate the category of motor disturbance. The next step consists of determining whether the movement disorder appears in isolation or is associated with other neurological signs. Finally, clues bearing on the etiology are sought (hereditary or sporadic; primary, or secondary to a known neurological disease).

Some movement disorders are known to be associated with pathological changes in the basal ganglia (e.g., PD and HD), whereas the pathology in many others is still unclear [e.g., idiopathic torsion dystonia (ITD), ET and Gilles de la Tourette syndrome (GTS)]. ET is the commonest movement disorder, followed by PD, dystonia, and drug-induced movement disorders.

▶ HYPERKINETIC PHENOMENA

To categorize abnormal movements (e.g., chorea, tremor, ballism, myoclonus), one must be able to recognize the pattern of the involuntary movements. This can be difficult when combinations of different movements occur in the same individual. The term "dyskinesia" can be applied to any type of involuntary movement.

There are certain characteristics, which can help one arrive at a diagnosis:

1. Topography
2. Symmetry: asymmetric or symmetric
3. Nature: for example, stereotyped or nonstereotyped
4. Overflow to other body parts
5. Velocity: slow, intermediate, or fast

▶ TABLE 1–1. OVERLAPPING SIGNS IN SOME MOVEMENT DISORDERS

	Parkinson's Disease	Progressive Supranuclear Palsy	Multiple System Atrophy	Huntington's Disease	Wilson's Disease	Essential Tremor	Drugs (Dopaminergic Receptor Blockers)
Resting tremor	++	+	+	+	+	+	+
Postural tremor	+	+	+	+	+	++	+

6. Rhythm: regular or irregular
7. Relation to general voluntary movement
8. Relation to specific tasks
9. Relation to posture
10. Relation to sleep
11. Associated sensory symptoms
12. Suppressibility
13. Aggravating factors: for example, stress and anxiety
14. Precipitating factors: for example, alcohol and voluntary movement
15. Ameliorating factors: for example, sleep and relaxation.
16. Distractibility and consistency: to distinguish functional movement disorders
17. Heredity

TREMOR

Tremor comprises involuntary rhythmic oscillations of a body part produced by alternating or synchronous contractions of reciprocally innervated muscles.[1] It may be fast or slow, coarse or fine, uniplanar or biplanar. Resting tremor is seen with the body part completely at rest. Postural tremor appears while a limb is maintaining a posture. Tremor produced during movement is referred to as action tremor. Intentional tremor is also present during goal-directed activity but, in addition, worsens toward the completion of the activity. Tremor may involve the upper or lower limbs, lips, tongue, neck, or voice.

Resting Tremor

1. Occurs with the body part completely at rest.
2. Subsides with action.
3. Subsides with the assumption of a posture.

Postural Tremor

Postural tremor is seen immediately following the assumption of a posture. Some tremor can be seen both at rest and with action or the assumption of a posture; for example, rubral tremors due to lesions of the cerebellar outflow pathways in the midbrain.

Intention Tremor

This is seen in involvement of the cerebellum or its connections. (See Chaps. 26, 40, 41, 44.) It is present during goal-directed movement and worsens terminally.

Wing-Beating Tremor

This is large-amplitude, slow proximal tremor, causing the arms to be thrown up and down when extended. Changing the posture of the extended arm may alter the severity of the tremor.

Nonorganic Tremor

Nonorganic tremor should be suspected when the clinical characteristics are not consistent with recognized forms of tremor. Good indicators include sudden onset, inconsistent patterns, fluctuations in frequency and direction, distractibility, secondary gain, and dramatic response to placebo.

CHOREA

The word "chorea" derives from the Greek word for dance. Chorea consists of irregular, unpredictable brief, jerky movements that are usually of low amplitude. The term "semipurposeful" is sometimes used to describe chorea to help to identify it.[2] Although choreatic movements are really purposeless, patients may incorporate them into a deliberate movement in order to make them less noticeable. The movements are usually distal and range from mild chorea resembling fidgetiness in children to severe chorea interfering with speech, swallowing, maintaining posture, and the ability to walk. Facial grimacing and abnormal respiratory sounds are other manifestations of chorea. Chorea may be associated with hypotonia of the limbs. The gait may resemble a waltz. Chorea can result in a "hung-up" tendon reflex due to muscle contraction immediately after the reflex contraction due to muscle stretch. Motor impersistence (e.g., inability to protrude the tongue in a sustained manner, sometimes referred to as "Jack-in-the-box tongue") and "milkmaid grip" due to contractions alternating with relaxations of grip may be seen.

Chorea may be the only neurological sign of disease, as in rheumatic chorea and thyrotoxicosis, or may be part of a constellation of other signs, as in HD or neuroacanthocytosis. Keeping the wide differential diagnosis of chorea in mind, it is vital to take a detailed history, paying particular attention to the family and birth history, anoxic insult, and exposure to drugs, in addition to looking for associated neurological signs.

The causes of chorea are listed in Table 1–2 (also in Chapter 36).

BALLISM

Ballism is a proximal high-amplitude, sometimes flailing, movement related to chorea. As patients recover from ballism due to stroke, they often go through a phase of chorea. Ballism is usually limited to one side of the body (hemiballism). However, it may occur bilaterally (biballism) or confined to a single limb (monoballism). The cause of ballism is usually vascular, but other structural

▶ TABLE 1–2. **CAUSES OF CHOREA**

Hereditary Dominant	HD (*IT15* gene on chromosome 4p) , Huntington-like disease-1 (*HDL1* gene on chromosome 20p), Huntington-like disease-2 (*HDL2* gene on chromosome 16q), paroxysmal choreoathetosis and spasticity (*CSE* gene on chromosome 1p), DRPLA (CAG repeat disorder, chromosome 12p), benign hereditary chorea (*TITF-1* gene on chromosome 14q), spinocerebellar ataxias, and others
Hereditary Recessive	Wilson's disease, Niemann–Pick disease, Pelizaeus–Merzbacher disease, neurodegeneration with iron deposition (pantothenate kinase deficiency) formerly known as Hallervorden–Spatz disease, ataxia telangiectasia, Lesch–Nyhan disease, neuroacanthocytosis (*CHAC* gene on chromosome 9q), and others
Maternal Inheritance	Mitochondrial encephalopathies
Autoimmune	Rheumatic chorea, chorea gravidarum, systemic lupus erythematosus (SLE), polyarteritis nodosa, Behçet's disease
Electrolyte and Endocrine	Hyponatremia or hypernatremia, hypocalcemia, hypoglycemia or hyperglycemia, renal failure, hypoparathyroidism
Toxins	Mercury, carbon monoxide
Inflammatory	Encephalitis, acquired immune deficiency syndrome (AIDS)
Drugs	Neuroleptics, metoclopramide, L-dopa, anticonvulsants, steroids, oral contraceptives
Vascular	Infarcts

DRPLA, dentato-rubro-pallido-luysian atrophy; HD, Huntington's disease.

lesions and metabolic disturbances such as nonketotic hyperosmolar hyperglycemia can also produce it.

DYSTONIA

Dystonia is an abnormal movement characterized by sustained muscle contractions, frequently causing twisting and repetitive movements or abnormal postures.[3] Dystonic movements that are slow, twisting, and distal were formerly referred to as athetosis. Dystonia can be associated with fast rhythmic tremulous movements (dystonic tremor).[4] Dystonic movements can also be rapid resembling myoclonus (myoclonic dystonia). Electromyography (EMG) shows prolonged bursts typical of dystonia rather than the characteristic short duration bursts seen in myoclonus.[5]

Dystonia can involve any body part. According to the site of involvement, dystonia is classified as:

1. Focal: one body part involved (blepharospasm, oromandibular dystonia, spasmodic dysphonia, cervical dystonia, and occupational cramp).
2. Segmental dystonia: two or more contiguous parts are involved (Meige syndrome).
3. Multifocal dystonia: two or more noncontiguous parts are involved.
4. Hemidystonia: one side of the body is affected.
5. Generalized dystonia (crural with involvement of other parts).

Dystonia may occur when a body part is at rest or only when a body part is used to perform a voluntary activity (action dystonia). Also, a dystonia at rest may worsen on action. Idiopathic torsion dystonia (ITD) most often starts as a specific action dystonia, particularly inversion of the foot. As the disease progresses, dystonia occurs with nonspecific movements of other body parts (overflow dystonia) and ultimately at rest. Thus, any dystonia at rest represents a more severe form of dystonia than pure action dystonia. Dystonia may be task specific (e.g., writer's or musician's cramp). Even in these conditions, as the disease progresses less specific actions provoke it. Some of these task-specific dystonias may be associated with an additional tremor or myoclonic component.[6] A subgroup of idiopathic dystonia with myoclonic spasms and responsiveness to alcohol is believed to be a variant of ITD.[7,8]

Dystonia can be aggravated by stress, anxiety, fatigue, specific postures, and action. It is frequently relieved by sleep and rest. A peculiar feature of dystonia is some patients' ability to relieve a movement by "sensory tricks" that are usually tactile or proprioceptive stimuli. For example, blepharospasm can sometimes be relieved by touching the area around the eyes. This phenomenon is unique to dystonia and can assist in the diagnosis. Dystonia can also be paroxysmal, as in the paroxysmal dyskinesias (see Chapter 36). Diurnal variation can be seen in dystonia as in "dopa-responsive dystonia" (DRD).[9,10] The onset is in the legs and usually begins in childhood. There can be problems with the gait and frequent falls. A characteristic worsening toward the end of the day is often observed. There may be associated features of parkinsonism, and the condition responds well to long-term small doses of L-dopa. DRD may be mistaken for cerebral palsy. Diagnosis is crucial because of the response to treatment.

ATHETOSIS

"Athetosis" was a term formerly used to describe distal, slow, writhing forms of dystonia. Pseudoathetosis refers to abnormal movements resembling athetosis due to proprioceptive sensory loss, most evident when visual compensation is removed. Unlike dystonia, pseudoathetosis can be suppressed by supporting the limb.[11]

MYOCLONUS

Myoclonus describes sudden shocklike movements due to muscle contractions or inhibition of ongoing muscle activity (negative myoclonus). Myoclonus is usually random and irregular in time as in chorea, but unlike chorea the spasm is more abrupt. On occasion myoclonus may be rhythmic or oscillatory. Tics may resemble myoclonus but they are voluntarily suppressible for short periods. Tics are also associated with an inner buildup of tension during the suppression. Myoclonus may be mild or sometimes severe enough to move the whole body. Topographically it may be focal, segmental, multifocal, or generalized. Myoclonus can occur spontaneously or it may be stimulus sensitive (light, touch, noise, etc.). Myoclonus can sometimes be precipitated by action, as in the Ramsay Hunt syndrome (see Chapter 37). The origin of myoclonus may be cortical or subcortical (brain stem or spinal) (see Chapters 37, 22). Cortical myoclonus is an epileptic phenomenon, and the technique of back-averaging the electroencephalogram (EEG), using EMG activity as a trigger, will demonstrate the transient time-locked cortical event preceding the myoclonic jerk.

TICS

Tics are brief, involuntary, rapid, nonrhythmic movements (motor tics) or sounds (vocal tics) (see Chapter 39). They can be severe and frequent.[12] They occur against a background of normal motor activity. Tics can be classified into simple and complex. A simple motor tic is an abrupt, brief, isolated movement like an eye blink, shoulder shrug, facial grimace, or head jerk (clonic tic). The movement may also be slower and sustained, as in neck turning (tonic or dystonic tic). Complex motor tics include stereotyped facial expressions or patterned coordinated movements, such as touching or grooming behavior, smelling objects or body parts, shaking hands, scratching, kicking or obscene gesturing. The appearance of the complex motor tic may make it difficult to distinguish it from voluntary movement and many of these overlap with obsessive-compulsive behavior. Simple vocal tics usually consist of throat clearing, grunting, coughing, snorting or animal sounds such as hissing, barking, crowing, etc. Complex vocal tics comprise words, phrases, and, on occasion, obscene utterances or religious profanities. Tics are worsened by stress, anxiety, and fatigue. They are relieved by concentration on a task or absorbing activities such as reading or playing a musical instrument. Tics vary in frequency, amplitude, duration, and location. They are usually multifocal and can migrate from one body part to another. The common sites of occurrence are the face, neck, and shoulders. Tics are usually first noticed by others such as parents, teachers, and friends. Characteristic features of tics include:[13,14]

1. Occurrence of an irresistible urge to move before the tic. The tension that mounts before the tic is relieved by execution of the tic. In contrast to tics, the sensory urge to move in akathasia and restless legs syndrome (RLS) is constant. Also, the movements in akathasia tend to be more stereotyped.
2. Tics can be voluntarily suppressed for a short time; however, this leads to a build-up of tension and a rebound exacerbation.

STEREOTYPY

Repetitive and continuous complex motor acts are known as stereotypies.

AKATHISIA

Akathisia refers to motor activity as a voluntary effort to relieve continuous uncomfortable sensations. It usually takes the form of standing, pacing, trunk-rocking while standing, and sometimes marching on the spot. In severe cases, the need for motor activity is irrepressible.

ASTERIXIS (NEGATIVE MYOCLONUS)

These sudden irregular displacements are due to brief lapses of tone in a limb held in a posture against gravity. EMG reveals irregular silent periods during these lapses.

▶ HYPERKINETIC SYNDROMES

PHYSIOLOGICAL TREMOR

Muscle fibers whose motor units are being recruited at subtetanic rates produce vibrations. This small amplitude tremor can be appreciated only by means of an accelometer or other system of amplification. When muscle contractions are maintained, as when the arms are held outstretched, the movement becomes visible to the naked eye.[15] This is referred to as enhanced physiological tremor. This can be caused or exacerbated by anxiety, fatigue, thyrotoxicosis, hypoglycemia, alcohol withdrawal, sympathomimetic drugs, lithium, sodium valproate, and methylxanthines such as caffeine. These causes should be excluded before arriving at a diagnosis of ET (see Chapters 25–27).

ESSENTIAL TREMOR (ET)

ET, the commonest movement disorder, is typically a postural tremor, but may be accentuated by goal-directed activity. In some patients, the tremor is only present when they assume certain postures or alter their posture. The upper limbs are most frequently involved and the tremor may initially be asymmetric. Some early PD patients may present with postural tremor, and this plus the asymmetry may confound a diagnosis.[16] The tremor is typically uniplanar with flexion–extension movements of the hand.

Abduction–adduction and pronation–supination movements of the hand are occasionally seen.[17] In general lips, tongue, chin tremor is more in favor of PD and head and neck tremor more in favor of ET, albeit all can be seen in ET.

With the passage of time, the frequency of the tremor decreases and the amplitude may increase.[18] Eventually there may be a resting tremor. In severe cases, the tremor may interfere with nutrition and hydration and for these patients the term benign essential tremor is completely misplaced. Stress, anxiety, and central nervous system stimulants can all worsen the tremor. Alcohol in small quantities improves ET in most patients. Although this is a characteristic of ET, other forms of tremor may also respond.[19] Although the neurological examination is normal in the majority of patients with ET, soft signs such as mild abnormalities of tone, posture and balance may be seen.[16] ET can begin at any age, but is called senile tremor if it begins after the age of 65 years. ET is inherited in more than 50% of patients and three loci (ETM1–ETM3) have been identified and many candidate genes suggested. The molecular genetic results on individual genes have not been consistently replicated. Therefore, at the present time, there are only nominated loci and no single causative gene has been discovered so far.[20–25]

Genomewide scans in North American families reveal genetic linkage of essential tremor to a region on chromosome 6p23.[25] Apart from these features, essential, senile, and familial tremor are clinically the same.[26]

ORTHOSTATIC TREMOR

A variant of ET, orthostatic tremor is a typical postural tremor, which begins soon after standing up. There is a tremor of the lower limbs, which may cause the patellae to move up and down. Any other postures alleviate it. Most patients have a family history of ET.[27]

PARKINSONIAN TREMOR

Characteristically this is a slow, resting, biplanar, pill-rolling tremor in the 4–5 Hz frequency range. However, postural and kinetic tremors in a higher frequency range may also be seen. Onset of tremor is usually in one of the hands and is asymmetric.[28] Rarely it may begin in the legs. It may also involve the jaw and lips. A tremor of the perioral and nasal muscles (rabbit syndrome) can occur as is sometimes observed with neuroleptic medication. The resting tremor (RT) may be intermittent early in the course of PD and can be precipitated by anxiety, stress, and contralateral hand clenching. RT is uncommon in other parkinsonian syndromes.[29] The appearance of RT in ET does not necessarily indicate an additional diagnosis of PD.[30] Resting tremor may be a prominent sign in drug-induced parkinsonism.

TARDIVE DYSKINESIA

TD is defined as abnormal involuntary movement appearing after treatment with a neuroleptic drug for three or more months in a patient with no other identifiable causes for a movement disorder.[31] (see Chapter 35). TD persists for long after the withdrawal of the offending drug and may indeed only appear for the first time after the drug is stopped. In addition, the movements may worsen briefly after the drug is withdrawn. The movements in TD are complex choreatic and dystonic movements that are classically orobuccolingual, resembling chewing movements, but may affect other body parts as well. They usually spare the forehead. TD may involve abdominal and pelvic muscles, producing truncal or thrusting movements, and may be associated with respiratory dyskinesias.[32] A distinctive feature of the choreatic movements in TD, as compared to chorea in other conditions, is their stereotyped appearance.[33] Rhythmic chewing movements, intermittent tongue protrusion and or pushing the inside of the cheek with the tongue (bon-bon sign) are common. The typical chorea in TD is brief but frequently may be associated with more sustained movements (tardive dystonia). In drug-induced tardive syndromes, the whole spectrum of chorea, dystonia, tics, and akathasia may be seen.

PRIMARY AND SECONDARY DYSTONIAS

Dystonia can be classified according to its etiology as idiopathic (primary) and symptomatic (secondary). Approximately 30% of dystonia is secondary. Both primary and secondary dystonia can be familial or sporadic.[34] (see Chapters 28–31).

In childhood, generalized dystonia may be primary or secondary. In adults, primary dystonia is usually focal. The age of onset of dystonia is important for prognosis, as young-onset dystonia tends to evolve into generalized dystonia, whereas adult-onset dystonia is likely to remain focal. Onset with dystonia at rest, early speech involvement (except spasmodic dysphonia), rapid course, and association with other neurological signs suggest a secondary dystonia.

Hemidystonia is mostly symptomatic and calls for investigations for vascular or other structural lesions.[35,36]

Secondary dystonia may be associated with a variety of neurological signs other than dystonia. Dystonia in association with parkinsonism can occur in PD, PSP, multiple system atrophy (MSA), corticobasal degteneration (CBD) certain forms of spinocerebellar ataxia (Machado–Joseph disease), rapid onset dystonia and parkinsonism,[37] and the dystonia parkinsonism syndrome of the Philippines (Lubag).[38] (See Chapters 13, 15, 20, 21, 22, 24, 32, 42, 45.)

Exposure to drugs (D2 dopamine receptor antagonists, chronic L-dopa therapy, anticonvulsants), anoxia, birth injury, toxic exposure [manganese, carbon monoxide (CO), carbon disulfide, methanol], head injury, stroke, and encephalitis can all cause dystonia (see Chapter 31). Metabolic and storage disorders such as WD, GM1 and GM2 gangliosidosis, Lesch–Nyhan syndrome, and dystonic lipidosis (Niemann–Pick type 3) can all be associated with dystonia (see Chapters 24, 31). Of these, the diagnosis of WD is especially important, because it is treatable.

Acute dystonic reactions consist of sustained painful muscle spasms, with twisting and pulling movements occurring within minutes to hours of exposure to dopaminergic blocking drugs. Cervical dystonia , retrocollis, trismus, blepharospasm, and ocular deviations may be seen. These idiosyncratic reactions to dopamine receptor (D2) blockers occur mainly in juveniles or young adults.

Genetic causes of dystonia are summarized in Table 1–3.[37,39–44]

NONORGANIC DYSTONIA

Nonorganic dystonia represents a major diagnostic challenge. Clinically inconsistent and incongruous postures and patterns of movement, give-away weakness, sensory complaints in the affected limb, multiple somatizations, presence of a psychiatric disorder, secondary gain, and amenability to suggestion are clues to this diagnosis.[45] However, some dystonias with an organic basis, such as cervical dystonia, may remit spontaneously.[46]

MYOCOLONIC SYNDROMES

Myoclonus can be physiological and can occur after exercise, in excessive fatigue or when falling asleep (hypnagogic jerks). As in other movement disorders, myoclonus may be idiopathic (essential myoclonus) (see Chapters. 37, 38). Onset of essential myoclonus can be at any age and there may be a positive family history. Epileptic (cortical) myoclonus is almost always associated with other forms of seizures and is more common in the younger age groups. Examples include juvenile myoclonic epilepsy of Janz, Rasmussen's encephalitis, and the progressive myoclonic epilepsy syndromes (PMEs). The PMEs are characterized by varying combinations of myoclonic and generalized seizures, ataxia, and dementia. The common causes are Lafora body disease, sialidosis, mitochondrial encephalopathy, neuronal ceroid lipofucsinosis (NCL), and dentato-rubro-pallido-luysian atrophy (DRPLA). Myoclonus can also have a myriad of symptomatic causes. These include trauma, anoxia (Lance–Adams syndrome), post stroke, metabolic (hepatic and renal failure, hyponatremia, hypoglycemia, nonketotic hyperglycemia), subacute sclerosing panencephalitis, CJD, drugs (anticonvulsants), degenerative diseases (Alzheimer's, MSA), storage disorders (GM2 gangliosidosis, NCL, Tay–Sachs), WD, and lesions.

▶ TABLE 1–3. GENETIC CAUSES OF DYSTONIA

Locus	Gene (Reference)	Inheritance	Age of Onset (y)	Phenotype	Pathology
DYT1	*Torsin A* (39)	AD	6–9 (up to 26)	Generalized dystonia	No cell/dopamine loss
DYT5	*GCH1* (40)	AD	Childhood (up to >50)	Dystonia, P, fluctuations	Hypomelanized SN neurons
DYT8	*MR1* (41)	AD	Childhood	PNKD-1	—
DYT11	*SGCE* (42)	AD	Childhood	Myoclonic dystonia	—
DYT12	*ATP1A3* (37)	AD	Childhood (up to 45)	Rapid onset dystonia – P	No cell loss or LB
DYT16	*PRKRA* (43)	AR	2–18	Dystonia, P, pyramidal signs	—
DYT18	*SLC2A1* (44)	AD	Infancy (through childhood)	PED, epilepsy, anemia, mild cognitive impairment	—

Loci only were omitted.
AD, autosomal dominant; AR, autosomal recessive; P, Parkinsonism; PED, paroxysmal exertion-induced dyskinesia; PNKD, paroxysmal nonkinesigenic dyskinesia.

THE LANCE–ADAMS SYNDROME

This comprises chronic action myoclonus after cerebral anoxia. It is often accompanied by cerebellar ataxia.[47] A dramatic response to 5-hydroxytryptophan (5-HTP) is a feature of this condition.

SPINAL MYOCLONUS

This is usually repetitive, in one limb. Spinal cord lesions such as those due to trauma, tumor, or inflammatory conditions may be responsible.[48]

PALATAL MYOCLONUS

This is characterized by rhythmic jerking of the soft palate, often in conjunction with the pharyngeal, laryngeal, and extraocular muscles and the diaphragm. These occur at a frequency of about 2 Hz and can persist in sleep. The site of the lesion is often the central tegmental tract (red nucleus to inferior olive), or occasionally the dentate nucleus. The cause is usually infarction, but the syndrome has been reported in neoplastic, inflammatory, and degenerative processes.[49] At autopsy, pathology has been found in the inferior olive.[50]

TIC SYNDROMES

Tics can be seen in the general population (habit spasms). Transient tic disorder occurs in up to 15% of children and usually takes the form of a simple motor or vocal tic. It usually remits within 1 year of occurrence, but may recur during periods of stress in adult life (see Chapter 39). Chronic tics persist throughout life. GTS represents the most severe form of the primary tic disorders. It has a hereditary basis, with the probable locus of the abnormal gene on chromosome 7.[51] The tics are chronic, multifocal, motor and vocal. TS is associated with attention-deficit hyperactivity disorder, obsessive-compulsive disorder, sleep disorders, echolalia (repeating sounds and words from an external source, usually the last sound), echopraxia (repeating movements of another person), palilalia (repeating own words or sounds with increasing speed and decreasing clarity), coprolalia (obscene utterances), and copropraxia (obscene gesturing) (see Chapter 39). A recently emphasized symptom of TS is the sensory tic.[12] These are uncomfortable somatic sensations such as tickle, touch, and pressure, which are localized to specific body parts. Patients relieve these sensations by movements that are interpreted as voluntary (e.g., scratching a body part to relieve an itch). Tics can be due to secondary causes that include head injury, stroke, as part of neuroacanthocytosis, or dopaminergic receptor–blocking drugs where they may occur as a tardive syndrome.[52]

STEREOTYPIC SYNDROMES

These occur in mental retardation, psychosis, Lesch–Nyhan syndrome, neuroacanthocytosis, and Rett's syndrome (RS). In RS, the movements are typically hand-wringing or hand-washing.[53] (see Chapters 24, 31, 35, 45).

AKATHISIC SYNDROMES

Akathisia is often seen in patients on neuroleptics. It can occur as an acute syndrome after administration of the first dose or after an increased dose, often in a young adult. It can also occur as a tardive syndrome more than 3 months after instituting treatment. Akathisia may also be seen in PD. When the lower limb movements in akathisia resemble choreatic movements, the patients' need to move differentiates akathisia from TD.

SYNDROMES DISPLAYING ASTERIXIS

Asterixis is commonly seen in metabolic encephalopathies, as a reaction to general anesthesia, and during anticonvulsant therapy.

PERIODIC LEG MOVEMENTS IN SLEEP (PLMS)

PLMS, or nocturnal myoclonus, is distinct from the hypnagogic jerks experienced by normal people while falling asleep. It comprises repetitive, stereotyped extensions of the big toes and sometimes flexion of the ankles, knees, and hips.[54] Occasionally, the movements are unilateral. The movements occur in clusters lasting from 10 minutes to several hours and sometimes throughout sleep. PLMS can be associated with RLS, narcolepsy, or sleep apnea syndrome.[55,56]

RESTLESS LEGS SYNDROME (RLS)

In RLS, or Ekbom's syndrome, patients experience sensory disturbances in the legs that are characteristically relieved by movement. The sensations are variously described as creeping, crawling, stretching or pulling, and are felt in the muscles, tendons, or bones. On occasion they may be felt in the upper limbs. The symptoms usually peak 15–20 minutes after lying down at night. Relief is obtained by moving the legs around or pacing. RLS differs from akathasia in that it occurs at night and is not associated with neuroleptic medication. RLS may be primary or occur in association with several conditions, including diabetes mellitus, uremia, carcinoma, pregnancy, malabsorption, and chronic obstructive airway disease. Many of these conditions are associated with sensory neuropathy and probably represent secondary RLS.[57] RLS has a strong genetic component and three RLS loci have been already been nominated, but no causative genes have been discovered so far RLS can be seen in patients with PD but recently described RLS susceptibility genes are not associated with PD 9.

PAINFUL LEGS AND MOVING TOES SYNDROME (PLMT)

In this disorder there is typically a deep boring pain in the lower limbs associated with continuous, stereotyped flexion–extension or abduction–adduction movements of the toes.[58] Involvement of the upper limbs has also been described.[59] The pain experienced may be mild to severe; immersing the feet in hot or cold water sometimes helps. The pain does not localize to any dermatome or peripheral nerve. In contrast to akathasia, movements do not relieve the sensation and there is no subjective desire to move the limbs. Indeed, patients often strive to stop the movements. The movements tend to disappear in sleep although they may occasionally persist. Some cases are associated with peripheral nerve or radicular lesions, but, in many, the neurological examination is normal. A similar disorder with moving toes but no associated pain has also been described.[60]

PHANTOM DYSKINESIA

This refers to involuntary movements of the stump associated with sensory phenomena such as paresthesiae and pain experienced by amputees. Phantom dyskinesia may occur spontaneously or as a result of neuroleptics.[61,62] Involuntary movements of the amputated stump without the associated sensory phenomena have also been described.[63]

PAROXYSMAL DYSKINESIAS

Paroxysmal dyskinesias are disorders characterized by episodes of involuntary movements lasting varying amounts of time with return to normality in between. Unlike seizures, there is no loss of consciousness, incontinence, or postictal confusion. Three types of paroxysmal dyskinesias have been recognized:[14]

1. Paroxysmal kinesigenic dyskinesia (PKD).
2. Paroxysmal nonkinesigenic dyskinesia (PNKD).
3. Paroxysmal exertional dyskinesia (PED).

PKD is precipitated by sudden movements, startle, or hyperventilation. Stress or excitement worsen it. The attacks are brief, lasting less than 5 minutes, and occur several times a day. The attacks are mainly dystonic in nature and may be unilateral, alternating unilateral, or bilateral. In some patients the movements may be choreatic or ballistic.[64] Rest, or pressure on the affected limb may relieve the attack. Sensory symptoms may precede the attack.[65,66] The familial form is dominantly inherited. Unlike PNKD, both the familial and sporadic forms of PKD respond to anticonvulsants.

The attacks in PNKD occur spontaneously at rest but may be precipitated by stress, fatigue, caffeine, or alcohol. They are of longer duration than in PKD and may last many minutes to hours. They are also less frequent. When bilateral, they may be of sufficient magnitude to cause postural instability and falls. Orofacial dystonia can result in dysarthria. Attacks may be partially suppressed by rest, physical activity, or rubbing the limb.[67,68] Primary PNKD may be sporadic or familial. The familial cases show dominant inheritance (Mount–Reback syndrome, chromosome 2q). Secondary PNKD can occur due to a variety of conditions, including head trauma, multiple sclerosis, vascular events, and myelopathy.[69]

PED is triggered by prolonged exercise and the attacks are protracted. Inheritance is autosomal dominant. Frontal lobe seizures are believed to be responsible for paroxysmal hypnogenic dyskinesias, particularly attacks of short duration.[70,71]

HEMIFACIAL SPASM (HS)

HS is a condition in which there is contraction of the facial muscles, which is most often unilateral. It usually starts with eyelid twitching and can later involve the lower part of the face. It may be intermittent or continuous, and is precipitated by contraction of the facial muscles as in speaking or chewing. When bilateral, the facial contractions on both sides are asynchronous. The etiology is often any irritative lesion of the facial nerve, such as an aberrant intracranial blood vessel, tumor, or multiple sclerosis plaque.

STIFF PERSON SYNDROME

This is an unusual condition, with continuous isometric contraction of axial and proximal muscles resulting in pain and often ophistotonus (see Chapter 43). The disorder can be malignant, culminating in death. Assessment for GAD65 antibodies may aid in diagnosis.

▶ HYPOKINETIC PHENOMENA

BRADYKINESIA

Bradykinesia refers to slowness and poverty of movement. This typically manifests as hypomimia, micrographia, hypophonia, monotonous speech, reduced blink rate, and generalized motor slowness. A reduced arm swing while walking, one of the earliest signs in PD, is a manifestation of bradykinesia. Initiation of movement is often difficult. Repetitive hand and foot movements reveal a reduction in speed and amplitude, and there may be brief arrests of ongoing movement. Often it is the demeanor and overall gestalt that conveys the sense of bradykinesia in a parkinsonian syndrome.

RIGIDITY

Rigidity is an increase in muscle tone, which is equal in the flexors and extensors; it is elicited during passive movement. Rigidity may be smooth (lead pipe) or ratchety (cogwheel). Assessment requires the patient to relax, and it is best detected in the more distal joints of a limb. Rigidity can be unmasked in mild cases by voluntary contralateral activation of the opposite limb (Froment's sign). Topographical distribution of rigidity may give a clue to diagnosis, as in the case of PSP, where axial rigidity is pronounced.

POSTURAL DISTURBANCES

In parkinsonian syndromes there can be significant postural disturbances. The trunk becomes flexed, resulting in a stooped posture, and the upper limbs may also assume a flexed posture. Marked flexion of the neck can be seen in MSA. In the majority of patients with PD, postural and gait abnormalities occur within the first 5 years.[72] There may be impairment of righting reflexes; this can be tested by asking the subject to balance with the feet together while the examiner pulls suddenly from behind. Postural instability is a major cause of falls.

▶ HYPOKINETIC SYNDROMES

PARKINSONIAN SYNDROMES

The tetrad of tremor, rigidity, bradykinesia, and postural disturbances constitutes parkinsonism. Although classically seen in PD (see Chapter 13), other degenerative diseases may present as a parkinsonian syndrome. These include PSP (see Chapter 21), MSA (see Chapter 20), CBGD (see Chapter 22), dementia with Lewy bodies (DLB, see Chapter 18), Westphal variant of HD (see Chapters 33, 45), DRD (see Chapters 28, 30), pallidal degeneration (see Chapter 24) and neuroacanthocytosis (see Chapter 24). Symptomatic causes include WD (see Chapter 42), dopaminergic receptor–blocking drugs (see Chapter 23), toxins, 1-methyl-4-phenyl-1,2,3,6-tetrahydropyridine (MPTP), manganese, carbon disulfide vascular events, head injury, postencephalitic sequelae, and hydrocephalus.

▶ TABLE 1–4. EXCLUSION CRITERIA FOR IDIOPATHIC PARKINSONISM

1. Neuroleptics, calcium channel-blocking drugs
2. Exposure to toxins: 1-methyl-4-phenyl-1,2,3,6-tetrahydropyridine (MPTP), carbon monoxide inhalation, manganese, methanol, *n*-hexane
3. Definite encephalitis
4. Strokes, and stepwise deterioration
5. Repeated head injury
6. Early and severe dementia or autonomic dysfunction
7. Cerebellar signs, supranuclear gaze palsy, and negative response to high doses of L-dopa

Idiopathic Parkinsonism (IP)/ Parkinson's Disease (PD)

PD is typically a disease of the elderly, but onset in the fourth or fifth decade is not unusual. The diagnosis can be considered when two of the three cardinal features of parkinsonism (i.e., tremor, rigidity, and bradykinesia) are present. Abnormal signs are usually asymmetric. Postural instability is best used as an adjunct to the diagnosis. Although postural instability may be seen early in a minority of PD patients, it can sometimes be seen in normal elderly subjects.[73,74] In addition to the motor abnormalities, there may be associated cognitive (bradyphrenia and dementia), autonomic, and mood (depression) abnormalities. Calne and colleagues have proposed stratifying patients into three groups of increasing diagnostic certainty: possible, probable, and definite.[75] Table 1–4 provides the exclusion criteria for IP.

Progressive Supranuclear Palsy (PSP)

The characteristic features of PSP are a symmetrical akinetic-rigid syndrome with increased axial rigidity, impaired vertical gaze, early frequent falls, dysarthria, dysphagia, frontal lobe dementia, and poor response to L-dopa (see Chapter 21).

Multiple System Atrophy (MSA)

MSA refers to parkinsonian syndromes with varying combinations of pyramidal, cerebellar, and autonomic involvement. Response to L-dopa is poor. When the parkinsonian component is most prominent, it is referred to as striatonigral degeneration (MSA-SND). When the parkinsonian and cerebellar involvement are both prominent, it is referred to as sporadic olivopontocerebellar atrophy (MSA-OPCA) (see Chapter 20).

▶ TABLE 1–5. GENETIC CAUSES OF PARKINSON'S DISEASE AND PARKINSONISM

Locus	Gene (Reference)	Inheritance	Age of Onset (y)	Phenotype	Pathology
PD					
PARK1/4	*SNCA* (79, 80)	AD	20–85 (point mutations) 38–65 (duplications) 24–48 (triplications)	PD, sometimes with dementia (point mutations) DLB (multiplications)	ND, LB (point mutations) DLB (multiplications)
PARK2	*PRKN* (81)	AR	16–72 (mean 30)	EOP	Pure ND (rare LB)
PARK6	*PINK1* (82)	AR	20–40	EOP	Unavailable
PARK7	*DJ-1* (83)	AR	20–40	EOP	Unavailable
PARK8	*LRRK2* (84)	AD	32–79	PD	ND, LB (rare pure ND, tau pathology)
Parkinsonism					
FTDP-17*T*	MAPT (85)	AD	25–76	FTD, P, O, CBS	Tau pathology
FTDP-17*U*	PGRN (86)	AD	45–83	FTD, P, CBS, FTD-MND	Ub/TDP-43+ inclusions
	DCTN1 (87)	AD	33–56	P, hypoventilation, depression, weight loss (Perry syndrome)	ND, Ub/TDP-43+ inclusions

PD-EOP refers to clinical phenotype, as most patients with EOP due to *PRKN* mutations do not meet pathological criteria of PD diagnosis.
AD, autosomal dominant; AR, autosomal recessive; CBS, corticobasal syndrome; D, dementia; DLB, diffuse Lewy body disease; EOP, early-onset parkinsonism; FTD, frontotemporal dementia; FTD-MND, frontotemporal dementia with motor neuron disease; LB, Lewy bodies; ND, nigrostriatal degeneration; O, oculomotor abnormalities; P, parkinsonism; PD, Parkinson's disease; SN, substantia nigra; Ub, ubiquitin.

Corticobasal Degeneration (CBD)

CBD is an asymmetric akinetic-rigid syndrome with cortical signs that include apraxia, cortical sensory loss, alien hand, stimulus-sensitive myoclonus, and poor response to L-dopa.[76] (see Chapter 22).

Dementia with Lewy Bodies (DLB)

The characteristic features of DLB are those of a parkinsonian syndrome with fluctuating dementia and psychosis. Hallucinations may be prominent (see Chapter 18).

Frontotemporal Dementias with Parkinsonism Linked to Chromosome 17 (FTDP-17)

FTDP-17 comprises hereditary dementia, associated with parkinsonism.[77,78] The inheritance is autosomal dominant and is due to the *MAPT* gene mutations (FTDP-17*T*) or due to the *GRN* gene mutations (FTDP-17*U*). The clinical picture is heterogeneous, and varies depending on the type of deletion or mutation. Parkinsonian symptoms are often present. Levodopa is either ineffective, or of limited therapeutic value.

▶ GENETICS OF PARKINSONISM

The current state of genetics of PD and parkinsonism is presented in Table 1–5,[79–87] (see Chapter 9) and the current state of genetics of ataxia is presented in Table 1–6.[88–113] (See Chapter 40).

Only loci with known gene mutations are included. It should be emphasized that SCA2 and to a lesser extent SCA3 mutation carriers can present with parkinsonism indistinguishable from other forms of genetic parkinsonism or even from cases of sporadic PD (other then positive family history). These patients may not have any features of ataxia and interestingly the parkinsonism can be levodopa responsive.

Much of this book deals with how patients with specific movement disorders present to the clinician and how they are managed. A systematic approach to the patient with a movement disorder will lead to a correct differential diagnosis and ultimately the correct diagnosis. The need for a comprehensive history with thorough and, if necessary, repeated physical examinations cannot be overemphasized. The clinical data thus obtained give direction to specific laboratory investigations when required. After this, a management protocol can be formulated, keeping in mind the unique characteristics of each patient.

▶ TABLE 1–6. **GENETIC CAUSES OF ATAXIA**

Locus	Gene (Reference)	Age of Onset (y)	Phenotype
Autosomal dominant			
SCA1	*ATXN1* (88)	4th decade (<10 to >60)	Ataxia, pyramidal signs, peripheral neuropathy
SCA2	*ATXN2* (89)	3rd–4th decade (<10 to >60)	Ataxia, slow saccades, peripheral neuropathy, dementia
SCA3/MJD	*ATXN3* (114)	4th decade (10–70)	Ataxia, pyramidal and extrapyramidal signs, nystagmus, slow saccades, amyotrophy, fasciculations, sensory loss
SCA, 16q22-linked	*PLEKHG* (91)	55	Ataxia, late onset hearing loss
SCA5	*SPTBN2* (92)	3rd–4th decade (10–68)	Ataxia, early onset, slow course
SCA6	*CACNA1A* (93)	5th–6th decade (19–71)	Ataxia, sometimes episodic, slow progression
SCA7	*ATXN* (94)	3rd–4th decade (0.5–60)	Ataxia, visual loss with retinopathy
SCA8	*ATXN8OS* (95)	39 (18–65)	Ataxia, slowly progressive, brisk reflexes, decreased vibration sense, rare cognitive impairment
SCA10	*ATXN10* (96)	36	Ataxia, occasional seizures
SCA11	*TTBK2* (97)	30 (15–70)	Ataxia, mild
SCA12	*PPP2R2B* (98)	33 (8–55)	Ataxia, action tremor, brisk reflexes, mild parkinsonism, cognitive impairment
SCA13	*KCNC3* (99)	Childhood	Ataxia, mild mental retardation, short stature
SCA14	*PRKCG* (100)	28 (12–42)	Ataxia, axial myoclonus
SCA15	*ITPR1* (101)	—	Ataxia, slow progression
SCA17	*TBP* (102)	6–34	Ataxia, cognitive impairment, chorea, dystonia, myoclonus, epilepsy
SCA27	*FGF14* (103)	11 (7–20)	Ataxia, tremor, dyskinesia, cognitive impairment
EA1	*KCNA1* (104)	1st decade (2–15)	Episodic ataxia, myokimia, attacks seconds to minutes
EA2	*CACNA1A* (105)	3–52	Episodic ataxia, nystagmus, vertigo, later permanent ataxia
Autosomal recessive			
ARSACS	*SACS* (106)	Early infancy	Spastic ataxia, dysarthria, neuropathy, nystagmus
Friedreich's ataxia	*FXN* (107)	10–15 (<25)	Ataxia, reduced reflexes, dysarthria, spasticity, optic atrophy, reduced vibration and position sense, hearing loss, diabetes, scoliosis, cardiomyopathy
Vitamin E deficiency	*TTPA* (108)	<20	Ataxia, sensory neuropathy, extensor plantar response, reduced reflexes, tremor, retinitis pigmentosa
Abetalipoproteinemia	*MTP* (109)	<20	Ataxia, nystagmus, sensory neuropathy, amyotrophy, reduced reflexes, retinitis pigmentosa, cardiomyopathy
Ataxia telangiectasia	*ATM* (110)	<3	Ataxia, nystagmus, sensory neuropathy, amyotrophy, oculomotor apraxia, extensor plantar response, reduced reflexes, tremor, myoclonus, dystonia, chorea, diabetes, oculocutaneous telangiectasias, immunodeficiency
Ataxia with oculomotor apraxia, type 1	*Aprataxin* (111)	<20	Ataxia, nystagmus, sensory neuropathy, amyotrophy, oculomotor apraxia, ophtalmoplegia, gaze instability, reduced reflexes, tremor, dystonia, chorea, cognitive impairment, optic atrophy
Ataxia with oculomotor apraxia, type 2	*Senataxin* (112)	<20	Ataxia, nystagmus, sensory neuropathy, amyotrophy, saccadic pursuit, spasticity, extensor plantar response, tremor, dystonia, chorea, cognitive impairment, scoliosis
IOSCA	*C10ORF2* (113)	<2	Ataxia, sensory neuropathy, amyotrophy, ophtalmoplegia, hypotonia, reduced reflexes, chorea, cognitive impairment, epilepsy, hearing loss, optic atrophy, hypogonadism

Some loci with unknown genes were omitted.
ARSACS, autosomal recessive spastic ataxia of Charlevoix–Saguenay; EA, episodic ataxia; IOSCA, infantile-onset spinocerebellar ataxia; SCA, spinocerebellar ataxia.

▶ ACKNOWLEDGEMENT

We thank Dr. Christian Wider, Susan Calne, and Katherine Purcell for assistance with the manuscript.

REFERENCES

1. Jankovic J, Fahn S. Physiologic and pathologic tremors. Diagnosis, mechanism, and management. Ann Intern Med 1980;93:460–465.
2. Kishore A, Calne D. Involuntary movements: An overview. In Joseph A, Young R (eds). Movement Disorders in Neurology and Neuropsychiatry. Boston, MA: Blackwell Scientific, 2000, pp.1–2.
3. Committee AH. Ad Hoc Committee of the Dystonia Medical Research Foundation meeting in February 1984; 1984.
4. Jedynak CP, Bonnet AM, Agid Y. Tremor and idiopathic dystonia. Mov Disord 1991;6:230–236.
5. Obeso JA, Rothwell JC, Lang AE, et al. Myoclonic dystonia. Neurology 1983;33:825–830.
6. Ravits J, Hallett M, Baker M, et al. Primary writing tremor and myoclonic writer's cramp. Neurology 1985;35: 1387–1391.
7. Kurlan R, Behr J, Medved L, et al. Myoclonus and dystonia: A family study. Adv Neurol 1988;50:385–389.
8. Quinn NP, Rothwell JC, Thompson PD, et al. Hereditary myoclonic dystonia, hereditary torsion dystonia and hereditary essential myoclonus: An area of confusion. Adv Neurol 1988;50:391–401.
9. Nygaard TG, Marsden CD, Duvoisin RC. Dopa-responsive dystonia. Adv Neurol 1988;50:377–384.
10. Segawa M, Hosaka A, Miyagawa F, et al. Hereditary progressive dystonia with marked diurnal fluctuation. Adv Neurol 1976;14:215–233.
11. Sharp FR, Rando TA, Greenberg SA, et al. Pseudochoreoathetosis. Movements associated with loss of proprioception. Arch Neurol 1994;51:1103–1109.
12. Kurlan R. Tic disorders: An overview. In Joseph A, Young R (eds). Movement Disorders in Neurology and Neuropsychiatry. Boston, MA: Blackwell Scientific, 1999, pp. 437–441.
13. Jankovic J. The neurology of tics. In Marsden C, Fahn S (eds). Movement Disorders 2 London Butterworth, 1987, pp. 383–405.
14. Fahn S. Involuntary Movements In Rowland L (ed). Merritt's Neurology. Philadelphia: Lippincott Williams and Wilkins, 2000, pp. 38–41.
15. Young R, Weigner A: Tremor, in Swash M, Kennard C (eds): Scientific Basis of Clinical Neurology. Edinburgh: Churchill Livingston, 1985, pp 116–132.
16. Larsen TA, Calne DB. Essential tremor. Clin Neuropharmacol 1983;6:185–206.
17. Critchley M. Observations on essential (heredofamial) tremor. Brain 1949;72:113–139.
18. Elble RJ. Essential tremor frequency decreases with time. Neurology 2000;55:1547–1551.
19. Rajput AH, Jamieson H, Hirsh S, et al. Relative efficacy of alcohol and propranolol in action tremor. Can J Neurol Sci 1975;2:31–35.
20. Deng H, Le W, Jankovic J. Genetics of essential tremor. Brain 2007;130:1456–1464.
21. Gulcher JR, Jonsson P, Kong A, et al. Mapping of a familial essential tremor gene, FET1, to chromosome 3q13. Nat Genet 1997;17:84–87.
22. Higgins JJ, Pho LT, Nee LE. A gene (ETM) for essential tremor maps to chromosome 2p22-p25. Mov Disord 1997;12:859–864.
23. Higgins JJ, Loveless JM, Jankovic J, et al. Evidence that a gene for essential tremor maps to chromosome 2p in four families. Mov Disord 1998;13:972–977.
24. Lucotte G, Lagarde JP, Funalot B, et al. Linkage with the Ser9Gly DRD3 polymorphism in essential tremor families. Clin Genet 2006;69:437–440.
25. Shatunov A, Sambuughin N, Jankovic J, et al. Genomewide scans in North American families reveal genetic linkage of essential tremor to a region on chromosome 6p23. Brain 2006;129:2318–2331.
26. Findley LJ. Epidemiology and genetics of essential tremor. Neurology 2000;54:S8–S13.
27. FitzGerald PM, Jankovic J. Orthostatic tremor: An association with essential tremor. Mov Disord 1991;6:60–64.
28. Findley LJ, Gresty MA. Tremor. Br J Hosp Med 1981;26: 16–32.
29. Rajput AH, Rozdilsky B, Ang L, et al. Clinicopathologic observations in essential tremor: Report of six cases. Neurology 1991;41:1422–1424.
30. Rajput AH, Rozdilsky B, Ang L. Occurrence of resting tremor in Parkinson's disease. Neurology 1991;41: 1298–1299.
31. Tardive dyskinesia: Summary of a Task Force Report of the American Psychiatric Association. By the Task Force on Late Neurological Effects of Antipsychotic Drugs. Am J Psychiatry 1980;137:1163–1172.
32. Faheem AD, Brightwell DR, Burton GC, et al. Respiratory dyskinesia and dysarthria from prolonged neuroleptic use: Tardive dyskinesia? Am J Psychiatry 1982;139: 517–518.
33. Shoulson I. On chorea. Clin Neuropharmacol 1986;9 (Suppl 2):S85–S99.
34. Fahn S. Concept and classification of dystonia. Adv Neurol 1988;50:1–8.
35. Marsden CD, Obeso JA, Zarranz JJ, et al. The anatomical basis of symptomatic hemidystonia. Brain 1985;108 (Pt 2):463–483.
36. Pettigrew LC, Jankovic J. Hemidystonia: A report of 22 patients and a review of the literature. J Neurol Neurosurg Psychiatry 1985;48:650–657.
37. de Carvalho Aguiar P, Sweadner KJ, Penniston JT, et al. Mutations in the Na+/K+-ATPase alpha3 gene ATP1A3 are associated with rapid-onset dystonia parkinsonism. Neuron 2004;43:169–175.
38. Lee LV, Kupke KG, Caballar-Gonzaga F, et al. The phenotype of the X-linked dystonia-parkinsonism syndrome. An assessment of 42 cases in the Philippines. Medicine (Baltimore) 1991;70:179–187.
39. Ozelius LJ, Hewett JW, Page CE, et al. The early-onset torsion dystonia gene (DYT1) encodes an ATP-binding protein. Nat Genet 1997;17:40–48.
40. Ichinose H, Ohye T, Takahashi E, et al. Hereditary progressive dystonia with marked diurnal fluctuation caused

by mutations in the GTP cyclohydrolase I gene. Nat Genet 1994;8:236–242.
41. Rainier S, Thomas D, Tokarz D, et al. Myofibrillogenesis regulator 1 gene mutations cause paroxysmal dystonic choreoathetosis. Arch Neurol 2004;61: 1025–1029.
42. Zimprich A, Grabowski M, Asmus F, et al. Mutations in the gene encoding epsilon-sarcoglycan cause myoclonus-dystonia syndrome. Nat Genet 2001;29:66–69.
43. Camargos S, Scholz S, Simon-Sanchez J, et al. DYT16, a novel young-onset dystonia-parkinsonism disorder: Identification of a segregating mutation in the stress-response protein PRKRA. Lancet Neurol 2008;7:207–215.
44. Weber YG, Storch A, Wuttke TV, et al. GLUT1 mutations are a cause of paroxysmal exertion-induced dyskinesias and induce hemolytic anemia by a cation leak. J Clin Invest 2008;118:2157–2168.
45. Fahn S, Williams DT. Psychogenic dystonia. Adv Neurol 1988;50:431–455.
46. Friedman A, Fahn S. Spontaneous remissions in spasmodic torticollis. Neurology 1986;36:398–400.
47. Lance JW, Adams RD. The syndrome of intention or action myoclonus as a sequel to hypoxic encephalopathy. Brain 1963;86:111–136.
48. Frenken CW, Notermans SL, Korten JJ, et al. Myoclonic disorders of spinal origin. Clin Neurol Neurosurg 1976;79:107–118.
49. Lapresle J. Palatal myoclonus. Adv Neurol 1986;43: 265–273.
50. Ronthal M, Greenstein P. Myoclonus and asterixis. In Joseph A, Young R (eds). Movement Disorders in Neurology and Neuropsychiatry. Boston, MA: Blackwell Scientific, 1999, pp. 449–456.
51. Kroisel PM, Petek E, Emberger W, et al. Candidate region for Gilles de la Tourette syndrome at 7q31. Am J Med Genet 2001;101:259–261.
52. Klawans HL, Falk DK, Nausieda PA, et al. Gilles de la Tourette syndrome after long-term chlorpromazine therapy. Neurology 1978;28:1064–1066.
53. Dure IV LS P. Rett syndrome: A clinical and neurobiologic review. In Joseph A, Young R (eds). Movement Disorders in Neurology and Neuropsychiatry. Boston, MA: Blackwell Scientific, 1999, pp. 613–622.
54. Colman R. Periodic movements in sleep (nocturnal myoclonus) and restless leg syndrome. In Guilleminault C (ed). Sleeping and Waking Disorders: Indications and Techniques Menlo Park: Addison Wesley, 1982, pp. 265–296.
55. Lugaresi E, Cirignotta F, Coccagna G, et al. Nocturnal myoclonus and restless legs syndrome. Adv Neurol 1986;43:295–307.
56. Wetter TC, Pollmacher T. Restless legs and periodic leg movements in sleep syndromes. J Neurol 1997;244: S37–S45.
57. Ekbom K. Restless Legs. Handbook of Clinical Neurology. In Vinken P, Bruyn G, eds. Diseases of Nerves. Amsterdam: Elsevier Science, 1970, pp. 311–320.
58. Spillane JD, Nathan PW, Kelly RE, et al. Painful legs and moving toes. Brain 1971;94:541–556.
59. Montagna P, Cirignotta F, Sacquegna T, et al. "Painful legs and moving toes" associated with polyneuropathy. J Neurol Neurosurg Psychiatry 1983;46:399–403.
60. Dressler D, Thompson PD, Gledhill RF, et al. The syndrome of painful legs and moving toes. Mov Disord 1994;9:13–21.
61. Barnes TR, Braude WM. Akathisia variants and tardive dyskinesia. Arch Gen Psychiatry 1985;42:874–878.
62. Jankovic J, Glass JP. Metoclopramide-induced phantom dyskinesia. Neurology 1985;35:432–435.
63. Kulisevsky J, Marti-Fabregas J, Grau JM. Spasms of amputation stumps. J Neurol Neurosurg Psychiatry 1992;55: 626–627.
64. Pryles CV, Livingston S, Ford FR. Familial paroxysmal choreoathetosis of Mount and Reback; study of a second family in which this condition is found in association with epilepsy. Pediatrics 1952;9:44–47.
65. Jung SS, Chen KM, Brody JA. Paroxysmal choreoathetosis. Report of Chinese cases. Neurology 1973;23: 749–755.
66. Stevens H. Paroxysmal choreo-athetosis. A form of reflex epilepsy. Arch Neurol 1966;14:415–420.
67. Walker ES. Familial paroxysmal dystonic choreoathetosis: A neurologic disorder simulating psychiatric illness. Johns Hopkins Med J 1981;148:108–113.
68. Weber MB. Familial paroxysmal dystonia. J Nerv Ment Dis 1967;145:221–226.
69. Bennet D, Goetz C. Acquired paroxysmal dyskinesias. In Joseph A, Young R (eds). Movement Disorders in Neurology and Neuropsychiatry. Boston, MA: Blackwell Scientific, 1992, pp. 540–556.
70. Meierkord H, Fish DR, Smith SJ, et al. Is nocturnal paroxysmal dystonia a form of frontal lobe epilepsy? Mov Disord 1992;7:38–42.
71. Oguni M, Oguni H, Kozasa M, et al. A case with nocturnal paroxysmal unilateral dystonia and interictal right frontal epileptic EEG focus: A lateralized variant of nocturnal paroxysmal dystonia? Brain Dev 1992;14: 412–416.
72. Marttila RJ, Rinne UK. Disability and progression in Parkinson's disease. Acta Neurol Scand 1977;56:159–169.
73. Jankovic J, McDermott M, Carter J, et al. Variable expression of Parkinson's disease: A base-line analysis of the DATATOP cohort. The Parkinson Study Group. Neurology 1990;40:1529–1534.
74. Weiner WJ, Nora LM, Glantz RH. Elderly inpatients: Postural reflex impairment. Neurology 1984;34:945–947.
75. Calne D, Snow B, Lee C. Criteria for diagnosing Parkinson's disease. AnnNeurol 1992;32:S125–S127.
76. Lang AE. Parkinsonism in corticobasal degeneration. Adv Neurol 2000;82:83–89.
77. Haugarvoll K, Wszolek ZK, Hutton M. The genetics of frontotemporal dementia. Neurol Clin 2007;25:697–715, vi.
78. Reed LA, Wszolek ZK, Hutton M. Phenotypic correlations in FTDP-17. Neurobiol Aging 2001;22:89–107.
79. Polymeropoulos MH, Lavedan C, Leroy E, et al. Mutation in the alpha-synuclein gene identified in families with Parkinson's disease. Science 1997;276:2045–2047.
80. Singleton AB, Farrer M, Johnson J, et al. alpha-Synuclein locus triplication causes Parkinson's disease. Science 2003;302:841.
81. Kitada T, Asakawa S, Hattori N, et al. Mutations in the parkin gene cause autosomal recessive juvenile parkinsonism. Nature 1998;392:605–608.

82. Valente EM, Abou-Sleiman PM, Caputo V, et al. Hereditary early-onset Parkinson's disease caused by mutations in PINK1. Science 2004;304:1158–1160.
83. Bonifati V, Rizzu P, van Baren MJ, et al. Mutations in the DJ-1 gene associated with autosomal recessive early-onset parkinsonism. Science 2003;299:256–259.
84. Zimprich A, Biskup S, Leitner P, et al. Mutations in LRRK2 cause autosomal-dominant parkinsonism with pleomorphic pathology. Neuron 2004;44:601–607.
85. Hutton M, Lendon CL, Rizzu P, et al. Association of missense and 5'-splice-site mutations in tau with the inherited dementia FTDP-17. Nature 1998;393:702–705.
86. Baker M, Mackenzie IR, Pickering-Brown SM, et al. Mutations in progranulin cause tau-negative frontotemporal dementia linked to chromosome 17. Nature 2006;442: 916–919.
87. Farrer MJ, Hulihan MM, Kachergus JM, et al. DCTN1 mutations in Perry syndrome. Nat Genet 2009;41:163–165.
88. Banfi S, Servadio A, Chung MY, et al. Identification and characterization of the gene causing type 1 spinocerebellar ataxia. Nat Genet 1994;7:513–520.
89. Imbert G, Saudou F, Yvert G, et al. Cloning of the gene for spinocerebellar ataxia 2 reveals a locus with high sensitivity to expanded CAG/glutamine repeats. Nat Genet 1996;14:285–291.
90. Gispert S, Twells R, Orozco G, et al. Chromosomal assignment of the second locus for autosomal dominant cerebellar ataxia (SCA2) to chromosome 12q23-24.1. Nat Genet 1993;4:295–299.
91. Ishikawa K, Toru S, Tsunemi T, et al. An autosomal dominant cerebellar ataxia linked to chromosome 16q22.1 is associated with a single-nucleotide substitution in the 5' untranslated region of the gene encoding a protein with spectrin repeat and Rho guanine-nucleotide exchange-factor domains. Am J Hum Genet 2005;77: 280–296.
92. Ikeda Y, Dick KA, Weatherspoon MR, et al. Spectrin mutations cause spinocerebellar ataxia type 5. Nat Genet 2006;38:184–190.
93. Riess O, Schols L, Bottger H, et al. SCA6 is caused by moderate CAG expansion in the alpha1A-voltage-dependent calcium channel gene. Hum Mol Genet 1997;6:1289–1293.
94. David G, Abbas N, Stevanin G, et al. Cloning of the SCA7 gene reveals a highly unstable CAG repeat expansion. Nat Genet 1997;17:65–70.
95. Koob MD, Moseley ML, Schut LJ, et al. An untranslated CTG expansion causes a novel form of spinocerebellar ataxia (SCA8). Nat Genet 1999;21:379–384.
96. Matsuura T, Yamagata T, Burgess DL, et al. Large expansion of the ATTCT pentanucleotide repeat in spinocerebellar ataxia type 10. Nat Genet 2000;26:191–194.
97. Houlden H, Johnson J, Gardner-Thorpe C, et al. Mutations in TTBK2, encoding a kinase implicated in tau phosphorylation, segregate with spinocerebellar ataxia type 11. Nat Genet 2007;39:1434–1436.
98. Holmes SE, O'Hearn EE, McInnis MG, et al. Expansion of a novel CAG trinucleotide repeat in the 5' region of PPP2R2B is associated with SCA12. Nat Genet 1999;23: 391–392.
99. Waters MF, Minassian NA, Stevanin G, et al. Mutations in voltage-gated potassium channel KCNC3 cause degenerative and developmental central nervous system phenotypes. Nat Genet 2006;38:447–451.
100. Al-Maghtheh M, Vithana EN, Inglehearn CF, et al. Segregation of a PRKCG mutation in two RP11 families. Am J Hum Genet 1998;62:1248–1252.
101. van de Leemput J, Chandran J, Knight MA, et al. Deletion at ITPR1 underlies ataxia in mice and spinocerebellar ataxia 15 in humans. PLoS Genet 2007;3:e108.
102. Nakamura K, Jeong SY, Uchihara T, et al. SCA17, a novel autosomal dominant cerebellar ataxia caused by an expanded polyglutamine in TATA-binding protein. Hum Mol Genet 2001;10:1441–1448.
103. van Swieten JC, Brusse E, de Graaf BM, et al. A mutation in the fibroblast growth factor 14 gene is associated with autosomal dominant cerebellar ataxia [corrected]. Am J Hum Genet 2003;72:191–199.
104. Browne DL, Gancher ST, Nutt JG, et al. Episodic ataxia/myokymia syndrome is associated with point mutations in the human potassium channel gene, KCNA1. Nat Genet 1994;8:136–140.
105. Ophoff RA, Terwindt GM, Vergouwe MN, et al. Familial hemiplegic migraine and episodic ataxia type-2 are caused by mutations in the Ca2+ channel gene CACNL1A4. Cell 1996;87:543–552.
106. Engert JC, Berube P, Mercier J, et al. ARSACS, a spastic ataxia common in northeastern Quebec, is caused by mutations in a new gene encoding an 11.5-kb ORF. Nat Genet 2000;24:120–125.
107. Campuzano V, Montermini L, Molto MD, et al. Friedreich's ataxia: Autosomal recessive disease caused by an intronic GAA triplet repeat expansion. Science 1996;271: 1423–1427.
108. Ouahchi K, Arita M, Kayden H, et al. Ataxia with isolated vitamin E deficiency is caused by mutations in the alpha-tocopherol transfer protein. Nat Genet 1995;9:141–145.
109. Sharp D, Blinderman L, Combs KA, et al. Cloning and gene defects in microsomal triglyceride transfer protein associated with abetalipoproteinaemia. Nature 1993;365: 65–69.
110. Savitsky K, Bar-Shira A, Gilad S, et al. A single ataxia telangiectasia gene with a product similar to PI-3 kinase. Science 1995;268:1749–1753.
111. Date H, Onodera O, Tanaka H, et al. Early-onset ataxia with ocular motor apraxia and hypoalbuminemia is caused by mutations in a new HIT superfamily gene. Nat Genet 2001;29:184–188.
112. Moreira MC, Klur S, Watanabe M, et al. Senataxin, the ortholog of a yeast RNA helicase, is mutant in ataxia-ocular apraxia 2. Nat Genet 2004;36:225–227.
113. Nikali K, Saharinen J, Peltonen L. cDNA cloning, expression profile and genomic structure of a novel human transcript on chromosome 10q24, and its analyses as a candidate gene for infantile onset spinocerebellar ataxia. Gene 2002;299:111–115.
114. Kawaguchi Y, Okamoto T, Taniwaki M, et al. CAG expansions in a novel gene for Machado-Joseph disease at chromosome 14q32.1. Nat Genet 1994;8:221–228.

CHAPTER 2

Assessing Disability in Movement Disorders: Quantitative Techniques and Rating Scales

Seth L. Pullman and Rachel Saunders-Pullman

▶ INTRODUCTION

Quantitative methods of assessing disability in patients with movement disorders provide measures that can be clinically relevant, reproducible, and allow for rigorous mathematical and statistical scrutiny. These techniques also can assist in diagnosis through precise determination of the timing and organization of movements,[1] and help in the understanding of underlying brain pathophysiology.[2] Methods for assessment have increased in scope and breadth over the last decade—with almost twice as many publications relating to clinical motor quantification methods and motion analysis in peer-reviewed journals since 2000 compared with the prior decade. Advances in the sensitivity and precision of sensors, improvements in processor speeds, computer graphics, and the development of neural interface systems[3] have all contributed to faster, more accurate, more meaningful methods of assessing motor disability, as well as uncovering the relationships between brain activity and motor behavior.

Importantly, quantitative techniques often contribute to improvement in quality of life or medical care,[4–6] not just assign numerical values to motor findings. For example, with the analysis of early or mild conditions such as Parkinson disease (PD),[7] methods have been developed with guidelines for their predictive utility[8] as well as general clinical use. Movement disorder laboratories now assess motor disabilities with proprietary hardware and software, and evaluate a multitude of questions in motor control for clinical investigations and routine clinical service. New devices are also available commercially, many of which are designed for ambulatory and home use[9–13], with the caveat that they should be monitored by health care professionals for accuracy and interpretation. As movement disorders may have overlapping or subtle clinical features, discerning the presence of and differentiating conditions, for example PD from essential tremor (ET) or dystonia (DYT), with more certainty and objectivity is important for therapeutic and prognostic reasons.

Descriptive comments or ratings with four-point (0–3) or five-point (0–4) scales are typically used clinically to characterize disabilities, such as tremors, and other motor signs and symptoms of movement disorders such as PD, e.g. 1+ (for mild) to 4+ (for severe). Multiple scores are rated in the various scales. While scales differ in length, with the shorter scales focused on decreasing subject burden and assessment time, many also include subscales of varying structures. Though validated and used by clinicians, rating scales are subjective, and are variable from examiner to examiner. Not all scales are easily reproducible and clinical scales may be insensitive to small changes—particularly in the "close to normal" range. Furthermore, while many scales are ordinal, they are not necessarily linear. A logarithmic relationship has been found between clinical rating scales of tremor and tremor amplitudes, suggesting that a one-point change in clinical scores represents a substantial change in tremor amplitude.[14]

This chapter first provides a brief overview of clinical rating scales and then describes some of the currently available techniques for quantitative and diagnostic measurement of movement disorders. These include uses of reaction and movement time, transcranial magnetic stimulation, tremor analysis, balance posture and gait measurements, polymyography and back-averaging, and computerized analysis of hand movements. This discussion of techniques is meant to be representative, not exhaustive. As these objective measures of motor behavior become more widely used, they may provide standards by which the efficacy of new therapeutic approaches could be assessed.

▶ CLINICAL RATING SCALES

Rating scales may focus on severity of disease, disability, or both. They vary with regard to overall metrics including validity, interrater reliability, and intrarater reliability. The most frequently used rating scale for PD, the Unified Parkinson Disease Rating scale (UPDRS)[15] focused on motor dysfunction, and had good validity and reliability.[16] However, early changes were not as well captured, and it was recently revised (MDS-UPDRS)[17] to better assess milder grades of early change. Further, while mood and cognition were included in the initial UPDRS, these sections and additional nonmotor features have been expanded in the revised version.

Among the rating scales for dystonia, measurement of affected sites as well as ease of use are paramount. The Fahn–Marsden rating scale (Burke–Fahn–Marsden or BFM) initially was utilized in testing the efficacy of anticholinergics for generalized dystonia. The BFM is characteristic of most movement disorder rating scales: It is organized in multiple categories, and within the categories an ordinal rating is given, from 0 = no clinical involvement to 4 = the most severe clinical manifestation (Table 2–1). It has been widely employed in deep brain stimulation (DBS) trials, in part because most trials involved generalized dystonia patients, and also because it has demonstrated good reliability. The Unified Dystonia Rating Scale (UDRS) and Global Dystonia Rating Scale (GDS), which are somewhat easier to administer, are also highly reliable,[18] and in a recent DBS study, improvement was similar on both the FMRS and the UDRS.[19] Of the other dystonia rating scales, the Toronto Western Spasmodic Torticollis Rating Scale (TWSTRS), which focuses on cervical dystonia, has been frequently applied in trials.[20]

Similarly, there are a range of tremor, myoclonus and ataxia rating scales, such as the Tremor Rating Scale,[21] the Unified Myoclonus Rating Scale,[22] and the Scale for the Assessment and Rating of Ataxia (SARA).[23] In these conditions, establishment of the scales may be challenged by their applicability to different diseases, particularly when multiple movement disorders may be present. For myoclonus-dystonia, no combined scale to evaluate both the myoclonus and the dystonia has been established, and a dystonia scale is usually combined with a myoclonus scale.[24] In contrast, for conditions such as Wilson's disease[25] Huntington's disease,[26] and Friedreich's ataxia,[27] disease specific-scales including the Unified Wilson's Disease Rating Scale and the Unified Huntington's Disease Rating Scale demonstrate good clinimetric properties, and encompass different aspects of the disease. Similar to the UPDRS, such scales are also challenged by the need to capture mild as well as more severe manifestations.[28]

Finally, while some scales, such as the UPDRS have been used to assess the presence of features, not just the severity, interpretation of the scales is markedly different when used for screening purposes. For example, factor subscores have been employed in using the UPDRS as a measure for assessment of presence of parkinsonism in the elderly.[29] In contrast, disease-specific methods designed solely as screening tools may be more predictive in this regard.[30] The electrophysiologic methods described below face similar challenges, as the measurement for the screening of various diseases may differ from those measures that capture severity.

▶ REACTION TIME AND MOVEMENT TIME

Physiologic measures related to movement initiation and execution are reaction time (RT) and movement time (MT). Motor tasks that measure RT and MT usually include a preparatory period during which information about the type of movement is presented[31] for ballistic, targeted movements, or as part of a repeating pattern or sequence of movements [serial reaction time task (SRTT)].[32,33] Defective initiation and execution of movement are principal abnormalities of PD and other movement disorders, and can be quantified with RT/MT tests. Abnormalities of RT/MT are interpreted within the context of the experimental setup, and are considered due to defective motor unit recruitment in PD,[34] alterations in processes involved in amplitude generation,[35–37] deficiency in the speed or accuracy operator,[38] or postulated reduced motivation and decreased energy in the basal ganglia.[39]

In the physiologic analysis of these motor deficits, voluntary tasks can be separated into "preparatory" and "executory" phases, which derive from early clinical work on motor control by SAK Wilson[40] and from animal studies that directly measured neuronal activity during specific motor behavior.[41,42] The preparatory phase is thought to represent premovement neural processing in (but not limited to) nonprimary motor regions of the brain. The executory phase relates to processing after the onset of movement and reflects activity in the primary motor cortex, spinal cord, peripheral nerve, and muscle.[43]

RT paradigms can be constructed in several ways depending on the kind of information given in the preparatory period (prior to the "go" signal), the options available after the "go" signal, the number, duration, and frequency of cues presented (Figure 2–1). Simple RT tasks present unambiguous information about the nature of the impending movement. Simple RT is a form of measuring "motor set" which can be defined as a state of readiness to make a movement.[41] SRTT is used to measure procedural learning and investigate brain plasticity mechanisms, often along with other tests such as transcranial magnetic stimulation.[44] Choice RT tasks utilize more than one preparatory cue, which results in the need to consider more than one option for the

▶ TABLE 2–1. **THE FAHN-MARSDEN (BFM) SCALE: MOVEMENT SCALE**

Region	Provoking factor	Severity	Weight factor	Product	
Eyes	0-4	X	0-4	0.5	0-8
Mouth	0-4	X	0-4	0.5	0-8
Speech					
Swallow	0-4	X	0-4	1.0	0-16
Neck	0-4	X	0-4	0.5	0-8
R arm	0-4	X	0-4	1.0	0-16
L arm	0-4	X	0-4	1.0	0-16
Trunk	0-4	X	0-4	1.0	0-16
R leg	0-4	X	0-4	1.0	0-16
L leg	0-4	X	0-4	1.0	0-16
				Sum:	
				Maximum = 120	

I. Provoking Factor
A. General

0. No dystonia at rest or with action
1. Dystonia only with particular action
2. Dystonia with many actions
3. Dystonia on action of distant part of body or intermittently at rest
4. Dystonia present at rest

B. Speech and swallowing

0. Occasional, either or both
1. Frequent either
2. Frequent one and occasional other
3. Frequent both

II. Severity Factors
Eyes

0. No dystonia
1. Slight. Occasional blinking
2. Mild. Frequent blinking without prolonged spasms of eye closure
3. Moderate. Prolonged spasms of eyelid closure, but eyes open most of the time
4. Severe. Prolonged spasms of eyelid closure, with eyes closed at least 30% of the time

Mouth

0. no dystonia present
1. Slight. Occasional grimacing or other mouth movements (e.g., jaw opened or clenched; tongue movement
2. Mild. Movement present less than 50% of the time
3. Moderate dystonic movements or contractions present most of the time
4. Severe dystonic movements or contractions present most of the time

Speech and swallowing

0. Normal
1. Slightly involved; speech easily understood or occasional choking
2. Some difficulty in understanding speech or frequent choking
3. Marked difficulty in understanding speech or inability to swallow firm foods
4. Complete or almost complete anarthria, or marked difficulty swallowing soft foods and liquids

Neck

0. No dystonia present
1. Slight. Occasional pulling
2. Obvious torticollis, but mild
3. Moderate pulling
4. Extreme pulling

Arm

0. No dystonia present
1. Slight dystonia. Clinically insignificant
2. Mild. Obvious dystonia, but not disabling
3. Moderate. Able to grasp, with some manual function
4. Severe. No useful grasp

Trunk

0. No dystonia present
1. Slight bending; clinically insignificant
2. Definite bending, but not interfering with standing or walking
3. Moderate bending; interfering with standing or walking
4. Extreme bending of trunk preventing standing or walking

Leg

0. No dystonia present
1. Slight dystonia, but not causing impairment; clinically insignificant
2. Mild dystonia. Walks briskly and unaided
3. Moderate dystonia. Severely impairs walking or requires assistance
4. Severe. Unable to stand or walk on involved leg

An example clinical severity rating scale, this case the five-point (0–4) Fahn–Marsden (BFM) rating scale for dystonia, from We Move (http://www.mdvu.org/library). As in most severity scales, specific components are added to equal a total severity score. (Reproduced with permission from http://www.mdvu.org/library/ratingscales. All contents copyright © WE MOVE 2005.)

The clinical scales for PD (UPDRS, MDS-UPDRS), the tremor scale, dystonia scales (UDRSr, FMRS, TWSTRS, GDS), myoclonus (UMRS), ataxia (SARA), and HD (UHDRS) typically include both rating definition and form for the scales. As with this table, most rating scales can be obtained on-line from We Move at: http://www.mdvu.org/library/ratingscales. The SARA can be found at: http://www.ataxia-study-group.net and the new MDS-UPDRS at http://www.movementdisorders.org.

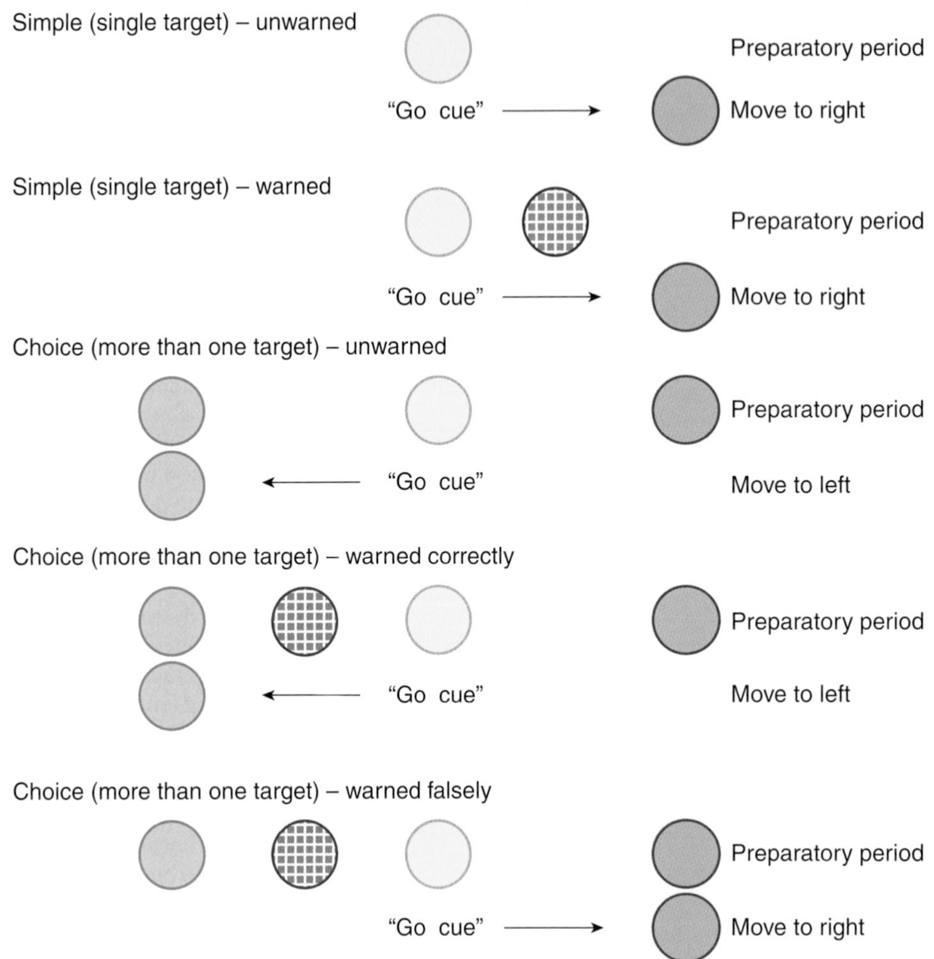

Figure 2–1. Examples of paradigms showing some of the possible simple and choice reaction time tests. The yellow center cue represents the start from which a subject moves (e.g., flexes the wrist or moves a finger) to a target after a "go" cue. In the simple (single target) set-up (at the top of the figure), the subject waits to move to a known target, generally after a variable preparatory time period. With more complex paradigms, warning signals (stippled) and more targets (for choice RT/MT) are utilized. Variable timing intervals as well as correct and false warning cues in the preparatory period are used for different experimental conditions.

impending movement, and to choose the correct one when the stimulus to move is given.[45–48] Studies have shown that simple RT and directional choice RT are significantly prolonged in PD.[43,47,49–52]

Although the target size has a strong influence over MT,[38,53] if the target size is kept constant MT is a useful quantitative motor test applied to PD.[47,54] MT has been shown to correlate with Hoehn and Yahr staging and UPDRS scores,[45,51,55] the Webster score,[56] global disability scores,[49,57] plasma levodopa levels,[45] rigidity,[55] and measures of asymmetry in hemiparkinsonism.[58] Combining RT and MT can be used for more global performance measures that have been applied in longitudinal studies such as those investigating dopaminergic tissue implantation in PD patients (Figure 2–2).[59]

▶ TRANSCRANIAL MAGNETIC STIMULATION

Transcranial magnetic stimulation (TMS) is a method of noninvasive stimulation of the central nervous system that was introduced for clinical use in the mid-1980s.[60] TMS quantifies motor output from the central nervous system and is used for studying the conductivity of the corticospinal system, excitation, and inhibition in disorders such as PD, stiff-person syndrome,[61] and the reorganization of brain circuitry after peripheral or central lesions.[44,62–65] TMS uses current stored in series capacitors, and discharged as a quick pulse through wire coils placed on the surface of the head. The coils induce a magnetic flux of short duration and high

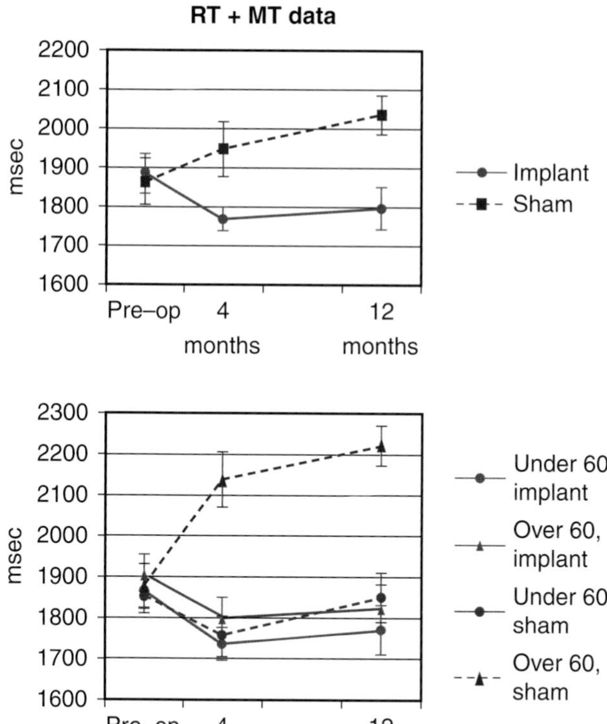

Figure 2–2. These graphs illustrate the utility of RT and MT measurements to study longitudinal changes in PD patients, in this case after dopamine tissue transplant and sham surgeries, modified from.[59] *Upper graph*: RT + MT means ±SD, grouped by type of transplant surgery. Note the deterioration in the sham surgery patients at 12 months, and the trend toward improvement in the implant patients. *Lower graph*: RT+ MT means ±SD, grouped by age. There is greater worsening in RT+ MT data in older patients who had sham surgery compared to all other groups, and no significant changes by 12 months in the other groups. (Modified with permission from Gordon PH, Yu Q, Qualls C, et al. Reaction time and movement time after embryonic cell implantation in Parkinson disease. Arch Neurol 2004;61:858–861.)

intensity that induce electrical current in the underlying cerebral cortex.[66] TMS delivery devices are embedded in a nonconductive plastic or rubber material and typically fashioned into figure eight, butterfly, or flat or concave circular shapes, and applied near the part of the brain under study. The various shapes and sizes are designed to distribute or focus the induced magnetic fields.

Stimulus intensity is expressed as a function of either the resting (or active) motor threshold, for example, 90% RMT (or AMT) or the percentage of the TMS machine output. Waveform recordings are usually obtained from a contralateral distal limb muscle, the motor evoked potential (MEP). Motor threshold is defined as the lowest stimulus intensity that evokes motor potentials of 50 μVin amplitude in five of 10 trials. Stimulus intensity is expressed as a percentage of the TMS device's maximum output. MEP amplitude is usually measured peak to peak, increases with stimulus intensity, and plateaus at 80% of the amplitude of the wave produced by peripheral stimulation. Unlike transcranial electrical stimulation, which directly excites cortical long tracts, the induced electrical fields of TMS preferentially stimulate neural elements oriented parallel to the surface of the brain. TMS pulses are associated with benign acoustic clicks and scalp or facial muscle activation. A momentary sense of disorientation at maximal stimulation may also be experienced. However, there are virtually no clinical cognitive or sensory effects at low intensities of TMS stimulation.

TMS may be delivered as a single pulse, in paired pulses, or as repetitive pulse trains (rTMS).[67,68] After a single-pulse TMS, prolongation of the central motor conduction time originates with the loss of large myelinated motor axons subsequent to degeneration, and the test assesses upper motor neuron dysfunction. Central motor conduction time, amplitude,[69] as well as other TMS measures are helpful in diagnosing and following progression in patients with upper motor neuron diseases, such as amyotrophic lateral sclerosis. Central motor conduction time alone may be of limited value when large diameter axons remain normal, or in diseases where long tract integrity is normal, such as with PD.

MEP amplitudes and latencies are influenced by multiple factors, including configuration and placement of the TMS coil, stimulus intensity, presence of conditioning pulses, muscle facilitation, and degree of phase cancellation. Suprasegmental modulation of MEPs may be inferred in several ways, including demonstration of relatively unchanged F-wave properties under the same stimulus conditions.

Paired pulse and rTMS are powerful ways to study human brain function, transiently stimulating or inhibiting different cortical areas. Paired pulses time-locked at precise interstimulus intervals (ISIs) may demonstrate changes in cortical excitability, specifically intracortical inhibition and facilitation.[70] Changes in cortical modulation of inhibitory and excitatory processes provide a window on motor control as well as maturation in the nervous system. The first pulse, or conditioning stimulus, is generally just subthreshold compared with the second or test pulse in studies using short ISIs between 1 and 15 milliseconds. At ISIs up to 6 milliseconds, an inhibition of the test MEP amplitude is normally found, while facilitation of MEP amplitudes may occur at ISIs between 6 and 15 milliseconds. Paired-pulse TMS at longer ISIs (100–250 milliseconds), using suprathreshold stimuli for both conditioning and test pulses, has been used to investigate longer-term effects.

Effects of rTMS on cortical excitability and inhibition outlast (for minutes to hours) the stimulation itself, a characteristic that could lead to therapeutic methods. Clinical applications are being considered in PD, depression, epilepsy, obsessive-compulsive disorders, and schizophrenia. Mostly for experimental purposes, rTMS from under 1 Hz to pulse trains up to 50 Hz have been shown to be safe in humans for up short periods.[71] rTMS at frequencies greater than 20 Hz increases cerebral blood flow and neuronal excitability, while low-frequency rTMS (1–2 Hz) has the opposite effect. The therapeutic potential of TMS is of interest as a safe and relatively lasting treatment for severe parkinsonism,[72] though some negative effects have been found.[73] In conjunction with somatosensory evoked potentials, TMS has been used to evaluate the disordered brain plasticity mechanisms as possible underlying causes of dystonia.[74]

▶ TREMOR ANALYSIS

Tremor is characterized by rhythmic oscillations around one or more joints, and can be a main cause of disability in PD.[75–78] Clinically, tremors are classified into those occurring (1) at rest, (2) while maintaining a posture, (3) with general actions, or (4) only during the execution of a specific task. Rest tremor is one of the hallmarks of PD, and even when mild, it may be problematic for PD patients. Action tremor, while not prominent early in the course of disease, occurs in up to 75% of PD patients.[79] Postural tremors typically occur in ET, or in PD with the arms outstretched or held close to the body ("sustention" tremors), and even task-related tremors occasionally affect PD patients.[80] Although tremor is among the most easily quantified movement disorder, there is no single thorough method of measuring tremors.[76] The clinical exam and rating scales are most important, but are nonetheless subjective and nonlinear.[14] Furthermore, clinical evaluation may not be sensitive enough to discern subtle changes over time, or objective enough to determine significant response to therapy.

Computerized tremor analysis is a method of evaluation using electronic motion or position transducers input to a computer usually through an analog-to-digital board. This technique objectively and reliably quantifies the important tremor characteristics: frequency and amplitude. Waveform properties, statistical analyses, and complex mathematical correlations can be determined off-line. Because tremors are quasi-sinusoidal, and as such, are amenable to mathematical analysis with a high degree of fidelity. However, tremors typically vary significantly throughout the day,[81] as well as from week to week, so multiple recording trials or longer recording durations are more likely to capture the true nature of most tremors.

Tremors can be classified by frequency (e.g., parkinsonian rest tremor from 3 to 6 Hz, ET from 4 to 12 Hz); frequency ranges for various disorders such as PD, ET, dystonia, and cerebellar disorders overlap considerably[82] and decrease with age.[83] Further, patients are not generally as bothered by tremor frequency as much as by amplitude and interference with voluntary activity. Large amplitude causes most of the morbidity associated with tremor in the context of the clinical situation in which tremor is present.[77,78] Therefore, while frequency is important nosologically, in terms of clinical disability and therapeutic effect, amplitude and other waveform characteristics are probably of more importance.

Different techniques exist for measuring tremor using devices constructed in clinical laboratories or available commercially.[9–13,84] One of the most common methods uses electronic motion detectors called accelerometers. These come in a variety of different designs from older, larger, and heavier (5 gm) models designed in the past to work with EEG amplifiers to smaller and lighter (<0.5 gm) miniature variety borrowed from the aerospace industry, and now used in smart phones, cameras, and other portable electronic devices. The smallest accelerometers are termed "piezoresistive" in that they incorporate a Wheatstone bridge measuring changes in resistance from strain gauges to which are attached a small seismic mass at the end of a miniature cantilever beam.[85] The beam is deflected in proportion to the amount of acceleration of the seismic mass, producing a voltage directly related to motion. These kinds of accelerometers are quite sensitive to sudden jerks if they are not critically damped and mechanically stopped. Other types of accelerometers are available but are larger and heavier than the piezoresistive devices. Variable-capacitance accelerometers contain a seismic disc that is accelerated between two fixed electrodes.

As an oscillatory movement, tremors have up to six degrees of freedom:[86] three translational (x, y, z planes) and three rotational (angular oscillations about axes in these planes). While dynamic collection of movement in all six degrees of freedom is possible, the amount of stored data becomes excessive. Furthermore, the added information by collecting in 3D or all six axes may not be significantly better for most investigations. Critical tremor features can usually be detected with uniaxial or biaxial devices with minimal loss of detail. Gyroscopes can be combined with accelerometers,[13] particularly for measuring angular movements such as the pill-rolling tremor of PD, but will add to the complexity of the data.

An advantage of miniature accelerometers is that they can be applied to almost any region of the body with minimal restrictions. The fingers, hands, or arms are typically involved in PD, but legs, jaw, forehead, and occasionally the neck or trunk may be useful recording sites. Because of their small size, miniature accelerometers do not to interfere with most voluntary or involuntary movements. Soft tissue motion may interfere with accurate recording, and movements with excessive rotational components will not be properly transduced by a linear uniaxial accelerometer. If these limitations are properly accounted for, however, accelerometry may be superior to other forms of tremor recording. Graphics tablets also have a role in evaluating action tremors, and their output can measure tremor in the x–y plane and pressure.[87–89] Torque motors provide very accurate means of recording tremors, but the body region under study (such as the wrist) must be secured, and usually one rotational axis is measured potentially restricting its clinical utility.

Accelerometer output, however, can be difficult to appreciate clinically because sinusoidal motion is not easily perceived in accelerometric units. These are usually given in terms of gravitational or "g" units (equal to 9.8 m/sec^2). With mathematical integration or software filters, however, true displacement of an oscillating body region can be derived from accelerometric data, provided low-frequency noise such as unwanted drift or higher frequency electronic interference are properly filtered.

The EMG should be recorded simultaneously with motion, using needle, wire, or more typically surface electrodes overlying active muscles. EMG can provide critically important information about motor unit recruitment and synchronization with the tremor activity.[76,83] This can also determine the relationship of the involved muscles to tremor movements and reveal whether antagonist muscles (e.g., flexion and extension of the wrist) are working at the same time, or alternately, to produce the tremor. To utilize EMG most appropriately in tremor analysis, the EMG signal has to be processed with rectification, integration, or smoothing to place its frequency profile into the tremor range.[76]

To record tremor activity, accelerometric, EMG, and other signals, such as force, are acquired through an analog-to-digital board, processed, and digitized in a clinical setting (Figure 2–3). Peak frequency and power are usually obtained using Fourier transform algorithms in which tremor signals are approximated by a series of sine and cosine waves. If the number of sampled points is N over a period of time T sec, then the sampling rate is N/T, the frequency resolution is $1/T$ Hz, and the maximum recordable frequency is $N/2T$ Hz (also known as the Nyquist frequency).[90] The power spectrum (or autospectrum), which is the Fourier transform multiplied by itself, effectively highlights the most prominent spectral peaks of tremors and improves signal-to-noise for analysis. Autospectra are described in terms of power or variance (hence the squared terms) against frequency, for example, g^2 vs. Hz. Fourier transforms are also used in cross-correlative analysis to determine the coherence or the frequency relationships between sets of waveforms.[91] Coherence is a measure of the magnitude of similarity and the phase differences between two signals. An ideal sine and cosine wave with identical frequency peaks would have a coherence magnitude of 1 at that frequency with a phase shift of 90°. Coherence is useful in determining relationships between any two clinical signals such as the agonist EMG and the tremor, or between tremors in right and left hands.

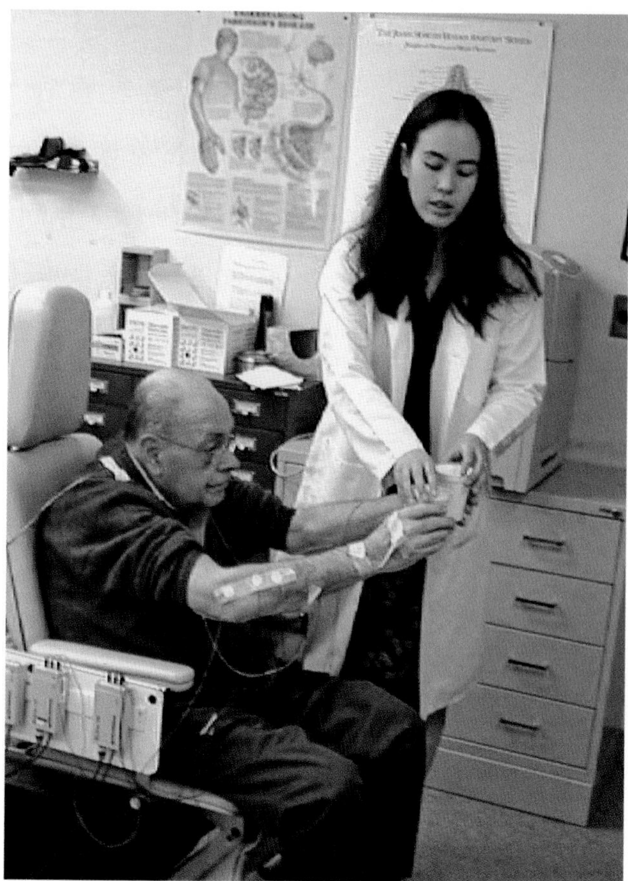

Figure 2–3. Picture of a subject undergoing a tremor analysis test. Tremor analysis uses specialized hardware to record the kinematics of tremors and other involuntary movements. The amplitude, frequency and underlying EMG activity of movements can be evaluated at rest, with postures and while performing those tasks which bring out the tremors. In this case, a subject is pouring water from hand to hand. Movements from any region of the body (the arms, legs, head, etc), side-to-side tremor relationships and associated EMG activity can be recorded and assessed in the time and frequency domains.

The objective findings of a tremor analysis test are most helpful when the clinical picture is complicated, or the response to medication or other treatment

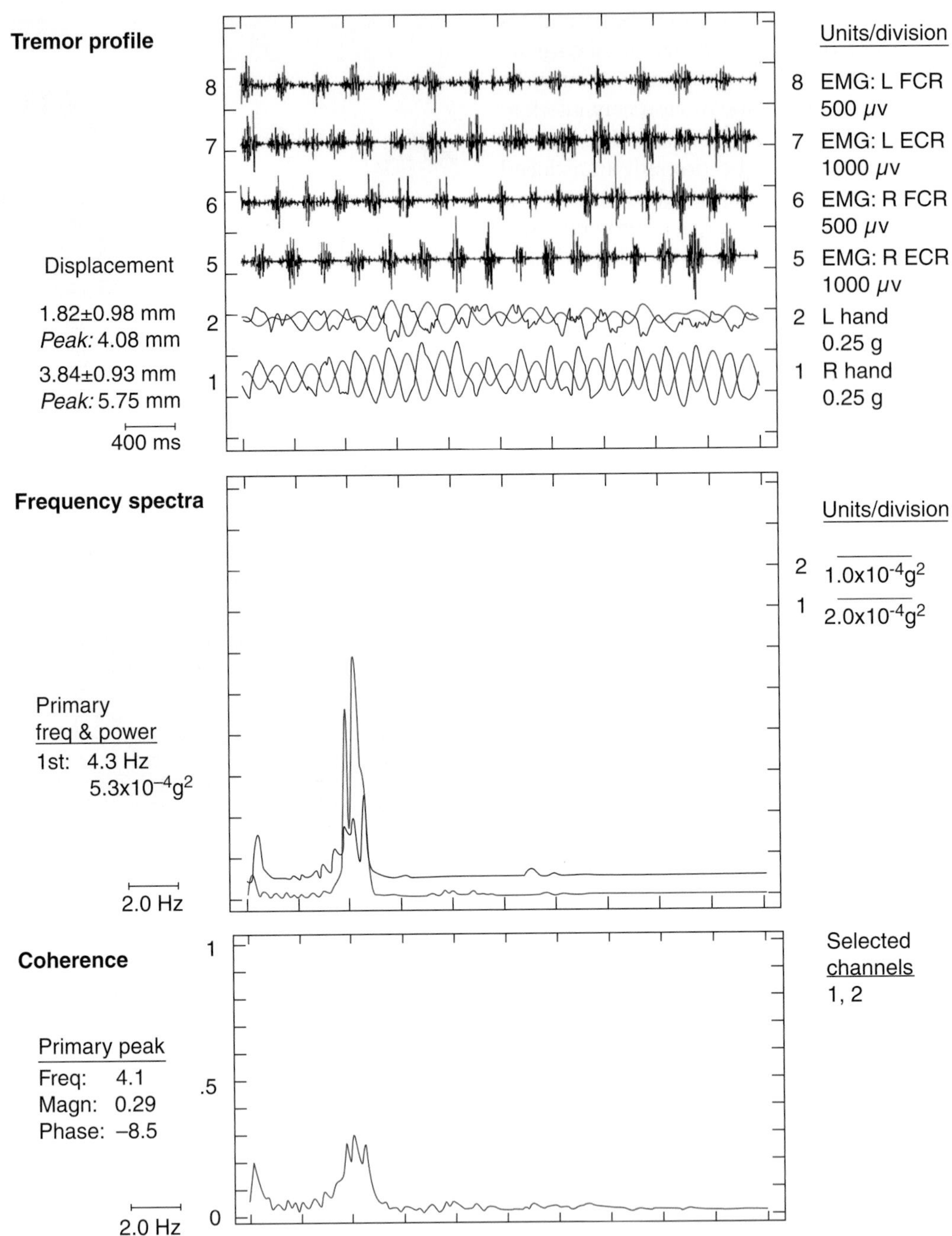

Figure 2–4. Tremor analysis of a patient with essential tremor just starting to pour water with both hands showing bilateral hand oscillations and related extensor and flexor forearm EMG activity. *Upper*: the tracings show surface EMG activity in forearm antagonist muscles, right and left flexor and extensor carpi radialis (FCR, ECR), and accelerometric with derived displacement data from both hands, indicating that the right hand is slightly worse (higher amplitudes). *Middle*: frequency spectra of both hands showing a main peak at 4.3 Hz. *Lower*: coherence tracings revealing cross-correlation relationships between the right and left sides (channels 1, 2).

needs to be monitored. Depending on recording circumstances, tremor frequencies can be reliably calculated to within 0.1 Hz, and tremor displacement amplitudes can be determined accurately to less than 0.5 mm (Figure 2–4). For example, parkinsonian action and essential tremors may be difficult to separate, but obviously important to distinguish for prognosis and treatment.[75,77,78,92] Both conditions occur with increasing age, and both may occur at rest or with actions. There are, however, some objective physiologic characteristics that may be used to separate the clinical phenomenology of these conditions.

In addition to its diagnostic utility, tremor analysis may be used to document the level of disability or the effect of medication, physical therapy, or surgery. The effect of intramuscular botulinum toxin injections in agonist muscles on PD tremors, for example, was shown to be insignificant on the basis of clinical rating scales and tremor measurements of amplitude.[93] Thus, results from the tremor analysis test can supplement the clinical examination in an objective and detailed manner. The diagnosis of psychogenic tremors, which should not be one of exclusion, is assisted with quantitative measurements where specific constellation of findings, such as an increased amplitude with inertial loading, distractibility, and inconsistency, can be objectively recorded.[94]

A typical tremor analysis test takes about 1 hour to complete, depending on the complexity of the clinical situation and the nature of the study. In most situations, patient is seated comfortably with a series of devices such as accelerometers and EMG electrodes attached over the appropriate limbs and muscles. The test should evaluate the patient during the same conditions as the clinical exam (e.g., at rest, with arms extended, or moving finger-to-nose) to allow for direct comparisons and for consistency, if the patient is evaluated multiple times. Specific maneuvers known to exaggerate or diminish tremor symptoms, such as writing or pouring a cup of water, can be used to further delineate and quantify the movement abnormalities caused by the tremor. Inertial loading can be used to help differentiate central from mechanical-reflex tremors. Several trials for each condition are taken over various epochs of time, task-specific data are then averaged and analyzed.

▶ BALANCE, POSTURE, AND GAIT MEASUREMENTS

Maintenance of balance in upright posture requires that a line drawn from the center of gravity perpendicular to the ground pass within the base of support between the feet. Gait is a combination of stance, stride, arm swing, and number of other subtle truncal adjustments. Voluntary movements may perturb the body off the support base so that it becomes mechanically unstable.[95–97] Compensatory axial and appendicular maneuvers accompany volitional movements to maintain stability. Unexpected perturbations in the forward or backward direction in young controls result in a stereotyped compensatory activation of the ankle joint musculature with a latency of just over 100 millisecond followed by synergistic activation of proximal leg muscles.[98] The normal elderly may use a proximal leg strategy with subsequent activation of distal musculature with reasonable results.[99]

Postural instability occurs among the elderly[100] and is a common symptom in idiopathic PD and parkinsonian syndromes.[101] It may not be responsive to pharmacotherapy.[102–105] Although the clinical exam serves as the most easily performed assessment, quantitative methods are used to more precisely determine underlying neuromuscular dysfunction.

A number of methodologies have been used to assess changes in postural stability and gait patterns,[106,107] including measurement of steadiness on quiet standing, ability to shift weight in forward/backward and lateral directions, and EMG responses to sudden destabilizing stimuli. Many investigators have measured steadiness during quiet standing.[108,109] This generally involves use of a balance platform with piezoelectric or mechanical force transducers to measure the position and path of the center of pressure. Studying potential mechanisms involving the cortical–basal ganglia-thalamo-cortical loops and effect of sudden destabilizing movements on long loop postural reflexes are other methods of analysis. Traub and coworkers analyzed anticipatory postural reflexes in the gastrocnemius to an unexpected change in torque on the arm in patients with PD.[110]

Elble and colleagues[111] have proposed that four core clinical features of gait: (1) interactions with the environment, (2) emotion, (3) hesitation and freezing, and (4) absent or inappropriate rescue reactions, can be used track the dysfunction of the cortical–basal ganglia-thalamo-cortical loops that result in gait disorders. These could also serve to develop a clinical rating scale that would avoid the ambiguities inherent in terms related to gait apraxia. Freezing of gait rating scales, particularly useful for in parkinsonism, can help determine the best treatment intervention.[112–114] Treatment for gait dysfunction and postural instability in PD has been considered using DBS in the pedunculopontine nucleus[115] and substantia nigra pars reticulata,[116] though the numbers of patients in these studies have been low.

Gait laboratories now routinely measure EMG responses in the lower extremities and trunk musculature, along with stride and stance kinemetrics.[97,117,118] Perturbations on a movable platforms such as treadmills, noninvasive limb measurements, pelvic tilt, and multiple joint measures[119] are all combined to provide quantitative assessment of balance and gait.

▶ POLYMYOGRAPHY AND BACK-AVERAGING

Myoclonus is defined as brief involuntary muscle contractions resulting in a quick body movements or limb jerks. Myoclonus may be focal, segmental, axial, multifocal, or generalized, rhythmic or arrhythmic. Focal and segmental myoclonus may originate at any level of the central or peripheral nervous system, whereas axial myoclonus frequently arises from the brain stem or spinal cord, multifocal myoclonus from the cerebral cortex, and generalized myoclonus from cerebral cortex or brain stem.[120–125] A remarkable number of different pathological conditions result in similar appearing jerks, yet no single biochemical or physiologic mechanism is common to all of them. Myoclonus is one of the most frequent neurologic signs in medicine. It occurs in many pathologic conditions and normal physiological states and is not associated with loss or change in consciousness.[123,125–128]

Cortical and subcortical myoclonic jerks characteristically are bursts of muscle activity, irregular in timing, separated by distinct pauses (distinguishing them from more continuous involuntary movements) and irregular in amplitude or force. Brief lapses in muscle tone, or asterixis, is a form of "negative" myoclonus because it phenomenologically appears as quick limb movements and physiologically may be caused by similar cerebral mechanisms as muscle jerks.[124,129] The brain Stem, spinal, and peripheral myoclonus represent different forms of myoclonus from the more typical quick irregular jerks. These types of myoclonus are composed of longer duration, more rhythmic muscle activity in segmental axial or limb myotomes, and may be generated by discrete spinal lesions or more diffusely in the propriospinal interneurons.[121,123]

Quantitative methods may be used to be differentiate myoclonus from other movement disorders and epilepsy.[22,121,130–132] Some presentations of myoclonus differ from epilepsy only in the extent of motor involvement. Myoclonus as well must be distinguished from forms of dystonia, chorea, tics, clonus, tremor, startle, and fasciculations for proper treatment and management. Although a long-standing controversy, animal models, and hippocampal slice preparations have shown that similar pathophysiologic mechanisms occur in both myoclonus originating from the cerebral cortex or brain stem and epilepsy.[133] Epilepsia partialis continua, therefore, is a form of continuous or repetitive focal myoclonus.[134]

Distinguishing myoclonus from other movement disorders may be difficult and requires both clinical examination and specialized physiologic tests to resolve. Dystonia is usually quite different phenomenologically from myoclonus, but some forms can be quick and termed "myoclonic dystonia."[135] Myoclonus dystonia is an alcohol-responsive autosomal dominant disorder characterized by a combination of myoclonus and dystonia with characteristic electrophysiological features.[136] Myoclonus does not present with the fluidity and proximal-to-distal randomness of chorea, or the urge, stereotypy, and partial voluntary control of tics. Myoclonus is different from clonus in that it is not sustained after tendon stretch and differs from tremor in that it is usually not sinusoidal and EMG recordings reveal discrete intervals between jerks. Some forms of brain stem or spinal myoclonus such as palatal myoclonus, however, can appear rhythmic and sinusoidal. Hemiballism is generally unilateral, irregular in timing and scaling, with long duration muscle bursts (>500 milliseconds) that are typically proximal, characteristics that, in their aggregate, are different from myoclonus of cortical or subcortical origin. Fasciculations and related conditions such as myokymia originate from single-motor units either in the anterior horn cell or its axons. While myoclonus may originate in the spinal cord or peripheral nervous system, it always involves the synchronous firing of more than single-motor units.[125]

Stimulus-sensitive myoclonus is also referred to as reflex or action myoclonus depending on whether external or internal afferent information triggers a jerk. These are either cortical or subcortical (reticular) in origin and can be distinguished clinically and with physiological tests. Nonstimulus sensitive myoclonus comprises the more rhythmic jerking of palatal or spinal myoclonus, the slower and more periodic discharges found in some acquired disorders such as Creutzfeldt–Jakob disease, and the faster but nonrepetitive irregular nonstimulus sensitive jerks of benign essential and physiologic myoclonus.[120]

A basic physiological method of investigation is multichannel polymyography (usually surface EMG) to determine muscle firing patterns, activation order, agonist/antagonist relationships, reflex responsiveness, EMG recruitment profiles, and EMG to jerk relationships. Polymyography is useful for determining the burst durations of myoclonic jerks as well as the patterns of antagonist actions and activation orders up or down the brain stem or spinal cord. While there are no absolute burst durations diagnostic of myoclonus, as a general rule, irregular co-contracting antagonist activity 10 to 50 milliseconds in duration is characteristic of cortical myoclonus while longer duration, more patterned or rhythmic EMG bursts up to 300 milliseconds may characterize brain stem, propriospinal, or spinal segmental myoclonus.

EEG is used to record concomitant cerebral cortical activity in patients with myoclonus or other movement disorders. Combined with EMG, back-averaging relates the EEG or sensory evoked potential with motor activity.[125] Back-averaging determines whether there are cortical transient potentials preceding involuntary movements that are time-locked to the EMG at an appropriate latency, providing strong evidence that the abnormal movements originate in the cerebral cortex.[132] An EMG electrode on the appropriate muscle serves as a trigger for averaging cortical potentials recorded over the scalp. The patient is tested at rest, during movement-inducing maneuvers or while subjected visual, audio or tactile stimuli. The test is often interpreted in conjunction with a standard EEG and somatosensory-evoked potentials. Additional types of quick involuntary movements, such as tics, chorea, and dystonia may be investigated with back-averaging to rule out conditions that may implicate higher centers in the brain. The Bereitschaftspotential, a relatively prolonged (500–1500 milliseconds) increase in EEG baseline, occurs prior to voluntary movement and is indicative of motor preparation. It is used to study to the extent to which motor behavior has voluntary cortical mechanisms, such as found in tic disorders.[137]

▶ COMPUTERIZED ANALYSIS OF HAND MOVEMENTS

Writing, drawing, or other hand movements can be used to quantify and study physiologic issues related to fine motor control. Referred to as graphonomics, this became a field of study in the early 1980s to investigate relationships between planning and execution of handwriting and drawing movements.[138] Interesting and testable concepts about writing and drawing that are relevant to movement disorders have evolved from graphonomics. One is the principle of isogony (quantified by the 2/3 power law[139]) and another is isochrony. These are two phenomena that have been robustly observed, with few exceptions, in the execution of continuous, planar drawing movements, independent of shape, size, and direction.[140,141] Isogony implies that drawing speed is inversely related to the curvature of the line drawn, and isochrony refers to the temporal invariance of drawing longer curved lines over the same angular displacement with increasing radius.

Among the more clinically useful methods in evaluating patients with movement disorders is analysis of writing and drawing using a digitizing tablet (Figure 2–5).[142–146] Other methods, such as using pads and keyboards connected to a computer, measure digital movements and can be used to study repetitive activity.[147–149] Advantages of all these methods are that no wires are attached and patients can write, draw, or move without restraints. Compared with handwriting, drawing requires subjects to execute standard figures, such as straight lines, circles, or spirals, so more comparable information, such as drawing shape and consistency, can be evaluated.[87,88,150] Freeform drawing also can also be recorded and used to study motor behavior and the relationship of line curvature to drawing velocity and other physiological issues.[151] Writing and drawing are multijointed tasks involving the distal and proximal upper limb and thus provide a window on a wide range of motor problems.[89,139]

One application using a digitizing table records circles or spirals.[87,88,145,150] It can quantify normal motor activity as well as measure dysfunction in patients with PD,[152] dystonia,[153] or ataxia from multiple sclerosis.[154] With an inking pen that also functions as a computer mouse, subjects draw spirals or other figures on plain paper, often with the starting point marked. Data are collected in the x, y, and z (pressure) axes and provide virtual triaxial recordings of kinematics and dynamics.

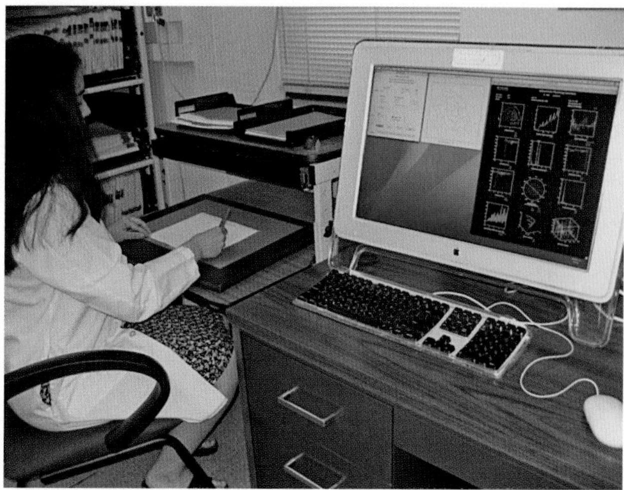

Figure 2–5. The spiral analysis test, a noninvasive graphonomics system of quantifying upper limb motor function. A digitizing tablet and writing pen are connected to a computer to record position, pressure, and time measurements of hand drawn spirals without wires or other attachments.

Quantification of handwritten spirals may be based on "unraveling" and averaging multiple spiral drawings that capture a range of spatial attributes related to spiral execution, and it provides data for computation of clinically relevant spiral indices (Figure 2–6). The indices correlate to clinical phenomena, such as tremor,[143] which are logarithmically related to tremor rating scales.[14] Spiral indices also measure drawing speed and acceleration, loop-to-loop width tightness and variation, drawing pressure over time, and can be used to develop an overall assessment of severity of motor execution.[155]

Drawing speed is calculated as the distance between consecutive x, y points, averaged over the length of the spiral, divided by the average time between sample points. Drawing acceleration and other derivatives are also calculated. Loop tightness, a measure of clinical micrographia, is a determination of the average distance between consecutive spiral loops over the entire drawing divided by the maximum spiral radius. Loop width variability, a mathematical correlate of limb ataxia, is calculated as the coefficient of variation of loop width. Spiral pressure data are evaluated over time and can assess unilateral asymmetry of drawing pressure by comparing the right and left sides of a spiral.

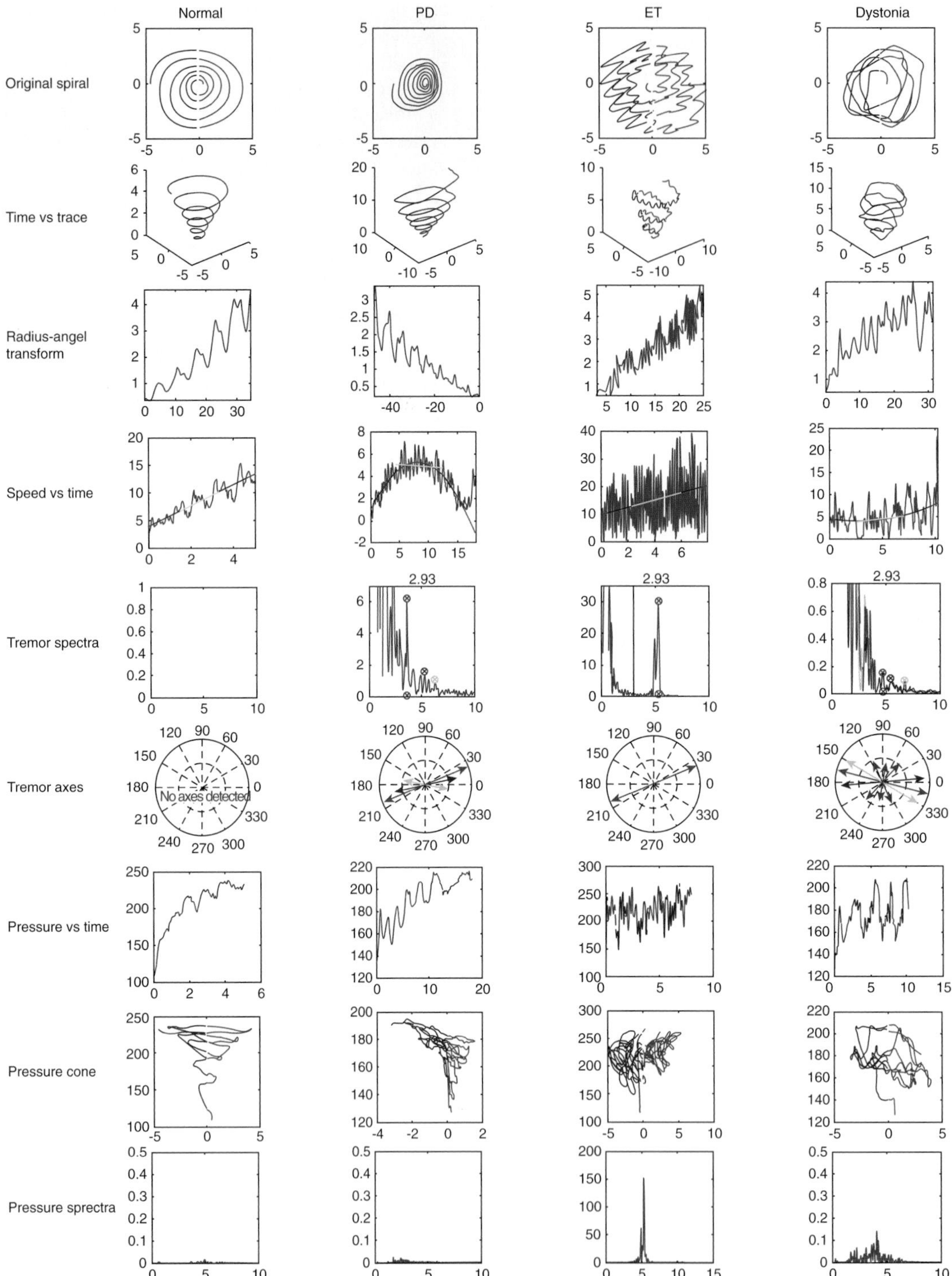

Figure 2–6. Example movement disorders quantified using spiral analysis. The spiral figures below are from one person without neurological or medical problems (normal), one with Parkinson's disease (PD), essential tremor (ET), and dystonia. The indices shown here highlight spatial, timing, and pressure features of spiral drawing. Characteristic of specific disorders are as follows: PD patients tend to have compressed spirals with side-to-side pressure asymmetry, multiple tremor axes, and decrement in speed of execution over time. ET patients have a single dominant frequency peak accompanied by a dominant direction of tremor. Pressure peaks in ET are also sharply peaked. Speeds can approach normal, but are consistently variable through time. Dystonia is characterized by multiple patterns of superimposed fluctuations in both spatial and pressure frequency, tremor direction, and speed. There are usually multiple frequencies and directions of tremor of comparable strength. The pressure spectrum is broad and asymmetric, and the speeds, in addition to their variability, may increase slightly or stay constant. (Modified with permission from Seth L. Pullman. Diagnostic tests of motor function. Available at: http://www.cmpl.columbia.edu/diagnostic.html, retrieved July 7, 2010.)

These extractions from spiral and other drawings have proven useful for specific motor control investigations as well for documenting changes after medical or surgical treatments.

REFERENCES

1. Elble RJ. Motion analysis to the rescue? Mov Disord 2000;15:595–597.
2. Leiguarda R, Merello M, Balej J, et al. Disruption of spatial organization and interjoint coordination in Parkinson's disease, progressive supranuclear palsy, and multiple system atrophy. Mov Disord 2000;15:627–640.
3. Hatsopoulos NG, Donoghue JP. The science of neural interface systems. Annu Rev Neurosci 2009;32:249–266.
4. Cooper RA, Dicianno BE, Brewer B, et al. A perspective on intelligent devices and environments in medical rehabilitation. Med Eng Phys 2008;30:1387–1398.
5. Hong M, Perlmutter JS, Earhart GM. A kinematic and electromyographic analysis of turning in people with Parkinson disease. Neurorehabil Neural Repair 2009;23:166–176.
6. Moore O, Peretz C, Giladi N. Freezing of gait affects quality of life of peoples with Parkinson's disease beyond its relationships with mobility and gait. Mov Disord 2007;22:2192–2195.
7. Montgomery EB, Jr., Koller WC, LaMantia TJ, et al. Early detection of probable idiopathic Parkinson's disease: I. Development of a diagnostic test battery. Mov Disord 2000;15:467–473.
8. Wasson JH, Sox HC, Neff RK, et al. Clinical prediction rules. Applications and methodological standards. N Engl J Med 1985;313:793–799.
9. van Someren EJ, van Gool WA, Vonk BF, et al. Ambulatory monitoring of tremor and other movements before and after thalamotomy: A new quantitative technique. J Neurol Sci 1993;117:16–23.
10. Hoff JI, van der Meer V, van Hilten JJ. Accuracy of objective ambulatory accelerometry in detecting motor complications in patients with Parkinson disease. Clin Neuropharmacol 2004;27:53–57.
11. Haeuber E, Shaughnessy M, Forrester LW, et al. Accelerometer monitoring of home- and community-based ambulatory activity after stroke. Arch Phys Med Rehabil 2004;85:1997–2001.
12. Caligiuri MP, Tripp RM. A portable hand-held device for quantifying and standardizing tremor assessment. J Med Eng Technol 2004;28:254–262.
13. Giuffrida JP, Riley DE, Maddux BN, et al. Clinically deployable Kinesia technology for automated tremor assessment. Mov Disord 2009;24:723–730.
14. Elble RJ, Pullman SL, Matsumoto JY, et al. Tremor amplitude is logarithmically related to 4- and 5-point tremor rating scales. Brain 2006;129:2660–2666.
15. Fahn S, Elton R, Members of the UPDRS Development Committee. Unified Parkinson's disease rating scale. In Fahn S, Marsden CD, Calne DB, Goldstein M (eds). Recent Developments in Parkinson's Disease, Volume 2. Floram Park, NJ: Macmillan Health Care Information, 1987, pp. 153–164.
16. Martinez-Martin P, Gil-Nagel A, Gracia LM, et al. Unified Parkinson's Disease Rating Scale characteristics and structure. The Cooperative Multicentric Group. Mov Disord 1994;9:76–83.
17. Goetz CG, Tilley BC, Shaftman SR, et al. Movement Disorder Society-sponsored revision of the Unified Parkinson's Disease Rating Scale (MDS-UPDRS): scale presentation and clinimetric testing results. Mov Disord 2008;23:2129–2170.
18. Comella CL, Leurgans S, Wuu J, et al. Rating scales for dystonia: a multicenter assessment. Mov Disord 2003;18: 303–312.
19. Susatia F, Malaty IA, Foote KD, et al. An evaluation of rating scales utilized for deep brain stimulation for dystonia. J Neurol 2009.
20. Comella CL, Jankovic J, Shannon KM, et al. Comparison of botulinum toxin serotypes A and B for the treatment of cervical dystonia. Neurology 2005;65:1423–1429.
21. Fahn S, Tolosa E, Martin C. Clinical rating scale for tremor. In Jankovic J, Tolosa E, (eds). Parkinson's Disease and Movement Disorders. Baltimore: Williams and Wilkins, 1993, pp. 271–280.
22. Frucht SJ, Leurgans SE, Hallett M, et al. The Unified Myoclonus Rating Scale. Adv Neurol 2002;89:361–376.
23. Schmitz-Hubsch T, du Montcel ST, Baliko L, et al. Scale for the assessment and rating of ataxia: Development of a new clinical scale. Neurology 2006;66:1717–1720.
24. Jog M, Kumar H. Bilateral pallidal deep brain stimulation in a case of myoclonus dystonia syndrome. Mov Disord 2009;24:1547–1549.
25. Leinweber B, Moller JC, Scherag A, et al. Evaluation of the Unified Wilson's Disease Rating Scale (UWDRS) in German patients with treated Wilson's disease. Mov Disord 2008;23:54–62.
26. Huntington Study Group. Unified Huntington's Disease Rating Scale: reliability and consistency. Mov Disord 1996;11:136–142.
27. Burk K, Malzig U, Wolf S, et al. Comparison of three clinical rating scales in Friedreich ataxia (FRDA). Mov Disord 2009.
28. Cano SJ, Riazi A, Schapira AH, et al. Friedreich's ataxia impact scale: a new measure striving to provide the flexibility required by today's studies. Mov Disord 2009;24: 984–992.
29. Benito-Leon J, Bermejo-Pareja F, Morales-Gonzalez JM, et al. Incidence of Parkinson disease and parkinsonism in three elderly populations of central Spain. Neurology 2004;62:734–741.
30. Saunders-Pullman R, Soto-Valencia J, Costan-Toth C, et al. A new screening tool for cervical dystonia. Neurology 2005;64:2046–2049.
31. Montgomery EB, Jr., Nuessen J, Gorman DS. Reaction time and movement velocity abnormalities in Parkinson's disease under different task conditions. Neurology 1991;41:1476–1481.
32. Philip BA, Wu Y, Donoghue JP, et al. Performance differences in visually and internally guided continuous manual tracking movements. Exp Brain Res 2008;190: 475–491.
33. Song S, Howard JH, Jr., Howard DV. Perceptual sequence learning in a serial reaction time task. Exp Brain Res 2008;189:145–158.

34. Grasso M, Mazzini L, Schieppati M. Muscle relaxation in Parkinson's disease: a reaction time study. Mov Disord 1996;11:411–420.
35. Hallett M, Khoshbin S. A physiological mechanism of bradykinesia. Brain 1980;103:301–314.
36. Chen R, Kumar S, Garg RR, et al. Impairment of motor cortex activation and deactivation in Parkinson's disease. Clin Neurophysiol 2001;112:600–607.
37. Espay AJ, Beaton DE, Morgante F, et al. Impairments of speed and amplitude of movement in Parkinson's disease: a pilot study. Mov Disord 2009;24:1001–1008.
38. Montgomery EB, Jr., Nuessen J. The movement speed/accuracy operator in Parkinson's disease. Neurology 1990;40:269–272.
39. Mazzoni P, Hristova A, Krakauer JW. Why don't we move faster? Parkinson's disease, movement vigor, and implicit motivation. J Neurosci 2007;27:7105–7116.
40. Wilson SAK. Some disorders of motility and of muscle tone, with special reference to the corpus striatum. Lancet 1925;2:1–10, 53–62, 169–178, 215–219, 268–276.
41. Evarts EV, Shinoda Y, Wise SP. Neurophysiological Approaches to Higher Brain Functions. New York: John Wiley and Sons, 1984.
42. Wise SP. The primate premotor cortex: past, present, and preparatory. Annu Rev Neurosci 1985;8:1–19.
43. Sheridan MR, Flowers KA, Hurrell J. Programming and execution of movement in Parkinson's disease. Brain 1987;110(Pt 5):1247–1271.
44. Pascual-Leone A, Tarazona F, Keenan J, et al. Transcranial magnetic stimulation and neuroplasticity. Neuropsychologia 1999;37:207–217.
45. Pullman SL, Watts RL, Juncos JL, et al. Dopaminergic effects on simple and choice reaction time performance in Parkinson's disease. Neurology 1988;38:249–254.
46. Cooper JA, Sagar HJ, Tidswell P, et al. Slowed central processing in simple and go/no-go reaction time tasks in Parkinson's disease. Brain 1994;117(Pt 3):517–529.
47. Evarts EV, Teravainen H, Calne DB. Reaction time in Parkinson's disease. Brain 1981;104:167–186.
48. Camicioli RM, Wieler M, de Frias CM, et al. Early, untreated Parkinson's disease patients show reaction time variability. Neurosci Lett 2008;441:77–80.
49. Heilman KM, Bowers D, Watson RT, et al. Reaction times in Parkinson disease. Arch Neurol 1976;33:139–140.
50. Rafal RD, Posner MI, Walker JA, et al. Cognition and the basal ganglia. Separating mental and motor components of performance in Parkinson's disease. Brain 1984;107(Pt 4):1083–1094.
51. Bloxham CA, Mindel TA, Frith CD. Initiation and execution of predictable and unpredictable movements in Parkinson's disease. Brain 1984;107(Pt 2):371–384.
52. Yokochi F, Nakamura R, Narabayashi H. Reaction time of patients with Parkinson's disease, with reference to asymmetry of neurological signs. J Neurol Neurosurg Psychiatry 1985;48:702–705.
53. Sanes JN. Information processing deficits in Parkinson's disease during movement. Neuropsychologia 1985;23:381–392.
54. Spirduso WW. Reaction and movement time as a function of age and physical activity level. J Gerontol 1975;30:435–440.
55. Ward CD, Sanes JN, Dambrosia JM, et al. Methods for evaluating treatment in Parkinson's disease. Adv Neurol 1983;37:1–7.
56. Rogers D, Lees AJ, Trimble M, et al. Concept of bradyphrenia: A neuropsychiatric approach. Adv Neurol 1987;45:447–450.
57. Marsden CD. The mysterious motor function of the basal ganglia: The Robert Wartenberg Lecture. Neurology 1982;32:514–539.
58. Rafal RD, Friedman JH, Lannon MC. Preparation of manual movements in hemiparkinsonism. J Neurol Neurosurg Psychiatry 1989;52:399–402.
59. Gordon PH, Yu Q, Qualls C, et al. Reaction time and movement time after embryonic cell implantation in Parkinson disease. Arch Neurol 2004;61:858–861.
60. Barker AT, Jalinous R, Freeston IL. Non-invasive magnetic stimulation of human motor cortex. Lancet 1985;1:1106–1107.
61. Sandbrink F, Syed NA, Fujii MD, et al. Motor cortex excitability in stiff-person syndrome. Brain 2000;123(Pt 11):2231–2239.
62. Di Lazzaro V, Oliviero A, Mazzone P, et al. Direct demonstration of long latency cortico-cortical inhibition in normal subjects and in a patient with vascular parkinsonism. Clin Neurophysiol 2002;113:1673–1679.
63. Rossini PM, Rossi S. Transcranial magnetic stimulation: diagnostic, therapeutic, and research potential. Neurology 2007;68:484–488.
64. Schneider SA, Talelli P, Cheeran BJ, et al. Motor cortical physiology in patients and asymptomatic carriers of parkin gene mutations. Mov Disord 2008;23:1812–1819.
65. Zanette G, Tamburin S, Manganotti P, et al. Different mechanisms contribute to motor cortex hyperexcitability in amyotrophic lateral sclerosis. Clin Neurophysiol 2002;113:1688–1697.
66. Kobayashi M, Pascual-Leone A. Transcranial magnetic stimulation in neurology. Lancet Neurol 2003;2:145–156.
67. Wassermann EM, Samii A, Mercuri B, et al. Responses to paired transcranial magnetic stimuli in resting, active, and recently activated muscles. Exp Brain Res 1996;109:158–163.
68. Romero JR, Anschel D, Sparing R, et al. Subthreshold low frequency repetitive transcranial magnetic stimulation selectively decreases facilitation in the motor cortex. Clin Neurophysiol 2002;113:101–107.
69. Floyd AG, Yu QP, Piboolnurak P, et al. Transcranial magnetic stimulation in ALS: utility of central motor conduction tests. Neurology 2009;72:498–504.
70. Kujirai T, Caramia MD, Rothwell JC, et al. Corticocortical inhibition in human motor cortex. J Physiol 1993;471:501–519.
71. Benninger DH, Lomarev M, Wassermann EM, et al. Safety study of 50 Hz repetitive transcranial magnetic stimulation in patients with Parkinson's disease. Clin Neurophysiol 2009;120:809–815.
72. Wassermann EM, Lisanby SH. Therapeutic application of repetitive transcranial magnetic stimulation: a review. Clin Neurophysiol 2001;112:1367–1377.

73. Boylan LS, Pullman SL, Lisanby SH, et al. Repetitive transcranial magnetic stimulation to SMA worsens complex movements in Parkinson's disease. Clin Neurophysiol 2001;112:259–264.
74. Tamura Y, Ueki Y, Lin P, et al. Disordered plasticity in the primary somatosensory cortex in focal hand dystonia. Brain 2009;132:749–755.
75. Critchley E. Clinical manifestations of essential tremor. J Neurol Neurosurg Psychiatry 1972;35:365–372.
76. Elble RJ, Koller WC. Tremor. In. Baltimore: The Johns Hopkins Press, 1990.
77. Findley LJ, Koller WC. Essential tremor: a review. Neurology 1987;37:1194–1197.
78. Marsden CD. Origins of normal and pathological tremor. In Findley LJ, Capildeo R (eds). Movement Disorders: Tremor. New York: Oxford University Press, 1984, pp. 37–84.
79. Lance JW, Schwab RS, Peterson EA. Action tremor and the cogwheel phenomenon in Parkinson's disease. Brain 1963;86:95–110.
80. Sanes JN, Hallett M. Limb positioning and magnitude of essential tremor and other pathological tremors. Mov Disord 1990;5:304–309.
81. Cleeves L, Findley LJ, Gresty M. Assessment of rest tremor in Parkinson's disease. Adv Neurol 1987;45:349–352.
82. Deuschl G, Raethjen J, Lindemann M, et al. The pathophysiology of tremor. Muscle Nerve 2001;24:716–735.
83. Elble RJ. Physiologic and essential tremor. Neurology 1986;36:225–231.
84. Boccagni C, Carpaneto J, Micera S, et al. Motion analysis in cervical dystonia. Neurol Sci 2008;29:375–381.
85. Budd JWG. Ultraminiature accelerometers and pressure transducers. Sensors 1984;1:12–15.
86. Frost JD, Jr. Triaxial vector accelerometry: a method for quantifying tremor and ataxia. IEEE Trans Biomed Eng 1978;25:17–27.
87. Elble RJ, Brilliant M, Leffler K, et al. Quantification of essential tremor in writing and drawing. Mov Disord 1996;11:70–78.
88. Pullman SL. Spiral analysis: A new technique for measuring tremor with a digitizing tablet. Mov Disord 1998;13 Suppl 3:85–89.
89. Wang S, Bain PG, Aziz TZ, et al. The direction of oscillation in spiral drawings can be used to differentiate distal and proximal arm tremor. Neurosci Lett 2005;384:188–192.
90. Glaser EM, Ruchkin DS. Principles of Neurobiological Signal Analysis. New York: Academic Press, 1976.
91. Bendat JS, Piersol AG. Random Data: Analysis and Measurement Procedures. New York: John Wiley & Sons, 1986.
92. Hubble JP, Busenbark KL, Koller WC. Essential tremor. Clin Neuropharmacol 1989;12:453–482.
93. Trosch RM, Pullman SL. Botulinum toxin A injections for the treatment of hand tremors. Mov Disord 1994;9:601–609.
94. Deuschl G, Koster B, Lucking CH, et al. Diagnostic and pathophysiological aspects of psychogenic tremors. Mov Disord 1998;13:294–302.
95. Knutsson E, Martensson A. Quantitative effects of L-dopa on different types of movements and muscle tone in Parkinsonian patients. Scand J Rehabil Med 1971;3:121–130.
96. Berg K, Norman KE. Functional assessment of balance and gait. Clin Geriatr Med 1996;12:705–723.
97. Ondo W. Gait and balance disorders. Med Clin North Am 2003;87:793–801, viii.
98. Nashner LM. Fixed patterns of rapid postural responses among leg muscles during stance. Exp Brain Res 1977;30:13–24.
99. Woolacott M, Shumway-Cook A, Nashner LM. Postural Reflexes and Aging. New York: Praeger, 1982.
100. Nayak US, Gabell A, Simons MA, et al. Measurement of gait and balance in the elderly. J Am Geriatr Soc 1982;30:516–520.
101. Suteerawattananon M, MacNeill B, Protas EJ. Supported treadmill training for gait and balance in a patient with progressive supranuclear palsy. Phys Ther 2002;82:485–495.
102. Lakke JP. Axial apraxia in Parkinson's disease. J Neurol Sci 1985;69:37–46.
103. Weinrich M, Koch K, Garcia F, et al. Axial versus distal motor impairment in Parkinson's disease. Neurology 1988;38:540–545.
104. Lew M. Overview of Parkinson's disease. Pharmacotherapy 2007;27:155S-160S.
105. Moore ST, MacDougall HG, Ondo WG. Ambulatory monitoring of freezing of gait in Parkinson's disease. J Neurosci Methods 2008;167:340–348.
106. Wang N, Ambikairajah E, Lovell NH, et al. Accelerometry based classification of walking patterns using time-frequency analysis. Conf Proc IEEE Eng Med Biol Soc 2007;2007:4899–4902.
107. IEEE. Computational Intelligence in Gait Research: A Perspective on Current Applications and Future Challenges. IEEE Trans Inf Technol Biomed 2009.
108. Stribley RF, Albers JW, Tourtellotte WW, et al. A quantitative study of stance in normal subjects. Arch Phys Med Rehabil 1974;55:74–80.
109. Seliktur R, Susak Z, Najenson T, et al. Dynamic features of standing and their correlation with neurologic disorders. Scand J Rehabil Med 1978;10:59–64.
110. Traub MM, Rothwell JC, Marsden CD. Anticipatory postural reflexes in Parkinson's disease and other akinetic-rigid syndromes and in cerebellar ataxia. Brain 1980;103:393–412.
111. Elble RJ. Gait and dementia: moving beyond the notion of gait apraxia. J Neural Transm 2007;114:1253–1258.
112. Giladi N, Huber-Mahlin V, Herman T, et al. Freezing of gait in older adults with high level gait disorders: association with impaired executive function. J Neural Transm 2007;114:1349–1353.
113. Giladi N, Tal J, Azulay T, et al. Validation of the freezing of gait questionnaire in patients with Parkinson's disease. Mov Disord 2009;24:655–661.
114. Golbe LI, Ohman-Strickland PA. A clinical rating scale for progressive supranuclear palsy. Brain 2007;130:1552–1565.
115. Weinberger M, Hamani C, Hutchison WD, et al. Pedunculopontine nucleus microelectrode recordings in movement disorder patients. Exp Brain Res 2008;188:165–174.
116. Chastan N, Westby GW, Yelnik J, et al. Effects of nigral stimulation on locomotion and postural stability in patients with Parkinson's disease. Brain 2009;132:172–184.

117. Wootten ME, Kadaba MP, Cochran GV. Dynamic electromyography. I. Numerical representation using principal component analysis. J Orthop Res 1990;8:247–258.
118. Wootten ME, Kadaba MP, Cochran GV. Dynamic electromyography. II. Normal patterns during gait. J Orthop Res 1990;8:259–265.
119. Collins TD, Ghoussayni SN, Ewins DJ, et al. A six degrees-of-freedom marker set for gait analysis: repeatability and comparison with a modified Helen Hayes set. Gait Posture 2009;30:173–180.
120. Obeso JA, Rothwell JC, Marsden CD. The spectrum of cortical myoclonus. From focal reflex jerks to spontaneous motor epilepsy. Brain 1985;108 (Pt 1):193–124.
121. Chokroverty S. Propriospinal myoclonus. Clin Neurosci 1995;3:219–222.
122. Rothwell JC. Brainstem myoclonus. Clin Neurosci 1995;3:214–218.
123. Rothwell JC. Pathophysiology of spinal myoclonus. Adv Neurol 2002;89:137–144.
124. Shibasaki H. Physiology of negative myoclonus. Adv Neurol 2002;89:103–113.
125. Shibasaki H, Hallett M. Electrophysiological studies of myoclonus. Muscle Nerve 2005;31:157–174.
126. Brown P, Thompson PD, Rothwell JC, et al. Axial myoclonus of propriospinal origin. Brain 1991;114(Pt 1A): 197–214.
127. Hallett M. Neurophysiology of brainstem myoclonus. Adv Neurol 2002;89:99–102.
128. Hallett M, Chadwick D, Marsden CD. Cortical reflex myoclonus. Neurology 1979;29:1107–1125.
129. Shibasaki H. Pathophysiology of negative myoclonus and asterixis. Adv Neurol 1995;67:199–209.
130. Hallett M. Myoclonus: relation to epilepsy. Epilepsia 1985;26 Suppl 1:S67–S77.
131. Ikeda A, Kakigi R, Funai N, et al. Cortical tremor: a variant of cortical reflex myoclonus. Neurology 1990;40: 1561–1565.
132. Shibasaki H. Neurophysiological classification of myoclonus. Neurophysiol Clin 2006;36:267–269.
133. Traub RD, Wong RK. Cellular mechanism of neuronal synchronization in epilepsy. Science 1982;216:745–747.
134. Watanabe K, Kuroiwa Y, Toyokura Y. Epilepsia partialis continua. Epileptogenic focus in motor cortex and its participation in transcortical reflexes. Arch Neurol 1984;41:1040–1044.
135. Ravits J, Hallett M, Baker M, et al. Primary writing tremor and myoclonic writer's cramp. Neurology 1985;35: 1387–1391.
136. Li JY, Cunic DI, Paradiso G, et al. Electrophysiological features of myoclonus-dystonia. Mov Disord 2008;23:2055–2061.
137. Berardelli A, Curra A, Fabbrini G, et al. Pathophysiology of tics and Tourette syndrome. J Neurol 2003;250: 781–787.
138. Van Gemmert AW, Teulings HL. Advances in graphonomics: studies on fine motor control, its development and disorders. Hum Mov Sci 2006;25:447–453.
139. Lacquaniti F, Terzuolo C, Viviani P. The law relating the kinematic and figural aspects of drawing movements. Acta Psychol (Amst) 1983;54:115–130.
140. Viviani P, McCollum G. The relation between linear extent and velocity in drawing movements. Neuroscience 1983;10:211–218.
141. Viviani P, Flash T. Minimum-jerk, two-thirds power law, and isochrony: converging approaches to movement planning. J Exp Psychol Hum Percept Perform 1995;21:32–53.
142. Elble RJ, Moody C, Higgins C. Primary writing tremor. A form of focal dystonia? Mov Disord 1990;5:118–126.
143. Elble RJ, Sinha R, Higgins C. Quantification of tremor with a digitizing tablet. J Neurosci Methods 1990;32: 193–198.
144. Liu X, Carroll CB, Wang SY, et al. Quantifying drug-induced dyskinesias in the arms using digitised spiral-drawing tasks. J Neurosci Methods 2005;144:47–52.
145. Louis ED, Yu Q, Floyd AG, et al. Axis is a feature of handwritten spirals in essential tremor. Mov Disord 2006;21:1294–1295.
146. Siebner HR, Ceballos-Baumann A, Standhardt H, et al. Changes in handwriting resulting from bilateral high-frequency stimulation of the subthalamic nucleus in Parkinson's disease. Mov Disord 1999;14:964–971.
147. Jabusch HC, Vauth H, Altenmuller E. Quantification of focal dystonia in pianists using scale analysis. Mov Disord 2004;19:171–180.
148. Taylor Tavares AL, Jefferis GS, Koop M, et al. Quantitative measurements of alternating finger tapping in Parkinson's disease correlate with UPDRS motor disability and reveal the improvement in fine motor control from medication and deep brain stimulation. Mov Disord 2005;20: 1286–1298.
149. Altenmuller E, Marco-Pallares J, Munte TF, et al. Neural reorganization underlies improvement in stroke-induced motor dysfunction by music-supported therapy. Ann N Y Acad Sci 2009;1169:395–405.
150. Miralles F, Tarongi S, Espino A. Quantification of the drawing of an Archimedes spiral through the analysis of its digitized picture. J Neurosci Methods 2006;152:18–31.
151. Viviani P, Burkhard PR, Chiuve SC, et al. Velocity control in Parkinson's disease: a quantitative analysis of isochrony in scribbling movements. Exp Brain Res 2009;194: 259–283.
152. Saunders-Pullman R, Derby C, Stanley K, et al. Validity of spiral analysis in early Parkinson's disease. Mov Disord 2007.
153. Zeuner KE, Peller M, Knutzen A, et al. How to assess motor impairment in writer's cramp. Mov Disord 2007;22:1102–1109.
154. Longstaff MG, Heath RA. Spiral drawing performance as an indicator of fine motor function in people with multiple sclerosis. Hum Mov Sci 2006;25:474–491.
155. Hsu AW, Piboolnurak PA, Floyd AG, et al. (2009), Spiral analysis in Niemann-Pick disease type C. Movement Disorders, 24: 1984–1990. doi: 10.1002/mds.22744.

CHAPTER 3

Neuroimaging of Movement Disorders

David J. Brooks and Nicola Pavese

▶ STRUCTURAL IMAGING IN PARKINSONISM

With the advent of high-field magnetic resonance imaging (MRI), volumetric acquisitions, and more sophisticated sequences, the role of structural imaging in the diagnosis of parkinsonian disorders is becoming more important. MRI can help exclude structural lesions such as basal ganglia tumors, hemorrhages, small vessel disease, and calcification, which have all been associated with parkinsonism, as has hydrocephalus. There is still debate concerning whether vascular parkinsonism is a distinct entity, although 5% of parkinsonian cases have no other evident pathology[1] (see Chapter 24). High-field MRI utilizing gray and white matter signal-suppressing inversion recovery sequences can show abnormal signal from the substantia nigra compacta in idiopathic Parkinson's disease (PD) patients.[2,3] Volumetric MRI has so far failed to detect a reduction in nigral volume in PD, possibly because of difficulties in accurately defining the border of the nigra compacta.[4] Interestingly, however, a reduction in putamen volume was noted by these workers, even in early cases. T_2-weighted MRI sequences directly reflect the iron content of brain areas. Michaeli and colleagues[5] have been able to detect increased nigral magnetic susceptibility in PD, although midbrain relaxation times overlapped considerably with those of healthy normals.

The striatum appears normal on T_2-weighted MRI in PD, but in striatonigral degeneration (SND) and multisystem atrophy (MSA), the putamen characteristically shows reduced signal running up the lateral extent due to iron deposition, and this may be covered by a rim of increased signal due to gliosis.[6–8] If concomitant pontocerebellar degeneration is also present, the lateral as well as longitudinal pontine fibers become evident as high signal on T_2 MRI, manifesting as the "hot cross bun" sign. Cerebellar and pontine atrophy may be visually obvious with increased signal evident in the cerebellar peduncles. Formal MR volumetry detects putamen and brain stem atrophy in most established cases.[9] Patients with progressive supranuclear palsy (PSP) do not show the putamen signal changes characteristic of MSA but may show third ventricular widening and midbrain atrophy. Recently, visual assessment of superior cerebellar peduncle atrophy has been shown to differentiate PSP patients from control, PD, and MSA patients with a sensitivity of 74% and a specificity of 94%.[10] In corticobasal degeneration (CBD), asymmetric hemispheric atrophy may be present, and MRI can usefully exclude multi-infarct disease and multifocal leukoencephalopathy. Putaminal hypointensity and hyperintense signal changes in the motor cortex or subcortical white matter on T_2-weighted images have also been reported.[11,12]

Diffusion-weighted imaging (DWI) and tensor MRI provide more sensitive modalities for discriminating atypical from typical parkinsonian disorders. Diffusion tensor imaging (DTI) detects altered water diffusibility as a raised apparent diffusion coefficient (ADC) and loss of directionality of diffusion as reduced fractional anisotropy (FA). To date only minor reductions in nigral FA have been reported in PD.[13] However, 90–100% of cases with clinically probable MSA and PSP have shown a raised putamen ADC across different series, whereas putamen ADCs are normal in PD.[14–16] MSA can be discriminated from PSP by the presence of an altered water diffusion signal in the middle cerebellar peduncle (MCP).[17] It remains to be seen how well DWI will perform with early gray cases in prospective series where clinical diagnostic uncertainty is still present.

Transcranial sonography (TCS) detects structural midbrain and striatal changes in parkinsonian disorders as hyperechogenic signals. Ninety-two percent of cases with clinically established PD were reported to have increased midbrain echogenicity with TCS in an initial large series.[18] However, with the threshold applied for abnormalitiy, 10% of elderly normals also showed hyperechogenicity. The increased TCS signal was more noticeable contralateral to the more clinically affected limbs but did not correlate with disability scores. In a more recent series, TCS was reported to have positive and negative predictive values of 86% and 83%, respectively, for clinically probable PD.[19]

While TCS sensitively detects nigral hyperechogenicity in idiopathic PD, 15% of essential tremor patients[20] and 40% of depressed patients[21] have also been reported to show such nigral hyperechogenicity, raising questions about the specificity of this finding. In a 5-year follow-up study of PD cases, there was no significant change in TCS findings while clinical disability progressed.[22] It has been suggested that the presence of midbrain hyperechogenicity is a trait rather than state marker for susceptibility to parkinsonism and may reflect the presence of midbrain iron deposition.[23] Abnormal nigral hyperechogenicity can also be detected in monogenic forms of parkinsonism, such as carriers of alpha synuclein, LRRK2, parkin, and DJ1 mutations. Interestingly, nigral hyperechogenicity does not appear to be associated with the atypical parkinsonian disorders MSA and PSP, although altered striatal signal can be detected in MSA.[24]

▶ MAGNETIC RESONANCE IMAGING IN HYPERKINETIC DISORDERS

MRI findings in nondegenerative movement disorders, such as idiopathic dystonia and Tourette's syndrome, tend to be normal, although cases of acquired dystonia may show structural lesions in the lentiform nucleus or posterior thalamus.[25] Magnetization transfer reflects the exchange of water protons between mobile and fixed compartments, such as free water in interstitial fluid and bound to proteins. It has been reported that idiopathic dystonia patients show abnormal central white matter and basal ganglia MT signals.[26]

Raised T_2-weighted MRI signal can be found in the lentiform nucleus and other gray matter areas in established neurological Wilson's disease, although the sensitivity of this modality for detecting subclinical cerebral involvement in the hepatic form is unclear.[27] Altered striatal T_2-weighted MRI signal and caudate atrophy are visually evident in cases of Huntington's disease (HD) with long-standing symptoms.[28] Premanifest HD gene carriers generally have normal MRI findings on inspection, but formal MR volumetry can detect subclinical caudate and putamen atrophy.[29] Striatal atrophy becomes more marked as they become symptomatic and develop motor signs.[30] Aylward et al. were able to predict time of conversion from preclinical to clinical HD by measuring caudate volumes.[31] These workers suggested that caudate volume may be a useful outcome measure for assessing treatment effectiveness in both presymptomatic and symptomatic subjects.

▶ FUNCTIONAL IMAGING APPROACHES

Functional imaging provides a robust means of detecting and characterizing the regional changes in brain metabolism and receptor binding associated with movement disorders. It can be of diagnostic value and also help to throw light on the pathophysiology underlying parkinsonian syndromes and involuntary movements. Functional imaging also provides a sensitive means of detecting subclinical disease in subjects at risk for degenerative disorders and of objectively following disease progression.

There are four main approaches to functional imaging. Positron emission tomography (PET) has the highest sensitivity, being able to detect femtomolar levels of positron-emitting radioisotopes at a spatial resolution of 2–3 mm. It allows quantitative in vivo examination of alterations in regional cerebral blood flow (rCBF); glucose, oxygen, and dopa metabolism; and brain receptor binding. Single photon emission tomography (SPECT) is a less-sensitive modality, but it is more widely available and provides measures of rCBF and receptor binding. Magnetic resonance spectroscopy (MRS) has lower sensitivity and spatial resolution than the two radioisotope imaging approaches, detecting millimolar metabolite levels (*N*-acetylaspartate, lactate, phospholipids, ATP) at a spatial resolution of around 1 cm. Finally, MRI can detect activation-induced changes in oxygenation of venous blood draining from brain regions when subjects perform tasks—the BOLD technique.

The changes in regional cerebral function that characterize different movement disorders can be examined in two main ways. First, focal changes in resting levels of regional cerebral metabolism, blood flow, and neuroreceptor availability can be measured. Second, abnormal patterns of brain activation or levels of neurotransmitter release can be detected when patients with movement disorders perform motor and cognitive tasks or are exposed to drug challenges. The majority of functional imaging research into brain function in movement disorders has, to date, concerned PET and SPECT, so this chapter will concentrate on these techniques but will address functional MRI and proton MRS findings where relevant.

▶ FUNCTIONAL IMAGING OF PD

INTRODUCTION

While the pathology of PD targets the dopamine cells in the substantia nigra in association with the formation of intraneuronal Lewy inclusion bodies, serotonergic cells in the median raphe and noradrenergic cells in the locus ceruleus are also involved, as are other pigmented and brain stem nuclei[32,33] (see Chapter 19). Loss of cells from the substantia nigra in PD results in profound dopamine depletion in the striatum, lateral nigral projections to putamen being most affected.[34,35] Lewy bodies are also found in the anterior cingulate and frontal, parietal, and temporal association cortex of non-demented PD cases at autopsy.[33] It remains uncertain whether dementia of

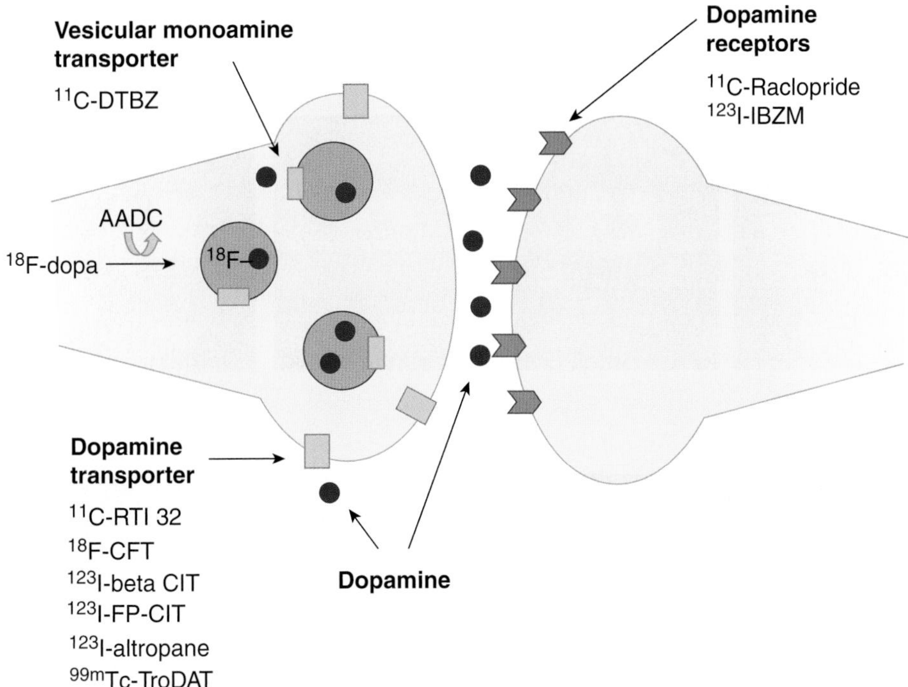

Figure 3–1. Schematic representation of a striatal presynaptic dopamine terminal showing neurobiological substrates of common PET and SPECT tracers. AADC, aromatic amino acid decarboxylase.

Lewy body type and PD represent opposite ends of a spectrum. Dementia of Lewy body type has overlapping features with Alzheimer's disease (AD), which is twice as prevalent in PD, although it is associated with a higher prevalence of fluctuating confusion, hallucinations, early-onset rigidity, and gait difficulties.[36]

IMAGING THE PRESYNAPTIC DOPAMINERGIC SYSTEM

The function of dopamine terminals in PD can be examined in vivo in several ways: first, terminal dopa decarboxylase activity can be measured with ^{18}F-dopa PET.[37,38] Second, the availability of presynaptic dopamine transporters (DATs) can be assessed with tropane-based PET and SPECT tracers.[39–43] Third, vesicle monoamine transporter density in dopamine terminals can be examined with ^{11}C-dihydrotetrabenazine (DHTBZ) PET[44] (Figs. 3–1 and 3–2). In early hemiparkinsonian cases, ^{18}F-dopa PET shows bilaterally reduced putamen tracer uptake, activity being most depressed in the putamen contralateral to the affected limbs.[45] ^{18}F-dopa PET can, therefore, detect subclinical disease evidenced as involvement of the "asymptomatic" putamen contralateral to clinically unaffected limbs. On average, PD patients show a 60% loss of specific putamen ^{18}F-dopa uptake in life compared to a 60–80% loss of ventrolateral nigra compacta cells and 95% loss of putamen dopamine at autopsy.[46] These findings suggest that striatal dopamine terminal dopa decarboxylase activity may be relatively upregulated in PD, presumably to boost dopamine turnover by remaining neurons. Cases of early hemi-PD (Hoehn and Yahr stage 1) show a 30–40% loss of ^{18}F-dopa uptake in the putamen contralateral to the affected limbs, suggesting that this loss of dopa decarboxylase activity may represent the threshold for onset of symptoms.

It is known that the pathology of PD is not uniform, ventrolateral nigral dopaminergic projections to the dorsal putamen being more affected than dorsomedial projections to the head of caudate.[35] ^{18}F-dopa PET reveals that, in patients with unilateral PD (Hoehn and Yahr stage 1), contralateral dorsal posterior putamen dopamine storage is first reduced.[47] As all limbs become clinically affected, ventral and anterior putamen and dorsal caudate dopaminergic function also become involved. Finally, when PD is well advanced, ventral head of caudate ^{18}F-dopa uptake starts to fall.

Significant changes in ^{18}F-dopa uptake throughout the whole brain volume can be localized in PD using statistical parametric mapping (SPM). This automated analysis at a voxel level makes it possible to detect dopamine terminal dysfunction in extrastriatal areas and explore possible compensatory responses at different stages of the disease. Increases in ^{18}F-dopa uptake have been reported in dorsolateral prefrontal cortex (DLPFC), anterior cingulate, and globus pallidus interna in early PD patients compared to normal controls, but not in more advanced cases.[48–50] It is likely that these early

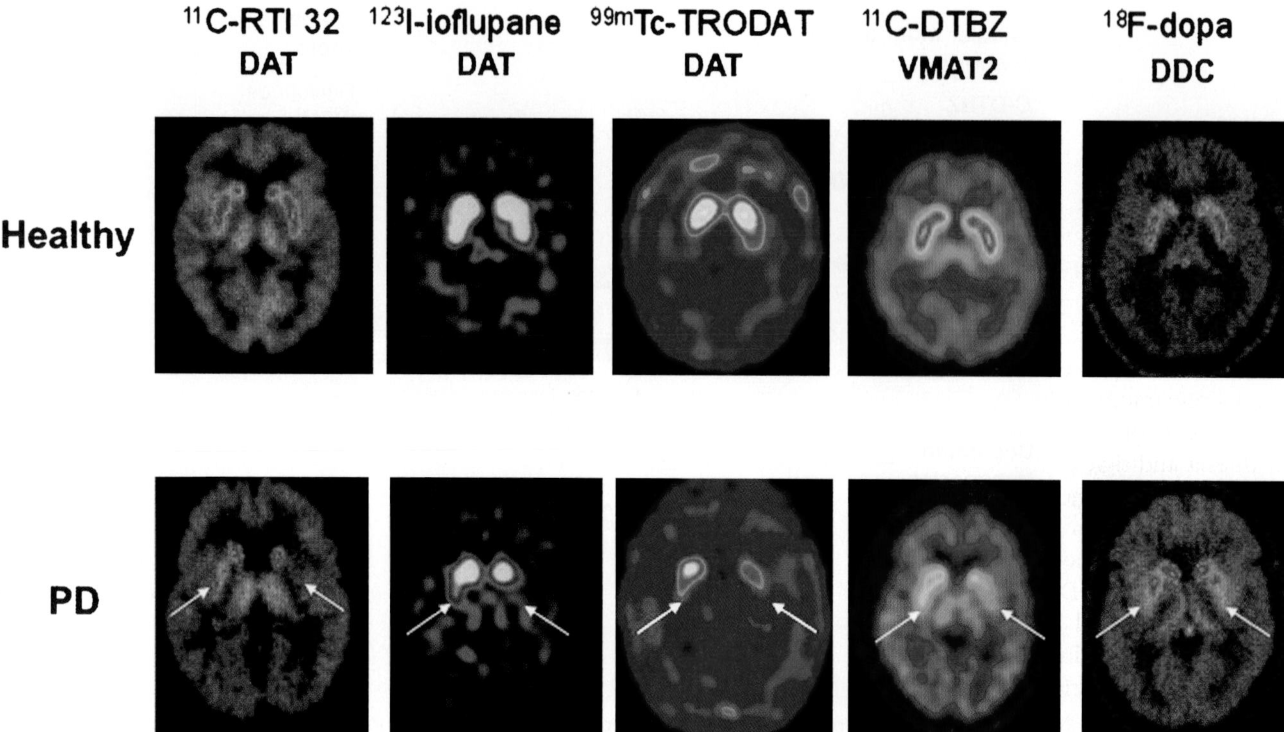

Figure 3–2. Imaging dopamine terminal function in healthy controls and early Parkinson's disease.

increases in frontal and pallidal ^{18}F-dopa uptake reflect a compensatory hyperactivity of dopa decarboxylase activity not only in the dopamine terminals present but also in innervating serotonin neurones. ^{18}F-dopa uptake in the globus pallidus interna is increased by 30–40% at the onset of PD symptoms when putaminal uptake is reduced by 30–40%. The enhanced function of the dopamine projections to the globus pallidus interna in early PD could represent an attempt to maintain a normal pattern of pallidal output to the ventral thalamus and motor cortex. The loss of this pallidal compensatory pathway in advanced stages of the disease, along with putamen dopaminergic function, could represent a critical step in the progression of the disease leading to the end of the "honeymoon period."[50]

There are now many radiotracers, mainly tropane-based, that are markers of DAT binding on nigrostriatal terminals and so provide a measure of integrity of dopaminergic function in PD. PET tracers include ^{11}C-CFT,[40] ^{18}F-CFT,[39] ^{11}C-RTI-32,[51] ^{11}C-nomifensine,[52] and ^{11}C-methyphenidate.[53] Available SPECT tracers include ^{123}I-beta-CIT,[41] ^{123}I-FP-CIT,[42] ^{123}I-altropane,[54] and ^{99m}Tc-TRODAT-1.[55] ^{123}I-beta-CIT gives the highest striatal:cerebellar uptake ratio of these SPECT tracers, but this reflects lower cerebellar nonspecific, rather than higher striatal specific, uptake and so this tracer provides a potentially noisy reference signal. Additionally, it binds nonselectively to dopamine, noradrenaline, and serotonin transporters and has the disadvantage that it takes 24 hours to equilibrate throughout the brain following intravenous injection, so scanning has to be delayed until the following day. For this reason, SPECT tracers such as ^{123}I-FP-CIT (Fig. 3–3) and ^{123}I-altropane have come into vogue because, despite their lower and time-dependent striatal:cerebellar uptake ratios, a diagnostic scan can be performed within 3 hours of tracer injection. The technetium-based tropane tracer, ^{99m}Tc-TRODAT-1, has the advantage that

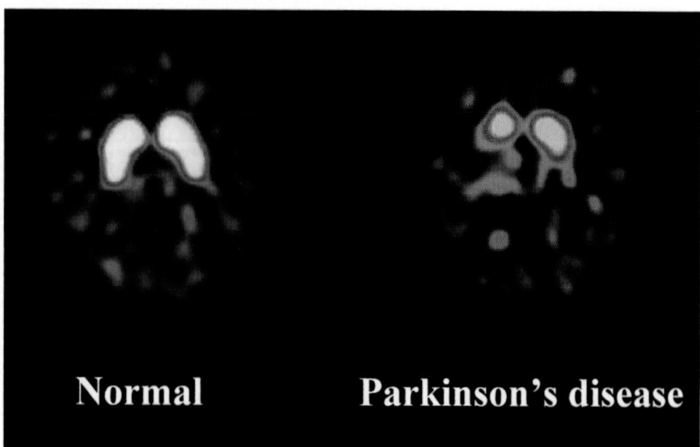

Figure 3–3. Single photon emission computed tomography images of ^{123}I-FP-CIT uptake in the brain of a control subject and in a patient with Parkinson's disease.

it is readily available in kit form but provides a lower striatal:cerebellar uptake ratio than the ^{123}I-based tracers and is less well extracted by the brain. All the above PET and SPECT tracers appear to differentiate clinically probable early PD from normal subjects or essential tremor patients with a sensitivity of 85–90%.[56,57] A positive PET or SPECT scan can thus be valuable for supporting a diagnosis of PD where there is diagnostic doubt. It is still not clear, however, that a negative PET or SPECT scan fully excludes this diagnosis, although the available evidence strongly supports this viewpoint.[58,59]

Putamen uptake of PET and SPECT presynaptic dopaminergic tracers shows an inverse correlation with the degree of locomotor disability in PD, reflecting limb bradykinesia and rigidity rather than rest tremor severity.[57,60]

The PET ligand ^{11}C-DHTBZ binds to the vesicular monoamine transporter type 2 (VMAT2). Recently, Lee et al. have measured striatal uptake of ^{11}C-DHTBZ, ^{18}F-dopa, and the DAT marker ^{11}C-methylphenidate in 35 PD patients and 16 age-matched healthy volunteers. ^{18}F-dopa Ki was reduced less than ^{11}C-DHTBZ binding in the parkinsonian striatum, whereas the ^{11}C-methylphenidate binding was reduced more than the ^{11}C-DHTBZ binding.[53] These results could indicate that putaminal ^{18}F-dopa uptake is relatively upregulated and binding of ^{11}C-methylphenidate relatively downregulated in PD. This finding makes physiological sense, as increased dopamine turnover and decreased uptake by DATs in a dopamine-deficiency syndrome should help to preserve synaptic transmitter levels. If this is the case, ^{11}C-DHTBZ PET signals may reflect most validly the density of dopaminergic terminals.

IMAGING THE POSTSYNAPTIC DOPAMINERGIC SYSTEM

Both PET and SPECT radioligands have been used to examine postsynaptic dopaminergic receptor binding. Dopamine receptors broadly fall into D1 (D1, D5) and D2 (D2, D3, D4) classes. The striatum contains mainly D1 and D2 receptor subtypes, and these both play a role in modulating locomotor function. PET with spiperone-based tracers and ^{123}I-IBZM SPECT studies have both reported normal levels of striatal D2 binding in untreated PD, while ^{11}C-raclopride PET has shown 10–20% increases in putamen D2 site availability.[61,62] As ^{11}C-raclopride competes with endogenous dopamine for D2 binding, the raised receptor availability in untreated PD seen with this ligand probably reflects the dopamine depletion present rather than a raised receptor density. Spiperone binding is not influenced by endogenous dopamine levels.

In chronically treated PD, ^{11}C-methylspiperone PET and ^{123}I-IBZM SPECT studies have reported normal or mildly reduced striatal D2 binding.[61] Serial ^{11}C-raclopride PET has shown that, after 6 months of exposure to L-dopa, the mildly increased putamen ^{11}C-raclopride binding seen in de novo PD patients normalizes.[63] Chronically L-dopa-exposed PD cases continue to show normal levels of putamen D2 binding, explaining their good locomotor response to L-dopa, while caudate D2 binding becomes 20% reduced.[64] ^{11}C-SCH23390 PET, a marker of D1 site binding, shows normal striatal uptake in de novo PD,[65] while patients who have been exposed to L-dopa for several years show a 20% reduction in striatal binding.[64] These findings are in good agreement with in vitro reports of striatal dopamine D1 and D2 receptor binding based on autopsy material from end-stage patients.

Similarly to idiopathic PD patients, drug-naive patients with parkinsonism associated with *parkin* gene mutations show increased putaminal ^{11}C-raclopride binding compared to normal subjects, while levodopa-treated patients show significant reductions in ^{11}C-raclopride binding in both caudate and putamen.[66]

^{11}C-FLB 457 PET is a very high-affinity marker of D2 and D3 receptors capable of quantitating their binding in extrastriatal as well as striatal areas. Advanced PD patients showed reduced ^{11}C-FLB 457 binding in thalamus, anterior cingulate, dorsolateral prefrontal and temporal cortex, although this was not seen in early cases.[67,68] Whether reductions in extrastriatal dopamine receptor binding lead to occurrence of cognitive and emotional deficits in PD patients remains to be ascertained.

MEASUREMENTS OF STRIATAL DOPAMINE LEVELS

Because of its sensitivity to endogenous dopamine levels, ^{11}C-raclopride PET potentially allows changes in synaptic levels of striatal dopamine induced by interventions to be monitored. A challenge with an intravenous bolus of 0.3 mg/kg metamphetamine caused a 24% reduction in putamen ^{11}C-raclopride binding in normal subjects due to competition for D2 receptor binding with the dopamine released.[69] It has been estimated that a 10% reduction in the availability of D2 receptors for ^{11}C-raclopride binding reflects a fivefold increase in synaptic dopamine levels.[70]

Piccini at al. have compared dopamine release induced by methamphetamine in striatal and cortical areas in patients with advanced PD and healthy volunteers.[71] The mean reductions in caudate and putamen ^{11}C-raclopride binding in PD patients were significantly attenuated compared with those observed in the normal subjects (8% vs 17% in caudate and 7% vs 25% in putamen). In individual patients, the percentage reduction in putamen ^{11}C-raclopride binding following methamphetamine correlated with disease severity as measured by both the Unified Parkinson's Disease Rating Scale (UPDRS) and putaminal ^{18}F-dopa uptake. Within-group SPM detected further areas of dopamine release in dorsal and ventrolateral prefrontal cortex and orbitofrontal cortex in both PD patients and normal subjects. Interestingly, dopamine release in frontal areas of PD patients was comparable to that observed in normal subjects, even though their striatal dopamine release was 60% reduced. These findings indicate that the capacity to release dopamine in frontal areas, at least after an acute pharmacological challenge, is preserved even in advanced stages of PD.

Several authors have used ^{11}C-raclopride PET to estimate changes in synaptic levels of dopamine induced by exogenous L-dopa in PD patients.[72–75] Striatal reductions in ^{11}C-raclopride binding induced by L-dopa become larger as motor disability increases and the disease progresses. The increasing synaptic dopamine levels generated by L-dopa as PD becomes more severe most probably reflect a failure of striatal terminals to store and buffer dopamine and may be responsible for the emergence of peak-dose dyskinesias.[74,75] In one study, individual improvements in UPDRS score induced by oral L-dopa (250 mg L-dopa/25 mg carbidopa) correlated significantly with reductions in putaminal ^{11}C-raclopride binding potential. Motor UPDRS sub-items were also examined. Improvements in rigidity and bradykinesia, but not in tremor or axial symptoms, correlated with putamen dopamine release, suggesting that relief of parkinsonian tremor and axial symptoms is not related to striatal synaptic dopamine levels and presumably occurs via extrastriatal mechanisms.[75]

Changes in synaptic levels of dopamine induced by oral L-dopa have also been assessed in PD patients who compulsively take far larger doses of levodopa than are clinically required (dopamine dysregulation syndrome, DDS).[76] Compared with PD patients who are not compulsively taking their medication, DDS patients showed enhanced L-dopa-induced dopamine release in ventral striatum. Interestingly, ventral striatal dopamine release in DDS patients correlated with self-reported compulsive drug "wanting" but not "liking," providing evidence that sensitization of ventral striatal circuitry links to craving for drugs.[77] The dissociation of craving for and enjoyment of stimuli fits with the Berridge hypothesis that these are mediated by separate circuitary.[78]

Finally, studies have been performed to detect endogenous release of dopamine during behavioral tasks performed by normal subjects and PD patients. Striatal dopamine release has been demonstrated during simple finger movements,[79] and repetitive transcranial magnetic stimulation over the motor cortex,[80] the performances of behavioral rewarded tasks,[81,82] and a spatial working memory task that also induced frontal ^{11}C-raclopride binding decreases.[83]

DETECTION OF PRECLINICAL PD

It has been estimated from postmortem studies that, for every patient who presents with clinical PD, there may be 10–15 subclinical cases with incidental brain stem Lewy body disease in the community.[84] Subjects likely to be at risk of developing PD include relatives of patients with the disorder.[85] Piccini et al.[86] used ^{18}F-dopa PET to study 32 asymptomatic adult relatives in seven kindreds with familial PD, each of which contained at least two affected individuals with L-dopa-responsive parkinsonism. In five of these kindreds, the pathology was unknown; the sixth kindred was subsequently found to have *parkin* gene mutations, while the seventh kindred was known to have diffuse Lewy body disease (DLBD). Affected individuals from the six non-*parkin* kindreds all showed the typical pattern of reduced striatal ^{18}F-dopa uptake associated with sporadic PD: putamen tracer uptake was more severely reduced than that of caudate. The *parkin* cases showed a severe loss of both caudate and putamen dopamine storage.

Of the asymptomatic adult relatives scanned, 25% showed levels of putamen ^{18}F-dopa uptake reduced more than 2.5 SD (standard deviation) below the normal mean. Three of the eight asymptomatic relatives with reduced putamen ^{18}F-dopa uptake subsequently developed clinical parkinsonism. Based on clinical surveys, a 15% prevalence is normally quoted for the presence of a positive family history in PD, although this approaches 40% if a fully informative history is available.[85] ^{18}F-dopa PET findings indicate that 25% of asymptomatic adult relatives of index cases with familial parkinsonism (i.e., 50% of the at-risk population) have evidence of subclinical dopaminergic dysfunction.

^{18}F-dopa PET findings for 34 asymptomatic and 2 clinically concordant co-twins of idiopathic sporadic PD patients aged 23–67 years have also been reported.[87] Eighteen co-twins were monozygotic (MZ), while 16 were dizygotic (DZ); 10 (55%) of the 18 MZ co-twins and 3 (18%) of the 16 DZ co-twins had levels of putamen ^{18}F-dopa uptake that were reduced more than 2.5 SD below the normal mean. The finding of a significantly higher concordance (55% vs 18%, $P = 0.03$) for dopaminergic dysfunction in MZ compared with DZ PD co-twins supports a genetic contribution toward this apparently sporadic disorder. Interestingly, when a subgroup of these co-twins was scanned serially, all 10 of the asymptomatic MZ co-twins scanned showed a decrease in putamen ^{18}F-dopa uptake on repeat scanning 4.0 ± 1.7 years after the first scan; the mean rate of the loss of putamen ^{18}F-dopa uptake was 4.5% per year. On the basis of their follow-up scans, three more MZ co-twins were classified as having subclinical PD. Nine asymptomatic DZ co-twins (mean age 56.7 ± 15.2 years) were also scanned twice over a period of 4.3 ± 2.2 years but showed no significant change in putamen ^{18}F-dopa uptake. The percentage annual loss in putamen ^{18}F-dopa uptake for MZ and DZ co-twins was significantly different ($P = 0.001$).

Over the 7 years of follow-up, two MZ co-twins and one DZ co-twin died without developing symptoms, while four MZ co-twins became clinically concordant for PD (at 65, 70, 72, and 78 years of age, 14, 2, 9, and 20 years after the onset of PD in their co-twins), resulting in a clinical concordance of 22.2% at follow-up. The clinical concordance within the MZ pairs over 60 years of age was higher (50%, 4 of 8). None of the DZ twin pairs became clinically concordant, and the difference in clinical concordance between the MZ and DZ twin pairs in the 60–70 age group was significant ($P = 0.04$; Fisher exact test).

Recently, Khan and colleagues[88] have reported reduction of ^{18}F-dopa uptake in caudate putamen, ventral and dorsal midbrain in asymptomatic carriers of a single *parkin* mutation compared to normal subjects. Whether these subjects will convert to clinical PD later on remains to be established.

While aging and a family history are still the greatest risk factors for PD, late-onset idiopathic hyposmia (reduced sense of smell) and REM behavior sleep disorder are also associated with neurodegenerative syndromes. Reduced ^{123}I-beta-CIT uptake has been reported in 7 out of 40 (17.5%) relatives of PD patients with no parkinsonian symptoms but with a complaint of hyposmia. Four out of seven (57%) of the subjects with reduced striatal ^{123}I-beta-CIT binding converted to clinical PD over a 2-year follow-up.[89] Hilker and colleagues[90] measured striatal and midbrain ^{18}F-dopa uptake in PD patients with a history of sleep disorders. They found a significant inverse correlation between mesopontine ^{18}F-dopa uptake and REM sleep duration, as measured by polysomnography. The authors suggested that increased monoaminergic activity in the rostral brain stem might result in the suppression of nocturnal REM sleep in PD. Eisensehr and coworkers[91] studied striatal presynaptic DATs with IPT SPECT, a DAT marker, in 8 patients with idiopathic subclinical RBD, 8 patients with idiopathic clinically manifest RBD, 11 controls, and 8 patients with PD Hoehn and Yahr stage 1. Striatal IPT uptake was reduced in patients with subclinical and clinical RBD, the latter having PD levels of binding.

FLUCTUATIONS AND DYSKINESIAS IN PD

PD patients with fluctuating responses to L-dopa show lower putamen ^{18}F-dopa uptake than those with early disease and sustained therapeutic responses. A confounder, however, when trying to compare presynaptic dopamine terminal function in these groups is that the former tend to have an earlier age of disease onset, more severe disease, longer disease duration, and a greater cumulative exposure to L-dopa. By using Analysis of Co-Variance (ANCOVA) to factor out effects of age at onset and disease duration in groups of fluctuators and nonfluctuators and also matching subgroups of these patients for age of onset and disease duration, de la Fuente-Fernandez et al. concluded that mean putamen ^{18}F-dopa uptake was 28% lower in PD patients with motor complications than in those without, but that there was considerable overlap of the two individual ranges.[92] While loss of putamen dopamine terminal function predisposes PD patients toward development of L-dopa-associated complications, it cannot be solely responsible for determining the timing of onset of fluctuations and involuntary movements.

Striatal dopamine D1 and D2 receptor availability has been examined in age-matched subgroups of 8 L-dopa-exposed dyskinetic patients and 10 nondyskinetic patients with similar clinical disease duration, disease severity, and daily L-dopa dosage.[64] Mean caudate and putamen D1 and putamen D2 bindings were normal for both the dyskinetic and the nondyskinetic PD subgroups, while caudate D2 binding was reduced in each by around 15%. Other series have also noted similar striatal dopamine D1 and D2 binding in fluctuating and dyskinetic PD patients compared with sustained responders.[93] These findings therefore suggest that onset of motor complications in PD is not primarily associated with alterations in striatal dopamine receptor availability.

When early nonfluctuating PD patients are given 3 mg/kg of L-dopa as an intravenous bolus, they show a mean 10% fall in posterior putamen ^{11}C-raclopride binding, while advanced cases with fluctuations show a 23% fall.[94] These reductions in putamen ^{11}C-raclopride binding correlate with disease severity assessed with the UPDRS when off medication and indicate that, as loss of dopamine terminals in PD increases, striatal buffering of dopamine fails when clinical doses of exogenous L-dopa are administered. This failure reflects a combination of upregulation of striatal dopamine synthesis and release of dopamine by the remaining terminals, along with severe loss of DATs preventing reuptake. It is this phenomenon, rather than changes in postsynaptic dopamine D1 and D2 receptor binding, that is likely to be the explanation for the more rapid response of advanced PD patients to oral L-dopa. This process will also result in high nonphysiological swings in synaptic dopamine levels, which may lead to excessive dopamine receptor internalization, again promoting fluctuating treatment responses.

de la Fuente-Fernandez et al.[73] have examined changes in ^{11}C-raclopride binding after an oral L-dopa challenge in advanced PD and shown that "off" episodes do not necessarily coincide with low synaptic dopamine levels. This finding is again in favor of fluctuations occurring either due to inappropriate levels of dopamine receptor internalization at times, making them unpredictably unavailable at the cell surface for stimulation, or due to aberrant downstream changes in basal ganglia transmission making them refractory, rather than due to a lack of dopaminergic tone at postsynaptic D2 receptors. Another study has examined changes in ^{11}C-raclopride binding after an oral L-dopa challenge in dyskinetic PD patients. Higher dyskinesia scores following a standard dose of oral L-dopa (250 mg L-dopa/25 mg carbidopa) were associated with larger putaminal ^{11}C-raclopride binding changes supporting the view that presynaptic mechanisms have an important role in the occurrence of L-dopa-induced dyskinesias.[75]

Medium spiny projection neurons in the caudate and putamen release opioids and substance P along with gamma-aminobutyric acid (GABA) into the external and internal pallidum.[95] Striatal projections to the external pallidum (GPe) contain enkephalin, which binds mainly to delta opioid sites and inhibits GABA release in the GPe. Striatal projections to the internal pallidum (GPi) transmit dynorphin, which binds to kappa opioid sites and inhibits glutamate release from subthalamic nucleus (STN) afferents to the GPi, and substance P, which binds to NK1 receptors. It is thought that phasic firing of striatopallidal projection neurons results primarily in GABA release, while sustained tonic firing causes additional modulatory opioid and substance P release. The caudate and the putamen also contain high densities of mu, kappa, and delta opioid sites. These receptors are located both presynaptically on dopamine terminals, where they regulate dopamine release, and postsynaptically on interneurons and medium spiny projection neurons to pallidum terminals. There is now strong evidence supporting the presence of deranged opioid and substance P transmission in the basal ganglia of PD patients both from postmortem studies and from lesion animal models of this disorder.[96,97] At autopsy, end-stage treated PD patients show raised levels of pallidal preproenkephalin. In rats lesioned with the nigral toxin 6-OHDA (6-hydroxydopamine), there are raised levels of striatal enkephalin and preproenkephalin expression while prodynorphin expression is suppressed.[95] When such animals are made hyperkinetic or frankly dyskinetic after chronic exposure to pulsatile doses of L-dopa, further overexpression of striatal preproenkephalin is seen along with raised expression of prodynorphin and substance P. L-dopa-naive MPTP (1-methyl-4-phenyl-1,2,3,6-tetrahydropyridine)-lesioned monkeys have also been reported to show raised striatal enkephalin and reduced substance P mRNA expression.[98] Exposure to L-dopa for 1 month failed to normalize striatal preproenkephalin mRNA expression while substance P mRNA expression became elevated.

^{11}C-Diprenorphine PET is a nonselective marker of mu, kappa, and delta opioid sites, and its binding is sensitive to levels of endogenous opioids. If raised basal ganglia levels of enkephalin and dynorphin are associated with levodopa-induced dyskinesias (LIDs), then PD patients with motor complications would be expected to show reduced binding of ^{11}C-diprenorphine compared to those with sustained treatment responses. Piccini et al.[99] have reported significant reductions in ^{11}C-diprenorphine binding in caudate, putamen, thalamus, and anterior cingulate in dyskinetic patients compared with sustained responders. Individual levels of putamen ^{11}C-diprenorphine uptake correlated inversely with severity of dyskinesia. ^{18}F-L829165 PET is a selective marker of NK1 site availability. In a preliminary study, thalamic NK1 availability has been shown to be reduced in dyskinetic PD patients but normal in nondyskinetic cases.[100] These in vivo findings support the presence of elevated levels of endogenous peptides in the basal ganglia of dyskinetic PD patients and suggest that this, rather than a primary alteration in dopamine receptor binding, may in part be responsible for the appearance of involuntary movements.

MODIFYING PROGRESSION OF PD

There are a number of difficulties that arise when attempting to assess the progression of PD clinically as rating scales are subjective, are nonlinear, consider multiple aspects of the disorder, and are biased toward particular symptoms—bradykinesia in the case of the UPDRS. More importantly, symptomatic therapy can mask disease progression, and it is difficult to achieve a full washout. PET and SPECT imaging and, potentially, MRI of the nigra provide complementary biological markers for objectively monitoring disease progression in vivo in PD. They are limited, however, to providing information concerning particular aspects of the disorder, such as dopamine terminal function or changes in nigral water environment.

Striatal ^{18}F-dopa uptake has been shown to correlate with subsequent postmortem dopaminergic cell densities in the substantia nigra and striatal dopamine levels of patients and of MPTP-lesioned monkeys.[101,102] It is also highly reproducible and, at least in human subjects with an intact dopamine system, does not appear to be influenced by dopaminergic medication.[103,104] ^{18}F-dopa PET can, therefore, be used as a marker of dopamine terminal function in PD, although it may overestimate terminal density due to a relative upregulation of dopa decarboxylase in remaining neurons as a response to nigral cell loss. Striatal ^{123}I-beta-CIT uptake has also been shown to be unaffected by several weeks of exposure to L-dopa[105] and dopamine agonists.[106,107] In contrast to ^{18}F-dopa, ^{123}I-beta-CIT uptake may underestimate terminal density due to a relative downregulation of DATs in remaining neurons as a response to nigral cell loss.

Several series have now shown that loss of striatal ^{18}F-dopa uptake occurs more rapidly in PD than in age-matched controls.[108–110] On average, in early L-dopa-treated PD, putamen ^{18}F-dopa uptake has been reported to decline by around 10% per annum while caudate uptake falls at about half that rate. Parallel rates of loss of putamen DAT binding have been reported with ^{18}F-CFT PET[111] and ^{123}I-beta-CIT,[112] ^{123}I-FP-CIT,[113] and ^{123}I-IPT

SPECT.[114] In one series, striatal ^{123}I-beta-CIT uptake in early PD correlated with initial levels of striatal transporter binding, suggesting an exponential disease process.[115]

As functional imaging can objectively follow loss of dopamine terminal function in PD, it provides a potential means of monitoring the efficacy of putative neuroprotective agents. Dopamine agonists are one such possible class as they suppress endogenous dopamine production in vivo, so attenuating its oxidative metabolism with potential free-radical formation. They are also weak antioxidants and free-radical scavengers in their own right, and may also act as mitochondrial membrane stabilizers, so blocking the apoptotic cascade. Two different trials have examined the relative rates of loss of dopamine terminal function in early PD in patients randomized to a dopamine agonist or L-dopa.

In the REAL PET 2-year double-blind multinational study, 186 de novo PD patients were randomized (1:1) to ropinirole or L-dopa.[116] The primary endpoint was changed in putamen ^{18}F-dopa uptake (Ki, influx constant) measured with PET. Scan data from six PET centers were transformed into standard stereotactic space at one center in order to normalize brain position and shape. Parametric Ki images were then generated and sampled with a standard region-of-interest (ROI) template. Ki images were also interrogated with SPM (SPM99) to localize voxel clusters where significant between-group differences in rates of loss of dopaminergic function were occurring; 74% of the ropinirole group and 73% of the L-dopa group completed the study. Mean (SD) daily doses of double-blind medication after 2 years were 12.2 (6.1) mg ropinirole and 558.7 (180.8) mg L-dopa. Only 14% of the ropinirole group and 8% of the L-dopa group required open supplementary L-dopa. Interestingly, 11% of the untreated patients thought to have PD were found to have normal caudate and putamen ^{18}F-dopa uptake at entry (identified by blinded review), and this group was analyzed separately. The ROI analysis found that loss of putamen Ki was significantly slower over 2 years with ropinirole (13.4%) than with L-dopa (−20.3%; $P = 0.022$). SPM revealed that falls in Ki were significantly slower in both putamen and substantia nigra with ropinirole compared with L-dopa (putamen: ropinirole, −14.1%; L-dopa, −22.9%; $P < 0.001$; substantia nigra: ropinirole, +4.3%; L-dopa, −7.5%; $P = 0.025$). Clinically, the incidence of dyskinesia was 26.7% with L-dopa but only 3.4% with ropinirole ($P < 0.001$). Improvements in mean UPDRS motor scores while taking medication were, however, superior (by 6.34 points) for the L-dopa cohort.

The other trial comprised a subgroup of the CALM-PD study in which a cohort of 82 early PD patients were randomized 1:1 to the dopamine agonist pramipexole (0.5 mg tds) or L-dopa (100 mg tds) and had serial ^{123}I-beta-CIT SPECT over a 4-year period.[117] Open supplementary L-dopa was allowed if there was lack of therapeutic effect. Patients initially treated with pramipexole demonstrated a significantly smaller loss of striatal ^{123}I-beta-CIT uptake from baseline than those in the L-dopa group (16% vs 25.5%) at 46 months. Again, the incidence of complications was significantly reduced in the pramipexole cohort, but improvement in UPDRS score while taking medication was greater in the L-dopa cohort.

These two trials, therefore, produced parallel findings, both suggesting that treatment with an agonist in early PD slows loss of dopamine terminal function by around one-third and delays treatment-associated complications. A difficulty is that the functional imaging findings favoring use of ropinirole and pramipexole as early treatment were not paralleled by a better clinical outcome in the PD agonist cohorts, as judged by UPDRS motor scores while receiving medication.

A similar clinical and imaging study with ^{18}F-dopa PET was performed to evaluate the neuroprotective effect of the anti-glutamatergic agent riluzole (50 and 100 mg) vs placebo in early PD. The trial was interrupted at the first ad interim analysis (when half of the patients had completed the 2-year trial) as no clinical differences were seen among the three groups. In agreement with the clinical data, ^{18}F-dopa PET showed similar annual decreases in mean putaminal Ki values in the patients treated with riluzole or placebo.[118]

Finally, a randomized, double-blind, placebo-controlled trial has recently been performed to assess the effect of levodopa itself on the rate of progression of PD (ELLDOPA study). Unfortunately, this study has failed to give a definitive answer. In fact, whereas from a clinical perspective, levodopa does not appear to hasten the progression of PD, the mean percent decline in the ^{123}I-beta-CIT uptake was significantly greater with levodopa than placebo.[119]

RESTORATIVE APPROACHES IN PD

Human Fetal Cell Implantation Trials

As well as providing a means of following natural disease progression and monitoring the effects of putative neuroprotective agents, functional imaging provides a means of examining the efficacy of restorative approaches to PD. Possible approaches include striatal implants of human and porcine fetal mesencephalic cells, retinal cells that release L-dopa/dopamine, and transformed cells that secrete dopamine, nerve growth factors, or express antiapoptotic genes, neural progenitor cells, and direct intrastriatal infusions of nerve growth factors.

There are now several open series detailing clinical and ^{18}F-dopa PET findings in advanced PD patients after implantation of fetal mesencephalic cells or tissue into striatum[120] (see Chapter 16). The Lund group has reported serial clinical and ^{18}F-dopa PET findings over a period of 10 years of two PD patients, following implantation of fetal midbrain cells into the putamen contralateral to their more affected limbs. Both of these patients have maintained a clinical improvement, particularly in "on" time, which went from 40% to all of the day in one unilaterally grafted case whose ^{18}F-dopa uptake into the implanted putamen reached the lower end of the normal range. It was subsequently demonstrated that the graft released normal synaptic levels of dopamine after an amphetamine challenge.[121]

Another four unilaterally transplanted PD patients showed ^{18}F-dopa PET evidence of graft function 1 year following surgery; three of them responded clinically to transplantation, but the fourth deteriorated and now has signs suggestive of MSA.[122] In a subsequent series of four bilaterally transplanted patients, a mean 50% improvement in UPDRS scores was demonstrated at 2 years, associated with a 60% increase in putamen and 30% increase in caudate ^{18}F-dopa uptake.[123]

Clinically successful transplantation of fetal tissue with corroborative serial ^{18}F-dopa PET findings has also been reported for five PD patients in a 2-year open follow-up French study,[124] and for six PD patients in a 2-year follow-up series from Tampa, Florida.[125] In the French study, grafted putamen Ki values correlated with percentage time "on" during the day and finger dexterity while in an "off" state. Two of the transplanted PD patients in the Florida series died from unrelated causes, and viable tyrosine hydroxylase-staining graft tissue forming connections with host neurons was found at autopsy.[126]

Given the encouraging findings of these pilot open series, two major double-blind controlled trials on the efficacy of implantation of human fetal cells in PD were sponsored by the NIH in the United States. The first of these involved 40 patients who were 34–75 years of age and had severe PD (mean duration 14 years).[127] These were randomized to receive either an implant of human fetal mesencephalic tissue or undergo sham surgery, and were followed for 1 year with a subsequent extension to 3 years. In the transplant recipients, mesencephalic tissue from four embryos cultured for up to 1 month was implanted into the putamen bilaterally (two embryos per side) via a frontal approach. In the patients who underwent sham surgery, holes were drilled in the skull but the dura was not penetrated. No immunotherapy was used. The transplanted patients showed no significant improvement in the primary endpoint, clinical global impression, at 1 year, but there was a significant improvement in the mean UPDRS motor score compared with the sham surgery group when tested in the morning before receiving medication (mean improvement 18%, $P = 0.04$). This improvement was more evident for patients under 60 years of age (34% improvement; $P = 0.005$). At 3 years, the mean total UPDRS score was improved 38% in the younger and 14% in the older transplanted groups (both $P < 0.01$); 16 out of 19 transplanted patients individually showed an increase in putamen ^{18}F-dopa uptake (group mean increase 40%), and increases were similar in the younger and older cohorts.[128] A drawback was that "off" dystonia and dyskinesias developed in 15% of the patients who received transplants in this series, even after reduction or discontinuation of L-dopa.

Subsequently, the second NIH trial was reported.[129] Here, 34 patients were randomized to receive bilateral implants of fetal mesencephalic tissue from four fetuses per side or from one fetus per side into posterior putamen, or had sham surgery (a partial burr hole without penetration of the dura). Fetal tissue was cultured for less than 48 hours before transplantation, and all patients received immunosuppression for 6 months after surgery. The trial duration was 2 years, and the primary outcome variable was the UPDRS motor score and quality of life. Putamen ^{18}F-dopa uptake was assessed with PET in a subset of patients; 31 patients completed and 2 patients died during the trial, while another 3 died subsequently from unrelated causes. At autopsy the transplanted patients showed significantly higher tyrosine hydroxylase staining in the putamen relative to the sham-grafted treated patients with graft innervation evident. Putamen ^{18}F-dopa uptake was unchanged in the control patients but showed a one-third increase in patients receiving tissue from four fetuses. Unfortunately, no significant differences were seen between the groups in clinical rating scores. The mean UPDRS motor score off medication for the controls deteriorated by 9.4, 3.5, and −0.7 points over 2 years for the controls, one fetus, and four fetus groups (four fetus vs controls, $P = 0.096$). Additionally, no significant differences in "on" time without dyskinesias, total "off" time, ADL (activities of daily living) scores, or L-dopa dose required were evident between the groups. Interestingly, those patients with lowest UPDRS scores responded significantly better to transplantation than to sham surgery. "Off" period dyskinesias were evident in 13 of 23 implanted patients but were not seen in the control arm.

In summary, despite both histological and ^{18}F-dopa PET evidences of graft function, neither of these controlled trials demonstrated clinical efficacy with their primary endpoints. There were indications, however, that younger, more severely affected patients benefited from intrastriatal implantation of human fetal dopamine cells. The other issue raised by these two trials is the occurrence of problematic "off" period dyskinesias in the implanted patients. It has been suggested that these involuntary movement are linked to a greater ^{18}F-dopa uptake in the ventral putamen.[130] Other studies, however, do not support the hypothesis that graft-induced dyskinesias are related to a dopaminergic overgrowth or an excess of dopamine production from the graft.[131,132]

A recent combined ^{18}F-dopa and ^{11}C-raclopride PET study has investigated factors that may influence the functional outcome after transplantation of fetal mesencephalic cells. Compared to the preoperative scan, serial postoperative PET scans showed sustained increases in striatal ^{18}F-dopa uptake, confirming long-term survival of the graft, whereas non-grafted regions showed a progressive reduction of ^{18}F-dopa uptake. Poor outcome after graft was associated with progressive dopaminergic denervation in areas outside the grafted regions.[132]

Intraputaminal Glial Cell Line–Derived Neurotrophic Factor (GDNF) Infusions

GDNF is a potent neurotrophic factor known to prevent the degeneration of dopamine neurons in rodent and primate models of PD where nigral degeneration is toxically induced with 6-OHDA or MPTP. The safety and efficacy of infusing GDNF directly into the posterior putamen has been recently studied in a small open trial.[133] Five PD patients had in-dwelling catheters inserted, and all have tolerated continuous GDNF delivery at a final level of 14 µg/day (6 µL/hour) for over 1 year, unilaterally in 1 patient and bilaterally in 4 patients, without serious side effects. Significant improvements were reported in UPDRS subscores: 39% and 61% improvements in the off-medication motor III and ADL II subscales, respectively, at 12 months. No change in cognitive status was detected on a battery of behavioral tests. Regions of interest sited in the vicinity of the catheter tip showed 18–24% increases in putaminal ^{18}F-dopa Ki, which were confirmed with SPM. Additionally, SPM detected 16–26% increases in nigral dopamine storage, suggesting that retrograde transport of GDNF may have occurred. These findings imply that putamen GDNF infusion is safe and may represent a potential restorative approach for PD. A more recent randomized placebo-controlled study, however, failed to show a clinical benefit of this procedure.[134]

MICROGLIAL ACTIVATION IN PD

Microglia constitute 10–20% of white cells in the brain and form their natural defence mechanism. They are normally in a resting state, but local injury causes them to activate and swell, expressing HLA antigens on the cell surface and releasing cytokines. The mitochondria of activated but not resting microglia express peripheral benzodiazepine sites, which may have a role in preventing apoptosis via membrane stabilization. Activated microglia, however, are also known to release a variety of immune cytokines and other neurotoxic factors that may lead to further neuronal death, particularly in those conditions characterized by extensive chronic microglial activation.[135] ^{11}C-PK11195 is an isoquinoline that binds selectively to peripheral benzodiazepine sites and so provides an in vivo PET marker of glial activation.

Loss of substantia nigra neurons in PD is known to be associated with microglial activation.[136] Two recent papers have reported significant increases in ^{11}C-PK11195 binding in nigral, striatal, and extrastriatal regions in PD patients compared to normal controls.[137,138] Ouchi et al. reported that nigral levels of ^{11}C-PK11195 uptake correlated with loss of striatal dopamine terminal function.[137] These findings therefore support the hypothesis that neuroinflammatory responses by activated microglia contribute to the neuronal loss in PD.

INVOLVEMENT OF NONDOPAMINERGIC SYSTEMS

Postmortem examinations of the brain in patients with different stages of PD have shown that serotonergic, noradrenergic, and cholinergic pathways are commonly involved in PD, although to a lesser extent than the dopaminergic system.[139] Lewy body pathology in nondopaminergic structures may be responsible for the development of nonmotor symptoms of PD, including depression, chronic fatigue, sleep disorders, and dementia.

The serotonergic system in PD patients has been investigated with PET and the 5-HT$_{1A}$ receptor ligand ^{11}C-WAY 100635.[140] In a group of patients with PD, decreases in median raphe 5-HT$_{1A}$ receptor binding, as measured by ^{11}C-WAY 100635, correlated with severity of both total tremor and resting tremor. The observation is in line with pathological findings showing neuronal loss in the dorsal raphe nuclei in PD[141] and suggests a possible role of serotonergic neurons in the pathogenesis of tremor. Alternatively, it may simply be that midbrain tegmental damage including the serotonergic cell bodies leads to onset of rest tremor.

It has been suggested that serotonergic loss might contribute to depression in PD. However, the results from neuroimaging studies so far do not support this view. PD patients with and without depression had similar midbrain uptake of ^{11}C-WAY 100635 binding.[142] Similarly, midbrain uptake of ^{123}I-beta-CIT, a SPECT ligand for the serotonin transporter, did not differ between PD patients with and without depression, and there were no correlations between radiotracer binding in this region and Hamilton Depression Rating Scale scores.[143]

^{11}C-RT132 is a PET tracer that binds with similar affinity to both dopamine and noradrenaline membrane transporters. In areas with low dopaminergic innervation, such as locus coeruleus, ^{11}C-RT132 mainly reflects the density of noradrenergic neurons. In other areas, however, a combined involvement of both dopaminergic and noradrenergic neurons is more likely. Remy et al.[144] have used ^{11}C-RT132 PET to assess PD patients with and without depression. The depressed PD patients were found to have lower ^{11}C-RT132 binding in locus coeruleus and several areas of the limbic system than nondepressed PD patients. This finding suggests that dopamine and noradrenaline rather than serotonin dysfunction may be important in the pathogenesis of depression in patients with PD.

Cholinergic function in PD patients has been assessed with the SPECT tracer ^{123}I-BMV, an acetylcholine vesicular transporter tracer, and more recently with ^{11}C-PMP PET, which provides a measurement of cortical acetylcholinesterase activity. Both techniques have been used to assess whether cholinergic deficiency plays a role in PD patients with dementia. A global reduction of cortical ^{123}I-BMV binding has been reported in both PD patients with dementia and AD patients, whereas PD patients without dementia showed selective reduced ^{123}I-BMV binding in the parietal and occipital cortex.[145] Cortical acetylcholinesterase activity, as measured by ^{11}C-PMP PET, is also reduced in PD patients with dementia.[146] These results support the therapeutic role of acetylcholinesterase inhibitors in PD dementia. Nevertheless, there is growing evidence that the pathogenesis of progressive cognitive impairment in PD is not confined to the cholinergic system.

Dementia is one of the most devastating nonmotor symptoms of PD and occurs in up to 40% of parkinsonian patients, a rate about six times higher than that in healthy people. Not surprisingly, neuroimaging techniques have increasingly been employed over the last years to elucidate the pathogenesis of dementia in PD. Non-demented PD patients show normal cortical metabolism, while ^{18}FDG (^{18}F-deoxyglucose) PET scans of frankly demented PD patients show an AD pattern of impaired brain glucose utilization, posterior parietal and temporal association areas being most affected.[147,148] It remains unclear whether the pattern of glucose hypometabolism in demented PD patients reflects coincidental AD, cortical Lewy body disease, loss of cholinergic projections, or some other degenerative process. Clinicopathological series suggest that there is considerable overlap in the cortical FDG PET findings of coincidental AD and cortical Lewy body disease, but that cortical Lewy body disease cases show a greater reduction in resting glucose metabolism of the primary visual cortex.[149] Interestingly, in one series, one-third of non-demented PD patients with established disease showed subclinical resting temporoparietal cortical metabolic dysfunction with both ^{18}FDG PET and ^{31}P-NMR spectroscopy.[150] Whether these are cases that will go on to become demented is still unclear.

Dementia in PD could also be associated with impaired mesolimbic, mesocortical, and caudate dopaminergic function. Ito et al.[151] assessed changes in dopaminergic function through the whole brain in PD patients with and without dementia matched for age disease duration and disease severity. Compared with PD patients without dementia, the patients with dementia showed reduced ^{18}F-dopa uptake in the right caudate and in the anterior cingulated and ventral striatum bilaterally. Finally, the PET ligand ^{11}C-PIB, a neutral thioflavin developed to image beta-amyloid plaques in AD, has been recently employed to assess PD patients with dementia.[152,153] Ahmed and colleagues[153] studied six PD patients with late dementia, using ^{11}C-PIB and ^{18}F-FDG PET to correlate in vivo regional brain beta-amyloid load with glucose metabolism. All patients had significantly reduced glucose metabolism in frontal, temporal, parietal, and occipital association areas compared to controls, but none showed any increase in beta-amyloid levels as measured by ^{11}C-PIB uptake (Fig. 3–4). These

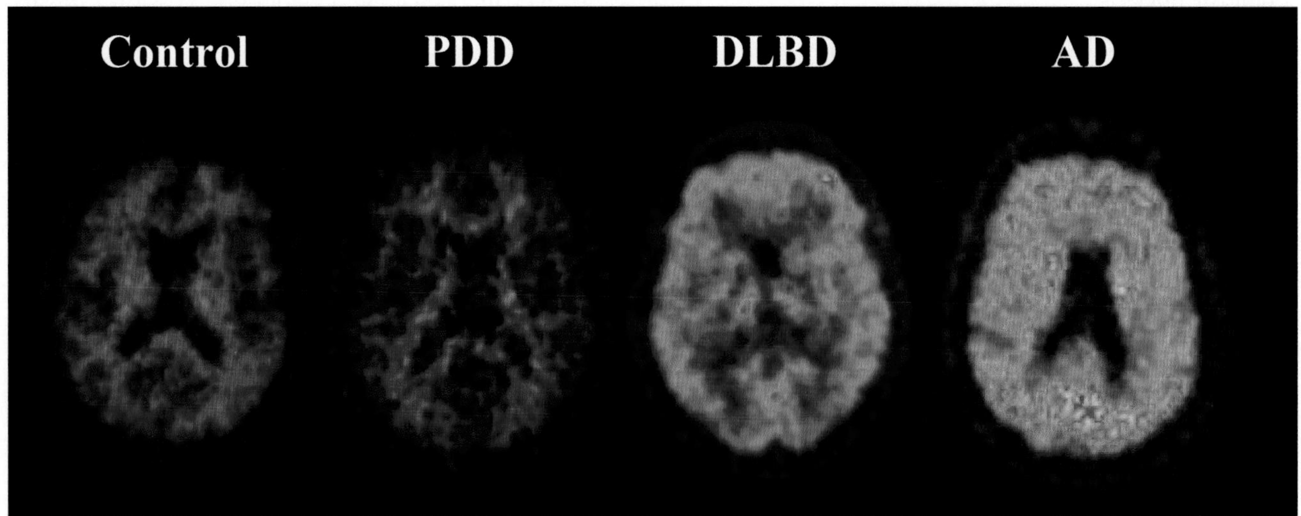

Figure 3–4. Positron emission tomography images of ^{11}C-PIB uptake in the brain of a control subject, in a patient with Parkinson's disease and later dementia (PDD), in a patient with diffuse Lewy body disease (DLBD), and in a patient with Alzheimer' disease (AD). Increased ^{11}C-PIB uptake is visible in the DLBD patient and in the AD patient.

findings suggest that beta-amyloid deposition does not contribute significantly to the pathogenesis of later dementia in PD.

RESTING BRAIN METABOLISM AND BRAIN ACTIVATION IN PD

PET studies have shown increased levels of resting oxygen and glucose metabolism in the contralateral lentiform nucleus of hemiparkinsonian patients with early disease, while PD patients with established bilateral involvement have normal levels of lentiform metabolism.[154,155] Covariance analysis reveals an abnormal profile of relatively raised resting lentiform nucleus and lowered frontal metabolism in PD patients with established disease even when absolute values are normal.[156] The degree of expression of this profile correlates with clinical disease severity. Amelioration of the parkinsonism with either levodopa or deep brain stimulation leads to reduction of the expression of the PD-related profile.[157,158]

While studies of resting CBF and metabolism provide insight into the cerebral dysfunction underlying movement disorders, measuring changes in rCBF while patients perform motor or cognitive tasks can be more revealing. When normal subjects move a joystick in freely selected directions with their right hand paced by a regular tone, $H_2^{15}O$ PET detects associated rCBF increases in contralateral sensorimotor cortex (SMC) and lentiform nucleus, and bilaterally in anterior cingulate, supplementary motor area (SMA), lateral premotor cortex (PMC), and dorsolateral prefrontal cortex (DLPFC).[159] Self-paced extensions of the index finger result in a similar pattern of activation.[160] When PD patients, scanned after stopping L-dopa for 12 hours, perform the same motor tasks, normal activation of SMC, PMC, and lateral parietal association areas are seen, but there is impaired activation of the contralateral lentiform nucleus and the anterior cingulate, SMA, and DLPFC—i.e., of those frontal areas that receive direct input from the basal ganglia. It is well recognized that, while patients with PD can perform isolated limb movements efficiently, attempts to perform repetitive or sequences of movements result in a fall in amplitude and motor arrest. Using $H_2^{15}O$ PET, Samuel et al.[161] demonstrated underactivity of mesial frontal areas and deactivation of dorsolateral prefrontal areas when patients perform prelearned sequential finger-thumb opposition movements with one or both hands. Lateral premotor and parietal areas were relatively overactivated, suggesting adaptive recruitment of a network normally used to facilitate externally cued rather than freely chosen movements. The cerebellum plays a primary role in coordination and accurate tracking. Rascol et al.[162] reported abnormally raised levels of cerebellar regional CBF when PD patients perform sequential finger-thumb opposition movements. Functional MRI has also demonstrated underactivity of the anterior SMA and DLPFC, and overactivity of lateral premotor and parietal areas in PD during sequential finger movements.[163] Additionally, overactivity of motor cortex and caudal SMA was also noted. The detection of motor area overactivity by these workers may, in part, reflect greater sensitivity of MRI compared with PET for activation studies, but may also reflect the more complex design of the paradigm employed. Here, the subjects had to perform fist-clenching in between sequential finger-thumb opposition movements. In support of the presence of primary motor cortex overactivation in PD, a second group has reported this finding when patients performed an externally cued reaching task.[164]

It has been proposed that (1) dorsal prefrontal cortex plays a crucial role in motor decision-making; (2) the SMA prepares and optimizes volitional motor programs once selected;[165] and (3) lateral PMC has a primary role in facilitating motor responses to external visual and auditory stimuli. An inability to activate DLPFC and SMA during freely selected and sequential movements could explain the difficulty that PD patients experience in initiating such actions. In contrast, their ability to overactivate lateral premotor and primary motor cortex allows them to respond well to visual and auditory cues, such as stepping over lines on the floor to aid their walking.

In a recent longitudinal study, 13 patients with recent-onset PD underwent $H_2^{15}O$ PET at baseline and again after a 2-year follow-up. On both occasions, subjects who were off medication were asked to perform paced reaching movements toward targets presented in a predictable order. As disease progressed, an increasing activation in the pallidum bilaterally and in the left putamen was observed. Motor-related activation increased in the right pre-SMA, anterior cingulate cortex, and the left postcentral gyrus. Increases in the right dorsal premotor cortex (DPMC) correlated well with progressive delays in movement initiation, whereas slowing of movement velocity was associated with declining activation in the left DLPFC and DPMC. These findings would indicate that as PD advances, motor performance is associated with the recruitment of brain regions normally involved in the execution of more complex tasks. The authors suggest that this may reflect a progressive loss of functional selectivity or inefficient compensatory activation.[166]

Effects of Treatment on Brain Activation

If loss of dopamine is responsible for the impaired activation of striatofrontal projections in PD, it should be possible to restore it by administering dopaminergic medication. Reduction of bradykinesia when PD patients performed paced joystick movements in freely chosen directions after subcutaneous injection of the nonselective dopamine D1 and D2 agonist, apomorphine, was associated with significant increases in both SMA and

DLPFC blood flow.[167,168] ^{133}Xe SPECT rCBF and event-related functional MRI studies have also demonstrated improvement in SMA flow during finger movements after PD patients are treated with apomorphine[169] and L-dopa.[170] Functional MRI was also able to detect a reduction in the overactivity of motor and lateral PMC during joystick movements after L-dopa administration.[171]

The effects of striatal fetal dopaminergic cell implantation on movement-related premotor and prefrontal activation in PD have been studied. Four PD patients who received bilateral human fetal mesencephalic transplants into caudate and putamen were studied with $H_2{}^{15}O$ PET at baseline and over the 2 years following surgery. Six months after transplantation, mean striatal dopamine storage capacity, measured with ^{18}F-dopa PET, was significantly elevated in these patients (putamen 78%, caudate 27%).[172] This was associated with a mean 12-point clinical improvement on the UPDRS but no significant change in cortical activation. By 18 months postsurgery, there was a 24-point reduction in UPDRS score, despite no further increase in striatal ^{18}F-dopa uptake. SMA and DLPFC activation during performance of joystick movements in freely chosen directions had now significantly improved. These findings suggest that the function of the graft goes beyond that of a simple dopamine delivery system and that functional integration of the grafted neurons into the host brain is necessary in order to produce substantial clinical recovery and restore cortical activation in PD.

Loss of striatal dopamine in PD leads to reduced inhibition of the GPi by striatum, resulting in excessive inhibitory pallidal output to the ventral thalamus and cortex and aberrant burst firing. By inhibiting motor GPi, either by lesioning or by high-frequency electrical deep brain stimulation (DBS), this excessive inhibition is reduced, so aiding volitional movement and improving frontal activation in PD patients. An alternative approach is to reduce the excitatory glutamatergic input to GPi from the STN with high-frequency DBS. A number of series have now established that pallidotomy, pallidal, and STN DBS all improve rigidity and bradykinesia in PD.

Grafton et al.[173] examined the regional cerebral activation in six PD patients associated with reaching out to grasp lighted targets before and after pallidotomy while withdrawn from medication. Surgery resulted in significantly increased SMA and lateral premotor activation, despite little change in patient performance. Significantly increased activation of SMA, lateral PMC, and dorsal prefrontal cortex after pallidotomy has also been demonstrated in PD patients off medication when performing joystick movements in freely selected directions.[174] There have been several $H_2{}^{15}O$ PET reports on the functional effects of DBS in PD. GPi stimulation improves contralateral bradykinesia and rigidity in association with increased resting levels of SMA and lentiform rCBF,[175] and increased contralateral sensorimotor, mesial premotor, and anterior cingulate cortex activation during performance of a visually guided reaching task.[176] STN DBS improves rostral SMA, lateral premotor, and DLPFC activation in PD during performance of joystick movements in freely chosen directions.[177–179] In contrast to pallidotomy, however, STN stimulation also results in increases in resting thalamic and decreases in resting motor cortex and caudal SMA rCBF, and reduced motor cortex activation. The decreased motor cortex activation may be a consequence of antidromic stimulation of direct projections to STN. It has been suggested that STN stimulation may also induce dopamine release in the striatum.[180,181] Results from three independent studies, however, do not support this view, as striatal ^{11}C-raclopride bindings in STN DBS "on" and "off" conditions were similar.[182–184]

The peduculopontine nucleus (PPN) plays an important role in locomotion and postural control and has therefore been proposed as a novel target for DBS, particularly for those PD patients with severe gait dysfunction and akinesia. Strafella et al.[185] have recently reported changes in rCBF at rest during off and on stimulation in an advanced PD patient with unilateral PPN-DBS. Interestingly, PPN stimulation increased rCBF in the thalamus bilaterally. Clinically, UPDRS motor score was reduced by approximately 20% when stimulator was on. Such improvement was mainly in relation to gait, contralateral tremor, and bradykinesia. These results need to be confirmed by larger studies; however, they indicate that PPN-DBS could represent an important therapeutic option for patients with postural instability and deterioration of gait.

Recently, inhibition of STN output has been attempted by the use of gene therapy. Genes for the enzyme glutamate decarboxylase (GAD), which converts glutamate to GABA, have been unilaterally transfected into the STN of 12 PD patients using an adenoassociated viral (AAV) vector. Significant reductions in thalamic metabolism on the operated side, along with concurrent metabolic increases in ipsilateral motor and premotor cortical regions, were observed. Abnormal elevations in the activity of metabolic networks associated with motor and cognitive functioning in PD patients were evident at baseline. The activity of the motor-related network declined after surgery and persisted at 1 year. These network changes correlated with improved clinical disability ratings.[186]

▶ ATYPICAL PARKINSONIAN SYNDROMES

MULTISYSTEM ATROPHY (MSA)

This condition is characterized pathologically by argyrophilic, alpha-synuclein-positive inclusions in glia and neurons in substantia nigra, striatum, brain stem, and cerebellar nuclei, and intermediolateral columns of the cord (see Chapter 20). It manifests as a parkinsonian syndrome with autonomic failure and ataxia, and includes striatonigral degeneration (SND), progressive autonomic failure (PAF), and olivopontocerebellar atrophy (OPCA) within its spectrum. Patients are often L-dopa nonresponsive. ^{18}FDG PET studies in patients with clinically probable SND show reduced levels of striatal glucose metabolism in 80–100% of cases, in contrast to PD, where striatal metabolism is preserved.[187–189] Eidelberg et al.[190] reported that parkinsonian patients with low levels of striatal glucose metabolism, irrespective of their L-dopa response, show little improvement after pallidotomy. Patients with the full syndrome of MSA have reduced mean levels of cerebellar, along with putamen and caudate, glucose hypometabolism. ^{18}FDG PET, therefore, provides a sensitive means of detecting the presence of striatal dysfunction where atypical parkinsonism is suspected.

Proton MRS can also help discriminate SND from PD.[191] *N*-acetyl-aspartate (NAA) is a metabolic marker of neuronal integrity present in millimolar concentrations. Reduced NAA:creatine proton MRS signal ratios were reported from the lentiform nuclei in six out of seven clinically probable SND cases, while eight out of nine probable PD cases showed normal levels of putamen NAA.

The function of both the pre- and postsynaptic dopaminergic systems is impaired in patients with SND. As in PD, putamen ^{18}F-dopa uptake is asymmetrically reduced, and individual levels of putamen ^{18}F-dopa uptake correlate with disability.[192] Patients with the full syndrome of MSA show a significantly greater reduction in mean caudate ^{18}F-dopa uptake than equivalently rigid PD patients (Fig. 3–5), although individual ranges overlap and a greater involvement of caudate only discriminates SND from PD with 70% specificity.[193] ^{18}FDG PET and proton MRS appear to be more robust than ^{18}F-dopa PET for discriminating typical from atypical parkinsonsm. Pirker et al.[194] recently examined striatal DAT binding in PD and MSA patients, and concluded that, while ^{123}I-beta-CIT SPECT reliably discriminates PD and MSA from normal, it cannot reliably discriminate between these two parkinsonian conditions.

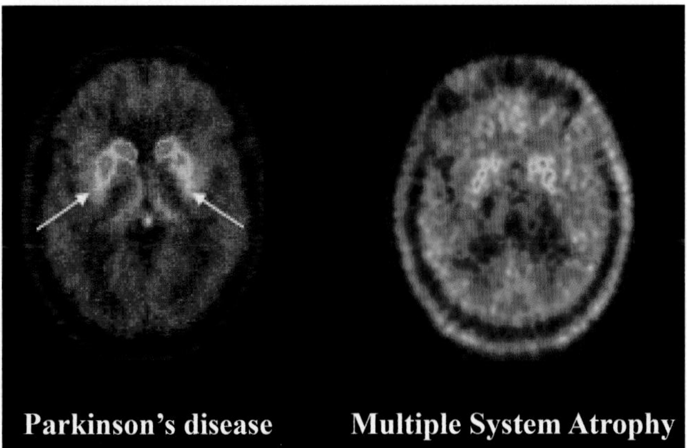

Figure 3–5. Positron emission tomography images of a patient with Parkinson's disease (PD) and a patient with multiple system atrophy. Arrows show reduced ^{18}F-dopa uptake in dorsal posterior putamen in PD.

SND patients show mild, but significant, reductions in their mean putamen ^{11}C-SCH23390 (D1) and ^{11}C-raclopride (D2) uptake, while this remains preserved in PD.[195–197] Again, there is an overlap between SND, normal, and PD ranges, so striatal D1 and D2 binding does not provide a sensitive discriminator of SND from PD. In support of this viewpoint, ^{123}I-IBZM SPECT found reduced striatal D2 binding in only two-thirds of de novo parkinsonian patients who showed a negative apomorphine response.[198] Given that a significant number of parkinsonian patients who respond poorly to L-dopa show normal levels of striatal D2 binding, it seems likely that degeneration of pallidal and brain stem rather than striatal projections is responsible for their refractory status. Seppi et al.[199] used ^{123}I-IBZM SPECT to follow striatal degeneration longitudinally in a group of early MSA cases. They found an annual 10% loss of striatal D2 binding in their 18-month study and concluded that ^{123}I-IBZM SPECT provides a valid future approach for testing the efficacy of putative neuroprotective agents in MSA.

The basal ganglia are rich in opioid peptides and binding sites, and these are differentially affected in SND and PD. ^{11}C-diprenorphine is a nonspecific opioid antagonist binding with equal affinity to mu, kappa, and delta sites. In nondyskinetic PD patients, caudate and putamen ^{11}C-diprenorphine uptake is preserved, whereas putamen uptake is reduced in 50% of patients thought to have SND.[200] ^{123}I-MIBG SPECT can be used to study functional integrity of cardiac sympathetic innervation in PD and MSA. Both these conditions show a reduction in mediastinal ^{123}I-MIBG signal, but this is significantly greater in PD, even in cases where no clinical evidence of autonomic failure is present.[201] This finding suggests a greater involvement of postganglionic sympathetic innervation of the myocardium in PD compared with MSA.

^{11}C-PK11195 PET has been used to study glial activation in MSA. More widespread subcortical increases in ^{11}C-PK11195 uptake are seen compared with PD, targeting the nigra, putamen, pallidum, thalamus, and brain stem.[202] It remains to be determined whether striatal ^{11}C-PK11195 uptake will provide a sensitive discriminator of MSA and PD.

In order to determine the overlap between pure autonomic failure, OPCA, and SND, groups of these patients have been studied with PET and proton MRS. Two out of seven PAF patients showed reduced putamen ^{18}F-dopa uptake in one series, suggesting that subclinical nigral dysfunction was present.[192] One of these patients subsequently developed MSA. In a series of 10 sporadic OPCA patients with autonomic failure but no rigidity, 7 showed reduced putamen ^{18}F-dopa uptake and 4 had reduced putamen ^{11}C-diprenorphine binding indicative of the presence of subclinical SND.[203] Reduced levels of striatal ^{18}F-dopa uptake,[204] striatal glucose hypometabolism,[205] and reduced lentiform NAA:creatine signal have also been reported in other series of sporadic OPCA cases.[191] In summary, the majority of sporadic OPCA cases with autonomic failure show functional imaging evidence of subclinical striatonigral dysfunction.

PROGRESSIVE SUPRANUCLEAR PALSY (PSP)

PSP is characterized pathologically by neurofibrillary tangle formation and neuronal loss in the substantia nigra, pallidum, superior colliculi, brain stem nuclei, and the periaqueductal gray matter (see Chapter 21). There is a lesser degree of cortical involvement. A number of series have reported changes in resting regional cerebral glucose metabolism in patients with clinically probable PSP, several of whom have later had the diagnosis confirmed at autopsy.[206–211] Cortical metabolism is globally depressed, and frontal areas are particularly targeted, levels of metabolism correlating with disease duration and performance on psychometric tests of frontal function. Hypofrontality is not specific for PSP; it can be seen in PD, SND, Pick's disease, HD, and depression. One case of clinically probable PSP with appropriate ^{18}FDG PET findings was subsequently reported to show progressive subcortical gliosis at autopsy.[212] Basal ganglia, cerebellar, and thalamic resting glucose metabolisms are also depressed in PSP, so distinguishing it from PD where metabolism is preserved. Proton MRS studies also show reduced lentiform nucleus NAA:creatine ratios in PSP, in contrast to PD.[213] While ^{18}FDG PET and proton MRS will discriminate at least 80% of PSP cases from PD, they are unable to reliably discriminate PSP from SND as striatal and frontal hypometabolism can be a feature of both these disorders. The pathology of PSP uniformly targets nigrostriatal dopaminergic projections, so in contrast to PD, putamen and caudate ^{18}F-dopa uptakes are equivalently reduced in PSP, levels correlating inversely with disease duration.[192,214,215] In one series, ^{18}F-dopa PET was able to discriminate 90% of PSP from PD cases on the basis of uniform caudate and putamen involvement in the former.[193]

Messa et al.[216] have also reported equivalent loss of putamen ^{123}I-beta-CIT uptake in PD and PSP but significantly greater caudate involvement in the latter. Pirker et al.,[194] however, found ^{123}I-beta-CIT SPECT less useful for discriminating PD from PSP. There is no clear correlation between levels of striatal ^{18}F-dopa uptake in PSP and the degree of disability.[192] Unlike PD and SND, where locomotor impairment appears to correlate with loss of dopaminergic fibers, loss of mobility in PSP is probably determined by degeneration of nondopaminergic pallidal and brain stem projections. Striatal D2 binding in PSP has been studied with both PET and SPECT; reductions have been consistently reported, although only 50–70% of patients individually show significant receptor loss.[197,217–219] It is likely that degeneration of downstream pallidal and brain stem projections is responsible for the poor L-dopa responsiveness of PSP rather than loss of dopamine receptors alone. Finally, a marked reduction of acetylcholinesterase activity as measured by ^{11}C-MP4A PET has been reported in the thalamus of patients with PSP.[220] The thalamus receives its main cholinergic inputs from the PPN and other brain stem cholinergic nuclei. It is, therefore, likely that the reduced thalamic acetylcholinesterase activity may reflect a significant neuronal loss in the brain stem structures. The PPN is involved in posture and gait control, eye movements, and attention, and its impairment may contribute to the motor and cognitive dysfunction typical of PSP.

CORTICOBASAL DEGENERATION (CBD)

This condition classically presents with an akinetic-rigid, apraxic limb that may exhibit alien behavior. Cortical sensory loss, dysphasia, myoclonus, supranuclear gaze problems, and bulbar dysfunction are also features, while intellect is spared until late. Eventually, all four limbs become involved, and the condition is invariably poorly L-dopa responsive. The pathology consists of collections of swollen, achromatic, tau-positive-staining Pick cells in the absence of argyrophilic Pick bodies, which target the posterior frontal, inferior parietal, and superior temporal lobes, the substantia nigra, and the cerebellar dentate nuclei[221] (see Chapter 22). PET and SPECT studies on patients with the clinical syndrome of CBD show greatest reductions in resting cortical oxygen and glucose metabolism in posterior frontal, inferior parietal, and superior temporal regions.[222–225] The thalamus and the striatum are also involved. The metabolic reductions are strikingly asymmetrical, being most severe contralateral to the more affected limbs. This contrasts with PD patients, who have preserved and symmetrical levels of striatal and thalamic glucose metabolism. In a recent study, ^{18}FDG PET has been reported to have 91% sensitivity and 99% specificity for the diagnosis of CBS when computer-assisted methodologies are applied.[226]

Striatal ^{18}F-dopa uptake is also reduced in CBD in an asymmetrical fashion, being most depressed contralateral to the more affected limbs.[222] Like PSP, but in contrast to PD, caudate and putamen ^{18}F-dopa uptakes are similarly depressed in CBD. ^{123}I-beta-CIT SPECT also shows an asymmetrical reduction in striatal DAT binding in CBD,[194] while ^{123}I-IBZM SPECT shows a severe asymmetrical reduction of striatal D2 binding.[227]

The above imaging findings may help discriminate CBD from Pick's disease where inferior frontal hypometabolism predominates, from PD where striatal metabolism is preserved and caudate ^{18}F-dopa uptake is relatively spared, and from PSP where frontal and striatal metabolisms tend to be more symmetrically involved.[228] Having said that, both Pick's and PSP pathology have been subsequently reported in clinically apparent CBD cases.

DIFFUSE LEWY BODY DISEASE (DLBD)

DLBD is the second most frequent cause of dementia after AD. Clinically, DLBD can be distinguished from AD by fluctuating cognition, occurrence of parkinsonism, and visual hallucinations, and from PD by the appearance of parkinsonian symptoms within 1 year of the onset of cognitive impairment. Whether DLBD, PD, and AD represent different components of a spectrum is unclear. DLBD patients show not only cerebral cortical neuronal loss, with Lewy bodies in surviving neurons, but also loss of nigrostriatal dopaminergic neurons. In contrast, nigral pathology is mild in AD. Using ^{123}I-FP-CIT SPECT, Walker et al.[229] have examined striatal DAT binding in 27 patients with clinically presumed DLBD, 17 with AD, 19 drug-naive patients with PD, and 16 controls. The presumed DLBD and PD patients had significantly lower uptake of caudate and putamen ^{123}I-FP-CIT than patients with AD ($P < 0.001$) and controls ($P < 0.001$). A problem, however, with the interpretation of this finding is that the DLBD and PD patient groups had equivalent parkinsonism on their UPDRS and Hoehn and Yahr ratings, while the AD patients and controls had slight or no rigidity. The SPECT findings could, therefore, simply have reflected clinical selection bias. The authors, however, were able to subsequently correlate their SPECT findings with 10 postmortem examinations. Nine of these 10 cases were thought to have DLBD in life, but only 4 had this diagnosis at autopsy. All four had reduced striatal ^{123}I-FP-CIT uptake. Five of the 10 cases had AD pathology and 4 of these 5 had normal ^{123}I-FP-CIT SPECT. These clinicoimaging correlations suggest that ^{123}I-FP-CIT SPECT may be helpful in discriminating DLBD from AD, but its role in patients with isolated dementia without parkinsonism remains unproven.

Yong et al.[230] have recently compared glucose metabolism in PD patients with and without dementia and patients with DLBD. Statistical comparisons between groups were performed with SPM. Compared to normal controls, both PD patients with dementia and DLBD patients showed significant metabolic decreases in the parietal lobe, occipital lobe, temporal lobe, frontal lobe, and anterior cingulate. When DLBD patients and PD patients with dementia were compared with PD patients without dementia, both groups showed a pattern of reduced glucose metabolism in the inferior and medial frontal lobe bilaterally and right parietal lobe. The metabolic deficit was greater in DLBD patients. The direct comparison between DLBD and PD with dementia showed a significant metabolic decrease in anterior cingulate in patients with DLBD. Taken together these findings support the view that PD with dementia and DBLD have similar underlying patterns of dysfunction.

The contribution of amyloid pathology to DLBD has been unclear. Two series have reported increased ^{11}C-PIB uptake in a majority of DLBD cases (Fig. 3–4), suggesting that DLBD is actually a condition with two underlying pathologies—Lewy body and amyloid—perhaps explaining the aggressive nature of the dementia relative to AD.[152,231]

▶ INVOLUNTARY MOVEMENT DISORDERS

HUNTINGTON'S DISEASE (HD) AND OTHER CHOREAS

HD is an autosomal-dominantly transmitted disorder associated with an excess of CAG triplet repeats (>38) in the IT15 gene on chromosome 4. The function of this gene is still uncertain, but the pathology of HD targets medium spiny projection neurons in the striatum, causing intranuclear and cytoplasmic inclusions to form. Patients with predominant chorea show a selective loss of striatal-external globus pallidal projections, which express GABA and enkephalin, while those with a predominant akinetic-rigid syndrome (the Westphal variant) show additional severe loss of striatal-internal pallidal fibers containing GABA and dynorphine.[232,233] A number of other degenerative disorders are also associated with chorea, including neuroacanthocytosis (NA), dentatorubropallidoluysian atrophy (DRPLA), and benign familial chorea (BFC).

The inflammatory disorders systemic lupus erythematosus (SLE) and Sydenham's chorea are also associated with chorea, as is chronic neuroleptic exposure. The mechanism underlying tardive dyskinesia (TD) is uncertain; postmortem studies have found low levels of subthalamic and pallidal GAD,[234] while neurochemical studies on a primate TD model have reported severe depletion of subthalamic and pallidal GABA.[235] These findings suggest that TD, like HD, may be associated with deranged GABA transmission.

Clinically affected HD patients show severely reduced levels of resting glucose and oxygen metabolism of their caudate and lentiform nuclei.[236–238] Levels of resting putamen metabolism correlate with locomotor function and caudate metabolism with performance on executive tests sensitive to frontal lobe function.[239,240] In early HD, cortical metabolism is preserved, but as the disease progresses and dementia becomes prominent, it also declines, the frontal cortex being targeted.[241] Caudate hypometabolism is not specific to HD, also being seen in NA, DRPLA, and some cases of BFC.[242–245] In contrast, striatal glucose metabolism is normal or elevated in inflammatory choreas, and TDs.[246–248]

Regional cerebral metabolism in HD has also been studied with proton MRS. NAA levels in the basal ganglia are reduced in affected patients, whereas lactate levels in the basal ganglia and cortex are elevated, suggesting that mitochondrial dysfunction is a feature of this disorder.[249] If the pathology of HD arises due to mitochondrial dysfunction, raised lactate levels in asymptomatic adult gene carriers should be expected. To date, lactate levels have been reported to be normal in asymptomatic gene carriers, more in favor of mitochondrial dysfunction representing an associated phenomenon rather than being causative. The medium spiny striatal neurons that degenerate in HD express D1, D2, opioid, and benzodiazepine receptors. PET and SPECT studies with benzamide- and spiperone-based tracers have all confirmed that striatal D2 binding is reduced by at least 30% in clinically affected HD patients.[250–252] ^{11}C-SCH23390 PET studies in HD have demonstrated reduced D1 binding in both striatum and temporal cortex.[253] Turjanski et al.[251] used ^{11}C-SCH23390 and ^{11}C-raclopride PET to study both D1 binding and D2 binding in HD. They found a parallel reduction in striatal binding to these receptor subtypes, irrespective of phenotype and levels of D1 and D2 binding correlating with severity of rigidity rather than chorea. Striatal opioid[254] and benzodiazepine[255] binding have also been shown to be reduced in clinically affected HD patients. The reductions are relatively small (20%), however, compared with the mean 60% loss of dopamine D1 and D2 receptor binding.

The finding of reduced striatal dopamine receptor binding in patients with HD is, however, not specific for this cause of chorea: a mean 70% reduction of striatal ^{11}C-raclopride binding has also been reported in NA.[256] In contrast, normal striatal D2 binding has been reported in SLE chorea[251] and TD.[257–259] This finding argues against the hypothesis that TD results from striatal D2 receptor supersensitivity following prolonged exposure to neuroleptics and suggests that the postmortem reports of downstream reductions in pallidal and subthalamic GABA levels are of greater relevance.

As clinically affected HD patients show at least a 30% loss of striatal glucose metabolism and dopamine receptor binding, ^{18}FDG, ^{11}C-SCH23390, and ^{11}C-raclopride PET should all be capable of detecting subclinical dysfunction, if present, in asymptomatic HD gene carriers. Reduced caudate glucose metabolism has been reported in 9 out of 12 and 3 out of 8 asymptomatic adult HD gene carriers in two different series,[260,261] while Weeks et al.[262] showed a significant parallel loss of striatal D1 and D2 binding in 4 out of 8 asymptomatic adults with the HD mutation.

The rate of progression of HD has also been followed with PET. Grafton et al.[263] found that caudate glucose metabolism declined annually by 3.1% in their cohort of HD patients, while Antonini et al.[264] reported an annual 6% change in striatal D2 binding. Andrews et al.[265] have reported an annual fall in striatal D1 and D2 binding of 3–4% in symptomatic HD gene carriers and 6% in asymptomatic HD gene carriers with active subclinical disease. Pavese et al.[266] found a linear 5% annual decline in striatal D2 binding in early HD measured serially on three occasions over 5 years. These workers were also able to detect early loss of frontal D2 binding with ^{11}C-raclopride PET. These findings all suggest that functional imaging provides an objective means of following HD progression in the event of effective neuroprotective or restorative interventions being found.

MICROGLIAL ACTIVATION IN HD

Postmortem studies of HD brains have shown a significant accumulation of activated microglia in regions affected by HD, such as the basal ganglia and the frontal cortex. Sapp et al.[267] reported a significant correlation between macroglia density and severity of HD pathology, suggesting a close association between microglial activation and neuronal death. ^{11}C-PK11195 PET has been used to investigate the extent of activated microglia in vivo in a cohort of HD patients. Compared to normal controls, HD patients showed significant increases in striatal ^{11}C-PK11195 binding, which significantly correlated with disease severity as reflected by the striatal reduction in ^{11}C-raclopride binding, the Unified Huntington's Disease Rating Scale (UHDRS), and the patients' CAG index. The HD patients also showed significant increases in microglia activation in cortical regions, including prefrontal cortex and anterior cingulated.[268] More recently, Tai et al.[269] have reported increased striatal and cortical ^{11}C-PK11195 binding in premanifest HD gene carriers, suggesting early accumulation of activated microglia in HD (Fig. 3–6). Individual levels of striatal ^{11}C-PK11195 binding in asymptomatic gene carriers significantly correlated with lower striatal ^{11}C-raclopride binding and with a higher probability of developing HD in 5 years.

Taken together, the findings from postmortem and neuroimaging studies support the view that activated microglia contribute to the ongoing neuronal degeneration in HD. Further studies in larger cohorts of patients and longitudinal assessments with serial PET scans are needed to establish whether ^{11}C-PK11195 PET is an effective marker of subclinical/active disease and whether the technique represents an objective tool to assess the efficacy of neuroprotection strategies in both premanifest HD gene carriers and clinically affected HD patients.

TRANSPLANTATION OF HD

Transplantation of embryonic striatal tissue into the degenerated striatum of rat and primate models of HD has

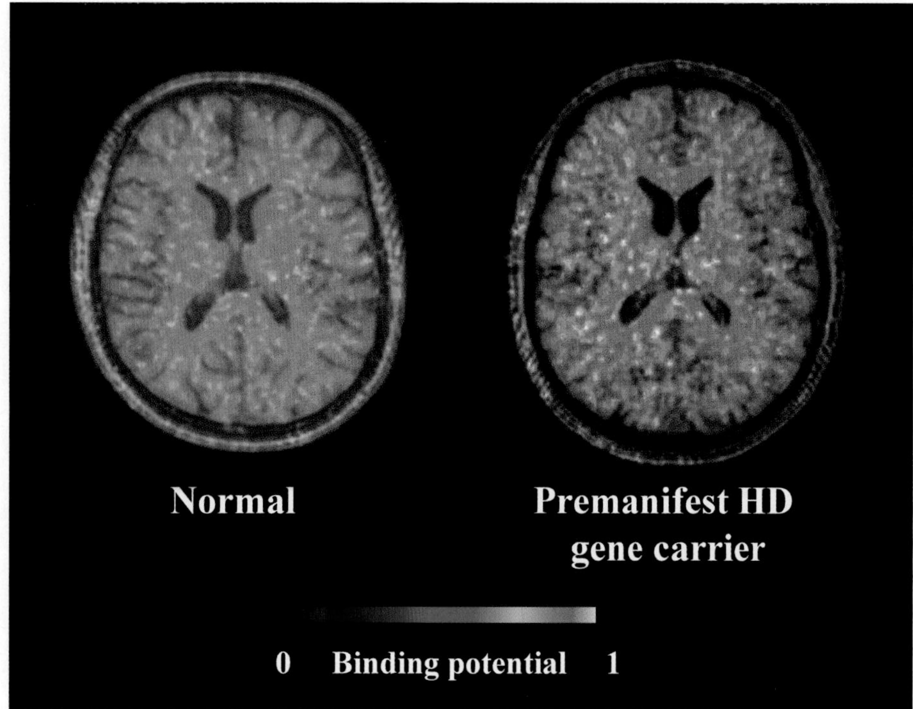

Figure 3–6. Positron emission tomography images of ^{11}C-PK11195 uptake in the brain of a control subject and in a premanifest Huntington's disease (HD) gene carrier. Increased ^{11}C-PK11195 binding is visible in the premanifest HD gene carrier.

been shown to be safe, and has demonstrated good graft survival with differentiation and integration of striatal grafts into host striatum. Recovery of striatal dopamine D2 binding in rats and marmosets lesioned with ibotenic acid after implantation of fetal striatal tissue has been detected with ^{11}C-raclopride PET.[270–272] In primate models, recovery of skilled motor and cognitive performance has been reported within 2 months, and improvements in dystonia scores within 4–5 months of grafting.[273] Physiological, neurochemical, and anatomical studies have shown that a partial restoration of striatal input and output circuitry by implanted striatal neurons does occur, but the time course of this in primates and humans remains unclear.

Clinical studies of the possible therapeutic effects of striatal allografts in patients with HD are now running in the United States, France, and England. To date, only three studies in humans have reported imaging findings. In the first of these studies, five HD patients received striatal implant in an open-label fashion. Three of the five patients showed a clinical improvement over a 12-month follow-up, and brain ^{18}FDG PET showed regional increases in glucose utilization.[274] The three patients with clinical improvement remained clinically stable at the end of a 2-year follow-up, and ^{18}FDG PET showed a further improvement of striatal and cortical metabolism, whereas the remaining two patients presented a further deterioration in both clinical symptoms and PET findings.[275] Reuter et al.[276] have recently reported two more HD patients with moderate disease who received bilateral fetal striatal allografts. One patient (Fig. 3–7) demonstrated prolonged clinical improvement over 5 years and increased striatal D2 receptor binding, evident with ^{11}C-raclopride PET, whereas the other patient did not improve clinically or radiologically. In contrast to these promising results, a clinical trial carried out in the United States failed to demonstrate any clinical or imaging improvement in HD patients after striatal graft.[277] Therefore, the role of striatal cells implantation in HD remains to be elucidated. Hopefully, the results of new clinical trials that are currently underway will help clarify this topic.

DYSTONIA

Dystonia is characterized by involuntary posturing and muscle spasms. The primary torsion dystonias (PTDs) range from severe, young-onset, generalized disorders to late-onset focal disease. The most common familial form of generalized PTD, DYT1 dystonia, is an autosomal-dominant disorder with around 40% penetrance and generally early-onset starting in a lower limb. All cases of DYT1 dystonia identified have a common mutation: a GAG deletion within the coding region

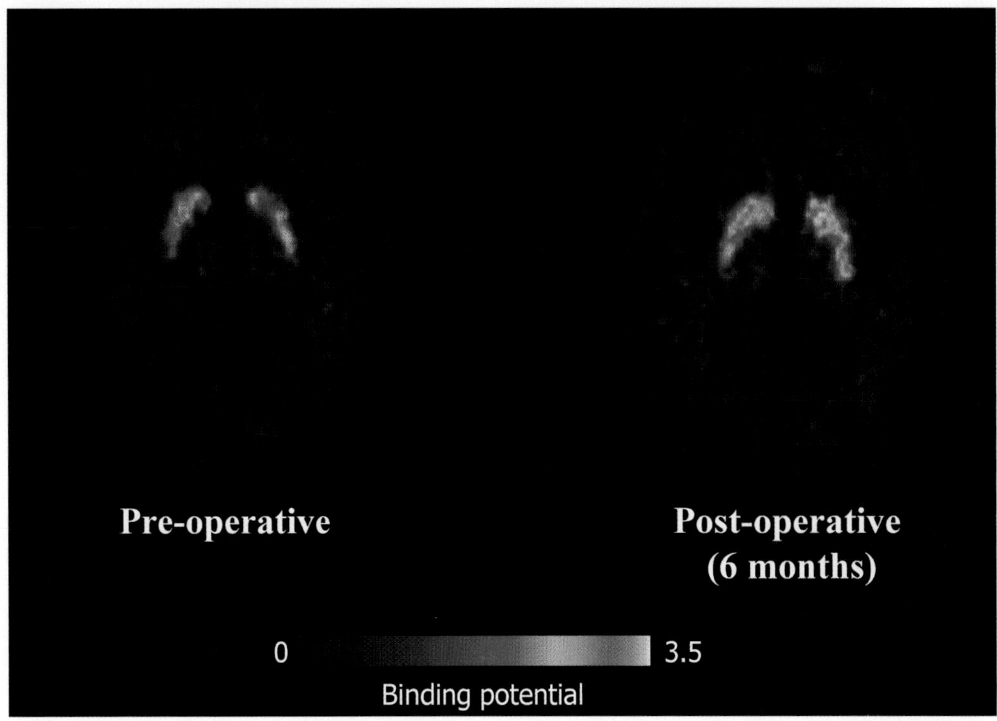

Figure 3–7. Positron emission tomography images of striatal ^{11}C-raclopride binding for a patient with Huntington's disease before and 6 months after bilateral implantation of fetal mesencephalic tissue into the caudate and putamen.

of the DYT1 gene on chromosome 9q34, which codes for torsin A, an ATP-binding protein of unknown function. A second generalized PTD locus has been mapped to chromosome 8p (DYT6); affected individuals have adult-onset generalized dystonia with craniocervical disease or focal dystonia. A third PTD gene (DYT13) has been mapped to chromosome 1p and has a phenotype of cranial–cervical and upper limb involvement with occasional generalization. Postmortem studies have shown that DYT1 mRNA is highly expressed in dopaminergic neurons of the substantia nigra pars compacta. This could conceivably result in abnormal dopaminergic neurotransmission in dystonia, although histopathological studies have failed to identify consistent structural or neurotransmitter abnormalities in idiopathic torsion dystonia (ITD). Regions affected in acquired dystonia include caudate, putamen, globus pallidus, and posterior thalamus.[278] It has been suggested that ITD arises due to a reduced inhibitory output from the basal ganglia to ventral thalamus and premotor areas, causing these to become inappropriately overactive. There have been a number of ^{18}FDG PET studies on resting levels of regional cerebral glucose metabolism in dystonia. A problem in interpreting the findings of early studies arises due to the heterogeneity of the patient groups recruited: familial, sporadic, and acquired dystonia have all been considered together, and patients with focal or hemidystonia have been favored in order to provide side-to-side comparisons of basal ganglia function. As a consequence, the relevance of some of these PET findings to PTD is uncertain. Additionally, some of these patients were clearly experiencing active muscular spasms while reportedly at rest. Resting lentiform nucleus metabolism in dystonia has been variously reported to be increased,[279,280] normal,[281–283] and decreased.[284]

Covariance analysis of ^{18}FDG PET findings in DYT1 carriers has produced more consistent and interpretable findings. In a series of reports, Eidelberg et al.[285] have shown an abnormal resting metabolic profile in DYT1 carriers, levels of lentiform nucleus glucose metabolism being relatively reduced and frontal metabolism raised. This pattern is seen whether DYT1 gene carriers are clinically affected or asymptomatic and is a pattern opposite to that seen in PD. A study on DYT1 dystonic patients while asleep has also shown preservation of this abnormal pattern of resting glucose metabolism and confirmed that it is not movement related. More recently, the same profile has been reported by these workers in other genetic mutations (e.g., DYT6) causing dystonia[259] and in essential blepharospasm.[286] These findings suggest a common imbalance of basal ganglia–frontal function may underlay the dystonias.

Cerebral activation studies in PTD have suggested an imbalance between sensorimotor and PMC function. If dystonia patients perform paced joystick movements with their right hands in freely selected directions, they show significantly increased levels of contralateral putamen, rostral SMA, lateral PMC, and dorsolateral prefrontal area activation.[287] In contrast, activation of contralateral SMC and caudal SMA is impaired; these are the motor cortical areas that send direct pyramidal tract projections to the spinal cord. Tempel[288,289] and Perlmutter[290] also noted attenuation of SMC and caudal SMA activation in PTD, and focal dystonia during vibrotactile stimulation. The pattern of activation in dystonia is, therefore, very different from the pattern associated with PD, where striatal, SMA, and prefrontal areas underfunction while primary motor cortex activation is either normal or increased.

It would seem, therefore, that dystonic limb movements in PTD are associated with inappropriate overactivation of basal ganglia–premotor area projections. Patients with acquired hemi- or focal dystonia due to basal ganglia and thalamic lesions also show increased levels of mesial and lateral PMC and dorsolateral prefrontal area activation during arm movement.[291] In contrast to PTD patients, however, acquired dystonia patients with basal ganglia lesions show raised rather than reduced primary motor cortex activation. This finding suggests that the pathology of PTD may have a direct inhibitory effect on primary SMC function not seen in secondary cases with focal basal ganglia lesions.

The question then arises: what is the significance of the frontal association area overactivity that is evident in both idiopathic and acquired dystonia? Three possibilities can be envisaged. First, the overactivity represents a primary dysfunction of motor planning circuitry. Second, the functional deficit in dystonia is at an executive level, and the prefrontal cortex becomes overactive in a conscious attempt to try and suppress the unwanted movements. Third, the frontal overactivity simply represents a secondary phenomenon reflecting primary basal ganglia overactivity.

Against the first hypothesis is the observation that ITD patients and normal subjects activate dorsolateral prefrontal and rostral SMAs equivalently when simply imagining joystick movements in freely chosen directions, but not performing them.[292] This suggests that the primary functional deficit in idiopathic dystonia must lie at an executive rather than planning level. Whether the frontal association area overactivity is simply secondary to primary basal ganglia overactivity or represents an adaptive phenomenon in a conscious attempt to suppress the syndrome, however, still remains unclear. In order to investigate this further, writer's cramp patients were studied while writing before and after treatment with botulinus toxin. These patients again demonstrated premotor overactivity and sensorimotor underactivity while writing continuously, and this pattern did not reverse after relief of the associated forearm cramp with botulinus toxin.[293] This would suggest that the frontal overactivity seen in dystonia during limb movement is part of the pathophysiology of the syndrome and is not simply an adaptive phenomenon to the presence of involuntary muscle spasms.

PET reports on dopaminergic function in dystonia have been confounded by inclusion of heterogeneous groups of patients. The only study to assess striatal ^{18}F-dopa uptake in purely familial PTD was by Playford et al.[294] These workers found that 8 out of 11 PTD patients had normal striatal dopamine storage but that the 3 with most severe disease and taking high doses of anticholinergics showed mild impairment of putamen ^{18}F-dopa uptake.[294] The authors concluded that dopamine terminal function was normal in the majority of PTD cases. Two asymptomatic obligate gene carriers were studied, and both had normal striatal ^{18}F-dopa uptake. Martin et al.[295] examined three PTD dystonic subjects with ^{18}F-dopa PET. One of these had normal and two reduced striatal ^{18}F-dopa uptake. In contrast, Otsuka et al.[282] found a mildly raised level of mean striatal ^{18}F-dopa uptake in eight patients with idiopathic dystonia. Most recently, a ^{123}I-beta-CIT SPECT study has reported normal striatal uptake in 10 patients with torticollis.[296] Combining the findings of these studies, it would appear likely that striatal dopamine terminal function is normal in the majority of PTD cases.

Striatal D2 binding has also been studied in idiopathic dystonia. An ^{18}F-spiperone PET study reported a mean 20% reduction putamen D2 binding in a collection of patients with either Meige syndrome or writer's cramp, but there was a wide overlap with the normal binding range.[290] A similar finding was reported in a ^{123}I-epidepride SPECT study involving 10 torticollis cases.[296] Reduced striatal D2 availability could conceivably result in decreased activity of the indirect striatopallidal pathway and breakthrough involuntary movements.

DOPA-RESPONSIVE DYSTONIA (DRD) AND DYSTONIA–PARKINSONISM

Dominantly inherited DRD is related to a mutation in the DYT5 gene coding for GTP cyclohydrolase 1. This enzyme constitutes part of the tetrahydrobiopterin synthetic pathway, the cofactor for tyrosine hydroxylase. Patients are unable to manufacture L-dopa, and hence dopamine, from endogenous tyrosine but can still convert exogenous L-dopa to dopamine. DRD cases generally present in childhood with diurnally fluctuating dystonia and later develop background parkinsonism. Occasionally, the condition presents as pure parkinsonism in adulthood. Asanuma et al.[297] have recently reported a specific pattern of regional metabolic covariation in DRD that differs from other inherited forms of dystonia. This pattern consisted in increases in the dorsal midbrain, cerebellum, and SMA and reductions in the motor and lateral PMC and basal ganglia. DRD has also been investigated with ^{123}I-beta-CIT SPECT and ^{18}F-dopa and ^{11}C- DHTBZ PET. ^{18}F-dopa PET and ^{123}I-beta-CIT SPECT findings are normal in the majority of DRD patients, so distinguishing this condition from early-onset dystonia–parkinsonism, where severely reduced putamen ^{18}F-dopa and ^{123}I-beta-CIT uptake is found.[298–301] Finally, ^{11}C-DHTBZ binding is increased in DRD compared to normal subjects. Increased VMAT2 expression in DRD could result from the combined effects of a dramatic decrease in intravesicular dopamine levels and possibly an increase in neuronal firing. However, upregulation of VMAT2 expression cannot be excluded.[302]

▶ CONCLUSIONS

Functional imaging:

- Provides a sensitive and objective means of detecting dopamine terminal dysfunction in PD where clinical doubt exists
- May be helpful in demonstrating striatal hypometabolism or reduced D2 binding in suspected atypical variants
- Can detect subclinical functional abnormalities when present in asymptomatic relatives at risk for PD and HD gene carriers
- Enables PD and HD progression to be objectively monitored and the efficacy of putative neuroprotective and restorative approaches to be evaluated
- Shows a common abnormal profile of resting glucose metabolism in the genetic dystonias
- Can detect microglial activation in subcortical degenerations

Blood flow and ligand activation studies have:

- Established that the akinesia of PD is associated with selective underfunctioning of the SMA and dorsal prefrontal cortex while inappropriate overactivity of these areas is associated with dystonia
- Found that parkinsonian "off" periods do not correlate well with basal ganglia synaptic dopamine levels, suggesting a postsynaptic contribution
- Shown that implants of fetal midbrain tissue can release normal amounts of dopamine after amphetamine challenges

REFERENCES

1. Hughes AJ, Daniel SE, Kilford L, et al. The accuracy of the clinical diagnosis of Parkinson's disease: A clinicopathological study of 100 cases. J Neurol Neurosurg Psychiatry 1992;55:181–184.
2. Hutchinson M, Raff U. Structural changes of the substantia nigra in Parkinson's disease as revealed by MR imaging. Am J Neuroradiol 2000;21:697–701.
3. Hu MT, White SJ, Herlihy AH, et al. A comparison of (18) F-dopa PET and inversion recovery MRI in the diagnosis of Parkinson's disease. Neurology 2001;56:1195–1200.
4. Geng DY, Li YX, Zee CS. Magnetic resonance imaging-based volumetric analysis of basal ganglia nuclei and substantia nigra in patients with Parkinson's disease. Neurosurgery 2006;58(2):256–262.
5. Michaeli S, Oz G, Sorce DJ, et al. Assessment of brain iron and neuronal integrity in patients with Parkinson's disease using novel MRI contrasts. Mov Disord 2007;22(3): 334–340.
6. Savoiardo M, Girotti F, Strada L, et al. Magnetic resonance imaging in progressive supranuclear palsy and other parkinsonian disorders. J Neural Transm Suppl 1994;42: 93–110.
7. Schrag A, Kingsley D, Phatouros C, et al. Clinical usefulness of magnetic resonance imaging in multiple system atrophy. J Neurol Neurosurg Psychiatry 1998;65:65–71.
8. Schrag A, Good CD, Miszkiel K, et al. Differentiation of atypical parkinsonian syndromes with routine MRI. Neurology 2000;54:697–702.
9. Schulz JB, Skalej M, Wedekind D, et al. Magnetic resonance imaging-based volumetry differentiates idiopathic Parkinson's syndrome from multiple system atrophy and progressive supranuclear palsy. Ann Neurol 1999;45: 65–74.
10. Paviour DC, Price SL, Stevens JM, et al. Quantitative MRI measurement of superior cerebellar peduncle in progressive supranuclear palsy. Neurology 2005;64(4):675–679.
11. Hauser RA, Murtaugh FR, Akhter K, et al. Magnetic resonance imaging of corticobasal degeneration. J Neuroimaging 1996;6(4):222–226.
12. Winkelmann J, Auer DP, Lechner C, et al. Magnetic resonance imaging findings in corticobasal degeneration. Mov Disord 1999;14(4):669–673.
13. Chan LL, Rumpel H, Yap K, et al. Case control study of diffusion tensor imaging in Parkinson's disease. J Neurol Neurosurg Psychiatry 2007;78(12):1383–1386.
14. Nicoletti G, Lodi R, Condino F, et al. Apparent diffusion coefficient measurements of the middle cerebellar peduncle differentiate the Parkinson variant of MSA from Parkinson's disease and progressive supranuclear palsy. Brain 2006;129:2679–2687.
15. Schocke MF, Seppi K, Esterhammer R, et al. Diffusion-weighted MRI differentiates the Parkinson variant of multiple system atrophy from PD. Neurology 2002;58(4): 575–580.
16. Seppi K, Schocke MF, Esterhammer R, et al. Diffusion-weighted imaging discriminates progressive supranuclear palsy from PD, but not from the parkinson variant of multiple system atrophy. Neurology 2003;60(6):922–927.
17. Paviour DC, Thornton JS, Lees AJ, et al. Diffusion-weighted magnetic resonance imaging differentiates Parkinsonian variant of multiple-system atrophy from progressive supranuclear palsy. Mov Disord 2007;22(1):68–74.
18. Berg D, Siefker C, Becker G. Echogenicity of the substantia nigra in Parkinson's disease and its relation to clinical findings. J Neurol 2001;248(8):684–689.
19. Prestel J, Schweitzer KJ, Hofer A, et al. Predictive value of transcranial sonography in the diagnosis of Parkinson's disease. Mov Disord 2006;21(10):1763–1765.
20. Stockner H, Sojer M, Klaus Seppi K, et al. Midbrain sonography in patients with essential tremor. Mov Disord 2007;22(3):414–417.

21. Walter U, Hoeppner J, Prudente-Morrissey L, et al. Parkinson's disease-like midbrain sonography abnormalities are frequent in depressive disorders. Brain 2007;130: 1799–1807.
22. Berg D, Merz B, Reiners K, et al. Five-year follow-up study of hyperechogenicity of the substantia nigra in Parkinson's disease. Mov Disord 2005;20:383–385.
23. Berg D, Roggendorf W, Schroder U, et al. Echogenicity of the substantia nigra: Association with increased iron content and marker for susceptibility to nigrostriatal injury. Arch Neurol 2002;59(6):999–1005.
24. Walter U, Dressler D, Probst T, et al. Transcranial brain sonography findings in discriminating between parkinsonism and idiopathic Parkinson disease. Arch Neurol 2007;64(11):1635–1640.
25. Bhatia KP, Marsden CD. The behavioural and motor consequences of focal lesions of the basal ganglia in man. Brain 1994;117:859–876.
26. Colosimo C, Pantano P, Calistri V, et al. Diffusion tensor imaging in primary cervical dystonia. J Neurol Neurosurg Psychiatry 2005;76(11):1591–1593.
27. Starosta-Rubinstein S, Young AB, Kluin K, et al. Clinical assessment of 31 patients with Wilson's disease: Correlations with structural changes on magnetic resonance imaging. Arch Neurol 1987;44:365–370.
28. Savoiardo M, Strada L, Oliva D, et al. Abnormal MRI signal in the rigid form of Huntington's disease. J Neurol Neurosurg Psychiatry 1991;54:888–891.
29. Antonini A, Leenders KL, Spiegel R, et al. Striatal glucose metabolism and dopamine D-2 receptor binding in asymptomatic gene carriers and patients with Huntington's disease. Brain 1996;119:2085–2095.
30. Paulsen JS, Magnotta VA, Mikos AE, et al. Brain structure in preclinical Huntington's disease. Biol Psychiatry 2006;59(1):57–63.
31. Aylward EH, Sparks BF, Field KM, et al. Onset and rate of striatal atrophy in preclinical Huntington disease. Neurology 2004;63(1):66–72.
32. Jellinger K. The pathology of parkinsonism. In Marsden CD, Fahn S (eds). Movement Disorders, 2nd ed. London: Butterworths, 1987, pp. 124–165.
33. Braak H, Tredici KD, Rub U, et al. Staging of brain pathology related to sporadic Parkinson's disease. Neurobiol Aging 2003;24:197–211.
34. Fearnley JM, Lees AJ. Ageing and Parkinson's disease: Substantia nigra regional selectivity. Brain 1991;114: 2283–2301.
35. Kish SJ, Shannak K, Hornykiewicz O. Uneven pattern of dopamine loss in the striatum of patients with idiopathic Parkinson's disease. N Engl J Med 1988;318:876–880.
36. McKeith IG, Galasko D, Kosaka K, et al. Consensus guidelines for the clinical and pathologic diagnosis of dementia with Lewy bodies (DLB): Report of the consortium on DLB international workshop. Neurology 1996;47: 1113–1124.
37. Brooks DJ, Ibañez V, Sawle GV, et al. Differing patterns of striatal ^{18}F-dopa uptake in Parkinson's disease, multiple system atrophy and progressive supranuclear palsy. Ann Neurol 1990;28:547–555.
38. Tedroff J, Aquilonius S-M, Hartvig P, et al. Cerebral uptake and utilisation of therapeutic [β-^{11}C]-L-dopa in Parkinson's disease measured by positron emission tomography. Relations to motor response. Acta Neurol Scand 1992;85: 95–102.
39. Rinne JO, Bergman J, Ruotinnen H, et al. Striatal uptake of a novel PET ligand, [^{18}F]β-CFT, is reduced in early Parkinson's disease. Synapse 1999;31:119–124.
40. Frost JJ, Rosier AJ, Reich SG, et al. Positron emission tomographic imaging of the dopamine transporter with ^{11}C-WIN 35,428 reveals marked declines in mild Parkinson's disease. Ann Neurol 1993;34:423–431.
41. Marek K, Seibyl JP, Zoghbi SS, et al. [I-123] beta-CIT SPECT imaging demonstrates bilateral loss of dopamine transporters in hemiparkinson's disease. Neurology 1996;46:231–237.
42. Benamer HTS, Patterson J, Wyper DJ, et al. Correlation of Parkinson's disease severity and duration with I-123-FP-CIT SPECT striatal uptake. Mov Disord 2000;15:692–698.
43. Seibyl JP, Marek KL, Quinlan D, et al. Decreased single-photon emission computed tomographic [^{123}I]β-CIT striatal uptake correlates with symptom severity in Parkinson's disease. Ann Neurol 1995;38:589–598.
44. Frey KA, Koeppe RA, Kilbourn MR, et al. Pre-synaptic monoaminergic vesicles in Parkinson's disease and normal aging. Ann Neurol 1996;40:873–884.
45. Nahmias C, Garnett ES, Firnau G, et al. Striatal dopamine distribution in Parkinsonian patients during life. J Neurol Sci 1985;69:223–230.
46. Leenders KL, Salmon EP, Tyrrell P, et al. The nigrostriatal dopaminergic system assessed in vivo by positron emission tomography in healthy volunteer subjects and patients with Parkinson's disease. Arch Neurol 1990;47:1290–1298.
47. Morrish PK, Sawle GV, Brooks DJ. Clinical and [^{18}F]dopa PET findings in early Parkinson's disease. J Neurol Neurosurg Psychiatry 1995;59:597–600.
48. Rakshi JS, Uema T, Ito K, et al. Frontal, midbrain and striatal dopaminergic function in early and advanced Parkinson's disease. A 3D [18F]Dopa-PET study. Brain 1999;122:1637–1650.
49. Kaasinen V, Nurmi E, Brück A, et al. Increased frontal [(18)F]fluorodopa uptake in early Parkinson's disease: Sex differences in the prefrontal cortex. Brain 2001;124: 1125–1130.
50. Whone AL, Moore RY, Piccini P, et al. Plasticity of the nigropallidal pathway in Parkinson's disease. Ann Neurol 2003;53:206–213.
51. Guttman M, Burkholder J, Kish SJ, et al. [^{11}C]RTI-32 PET studies of the dopamine transporter in early dopa-naive Parkinson's disease: Implications for the symptomatic threshold. Neurology 1997;48:1578–1583.
52. Tedroff J, Aquilonius S-M, Laihinen A, et al. Striatal kinetics of [11C]-(+)-nomifensine and 6-[18F]fluoro-L-dopa in Parkinson's disease measured with positron emission tomography. Acta Neurol Scand 1990;81:24–30.
53. Lee CS, Samii A, Sossi V, et al. In vivo positron emission tomographic evidence for compensatory changes in presynaptic dopaminergic nerve terminals in Parkinson's disease. Ann Neurol 2000;47:493–503.
54. Fischman AJ, Bonab AA, Babich JW, et al. [C-11, I-127] altropane: A highly selective ligand for PET imaging of dopamine transporter sites. Synapse 2001;39:332–342.

55. Mozley PD, Schneider JS, Acton PD, et al. Binding of [Tc-99m]TRODAT-1 to dopamine transporters in patients with Parkinson's disease and in healthy volunteers. J Nucl Med 2000;41:584–589.
56. Brooks DJ, Playford ED, Ibanez V, et al. Isolated tremor and disruption of the nigrostriatal dopaminergic system: An [18]Fdopa PET study. Neurology 1992;42:1554–1560.
57. Benamer TS, Patterson J, Grosset DG, et al. Accurate differentiation of parkinsonism and essential tremor using visual assessment of [^{123}I]-FP-CIT imaging: The [^{123}I]-FP-CIT Study Group. Mov Disord 2000;15:503–510.
58. Marshall VL, Patterson J, Hadley DM, Grosset KA, Grosset DG. Two-year follow-up in 150 consecutive cases with normal dopamine transporter imaging. Nucl Med Commun 2006;27(12):933–937.
59. Tolosa E, Borght TV, Moreno E. Accuracy of DaTSCAN ((123)I-ioflupane) SPECT in diagnosis of patients with clinically uncertain parkinsonism: 2-Year follow-up of an open-label study. Mov Disord 2007;22(16): 2346–2351.
60. Vingerhoets FJG, Schulzer M, Caine DB, et al. Which clinical sign of Parkinson's disease best reflects the nigrostriatal lesion? Ann Neurol 1997;41:58–64.
61. Playford ED, Brooks DJ. In vivo and in vitro studies of the dopaminergic system in movement disorders. Cerebrovasc Brain Metab Rev 1992;4:144–171.
62. Rinne UK, Laihinen A, Rinne JO, et al. Positron emission tomography demonstrates dopamine D2 receptor supersensitivity in the striatum of patients with early Parkinson's disease. Mov Disord 1990;5:55–59.
63. Antonini A, Schwarz J, Oertel WH, et al. [^{11}C]Raclopride and positron emission tomography in previously untreated patients with Parkinson's disease: Influence of L-dopa and lisuride therapy on striatal dopamine D_2-receptors. Neurology 1994;44:1325–1329.
64. Turjanski N, Lees AJ, Brooks DJ. PET studies on striatal dopaminergic receptor binding in drug naive and L-dopa treated Parkinson's disease patients with and without dyskinesia. Neurology 1997;49:717–723.
65. Rinne JO, Laihinen A, Nagren K, et al. PET demonstrates different behaviour of striatal dopamine D1 and D2 receptors in early Parkinson's disease. J Neurosci Res 1990;27:494–499.
66. Scherfler C, Khan NL, Pavese N, et al. Upregulation of dopamine D2 receptors in dopaminergic drug-naive patients with Parkin gene mutations. Mov Disord 2006;21(6):783–788.
67. Kaasinen V, Någren K, Hietala J, et al. Extrastriatal dopamine D2 and D3 receptors in early and advanced Parkinson's disease. Neurology 2000;54(7):1482–1487.
68. Kaasinen V, Aalto S, NAgren K, et al. Extrastriatal dopamine D(2) receptors in Parkinson's disease: A longitudinal study. J Neural Transm 2003;110(6):591–601.
69. Piccini P, Brooks DJ, Bjorklund A, et al. Dopamine release from nigral transplants visualized in vivo in a Parkinson's patient. Nat Neurosci 1999;2:1137–1140.
70. Breier A, Su TP, Saunders R, et al. Schizophrenia is associated with elevated amphetamine-induced synaptic dopamine concentrations: Evidence from a novel positron emission tomography method. Proc Natl Acad Sci U S A 1997;94:2569–2574.
71. Piccini P, Pavese N, Brooks DJ. Endogenous dopamine release after pharmacological challenges in Parkinson's disease. Ann Neurol 2003;53:647–653.
72. Tedroff J, Pedersen M, Aquilonius SM, et al. Levodopa-induced changes in synaptic dopamine in patients with Parkinson's disease as measured by [11C]raclopride displacement and PET. Neurology 1996;46:1430–1436.
73. de la Fuente-Fernandez R, Lu JQ, Sossi V, et al. Biochemical variations in the synaptic level of dopamine precede motor fluctuations in Parkinson's disease: PET evidence of increased dopamine turnover. Ann Neurol 2001;49:298–303.
74. de la Fuente-Fernandez R, Sossi V, Huang Z, et al. Levodopa-induced changes in synaptic dopamine levels increase with progression of Parkinson's disease: Implications for dyskinesias. Brain 2004;127:2747–2754.
75. Pavese N, Evans AH, Tai YF, et al. Clinical correlates of levodopa-induced dopamine release in Parkinson disease: A PET study. Neurology 2006;67:1612–1617.
76. Giovannoni G, O'Sullivan JD, Turner K, et al. Hedonistic homeostatic dysregulation in patients with Parkinson's disease on dopamine replacement therapies. J Neurol Neurosurg Psychiatry 2000;68(4):423–428.
77. Evans AH, Pavese N, Lawrence AD, et al. Compulsive drug use linked to sensitized ventral striatal dopamine transmission. Ann Neurol 2006;59(5):852–858.
78. Robinson TE, Berridge KC. The neural basis of drug craving: An incentive-sensitization theory of addiction. Brain Res Brain Res Rev 1993;18(3):247–291.
79. Goerendt IK, Messa C, Lawrence AD, et al. Dopamine release during sequential finger movements in Parkinson's disease: A PET study. Brain 2003;126:312–325.
80. Strafella AP, Paus T, Fraraccio M, et al. Striatal dopamine release induced by repetitive transcranial magnetic stimulation of the human motor cortex. Brain 2003;126:2609–2615.
81. Koepp MJ, Gunn RN, Lawrence AD, et al. Evidence for striatal dopamine release during a video game. Nature 1998;393:266–268.
82. Lawrence AD, Brooks DJ. Neural correlates of reward processing in the human brain: A PET study. Neurology 1999;52(suppl 2):A307.
83. Sawamoto N, Piccini P, Hotton G, et al. Cognitive deficits and striato-frontal dopamine release in Parkinson's disease. Brain 2008;131:1294–302.
84. Golbe LI. The genetics of Parkinson's disease: A reconsideration. Neurology 1990;40(suppl 3):7–16.
85. Lazzarini AM, Myers RH, Zimmerman TRJ, et al. A clinical genetic study of Parkinson's disease: Evidence for dominant transmission. Neurology 1994;44:499–506.
86. Piccini P, Morrish PK, Turjanski N, et al. Dopaminergic function in familial Parkinson's disease: A clinical and ^{18}F-dopa PET study. Ann Neurol 1997;41:222–229.
87. Piccini P, Burn DJ, Ceravalo R, et al. The role of inheritance in sporadic Parkinson's disease: Evidence from a longitudinal study of dopaminergic function in twins. Ann Neurol 1999;45:577–582.
88. Khan NL, Scherfler C, Graham E, et al. Dopa minergic dysfunction in unrelated, asymptomatic carriers of a single parkin mutation. Neurology 2005;64: 134–136.

89. Ponsen MM, Stoffers D, Booij J, et al. Idiopathic hyposmia as a preclinical sign of Parkinson's disease. Ann Neurol 2004;56:173–181.
90. Hilker R, Razai N, Ghaemi M, et al. [18F]fluorodopa uptake in the upper brainstem measured with positron emission tomography correlates with decreased REM sleep duration in early Parkinson's disease. Clin Neurol Neurosurg 2003;105(4):262–269.
91. Eisensehr I, Linke R, Tatsch K, et al. Increased muscle activity during rapid eye movement sleep correlates with decrease of striatal presynaptic dopamine transporters. IPT and IBZM SPECT imaging in subclinical and clinically manifest idiopathic REM sleep behavior disorder, Parkinson's disease, and controls. Sleep 2003;26(5):507–512.
92. de la Fuente-Fernandez R, Pal PK, Vingerhoets FJG, et al. Evidence for impaired presynaptic dopamine function in parkinsonian patients with motor fluctuations. J Neural Transm 2000;107:49–57.
93. Kishore A, de la Fuente-Fernandez R, Snow BJ, et al. Levodopa-induced dyskinesias in idiopathic parkinsonism (IP): A simultaneous PET study of dopamine D1 and D2 receptors. Neurology 1997;48:A327 (abstract).
94. Torstenson R, Hartvig P, Långström B, et al. Differential effects of levodopa on dopaminergic function in early and advanced Parkinson's disease. Ann Neurol 1997;41: 334–340.
95. Henry B, Brotchie JM. Potential of opioid antagonists in the treatment of levodopa-induced dyskinesias in Parkinson's disease. Drugs Aging 1996;9:149–158.
96. Nisbet AP, Foster OJF, Kingsbury A, et al. Preproenkephalin and preprotachykinin messenger-RNA expression in normal human basal ganglia and in Parkinson's disease. Neuroscience 1995;66:361–376.
97. Jolkkonen J, Jenner P, Marsden CD. L-Dopa reverses altered gene expression of substance P but not enkephalin in the caudate-putamen of common marmosets treated with MPTP. Mol Brain Res 1995;32:297–307.
98. Lavoie B, Parent A, Bedard PJ. Effects of dopamine denervation on striatal peptide expression in parkinsonian monkeys. Can J Neurol Sci 1991;18:373–375.
99. Piccini P, Weeks RA, Brooks DJ. Opioid receptor binding in Parkinson's patients with and without levodopa-induced dyskinesias. Ann Neurol 1997;42:720–726.
100. Whone AL, Rabiner EA, Arahata Y, et al. Reduced substance P binding in Parkinson's disease complicated by dyskinesias: An F-18-L829165 PET study. Neurology 2002;58(suppl 3):A488–A489.
101. Snow BJ, Tooyama I, McGeer EG, et al. Human positron emission tomographic [^{18}F]fluorodopa studies correlate with dopamine cell counts and levels. Ann Neurol 1993;34:324–330.
102. Pate BD, Kawamata T, Yamada T, et al. Correlation of striatal fluorodopa uptake in the MPTP monkey with dopaminergic indices. Ann Neurol 1993;34:331–338.
103. Ceravolo R, Piccini P, Bailey DL, et al. 18F-dopa PET evidence that tolcapone acts as a central COMT inhibitor in Parkinson's disease. Synapse 2002;43:201–207.
104. Turjanski N, Lees AJ, Brooks DJ. Striatal dopaminergic receptor dysfunction in patients with restless legs syndrome: ^{18}F-dopa and ^{11}C-raclopride PET studies. Neurology 1999;52:932–937.
105. Innis RB, Marek KL, Sheff K, et al. Effect of treatment with L-dopa/carbidopa or L-selegiline on striatal dopamine transporter SPECT imaging with [I-123]beta-CIT. Mov Disord 1999;14:436–442.
106. Ahlskog JE, Uitti RJ, O'Connor MK, et al. The effect of dopamine agonist therapy on dopamine transporter imaging in Parkinson's disease. Mov Disord 1999;14: 940–946.
107. Marek K, Jennings D, Tabamo R, et al. InSPECT: An investigation of the effect of short-term treatment with pramipexole or levodopa on [123I] B-CIT and SPECT imaging in early Parkinson disease. Neurology 2006;66(5):A112–A112.
108. Vingerhoets FJG, Snow BJ, Lee CS, et al. Longitudinal fluorodopa positron emission tomographic studies of the evolution of idiopathic parkinsonism. Ann Neurol 1994;36:759–764.
109. Morrish PK, Rakshi JS, Sawle GV, et al. Measuring the rate of progression and estimating the preclinical period of Parkinson's disease with [^{18}F]dopa PET. J Neurol Neurosurg Psychiatry 1998;64:314–319.
110. Nurmi E, Ruottinen HM, Bergman J, et al. Rate of progression in Parkinson's disease: A 6-[18F]fluoro-L-dopa PET study. Mov Disord 2001;16:608–615.
111. Nurmi E, Ruottinen HM, Kaasinen V, et al. Progression in Parkinson's disease: A positron emission tomography study with a dopamine transporter ligand. Ann Neurol 2000;47:804–808.
112. Marek K, Innis R, van Dyck C, et al. [123I]beta-CIT SPECT imaging assessment of the rate of Parkinson's disease progression. Neurology 2001;57:2089–2094.
113. Winogrodzka A, Bergmans P, Booij J, et al. [123I]FP-CIT SPECT is a useful method to monitor the rate of dopaminergic degeneration in early-stage Parkinson's disease. J Neural Transm 2001;108:1011–1019.
114. Schwarz J, Tatsch K, Linke R, et al. Measuring the decline of dopamine transporter binding in patients with Parkinson's disease using 123I-IPT and SPECT. Neurology 1997;48(suppl 2):A208 (abstract).
115. Marek KL, Innis R, Seibyl J. -CIT/SPECT assessment of determinants of variability in progression of Parkinson's disease. Neurology 1999;52(suppl 2):A91–A92 (abstract).
116. Whone AL, Watts RL, Stoessl J, et al. Slower progression of PD with ropinirol versus L-dopa: The REAL-PET study. Ann Neurol 2003;54:403–414.
117. Parkinson Study Group. Dopamine transporter brain imaging to assess the effects of pramipexole vs levodopa on Parkinson disease progression. JAMA 2002;287: 1653–1661.
118. Pavese N, Rascol O, Olanow WC, et al. The effects of riluzole on progression of early Parkinson's disease: An 18F-fluorodopa PET study. Parkinsonism Relat Disord 2005;11(suppl 2):229 (abstract).
119. Fahn S, Oakes D, Shoulson I, et al. Levodopa and the progression of Parkinson's disease. N Engl J Med 2004;351:2498–2508.
120. Lindvall O. Cerebral implantation in movement disorders: State of the art. Mov Disord 1999:14:201–205.
121. Piccini P, Brooks DJ, Bjorklund A, et al. Dopamine release from nigral transplants visualised in vivo in a Parkinson's patient. Nat Neurosci 1999;2:1137–1140.

122. Wenning GK, Odin P, Morrish PK, et al. Short- and long-term survival and function of unilateral intrastriatal dopaminergic grafts in Parkinson's disease. Ann Neurol 1997;42:95–107.
123. Hagell P, Schrag AE, Piccini P, et al. Sequential bilateral transplantation in Parkinson's disease: Effects of the second graft. Brain 1999;122:1121–1132.
124. Remy P, Samson Y, Hantraye P, et al. Clinical correlates of [^{18}F]fluorodopa uptake in five grafted parkinsonian patients. Ann Neurol 1995;38:580–588.
125. Hauser RA, Freeman TB, Snow BJ, et al. Long-term evaluation of bilateral fetal nigral transplantation in Parkinson disease. Arch Neurol 1999;56:179–187.
126. Kordower JH, Freeman TB, Chen EY, et al. Fetal nigral grafts survive and mediate clinical benefit in a patient with Parkinson's disease. Mov Disord 1998;13:383–393.
127. Freed CR, Greene PE, Breeze RE, et al. Transplantation of embryonic dopamine neurons for severe Parkinson's disease. N Engl J Med 2001;344:710–719.
128. Nakamura T, Dhawan V, Chaly T, et al. Blinded positron emission tomography study of dopamine cell implantation for Parkinson's disease. Ann Neurol 2001;50: 181–187.
129. Olanow CW, Goetz CG, Kordower JH, et al. A double-blind controlled trial of bilateral fetal nigral transplantation in Parkinson's disease. Ann Neurol 2003;54: 403–414.
130. Ma Y, Feigin A, Dhawan V, et al. Dyskinesia after fetal cell transplantation for parkinsonism: A PET study. Ann Neurol 2002;52:628–634.
131. Hagell P, Piccini P, Bjorklund A, et al. Dyskinesias following neural transplantation in Parkinson's disease. Nat Neurosci 2002;5:627–628.
132. Piccini P, Pavese N, Hagell P, et al. Factors affecting the clinical outcome after neural transplantation in Parkinson's disease. Brain 2005;128:2977–2986.
133. Gill SS, Patel NK, Hotton GR, et al. Direct brain infusion of glial cell line-derived neurotrophic factor (GDNF) in Parkinson's disease. Nat Med 2003;9:589–595.
134. Lang AE, Gill S, Patel NK, et al. Randomized controlled trial of intraputamenal glial cell line-derived neurotrophic factor infusion in Parkinson disease. Ann Neurol 2006;59:459–466.
135. Wilms H, Sievers J, Dengler R, et al. Intrathecal synthesis of monocyte chemoattractant protein-1 (MCP-1) in amyotrophic lateral sclerosis: Further evidence for microglial activation in neurodegeneration. J Neuroimmunol 2003;144:139–142.
136. McGeer PL, Itagaki S, Boyes BE, et al. Reactive microglia are positive for HLA-DR in the substantia nigra of Parkinson's and Alzheimer's disease brains. Neurology 1988;38:1285–1291.
137. Ouchi Y, Yoshikawa E, Sekine Y, et al. Microglial activation and dopamine terminal loss in early Parkinson's disease. Ann Neurol 2005;57:168–175.
138. Gerhard A, Pavese N, Hotton G, et al. In vivo imaging of microglial activation with [11C](R)-PK11195 PET in idiopathic Parkinson's disease. Neurobiol Dis 2006;21: 404–412.
139. Hornykiewicz O. Biochemical aspects of Parkinson's disease. Neurology 1998;51(suppl 2):S2-S9.
140. Doder M, Rabiner EA, Turjanski N, et al. Tremor in Parkinson's disease and serotonergic dysfunction: An ^{11}C-WAY 100635 PET study. Neurology 2003;60:601–605.
141. Halliday GM, Blumbergs PC, Cotton RG, et al. Loss of brainstem serotonin- and substance P-containing neurons in Parkinson's disease. Brain Res 1990;510:104–107.
142. Doder M, Rabiner EA, Turjanski N, et al. Brain Serotonin $5HT_{1A}$ receptor in Parkinson's disease with and without depression measured with positron emission tomography with 11C-WAY100635. Mov Disord 2000;15:213 (abstract).
143. Kim SE, Choi JY, Choe YS, et al. Serotonin transporters in the midbrain of Parkinson's disease patients: A study with 123I-beta-CIT SPECT. J Nucl Med 2003;44(6):870–876.
144. Remy P, Doder M, Lees A, et al. Depression in Parkinson's disease: Loss of dopamine and noradrenaline innervation in the limbic system. Brain 2005;128(6):1314–1322.
145. Kuhl DE, Minoshima S, Fessler JA, et al. In vivo mapping of cholinergic terminals in normal aging, Alzheimer's disease, and Parkinson's disease. Ann Neurol 1996;40(3): 399–410.
146. Bohnen NI, Kaufer DI, Hendrickson R, et al. Cognitive correlates of cortical cholinergic denervation in Parkinson's disease and parkinsonian dementia. J Neurol 2006;253(2):242–247.
147. Kuhl DE, Metter EJ, Benson DF. Similarities of cerebral glucose metabolism in Alzheimer's and Parkinsonian dementia. J Cereb Blood Flow Metab 1985;5:S169–S170.
148. Peppard RF, Martin WRW, Guttman M, et al. The relationship of cerebral glucose metabolism to cognitive deficits in Parkinson's disease. Neurology 1988;38(suppl 1):364.
149. Bohnen NI, Minoshima S, Giordani B, et al. Motor correlates of occipital glucose hypometabolism in Parkinson's disease without dementia. Neurology 1999;52:541–546.
150. Hu MTM, Taylor-Robinson SD, Chaudhuri KR, et al. Cortical dysfunction in non-demented Parkinson's disease patients: A combined ^{31}Phosphorus MRS and ^{18}FDG PET study. Brain 2000;123:340–352.
151. Ito K, Nagano-Saito A, Kato T, et al. Striatal and extrastriatal dysfunction in Parkinson's disease with dementia: A 6-[18F]fluoro-L-dopa PET study. Brain, 2002;125(6): 1358–1365.
152. Edison P, Rowe CC, Rinne JO, et al. Amyloid load in Parkinson's disease dementia and Lewy body dementia measured with [11C]PIB positron emission tomography. J Neurol Neurosurg Psychiatry 2008;79(12):1331–1338.
153. Ahmed I, Edison P, Quinn NP, et al. Amyloid deposition and glucose metabolism in Parkinson's disease dementia (PDD). An [11C]PIB and [18 F]FDG PET study. Mov Disord 2007;22(suppl 16):S139–S140.
154. Miletich RS, Chan T, Gillespie M, et al. Contralateral basal ganglia metabolism is abnormal in hemiparkinsonian patients. An FDG-PET study. Neurology 1988;38:S260.
155. Wolfson LI, Leenders KL, Brown LL, et al. Alterations of regional cerebral blood flow and oxygen metabolism in Parkinson's disease. Neurology 1985;35:1399–1405.
156. Eidelberg D, Moeller JR, Dhawan V, et al. The metabolic topography of parkinsonism. J Cereb Blood Flow Metab 1994;14:783–801.
157. Feigin A, Fukuda M, Dhawan V, et al. Metabolic correlates of levodopa response in Parkinson's disease. Neurology 2001;57(11):2083–2088.

158. Lin TP, Carbon M, Tang C, et al. Metabolic correlates of subthalamic nucleus activity in Parkinson's disease. Brain 2008;131(Pt 5):1373–1380.
159. Playford ED, Jenkins IH, Passingham RE, et al. Impaired mesial frontal and putamen activation in Parkinson's disease: A PET study. Ann Neurol 1992;32:151–161.
160. Jahanshahi M, Jenkins IH, Brown RG, et al. Self-initiated versus externally-triggered movements: Measurements of regional cerebral blood flow and movement-related potentials in normals and Parkinson's disease. Brain 1995;118:913–933.
161. Samuel M, Ceballos-Baumann AO, Blin J, et al. Evidence for lateral premotor and parietal overactivity in Parkinson's disease during sequential and bimanual movements: A PET study. Brain 1997;120:963–976.
162. Rascol O, Sabatini U, Fabre N, et al. The ipsilateral cerebellar hemisphere is overactive during hand movements in akinetic parkinsonian patients. Brain 1997;120: 103–110.
163. Sabatini U, Boulanouar K, Fabre N, et al. Cortical motor reorganization in akinetic patients with Parkinson's disease: A functional MRI study. Brain 2000;123:394–403.
164. Thobois S, Dominey P, Decety J, et al. Overactivation of primary motor cortex is asymmetrical in hemiparkinsonian patients. Neuroreport 2000;11:785–789.
165. Mushiake H, Inase M, Tanji J. Selective coding of motor sequence in the supplementary motor area of the monkey cerebral cortex. Exp Brain Res 1990;82:208–210.
166. Carbon M, Felice Ghilardi M, Dhawan V, et al. Correlates of movement initiation and velocity in Parkinson's disease: A longitudinal PET study. Neuroimage 2007;34: 361–370.
167. Jenkins IH, Fernandez W, Playford ED, et al. Impaired activation of the supplementary motor area in Parkinson's disease is reversed when akinesia is treated with apomorphine. Ann Neurol 1992;32:749–757.
168. Brooks DJ, Jenkins IH, Passingham RE. Positron emission tomography studies on regional cerebral control of voluntary movement. In Mano N, Hamada I, DeLong MR (eds). Role of the Cerebellum and Basal Ganglia in Voluntary Movement. Amsterdam: Excerpta Medica, 1993, pp. 267–274.
169. Rascol O, Sabatini U, Chollet F, et al. Supplementary and primary sensory motor area activity in Parkinson's disease. Regional cerebral blood flow changes during finger movements and effects of apomorphine. Arch Neurol 1992;49:144–148.
170. Rascol O, Sabatini U, Chollet F, et al. Normal activation of the supplementary motor area in patients with Parkinson's disease undergoing long-term treatment with levodopa. J Neurol Neurosurg Psychiatry 1994;57:567–571.
171. Haslinger B, Erhard P, Kampfe N, et al. Event-related functional magnetic resonance imaging in Parkinson's disease before and after levodopa. Brain 2001;124: 558–570.
172. Piccini P, Lindvall O, Bjorklund A, et al. Delayed recovery of movement-related cortical function in Parkinson's disease after striatal dopaminergic grafts. Ann Neurol 2000;48:689–695.
173. Grafton ST, Waters C, Sutton J, et al. Pallidotomy increases activity of motor association cortex in Parkinson's disease: A positron emission tomographic study. Ann Neurol 1995;37:776–783.
174. Samuel M, Ceballos-Baumann AO, Turjanski N, et al. Pallidotomy in Parkinson's disease increases SMA and prefrontal activation during performance of volitional movements: An $H_2^{15}O$ PET study. Brain 1997;120:1301–1313.
175. Davis KD, Taub E, Houle S, et al. Globus pallidus stimulation activates the cortical motor system during alleviation of parkinsonian symptoms. Nat Med 1997;3:671–674.
176. Fukuda M, Mentis M, Ghilardi MF, et al. Functional correlates of pallidal stimulation for Parkinson's disease. Ann Neurol 2001;49:155–164.
177. Limousin P, Greene J, Polak P, et al. Changes in cerebral activity pattern due to subthalamic nucleus or internal pallidum stimulation in Parkinson's disease. Ann Neurol 1997;42:283–291.
178. Ceballos-Baumann AO, Boecker H, Bartenstein P, et al. A positron emission tomographic study of subthalamic nucleus stimulation in Parkinson disease: Enhanced movement-related activity of motor-association cortex and decreased motor cortex resting activity. Arch Neurol 1999;56:997–1003.
179. Strafella AP, Dagher A, Sadiko, AF. Cerebral blood flow changes induced by subthalamic stimulation in Parkinson's disease. Neurology 2003;60:1039–1042.
180. Benazzouz A, Gao D, Ni Z, et al. High frequency stimulation of the STN influences the activity of dopamine neurons in the rat. Neuroreport 2000;11:1593–1596.
181. Bruet N, Windels F, Bertrand A, et al. High frequency stimulation of the subthalamic nucleus increases the extracellular contents of striatal dopamine in normal and partially dopaminergic denervated rats. J Neuropathol Exp Neurol 2001;60:15–24.
182. Thobois S, Fraix V, Savasta M, et al. Chronic subthalamic nucleus stimulation and striatal D2 dopamine receptors in Parkinson's disease—A [(11)C]-raclopride PET study. J Neurol 2003;250:1219–1223.
183. Strafella AP, Sadikot AF, Dagher A. Subthalamic deep brain stimulation does not induce striatal dopamine release in Parkinson's disease. Neuroreport 2003;14: 1287–1289.
184. Hilker R, Voges J, Ghaemi M, et al. Deep brain stimulation of the subthalamic nucleus does not increase the striatal dopamine concentration in parkinsonian humans. Mov Disord 2003;18:41–48.
185. Strafella AP, Lozano AM, Ballanger B, et al. rCBF changes associated with PPN stimulation in a patient with Parkinson's disease: A PET study. Mov Disord 2008;23: 1051–1054.
186. Feigin A, Kaplitt MG, Tang C, et al. Free in PMC Modulation of metabolic brain networks after subthalamic gene therapy for Parkinson's disease. Proc Natl Acad Sci U S A 2007;104:19559–19564.
187. De Volder AG, Francard J, Laterre C, et al. Decreased glucose utilisation in the striatum and frontal lobe in probable striatonigral degeneration. Ann Neurol 1989;26: 239–247.
188. Otsuka M, Ichiya Y, Hosokawa S, et al. Striatal blood flow, glucose metabolism, and ^{18}F-dopa uptake: Difference in Parkinson's disease and atypical parkinsonism. J Neurol Neurosurg Psychiatry 1991;54:898–904.

189. Eidelberg D, Takikawa S, Moeller JR, et al. Striatal hypometabolism distinguishes striatonigral degeneration from Parkinson's disease. Ann Neurol 1993;33:518–527.
190. Eidelberg D, Moeller JR, Ishikawa T, et al. Regional metabolic correlates of surgical outcome following unilateral pallidotomy for Parkinson's disease. Ann Neurol 1996;39:450–459.
191. Davie CA, Wenning GK, Barker GJ, et al. Differentiation of multiple system atrophy from idiopathic Parkinson's disease using proton magnetic resonance spectroscopy. Ann Neurol 1995;37:204–210.
192. Brooks DJ, Salmon EP, Mathias CJ, et al. The relationship between locomotor disability, autonomic dysfunction, and the integrity of the striatal dopaminergic system, in patients with multiple system atrophy, pure autonomic failure, and Parkinson's disease, studied with PET. Brain 1990;113:1539–1552.
193. Burn DJ, Sawle GV, Brooks DJ. The differential diagnosis of Parkinson's disease, multiple system atrophy, and Steele-Richardson-Olszewski syndrome: Discriminant analysis of striatal 18F-dopa PET data. J Neurol Neurosurg Psychiatry 1994;57:278–284.
194. Pirker W, Asenbaum S, Bencsits G, et al. [I-123]beta-CIT SPECT in multiple system atrophy, progressive supranuclear palsy, and corticobasal degeneration. Mov Disord 2000;15:1158–1167.
195. Shinotoh H, Aotsuka A, Yonezawa H, et al. Striatal dopamine D_2 receptors in Parkinson's disease and striatonigral degeneration determined by positron emission tomography. In Nagatsu T, Fisher A, Yoshida M (eds). Basic, Clinical, and Therapeutic Advances of Alzheimer's and Parkinson's Diseases. New York: Plenum Press, 1990, vol. 2, pp. 107–110.
196. Shinotoh H, Inoue O, Hirayama K, et al. Dopamine D_1 receptors in Parkinson's disease and striatonigral degeneration: A positron emission tomography study. J Neurol Neurosurg Psychiatry 1993;56:467–472.
197. Brooks DJ, Ibanez V, Sawle GV, et al. Striatal D_2 receptor status in Parkinson's disease, striatonigral degeneration, and progressive supranuclear palsy, measured with ^{11}C-raclopride and PET. Ann Neurol 1992;31:184–192.
198. Schwarz J, Tatsch K, Arnold G, et al. ^{123}I-iodobenzamide-SPECT predicts dopaminergic responsiveness in patients with de-novo parkinsonism. Neurology 1992;42: 556–561.
199. Seppi K, Donnemiller E, Riccabona G, et al. Disease progression in PD vs MSA: A SPECT study using 123-I IBZM. Parkinsonism Relat Disord 2001;7:S24 (abstract).
200. Burn DJ, Rinne JO, Quinn NP, et al. Striatal opioid receptor binding in Parkinson's disease, striatonigral degeneration, and Steele-Richardson-Olszewski syndrome: An ^{11}C-diprenorphine PET study. Brain 1995;118:951–958.
201. Druschky A, Hilz MJ, Platsch G, et al. Differentiation of Parkinson's disease and multiple system atrophy in early disease stages by means of I-123-MIBG-SPECT. J Neurol Sci 2000;175:3–12.
202. Gerhard A, Banati RB, Goerres GB, et al. [11C](R)PK11195 PET imaging of microglial activation in multiple system atrophy. Neurology 2003;61:686–689.
203. Rinne JO, Burn DJ, Mathias CJ, et al. PET studies on the dopaminergic system and striatal opioid binding in the olivopontocerebellar atrophy variant of multiple system atrophy. Ann Neurol 1995;37:568–573.
204. Otsuka M, Ichiya Y, Kuwabara Y, et al. Striatal ^{18}F-dopa uptake and brain glucose metabolism by PET in patients with syndrome of progressive ataxia. J Neurol Sci 1994;124:198–203.
205. Gilman S, Koeppe RA, Junck L, et al. Patterns of cerebral glucose metabolism detected with positron emission tomography differ in multiple system atrophy and olivopontocerebellar atrophy. Ann Neurol 1994;36:166–175.
206. D'Antona R, Baron JC, Samson Y, et al. Subcortical dementia: Frontal cortex hypometabolism detected by positron tomography in patients with progressive supranuclear palsy. Brain 1985;108:785–800.
207. Blin J, Baron JC, Dubois P, et al. Positron emission tomography study in progressive supranuclear palsy. Arch Neurol 1990;47:747–752.
208. Goffinet AM, De Volder AG, Gillain C, et al. Positron tomography demonstrates frontal lobe hypometabolism in progressive supranuclear palsy. Ann Neurol 1989;25: 131–139.
209. Foster NL, Gilman S, Berent S, et al. Cerebral hypometabolism in progressive supranuclear palsy studied with positron emission tomography. Ann Neurol 1988;24: 399–406.
210. Otsuka M, Ichiya Y, Kuwabara Y, et al. Cerebral blood flow, oxygen and glucose metabolism with PET in progressive supranuclear palsy. Ann Nucl Med 1989;3: 111–118.
211. Goffinet A, De Volder AG, Gillain C, et al. Positron tomography demonstrates frontal lobe hypometabolism in progressive supranuclear palsy. Ann Neurol 1989;25: 131–139.
212. Foster NL, Gilman S, Berent S, et al. Progressive subcortical gliosis and progressive supranuclear palsy can have similar clinical and PET abnormalities. J Neurol Neurosurg Psychiatry 1992;55:707–713.
213. Davie CA, Barker GJ, Machado C, et al. Proton magnetic resonance spectroscopy in Steele-Richardson-Olszewski syndrome. Mov Disord 1997;12:767–771.
214. Leenders KL, Frackowiak RS, Lees AJ. Steele-Richardson-Olszewski syndrome. Brain energy metabolism, blood flow and fluorodopa uptake measured by positron emission tomography. Brain 1988;111:615–630.
215. Bhatt MH, Snow BJ, Martin WRW, et al. Positron emission tomography in progressive supranuclear palsy. Arch Neurol 1991;48:389–391.
216. Messa C, Volonte MA, Fazio F, et al. Differential distribution of striatal [^{123}I]β-CIT in Parkinson's disease and progressive supranuclear palsy, evaluated with single-photon emission tomography. Eur J Nucl Med 1998;25:1270–1276.
217. Baron JC, Maziere B, Loc'h C, et al. Progressive supranuclear palsy: Loss of striatal dopamine receptors demonstrated in vivo by positron tomography and 76Br-bromospiperone. Lancet 1983;ii:1–7.
218. Wienhard K, Coenen HH, Pawlik G, et al. PET studies of dopamine receptor distribution using [18F]fluoroethylspiperone: Findings in disorders related to the dopaminergic system. J Neural Transm 1990;81:195–213.
219. Brucke T, Podreka I, Angelberger P, et al. Dopamine D2 receptor imaging with SPECT: Studies in different

neuropsychiatric disorders. J Cereb Blood Flow Metab 1991;11:220–228.
220. Shinotoh H, Namba H, Yamaguchi M, et al. Positron emission tomographic measurement of acetylcholinesterase activity reveals differential loss of ascending cholinergic systems in Parkinson's disease and progressive supranuclear palsy. Ann Neurol 1999;46(1):62–69.
221. Feaney MB, Dickson DW. Widespread cytoskeletal pathology characterizes corticobasal degeneration. Am J Pathol 1995;146:1388–1396.
222. Sawle GV, Brooks DJ, Marsden CD, et al. Cortico-basal degeneration: A unique pattern of regional cortical oxygen metabolism and striatal fluorodopa uptake demonstrated by positron emission tomography. Brain 1991;114:541–556.
223. Eidelberg D, Dhawan V, Moeller JR, et al. The metabolic landscape of cortico-basal ganglionic degeneration: Regional asymmetries studied with positron emission tomography. J Neurol Neurosurg Psychiatry 1991;54:856–862.
224. Blin J, Vidhailhet M-J, Pillon B, et al. Corticobasal degeneration: Decreased and asymmetrical glucose consumption as studied by PET. Mov Disord 1992;7:348–354.
225. Markus HS, Lees AJ, Lennox G, et al. Patterns of regional cerebral blood flow in corticobasal degeneration studied using HMPAO SPECT: Comparison with Parkinson's disease and normal controls. Mov Disord 1995;10:179–187.
226. Eckert T, Barnes A, Dhawan V, et al. FDG PET in the differential diagnosis of parkinsonian disorders. Neuroimage 2005;26:912–921.
227. Frisoni GB, Pizzolato G, Zanetti O, et al. Corticobasal degeneration: Neuropsychological assessment and dopamine D-2 receptor SPECT analysis. Eur Neurol 1995;35:50–54.
228. Nagahama Y, Fukuyama H, Turjanski N, et al. Cerebral glucose metabolism in corticobasal degeneration: Comparison with progressive supranuclear palsy and normal controls. Mov Disord 1997;12:691–696.
229. Walker Z, Costa DC, Walker RW, et al. Differentiation of dementia with Lewy bodies from Alzheimer's disease using a dopaminergic presynaptic ligand. J Neurol Neurosurg Psychiatry 2002;73:134–140.
230. Yong SW, Yoon JK, An YS, et al. A comparison of cerebral glucose metabolism in Parkinson's disease, Parkinson's disease dementia and dementia with Lewy bodies. Eur J Neurol 2007;14(12):1357–1362.
231. Gomperts SN, Rentz DM, Moran E, et al. Imaging amyloid deposition in Lewy body diseases. Neurology 2008;71(12):903–910.
232. Albin RL, Qin Y, Young AB, et al. Preproenkephalin messenger RNA-containing neurons in striatum of patients with symptomatic and presymptomatic Huntington's disease: An in situ hybridisation study. Ann Neurol 1991;30:542–549.
233. Albin RL, Reiner A, Anderson KD, et al. Striatal and nigral neuron subpopulations in rigid Huntington's disease: Implications for the functional anatomy of chorea and rigidity-akinesia. Ann Neurol 1990;27:357–365.
234. Andersson U, Haggstrom J-E, Levin ED, et al. Reduced glutamate decarboxylase activity in the subthalamic nucleus of patients with tardive dyskinesia. Mov Disord 1989;4:37–46.
235. Gunne LM, Haggstrom J-E, Sjoquist B. Association with persistent neuroleptic-induced dyskinesia of regional changes in brain GABA synthesis. Nature 1984;309:347–349.
236. Kuhl DE, Phelps ME, Markham CH, et al. Cerebral metabolism and atrophy in Huntington's disease determined by 18FDG and computed tomographic scans. Ann Neurol 1982;12:425–434.
237. Hayden MR, Martin WRW, Stoessl AJ, et al. Positron emission tomography in the early diagnosis of Huntington's disease. Neurology 1986;36:888–894.
238. Leenders KL, Frackowiak RSJ, Quinn N, et al. Brain energy metabolism and dopaminergic function in Huntington's disease measured in vivo using positron emission tomography. Mov Disord 1986;1:69–77.
239. Young AB, Penney JB, Starosta-Rubinstein S, et al. PET scan investigations of Huntington's disease: Cerebral metabolic correlates of neurological features and functional decline. Ann Neurol 1986;20:296–303.
240. Berent S, Giordani B, Lehtinen S, et al. Positron emission tomographic scan investigations of Huntington's disease: Cerebral metabolic correlates of cognitive function. Ann Neurol 1988;23:541–546.
241. Kuwert T, Lange HW, Langen KJ, et al. Cortical and subcortical glucose consumption measured by PET in patients with Huntington's disease. Brain 1990;113:1405–1423.
242. Dubinsky RM, Hallett M, Levey R, et al. Regional brain glucose metabolism in neuroacanthocytosis. Neurology 1989;39:1253–1255.
243. Hosokawa S, Ichiya Y, Kuwabara Y, et al. Positron emission tomography in cases of chorea with different underlying diseases. J Neurol Neurosurg Psychiatry 1987;50:1284–1287.
244. Kuwert T, Lange HW, Langen KJ, et al. Normal striatal glucose consumption in two patients with benign hereditary chorea as measured by positron emission tomography. J Neurol 1990;237:80–84.
245. Suchowersky O, Hayden MR, Martin WRW, et al. Cerebral metabolism of glucose in benign hereditary chorea. Mov Disord 1986;1:33–45.
246. Guttman M, Lang AE, Garnett ES, et al. Regional cerebral glucose metabolism in SLE chorea: Further evidence that striatal hypometabolism is not a correlate of chorea. Mov Disord 1987;2:201–210.
247. Weindl A, Kuwert T, Leenders KL, et al. Increased striatal glucose consumption in Sydenham chorea. Mov Disord 1993;8:437–444.
248. Pahl JJ, Mazziotta JC, Cummings J, et al. Positron emission tomography in tardive dyskinesia and Huntington's disease. J Cereb Blood Flow Metabol 1987;7:1253–1255.
249. Jenkins BG, Koroshetz WJ, Beal MF, et al. Evidence for impairment of energy metabolism in vivo in Huntington's disease using localised ^{1}H NMR spectroscopy. Neurology 1993;43:2689–2695.
250. Hägglund J, Aquilonius S-M, Eckernäs S, et al. Dopamine receptor properties in Parkinson's disease and Huntington's chorea evaluated by positron emission tomography using [11C]-N-methyl-spiperone. Acta Neurol Scand 1987;75:87–94.
251. Turjanski N, Weeks R, Dolan R, et al. Striatal D_1 and D_2 receptor binding in patients with Huntington's disease and other choreas: A PET study. Brain 1995;118:689–696.

252. Pirker W, Asenbaum S, Wenger S, et al. Iodine-123-epidepride-SPECT: Studies in Parkinson's disease, multiple system atrophy and Huntington's disease. J Nucl Med 1997;38:1711–1717.
253. Karlsson P, Lundin A, Anvret M, et al. Dopamine D1 receptor number: A sensitive PET marker for early brain degeneration in Huntington's disease. Eur Arch Psychiatry Clin Neurosci 1994;243:249–255.
254. Weeks RA, Cunningham VJ, Piccini P, et al. ^{11}C-Diprenorphine binding in Huntington's disease: A comparison of region of interest analysis and statistical parametric mapping. J Cereb Blood Flow Metabol 1997;17:943–949.
255. Holthoff VA, Koeppe RA, Frey KA, et al. Positron emission tomography measures of benzodiazepine receptors in Huntington's disease. Ann Neurol 1993;34:76–81.
256. Brooks DJ, Ibanez V, Playford ED, et al. Presynaptic and postsynaptic striatal dopaminergic function in neuroacanthocytosis: A positron emission tomographic study. Ann Neurol 1991;30:166–171.
257. Andersson U, Eckernas SA, Hartvig P, et al. Striatal binding of ^{11}C-NMSP studied with positron emission tomography in patients with persistent tardive dyskinesia: No evidence for altered dopamine receptor binding. J Neural Transm 1990;79:215–226.
258. Blin J, Baron JC, Cambon H, et al. Striatal dopamine D2 receptors in tardive dyskinesia: PET study. J Neurol Neurosurg Psychiatry 1989;52:1248–1252.
259. Trost M, Carbon M, Edwards C, et al. Primary dystonia: Is abnormal functional brain architecture linked to genotype? Ann Neurol 2002;52:853–856.
260. Grafton ST, Mazziotta JC, Pahl JJ, et al. A comparison of neurological, metabolic, structural, and genetic evaluations in persons at risk for Huntington's disease. Ann Neurol 1990;28:614–621.
261. Hayden MR, Hewitt J, Martin WRW, et al. Studies in persons at risk for Huntington's disease. N Engl J Med 1987;317:382–383.
262. Weeks RA, Piccini P, Harding AE, et al. Striatal D_1 and D_2 dopamine receptor loss in asymptomatic mutation carriers of Huntington's disease. Ann Neurol 1996;40:49–54.
263. Grafton ST, Mazziotta JC, Pahl JJ, et al. Serial changes of cerebral glucose metabolism and caudate size in persons at risk for Huntington's disease. Arch Neurol 1992;49:1161–1167.
264. Antonini A, Leenders KL, Eidelberg D. [C-11]Raclopride-PET studies of the Huntington's disease rate of progression: Relevance of the trinucleotide repeat length. Ann Neurol 1998;43:253–255.
265. Andrews TC, Weeks RA, Turjanski N, et al. Huntington's disease progression: PET and clinical observations. Brain 1999;122:2353–2363.
266. Pavese N, Andrews TC, Brooks DJ, et al. Progressive striatal and cortical dopamine receptor dysfunction in Huntington's disease: A PET study. Brain 2003;126: 1127–1135.
267. Sapp E, Kegel KB, Aronin N, et al. Early and progressive accumulation of reactive microglia in the Huntington disease brain. J Neuropathol Exp Neurol 2001;60(2):161–172.
268. Pavese N, Gerhard A, Tai YF, et al. Microglial activation correlates with severity in Huntington disease: A clinical and PET study. Neurology 2006;66(11):1638–1643.
269. Tai YF, Pavese N, Gerhard A, et al. Microglial activation in presymptomatic Huntington's disease gene carriers. Brain 2007;130:1759–1766.
270. Fricker RA, Torres EM, Hume SP, et al. The effects of donor stage on the survival and function of embryonic striatal grafts in the adult rat brain. II. Correlation between positron emission tomography and reaching behaviour. Neuroscience 1997;79:711–722.
271. Kendall L, Rayment D, Aigbirhio F, et al. In vivo PET analysis of the status of striatal allografts in the common marmoset. Eur J Neurosci 1998;10:15604.
272. Torres EM, Fricker RA, Hume SP, et al. Assessment of striatal graft viability in the rat in vivo using a small diameter PET scanner. Neuroreport 1995;6:2017–2021.
273. Brasted PJ, Watts C, Torres EM, et al. Behavioural recovery following striatal transplantation: Effects of postoperative training and P-zone volume. Exp Brain Res 1999;128:535–538.
274. Bachoud-Levi A, Remy P, Nguyen JP, et al. Motor and cognitive improvements in patients with Huntington's disease after neural transplantation. Lancet 2000;356: 1975–1979.
275. Gaura V, Bachoud-Levi AC, Ribeiro MJ, et al. Striatal neural grafting improves cortical metabolism in Huntington's disease patients. Brain 2004;127:65–72.
276. Reuter I, Tai YF, Pavese N, et al. Long-term clinical and positron emission tomography outcome of fetal striatal transplantation in Huntington's disease. J Neurol Neurosurg Psychiatry 2008;79(8):948–951.
277. Hauser RA, Furtado S, Cimino CR, et al. Bilateral human fetal striatal transplantation in Huntington's disease. Neurology 2002;158(5):687–695.
278. Bhatia KP, Marsden CD. The behavioural and motor consequences of focal lesions of the basal ganglia in man. Brain 1994;117:859–876.
279. Chase T, Tamminga CA, Burrows H. Positron emission studies of regional cerebral glucose metabolism in idiopathic dystonia. Adv Neurol 1988;50:237–241.
280. Eidelberg D, Dhawan V, Cedarbaum J, et al. Contralateral basal ganglia hypermetabolism in primary unilateral limb dystonia. Neurology 1990;40(suppl 1):399.
281. Gilman S, Junck L, Young AB, et al. Cerebral metabolic activity in idiopathic dystonia studied with positron emission tomography. Adv Neurol 1988;50:231–236.
282. Stoessl AJ, Martin WRW, Clark C, et al. PET studies of cerebral glucose metabolism in idiopathic torticollis. Neurology 1986;36:653–657.
283. Otsuka M, Ichiya Y, Shima F, et al. Increased striatal ^{18}F-dopa uptake and normal glucose metabolism in idiopathic dystonia syndrome. J Neurol Sci 1992;111:195–199.
284. Karbe H, Holthoff VA, Rudolf J, et al. Positron emission tomography demonstrates frontal cortex and basal ganglia hypometabolism in dystonia. Neurology 1992;42: 1540–1544.
285. Eidelberg D, Moeller JR, Antonini A, et al. Functional brain networks in DYT1 dystonia. Ann Neurol 1998;44: 303–312.
286. Hutchinson M, Nakamura T, Moeller JR, et al. The metabolic topography of essential blepharospasm: A focal dystonia with general implications. Neurology 2000;55: 673–677.

287. Ceballos-Baumann AO, Passingham RE, Warner T, et al. Over-activity of rostral and underactivity of caudal frontal areas in idiopathic torsion dystonia: A PET activation study. Ann Neurol 1995;37:363–372.
288. Tempel LW, Perlmutter JS. Abnormal vibration-induced cerebral blood flow responses in idiopathic dystonia. Brain 1990;113:691–707.
289. Tempel LW, Perlmutter JS. Abnormal cortical responses in patients with writer's cramp. Neurology 1993;43:2252–2257.
290. Perlmutter JS, Stambuk MK, Markham J, et al. Decreased [F-18] spiperone binding in putamen in idiopathic focal dystonia. J Neurosci 1997;17:843–850.
291. Ceballos-Baumann AO, Passingham RE, et al. Overactivity of primary and accessory motor areas after motor reorganisation in acquired hemi-dystonia: A PET activation study. Ann Neurol 1995;37:746–757.
292. Ceballos-Baumann AO, Marsden CD, Passingham RE, et al. Cerebral activation with performing and imagining movement in idiopathic torsion dystonia (ITD): A PET study. Neurology 1994;44(suppl 2):A338 (abstract).
293. Ceballos-Baumann AO, Sheean G, Marsden CD, et al. Botulinum toxin does not reverse the cortical dysfunction associated with writer's cramp. Brain 1997;120:571–582.
294. Playford ED, Fletcher NA, Sawle GV, et al. Integrity of the nigrostriatal dopaminergic system in familial dystonia: An ^{18}F-dopa PET study. Brain 1993;116:1191–1199.
295. Martin WRW, Stoessl AJ, Palmer M, et al. PET scanning in dystonia. Adv Neurol 1988;50:223–229.
296. Naumann M, Pirker W, Reiners K, et al. Imaging the pre- and postsynaptic side of striatal dopaminergic synapses in idiopathic cervical dystonia: A SPECT study using [^{123}I] Epidepride and [^{123}I]β-CIT. Mov Disord 1998;13:319–323.
297. Asanuma K, Ma Y, Huang C, et al. The metabolic pathway of dopa responsive dystonia. Ann Neurol 2005;57:596–600.
298. Sawle GV, Leenders KL, Brooks DJ, et al. Dopa-responsive dystonia: [^{18}F]Dopa positron emission tomography. Ann Neurol 1991;30:24–30.
299. Snow BJ, Nygaard TG, Takahashi H, et al. Positron emission tomography studies of dopa-responsive dystonia and early-onset idiopathic parkinsonism. Ann Neurol 1993;34:733–738.
300. Turjanski N, Bhatia K, Burn DJ, et al. Comparison of striatal ^{18}F-dopa uptake in adult-onset dystonia-parkinsonism, Parkinson's disease, and dopa-responsive dystonia. Neurology 1993;43:1563–1568.
301. Naumann M, Pirker W, Reiners K, et al. [123I]beta-CIT single-photon emission tomography in DOPA-responsive dystonia. Mov Disord 1997;12:448–451.
302. de la Fuente-Fernandez R, Furtado S, Guttman M, et al. VMAT2 binding is elevated in dopa-responsive dystonia: Visualizing empty vesicles by PET. Synapse 2003;49(1):20–28.

SECTION II

NEUROSCIENTIFIC FOUNDATIONS

CHAPTER 4

Functional Anatomy of the Basal Ganglia

Yoland Smith

▶ INTRODUCTION

Although the basal ganglia nuclei have first been recognized more than 300 years ago by the English anatomist Thomas Willis, our modern view of the basal ganglia circuitry dates back from the mid-1950s after the introduction of tract-tracing methods that allowed investigators to dissect out at the macroscopic and microscopic levels the main constituents and neural connections involved in the transmission and processing of information through these brain regions. In the early 1990s, these efforts led to the development of working models of basal ganglia function and dysfunction (the so-called "direct and indirect basal ganglia pathways"), which, since then, have been the basis for our current view of the basal ganglia circuitry and the framework for the development of modern surgical approaches aimed at lesioning or stimulating the subthalamic nucleus (STN) or the internal globus pallidus (GPi) for basal ganglia diseases. Based on their close anatomical and functional relationships with the basal ganglia, new deep brain stimulation (DBS) targets will be discussed in this chapter.

In light of their clear involvement in neurodegenerative diseases characterized symptomatically by movement disorders, such as Parkinson's disease (PD) and Huntington's chorea, the basal ganglia are commonly seen as integral constituents of the extrapyramidal motor system. Although they, indeed, play significant roles in regulating motor behaviors, basal ganglia functions extend far beyond the motor systems and also include high-order processing of cognitive- and limbic-related information. The functional anatomy of the neural circuits and synaptic networks that underlie motor and non-motor functions of the basal ganglia will be presented and discussed in this chapter.

Because of space constraints, this chapter does not aim at covering the whole literature on basal ganglia anatomy. The readers are referred to other comprehensive reviews and compendiums for a survey of the early literature and a more general overview of this field.[1–41]

▶ FUNCTIONAL CIRCUITRY OF THE BASAL GANGLIA

In primates, the basal ganglia are made up of the caudate nucleus and putamen, which form the dorsal striatum and the nucleus accumbens and olfactory tubercle commonly referred to as the ventral striatum. In rats and mice, a single mass of gray matter, called the caudate–putamen complex, forms the dorsal striatum. The other basal ganglia structures include the GP, which is made up of the internal and external segments commonly named GPi and GPe (external GP), in primates. In rodents, the entopeduncular nucleus is the homologue of GPi, while the GP is the homologue of the GPe. Another key basal ganglia structure, often considered as the "pacemaker" of the basal ganglia is the STN, a small almond-shaped nucleus ventral to the thalamus between the diencephalon and midbrain.[10,20,21,30,31] The importance of the STN in the normal and pathological circuitry of the basal ganglia is highlighted by the fact that it is a prime surgical target in PD.[42–52] Finally, the substantia nigra, located at the basis of the midbrain, is another key component of the basal ganglia network. It comprises two major parts; the substantia nigra pars compacta (SNc) is made up of densely packed dopaminergic neurons, while the substantia nigra pars reticulata (SNr) comprises GABAergic projection neurons. Neighboring dopaminergic cell groups include the medially located ventral tegmental area (VTA) and the caudal retrorubral field (RRF). Extrinsic information to the basal ganglia circuitry flows through the striatum and the STN, known as the main entry stations of the basal ganglia. Once the information has been processed and integrated, it is forwarded to the frontal cortical regions or brain stem pedunculopontine nucleus (PPN) via functionally segregated basal

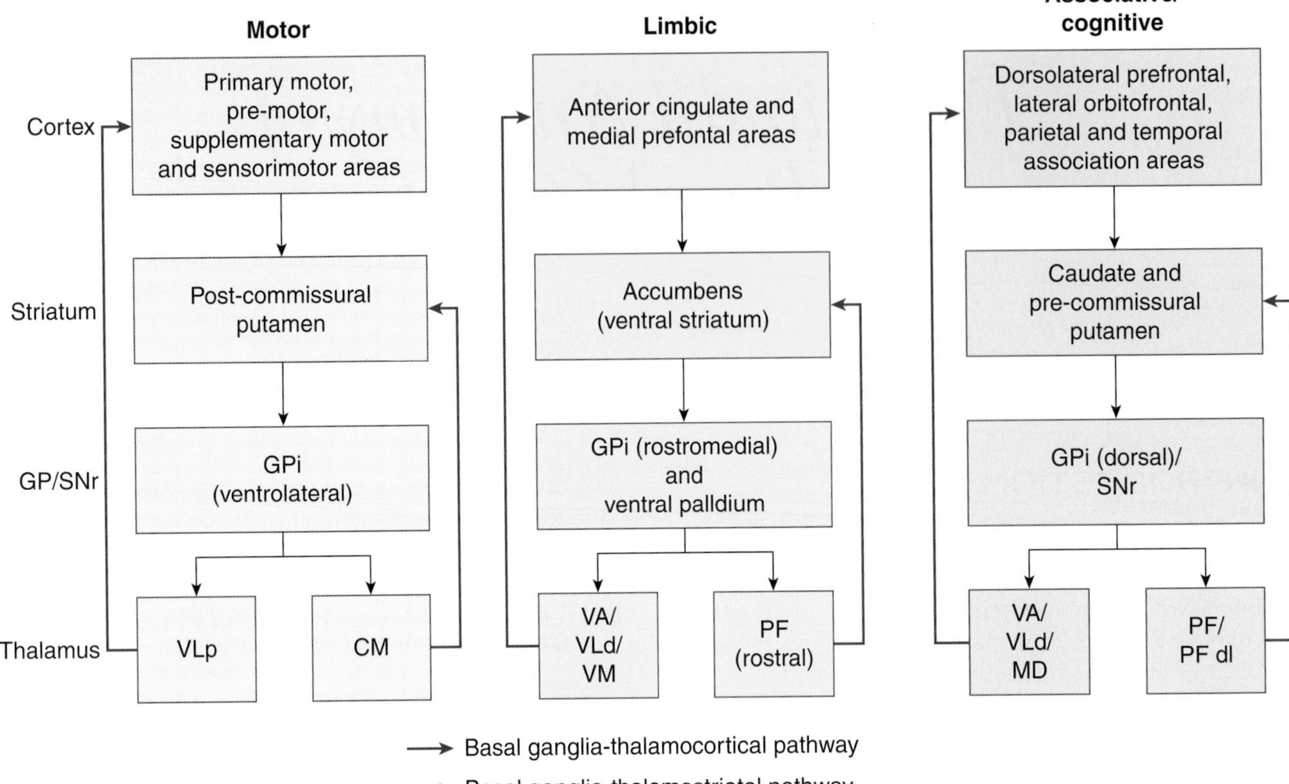

Figure 4–1. Segregated basal ganglia–thalamocortical and thalamostriatal functional loops. Each functional modality is processed and travels through segregated regions of basal ganglia and thalamic nuclei (VA/VL and CM/PF) involved in motor, limbic, and associative/cognitive functions.

ganglia–tegmental or thalamocortical channels of information (Fig. 4–1).

▶ THE STRIATUM IS THE MAIN ENTRANCE TO THE BASAL GANGLIA CIRCUITRY

The dorsal and the ventral striatum receive their main extrinsic inputs from functionally segregated regions of the cerebral cortex; inputs from associative and sensorimotor areas terminate predominantly in the caudate nucleus and putamen, whereas limbic cortices innervate the ventral striatum.[1]

The striatum is compartmentalized into the patch (or striosomes) and the extrastriosomal matrix, recognized as two distinct striatal compartments that receive different extrinsic inputs, project to different targets, and display distinct neurochemistry.[2,53] Imbalanced activity between the patch and matrix compartments likely underlies abnormal repetitive motor behaviors known as stereotypies.[54–57] Striosomal neurons are preferentially recruited following chronic exposure to psychostimulants, thereby indicating neural endpoints of the transmission from action–outcome associative behavior to conditioned habitual responding.[57] The differential regulation of the Ras/Rap/ERK MAP kinase signal transduction cascades between the patch and matrix compartments predicts the severity of motor side effects induced by chronic dopaminergic therapy in parkinsonism.[58] Striatal patch projection neurons are preferentially lost in X-linked progressive dystonia–parkinsonism.[59,60] Differential changes in GABA-A receptor subunit expression between the patch and matrix compartments likely underlie changes in mood in Huntington's disease.[61]

CELLULAR ORGANIZATION OF THE STRIATUM

The GABAergic medium spiny projection neurons are the main subtype of striatal neurons accounting for more than 95% of the total striatal neuronal population.[62] These neurons have a small- to medium-sized cell body from which originates a heavily spiny dendritic tree. Two main subtypes of striatal projection neurons have been identified based on dopamine receptor expression, neuropeptide content, and main projection sites: the "direct pathway neurons" mainly express D1 dopamine receptors, contain substance P and dynorphin, and project directly to the basal ganglia output nuclei, GPi and SNr. On the other hand, "indirect pathway" neurons strongly express D2 dopamine receptors, display enkephalin immunoreactivity, and target the GPe.[2] Striatal D1 projection neurons have a larger dendritic tree and are less excitable than D2 indirect pathway neurons in mice.[63–66]

On average, single striatal projection neurons harbor about 5000 spines distributed homogeneously at about 1 spine/μm on distal dendrites in primate and nonprimate species.[67–70] PD is characterized by a prominent loss of striatal spines, reaching as much as 50% in the post-commissural sensorimotor putamen in MPTP-treated parkinsonian monkeys.[67–70] In transgenic mice, striatal spine loss affects exclusively D2-containing indirect pathway neurons.[68] These observations have not been confirmed in MPTP-treated monkeys and human parkinsonians, which both display a more homogeneous spine loss between the two populations of striatal projection neurons.[33,70]

The medium spiny neurons give rise to a rich network of intrastriatal axon collaterals that contact neighboring projection neurons within the vicinity of the parent cell bodies.[71] On the basis of paired recording electrophysiological studies in the rat striatum, these lateral connections have been characterized as sparse, distal, and poorly influential on striatal projection neurons activity.[72,73] However, these connections display a high degree of specificity and allow communication between direct and indirect pathway neurons. Unidirectional connections between pairs of D1- or D2-positive neurons, or from D2- to D1-containing projection neurons,[74] have been identified, while connections from D1- to D2-positive neurons are infrequent. The strength of these intrastriatal connections is substantially reduced in parkinsonism.[74]

Four main populations of interneurons have been identified in the striatum. In rats, they represent about 2–3% of the total striatal neuronal population, while in nonhuman primates as much as 20–25% of all striatal neurons are accounted for by interneurons.[15,16,75,76] The *cholinergic interneurons*, also referred to as the "tonically active" neurons (TANs),[76–79] display a significant degree of co-localization with calretinin in primates.[80] These neurons, which receive a significant innervation from GABAergic axon collaterals of substance P–positive projection neurons in rats,[81] play a key role in regulating motivated behaviors and reward-related learning.[77,78,82–89] A rich network of interconnections with GABAergic interneurons allows cross-talk between populations of cholinergic interneurons, thereby providing a mechanism for their widespread recurrent inhibition via nicotinic excitation.[90] The cholinergic interneurons play key roles in mediating dopamine-dependent plasticity and learning in the mammalian striatum.[24,91–95]

The *GABA/PV (parvalbumin) interneurons,* also called "fast spiking interneurons," form pericellular symmetric synapses on the proximal part of striatal output neurons. These neurons are electrotonically coupled through gap junctions, and control spike timing in output neurons, thereby facilitating fast-forward intrastriatal inhibition of projection neurons in response to cortical activation.[15,16,76,96]

The *GABA/nitric oxide synthase/neuropeptide Y/ somatostatin interneurons* are categorized electrophysiologically as "persistent and low-threshold spike" neurons.[15,16,76] These neurons generate large inhibitory currents in output neurons and modulate plasticity at glutamatergic synapses through nitric oxide release.[16] In addition, somatostatin can modify the processing and output of the striatum because it entrains projection neurons into the rhythms generated by some interneurons.[97]

The *medium-sized GABA/calretinin interneurons,* considered as the largest population of striatal interneurons in humans,[80] display physiological characteristics similar to the persistent- and low-threshold spike neurons, and strongly inhibit output neurons.[76]

EXTRINSIC CONNECTIVITY OF THE STRIATUM

The Corticostriatal Projections

The cerebral cortex is a major source of striatal glutamatergic innervation. The corticostriatal system, which arises from all cortical regions, is highly topographic, thereby imposing functionally segregated maps upon the striatum (Fig. 4–1).[98] Based on findings from various species, including humans, a basic scheme of functional connectivity between the cerebral cortex and the striatum has been recognized.[99–119] Striatal inputs from the somatosensory, motor, and pre-motor cortices are somatotopic and terminate in a band-like fashion in the post-commissural putamen while associative cortical regions from frontal, parietal, and temporal lobes innervate the caudate nucleus and the pre-commissural putamen. The limbic cortices, the amygdala, and the hippocampus innervate the ventral striatum (Fig. 4–1).[1,98] Functionally related associative or sensorimotor cortical inputs from areas connected through cortico-cortical projections either overlap or remain segregated in the striatum.[116–119]

Two distinct populations of corticostriatal neurons have been identified in rats; the "intratelencephalic neurons (IT)" are located in superficial cortical lamina, project solely to the striatum and the cerebral cortex, and target preferentially "direct" pathway neurons. On the other hand, the "pyramidal tract (PT)" neurons are located deeper within the cortex, project to the brain stem and spinal cord with collaterals to the striatum, and target preferentially "indirect" pathway neurons.[120,121] Recent electrophysiological data challenged the physiological significance of these anatomical observations, suggesting that IT neurons are the main source of functional excitatory inputs to both populations of striatal projection neurons in rats.[122] The existence of PT corticostriatal neurons remains controversial in primates.[123–125]

GABA/PV interneurons receive strong cortical inputs, setting up the stage for feed-forward inhibition of striatal projection neurons in response to activation of corticostriatal afferents.[15,16,128] In the 6-hydroxydopamine (OHDA)-treated rat model of PD, the feed-forward inhibition from GABA/PV interneurons possibly contributes to the imbalance of activity between the two populations of striatofugal neurons,[129] a hypothesis that was recently challenged by electrophysiological data showing a lack of correlation between cortical information flowing to GABA/PV neurons versus projection neurons.[96]

The Thalamostriatal Projections

The thalamus also significantly contributes to the extrinsic glutamatergic innervation of the striatum. Although the role of the thalamostriatal system has long been neglected in the functional circuitry of the basal ganglia, the recent evidence that DBS of the caudal intralaminar nuclei, the main sources of thalamostriatal projections, alleviates some symptoms of PD and Tourette's syndrome (see below) has generated significant interest in this projection system. Although the caudal intralaminar nuclei are the main sources of thalamostriatal projections, most thalamic nuclei contribute to this projection. The origin and functional anatomy of these different thalamostriatal systems will now be discussed.

The Caudal Intralaminar Nuclei: Main Sources of the Thalamostriatal System

In primates, the centromedian (CM) and parafascicular (PF) nuclei are the main sources of thalamostriatal projections that largely terminate in different functional regions of the striatum. The medial part of the CM projects to the post-commissural sensorimotor putamen, while the PF innervates preferentially associative regions of the caudate nucleus and limbic-related areas in the ventral striatum.[14,37] The dorsolateral PF is specifically connected with the pre-commissural putamen. The degree of striatal innervation from the CM/PF is far more prominent than the sparse projections to the cerebral cortex.[130] At the ultrastructural level, CM and PF terminals form asymmetric synapses mainly with the dendrites of striatal projection neurons.[131–133] A significant CM innervation of cholinergic, parvalbumin-containing, and somatostatin-positive striatal interneurons, but not calretinin-positive neurons, has also been described in monkeys.[134] In keeping with these anatomical data, CM/PF modulation affects the physiological activity and neurotransmitter release from cholinergic interneurons.[135–137] In addition, striatal inputs from the CM/PF are essential regulators of sensory responses of TANs (likely cholinergic) acquired during sensorimotor learning in primates.[138–140]

Thalamostriatal Projections from Anterior Intralaminar and Other Thalamic Nuclei

The CM/PF complex is not the sole origin of the thalamostriatal system. Many other thalamic nuclei also provide topographic and functionally organized projections to the striatum.[14,37,141–145] However, there is a striking difference between the synaptic organization of striatal projections from CM/PF versus other thalamic nuclei, that is, CM/PF terminals mainly establish axo-dendritic synapses with medium spiny neurons and interneurons, whereas projections from other thalamic nuclei are almost exclusively involved in axo-spinous synapses with projection neurons.[14,37,141–145] The extent and axon collateralization of cortical versus striatal projections from CM/PF compared with other thalamic nuclei is significantly different. In contrast to the CM/PF, which are mainly linked with the striatum, providing only sparse inputs to frontal cortical areas, other thalamostriatal neurons project mainly to the cerebral cortex with modest striatal innervation.[14,37,131,133,144,146] At the striatal level, thalamic inputs from single CM/PF neurons are much more focused and generate a more profuse field of terminals than individual cortical axons.[37,125,130] So far, there is no clear indication of the functional significance of such anatomical differences between the two main sources of striatal glutamatergic innervation.

Vesicular Glutamate Transporters as Specific Markers of Thalamostriatal versus Corticostriatal Projections

In rats and primates, the vesicular glutamate transporters 1 and 2 (vGluT1 and vGluT2) are specifically expressed in corticostriatal and thalamostriatal glutamatergic terminals, respectively.[14,37,145,147] In nonhuman primates, more than 95% vGluT1 terminals form axo-spinous synapses in the striatum, whereas only 50–60% vGluT2 terminals display such synaptic arrangement, a pattern that remains unaltered in the nonhuman primate model of PD.[145] Consistent with the idea that the CM/PF complex is the main source of axo-dendritic glutamatergic inputs to the striatal matrix, there is a significant increase in the proportion of vGluT2 terminals forming axo-dendritic synapses in the matrix compared with patch compartments in rats.[14,37,133]

Functions of the Thalamostriatal Systems

Based on their origin and relative degree of striatal versus cortical innervation, it is reasonable to believe that the functions of CM/PF projections to the striatum are most likely different from those of other thalamostriatal systems. In monkeys, CM/PF neurons supply striatal neurons with attentional value stimuli that act as detectors of contralateral behaviorally significant events.[138,139] Changes in CM/PF activity are, indeed, induced in response to attention-demanding reaction-time task in humans.[148] In monkeys, the physiological consequences of CM/PF stimulation upon striatal projection neurons and cholinergic interneurons activity are complex and likely involve intrastriatal GABAergic microcircuits,[135–137] whereas stimulation of rostral intralaminar nuclei elicits complex changes in cognitive functions, probably through modulation of both cortical and striatal activities.[149–150] Other thalamostriatal systems may act as positive reinforcers of specific populations of striatal neurons involved in performing a selected cortically driven behavior.[14,37,151]

The CM/PF Degenerates in Parkinson's Disease

Postmortem studies have revealed as much as 50% cells loss in the CM/PF complex of patients with progressive supranuclear palsy, Huntington's disease, or PD.[152,153] In patients with PD, neurons devoid of parvalbumin or calbindin immunoreactivity are specifically affected in the CM, while parvalbumin neurons are mainly affected in the PF.[153] Changes in the shape of thalami between patients with PD and healthy controls have also been described.[154] There is controversy regarding the development of these thalamic pathologies in animal models of parkinsonism. For instance, although some studies described a loss of PF neurons in 6-OHDA-treated rats and MPTP-treated mice, others could not replicate these findings under similar conditions.[14,37] In MPTP-treated parkinsonian monkeys, there is a significant reduction in the relative abundance of vGluT2-positive terminals forming axo-dendritic synapses in the putamen, suggesting a possible degeneration of CM-striatal neurons in this animal model.[145]

The Mesostriatal Dopaminergic Systems

Three main populations of ventral midbrain dopaminergic neurons have been recognized: the A8 (RRF), A9 (SNc), and A10 (VTA) cell groups. Each sub-nucleus is made up of dopaminergic neurons and small populations of GABAergic interneurons, except in the VTA, which includes a modest population of GABAergic projection neurons.[9] Neurotensin and cholecystokinin are co-expressed in subpopulations of dopaminergic neurons in the medial SNc and VTA.[155–158] The level of dopamine transporter is higher in ventral tier SNc (SNc-v) than in other ventral midbrain dopaminergic neurons,[159] a feature that likely accounts for the increased sensitivity of SNc-v neurons to the toxic effects of MPTP.[160,161] Calbindin D28K (CB) is expressed in VTA, RRF, and dorsal tier SNC (SNc-d) neurons, but not in the SNc-v,[9,162] a neurochemical feature that may account for the relative sparing of SNc-d and VTA neurons in PD.[163–165] The relative expression level of CB in the striatum and the SN is correlated with the pattern of nigrostriatal dopaminergic denervation in PD. For instance, the sensorimotor post-commissural putamen, considered as the most sensitive striatal region to dopaminergic denervation in PD (see below), does not express calbindin immunoreactivity.[166] In the substantia nigra, the CB-enriched SNc-d and VTA neurons are relatively spared,[159,167] while SNc neurons that receive CB-containing striatal inputs are more resistant to neurodegeneration and MPTP-induced toxicity than SNc neurons in the CB-poor nigrosomes.[164] In light of these findings, it is reasonable to suggest that CB likely plays a neuroprotective role in the dopaminergic pathogenesis of PD.

In primates, the following features characterize the sources and topography of the nigrostriatal dopaminergic system: (1) the neuronal columns in the SNc-v target preferentially the sensorimotor striatum (i.e., post-commissural putamen), (2) VTA and SNc-d neurons project mainly to the limbic striatum (i.e., nucleus accumbens), and (3) dopaminergic neurons in the densocellular part of SNc-v innervate the associative striatum (i.e., caudate nucleus and pre-commissural putamen).[9,33] In rats, SNc-d neurons project predominantly to the dorsal striatum.[168]

Two main types of nigrostriatal axons have been identified in single cell filling studies: (1) a population of thin, varicose, and widely distributed fibers that originate from SNc-d, VTA, and RRF neurons, and terminate preferentially in the matrix striatal compartment and (2) thick varicose fibers from the SNc-v that innervate mostly the patch striatal compartment.[169] This concept of dual nigrostriatal fiber systems was recently challenged using a more sensitive viral tracing method, which suggests a profuse axonal arborization of individual nigrostriatal dopaminergic axons that do not display any specific compartmental organization in rats.[170]

In addition to the regional pattern of dopaminergic denervation described above suggesting that the sensorimotor striatal territory is the most sensitive striatal region in PD, while the ventral striatum is less susceptible to the parkinsonian pathology,[171–174] a preferential dopaminergic denervation of striosomes over the extrastriosomal matrix has been described in MPTP-treated monkeys.[165,175]

Dopamine mediates its pre- and postsynaptic neuromodulatory effects through activation of five dopamine receptor subtypes, all of which being expressed to varying degree in striatal output neurons and interneurons. The loss of dopamine-mediated regulation of striatal glutamatergic and cholinergic transmission is a key feature of the neurochemical pathology of PD.

Another pathological hallmark of PD is the massive loss and morphological changes of spines in the striatum, a phenomenon dependent on dopaminergic and glutamatergic transmission that likely affects the integration and processing of extrinsic information to the basal ganglia circuitry.[6,9,33,70]

The serotonergic system from the raphe nuclei and the noradrenergic ascending projections from the locus coeruleus are two other important modulatory systems of the basal ganglia but, for the sake of space, will not be discussed in detail in this chapter. However, it is important to note that these two neurotransmitters regulate the physiological activity of various basal ganglia nuclei and possibly contribute to the loss of midbrain dopaminergic neurons and the development of depression, mood disorders, and motor side effects of long-term dopaminergic therapy in PD.[176–182]

Striatal Dopamine Interneurons in PD

A population of striatal dopaminergic interneurons has been characterized in dopamine-depleted rats and monkeys, and in the dorsal striatum of PD patients.[183–187] These small aspiny neurons, which express various markers of dopaminergic neurons, also co-localize with GABAergic markers and, for a small subset, calretinin.[183,186] They are mainly distributed in the pre-commissural putamen and caudate nucleus, and receive scarce synaptic inputs in MPTP-treated monkeys.[186] Their density increases after nigrostriatal dopamine denervation and striatal administration of glial-cell line derived neurotrophic factor (GDNF),[188] suggesting a potential compensatory role in PD.

Extrastriatal Dopaminergic Systems

In addition to the striatum, extrastriatal dopamine acts directly at the level of the GP, STN, and SNr.[9,33] The existence of dopaminergic thalamic afferents has recently been described, a system that may fine regulate the information flow through the basal ganglia–thalamocortical loops in normal and parkinsonian conditions.[9,33,189–191,191a]

▶ THE DIRECT AND INDIRECT PATHWAYS OF THE BASAL GANGLIA

The direct and indirect pathway model of the basal ganglia has been the platform for tremendous developments in basic and clinical basal ganglia research for the past decades. This model, which has been challenged, revised, and updated based on gain in new knowledge of the basal ganglia circuitry, remains the most reliable working model of the normal and abnormal basal ganglia circuitry. According to this model, the striatal information flows along two main pathways to reach the basal ganglia output nuclei: the "direct pathway" characterized as a monosynaptic connection between the striatum and the basal ganglia output nuclei, the GPi, and the SNr, and the "indirect pathway," which comprises polysynaptic connections that link the striatum and GPi/SNr via the GPe and the STN.[2,192–194] The populations of GABAergic striatal neurons that give rise to these pathways are segregated by their peptide content (substance P, direct; enkephalin, indirect) and their preferential expression of dopamine receptor subtypes (D1, direct; D2, indirect).[194] An imbalance of activity between these two pathways, in favor of the indirect pathway, underlies some of the main motor symptoms of parkinsonism. Because of functionally opposite effects of D1 and D2 dopamine receptor activation upon striatal neurons, the striatal dopamine denervation leads to increased activity of indirect striatofugal neurons and decreased output from direct striatofugal neurons in PD. Together, these opposite changes lead to increased GABAergic basal ganglia outflow to the thalamus, which, in turn, may reduce cortical excitability and decrease motor behaviors (Fig. 4–2).

This traditional scheme of the basal ganglia connectivity has been challenged and revisited in light of data, suggesting that the two pathways may not be as segregated as originally thought. For instance, it appears that most striatofugal neurons of the direct pathway give off collaterals to the GPe[8,195–197] and that D1 and D2 receptor mRNAs may not be as segregated as originally thought.[198–204] The degree of segregation of D1 and D2 receptor protein immunoreactivity is controversial. On the one hand, some groups reported an almost complete segregation of the two receptor subtypes in distinct populations of striatal spines,[121,205] while others showed significant co-localization of dopamine receptor immunoreactivity at the single cell level in the rat striatum.[206,207]

These controversies were recently revisited following the development of bacterial artificial chromosome (BAC) transgenic mice[208,209] that display a complete segregation of D1 and D2 receptor mRNAs, even when measured with the highly sensitive single cell mRNA amplification method, an approach that revealed significant D1/D2 co-localization in normal rats.[25,68,199,200,204] However, an important fact to keep in mind while interpreting dopamine-mediated effects in individual striatofugal neurons is the possible expression of other D1 or D2 receptor family subtypes (i.e., D3, D4, and D5 receptors) in the two main populations of striatofugal neurons,[210–215] an unknown information in BAC-D1/EGFP or BAC-D2/EGFP transgenic mice. However, we believe that such information is essential to characterize the chemical phenotype of striatofugal neurons in these transgenic animals, and ensure that functional data gathered from these mice can be translated to normal brains.

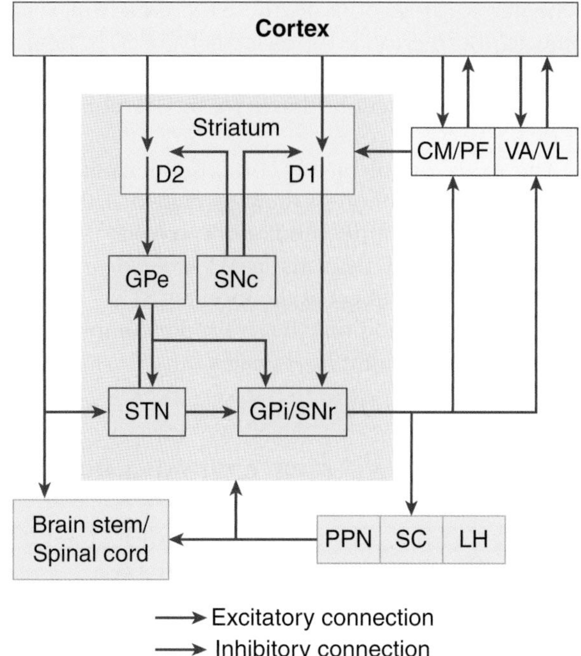

Figure 4–2. Direct and indirect pathway model of the basal ganglia. The blue box indicates tightly interconnected basal ganglia nuclei that receive extrinsic inputs from cortical, thalamic, and brainstem regions. The extrastriatal SNc dopaminergic projections to GPe, STN, and GPi/SNr have been omitted from this diagram. The connections between the basal ganglia and the PPN/SC/LH are depicted in more detail in Fig. 4–4. Abbreviations: CM, centromedian nucleus of the thalamus; D1 and D2, dopamine D1-type and D2-type receptors; GPe, globus pallidus external segment; GPi, globus pallidus internal segment; LH, lateral habenula; PF, parafascicular nucleus of thalamus; PPN, pedunculopontine nucleus; SC, superior colliculus; SNc, substantia nigra pars compacta; SNr, substantia nigra pars reticulata; STN, subthalamic nucleus; VA/VL, ventral anterior and ventrolateral nuclei of thalamus.

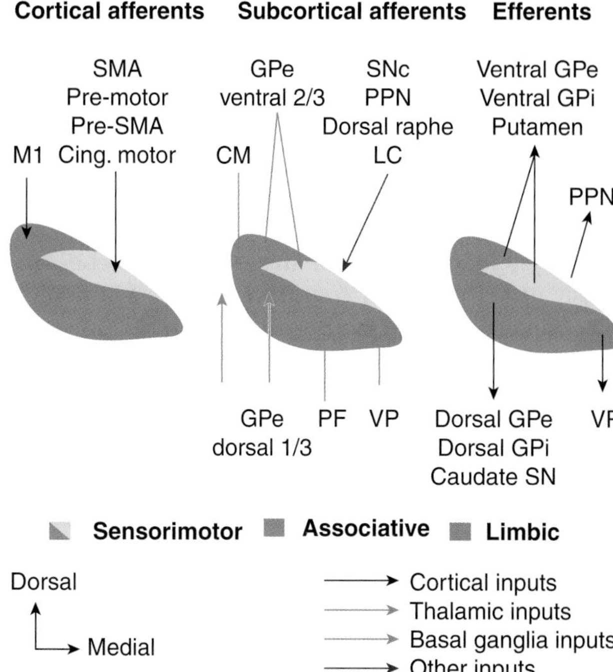

Figure 4–3. Afferent and efferent connections of functional subregions of the subthalamic nucleus. The sensorimotor region is further subdivided according to the source of primary motor versus pre-motor, supplementary, and cingulate motor cortical inputs. Abbreviations: Cing. mot., cingulate motor area of cortex; CM, centromedian nucleus of the thalamus; GPe, globus pallidus external segment; GPi, globus pallidus internal segment; LC, locus coeruleus; M1, primary motor area of cortex; PF, parafascicular nucleus of thalamus; PPN, pedunculopontine nucleus; Pre-motor, pre-motor area of cortex; SMA, supplementary motor area of cortex; SN, substantia nigra; SNc, substantia nigra compacta.

▶ FUNCTIONAL ANATOMY OF THE HYPERDIRECT CORTICOSUBTHALAMIC PROJECTION

Extrinsic cortical information also reaches the basal ganglia circuitry through the STN. The conduction speed of the information flow through the corticosubthalamic tract to the SNr and GPi is faster than information traveling along the direct and indirect corticostriatofugal pathways.[216] Fast excitatory responses that are abolished after excitotoxic lesion of the STN are induced in basal ganglia output neurons following electrical stimulation of motor cortices.[216–218] Motor cortical inputs to the STN are topographically organized so that projections from M1 innervate mainly the dorsolateral tier of the nucleus, while projections from the supplementary motor area (SMA), pre-motor cortices (PM), and the cingulate motor cortex (CM) converge to the dorsomedial STN. There is a reversed somatotopic arrangement of M1 projections to the dorsolateral STN compared with SMA projections the dorsomedial STN.[216–218] The frontal and supplementary eye field cortical areas terminate in the ventrolateral half of the STN, while the medial-most STN region is related to the processing of limbic-related information (Fig. 4–3). However, the exact sources and pattern of termination of non-motor cortical inputs to the ventral sectors of STN remain poorly characterized.

A center-surround model of functional interactions between hyperdirect and direct/indirect pathway projections at the level of GPi has been proposed as the substrate for proper selection of motor programs.[216] According to this hypothesis, hyperdirect cortical information flowing through the STN is sent to a large pool of GPi neurons, thereby exciting a large group of basal ganglia output neurons unrelated to the selected motor act (i.e., the "surround neurons"). Simultaneously, corollary and highly focused signals transmitted along the corticostriatal system influence a restricted pool of GPi neurons (i.e., the "center neurons").[216]

Despite its significant interest, the anatomical and physiological basis for this model must be cautiously examined. First, tract-tracing studies in nonhuman primates have demonstrated that the relationships between the STN, GPe, and GPi are topographic and highly specific, connecting functionally related neurons in GPe, GPi, and STN.[219,220] This pattern is not consistent with the assumption made by the model that the STN sends diffuse projections to the GPi that target neurons unrelated to the selected motor programs. Second, most STN neurons increase their activity at or after the onset of motor acts during active step-tracking movements in monkeys,[221] thereby reducing the possibility that the corticosubthalamic projection participates in the preparation of movements as suggested by the center-surround hypothesis. However, pre-movement-related local field potentials have been recorded with DBS electrodes in the STN of parkinsonian patients a few seconds prior to electromyographic onset, suggesting a potential role for the hyperdirect pathway in movement preparation.[222,222a] Whether this indicates a normal or pathological feature of the STN in PD remains to be determined. Thus, the exact functional relationships between the hyperdirect, direct, and indirect pathways of basal ganglia outflow to regulate proper selection of motor behaviors remain a matter of debate that should be addressed in future studies.

Although the functional anatomy of the motor corticosubthalamic system has been studied in detail, such is not the case for non-motor cortical inputs to the STN. However, recent rodent studies have established that the corticosubthalamic projections from the prefrontal cortex play a role in the preparatory processes, attention, perseveration, and other important cognitive or limbic functions,[223–232] but the sources of non-motor cortical afferents to the STN remain poorly characterized in primates. In humans, connections between high-order associative areas of the frontal lobe and the STN have been suggested by means of diffusion-weighed magnetic resonance imaging methods.[233] It is also important to keep in mind that cognitive changes are sometimes induced by misplaced DBS electrodes in the STN of PD patients.[234–241] It is worth noting that the ventromedial STN is closely linked with the caudate nucleus and associative regions of GPe and GPi, providing another substrate for STN stimulation-mediated effects on complex cognitive functions.[219,220,242,243] The caudal intralaminar nuclei and the tegmental PPN also send glutamatergic projections to the STN, which may contribute to the increased firing activity of STN neurons in parkinsonian conditions[220] (Fig. 4–3). The STN sends glutamatergic projections back to the cerebral cortex and PPN.[220,242–244]

The exact origin of the corticosubthalamic system remains unclear. Although there is evidence that these may be collaterals of descending PT axons,[245,246] the filling of individual PT neurons in M1 labeled only a few scarcely distributed fibers in the monkey STN,[125] suggesting that this projection may have a more complex origin than previously thought in primates.

▶ FUNCTIONAL RELATIONSHIPS BETWEEN THE PEDUNCULOPONTINE NUCLEUS AND THE BASAL GANGLIA

CELLULAR ORGANIZATION AND CONNECTIVITY OF THE PPN

The PPN comprises a rich network of chemically heterogeneous neurons around the superior cerebellar peduncle. It lies medial to the medial lemniscus, lateral to the decussation of the superior cerebellar peduncle, dorsal to the RRF, caudal to the dorsomedial region of the caudalmost part of the substantia nigra, and rostral by the cuneiform nuclei. Two major sub-nuclei have been identified: the PPN pars compacta (PPNc), made up of densely packed cholinergic neurons in the caudolateral half of the nucleus, and the PPN pars diffusa (PPNd), which comprises loosely distributed non-cholinergic neurons located more medially along the dorsoventral extent of the superior cerebellar peduncle. About 10,000–15,000 cholinergic neurons[247,248] make up 90% of the human PPNc.[249] In monkeys, 40% cholinergic neurons in the PPN co-express glutamate immunoreactivity.[250] Dopaminergic, noradrenergic, GABAergic, and various peptidergic neurons are also present within the boundaries of the PPN.[251–256]

The PPN is closely related to the basal ganglia. It receives major inputs from the GPi and SNr (see below) and a more modest afferent projection from the STN. Additional inputs from the spinal cord, raphe nuclei, locus coeruleus, deep cerebellar nuclei, superior colliculus, and SNc have also been reported.[245–256] In turn, the PPN innervates most basal ganglia nuclei, although the SNc and the STN are the preferential targets of these ascending projections that use glutamate and acetylcholine as neurotransmitters.[257,258] The PPN also sends descending projections to pontine, medullary, and spinal structures, thereby providing a route through which basal ganglia outflow could bypass the thalamocortical loop to directly influence the reticular formation and spinal cord (see below).

The PPN is also a major source of cholinergic and non-cholinergic projections to the thalamus, an ascending system that mediates cortical desynchronization during waking and rapid eye movement (REM) sleep. Both cholinergic and glutamatergic PPN inputs target thalamostriatal neurons in the caudal intralaminar thalamic nuclei in monkeys,[259] providing an additional indirect route via which the PPN may regulate basal ganglia activity. The PPN is, thus, in a strategic position to regulate activity of both basal ganglia–thalamocortical and basal ganglia–thalamostriatal loops.[252,256,259]

Despite the obvious limitations of the diffusion tensor imaging (DTI) method to differentiate afferent from efferent fiber pathways and small fiber tracts, this approach was recently used to confirm and extend our knowledge of PPN connectivity in humans.[260–263]

THE PPN IS A TARGET FOR FUNCTIONAL DEEP BRAIN STIMULATION IN MOVEMENT DISORDERS

The PPN is involved in the initiation and modulation of gait and other stereotyped movements in animals.[254,264–266] Bilateral lesion of the PPN induces bradykinesia in monkeys.[266–268] As much as 50% loss of cholinergic neurons has been reported in the PPN of parkinsonian patients.[269,270] GABA-A receptor blockade or low-frequency stimulation in the PPN reverses akinesia in MPTP-treated parkinsonian monkeys.[271–273] DBS in the PPN area appears to be a suitable antiparkinsonian strategy for patients with gait freezing and poor balance, two late-onset symptoms of PD unresponsive to dopamine therapy.[254,274–280] Despite early promising results of PPN DBS,[274–280] the exact brain stem site of stimulation and the mechanisms underlying the benefit of this procedure remain poorly understood. Some investigators have argued that the peripeduncular nucleus, a cell group located rostral and lateral to the PPN, has been the predominant target of DBS performed so far in some PD patients.[279–283]

▶ BASAL GANGLIA OUTFLOW TO THE THALAMUS AND BRAIN STEM

The GPi and the SNr are known as the main output nuclei of the basal ganglia. They receive functionally segregated striatal inputs and send this information through axonal projections that collateralize to thalamic and brain stem targets (Fig. 4–4). The anatomical organization of GPi and SNr outflow will now be discussed, and the role of these projections in the transmission and processing of basal ganglia information through cortical and subcortical loops in normal and pathological conditions will be examined.

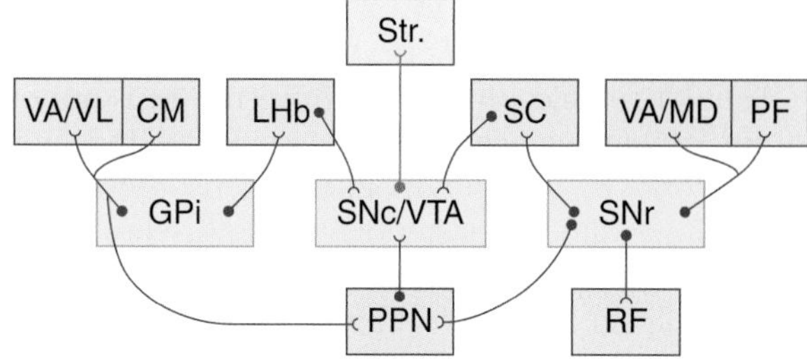

Figure 4–4. Main output projections of the GPi and SNr. This diagram also illustrates some of the subcortical inputs to SNc/VTA dopaminergic neurons that have been considered as sources of reward- or sensory-related influences to midbrain dopaminergic neurons. Abbreviations: CM, centromedian nucleus; GPi, globus pallidus internal segment; LHb, lateral habenular nucleus; MD, mediodorsal nucleus; PF, parafascicular nucleus; PPN, pedunculopontine nucleus; RF, reticular formation; SC, superior colliculus; SNc, substantia nigra compacta; SNr, substantia nigra pars reticulata; Str, striatum; VA, ventral anterior nucleus; VL, ventral lateral nucleus; VTA, ventral tegmental area.

EFFERENT PROJECTIONS OF GPi

The primate GPi comprises two major types of projection neurons; the type I neurons project to the thalamus and PPN, whereas the type II neurons that lie along the border of GPi project to the lateral habenula with rare collaterals to the anterior thalamic nuclei (see below).[284] The organization of these projections will now be discussed in further detail.

The Pallidothalamic Projection

The pallidothalamic projection travels via the ansa lenticularis and lenticular fasciculus to the ventral anterior/ventral lateral (VA/VL) nuclei,[1,285,286] where it arborizes in a topographic fashion. There is some controversy regarding the exact origin of axons that make up the two major pallidal outflow systems. Some studies concluded that neurons in the caudal sensorimotor portion of the GPi travel medially through the lenticular fasciculus to reach their thalamic target, whereas axonal projections from rostral GPi neurons form the ansa lenticularis.[287] This scheme is far simpler than that proposed in other studies, suggesting that fibers coursing through the ansa lenticularis frequently follow lengthy courses through the caudorostral extent of GPi to reach the thalamus.[284,288] This discrepancy may result from the high degree of neuronal heterogeneity in the primate GPi.[284]

The delineation is critical toward effective surgical treatment of various movement disorders.[287]

Pallidothalamic projections from the sensorimotor GPi are largely segregated from associative and limbic GPi outflow. In squirrel monkeys, sensorimotor GPi neurons innervate the posterior VL (VLp), whereas projections from the associative and limbic GPi terminate preferentially in the parvocellular VA (VApc) and the dorsal VL (VLd). The limbic GPi also projects to the ventromedial nucleus.[98,285,286]

The pallidal-, nigral-, and cerebellar-receiving territories are largely segregated in the primate thalamus, while they slightly overlap in rodents.[289–291] Although both pallidothalamic and cerebellothalamic outflow gains access to primary, supplementary, and pre-motor cortices,[1,3–5,292–294] the sources of GPi or cerebellar projections to specific motor cortical areas are largely segregated and quantitatively different, so that the degree of GPi innervation of thalamocortical neurons that project to the supplementary and presupplementary motor areas is more prominent than that of projections from the cerebellar dentate nucleus to these cortical regions.[292] The differential level of calbindin D28K immunoreactivity serves as landmarks between GPi and cerebellar termination sites in VL.[285] The pallidothalamic projection is mainly ipsilateral, although a significant 10–20% of pallidothalamic neurons project to the contralateral VA/VL.[295]

The axonal projections of most sensorimotor GPi neurons that project to the VA/VL collateralize to the CM (Figs. 4–1 and 4–4) where they target thalamostriatal neurons projecting back to the sensorimotor striatal territory (i.e., the post-commissural putamen). Similarly, the associative GPi innervates the dorsolateral extension of PF (PFdl), which projects back to the pre-commissural associative territory of the putamen, while the limbic GPi innervates the rostrodorsal PF, which, in turn, sends projections to the nucleus accumbens. Through these projections, the CM/PF is integrated into closed and open basal ganglia–thalamostriatal loops that run in parallel with the basal ganglia–thalamocortical system[14,37,296] (Fig. 4–1).

The Pallidotegmental Projection

The PPN is the main target of descending pallidotegmental fibers. In nonhuman primates, as much as 80% of GPi neurons projecting to the PPN send axon collaterals to the VA/VL (Fig. 4–4). In contrast to the thalamus, where motor, associative, and limbic information is largely segregated, a higher degree of functional convergence at the level of individual PPN neurons has been described in the PPN.[297] The medial pars diffusa of the PPN is the principal site of termination of basal ganglia outflow from GPi and SNr, suggesting that some of these PPN neurons may send the projection back to the basal ganglia, thereby forming additional subcortical loops integrated within the basal ganglia circuitry.[254,256,258,297]

The Pallidohabenular Projection

The pallidohabenular projection originates from a distinct population of neurons located along the borders of GPi in nonhuman primates.[1,284] In light of recent tracing studies in primates, the pallidohabenular projection is functionally organized and more massive than previously thought.[284] The sensorimotor GPi projects to the centrolateral part of the lateral habenular nucleus, whereas the limbic and the associative GPi innervate the medial part of the nucleus.[297a] Although the pallidohabenular projection is mainly GABAergic like other GPi output systems, a subset of cholinergic neurons also give rise to this projection in rats.[298,299] In light of its close connections with the GPi and various limbic structures, the lateral habenula is considered as a functional interface between the limbic system and the basal ganglia.[300–306,306a]

The lateral habenula is a significant source of glutamatergic projections to VTA dopaminergic neurons.[300,307,307a] Although the functional anatomy of this network has been carefully studied in rodents, much remains to be characterized in primates (Fig. 4–4). In primates, GPi neurons convey reward-related signals to the lateral habenula, which then influences the striatum and other basal ganglia nuclei through regulation of dopaminergic and serotonergic systems[305] (Fig. 4–4). The lateral habenula is also involved in learning, memory, and attention.[308,309] Because of its close relationships with monoaminergic systems, the lateral habenula is considered as a potential target site for DBS in patients with severe depression.[310]

EFFERENT PROJECTIONS OF SNr

The Nigrothalamic Projection

In primates, SNr and GPi inputs to the ventral thalamus are largely segregated from each other and from cerebellar projections.[289] In nonhuman primates, the nigrothalamic cells account for the largest population of nigrofugal neurons. Projections from the medial part of the SNr terminate mostly in the medial magnocellular division of the VA (VAmc) and the mediodorsal nucleus (MDmc) that, in turn, project to anterior regions of the frontal lobe, including the principal sulcus and the orbital cortex.[1,11,311–316]

Neurons in the lateral SNr innervate preferentially to the lateral posterior sector of the VAmc and different parts of MD mostly related to posterior regions of the frontal lobe, including the frontal eye field areas of the pre-motor cortex (Fig. 4–4). SNr outflow also targets thalamocortical neurons that project to the area TE in the inferotemporal cortex, providing a substrate through which basal ganglia can influence high-order visual processing.[315] Dysfunctions in this system may, therefore, result in alterations in visual perceptions, including visual hallucinations in some basal ganglia disorders.

In rats, functionally segregated striatal neurons innervate different lamella of SNr neurons, which, in turn, project to different thalamic nuclei. The dendrites of individual SNr neurons largely conform to the geometry of striatonigral projections, which strongly supports the concept of a parallel architecture of striatonigral circuits.[317–319] SNr neurons also innervate rostral and caudal intralaminar thalamic nuclei. In monkeys, SNr projections terminate in PF where they form synapses with thalamostriatal neurons that project to the caudate nucleus.[14,37,296]

The Nigrotegmental Projection

The nigrotegmental projection has not been studied in detail in primates, but in rats it displays a dorsoventral topography and terminates preferentially on non-cholinergic neurons in the medial two-thirds of the PPNd.[320,321] In monkeys, nigrotegmental cells are found throughout the mediolateral extent of the SNr, and most send axon collaterals to the ventral anterior thalamic nucleus[1,311] (Fig. 4–4).

The Nigrocollicular Projection

The nigrocollicular projection is massive and terminates in the intermediate layer of the superior colliculus where nigral terminals form distinctive clusters that innervate neurons that project to the spinal cord, medulla, and periabducens area (Fig. 4–4). This projection controls saccadic eye movements toward auditory or visual stimuli,[18,32,322–324] which is consistent with the fact that collicular neurons targeted by SNr projections also receive visual inputs from the cerebral cortex and project to tegmental regions that control eye movements.

In turn, the superior colliculus projects to SNc dopaminergic neurons in rats and primates.[325–330] This projection is considered as a prime source of sensory-related events to dopaminergic nigrostriatal neurons, thereby suggesting that the phasic responses of midbrain dopaminergic neurons in complex tasks may be related to "sensory prediction errors" instead of "reward prediction errors"[331–339] (Fig. 4–4).

The Nigroreticular Projection

The SNr also sends projections to the medullary reticular formation. In rats, this projection originates from neurons in the dorsolateral SNr and terminates in the parvicellular reticular formation. Nigroreticular neurons receive GABAergic inputs from the striatum and the GP. This projection most likely plays a role in controlling orofacial movements because reticular neurons that receive SNr inputs project to orofacial motor nuclei.[340–342]

▶ CONCLUDING REMARKS

Our understanding of the functional anatomy of the basal ganglia has grown substantially over the past decades, which led to significant changes in our current view of basal ganglia functioning under normal and pathological conditions. Although the exact role of basal ganglia remains highly speculative, there is a general consensus that these brain regions are endowed with highly complex integrative properties of information that extends far beyond the sensorimotor domain. The close interconnections between basal ganglia nuclei and associative or limbic cortical areas provide a solid substrate through which integration and processing of non-motor information can be performed. The complex non-motor symptomatology of basal ganglia diseases is another indication that functional changes in cortical and subcortical basal ganglia–related networks may encompass multifarious motor and non-motor deficits, which, in many cases, also include complex neuropsychiatric symptoms. The recent evidence that DBS of the STN in PD may result in complex neuropsychiatric and cognitive changes is another evidence for basal ganglia regulation of non-motor functional modalities. The continued development of sensitive neuroanatomical tracing methods and brain imaging techniques should provide the necessary tools to deepen our understanding of the neuronal micro- and macrocircuits that should be targeted to further improve the outcome of basal ganglia disorder therapies.

▶ ACKNOWLEDGMENTS

The author thanks Adriana Galvan for her help in the preparation of figures and various members of my laboratory who have contributed to the original publication of some of the data discussed in this chapter. Thanks are also due the various funding agencies that have contributed to the support of research from my laboratory, discussed in this chapter, including the National Institute of Neurologic Disease and Stroke (NINDS), National Parkinson Foundation and Tourette Syndrome Association. I am also grateful to the continued support from the Yerkes National Primate Research Center NIH base grant.

REFERENCES

1. Parent A, Hazrati LN. Functional anatomy of the basal ganglia. I. The cortico-basal ganglia-thalamo-cortical loop. Brain Res Rev 1995;20:91.
2. Gerfen CR, Wilson CJ. The basal ganglia. In Björklund A, Hökfelt T, Swanson L (eds). Handbook of Chemical Neuroanatomy, Integrated Systems of the CNS, Part iii. Amsterdam: Elsevier, 1996, p. 369.
3. Middleton FA, Strick PL. New concepts about the organization of basal ganglia output. Adv Neurol 1997;74:57.

4. Middleton FA, Strick PL. Basal ganglia output and cognition: Evidence from anatomical, behavioral, and clinical studies. Brain Cogn 2000;42:183.
5. Middleton FA, Strick PL. Basal ganglia and cerebellar loops: Motor and cognitive circuits. Brain Res Rev 2000;31:236.
6. Nicola SM, Surmeier J, Malenka RC. Dopaminergic modulation of neuronal excitability in the striatum and nucleus accumbens. Annu Rev Neurosci 2000;23:185.
7. Gerfen CR. Dopamine-mediated gene regulation in models of Parkinson's disease. Ann Neurol 2000;47:S42.
8. Parent A, Sato F, Wu Y, et al. Organization of the basal ganglia: The importance of axonal collateralization. Trends Neurosci 2000;23:S20.
9. Smith Y, Kieval JZ. Anatomy of the dopamine system in the basal ganglia. Trends Neurosci 2000;23:S28.
10. Bevan MD, Magill PJ, Terman D, et al. Move to the rhythm: Oscillations in the subthalamic nucleus-external globus pallidus network. Trends Neurosci 2002; 25:525.
11. Afifi AK. The basal ganglia: A neural network with more than motor function. Semin Pediatr Neurol 2003;10:3.
12. Graybiel AM. Network-level neuroplasticity in cortico-basal ganglia pathways. Parkinsonism Relat Disord 2004;10:293.
13. Kelly RM, Strick PL. Macro-architecture of basal ganglia loops with the cerebral cortex: Use of rabies virus to reveal multisynaptic circuits. Prog Brain Res 2004;143:449.
14. Smith Y, Raju DV, Pare JF, et al. The thalamostriatal system: A highly specific network of the basal ganglia circuitry. Trends Neurosci 2004;27:520.
15. Tepper JM, Bolam JP. Functional diversity and specificity of neostriatal interneurons. Curr Opin Neurobiol 2004;14:685.
16. Tepper JM, Koos T, Wilson CJ. GABAergic microcircuits in the neostriatum. Trends Neurosci 2004;27:662.
17. Tepper JM, Abercrombie ED, Bolam JP. Basal ganglia macrocircuits. Prog Brain Res 2007;160:3.
18. McHaffie JG, Stanford TR, Stein BE, et al. Subcortical loops through the basal ganglia. Trends Neurosci 2005;28:401.
19. Boyes J, Bolam JP. Localization of GABA receptors in the basal ganglia. Prog Brain Res 2007;160:229.
20. Hammond C, Bergman H, Brown P. Pathological synchronization in Parkinson's disease: Networks, models and treatments. Trends Neurosci 2007; 30:357.
21. Wichmann T, Delong MR. Anatomy and physiology of the basal ganglia: Relevance to Parkinson's disease and related disorders. Handb Clin Neurol 2007;83:1.
22. Graybiel AM. The basal ganglia: Learning new tricks and loving it. Curr Opin Neurobiol 15:638.
23. Graybiel AM. Habits, rituals, and the evaluative brain. Annu Rev Neurosci 2008;31:359.
24. Pisani A, Bernardi G, Ding J, et al. Re-emergence of striatal cholinergic interneurons in movement disorders. Trends Neurosci 2007;30:545.
25. Surmeier DJ, Ding J, Day M, et al. D1 and D2 dopamine-receptor modulation of striatal glutamatergic signaling in striatal medium spiny neurons. Trends Neurosci 2007;30:228.
26. Wilson CJ. GABAergic inhibition in the neostriatum. Prog Brain Res 2007;160:91.
27. Haber SN. The primate basal ganglia: Parallel and integrative networks. J Chem Neuroanat 2003;26:317.
28. Haber S. Parallel and integrative processing through the Basal Ganglia reward circuit: Lessons from addiction. Biol Psychiatry 2008;64:173.
29. Braak H, Del Tredici K. Cortico-basal ganglia-cortical circuitry in Parkinson's disease reconsidered. Exp Neuro 2008;212:226.
30. Israel Z, Bergman H. Pathophysiology of the basal ganglia and movement disorders: From animal models to human clinical applications. Neurosci Biobehav Rev 2008;32:367.
31. Obeso JA, Rodriguez-Oroz MC, Benitez-Temino B, et al. Functional organization of the basal ganglia: Therapeutic implications for Parkinson's disease. Mov Disord 2008;23(suppl 3):S548.
32. Redgrave P, Gurney K, Reynolds J. What is reinforced by phasic dopamine signals? Brain Res. Rev 2008;58:322.
33. Smith Y, Villalba R. Striatal and extrastriatal dopamine in the basal ganglia: An overview of its anatomical organization in normal and Parkinsonian brains. Mov Disord 2008;23(suppl 3):S534.
34. Tepper JM, Wilson CJ, Koos T. Feedforward and feedback inhibition in neostriatal GABAergic spiny neurons. Brain Res Rev 2008;58:272.
35. Yelnik J. Modeling the organization of the basal ganglia. Rev Neurol (Paris) 2008;164:969.
36. Nambu A. Seven problems on the basal ganglia. Curr Opin Neurobiol 2008;18:595.
37. Smith Y, Raju D, Nanda B, et al. The thalamostriatal systems: Anatomical and functional organization in normal and parkinsonian states. Brain Res Bul 2009;78:60.
38. Haber SN, Gdowski MJ. The basal ganglia. In Paxinos G, Mai JK (eds). The Human Nervous System, 2nd ed. Amsterdam: Elsevier Academic Press, 2004, p. 677.
39. Schultz W. Behavioral theories and the neurophysiology of reward. Annu Rev Psychol 2006;57:87.
40. Schultz W. Multiple dopamine functions at different time courses. Annu Rev Neurosci 2007;30:259.
41. Schultz W. Behavioral dopamine signals. Trends Neurosci 2007;30:203.
42. Balaz M, Rektor I, Pulkrabek J. Participation of the subthalamic nucleus in executive functions: An intracerebral recording study. Mov Disord 2008;23:553.
43. Benabid AL, Chabardes S, Mitrofanis J, et al. Deep brain stimulation of the subthalamic nucleus for the treatment of Parkinson's disease. Lancet Neurol 2009;8:67.
44. Benarroch EE. Subthalamic nucleus and its connections: Anatomic substrate for the network effects of deep brain stimulation. Neurology 2009;70:1991,2008
45. DeLong MR, Wichmann T. Deep brain stimulation for Parkinson's disease. Ann Neurol 2001;49:142.
46. Limousin P, Martinez-Torres I. Deep brain stimulation for Parkinson's disease. Neurotherapeutics 2008;5:309.
47. Lozano AM, Snyder BJ. Deep brain stimulation for parkinsonian gait disorders. J Neurol 2008;255(suppl 4):30.
48. Temel Y. Subthalamic nucleus stimulation in Parkinson's disease: The other side of the medallion. Exp Neurol 2008;211:321.
49. Tommasi G, Krack P, Fraix V, et al. Pyramidal tract side effects induced by deep brain stimulation of the

subthalamic nucleus. J Neurol Neurosurg. Psychiatry 2008; 79:813.

50. Videnovic A, Metman LV. Deep brain stimulation for Parkinson's disease: Prevalence of adverse events and need for standardized reporting. Mov Disord 2008;23:343.
51. Wichmann T, Delong MR. Deep brain stimulation for neurologic and neuropsychiatric disorders. Neuron 2006;52:197.
52. Yu H, Neimat JS. The treatment of movement disorders by deep brain stimulation. Neurotherapeutics 2008;5:26.
53. Graybiel AM. Neurotransmitters and neuromodulators in the basal ganglia. Trends Neurosci 1990;13:244.
54. Saka E, Graybiel AM. Pathophysiology of Tourette's syndrome: Striatal pathways revisited. Brain Dev 2003;25(suppl 1):S15.
55. Saka E, Goodrich C, Harlan P. Repetitive behaviors in monkeys are linked to specific striatal activation patterns. J Neurosci 2004;24:7557.
56. Canales JJ, Graybiel AM. A measure of striatal function predicts motor stereotypy. Nat Neurosci 2000;3:377.
57. Canales JJ. Stimulant-induced adaptations in neostriatal matrix and striosome systems: Transiting from instrumental responding to habitual behavior in drug addiction. Neurobiol Learn Mem 2005;83:93.
58. Crittenden JR, Cantuti-Castelvetri I, Saka E, et al. Dysregulation of CalDAG-GEFI and CalDAG-GEFII predicts the severity of motor side-effects induced by anti-parkinsonian therapy. Proc Natl Acad Sci USA 2009;106:2973.
59. Goto S, Lee LV, Munoz EL, et al. Functional anatomy of the basal ganglia in X-linked recessive dystonia-parkinsonism. Ann Neurol 2005;58:7.
60. Sato K, Sumi-Ichinose C, Kaji R, et al. Differential involvement of striosome and matrix dopamine systems in a transgenic model of dopa-responsive dystonia. Proc Natl Acad Sci USA 2008;105:12551.
61. Tippett LJ, Waldvogel HJ, Thomas SJ, et al. Striosomes and mood dysfunction in Huntington's disease. Brain 2007;130:206.
62. Oorschot DE. Total number of neurons in the neostriatal, pallidal, subthalamic, and substantia nigral nuclei of the rat basal ganglia: A stereological study using the cavalieri and optical dissector methods. J Comp Neurol 1996; 366:580.
63. Gertler TS, Chan CS, Surmeier DJ. Dichotomous anatomical properties of adult striatal medium spiny neurons. J Neurosci 2008;28:10814.
64. Kreitzer AC, Malenka RC. Endocannabinoid-mediated rescue of striatal LTD and motor deficits in Parkinson's disease models. Nature 2007;445:643.
65. Cepeda C, Andre VM, Yamazaki I, et al. Differential electrophysiological properties of dopamine D1 and D2 receptor-containing striatal medium-sized spiny neurons. Eur J Neurosci 2008;27:671.
66. Day M, Wokosin D, Plotkin JL, et al. Differential excitability and modulation of striatal medium spiny neuron dendrites. J Neurosci 2008;28:11603.
67. Ingham CA, Hood SH, Arbuthnott GW. Spine density on neostriatal neurones changes with 6-hydroxydopamine lesions and with age. Brain Res 1989;503:334.
68. Day M, Wang Z, Ding J, et al. Selective elimination of glutamatergic synapses on striatopallidal neurons in Parkinson disease models. Nat Neurosci 2006;9:251.
69. Wickens JR, Arbuthnott GW, Shindou T. Simulation of GABA function in the basal ganglia: Computational models of GABAergic mechanisms in basal ganglia function. Prog Brain Res 2007;160:313.
70. Villalba RM, Lee H, Smith Y. Dopaminergic denervation and spine loss in the striatum of MPTP-treated monkeys. Exp Neurol 2009;215:220.
71. Wilson CJ, Groves PM. Fine structure and synaptic connections of the common spiny neuron of the rat neostriatum: A study employing intracellular inject of horseradish peroxidase. J Comp Neurol 1980;194:599.
72. Jaeger D, Kita H, Wilson CJ. Surround inhibition among projection neurons is weak or nonexistent in the rat neostriatum. J Neurophysiol 1994;72:2555.
73. Koos T, Tepper JM, Wilson CJ. Comparison of IPSCs evoked by spiny and fast-spiking neurons in the neostriatum. J Neurosci 2004;24:7916.
74. Taverna S, Ilijic E, Surmeier DJ. Recurrent collateral connections of striatal medium spiny neurons are disrupted in models of Parkinson's disease. J Neurosci 2008;28:5504.
75. Graveland GA, DiFiglia M. The frequency and distribution of medium-sized neurons with indented nuclei in the primate and rodent neostriatum. Brain Res 1985;327:307.
76. Kawaguchi Y, Wilson CJ, Augood SJ, et al. Striatal interneurones: Chemical, physiological and morphological characterization. Trends Neurosci 1995;18:527.
77. Aosaki T, Graybiel AM, Kimura M. Effect of the nigrostriatal dopamine system on acquired neural responses in the striatum of behaving monkeys. Science 1994;265:412.
78. Aosaki T, Tsubokawa H, Ishida A, et al. Responses of tonically active neurons in the primate's striatum undergo systematic changes during behavioral sensorimotor conditioning. J Neurosci 1994;14:3969.
79. Bennett BD, Wilson CJ. Spontaneous activity of neostriatal cholinergic interneurons in vitro. J Neurosci 1999;19:5586.
80. Cicchetti F, Beach TG, Parent A. Chemical phenotype of calretinin interneurons in the human striatum. Synapse 1998;30:284.
81. Smith AD, Bolam JP. The neural network of the basal ganglia as revealed by the study of synaptic connections of identified neurones. Trends Neurosci 1990;13:259.
82. Graybiel AM, Aosaki T, Flaherty AW. The basal ganglia and adaptive motor control. Science 1994;265:1826.
83. Kimura M, Yamada H, Matsumoto N. Tonically active neurons in the striatum encode motivational contexts of action. Brain Dev 2003;25(suppl 1):S20.
84. Kimura M, Matsumoto N, Okahashi K. Goal-directed, serial and synchronous activation of neurons in the primate striatum. Neurorepor 2003;14:799.
85. Yamada H, Matsumoto N, Kimura M. Tonically active neurons in the primate caudate nucleus and putamen differentially encode instructed motivational outcomes of action. J Neurosci 2004;24:3500.
86. Apicella P. Leading tonically active neurons of the striatum from reward detection to context recognition. Trends Neurosci 2007;30:299.
87. Tan CO, Bullock D. A dopamine-acetylcholine cascade: Simulating learned and lesion-induced behavior of striatal cholinergic interneurons. J Neurophysiol 2008;100:2409.

88. Joshua M, Adler A, Mitelman R. Midbrain dopaminergic neurons and striatal cholinergic interneurons encode the difference between reward and aversive events at different epochs of probabilistic classical conditioning trials. J Neurosci 2008;28:11673.
89. Joshua M, Adler A, Rosin B. Encoding of probabilistic rewarding and aversive events by pallidal and nigral neurons. J Neurophysiol 2009;101:758.
90. Sullivan MA, Chen H, Morikawa H. Recurrent inhibitory network among striatal cholinergic interneurons. J Neurosci 2008;28:8682.
91. Wang Z, Kai L, Day M, et al. Dopaminergic control of corticostriatal long-term synaptic depression in medium spiny neurons is mediated by cholinergic interneurons. Neuron 2006;50:443.
92. Shen W, Tian X, Day M, et al. Cholinergic modulation of Kir2 channels selectively elevates dendritic excitability in striatopallidal neurons. Nat Neurosci 2007;10:1458.
93. Ding J, Guzman JN, Tkatch T, et al. RGS4-dependent attenuation of M4 autoreceptor function in striatal cholinergic interneurons following dopamine depletion. Nat Neurosci 2006;9:832.
94. Maurice N, Mercer J, Chan CS, et al. D2 dopamine receptor-mediated modulation of voltage-dependent Na+ channels reduces autonomous activity in striatal cholinergic interneurons. J Neurosci 2004;24:10289.
95. Cabrera-Vera TM, Hernandez S, Earls LR, et al. RGS9-2 modulates D2 dopamine receptor-mediated Ca^{2+} channel inhibition in rat striatal cholinergic interneurons. Proc Natl Acad Sci USA 2004;101:16339.
96. Berke JD. Uncoordinated firing rate changes of striatal fast-spiking interneurons during behavioral task performance. J Neurosci 2008;28:10075.
97. Galarraga E, Vilchis C, Tkatch T, et al. Somatostatinergic modulation of firing pattern and calcium-activated potassium currents in medium spiny neostriatal neurons. Neuroscience 2007;146:537.
98. Alexander GE, DeLong MR, Strick PL. Parallel organization of functionally segregated circuits linking basal ganglia and cortex. Annu Rev Neurosci 1986;9:357.
99. Gerfen CR. The neostriatal mosaic: Compartmentalization of corticostriatal input and striatonigral output systems. Nature 1984;311:461.
100. McGeorge AJ, Faull RL. The organization of the projection from the cerebral cortex to the striatum in the rat. Neuroscience 1989;29:503.
101. Reep RL, Cheatwood JL, Corwin JV. The associative striatum: Organization of cortical projections to the dorsocentral striatum in rats. J Comp Neurol 2003;467:271.
102. Alloway KD, Lou L, Nwabueze-Ogbo F, et al. Topography of cortical projections to the dorsolateral neostriatum in rats: Multiple overlapping sensorimotor pathways. J Comp Neurol 2006;499:33.
103. McHaffie JG, Thomson CM, Stein BE. Corticotectal and corticostriatal projections from the frontal eye fields of the cat: An anatomical examination using WGA-HRP. Somatosens Mot Res 2001;18:117.
104. Gerardin E, Lehericy S, Pochon JB, et al. Foot, hand, face and eye representation in the human striatum. Cereb Cortex 2003;13:162.
105. Lehericy S, Ducros M, Krainik A, et al. 3-D diffusion tensor axonal tracking shows distinct SMA and pre-SMA projections to the human striatum. Cereb Cortex 2004;14:1302.
106. Lehericy S, Ducros M, Van de Moortele PF, et al. Diffusion tensor fiber tracking shows distinct corticostriatal circuits in humans. Ann Neurol 2004;55:522.
107. Wiesendanger E, Clarke S, Kraftsik R, et al. Topography of cortico-striatal connections in man: Anatomical evidence for parallel organization. Eur J Neurosci 2004;20:1915.
108. Postuma RB, Dagher A. Basal ganglia functional connectivity based on a meta-analysis of 126 positron emission tomography and functional magnetic resonance imaging publications. Cereb Cortex 2006;16:1508.
109. Dominey PF, Inui T, Hoen M. Neural network processing of natural language: II. Towards a unified model of corticostriatal function in learning sentence comprehension and non-linguistic sequencing. Brain Lang 2009; 109:80.
110. Nagano-Saito A, Leyton M, Monchi O. Dopamine depletion impairs frontostriatal functional connectivity during a set-shifting task. J Neurosci 2008;28:3697.
111. Seger CA. How do the basal ganglia contribute to categorization? Their roles in generalization, response selection, and learning via feedback. Neurosci. Biobehav. Rev 2008;32:265.
112. Nakano K, Kayahara T, Tsutsumi T. Neural circuits and functional organization of the striatum. J Neurol 2000;247(suppl 5):V1.
113. Nakano K. Neural circuits and topographic organization of the basal ganglia and related regions. Brain Dev 2000;22(suppl 1):S5.
114. Haber SN, Kim KS, Mailly P, et al. Reward-related cortical inputs define a large striatal region in primates that interface with associative cortical connections, providing a substrate for incentive-based learning. J Neurosci 2006;26:8368.
115. Calzavara R, Mailly P, Haber SN. Relationship between the corticostriatal terminals from areas 9 and 46, and those from area 8A, dorsal and rostral premotor cortex and area 24c: An anatomical substrate for cognition to action. Eur J Neurosci 2007;26:2005.
116. Yeterian EH, Van Hoesen GW. Cortico-striate projections in the rhesus monkey: The organization of certain cortico-caudate connections. Brain Res 1978;139:43.
117. Selemon LD, Goldman-Rakic PS. Longitudinal topography and interdigitation of corticostriatal projections in the rhesus monkey. J Neurosci 1985;5:776.
118. Parthasarathy HB, Schall JD, Graybiel AM. Distributed but convergent ordering of corticostriatal projections: Analysis of the frontal eye field and the supplementary eye field in the macaque monkey. J Neurosci 1992;12:4468.
119. Flaherty AW, Graybiel AM. Two input systems for body representations in the primate striatal matrix: Experimental evidence in the squirrel monkey. J Neurosci 1993;13:1120.
120. Reiner A, Jiao Y, Del Mar N, et al. Differential morphology of pyramidal tract-type and intratelencephalically projecting-type corticostriatal neurons and their intrastriatal terminals in rats. J Comp Neurol 2003;457:420.
121. Lei W, Jiao Y, Del Mar N, et al. Evidence for differential cortical input to direct pathway versus indirect

pathway striatal projection neurons in rats. J Neurosci 2004;24:8289.

122. Ballion B, Mallet N, Bezard E, et al. Intratelencephalic corticostriatal neurons equally excite striatonigral and striatopallidal neurons and their discharge activity is selectively reduced in experimental parkinsonism. Eur J Neurosci 2008;27:2313.
123. Jones EG, Coulter JD, Burton H, et al. Cells of origin and terminal distribution of corticostriatal fibers arising in the sensory-motor cortex of monkeys. J Comp Neurol 1997;173:53.
124. Turner RS, DeLong MR. Corticostriatal activity in primary motor cortex of the macaque. J Neurosci 2000;20:7096.
125. Parent M, Parent A. Single-axon tracing study of corticostriatal projections arising from primary motor cortex in primates. J Comp Neurol 2006;496:202.
126. Kemp JM, Powell TP. The termination of fibres from the cerebral cortex and thalamus upon dendritic spines in the caudate nucleus: A study with the Golgi method. Philos Trans R Soc Lond B Biol Sci 1971;262:429.
127. Lapper SR, Smith Y, Sadikot AF, et al. Cortical input to parvalbumin-immunoreactive neurones in the putamen of the squirrel monkey. Brain Res 1992;580:215.
128. Mallet N, Le Moine C, Charpier S, et al. Feedforward inhibition of projection neurons by fast-spiking GABA interneurons in the rat striatum in vivo. J Neurosci 2005;25:3857.
129. Mallet N, Ballion B, Le Moine C, et al. Cortical inputs and GABA interneurons imbalance projection neurons in the striatum of parkinsonian rats. J Neurosci 2006;26:3875.
130. Parent M, Parent A. Single-axon tracing and three-dimensional reconstruction of centre median-parafascicular thalamic neurons in primates. J Comp Neurol 2005;481:127.
131. Sadikot AF, Parent A, Francois C. Efferent connections of the centromedian and parafascicular thalamic nuclei in the squirrel monkey: A PHA-L study of subcortical projections. J Comp Neurol 1992;315:137.
132. Sidibe M, Smith Y. Differential synaptic innervation of striatofugal neurones projecting to the internal or external segments of the globus pallidus by thalamic afferents in the squirrel monkey. J Comp Neurol 1996;365:445.
133. Raju DV, Shah DJ, Wright TM, et al. Differential synaptology of vGluT2-containing thalamostriatal afferents between the patch and matrix compartments in rats. J Comp Neurol 2006;499:231.
134. Sidibe M, Smith Y. Thalamic inputs to striatal interneurons in monkeys: Synaptic organization and co-localization of calcium binding proteins. Neuroscience 1999;89:1189.
135. Wilson CJ, Chang HT, Kitai ST. Origins of post synaptic potentials evoked in spiny neostriatal projection neurons by thalamic stimulation in the rat. Exp Brain Res 1983;51:217.
136. Zackheim J, Abercrombie ED. Thalamic regulation of striatal acetylcholine efflux is both direct and indirect and qualitatively altered in the dopamine-depleted striatum. Neuroscience 2005;131:423.
137. Nanda B, Galvan A, Smith Y, et al. Effects of stimulation of the centromedian nucleus of the thalamus on the activity of striatal cells in awake rhesus monkeys. Eur J Neurosci 2009;29:588.
138. Minamimoto T, Kimura M. Participation of the thalamic CM-Pf complex in attentional orienting. J Neurophysiol 2002; 87:3090.
139. Minamimoto T, Hori Y, Kimura M. Complementary process to response bias in the centromedian nucleus of the thalamus. Science 2005;308:1798.
140. Kimura M, Minamimoto T, Matsumoto N, et al. Monitoring and switching of cortico-basal ganglia loop functions by the thalamo-striatal system. Neurosci Res 2004;48:355.
141. Groenewegen HJ, Berendse HW. The specificity of the 'nonspecific' midline and intralaminar thalamic nuclei. Trends Neurosci 1994;17:52
142. McFarland NR, Haber SN. Convergent inputs from thalamic motor nuclei and frontal cortical areas to the dorsal striatum in the primate. J Neurosci 1994;20:3798.
143. Haber SN, Calzavara R. The cortico-basal ganglia integrative network: The role of the thalamus. Brain Res Bull. 2009;78:69.
144. Lacey CJ, Bolam JP, Magill PJ. Novel and distinct operational principles of intralaminar thalamic neurons and their striatal projections. J Neurosci 2007;27:4374.
145. Raju DV, Ahern TH, Shah DJ, et al. Differential synaptic plasticity of the corticostriatal and thalamostriatal systems in an MPTP-treated monkey model of parkinsonism. Eur J Neurosci 2008;27:1647.
146. Sadikot AF, Parent A, Smith Y, et al. Efferent connections of the centromedian and parafascicular thalamic nuclei in the squirrel monkey: A light and electron microscopic study of the thalamostriatal projection in relation to striatal heterogeneity. J Comp Neurol 1992;320:228.
147. Raju DV, Smith Y. Differential localization of vesicular glutamate transporters 1 and 2 in the rat striatum. In Bolam JP, Ingham CA, Magill P J (eds). The Basal Ganglia VIII. New York: Springer, 2005 p. 601.
148. Kinomura S, Larsson J, Gulyas B, et al. Activation by attention of the human reticular formation and thalamic intralaminar nuclei. Science 1996;271:512.
149. Schiff ND, Giacino JT, Kalmar K A, et al. Behavioural improvements with thalamic stimulation after severe traumatic brain injury. Nature 2007;448:600.
150. Mair RG, Hembrook JR. Memory enhancement with event-related stimulation of the rostral intralaminar thalamic nuclei. J Neurosci 2008;28:14293.
151. Haber S, McFarland NR. The place of the thalamus in frontal cortical-basal ganglia circuits. Neuroscientist 2001;7:315.
152. Henderson JM, Carpenter K, Cartwright H, et al. Loss of thalamic intralaminar nuclei in progressive supranuclear palsy and Parkinson's disease: Clinical and therapeutic implications. Brain 2000;123 (Pt 7):1410.
153. Henderson JM, Carpenter K, Cartwright H, et al. Degeneration of the centre median-parafascicular complex in Parkinson's disease. Ann Neurol 2000;47:345.
154. McKeown MJ, Uthama A, Abugharbieh R, et al. Shape (but not volume) changes in the thalami in Parkinson disease. BMC Neurol 2008;8:8.
155. Seroogy K, Ceccatelli S, Schalling M, et al. A subpopulation of dopaminergic neurons in rat ventral mesencephalon contains both neurotensin and cholecystokinin. Brain Res 1988;455:88.

156. Seroogy KB, Dangaran K, Lim S, et al. Ventral mesencephalic neurons containing both cholecystokinin- and tyrosine hydroxylase-like immunoreactivities project to forebrain regions. J Comp Neuro 1989;279:397.
157. Seutin V. Dopaminergic neurones: Much more than dopamine? Br J Pharmacol 2005;146:167.
158. Binder EB, Kinkead B, Owens MJ, et al. Neurotensin and dopamine interactions. Pharmacol Rev 2001;53:453.
159. Haber SN, Ryoo H, Cox C, et al. Subsets of midbrain dopaminergic neurons in monkeys are distinguished by different levels of mRNA for the dopamine transporter: Comparison with the mRNA for the D2 receptor, tyrosine hydroxylase and calbindin immunoreactivity. J Comp Neuro 1995;362:400.
160. Sanghera MK, Manaye K, McMahon A, et al. Dopamine transporter mRNA levels are high in midbrain neurons vulnerable to MPTP. Neuroreport 1997;8:3327.
161. Bezard E, Gross CE, Fournier MC, et al. Absence of MPTP-induced neuronal death in mice lacking the dopamine transporter. Exp Neurol 1999;155:268.
162. Gerfen CR, Baimbridge KG, Miller JJ. The neostriatal mosaic: compartmental distribution of calcium-binding protein and parvalbumin in the basal ganglia of the rat and monkey. Proc Natl Acad Sci USA 1985;82:8780.
163. Yamada T, McGeer PL, Baimbridge KG, et al. Relative sparing in Parkinson's disease of substantia nigra dopamine neurons containing calbindin-D28K. Brain Res 1990;526:303.
164. Damier P, Hirsch EC, Agid Y, et al. The substantia nigra of the human brain. II. Patterns of loss of dopamine-containing neurons in Parkinson's disease. Brain 1999;122(Pt 8):1437.
165. Iravani MM, Syed E, Jackson MJ, et al. A modified MPTP treatment regime produces reproducible partial nigrostriatal lesions in common marmosets. Eur J Neurosci 2005;21:841.
166. Karachi C, Francois C, Parain K, et al. Three-dimensional cartography of functional territories in the human striatopallidal complex by using calbindin immunoreactivity. J Comp Neurol 2002;450:122.
167. Iacopino A, Christakos S, German D, et al. Calbindin-D28K-containing neurons in animal models of neurodegeneration: Possible protection from excitotoxicity. Mol Brain Res 1992;13:251.
168. Gerfen CR, Herkenham M, Thibault J. The neostriatal mosaic: II. Patch- and matrix-directed mesostriatal dopaminergic and non-dopaminergic systems. J Neurosci 1987;7:3915.
169. Prensa L, Parent A. The nigrostriatal pathway in the rat: A single-axon study of the relationship between dorsal and ventral tier nigral neurons and the striosome/matrix striatal compartments. J Neurosci 2001; 21:7247.
170. Matsuda W, Furuta T, Nakamura KC, et al. Single nigrostriatal dopaminergic neurons form widely spread and highly dense axonal arborizations in the neostriatum. J Neurosci 2009;29:444.
171. Kish SJ, Shannak K, Hornykiewicz O. Uneven pattern of dopamine loss in the striatum of patients with idiopathic Parkinson's disease. Pathophysiologic and clinical implications. N Engl J Med 1998;318:876.
172. Brooks DJ, Ibanez V, Sawle GV, et al. Differing patterns of striatal 18F-dopa uptake in Parkinson's disease, multiple system atrophy, and progressive supranuclear palsy. Ann Neurol 1990;28:547.
173. Damier P, Hirsch EC, Agid Y, et al. The substantia nigra of the human brain. I. Nigrosomes and the nigral matrix, a compartmental organization based on calbindin D(28K) immunohistochemistry. Brain 1999;122(Pt 8):1421.
174. Gibb WR, Lees AJ. Anatomy, pigmentation, ventral and dorsal subpopulations of the substantia nigra, and differential cell death in Parkinson's disease. J Neurol Neurosurg Psychiatry 1991;54:388.
175. Moratalla R, Quinn B, DeLanney LE, et al. Differential vulnerability of primate caudate-putamen and striosome-matrix dopamine systems to the neurotoxic effects of 1-methyl-4-phenyl-1,2,3,6-tetrahydropyridine. Proc Natl Acad Sci USA 1992;89:3859.
176. Fornai F, Ruffoli R, Soldani P, et al. The "Parkinsonian heart": From novel vistas to advanced therapeutic approaches in Parkinson's disease. Curr Med Chem 2007;14:2421.
177. Fornai F, di Poggio AB, Pellegrini A, et al. Noradrenaline in Parkinson's disease: From disease progression to current therapeutics. Curr Med Chem 2007;14:2330.
178. Rommelfanger KS, Edwards GL, Freeman KG, et al. Norepinephrine loss produces more profound motor deficits than MPTP treatment in mice. Proc Natl Acad Sci USA 2007;104:13804.
179. Rommelfanger KS, Weinshenker D. Norepinephrine: The redheaded stepchild of Parkinson's disease. Biochem Pharmacol 2007;74:177.
180. Carta M, Carlsson T, Munoz A, et al. Serotonin-dopamine interaction in the induction and maintenance of L-DOPA-induced dyskinesias. Prog Brain Res 2008;172:465.
181. Carta AR, Frau L, Pontis S, et al. Direct and indirect striatal efferent pathways are differentially influenced by low and high dyskinetic drugs: Behavioural and biochemical evidence. Parkinsonism Relat Disord 2008;14(suppl 2):S165.
182. Fox SH, Chuang R, Brotchie JM. Parkinson's disease—Opportunities for novel therapeutics to reduce the problems of levodopa therapy. Prog Brain Res 2008;172:479.
183. Betarbet R, Turner R, Chockkan V, et al. Dopaminergic neurons intrinsic to the primate striatum. J Neurosci 1997;17:6761.
184. Cossette M, Levesque D, Parent A. Neurochemical characterization of dopaminergic neurons in human striatum. Parkinsonism Relat Disord 2005;11:277.
185. Cossette M, Lecomte F, Parent A. Morphology and distribution of dopaminergic neurons intrinsic to the human striatum. J Chem Neuroanat 2005;29:1.
186. Mazloom M, Smith Y. Synaptic microcircuitry of tyrosine hydroxylase-containing neurons and terminals in the striatum of 1-methyl-4-phenyl-1,2,3,6-tetrahydropyridine-treated monkeys. J Comp Neurol 2006;495:453.
187. Tande D, Hoglinger G, Debeir T, et al. New striatal dopamine neurons in MPTP-treated macaques result from a phenotypic shift and not neurogenesis Brain 2006;129:1194.
188. Palfi S, Leventhal L, Chu Y, et al. Lentivirally delivered glial cell line-derived neurotrophic factor increases the number

of striatal dopaminergic neurons in primate models of nigrostriatal degeneration. J Neurosci 2002;22:4942.
189. Freeman A, Ciliax B, Bakay R, et al. Nigrostriatal collaterals to thalamus degenerate in parkinsonian animal models. Ann Neurol 2001;50:321.
190. Sanchez-Gonzalez MA, Garcia-Cabezas MA, Rico B, et al. The primate thalamus is a key target for brain dopamine. J Neurosci 2005;25:6076.
191. Garcia-Cabezas MA, Rico B, Sanchez-Gonzalez MA, et al. Distribution of the dopamine innervation in the macaque and human thalamus. Neuroimage 2007;34:965.
191a. Garcia-Cabezas MA, Martinez-Sanchez P, Sanchez-Gonzalez MA, et al. Dopamine innervation in the thalamus: Monkey versus rat. Cereb Cortex 2009;19:424.
192. Albin RL, Young AB, Penney JB. The functional anatomy of basal ganglia disorders. Trends Neurosci 1989;12:366.
193. Bergman H, Wichmann T, DeLong MR. Reversal of experimental parkinsonism by lesions of the subthalamic nucleus. Science 1990;249:1436.
194. Gerfen CR, Engber TM, Mahan LC, et al. D1 and D2 dopamine receptor-regulated gene expression of striatonigral and striatopallidal neurons. Science 1990;250:1429.
195. Kawaguchi Y, Wilson CJ, Emson PC. Projection subtypes of rat neostriatal matrix cells revealed by intracellular injection of biocytin. J Neurosci 1990;10:3421.
196. Parent A, Charara A, Pinault D. Single striatofugal axons arborizing in both pallidal segments and in the substantia nigra in primates. Brain Res 1995;698:280.
197. Levesque M, Parent A. The striatofugal fiber system in primates: A reevaluation of its organization based on single-axon tracing studies. Proc Natl Acad Sci USA 2005;102:11888.
198. Le Moine C, Normand E, Bloch B. Phenotypical characterization of the rat striatal neurons expressing the D1 dopamine receptor gene. Proc Natl Acad Sci USA 1991;88:4205.
199. Surmeier DJ, Eberwine J, Wilson CJ, et al. Dopamine receptor subtypes colocalize in rat striatonigral neurons. Proc Natl Acad Sci USA 1992;89:10178.
200. Surmeier DJ, Reiner A, Levine MS, et al. Are neostriatal dopamine receptors co-localized? Trends Neurosci 1993;16:299.
201. Gerfen CR, Keefe KA. Neostriatal dopamine receptors. Trends Neurosci 1994;17:2; author reply 4-5.
202. Le Moine C, Bloch B. D1 and D2 dopamine receptor gene expression in the rat striatum: Sensitive cRNA probes demonstrate prominent segregation of D1 and D2 mRNAs in distinct neuronal populations of the dorsal and ventral striatum. J Comp Neurol 1995;355:418.
203. Svenningsson P, Le Moine C, Aubert I, et al. Cellular distribution of adenosine A2A receptor mRNA in the primate striatum. J Comp Neuro 1998;399:229.
204. Surmeier DJ, Song WJ, Yan Z. Coordinated expression of dopamine receptors in neostriatal medium spiny neurons. J Neurosci 1996;16:6579.
205. Hersch SM, Ciliax BJ, Gutekunst CA, et al. Electron microscopic analysis of D1 and D2 dopamine receptor proteins in the dorsal striatum and their synaptic relationships with motor corticostriatal afferents. J Neurosci 1995;15:5222.
206. Aizman O, Brismar H, Uhlen P, et al. Anatomical and physiological evidence for D1 and D2 dopamine receptor colocalization in neostriatal neurons. Nat Neurosci 2000;3:226.
207. Deng YP, Lei WL, Reiner A. Differential perikaryal localization in rats of D1 and D2 dopamine receptors on striatal projection neuron types identified by retrograde labeling. J Chem Neuroanat 2006;32:101.
208. Heintz N. BAC to the future: The use of bac transgenic mice for neuroscience research. Nat Rev Neurosci 2001;2:861.
209. Gong S, Zheng C, Doughty ML, et al. A gene expression atlas of the central nervous system based on bacterial artificial chromosomes. Nature 2003;425:917.
210. Le Moine C, Bloch B. Expression of the D3 dopamine receptor in peptidergic neurons of the nucleus accumbens: Comparison with the D1 and D2 dopamine receptors. Neuroscience 1996;73:131.
211. Gurevich EV, Joyce JN. Distribution of dopamine D3 receptor expressing neurons in the human forebrain: Comparison with D2 receptor expressing neurons. Neuropsychopharmacology 1999;20:60.
212. Khan ZU, Gutierrez A, Martin R, et al. Dopamine D5 receptors of rat and human brain. Neuroscience 2000;100:689.
213. Rivera A, Alberti I, Martin AB, et al. Molecular phenotype of rat striatal neurons expressing the dopamine D5 receptor subtype. Eur. J Neurosci 2002;16:2049.
214. Noain D, Avale ME, Wedemeyer C, et al. Identification of brain neurons expressing the dopamine D4 receptor gene using BAC transgenic mice. Eur J Neurosci 2006;24:2429.
215. Araki KY, Sims JR, Bhide PG. Dopamine receptor mRNA and protein expression in the mouse corpus striatum and cerebral cortex during pre- and postnatal development. Brain Res 2007;1156:31.
216. Nambu A, Tokuno H, Takada M. Functional significance of the cortico-subthalamo-pallidal 'hyperdirect' pathway. Neurosci Res 2002;43:111.
217. Nambu A, Takada M, Inase M, et al. Dual somatotopical representations in the primate subthalamic nucleus: Evidence for ordered but reversed body-map transformations from the primary motor cortex and the supplementary motor area. J Neurosci 1996;16:2671.
218. Strafella AP, Vanderwerf Y, Sadikot AF. Transcranial magnetic stimulation of the human motor cortex influences the neuronal activity of subthalamic nucleus. Eur. J Neurosci 2004;20:2245.
219. Shink E, Bevan MD, Bolam JP, et al. The subthalamic nucleus and the external pallidum: Two tightly interconnected structures that control the output of the basal ganglia in the monkey. Neuroscience 1996;73:335.
220. Smith Y, Bevan MD, Shink E, et al. Microcircuitry of the direct and indirect pathways of the basal ganglia. Neuroscience 1998;86:353.
221. Wichmann T, Bergman H, DeLong MR. The primate subthalamic nucleus. III. Changes in motor behavior and neuronal activity in the internal pallidum induced by subthalamic inactivation in the MPTP model of parkinsonism. J Neurophysiol 1994;72:521.
222. Paradiso G, Cunic D, Saint-Cyr JA, et al. Involvement of human thalamus in the preparation of self-paced movement. Brain 2004;127:2717.
222a. Purzner J, Paradiso GO, Cunic D, et al. Involvement of the basal ganglia and cerebellar motor pathways in

the preparation of self-initiated and externally triggered movements in humans. J Neurosci 2007;27:6029.
223. Baunez C, Humby T, Eagle DM, et al. Effects of STN lesions on simple vs choice reaction time tasks in the rat: Preserved motor readiness, but impaired response selection. Eur. J Neurosci 2001;13:1609.
224. Chudasama Y, Baunez C, Robbins TW. Functional disconnection of the medial prefrontal cortex and subthalamic nucleus in attentional performance: Evidence for corticosubthalamic interaction. J Neurosci.2003;23:5477.
225. Winstanley CA, Baunez C, Theobald DE, et al. Lesions to the subthalamic nucleus decrease impulsive choice but impair autoshaping in rats: The importance of the basal ganglia in Pavlovian conditioning and impulse control. Eur J Neurosci 2005;21:3107.
226. Blandini F, Fancellu R, Armentero MT, et al. Unilateral lesion of the subthalamic nucleus enhances cortical fos expression associated with focally evoked seizures in the rat. Brain Res 2006;1101:145.
227. Eagle DM, Baunez C, Hutcheson DM, et al. Stop-signal reaction-time task performance: Role of prefrontal cortex and subthalamic nucleus. Cereb Cortex 2008;18:178.
228. Le Jeune F, Peron J, Biseul I, et al. Subthalamic nucleus stimulation affects orbitofrontal cortex in facial emotion recognition: A PET study. Brain 2008;131:1599.
229. Tzagournissakis M, Dermon CR, Savaki HE. Functional metabolic mapping of the rat brain during unilateral electrical stimulation of the subthalamic nucleus. J Cereb Blood Flow Metab 1994;14:132.
230. Maurice N, Deniau JM, Glowinski J. Relationships between the prefrontal cortex and the basal ganglia in the rat: Physiology of the corticosubthalamic circuits. J Neurosci 1998;18:9539.
231. Kolomiets BP, Deniau JM, Mailly P. Segregation and convergence of information flow through the cortico-subthalamic pathways. J Neurosci 2001;21:5764.
232. Kolomiets BP, Deniau JM, Glowinski J. Basal ganglia and processing of cortical information: Functional interactions between trans-striatal and trans-subthalamic circuits in the substantia nigra pars reticulata Neuroscience 2003;117:931.
233. Aron AR, Behrens TE, Smith S, et al. Triangulating a cognitive control network using diffusion-weighted magnetic resonance imaging (MRI) and functional MRI. J Neurosci 2007;27:3743.
234. Gerschlager W, Alesch F, Cunnington R. Bilateral subthalamic nucleus stimulation improves frontal cortex function in Parkinson's disease. An electrophysiological study of the contingent negative variation. Brain 1999;122(Pt 12):2365.
235. Schroeder U, Kuehler A, Haslinger B, et al. Subthalamic nucleus stimulation affects striato-anterior cingulate cortex circuit in a response conflict task: A PET study. Brain 2002;125:1995.
236. Hershey T, Revilla FJ, Wernle A, et al. Stimulation of STN impairs aspects of cognitive control in PD. Neurology 2004;62:1110.
237. Haegelen C, Verin M, Broche BA. Does subthalamic nucleus stimulation affect the frontal limbic areas? A single-photon emission computed tomography study using a manual anatomical segmentation method. Surg. Radiol Anat 2005;27:389.
238. Funkiewiez A, Ardouin C, Caputo E. Long term effects of bilateral subthalamic nucleus stimulation on cognitive function, mood, and behaviour in Parkinson's disease. J Neurol Neurosurg Psychiatry 2004;75:834.
239. Funkiewiez A, Ardouin C, Cools R. Effects of levodopa and subthalamic nucleus stimulation on cognitive and affective functioning in Parkinson's disease. Mov Disord 2006;21:1656.
240. Campbell MC, Karimi M, Weaver PM. Neural correlates of STN DBS-induced cognitive variability in Parkinson disease. Neuropsychologia 2008;46:3162.
241. Kalbe E, Voges J, Weber T. Frontal FDG-PET activity correlates with cognitive outcome after STN-DBS in Parkinson disease. Neurology 2009;72:42.
242. Parent A, Smith Y. Organization of efferent projections of the subthalamic nucleus in the squirrel monkey as revealed by retrograde labeling methods. Brain Res. 1987;436:296.
243. Smith Y, Hazrati LN, Parent A. Efferent projections of the subthalamic nucleus in the squirrel monkey as studied by the PHA-L anterograde tracing method. J Comp Neurol 1990;294:306.
244. Degos B, Deniau JM, Le Cam J, et al. Evidence for a direct subthalamo-cortical loop circuit in the rat. Eur. J Neurosci 2008;27:2599.
245. Kitai ST, Deniau JM. Cortical inputs to the subthalamus: Intracellular analysis. Brain Res 1981;214:411.
246. Giuffrida R, Li Volsi G, Maugeri G, et al. Influences of pyramidal tract on the subthalamic nucleus in the cat. Neurosci Lett 1985;54:231.
247. Garcia-Rill E, Biedermann JA, Chambers T, et al. Mesopontine neurons in schizophrenia. Neuroscience 1995;66:321.
248. Garcia-Rill E, Reese NB, Skinner RD. Arousal and locomotion: From schizophrenia to narcolepsy. Prog Brain Res 1996;107:417.
249. Mesulam MM, Geula C, Bothwell MA, et al. Human reticular formation: Cholinergic neurons of the pedunculopontine and laterodorsal tegmental nuclei and some cytochemical comparisons to forebrain cholinergic neurons. J Comp Neurol 1989;283:611.
250. Lavoie B, Parent A. Pedunculopontine nucleus in the squirrel monkey: Distribution of cholinergic and monoaminergic neurons in the mesopontine tegmentum with evidence for the presence of glutamate in cholinergic neurons. J Comp Neurol 1994;344:190.
251. Inglis WL, Winn P. The pedunculopontine tegmental nucleus: Where the striatum meets the reticular formation. Prog Neurobiol 1995;47:1.
252. Rye DB. Contributions of the pedunculopontine region to normal and altered REM sleep. Sleep 1997;20:757.
253. Winn P, Brown VJ, Inglis WL. On the relationships between the striatum and the pedunculopontine tegmental nucleus. Crit Rev Neurobiol 1997;11:241.
254. Pahapill PA, Lozano AM. The pedunculopontine nucleus and Parkinson's disease. Brain 2000;123 (Pt 9):1767.
255. Winn P. Experimental studies of pedunculopontine functions: Are they motor, sensory or integrative? Parkinsonism Relat. Disord 2008;14(suppl 2):S194.

256. Mena-Segovia J, Bolam JP, Magill PJ. Pedunculopontine nucleus and basal ganglia: Distant relatives or part of the same family? Trends Neurosci 2004; 27:585.
257. Charara A, Smith Y, Parent A. Glutamatergic inputs from the pedunculopontine nucleus to midbrain dopaminergic neurons in primates: Phaseolus vulgaris-leucoagglutinin anterograde labeling combined with postembedding glutamate and GABA immunohistochemistry. J Comp Neurol 1996;364:254.
258. Mena-Segovia J, Winn P, Bolam JP. Cholinergic modulation of midbrain dopaminergic Systems. Brain Res Rev 2008;58:265.
259. Sidibe M, Pare JF, Raju DV, et al. Anatomical and functional relationships between intralaminar thalamic nuclei and basal ganglia in monkeys. In Nicholson LFB, Faull RLM (eds). The Basal Ganglia VII. New York: Kluwer Academic/Plenum, 2002, p.409.
260. Muthusamy KA, Aravamuthan BR, Kringelbach, et al. Connectivity of the human pedunculopontine nucleus region and diffusion tensor imaging in surgical targeting. J Neurosurg 2007;107:814.
261. Aravamuthan BR, Muthusamy KA, Stein JF, et al. Topography of cortical and subcortical connections of the human pedunculopontine and subthalamic nuclei. Neuroimage 2007,37:694.
262. Aravamuthan BR, Stein JF, Aziz TZ. The anatomy and localization of the pedunculopontine nucleus determined using probabilistic diffusion tractography. Br. J Neurosurg 2008;22(suppl 1):S25.
263. Aravamuthan BR, McNab JA, Miller KL, et al. Cortical and subcortical connections within the pedunculopontine nucleus of the primate Macaca mulatta determined using probabilistic diffusion tractography. J Clin. Neurosci 2009;16:413.
264. Garcia-Rill E, Houser CR, Skinner RD, et al. Locomotion-inducing sites in the vicinity of the pedunculopontine nucleus. Brain Res Bull 1987;18:731.
265. Piallat B, Chabardes S, Torres N, et al. Gait is associated with an increase in tonic firing of the sub-cuneiform nucleus neurons. Neuroscience 2009;158:1201.
266. Weinberger M, Hamani C, Hutchison WD, et al. Pedunculopontine nucleus microelectrode recordings in movement disorder patients. Exp Brain Res 2008;188:165.
267. Kojima J, Yamaji Y, Matsumura M, et al. Excitotoxic lesions of the pedunculopontine tegmental nucleus produce contralateral hemiparkinsonism in the monkey. Neurosci Lett 1997;226:111.
268. Munro-Davies L, Winter J, Aziz TZ, et al. Kainate acid lesions of the pedunculopontine region in the normal behaving primate. Mov Disord 2001;16:150.
269. Hirsch EC, Graybiel AM, Duyckaerts C, et al. Neuronal loss in the pedunculopontine tegmental nucleus in Parkinson disease and in progressive supranuclear palsy. Proc Natl Acad Sci USA 1987;84:5976.
270. Jellinger KA. Neuropathology of movement disorders. Neurosurg Clin N Am 1998;9:237.
271. Jenkinson N, Nandi D, Muthusamy K, et al. Anatomy, physiology, and pathophysiology of the pedunculopontine nucleus. Mov Disord 2009;24:319.
272. Nandi D, Aziz TZ, Giladi N, et al. Reversal of akinesia in experimental parkinsonism by GABA antagonist microinjections in the pedunculopontine nucleus. Brain 2002;125:2418.
273. Jenkinson N, Nandi D, Miall RC, et al. Pedunculopontine nucleus stimulation improves akinesia in a Parkinsonian monkey. Neuroreport 2004;15:2621.
274. Pierantozzi M, Palmieri MG, Galati S. Pedunculopontine nucleus deep brain stimulation changes spinal cord excitability in Parkinson's disease patients. J Neural Transm 2008;115:731.
275. Ferraye MU, Debu B, Pollak P. Deep brain stimulation effect on freezing of gait. Mov Disord 2008;23(suppl 2):S489.
276. Lozano AM, Snyder BJ. Deep brain stimulation for parkinsonian gait disorders. J Neurol 2008;255(suppl 4):30.
277. Nandi D, Liu X, Winter JL, et al. Deep brain stimulation of the pedunculopontine region in the normal non-human primate. J Clin Neurosci 2002;9:170.
278. Nandi D, Jenkinson N, Stein J, et al. The pedunculopontinhe nucleus in Parkinson's disease: Primate studies. Br J Neurosurg 2008;22(suppl 1):S4.
279. Mazzone P, Lozano A, Stanzione P, et al. Implantation of human pedunculopontine nucleus: A safe and clinically relevant target in Parkinson's disease. Neuroreport 2005;16:1877.
280. Stefani A, Lozano AM, Peppe A, et al. Bilateral deep brain stimulation of the pedunculopontine and subthalamic nuclei in severe Parkinson's disease. Brain 2007; 130:1596.
281. Yelnik J. PPN or PPD, what is the target for deep brain stimulation in Parkinson's disease? Brain 2007;130:e79; author reply e80.
282. Zrinzo L, Zrinzo LV, Hariz M. The peripeduncular nucleus: A novel target for deep brain stimulation? Neuroreport 2007;18:1301.
283. Zrinzo L, Zrinzo LV. Surgical anatomy of the pedunculopontine and peripeduncular nuclei. Br J Neurosurg 2008;22(suppl 1):S19.
284. Parent M, Levesque M, Parent A. Two types of projection neurons in the internal pallidum of primates: Single-axon tracing and three-dimensional reconstruction. J Comp Neurol 2001;439:162.
285. Percheron G, Francois C, Talbi B, et al. The primate motor thalamus. Brain Res Rev 1996;22:93.
286. Sidibe M, Bevan MD, Bolam JP, et al. Efferent connections of the internal globus pallidus in the squirrel monkey: I. Topography and synaptic organization of the pallidothalamic projection. J Comp Neurol 1997;382:323.
287. Baron MS, Sidibe M, DeLong MR, et al. Course of motor and associative pallidothalamic projections in monkeys. J Comp Neurol 2001;429:490.
288. Kuo JS, Carpenter MB. Organization of pallidothalamic projections in the rhesus monkey. J Comp Neurol 1973;151:201.
289. Ilinsky IA, Tourtellotte WG, Kultas-Ilinsky K. Anatomical distinctions between the two basal ganglia afferent territories in the primate motor thalamus. Stereotact Funct Neurosurg 1993;60:62.
290. Sakai ST, Stepniewska I, Qi HX, et al. Pallidal and cerebellar afferents to pre-supplementary motor area thalamocortical neurons in the owl monkey: A multiple labeling study. J Comp Neurol 2000;417:164.

291. Gallay MN, Jeanmonod D, Liu J. Human pallidothalamic and cerebellothalamic tracts: Anatomical basis for functional stereotactic neurosurgery. Brain Struct Funct 2008;212:443.
292. Akkal D, Dum RP, Strick PL. Supplementary motor area and presupplementary motor area: Targets of basal ganglia and cerebellar output. J Neurosci 2007; 27:10659.
293. Schell GR, Strick PL. The origin of thalamic inputs to the arcuate premotor and supplementary motor areas. J Neurosci 1984;4:539.
294. Strick PL. How do the basal ganglia and cerebellum gain access to the cortical motor areas? Behav Brain Res 1985;18:107.
295. Hazrati LN, Parent A. Contralateral pallidothalamic and pallidotegmental projections in primates: An anterograde and retrograde labeling study. Brain Res 1991; 567:212.
296. Sidibe M, Pare JF, Smith Y. Nigral and pallidal inputs to functionally segregated thalamostriatal neurons in the centromedian/parafascicular nuclear compex in monkey. J Comp Neurol 2002;447:286.
297. Shink E, Sidibe M, Smith Y. Efferent connections of the internal globus pallidus in the squirrel monkey: II. Topography and synaptic organization of pallidal efferents to the pedunculopontine nucleus. J Comp Neurol 1997;382:348.
297a. Pare JF, Smith Y. Functional segregation of basal ganglia circuits through the lateral habenula in primates. Soc Neurosci 2009.
298. Moriizumi, T, Hattori, T. Choline acetyltransferase-immunoreactive neurons in the rat entopeduncular nucleus. Neuroscience 1992;46:721.
299. Kha HT, Finkelstein DI, Pow DV, et al. Study of projections from the entopeduncular nucleus to the thalamus of the rat. J Comp Neuro 2000;426:366.
300. Matsumoto M, Hikosaka O. Lateral habenula as a source of negative reward signals in dopamine neurons. Nature 2007;447:1111.
301. Matsumoto M, Hikosaka O. Negative motivational control of saccadic eye movement by the lateral habenula. Prog Brain Res 2008;171:399.
302. Matsumoto M, Hikosaka O. Representation of negative motivational value in the primate lateral habenula. Nat Neurosci 2009;12:77.
303. Hikosaka O, Sesack SR, Lecourtier L, et al. Habenula: Crossroad between the basal ganglia and the limbic system. J Neurosci 2008;28:11825.
304. Hikosaka O. [Decision-making and learning by cortico-basal ganglia network]. Brain Nerve 2008;60:799.
305. Hong S, Hikosaka O. The globus pallidus sends reward-related signals to the lateral habenula Neuron 2008;60:720.
306. Geisler S, Trimble M. The lateral habenula: No longer neglected. CNS Spectr 2008;13:484.
306a. Matsumoto M. Role of the lateral habenula and dopamine neurons in reward processing. Brain Nerve 2009; 61:389.
307. Ji H, Shepard PD. Lateral habenula stimulation inhibits rat midbrain dopamine neurons through a GABA(A) receptor-mediated mechanism. J Neurosci 2007;27:6923.
307a. Kim U. Topographic commissural and descending habenula projections in the rat. J Comp Neurol 2009;513:173.
308. Klemm WR. Habenular and interpeduncularis nuclei: Shared components in multiple-function networks. Med Sci Monit 2004;10:RA261.
309. Lecourtier L, Kelly PH. A conductor hidden in the orchestra? Role of the habenular complex in monoamine transmission and cognition. Neurosci Biobehav Rev 2007;31:658.
310. Sartorius A, Henn FA. Deep brain stimulation of the lateral habenula in treatment resistant major depression. Med Hypotheses 2007;69:1305.
311. Parent A, Mackey A, Smith Y, et al. The output organization of the substantia nigra in primate as revealed by a retrograde double labeling method. Brain Res Bull 1983;10:529.
312. Kultas-Ilinsky K, Ilinsky IA. Fine structure of the magnocellular subdivision of the ventral anterior thalamic nucleus (VAmc) of Macaca mulatta: II. Organization of nigrothalamic afferents as revealed with EM autoradiography. J Comp Neurol 1990;294:479.
313. Francois C, Tande D, Yelnik J, et al. Distribution and morphology of nigral axons projecting to the thalamus in primates. J Comp Neurol 2002;447:249.
314. Middleton FA, Strick PL. Anatomical evidence for cerebellar and basal ganglia involvement in higher cognitive function. Science 1994;266:458.
315. Middleton FA, Strick PL. The temporal lobe is a target of output from the basal ganglia. Proc Natl Acad Sci USA 1996;93:8683.
316. Middleton FA, Strick PL. Basal-ganglia 'projections' to the prefrontal cortex of the primate. Cereb Cortex 2002;12:926.
317. Deniau JM, Menetrey A, Charpier S. The lamellar organization of the rat substantia nigra pars reticulata: segregated patterns of striatal afferents and relationship to the topography of corticostriatal projections. Neuroscience 1996;73:761.
318. Deniau JM, Mailly P, Maurice N, et al. The pars reticulata of the substantia nigra: a window to basal ganglia output. Prog Brain Res 2007;160:151.
319. Mailly P, Charpier S, Menetrey A, et al. Three-dimensional organization of the recurrent axon collateral network of the substantia nigra pars reticulata neurons in the rat. J Neurosci 2003;23:5247.
320. Grofova I, Zhou M. Nigral innervation of cholinergic and glutamatergic cells in the rat mesopontine tegmentum: Light and electron microscopic anterograde tracing and immunohistochemical studies. J Comp Neuro 1998;395:359.
321. Spann BM, Grofova I. Nigropedunculopontine projection in the rat: An anterograde tracing study with phaseolus vulgaris-leucoagglutinin (PHA-L). J Comp Neurol 1991;311:375.
322. Hikosaka O. Basal ganglia mechanisms of reward-oriented eye movement. Ann N Y Acad Sci 2007;1104: 229.
323. Hikosaka O, Takikawa Y, Kawagoe R. Role of the basal ganglia in the control of purposive saccadic eye movements. Physiol Rev 2000;80:953.
324. Sato M, Hikosaka O. Role of primate substantia nigra pars reticulata in reward-oriented saccadic eye movement. J Neurosci 2002;22:2363.

325. Coizet V, Comoli E, Westby GW, et al. Phasic activation of substantia nigra and the ventral tegmental area by chemical stimulation of the superior colliculus: An electrophysiological investigation in the rat. Eur J Neurosci 2003;17:28.
326. Coizet V, Overton PG, Redgrave P. Collateralization of the tectonigral projection with other major output pathways of superior colliculus in the rat. J Comp Neurol 2007;500:1034.
327. Comoli E, Coizet V, Boyes J, et al. A direct projection from superior colliculus to substantia nigra for detecting salient visual events. Nat Neurosci 2003;6:974.
328. Dommett E, Coizet V, Blaha, et al. How visual stimuli activate dopaminergic neurons at short latency. Science 2005;307:1476.
329. May PJ, McHaffie JG, Stanford TR, et al. Tectonigral projections in the primate: A pathway for pre-attentive sensory input to midbrain dopaminergic neurons. Eur J Neurosci 2009;29:575.
330. McHaffie JG, Jiang H, May PJ, et al. A direct projection from superior colliculus to the substantia nigra pars compacta in the cat. Neuroscience 2006;138:221.
331. Redgrave P, Prescott TJ, Gurney K. Is the short-latency dopamine response too short to signal reward error? Trends Neurosci 1999;22:146.
332. Redgrave P, Gurney K. The short-latency dopamine signal: A role in discovering novel actions? Nat Rev Neurosci 2006;7:967.
333. Newsome WT, Schultz W, Fiorillo CD: The temporal precision of reward prediction in dopamine neurons. Nat Neurosci 2008;11:966.
334. Redgrave P, Gurney K, Reynolds J. What is reinforced by phasic dopamine signals? Brain Res Rev 200858:322.
335. Laurent PA. The emergence of saliency and novelty responses from Reinforcement Learning principles. Neural Netw 2008;21:1493.
336. Kobayashi S, Schultz W. Influence of reward delays on responses of dopamine neurons. J Neurosci 2008;28:7837.
337. Schultz W. Multiple dopamine functions at different time courses. Annu Rev. Neurosci 2007;30:259.
338. Schultz W. Behavioral dopamine signals. Trends Neurosci 2007;30:203.
339. Schultz W, Preuschoff K, Camerer C. Explicit neural signals reflecting reward uncertainty Philos. Trans R Soc Lond B Biol Sci 2008;363:3801.
340. Mogoseanu D, Smith AD, Bolam JP. Monosynaptic innervation of trigeminal motor neurones involved in mastication by neurones of the parvicellular reticular formation. J Comp Neurol 1993;336:53.
341. Mogoseanu D, Smith AD, Bolam JP. Monosynaptic innervation of facial motoneurones by neurones of the parvicellular reticular formation. Exp Brain Res 1994;101:427.
342. Fay RA, Norgren R. Identification of rat brainstem multisynaptic connections to the oral motor nuclei using pseudorabies virus. III. Lingual muscle motor systems. Brain Res Rev 1997;25:291.

CHAPTER 5

Pathophysiology of the Basal Ganglia and Movement Disorders

José A. Obeso, María C. Rodríguez-Oroz, Inés Trigo-Damas, and M. Rodríguez

The term "basal ganglia" (BG) is applied to several gray matter structures located at the base of the cerebral hemispheres. Nowadays, it is commonly used to refer to the striatum (caudate and putamen), the globus pallidus pars externa (GPe) and pars interna (GPi), the subthalamic nucleus (STN) and, the substantia nigra pars compacta (SNc) and pars reticulata (SNr). Traditionally, the BG have been associated with the control of movement and their dysfunction is the origin of movement disorders such as the parkinsonian syndrome, hemichorea-ballismus, and dystonia.[1]

Currently (see Chapter 4), the BG are functionally subdivided as motor, oculomotor, associative, limbic, and orbitofrontal according to the main cortical projection areas, which form loops through the posterior putamen, caudate nucleus, anterior, and ventral striatum.[2–4] These connections engage in motor control and other functions such as explicit and implicit learning, reward-related behavior, habit formation and attention to stimuli.[5–7] Accordingly, the traditional view that the BG are related only with movement and motor learning is no longer tenable.

This chapter reviews the main physiological features of the BG, common to all functional domains and, the pathophysiology of movement disorders according to their clinical relevance. More recently recognized clinical manifestations of BG dysfunction, i.e., behavioral and mood disorders, are considered in detail elsewhere.[8,9]

▶ PHYSIOLOGICAL FEATURES OF THE BASAL GANGLIA

In this section, we discuss the main characteristics of neuronal activity in the normal BG and more recent functional studies on brain imaging in humans. We then conclude with a general appraisal of the operational mode of the BG. In order to achieve our objective, we start by providing a summary of the classic pathophysiological model, and also discuss the architectonic features of the BG. The latter are important inasmuch as anatomy is the substrate of function and provides constraints for any analysis regarding the physiological role of a structure. Details about connectivity and functional organization are in Chapter 4.

GENERAL ANATOMOPHYSIOLOGICAL ORGANIZATION

The Classic Model

Cortical inputs reach the BG through the striatum and rely back to the cortex via the thalamus, through the GPi and SNr, the output nuclei of the BG (Fig. 5–1A). Striatal medium spiny neuron (MSN) activity is conveyed to the GPi/SNr through a monosynaptic GABAergic projection ("direct" pathway), and polysynaptic ("indirect" pathway) connections which involve the external GPe and the STN.[10,11,12] Neuronal activity in the GPi/SNr is mainly tonic and inhibitory onto their projection targets in the thalamus and brain stem; phasic reduction ("pausing") of BG output is the key physiological feature underlying facilitation, i.e., movement or action, of cortical and brain stem motor regions.[13,14] Dopamine modulates glutamatergic effects on corticostriatal inputs by exerting a dual effect on striatal neurons, exciting D1 neurons in the direct pathway and inhibiting D2 neurons in the indirect pathway.[15] Accordingly, a general functional scheme is that activation of the "indirect circuits" leads to movement inhibition or arrest, while activation of the "direct" circuit facilitates movement execution.[11,16]

In the *parkinsonian state*, striatal dopamine (DA) deficiency reduces inhibition of MSN in the indirect pathway and decreased excitation of MSN giving rise to the direct pathway. Increased inhibition from the striatum to GPe leads to disinhibition of STN, which then overdrives the GPi/SNr.[16,17] In parallel, decreased activation of MSN in the direct pathway reduces its inhibitory influence on GPi/SNr, and contributes to excessive neuronal activity in these output neurons (Fig. 5–1B). The *dyskinetic* state is characterized by reduction in the output

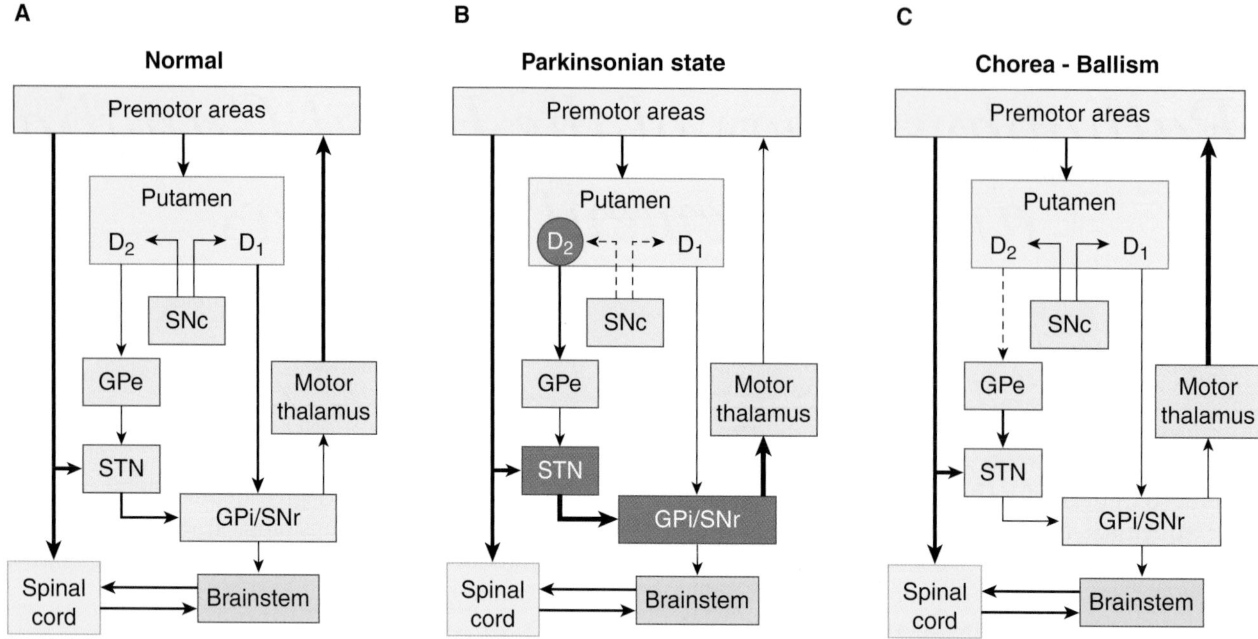

Figure 5–1. Schematic diagram of the classic BG ganglia model for the motor circuit. (A) Normal state. The "direct" and "indirect" circuits form the major striatopallidal projection systems. MSNs giving rise to the "indirect" circuit express D2 receptors, while those in the "indirect" circuit express D1 receptors. Dopamine (DA) excites D1 and inhibits D2 containing MSN. The "direct" circuit is GABAergic and inhibits the GPi, while activation of the "indirect" circuit induces excitation of the GPi via dishinhibition of the STN from the GPe. (B) Parkinsonian state. DA loss provokes inhibition of MSN, which increase their GABAergic activity onto the GPe. The latter becomes hypoactive and therefore, there is reduced inhibition of the STN, which increases its efferent glutamatergic activity, overdriving the GPi. In addition, DA depletion causes hypoactivation of MSN in the direct circuit. The net result is excessive efferent activity in the GPi onto the motor thalamus and cortical motor areas. (C) Chorea-ballism. Essentially the opposite functional changes than in the parkinsonian state occur. Lesion of the STN in normal subjects reduces glutamatergic activity onto the GPi causing reduced efferent inhibition onto the thalamocortical projection. BG, basal ganglia; DA, dopamine; MSN, Medium spiny neuron; D1, dopamine D1 receptor; D2, dopamine D2 receptor; SNc, substantia nigra pars compacta; SNr, substantia nigra pars reticulate; GPe, globus pallidus pars externa; Gpi, globus pallidus pars interna; STN, subthalamic nucleus. (Data Modified from DeLong MR. Primate models of movement disorders of basal ganglia origin. Trend Neurosci 1990;13:281–285.)

of the BG, essentially due to changes in the opposite direction to the ones underlying the parkinsonian states (Fig. 5–1C); accordingly, reduced STN activity and decreased BG output facilitate involuntary movements.[16,17] Altogether, this classic model is based on the idea that activity in the direct circuit facilitates movement, while increased activity in the indirect circuit halts movement. The essential determinant of the motor state is the firing rate in the STN and GPi, whose degree of activity (hyper/hypo) predicts the clinical state of Parkinsonism and dyskinesias.

Newer Anatomical and Physiological Concepts

The BG is a complex network with two entry points,[18] the striatum and STN, several internal or horizontal circuits that guarantee that neuronal activity in the efferent arm, the GPi/SNr (Fig. 5–2) is maintained within normal levels. Important projections to the brain stem (i.e., to the midbrain tegmentum and the superior colliculus)[19] are also recognized. Neuronal activity arrives at the BG via two different projection systems:

1. Direct disynaptic projections to the GPi via the striatum and STN, which have an opposite physiological effect. Activation of the corticostriatal-GPi/SNr projection (the "direct" circuit) induces inhibition of BG ouput; contrariwise, activation of the cortico-STN-GPi projection (the "hyperdirect pathway") causes excitation.
2. Indirect trisynaptic projections, which include corticostriatal–GPe-GPi connections and also the corticostriatal–GPe/STN-GPi ("classic indirect circuit") pathway.[20]

A newly recognized feature of BG connectivity is the reciprocity of projections (Fig. 5–2), so that the

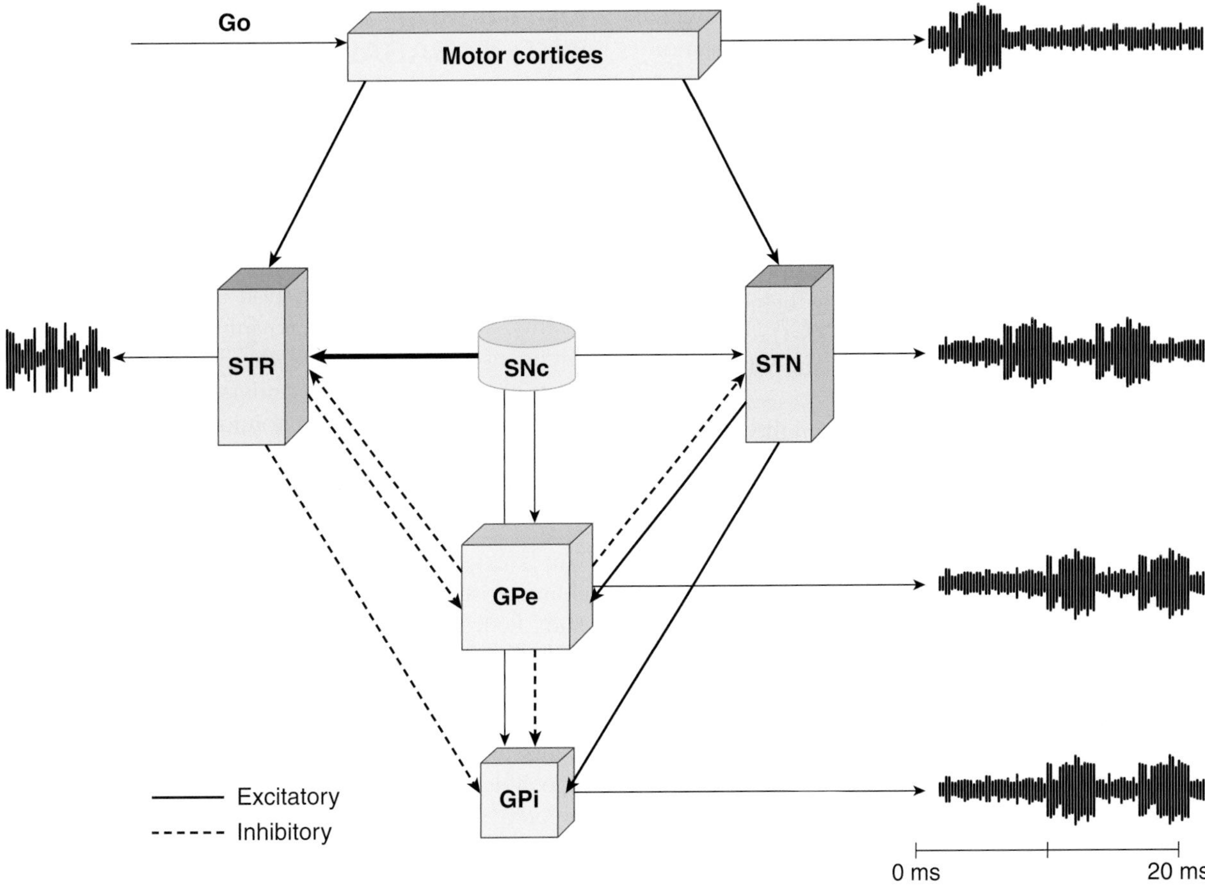

Figure 5–2. Scheme of the main cortico-BG projections and intra BG nuclei circuitry. The principal network is based on a series of disynaptic and trisynaptic bidirectional connections. The striatum and STN are excited by the cortical projections and they project to the GPe and GPi in both inhibitory and excitatory manner, respectively. The central location of the GPe plays a key role in the modulation of BG output projections, either directly via the GPi or indirectly via the STN and eventually the striatum. Neuronal firing activity related to a simple movement is schematically depicted. Following a "go" signal, the motor areas become phasically activated and dispatch a simultaneous volley to the motor striatum and STN. Note that GPe receives activity of opposite functional (excitatory or inhibitory) sign by disynaptic connections and it is in a central position to modulate GPi output activity. BG, basal ganglia; SNc, substantia nigra pars compacta; GPe, globus pallidus pars externa; Gpi, globus pallidus pars interna; STN, subthalamic nucleus; STR, striatum.

flow of neuronal activity can no longer be considered unidirectionally within a given loop. Thus, the classic model implicitly regarded the BG as a "go through" structure, but current data do not support such a conception.

Whereas the striatum and STN are the main structures receiving cortical and thalamic efferent activity onto the BG, the physiological features of these entry points are quite distinct, and probably have a different underlying functional role. The excitability of MSNs, which are the projection neurons, is strongly influenced by the following mechanisms:

1. Recurrent collateral and GABAergic interneurons, which together exert a powerful inhibition on MSN.
2. Cholinergic tonic activity interneurons.
3. GABAergic efferents from the GPe.
4. The ascending nigrostriatal dopaminergic system, which plays a critically important role in modulating striatal input and also serotonin afferents from the raphe nuclei.

All of these intervene to regulate the MSN membrane's potential threshold and "up and down" excitability states and, ultimately, the firing activity. Noticeably, there is a net predominance of inhibition on MSN, which probably explains why MSN typically fires at very low frequency (1–3 Hz) and high-frequency firing associated with local stimulation is very short lasting. The relevance of this feature is discussed at the end of this section.

STN neurons fire spontaneously at around 30 Hz in the awake primate. These neurons are rapidly and robustly excited by afferent cortical activity, which induces a short latency and brief duration excitation–inhibition response and a late excitation; the same pattern of activity is subsequently mirrored in the GPe and GPi,[20] indicating a tight reciprocal excitatory-inhibitory connection between STN and GPe.[4] Interneurons are scarce in the STN and mainly present in the limbic region.[21] The excitability of the STN is also modulated by dopaminergic terminals (a modest projection from the SNc) but particularly, and powerfully by the GPe inhibitory projection (Fig. 5–2). In fact, the STN-GPe-GPi form an internal circuit that governs BG output, whereby the GPe plays a pivotal role.[22]

There has been much debate over the extent to which these parallel lines of communication between cortex and BG should be considered closed or open loops. It appears that the existence of synaptic relays at strategic locations in the striatum, output nuclei, thalamus, and cerebral cortex enables signals within any particular loop to be modified by extraneous inputs. Indeed, there are several newer indications against considering the corticostriatal projection only as a closed loop system. For instance, projections to the striatum from a local area of cortex comprise several probably independent functional components;[23] input from different cortical layers makes differential contacts with the neurochemically distinguished patch and matrix compartments of the striatum[24] and collateral of cortical motoneurones (layer V), giving rise to the pyramidal tract mainly contact with MSN expressing D2-type receptors, whereas cortical neurons projecting only to striatum and cortex connect with MSN expressing D-1 receptors.[25] Thus, arguments about whether the loops are open or closed may be considered fruitless as circuits and connections through the BG have multiple sites where modulation can occur.

NEURONAL ACTIVITY IN THE BASAL GANGLIA

Classic physiological studies of the BG consisted of single-cell extracellular recording "in vivo" and intracellular recording in slice preparation. More recently, it has been possible to record groups of cells simultaneously from one or several BG nuclei and also local field potentials (LFP) from implanted macroelectrodes. Signals recorded in the BG provide information about the source of afferents, and the nature (i.e., inhibition, excitation) and timing of output activity with respect to specific tasks. They also allow a better understanding of the relative functional relevance of anatomical connections.

Extracellular Recording. Single-Cell Activity.

The background spiking activity of BG neurons is very characteristic and different among nuclei[26] (Table 5–1). The low-frequency discharge of MSN and striatal cholinergic interneurons and midbrain dopaminergic neurons, contrasts strikingly with the high (30–50 spikes/s) frequency discharge of the neurons in both pallidal segments and SNr. The high spontaneous discharge rate of pallidal and SNr neurons enables them to influence targeted structures bi-directionally with both increases and decreases in discharge rate.

The relationship between movement and cell discharges has been examined in depth over the years. Combining data from recordings in nonanesthetized monkeys and patients (during surgery), this may be summarized as:

1. Neuronal discharges are elicited in response to active or passive manipulation of specific body parts (Fig. 5–3B) revealing a somatotopic arrange-

▶ TABLE 5–1. RELATIONSHIP BETWEEN MOVEMENT AND CELL DISCHARGES AMONG NUCLEI OF BG

Location	Normal Rates (s^{-1})	Pattern	MPTP-Treated Monkeys	Response to Passive Limb Manipulation/ Active Movements
Striatum	4–7	Short bursting	– / ↓	+
GPe	40–70	Irregular	↓	+
GPi	60–90	Tonic	↑	++
STN	20–30	Irregular	↑	+++
SNr	50–70	Tonic	–	–
SNc	0.2–6	Irregular	–	–

Average firing rates and firing patterns of different BG nuclei in the healthy state and changes in the parkinsonian state in MPTP-treated monkeys (↑ elevated, – no change, ↓ reduced). Motor responses to either passive or active manipulation of the limbs are indicated as increases in the firing rate of the different BG nuclei (+ small increase, ++ medium increase, +++ large increase, – no increase). BG, basal ganglia; SNc, substantia nigra pars compacta; SNr, substantia nigra pars reticulate; GPe, globus pallidus pars externa; Gpi, globus pallidus pars interna; STN, subthalamic nucleus. (Modified with permission from van Albada SJ and Robinson PA. Mean field modeling of the basal ganglia-thalamocortical system. I Firing rates in healthy and parkinsonian states. J Theor Biol 2009;257:642–663. Copyright © Elsevier.)

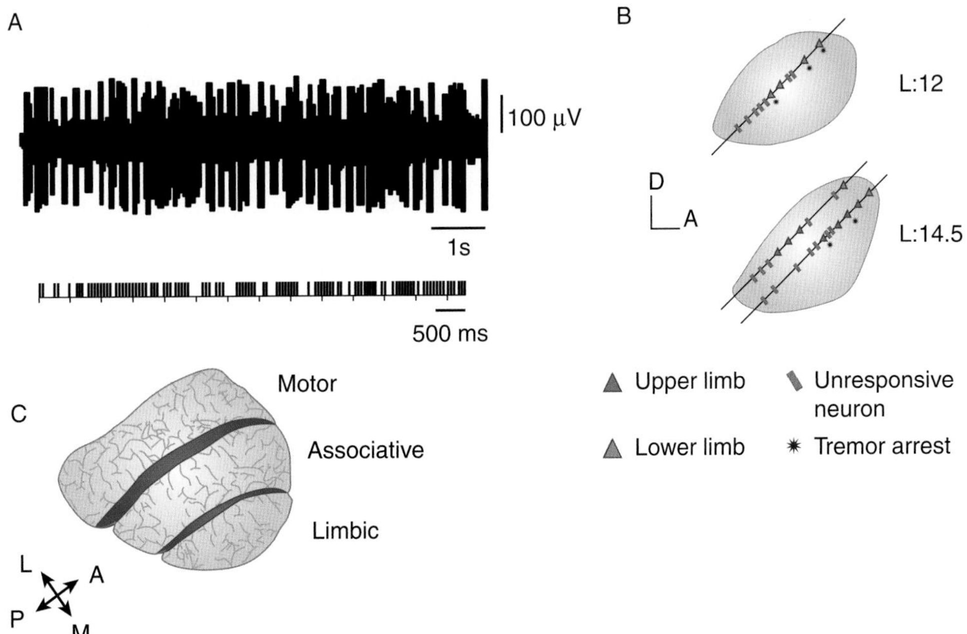

Figure 5–3. Physiological and functional overview of the subthalamic nucleus (STN). (A) Spontaneous discharge of a typical irregular neuron in STN in a patient with Parkinson's disease. Extracellular recorded action potentials (*top*) and digitized spike activity (*bottom*). (Modified with permission from Rodriguez-Oroz MC, Rodriguez M, Guridi J, et al. The subthalamic nucleus in Parkinson's disease: somatotopic organization and physiological characteristics. Brain 2001;124:1777–1790. Copyright © Oxford University Press.) (B) Somatotopic arrangement of STN neurons responding to passive or active movements in patients with Parkinson's disease. Two parasagittal planes (Data from Schaltenbrand G, Wahren W. Atlas for Stereotaxy of the Human Brain. 2nd ed. Stuttgart: Thieme, 1977.) are represented at laterality 12 and 14.5 mm with respect to the AC–PC line. Comparison of the two slices shows a clear medial bias of the representation of the leg with respect to the arm. D, dorsal; A, anterior; *Microstimulation in the indicated points selectively stopped tremor of the leg or the arm. (Modified with permission from Rodriguez-Oroz MC, Rodriguez M, Guridi J, et al. The subthalamic nucleus in Parkinson's disease: somatotopic organization and physiological characteristics. Brain 2001;124:1777–1790. Copyright © Oxford University Press.) (C) The STN shows three anatomical as well as functional subdivisions: The dorsolaterally located somatomotor part, the ventromedially located associative part, and the medial tip, which represents the limbic part. Each circuit is processed within the corresponding functional part of the STN. (Modified with permission from Temel Y, Blokland A, Steinbusch HWM, Visser-Vandewalle VV. The functional role of the subthalamic nucleus in cognitive and limbic circuits. Prog Neurobiol 2005;76:393–413. Copyright © Elsevier.)

ment that coincides with histological studies using anterograde/retrograde tracer.[27,28] For the "motor loop", neurons related with movement are mainly in the posterolateral region of each nuclei and exhibit a dorsoventral somatotopic organization. This has been worked out in detail in the monkey and in patients submitted to surgical treatments for the GPi and STN. Motor-related activity (Fig. 5–3A) is recorded from the dorsolateral region of the STN (and other BG nuclei) but not from the associative or limbic regions (Fig. 5–3C). Neurons responding to movements of the leg are placed in the dorsal region, face-related neurons are ventrally and arm-related neurons lie in between.

2. BG activity may precede movement initiation in the striatum,[29] STN[30] and both GP segments[31,32] but in a higher proportion of cells, neural changes coincide with the onset of muscle contraction.[33] Importantly, cell firing in output nuclei can go up and down before and during task performance. Pallidal neurons change their firing activity according to specific kinematics of movement, like duration and amplitude, but not in relation to patterns of muscle recruitment.[34]
3. SNc firing in the awake primate is characterized by irregular firing patterns at a low frequency (6–8 Hz) and occasional bursting activity. The latter typically occurs in association with cues predicting reward, but also aversive events. Such activity is thought to indicate to dopaminergic neurons how to encode complex information patterns, like novelty or the prediction error for a future action.[35,36]

Intracellular Recordings

Slice studies allow to record with intracellular electrodes and therefore, provide further detail about physiological features of given structures. Striatal recordings have revealed a functional bias toward excitation of MSNs expressing D2 receptors (striato-GPe projection) in response to cortical stimulation. These MSNs make synaptic connections with other D2-MSNs and also with MSN expressing D1 receptors, whereas D1-MSNs make synaptic connections only with other D1-MSNs.[37] Synapses from D2-MSNs have a larger postsynaptic GABA receptor area[38] and larger dendritic tree[39] than D1-MSNs. Thus, a cortical (or thalamic) afferent volley is more likely to facilitate activity in the "indirect pathway" than in the "direct" pathway. The motor efferent copy signals from the cortex also appear, preferentially, to target the D2-MSNs.[25]

Intracellular recording allows us to study plastic changes in MSN synapses. Thus, cortical high frequency stimulation[40,41] induces long-term potentiation (LTP) or long-term depression (LTD) on MSN, depending on the frequency and duration of the stimulus. Corticostriatal synapses also exhibit bidirectional synaptic plasticity, which means that they can be either potentiated or depressed depending on the information arriving from the cortex. Cortical low-frequency stimulation reverses previously induced corticostriatal LTP and evokes LTD, in a process known as depotentiation, which seems to be crucial for the storage of memory and the elimination of incorrect or useless information.[42]

Firing Synchrony and Oscillatory Activity

Multiunit recordings in animals have shown no synchrony of neuronal activity throughout the BG[43] in the normal state but a marked increment in deep sleep, under anesthesia, and after severe DA depletion.[44] This has been further documented by recording LFP through electrodes implanted in patients into the STN or GPi for deep brain stimulation (DBS) in patients operated to treat Parkinson's disease (PD) and other movement disorders. The time evolution of this activity is very similar to that recorded from the motor cortex in normal subjects. Time-locked changes in STN activity have been recorded during simple sensorimotor and more complex tasks requiring decisions between relevant or non-relevant stimuli,[45] as well as during movement observation[46,47] and with emotional stimuli such as showing emotionally laden and neutral pictures.[48] The data may thus be taken in support for activation of the BG both before and after movement onset and also during cognitive and emotionally related tasks.

Functional Imaging Studies

Studies in humans have confirmed by and large the basic subdivisions of the BG in motor, associative, and limbic.[49–51] Tractography-based studies using diffusion tensor imaging have reported a strong correlation between corticostriatal connections and anatomical data from tracing studies in nonhuman primates.[10,11]

A meta-analysis of 126 functional magnetic resonance imaging (fMRI) and positron emission tomography (PET) in normal volunteers[52] revealed the five segregated loops as predicted from monkey studies. Activation studies (fMRI and PET) have revealed a topographical segregation according to the requested task and underlying functions. Activation in the posterior (i.e., sensorimotor) putamen was consistently reported for any movement and presented a somatotopical organization,[53,54] with the leg lying dorsal, face ventral and arm in-between, as expected.[15,17,18] Preparatory activation as well as finger movement sequencing was located more rostrally in the anterior putamen,[54] while activation of the associative territory was observed during tasks such as motor internal representation[4,55] selection and planning of sequential actions.[56–62] Interestingly, one fMRI study has shown a network including the inferior frontal cortex, the STN and the presuplementary motor area (preSMA) in the right hemisphere implicated in inhibiting a movement immediately after its onset or when stopping the order to move.[63]

ESSENTIAL MECHANISMS OF BASAL GANGLIA FUNCTION

The BG appeared early and has been conserved throughout the evolution of vertebrates. Thus the problem(s) that these nuclei evolved to solve must be enduring and relevant to all vertebrates. The general organization of afferent/efferent connections is fairly homogenous interspecies and the different functional domains, i.e., motor, associative, and emotional, seem to be ruled by similar anatomofunctional organization. All of these aspects point to a basic and common operational mode. Currently, a favored view is that the BG is critical in the process of selection, i.e., it aids the brain to choose a given action among several ongoing options, and learning, particularly implicit learning. Indeed, the essential features of BG organization are in keeping with this approach.[64]

Firstly, let us consider the anatomical data. MSN receive large numbers (tens of thousands) of glutamatergic inputs from the cortex and thalamus, which predominantly form asymmetric contacts on the heads of dendritic spines.[65] It has been estimated that approximately 5000 glutamatergic afferents project to each striatal MSN, and 100 MSNs project onto each pallidal neuron. Such a convergence of activity from input to output requires a precise mechanism to filter incoming and outgoing signals to select the required movement or behavior. This activity is largely mediated by dopamine and to some extent by GABAergic interneurons.

Indeed, the main function of dopamine appears to be to modulate (both presynaptically and postsynaptically) the effects of afferent glutamatergic terminals on MSNs.[66] In addition, GABAergic interneurons and axon collaterals from MSNs exert a powerful intrastriatal inhibition.[67] Together, these mechanisms permit to facilitate cortical afferent activity corresponding to a given movement, task or behavior, while competing stimuli are canceled out. This is supported by experimental evidence indicating that dopamine enhances synchronous corticostriatal afferent volleys while simultaneously inhibiting other inputs.[68]

Secondly, physiological features. A fundamental finding is that tonic output from GABAergic GPi/SNr neurons inhibits their projection targets in the thalamus and brain stem, while phasic reduction ("pausing") of BG output activity disinhibits thalamocortical/brain stem regions, allowing movement (Fig. 5–4).[13,14] Thus, the removal of inhibition from the projection targets, i.e., motor thalamus for the limbs or superior colliculus for eye movements, is the output signal facilitating a given action, i.e., "the winner" activity. Before that, major internal computing occurs within BG, so that a given functional channel is facilitated while the rest are inhibited. The proportional increase/decrease ratio for GPi neurons is normally >1 and for SNr it is about 2:1, which is the one expected if a selected targeted structure is disinhibited while inhibition is maintained or increased on targets that might distort the selected action/movement.[64]

Thirdly, neuroimaging studies in healthy volunteers with fMRI have unraveled engagement and changes in activity of the BG related to the acquisition and learning of new motor tasks (Fig. 5–5).[59] These observations suggest a dynamic transfer of information during learning from rostral associative premotor striatal areas to sensorimotor regions.[69] The striatum[70] as well as the functional interactions between the striatum and the hippocampus[71] have also been implicated in the consolidation of procedural memory, a process that characterizes the spontaneous performance gains that occur in the immediate posttraining period.[72]

In conclusion, the BG are arranged to favor a given task or behavior according with context and past experience, while suppressing all other options.[73,74] Under normal circumstances, behavior mainly consists of routine actions, which require minimal selection and facilitation, as both external and internal factors are predictable as long as all circumstances remain constant. In such routine daily activities, we envisage that the BG are predominantly shifted to allow activity to proceed as learned and planned without interference, which physiologically should equate to maintaining tonic discharging activity in the GPi/SNr probably by preferential activation of the-STN-via the "indirect" and hyperdirect circuits. In the next section, we shall examine the outcome of derangement of these general functions.

▶ BASAL GANGLIA PATHOPHYSIOLOGY AND MOVEMENT DISORDERS

There are three established movement disorders definitely associated with dysfunction of the BG:

1. The cardinal motor features of PD, i.e., resting tremor, akinesia, and rigidity giving rise to the parkinsonian syndrome.
2. Dystonic movements and postures.
3. Chorea-ballism. From a practical view, chorea-ballism may also be extended to levodopa-induced dyskinesias in PD patients, which represents the most frequent cause of this manifestation.

In other movement disorders, like tics or restless legs, the putative role of the BG is still pending definitive ascertainment or there is no definitive involvement, as, for instance, is the case in myoclonus, postural and action tremor or ataxia. In this section, we shall focus mainly on the pathophysiology of the parkinsonian and dyskinetic (i.e., chorea-ballism) states.

THE PARKINSONIAN STATE

The parkinsonian state can be functionally characterized by two main features:[75] (1) Striatal DA depletion.[76] (2) Increased neuronal activity in the STN and GPi/SNr leading to over-inhibition of the thalamocortical and brain stem motor systems.[77]

Dopaminergic Deficit and Striatal Mechanisms

The classic motor features that allow the diagnosis of PD typically have a focal onset, spreading to affect the hemibody within 1–2 years to become generalized in less than 5 years[78] on average. Striatal DA depletion is around 70–80% in the posterior putamen, when initial motor features appear, both in the MPTP monkey model and in patients, as assessed by 18-fluoro-dopa PET and SPECT-DAT scans[79–81] that show a typical rostrocaudal gradient, with the caudate least and the posterior putamen most denervated. Disease progression is associated with loss of DA in the anterior striatum and also reduction in the asymmetry of the deficit between the initially affected side and the secondarily affected striatum.[82]

DA depletion causes profound changes in striatal physiological functions. Studies in rats and monkeys using molecular markers (i.e., enkephalin, dynorphin, substance P, D1, and D2 expression) led to the general concept that DA depletion caused decreased activation of D1 bearing striatal neurons and consequently, reduced activity in the "direct" pathway and, on the

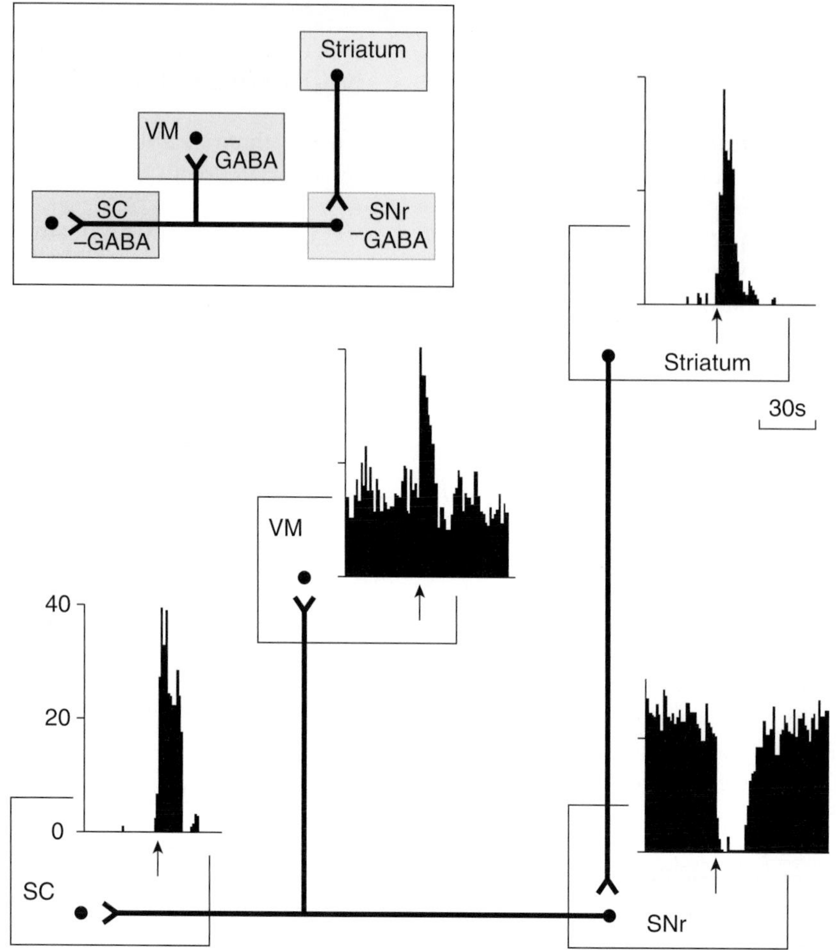

Figure 5-4. Anatomo-physiological organization of the classic "direct" and "indirect" circuits to illustrate the concept of "pausing" or disinhibition of basal ganglia (BG) ouput as main mechanism facilitating movement.Normally, the striatonigrofugal projection maintains tonic inhibition onto the ventromedial thalamic nucleus (V/M) and the superior colliculus (SC). Phasic firing of a striatal neuron induces a clear cut silencing of the tonically active nigral neurones (SNr), which reduces tonic output inhibition. This allows a phasic, time-locked (to an event or action) discharge in SC and thalamic cells. Calibration of spike frequency is given in spikes per second. The arrow in each histogram indicates the onset of glutamate injection in the striatum. (Adapted with permission from Chevalier G and Deniau JM.[14] Copyright © Elsevier.)

other hand, reduced inhibition of D2 bearing striatal neurons resulting in increased activity in striatopallidal (GPe) projections.[15,83,84] In keeping with this, voltage-clamp recordings revealed that in response to cortical stimulation, MSN in the "indirect" pathway are more likely to release glutamate and activate their target neurons.[85]

DA depletion also modifies striatal synaptic plasticity. The best known effect is blockade of LTP induced in MSN by cortical high frequency stimulation.[40,41] Corticostriatal synapses also exhibit bidirectional synaptic plasticity, where LTP or LTD is induced depending on the information arriving from the cortex. This capacity to reverse and shift from facilitation to inhibition, a process known as depotentiation, is lost in rats with 6-OHDA lesions that have developed dyskinesias in response to levodopa.[86]

A more recently recognized feature of the DA denervated striatum is a loss in the number and length of dendritic spines of MSN.[87,88] This has now been verified in several models in rodents, monkeys with MPTP lesion, and patients with PD. A recent study in the monkey showed a direct relationship between the severity and topography of DA depletion and the loss of spines.[89] This study, contrary to previous claims in mice, failed to reveal a differential reduction in spines according to the presence of D1 or D2 bearing MSN.

Striatal interneurons are also functionally changed by DA depletion. A classic concept stated that activity of tonically active neurons (TAN), generally considered

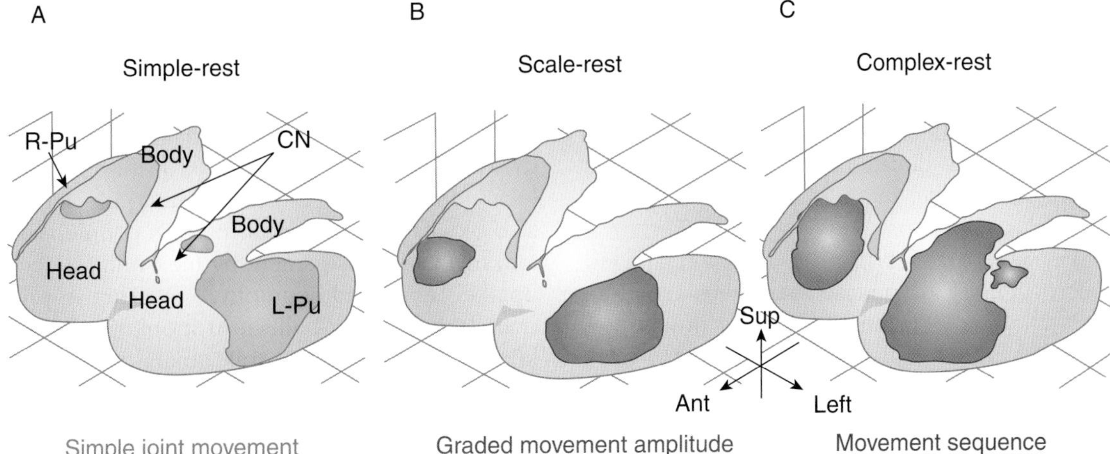

Figure 5–5. Three-dimensional views of striatal activation during the performance of motor tasks of different frequencies and complexity compared with rest (random effect group study, cluster activated at $p < 0.05$, corrected for the volume of the striatum). (A) Simple task consisting in a simple repetitive flexion of the index finger. (B) Scale task consisting in simple sequences of finger tapping under different frequencies. (C) Complex task consisting in a complex sequence of 10 moves. Ant, anterior; CN, caudate nucleus; L-Pu, left putamen; R-Pu, right putamen; Sup, superior. (Adapted with permission from Lehéricy S, Bardinet E, Tremblay L, et al.[49] Copyright © Oxford University Press.)

the prototype of cholinergic interneurons, is increased in the parkinsonian state. This was based on the clinical observation that anticholinergic drugs may improve parkinsonian signs. However, modern studies have produced heterogeneous results. In MPTP monkeys, there is an increase in the proportion of TANs discharging at ~16 Hz,[90] but no change in the basal firing rate or in their degree of synchronization of TANs.[91] The other major type of striatal interneurons, the fast-spiking GABAergic interneurons, appears to become less excitable after DA depletion.[92] However, in vivo recordings from DA-depleted rats show that these neurons do not change their firing rate in response to cortical stimulation. Studies with striatal interneurons may produce conflicting results because there is a complex and reciprocal interaction between DA, TANs, and GABA interneurons,[67,93–95] and the compensatory changes occurring in an attempt to compensate for DA depletion. In general, it may be said that in the parkinsonian state there is an increase in the excitability of cholinergic interneurons and reduction in the activity of GABA-interneurons. These changes result in impaired corticostriatal transmission and reduced feed-forward intrastriatal inhibition.

Altogether, DA depletion caused a shift in corticostriatal transmission whereby GABAergic-MSNs in the "indirect" circuit are preferentially activated, leading to overinhibition of the GPe. This, in turns, facilitates activity in the STN by disinhibition from the GPe, and increases GPi activity. The latter occurs by a dual mechanism, reduced GABAergic activity in the "direct circuit" and increased STN excitation. In sum, striatal DA depletion modulates striatopallidal activity leading to overactivity in the output nuclei of the BG.

The Parkinsonian State and Output Activity of the Basal Ganglia

Dysfunction of the BG leading to movement disorders or other nonmotor manifestations[9] depends on abnormalities in neuronal activity in the output nuclei. The most relevant example illustrating this basic concept comes from functional neurosurgery both experimentally and in patients. Lesions of the STN in monkeys who subsequently received systemic MPTP led to profound bilateral DA striatal depletion but Parkinsonism only arose in the nonoperated side. Markers of neuronal activity in the GPi and SNr showed that the previous STN lesion kept BG output in that hemisphere within or near normal limits,[96] explaining the absence of parkinsonian features on that side despite severe striatal DA loss. Similarly, lesion of the STN or GPi in PD patients or DBS regularizes BG-cortical activity on the operated hemisphere.[97,98] Maintaining BG output within normal limits is therefore the ultimate therapeutic goal of any symptomatic therapy for PD.

DA modulates output excitability indirectly, through striatopallidal circuits, as explained aforementioned, but also by way of direct nigral dopaminergic innervation of extrastriatal BG nuclei.[99] Thus, the GPe and GPi have a nigropallidal dopaminergic direct projection and also receive collaterals from nigrostriatal axons.[100] D2 expressing neurons are found in about 40–50% of all pallidal neurons[101] and local administration of DA into the GP (in the rat) modifies the neuronal firing rate.[102] Similarly, the STN is also innervated by dopaminergic axons and STN neurons express D1 and D2 receptors.[103] Indeed, DA depletion has a direct effect on STN activity,[104] and direct denervation of terminals directed to the STN increases its activity, indicating a direct modulatory effect of DA on the STN.[104]

The GPe, STN, and GPi form a highly organized internal microcircuit with precise anatomical connections (Fig. 5–2).[4] The GPe inhibitory projection to the GPi accounts for about half of GPi afferents,[105] while the STN exerts a powerful excitatory drive onto both GPe and GPi. Normally, stimulation of the STN[20] induces strong excitation of the GPe, which becomes activated and induces inhibition of the GPi and STN. Such GPi inhibition, which induces movement facilitation, predominates over the short latency excitatory response evoked in the GPi from the STN. In other words, movement-related cortical activation will produce a fast conducting excitatory volley onto the STN, which via disynaptic connection GPe-STN-GPi connection will mainly produce inhibition of tonic GPi activity and may therefore facilitate a given movement or behavior. This dual and reciprocal connectivity provides a large capacity to the GPe-STN-GPi network for modulating BG output. This allows functional compensation of striatal DA loss in the early, presymptomatic state, of PD.[106] Once the dopaminergic deficit surpasses the threshold for the available compensatory mechanisms, the GPe-STN-GPi network becomes hyperactive and loses its normal physiological tuning.

Accordingly, the parkinsonian state is mainly characterized by a shift in the internal equilibrium of the BG, whereby overactivity in the excitatory STN–GPi pathway predominates and overwhelms the reduced inhibitory effects from the GPe (which is hypoactive).[107] This leads to excessive spontaneous firing of the GPi as well as increased responsiveness to peripheral stimuli[108] and a decreased signal to noise ratio,[109] thereby acting against the normal facilitation of a desired movement.[8]

PATHOPHYSIOLOGY OF DYSKINESIAS

According to the classic model, dyskinesias (i.e., chorea or ballism) result from reduced activity in the STN-GPi projection leading to decreased firing in GPi output.[11,16,17] Choreatic or ballic movements can be seen as secondary to a focal lesion of the BG, i.e., more often but not exclusively with lesion of the STN, and also when induced by levodopa (LID) in patients with PD. Essentially, chorea-ballism represents the abnormal release of fragments of normal movement. Thus, the actual movements are not qualitatively abnormal; it is their spontaneous, purposeless, and involuntary nature that confers abnormality.[110] In either instance the underlying pathophysiological mechanisms are similar.[110,111] Thus, in simple terms, the pathophysiology of this type of dyskinetic movements can be seen as the opposite of Parkinsonism.[16,112]

The fundamental work on the pathophysiology of dyskinesias was first performed in normal monkeys by local administration of bicuculline to block the GPe and also blockade or lesion of the STN coupled to postmortem metabolic assessment by measuring 2-deoxiglucose uptake by autoradiography.[113–115] This approach produced hemichorea-ballism in monkeys due to bicuculline inhibition of GABAergic striatal projection onto the GPe, leading to increased GPe efferent activity and over-inhibition of the STN and, as a consequence, decreased glutamatergic excitatory activity onto the GPi.[115,116] Neuronal recording of extracellular activity in the GPi of normal monkeys with chorea induced by injection of bicuculline into the GPe showed reduced firing rate and abnormal pattern of neuronal synchronization.[108] Evidence, therefore, supported a major role of the "indirect pathway" in the induction of dyskinesias.

Subsequently, studies were expanded to monkeys with MPTP-induced Parkinsonism treated with dopaminergic drugs and also to the rat model with 6-OHDA unilateral lesion where it was shown that low (6 mg/Kg) levodopa doses also triggered involuntary movements.[117] Here, the following mechanism was proposed for LID: Levodopa administration (2–3 times/day) leads to large and frequent (hourly) changes in striatal DA availability, thus producing discontinuous and abnormal activation of dopaminergic receptors on MSN. This leads to abnormal plastic synaptic changes and a cascade of intracellular signaling alterations.[118] Physiologically, this is translated into excessive inhibition of MSN giving rise to the indirect striato-GPe projection, disinhibition of the GPe, over inhibition of STN and reduced STN excitatory drive, and consequently, hypoactivity in GPi/SNr output neurons (see Fig. 5–1C). It is believed that LID in PD follows the same chain of events as described previously for chorea-ballism secondary to GPe/STN blockade. Recording of neuronal activity in the GPe and GPi in MPTP monkeys[119] and PD patients[120] exhibiting LIDs during surgery corroborated the increment and reduction of GPe and GPi neuronal activity, respectively.[119–121]

In addition, in recent years, evidence has accumulated for abnormal D1 receptor activation in the striatum of dyskinetic animals, and interest has been centered on the "direct circuit" as a mediator of LID. While expression of D1 striatal receptors is unchanged in LID in MPTP monkeys, new data have shown increased binding of [35S]GTP gamma-S, indicating increased efficiency of receptor signaling.[122] Levels of Cdk5 (cyclin-dependent protein kinase 5) and DARP-32 (dopamine-regulated and cAMP-regulated phosphoprotein of 32kDa), two pivotal players in D1 signal transduction pathway are also increased in the striatum of dyskinetic monkeys.[122]

Furthermore, LID in MPTP monkeys correlated linearly with D 3 receptor binding levels.[123]

One major interpretation difficulty of the aforementioned findings is that it is impossible to separate out the consequences of the involuntary movements into striatal mechanisms and the putative causes of LID. In other words, many (if not all) of the plastic and molecular changes associated with LID experimentally could be the consequence, not the cause, of the movements which via cortical somesthetic afferents and corticostriatal projections could activate MSN.[118] Regardless of the origin and significance of these striatal changes, LID are certainly associated with abnormal GPi output activity as pallidotomy consistently eliminates LID and also chorea-ballism dyskinesias of any cause (see Chapter 18). This effect goes against the prediction of the classic model, whereby lesion or blockade of BG output should reduce thalamic inhibition and lead to dyskinesias. Accordingly, other physiological features apart from the reduced firing rate of GPi neurons have been considered relevant in the origin of LID.[109] These include firing patterns, particularly the duration and frequency of pauses,[124] and more recently, oscillatory patterns. Thus, it has been recognized that PD patients with LID exhibit low-frequency (6–8 Hz) oscillations in the STN[125] and GPi[126] that correlate with the presence of LIDs in the limbs. Pallidotomy probably abolishes LIDs by blocking these abnormal patterns of neuronal synchronization.

▶ CONCLUSIONS

The functional organization of the BG seems to be designed to serve a selection function, a basic strategy to facilitate or inhibit particular actions. Indeed, the scope of this fundamental BG function has now been expanded to apply a similar principle for the control of behavior and emotions.[9] Slowness and reduced spontaneous movement in PD are associated with DA reduction in the posterior putamen and functional abnormalities in the motor circuit. In PD, DA deficit progresses rostrally to alter executive and learning functions and eye movements (i.e., slow and hypometric saccade movements). DA loss in the ventral striatum is associated with apathy, depression, and deficits in reward processing and novelty seeking. Excessive or inadequate dopaminergic activation, as seen in PD patients under treatment with levodopa and DA agonists, improves motor features but can be associated with involuntary movements, impaired associative learning and a variety of behavioural problems (hypersexuality, increased eating, pathological gambling and shopping, etc.), euphoria and psychosis (hallucinations and delirium). Both bradykinesia and LIDs in PD may be understood as a defect in BG selection mechanisms, whereby there is excessive or reduced inhibition of movements and actions.[8,9] A similar concept may be thought to apply to the whole spectrum of BG domains and the associated pathological manifestations.

REFERENCES

1. Denny-Brown D: The midbrain and motor integration. Proc R Soc Med 1962;55:527–538.
2. Alexander GE, DeLong MR, an dStrick PL. Parallel organization of functionally segregated circuits linking basal ganglia and cortex. Ann Rev Neurosci 9:357–381.
3. Middleton FA, Strick PL: Basal ganglia and cerebellar loops: motor and cognitive circuits. Brain Res Rev 2000;31:236–250.
4. Smith Y, Bevan MD, Shink E, Bolam JP: Microcircuitry of the direct and indirect pathways of the basal ganglia. Neuroscience 1998;86:353–358.
5. Pasupathy A and Miller EK: Different time courses of learning-related activity in the prefrontal cortex and striatum. Nature 2005;433:873–876.
6. Yin HH and Knowlton B. The role of the basal ganglia in habit formation. Nat Neurosci Rev 2006;7:464–476.
7. Hikosaka O, Nakamura K, Sakai K, et al. Central mechanisms of motor learning. Curr Opin Neurobiol 2002;12:217–222.
8. Rodriguez-Oroz MC, Jahansahi M, Krack P, et al. Initial clinical manifestations of Parkinson's disease: Features and pathophysiological mechanisms. Lancet Neurol 2009;8:1128–1139.
9. Voon V, Fernagut PO, Wickens J, et al. Chronic dopaminergic stimulation in Parkinson's disease: From dyskinesias to impulse control disorders. Lancet Neurol 2009;8: 1140–1149.
10. Penney JB Jr, and Young AB. Striatal inhomogeneities and basal ganglia function. Mov Disord 1986;1:3–15.
11. Albin RL, Young AB, and Penney JB. The functional anatomy ofbasal ganglia disorders. Trends Neurosci 1989;12:366–375.
12. Alexander GE and Crutcher MD. Functional architecture of basal ganglia circuits: Neural substrates of parallel processing. Trends Neurosci 1990;13:266–271.
13. Hikosaka O and Wurtz RH. Visual and oculomotor functions of monkey substantia nigra pars reticulata. III. Memory-contingent visual and saccade responses. J Neurophysiol 1983;49:1268–1284.
14. Chevalier G and Deniau JM. Disinhibition as a basic process in the expression of striatal functions. Trends Neurosci 1990;13:277–280.
15. Gerfen CR, Engber TM, Mahan LC, et al. D1 and D2 dopamine receptor-regulated gene expression of striatonigral and striatopallidal neurons. Science 1990;250:1429–1432.
16. DeLong MR. Primate models of movement disorders of basal ganglia origin. Trend Neurosci 1990;13:281–285.
17. Crossman AR. Primate models of dyskinesia: the experimental approach to the study of basal ganglia-related involuntary movement disorders. Neuroscience 1987;21:1–40.
18. DeLong MR and Wichmann T. Circuits and circuit disorders of the basal ganglia. Arch Neurol 2007;64:20–24.

19. Soda M and Hikosaka O. Role for subthalamic nucleus neurons in switching from automatic to controlled eye movement. J Neurosci 2008;28:7209–7218.
20. Kita H, Tachibana Y, Nambu A, et al. Balance of monosynaptic excitatory and disynaptic inhibitory responses of the globus pallidus induced after stimulation of the subthalamic nucleus in the monkey. J Neurosci 2005;25:8611–8619.
21. Lévesque JC and Parent A. GABAergic interneurons in human subthalamic nucleus. Mov Disord 2005;20:574–584.
22. Obeso JA, Rodriguez-Oroz MC, Blesa FJ, et al. The globus pallidus pars externa and Parkinson's disease. Ready for prime time? Exp Neurol 2006;202:1–7.
23. Haber, S.N. The primate basal ganglia: parallel and integrative networks. J Chem Neuroanat 2003;26:317–330.
24. Gerfen CR. The neostriatal mosaic: multiple levels of compartmental organization. Trends Neurosci 1992;15: 132–139.
25. Lei W, Jiao Y, Del Mar N, et al. Evidence for differential cortical input to direct pathway versus indirect pathway striatal projection neurons in rats. J Neurosci 2004;24:8289–8299.
26. van Albada SJ and Robinson PA. Mean field modelling of the basal ganglia-thalamocortical system. I Firing rates in healthy and parkinsonian states. J Theor Biol 2009;257:642–663.
27. Nambu A, Takada M, Inase M, et al. Dual somatotopical representations in the primate subthalamic nucleus: evidence for ordered but reversed body-map transformations from the primary motor cortex and the supplementary motor area. J Neurosci 1996;16:2671–2683.
28. Miyachi S, Lu X, Imanishi M, et al. Somatotopically arranged inputs from putamen and subthalamic nucleus to primary motor cortex. Neurosci Res 2006;56:300–308.
29. Schultz W and Romo R. Role of primate basal ganglia and frontal cortex in the internal generation of movements. I. Preparatory activity in the anterior striatum. Exp Brain Res 1992;91:363–384.
30. Rodriguez-Oroz MC, Rodriguez M, Guridi J, et al. The subthalamic nucleus in Parkinson's disease: Somatotopic organization and physiological characteristics. Brain 2001;124:1777–1790.
31. Anderson ME, Turner RS: Activity of neurons in cerebellar-receiving and pallidal-receiving areas of the thalamus of the behaving monkey. J Neurophysiol 1991;66: 879–893.
32. Brotchie P, Iansek R, and Horne MK. Motor function of the monkey globus pallidus. 1. Neuronal discharge and parameters of movement. Brain 1991;114: 1667–1683.
33. DeLong MR and Georgopoulos AP. Motor functions of the basal ganglia as revealed by studies of single cell activity in the behaving primate. Adv Neurol 1979;24:131–140.
34. Turner RS and Anderson ME. Context-dependent modulation of movement-related discharge in the primate globus pallidus. J Neurosci 2005;25:2965–2976.
35. Redgrave P, Gurney K, an dReynolds J. What is reinforced by phasic dopamine signals? Brain Res Rev 2008;58: 322–339.
36. Joshua M, Adler A, Rosin B, et al. Encoding of probabilistic rewarding and aversive events by pallidal and nigral neurons. J Neurophysiol 2009;101:758–772.
37. Surmeier DJ, Ding J, Day M, et al. D1 and D2 dopamine-receptor modulation of striatal glutamatergic signaling in striatal medium spiny neurons. Trends Neurosci 2007;30:228–235.
38. Taverna S, Ilijic E, Surmeier DJ. Recurrent collateral connections of striatal medium spiny neurons are disrupted in models of Parkinson's disease. J Neurosci 2008;28: 5504–5512.
39. Gertler TS, Chan CS, Surmeier DJ. Dichotomous anatomical properties of adult striatal medium spiny neurons. J Neurosci 2008;28:10814–10824.
40. Calabresi P, Maj R, Pisani A, et al. Long-term synaptic depression in the striatum: Physiological and pharmacological characterization. J Neurosci 1992;12:4224–4233.
41. Calabresi P, Pisani A, Mercuri NB, et al. Long-term potentiation in the striatum is unmasked by removing the voltage-dependent magnesium block of NMDA receptor channels. Eur J Neurosci 1992;4:929–935.
42. Fino E, Glowinski J, Venance L. Bidirectional activity-dependent plasticity at corticostriatal synapses. J Neurosci 2005;25:11279–11287.
43. Goldberg JA, Rokni U, Boraud T, et al. Spike synchronization in the cortex/basal-ganglia networks of Parkinsonian primates reflects global dynamics of the local field potentials. J Neurosci 2003;24:6003–6010.
44. Rodríguez M, Pereda E, González J, et al. Neuronal activity in the substantia nigra in the anaesthetized rat has fractal characteristics. Evidence for firing-code patterns in the basal ganglia. Exp Brain Res 2003;151:167–172.
45. Sauleau P, Eusebio A, Tewathasan W, et al. Involvement of the subthalamic nucleus in engagement with behaviourally relevant stimuli. Eur J Neurosci 2009;29:931–942.
46. Marceglia S, Fiorio M, Foffani G, et al. Modulation of beta oscillations in the subthalamic area during action observation in Parkinson's disease. Neuroscience 2009;161:1027–1036.
47. Alegre M, Rodriguez-Oroz MC, Valencia M, et al. Changes in subthalamic activity during movement observation in Parkinson's disease: Is the mirror system mirrored in the basal ganglia? Clin Neurophysiol 2010;121:414–425.
48. Brücke C, Kupsch A, Schneider GH, et al. The subthalamic region is activated during valence-related emotional processing in patients with Parkinson's disease. Eur J Neurosci 2007;26:767–774.
49. Lehéricy S, Bardinet E, Tremblay L, et al. Motor control in basal ganglia circuits using fMRI and brain atlas approaches. Cereb Cortex 2006;16:149–161.
50. Draganski B, Khefir F, Klöppel S, et al. Evidence for segregated and integrative connectivity patterns in the human basal ganglia. J Neurosci 2008;28:7143–7152.
51. Lehéricy S, Ducros M, Van de Moortele PF, Francois C, et al. Diffusion tensor fiber tracking shows distinct corticostriatal circuits in humans. Ann Neurol 2004;55:522–529.
52. Postuma RB and Dagher A. Basal ganglia functional connectivity based on a meta-analysis of 126 positron emission tomography and functional magnetic resonance imaging publications. Cereb Cortex 2006;16:1508–1521.
53. Decety J, Perani D, Jeannerod M, et al. Mapping motor representations with positron emission tomography. Nature 1994;371:600–602.
54. Lehéricy S, van de Moortele PF, Lobel E, et al. Somatotopical organization of striatal activation during finger

and toe movement: A 3-T functional magnetic resonance imaging study. Ann Neurol 1998;44:398–404.
55. Jenkins IH, Brooks DJ, Nixon PD, et al. Motor sequence learning: a study with positron emission tomography. J Neurosci 1994;14:3775–3790.
56. Jueptner M, Frith CD, Brooks DJ, et al. Anatomy of motor learning. II. Subcortical structures and learning by trial and error. J Neurophysiol 1997;77:1325–1337.
57. Jenkins IH, Jahanshahi M, Jueptner M, et al. Self-initiated versus externally triggered movements. II. The effect of movement predictability on regional cerebral blood flow. Brain 2000;123:1216–1228.
58. Gerardin E, Pochon JB, Poline JB, et al. Distinct striatal regions support movement selection, preparation, and execution. Neuroreport 2004;15:2327–2331.
59. Lehéricy S, Benali H, Van de Moortele PF, et al: Distinct basal ganglia territories are engaged in early and advanced motor sequence learning. Proc Natl Acad Sci U S A 2005;102:12566–12571.
60. Floyer-Lea A and Matthews PM. Changing brain networks for visuomotor control with increased movement automaticity. J Neurophysiol 2004;92:2405–2412.
61. Wu T, Kansaku K, and Hallett M. How self-initiated memorized movements become automatic: a functional MRI study. J Neurophysiol 2004;91:1690–1698.
62. Grafton ST, Mazziotta JC, Presty S, et al. Functional anatomy of human procedural learning determined with regional cerebral blood flow and PET. J Neurosci 1992;12:2542–2548.
63. Aron AR, Behrens TE, Smith S, et al. Triangulating a cognitive control network using diffusion-weighted magnetic resonance imaging (MRI) and functional MRI. J Neurosci 2007;27:3743–3752.
64. Redgrave P: Basal ganglia. Scholarpedia 2007;2:1825.
65. Wilson CJ. Basal ganglia. In GM Shepherd, (ed). The Synaptic Organization of the Brain. New York, NY: Oxford University Press, 2004, pp. 361–414.
66. Bamford NS, Robinson S, Palmiter R, et al. Dopamine modulates release from corticostriatal terminals. J Neurosci 2004;24:9541–9552.
67. Tepper MJ, Koós T, Wilson CJ. GABAergic microcircuits in the neostriatum. Trends Neurosci 2004;27: 662–669.
68. Bamford NS, Zhang H, Schmitz Y, et al. Heterosynaptic dopamine neurotransmission selects sets of corticostriatal terminals. Neuron 2004;42:653–663.
69. Hikosaka O, Nakamura K, Sakai K, et al. Central mechanisms of motor skill learning. Curr Opin Neurobiol 2002;12:217–222.
70. Rauch SL, Whalen PJ, Savage CR, et al. Striatal recruitment during an implicit sequence learning task as measured by functional magnetic resonance imaging. Hum Brain Mapp 1997;5:124–132.
71. Albouy G, Sterpenich V, Balteau E, et al. Both the hippocampus and striatum are involved in consolidation of motor sequence memory. Neuron 2008;58: 261–272.
72. Maquet P, Schwartz S, Passingham R, et al. Sleep-related consolidation of a visuomotor skill: Brain mechanisms as assessed by functional magnetic resonance imaging. J Neurosci 2003;23:1432–1440.
73. Redgrave P, Prescott TJ, Gurney K. The basal ganglia: A vertebrate solution to the selection problem? Neuroscience 1999;89:1009–1023.
74. Mink JW. The basal ganglia and involuntary movements: Impaired inhibition of competing motor patterns. Arch Neurol 2003;60:1365–1368.
75. Obeso JA, Marin C, Rodriguez-Oroz C, et al. The basal ganglia in Parkinson's disease: Current concepts and unexplained observations. Ann Neurol 2008;64: S30–S46.
76. Bezard E, Dovero S, Prunier C, et al. Relationship between the appearance of symptoms and the level of nigrostriatal degeneration in a progressive 1-methyl-4-phenyl-1,2,3,6-tetrahydropyridine-lesioned macaque model of Parkinson's disease. J Neurosci 2001;21: 6853–6861.
77. Vila M, Levy R, Herrero MT, et al. Consequences of nigrostriatal denervation on the functioning of the basal ganglia in human and nonhuman primates: An in situ hybridization study of cytochrome oxidase subunit I mRNA. J Neurosci 1997;17:765–773.
78. Poewe W. Clinical measures of progression in Parkinson's disease. Mov Disord 2009;24:S671–S676.
79. Blesa J. et al: Progression of Dopaminergic Depletion in a Model of MPTP-InducedParkinsonism in Non-Human Primates. An ^{18}F-DOPA and ^{11}C-DTBZ PET study. Neurobio Dis 2010. (In press).
80. Pavese N, Khan NL, Scherfler C, et al. Nigrostriatal dysfunction in homozygous and heterozygous parkin gene carriers: An 18F-dopa PET progression study. Mov Disord 2009;24:2260–2266.
81. Marek K, Jennings D, and Seibyl J. Single-photon emission tomography and dopamine transporter imaging in Parkinson's disease. Adv Neurol 2003;91:183–191.
82. Nandhagopal R, Kuramoto L, Schulzer M, et al. Longitudinal progression of sporadic Parkinson's disease: A multi-tracer positron emission tomography study. Brain 2009;132:2970–2979.
83. Herrero MT, Augood SJ, Asensi H, et al. Effects of l-dopa therapy on dopamine D-2 receptor mRNA expression in the striatum of MPTP-intoxicated parkinsonian monkeys. Mol Brain Res 1996;42:149–155.
84. Soghomonian JJ and Chesselet MF. Effects of nigrostriatal lesions on the levels of messenger RNAs encoding two isoforms of glutamate decarboxylase in the globus pallidus and entopeduncular nucleus of the rat. Synapse 1992;11:124–133.
85. Kreitzer AC and Malenka RC. Endocannabinoid-mediated rescue of striatal LTD and motor deficits in Parkinson's disease models. Nature 2007;445:643–647.
86. Picconi B, Centonze D, Hakansson K, et al. Loss of bidirectional striatal synaptic plasticity in L-Dopa-induced dyskinesia. Nat Neurosci 2003;6:501–506, 2003.
87. Day M, Wang Z, Ding J, An X, et al. Selective elimination of glutamatergic synapses on striatopallidopaminel neurons in Parkinson disease models. Nat Neurosci 2006;9:251–259.
88. Stephens B, Mueller AJ, Shering AF, et al. Evidence of a breakdown of corticostriatal connections in Parkinson's disease. Neuroscience 2005;32:741–754.

89. Villalba RM, Lee H, and Smith Y. Dopaminergic denervation and spine loss in the striatum of MPTP-treated monkeys. Exp Neurol 2009;215:220–227.
90. Raz A, Frechter-Mazar V, Feingold A, et al. Activity of pallidal and striatal tonically active neurons is correlated in MPTP-treated monkeys but not in normal monkeys. J Neurosci 2001;21:RC128, 1–5.
91. Aosaki T, Kimura M, and Graybiel AM. Temporal and spatial characteristics of tonically active neurons of the primate's striatum. J Neurophysiol 1995;73: 1234–1252.
92. Fino E, Glowinski J, and Venance L. Effects of acute dopamine depletion on the electrophysiological properties of striatal neurons. Neurosci Res 2007;58:305–316.
93. Calabresi P Centonze D, Gubellini P, et al. Acetylcholine-mediated modulation of striatal function. Trends Neurosci 2000;23:120–126.
94. Pakhotin P and Bracci E. Cholinergic interneurons control the excitatory input to the striatum. J Neurosci 2007;27:391–400.
95. Tecuapetla F, Koós T, Tepper JM, et al. Differential dopaminergic modulation of neostriatal synaptic connections of striatopallidal axon collaterals. J Neurosci 2009;29:8977–8990.
96. Guridi J, Herrero MT, Luquin MR, et al. Subthalamotomy in parkinsonian monkeys. Behavioural and biochemical analysis. Brain 1996;119:1717–1727.
97. Ceballos-Baumann AO, Obeso JA, Vitek JL, et al. Restoration of thalamocortical activity after posteroventral pallidotomy in Parkinson's disease. Lancet 1994;344:814.
98. Eidelberg D, Moeller JR, Ishikawa T, et al. Regional metabolic correlates of surgical outcome following unilateral pallidotomy for Parkinson's disease. Ann Neurol 1996;39:350–359.
99. Smith Y and Villalba R. Striatal and extrastriatal dopamine in the basal ganglia: An overview of its anatomical organization in normal and Parkinsonian brains. Mov Disord 2008; 23:S534–S547.
100. Parent A and Hazrati LN. Functional anatomy of the basal ganglia. I. The cortico-basal ganglia-thalamo-cortical loop. Brain Res Brain Res Rev 1995;20:91–127.
101. Floran B, Floran L, Sierra A, et al. D2 receptor-mediated inhibition of GABA release by endogenous dopamine in the rat globus pallidus. Neurosci Lett 1997;237:1–4.
102. Galvan A, Floran B, Erlij D, et al. Intrapallidal dopamine restores motor deficits induced by 6-hydroxydopamine in the rat. J Neural Transm 2001;108:153–166.
103. Francois C, Savy C, Jan C, et al. Dopaminergic innervation of the subthalamic nucleus in the normal state, in MPTP-treated monkeys, and in Parkinson's disease patients. J Comp Neurol 2000;425:121–129.
104. Kreiss DS, Anderson LA, Walters JR. Apomorphine and dopamineD-1 receptor agonists increase the firing rates of subthalamic nucleus neurons. Neuroscience 1996;72:863–867.
105. Smith Y, Wichmann T, DeLong MR. Synaptic innervation of neurones in the internal pallidal segment by the subthalamic nucleus and the external pallidum in monkeys. J Comp Neurol 1994;343:297–318.
106. Bezard E, Dovero S, Prunier C, et al. Relationship between the appearance of symptoms and the level of nigrostriatal degeneration in a progressive 1-methyl-4-phenyl-1,2,3,6-tetrahydropyridine-lesioned macaque model of Parkinson's disease. J Neurosci 2001;21: 6853–6861.
107. Rubchinsky LL, Kopell N, Sigvardt KA. Modeling facilitation and inhibition of competing motor programs in basal ganglia subthalamic nucleus-pallidopaminel circuits. Proc Natl Acad Sci U S A 2003;100:14427–14432.
108. Filion M, Tremblay L, Bedard PJ. Abnormal influences of passive limb movement on the activity of globus pallidus neurons in parkinsonian monkeys. Brain Res 1988;444:165–176.
109. Boraud T, Bezard E, Bioulac B, et al. Ratio of inhibited-to-activated pallidal neurons decreases dramatically during passive limb movement in the MPTP-treated monkey. J Neurophysiol 2000;83:1760–1763.
110. Obeso JA, Rodriguez-Oroz MC, Rodriguez M, et al. Pathophysiology of levodopa-induced dyskinesias in Parkinson's disease: Problems with the current model. Ann Neurol 2000;47:S22–S32; discussion S32–S34.
111. Suarez JI, Metman LV, Reich SG, et al. Pallidotomy for hemiballismus: Efficacy and characteristics of neuronal activity. Ann Neurol 1997;42:807–811, 1997.
112. Guridi J and Obeso JA. The subthalamic nucleus, hemiballismus and Parkinson's disease: reappraisal of a neurosurgical dogma. Brain 2001;124:5–19.
113. Mitchell IJ, Jackson A, Sambrook MA, et al. Common neural mechanisms in experimental chorea and hemiballismus in the monkey. Evidence from 2-deoxyglucose autoradiography. Brain Res 1985;339: 346–350.
114. Carpenter MB, Whittier JR, Mettler FA. Analysis of choreoid hyperkinesia in the Rhesus monkey: Surgical and pharmacological analysis of hyperkinesia resulting from lesions in the subthalamic nucleus of Luys. J Comp Neurol 1950;92:293–331.
115. Crossman AR, Sambrook MA, et al. Experimental hemichorea/hemiballismus in the monkey: Studies on the intracerebral site of action in a drug-induced dyskinesia. Brain 1987;107:579–596.
116. Mitchell IJ, Jackson A, Sambrook MA, et al. The role of the subthalamic nucleus in experimental chorea: evidence from 2-deoxyglucose metabolic mapping and horseradish peroxidase tracing studies. Brain 1989;112: 1533–1548.
117. Cenci MA, Whishaw IQ, Schallert T. Animal models of neurological deficits: how relevant is the rat? Nat Rev Neurosci 2002;3:574–579.
118. Jenner P. Molecular mechanisms of L-DOPA-induced dyskinesia. Nat Rev Neurosci 2008;9:665–677.
119. Papa SM, Desimone R, Fiorani M, et al. Internal globus pallidus discharge is nearly suppressed during levodopa-induced dyskinesias. Ann Neurol 1999;46: 732–738.
120. Merello M, Balej J, Delfino M, et al. Apomorphine induces changes in GPi spontaneous outfl ow in patients with Parkinson's disease. Mov Disord 1999;14:45–49.
121. Boraud T, Bezard E, Bioulac B, et al. Dopamine agonist-induced dyskinesias are correlated to both firing pattern and frequency alterations of pallidal neurones in the MPTP-treated monkey. Brain 2001;124:546–557.

122. Aubert I, Guigoni C, Hakansson K, et al. Increased D1 dopamine receptor signaling in levodopa-induced dyskinesia. Ann Neurol 2005;57:17–26.
123. Bezard E, Ferry S, Mach U, et al. Attenuation of levodopa-induced dyskinesia by normalizing dopamine D3 receptor function. Nat Med 2003;9:762–767.
124. Vitek JL, Giroux M. Physiology of hypokinetic and hyperkinetic movement disorders: Model for dyskinesia. Ann Neurol 2000;47:S131–S140.
125. Alonso-Frech F, Zamarbide I, Alegre M, Rodriguez-Oroz MC, Guridi J, Manrique M, Valencia M, Artieda J, et al. Slow oscillatory activity and levodopa-induced dyskinesias in Parkinson's disease. Brain 2006;129:1748–1757.
126. Foffani G, Ardolino G, Meda B, et al. Altered subthalamo-pallidal synchronisation in parkinsonian dyskinesias. J Neurol Neurosurg Psychiatry 2005;76:426–428.

CHAPTER 6

Functional Neurochemistry of the Basal Ganglia

Anthony P. Nicholas and David G. Standaert

Progressive degeneration of neurons of the various nuclei of the basal ganglia leads to many clinical disorders manifesting in severe disabling motor, autonomic, and cognitive problems. The different nuclei of the basal ganglia, especially the striatum, are the sites of actions of diverse neurotransmitters and neuropeptides.[1] Classic and modern neuroanatomical and neurochemical studies have enabled us to draw a working model of the circuits of the basal ganglia.[2–4] Although very much simplified, these models have been valuable and have advanced our understanding of the molecular circuitries as well as the role played by the individual neurotransmitters and neuropeptides in the functions of the basal ganglia.

This chapter reviews the information relevant to the patterns of organization of five major neurotransmitters, namely, dopamine, acetylcholine (ACh), glutamate, serotonin, and noradrenaline, and their receptors in the basal ganglia and briefly relates to the changes that occur in the diseases of the basal ganglia.

▶ OVERVIEW OF THE CIRCUITS OF THE BASAL GANGLIA

The basal ganglia may be divided into several functional subcompartments. The primary input structures are the caudate, putamen, and the nucleus accumbens, which are collectively termed the "striatum." The putamen processes the motor component of basal ganglia-thalamocortical circuits, whereas caudate and nucleus accumbens mediate cognitive, emotive, and limbic inputs. The spiny neurons, the principal input and output cells accounting for more than three quarters of the total striatal neuronal population, receive the excitatory synaptic inputs from neocortex as well as thalamus and the dopaminergic input from substantia nigra pars compacta (SNc).[5] Two neurochemically and anatomically distinct populations of spiny neurons of the striatum project downstream to the globus pallidus internal segment (GPi) and substantia nigra pars reticulata (SNr), which are the basal ganglia output nuclei (GPi/SNr). A specific subpopulation of γ-aminobutyric acid (GABA)- and substance P-containing spiny neurons that project directly to the GPi and SNr forms the direct pathway. The indirect pathway arises from a separate subpopulation of spiny neurons that coexpress GABA and enkephalin and project to the external segment of globus pallidus (GPe).[6] GPe sends a GABAergic projection to the subthalamus (STN), which in turn provides glutamatergic innervations of GPi/SNr. The high basal discharge of the GABAergic GPi neurons, the major output nucleus of the basal ganglia circuit, results in tonic inhibitory control over the nonmotor and motor thalamus, and the mesopontine tegmentum.

This working model of basal ganglia circuits (Fig. 6–1) suggests that the basal activity of the pallidal neurons is kept in check by a balance of the direct inhibitory pathway tending to reduce basal ganglia output and the excitatory indirect pathway tending to increase the output. During normal movement, changes in the balance of the direct and indirect pathways reduce GPi/SNr inhibition of thalamus, allowing engagement of thalamocortical circuits necessary for the speed and guidance of movements. An imbalance of activity, however, in the direct and indirect pathways can perturb the normal degree of GPi/SNr inhibition of thalamocortical activity, producing either hypokinetic or hyperkinetic movement disorders.[7,8] For example, in Parkinson's disease (PD), models suggest that activity is reduced in the direct pathway and increased in the indirect pathway, both leading to enhanced GPi/SNr activity and excessive inhibition of thalamus.[7,8] These models are necessarily greatly simplified, and emphasize the *quantity* of activity in specific pathways while neglecting the *patterns* and *content* of such activity. Despite these deficiencies, the models are a useful starting point, and have led to substantial new insights and the development of new treatments.

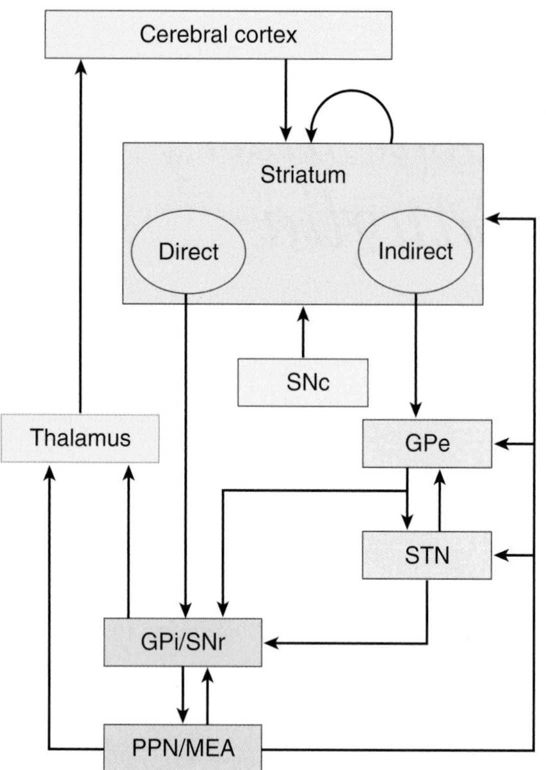

Figure 6–1. Schematic of basal ganglia circuitry model. Direct and indirect pathways originating from striatum are named according to the immediacy of their regulation of the basal ganglia output nuclei, GPi/SNr. The projections from each region are color coded by their major neurotransmitters in the Color Gallery. GPe, globus pallidus external segment; GPi/SNr, globus pallidus internal segment/substantia nigra pars reticulata; PPN/MEA, pedunculopontine nucleus/midbrain extrapyramidal area; SNc, substantia nigra pars compacta; STN, subthalamic nucleus.

The remainder of the chapter focuses on the major neurotransmitter systems in the basal ganglia: dopamine, ACh, glutamate, serotonin, and noradrenaline.

▶ NEUROCHEMICAL ORGANIZATION OF THE DOPAMINERGIC SYSTEM IN THE BASAL GANGLIA

SOURCE OF DOPAMINE IN THE BASAL GANGLIA

About 80% of the total brain dopamine is in the striatum, with the next highest level in the substantia nigra followed by the GP and STN. Even within the striatum, dopamine levels are uneven. The caudal head and the rostral body of the caudate contain more dopamine than the rostral head, the caudal regions, and the tail of the caudate nucleus. Within the putamen, the caudal regions have more dopamine than the rostral regions. Dopamine levels in SNc are three times more than in SNr, and GPe has more dopamine than GPi.[9]

Dopaminergic innervations of the nucleus accumbens arise from the ventral tegmental area (VTA; A8) group of dopaminergic neurons of the mesencephalon and that of the caudate nucleus and the putamen from the A9 cell group in SNc.[10] The dopaminergic neurons of SNc are organized into dorsal and ventral tiers.[11] The ventral tier of SNc neurons projects to the dorsolateral motor striatum; the dorsal tier projects to the associative striatum. The ventrally located dopaminergic neurons are the most vulnerable in PD, and in MPTP and rotenone toxicity.[12–17] The different subdivisions of the VTA project to the nucleus accumbens, and the fundus striatum.[18] The effects of dopamine released from SNc neurons are further regulated by cholecystokinin and neurotensin; two neuropeptides that are colocalized within these midbrain dopaminergic neurons and may be coreleased with dopamine.[19]

The tyrosine hydroxylase (TH)-immunopositive fibers from the midbrain dopaminergic neurons are distributed throughout the striatum, but in a heterogeneous pattern[20,21] that is consistent with the fact that levels of dopamine vary in different regions of the striatum.[9] TH-immunoreactive fibers are more dense in the dorsal and ventral caudate nucleus and the nucleus accumbens than in the dorsolateral striatum. Throughout the striatum there are many TH-poor patches intermixed with TH-rich matrix regions. Collaterals from the nigrostriatal fibers also innervate GPi and GPe, and STN densely.[20] GPi has more dense dopaminergic innervation than GPe.

Another important source of dopamine to the human striatum is the TH-immunopositive interneurons that reside within the striatum.[20] These neurons express mRNA for the dopamine transporter, suggesting that dopamine is actively transported into these neurons.[22,23] The number of these neurons increases in 1-methyl-4-phenyl-1,2,3,6-tetrahydropyridine (MPTP) models of PD in primates, suggesting that these striatal dopaminergic neurons are enhanced as a consequence of striatal dopamine denervation and may play a compensatory role in dopamine deficiency states.[20]

Dopaminergic terminals synapse predominantly on dendritic shafts and spines of striatal medium spiny neurons,[24,25] where they appear to regulate responsiveness to cortical and thalamic excitatory drive.[26,27] Distinct subpopulations of dopaminergic neurons project to the "striosomes" and "matrix" compartments of the striatum.[28] These compartments represent separate subchannels of afferent and efferent circuits through basal ganglia. Based on corticostriatal connections, the striosome compartment processes limbic information, whereas the striatal matrix processes sensorimotor information.[28] SNc neurons also extend dendrites into pars reticulata, where they release dopamine, modulating

GABA release, neuronal activity in pars reticulata and, subsequently, basal ganglia output to thalamus.[29]

MOLECULAR DIVERSITY OF DOPAMINE RECEPTORS AND THEIR SIGNAL TRANSDUCTION

The diverse effects of dopamine are mediated by D1 and D2 subfamilies of dopamine receptors, which are defined by pharmacological, anatomical, and biochemical criteria.[30–34] All dopamine receptors identified to date are members of the superfamily of G protein-coupled receptors (GPCR).[35] All GPCRs have a seven transmembrane spanning structure linked by three alternating extracellular and intracellular domains, an extracellular N-terminal, and a cytoplasmic C-terminal. More than 1000 GPCRs, accounting for more than 1% of the total human genome, have been identified. Besides the well-established role of triggering the second messenger functions, activation of G proteins may also trigger molecular cascades that are responsible for cell survival, cell death, and neoplasia.[36] On the basis of their structure, the GPCRs are classified into families A, B, and C.[35] Dopamine receptors have structural and functional similarities to G protein receptors of other monoamines and rhodopsin, and belong to the A family of GPCRs. The genes coding for the D1 subfamily are intronless, and have a shorter third cytoplasmic loop, but have an intracellular C-terminal, which is seven times longer than in D2 receptors.[34]

The D1 subfamily consists of D1 and D5 receptors. They are coupled to the G proteins Gs and Golf, and when activated result in an increase in adenylyl cyclase and cyclic AMP levels postsynaptically. Dopamine has 10 times more affinity to D5 receptor than for D1, but pharmacologically D1 and D5 are otherwise indistinguishable.[34]

The D2 subfamily consists of D2, D3, and D4 receptors, which are coupled to the inhibitory Gi, Go class of G proteins, and when stimulated result in a decrease in adenylyl cyclase and cyclic AMP levels, and modulate ion channels. The D2 receptors are further divided into D2S and D2L, but both receptors have similar pharmacology and distribution patterns.[34] The D4 receptors show polymorphism,[37] but the significance of the polymorphic variants remains to be explored.

The classification of the dopamine receptor gene family, including binding properties, selective agonists and antagonists, and general distributions in brain are summarized in Table 6–1.

TABLE 6–1. DOPAMINE RECEPTOR SUBTYPES

Receptor Class	Receptor Subtype	Isoforms	Second Messenger	Selective Agonists	Selective Antagonists	Localization
D1 subfamily			Increase cyclic AMP			
	D1 (DIA)			SKF 38393 CY 208–243 (partial agonists) A 77636, SKF 82958 (full agonists)	SCH 23390 (some 5-HT effects) SCH-39166 (no 5-HT effects)	Striatal spiny neurons (direct pathway)
	D5 (DIB)	Pseudogenes on chromosomes 1 and 2 polymorphisms				Cortex, thalamus, cholinergic striatal neurons, SNc
D2 subfamily			Decrease cyclic AMP			
	D2 (D2A)	Short/long splice variants, six introns		Bromocriptine Quinpirole	Spiroperidol (some 5-HT effects) Raclopride	Striatal spiny neurons[34] (indirect pathway)
	D3 (D2B)	Two splice variants (truncated), five introns		7-OH-DPAT PD 128,907		SNc (autoreceptor) Ventral striatum, limbic regions
	D4 (D2C)	Polymorphisms (2–10 repeats)			Clozapine (some muscarinic + 5-HT effects) L 745870 U 101958	Frontal cortex, midbrain, striatum

7-OH-DPAT, 7-hydroxy-*N*,*N*-di-*n*-propyl-2-aminotetralin; SNc, substantia nigra pars compacta.

DOPAMINE RECEPTOR DISTRIBUTION IN THE BASAL GANGLIA

All the dopamine receptor subtypes have been localized to different nuclei of the basal ganglia.[38] The striatum shows the maximum expression of D1 receptors in the human brain.[34,39,40] D1 receptor mRNA is found throughout the nucleus accumbens, caudate nucleus, and the putamen. The labeling for D1 receptor mRNA is more dense in the nucleus accumbens and the medial caudate than in the lateral regions of the putamen, thereby suggesting a pattern of decreasing intensity from a medial to a lateral direction.[40] The mRNA for D1 receptor is expressed in the GABA- and substance P-containing neurons that project directly to GPi and SNr; accordingly, the D1 receptor protein, but not mRNA, for D1 receptor is highly expressed in GPi and SNr.[28] D1 receptors are also expressed highly in the prefrontal cortex,[41] in contrast to barely detectable levels of D2 binding in these cortical areas.

D2 receptor mRNA is highly expressed in spiny neurons that express GABA and enkephalin and project to GPe and indirectly to GPi through STN.[42] GPe shows significant D2 immunoreactivity. The D2 receptor protein is localized to the dendrites and spine heads more than to the soma of these striatal input–output neurons. The D1 and D2 receptors are expressed mostly in separate subpopulations of the striatal spiny neurons, but there are a small number of medium spiny neurons that express both D1 and D2 receptors.[43,44] The dendrites of SNc cells contain D2 autoreceptors.

The nucleus accumbens shows the highest concentration of D3 receptors of all brain regions. D3 mRNA is localized in the spiny neurons of nucleus accumbens that show colocalization of neurotensin and substance P.[45–47]

The D4 receptors are expressed in the soma, dendritic shaft, and spines of the medium spiny neurons of the striatum, more so in the striosomes than in the matrix.[48,49] D4 receptor labeling is more dense in the dorsolateral compartment than in the ventromedial caudate nucleus and the nucleus accumbens, a pattern that is opposite to that of D1 distribution in the striatum. The external and internal segments of GP and SNr demonstrate labeling for D4 receptors.[48,49]

D5 receptor mRNAs have been localized within the medium spiny neurons as well as in the large cholinergic interneurons of the striatum and in the terminals of the GABA/striatopallidal neurons. Dense labeling of D5 receptors is also noted in SNc and SNr.[50]

FUNCTIONS OF DOPAMINE RECEPTOR SUBTYPES

Pharmacological, behavioral, and gene manipulation (knockout) techniques have recently begun to unravel the role played by the individual subtypes of dopamine receptors.[34,51,52] These studies suggest that D1 receptors may be involved in locomotor activity in novel environment; spatial and working memory, especially cortical D1 receptors; and locomotor responses to psychostimulant drugs.[52–54] D2 receptors play a major role in initiating and maintaining normal locomotor behavior.[52] D2 autoreceptors when activated by agonists cause a decreased release of dopamine and resultant decrease in motor activity, whereas agonists of postsynaptic D2 receptors induce hyperactivity.[52] Mice lacking D2 receptors have a prominent hunched posture and delay in initiating movements, as well as other locomotor and postural features of PD.[55] D2 receptors, when coactivated with D1 receptors, play a major role in locomotor responses to drugs of abuse. D3 receptors, located mostly in the limbic striatum, when stimulated specifically, induced hypolocomotion, and antagonists of D3 receptors induced hyperlocomotion.[34,51,52] D3 receptors may also have a role in drug-seeking behavior.[56] The D4 receptor has been speculated to play a role in novelty-seeking behavior.[57] The D5 receptors may inhibit locomotor behavior.[51,52]

▶ NEUROCHEMICAL ORGANIZATION OF THE ACETYLCHOLINERGIC SYSTEM IN THE BASAL GANGLIA

SOURCE OF ACETYLCHOLINE IN THE BASAL GANGLIA

The dense cholinergic input to the different subnuclei of the basal ganglia is from two different sources. The striatum contains exceptionally high levels of ACh, and acetylcholinesterase.[5] Striatal ACh is derived almost exclusively from giant aspiny interneurons, which constitute 2% of total striatal neurons.[58] These cholinergic neurons are tonically active and fire at about 5 Hz; they pause their tonic firing during learning of conditioned motor tasks.[58,59] The cholinergic terminals derived from these neurons ramify densely and extensively and synapse predominantly on spiny neurons,[60] where ACh modulates, postsynaptically, the responsiveness of the spiny neurons to the excitatory cortical and thalamic inputs located on the spine heads.[61] These large cholinergic interneurons receive glutamatergic input from the cerebral cortex and thalamus,[62] and dopaminergic input from SN and VTA.[63]

The GP, STN, SN, and thalamus receive significant cholinergic projections from the ascending outputs of the pedunculopontine nucleus (PPN).[64–66] The PPN projection to the GPi is less dense than its projection to the SN and STN. The PPN, representing the Ch5 subgroup of cholinergic neurons of the brain, is located in the mesopontine tegmentum, and contains both cholinergic and glutamatergic components. The PPN itself receives direct projections from GPi[67] and SNr, and projects caudally to motor structures in brainstem.[68] The pallido-PPN projections may terminate preferentially in the cholinergic subdivision of PPN.[69,70] In PD, there is pathological involvement of the PPN.[71] Moreover, there is a dramatic increase (>200%) in muscarinic-binding sites in GPi in this disease, possibly reflecting compensatory upregulation of the receptors in the face of reduced cholinergic activity.[72] Thus, in addition to the intrinsic cholinergic system in striatum, the PPN mediates cholinergic effects on other extrastriatal sites of the basal ganglia.

MOLECULAR DIVERSITY OF CHOLINERGIC RECEPTORS AND THEIR SIGNAL TRANSDUCTION

The cholinergic effects are mediated by the ligand-gated ion channel nicotinic acetylcholinergic receptor family (nAChR),[73,74] and the G protein-coupled muscarinic acetylcholinergic (mAChR) family.[75,76] Both classes of receptors are abundant in the brain and basal ganglia structures.

Nicotinic Receptors

The ionotropic nAChR has a pentameric structure consisting of two copies of one of the many subtypes of α subunits, separated by a copy of one of the β subunits and/or γ subunit and a δ subunit. Eight α (α2–α10) and three β subunits (β2–β4) of the nAChRs have been cloned. Different combinations of these α and β subunits form varieties of functional nAChRs with pharmacological and physiological properties that are distinct to each of them.[73,74] The α4–β2-containing nAChR, a receptor with very high binding affinity to nicotine, is the most common type observed in the brain and in some nuclei of the basal ganglia. The mRNA for α4–β2 nAChR is very densely expressed in SNc, and these receptors are found on the dopaminergic terminals in the striatum.[74]

Muscarinic Receptors

The five distinct subtypes of mAChRs are members of the A family group of the GPCR superfamily. The m1, m3, and m5 receptors are functionally related and are coupled to Gαq11 and Gα13 subtypes of G proteins, which lead to activation of phospholipase C and phospholipase D. The m2 and m4 receptors couple to the inhibitory Gi and Go proteins, leading to inhibition of adenylyl cyclase and decrease in cyclic AMP levels.[75,76]

The classification of the mAChR gene family, including binding properties, signal transduction mechanisms, and distributions in brain, is summarized in Table 6–2.

CHOLINERGIC RECEPTOR DISTRIBUTION IN THE BASAL GANGLIA

Nicotinic Receptors

The α4 and β2 subunits containing nAChR are the most common in the brain and the basal ganglia. Bungarotoxin-binding α7 is the next most commonly found subunit of nAChR. The mRNA for α 3, 4, 5, 6, and 7 subunits and β 2, 3, and 4 subunits has been localized to the SN and VTA. α7 expression may be more prominent in VTA than in SN. β2 is expressed in all the neurons of VTA and SN. The mRNA for nAChRs has not been localized convincingly in any of the striatal neurons. The α4–β2 nAChR is very densely expressed in SNc, and the protein for these receptors is found on the dopaminergic terminals in the striatum. Nicotinic receptors in the basal ganglia appear to be mostly located in the presynaptic

▶ TABLE 6–2. MUSCARINIC ACETYLCHOLINE RECEPTOR SUBTYPES

Molecular Subtype	Pharmacological Subclass	Isoforms	Second Messenger	Basal Ganglia Localization
m1	M1	None	Increase PI hydrolysis	Striatal spiny neurons (direct and indirect pathways)
m2	M2	None	Decrease cyclic AMP	Cholinergic striatal interneurons, PPN, cortex, thalamus
m3	M3 > M1 > M2	None	Increase PI hydrolysis	Subthalamus and widespread regions outside striatum
m4	M1 and M2	None	Decrease cyclic AMP	Striatal spiny neurons (direct pathway)
m5	M1 > M2	None	Increase PI hydrolysis	SNc (nigrostriatal terminals?)

PI, phosphatidylinositol; PPN, pedunculopontine nucleus; SNc, substantia nigra pars compacta.

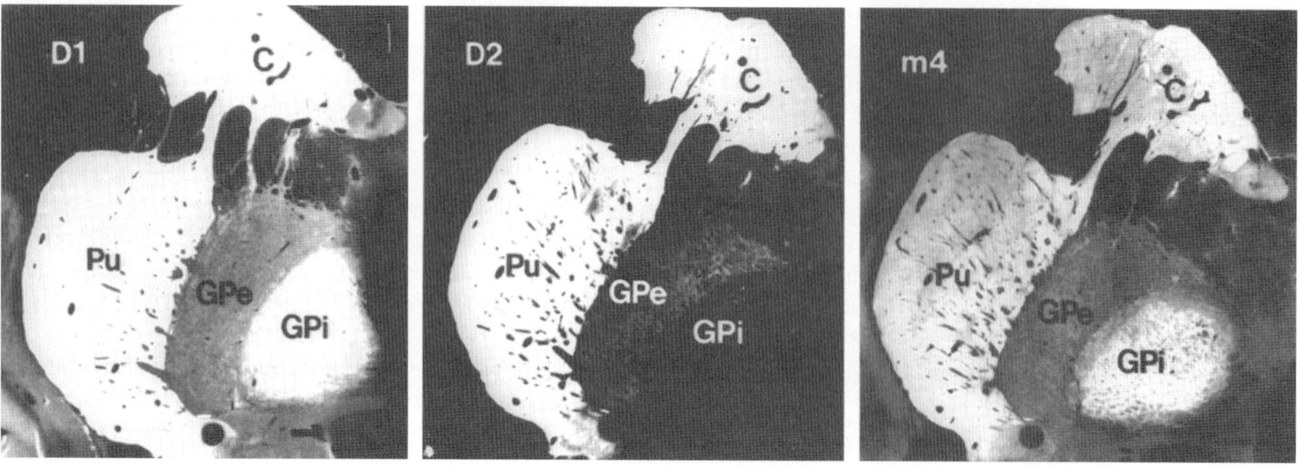

Figure 6–2. Immunocytochemical localization of dopaminergic (D1 and D2) and muscarinic cholinergic (m4) receptor subtypes in monkey basal ganglia. Low-power darkfield micrograph of immunoperoxidase-stained brain tissue sections through neostriatum and globus pallidus. Note intense staining (white areas) of all three receptors in caudate (C) and putamen (Pu), and selective localization to either globus pallidus interna (GPi) for D1 and m4 or globus pallidus externa (GPe) for D2, suggesting selective expression of the subtypes in the striatofugal neurons and terminals of the direct or indirect pathways, respectively. Coronal sections; lateral portion positioned on the left and medial on the right; scale bars = 100 μm.

nerve terminals and facilitate the release of dopamine in the striatum.[73,74]

Muscarinic Receptors

All mAChR mRNAs and proteins have been detected in basal ganglia.[77–86] The m1, m2, and m4 receptors account for the vast majority of striatal muscarinic-binding sites,[79–81] and are distributed heterogeneously in the patch and matrix compartments of the striatum.[82] The m4 subtype (Figs. 6–2 and 6–3) is the most abundant mAChR in neostriatum, accounting for 50% of total mAChR, and may be the key target for anticholinergic drugs used in movement disorders. The m4 immunoreactivity is dense in patches and corresponds to patches high in D1 and glutamate receptor subunit GluR1 (Fig. 6–3). The other muscarinic receptor proteins do not show such differential localization in patch and matrix divisions. The m4 mRNA and protein are present in about 70% of spiny neurons of striatum,[77,82,83] particularly those that express substance P,[84] and, thus, probably project via the direct pathway to basal ganglia output nuclei. Figure 6-2 shows intense m4 immunoreactivity in the caudate and putamen, and in the terminal zone of the direct pathway projection neurons in GPi. m4 mRNA is also noted in 50% of D2/enkephalin spiny neurons of the striatum, which contribute to the indirect pathway. This finding suggests the possibility that m4, like D1, is localized on the terminals of direct pathway projection neurons. The m1 subtype is expressed in all of the spiny projection neurons, whereas in the striatum the m2 receptor (Fig. 6–4) is expressed in the cholinergic interneurons only, where it serves as an autoreceptor.[83,84]

The m1 subtype is mostly postsynaptic on the dendrites and spines of all spiny neurons; m4 is postsynaptic in the spines of a subset of spiny neurons, as well as presynaptically localized in axon terminals, many of which appear to be GABAergic and are probably from the axon collaterals of the direct pathway projection neurons.[82] In contrast, m2 is abundant in cholinergic nerve terminals,

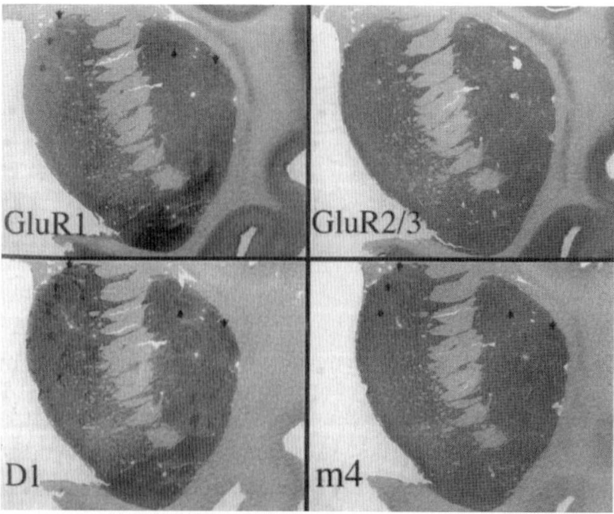

Figure 6–3. Comparison of the distributions of GluR1, GluR2/3, D1, and m4 proteins in human striatum. Note that GluR1, D1, and m4 are all enriched in patches (arrows), but GluR2/3 is not.

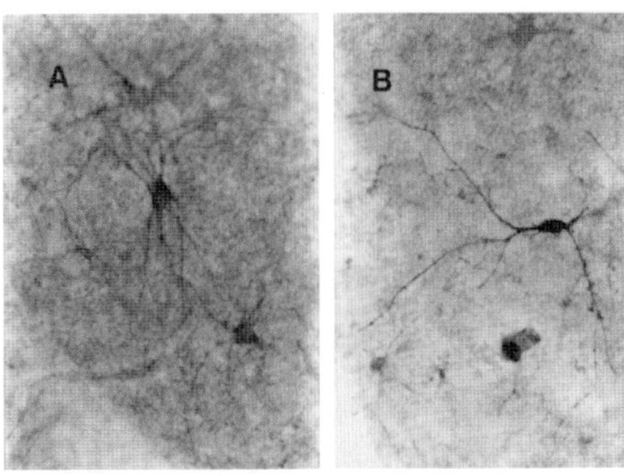

Figure 6–4. Immunocytochemical localization of muscarinic cholinergic m2 receptor subtype in large striatal interneurons. Several examples of human striatal interneurons expressing m2. These neurons have the same frequency, size, and morphology as giant aspiny interneurons, and m2 colocalizes with choline acetyltransferase immunoreactivity, a marker for cholinergic neurons.

where the presynaptic receptor controls transmitter release. Thus, differential expression and trafficking of the mAChR subtypes allows ACh to have different effects on direct and indirect pathway spiny neurons, as well as on interneurons.

Among other basal ganglia structures, the m4 receptor protein is highly enriched in GPi (Fig. 6–2). Because mAChR mRNAs are not detected in GPi,[77] the protein is probably synthesized and transported to the GABAergic terminals of the striatal projection neurons, which express m4 mRNA[77] and protein.[83] Another possibility, however, is that m4 is present on glutamatergic terminals derived from subthalamus, which also expresses the m4 mRNA.[77] The mAChR-binding sites in GPi are upregulated substantially in PD, perhaps secondary to reduced cholinergic transmission from PPN.[72] The subthalamus also expresses relatively high levels of m3 mRNA[77] and protein.[80] The PPN expresses high levels of m2 protein,[13] where it probably functions as an autoreceptor. Finally, the dopaminergic neurons in SN are one of few sites in the brain with m5 mRNA[77] and with no other reported receptor subtypes. Although there are only very low levels of m5 protein (e.g., where detectable, accounting for less than 2% of total mAChR), this receptor might be localized on nigrostriatal terminals, because dopamine release in striatum is known to be regulated by a muscarinic receptor.[86]

FUNCTIONS OF THE ACETYLCHOLINERGIC RECEPTORS

The central cholinergic system has been speculated to play a role in reward and reinforcement,[87] memory,[88] attention mechanisms,[88] neuroprotection,[89] locomotor activity, analgesia, and neurotransmitter release.[90] The cholinergic system of the central nervous system (CNS) may be classified broadly into two major subdivisions: the rostral division, consisting of the septohippocampal system, the nucleus basalis of Meynert, and related nuclei; and the caudal group of cholinergic neurons in the PPN, and lateral dorsal tegmental nucleus. Although the rostral group plays a prominent role in memory and attention mechanisms, the caudal PPN group has a role in locomotor, reward and reinforcement behavior, and in arousal and alerting phenomenon.[88] These diverse functions of the cholinergic system are mediated by both nAChR and mAChR. In the absence of specific agonists and antagonists, our understanding of the roles of these individual AChRs in the functions of basal ganglia is derived from knockout studies.[91–104]

NICOTINIC RECEPTORS

The most important function of presynaptic nAChR in the basal ganglia is to modulate neurotransmitter release.[90] However, knockout studies have provided additional information of the specific role that the individual subunits may play in other functions of nAChR.[91,92] The β2 subunit appears to play a major role in many of the speculated effects of nicotine. Mice lacking the β2 subunit not only lose high-affinity nicotine binding but also nicotine-induced dopamine but not ACh release, as well as the reinforcing properties of nicotine, suggesting that the β2 subunit is critical for nicotine, and possibly cocaine, addiction.[92–95] The α5-deficient mice demonstrate significant decrease in the short-term effects of nicotine.[96]

MUSCARINIC RECEPTORS

In the striatum, m1 mAChRs play a facilitatory role.[97–99] In m1-deficient mice, there is an increased extracellular dopamine level, and consequently increased locomotor activity.[99,100] The increased dopamine level in the striatum has been speculated to be due to decreased inhibition of the nigrostriatal dopaminergic neurons by the m1-deficient striatonigral direct pathway.[99]

Almost all D1 receptor-expressing medium spiny striatal projection neurons that give rise to the direct pathway to GPi also express m4 (as well as m1) muscarinic receptors, whereas less than half of the D2 receptor-expressing striatal projection neurons that send efferents to GPe and form part of the indirect pathway express the m4 subtype. Mice deficient in m4 nAChRs have increased spontaneous locomotor activity and, when D1 receptor are stimulated with agonists, the hyperactivity is further enhanced, suggesting that the D1 receptor and m4 mAChR have opposing effects on the direct pathway.[101] This is reflected at the cellular level by the fact that D1 receptor stimulation leads to an increase in adenylyl cyclase, whereas m4 stimulation decreases adenylyl cyclase, within the spiny neurons.[101]

The m5 nAChRs, which are prominently expressed in the dopaminergic neurons of SN and VTA, regulate the release of dopamine in the striatum, and may play an active role in drug-seeking behavior, especially reward and withdrawal of opiates.[102]

The m2 and m3 receptors, which are not expressed prominently in the basal ganglia, may mediate analgesia,[103] salivary gland secretion, food intake, and weight gain,[104] respectively.

▶ NEUROCHEMICAL ORGANIZATION OF THE GLUTAMATERGIC SYSTEM IN THE BASAL GANGLIA

SOURCE OF GLUTAMATE IN THE BASAL GANGLIA

Glutamate is the principal excitatory neurotransmitter in the brain. Within the basal ganglia circuitry, it plays a prominent role in the physiology of the cortex, striatum, GP, STN, SN, and thalamus. The striatum receives a massive glutamatergic projection from virtually all areas of the neocortex.[105,106] In addition, the centromedian and parafascicular thalamic nuclei send glutamatergic projections to the striatum.[107] Terminals from cortex synapse almost exclusively on heads of dendritic spines, whereas those from thalamus synapse mostly with dendrites and, less frequently, with spines.[107] Individual dendritic spines of striatal neurons receive convergent input from cortical glutamatergic afferents and dopaminergic nigrostriatal cells. Cortical glutamatergic neurons also send projections to STN, SN, and thalamus. Other regions of the basal ganglia (GPe, GPi, and SNc/SNr) receive excitatory glutamatergic input from the STN.[107] In short, all nuclei of the basal ganglia either receive and/or send glutamatergic projections. There are significant alterations in glutamatergic neurotransmission in disorders of the basal ganglia, and the glutamate system is an important target for therapeutic intervention as well as for potential neuroprotective agents.[108]

MOLECULAR DIVERSITY OF GLUTAMATE RECEPTORS AND THEIR SIGNAL TRANSDUCTION

Glutamate receptors are classified into ionotropic receptors (iGluR), and metabotropic receptors (mGluR).[109] The cation-specific iGluRs are named for the agonist compounds that elicit specific physiological responses, and are called *N*-methyl-D-aspartate (NMDA), α-amino-3-hydroxy-5-methyl-4-isoxazole-propionic acid (AMPA), and kainate (KA) receptors.

NMDA Receptors

NMDA receptors are heteromeric, and their pharmacological and physiological properties are largely determined by their subunit composition. Most current evidence suggests that they are composed of four subunits derived from three distinct families of proteins.[109–114] All NMDA receptors contain one, and perhaps two, members of the NMDAR1 subunit family. The NMDAR1 family consists of at least eight variants derived from alternative splicing of a single gene (NMDAR 1a–h). The NMDAR1 receptors proteins contain most of the regulatory sites found on native NMDA receptors, but if assembled without other subunits they conduct only a very small amount of current. The second major family of NMDA receptor subunits, NMDAR 2A–D, are the product of four separate genes and each shows a more restricted anatomical distribution. The NMDAR3 proteins are a third family, with a much more limited pattern of expression. NMDAR2 and NMDAR3 subunits are combined with the NMDAR1 subunits to form native NMDA receptors, which have characteristic properties that include activation by glutamate or NMDA analogues, blockade by drugs such as phencylidine, voltage-dependent blockade by magnesium ion, and the ability when activated to allow both sodium and calcium currents to pass. These last two properties give NMDA receptors a special role in the regulation of neuronal plasticity: voltage-dependent blockade by magnesium ion means that NMDA receptors require not only the presence of glutamate, but also depolarization of the neuronal membrane (cause, e.g., by activation of an AMPA receptor) to activate. Thus, they are "coincidence detectors," and can trigger plastic events. The mechanism by which they lead to plasticity is through their ability to flux calcium ions which can in turn activate a variety of signaling cascades.

AMPA/KA Receptors

The AMPA receptor subunits were the first of the glutamate receptors to be cloned.[115,116] Like the NMDA receptors and other ligand-gated ion channels, the AMPA receptors are multimeric heteromers composed of several distinct subunits. GluR1–4 (also known as GluR A–D) are AMPA receptor subunits, which can assemble in various combinations to form functional receptors.[109] Alternative splicing of the RNA of each of the four AMPA receptor subunits (GluR1–4), termed "flip" and "flop," add further to the complexity in the composition of AMPA receptors.[117] KA receptors are closely related to the AMPA family, and are composed of five distinct subunits (GluR5–7, KA1, and KA2). The specific subunit composition of a given AMPA or KA receptor determines its precise physiological, and pharmacological properties.

The primary action of AMPA and KA receptors is that when activated by glutamate they produce a fast sodium-dependent inward current that leads to neuronal depolarization. Most of the AMPA and KA receptors found in the normal brain are impermeable to calcium. In the case of the AMPA receptors, this permeability to Ca^{2+} is dependent on receptor subunit composition; the inclusion of a GluR2 subunit in the receptor assembly, present in most native AMPA receptors, prevents Ca^{2+} permeability.[118] Interestingly, the ability of GluR2 to block Ca^{2+} flux is the result of an unusual molecular mechanisms known as "RNA editing," in which an enzyme modified the structure of one base of the messenger RNA for GluR2. This may be important because there is some evidence that this editing process may be deficient in some disease states, leading to AMPA receptors with abnormally high permeability to calcium.

Metabotropic Receptors

The metabotropic receptors are coupled to G proteins and belong to the family C type of GPCRs. Characteristic of this family of GPCRs, mGluRs have an exceptionally long N-terminal. Molecular cloning studies have demonstrated the existence of at least eight distinct metabotropic receptor genes (mGluR1–8). All of these are found in the brain except mGluR6, which is expressed in the retina.[109,119] The mGluRs are further divided into three groups. Group I mGluRs, consisting of mGluR1 and mGluR5, stimulate phospholipase C, and increase levels of inositol triphosphate and intracellular calcium. In contrast, groups II (mGluR2, and mGluR3) and III (mGluR4–8) inhibit adenylyl cyclase, and thus decrease cyclic AMP levels.

Metabotropic receptors are likely to have a wide variety of modulatory roles in brain function. Members of the metabotropic receptor families are found at nearly all excitatory synapses in the brain, both postsynaptically (often Group I receptors) and presynaptically (often Group II and/or Group III). They may also be found on the presynaptic terminals of nonglutamatergic neurons, and participate in regulation of the release of GABA and other transmitters. The mGluRs have a rich pharmacology, with many drugs that have selective actions on different receptor types. A number of these mGluR-targeted drugs are currently in development as treatments for movement disorders and other neurological conditions.

GLUTAMATERGIC RECEPTOR DISTRIBUTION IN THE BASAL GANGLIA

NMDA Receptors

Receptor-binding studies indicate that NMDA receptors are found throughout the basal ganglia but are most abundant in striatum.[120,121] Lower levels are seen in GP, STN, SN, and thalamus. Among the different subtypes, the NMDAR 1 gene product shows an extremely widespread distribution, with moderate to intense staining in striatum, and lower but detectable levels in GP, STN, SNc/SNr, and thalamus.[122,123] There is also specificity in the expression of the NMDA R1 subtypes, with distinct patterns of splice forms present in the different basal ganglia nuclei.[124,125]

The mRNAs for the NMDAR 2 family of subunits are differentially distributed in basal ganglia structures.[123] In the striatum, NMDAR 2B is the predominant species, but NMDAR 2A is also detectable. Elsewhere, in the GP, STN, and SN, NMDAR 2D is most abundant. Interestingly, NMDAR 2C, generally considered a cerebellar subunit, is relatively enriched in SNc. Within the striatum, differences in cellular expression of NMDA receptor subunit genes and isoforms have been described.[124] Striatal projection neurons have higher levels of NMDAR 1 and NMDAR 2B message than intrinsic somatostatin and cholinergic neurons. In contrast, these interneurons express NMDAR 2D mRNA, but the projection neurons do not. Thus, there is evidence that different populations of striatal neurons express distinct heteromeric forms of the NMDA receptor.[125]

In PD and models of parkinsonism, there is substantial evidence for modulation of the structure and function of NMDA receptors. In particular, striatal dopamine depletion appears to lead to a reduction in striatal NMDA R2B subunits, whereas chronic levodopa therapy leading to dyskinesia causes an increase in NMDA R2B along with hyperphosphorylation of striatal NMDA receptor subunits (reviewed in Hallett and Standaert). These effects may be important in the pathogenesis of levodopa-induced dyskinesias (LIDs).

AMPA Receptors

Proteins from the AMPA receptor family are also widely distributed in the basal ganglia. Antibodies recognizing GluR1 label medium spiny, medium aspiny, and large aspiny, neurons of the striatum.[126,127] Moreover, the GluR1 subunit appears to be enriched in striosomes corresponding to substance P-enriched and calbindin-poor regions. In addition, in the human striatum, GluR1 patches colocalize with dopamine D1 receptor patches (Fig. 6–3). In contrast, antibodies that recognize GluR2/3 and GluR4 do

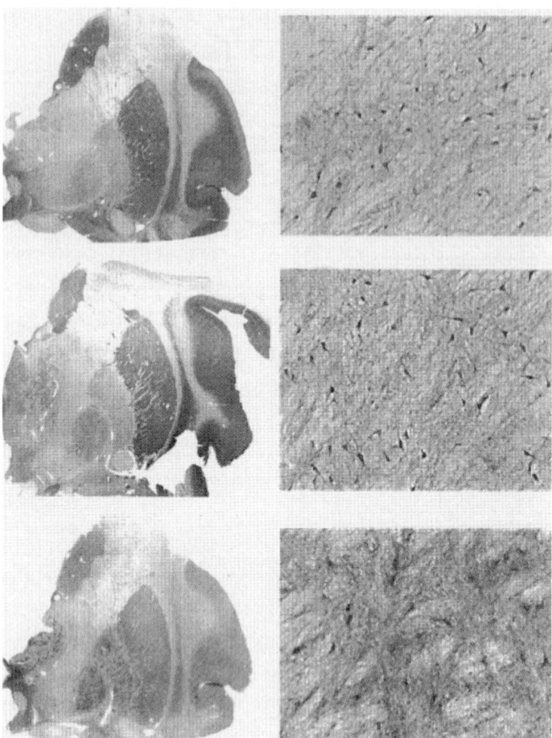

Figure 6–5. Distribution of GluR1, GluR2/3, and GluR4 in human basal ganglia; panels on right show higher magnification of cells in the GPi. Note that each of the subunits shows both cellular and neuropil staining in this nucleus.

not show differential striosomal versus matrix staining. GluR2/3 antibodies primarily label medium spiny neurons, and GluR4 antibodies do not label striatal neurons. In the rat striatum, GluR1 does not colocalize with striatopallidal or striatonigral projection neurons, but it does colocalize with parvalbumin-positive interneurons.[126] In contrast, GluR2/3 is localized to most projection neurons.

GluR1 is also found in GPe, GPi, STN, and SNc/SNr.[128] Fig. 6–5 shows GluR1 immunoreactivity in striatum and GPe/GPi in the human brain, and demonstrates stained neurons in the GPi. Fig. 6–6 shows the intense GluR1 immunoreactivity in monkey STN, and Fig. 6–7 shows labeled neurons in SN.[129] Neurons enriched in GluR2/3 are found in GPi (Fig. 6–5), and in SNc/SNr (Fig. 6–7), and there are GluR4-immunoreactive neurons in SNr. Finally, it should be noted that GluR4 and, to a lesser extent, GluR1 may be located in glial cells in some brain regions.[128]

Metabotropic Receptors

Analysis of the regional and cellular distributions of mGluR message in the basal ganglia reveals that these receptors have distinct localizations.[130–133] Both substance P- and enkephalin-containing medium-sized projection neurons and the large interneurons of the striatum ex-

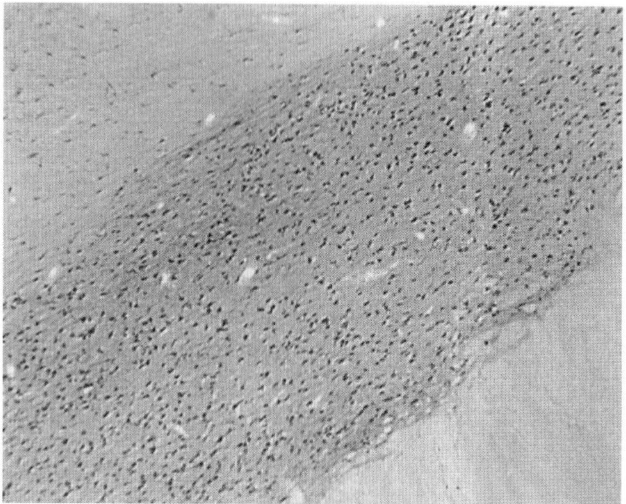

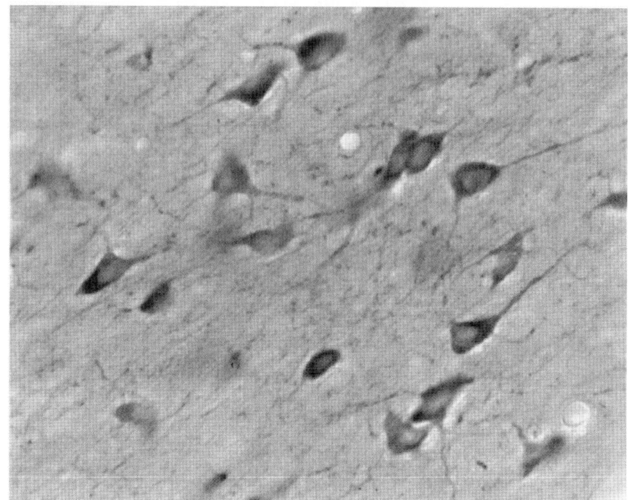

Figure 6–6. GluR1 immunoreactivity in the monkey subthalamic nucleus (top panel). Bottom panel shows a higher magnification (×40).

press mRNA and proteins for mGluR1 and mGluR5.[131] Intense immunolabeling for mGluR1 and mGluR5 is seen in both pallidal segments, as well as preferentially in the glutamatergic subthalamopallidal synapses.[132] Among the group II mGluRs, mGluR2 mRNA is expressed mostly in the large striatal interneurons and by the neurons of the STN, and mGluR3 mRNA in most striatal neurons as well as some glial cells.[133] Although the abundance of mGluR2 mRNA in the striatum overall is low, mGluR2 protein is present within the striatum on corticostriatal axons, arising from mGluR2-expressing cortical neurons. Only moderate levels of the group III family members are expressed in the striatum and the pallidal segments, but proteins of these receptors are strongly expressed on the GABAergic striatopallidal and striatonigral terminals. This localization of group III mGluRs may be of therapeutic relevance, as they are positioned to modulate striatal outflow and potentially

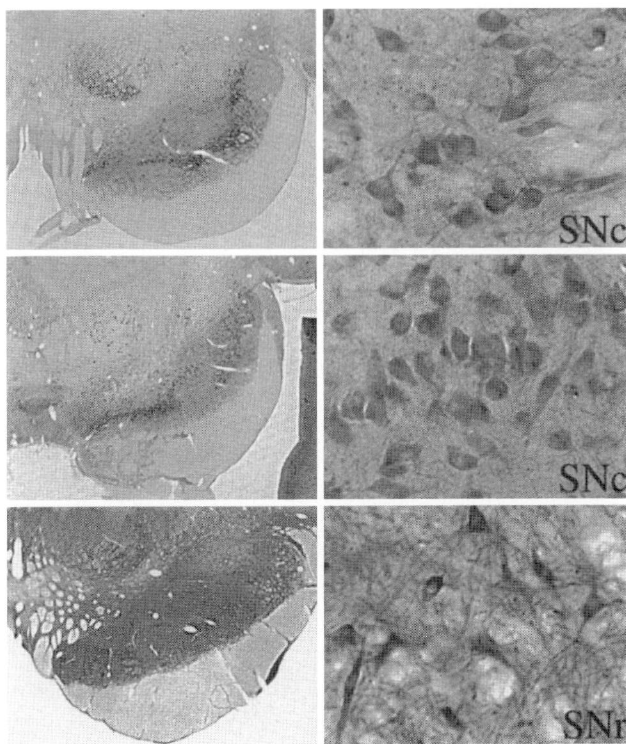

Figure 6–7. Immunocytochemistry of glutamate receptor subunits in monkey substantia nigra. GluR1 (top) and GluR2/3 (middle) immunoreactive neurons are relatively concentrated in the SNc. In contrast, the NMDAR 1 (bottom) subunit is more abundant in SNr, where much of the immunoreactivity is found in dendrites.

modulate the balance of activity in the direct and indirect pathways.

The distributions of glutamate receptors in the basal ganglia are summarized in Table 6–3.

▶ NEUROCHEMICAL ORGANIZATION OF THE SEROTONERGIC SYSTEM IN THE BASAL GANGLIA

SOURCE OF SEROTONIN IN THE BASAL GANGLIA

The serotonin-producing neurons, based on their anatomical locations and connectivity, are grouped into nine (B1–B9) subdivisions.[134,135] The basal ganglia receive dense serotonergic innervations (B5) from the dorsal raphe nucleus (DRN).[136] About 35% of DRN neurons project to the striatum and 80–90% of these projections arise from the rostral and dorsomedial region of DRN.[136] The DRN neurons that project to the basal ganglia are functionally distinct and belong to a group of neurons that respond physiologically to altered muscle tone and sleep–wake/arousal states.[137] In contrast, the caudal "autonomic" subdivision of DRN projects to the hypothalamic-pituitary axis and plays a role in the neuroendocrine response to stress.[138]

The different subnuclei of the basal ganglia receive varying densities of serotoninergic innervations. Earlier neurochemical studies suggested that serotonin levels are higher in the SN and GP than in the striatum.[139] Immunocytochemical studies confirm that the SN receives the heaviest serotonergic innervation.[136,140] Axons from DRN terminate more densely in the caudal and lateral third than in the rostral and medial substantia nigra. The dense region of serotonergic innervations of caudal and lateral nigra may correspond to the region of SN that degenerates the earliest in PD, and is vulnerable to the mitochondrial toxins MPTP and rotenone.[11,15–17] In the SN, serotonergic fibers terminate mostly in SNr, where the dendrites of the dopaminergic neurons of SNc reside. The DRN neurons that project to the SN also project to the striatum by axon collaterals.

Within the GP, the medial pallidal segment stains more intensely for serotonin-immunopositive terminals than the lateral pallidal segment. The STN receives moderately dense serotonergic innervations from the dorsal raphe.[140]

The caudate and putamen receive less dense serotonergic innervations than the SN and GP, and the distribution pattern of the serotonergic terminals is heterogeneous. The nucleus accumbens and the ventro- and dorsomedial limbic striatum receive denser serotonergic innervations than the associative striatum and the dorsolateral motor striatum.[140]

There are many significant patches of dorsolateral striatum that stain poorly for serotonergic terminals and these serotonin-poor patches correspond to TH-poor patches and striosomes. The matrix areas of the striatum receive significantly more dense serotonin immunostaining and correspond to TH-rich matrix compartment of the striatum. These findings suggest that the limbic and nonlimbic compartments of the striatum may be influenced by different serotonergic mechanisms.[140] The serotonergic terminals terminate predominantly on the dendritic spines or the shaft of the output neurons of the striatum, GP, and SN.[140]

MOLECULAR DIVERSITY OF SEROTONIN RECEPTORS AND THEIR SIGNAL TRANSDUCTION

Modern molecular biological and pharmacological techniques have identified seven different families of serotonin (5-HT) receptors (5-HT$_1$ to 5-HT$_7$), and 14 different 5-HT receptors.[141,142] All but one family, the 5-HT$_3$ family, which is a ligand-gated cation channel, are G protein-linked metabotropic receptors. Members of the 5-HT$_1$ family, consisting of 5-HT$_{1A}$, 5-HT$_{1B}$, 5-HT$_{1D}$, 5-HT$_{1E}$, and 5-HT$_{1F}$ subtypes, are coupled mostly to Gi/o/z proteins, and, when activat-

▶ **TABLE 6–3. GLUTAMATE RECEPTOR SUBTYPES IN THE BASAL GANGLIA**

Receptor Type	Basal Ganglia Localization
NMDA	*Predominantly post-synaptic*
NMDAR 1	Striatum: *projection neurons > intrinsic neurons*; GPe; GPi; STN; SNc; SNr
NMDAR 2A	Striatum
NMDAR 2B	Striatum: *projection neurons > intrinsic neurons*
NMDAR 2C	SNc
NMDAR 2D	Striatum: *intrinsic neurons » projection neurons*; GPe; GPi; STN; SNc; SNr
AMPA	*Predominantly post-synaptic*
GluR1	Striatum: *patch > matrix; intrinsic neurons » projection neurons; medium spiny, medium aspiny & large aspiny neurons*; GPe; GPi; STN; SNc; SNr
GluR2/3	Striatum: *medium spiny neurons*; GPi; SNc
GluR4	GPi; SNr; glia
Metabotropic	*Pre and post-synaptic, as noted below*
mGluR1	Mostly post-synaptic, Striatum < GPe < GPi < STN < SNc < SNr
mGluR2	Pre-synaptic, corticostriatal axons; postsynaptic, STN, cholinergic neurons
mGluR3	Mostly post-synaptic, striatal neurons; glia
mGluR4	Mostly pre-synaptic; striatum, striato-pallidal terminals
mGluR5	Mostly post-synaptic; striatum: *projection neurons » intrinsic neurons*; » GPe; GPi; STN; SNc; SNr
mGluR7	Mostly pre-synaptic; striatum, striato-pallidal and striato-nigral terminals

ed, inhibit adenylyl cyclase activity, decrease cyclic AMP postsynaptically, and open K$^+$ channels. The 5-HT$_2$ family members (5-HT$_{2A}$, 5-HT$_{2B}$, 5-HT$_{2C}$) are coupled to Gq/11 proteins, and result in an increase in phospholipase C activity, an increase in inositol trisphosphate and diacylglycerol levels postsynaptically, and also close K$^+$ channels. The rest of the members of 5-HT receptor families, 5-HT$_3$ to 5-HT$_7$, are coupled to Gs proteins, and, when activated, stimulate adenylyl cyclase activity and lead to increased levels of cyclic AMP postsynaptically.

SEROTONERGIC RECEPTOR DISTRIBUTION IN THE BASAL GANGLIA

The various 5-HT receptors are distributed throughout the various nuclei of the basal ganglia (Table 6–4).[142] Most are found postsynaptically at the target site of different nuclei of the basal ganglia. The 5-HT$_{1B/1D}$ receptors are localized to the soma, dendrite, and axon terminals of the DRN neurons as autoreceptors, and, when stimulated, decrease the firing rate and/or decrease release of serotonin at their terimals.[142,143]

The different subtypes of the 5-HT receptor family have been identified in the caudate-putamen, SN, and the pallidal segments.[142] The mRNAs for several of these receptors (5-HT$_{1A,1B/1D}$, 5-HT$_{2A,2C}$, 5-HT$_3$, 5-HT$_4$, 5-HT$_5$) are localized predominantly postsynaptically in the GABAergic output neurons of the striatum, and the proteins of these receptors are found in the target sites of the terminals of the striatal output neurons, namely GPe and SNr.[142] The 5-HT$_{2C}$ subtype is more dense in the medial GP than in any other basal ganglia structure, and this receptor is upregulated in PD.[144] The 5-HT$_{2C}$ receptor mRNA is localized to the GABAergic output neurons of GPi. Of the most recently identified 5-HT$_6$ and 5-HT$_7$ families, the 5-HT$_6$ family of receptors, located in the dendrites of the GABAergic striatopallidal and striatonigral output neurons, appear to have significant interaction with the dopaminergic system. The 5-HT$_{2B}$ and 5-HT$_7$ receptors have not yet been localized to any nucleus of the basal ganglia.[142]

FUNCTIONS OF THE SEROTONERGIC RECEPTORS

Serotonin plays an important role in neurobiological mechanisms of anxiety, sleep–wake cycle, mood regulation, neuroendocrine and locomotor response to stress, and pain. Recently, gene knockout technology has been used to understand the specific role played by individual 5-HT receptor subtypes in various functions of the serotonergic system.[145,146] The 5-HT$_{1A}$ knockouts exhibit a heightened anxiety response,[146] and pharmacological studies suggest that 5-HT$_{1A}$ agonists have anxiolytic and antidepressant properties, thereby suggesting a role of 5-HT$_{1A}$ in anxiety response.[142] The 5-HT$_{1B}$ knockouts have increased locomotor activity, increased aggressiveness, and a tendency to self-administer cocaine.[146] This behavior has been speculated to be due to a lack of expression of 5-HT$_{1B}$ receptor in the inhibitory GABAergic output neurons of the stria-

▶ TABLE 6–4. SEROTONERGIC RECEPTOR SUBTYPES IN THE BASAL GANGLIA

Receptor Family	Type of Receptor	Effector Mechanisms	Subtypes	Location in the Basal Ganglia	Speculated Function in
5-HT_1	G protein-linked	Inhibits adenylyl cyclase Opens K^+ channels	5-HT_{1A}	Caudate–putamen Subthalamic nucleus	Anxiety, depression
			5-HT_{1B}	Caudate–putamen Substantia nigra Globus pallidus	Locomotion
			$5\text{-HT}_{1D\alpha}$	Substantia nigra	
			$5\text{-HT}_{1D\beta}$		
			5-HT_{1E}	Caudate–putamen	
			5-HT_{1F}	Caudate–putamen	
5-HT_2	G protein-linked	Stimulation of phospholipase C Closing of K^+ channels	5-HT_{2A}	Nucleus accumbens Caudate–putamen	
			5-HT_{2B}	None detected in the basal ganglia	
			5-HT_{2C}	Nucleus accumbens	
				Caudate–putamen	
				Substania nigra	
5-HT_3	Ligand-gated cation channel			GABAergic projections neurons of caudate–putamen	Anxiety, depression Emesis
5-HT_4	G protein-linked	Stimulation of adenylyl cyclase		GABAergic projections neurons of caudate–putamen	Anxiety, depression
5-HT_{5A}	G protein-linked	Inhibits adenylyl cyclase		Caudate–putamen	
5-HT_{5B}	G protein-linked			Caudate–putamen	
5-HT_6	G protein-linked	Stimulation of adenylyl cyclase		Dendrites of GABAergic striatopallidal and strlatonigral neurons	Dopamine transmission
5-HT_7	G protein-linked	Stimulation of adenylyl cyclase		None detected in the basal ganglia	Circadian rhythms

tum, so that the mesencephalic neurons go unchecked, resulting in increased release of dopamine and leading to a heightened addictive behavior.[146] The $5\text{-HT}_{1B/D/F}$ receptor agonists, the triptans, cause vasoconstriction, and reduce inflammatory response and pain of migraine attacks.[147] Several atypical and typical antipsychotic drugs have high affinity to $5\text{-HT}_{2C/A}$ receptors.[142] The 5-HT_3 receptors facilitate dopamine transmission, and antagonsits of these receptors are anxiolytics and antiemetics.[142] The recently identified 5-HT_6 receptor may interact significantly with the GABAergic medium spiny neurons of the striatum,[142] and the 5-HT $_7$ receptor may play a role in circadian rhythms.[142]

The pioneering biochemical studies of Hornykiewicz et al. clearly demonstrated that brain serotonin levels are 40% decreased in human PD.[148] Subsequent studies by several other groups showed that serotonin levels are indeed decreased in PD, more so in the depressed PD patients than in the nondepressed patients.[148] Neuropathological studies using traditional techniques, and immunocytochemical methods using antibodies specific to phenylalanine hydroxylase, have confirmed that DRN neurons do degenerate in PD.[149,150] The DRN neuron counts may be normal in the early stages of PD, but the loss is significant in patients in late stages of PD, although not as severe as the dopaminergic neurons of SN. The 5-HT neuronal loss in multisystem atrophies may be more predominant in raphe magnus, raphe pallidus, and raphe obscurus, which send descending serotonergic projections to the autonomic and motor nuclei of the brainstem and spinal cord.[151]

As the enzyme aromatic acid decarboxylase (AADC) is present in both 5-HT and catecholamine neurons, it has long been suspected that the efficacy of levodopa as one of the best pharmacological treatments for PD, depends on surviving striatal serotonergic pathways to convert a significant amount of exogenous levodopa into DA [Everett, 1970 #76]. These experiments suggested that AADC in serotonergic neurons, if overwhelmed by large amounts of exogenous levodopa, can produce DA and that this would be done at the expense of 5-HT production [Arai, 1995 #73; Arai, 1994 #74; Nicholas, 2008 #53]. In animal models and humans with LID, antidyskinetic effects utilizing serotonergic mechanisms have been shown with various drugs, although most of these agents also bind to other monoamine receptors as well [Nicholson, 2002 #77]. However, using more specific 5-HT-receptor-binding drugs, recent evidence suggests that in a 6-hydroxydopamine rat model of PD, levodopa exposure results in upregulation of striatal 5-HT_{1B} receptors [Zhang, 2008 #78] independent from DA depletion and an antidyskinetic effect can be obtained with 5-HT_{1A} [Carta, 2007 #75] and 5-HT_{1B} agonists [Carta, 2007 #75; Zhang, 2008 #78], believed to be working at autoreceptors on serotonergic neuronal cell bodies/dendrites and terminals, respectively [Carta, 2007 #75].

▶ NEUROCHEMICAL ORGANIZATION OF THE NORADRENERGIC SYSTEM IN THE BASAL GANGLIA

SOURCE OF NORADRENALINE IN THE BASAL GANGLIA

Using formaldehyde-induced fluorescence, noradrenaline neurons in the pons and caudal medulla oblongata were at first difficult to distinguish from other catecholamine producing cells present in the brain.[152] The synthesis of noradrenaline starts in a process similar to what is seen in dopaminergic neurons, where tyrosine is converted to L-DOPA by TH. AADC then converts L-DOPA into dopamine, which is then transported into synaptic vesicles by the vesicular monoamine transporter. In noradrenergic neurons, dopamine β-hydroxylase (DBH) acts within synaptic vesicles to then convert dopamine into noradrenaline. Using an antibody derived from bovine adrenal gland DBH, the noradrenaline system was finally mapped in rat CNS, but virtually no DBH-immunoreactive terminal staining was seen in the rat SNc and caudate/putamen in this study,[153] suggesting that noradrenaline was not an important neurotransmitter in basal ganglia functioning. However, this finding was in contrast to other studies in various species showing evidence that DBH[154,155] and noradrenaline[155–159] was indeed present in the striatum, but in low levels as compared to serotonin and dopamine.

Formaldehyde-induced fluorescence techniques combined with brainstem lesions finally delineated noradrenaline CNS pathways[160] from the rest of the catecholamine cell groups that were first mapped in the rat brain by Dahlström and Fuxe.[152] Out of the 12 originally identified catecholamine neuronal nuclei, the A1–A7 cell groups were deemed to primarily produce noradrenaline.[160] Furthermore, these cells were grouped into two major noradrenergic systems, including a lateral tegmental (LT) group (A1–A3, A5, A7) and a subcoeruleus/LC group (A4, A6). Although there is some overlap between projections, noradrenergic neurons of the LT group primarily innervate ventral areas of the spinal cord, most motor and reticular brainstem nuclei, as well as selected areas of the hypothalamus and basal forebrain. The LC group also projects to ventral spinal cord, but in addition innervates sensory brainstem nuclei, especially the dorsal thalamus, and the cerebral and cerebellar cortices. As noradrenaline content was considered sparse, innervation of basal ganglia structures was more difficult to ascertain. Using retrograde track-tracing methods in the rat, the LC was first shown to project to the reticular formation dorsal to the SN, but not to the SN itself.[161] However, anterograde tracing from the rat LC did suggest a modest projection to the SNc, but not to the caudate/putamen.[162] In monkeys, combined track-tracing methods clearly showed that the noradrenergic innervation to the striatum[163] and both segments of the globus pallidus[164] originated from the LC. However, when the LC was lesioned in rats, DBH activity decreased in many brain areas, but only negligibly in the SNc and striatum, suggesting that the origin of noradrenaline in rodent basal ganglia structures was not principally from the LC.[154] These findings were contrasted by combination lesioning/retrograde tracing studies in rats, showing a distinct projection from the LC to caudate/putamen.[165] Because it was suggested that the basal ganglia and SN are poorly innervated by noradrenergic pathways, the volume transmission theory provides another explanation for how monoamines such as noradrenaline may have effects on distant basal ganglia structures after diffusing long distances in the brain (10 mm in rats, 7 mm in cats).[166] Indeed, there is evidence that both dopamine[167] and noradrenaline[168] may influence neurons from distant sites using this process.

MOLECULAR DIVERSITY OF NORADRENALINE RECEPTORS AND THEIR DISTRIBUTION IN THE BASAL GANGLIA

The diverse effects of noradrenaline are mediated by the α-1 (A-1), α-2 (A-2), and β (B) subfamilies of noradrenergic receptors, which are defined by pharmacological, anatomical, and biochemical criteria.[169] Similar to dopamine receptors, all noradrenaline receptors identified to date are members of the GPCR superfamily, consisting of seven transmembrane spanning structures linked by three alternating extracellular and intracellular domains, an extracellular N-terminal, and a cytoplasmic C-

▶ **TABLE 6–5. NORADRENALINE RECEPTOR SUBTYPES IN THE CNS**

Receptor Subtype	Sequence/ Species	Radioligand Affinity Profile	Major mRNA Localizations	Intracellular Function(s)
Alpha 1 subfamily				Increase intracellular calcium and/or activate protein kinase C and/or phospholipase A2, C, D
A-1a(c)	Rat and human	Prazosin = WB4101 > phentolamine > oxymetazoline > adrenaline > noradrenaline	Brainstem motor nuclei, hippocampus	
A-1b	Rα1B—Rat	Prazosin > WB4101 > phentolamine > oxymetazoline > adrenaline > noradrenaline	Cerebral cortex, thalamus, spinal cord, dorsal raphe, pineal	
A-1d	RA42—Rat	Prazosin = WB4101 > noradrenaline > phentolamine > adrenaline > oxymetazoline	Hippocampus, olfactory bulb, cerebral cortex	
Alpha 2 subfamily				Decrease cyclic AMP or activate K^+ channels, phospholipase A2, Na^+/H^+ exchange or increase intracellular calcium
A-2a	C10—Human	Yohimbine > phentolamine > oxymetazoline > adrenaline > prazosin > noradrenaline	Locus coeruleus, cerebral cortex, hypothalamus, medulla oblongata	
	RG20—Rat	Phentolamine > oxymetazoline > yohimbine > (adrenaline > noradrenaline)		
A-2b	C2—Human RNG—Rat	Yohimbine > phentolamine > prazosin > noradrenaline > oxymetazoline > adrenaline	Thalamus	
A-2c	C4 – Human RG10—Rat	Yohimbine > phentolamine > prazosin > oxymetazoline > adrenaline > noradrenaline	Striatum, cerebral cortex, hippocampus, olfactory bulb, cerebellum	
Beta subfamily				Increase cyclic AMP
B-1	Rat and human	CGP20712>betaxolol = metroprolol > isoprenaline > atenolol > ICI118551	Cerebral cortex, pineal	
B-2	Rat and human	ICI118551 > isoprenaline >> betaxolol > atenolol > CGP20712 > metroprolol	Cerebral cortex, olfactory bulb	

terminal. Each subfamily of noradrenergic receptors has been further subdivided into individual subtypes and their distinct genetic locations were mapped within the rat brain using in situ hybridization techniques.[170–175]

The classification of the noradrenaline receptor gene family, including binding properties of agonists and antagonists and general distributions of mRNA for these subsets in the brain are summarized in Table 6–5. Note that human and rat A-2a receptors have different pharmacological profiles and B-3 receptors were not included because they are not present in the brain.

Due to the lack of specificity of subset-specific noradrenergic drugs for use in autoradiographic localization, in situ hybridization was the first method of choice to determine areas of the brain containing mRNA for distinct noradrenergic receptor subtypes.[169] Of note, these studies determined that the mRNA for the A-2a noradrenaline receptor was most abundant in the LC, whereas A-2c noradrenaline receptor mRNA was most prevalent in the striatum,[172,175,176] but could not demonstrate the receptors themselves (Fig. 6–8). Although mRNA for adrenergic receptors was not detected in the SN using these methods, autoradiographic labeling of nonspecific A-2 adrenergic drugs did showing binding in this area,[177–179] suggesting that these receptors were primarily presynaptic in location.[175] Later, subset-specific antibodies were made to some of these receptors, demonstrating specific cellular localizations in basal ganglia structures. For example, strong A-2c immunoreactivity was seen in the rat SN, striatum, GPi and STN.[180] A-2a immunoreactivity was also seen in the rat STN and large fusiform cells in the striatum, although this receptor is more abundant in catecholamine neurons of the brainstem,[181] including the LC and a few TH-dual labeled cells in the SNc.[182] In the rat, dual immunolabeling of TH with A-2c receptors was also demonstrated in 77–83% of SNc and 92% of LC neurons.[183] In rat striatum, 94% of medium-sized spiny GABAergic projection neurons were found to contain A-2c immunoreactivity, whereas GABAergic striatal interneurons were devoid of these adrenoceptors.[184]

Recently, transgenic mice that endogenously overexpress A-1 adrenoceptor subtypes fused with enhanced

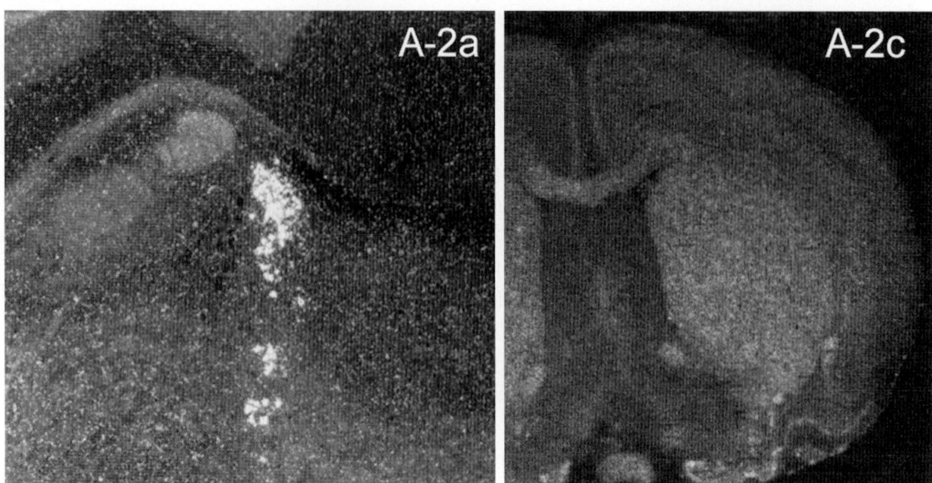

Figure 6–8. In situ hybridization of A-2a and A-2c noradrenergic receptor mRNAs in the rat LC and striatum, respectively.

green fluorescent protein were used to determine the cellular localizations of A-1a and -b noradrenaline receptors in the brain. Small amounts of A-1a[185] and -b[186] receptor labeling were found in neurons of the SN and striatum, but not the LC and globus pallidus. The significance of these findings as it relates to basal ganglia functioning is not yet known.

FUNCTIONS OF NORADRENALINE RECEPTOR SUBTYPES

Pharmacological, behavioral, and gene manipulation (knockout) techniques have also been used to study the phenotypic roles of noradrenaline receptors. For example, mice that lack A-2a receptors had increased heart rate and piloerection, impaired motor coordination skills, increased anxiety-like behavior, and an abnormal diurnal activity pattern. In addition, neurochemical analysis of monoamine neurotransmitters revealed a considerable increase in brain noradrenaline turnover in these mice.[187] In contrast, lack of A-2c receptors decreased the rate of monoamine turnover in the brain, whereas overexpression of this receptor increased dopamine metabolism and storage.[188] In contrast to A-2a receptors, alteration of A-2c receptors did not have any major effect on spontaneous locomotor activity or diurnal rhythm, although the amount of brain A-2c receptors were proportional to the hypothermic response caused by the nonspecific A-2 agonist dexmedetomidine.[188] Injections of the A-2 agonist clonidine in the SNc caused decreased burst firing and regularized the firing pattern of dopamine neurons with no change in firing rate, whereas the A-2c antagonist yohimbine deregularized the firing pattern and increased both the firing rate and burst firing of these neurons.[189] In the striatum, noradrenaline release is believed to be controlled by both A-2a and -c autoreceptors.[190–192] As a result, lesions of the LC or chronic noradrenaline depletion resulted in decreased striatal dopamine release[193] and compensatory upregulation of striatal D2 receptors.[194,195] There is also some evidence that dopamine can act as an additional substrate on striatal A-2c receptors.[196] Collectively, these studies suggest that A-2a and -c noradrenaline receptors play a critical role in dopamine metabolism, not only within the SN itself but also at the level of their terminal fields within the striatum as well.

In most patients with PD, the LC is severely damaged with the presence of Lewy bodies, similar to dopamine neurons of the SNc.[197] In addition, striatal noradrenaline can be decreased as much as 80% in PD patients.[157] Recently, it has been shown that, similar to 5-HT, exogenous levodopa causes further decreases in striatal noradrenaline, and this is further reduced in a MPTP mouse model of LID.[158] The importance of noradrenaline and its receptors in basal ganglia functioning is highlighted by the fact that some of the most effective treatments in monkey models[198–200] and humans with LID[201] are drugs that antagonize A-2 noradrenergic receptors.

▶ SUMMARY

The striatum, the entry point of all major information to the basal ganglia, receives converging inputs from several neurotransmitter systems. Of these, dopamine is the predominant neurotransmitter, as supported by the observation that 80% of all brain dopamine is found in the striatum. Dopamine provides an input to almost every striatal neuron. The limbic and associative cortical areas send excitatory glutamatergic input to the striatum. The intralaminar and other thalamic nuclei also convey their information through the glutamatergic projections to the striatum. Along with the cortical and thalamic glutamater-

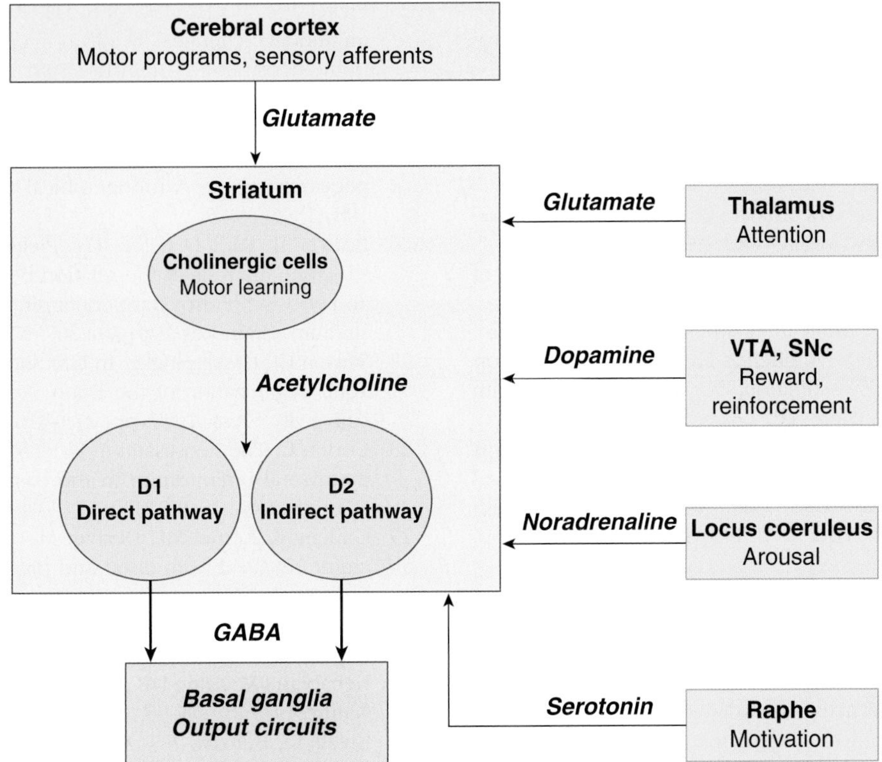

Figure 6–9. Schematic illustrating the convergence of neurotransmitter systems in the striatum. The striatum receives extrinsic input from cortex and thalamus (glutamate), VTA and SNc (dopamine), locus coerulus (noradrenaline), and the raphe (serotonin) as well as intrinsic input from cholinergic interneurons (ACh). The outputs of the striatum are GABAergic. The diagram also illustrates some of the potential functions of these inputs. VTA, ventral tegmental area; GABA, γ-aminobutyric acid.

gic afferents, serotonergic and noradrenergic inputs are believed to converge onto the dendritic spines and shafts of the same medium spiny input–output neuron of the striatum where the dopaminergic terminals also terminate. The activity of the medium spiny neuron is further modified by the giant cholinergic and other interneurons. Dopamine, as the predominant neurotransmitter, is in a position to reinforce, either positively or negatively, learning, initiating, consolidating, memorizing, and retrieving the information provided by the glutamatergic and serotonergic systems[202] (Fig. 6–9). This basic structural and neurochemical unit of the striatum is preserved in both the ventral and dorsal striatum.[203] There is overwhelming evidence from clinical and basic science literature that hyper- and hypodopaminergic states in the striatum manifest in hyper- or hypokinetic syndromes. Dysfunctions of this basic neurochemical unit in the motor compartment of the striatum may be responsible for the spectrum of abnormal movements that are noted in disorders of the basal ganglia. However, it must be emphasized that, besides their role in locomotor behavior, the basal ganglia have been speculated to be involved in procedural memory,[204–207] attentional mechanisms,[208,209] learning, and addictive behavior.[209,210] The next wave of information relating to the molecular cascades that are responsible for interactions between dopamine and other neurotransmitters and neuropeptides will further consolidate our understanding of the functions of the basal ganglia.

▶ ACKNOWLEDGMENTS

This chapter was supported by The University of Alabama at Birmingham Department of Neurology, the Parkinson Association of Alabama, Inc., and the American Parkinson's Disease Association.

REFERENCES

1. Graybiel A. Neurotransmitters and neuromodulators in the basal ganglia. Trends Neurosci 1990;13:244–254.
2. Alexander G, Delong M, Strick P. Parallel organization of functionally segregated circuits linking basal ganglia and cortex. Annu Rev Neurosci 1986;9:357–381.
3. Albin RL, Young AB, Penney JB. The functional anatomy of basal ganglia disorders. Trends Neurosci 1989;12:366–375.
4. Alexander GE, Crutcher MD. Functional architecture of basal ganglia circuits: Neural substrates of parallel processing. Trends Neurosci 1990;13:266–271.

5. Smith Y, Bevan MD, Shink E, et al. Microcircuitry of the direct and indirect pathways of the basal ganglia. Neuroscience 1998;86:353–387.
6. Reiner A, Anderson KD. The patterns of neurotransmitter and neuropeptide co-occurrence among striatal projection neurons: Conclusions based on recent findings. Brain Res Rev 1990;15:251–265.
7. Penney JBJ, Young AB. Striatal inhomogeneities and basal ganglia function. Mov Disord 1986;1:3–15.
8. DeLong MR. Primate models of movement disorders of basal ganglia origin. Trends Neurosci 1990;13:281–285.
9. Hornykiewicz O. Brain monoamines and parkinsonism. In Bernard BK (ed). Aminergic Hypothesis of Behavior: Reality or Cliché? Washington, DC: Department of Health Education and Welfare, 1975, vol 3, pp. 13–21.
10. Bjorklund A, Lindvall O. Dopamine-containing systems in the CNS. In Bjorklund A, Hokfelt T (eds). Classical Transmitters in the CNS: Handbook of Chemical Neuroanatomy. New York, NY: Elsevier, 1984, part 1, pp. 55–122.
11. Forno LS. Pathology of parkinsonism. J Neurosurg 1966;24(Suppl 2):266–271.
12. German DC, Dubach M, Askari S, et al. 1-Methyl-4-phenyl-1,2,3,6-tetrahydropyridine-induced parkinsonian syndrome in *Macaca fascicularis*: Which midbrain dopaminergic neurons are lost? Neuroscience 1988;24:161–174.
13. Hirsch EC, Graybiel AM, Agid Y. Selective vulnerability of pigmented dopaminergic neurons in Parkinson's disease. Acta Neurol Scand Suppl 1989;126:19–22.
14. German DC, Manaye KF, Sonsalla PK, Brooks BA: Midbrain dopaminergic cell loss in Parkinson's disease and MPTP-induced parkinsonism: Sparing of calbindin-D28k-containing cells. Ann N Y Acad Sci 1992;648:42–62.
15. Graybiel AM, Moratalla R, Quinn B, et al. Early-stage loss of dopamine uptake-site binding in MPTP-treated monkeys. Adv Neurol 1993;60:34–39.
16. Hirsch E, Graybiel AM, Agid YA. Melanized dopaminergic neurons are differentially susceptible to degeneration in Parkinson's disease. Nature 1988;334:345–348.
17. Betarbet R, Sherer TB, MacKenzie G, et al. Chronic systemic pesticide exposure reproduces features of Parkinson's disease. Nat Neurosci 2000;3:1301–1306.
18. Parent A, Mackey A, De Bellefeuille L. The subcortical afferents to caudate nucleus and putamen in primate: A fluorescence retrograde double labeling study. Neuroscience 1983;10:1137–1150.
19. Jayaraman A, Nishimori T, Dobner P, et al. Cholecystokinin and neurotensin mRNAs are differentially expressed in subnuclei of the ventral tegmental area. J Comp Neurol 1990;296:291–302.
20. Prensa L, Cossette M, Parent A. Dopaminergic innervation of human basal ganglia. J Chem Neuroanat 2000;20: 207–213.
21. Holt DJ, Graybiel AM, Saper CB. Neurochemical architecture of the human striatum. J Comp Neurol 1997;384:1–25.
22. Betarbet R, Turner R, Chockkan V, et al. Dopaminergic neurons intrinsic to the primate striatum. J Neurosci 1997;17:6761–6768.
23. Betarbet R, Greenamyre JT. Differential expression of glutamate receptors by the dopaminergic neurons of the primate striatum. Exp Neurol 1999;159:401–408.
24. Pickel VM, Beckley SC, Joh TH, Reis DJ. Ultrastructural immunocytochemical localization of tyrosine hydroxylase in the neostriatum. Brain Res 1981;225:373–385.
25. Arluison M, Dietl M, Thibault J. Ultrastructural morphology of dopaminergic nerve terminals and synapses in the striatum of the rat using tyrosine hydroxylase immunocytochemistry: A topographical study. Brain Res Bull 1984;13:269–285.
26. Bouyer JJ, Park DH, Joh TH, Pickel VM. Chemical and structural analysis of the relation between cortical inputs and tyrosine hydroxylase-containing terminals in rat neostriatum. Brain Res 1984;302:267–275.
27. Wilson CJ. Basal ganglia. In GM Shepherd (ed). The Synaptic Organization of the Brain. New York, NY: Oxford University Press, 1990, pp. 279–316.
28. Gerfen C. The neostriatal mosaic: Multiple levels of compartmental organization in the basal ganglia. Annu Rev Neurosci 1992;15:285–320.
29. Gauchy C, Kemel ML, Desban M, et al. The role of dopamine released from distal and proximal dendrites of nigrostriatal dopaminergic neurons in the control of GABA transmission in the thalamic nucleus ventralis medialis in the cat. Neuroscience 1987;22:935–946.
30. Kebabian JW, Calne DB. Multiple receptors for dopamine. Nature 1979;277:93–96.
31. Civelli O, Bunzow JR, Grandy DK. Molecular diversity of the dopamine receptors. Annu Rev Pharmacol Toxicol 1993;33:281–307.
32. Jackson DM, Westlind-Danielsson A. Dopamine receptors: Molecular biology, biochemistry and behavioural aspects. Pharmacol Ther 1994;64:291–370.
33. Hartman DS, Civelli O. Dopamine receptor diversity: Molecular and pharmacological perspectives. Prog Drug Res 1997;48:173–194.
34. Missale C, Nash SR, Robinson SW, et al. Dopamine receptors: From structure to function. Physiol Rev 1998;78: 189–225.
35. Gether U. Uncovering molecular mechanisms involved in activation of G protein-coupled receptors. Endocr Rev 2000;21:90–113.
36. Marinissen MJ, Gutkind JS. G-protein-coupled receptors and signalling networks: Emerging paradigms. Trends Pharmacol Sci 2001;22:368–376.
37. Van Tol HHM, Wu CM, Guan H-C, et al. Multiple dopamine D4 receptor variants in the human population. Nature 1992;358:149–152.
38. Meador-Woodruff JH, Damask SP, Wang J, et al. Dopamine receptor mRNA expression in human striatum and neocortex. Neuropsychopharmacology 1996;15:17–29.
39. Dearry A, Gingrich JA, Falardeau P, et al. Molecular cloning and expression of the gene for a human D1 dopamine receptor. Nature 1990;347:72–76.
40. Hurd YL, Suzuki M, Sedvall GC. D1 and D2 dopamine receptor mRNA expression in whole hemisphere sections of the human brain. J Chem Neuroanat 2001;22:127–137.
41. Lidow MS, Koh PO, Arnsten AF. D1 dopamine receptors in the mouse prefrontal cortex: Immunocytochemical and cognitive neuropharmacological analyses. Synapse 2003;47:101–108.
42. Khan ZU, Gutierrez A, Martin R, et al. Differential regional and cellular distribution of dopamine D2-like

receptors: An immunocytochemical study of subtype-specific antibodies in rat and human brain. J Comp Neurol 1998;402:353–371.

43. Lester J, Fink S, Aronin N, et al. Colocalization of D1 and D2 dopamine receptor mRNAs in striatal neurons. Brain Res 1993;621:106–110.
44. Surmeier DJ, Eberwine J, Wilson CJ, et al. Dopamine receptor subtypes colocalize in rat striatonigral neurons. Proc Natl Acad Sci U S A 1992;89:10178–10182.
45. Landwehrmeyer B, Mengod G, Palacios JM. Dopamine D3 receptor mRNA and binding sites in human brain. Brain Res Mol Brain Res 1993;18:187–192.
46. Murray AM, Ryoo HL, Gurevich E, et al. Localization of dopamine D3 receptors to mesolimbic and D2 receptors to mesostriatal regions of human forebrain. Proc Natl Acad Sci U S A 1994;91:11271–11275.
47. Gurevich EV, Joyce JN. Distribution of dopamine D3 receptor expressing neurons in the human forebrain: Comparison with D2 receptor expressing neurons. Neuropsychopharmacology 1999;20:60–80.
48. Mrzljak L, Bergson C, Pappy M, et al. Localization of dopamine D4 receptors in GABAergic neurons of the primate brain. Nature 1996;381:245–248.
49. Rivera A, Cuellar B, Giron FJ, et al. Dopamine D4 receptors are heterogeneously distributed in the striosomes/matrix compartments of the striatum. J Neurochem 2002;80:219–229.
50. Khan ZU, Gutierrez A, Martin R, et al. Dopamine D5 receptors of rat and human brain. Neuroscience 2000;100: 689–699.
51. Sibley DR. New insights into dopaminergic receptor function using antisense and genetically altered animals. Annu Rev Pharmacol Toxicol 1999;39:313–341.
52. Glickstein SB, Schmauss C. Dopamine receptor functions: Lessons from knockout mice. Pharmacol Ther 2001;91:63–83.
53. El-Ghundi M, Fletcher PJ, Drago J, et al. Spatial learning deficit in dopamine D(1) receptor knockout mice. Eur J Pharmacol 1999;383:95–106.
54. Williams GV, Goldman-Rakic PS. Modulation of memory fields by dopamine D1 receptors in prefrontal cortex. Nature 1995;376:572–575.
55. Baik JH, Picetti R, Saiardi A, et al. Parkinsonian-like locomotor impairment in mice lacking dopamine D2 receptors. Nature 1995;377:424–428.
56. Caine SB, Koob GF. Modulation of cocaine self-administration in the rat through D-3 dopamine receptors. Science 1993;260:1814–1816.
57. Dulawa SC, Grandy DK, Low MJ, et al. Dopamine D4 receptor-knock-out mice exhibit reduced exploration of novel stimuli. J Neurosci 1999;19:9550–9556.
58. Zhou FM, Wilson CJ, Dani JA. Cholinergic interneuron characteristics and nicotinic properties in the striatum. J Neurobiol 2002;53:590–605.
59. Pisani A, Bonsi P, Picconi B, et al. Role of tonically-active neurons in the control of striatal function: Cellular mechanisms and behavioral correlates. Prog Neuropsychopharmacol Biol Psychiatry 2001;25:211–230.
60. Izzo PN, Bolam JP. Cholinergic synaptic input to different parts of spiny striatonigral neurons in the rat. J Comp Neurol 1988;269:219–234.
61. Kemp JM, Powell TPS. The termination of fibres from the cerebral cortex and thalamus upon dendritic spines in the caudate nucleus: A study with the Golgi method. Philos Trans R Soc Lond Biol Sci 1971;262:429–439.
62. Contant C, Umbriaco D, Garcia S, et al. Ultrastructural characterization of the acetylcholine innervation in adult rat neostriatum. Neuroscience 1996;71:937–947.
63. Kubota Y, Inagaki S, Shimada S, et al. Neostriatal cholinergic neurons receive direct synaptic inputs from dopaminergic axons. Brain Res 1987;413:179–184.
64. Mesulam M-M, Mash D, Hersh L, et al. Cholinergic innervation of the human striatum, globus pallidus, subthalamic nucleus, substantia nigra, and red nucleus. J Comp Neurol 1992;323:252–268.
65. Rye DB, Saper CB, Lee HJ, Wainer BH. Pedunculopontine tegmental nucleus of the rat: Cytoarchitecture, cytochemistry, and some extrapyramidal connections of the mesopontine tegmentum. J Comp Neurol 1987;259:483–528.
66. Pahapill PA, Lozano AM. The pedunculopontine nucleus and Parkinson's disease. Brain 2000;123(Pt 9): 1767–1783.
67. Kim R, Nakano K, Jayaraman A, et al. Projections of the globus pallidus and adjacent structures: An autoradiographic study in the monkey. J Comp Neurol 1976;169:263–290.
68. Rye DB, Lee HJ, Saper CB, Wainer BH. Medullary and spinal efferents of the pedunculopontine tegmental nucleus and adjacent mesopontine tegmentum in the rat. J Comp Neurol 1988;269:315–341.
69. Rye D, Thomas J, Levey A. Distribution of molecular muscarinic (m1-m4) receptor subtypes and choline acetyltransferase in the pontine reticular formation of man and non-human primates. Sleep Res Abstr 1995;24:59.
70. Shink E, Sidibe M, Smith Y. Efferent connections of the internal globus pallidus in the squirrel monkey: II. Topography and synaptic organization of pallidal efferents to the pedunculopontine nucleus. J Comp Neurol 1997;382:348–363.
71. Zweig RM, Jankel WR, Hedreen JC, et al. The pedunculopontine nucleus in Parkinson's disease. Ann Neurol 1989;26:41–46.
72. Griffiths PD, Sambrook MA, Perry R, Crossman AR. Changes in benzodiazepine and acetylcholine receptors in the globus pallidus in Parkinson's disease. J Neurol Sci 1990;100:131–136.
73. Changeux JP, Bertrand D, Corringer PJ, et al. Brain nicotinic receptors: Structure and regulation, role in learning and reinforcement. Brain Res Brain Res Rev 1998;26:198–216.
74. Klink R, de Kerchove d'Exaerde A, Zoli M, et al. Molecular and physiological diversity of nicotinic acetylcholine receptors in the midbrain dopaminergic nuclei. J Neurosci 2001;21:1452–1463.
75. Caulfield MP, Birdsall NJ. International Union of Pharmacology. XVII. Classification of muscarinic acetylcholine receptors. Pharmacol Rev 1998;50:279–290.
76. van Koppen CJ, Kaiser B. Regulation of muscarinic acetylcholine receptor signaling. Pharmacol Ther 2003;98: 197–220.
77. Weiner DM, Levey AI, Brann MR. Expression of muscarinic acetylcholine and dopamine receptor mRNAs in rat basal ganglia. Proc Natl Acad Sci U S A 1990;87: 7050–7054.

78. Vilaro MT, Mengod G, Palacios JM. Advances and limitations of the molecular neuroanatomy of cholinergic receptors: The example of multiple muscarinic receptors. Prog Brain Res 1993;98:95–101.
79. Levey A, Kitt C, Simonds W, et al. Identification and localization of muscarinic acetylcholine receptor proteins in brain with subtype-specific antibodies. J Neurosci 1991;11:3218–3226.
80. Levey AI, Edmunds SM, Heilman CJ, et al. Localization of muscarinic m3 receptor protein and m3 receptor binding in rat brain. Neuroscience 1994;63:207–221.
81. Flynn D, Ferrari-DiLeo G, Mash D, Levey A. Differential regulation of molecular subtypes of muscarinic receptors in Alzheimer's disease. J Neurochem 1995;64:1888–1891.
82. Hersch SM, Gutekunst CA, Rees HD, et al. Distribution of m1-m4 muscarinic receptor proteins in the rat striatum: Light and electron microscopic immunocytochemistry using subtypespecific antibodies. J Neurosci 1994;14:3351–3363.
83. Bernard V, Normand E, Bloch B. Phenotypical characterization of the rat striatal neurons expressing muscarinic receptor genes. J Neurosci 1992;12:3591–3600.
84. Yan Z, Flores-Hernandez J, Surmeier DJ. Coordinated expression of muscarinic receptor messenger RNAs in striatal medium spiny neurons. Neuroscience 2001;103:1017–1024.
85. Rye D, Thomas J, Levey A. Distribution of molecular muscarinic (m1-m4) receptor subtypes and choline acetyltransferase in the pontine reticular formation of man and non-human primates. Sleep Res Abstr 1995;24:59.
86. Yasuda RP, Ciesla W, Flores LR, et al. Development of antisera selective for m4 and m5 muscarinic cholinergic receptors: Distribution of m4 and m5 receptors in rat brain. Mol Pharmacol 1993;43:149–157.
87. Kitabatake Y, Hikida T, Watanabe D, et al. Impairment of reward-related learning by cholinergic cell ablation in the striatum. Proc Natl Acad Sci U S A 2003;100:7965–7970.
88. Everitt BJ, Robbins TW. Central cholinergic systems and cognition. Annu Rev Psychol 1997;48:649–684.
89. Belluardo N, Mudo G, Blum M, et al. Neurotrophic effects of central nicotinic receptor activation. J Neural Transm Suppl 2000;60:227–245.
90. Dani JA. Overview of nicotinic receptors and their roles in the central nervous system. Biol Psychiatry 2001;49:166–174.
91. Cordero-Erausquin M, Marubio LM, Klink R, et al. Nicotinic receptor function: New perspectives from knockout mice. Trends Pharmacol Sci 2000;21:211–217.
92. Picciotto MR, Caldarone BJ, King SL, et al. Nicotinic receptors in the brain. Links between molecular biology and behavior. Neuropsychopharmacology 2000;22:451–465.
93. Picciotto MR, Caldarone BJ, Brunzell DH, et al. Neuronal nicotinic acetylcholine receptor subunit knockout mice: Physiological and behavioral phenotypes and possible clinical implications. Pharmacol Ther 2001;92:89–108.
94. Marubio LM, Gardier AM, Durier S, et al. Effects of nicotine in the dopaminergic system of mice lacking the alpha4 subunit of neuronal nicotinic acetylcholine receptors. Eur J Neurosci 2003;17:1329–1337.
95. Zachariou V, Caldarone BJ, Weathers-Lowin A, et al. Nicotine receptor inactivation decreases sensitivity to cocaine. Neuropsychopharmacology 2001;24:576–589.
96. Salas R, Orr-Urtreger A, Broide RS, et al. The nicotinic acetylcholine receptor subunit alpha 5 mediates short-term effects of nicotine in vivo. Mol Pharmacol 2003;63:1059–1066.
97. Bymaster FP, McKinzie DL, Felder CC, et al. Use of M1-M5 muscarinic receptor knockout mice as novel tools to delineate the physiological roles of the muscarinic cholinergic system. Neurochem Res 2003;28:437–442.
98. Zhang W, Yamada M, Gomeza J, et al. Multiple muscarinic acetylcholine receptor subtypes modulate striatal dopamine release, as studied with M1-M5 muscarinic receptor knock-out mice. J Neurosci 2002;22:6347–6352.
99. Hamilton SE, Nathanson NM. The M1 receptor is required for muscarinic activation of mitogen-activated protein (MAP) kinase in murine cerebral cortical neurons. J Biol Chem 2001;276:15850–15853.
100. Gerber DJ, Sotnikova TD, Gainetdinov RR, et al. Hyperactivity, elevated dopaminergic transmission, and response to amphetamine in M1 muscarinic acetylcholine receptor-deficient mice. Proc Natl Acad Sci U S A 2001;98:15312–15317.
101. Gomeza J, Zhang L, Kostenis E, et al. Enhancement of D1 dopamine receptor-mediated locomotor stimulation in M(4) muscarinic acetylcholine receptor knockout mice. Proc Natl Acad Sci U S A 1999;96:10483–10488.
102. Basile AS, Fedorova I, Zapata A, et al. Deletion of the M5 muscarinic acetylcholine receptor attenuates morphine reinforcement and withdrawal but not morphine analgesia. Proc Natl Acad Sci U S A 2002;99:11452–11457.
103. Wess J, Duttaroy A, Gomeza J, et al. Muscarinic receptor sub-types mediating central and peripheral antinociception studied with muscarinic receptor knockout mice: A review. Life Sci 2003;72:2047–2054.
104. Yamada M, Miyakawa T, Duttaroy A, et al. Mice lacking the M3 muscarinic acetylcholine receptor are hypophagic and lean. Nature 2001;410:207–212.
105. Divac I, Fonnum F, Storm-Mathisen J. High affinity uptake of glutamate in terminals of corticostriatal axons. Nature 1977;266:377–378.
106. Young A, Bromberg M, Penney J. Decreased glutamate uptake in subcortical areas deafferented by sensorimotor cortical ablation in the cat. J Neurosci 1981;1:241–249.
107. Parent A. Extrinsic connections of the basal ganglia. Trends Neurosci 1990;13:254–258.
108. Blandini F, Porter R, Greenamyre J. Glutamate and Parkinson's disease. Mol Neurobiol 1996;12:73–94.
109. Ozawa S, Kamiya H, Tsuzuki K. Glutamate receptors in the mammalian central nervous system. Prog Neurobiol 1998;54:581–618.
110. Ishii T, Moriyoshi K, Sugihara H, et al. Molecular characterization of the *N*-methyl-D-aspartate receptor subunits. J Biol Chem 1993;268:2836–2843.
111. Kutsuwada T, Kashiwabuchi N, Mori H, et al. Molecular diversity of the NMDA receptor channel. Nature 1992;358:36–41.
112. Meguro H, Mori H, Araki K, et al. Functional characterization of a heteromeric NMDA receptor channel expressed from cloned cDNAs. Nature 1992;357:70–74.
113. Monyer H, Sprengel R, Schoepfer R, et al. Heteromeric NMDA receptors: Molecular and functional distinction of subtypes. Science 1992;256:1217–1221.

114. Moriyoshi K, Masu M, Ishii T, et al. Molecular cloning and characterization of the rat NMDA receptor. Nature 1991;354:31–37.
115. Keinanen K, Wisden W, Sommer B, et al. A family of AMPA-selective glutamate receptors. Science 1990;249: 556–560.
116. Hollmann M, O'Shea-Greenfield A, Rogers S, Heinemann S. Cloning by functional expression of a member of the glutamate receptor family. Nature 1989;342:643–648.
117. Hollmann M, Hartley M, Heineman S. Ca2+ permeability of KA-AMPA-gated glutamate receptor channels depends on subunit composition. Science 1991;252:851–853.
118. Sommer B, Keinanen K, Verdoorn T, et al. Flip and flop: A cell specific functional switch in glutamate-operated channels. Science 1990;249:1580–1585.
119. Pin J-P, Duvoisin R. The metabotropic glutamate receptors: Structure and functions. Neuropharmacology 1995;34:1–26.
120. Albin RL, Makowiec RL, Hollingsworth ZR, et al. Excitatory amino acid binding sites in the basal ganglia of the rat: A quantitative autoradiographic study. Neuroscience 1992;46:35–48.
121. Ravenscroft P, Brotchie J. NMDA receptors in the basal ganglia. J Anat 2000;196(Pt 4):577–585.
122. Petralia R, Yokotani N, Wenthold R. Light and electron microscope distribution of the NMDA receptor subunit NMDAR1 in the rat nervous system using a selective anti-peptide antibody. J Neurosci 1994;14:667–696.
123. Nash N, Heilman C, Rees H, Levey A. Novel human NMDA receptor subunits: Cloning and immunological characterization of exon 5 containing isoforms. Soc Neurosci Abstr 1995;21:1111.
124. Standaert D, Testa C, Young A, Penney J. Organization of *N*-methyl-D-aspartate glutamate receptor gene expression in the basal ganglia of the rat. J Comp Neurol 1994;343: 1–16.
125. Landwehrmeyer G, Standaert D, Testa C, et al. NMDA receptor subunit mRNA expression by projection neurons and interneurons in rat striatum. J Neurosci 1995;15: 5297–5307.
126. Martin LJ, Blackstone CD, Levey AI, et al. AMPA glutamate receptor subunits are differentially distributed in rat brain. Neuroscience 1993;53:327–358.
127. Petralia RS, Wenthold RJ. Light and electron immunocytochemical localization of AMPA-selective glutamate receptors in the rat brain. J Comp Neurol 1992;318: 329–354.
128. Paquet M, Smith Y. Differential localization of AMPA glutamate receptor subunits in the two segments of the globus pallidus and the substantia nigra pars reticulata in the squirrel monkey. Eur J Neurosci 1996;8:229–233.
129. Paquet M, Tremblay M, Soghomonian JJ, et al. AMPA and NMDA glutamate receptor subunits in midbrain dopaminergic neurons in the squirrel monkey: An immunohistochemical and in situ hybridization study. J Neurosci 1997;17:1377–1396.
130. Testa C, Standaert D, Young A, Penney J. Metabotropic glutamate receptor mRNA expression in the basal ganglia of the rat. J Neurosci 1994;14:3005–3018.
131. Testa C, Standaert D, Landwehrmeyer G, et al. Differential expression of mGluR5 metabotropic glutamate receptor mRNA by rat striatal neurons. J Neurosci 1995;354: 241–252.
132. Hubert GW, Paquet M, Smith Y. Differential subcellular localization of mGluR1a and mGluR5 in the rat and monkey substantia nigra. J Neurosci 2001;21:1838–1847.
133. Smith Y, Charara A, Hanson JE, et al. GABA(B) and group I metabotropic glutamate receptors in the striatopallidal complex in primates. J Anat 2000;196(Pt 4):555–576.
134. Dahlstrom A, Fuxe K. Evidence for the existence of monoamine neurons in the central nervous system. I. Demonstration of monoamines in the cell bodies of brainstem neurons. Acta Physiol Scand 1964;62(Suppl 232):1–55.
135. Tork I. Anatomy of the serotonergic system. Ann N Y Acad Sci 1990;600:9–35.
136. Steinbusch HW, Nieuwenhuys R, Verhofstad AA, et al. The nucleus raphe dorsalis of the rat and its projection upon the caudatoputamen. A combined cytoarchitectonic, immunohistochemical and retrograde transport study. J Physiol (Paris) 1981;77:157–174.
137. Jacobs BL, Fornal CA. Serotonin and motor activity. Curr Opin Neurobiol 1997;7:820–825.
138. Lowry CA. Functional subsets of serotonergic neurones: Implications for control of the hypothalamic-pituitary-adrenal axis. J Neuroendocrinol 2002;14:911–923.
139. Bacopoulos NG, Redmond DE, Roth RH. Serotonin and dopamine metabolites in brain regions and cerebrospinal fluid of a primate species: Effects of ketamine and fluphenazine. J Neurochem 1979;32:1215–1218.
140. Lavoie B, Parent A. Immunohistochemical study of the serotonergic innervation of the basal ganglia in the squirrel monkey. J Comp Neurol 1990;299:1–16.
141. Hoyer D, Clarke DE, Fozard JR, et al. International Union of Pharmacology classification of receptors for 5-hydroxytryptamine (serotonin). Pharmacol Rev 1994;46:157–203.
142. Barnes NM, Sharp T. A review of central 5-HT receptors and their function. Neuropharmacology 1999;38: 1083–1152.
143. Gothert M. Presynaptic serotonin receptors in the central nervous system. Ann N Y Acad Sci 1990;604:102–112.
144. Fox SH, Brotchie JM. 5-HT2C receptor binding is increased in the substantia nigra pars reticulata in Parkinson's disease. Mov Disord 2000;15:1064–1069.
145. Gingrich JA, Hen R. The broken mouse: The role of development, plasticity and environment in the interpretation of phenotypic changes in knockout mice. Curr Opin Neurobiol 2000;10:146–152.
146. Gingrich JA, Hen R. Dissecting the role of the serotonin system in neuropsychiatric disorders using knockout mice. Psychopharmacology (Berl) 2001;155:1–10.
147. Tepper SJ, Rapoport AM, Sheftell FD. Mechanisms of action of the 5-HT1B/1D receptor agonists. Arch Neurol 2002;59:1084–1088.
148. Kish SJ. Biochemistry of Parkinson's disease: Is a brain serotonergic deficiency a characteristic of idiopathic Parkinson's disease? Adv Neurol 2003;91:39–49.
149. Paulus W, Jellinger K. The neuropathologic basis of different clinical subgroups of Parkinson's disease. J Neuropathol Exp Neurol 1991;50:743–755.
150. Halliday GM, Blumbergs PC, Cotton RG, et al. Loss of brainstem serotonin- and substance P-containing neurons in Parkinson's disease. Brain Res 1990;510:104–107.

151. Kovacs GG, Kloppel S, Fischer I, et al. Nucleus-specific alteration of raphe neurons in human neurodegenerative disorders. Neuroreport 2003;14:73–76.
152. Dahlström A, Fuxe K. Evidence for the existence of monoamine neurons in the central nervous system. I. Demonstration of monoamines in the cell bodies of brainstem neurons. Acta Physiol Scand 1964;62(Suppl 232):1–55.
153. Swanson LW, Hartman BK. The central adrenergic system. An immunofluorescence study of the localization of cell bodies and their efferent connections in the rat utilizing dopamine-b-hydroxylase. J Comp Neurol 1975;163:467–506.
154. Ross RA, Reis DJ. Effects of lesions of locus coeruleus on regional distribution of dopamine-b-hydroxylase activity in rat brain. Brain Res 1974;73:161–166.
155. Udenfriend S, Creveling CR. Localization of dopamine-b-oxidase in brain. J Neurochem 1959;4:350–352.
156. Glowinski J, Iversen LL. Regional studies of catecholamines in the rat brain—I. The deposition of [3H] norepinephrine, [3H]dopamine and [3H]dopa in various regions of the brain. J Neurochem 1966;13:655–669.
157. Hornykiewicz O. Brain monoamines and parkinsonism. In Bernard BK (ed). Aminergic Hypothesis of Behavior: Reality or Cliché?. Washington, DC: Department of Health Education and Welfare, 1975, pp. 13–21.
158. Nicholas AP, Buck K, Ferger B. Effects of levodopa on striatal monoamines in mice with levodopa-induced hyperactivity. Neurosci Lett 2008;443:204–208.
159. Nishi K, Kondo T, Narabayashi H. Destruction of norepinephrine terminals in 1-methyl-4-phenyl-1,2,3,6-tetrahydropyridine (MPTP)-treated mice reduces locomotor activity induced by L-DOPA. Neurosci Lett 1991;123:244–247.
160. Moore RY, Card JP. Noradrenaline-containing neuron systems. In Björklund A, Hökfelt T (eds). Handbook of Chemical Neuroanatomy: Classical Transmitters in the CNS. Part I. Elsevier: Amsterdam, 1984, pp. 123–156.
161. Bunney BS, Aghajanian GK. The precise localization of nigral afferents in the rat as determined by a retrograde tracing technique. Brain Res 1976(117):423–435.
162. Jones BE, Moore RY. Ascending projections of the locus coeruleus in the rat. II. Autoradiographic study. Brain Res 1977;127:23–53.
163. Parent A, Mackey A, De Bellefeuille L. The subcortical afferents to caudate nucleus and putamen in primate: A fluorescence retrograde double labeling study. Neuroscience 1983;10:1137–1150.
164. DeVito JL, Anderson ME, Walsh KE. A horseradish peroxidase study of afferent connections of the globus pallidus in Macaca mulatta. Exp Brain Res 1980;38:65–73.
165. Mason ST, Fibiger HC. Regional topography within noradrenergic locus coeruleus as revealed by retrograde transport of horseradish peroxidase. J Comp Neurol 1979;187:703–724.
166. Fuxe K, Agnati LF. Volume Transmission in the Brain. New York: Raven Press, 1991.
167. Schneider JS, Rothblat DS, DiStefano L. Volume transmission of dopamine over large distances may contribute to recovery from experimental parkinsonism. Brain Res 1994;643:86–91.
168. Callado LF, Stamford JA. Spatiotemporal interaction of α2 autoreceptors and noradrenaline transporters in the rat locus coeruleus: Implications for volume transmission. J Neurochem 2002;74:2350–2358.
169. Nicholas AP, Hökfelt T, Pieribone VA. The distribution and significance of specific central nervous system adrenoceptors examined with in situ hybridization. Trends Pharmacol Sci 1996;17:245–255.
170. Domyancic AV, Morilak DA. Distribution of α1A adrenergic receptor mRNA in the rat brain visualized by in situ hybridization. J Comp Neurol 1997;386:358–378.
171. McCune SK, Voigt MM, Hill JM. Expression of multiple alpha adrenergic receptor subtype messenger RNAs in the adult rat brain. Neuroscience 1993;57:143–151.
172. Nicholas AP, Pieribone VA, Hökfelt T. Distribution of mRNAs for alpha-2 adrenergic receptor subtypes in rat brain: An in situ hybridization study. J Comp Neurol 1993;328:575–594.
173. Nicholas AP, Pieribone VA, Hökfelt T. Cellular localization of mRNA for beta-1 and beta-2 adrenergic receptors in rat brain: An in situ hybridization study. Neuroscience 1993;56:1023–1039.
174. Pieribone VA, et al. Distribution of a1 adrenoceptors in rat brain revealed by in situ hybridization experiments utilizing subtype-specific probes. J Neurosci 1994;14(7): 4252–4268.
175. Scheinin M, et al. Distribution of α2-adrenergic receptor subtype gene expression in rat brain. Mol Brain Res 1994;21:133–149.
176. Nicholas AP, et al. In situ hybridization. A complementary method to radiolgand-mediated autoradiography for localizing adrenergic, alpha-2 receptor-producing cells. Ann NY Acad Sci 1995;763:222–242.
177. Boyajian CL, Loughlin SE, Leslie FM. Anatomical evidence for alpha-2 adrenoceptor heterogeneity: Differential autoradiographic distributions of [3H]rauwolscine and [3H]idazoxan in rat brain. J Pharmacol Exp Ther 1987;241:1079–1091.
178. Hudson AL, et al. 3H-RX821002: A highly selective ligand for the identification of α2-adrenoceptors in the rat brain. Mol Neuropharmacol 1992;1:219–229.
179. Unnerstall JR, Kopajtic TA, Kuhar MJ. Distribution of a2 agonist binding sites in the rat and human central nervous system: Analysis of some functional, anatomical correlates of the pharmacological effects of clonidine and related adrenergic agents. Brain Res Rev 1984;7:69–101.
180. Rosin DL, et al. Distribution of alpha 2C-adrenergic receptor-like immunoreactivity in the rat central nervous system. J Comp Neurol 1996;372:135–165.
181. Talley EM, et al. Distribution of alpha 2A-adrenergic receptor-like immunoreactivity in the rat central nervous system. J Comp Neurol 1996;372:111–134.
182. Rosin DL, et al. Immunohistochemical localization of α2A-adrenergic receptors in catecholaminergic and other brainstem neurons in the rat. Neuroscience 1993;56:139–155.
183. Lee A, et al. Localization of α2C-adrenergic receptor immunoreactivity in catecholaminergic neurons in the rat central nervous system. Neuroscience 1998;84: 1085–1096.
184. Holmberg M, et al. Adrenergic α2C-receptors reside in rat striatal GABAergic projection neurons: Comparison of radioligand binding and immunohistochemistry. Neuroscience 1999;93:1323–1333.

185. Papay R, et al. Localization of the mouse alpha1A-adrenergic receptor (AR) in the brain: Alpha1aar is expressed in neurons, GABAergic interneurons, and NG2 oligodendrocyte progenitors. J Comp Neurol 2006;497:209–222.
186. Papay R, et al. Mouse alpha1B-adrenergic receptor is expressed in neurons and NG2 oligodendrocytes. J Comp Neurol 2004;478:1–10.
187. Lähdesmäki J, et al. Behavioral and neurochemical characterization of α2A-adrenergic receptor knockout mice. Neuroscience 2002;113:289–299.
188. Sallinen J, et al. Genetic alteration of α2C-adrenoceptor expression in mice: Influence on locomotor, hypothermic, and neurochemical effects of dexmedetomidine, a subtype-nonselective α2-adrenoceptor agonist. Mol Pharmacol 1997;51:36–46.
189. Grenhoff J, Svensson TH. Clonidine regularizes substantia nigra dopamine cell firing. Life Sci 1988;42:2003–2009.
190. Gobert A, et al. Quantification and pharmacological characterization of dialysate levels of noradrenaline in the striatum of freely-moving rats: Release from adrenergic terminals and modulation by α2-autoreceptors. J Neurosci Meth 2004;140:141–152.
191. Yavich L, et al. α2-Adrenergic control of dopamine overflow and metabolism in mouse striatum. Eur J Pharmacol 1997;339:113–119.
192. Yavich L, et al. Atipamezole, an α2-adrenoceptor antagonist, augments the effects of image-DOPA on evoked dopamine release in rat striatum. Eur J Pharmacol 2003;462:83–89.
193. Lategan AJ, Marien MR, Colpaert FC. Effects of locus coeruleus lesions on the release of endogenous dopamine in the rat nucleus accumbens and caudate nucleus as determined by intracerebral microdialysis. Brain Res 1990;523:134–138.
194. Harro J, et al. Effect of denervation of the locus coeruleus projections by DSP-4 treatment on [3H]-raclopride binding to dopamine D2 receptors and D2 receptor–G protein interaction in the rat striatum. Brain Res 2003;976:209–216.
195. Schank JR, et al. Dopamine beta-hydroxylase knockout mice have alterations in dopamine signaling and are hypersensitive to cocaine. Neuropsychopharmacology 2006;31:2221–2230.
196. Zhang W, et al. α2C Adrenoceptors inhibit adenylyl cyclase in mouse striatum: Potential activation by dopamine. J Pharmacol Exp Ther 1999;289:1286–1292.
197. Forno LS. Pathology of parkinsonism. J Neurosurg 1966;24(Suppl 2):266–271.
198. Grondin R, et al. Noradrenoceptor antagonism with idazoxan improves L-dopa-induced dyskinesias in MPTP monkeys. Nauyn-Schm Arch Pharmacol 2000;361:181–186.
199. Henry B, et al. The α2-adrenergic receptor antagonist idazoxan reduces dyskinesia and enhances antiparkinsonian actions of L-dopa in the MPTP-lesioned primate model of Parkinson's disease. Mov Disord 1999;14: 744–753.
200. Savola J-M, et al. Fipamezole (JP-1730) is a potent α2-adrenergic receptor antagonist that reduces levodopa-induced dyskinesia and enhances anti-parkinsonian actions of L-dopa in the MPTP-lesioned primate model of Parkinson's disease. Mov Disord 2003;18:872–883.
201. Rascol O, et al. L-Dopa-induced dyskinesias improvement by an α2 antagonist, idazoxan, in patients with Parkinson's disease. Mov Disord 1997;12(Suppl 1):111.
202. Schultz W. Predictive reward signal of dopamine neurons. J Neurophysiol 1998;80:1–27.
203. Nicola SM, Malenka RC. Modulation of synaptic transmission by dopamine and norepinephrine in ventral but not dorsal striatum. J Neurophysiol 1998;79:1768–1776.
204. Phillips AG, Carr GD. Cognition and the basal ganglia: A possible substrate for procedural knowledge. Can J Neurol Sci 1987;14:381–385.
205. Knowlton BJ, Mangels JA, Squire LR. A neostriatal habit learning system in humans. Science 1996;273:1399–1402.
206. Squire LR, Zola SM. Structure and function of declarative and nondeclarative memory systems. Proc Natl Acad Sci U S A 1996;93:13515–13522.
207. Squire LR. Memory systems. CR Acad Sci III 1998;321: 153–156.
208. Jayaraman A. The basal ganglia and cognition: An interpretation of anatomical connectivity pattern. In Schneider JS, Lidsky T (eds). Basal Ganglia and Behavior: Sensory Aspects of Motor Functioning. Toronto: Hans Huber Publications, 1987, pp. 149–160.
209. Nieoullon A. Dopamine and the regulation of cognition and attention. Prog Neurobiol 2002;67:53–83.
210. Nestler EJ. Common molecular and cellular substrates of addiction and memory. Neurobiol Learn Mem 2002;78:637–647.

CHAPTER 7

Neurotrophic Factors

Mart Saarma, Päivi Lindholm, and Urmas Arumäe

▶ INTRODUCTION TO NEUROTROPHIC FACTORS

NEUROTROPHIC FACTORS IN DEVELOPMENT AND PROGRAMMED CELL DEATH

During animal development, neurons are overproduced, but when contacts with other cells and neurons are formed, the excess of neurons is removed by genetically controlled programmed cell death (PCD). This process ensures correct formation of neuronal contacts and the system match between the neurons and their targets, which are critically important for the development of vertebrate nervous system.[1] Experimental data demonstrate that different cell-intrinsic and cell-extrinsic factors regulate this process, including cell-intrinsic transcriptional programs, as well as growth factors secreted in the autocrine manner. Cell-extrinsic factors include secreted or cell-surface-bound molecules provided by the neighboring cells, tissues and extracellular matrix. Neurotrophic factors (NTFs) are important groups of proteins secreted by the target tissues and inhibiting PCD of the neurons innervating these targets. NTFs provide trophic support for the neurons by keeping them alive and maintaining their phenotype.

During developmental periods of PCD, from 20% to 80% of neurons in a given population die by apoptosis.[2] NTFs play a key role in preventing apoptotic death, thereby regulating the number of target-innervating neurons and the density of innervation.

MECHANISMS OF NEUROTROPHIC FACTORS

The concept of NTFs was formulated by Rita Levi-Montalcini and Victor Hamburger and was based on the studies on nerve growth factor (NGF). It is interesting to note that NGF was the first discovered growth factor and NTF that opened a completely new field in biology.[3,4] According to the target-field model,[5] neurons are intrinsically apoptotic at PCD and compete for the anti-apoptotic NTFs that are secreted by the target tissues in limited amounts. As a result, only those neurons that first reach the target and receive proper neurotrophic support are rescued, whereas those neurons that are late or form synapses with wrong target tissues remain without NTFs and die by default apoptosis (Fig. 7–1). Active killing of the neurons by target-derived NTFs or pro-NTFs has also been postulated as a part of target control upon the number of innervating neurons.[6] The NTFs bind to their cognate receptors at neurite terminals, followed by the endocytosis of the ligand-receptor complex. Thereafter, the complex is retrogradely transported along the axon to the cell soma.[7] Binding of the ligand triggers the receptor activation, which usually means phosphorylation on tyrosine, serine, or threonine residues in the intracellular part of the transmembrane receptors. Phosphorylated amino acids form docking sites for the adaptor proteins or enzymes that activate downstream survival, promoting signaling pathways, and thereby

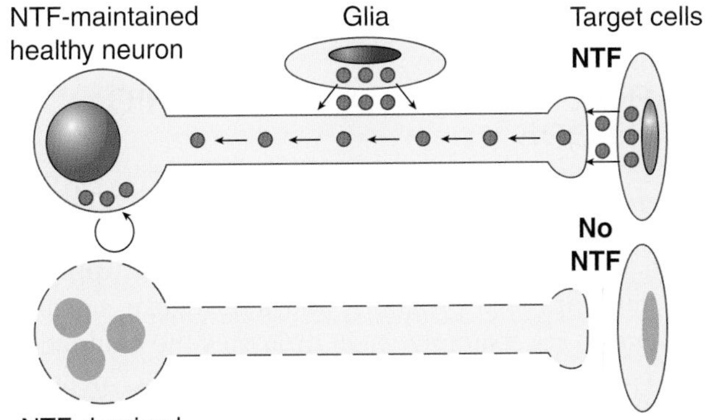

Figure 7-1. Target dependence of the neurons during PCD. Neurotrophic factors (NTF) are secreted by the target cells and transported retrogradely from the neurite terminals to the somae. NTFs suppress the apoptotic program, whereas in the neurons that are left without NTFs, the apoptotic program remains unsuppressed and kills the cell. Target tissues produce NTFs in the limited amounts, but NTFs can be provided also by glial cells or in the autocrine manner by the neurons themselves.

suppress the apoptotic program. The role of NTF in the development of the peripheral nervous system, (PNS) is well established, but the role of NTFs in the development and maintenance of the central nervous system (CNS) is less clear, although currently actively studied.

CLASSES OF NEUROTROPHIC FACTORS

Many growth factors have effects on the nervous systems at different stages of development, and, therefore, can be called NTFs. If this broader classification of "neurotrophic factors" is used, a wide range of growth factor proteins with different functional specificities would be included. However, it is now commonly accepted that NTFs consist of four main growth factor protein families: (1) neurotrophins,[8,9] (2) glial cell line–derived neurotrophic factor (GDNF) family ligands (GFL),[10,11] (3) the neuropoietic cytokine family (also known as interleukin-6 [IL-6] or glycoprotein 130 (g130) family),[12] (4) and finally, the conserved dopamine neurotrophic factor (CDNF)/mesencephalic astrocyte–derived neurotrophic factor (MANF) family.[13,14] Neurotrophin, GFL, and neurokine family members signal via transmembrane receptor tyrosine kinases (RTKs), or have receptors associated with kinases.[11] The receptor system for CDNF/MANF family members is currently unclear. As mentioned earlier, various growth factors from other families have also neurotrophic activities. Examples of these include members of the vascular endothelial growth factor (VEGF), transforming growth factor-beta (TGF-β), insulinlike growth factor, fibroblast growth factor (FGF) families, erythropoietin, ephrins, and many others.

TARGETS OF NEUROTROPHIC FACTORS

NTFs affect specific sets of neuronal subpopulations that are genetically competent to respond, i.e., express cognate receptors on their surface and have appropriate transcriptional programs and intracellular signaling pathways. For example, NGF promotes the maturation, survival, and maintenance of sympathetic neurons, GDNF regulates the migration of enteric neurons, ciliary neurotrophic factor (CNTF) supports the survival of ciliary parasympathetic neurons and CDNF maintains the DA neurons. In addition to survival-promoting activity on postmitotic neurons,[1] NTFs affect proliferation, migration, differentiation, and maturation of neuronal precursors.[15] They also regulate neuritogenesis, formation, and maintenance of synaptic contacts, axonal sprouting, dendritic arborization, and synaptic plasticity (for review—[9]). It is well established that NTFs also affect the non-neuronal cells and tissues; for example, brain-derived neurotrophic factor (BDNF) regulates heart development, GDNF controls kidney development and spermatogenesis, and IL-6, secreted by T cells and macrophages, stimulates immune response to trauma.

▶ NTFs AND MOVEMENT DISORDERS

NTFs AS TREATMENT FOR NEURODEGENERATIVE DISEASE

Soon after recognition of the potency of NTFs to promote the survival of neurons, they were seen as useful tools for the treatment of the neurological and particularly the neurodegenerative diseases. During the last decade, it has been clearly shown that NTFs have positive effects in the animal models of neurological diseases and trauma (for review—[16–18]); for example, NGF has beneficial effects in animal models of Alzheimer's disease, BDNF has been successfully tested in animal models of Parkinson's disease (PD), as well as in stroke. GDNF, its homolog neurturin (NRTN), and CNTF have been efficient in animal models of amyotrophic lateral sclerosis (ALS). These studies have also revealed several limitations, including poor bioavailability, inability to pass the blood–brain barrier, and high molecular weight. Clinical trials of NTF in neurodegenerative disease have so far produced controversial results. For example, GDNF and NRTN have successfully passed phase 1 clinical trials of PD, but more recent phase 2 clinical trials have been less impressive. Since most of the preclinical and clinical data with NTFs have been accumulated from trials on animal models and patients with PD, in this chapter we mostly focus on the mechanisms of action and effects of NTFs that may be useful in this disease.

NEUROTROPHIC FACTORS: THE NEUROTROPHIN CLASS

Neurotrophin Ligands

Neurotrophins are the best studied and characterized trophic factors in the nervous system (for review—[8,9,19,20]). They regulate the proliferation, differentiation, survival/death, adult maintenance, and such of several types of neurons, but also many non-neuronal cells. They are critically important for the development, physiological regulation, and maintenance of the nervous system.

The family of neurotrophins includes four members in the mammals: (1) NGF, (2) BDNF, (3) neurotrophin-3 (NT-3), and (4) neurotrophin-4 (NT-4). Neurotrophins are initially synthesized as pre-pro-neurotrophin (pro-NT) precursors and the pre-part is cleaved off during protein synthesis. The pro-NTs are usually cleaved inside the cells to release the mature active proteins; however, it has been recently documented that pro-NGF, pro-BDNF, and pro-NT-3 can be secreted as pro-NTs that have biological activities different from the mature neurotrophins.[21,22] Neurotrophins are thus secreted as both mature and pro-NTs. In addition to the constitutive secretion that usually occurs in non-neuronal cells, both mature and pro-NTs can be secreted in a regulated manner by the neurons too. In the nervous system, the common physiological regulator of neurotrophin secretion is neuronal activity.[19,23] Structurally neurotrophins are classified as cystine-knot cytokines, and they function as homodimers.

Neurotrophin Receptors

Neurotrophins are unique in that they signal through three different types of transmembrane receptor systems: (1) receptor tyrosine kinases (RTKs), which are a members of the tropomyosin-related kinase (Trk) family; (2) the p75 neurotrophin receptor ($p75^{NTR}$), a member of tumor necrosis factor receptor superfamily; and (3) the trafficking receptor sortilin, a member of the Vps10p domain receptor family (for review—[19,22,24,25]) (Fig. 7–2). NGF binds specifically to TrkA, BDNF and NT-4 to TrkB, and NT-3 mainly to TrkC (but more weakly also to TrkA and TrkB). All four neurotrophins can bind to $p75^{NTR}$ with similar affinity. Although $p75^{NTR}$ and Trk receptors do not interact directly, there is evidence that a complex forms between these receptors in the presence of neurotrophin ligands.[26] As a rule, neurotrophins promote cell survival and differentiation during development through the activation of Trk receptors. On neurotrophin binding, Trk receptors dimerize, become autophosphorylated and recruit adaptor proteins such as Shc, FRS2, and effector molecules such as phospholipase C-gamma (PLC)-γ and phosphatidylinositol (PI)-3 kinase. The key docking site in TrkA is phosphotyrosine Tyr^{490} that recruits either Shc or FRS2 and activates MAPK and AKT pathways that stimulate the neurite outgrowth and cell survival, respectively. Phosphorylated Tyr^{790} in turn recruits PLC-γ that regulates various cellular activities, including neurotrophin secretion (for review—[25,27,28]).

The biological activity of neurotrophins can be regulated by posttranslational processing of the proteins. As noted earlier, pro-NTs are converted to mature proteins by proteolytic cleavage. Both pro- and mature forms are secreted and are active in signaling, although their biological effects can be opposite: pro-NGF and pro-BDNF signaling via $p75^{NTR}$ and sortilin mediates apoptotic cell death, whereas mature neurotrophins signaling via Trk receptors and $p75^{NTR}$ promotes cell survival.

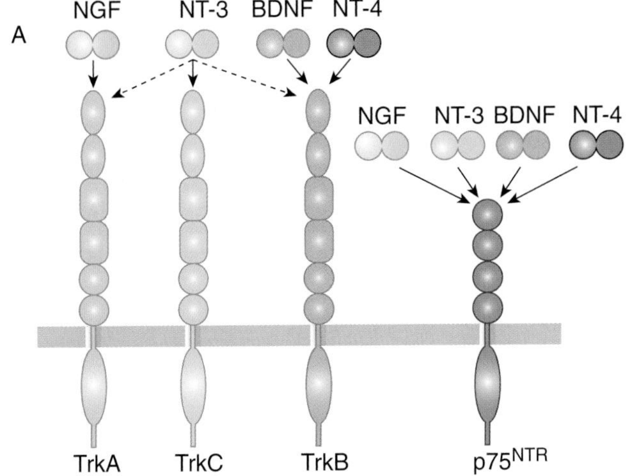

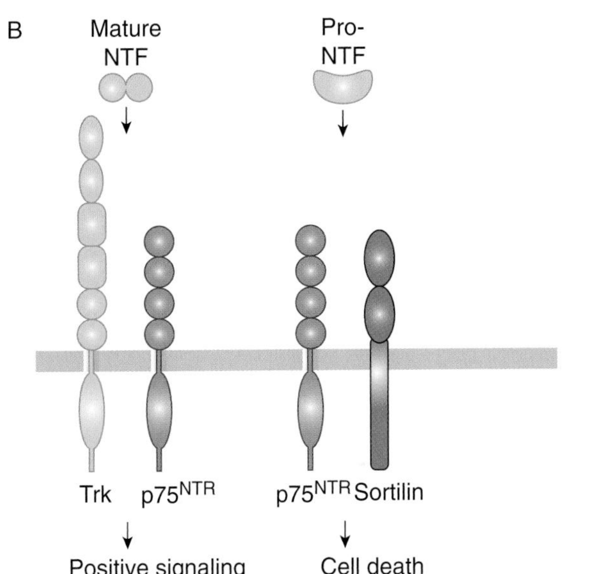

Figure 7-2. Ligand-receptor complexes of neurotrophins. (A) Neurotrophins bind to specific Trk receptors as indicated either with high (*solid arrows*) or low (*dashed arrows*) affinity, whereas all neurotrophins bind $p75^{NTR}$. (B) Mature neurotrophins bind receptor complexes consisting of $p75^{NTR}$ and the respective Trk, resulting in the positive signals, whereas pro-NTs bind receptor complexes consisting of $p75^{NTR}$ and sortilin, resulting in the cell death.

Effects of Neurotrophins on Neurons

Neurotrophins support various neuronal populations in the PNS and CNS (for review—[8,9,29]). NGF acts on sympathetic and sensory neurons and regulates, for example, nociception and temperature sensation. In the brain, NGF promotes the survival of cholinergic neurons in the basal forebrain that project to the hippocampus and are believed to play an important role on the memory process that is affected in Alzheimer's disease. BDNF and NT-3 are more widely expressed in the brain and are linked to the survival and physiological regulation of multiple CNS neuronal populations. BDNF was the first NTF described to promote the survival and dopamine uptake of midbrain DA neurons in vitro. Also, NT-3 and NT-4 have been reported to promote the survival of midbrain DA neurons.[30]

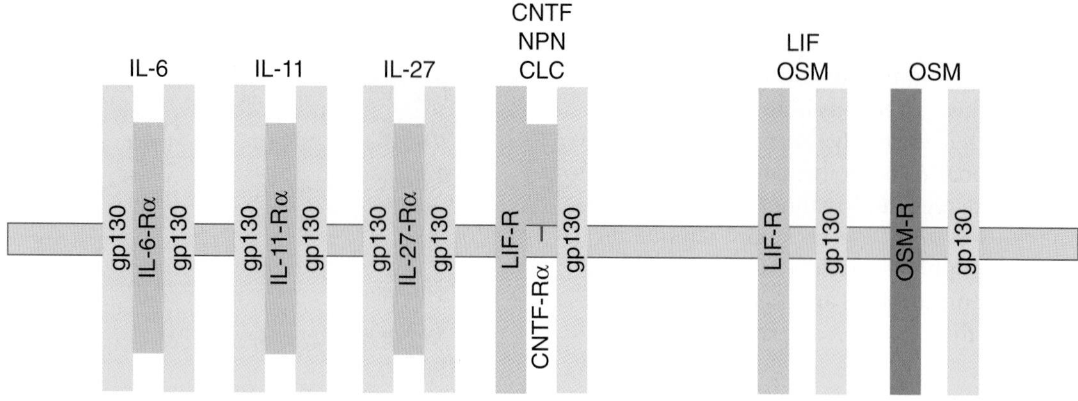

Figure 7-3. Receptor complexes of the neurokines. Neurokines bind to either tri- or bipartite receptor complexes as indicated. The tripartite complexes contain a ligand-specific non-signaling co-receptor α that is either a transmembrane or GPI-anchored (CNTF-Rα) protein.

The receptor for BDNF, TrkB, is expressed in the DA neurons of the substantia nigra (SN) pars compacta[31] and the ligand can be retrogradely transported from the striatum to the cell bodies of DA neurons in SN.[32] Whether BDNF signaling via TrkB receptor is involved in regulating the development and maintenance of DA neurons in vivo is controversial. BDNF-deficient mice, which die at the age of 3–4 weeks, do not have significant alterations in the nigrostriatal DA system suggesting that BDNF does not have crucial role in the survival and maturation of DA neurons during embryonic and early postnatal development in vivo. In line with that, conditional removal of the BDNF receptor TrkB from murine DA neurons did not affect the number of nigral DA neurons even at 2 years of age, indicating only a minor role for TrkB in the maintenance of target innervation of DA neurons in the SN of aged mice.[33] Interestingly, analyzing BDNF knockout mice Baker and colleagues found reduction of DA dendrites,[34] suggesting that BDNF has a role in the phenotypic maturation of DA neurons. Thus, in vivo experiments indicate only a minor role for BDNF-TrkB signaling in the development and adult maintenance of DA neurons. This does not, however, preclude the possibility that BDNF may be important in protecting or promoting the recovery of DA neurons in neurodegenerative disorders. In addition, BDNF may exert its effects on DA neurons through synergistic cross-talk with other trophic factors regulating DA neuron survival.[30,35]

NEUROTROPHIC FACTORS: THE NEUROKINE CLASS

Neurokine Ligands and Receptor Systems

Neurokines (for review—[12]) are a group of small structurally related pleiotrophic cytokines that all activate a common gp130 receptor. They include CNTF, leukemia inhibitory factor (LIF), cardiotrophin 1 (CT-1), neuropoietin (NPN), cardiotrophin-like cytokine (CLC), oncostatin M (OSM), IL-6, IL-11, and IL-27. Neurokines are alternatively called the neuropoietic cytokine family, IL-6 family, or gp130 family. Neurokines bind to receptor complexes on the plasma membrane that are formed by combinations of different subunits of the class 1 cytokine receptors (for review—[36,37]).

The neurokine receptors can be divided into two types: (1) signal-transducing receptors, including gp130, LIF receptor (LIF-R) and OSM receptor (OSM-R); and (2) the non-signaling α-receptors CNTF-Rα (a GPI-anchored protein), IL-6-Rα, IL-11-Rα, and IL-27-Rα (transmembrane proteins). Each ligand recruits the receptor subunits in the combination specific for it, but gp130 is always included (Fig. 7–3). Sometimes, two gp130 proteins (IL-6, IL-11) are recruited to the receptor complex. In other cases, gp130 heterodimerizes with either LIF-R or OSM-R. Some neurokines (LIF, OSM) can directly bind their respective signaling receptors and as a result form the bipartite heterodimeric receptor complexes. Other neurokines (CNTF, IL-6, IL-11, IL-27) bind first to the ligand-specific α-receptor and only thereafter recruit the signaling receptor subunits, resulting in the tripartite receptors. The α-receptors are not involved in the signaling but only give the ligand-specificity to the common gp130. The gp130 is expressed ubiquitously, but the other receptor subunits are expressed in the more restricted and regulated manner; thereby, the presence or absence of other subunits, especially the ligand-specific α-receptors, do not allow the activation of gp130 in the inappropriate tissues. OSM can activate two different receptor complexes (OSMR/gp130 or LIFR/gp130). Although less studied, NPN and CLC are proposed to bind the same tripartite receptor complex as CNTF (CNTF-Rα/LIF-R/gp130).[38] A specific α-receptor has also been proposed for CT-1, but its existence is still elusive.

Signaling by Neurokines

Gp130, LIFR and OSMR are recruiter receptors that lack the signal-transducing capacity of their own. On ligand binding, they recruit cytoplasmic signaling proteins of the Janus kinase (JAK) and signal transducer and activator of transcription (STAT) families (for review—[37,39,40]). When recruited to the receptors, JAK kinases autoactivate and phosphorylate specific tyrosine residues on the receptors that then act as the docking sites for the other signaling proteins. STATs are an essential class of the proteins recruited to the activated neurokine receptors. They also become phosphorylated by JAKs at specific tyrosine residues. STATs are the transcription factors that, on tyrosine phosphorylation, are translocated to the nucleus, where they regulate the activity of specific genes. In addition to the STAT pathway, the MAPK pathway is activated on ligand binding to the neurokine receptors.

Because they use the common signaling receptor gp130, the effects of the neurokines are often pleiotrophic and redundant in manner.[41] Indeed, deletion of a single neurokine in knockout mice generally causes mild defects, whereas knockout of gp130 or LIFR receptors leads to a much more severe phenotype (for review—[42]). The biology of neurokines in the nervous system is less studied than that of other NTFs (reviewed in [12]). Spinal motoneurons, several parasympathetic neurons, and also DA neurons are maintained by CNTF in vitro, whereas LIF maintains sensory neurons and motoneurons. CT-1 may act as the target-derived NTFs for the embryonic spinal motoneurons, as suggested by the loss of motoneurons in the mice deficient in CT-1 or CNTFRα. CNTF and LIF are essential in the maintenance and differentiation of neural progenitor cells. Neurokines, in particular LIF, CNTF and IL-6 are upregulated in the axotomized motoneurons and can rescue these neurons from axotomy-induced death and promote axonal regeneration. Hence, neurokines are essential factors in the biology and pathology of the nervous system, and further studies are needed to better understand their functions in the nervous systems.

NEUROTROPHIC FACTORS: THE GDNF FAMILY

GDNF Family Ligands

GDNF is a potent NTF for midbrain DA neurons. It was originally isolated from the culture medium of a rat B49 glial cell line because of its ability to promote dopamine uptake, survival, and morphological differentiation of embryonic midbrain DA neurons in culture.[43] GDNF together with the related proteins artemin (ARTN), neurturin (NRTN), and persephin (PSPN) constitute the GDNF family ligands (GFLs) (for review—[10]). GDNF and NRTN are expressed in the developing and adult brain, but also in the PNS, as well as in the non-neuronal organs. Notably GDNF is expressed in the developing kidney and testis. ARTN and PSPN are mostly expressed in the PNS and non-neuronal organs.[10]

GFLs are synthesized in the form of pre-pro-GFL proteins that are cotranslationally processed to a pro-GFL in the endoplasmic reticulum (ER). GFLs are secreted from the cells, usually as the mature GFL, but sometimes also as a pro-GFL. The monomeric mature GFLs are biologically inactive, and they must form homodimers to become biologically active.

GNDF Family Receptor Systems

GFLs can signal via two independent receptors systems—the receptor tyrosine kinase (RTK) RET and the neural cell adhesion molecule (NCAM). The major GFL-signaling receptor is RET. Although RET is similar to other RTKs, it has several special features. Firstly, it requires Ca^{2+} ions for full activity.[44] Secondly, GFL does not bind and activate RET directly.[10,11,45] It is activated by binding to a complex formed by a GFL bound to its cognate glycosylphosphatidylinositol (GPI)-anchored coreceptor GFRα. Consequently, GFLs interact with RET, but only in the presence of specific GFRα coreceptors. According to the current understanding, homodimeric GFLs bind to monomeric GFRα molecules inducing their homodimerization. Thereafter, the dimeric GFL–GFRα complex brings two RET molecules together, triggering transphosphorylation of specific tyrosine residues in their tyrosine kinase domains and activating intracellular signaling. Four different GFL–GFRα pairs exist in mammals: (1) GDNF–GFRα1, (2) NRTN–GFRα2, (3) ARTN–GFRα3, and (3) PSPN–GFRα4 (Fig. 7–4A). These interactions are physiologically significant and are characterized by high-affinity kinetics. There is evidence of cross-talk in this system, in that, GDNF can interact with GFRα2 and GFRα3, and NRTN and ARTN with GFRα1, but the affinity of these alternative interactions is significantly lower and the neurophysiologic importance is unclear.

In addition to RET, GFL can also signal through NCAM, a molecule that is better known as the homophilic cell adhesion molecule[46–48] (Fig. 7–4B). In vitro and in vivo data clearly show that $p140^{NCAM}$ can function as the alternative signaling receptor for all four GDNF family ligands. In the presence of specific GFRα coreceptors, GFLs can bind to $p140^{NCAM}$ with higher affinity and activate Src-like kinase, Fyn, and focal adhesion kinase (FAK). Interestingly, GFRα1 interaction with NCAM even in the absence of GDNF can inhibit NCAM-mediated cell adhesion. It is possible that GDNF–GFRα1–NCAM and GFRα1–NCAM interactions have different biological readouts and physiological consequences. Current experiments indicate that GDNF, by binding to GFRα1 and activating NCAM, stimulates Schwann cell migration,

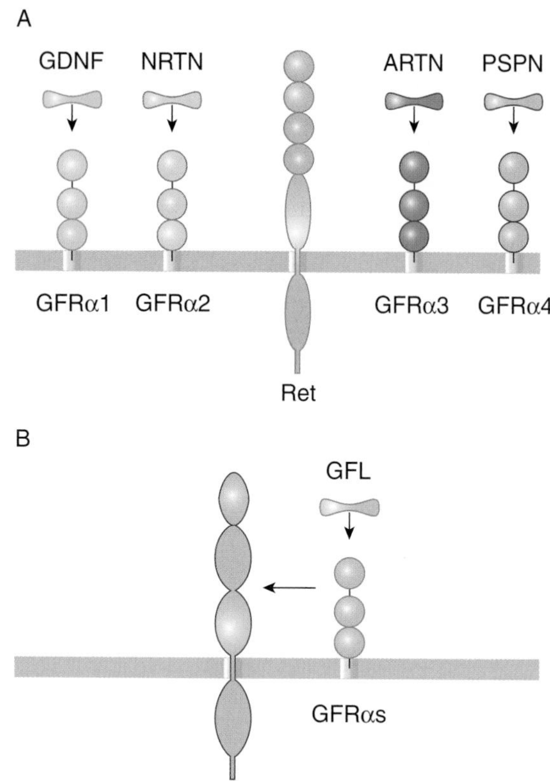

Figure 7-4. Ligand-receptor complexes of the GDNF family ligands. (A) GFL bind specific GFRα co-receptors as indicated that thereafter bind the signaling receptor tyrosine kinase Ret. (B) Specific GFL-GFRα complexes can also bind NCAM as an alternative signaling receptor.

hippocampal neurite outgrowth, and development of olfactory neurons in RET-independent manner.[47,48]

Signaling Pathways Triggered by GDNF Family Ligands

In most cases RET is activated by GFLs through binding to GFRα receptors leading to RET tyrosine phosphorylation (for review—[10,11,49]). The GFL–GFRα homodimeric complex brings two molecules of RET together, triggering transphosphorylation of specific tyrosine residues, in particular Tyr^{905}, Tyr^{981}, Tyr^{1015}, Tyr^{1062}, and Tyr^{1096} in the intracellular part of RET. Several signal-transducing proteins bind to phosphotyrosines and trigger the intracellular signaling cascades, which regulate cell survival, differentiation, proliferation, migration, chemotaxis, branching morphogenesis, neurite outgrowth, synaptic plasticity, and so on. Of the best-characterized pathways, the MAP kinase pathway is involved in the neurite outgrowth of the neurons, whereas the PI-3K–Akt pathway is responsible for both neuronal survival and neurite outgrowth. Both these pathways are activated from Tyr^{1062}. GFLs also phosphorylate Tyr^{981} that activates Src-family kinases, which promotes neurite outgrowth, and neuronal survival.

NEUROTROPHIC FACTORS: THE CDNF/MANF FAMILY

CDNF/MANF Ligands

The CDNF/MANF family is the most recently discovered and therefore least studied family of NTFs. MANF was originally identified from the culture medium of the rat type-1 astrocyte cell line based on its trophic effects on cultured DA neurons.[13] The family consists of two mammalian proteins: (1) MANF (also known as arginine-rich mutated in early stage tumors [ARMET]) and (2) CDNF. Human CDNF shows 59% amino acid identity with human MANF, while invertebrate animals encode a single protein that is homologous to CDNF and MANF (Fig. 7–5A). Thus, CDNF and MANF proteins form a novel evolutionarily conserved CDNF/MANF family of secreted factors with eight cysteine residues of similar spacing (Fig. 7–5A). Unlike the neurotrophins and GFLs, the CDNF/MANF family proteins lack a higher molecular weight prosequence, and consist simple of the signal sequence followed by the mature part of the protein (for review—[50]).

Crystal structures of mammalian MANF and CDNF do not resemble any other known growth factors (Fig. 7–5B). The proteins consist of two domains: (1) the N-terminal domain with five α-helices and three S–S bridges and (2) the short C-terminal domain that is also natively unfolded. Remarkably, the N-termini of MANF and CDNF have a saposin-like (SAPLIP) domain, suggesting that they, like other SAPLIPs, may bind lipids or membranes. The unique MANF C-terminus contains a CKGC disulfide bridge similar to reductases and disulfide isomerases, consistent with a role in ER stress response.[51]

Cellular Effects of CDNF and MANF Neurotrophic Factors

Recombinant human MANF promotes the survival and induced sprouting of E14 rat DA neurons in culture, but has no effects on GABAergic or serotonergic neurons in culture.[13] In animal models of PD, CDNF can very efficiently protect and repair nigrostriatal DA neurons.[14] MANF also has neuroprotective, as well as neurorestorative effects in the rat 6-hydroxydopamine (6-OHDA) model of PD in vivo.

Although mammalian CDNF and MANF can effectively support the survival of DA neurons in vivo, their receptors and respective signaling pathways remain unclear. As MANF is also an ER-stress-induced protein with cytoprotective roles, it may activate completely different signaling pathways than other known NTFs.

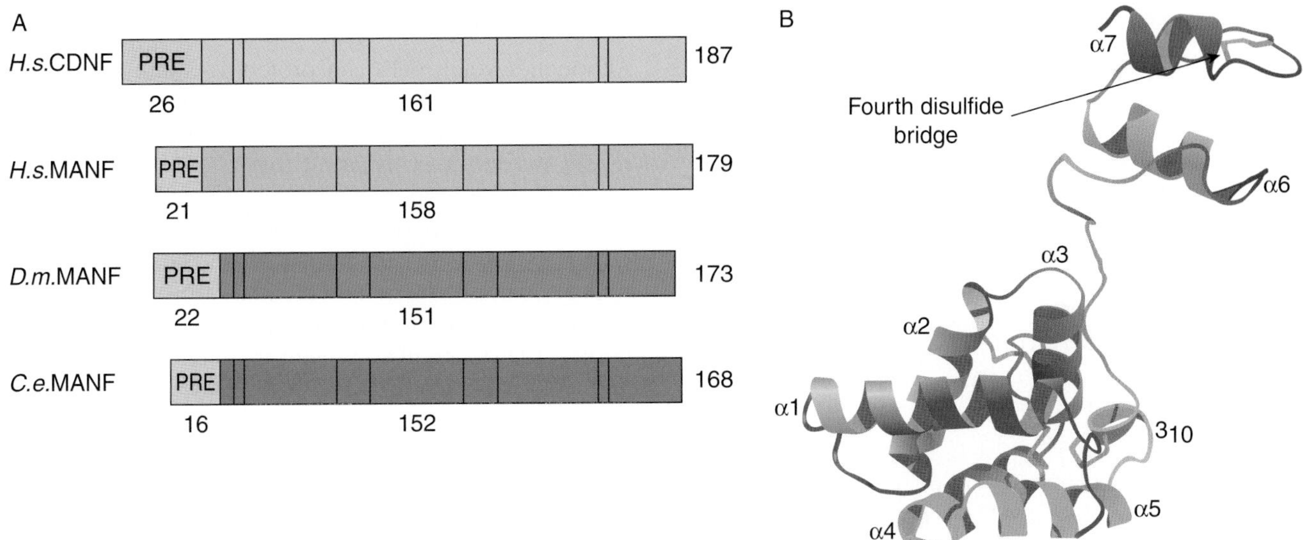

Figure 7-5. The CDNF/MANF family. (A) The CDNF/MANF family factors from human, *Drosophila melanogaster* (Dm) and *Caenorhabditis elegans* (Ce). Shown are the lengths of the prodomains and mature domains, and the positions of conserved cysteines (*arrows*). (B) The crystal structure of MANF. All α-helices are shown and labeled by numbers. Disulfide (S–S) bridges are shown in sticks with carbon in magenta and sulfur in yellow. The N-terminal regions of MANF and CDNF have three S–S bridges and form a saposin-like (SAPLIP) domain. The C-terminal domain is composed of helices α6-α7 and is connected to the N-terminal domain by a flexible loop. An arrow marks the position of the fourth disulfide bridge.

▶ NTFs IN MODELS OF PARKINSON'S DISEASE

ROLE OF NTFs IN MAINTENANCE OF DOPAMINERGIC NEURONS

The question of whether there are specific NTFs that are required in order to keep adult DA neurons alive is still under debate. Conditional removal of the GDNF receptor RET specifically from the CNS DA system causes progressive and adult-onset loss of DA neurons in the SN and degeneration of DA nerve terminals in the striatum.[33] Interestingly, other GDNF-dependent neurons, such as the DA neurons in the ventral tegmental area (VTA) and noradrenergic neurons of the *locus coeruleus* were not affected. Similarly, mice with conditionally reduced levels of GDNF in adult animals had a significantly different phenotype, showing pronounced catecholaminergic cell death in the *locus coeruleus*, along with significant loss of DA neurons in the SN and in the VTA.[52] Together, these results suggest that GDNF signaling via RET is essential for the long-term maintenance of SN DA neurons, but not for VTA and *locus coeruleus*, where GDNF likely signals via alternative receptors.

Deletion of the BDNF receptor TrkB has no significant effect on the DA system,[33] nor does the ablation of single genes of BDNF, NT-3, or NT-4 or their respective Trk receptors However, double haploinsufficiency for NT-3 and NT-4 receptors TrkC and TrkB, respectively, does lead to the loss of DA neurons.[53,54] Thus, neurotrophin signaling does appear to be important to DA neuron survival, but there is substantial redundancy in this system. At present, little is known about the potential role of the CDNF/MANF family in the development and adult maintenance of the DA system.

THERAPEUTIC EFFECTS OF NTFs IN MODEL SYSTEMS

GDNF Family Ligands

The trophic activity of GDNF has been intensively studied in rodent (Fig. 7–6A) and primate models of PD. In rodent models, neuroprotective and neurorestorative effects as measured by dopamine levels, fiber densities, and motor behavior have been seen after GDNF was injected into the striatum in a mouse 1-methyl-4-phenyl-1,2,3,6-tetrahydropyridine (MPTP) model of PD[55] and after injection into the SN before the nigral 6-OHDA injection.[56] Protection against 6-OHDA has also been observed after striatal and intraventricular injection and continuous GDNF infusion.[57–61] GDNF-secreting intranigral grafts are also protective against 6-OHDA lesions.[62] Comparable protective and neurorestorative effects of GDNF have also been shown in the nonhuman primate models of PD.[57,58,63,64]

The GDNF family member neurturin (NRTN) also has protective and restorative effects on DA neurons in animal models of PD, when delivered either by injection or

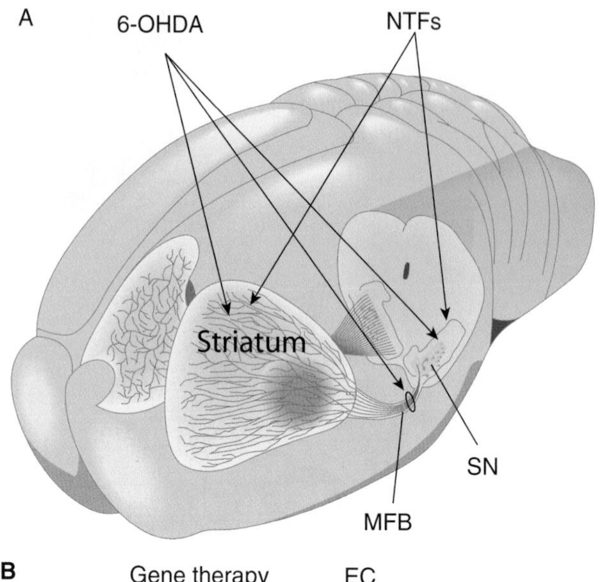

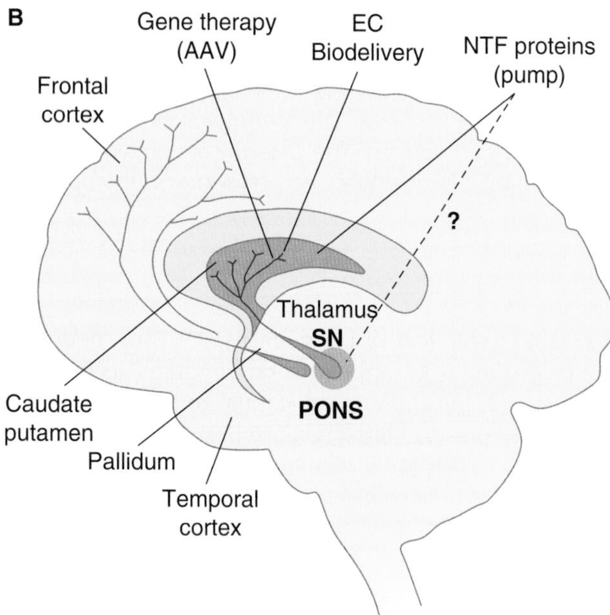

Figure 7-6. Principal designs of NTF application to the Parkinsonian brain. (A) Rodent experiments where the neurotoxin 6-OHDA is injected into the striatum, substantia nigra (SN) or medial forebrain bundle (MFB). The NTFs could be injected to the striatum or SN either before (neuroprotection) or after (neurorestoration) the toxins. (B) For patient treatments, the NTFs can be delivered to the caudate putamen either as the recombinant proteins using the peristaltic pumps, genes encoding NTFs using the adeno accociated viral vectors (AAV), or the engineered cells using encapsulated cell biodelivery (ECB). Application to the SN could also be considered.

by NRTN-secreting intranigral grafts.[62,65] NRTN expressing adeno-associated virus (AAV) serotype 2 (CERE-120) induces functional recovery and preservation of DA neurons in MPTP-treated monkeys.[66] Neuroprotection has also been observed with the related proteins ARTN and PSPN.[67–69]

CDNF/MANF Family Factors

Although several NTFs can protect DA neurons against the toxic injury, until recently only GDNF and NRTN had been shown to have neurorestorative effects. Therefore, recent results demonstrating that CDNF possibly also has restorative properties may be of great importance.[14] In the 6-OHDA model, CDNF is at least as efficient as GDNF, but its effect is specific for the central DA neurons in contrast to GDNF, which has a broader scope of targets. In addition to the protection of DA neuronal cell bodies, CDNF can also prevent the degeneration of DA fibers more efficiently than GDNF. MANF also has strong neuroprotective and neurorestorative effect in a similar rat PD model.[70] After striatal injection, MANF produces a larger diffusion volume at the injection site than GDNF,[70] a property that may reflect the differences in the density of their transport machineries and/or receptors, and may be important in maximizing the therapeutic effect. In marked contrast to all other NTFs described, CDNF and MANF have no survival-promoting activity for peripheral sympathetic and sensory neurons in vitro, which may give them a better side effect profile in clinical use. Together, these properties make CDNF and MANF promising candidates for the therapy of PD.

▶ NTFs IN HUMAN PARKINSON'S DISEASE

CLINICAL TRIALS WITH NTF PROTEINS: GDNF INFUSION

Discovery of NTFs, such as GDNF, CDNF, and MANF, which strongly promote the survival, axon regeneration, and synapse formation of DA neurons in vivo opened new avenues for developing effective treatment for PD. The first clinical trials with NTFs in PD patients started more than 10 years ago. However, the major problem in the clinical use of the NTFs is their inability to cross the blood–brain barrier, and therefore the need to deliver them intracerebrally. In addition, systemic delivery of NTFs increases the risk of adverse effects resulting from activating the receptor signaling in other tissues/organs of the body.

To overcome the aforementioned bottlenecks, techniques for local delivery of NTFs into the caudate and putamen have been developed (Fig. 7–6B). While several NTFs are effective when delivered this way in animal models, only GDNF has reached human clinical trials, and results have been conflicting. In open-label trials,[71,72] GDNF was delivered via intraputaminally inserted ultrathin catheter accompanied with an abdominally mounted pump that dosed the daily GDNF delivery. A phase 1 safety trial on five patients revealed highly significant improvements of the PD symptoms and no significant clinical side effects after one year period.[71] A second open-label study on 10 patients showed similar improvements in the motor functions that continued after GDNF washout, and again no significant adverse effects.[72] In contrast, a double-blind clinical study showed no significant improvement in the GDNF-treated PD patients, compared with sham surgery and vehicle infusion, and the development of anti-GDNF antibodies was observed in three patients.[73] The appearance of these GDNF function–blocking antibodies poses great potential risk, because these antibodies may block endogenous GDNF and conceivably worsen patient's condition.

These contradictory results have drawn attention to several technical aspects that should be taken into account. Many researchers believe that the failure of the double-blind GDNF trial may relate to poor delivery systems.[74–76] In addition to the complexities of the methods of delivery, attention must also be paid to the properties of the recombinant protein. Recombinant GDNF protein prepared in *Escherichia coli* was used; because bacterially produced mammalian secretory proteins must be renaturated in vitro, there is always a risk that a fraction of the protein could remain inactive. This potential problem could be overcome by using GDNF or other NTFs produced in mammalian cells. The site of NTF delivery must also be carefully considered. Although striatal delivery of GDNF has produced good results in animal models, the human brain is much larger, and one could also consider simultaneous delivery at multiple sites, e.g., both striatum and SN. Finally, other factors such as CDNF and MANF may offer several advantages, because they diffuse more widely and their actions are more specific for dopamine neurons.[70]

CLINICAL TRIALS: GENE THERAPY WITH NEUROTROPHIC FACTORS

Gene therapy, the delivery of genetic material that drives the expression of specific proteins, offers an alternative to direct infusion of neurotrophic proteins. This has been accomplished in human trials using an AAV engineered to express NRTN (CERE-120) (Fig. 7–6B). Studies in aging monkeys showed clear functional and structural benefits of the AAV–NRTN on the DA system.[77] A phase 1, open-label clinical trial was conducted in 12 human patients, which demonstrated good safety and showed significant beneficial effects.[78] A larger double-blind, controlled phase 2 trial of CERE-120 in 58 patients with advanced PD confirmed the safety and tolerability of this approach, but unfortunately did not demonstrate an appreciable difference between patients treated with CERE-120 versus those in the control group; both groups had a substantial number of patients who demonstrated a meaningful clinical improvement from baseline.

There are several reasons why the double-blind trial of CERE-120 may have failed. One possibility is that NRTN, when compared with GDNF, MANF, and CDNF, is not optimal for PD treatment. Firstly, NRTN is a very basic protein, and its diffusion in the brain is even more restricted than that of GDNF.[79] In addition, in contrast to CDNF, MANF, or GDNF, NRTN is not readily secreted from the brain cells.[80] It should also be noted that at least in mouse and rat, DA neurons do not express the GFRα2, the cognate coreceptor for NRTN, and most likely NRTN signals into DA neurons via GDNF receptor GFRα1 and RET, reducing its potency. Future efforts at gene therapy for PD are likely to focus on the growth factors GDNF, CDNF, and MANF, all of which are expressed in the caudate putamen and show neurorestorative effects in the animal models of PD as well as improved delivery of NRTN.

CELL THERAPIES WITH NEUROTROPHIC FACTORS

A disadvantage of the existing viral gene delivery systems is that once activated, the expression cannot be turned off when undesired effects occur. One of the most promising approaches of NTF-based therapy that overcomes this problem is encapsulated cell biodelivery (ECB) (Fig. 7–6B). In that method, NTF-producing mammalian cells are mounted into nonadherent hollow-fiber membrane catheters of less than 1 mm in diameter, which are then placed into the striatum. NTF-producing cells are immune isolated by a membrane, yet nutrients from the surrounding and NTF from the cells are free to diffuse. ECB approach has several advantages.[81] Firstly, inconvenient intra-abdominal pumps that are used for GDNF protein delivery and may cause complications are avoided. Secondly, GDNF is produced by mammalian cells that warrant correct posttranslational modifications and rigorous cellular quality control. Indeed, it is generally known that recombinant NTFs produced in mammalian cells are usually more bioactive than are their bacterial counterparts. And thirdly, catheters are easy to remove when adverse effects are noted.

Although the cell delivery approach has been successful in animal models, clinical experience with this approach is limited. A Danish biotechnology company, NsGene A/S, has announced that its encapsulated cell biodelivery product, NsG0202, has been successfully implanted in six patients with Alzheimer's disease (AD) as a part of an ongoing phase 1b clinical trial. The NsG0202 product consists of human cells genetically modified to secrete NGF to the surrounding brain. This is likely to be an important first step in the broader development of this approach.

SMALL MOLECULE NTF MIMETICS

Are there alternative approaches to the current NTF-based therapies? It is obvious that despite great potential,

NTFs have also limitations as therapeutic proteins. Firstly, these large molecules do not pass blood–brain barrier and therefore they must be delivered intracerebrally. Secondly, compared with small molecules NTFs have poor bioavailability and pharmacokinetics. And finally, the therapeutic use of NTFs is expensive.

One of the promising approaches toward overcoming these problems is the development of low-molecular-weight NTF mimetics—small-molecule agonists capable of activating specific NTF receptors and triggering the prosurvival signaling without the natural ligand. Interestingly, several small-molecule inhibitors of RTKs have been developed, but there has been very little progress in developing RTK agonists. Two significant steps toward the creation of efficient NTF mimetics have already been made. First, small-molecule agonists (<600 Da) have been synthesized that specifically activate the Trk receptor, thereby mimicking neurotrophin signaling.[82,83] These peptidyl Trk agonists bind to the natural ligand-binding site with nanomolar affinity, triggering neurotrophin-like intracellular signaling and relevant biological responses. Most importantly, these agonists are truly monovalent and thus activate the receptors directly without dimerization. The second significant study[84] demonstrated that a quinol-type small molecule binds with 10 μM affinity to GFRα1 and activates RET phosphorylation. This molecule of 456.5 Da is monovalent and therefore clearly unable to bring the two separate RET receptor complexes together, which is required for RET activation. The GFRα1/RET agonist might bind to a 'hot spot' on a preformed GFRα1-RET receptor complex or triggering a conformational change in GFRα1, leading to the RET activation. Clearly, more NTF mimetics will be developed and their therapeutic potencies studied in the future.

▶ SUMMARY AND PROSPECTS

NTFs have potent effects on the survival and recovery of neurons. The most extensively studied system is the dopaminergic nigrostriatal pathway, affected in PD. Several NTFs have been shown to have powerful and specific effects on DA neurons in animal models. Human clinical trials with NTFs are at an early stage, and are yet to result in unequivocal success. However, there are clear directions in which this approach may move forward. NTFs offer great hope for patients with PD and neurodegenerative disorders, because they have the potential to not only halt the progression of these diseases but also to induce recovery.

REFERENCES

1. Buss RR, Sun W, and Oppenheim RW. Adaptive roles of programmed cell death during nervous system development. Annu Rev Neurosci 2006;29:1–35.
2. Oppenheim RW. Cell death during development of the nervous system. Annu Rev Neurosci 1991;14:453–501.
3. Levi-Montalcini R. The nerve growth factor: thirty-five years later. EMBO J 1987;6:1145–1154.
4. Levi-Montalcini R. The saga of the nerve growth factor. Neuroreport 1998;9:R71–R83.
5. Barde YA. Trophic factors and neuronal survival. Neuron 1989; 2:1525–1534.
6. Deppmann CD, Mihalas S, Sharma N, et al. A model for neuronal competition during development. Science 2008;320:369–373.
7. Zweifel LS, Kuruvilla R, and Ginty DD. Functions and mechanisms of retrograde neurotrophin signalling. Nat Rev Neurosci 2005;6:615–625.
8. Bibel M and Barde YA. Neurotrophins: Key regulators of cell fate and cell shape in the vertebrate nervous system. Genes Dev 2000;14:2919–2937.
9. Huang EJ and Reichardt LF. Neurotrophins: Roles in neuronal development and function. Annu Rev Neurosci 2001;24:677–736.
10. Airaksinen MS, Saarma M. The GDNF family: Signalling, biological functions and therapeutic value. Nat Rev Neurosci 2002;3:383–394.
11. Bespalov MM and Saarma M. GDNF family receptor complexes are emerging drug targets. Trends Pharmacol Sci 2007;28:68–74.
12. Bauer S, Kerr BJ, and Patterson PH. The neuropoietic cytokine family in development, plasticity, disease and injury. Nat Rev Neurosci 2007;8:221–232.
13. Petrova P, Raibekas A, Pevsner J, et al. MANF: A new mesencephalic, astrocyte-derived neurotrophic factor with selectivity for dopaminergic neurons. J Mol Neurosci 2003;20:173–188.
14. Lindholm P, Voutilainen MH, Lauren J, et al. Novel neurotrophic factor CDNF protects and rescues midbrain dopamine neurons in vivo. Nature 2007;448:73–77.
15. Bernd P. The role of neurotrophins during early development. Gene Expr 2008;14:241–250.
16. Thoenen H and Sendtner M. Neurotrophins: From enthusiastic expectations through sobering experiences to rational therapeutic approaches. Nat Neurosci 2002;5 Suppl:1046–1050.
17. Chiocco MJ, Harvey BK, Wang Y, et al. Neurotrophic factors for the treatment of Parkinson's disease. Parkinsonism Relat Disord 2007;13(suppl 3):S321–S328.
18. Fumagalli F, Molteni R, Calabrese F, et al. Neurotrophic factors in neurodegenerative disorders: potential for therapy. CNS Drugs 2008;22:1005–1019.
19. Lu B, Pang PT, and Woo NH. The yin and yang of neurotrophin action. Nat Rev Neurosci 2005;6:603–614.
20. Chao MV, Rajagopal R, and Lee FS. Neurotrophin signalling in health and disease. Clin Sci (Lond) 2006;110:167–173.
21. Lee R, Kermani P, Teng KK, et al. Regulation of cell survival by secreted proneurotrophins. Science 2001;294:1945–1948.
22. Nykjaer A, Willnow TE, Petersen CM. p75NTR: Live or let die. Curr Opin Neurobiol 2005;15:49–57.
23. Kuczewski N, Porcher C, Lessmann V, et al. Activity-dependent dendritic release of BDNF and biological consequences. Mol Neurobiol 2009;39:37–49.

24. Patapoutian A and Reichardt LF. Trk receptors: Mediators of neurotrophin action. Curr Opin Neurobiol 2001;11: 272–280.
25. Zampieri N and Chao MV. Mechanisms of neurotrophin receptor signalling. Biochem Soc Trans 2006;34:607–611.
26. Wehrman T, He X, Raab B, et al. Structural and mechanistic insights into nerve growth factor interactions with the TrkA and p75 receptors. Neuron 2007;53:25–38.
27. Kaplan DR and Miller FD. Neurotrophin signal transduction in the nervous system. Curr Opin Neurobiol 2000;10:381–391.
28. Miller FD and Kaplan DR. Neurotrophin signalling pathways regulating neuronal apoptosis. Cell Mol Life Sci 2001;58:1045–1053.
29. Davies AM. Regulation of neuronal survival and death by extracellular signals during development. EMBO J 2003;22:2537–2545.
30. Krieglstein K. Factors promoting survival of mesencephalic dopaminergic neurons. Cell Tissue Res 2004;318: 73–80.
31. Numan S, Gall CM, and Seroogy KB. Developmental expression of neurotrophins and their receptors in postnatal rat ventral midbrain. J Mol Neurosci 2005;27:245–260.
32. Mufson EJ, Kroin JS, Liu YT, et al. Intrastriatal and intraventricular infusion of brain-derived neurotrophic factor in the cynomologous monkey: Distribution, retrograde transport and co-localization with substantia nigra dopamine-containing neurons. Neuroscience 1996;71:179–191.
33. Kramer ER, Aron L, Ramakers GM, et al. Absence of Ret signaling in mice causes progressive and late degeneration of the nigrostriatal system. PLoS Biol 2007;5:e39.
34. Baker SA, Stanford LE, Brown RE, et al. Maturation but not survival of dopaminergic nigrostriatal neurons is affected in developing and aging BDNF-deficient mice. Brain Res 2005;1039:177–188.
35. Krieglstein K, Strelau J, Schober A, et al. TGF-[beta] and the regulation of neuron survival and death. J Physiol-Paris 2002;96:25–30.
36. Ben Shlomo I, Yu Hsu S, Rauch R, et al. Signaling receptome: A genomic and evolutionary perspective of plasma membrane receptors involved in signal transduction. Sci STKE 2003;2003:re9.
37. Heinrich PC, Behrmann I, Haan S, et al. Principles of interleukin (IL)-6-type cytokine signalling and its regulation. Biochem J 2003;374:1–20.
38. Rousseau F, Chevalier S, Guillet C, et al. Ciliary neurotrophic factor, cardiotrophin-like cytokine, and neuropoietin share a conserved binding site on the ciliary neurotrophic factor receptor {alpha} chain. J Biol Chem 2008;283: 30341–30350.
39. Haan C, Kreis S, Margue C, Behrmann I. Jaks and cytokine receptors: An intimate relationship. Biochem Pharmacol 2006;72:1538–1546.
40. Schindler C, Levy DE, and Decker T. JAK-STAT signaling: From interferons to cytokines. J Biol Chem 2007;282:20059–20063.
41. Muller-Newen G. The cytokine receptor gp130: Faithfully promiscuous. Sci STKE 2003;2003:E40.
42. Fasnacht N, and Mnller W. Conditional gp130 deficient mouse mutants. Semin Cell Dev Biol 2008;19:379–384.
43. Lin LF, Doherty DH, Lile JD, et al. GDNF: A glial cell line-derived neurotrophic factor for midbrain dopaminergic neurons. Science 1993;260:1130–1132.
44. Nozaki C, Asai N, Murakami H, et al. Calcium-dependent Ret activation by GDNF and neurturin. Oncogene 1998;16:293–299.
45. Takahashi M. The GDNF/RET signaling pathway and human diseases. Cytokine Growth Factor Rev 2001;12:361–373.
46. Paratcha G, Ledda F, and Ibanez CF. The neural cell adhesion molecule NCAM is an alternative signaling receptor for GDNF family ligands. Cell 2003;113:867–879.
47. Sjostrand D, Carlsson J, Paratcha G, et al. Disruption of the GDNF binding site in NCAM dissociates ligand binding and homophilic cell adhesion. J Biol Chem 2007;282:12734–12740.
48. Sjostrand D and Ibanez CF. Insights into GFRalpha1 regulation of neural cell adhesion molecule (NCAM) function from structure-function analysis of the NCAM/GFRalpha1 receptor complex. J Biol Chem 2008;283:13792–13798.
49. Runeberg-Roos P, Saarma M. Neurotrophic factor receptor RET: Structure, cell biology, and inherited diseases. Ann Med 2007;39:572–580.
50. Andressoo JO and Saarma M. Signalling mechanisms underlying development and maintenance of dopamine neurons. Curr Opin Neurobiol 2008;18:297–306.
51. Airavaara M, Shen H, Kuo C-C, et al. Mesencephalic astrocyte-derived neurotrophic factor (MANF) reduces ischemic brain injury and promotes behavioral recovery in rats. Exp Neurol 2009, in press.
52. Pascual A, Hidalgo-Figueroa M, Piruat JI, et al. Absolute requirement of GDNF for adult catecholaminergic neuron survival. Nat Neurosci 2008;11:755–761.
53. Bohlen und HO, Minichiello L, and Unsicker K. Haploinsufficiency for trkB and trkC receptors induces cell loss and accumulation of alpha-synuclein in the substantia nigra. FASEB J 2005;19:1740–1742.
54. Zaman V, Nelson ME, Gerhardt GA, et al. Neurodegenerative alterations in the nigrostriatal system of trkB hypomorphic mice. Exp Neurol 2004;190:337–346.
55. Tomac A, Lindqvist E, Lin L-FH, et al. Protection and repair of the nigrostriatal dopaminergic system by GDNF in vivo. Nature 1995;373:335–339.
56. Kearns CM, Cass WA, Smoot K, et al. GDNF protection against 6-OHDA: Time dependence and requirement for protein synthesis. J Neurosci 1997;17:7111–7118.
57. Aoi M, Date I, Tomita S, et al. Single or continuous injection of glial cell line-derived neurotrophic factor in the striatum induces recovery of the nigrostriatal dopaminergic system. Neurol Res 2000;22:832–836.
58. Rosenblad C, Martinez-Serrano A, and Bjorklund A. Intrastriatal glial cell line-derived neurotrophic factor promotes sprouting of spared nigrostriatal dopaminergic afferents and induces recovery of function in a rat model of Parkinson's disease. Neuroscience 1998;82:129–137.
59. Kirik D, Georgievska B, Rosenblad C, et al. Delayed infusion of GDNF promotes recovery of motor function in the partial lesion model of Parkinson's disease. Eur J Neurosci 2001;13:1589–1599.
60. Sauer H, Rosenblad C, and Bjorklund A. Glial cell line-derived neurotrophic factor but not transforming growth

factor beta 3 prevents delayed degeneration of nigral dopaminergic neurons following striatal 6-hydroxydopamine lesion. Proc Natl Acad Sci U S A 1995;92:8935–8939.
61. Rosenblad C, Kirik D, and Bjorklund A. Sequential administration of GDNF into the substantia nigra and striatum promotes dopamine neuron survival and axonal sprouting but not striatal reinnervation or functional recovery in the partial 6-OHDA lesion model. Exp Neurol 2000;161:503–516.
62. Akerud P, Alberch J, Eketjall S, et al. Differential effects of glial cell line-derived neurotrophic factor and neurturin on developing and adult substantia nigra dopaminergic neurons. J Neurochem 1999;73:70–78.
63. Hoffer BJ, Hoffman A, Bowenkamp K, et al. Glial cell line-derived neurotrophic factor reverses toxin-induced injury to midbrain dopaminergic neurons in vivo. Neurosci Lett 1994;182:107–111.
64. Bowenkamp KE, Hoffman AF, Gerhardt GA, et al. Glial cell line-derived neurotrophic factor supports survival of injured midbrain dopaminergic neurons. J Comp Neurol 1995;355:479–489.
65. Rosenblad C, Kirik D, and Bjorklund A. Neurturin enhances the survival of intrastriatal fetal dopaminergic transplants. Neuroreport 1999;10:1783–1787.
66. Kordower JH, Herzog CD, Dass B, et al. Delivery of neurturin by AAV2 (CERE-120)-mediated gene transfer provides structural and functional neuroprotection and neurorestoration in MPTP-treated monkeys. Ann Neurol 2006;60:706–715.
67. Rosenblad C, Gronborg M, Hansen C, et al. In vivo protection of nigral dopamine neurons by lentiviral gene transfer of the novel GDNF-family member neublastin/artemin. Mol Cell Neurosci 2000;15:199–214.
68. Milbrandt J, de Sauvage FJ, Fahrner TJ, et al. Persephin, a novel neurotrophic factor related to GDNF and neurturin. Neuron 1998;20:245–253.
69. Akerud P, Holm PC, Castelo-Branco G, et al. Persephin-overexpressing neural stem cells regulate the function of nigral dopaminergic neurons and prevent their degeneration in a model of Parkinson's disease. Mol Cell Neurosci 2002;21:205–222.
70. Voutilainen MH, Bäck S, Pörsti E, et al. Neurotrophic factor MANF is neurorestorative in rat model of Parkinson's disease. J Neurosci, 2009, in press.
71. Gill SS, Patel NK, Hotton GR, et al. Direct brain infusion of glial cell line-derived neurotrophic factor in Parkinson disease. Nat Med 2003;9:589–595.
72. Slevin JT, Gerhardt GA, Smith CD, et al. Improvement of bilateral motor functions in patients with Parkinson disease through the unilateral intraputaminal infusion of glial cell line-derived neurotrophic factor. J Neurosurg 2005;102:216–222.
73. Lang AE, Gill S, Patel NK, et al. Randomized controlled trial of intraputamenal glial cell line-derived neurotrophic factor infusion in Parkinson disease. Ann Neurol 2006;59:459–466.
74. Chebrolu H, Slevin JT, Gash DA, et al. MRI volumetric and intensity analysis of the cerebellum in Parkinson's disease patients infused with glial-derived neurotrophic factor (GDNF). Exp Neurol 2006;198:450–456.
75. Sherer TB, Fiske BK, Svendsen CN, et al. Crossroads in GDNF therapy for Parkinson's disease. Mov Disord 2006;21:136–141.
76. Patel NK and Gill SS. GDNF delivery for Parkinson's disease. Acta Neurochir Suppl 2007;97:135–154.
77. Herzog CD, Dass B, Holden JE, et al. Striatal delivery of CERE-120, an AAV2 vector encoding human neurturin, enhances activity of the dopaminergic nigrostriatal system in aged monkeys. Mov Disord 2007;22:1124–1132.
78. Check E. Second chance. Nat Med 2007;13:770–771.
79. Hamilton JF, Morrison PF, Chen MY, et al. Heparin coinfusion during convection-enhanced delivery (CED) increases the distribution of the glial-derived neurotrophic factor (GDNF) ligand family in rat striatum and enhances the pharmacological activity of neurturin. Exp Neurol 2001;168:155–161.
80. Fjord-Larsen L, Johansen JL, Kusk P, et al. Efficient in vivo protection of nigral dopaminergic neurons by lentiviral gene transfer of a modified Neurturin construct. Exp Neurol 2005;195:49–60.
81. Lindvall O and Wahlberg LU. Encapsulated cell biodelivery of GDNF: A novel clinical strategy for neuroprotection and neuroregeneration in Parkinson's disease? Exp Neurol 2008;209:82–88.
82. Zaccaro MC, Lee HB, Pattarawarapan M, et al. Selective small molecule peptidomimetic ligands of TrkC and TrkA receptors afford discrete or complete neurotrophic activities. Chem Biol 2005;12:1015–1028.
83. Ivanisevic L, Zheng W, Woo SB, et al. TrkA receptor "hot spots" for binding of NT-3 as a heterologous ligand. J Biol Chem 2007;282:16754–16763.
84. Tokugawa K, Yamamoto K, Nishiguchi M, et al. XIB4035, a novel nonpeptidyl small molecule agonist for GFRalpha-1. Neurochem Int 2003;42:81–86.

CHAPTER 8

Neuropathology of Parkinsonian Syndrome

Dennis W. Dickson

▶ INTRODUCTION

The common denominator of virtually all disorders associated with clinical parkinsonism is neuronal loss in the substantia nigra, particularly of dopaminergic neurons in the *pars compacta* (A9) that project to the striatum (Fig. 8–1). The exception to this concept is parkinsonism due to direct injury to the striatum, such as that seen in vascular parkinsonism, in which infarcts or hemorrhages are present in the basal ganglia, especially the globus pallidus, without necessarily affecting the substantia nigra.[1] The ventrolateral tier of neurons appears to be the most vulnerable in many parkinsonian disorders, and these project heavily to the putamen.[2] The more medial group of dopaminergic neurons (A10) send projections to the forebrain and medial temporal lobe and are less affected. The basis for selective vulnerability between A9 and A10 neurons has been explored with microarray expression studies, which show different patterns of gene expression in A9 and A10 neurons,[3] but much remains to be learned how this translates into selective neuronal loss of A9 neurons in parkinsonian disorders. The dorsal tier of neurons may be most vulnerable to neuronal loss associated with aging.[4]

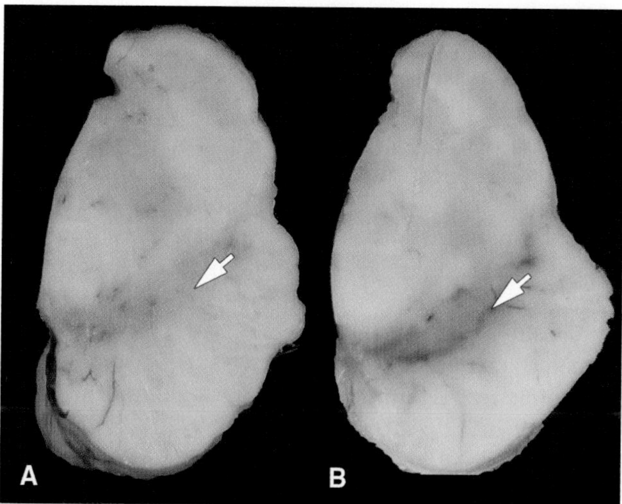

Figure 8–1. Macroscopic findings in PD. Transverse sections of the hemi-midbrain at the level of the third nerve in a patient with long-standing PD (A) and an elderly normal individual (B). The major difference is loss of neuromelanin pigment that is most marked in the ventrolateral parts of the substantia nigra (arrow).

▶ NEUROPATHOLOGY OF PARKINSON'S DISEASE (PD)

The clinical features of PD are bradykinesia, rigidity, tremor, postural instability, autonomic dysfunction, and bradyphrenia. The most frequent pathologic substrate for PD is Lewy body (LB) disease.[5] Some cases of clinically typical PD have other pathologic processes at autopsy, such as progressive supranuclear palsy (PSP), multiple system atrophy (MSA), or vascular disease, but these are uncommon, especially when the clinical diagnosis is made after several years of clinical follow-up.[6,7] The diagnostic accuracy rate can approach as high as 90% in some series.[8]

The brain in PD is usually grossly normal when viewed from the outer surface. There may be mild frontal atrophy is some cases, but this is variable. The most obvious morphologic change in PD is visible after the brain stem is sectioned. The loss of neuromelanin pigmentation in the substantia nigra and locus ceruleus is usually apparent (Fig. 8–1). Neuromelanin pigment is an oxidized by-product of di-oxy-phenylalanine, a precursor to dopamine, norepinephrine, and epinephrine, which accumulates with increasing age in neurons that produce these neurotransmitters. Histologically, there is neuronal loss in the substantia nigra *pars compacta* along with compensatory astrocytic and microglial proliferation, with the degree of neuronal loss correlating with disease duration.[9] Neuromelanin pigment may be found in the cytoplasm of macrophages, a marker of neuronal loss.[10] It is less common to find neurons undergoing active neuronophagia (i.e., phagocytosis by macrophages).

Neuronal loss in the substantia nigra is associated with loss of dopaminergic nerve termini in the striatum, especially the posterior putamen, and some experimental studies suggest that striatal nerve termini degenerate prior to neuronal loss in the substantia nigra, consistent with a dying back-type disease process.[11] Functional imaging studies also show posterior putamen dopamine deficiencies in presymptomatic, at-risk individuals.[12]

The hallmark histopathologic finding in PD is the LB, which appears as a hyaline cytoplasmic inclusion in vulnerable brain stem nuclei, but also as less well-defined "pale bodies" or "cortical-type" LBs, which have a much wider distribution, including the basal forebrain (especially the basal nucleus of Meynert) and amygdala (Fig. 8–2). In PD the convexity neocortex usually has a few or no LBs, but the limbic cortex and the amygdala may be affected. Depending upon the age of the individual, varying degrees of Alzheimer-type pathology may be detected, but if the person is not demented, this usually falls within the range that is common for that age. Some cases may have abundant senile plaques, but few or no neurofibrillary tangles (NFTs).

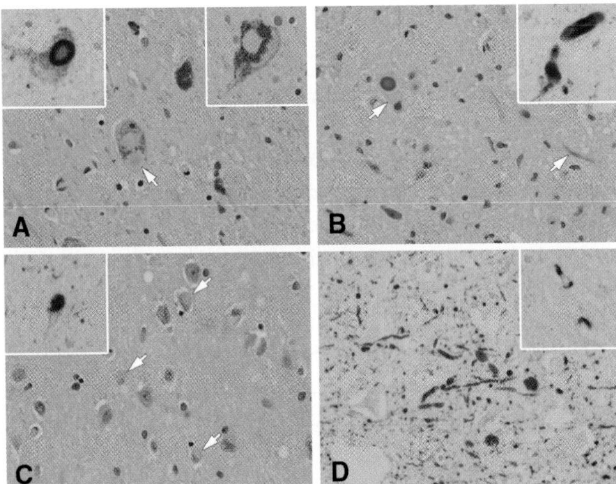

Figure 8–2. Microscopic findings in PD include Lewy bodies (arrow in A) that appear as hyaline intracytoplasmic inclusions or "pale bodies" (right inset in A) that show α-synuclein immunoreactivity (left inset in A). Swollen neuronal processes, most notably in the dorsal motor nucleus of the vagus (arrow in B), also contain compact dense α-synuclein immunoreactive inclusions (so-called "intra-neuritic Lewy bodies" (inset in B)). In the cortex less-well-defined cytoplasmic inclusions, so-called "cortical Lewy bodies" (arrows in C), also have α-synuclein immunoreactivity (inset in C). In some regions such as the hippocampus and amygdala, there are many α-synuclein immunoreactive neuritic processes (Lewy neurites) (D). Less common are glial inclusions, most often detected in white matter in the basal ganglia and the midbrain (inset in D).

LBs are proteinaceous neuronal cytoplasmic inclusions composed of α-synuclein.[13] In some regions of the brain, such as the dorsal motor nucleus of the vagus, LBs tend to form within neuronal processes (Fig. 8–2) referred to as intra-neuritic LBs. In most cases, LBs are accompanied by a variable number of abnormal neuritic profiles, referred to as Lewy neurites (LNs). LNs were first described in the hippocampus (Fig. 8–2),[14] but are also found in other regions of the brain, including the amygdala, cingulate gyrus, and temporal cortex. At the electron microscopic level, LBs are composed of densely aggregated filaments[15] and LNs also are filamentous, but they are usually not as densely packed.[14] The chemical composition of LBs has been inferred from immunohistochemical studies. While antibodies to neurofilament were first shown to label LBs,[16] ubiquitin[17] and more recently α-synuclein[13] (Fig. 8–2) antibodies are better markers for LBs, and α-synuclein appears to be the most specific marker currently available. LNs have the same immunoreactivity profile as LBs.

Neurons that are most vulnerable to LBs include the monoaminergic neurons of the substantia nigra, locus ceruleus, and dorsal motor nucleus of the vagus, as well as cholinergic neurons in the basal forebrain (Table 8–1). LBs are rarely detected in the basal ganglia or thalamus, but are common in the hypothalamus, especially the posterior and lateral hypothalamus, and the brain stem reticular formation. LNs are not uncommon in the striatum, especially in late stages of PD.[18] The oculomotor nuclear complex is also vulnerable. In the pons, the raphe and pedunculopontine nuclei are often affected, but neurons of the pontine base are not. LBs have not been described in the cerebellar cortex. In the spinal cord, the neurons of the intermediolateral cell column are most vulnerable. LBs can be found in the autonomic ganglia, including sympathetic ganglia[15] and in the intramural parasympathetic ganglia of the esophagus, stomach, and urinary bladder.[19] LNs are also found in autonomic nerve termini in the intestine[20] and heart.[21,22] While not usually numerous in typical PD, LBs can be found in cortical neurons, especially in the limbic lobe. Cortical LBs can be difficult to detect with routine histology, but are visible with special staining techniques, such as immunohistochemistry for α-synuclein (Fig. 8–2), and are usually most numerous in small neurons in lower cortical layers.

Recently, Braak and coworkers proposed a pathologic staging system for PD.[23,24] In this system, early pathologic manifestations of PD are detected in the

▶ **TABLE 8–1. DISTRIBUTION OF α-SYNUCLEIN PATHOLOGY IN TYPICAL PD**

Anatomical Region	α-Synuclein Pathology	Neuronal Loss	Braak PD Stage
Autonomic nervous system			
Sympathetic ganglia	LN, LB	+	0
Gastroesophageal	LN, LB	–	0
Cardiac	LN	–	0
Adrenal	LN	–	0
Olfactory bulb			
Anterior olfactory n.	LN, LB	++	1
Medulla			
Dorsal motor n. vagus	LB, iLB	++	1
Pons			
Locus ceruleus	LB, LN	+++	2
Midbrain			
Substantia nigra (A9)	LB, LN, GCI, Sph	+++	3
Basal forebrain			
Basal n. Meynert	cLB, iLB	++	3
Amygdala	cLB, LN	–	4
Medial temporal lobe			
Hippocampus (CA2)	LN	–	4
Hippocampus (CA4)	cLB	–	4
Convexity neocortex			
Frontal cortex	cLB, LN	–	5
Parietal cortex	cLB, LN	–	6
Basal ganglia			
Putamen	LN, GCI	–	5-6
Globus pallidus	Sph	–	5-6

LB, Lewy bodies; LN, Lewy neurites; GCI, glial cytoplasmic inclusions; iLB, intraneurites lewy body; cLB, cortical lewy body; Sph, spheroids; neuronal loss: +++, severe; ++, moderate; +, documented; –, negative or not documented.

dorsal motor nucleus of the vagus and anterior olfactory nucleus, with subsequent spread of the pathology to locus ceruleus, substantia nigra, and basal forebrain. The scheme was based upon screening of cases for initial pathology in the medulla, which has been faulted by some.[25] In the final stages, pathology extends to the neocortex, particularly limbic cortices and multimodal association cortices of frontal and temporal lobes (Table 8–1). This progression of pathology in the cortex is similar to that originally described by Kosaka and coworkers for LB dementia.[26] Although the staging system fits in most cases, it does not fit all disorders associated with LBs. The staging scheme does not have relevance to LBs that occur in the setting of Alzheimer's disease (AD),[27] where many cases have LBs confined to the amygdala.[28] Involvement of the spinal cord intermediolateral column is relatively early in the disease process, possibly after the dorsal motor nucleus of the vagus, but before the SN.[29] In addition some individuals with possibly preclinical PD have LBs in autonomic ganglia.[30] The basal ganglia have α-synuclein pathology, mostly LNs, in many cases of PD, and evidence suggests that it is involved relatively late in the disease process.[18,31]

If the staging system proposed by Braak is correct, non-motor, non-dopaminergic symptoms should precede motor symptoms.[32] For example, one might predict that early PD may be characterized by autonomic dysfunction, olfactory dysfunction, sleep disorder, and depression, given the roles of lower brain stem monoaminergic nuclei and spinal and enteric ganglia in those processes. Later stages of PD, associated with involvement of limbic cortices and multimodal association cortices, would be predicted to be associated with cognitive and psychiatric symptoms.[33]

LBs are found in about 10% of brains from normal elderly individuals over age 65 years,[34] a process referred to as "incidental" LB disease.[35–37] These cases may represent the earliest stages of PD, and the distribution of LBs and the non-motor clinical manifestations in some cases seem to favor this argument.[29,38–43] In particular, such cases have LBs, albeit in small numbers and not accompanied by neuronal loss or gliosis, in brain regions that are vulnerable to pathology in full-blown PD. It is impossible to know whether these individuals, who may or may not have non-motor prodromal features of PD, would eventually progress to PD; however, it is intriguing to note that for the most part they share a similar risk factor profile with PD.[44] It is also possible that some of these cases may represent preclinical dementia with LBs.[45]

▶ NEUROPATHOLOGY OF DEMENTIA IN PD

Formal clinical guidelines for the diagnosis of PD-related dementia have only recently been proposed[33] with operational procedures suggested shortly thereafter.[46] Pathological findings that likely account for dementia in PD are mixed and have been reviewed.[33] In an early study from the Queen Square parkinson brain bank, the pathologic substrates for dementia included severe pathology in monoaminergic and cholinergic nuclei that project to the cortex in the absence of Alzheimer-type pathology, producing a "subcortical dementia" (39%); coexistent Alzheimer's disease (29%); and diffuse cortical LBs (26%).[47] More recent studies place greater emphasis on cortical LBs. Given that cortical LBs virtually always occur in the setting of pathology affecting subcortical monoaminergic and cholinergic nuclei that project to the cortex,[48,49] it is difficult to ascribe clinical features to one or the other. While some cases have coexistent AD, in many cases the Alzheimer-type pathology is insufficient to confidently warrant diagnosis of AD.[50] Most cases have plaque-predominant pathology, a process that has been referred to as pathological aging.[51] The recent development of amyloid imaging methods confirms the presence of cortical amyloid deposits in many individuals with PD and dementia.[52]

Virtually all brains of patients with PD have a few cortical LBs, and several recent studies have shown that cortical LBs are numerous in cases of PD with dementia[50,53,54] and that the density of cortical LBs and LNs, especially in medial temporal lobe structures,[55] correlates with the severity of dementia. There are exceptions to this, however, with occasional reports of neurologically normal individuals with cortical LBs.[56,57]

Dementia with Lewy bodies (DLB) is a clinicopathologic entity with a specific constellation of clinical features, including cognitive impairment, visual hallucinations, fluctuating cognition, and parkinsonism.[58] Other common clinical features are rapid eye movement behavior disorder (RBD), severe neuroleptic sensitivity, and reduced striatal dopamine transporter activity on functional neuroimaging.[59] There is considerable overlap between clinical features of DLB and PD with dementia, the major difference being the timing of the major clinical features. Parkinsonism is a necessary and early clinical feature preceding dementia in PD with dementia, but it is not required and when present is often mild (akinetic rigid type) in DLB. At present there are no defining pathologic differences between DLB and PD with dementia for individual cases, but on average neuronal loss is less in the substantia nigra in DLB compared to PD with dementia,[31] which reflects the fact that motor signs are necessary and early for PD with dementia, but not required for clinical diagnosis of DLB.

The research neuropathologic criteria for DLB emphasize the likelihood that the pathologic findings would be associated with clinical features of DLB.[60] These criteria describe a matrix in which the likelihood of the DLB syndrome is directly related to the severity of LBs and is inversely related to the severity of AD pathology.[60] This is based upon evidence that when Alzheimer pathology is severe, the usual clinical presentation is Alzheimer-type dementia, not DLB.[61] Severity of LB pathology is based on the distribution of LBs—brain stem–predominant LBs, LBs in mostly limbic cortices, and LBs in multimodal association cortices. Severity of AD-type pathology is assessed using methods to score the severity of cortical plaques and the topography of neurofibrillary degeneration.

▶ NEUROPATHOLOGY OF MULTIPLE SYSTEM ATROPHY

Multiple system atrophy (MSA) is a neurodegenerative disease characterized by Parkinsonism, cerebellar ataxia, and idiopathic orthostatic hypotension.[62] It is thought to be a sporadic disease, but variants in the α-synuclein gene have recently been implicated as a genetic risk factor.[63,64] The MSA brain shows varying degrees of atrophy of cerebellum, cerebellar peduncles, pons and medulla, as well as atrophy and discoloration of the posterolateral putamen and pigment loss in the substantia nigra (Fig. 8–3). The histopathological findings include neuronal loss, gliosis, and microvacuolation, involving the putamen, substantia nigra,

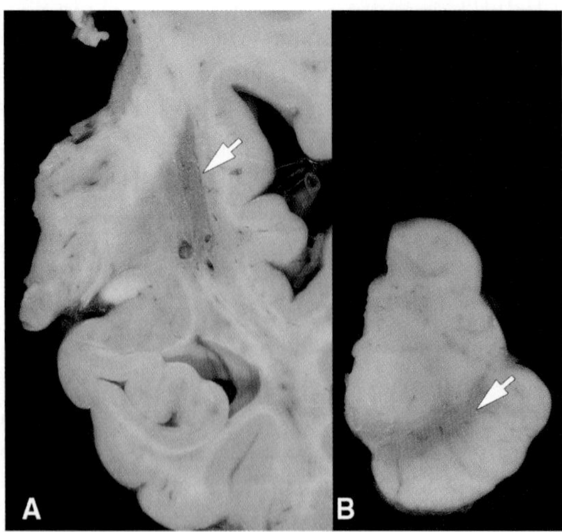

Figure 8–3. Macroscopic findings in MSA. Severe atrophy and granular softening in the posterior putamen (arrow in A) is usually associated with loss of neuromelanin pigment in the substantia nigra, most severe in the ventrolateral region (arrow in B).

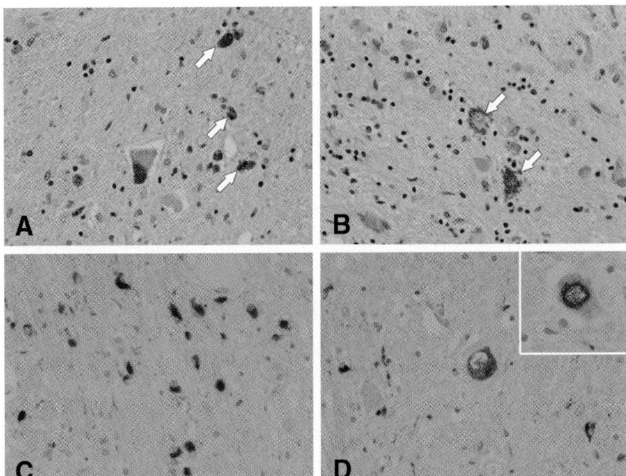

Figure 8–4. Microscopic findings in MSA. There is neuronal loss and gliosis, with extraneuronal neuromelanin (arrows in A) in the substantia nigra. In the putamen, neuronal loss and gliosis is accompanied by iron pigment in neurons and glia (arrows in B). The hallmark lesion of MSA is the glial cytoplasmic inclusions, many of which are shown here with α-synuclein immunohistochemistry in pontocerebellar fiber tract in the pons (C). In pontine base neurons may have cytoplasmic inclusions with α-synuclein inmunohistochemistry and some have intranuclear inclusions (inset in D).

cerebellum, olivary nucleus, pontine base, and intermediolateral cell column of the spinal cord. White matter inevitably shows demyelination, with the brunt of the changes affecting white matter tracts in the cerebellum and pons.

The most definitive histopathologic finding in MSA is the oligodendroglial glial cytoplasmic inclusion (GCI).[65] GCIs can be detected with silver stains, such as the Gallyas silver stain, but are best seen with antibodies to synuclein, where they appear as flame- or sickle-shaped inclusions in oligodendrocytes (Fig. 8–4). At the ultrastructural level, GCIs are non-membrane-bound cytoplasmic inclusions composed of filaments (7–10 nm) and granular material that often coats the filaments.[66] They are specific for MSA and have not been found in other neurodegenerative diseases. In addition to GCI, synuclein immunoreactive lesions are also detected in some neurons in MSA (Fig. 8–4). Neurons that are vulnerable to cytoplasmic and nuclear inclusions in MSA are found in the putamen, pontine base, and inferior olive. Less often neurons in the nucleus accumbens, hippocampus, basal nucleus of Meynert, substantia nigra, and locus ceruleus are affected. Biochemical studies of synuclein in MSA have shown changes in its solubility,[67] which have also been reported in LB disease.[68,69]

▶ NEUROPATHOLOGY OF PROGRESSIVE SUPRANUCLEAR PALSY (PSP)

PSP is an atypical parkinsonian disorder associated with progressive axial rigidity, vertical gaze palsy, dysarthria, and dysphagia first described by Steele–Richardson–Olszewski.[70] Some patients with PSP present initially with clinical features similar to PS before developing characteristic signs of Richardson's syndrome.[71] Frontal lobe dementia or speech apraxia are present in some cases,[72,73] while other patients present with primary freezing of gait and akinesia.[74,75] In some other patients the clinical features of corticobasal ganglionic degeneration are the initial manifestations.[76] In contrast to PD, gross examination of the brain often has distinctive features. Most cases have varying degrees of frontal atrophy that may involve the pre-central gyrus, especially in those with long tract signs.[76] The midbrain, especially the midbrain tectum, and to a lesser extent the pons shows atrophy. The third ventricle and aqueduct of Sylvius may be dilated. The substantia nigra shows loss of pigment, while the locus ceruleus is often better preserved. The macroscopic feature that is of most differential diagnostic value for the parkinsonian disorders is atrophy of the subthalamic nucleus, which is consistent in PSP and not a feature of other parkinsonian disorders (Fig. 8–5). The superior cerebellar peduncle and the hilus of the cerebellar dentate nucleus are usually atrophic and have a gray color due to myelinated fiber loss.[77] This finding has been shown to be clinically useful in differential diagnosis of atypical parkinsonism[78,79] and preliminary studies using diffusion tensor imaging highlight these differences.[80]

Microscopic findings include neuronal loss, gliosis, and NFTs affecting basal ganglia, diencephalon, brain stem, and cerebellum (Fig. 8–6). The nuclei most affected

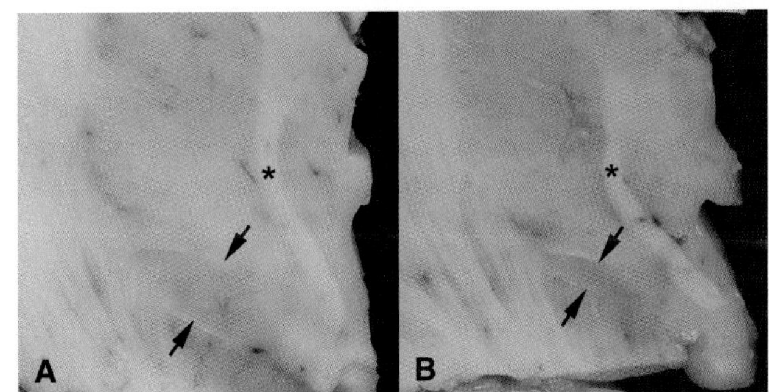

Figure 8–5. Macroscopic feature in PSP. The most distinctive finding in PSP is atrophy of the subthalamic nucleus (STN) atrophy. In these two sections of the thalamus at the level of the mammillothalamic tract (*), the normal brain (A) has an STN that is nearly twice the diameter as that in PSP (B).

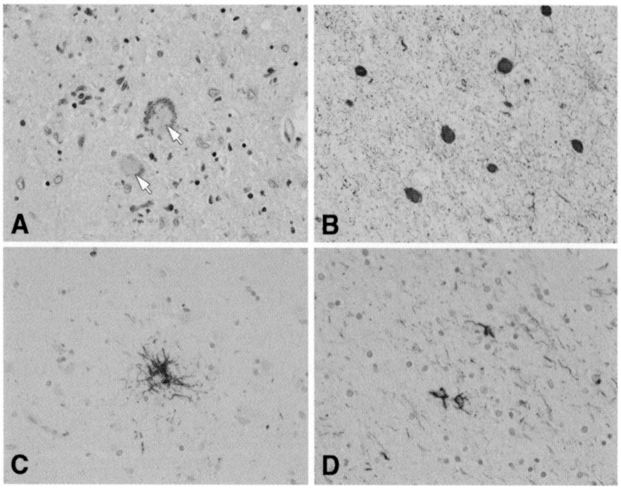

Figure 8–6. Microscopic features of PSP. Neurons in the substantia nigra have globus neurofibrillary tangles (arrows in A). Tangles such as these in the subthalamic nucleus have prominent phospho-tau immunoreactivity (B). Phospho-tau immunohistochemistry also reveals glia lesions in PSP, including tufted astrocytes in the basal ganglia (C) and oligodendroglial coiled bodies and threads in the white matter of the thalamic fasciculus (D).

are the globus pallidus, subthalamic nucleus, and substantia nigra.[81] The cerebral cortex is relatively spared, but lesions are common in the peri-Rolandic region.[82] Recent studies suggest that cortical pathology may be more widespread in cases of PSP with atypical features, such as dementia, corticobasal syndrome, or speech apraxia.[83,84]

The striatum and the thalamus often have some degree of neuronal loss and gliosis, especially ventral anterior and lateral thalamic nuclei. The basal nucleus of Meynert usually has mild cell loss, but more extensive tau pathology. The brain stem regions that are affected include the superior colliculus, periaqueductal gray matter, oculomotor nuclei, red nucleus, locus ceruleus, pontine nuclei, pontine tegmentum, vestibular nuclei, medullary tegmentum, and inferior olives. The cerebellar dentate nucleus is frequently affected and may show grumose degeneration, a type of neuronal degeneration associated with clusters of degenerating presynaptic terminals around dentate neurons.[85] The dentatorubrothalamic pathway consistently shows fiber loss. The cerebellar cortex is preserved, but there may be mild Purkinje loss with scattered axonal torpedoes. The spinal cord is often affected, where neuronal inclusions can be found in the anterior horn and intermediolateral cell column.

Silver stains (e.g., Gallyas stain) or immunostaining for tau reveal NFTs in residual neurons in the basal ganglia, diencephalon, brain stem and spinal cord. In addition to NFT, special stains demonstrate argyrophilic, tau-positive inclusions in both astrocytes and oligodendrocytes. Tufted astrocytes are increasingly recognized as a characteristic feature of PSP and are commonly found in the motor cortex and striatum. They are fibrillary lesions within astrocytes based upon double immunolabeling of tau and glial fibrillary acidic protein. Oligodendroglial lesions appear as argyrophilic and tau-positive perinuclear fibers, so-called "coiled bodies,"[86] and they are often accompanied by threadlike processes in the white matter, especially in the diencephalon and cerebellar white matter.

The tau protein in PSP is distinct from that which is found in neurofibrillary pathology in AD. In AD the abnormal insoluble tau migrates as three major bands (68, 64 and 60 kDa) on Western blots, while in PSP it migrates as two bands (68 and 64 kDa) corresponding to selective involvement of tau with four repeats in the microtubule binding domain of tau (4R tau), which is generated by alternative splicing of exon 10 of the tau gene.[87] Similar changes are noted in tau in corticobasal degeneration (CBD), while lower molecular weight tau fragments may differentiate tau pathology in PSP and CBD.[88]

▶ NEUROPATHOLOGY OF CORTICOBASAL DEGENERATION (CBD)

Corticobasal degeneration is only rarely mistaken for PD due to characteristic focal cortical signs that are the clinical hallmark of this disorder. Common clinical presentations include progressive asymmetrical rigidity and apraxia, progressive aphasia, and progressive frontal lobe dementia.[89–91] Most cases also have some degree of parkinsonism, with bradykinesia, rigidity, and dystonia more common than tremor. Given the prominent cortical findings on clinical evaluations, it is not surprising that gross examination of the brain often reveals focal cortical atrophy. The atrophy may be severe in some cases or more often subtle and hardly noticeable in others. It may be asymmetrical. Atrophy is often most marked in the medial superior frontal gyrus, parasagittal pre- and post-central gyri, and the superior parietal lobule (Fig. 8–7). The temporal and occipital lobes are usually preserved. The brain stem does not have gross atrophy as in PSP, but neuromelanin pigment loss is common in the substantia nigra. In contrast to PSP, the superior cerebellar peduncle and the subthalamic nucleus are not grossly atrophic. The cerebral white matter in affected areas is often attenuated and may have a gray discoloration. The corpus callosum is sometimes thinned, and the frontal horn of the lateral ventricle is frequently dilated. The caudate head may have flattening. The thalamus may be smaller than usual.

Microscopic examination of atrophic cortical sections shows neuronal loss with superficial spongiosis, gliosis, and usually many achromatic or ballooned neurons. Ballooned neurons are swollen and vacuolated

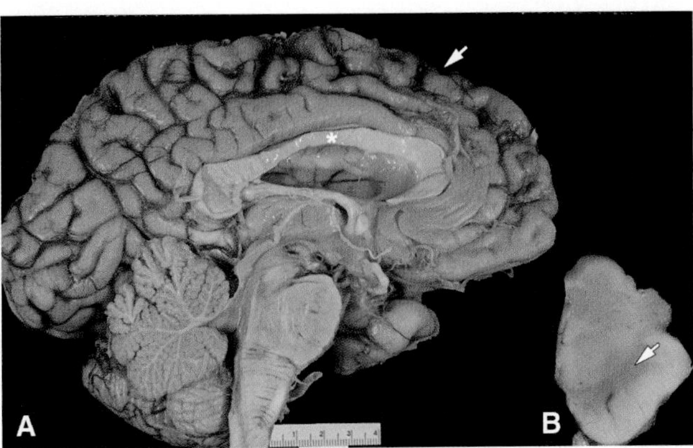

Figure 8–7. Macroscopic feature in CBD. The medial superior frontal gyrus (arrow in A) has atrophy and there is thinning of the corpus callosum (* in A). The substantia nigra has loss of neuromelanin pigment (arrow in B).

neurons found in middle and lower cortical layers, which are variably positive with silver stains and tau immunohistochemistry, but intensely stained with immunohistochemistry for alpha-B-crystallin, a small heat shock protein, and for neurofilament (Fig. 8–8).

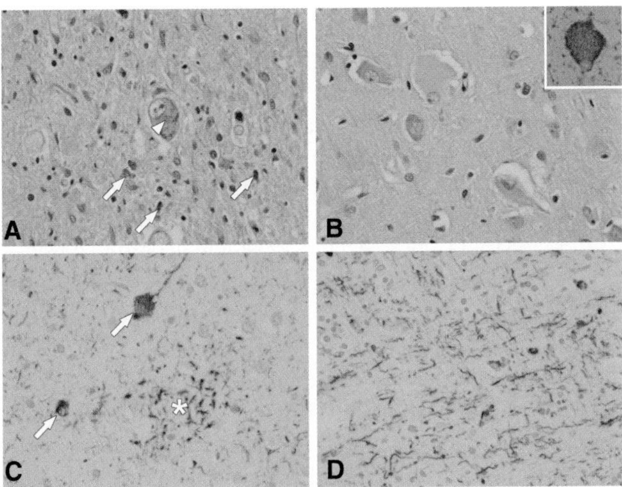

Figure 8–8. Microscopic features of CBD. The substantia nigra has neuronal loss, gliosis and extraneuronal neuromelanin (arrows in A), as well as neurons with tangles (arrowhead in A). In the cortex, ballooned neurons are a characteristic, although nonspecific, feature of CBD (B). They are immunoreactive for phosphorylated neurofilament (inset in B). Immunohistochemistry for phospho-tau reveals threadlike processes, small neuronal inclusions (arrows in C) and astrocytic plaques (* in C). Another diagnostic significant feature of CBD is the presence of numerous threadlike processes with phospho-tau immunohistochemistry in white matter of the cerebrum (D) and basal ganglia.

Cortical neurons in atrophic areas also have tau-immunoreactive lesions. In some neurons tau is densely packed into a small inclusion body somewhat reminiscent of a Pick body or a small NFT. In other neurons the filamentous inclusions are more dispersed and diffuse, consistent with so-called "pretangles." As in PSP, neurofibrillary lesions in CBD are not detected well with most diagnostic silver stains and thioflavin fluorescent microscopy. Neurofibrillary lesions in brain stem monoaminergic nuclei, such as the locus ceruleus and substantia nigra, sometimes resemble globose NFT.

In addition to fibrillary lesions in the perikarya of neurons, the neuropil of CBD invariably contains a large number of threadlike tau-immunoreactive processes. They are usually profuse in both gray and white matter, and this latter feature is an important attribute of CBD and a useful feature in differentiating it from other disorders.[92]

The most characteristic tau-immunoreactive lesion in the cortex in CBD is an annular cluster of short, stubby processes with fuzzy outlines that may be highly suggestive of a neuritic plaque of AD[93] (Fig. 8–8). In contrast to Alzheimer plaques they do not contain amyloid, but rather tau-positive astrocytes, and have been referred to as "astrocytic plaques." Astrocytic plaques differ from the tufted astrocytes seen in PSP and the two lesions do not coexist in the same brain.[94] The *astrocytic plaque* may be the most specific *histopathologic lesion of CBD.*

In addition to cortical pathology, deep gray matter is consistently affected in CBD. The globus pallidus and the putamen show mild neuronal loss with gliosis. Thalamic nuclei may also be affected. In the basal ganglia, threadlike processes are often extensive, often in the pencil fibers of the striatum. Tau-positive neurons, but not NFT, are common in the striatum and globus pallidus. The internal capsule and the thalamic fasciculus often have many threadlike processes. The subthalamic nucleus usually has a normal neuronal population, but neurons may have tau inclusions and there may be many threadlike lesions in the nucleus. Fibrillary gliosis typical of PSP is not seen in the subthalamic nucleus in CBD.

The substantia nigra usually shows moderate to severe neuronal loss with extraneuronal neuromelanin and gliosis. Many of the remaining neurons contain NFTs, which have also been termed "corticobasal bodies"[95] (Fig. 8–8). The locus ceruleus and raphe nuclei have similar inclusions. In contrast to PSP where neurons in the pontine base almost always have at least a few NFTs, the pontine base is largely free of NFT in CBD. On the other hand, tau inclusions in glia and threadlike lesions are frequent in the pontine base. The cerebellum has mild Purkinje cell loss and axonal torpedoes. There is also mild neuronal loss in the dentate nucleus, but grumose degeneration is much less common than in PSP.

In CBD the filaments have a paired helical appearance at the electron microscopic level, but the diameter

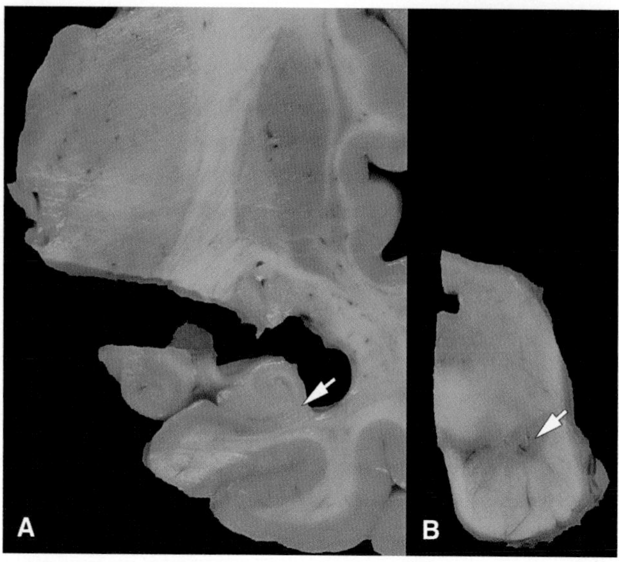

Figure 8–9. Macroscopic feature in Guam PDC. In addition to cortical atrophy (not shown), coronal sections of the brain show marked hippocampal atrophy, especially affecting CA1 sector (arrow in A). There is also loss of neuromelanin pigment in the substantia nigra (arrow in B).

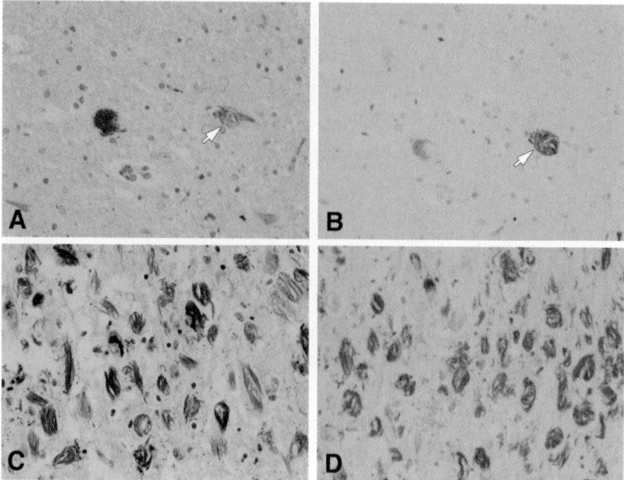

Figure 8–10. Microscopic features of Guam PDC. The substantia nigra has severe neuronal loss with only a few residual pigmented neurons and argyrophilic extracellular NFT (arrow in A) that are positive for phospho-tau (arrow in B). In the hippocampus, there are numerous NFTs, many of which are extracellular and are positive for Gallyas silver stain (black inclusions, C) and phospho-tau (brown inclusions, D).

is wider and the periodicity is longer than the paired helical filaments of AD.[96] These structures have been referred to as twisted ribbons. Similar to PSP, abnormal insoluble tau in CBD migrates as two prominent bands (68 and 64 kDa) on Western blots.[97]

▶ NEUROPATHOLOGY OF GUAM PARKINSON–DEMENTIA COMPLEX

A characteristic parkinsonism with dementia (Parkinson–dementia complex, PDC) with a number of features that overlap with PSP has been reported in the native Chamorro population of Guam since the 1950s.[98] The frequency of PDC is declining in recent years for unknown reasons, and the etiology is unknown.[99-101] The gross findings in PDC are notable for cortical atrophy affecting frontal and temporal lobes, as well as atrophy of the hippocampus (Fig. 8–9) and the tegmentum of the rostral brain stem. The substantia nigra usually has loss of neuromelanin pigment (Fig. 8–9). These areas typically have neuronal loss and gliosis with many NFTs in residual neurons; extracellular NFTs are also numerous (Fig. 8–10). In the cortex NFTs show a different laminar distribution from AD, with more NFTs in superficial cortical layers in Guam PDC and in lower cortical layers in AD.[102] The hippocampus has numerous NFTs. The substantia nigra and the locus ceruleus also have marked neuronal loss and NFT in the few residual neurons (Fig. 8–10). The basal nucleus and large neurons in the striatum are also vulnerable to NFT. Biochemically and morphologically, NFTs in Guam PDC are indistinguishable from those in AD.[103,104] In both conditions, tau is composed of a mixture of tau with three repeats (3R) and four repeats (4R) in the microtubule domain.[87] Some patients with PDC have concomitant motor neuron disease with clinical and pathologic features similar to amyotrophic lateral sclerosis (ALS).[105] A recently identified marker for neurodegeneration in ALS is TAR DNA binding protein of 43 kDa (TDP-43),[106] and TDP-43 is consistently found in Guam cases with motor neuron disease,[107,108] but also in cases with just PDC.[109] A subset of LB PD cases also has TDP-43 immunoreactivity,[110] but in most cases this can be linked to presence of concurrent Alzheimer pathology. In AD anywhere from 20–50% of cases have TDP-43 immunoreactivity,[111–113] with TDP-43 deposited in neurons with neurofibrillary pathology.[113] These results suggest that TDP-43 pathology is innately associated with 3R + 4R tau as seen in Guam PDC and AD.

REFERENCES

1. Zijlmans JC, Daniel SE, Hughes AJ, et al. Clinicopathological investigation of vascular parkinsonism, including clinical criteria for diagnosis. Mov Disord 2004;19:630.
2. Gibb WR, Lees AJ. Anatomy, pigmentation, ventral and dorsal subpopulations of the substantia nigra, and differential cell death in Parkinson's disease. J Neurol Neurosurg Psychiatry 1991;54:388.

3. Chung CY, Seo H, Sonntag KC, et al. Cell type-specific gene expression of midbrain dopaminergic neurons reveals molecules involved in their vulnerability and protection. Hum Mol Genet 2005;14:1709.
4. Fearnley JM, Lees AJ. Ageing and Parkinson's disease: substantia nigra regional selectivity. Brain 1991;114(Pt 5):2283.
5. Hughes AJ, Daniel SE, Blankson S, et al. A clinicopathologic study of 100 cases of Parkinson's disease. Arch Neurol 1993;50:140.
6. Rajput AH, Rozdilsky B, Rajput A. Accuracy of clinical diagnosis in parkinsonism—A prospective study. Can J Neurol Sci 1991;18:275.
7. Rajput AH, Voll A, Rajput ML, et al. Course in Parkinson disease subtypes: A 39-year clinicopathologic study. Neurology 2009;73:206.
8. Hughes AJ, Daniel SE, Lees AJ. Improved accuracy of clinical diagnosis of Lewy body Parkinson's disease. Neurology 2001;57:1497.
9. Greffard S, Verny M, Bonnet AM, et al. A stable proportion of Lewy body bearing neurons in the substantia nigra suggests a model in which the Lewy body causes neuronal death. Neurobiol Aging 2010 Jan;31(1):99–103. Epub 2008 May 23.
10. McGeer PL, Itagaki S, Akiyama H, et al. Rate of cell death in parkinsonism indicates active neuropathological process. Ann Neurol 1988;24:574.
11. Betarbet R, Sherer TB, MacKenzie G, et al. Chronic systemic pesticide exposure reproduces features of Parkinson's disease. Nat Neurosci 2000;3:1301.
12. Brooks DJ. The early diagnosis of Parkinson's disease. Ann Neurol 1998;44:S10.
13. Spillantini MG, Schmidt ML, Lee VM, et al. Alpha-synuclein in Lewy bodies. Nature 1997;388:839.
14. Dickson DW, Ruan D, Crystal H, et al. Hippocampal degeneration differentiates diffuse Lewy body disease (DLBD) from Alzheimer's disease: Light and electron microscopic immunocytochemistry of CA2-3 neurites specific to DLBD. Neurology 1991;41:1402.
15. Forno LS, Norville RL. Ultrastructure of Lewy bodies in the stellate ganglion. Acta Neuropathol 1976;34:183.
16. Galvin JE, Lee VM, Baba M, et al. Monoclonal antibodies to purified cortical Lewy bodies recognize the mid-size neurofilament subunit. Ann Neurol 1997;42:595.
17. Kuzuhara S, Mori H, Izumiyama N, et al. Lewy bodies are ubiquitinated. A light and electron microscopic immunocytochemical study. Acta Neuropathol (Berl) 1988;75:345.
18. Tsuboi Y, Uchikado H, Dickson DW. Neuropathology of Parkinson's disease dementia and dementia with Lewy bodies with reference to striatal pathology. Parkinsonism Relat Disord 2007;13(suppl 3):S221.
19. Braak H, de Vos RA, Bohl J, et al. Gastric alpha-synuclein immunoreactive inclusions in Meissner's and Auerbach's plexuses in cases staged for Parkinson's disease-related brain pathology. Neurosci Lett 2006;396:67.
20. Lebouvier T, Chaumette T, Damier P, et al. Pathological lesions in colonic biopsies during Parkinson's disease. Gut 2008;57:1741.
21. Fujishiro H, Frigerio R, Burnett M, et al. Cardiac sympathetic denervation correlates with clinical and pathologic stages of Parkinson's disease. Mov Disord. 2008 Jun 15;23(8):1085–1092.
22. Orimo S, Amino T, Itoh Y, et al. Cardiac sympathetic denervation precedes neuronal loss in the sympathetic ganglia in Lewy body disease. Acta Neuropathol (Berl) 2005;109:583.
23. Braak H, Ghebremedhin E, Rub U, et al. Stages in the development of Parkinson's disease-related pathology. Cell Tissue Res 2004;318:121.
24. Braak H, Del Tredici K: Neuroanatomy and pathology of sporadic Parkinson's disease. Adv Anat Embryol Cell Biol 2009;201:1.
25. Kalaitzakis ME, Graeber MB, Gentleman SM, et al. The dorsal motor nucleus of the vagus is not an obligatory trigger site of Parkinson's disease: A critical analysis of alpha-synuclein staging. Neuropathol Appl Neurobiol 2008;34:284.
26. Katsuse O, Iseki E, Marui W, et al. Developmental stages of cortical Lewy bodies and their relation to axonal transport blockage in brains of patients with dementia with Lewy bodies. J Neurol Sci 2003;211:29.
27. Dickson DW, Uchikado H, klos KJ, et al. A critical review of the Braak staging scheme for Parkinson's disease. Mov Disord 2006;21:S559.
28. Uchikado H, Lin WL, DeLucia MW, et al. Alzheimer disease with amygdala Lewy bodies: a distinct form of alpha-synucleinopathy. J Neuropathol Exp Neurol 2006; 65:685.
29. Klos KJ, Ahlskog JE, Josephs KA, et al. Alpha-synuclein pathology in the spinal cords of neurologically asymptomatic aged individuals. Neurology 2006;66:1100.
30. Saito Y, Kawashima A, Ruberu NN, et al. Accumulation of phosphorylated alpha-synuclein in aging human brain. J Neuropathol Exp Neurol 2003;62:644.
31. Tsuboi Y, Dickson DW. Dementia with Lewy bodies and Parkinson's disease with dementia: are they different? Parkinsonism Relat Disord 2005;11(suppl 1):S47.
32. Langston JW. The Parkinson's complex: Parkinsonism is just the tip of the iceberg. Ann Neurol 2006;59:591.
33. Emre M, Aarsland D, Brown R, et al. Clinical diagnostic criteria for dementia associated with Parkinson's disease. Mov Disord 2007;22:1689.
34. Forno LS: Concentric hyalin intraneuronal inclusions of Lewy type in the brains of elderly persons (50 incidental cases): Relationship to parkinsonism. J Am Geriatr Soc 1969;17:557.
35. Beach TG, Adler CH, Lue L, et al. Unified staging system for Lewy body disorders: correlation with nigrostriatal degeneration, cognitive impairment and motor dysfunction. Acta Neuropathol 2009;117:613.
36. Markesbery WR, Jicha GA, Liu H, et al. Lewy body pathology in normal elderly subjects. J Neuropathol Exp Neurol 2009;68:816.
37. Dickson DW, Fujishiro H, Delledonne A, et al. Evidence that incidental Lewy body disease is pre-symptomatic Parkinson's disease. Acta Neuropathol 2008.
38. Bloch A, Probst A, Bissig H, et al. Alpha-synuclein pathology of the spinal and peripheral autonomic nervous system in neurologically unimpaired elderly subjects. Neuropathol Appl Neurobiol 2006;32:284.
39. Del Tredici K, Rub U, De Vos RA, et al. Where does parkinson disease pathology begin in the brain? J Neuropathol Exp Neurol 2002;61:413.

40. Iwanaga K, Wakabayashi K, Yoshimoto M, et al. Lewy body-type degeneration in cardiac plexus in Parkinson's and incidental Lewy body diseases. Neurology 1999;52:1269.
41. Jellinger KA. Alpha-synuclein pathology in Parkinson's and Alzheimer's disease brain: Incidence and topographic distribution—A pilot study. Acta Neuropathol (Berl) 2003;106:191.
42. Parkkinen L, Soininen H, Alafuzoff I. Regional distribution of alpha-synuclein pathology in unimpaired aging and Alzheimer disease. J Neuropathol Exp Neurol 2003;62:363.
43. Uchiyama M, Isse K, Tanaka K, et al. Incidental Lewy body disease in a patient with REM sleep behavior disorder. Neurology 1995;45:709.
44. Frigerio R, Fujishiro H, Maraganore DM, et al. Comparison of risk factor profiles in incidental Lewy body disease and Parkinson disease. Arch Neurol 2009; 66:1114.
45. Frigerio R, Fujishiro H, Ahn TB, et al. Incidental Lewy body disease: Do some cases represent a preclinical stage of dementia with Lewy bodies? Neurobiol Aging 2009.
46. Dubois B, Burn D, Goetz C, et al. Diagnostic procedures for Parkinson's disease dementia: recommendations from the movement disorder society task force. Mov Disord 2007;22:2314.
47. Hughes AJ, Daniel SE, Kilford L, et al. Accuracy of clinical diagnosis of idiopathic Parkinson's disease: a clinico-pathological study of 100 cases. J Neurol Neurosurg Psychiatry 1992;55:181.
48. Nakano I, Hirano A. Parkinson's disease: Neuron loss in the nucleus basalis without concomitant Alzheimer's disease. Ann Neurol 1984;15:415.
49. Whitehouse PJ, Hedreen JC, White CL, 3rd, et al. Basal forebrain neurons in the dementia of Parkinson disease. Ann Neurol 1983;13:243.
50. Apaydin H, Ahlskog JE, Parisi JE, et al. Parkinson disease neuropathology: later-developing dementia and loss of the levodopa response. Arch Neurol 2002;59:102.
51. Dickson DW, Crystal HA, Mattiace LA, et al. Identification of normal and pathological aging in prospectively studied nondemented elderly humans. Neurobiol Aging 1992;13:179.
52. Edison P, Rowe CC, Rinne JO, et al. Amyloid load in Parkinson's disease dementia and Lewy body dementia measured with [11C]PIB positron emission tomography. J Neurol Neurosurg Psychiatry 2008;79:1331.
53. Hurtig HI, Trojanowski JQ, Galvin J, et al. Alpha-synuclein cortical Lewy bodies correlate with dementia in Parkinson's disease. Neurology 2000;54:1916.
54. Aarsland D, Perry R, Brown A, et al. Neuropathology of dementia in Parkinson's disease: A prospective, community-based study. Ann Neurol 2005;58:773.
55. Churchyard A, Lees AJ. The relationship between dementia and direct involvement of the hippocampus and amygdala in Parkinson's disease. Neurology 1997; 49:1570.
56. Parkkinen L, Kauppinen T, Pirttila T, et al. Alpha-synuclein pathology does not predict extrapyramidal symptoms or dementia. Ann Neurol 2005;57:82.
57. Zaccai J, Brayne C, McKeith I, et al. Patterns and stages of alpha-synucleinopathy: Relevance in a population-based cohort. Neurology 2008;70:1042.
58. McKeith I, Mintzer J, Aarsland D, et al. Dementia with Lewy bodies. Lancet Neurol 2004;3:19.
59. McKeith I, O'Brien J, Walker Z, et al. Sensitivity and specificity of dopamine transporter imaging with 123I-FP-CIT SPECT in dementia with Lewy bodies: A phase III, multicentre study. Lancet Neurol 2007;6:305.
60. McKeith IG, Dickson DW, Lowe J, et al. Diagnosis and management of dementia with Lewy bodies: Third report of the DLB Consortium. Neurology 2005;65:1863.
61. Lopez OL, Becker JT, Kaufer DI, et al. Research evaluation and prospective diagnosis of dementia with Lewy bodies. Arch Neurol 2002;59:43.
62. Wenning GK, Tison F, Ben Shlomo Y, et al. Multiple system atrophy: A review of 203 pathologically proven cases. Mov Disord 1997;12:133.
63. Scholz SW, Houlden H, Schulte C, et al. SNCA variants are associated with increased risk for multiple system atrophy. Ann Neurol 2009;65:610.
64. Al-Chalabi A, Durr A, Wood NW, et al. Genetic variants of the alpha-synuclein gene SNCA are associated with multiple system atrophy. PLoS ONE 2009;4:e7114.
65. Papp MI, Kahn JE, Lantos PL. Glial cytoplasmic inclusions in the CNS of patients with multiple system atrophy (striatonigral degeneration, olivopontocerebellar atrophy and Shy-Drager syndrome). J Neurol Sci 1989;94:79.
66. Lin WL, DeLucia MW, Dickson DW. Alpha-synuclein immunoreactivity in neuronal nuclear inclusions and neurites in multiple system atrophy. Neurosci Lett 2004;354:99.
67. Dickson DW, Liu W, Hardy J, et al. Widespread alterations of alpha-synuclein in multiple system atrophy. Am J Pathol 1999;155:1241.
68. Kahle PJ, Neumann M, Ozmen L, et al. Hyperphosphorylation and insolubility of alpha-synuclein in transgenic mouse oligodendrocytes. EMBO Rep 2002;3:583.
69. Klucken J, Ingelsson M, Shin Y, et al. Clinical and biochemical correlates of insoluble alpha-synuclein in dementia with Lewy bodies. Acta Neuropathol 2006;111:101.
70. Steele JC, Richardson JC, Olszewski J. Progressive supranuclear palsy. A heterogeneous degeneration involving the brain stem, basal ganglia and cerebellum with vertical gaze and pseudobulbar palsy, nuchal dystonia and dementia. Arch Neurol 1964;10:333.
71. Williams DR, Holton JL, Strand C, et al. Pathological tau burden and distribution distinguishes progressive supranuclear palsy-parkinsonism from Richardson's syndrome. Brain 2007;130:1566.
72. Josephs KA, Duffy JR. Apraxia of speech and nonfluent aphasia: a new clinical marker for corticobasal degeneration and progressive supranuclear palsy. Curr Opin Neurol 2008;21:688.
73. Josephs KA, Petersen RC, Knopman DS, et al. Clinicopathologic analysis of frontotemporal and corticobasal degenerations and PSP. Neurology 2006;66:41.
74. Ahmed Z, Josephs KA, Gonzalez J, et al. Clinical and neuropathologic features of progressive supranuclear palsy with severe pallido-nigro-luysial degeneration and axonal dystrophy. Brain 2008;131:460.

75. Williams DR, Holton JL, Strand K, et al. Pure akinesia with gait freezing: a third clinical phenotype of progressive supranuclear palsy. Mov Disord 2007;22:2235.
76. Josephs KA, Katsuse O, Beccano-Kelly DA, et al. Atypical progressive supranuclear palsy with corticospinal tract degeneration. J Neuropathol Exp Neurol 2006;65:396.
77. Tsuboi Y, Slowinski J, Josephs KA, et al. Atrophy of superior cerebellar peduncle in progressive supranuclear palsy. Neurology 2003;60:1766.
78. Paviour DC, Price SL, Stevens JM, et al. Quantitative MRI measurement of superior cerebellar peduncle in progressive supranuclear palsy. Neurology 2005;64:675.
79. Slowinski J, Imamura A, Uitti RJ, et al. MR imaging of brainstem atrophy in progressive supranuclear palsy. J Neurol 2008;255:37.
80. Nilsson C, Markenroth Bloch K, Brockstedt S, et al. Tracking the neurodegeneration of parkinsonian disorders—A pilot study. Neuroradiology 2007;49:111.
81. Hauw JJ, Daniel SE, Dickson D, et al. Preliminary NINDS neuropathologic criteria for Steele-Richardson-Olszewski syndrome (progressive supranuclear palsy). Neurology 1994;44:2015.
82. Hauw JJ, Verny M, Delaere P, et al. Constant neurofibrillary changes in the neocortex in progressive supranuclear palsy. Basic differences with Alzheimer's disease and aging. Neurosci Lett 1990;119:182.
83. Tsuboi Y, Josephs KA, Boeve BF, et al. Increased tau burden in the cortices of progressive supranuclear palsy presenting with corticobasal syndrome. Mov Disord 2005;20:982.
84. Josephs KA, Boeve BF, Duffy JR, et al. Atypical progressive supranuclear palsy underlying progressive apraxia of speech and nonfluent aphasia. Neurocase 2005; 11:283.
85. Ishizawa K, Lin WL, Tiseo P, et al. A qualitative and quantitative study of grumose degeneration in progressive supranuclear palsy. J Neuropathol Exp Neurol 2000;59:513.
86. Braak H, Braak E: Cortical and subcortical argyrophilic grains characterize a disease associated with adult onset dementia. Neuropathol Appl Neurobiol 1989;15:13.
87. de Silva R, Lashley T, Gibb G, et al. Pathological inclusion bodies in tauopathies contain distinct complements of tau with three or four microtubule-binding repeat domains as demonstrated by new specific monoclonal antibodies. Neuropathol Appl Neurobiol 2003;29:288.
88. Arai T, Ikeda K, Akiyama H, et al. Identification of amino-terminally cleaved tau fragments that distinguish progressive supranuclear palsy from corticobasal degeneration. Ann Neurol 2004;55:72.
89. Litvan I, Campbell G, Mangone CA, et al. Which clinical features differentiate progressive supranuclear palsy (Steele-Richardson-Olszewski syndrome) from related disorders? A clinicopathological study. Brain 1997;120(Pt 1:65.
90. Rinne JO, Lee MS, Thompson PD, et al. Corticobasal degeneration. A clinical study of 36 cases. Brain 1994;117(Pt 5):1183.
91. Litvan I, Grimes DA, Lang AE, et al. Clinical features differentiating patients with postmortem confirmed progressive supranuclear palsy and corticobasal degeneration. J Neurol 1999;246(suppl 2):II1.
92. Dickson DW, Bergeron C, Chin SS, et al. Office of Rare Diseases neuropathologic criteria for corticobasal degeneration. J Neuropathol Exp Neurol 2002;61:935.
93. Feany MB, Dickson DW. Widespread cytoskeletal pathology characterizes corticobasal degeneration. Am J Pathol 1995;146:1388.
94. Komori T, Arai N, Oda M, et al. Astrocytic plaques and tufts of abnormal fibers do not coexist in corticobasal degeneration and progressive supranuclear palsy. Acta Neuropathol (Berl) 1998;96:401.
95. Gibb WR, Luthert PJ, Marsden CD. Corticobasal degeneration. Brain 1989;112(Pt 5):1171.
96. Ksiezak-Reding H, Morgan K, Mattiace LA, et al. Ultrastructure and biochemical composition of paired helical filaments in corticobasal degeneration. Am J Pathol 1994;145:1496.
97. Dickson DW. Neuropathologic differentiation of progressive supranuclear palsy and corticobasal degeneration. J Neurol 1999;246(suppl 2):II6.
98. Hirano A, Malamud N, Elizan TS, et al. Amyotrophic lateral sclerosis and Parkinsonism-dementia complex on Guam. Further pathologic studies. Arch Neurol 1966;15:35.
99. Galasko D, Salmon DP, Craig UK, et al. Clinical features and changing patterns of neurodegenerative disorders on Guam, 1997-2000. Neurology 2002;58:90.
100. Plato CC, Garruto RM, Galasko D, et al. Amyotrophic lateral sclerosis and parkinsonism-dementia complex of Guam: Changing incidence rates during the past 60 years. Am J Epidemiol 2003;157:149.
101. Steele JC, McGeer PL. The ALS/PDC syndrome of Guam and the cycad hypothesis. Neurology 2008;70:1984.
102. Hof PR, Perl DP, Loerzel AJ, et al. Amyotrophic lateral sclerosis and parkinsonism-dementia from Guam: Differences in neurofibrillary tangle distribution and density in the hippocampal formation and neocortex. Brain Res 1994;650:107.
103. Buee-Scherrer V, Buee L, Hof PR, et al. Neurofibrillary degeneration in amyotrophic lateral sclerosis/parkinsonism-dementia complex of Guam. Immunochemical characterization of tau proteins. Am J Pathol 1995;146:924.
104. Mawal-Dewan M, Schmidt ML, Balin B, et al. Identification of phosphorylation sites in PHF-TAU from patients with Guam amyotrophic lateral sclerosis/parkinsonism-dementia complex. J Neuropathol Exp Neurol 1996;55:1051.
105. Oyanagi K, Wada M. Neuropathology of parkinsonism-dementia complex and amyotrophic lateral sclerosis of Guam: An update. J Neurol 1999;246(suppl 2):II19.
106. Neumann M, Sampathu DM, Kwong LK, et al. Ubiquitinated TDP-43 in frontotemporal lobar degeneration and amyotrophic lateral sclerosis. Science 2006;314:130.
107. Hasegawa M, Arai T, Akiyama H, et al. TDP-43 is deposited in the Guam parkinsonism-dementia complex brains. Brain 2007;130:1386.
108. Geser F, Winton MJ, Kwong LK, et al. Pathological TDP-43 in parkinsonism-dementia complex and amyotrophic lateral sclerosis of Guam. Acta Neuropathol 2008;115:133.
109. Miklossy J, Steele JC, Yu S, et al. Enduring involvement of tau, beta-amyloid, alpha-synuclein, ubiquitin and

TDP-43 pathology in the amyotrophic lateral sclerosis/parkinsonism-dementia complex of Guam (ALS/PDC). Acta Neuropathol 2008;116:625.

110. Nakashima-Yasuda H, Uryu K, Robinson J, et al. Co-morbidity of TDP-43 proteinopathy in Lewy body related diseases. Acta Neuropathol 2007;114:221.

111. Arai T, Hasegawa M, Akiyama H, et al. TDP-43 is a component of ubiquitin-positive tau-negative inclusions in frontotemporal lobar degeneration and amyotrophic lateral sclerosis. Biochem Biophys Res Commun 2006;351:602.

112. Hu WT, Josephs KA, Knopman DS, et al. Temporal lobar predominance of TDP-43 neuronal cytoplasmic inclusions in Alzheimer disease. Acta Neuropathol 2008;116:215.

113. Amador-Ortiz C, Lin WL, Ahmed Z, et al. TDP-43 immunoreactivity in hippocampal sclerosis and Alzheimer's disease. Ann Neurol 2007;61:435.

SECTION III

CLINICAL DISORDERS

I. PARKINSONIAN STATES: PARKINSON'S DISEASE

CHAPTER 9

Genetics of Parkinson's Disease and Parkinsonian Disorders

Andrew B. West

▶ INTRODUCTION TO THE GENETICS OF PARKINSON DISEASE

Parkinson's disease (PD) is the second most common neurodegenerative disease, with some estimates suggesting over one million Americans suffering with symptoms. The pathological hallmark of PD that gives rise to the trademark motor complications is the loss of melanized tyrosine-hydroxylase-positive dopaminergic neurons in the substantia nigra pars compacta. The fundamental mechanisms underlying the loss of this indispensable nucleus of neurons remain largely a mystery. Additional lesions and cell loss likewise occur in many regions throughout the central and peripheral nervous system, probably responsible for the diverse and debilitating non-motor symptoms associated with the disease.[1,2]

PHENOTYPES OF PARKINSONISM

PD is a complex disease with variable clinical presentation. Although an idea of what typical late-onset PD encompasses, both clinically and pathologically, has formed over the last century, it is likely that PD and related disorders encompass a number of distinct but overlapping etiologies.[3] This spectrum includes many cases that can be said to suffer with parkinsonism but not necessarily PD. In most cases the approach used to separate these different phenotypes is clinical assessment, an imperfect tool at best. As this chapter delves into the molecular genetics of PD and closely related disorders, it is critically important to recognize that what is currently classified as "PD" may include diseases of different origins and causes. Ultimately, an accurate classification may demand identification of the specific cause(s) of disease, and genetic-based approaches are likely to play a central role in the development of better diagnostic approaches.

The goal of this chapter is to highlight advances in human genetic studies with the goal of placing each seminal study into a conceptual framework whereby appropriate future downstream studies, derived from criteria clearly justified from human genetic studies, can be designed for clarifying disease etiology and the development of a cure.

▶ HISTORICAL BACKGROUND OF PD GENETICS

For much of the 20th century, PD was regarded as the archetypal neurodegenerative disorder with little or no genetic cause of disease. Indeed, most PD patients seen in modern movement disorder clinics do not report a family history of disease, in contrast to other rarer movement disorders such as Huntington's disease and frontal–temporal dementia. In James Parkinson's initial descriptions of the disease, a familial component was not mentioned, in line with Charcot's testament that "paralysis agitans is not a family disease."[4] Nevertheless, descriptions of families that pass disease from one generation to the next have been described since shortly after the recognition of PD as a distinct clinical entity.

DISCOVERIES OF PD KINDREDS

PD kindreds were described by Gowers, and later Mjönes, among others, but these kindreds harbored a disease with comorbidities not usually associated with sporadic PD, and hence characterized as a "Parkinson's plus syndrome," or other variable nomenclature that typically includes the term parkinsonism as opposed to PD (see Fig. 9–1). These families often pass a highly penetrant mutation compatible with Mendelian autosomal-dominant inheritance. Considering the lack of diagnostic and pathological tools available at the time, the controversy centered on whether these kindreds possessed enough phenotypic overlap to be considered related to typical late-onset PD, and intra-familial variability in disease presentation further confounded the analysis. In general, many of these large kindreds with apparent autosomal dominant inheritance are marked by early-onset akinetic-rigid disease

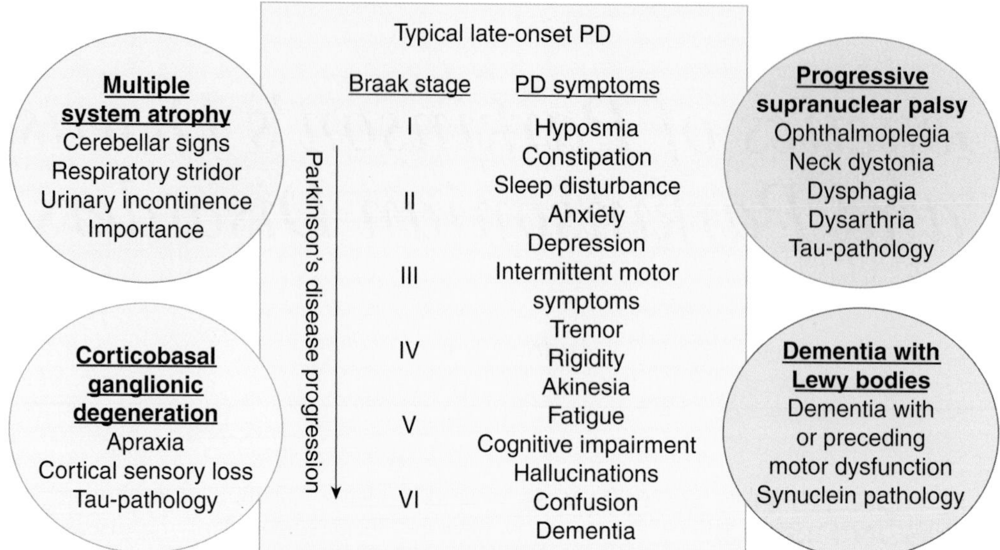

Figure 9–1. Symptoms commonly associated with typical late-onset PD are indicated in a chronological progression together with proposed Braak pathological staging, where Braak stage I precedes motor symptoms but might correlate with hyposmia and constipation, for example. Most genetic studies require a diagnosis that includes motor symptoms (e.g., resting tremor, rigidity, bradykinesia) that are generally thought to occur in the mid-stages of disease, and hence early stage disease is often missed. Disorders generally thought as distinct from typical PD are defined by characteristic symptoms not associated with typical PD (e.g., early dementia in DLB, or ophthalmoplegia in PSP) and are less frequent in the population than symptoms associated with PD, although parkinsonian features (listed as PD symptoms in this figure) often accompany these disorders, hence the term Parkinson's plus syndromes (PPS). Familial PD encompasses widely variable phenotypes, even within the same family and due to the same mutation. Human genetic studies are helping to refine etiology and separate symptoms and diseases that might have distinct origins.

and accompanied by a variety of additional characteristics, including early cognitive disturbance. Although the molecular defects responsible for a number of these kindreds have been discovered, the issue of whether these forms of parkinsonism share the same etiology as sporadic PD is still largely an open question, and has not been clarified to a great degree even by modern genetic and pathologic studies.

▶ EARLY MOLECULAR GENETIC STUDIES: THE CONTURSI KINDRED

Substantial advances in the study of PD genetics were made in the 1980s and 1990s. Through the development of large movement disorder centers where astute clinical observations were coupled with more detailed patient histories, additional large kindreds became available for analysis. At the same time, major advances in the methods for molecular genetics and linkage analysis were occurring.

A key development was the analysis of a large Italian–American family called the "Contursi kindred." This family was exceptional in the number of affected and unaffected cases across several generations available for genetic studies. As with other kindreds with inherited forms of parkinsonism, the affected individuals have a complex phenotype, typically demonstrating early-onset disease accompanied by features of dementia with Lewy bodies (DLB). However, the symptoms in the Contursi kindred also demonstrate remarkable intra-familial variability, with age of disease onset ranging from 18 to 81 years.[5] Using linkage analysis, a large region of chromosome 4p14 was associated with disease. Of the genes present at the disease locus, one was an obvious choice for further study: alpha-synuclein. This protein had previously been associated with the pathological structures in Alzheimer's disease (AD) plaques. A non-synonymous missense mutation was detected in the alpha-synuclein gene in affected individuals from the Contursi kindred but not in unaffected individuals, and the clear segregation of the mutation through the family suggested the pathogenicity of this variant (or one in complete disequilibrium nearby) within reasonable doubt.[6] Interestingly, the family that Mjönes described in 1949 was later found to also have mutations in the alpha-synuclein gene.[7]

EVIDENCE FOR INHERITANCE OF PD FROM TWIN STUDIES

Analysis of twin siblings is a classical method to discern inheritance of disease, and the comparative analysis of monozygotic (MZ) and dizygotic (DZ) pairs is often used to analyze the comparative effects of genetics and environment. In PD, early twin studies demonstrated no significant difference in the rate of PD between MZ and DZ twins,[8,9] suggesting that genetic variability might not play a significant role in disease susceptibility. Thus, for the majority of the 20th century, the available evidence largely supported the view that heredity does not play a role in the etiology of PD.

As the understanding of PD as a progressive neurodegenerative disorder improved and it became clear that cell loss in the substantia nigra might precede clinical symptoms by many years, it was recognized that the original twin studies may be confounded by twin pairs with preclinical disease (e.g., a lack of obvious tremor and/or motor complications) coupled with variability at age of disease onset. Follow-up studies were conducted using imaging technology capable of measuring dopaminergic input in the nigral–striatal pathway. These studies revealed that in MZ twin pairs where one twin had PD, the clinically unaffected siblings in fact frequently had significant loss of dopamine in the striatum, indicative of preclinical disease.[10–12] These results were augmented by very large-scale studies in twin registries, which suggested that an increased risk of clinical PD was in fact detectable among younger onset MZ twins.[13] Collectively, these more modern twin studies have provided clear evidence for a genetic contribution to the etiology of at least some cases of typical PD.

▶ MENDELIAN PARKINSONISM

With the discovery of alpha-synuclein, the first genetic variant causative for parkinsonism, a renewed interest gripped the field of PD genetics. It is important to understand the limits of current methodology: for linkage analysis approaches, DNA derived from a minimum of four or five affected individuals from one family are usually necessary for a chance at detecting disease loci of manageable size. Given the late-onset nature of PD and rarity of familial disease, there are relatively few families available for genetic analysis. However, through the dedication of clinicians and geneticists and their teams of scientists, a tremendous amount of effort has resulted in the collection of dozens of families around the world that fulfill criteria for possible linkage analysis and discovery of Mendelian PD genes. Alleles that segregate with parkinsonism in families, even when a specific gene or mutation has not yet been identified, are designated as *PARK* loci, nominated by clinicians and geneticists.

Currently, 13 *PARK* loci have been defined, although not all *PARK* loci are as clearly linked to typical late-onset PD as others. Mutations in five of these genes have proven pathogenicity defined by extensive segregation analyses in multiple families. The evidence for the involvement of the remaining eight *PARK* loci is at present incomplete, and it is possible, indeed likely, that some of the remaining loci are erroneously assigned or have no direct relevance to PD pathogenesis. Most *PARK* loci can be split into dominant or recessive disease modalities (see Table 9–1).

AUTOSOMAL-DOMINANT DISEASE

PARK1 and *PARK4*: Alpha-Synuclein

The *PARK1* locus encodes the alpha-synuclein gene. The *PARK1* locus has been studied extensively, and mutations in this locus are quite rare. An A53T mutation was found in the Contursi kindred, and causes a highly penetrant early-onset parkinsonism with several cases displaying features of DLB. Outside of the Contursi kindred, the vast majority of individuals with PD do not possess coding mutations in alpha-synuclein, although missense mutations in several other families beside the Contursi kindred have been described, including an A30P mutation and an E46K mutation.[14,15] Autosomal-dominant inheritance of disease in these families with alpha-synuclein point mutations suggests toxic "gain of function" mechanisms, whereby alpha-synuclein gains a toxic property when mutated. The exact nature of this property remains obscure.

Additional support for the key role of alpha-synuclein in parkinsonism came from the discovery of the *PARK4* locus. Originally thought to be a separate gene, surprisingly, this "locus" in fact turned out to be a gene multiplication of alpha-synuclein, leading to increased expression of the normal alpha-synuclein protein. Thus, an exotic "gain of function" is not required; rather, simple overexpression of normal alpha-synuclein is sufficient for early-onset parkinsonism.[16]

Nearly concurrent with the identification of mutations in alpha-synuclein in families with parkinsonism, biochemical studies using PD-affected brain tissue demonstrated that alpha-synuclein protein was the major protein constituent forming Lewy body structures.[17,18] This was true of sporadic cases, with typical PD features and no family history, and redefined the classification of PD as a *synucleinopathy*. This approach emphasizes the central role of the alpha-synuclein gene and protein in pathogenic mechanisms. It has also led to a reexamination of the pathology of PD and revealed a much more extensive pattern of pathology than previously appreciated.[2]

These genetic studies would seem to point to alpha-synuclein as a target of therapy for PD, but it presents several challenges. The protein possesses a natively unfolded structure reminiscent of a small protein chaperone and is therefore not an ideal drug target or

▶ **TABLE 9–1. PARK LOCI AND GENES LINKED TO FAMILIAL PD**

Locus	Location	Gene	Inheritance	Clinical Phenotype	Response to L-Dopa	Pathology
PARK1 and PARK4	4q21	*α-synuclein*	AD	Early-onset PD, dementia common (DLB)	Good	Extensive LBs beyond typical PD, SNpc loss
PARK2	6q25	*parkin*	Usually AR	Juvenile and early-onset PD, relative benign course of disease	Good	Profound loss of SNpc neurons, often without LBs
PARK3	2p13	Unknown	AD	Late-onset PD, some dementia	Good	Unknown
PARK5	4p14	*UchL1*	Unclear	Late-onset PD (only two patients described)	Good	Unknown
PARK 6	1p36	*PINK1*	AR	Early-onset PD	Good	Unknown
PARK7	1p36	*DJ-1*	AR	Early-onset PD	Good	Unknown
PARK8	12q12	*LRRK2*	AD	Typical late-onset PD	Good	Typical LB and SNpc loss, some familial variation
PARK9	1p36	*ATP13A2*	AR	Kufor–Rakeb syndrome, dominant pyramidal signs	Fair	Unknown
PARK10	1p32	Unknown	Possible susceptibility gene for PD	Not applicable Late-onset population	Not applicable	Not applicable
PARK11	2q36-37	*GIGYF2*	Unclear	Early and late-onset PD	Good	Unknown
PARK12	Xq21-25	Unknown	Possible susceptibility gene for PD	Not applicable Familial PD	Not applicable	Not applicable
PARK13	2p12	*HTRA2*	Unclear	Late-onset PD	Good	Unknown

AR = Autosomal-recessive, AD = Autosomal Dominant, LB = Lewy bodies,

part of an obvious pathway modifiable by therapeutics. Producing models of alpha-synuclein toxicity has proved challenging. The formation of alpha-synuclein aggregates is protective in some models while detrimental in others, leaving fundamental questions about the role of alpha-synuclein in cell death largely unanswered.[19] In whole animal models, neither mutations of alpha-synuclein nor overexpressions of the native protein have reliably recapitulated the PD phenotype, leaving an impression that additional models need to be developed.[20]

PARK8: Leucine-Rich Repeat Kinase 2

Characterization of a large Japanese family with late-onset PD led to the identification of the *PARK8* locus,[21] with missense mutations subsequently identified in conserved protein domains in the leucine-rich repeat kinase 2 (LRRK2) gene.[22,23] Screening for mutations in conserved enzymatic domains led to the identification of the most common known LRRK2 mutation, G2019S, occurring in the activation loop of the kinase domain.[24–26] As opposed to alpha-synuclein point mutations and multiplications that affect only a handful of PD-associated cases, LRRK2 mutations are responsible for 1–2% of typical late-onset sporadic PD and ~5% of PD compatible with dominant transmission in most Caucasian cohorts.

In some populations such as the Ashkenazi Jews and North African Arabs, the G2019S mutation causes 29% and 39% of late-onset PD, respectively.[25,27] In other Asian populations, LRRK2 mutations appear very rare. Due to the relatively high penetrance (compared with other genetic diseases) of LRRK2 mutations and the corresponding low frequency of LRRK2 mutations in control populations, LRRK2 is considered a Mendelian PD gene and not a susceptibility factor in most populations. Many genetic variants that cause changes in amino acid sequence have been identified in LRRK2 (see Table 9–2), but only a handful are considered pathogenic. Future animal models and biochemical assays may help further refine pathogenic versus benign genetic alterations.

In contrast to the other known Mendelian PD genes, LRRK2 mutations cause a late-onset disease similar or identical to late-onset sporadic PD in most cases.[28] Pathological analysis of LRRK2 cases shows overlap with typical PD with nigral cell loss and the formation of Lewy bodies. Interestingly, there is some variation in different populations, with the original Spanish and Japanese

▶ **TABLE 9–2. GENETIC VARIANTS WITHIN THE LRRK2 GENE**

Possible LRRK2 Mutations		
Missense Mutation	**Exon**	**Conserved domain**
E10K	1	LRRK2 repeats
A211V	5	LRRK2 repeats
E334K	8	LRRK2 repeats
K544V	13	LRRK2 repeats
M712V	17	Ankyrin-like
R793M	18	Ankyrin-like
Q930R	20	None
S973N	22	None
R1067Q	23	LRR
S1096C	23	LRR
Q1111H	23	LRR
L1114L	23	LRR
L1122V	24	LRR
A1151T	24	LRR
L1165P	24	LRR
I1192V	25	LRR
S1228T	26	LRR
R1325Q	28	GTPase
K1468E	30	GTPase
R1483Q	30	GTPase
R1514Q	31	GTPase
P1542S	31	COR
V1613A	33	COR
R1628P	33	COR
R1728L/H	35	COR
L1795F	36	COR
M1869T/V	37	COR
R1941H	39	Kinase
Y2006H	40	Kinase
I2012T	40	Kinase
T2031S	40	Kinase
N2081D	41	Kinase
T2141M	43	Kinase
R2143H	43	Kinase
Y2189C	43	WD-40 like
T2356I	47	WD-40 like
V2390M	47	WD-40 like
M2397T	48	WD-40 like
L2466H	49	WD-40 like
Pathogenic LRRK2 Mutations		
Missense Mutation	**Exon**	**Conserved domain**
R1441C	30	GTPase
R1441G	30	GTPase
R1441H	30	GTPase
Y1699C	34	COR
G2019S	40	Kinase
I2020T	40	Kinase
Variant Associated with PD		
G2385R	47	WD-40 like

kindreds with LRRK2 mutations showing marked clinical and pathological divergence from typical PD.

LRRK2 may be an important target for the therapy of PD. Since LRRK2 is a protein kinase and part of the proteome is considered modifiable by small molecules, LRRK2 itself may represent a robust therapeutic target for disease intervention. This view is supported by the observation that several of the most common mutant forms of LRRK2 seem to have increased kinase activity. Thus, inhibitors of LRRK2 may be beneficial in these genetic forms of PD. Because of the high frequency of LRRK2 mutations and sheer number of identified individuals with mutations, sometimes in presymptomatic cases, it is feasible to assemble cohorts with LRRK2 mutation for longitudinal studies and clinical trials. It is, however, unclear at this point what role the LRRK2 protein plays in sporadic PD, and whether an inhibitor of LRRK2 activity would be beneficial in individuals who do not have an LRRK2 mutation.

AUTOSOMAL-RECESSIVE DISEASE

PARK2: Parkin

The first recessive PD locus (*PARK2*) was mapped in a large Japanese family characterized by juvenile onset PD.[29] Although these patients had levodopa-responsive parkinsonism, pathological analysis showed dramatic depletion of SNpc cells without the overt presence of Lewy bodies. Amplification of microsatellite markers near the MnSOD gene identified probands with homozygous deletions, and fine mapping identified large genomic deletions segregating with disease in a large previously undescribed gene the investigators dubbed "parkin." Follow-up analysis demonstrated that mutations in parkin are the major cause of juvenile-onset PD, and the most common known cause of early-onset PD.[30] Whole-genome scans reveal that parkin genetic variability is uniquely linked to early-onset PD, and there is no single clinical feature that delineates patients with mutations from early-onset patients without mutations.[31]

Parkin mutations range from single base pair deletions in coding exons to deletions spanning over a million base pairs, often coupled in the heterozygous state with missense mutations in conserved domains.[32] It is not known why the *PARK2* locus and the parkin gene are hotspots for recombination events and mutations. The parkin gene is one of the largest genes in the human genome, despite encoding a protein of average size, and comprises much of a common fragile site identified in cancer research.[33] The mechanism by which parkin mutation leads to disease is almost certainly "loss of function." Large and small deletions and insertions destabilize the mRNA transcript, while point mutations cause solubility and protein stability problems.[34] Heterozygous single parkin mutations have been described in patients with PD, although their role in disease causation remains uncertain. They may represent a susceptibility factor for disease or may simply be coincidental with disease.[35]

The pathological effects of parkin mutations remain inconclusive since less than 10 cases have been available for postmortem analysis; fewer than five cases are described with any depth in the literature. Initial postmortem descriptions in the Japanese juvenile-onset PD cases suggest nigral degeneration without the formation of Lewy bodies. Similar to alpha-synuclein, mouse modeling of the effects of parkin mutations has not revealed the function of parkin in a straightforward way, but several lines of evidence are converging on the idea that parkin participates in the health of mitochondria in some fashion.[36]

PARK6 (PINK1) and *PARK7* (DJ-1)

The PARK6 and PARK7 loci are rare causes of autosomal-recessive parkinsonism. In families with a recessive pattern of inheritance, linkage analysis and positional cloning approaches identified mutations in the PINK1 gene (*PARK6*),[37] and mutations in the DJ-1 gene (*PARK7*).[38] Similar to parkin mutations, loss of function mutations that include deletions and nonsense mutations are common in PINK1- and DJ-1-associated families. Again similar to parkin mutations, mutations in PINK1 and DJ-1 cause early-onset parkinsonism, although neither PINK1 nor DJ-1 cases have been available for postmortem analysis. Thus, a definitive assessment of overlap between PINK1 and DJ-1 cases and other forms of parkinsonism awaits further study and the opportunity to examine directly the effects of these mutations on brain pathology.

PINK1 protein contains a canonical mitochondrial localization signal and appears to function downstream of parkin in the maintenance of mitochondria, at least in invertebrate animal model systems.[39,40] DJ-1 appears to function in oxidative stress-sensitive pathways, and is similar to all other Mendelian PD genes in that expression is not restricted to the brain or neurons affected in PD. Loss of expression of these genes and their protein products (parkin, DJ-1, and PINK1) seems well tolerated in most cells in the body, with the exception of those capable of generating parkinsonism phenotypes in humans. Functional studies involving the recessive Mendelian PD genes might help uncover biochemical pathways important for PD or at least important for neurons susceptible to PD pathobiology, even though patients harboring the recessive mutations have divergent phenotypes from typical late-onset PD.

OTHER PARK LOCI

Recessive mutations in the ATP13A2 gene have been described in patients with early-onset parkinsonism with spasticity and dementia.[41] Although this was assigned to the PARK9 locus, the clinical features differ enough from typical sporadic PD that controversy has developed as to whether this is in fact a gene for parkinsonism, or best considered as a different disorder. There is at present no clear evidence for the involvement of PARK9 in typical late-onset PD.

In candidate screening approaches, a missense mutation was identified in a sib pair in the UCH-L1 gene,[42] and this mutation has not been identified in other affected or control individuals. This sib pair is the only known example of familial disease linked to this locus, and controversy around UCH-L1 as a PARK locus revolves around whether pathogenicity and causation can be proven without convincing familial segregation evidence. Rare coding mutations identified in candidate screening approaches are now commonplace events in high-throughput sequencing projects, and poor evidence of pathogenicity. On the other hand, another non-synonymous variant S18Y within the gene demonstrated a modest association with PD in meta-analysis studies,[43] but not in direct single studies that involve several thousand cases and controls.[44]

Mutations in the mouse Omi/HtrA2 gene underlie the motor neuron disease 2 (MND2) mutant mouse, and screening of this gene in a PD case and control population identified a non-synonymous alteration found in four PD patients but no controls .[45] This was assigned to the PARK13 locus, but follow-up screening in larger cohorts showed no difference in the frequency of this mutation in cases and controls.[46] Thus the genetic basis of Omi/HtrA2 involvement in PD remains tentative and awaits further study. Similarly, rare missense mutations in GIGYF2, described as the PARK11 locus, have been described,[47] although the association remains circumstantial.[48]

▶ GENETIC SUSCEPTIBILITIES IN PARKINSON'S DISEASE

Mutations in the known Mendelian PD genes likely account for only a small proportion of PD cases worldwide. Most cases of PD are sporadic and lack a clear family history. Genetic susceptibilities, or genetic risk factors, are variations in genes that modify the probability of developing disease, but are not directly causative. One hypothesis for the development of PD is that underlying genetic backgrounds combine with cellular events related to aging and exposure that initiate neurodegeneration in an apparent cascade through the nervous system. Understanding the genetic susceptibility component to PD may provide a straightforward approach to deciphering the rest of the puzzle.

The search for genetic risk factors for sporadic PD has grown in magnitude and scope in recent years. In the 1990s, PD case and control populations reported in the literature rarely involved more than a hundred cases and controls at individual institutes, and investigators were grossly underpowered to identify associations of low to moderate effect in disease. Recent studies and meta-analyses that involve thousands of PD patients and controls have helped clarify the role of genetic susceptibilities in PD and have identified both variation within the known Mendelian PD genes and pathways not previous indentified. It is important to note that despite the degree of effort invested, the effect size of most of the PD genetic risk factors identified so far is small. No single risk factor approaches the strength, for example, of the ApoE4 risk allele in AD, and thus if risk factors play an important role in the etiology of PD, they may do so in tandem with other genes or environmental triggers, rather than as single gene effects.

RISK FACTORS WITHIN THE *PARK* LOCI

Pathogenic mutations in the Mendelian PD genes lead directly to the development of parkinsonism, often of early onset and with atypical features. It is also possible for Mendelian PD genes to contain genetic variants that, in combination with other factors, may enhance PD risk, leading to late onset of typical disease. When a Mendelian PD gene is found, genetics laboratories with PD cases, controls, and extended kindreds initially screen for pathogenic mutations in newly described PD-associated (e.g., PARK loci) genes and inevitably identify common genetic variation present in both case and control populations. Sometimes, a particular genetic variant is overrepresented in cases versus controls, thereby highlighting a particular risk allele for PD susceptibility.

One of the first such instances of an association of variation in a PARK gene with late-onset PD involves the promoter region of the *PARK1* gene alpha-synuclein, where a particular length of a dinucleotide repeat structure upstream of the first exon is overrepresented in PD cases versus controls.[49] Follow-up studies suggest that single nucleotide polymorphisms (SNPs) in the 3′ UTR of alpha-synuclein likewise associate with PD.[50] Whether the variants themselves represent functional disease modifiers or the associated variants are in disequilibrium with other functional variants as part of a risk allele is difficult to discern without extensive functional and genetic studies. Nevertheless, common variation in alpha-synuclein consistently associated with disease susceptibility further places the alpha-synuclein gene as central to PD.

In contrast to alpha-synuclein, common genetic variation in *PARK8* (LRRK2) does not appear to modify risk for PD in Caucasian populations.[51] Some evidence for a LRRK2 non-synonymous variant G2385R overrepresented in some Asian PD cohorts suggests LRRK2 common variation may affect disease susceptibility.[52] Whether G2385R represents the functional variant responsible for disease susceptibility or the variant is in disequilibrium with other functional variants remains an open question.

Common variation in the *PARK2* locus and parkin gene has not faithfully demonstrated association with late-onset PD. Accounts of promoter variation associating with disease seem refined to particular populations,[53,54] and nonpathogenic non-synonymous coding variants are also not consistently associated with disease. The other recessive *PARK* loci encoding DJ-1 and PINK1 likewise do not contain common variation consistently associated with PD. Loss of function variation in the recessive PARK genes may be responsible for a significant proportion of early-onset disease, but the relationship to typical late-onset PD becomes hard to discern on a genetic level. Because of the lack of genetic variation associated with PD within the recessive Mendelian PD genes, coupled with the lack of clinical overlap between cases harboring mutations in these genes and typical sporadic PD, the etiological connection between recessive PD genes and typical PD remains unclear.

RISK FACTORS IN OTHER GENES

Genetic variation in the microtubule binding protein tau has been linked to PD risk. The gene for tau spans part of chromosome 17q21 that displays marked reduced recombination rates and unusually large blocks of disequilibrium. Tau protein is implicated in a number of neurodegenerative disorders such as AD, where intraneuronal tau-positive tangles correlate with clinical severity of disease. Mutations in tau that affect mRNA splicing and isoform production cause frontal–temporal dementia with parkinsonism.[55] SNPs within tau largely segregate into two haplotypes in humans dubbed H1 and H2 10072441. The H1 allele is overrepresented in PD cases versus controls, and detailed studies demonstrate that variations near the 5′ exons and promoter region show the strongest association with disease.[56–58]

The glucocerebrosidase gene (GBA) has also been implicated as a PD risk factor. Recessive loss of function mutation in GBA causes Gaucher disease, a lysosomal storage disorder. Similar to loss of function variation in the parkin gene that causes early-onset parkinsonism, a wide variety of mutations have been described in GBA that cause Gaucher disease, including point mutations, rearrangements, and deletions. The mechanism for genetic instability in the GBA locus is thought to arise from the presence of an inactive pseudo-GBA gene nearby the active and required GBA gene.[59] Thus, hyper-recombination events are likely spurred by nearby homologous sequences. Reports of patients with Gaucher disease with early-onset parkinsonism above and beyond what would be expected based on coincidence suggested a link between GBA and early-onset PD.[60] Based on these clinical observations, the GBA gene was screened for mutations in small cohorts of PD cases and controls. As with dominant missense mutations in the LRRK2 gene, the highest known frequencies of GBA mutations in PD cases versus controls are found in the Ashkenazi Jew population.[61] Larger late-onset PD populations demonstrate no significant difference in GBA mutations in cases versus controls.[62] In contrast, the limited available datasets show GBA mutations are enriched in early-onset parkinsonism populations.[63] Future studies are required for more definitive evidence of the involvement of GBA function in typical late-onset PD.

GENOME-WIDE ASSOCIATION STUDIES IN PD

In recent years, technological advances have provided the capability to study genetic variation on a genome-wide scale. The most widely used method relies on the assessment of hundreds of thousands of SNPs. Although the genetic variants that are directly assessed may not likely be causative for disease themselves (since they are, by definition, common genetic variants), they may provide insight into genetic variation that is pathogenic since the assessed variants may be in disequilibrium with variation of interest. The general requirement for the identification of variation that is significant on a genome-wide level is that disease-causing alleles have similar genetic backgrounds and that particular disease alleles possess modest to high effect sizes. Most genome-wide studies are different from standard linkage approaches in that they do not necessarily require extended families that pass disease from one generation to the next; rather, genome-wide studies usually require case and control series that number in thousands, to potentially tens of thousands of cases to have the power to detect associated genetic variation.

Initial genome-wide studies in PD have yet to yield new information about the genetic basis of disease. The first genome-wide study largely failed to identify any genetic variation significant on a genome-wide level, and the variants that showed a trend for association failed to replicate association in further studies.[64,65] Much larger studies have been undertaken, but they have for the most part confirmed the existing PARK loci and reinforced the idea that individual common genetic variants do not have a large role in causing sporadic PD. Future larger studies promise to identify associated variation of subtle effect as well as rare variants and effects operating in tandem with other factors in defining the role of heritability in PD.

▶ CONCLUSIONS

The identification of specific genes and individual genetic variants capable of causing the complex phenotype of PD are among the most important advances in PD research. They have provided important insight into the underlying disease mechanisms. The next challenge is to translate these discoveries into therapies for the disease. One of the fundamental problems with PD and other neurological disorders is the lack of successful models of disease where hypotheses might be generated and tested. Human genetics studies provide a foundation to move cellular and biochemical studies forward in a direction relevant to disease processes. Genetic variants that segregate with disease in large families provide the most straightforward and conclusive evidence of pathogenicity of particular genetic alterations.

The complex and varied phenotype of PD is a challenge for the studies of genetics of the disorders. If clinical criteria for PD relevance demands high similarity to typical late-onset disease in cases that carry mutations, only one Mendelian PD gene would qualify: LRRK2. The other genes might be considered parkinsonism-related or early-onset PD genes. But genetic data must be combined with pathological data in addition to clinical data, and since alpha-synuclein is the major protein component of Lewy bodies in PD, it must also be central for disease processes. A biochemical link between alpha-synuclein and LRRK2 has not been identified, but if one is found, it could represent a major advance in understanding PD.

Rare mutations in genes without conclusive evidence of familial segregation with disease still remain controversial in regard to relevance to the pathogenesis of PD. The so-called Mendelian genes (that demonstrate clear segregation) include alpha-synuclein, parkin, DJ-1, PINK1, and LRRK2. The conserved protein domains encoded within the PD genes associate with a wide range of cellular functions (see Fig. 9–2) and have presented challenges in the reconciliation of common pathways of disease. Mechanisms of vesicle release and transport, the ubiquitin proteasome pathway and protein turnover, mitochondrial function, oxidative stress, and signal transduction pathways have all been implicated through the study of these proteins. Of note, all genes encode proteins expressed in substantia nigra neurons, and most proteins demonstrate highest expression in neurons in the human brain, with the possible exception of DJ-1.

Apart from pathogenic mutations in Mendelian PD genes, genetic susceptibilities that involve more common variation in defining a genetic background with heightened risk for the development of PD also promise to reveal the molecular basis of disease. The most consistent and robust associations involve variants in the alpha-synuclein gene and the tau gene, and promising initial associations with rare GBA mutations. Both alpha-synuclein and tau have implications in a number of neurodegenerative disorders, including AD, MSA, PSP, FTDP-17, and others, and susceptibility studies

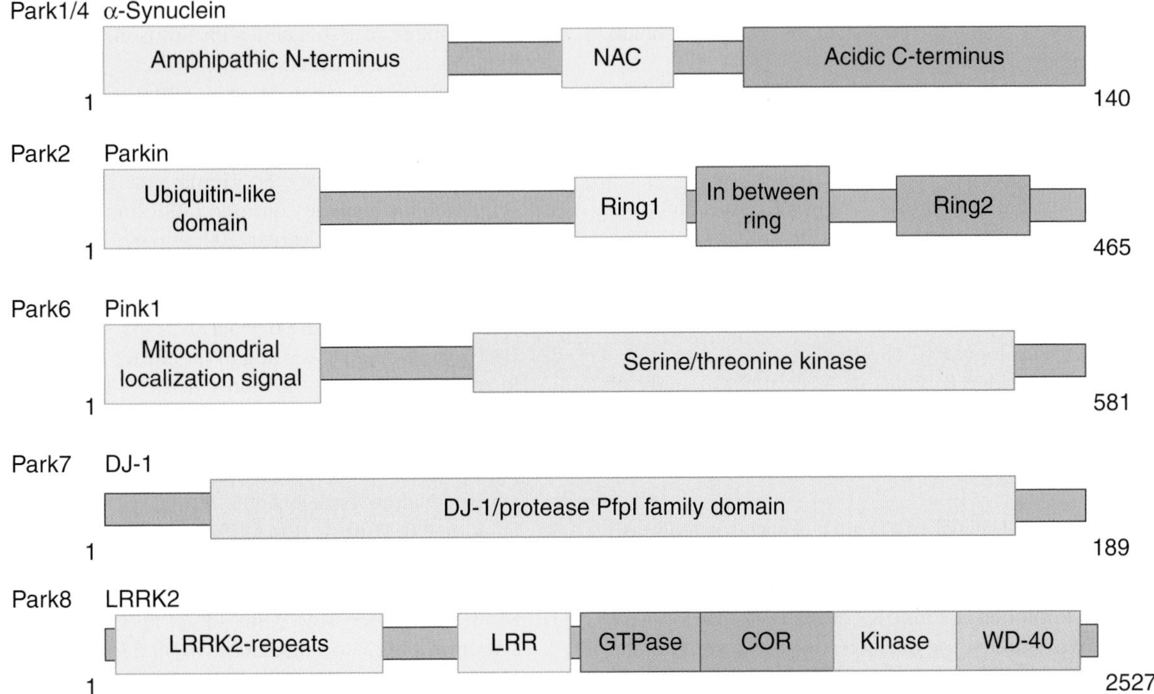

Figure 9–2. Conserved protein domains associated with the encoded proteins of the PARK family of genes. The number of amino acids that comprise each protein is listed at the terminus of each representation, and the size of each domain is not to scale. Alpha-synuclein encodes a small chaperone-like protein with structural similarities to the 14-3-3 family of proteins, and encodes a "non-amyloid component" found in senile plaques in AD. The parkin protein encodes a rare ubiquitin-like domain, unusual for RING domain (really interesting new gene) protein, and RING domain proteins often associate with E3-ligase proteins that function in ubiquitin-dependent pathways. The PINK1 protein encodes a canonical mitochondrial localization signal sequence that is cleaved inside mitochondria, together with a serine/threonine kinase domain. The proto-oncogene DJ-1 encodes an evolutionarily conserved domain similar to domains found in PfpI family proteins. Finally, the large LRRK2 protein encodes two conserved enzymatic domains, a GTPase domain, and a serine/threonine kinase domain, an unusual arrangement unique in mammals with the exception of the LRRK1 protein. Additionally, LRRK2 encodes a series of sequence repeats at the N-terminus, and other potential interaction and structure domains that include a leucine-rich-repeat domain, a c-terminal of RAS domain, and a WD-40-like domain. The diversity of the protein domains within the PARK proteins are difficult to reconcile into a single pathway, and suggest the possibility of distinct etiologies associated with each gene. The relationship between the activity of these proteins and typical late-onset PD is largely unknown.

that demonstrate the involvement of common variation in alpha-synuclein and tau in PD are not necessarily unexpected. However, tau tangles, which are typical of AD, are only rarely observed in PD, suggesting that the involvement of tau in PD-linked neurodegeneration is different from that which occurs in AD. The involvement of GBA mutations in PD are less well understood and more speculative, but have exciting implications for understanding novel aspects of PD pathogenesis.

It is possible that individual genes with the highest effect on PD susceptibility are already known, for example, LRRK2 and alpha-synuclein, but it seems just as likely that identification of major pathways and important genes will require technology not yet available and studies only now being conceived. The future of genetic research in PD will involve studies that genotype or completely sequence the genome of thousands to tens of thousands of cases and controls. With this large-scale effort, the hope is that we begin to uncover the tip of the iceberg in understanding the heritability of PD.

REFERENCES

1. Braak H, Del Tredici K. Neuroanatomy and pathology of sporadic Parkinson's disease. Adv Anat Embryol Cell Biol 2009;201:1.
2. Braak H, Ghebremedhin E, Rub U, et al. Stages in the development of Parkinson's disease-related pathology. Cell Tissue Res 2004;318:121.
3. Fahn S. Description of Parkinson's disease as a clinical syndrome. Ann N Y Acad Sci 2003;991:1.

4. Charcot JM. Lectures on the diseases of the nervous system. Translated by G Sigerson. Published by New Sydonham Society, London, England, 1877.
5. Golbe LI, Di Iorio G, Lazzarini A, et al. The Contursi kindred, a large family with autosomal dominant Parkinson's disease: Implications of clinical and molecular studies. Adv Neurol 1999;80:165.
6. Polymeropoulos MH, Lavedan C, Leroy E, et al. Mutation in the alpha-synuclein gene identified in families with Parkinson's disease. Science 1997;276:2045.
7. Fuchs J, Nilsson C, Kachergus J, et al. Phenotypic variation in a large Swedish pedigree due to SNCA duplication and triplication. Neurology 2007;68:916.
8. Duvoisin RC, Eldridge R, Williams A, et al. Twin study of Parkinson disease. Neurology 1981;31:77.
9. Ward CD, Duvoisin RC, Ince SE, et al. Parkinson's disease in 65 pairs of twins and in a set of quadruplets. Neurology 1983;33:815.
10. Burn DJ, Mark MH, Playford ED, et al. Parkinson's disease in twins studied with 18F-dopa and positron emission tomography. Neurology 1992;42:1894.
11. Laihinen A, Ruottinen H, Rinne JO, et al. Risk for Parkinson's disease: Twin studies for the detection of asymptomatic subjects using [18F]6-fluorodopa PET. J Neurol 2000;247 (suppl 2):II110.
12. Menza MA, Mark MH, Burn DJ, et al. Personality correlates of [18F]dopa striatal uptake: Results of positron-emission tomography in Parkinson's disease. J Neuropsychiatry Clin Neurosci 1995;7:176.
13. Tanner CM, Ottman R, Goldman S, et al. Parkinson Disease in twins; an etiologic study JAMA, 1999;281(4) 341–346. [PMD: 9929087]
14. Kruger R, Kuhn W, Muller T, et al. Ala30Pro mutation in the gene encoding alpha-synuclein in Parkinson's disease. Nat Genet 1998;18:106.
15. Zarranz JJ, Alegre J, Gomez-Esteban JC, et al. The new mutation, E46K, of alpha-synuclein causes Parkinson and Lewy body dementia. Ann Neurol 2004;55:164.
16. Singleton AB, Farrer M, Johnson J, et al. Alpha-synuclein locus triplication causes Parkinson's disease. Science 2003; 302:841.
17. Spillantini MG, Crowther RA, Jakes R, et al. Alpha-synuclein in filamentous inclusions of Lewy bodies from Parkinson's disease and dementia with Lewy bodies. Proc Natl Acad Sci U S A 1998;95:6469.
18. Spillantini MG, Schmidt ML, Lee VM, et al. Alpha-synuclein in Lewy bodies. Nature 1997;388:839.
19. Waxman EA, Giasson BI. Molecular mechanisms of alpha-synuclein neurodegeneration. Biochim Biophys Acta 2009; 1792(7):616–624.
20. Melrose HL, Lincoln SJ, Tyndall GM, et al. Parkinson's disease: A rethink of rodent models. Exp Brain Res 2006;173:196.
21. Funayama M, Hasegawa K, Kowa H, et al. A new locus for Parkinson's disease (PARK8) maps to chromosome 12p11.2-q13.1. Ann Neurol 2002;51:296.
22. Zimprich A, Biskup S, Leitner P, et al. Mutations in LRRK2 cause autosomal-dominant parkinsonism with pleomorphic pathology. Neuron 2004;44:601.
23. Paisan-Ruiz C, Jain S, Evans EW, et al. Cloning of the gene containing mutations that cause PARK8-linked Parkinson's disease. Neuron 2004;44:595.
24. Di Fonzo A, Rohe CF, Ferreira J, et al. A frequent LRRK2 gene mutation associated with autosomal dominant Parkinson's disease. Lancet 2005;365:412.
25. Lesage S, Durr A, Tazir M, et al. LRRK2 G2019S as a cause of Parkinson's disease in North African Arabs. N Engl J Med 2006;354:422.
26. Nichols WC, Pankratz N, Hernandez D, et al. Genetic screening for a single common LRRK2 mutation in familial Parkinson's disease. Lancet 2005;365:410.
27. Ozelius LJ, Senthil G, Saunders-Pullman R, et al. LRRK2 G2019S as a cause of Parkinson's disease in Ashkenazi Jews. N Engl J Med 2006;354:424.
28. Biskup S, West AB. Zeroing in on LRRK2-linked pathogenic mechanisms in Parkinson's disease. Biochim Biophys Acta 2009;1792(7):625–633.
29. Kitada T, Asakawa S, Hattori N, et al. Mutations in the parkin gene cause autosomal recessive juvenile parkinsonism. Nature 1998;392:605.
30. Lucking CB, Durr A, Bonifati V, et al. Association between early-onset Parkinson's disease and mutations in the parkin gene. N Engl J Med 2000;342:1560.
31. Scott WK, Nance MA, Watts RL, et al. Complete genomic screen in Parkinson disease: Evidence for multiple genes. JAMA 2001;286:2239.
32. West AB, Maidment NT. Genetics of parkin-linked disease. Hum Genet 2004;114:327.
33. West AB, Dawson VL, Dawson TM. To die or grow: Parkinson's disease and cancer. Trends Neurosci 2005; 28:348.
34. Sriram SR, Li X, Ko HS, et al. Familial-associated mutations differentially disrupt the solubility, localization, binding and ubiquitination properties of parkin. Hum Mol Genet 2005;14:2571.
35. West A, Periquet M, Lincoln S, et al. Complex relationship between Parkin mutations and Parkinson disease. Am J Med Genet 2002;114:584.
36. Dodson MW, Guo M. Pink1, Parkin, DJ-1 and mitochondrial dysfunction in Parkinson's disease. Curr Opin Neurobiol 2007;17:331.
37. Valente EM, Abou-Sleiman PM, Caputo V, et al. Hereditary early-onset Parkinson's disease caused by mutations in PINK1. Science 2004;304:1158.
38. Bonifati V, Rizzu P, van Baren MJ, et al. Mutations in the DJ-1 gene associated with autosomal recessive early-onset parkinsonism. Science 2003;299:256.
39. Poole AC, Thomas RE, Andrews LA, et al. The PINK1/Parkin pathway regulates mitochondrial morphology. Proc Natl Acad Sci U S A 2008;105:1638.
40. Deng H, Dodson MW, Huang H, et al. The Parkinson's disease genes pink1 and parkin promote mitochondrial fission and/or inhibit fusion in Drosophila. Proc Natl Acad Sci U S A 2008;105:14503.
41. Ramirez A, Heimbach A, Grundemann J, et al. Hereditary parkinsonism with dementia is caused by mutations in ATP13A2, encoding a lysosomal type 5 P-type ATPase. Nat Genet 2006;38:1184.
42. Leroy E, Boyer R, Auburger G, et al. The ubiquitin pathway in Parkinson's disease. Nature 1998;395:451.
43. Maraganore DM, Lesnick TG, Elbaz A, et al. UCHL1 is a Parkinson's disease susceptibility gene. Ann Neurol 2004; 55:512.

44. Hutter CM, Samii A, Factor SA, et al. Lack of evidence for an association between UCHL1 S18Y and Parkinson's disease. Eur J Neurol 2008;15:134.
45. Strauss KM, Martins LM, Plun-Favreau H, et al. Loss of function mutations in the gene encoding Omi/HtrA2 in Parkinson's disease. Hum Mol Genet 2005;14:2099.
46. Simon-Sanchez J, Singleton AB. Sequencing analysis of OMI/HTRA2 shows previously reported pathogenic mutations in neurologically normal controls. Hum Mol Genet 2008;17:1988.
47. Lautier C, Goldwurm S, Durr A, et al. Mutations in the GIGYF2 (TNRC15) gene at the PARK11 locus in familial Parkinson disease. Am J Hum Genet 2008;82:822.
48. Bras J, Simon-Sanchez J, Federoff M, et al. Lack of replication of association between GIGYF2 variants and Parkinson disease. Hum Mol Genet 2009;18:341.
49. Maraganore DM, de Andrade M, Elbaz A, et al. Collaborative analysis of alpha-synuclein gene promoter variability and Parkinson disease. JAMA 2006;296:661.
50. Myhre R, Toft M, Kachergus J, et al. Multiple alpha-synuclein gene polymorphisms are associated with Parkinson's disease in a Norwegian population. Acta Neurol Scand 2008;118:320.
51. Biskup S, Mueller JC, Sharma M, et al. Common variants of LRRK2 are not associated with sporadic Parkinson's disease. Ann Neurol 2005;58:905.
52. Funayama M, Li Y, Tomiyama H, et al. Leucine-rich repeat kinase 2 G2385R variant is a risk factor for Parkinson disease in Asian population. Neuroreport 2007;18:273.
53. Tan EK, Puong KY, Chan DK, et al. Impaired transcriptional upregulation of Parkin promoter variant under oxidative stress and proteasomal inhibition: Clinical association. Hum Genet 2005;118:484.
54. West AB, Maraganore D, Crook J, et al. Functional association of the parkin gene promoter with idiopathic Parkinson's disease. Hum Mol Genet 2002;11:2787.
55. Hutton M, Lendon CL, Rizzu P, et al. Association of missense and 5′-splice-site mutations in tau with the inherited dementia FTDP-17. Nature 1998;393:702.
56. Tobin JE, Latourelle JC, Lew MF, et al. Haplotypes and gene expression implicate the MAPT region for Parkinson disease: The gene PD study. Neurology 2008; 71:28.
57. Skipper L, Wilkes K, Toft M, et al. Linkage disequilibrium and association of MAPT H1 in Parkinson disease. Am J Hum Genet 2004;75:669.
58. Kwok JB, Teber ET, Loy C, et al. Tau haplotypes regulate transcription and are associated with Parkinson's disease. Ann Neurol 2004;55:329.
59. Winfield SL, Tayebi N, Martin BM, et al. Identification of three additional genes contiguous to the glucocerebrosidase locus on chromosome 1q21: Implications for Gaucher disease. Genome Res 1997;7:1020.
60. Bembi B, Zambito Marsala S, Sidransky E, et al. Gaucher's disease with Parkinson's disease: Clinical and pathological aspects. Neurology 2003;61:99.
61. Gan-Or Z, Giladi N, Rozovski U, et al. Genotype-phenotype correlations between GBA mutations and Parkinson disease risk and onset. Neurology 2008;70:2277.
62. Toft M, Pielsticker L, Ross OA, et al. Glucocerebrosidase gene mutations and Parkinson disease in the Norwegian population. Neurology 2006;66:415.
63. Clark LN, Ross BM, Wang Y, et al. Mutations in the glucocerebrosidase gene are associated with early-onset Parkinson disease. Neurology 2007;69:1270.
64. Evangelou E, Maraganore DM, Ioannidis JP. Meta-analysis in genome-wide association datasets: Strategies and application in Parkinson disease. PLoS ONE 2007; 2:e196.
65. Maraganore DM, de Andrade M, Lesnick TG, et al. High-resolution whole-genome association study of Parkinson disease. Am J Hum Genet 2005;77:685.

CHAPTER 10

Epidemiology of Parkinson's Disease

Connie Marras and Caroline M. Tanner

▶ INTRODUCTION

Epidemiologic investigation plays an important role in health planning, by providing estimates of disease frequency, including regional and temporal variations. In the 1950s, Kurland and his colleagues[1] in Rochester, Minnesota, and Gudmundsson[2] in Iceland provided the first community-based estimates of Parkinson's disease (PD) prevalence, finding it to be one of the most common neurodegenerative disorders of the elderly. This chapter reviews the worldwide incidence and prevalence of PD and provides the reader with tools for interpreting such studies.

Epidemiology is also a powerful method for investigating disease etiology. Observational studies have revealed numerous factors that are associated, positively or negatively, with the occurrence of PD. These associations include both environmental and genetic factors. Prevailing thought as to whether genetic or environmental factors are more important in causing PD has fluctuated multiple times since PD was first described in 1817.[3] The etiology remains largely unknown, and this may reflect a complex interaction of environmental and genetic factors that combine to cause disease. These factors could also vary from individual to individual or population to population. Epidemiologic studies thus continue to be a cornerstone of our search for the determinant(s) of PD. We review the associations, both direct and indirect, of PD with demographic and environmental factors. We also consider familial factors, as these have been revealed using observational study designs. First, we emphasize some methodologic considerations important to the interpretation of this continually expanding literature.

DIAGNOSTIC CONSIDERATIONS

The diagnosis of PD is currently based on clinical examination. The cardinal signs of PD (bradykinesia, resting tremor, cogwheel rigidity, and postural reflex impairment) are not unique to PD, but are seen in several possibly related but clinically distinct disorders such as progressive supranuclear palsy, multiple system atrophy, or diffuse Lewy body disease. Particularly early in the course, clinical distinction among these disorders is difficult. The overlap in clinical features between multiple disorders that do not have premortem biological markers creates a challenge for epidemiologic studies. Attempts to discover the determinants of disease will be confounded if samples of "cases" include patients with clinically similar disorders but with different risk factors. In one series, 20% of cases diagnosed in life as having PD had some other diagnosis, usually some form of atypical parkinsonism, at autopsy.[4] Because cases in which the clinical diagnosis is in question are more likely to be referred for autopsy, this rate is likely higher than would be found if all cases could be evaluated pathologically.[5] Nonetheless, these results highlight the possibility that some cases of atypical parkinsonism may be erroneously diagnosed as PD. Inclusion of these cases in etiologic studies may obscure an association between risk factors and PD. In epidemiologic studies, the frequency of PD will be overestimated. Also, their inclusion in genetic studies may lead to erroneous conclusions about the contribution of heredity. As PD is a relatively uncommon disorder, and most studies are based on relatively small numbers of cases, the error introduced by misclassification can be significant.

Imaging (positron emission tomography [PET] or single photon emission tomography and ultrasound) may help to confirm the diagnosis in some; however, the interpretation of borderline or normal scans is still under some debate.[6] Moreover, these techniques are not widely available and are too expensive for use in large-scale epidemiologic studies. Investigations of the value of neuroimaging as part of staged screening in populations are underway.[7,8]

There are currently several different sets of clinical diagnostic criteria that are commonly used,[9,10] and none has perfect accuracy. Estimates of disease frequency will vary according to the diagnostic criteria used. For example, a study using the presence of parkinsonism as the only diagnostic criterion for PD will likely include many persons with other disorders. Strict diagnostic criteria, therefore, are desirable to ensure homogeneity of a study sample, but often are difficult to employ, particularly in a retrospective fashion.

While diagnostic criteria are not uniformly applied in contemporary studies of PD, differences in case ascertainment and diagnosis were even greater in the past. Studies including secondary cases of parkinsonism such as postencephalitic, vascular, or drug-induced parkinsonism were common.[1,2,11,12]

As genetic factors associated with the development of parkinsonism are elucidated, further challenges in classification arise. In recent years, gene mutations associated with phenotypes very similar and in some cases indistinguishable from classical PD have been identified.[13] In the case of mutations of the gene encoding alpha-synuclein, the associated pathology is consistent with classical PD.[14] However, in the majority of pathologically examined cases of PD associated with mutations of the *parkin* gene the characteristic Lewy bodies of PD are not found.[15,16] Pathological examination of cases of PD associated with *LRRK2* mutations have shown considerable heterogeneity; cases both with and without Lewy body pathology have been reported.[17] This creates a challenging problem of classification, as the degree to which a genetically defined subset is distinct from the original clinically defined disorder is unclear. To date, genetic mutations have been found to account for a minority of cases of PD in most populations. Mutations in the *LRRK2* gene are most common. In North America, 1–2% of PD cases have *LRRK2* gene mutations, but in North Africa and the Middle East, as many as 30% of PD cases may be due to this mutation.[18]

Genetic testing has not been a routine part of epidemiologic studies. As the genetic heterogeneity of "PD" is revealed, however, epidemiologic studies can be limited to specific genetically defined entities. Environmental or genetic modifying factors that were previously obscured could become evident if environmental factors influencing the penetrance and/or expression of each genetic form of parkinsonism are different. Genetic differences between patients may determine susceptibility to individual environmental factors, or may influence clinical features such as age of onset or severity. Studies of genetically homogeneous subsets will require large populations. In most cases, this will involve multicenter, international collaborations.

CONSIDERATIONS IN RISK FACTOR ASSESSMENT

Risk factor assessment can be affected by the diagnostic difficulties aforementioned, by the uncertain length of a presymptomatic period, and by the fact that PD is a disorder of late life and relatively rare. The clinical manifestations of PD may be preceded by a long "latent" stage.[19] The existence of presymptomatic PD is suggested by the finding of reduced striatal fluorodopa uptake consistent with degeneration of nigrostriatal pathways in asymptomatic individuals who later have developed symptoms of PD.[20,21] The finding of Lewy bodies in the brains of persons not known to have clinical evidence of PD during life lends further support to the concept of a presymptomatic period. "Incidental Lewy bodies" and clinical PD are both age-related phenomena.[22,23] Recent clinical and pathological studies suggest that parkinsonism may be a late manifestation of a chronic process beginning with symptoms of autonomic dysfunction (constipation, urinary symptoms), sleep disorders (REM sleep behavior disorder, excessive daytime sleepiness) or olfactory deficits.[24–27] If this is correct, then many people with "premotor" parkinsonism will be missed using current diagnostic methods in which biological disease markers are lacking. This makes the identification of environmental risk factors difficult for several reasons. An uncertain proportion of exposed but as yet not clinically manifest cases may be "misclassified" as unaffected, reducing the ability to detect associations. Moreover, the length of the latent period is unknown. A latent period of uncertain length makes it impossible to target exposure histories to a specific period, and potential measurement error is further increased.

Because PD is a disorder of late life, historical information may be inaccurate. Identifying familial patterns of disease is difficult if pathologically affected family members die before clinical signs are apparent. Clinical information and diagnostic accuracy is limited for ancestral generations, and DNA will be scarce. Ascertaining exposures will also be dependent on recall. Rarely will objective measures of exposure be available. These issues are addressed in the specific sections on risk factors to which they apply.

Each of these challenges is magnified by the fact that PD is a relatively rare disorder. Thus, large base populations are needed from which cases can be identified, meaning that epidemiologic studies are expensive and logistically difficult. Despite the challenges, epidemiologic investigations have added considerably to our understanding of PD and serve as an impetus for future study. These results are summarized in the remainder of this chapter.

▶ EPIDEMIOLOGY OF PARKINSON'S DISEASE

MEASURES OF DISEASE FREQUENCY

Disease frequency can be described in terms of either prevalence or incidence. Prevalence describes the number of cases of a condition in a population at one point in time. Incidence is the number of new cases occurring in a given time period for a specific location. Incidence is the more informative estimate of disease frequency as it is relatively unaffected by factors affecting disease survival and allows a more useful comparison of disease frequency over time or between populations. This is particularly important for a disorder with long survival, such as PD. Both incidence and prevalence are affected by the age distribution of the population from which the sample is derived. Therefore, crude total incidence or prevalence estimates must be compared considering the age structure of the populations under study. Incidence or prevalence estimates are comparable across populations when age-adjusted to a reference population, or when compared within small age strata. Gender adjustment is useful when the proportions of men and women vary among populations, or when study methods bias the sample in favor of men or women.

Studies of disease frequency may identify cases using different techniques. Most studies identify cases through contact with health care professionals who care for patients with PD or through review of health care service and/or pharmacy records. Alternatively, direct surveys of individuals can be done. Identifying cases through health care professionals or health record systems provides increased efficiency and allows a larger population to be included in the study, although such methods will not identify undiagnosed PD. Some studies have used pharmacy records alone, but this approach has been demonstrated to have low sensitivity.[28] This can be expected given that PD patients usually remain untreated for one or more years after diagnosis. Surveys of individuals (door-to-door surveys) allow more complete ascertainment, including undiagnosed cases, if the process used (usually a screening questionnaire followed by an examination in those who screen positive) is sensitive. The time and expense involved in this process limit its widespread application. Even considering only examination-verified cases consistent with idiopathic PD, estimates of incidence and prevalence can vary significantly by minor alterations in diagnostic criteria.[29]

INCIDENCE

Most incidence studies of PD have identified cases through health care professionals, either by asking physicians to report diagnosed cases or by reviewing medical records. [30] Door-to-door surveys are less common, particularly for incidence studies, as the prospective follow-up necessary to identify new cases is very labor intensive. As a result, most reported incidence rates include only PD patients diagnosed by health care professionals. Also, it has been common for these studies not to confirm the diagnosis by examination, and medical notes often provide incomplete information to apply formal diagnostic criteria. Therefore, inclusion of some cases that do not actually have PD is likely.

Crude incidence rates of idiopathic PD in studies which consider the entire age range and both sexes range from 4.5–19/100,000 population/year, reflecting, at least in part, variations in study design such as ascertainment methods, case definition, and age distribution of the sample population.[31–44] More uniform rates (6.7–10.2/100,000 population/year)[11,31–33,35–37,41–43,45–51] are obtained when the results are age-adjusted to a reference population (Table 10–1). One study performed in China found a much lower incidence rate (1.6/100,000 person-years) age-adjusted to the WHO standard population.[45] This study used a door-to-door survey to identify cases, which would have been expected to identify more cases if the survey instrument was sufficiently sensitive. This result suggests a lower frequency of PD in China, however, recent prevalence data does not bear this out (see "Prevalence," later). In general, higher crude incidence values, ranging from 7–23.8/100,000 population/year were obtained in earlier studies, which did not distinguish secondary parkinsonism from PD.[1,2,11,52,53] Some studies made the diagnosis of parkinsonism solely based on medical records, and may have included persons with other disorders, such as essential tremor. A study conducted in Finland found that 201 of 775 patients who carried the diagnosis of PD on the basis of medical records were considered to have essential tremor when examined. Incidence rates can be used to predict lifetime risk of the occurrence of a disease for individuals given a specific expected mortality rate. When the incidence rates for PD were applied to a hypothetical cohort in Olmsted County, Minnesota, United States, the lifetime risk for PD was calculated to be 4.4% for men and 3.7% for women.[54]

PREVALENCE

Most persons with PD live many years before death. Consequently, the prevalence of PD is much higher than incidence, and prevalence estimates can be more precise. Because prevalence can be obtained in a cross-sectional fashion without longitudinal observation, it is also easier to obtain. The cases identified in prevalence studies are not necessarily representative of all patients with PD, however, as long-surviving cases are more likely to be identified. Interpretations of observations on disease characteristics or risk factors based on prevalence data must take this into account.

Three general approaches have been used to estimate the prevalence of PD. The first method estimates prevalence based on clinic populations, often at an academic referral center. This technique is inherently inaccurate as social or economic factors may determine who seeks medical care at a given clinical site. In addition, there may be an overrepresentation of mid-stage disease cases with mildly affected individuals not requiring or seeking care at a referral center and end-stage patients being unable to travel to the clinic. The second approach estimates prevalence from health service records of diagnosed cases or drug utilization. Records of physician diagnosis are more reliable; using only drug-prescribing information typically results in significant misclassification.

TABLE 10–1. AGE-ADJUSTED TOTAL* AND AGE-SPECIFIC INCIDENCE OF PARKINSON'S DISEASE PER 100,000 PERSON-YEARS

<table>
<tr><th rowspan="2">Reference</th><th rowspan="2">Population Studied</th><th rowspan="2">Total Age-Adjusted* Incidence (Person-yrs of Observation)</th><th colspan="11">Age Strata</th></tr>
<tr><th><40</th><th>40–44</th><th>45–49</th><th>50–54</th><th>55–59</th><th>60–64</th><th>65–69</th><th>70–74</th><th>75–79</th><th>80–84</th><th>≥85</th></tr>
<tr><td>Brewis, 1966[11]</td><td>Carlisle, UK</td><td>8.7 (497,707)</td><td>0</td><td colspan="2">7.1</td><td colspan="2">20.0</td><td colspan="2">43.1</td><td colspan="2">65.0</td><td colspan="2">37.3</td></tr>
<tr><td>Wang, 1991[44]</td><td>China</td><td>1.6 (3,869,162)</td><td>0</td><td colspan="2">0.3</td><td colspan="2">3.0</td><td colspan="2">2.8</td><td colspan="2">18.7</td><td colspan="2">16.5</td></tr>
<tr><td>Granieri, 1991[41]</td><td>Ferrara, Italy</td><td>6.7 (3,747,620)</td><td>1.1</td><td>4.4</td><td>6.9</td><td>13.9</td><td>21.0</td><td>43.7</td><td>29.3</td><td>32.5</td><td colspan="3">13.1</td></tr>
<tr><td>Mayeux, 1995[37]</td><td>New York City, USA</td><td>7.2 (639,294)</td><td></td><td>0</td><td colspan="4">10.7</td><td colspan="2">54.2</td><td colspan="2">132.6</td><td>212.8</td></tr>
<tr><td>Morens, 1996[46]</td><td>Hawaii, USA</td><td>NA (173,337)</td><td colspan="2">NA</td><td>0</td><td>6.1</td><td>33.8</td><td>27.6</td><td>45.4</td><td>67.0</td><td>139.1</td><td>116.9</td><td>77.8</td></tr>
<tr><td>Kusumi, 1996[35]</td><td>Yonago City, Japan</td><td>7.8 (526,814)</td><td>0</td><td>0</td><td>4.2</td><td>2.3</td><td>16.7</td><td>27.2</td><td>51.5</td><td>81.1</td><td>76.8</td><td>113.7</td><td>26.0</td></tr>
<tr><td>Fall, 1996[33]</td><td>Ostergotland County, Sweden</td><td>7.3 (85,331)</td><td>1.6</td><td colspan="2">3.3</td><td colspan="2">9.0</td><td colspan="2">22.4</td><td colspan="2">59.4</td><td colspan="2">79.5</td></tr>
<tr><td>Bower, 1999[31]</td><td>Olmsted County, Minnesota, USA</td><td>10.2 (1,424,474)</td><td colspan="3">0.44</td><td colspan="2">17.4</td><td colspan="2">52.5</td><td colspan="2">93.1</td><td colspan="2">79.1</td></tr>
<tr><td>Baldereschi, 2000[29]</td><td>Italy</td><td>NA (12,152)</td><td colspan="6">NA</td><td>221</td><td>239</td><td>353</td><td>678</td><td>NA</td></tr>
<tr><td>MacDonald, 2000[36]</td><td>United Kingdom</td><td>NA (150,345)</td><td colspan="2">0</td><td>20</td><td colspan="2">0</td><td>50</td><td>37</td><td>222</td><td>100</td><td>0</td><td>116</td></tr>
<tr><td>Chen, 2001[32]</td><td>Taiwan</td><td>8.7** (49,830)</td><td>NA</td><td colspan="2">0</td><td colspan="2">18.5</td><td colspan="2">47.4</td><td colspan="2">100.2</td><td colspan="2">0</td></tr>
<tr><td>Morioka, 2002[42]</td><td>Japan</td><td>9.1 (1,082,000)</td><td colspan="3">1.2</td><td colspan="2">10.2</td><td colspan="2">36.1</td><td colspan="2">94.5</td><td colspan="2">80.6</td></tr>
<tr><td>Van den Eeden 2003[43]</td><td>California, USA</td><td>9.7 (4,776,038)</td><td>0.3</td><td colspan="2">2.5</td><td colspan="2">9.8</td><td colspan="2">38.8</td><td colspan="2">107.2</td><td colspan="2">119.0</td></tr>
<tr><td>De Lau 2004[48‡]</td><td>Netherlands</td><td>NA (39,878)</td><td colspan="4">NA</td><td colspan="2">30</td><td colspan="2">140</td><td colspan="2">330</td><td>430</td></tr>
<tr><td>Benito-Leon 2004[49‡]</td><td>Spain</td><td>NA (12,710)</td><td colspan="6">NA</td><td>135</td><td>293</td><td>476</td><td>797</td><td>1342</td></tr>
<tr><td>Tan, 2007[50‡]</td><td>Singapore</td><td>NA (31,426)</td><td colspan="3">NA</td><td colspan="2">10</td><td colspan="2">54</td><td colspan="2">56</td><td colspan="2">0</td></tr>
<tr><td>Mehta, 2007[51b]</td><td>Australia</td><td>NA (3509)</td><td colspan="5">NA</td><td colspan="2">480</td><td colspan="2">820</td><td colspan="2">560</td></tr>
</table>

*Adjusted to the World Health Organization standard population 2001, NA = not available.
**Assumes no cases below age 40.
‡door-to-door survey or random sample.

In settings where health care is universally available and uniformly delivered and physician recognition of parkinsonism is high, reasonable estimates can be obtained using this method. However, even in developed nations, the prevalence of undiagnosed PD appears to be high enough that methods that do not detect this group significantly underestimate the prevalence of the disorder.[55] The third method estimates prevalence based on direct screening of a target population, followed by a physician examination of screen positive individuals. Assuming full participation in the screening assessment and high sensitivity of the screening procedure, direct evaluation would yield the most accurate estimate. The time and expense involved in direct screening limit its use.

Crude estimates of PD prevalence have been reported to vary from 18/100,000 persons in a Shanghai, China, population survey[56] to 328/100,000 in a door-to-door survey of the Parsi community in Bombay, India (a population in which 44% of persons are aged 50 or older). When results are age-adjusted to the 2001 WHO standard population the estimates range from 17 to 227 per 100,000[11,32,35,37–39,41,45,51,57–96] (Table 10–2A–D). Most estimates of overall crude prevalence (males and females, entire age range) fall between 100 and 200 per 100,000 people, although as might be predicted, the prevalence estimates derived by door-to-door methods are greater than those derived by other methods for comparable populations (see Table 10–2A–D).

Variations in case ascertainment and diagnostic criteria can only account for some of the variability in disease frequency observed. For example, studies of PD prevalence between the Island of Als and the Faroe Islands, two geographically and genetically distinct areas of Denmark, found a two-fold higher disease prevalence in the Faroe Islands despite using the same study methods.[97,98] Temporal variation is suggested when comparing overall estimates for China across decades.[44,88] The increased prevalence in recent years may reflect a true increase in PD frequency, particularly as earlier estimates were based on the usually reliable door-to-door screening method.

MORTALITY

In the case of PD, mortality rates are more readily available than other measures of disease frequency (incidence and prevalence); nevertheless, death rates do not accurately reflect the true distribution of disease. This is because PD is not a direct cause of death, and often is not even a contributing cause. PD is recorded on half or fewer of the death certificates of known cases,[99,100] and the likelihood of PD being mentioned on the death certificate varies substantially by sociodemographic factors.[101] Also, reported rates vary depending on whether PD must be noted on the death certificate as an underlying cause of death or can be a contributing cause to be counted. Mortality rates are also influenced by variability in diagnostic accuracy, temporal and geographic differences in death statistics reporting, and the age distribution of the source population. Nonetheless, mortality rate represents a unique population-based statistic because the information is accrued over long time periods in virtually all communities. Although of limited usefulness for estimating absolute values of disease frequency, comparisons of mortality rates between subgroups of patients and over time may show important trends, when mortality statistics have been collected using similar methods.

In general, higher mortality rates from PD have been reported for the United States and Northern Europe.[100,102–111] Mortality rates increase with age in all reports, rising sharply after age 60 to rates of 100/100,000 or more in those aged 80 or greater at death. Mortality rates, like incidence and prevalence, are slightly higher for men than for women (see also "Gender-Specific Distribution"). Reported PD mortality increased from the early 1920s to the 1950s in all countries studied.[112] In subsequent years, rates increased in the older age groups, but decreased or were stable at younger ages at death. Longer survival, fewer cases of postencephalitic parkinsonism, as well as improved ascertainment likely contribute to these trends. In more recent years (1985–2004), mortality rates from PD were found to be stable in the United Kingdom.[113]

Compared with persons without PD, mortality is increased approximately twofold after adjusting for age.[46,97,114–122] The standardized mortality rates (standardized for age and gender to a reference population) appear to increase with increasing duration of disease[118,122,123] although after comparing with a group with similar levels of co morbidity, the mortality rates compared with non-PD were stable across the spectrum of disease duration.[124] The standardized mortality rates have been found to be similar for men and women with PD in some studies[119,125] and higher for men in others.[121] The effect of PD on life expectancy is most marked in individuals with a young age at onset.[126]

Examination of mortality rates by state within the United States found as much as twofold variation from state to state, with a significant south to north increasing gradient, which was particularly evident in whites.[127] Regional variation in mortality from PD has also been reported in other countries.[102,128] If this does not reflect variation in ascertainment or reporting practices for cause of death, then these patterns may provide clues to environmental or other risk factors for PD.

AGE-SPECIFIC DISTRIBUTION

Both the incidence and the prevalence of PD increase with increasing age of the population surveyed. (Tables 10–1 and 10–2A–D) PD is rare before age 50, and incidence and prevalence increase steadily until the eighth or

▶ **TABLE 10-2A. AGE-ADJUSTED TOTAL* AND AGE-SPECIFIC PREVALENCE OF PARKINSON'S DISEASE PER 100,000 IN EUROPE**

Reference	Location	Age-Adjusted* Prevalence (Population Size)	Age Strata										
			<40	40-44	45-49	50-54	55-59	60-64	65-69	70-74	75-79	80-84	≥85
Brewis, 1966[11]	Carlisle, UK	84.9 (71,101)	0	144.6		161.8		315.2		613.7		443.9	
Marttila, 1976[57]	Finland	82.7 (402,988)	0.8	27.8		136.2		503.5		736.1		464.8	
Rosati, 1980[58]	Italy	61.4 (1,473,800)	3.3	38.6		204.5		342.1		311.3		82.6	
Sutcliffe, 1985[59]	England	70.3 (208,000)	3			4.0		277.0		702.0		1136	
Mutch, 1986[60]	Scotland	90.9 (151,616)	0	46.6		77.9		254.0		839.6		1925	
D'Alessandro 1987[65]	San Marino	100.4 (22,322)	0				80.3	380.2	573.3	1236.0	1950.3	949.3	0
Granieri, 1991[41]	Italy	120.3 (176,621)	42.8	103.9		186.8		381.5		624.3		783.2	
Morgante, 1992[73]**	Italy	NA (24,496)	NA	0		115.6		621.4		1978.3		3055	
Dias, 1994[69]	Portugal	78.7 (219,928)	0	0	36		169		652		890		
Tison, 1994[77]**	France	NA (3149)	NA				500			400	1800	2200	4800
De Rijk, 1995[66]**	Netherlands	NA (6969)	NA				300		1000		3100		4300
Sutcliffe, 1995[38]	England	73.1 (302,500)	0.6	4	10	76	111	159	343	664	856	1400	1044
Trenkwalder, 1995[79]**	Germany	NA (982)	NA						713				
DeRijk, 1997[68]**	Europe, 5 countries	NA (17,205)	NA						600	100	2800	3600	3400
Chio, 1998[63]	Italy	75.3 (61,830)	0			115.3		288.2		835.1		894.0	
Errea, 1999[70]	Spain	92.3 (60,724)	3.3	16.5		100.2		435.6		953.3		892.9	
De Rijk, 2000[67]**	Europe, 7 countries	NA (18506)	NA						600	1000	2400	3000	2580
Schrag, 2000[75]	England	90.1‡ (121,608)	NA	12		109		342		961		1265	
Claveria, 2002 [64]**	Spain	227.0‡ (1579)	NA	0		0		626		1258		9154	
Benito-Leon, 2003 [61]**	Spain	NA (5,278)	NA						485	1633	1878	3247	1532
Kis, 2002 [72]**	Italy	NA (750)	NA					500	1000	600	6500	1000	NA
Bergaereche, 2004[62]**	Spain	NA (2000)	NA						109		2494		2068
Taba, 2002[76]	Estonia	111.1 (153,240)	0	22		127		493		1232		1109	
Totaro, 2005[78]	Italy	89.2 (297,424)	1.9		49.1		145.2		583.7		1289.3		1705.5
Hobson, 2005[71]	UK	55.4 (77,388)	0	32		63		228		537		653	
Porter 2006[74]	UK	71.9 (108,597)	0	7		51	65	228	369	724	1115	814	928

*Adjusted to the World Health Organization standard population 2001.
**Door-to-door surveys or random sample from population registers.
‡Assumes no cases under age 40, NA = not available.

TABLE 10-2B. AGE-ADJUSTED TOTAL* AND AGE-SPECIFIC PREVALENCE OF PARKINSON'S DISEASE PER 100,000 IN ASIA

Reference	Location	Age-Adjusted* Prevalence (Denominator)	Age Strata										
			<40	40-44	45-49	50-54	55-59	60-64	65-69	70-74	75-79	80-84	≥85
Harada, 1983[80]	Japan	70.1 (125,291)	4.7	39.9		85.8		245.1		698.4		752.7	
Li, 1985[81]**	China	NA (63,195)	NA			92		145		615			
Okada, 1990[82]	Japan	58.6 (80,639)	23.2	19.6		63.6		338.6		478.7		335.7	
Wang, 1991[45]	China	16.6 (3,869,162)	0.7			22.5		89.4		157.6		132.4	
Wang, 1994[84]**	China	NA (2.205)	NA			0		780.0		1750		2500	
Kusumi, 1996[35]	Japan	73.3 (132,315)	0	8.39	41.84	23.29	71.52	210.01	457.93	669.1	850.48	750.0	
Wang, 1996[85]	Taiwan	NA (3915)	NA			273		535		565		1839	
Chen, 2001[32]	Taiwan	117.2 (10,058)‡	NA	37.8		122.5		546.7		819.7		2197.8	
Zhang 2003[87]**	China	NA (5,743)	NA				290		1157		3534		3472
Tan 2004[158]**	Singapore	NA (14,906)	NA			50		280		510		1250	
Zhang 2005[86]** (rural)	China	NA (16,488)	NA			103		621		902		1744	
Zhang 2005 [88]**	China	NA (29,454)	NA				320		1130		2740		4030

*Adjusted to the World Health Organization standard population 2001.
**Door-to-door surveys or random sample from population registers.
NA = not available.
‡Assumes no cases under 40 years of age.

TABLE 10-2C. AGE-ADJUSTED TOTAL* AND AGE-SPECIFIC PREVALENCE OF PARKINSON'S DISEASE PER 100,000 IN NORTH AND SOUTH AMERICA

Reference	Location	Age-Adjusted* Prevalence (Denominator)	Age Strata										
			<40	40–44	45–49	50–54	55–59	60–64	65–69	70–74	75–79	80–84	≥85
Svenson, 1991[94]	Alberta, Canada	NA (2,400,000)	NA	46.6		77.9		254.0		839.6		1925	
Mayeux, 1992[91]	New York, USA	87.0 (179,941)	23			45.7		234.8		525.6		1145	
Mayeux, 1995[37]	New York, USA	62.6 (213,302)	1.3		99.3				509.5		1192.9		823.8
Chouza, 1996[90]**	Uruguay	138.7 (4,468)‡	NA	163					270		2703		
Melcon, 1997[92]**	Argentina	173.2 (7,765)‡	NA	0		152.9		636.9		1727.0		3385.4	
Nicoletti 2003[93]**	Bolivia	106.4 (9955)	0	133		371		443					
Barbosa 2006[89]**	Brazil	NA (1,186)	NA						800	2900	2800	8500	14300

*Adjusted to the World Health Organization standard population 2001.
**Door-to-door survey or random sample from population registers, NA = not available.

▶ **TABLE 10–2D. AGE-ADJUSTED TOTAL* AND AGE-SPECIFIC PREVALENCE OF PARKINSON'S DISEASE PER 100,000 IN AFRICA**

Reference	Location	Age-Adjusted* Prevalence (Denominator)	Age Strata										
			<40	40-44	45-49	50-54	55-59	60-64	65-69	70-74	75-79	80-84	≥85
Ashok, 1986[39]	Libya	51.9 (518,745)	0.2	22.8		91.5		185.7		524.6			

*Adjusted to the World Health Organization standard population 2001, NA = not available.

ninth decade for incidence or the tenth decade for prevalence, when rates appear to decline. This apparent decline among the most elderly likely represents an artifact resulting from poor ascertainment and the very few people in these age groups. It may also reflect diagnostic uncertainty separating PD from other types of parkinsonism, particularly in persons with coexisting dementia.[29]

GENDER-SPECIFIC DISTRIBUTION

Parkinson's disease appears to be more common in men than in women in most studies. Most dramatic is the finding of a more than threefold higher prevalence in men compared with women in China.[81] More typically, prevalence rates in men are higher, but less than twice the rates in women. The observed male preponderance is less robust than the association with increasing age, and there is some variability across studies. A systematic review of incidence studies found that of nine studies that reported age-standardized male:female ratios, six found a male predominance.[30] The male:female ratio ranged from 0.9 to 2.0 across the nine studies. A meta-analysis of seven incidence studies that provided gender-specific incidence data calculated a weighted average male: female ratio of 1.49.[129] Given that the male predominance is seen in incidence studies and persists after age standardization, the association does not appear to be due to differences in survival or in the underlying age composition of the populations sampled. However, differences in access to health care, diagnostic practices or attitudes toward seeking health care may contribute to this apparent increased risk of PD for men.

Several studies conducted in Japan, including both incidence and prevalence studies, have found a female preponderance of PD.[130] This preponderance was found not only when cases were identified using health care service sources, but also when direct surveys of individuals were used, suggesting that higher health care use in women did not explain this pattern. The authors speculate that an environmental exposure relevant to women in Japan and men in other countries may be responsible for this frequency pattern.

RACE-SPECIFIC DISTRIBUTION

The prevalence of PD appears to vary internationally (Table 10–2A–E). The differences in disease frequency may reflect variations in risk determined by the genetic composition of the populations surveyed, and/or differences in exposure to environmental risk factors.

▶ **TABLE 10–2E. AGE-ADJUSTED TOTAL* AND AGE-SPECIFIC PREVALENCE OF PARKINSON'S DISEASE PER 100,000 IN NEW ZEALAND AND AUSTRALIA**

Reference	Location	Age-Adjusted* Prevalence (Denominator)	Age Strata										
			<40	40-44	45-49	50-54	55-59	60-64	65-69	70-74	75-79	80-84	≥85
Caradoc-Davies, 1992[95]	New Zealand	109.6 (105,075)	3.7				91.1		476.0		999		1994.6
McCann, 1998[96]**	Australia	NA (1207)	414										
Chan, 2001[141]**	Australia	NA (527)	NA					3600					
Mehta, 2007[51]**	Australia	NA (3509)	NA			0		480		820			

*Adjusted to the World Health Organization standard population 2001.
**Door-to-door survey or random sample from population registers.
NA = not available.

Alternatively, differences in study methods, diagnostic patterns, or survival with disease may account for the differences. Caucasians in Europe and North America are usually reported to have a higher prevalence, while rates are intermediate for Asians in Japan and China and lowest for blacks in Africa and in some US populations. These data have been interpreted as an indication that whites have a higher risk for PD. However, more recent studies from Asia do not show striking differences in disease prevalence compared with studies in Caucasians. Whether this reflects an actual change in the frequency of disease, improved survival with disease, or improved identification of cases is not known.

Studies using the same case ascertainment methods for samples of different ethnic groups or to sample multiethnic populations can provide more informative comparisons across ethnic groups by eliminating methodologic differences. Most of these studies suggest significant differences in prevalence across populations. As shown in Table 10–3, several hospital-based studies conducted in the United States and Africa found lower rates of PD in blacks.[131–136] These observations are subject to biases, including those resulting from differences in access to health care, health care seeking behavior and differences in survival. A study of PD frequency in New York City found similar *incidence* rates across white, black, and Hispanic patients despite significantly lower prevalence in blacks, especially young men, suggesting poor survival in this group.[37] A second study found lower incidence in blacks.[43] Because, the first study used estimates from census data as the "denominator" in calculating incidence, while the second study used an actual count of the base population, these apparent differences in incidence may be due instead to different methods.

Estimates of prevalence vary so widely even within ethnically similar populations that any conclusions regarding a racial (or genetic) basis to differences in PD prevalence across studies should be made with caution. For example, Chio and colleagues[63] compared age and sex-adjusted prevalence figures derived from nine Italian studies and found a twofold variation in prevalence rates. Methodologic differences between studies may account for some of the variation. However, insight into the relative importance of genetic and environmental factors can be obtained by comparing disease frequency in genetically similar populations separated geographically, being careful to use comparable sampling methods. Such studies suggest a stronger environmental than genetic contribution to variations in disease frequency by race. For example, using the same case ascertainment methods and with standardized training, Schoenberg and colleagues demonstrated a fivefold greater age-standardized prevalence among African Americans in Copiah County, Mississippi, than in Ibadan, Nigeria.[137] This is in keeping with the similar prevalence of PD

TABLE 10–3. CRUDE PREVALENCE OR INCIDENCE OF PARKINSON'S DISEASE IN STUDIES REPORTING MORE THAN ONE ETHNIC OR RACIAL GROUP

	Prevalence (per 100,000)	Incidence (per 100,000)
Location		
Johannesburg, South Africa[101]		
Whites	159	
Blacks	4	
Baltimore, USA[102]		
Whites	125	
Blacks	21	
Mississippi, USA[103]		
Whites	159	
Blacks	103	
New Orleans, USA[104]		
Whites	146	
Blacks	22	
Harare, Zimbabwe[105]		
Whites	94	
Blacks	21	
California, USA[43]		
Hispanics		16.6 (12.0, 21.3)
Whites		13.6 (11.5, 15.7)
Asians		11.3 (7.2, 15.3)
Blacks		10.2 (6.4, 14.0)
Singapore[50]		
Chinese	330 (220, 480)	
Malays	290 (130, 670)	
Indians	270 (120, 670)	
Bangalore, India[137]		
Indians	19600*	
Anglo-Indians	3900*	
Pennsylvania, USA[136]**		
Latinos		40
Whites		54
Blacks		23

*Among residents of elder care homes. Odds ratio for Indian/Anglo-Indian = 3.9 (95% CI 1.3, 12.9).
**Relative risk of PD Blacks/Whites = 0.43 (95% CI 0.31 – 0.60), for Latinos/Whites = 0.74 (95% CI 0.41 – 1.31).

between whites and African-Americans found in their door-to-door survey in Copiah County, Mississippi. The same pattern of findings is seen in a study by Morens and colleagues, who found an incidence of PD in a cohort of Japanese-American men (11 per 100,000 adjusted to the 1970 US population)[46] more in keeping with other American frequency studies than Asian studies. This pattern would suggest that racial differences are due to environmental factors affecting incidence or survival. Tan and colleagues compared the prevalence of PD between Chinese, Malays, and Indians in a single door-to-door survey.[83] Similar prevalence rates were found across the three ethnic groups (see Table 10–3), suggesting that genetic differences play a minor role in PD frequency among these three groups.

In contrast, a study of PD prevalence in elder care homes in India found a fourfold higher prevalence of PD among Indians than Anglo-Indians[138] (Table 10–3). A prevalence study simultaneously comparing Bulgarian Gypsies to Bulgarian Caucasians and using more intensive methods to ascertain PD in Gypsies found a considerably lower prevalence in Gypsies (16.2 versus 136.7), albeit with wide confidence intervals.[139] The two groups had no identified differences in environmental exposures; however, it is impossible to be certain that all relevant exposures were considered. This is consistent with a genetic origin to racial differences in prevalence estimates. Gypsies are thought to be of North Indian descent, with closer genetic background to Asians than Europeans. Because Gypsies are genetically and ethnically isolated, generalizing to other Asians may not be appropriate. Apparently contradictory results regarding the influence of race on the distribution of disease could reflect variable contributions of genetic and environmental factors in determining the occurrence of PD across different ethnic groups. The clarification of the true differences in disease risk associated with race require confirmation in prospective incidence studies in racially diverse populations, similar to the studies conducted in New York City[37] or in Northern California.[43] Ideally, these would be conducted using survey methods that identify all members of a population, such as door-to-door surveys, to minimize bias due to health care related factors and obtain more accurate estimates of disease frequency. It must be recognized, however, that the resources needed for such intensive ascertainment restrict investigations to the study of small populations. This limits the precision of the estimates that can be obtained.

TEMPORAL TRENDS

Whether the incidence of PD has changed since 1817 is unknown due to the paucity of longitudinal data. In general, studies show slightly increasing or stable incidence and prevalence over time. PD incidence was studied in Olmsted County, Minnesota, during the 50-year period 1935–1988.[140] To minimize variability resulting from differences in diagnostic criteria over time, all cases were classified by a single neurologist using existing diagnostic criteria. Estimated incidence increased from 9.2/100,000 annually for the interval 1935-1944 to 16.3/ 100,000 for the interval 1975-1984. More recently, a comparison of age-adjusted prevalence rates in Finland between 1971 and 1992 using comparable methods showed an increased overall prevalence (from 139 to 166) which was entirely accounted for by an increase in the prevalence among men (from 138 to 228). Incidence rates followed the same trends.[34] In a door-to-door survey in Australia, the prevalence estimate in 2001 was at least 42.5% higher than a 1966 survey when methodologic differences between the studies were taken into account.[141] Using comparable methods based on identification of cases through general practitioners in Northampton, England, a moderate increase in prevalence, 108 to 121 per 100,000, was found between 1982 and 1990.[38] These results could be attributed to changing awareness of the symptoms of PD, changing attitudes toward making a diagnosis of the disorder, as well as evolving diagnostic criteria.

In contrast, other studies have shown stable disease frequency. A prospective cohort study of Japanese-American men in Hawaii found no significant trends in prevalence at three time points between 1982 and 1992. Another study comparing prevalence and incidence in Yonago City, Japan, between 1980 and 1992 found stable disease frequency.[35] Similarly, using health service records the incidence of PD was found to be relatively stable over 15 years in Minnesota.[142] It is possible that, in these more recent studies, the time intervals considered are too short to reasonably expect changes in disease frequency. In a meta-analysis using age adjustment and gender adjustment for comparison purposes, Zhang and Roman found no significant temporal fluctuations in the incidence and prevalence in Europe and the United States over the past 50 years.[143] Because the studies included employed a broad range of methods and diagnostic criteria, many including atypical cases or postencephalitic cases, conclusions drawn from this analysis may be misleading. Whether or not the incidence and prevalence of PD is increasing or stable is not clear.

GEOGRAPHIC DISTRIBUTION

The reported rates of PD show marked geographic variation. For comparison, Zhang and Roman age-adjusted rates to the 1970 U.S. population[143] and found that reported incidence rates varied worldwide from 1.9/100,000 in China to 22.1/100,000 in Rochester, Minnesota. Age-adjusted prevalence ranged from 18/100,000 in China to 234/100,000 in Montevideo, Uruguay. Similar variation is seen in the age-adjusted prevalence rates of Table 10–2A–D. Even within the same country, epidemiologic studies have documented significant regional variation in the mortality rates[102,127,128] and prevalence[144] of PD. In the United States, for example, higher mortality rates with increasing latitude have been suggested.[127] Any of the reported differences in PD frequency could be artifacts of differences in study design, including diagnostic criteria and case ascertainment. Socioeconomic factors likely have a greater impact on the estimated prevalence than on the incidence of PD. Lower prevalence rates may simply reflect poor socioeconomic conditions and consequently shortened survival. Because most reported rates are of prevalence, rather than incidence, this qualification is important. However, if these differences represent true variations in disease frequency, they indicate differences in the distribution of genetic and environmental risk factors for PD between the populations studied. Identification of these would provide important direction for clinical and basic scientists investigating PD etiology.

RISK FACTORS

Methodologic Considerations

Many studies have investigated factors associated with the occurrence of PD, and numerous environmental exposures, behavioral factors, and demographic factors have been identified as being directly or indirectly associated with PD. Those directly associated may be related to the cause of PD, while those inversely associated could be protective factors. These studies are invaluable for the clues to disease etiology that they provide; however, there are limitations to the conclusions that can be drawn from them. The vast majority of these studies have been case-control studies collecting retrospective information on exposures, often over the lifetime of the participants. This method generates a measure of association between an exposure and disease, but causality cannot be proven.

Retrospective studies are limited by uncertainty and bias in measurement due to several factors. Because of the retrospective nature of the data collection, it is not always clear that the exposure preceded the onset of the disease. Even when the proper temporal relationship seems obvious, such as a childhood exposure and late-life onset of symptoms, or in a prospective study of disease incidence, the suspected presymptomatic period is of unknown duration (see "Introduction"), making it impossible to know whether or not an exposure has predated the beginning of the pathological process. The retrospective nature of the data collection also makes the exposure difficult to confirm. This is particularly true for a late-life disorder when the timing of the determining events is unknown. Early-life exposures can rarely be verified. Even most midlife exposures are obtained by self-report and are rarely confirmed by written records or biological assays such as blood tests for environmentally persistent chemicals or metals. Case-control studies are susceptible to recall bias, where affected individuals are more likely to think about and recall unusual exposures than controls as they search themselves for reasons that they have PD. This potential bias is particularly important when the exposures cannot be objectively confirmed. It is also important to remember that case-control studies of prevalent cases may be detecting factors associated with long survival, or early onset of disease. Lastly, in observational studies, there is no way to distinguish the influential environmental factor from among several factors that are usually found together. Examples of this are rural living and well water consumption, or the many chemicals found in cigarette smoke. For all of these reasons, complementary investigations to support causality must be performed. This includes collaboration with basic scientists to confirm biological plausibility, looking for dose–response relationships between exposure and disease frequency or severity, and consistency of association across studies.

Factors Directly Associated with Parkinson's Disease

Demographic Factors

Increasing age is the factor most consistently associated with an increased risk of PD (Tables 10–1, 10–2A–D). When considered as a clue to the cause of PD, this association may reflect age-related neuronal vulnerability. However, other time-dependent factors such as duration of exposure to a toxicant or the accumulation of a genetically determined biologic defect cannot easily be separated from age-related changes. Overall, men appear to be at slightly greater risk (about 1.5 times) of developing PD than do women. (See "Gender-Specific Distribution") Whether these reported differences reflect differences in ascertainment, inherent biologic differences in susceptibility, or gender-associated behavioral differences resulting in greater toxicant exposures is unknown.

Familial Factors

Epidemiologic studies of familial patterns of disease can provide valuable clues to the importance of genetic factors to PD. It must be remembered, however, that since families also share behaviors and environments, familial clustering may sometimes have nongenetic causes. Multiple case-control studies have implicated a genetic component to PD by finding that cases more frequently have affected family members than controls. The odds ratio for PD associated with having a family member affected with PD versus those not affected has ranged from 2.4 to 14.6 using patients identified at specialty clinics.[145–159] Community-based studies have also shown an increased risk, but of lower magnitude (odds ratios 2.3:3.7)[160–167] A meta-analysis of studies assessing the relative risk of PD in individuals with an affected first-degree relative, calculated the best summary estimate for relative risk of PD to be 2.9 (95% CI 2.2–3.8).[168] This estimate was based on six studies that had all of the following four methodologically rigorous attributes: (1) Enumerated all first-degree relatives and classified each individually for the presence or absence of PD, (2) confirmed the presence or absence of PD by either direct examination or review of medical records, (3) identified cases from a defined population and randomly sampled controls from the same population, and (4) used a reconstructed cohort analysis instead of a case-control analysis. Having a sibling with PD appears to confer the highest risk (summary relative risk = 4.4 compared with 2.7 for a parent–child pair).[168] In a single prospective community-based study, the relative risk of developing PD over a mean follow-up time of 2 years was 2.5 in those with an affected first-degree relative compared with those without. Among persons with at least two affected relatives, the relative risk was 10.4, although the confidence interval was wide (1.2–89.2).[169]

The population of Iceland provides a unique means for investigating the role of genetics in PD because of their long-standing database of genealogic information in a relatively genetically and environmentally isolated population. After identifying 772 living and dead persons with parkinsonism over the preceding 50 years, genealogic information over 11 centuries was used to determine relatedness of those with parkinsonism and a control group.[170] PD cases were more closely related than the controls, and PD risk was increased most in siblings; less so in offspring. This pattern supports a role for a common early environmental factor or, alternatively, recessively inherited modifying genes. Analysis of familial patterns of PD in Finland, a similarly isolated population, also concluded that genetic factors were important in the pathogenesis of PD, more so in early-onset disease, and that contributing genetic factors were likely to be heterogeneous.[171] One of the significant limitations of studies in such isolated populations is uncertain generalizability. If susceptibility to PD is determined by a combination of genetic and environmental factors, then genetic risk factors identified in a genetically isolated population may not be relevant to other populations.

A genetic contribution to PD is suggested by the discovery of families with parkinsonism inherited in an autosomal dominant or recessive pattern. The clinical or pathological features of at least some of the cases in most of these families are not fully consistent with those of typical PD. However, in many the disorder is indistinguishable from idiopathic PD. Genetic linkage analysis has revealed causative mutations in some families, but these mutations have been found to be uncommon causes of PD in most populations. Notable exceptions are the high prevalence of PD associated with *LRRK2* mutations in the Ashkenazi Jewish[172] and North African Arabic[173] populations. The pathologic mechanisms of these mutations may provide important avenues of research. These mutations are discussed in Chapter 10.

Twin studies have also been used to test the hypothesis of a genetic contribution to the etiology of PD, with their results failing to support a major effect. Intrapair concordance rates should be much higher in monozygotic (MZ) twins than in dizygotic (DZ) twins if a genetic factor is an important causative component of PD. Twin studies have shown similar rates of concordance in MZ and DZ twin pairs.[174–180] The overall similarity in concordance in MZ and DZ pairs is not consistent with a significant genetic contribution to PD. Yet, in a late-life disorder with a potentially long presymptomatic period, it is possible that a cross-sectional study underestimates twin concordance by failure to identify pre symptomatic individuals and individuals that have already died but were destined to manifest the disease. Discrepancies of up to 28 years in age of onset between MZ twins has been reported.[176] In a small number of twin pairs discordant for PD clinically, many of the asymptomatic co-twins had significantly decreased putamenal 18F-dopa uptake measured by PET-scan,[181,182] suggesting concordance for dopamine system deficits. Additionally, a pattern of higher dopamine deficit concordance in MZ than DZ twin pairs has been found in one study.[20] Longitudinal clinical follow-up in such cohorts will be important to confirm the relevance of such findings. Even if there is greater dopamine deficit concordance than clinical concordance, variability in age at clinical onset between MZ twins indicates nongenetic influences on the biological processes involved in PD.

One twin study found that concordance rates were much higher when symptoms began before the age of 50.[176] This has suggested that the importance of genetic factors is not uniform across the age range, and in the less common young onset parkinsonism, genetic factors appear to be primary.

Associations between PD and other diseases can give clues to common pathogenesis. A family history of essential tremor has also been found to be more common in patients with PD than in controls.[147,151] This observation is also susceptible to bias in that persons with PD are likely to be particularly observant of tremor in others. There is also the potential for diagnostic confusion between PD and essential tremor, particularly if the reported cases were not examined by study personnel. If there truly is a positive association between PD and essential tremor, it suggests shared determinants between the two diseases.

Chemical Exposures

Following the description of a cluster of toxicant-induced parkinsonism strikingly similar to PD,[183] interest in an environmental cause of PD burgeoned. The responsible compound, the pyridine 1-methyl-4-phenyl-1,2,3,6-tetrahydropyridine (MPTP), induces clinical, pathological, and biochemical changes in humans and primates remarkably like those of PD.[184–186] Whereas MPTP is unlikely to be environmentally present in sufficient quantities to cause most cases of PD, chemically similar compounds more commonly present might theoretically be causative. For example, the herbicide paraquat is a structural analog of MPTP and the pesticide rotenone shares with MPTP the common function of inhibiting mitochondrial complex 1. In rats, chronic exposure to rotenone results in a progressive nigral lesion,[187] and paraquat depletes dopamine in frogs.[188]

Multiple case-control studies have investigated the association between pesticide exposure and PD. Most have found positive associations. A meta-analysis of 19 such studies from North America, Europe, and Asia until 1999 found a combined odds ratio of 1.94 (95% CI 1.49–2.53) for PD in the presence of a positive history of pesticide exposure.[189] Across studies, a dose–response relationship was also suggested, and within a study of licensed pesticide applicators, PD risk increased with more days of pesticide use.[190] A population-based study of PD mortality found a significantly higher rate in California counties using pesticides than in counties with negligible pesticide use.[191] To date, most studies have investigated occupational pesticide use; however, one study has also implicated home pesticide and herbicide use (OR 1.9, 95% CI 1.3–2.9).[192] It is interesting that rural living, drinking well water, and farming have also been identified as associated with the occurrence of PD in multiple studies.[189] It is possible that these findings represent co-occurrence with pesticide exposure or other as yet unidentified pathogenic factors.

Most epidemiological studies have not investigated associations between individual agents or even classes of agents and PD. Pesticides have different, often poorly defined mechanisms of toxicity, and it is not clear which mechanisms are relevant to PD. If there truly is a causative association between some pesticides or herbicides and PD, then the odds ratios reported thus far are likely an underestimation of the effect of the pathogenic agent(s). Exposure to paraquat, organochlorines, and carbamates have been specifically associated with PD.[190,193] Dieldrin has been shown to produce nigral injury in vitro and post mortem levels of dieldrin were elevated compared with controls.[194,195] Such observations complement epidemiologic studies of associations between pesticides and PD.

Despite the consistency of the association with pesticide exposure and the supporting laboratory evidence, case-control studies are still unable to demonstrate causality unequivocally, for the reasons discussed earlier. The findings to date await replication in unselected, prospectively followed cohorts. Once specific agents are identified, further investigation in the laboratory will be essential to identifying mechanisms of injury.

Pesticides are not the only chemicals to be implicated. Studies have detected positive associations between PD and history of exposure to "any chemicals,"[153,196] industrial exposure,[197,198] solvents,[196,199] wood preservatives,[199] glues, paints, or lacquers,[199] carbon monoxide,[199] and general anesthesia.[199] Most of these observations await confirmation in other studies and the associations remain tentative at present.

Metal Exposures

Exposure to metals has been investigated as a risk factor for PD, prompted in part by the long-known ability of manganese toxicity to produce parkinsonism,[200] the finding of elevated iron levels in the substantia nigra of patients with PD,[201] and epidemiologic associations between industrial activities involving metal exposure and elevated rates of PD.[197] The results of studies of specific metal exposure have been inconsistent,[202] although some studies have suggested a positive association between PD and manganese, mercury,[202] or lead[203] exposure. The relationship between manganese exposure in welding and PD has been highly controversial recently.[204] In a clinic series and an occupational group referred for medicolegal evaluation, welding has been associated with either high prevalence or earlier onset of PD.[205,206] However, neither welding nor manganese exposure have been associated with PD risk in other studies using clinic or industry-based samples or in studies linking occupational and disease registries.[155,206–216]

Variations in methods of determining exposure status, as well as frequency and levels of exposure in the population studied may contribute to the inconsistencies. For example, in one case-control study, positive associations with multiple exposures elicited by subjective assessment could not be confirmed by a more objective job exposure matrix method.[199] This could be because subjective assessments are prone to recall bias. On the other hand, job exposure matrices are unable to individualize exposure assessment beyond that usual for the stated occupation, so such assessments tend to be imprecise, even though more objective. Further complicating the study of risk factors is the finding that certain exposure combinations may be associated with increased risk, yet where each single exposure at similar levels is not. This may be the case for exposure to combinations of lead–copper, lead–iron, and iron–copper.[202]

Dietary and Metabolic Factors

A number of foods and nutrients have been investigated for their association, both direct and indirect, with PD. The most consistent finding to date has been an increased risk with higher intake of dairy products.[217–219] Potential mechanisms for this association include neurotoxins contaminating dairy products and reduction in uric acid levels. (Higher uric acid levels appear to protect against PD, see "Other Inverse Associations"). Increased risk with total fat,[220,221] in particular animal fat,[221,222] has also been found in several studies.[223] This has been hypothesized to the result of oxidative stress, as lipids are a source of oxygen radicals through peroxidation. Other dietary factors have not yet been consistently associated with PD. The imprecise nature of estimating food intake over long periods (as in the period before the onset of PD) makes the accurate study of dietary risk factors very difficult. The challenges are compounded by the fact that any one of a number of components of each food may be the factor of interest. It is still uncertain whether any of the associations observed to date indicate a specific effect of a dietary constituent, an effect of a co existing toxicant or are markers of a lifestyle pattern predisposing to (or protecting from) PD.

Obesity in mid life has been associated with increased disease risk and a dose-dependent association of PD and increasing body mass index has been found.[224–226] These observations could be explained by either early PD-related behavioral changes or metabolic states representing risk factors for PD. Lower total or LDL cholesterol levels have also been associated with a higher risk of PD in most studies that have assessed the relationships.[227–229]

Other Potential Risk Factors

Because infection (probably viral) resulted in an epidemic of parkinsonism following encephalitis early in this century, the belief that PD was the result of infection persisted for decades, despite the clear differences clinically and pathologically between the postencephalitic disease and PD.[230] While an infectious agent has never been identified in PD,[231–235] and the insidious onset and slowly progressive course make traditional agents unlikely, the ubiquitous soil pathogen *Nocardia asteroides* has been reported to cause a nigral lesion in animals and has been proposed as a cause of PD.[236] Evidence supporting this hypothesis, however, was not found in a serological study in humans.[237] An inverse association between childhood measles infection and PD has been found in one study.[238] Whether this finding represents a protective effect, an adverse effect of previous measles infection in adulthood causing reduced survival or an association between measles and another factor inversely associated with PD cannot be determined from the present data.

Several factors related to life experience or behavioral factors have been associated with the occurrence of PD. Emotional stress, which may cause increased dopamine turnover resulting in increased risk of oxidative nerve cell death[239,240] has been associated with an increased disease risk in two studies of persons surviving extreme emotional and physical hardship.[241–243] Heavy physical work has also been implicated.[244] A positive association with head trauma has been reported in several studies,[147,151,153,196,199,245–248] and there is a higher risk with more frequent injuries.[209,247,248] Head injury could act through inducing inflammation or compromising the blood brain barrier, exposing the central nervous system to toxins.

A particular personality type has been identified as more common before the onset of PD than among controls in multiple studies, including twin studies.[249] The features of this personality include shyness, cautiousness, inflexibility, punctuality, and depressiveness. Whether this represents the earliest feature of the neurochemical changes of PD, or an association between such a personality and causative environmental exposures or genetic factors is not known.

Various occupational risk factors have also been proposed. The types of work that have been associated with PD in one or more studies are numerous and diverse and a common underlying factor is not obvious. The most consistently observed occupational risk factor is agricultural work. This may be due to exposure to pesticides or to other toxic agents such as endotoxin. Endotoxin in the walls of gram negative bacteria has been shown to be capable of causing nigral injury in laboratory studies.[250] Increased risk of PD in teachers and health care workers has also been suggested to reflect increased exposure to infectious agents that could contribute to a heightened inflammatory state.[190,250] As with many other proposed risk factors, the associations await confirmation in other studies. Regarding clues to etiology that these associations provide, exposures inherent in the type of work must be considered. This is difficult, however, as job titles are usually associated with varied job tasks and environments. Detailed job task histories are thus usually more revealing. Occupational associations must also consider the lifestyle that the occupation demands that accompany certain jobs. Occupations involving shift work and greater physical activity have been inversely associated with PD.[207,251] It is also possible, however, that certain occupations are chosen on the basis of suitability to the personality type that is associated with PD. Therefore, not all occupational associations may represent clues to etiology.

Putative risk factors for PD lead to important hypotheses regarding disease etiology and pathophysiology, which may launch large efforts of investigation by basic and clinical researchers. With the numerous associations that have been observed, it is important to find ways to focus attention for further investigation on those most likely to be genuine and relevant. Thus, attention to biological plausibility, dose–response relationships, and consistency of association are important considerations.

Factors Inversely Associated with Parkinson's Disease

Cigarette Smoking

The inverse association between PD and both active and passive cigarette smoking, has been reported in many studies.[252–254] A meta-analysis estimated the magnitude of risk reduction from active cigarette smoking to be approximately 40%.[252] A pooled analysis confirmed a dose-dependent inverse association between smoking and PD. The relationship appears to be less strong in individuals with age of onset older than 75 years.[255] A recent study found that male smokers with PD had no increase in mortality compared with male nonsmokers with PD, suggesting that smoking may have a beneficial effect on the course of the disease.[122]

The inverse association between cigarette smoking and PD risk may be due to a direct effect of cigarette smoke or to a confounding factor associated with both PD risk and aversion to smoking. The so-called "parkinsonian personality," which is proposed to be a reflection of an underlying dopamine deficiency, may result in the avoidance of novelty-seeking behaviors such as smoking[256] or in a lack of propensity for addiction.

Earlier mortality in smokers (thus dying before manifesting PD) has also been proposed as an explanation for the observed inverse association. However, a large cohort study demonstrated a reduced incidence of PD in cigarette smokers even at young ages when mortality from any cause is low, and found insufficient mortality differences between smokers and non-smokers to account for the reduction in incident PD cases.[257]

A direct effect of cigarette smoking on PD risk is supported by a recent study finding that the gender ratio of PD prevalence has changed in kind with changing demographics of cigarette smoking behavior internationally.[258] As more women have taken up smoking, the relative frequency of PD among women compared with men has declined in those same regions. The degree of correlation suggested that smoking reduces PD risk by approximately 74%. Twin studies also support a direct effect of cigarette smoke. Cigarette smoking was less frequent in the affected twins of discordant MZ twin pairs in two studies.[176,259] Monozygotic twins are particularly powerful for investigating environmental factors as genetic factors influencing disease occurrence are eliminated; thus, it does not appear that genetic factors that influence both smoking behavior and PD risk are responsible for the association. When twins have lived together much of their lives, many environmental factors are controlled as well, allowing discrimination among putative risk factors.

An interaction between smoking status (in pack-years) and monoamine oxidase B genotype has been found in one study. The inverse relationship between smoking and the occurrence of PD was smaller for those with the G allele of the dopamine metabolizing enzyme monoamine oxidase B than for those with the A allele. Observing such interactions may provide additional clues to the mechanisms by which cigarette smoking and PD are related. Together, these results support a biologic effect of smoking on risk for PD, and several lines of laboratory evidence suggest that nicotine may be the protective factor.[260] Alternatively, nicotine or other components of cigarette smoke may induce xenobiotic metabolizing enzymes enabling more rapid detoxification of a parkinsonism-causing toxicant.[261,262]

Coffee Consumption and Other Dietary Factors

Coffee drinking is also inversely associated with PD risk, a relationship seen in case-control and prospective cohort studies and supported by a large meta-analysis.[252,263,264] The magnitude of risk reduction is similar to that seen with cigarette smoking. This relationship does not appear to extend to decaffeinated coffee, and extends to caffeine from non-coffee sources, suggesting that caffeine is the determining factor in the relationship.[263,265,266] Protection may occur through adenosine A2A antagonism, and laboratory studies have shown that caffeine can block MPTP toxicity in animal models, providing biological plausibility for a direct protective action against PD.[267,268] However, if caffeine is considered to be "addictive," one could still propose a lack of propensity for addiction in people with PD as being responsible for the observed relationships.

An inverse association between PD and the amount of antioxidants consumed in the diet, including vitamin E, has been a topic of particular interest among dietary factors. Such an association would support a role for oxidative stress in the degeneration of nigral neurons and have potential implications for disease prevention. Several case-control studies have suggested an inverse association but most recent studies have not supported this.[220–222,269–274] Recently, however, diets high in uric acid, a potent antioxidant, have been inversely associated with risk for PD.[275] That this is a true effect is supported by several lines of evidence (see "Other Inverse Associations").

Other Inverse Associations

Higher plasma uric acid levels have been consistently found to be associated with a reduced risk of PD in prospective studies.[276–278] Diets high in uric acid have similarly been inversely associated with risk[275] as mentioned earlier, as has a history of gout in men.[279] A favorable effect of high uric acid levels on the course of PD has been suggested.[280] Uric acid is a potent antioxidant, which may explain the association. There is interest in investigating ways to safely elevate uric acid levels as a neuroprotective intervention for PD.

Several pharmacologic agents have been associated with reduced risk of PD. Such findings are particularly interesting due to the potential for disease prevention or modification. Most, but not all studies have found PD risk to be reduced in habitual users of nonsteroidal anti-inflammatory drugs.[281–287] A dose-dependent association has also been found. This finding supports a role of inflammation in PD pathogenesis. Levels of the inflammatory biomarker interleukin (IL)-6 were found to be elevated prior to the diagnosis of PD in one study, also suggesting a role for inflammation early in the disease process.[288] Calcium channel blockers have been of interest as neuroprotective agents because of the potential to reduce apoptosis and glutamate-mediated excitotoxicity, and more recent evidence suggests that L-type calcium channel blockers may have the potential to confer resistance to MPTP-induced degeneration upon dopaminergic cells of the substantia nigra.[289] Epidemiologic studies have been conflicting,[290–292] but a recent case-control study found an inverse association between PD and current users of calcium channel blockers.[292] Long-term use before onset was not reported, however, limiting causal inference. Treatment with cholesterol-lowering agents has been associated with PD in case-control studies.[293,294] The significance of this is unclear given the association of lower cholesterol levels with higher PD risk (see "Factors Directly Associated with PD").

Greater levels of physical activity in midlife have been associated with lower risk of PD in two of three prospective studies[251,295,296] Physical activity could act to reduce risk for neurodegeneration by counteracting oxidative stress or increasing trophic factor release.[297]

Because of the increased risk of PD in men, estrogen has been proposed as a protective factor. Results to date have been conflicting, but recently a study investigating the risk of PD related to oophorectomy before menopause within the medical records linkage system of Olmsted County found a higher risk of parkinsonism associated with oophorectomy and greater risk with younger age at oophorectomy.[298] Similar results were obtained for PD but did not reach statistical significance. This result is consistent with a protective effect of endogenous estrogen.

In summary, among environmental factors, exposure to pesticides as a risk factor and cigarette smoking, and caffeine consumption as factors associated with decreased risk have the most support in the literature thus far. There is also support for the role of genetic factors in determining susceptibility to PD. The role of genetic susceptibility in PD is a rapidly expanding field, and genetic factors may modify the effect of environmental and demographic factors on the risk of disease. Such interactions represent an additional challenge to understanding the various contributions to the cause of PD. The roles of specific genes in the susceptibility to PD are discussed in Chapter 10.

▶ CONCLUSION

Epidemiologic investigations of the patterns of disease occurrence have given many clues to the cause(s) of PD. Multiple associations with genetic and environmental factors have been identified, and various studies have also suggested interactions between the environment and genes in the process leading to PD. The challenge over the coming years will be to discern which associations are etiologically relevant. This will involve reciprocal communication between clinical and basic scientists. The biological plausibility of associations identified through epidemiologic studies can be tested in the laboratory. Contributions from basic science about mechanisms of toxicity of compounds or insights from animal models can guide future epidemiologic studies to confirm relevance to human disease. Such collaboration will be essential given the evolving picture of multiple contributing factors to the cause of PD.

REFERENCES

1. Kurland LT. Epidemiology: Incidence, geographic distribution and genetic considerations. In Field WS (ed). Pathogenesis and Treatment of Parkinsonism. Springfield: Thomas, 1958, pp. 5–43.
2. Gudmundsson K. A clinical survey of parkinsonism in Iceland. Acta Neurol Scand1967;33:9–61.
3. Parkinson J. An Essay on the Shaking Palsy. London: Sherwood, Neeley, and Jones, 1817.
4. Hughes AJ, Daniel SE, Kilford L, et al. Accuracy of clinical diagnosis of idiopathic Parkinson's disease: A clinico-pathological study of 100 cases. J Neurol Neurosurg Psychiatry 1992;55:181–184.
5. Maraganore D, Anderson DW, Bower H, et al.. Autopsy patterns for Parkinson's disease and related disorders in Olmsted County, Minnesota. Neurology 1999;53: 1342–1344.
6. Silveira-Moriyama L, Schwingenschuh P, O'Donnell A, et al. Olfaction in patients with suspected parkinsonism and scans without evidence of dopaminergic deficit (SWEDDs). J Neurol Neurosurg Psychiatry 2009;80(7):744–748.
7. Marek K. Pramipexole versus levodopa: Effects on Parkinson disease progression assessed by dopamine transporter imaging. Neurology 2002;58(suppl 3):A82–A82.
8. Berg D. Ultrasound in the (premotor) diagnosis of Parkinson's disease. Parkinsonism Relat Disord2007;13(suppl 3):S429–S433.
9. Albanese A. Diagnostic criteria for Parkinson's disease. J Neurol Sci 2003;24(suppl 1):S23–S26.
10. Litvan I, Bhatia KP, Burn DJ, et al. Movement Disorders Society Scientific Issues Committee report: SIC Task Force appraisal of clinical diagnostic criteria for Parkinsonian disorders. Mov Disord 2003;18(5):467–486.
11. Brewis M, Poskanzer MD, Rolland H, et al. Neurological disease in an English city. Acta Neurol Scand Suppl 1966.
12. Rajput AH. Epidemiology of Parkinson's disease. Can J Neurol Sci 1984;11(1 suppl):156–159.
13. Klein C, Lohmann-Hedrich K. Impact of recent genetic findings in Parkinson's disease. Curr Opin Neurol 2007;20:453–464.
14. Langston JW, Sastry S, Chan P, et al. Novel alpha-synuclein-immunoreactive proteins in brain samples from the Contursi kindred, Parkinson's, and Alzheimer's disease. Exp Neurol 1998;154:684–690.
15. Takahashi H, Ohama E, Suzuki S, et al. Familial juvenile parkinsonism: Clinical and pathologic study in a family. Neurology 1994;44:437–441.
16. Yamamura Y, Hattori N, Matsumine H, et al. Autosomal recessive early-onset parkinsonism with dirunal fluctuation: Clinicopathologic characteristics and molecular genetic identification. Brain Dev Suppl 2000;22:87–91.

17. Wszolek ZK, Pfeiffer RF, Tsuboi Y, et al. Autosomal dominant parkinsonism associated with variable synuclein and tau pathology. Neurology 2004;62(9):1619–1622.
18. Paisan-Ruiz C. LRRK2 gene variation and its contribution to Parkinson disease. Hum Mutat 2009;30(8):1153–1160.
19. Koller WC, Langston JW, Hubble JP, et al. Does a long preclinical period occur in Parkinson's disease. Neurol Suppl 1991;41:8–13.
20. Piccini P, Burn DJ, Ceravolo R, et al. The role of inheritance in sporadic Parkinson's disease: Evidence from a longitudinal study of dopaminergic function in twins. Ann Neurol 1999;45:577–582.
21. Sawle GV, Wroe SJ, Lees AJ, et al. The identification of presymptomatic parkinsonism: Clinical and [18F]dopa positron emission tomography studies in an Irish kindred. Ann Neurol 1992;32:609–617.
22. Forno LS. Concentric hyalin intraneuronal inclusions of Lewy type in brains of elderly persons (60 incidental cases): Relationships to parkinsonism. J Am Geriatr Soc 1969;17:557–575.
23. Gibb WR, Lees AJ. The relevance of the Lewy body to the pathogenesis of idiopathic Parkinson's disease. J Neurol Neurosurg Psychiatry 1988;51(6):745–752.
24. Ross GW, Petrovitch H, Abbott RD, et al. Association of olfactory dysfunction with risk for future Parkinson's disease. Ann Neurol 2008;63(2):167–173.
25. Braak H Bohl JR, Muller CM, et al. E. Stanley Fahn Lecture 2005: The staging procedure for the inclusion body pathology associated with sporadic Parkinson's disease reconsidered. Mov Disord 2006;21(12):2042–2051.
26. Langston JW. The Parkinson's complex: Parkinsonism is just the tip of the iceberg. Ann Neurol 2006;59(4):591–596.
27. Lim SY, Fox SH, Lang AE. Overview of the extranigral aspects of Parkinson disease. Arch Neurol 2009;66(2): 167–172.
28. van de Vijver DA, Stricker BH, Breteler MM, et al. Evaluation of antiparkinsonian drugs in pharmacy records as a marker for Parkinson's disease. Phar World Sci 2001;23(4):148–152.
29. Bower JH, Maraganore DM, McDonnell SK, et al. Influence of strict, intermediate, and broad diagnostic criteria on the age- and sex-specific incidence of Parkinson's disease. Mov Disord 2000;15(5):819–825.
30. Twelves D, Perkins KS, Counsell C. Systematic review of incidence studies of Parkinson's disease. Mov Disord 2003;18(1):19–31.
31. Bower JH, Maraganore DM, McDonnell SK, et al. Incidence and distribution of parkinsonism in Olmsted County, Minnesota, 1976–1990. Neurology 1999;52(6):1214–1220.
32. Chen RC, Chang SF, Su CL, et al. Prevalence, incidence, and mortality of PD: A door-to-door survey in Ilan county, Taiwan. Neurology 2001;57(9):1679–1686.
33. Fall PA, Axelson O, Fredriksson M, et al. Age-standardized incidence and prevalence of Parkinson's disease in a Swedish community. J Clin Epidemiol 1996;49(6): 637–641.
34. Kuopio AM, Marttila RJ, Helenius H, et al. Changing epidemiology of Parkinson's disease in southwestern Finland. Neurology 1999;52(2):302–308.
35. Kusumi M, Nakashima K, Harada H, et al. Epidemiology of Parkinson's disease in Yonago City, Japan: Comparison with a study carried out 12 years ago. Neuroepidemiology 1996;15(4):201–207.
36. MacDonald BK, Cockerell OC, Sander JW, et al. The incidence and lifetime prevalence of neurological disorders in a prospective - study in the UK. Brain 2000;123: 665–676.
37. Mayeux R, Marder K, Cote L, et al. The frequency of idiopathic Parkinson's disease by age, ethnic group, sex in northern Manhattan, 1988–1993. Am J Epidemiol 1995;142:820–827.
38. Sutcliffe RL, Meara JR. Parkinson's disease epidemiology in the Northampton District, England, 1992. Acta Neurol Scand 1995;92(6):443–450.
39. Ashok PP, Radhakrishnan K, Sridharan R, et al. Epidemiology of Parkinson's disease in Benghazi, North-East Libya. Clin Neurol Neurosurg 1986;88(2):109–113.
40. Cockerell OC, Goodridge DM, Brodie D, Sander JW, Shorvon SD. Neurological disease in a defined population: The results of a pilot study in two general practices. Neuroepidemiology 1996;15(2):73–82.
41. Granieri E, Carreras M, Casetta I, et al. Parkinson's disease in Ferrara, Italy, 1967 through 1987. Arch Neurol 1991;48(8):854–857.
42. Morioka S, Sakata K, Yoshida S, et al. Incidence of Parkinson disease in Wakayama, Japan. J Epidemiol 2002;12(6):403–407.
43. Van Den Eeden SK, Tanner CM, Bernstein AL, et al. Incidence of Parkinson's disease: Variation by age, gender, and race/ethnicity. Am J Epidemiol 2003;157(11): 1015–1022.
44. Wang YS, Shi YM, Wu ZY, et al. Parkinson's disease in China. Coordinational Group of Neuroepidemiology, PLA. Chinese Medical Journal 1991;104(11): 960–964.
45. Wang Y. [The incidence and prevalence of Parkinson's disease in the People's Republic of China]. Chung-Hua Liu Hsing Ping Hsueh Tsa Chih Chinese J Epidemiol 1991;12(6):363–365.
46. Morens DM, Davis JW, Grandinetti A, et al. Epidemiologic observations on Parkinson's disease: Incidence and mortality in a prospective study of middle-aged men. Neurology 1996;46(4):1044–1050.
47. Baldereschi M, Di Carlo A, Rocca WA, et al. Parkinson's disease and parkinsonism in a longitudinal study: Two-fold higher incidence in men. ILSA Working Group. Italian Longitudinal Study on Aging. Neurology 2000;55(9): 1358–1363.
48. de Lau LM, Giesbergen PC, de Rijk MC, et al. Incidence of parkinsonism and Parkinson disease in a general population: The Rotterdam Study. Neurology 2004;63(7): 1240–1244.
49. Benito-Leon J, Bermejo-Pareja F, Morales-Gonzalez JM, et al. Incidence of Parkinson disease and parkinsonism in three elderly populations of central Spain. Neurology 2004;62(5):734–741.
50. Tan LC, Venketasubramanian N, Jamora RD, et al. Incidence of Parkinson's disease in Singapore. Parkinsonism Relat Disord 2007;13(1):40–43.
51. Mehta P, Kifley A, Wang JJ, et al. Population prevalence and incidence of Parkinson's disease in an Australian community. Intern Med J 2007;37(12):812–814.

52. Rajput AH, Offord KP, Beard CM, Kurland LT. Epidemiology of parkinsonism: Incidence, classification, and mortality. Ann Neurol 1984;16(3):278–282.
53. Jenkins AC. Epidemiology of parkinsonism in Victoria. Med J Australia 1966;2(11):496–502.
54. Elbaz A, Bower JH, Maraganore DM, et al. Risk tables for parkinsonism and Parkinson's disease. J Clin Epidemiol 2002;55(1):25–31.
55. Taylor KS, Counsell CE, Harris CE, et al. Screening for undiagnosed parkinsonism in people aged 65 years and over in the community. Parkinsonism Relat Disord 2006;12(2):79–85.
56. Shi YM. Study on the prevalence of Parkinson's disease in Hongkou District, Shanghai. Chung-Hua Liu Hsing Ping Hsueh Tsa Chih Chinese J Epidemiol 1987;8(4):205–207.
57. Marttila RJ, Rinne UK. Epidemiology of Parkinson's disease in Finland. Acta Neurol Scand1976;53(2):81–102.
58. Rosati G, Granieri E, Pinna L, et al. The risk of Parkinson disease in Mediterranean people. Neurology 1980;30(3):250–255.
59. Sutcliffe RL, Prior R, Mawby B, et al. Parkinson's disease in the district of the Northampton Health Authority, United Kingdom. A study of prevalence and disability. Acta Neurol Scand1985;72(4):363–379.
60. Mutch WJ, Dingwall-Fordyce I, Downie AW, et al. Parkinson's disease in a Scottish city. Brit Med J (Clin Res Ed) 1986;292(6519):534–536.
61. Benito-Leon J, Bermejo-Pareja F, Rodriguez J, et al. Prevalence of PD and other types of parkinsonism in three elderly populations of central Spain. Mov Disord 2003;18(3):267–274.
62. Bergareche A, De La Puente E, Lopez de Munain A, et al. Prevalence of Parkinson's disease and other types of Parkinsonism. A door-to-door survey in Bidasoa, Spain. J Neurol 2004;251(3):340–345.
63. Chio A, Magnani C, Schiffer D. Prevalence of Parkinson's disease in Northwestern Italy: Comparison of tracer methodology and clinical ascertainment of cases. Mov Disord 1998;13(3):400–405.
64. Claveria LE, Duarte J, Sevillano MD, et al. Prevalence of Parkinson's disease in Cantalejo, Spain: A door-to-door survey. Mov Disord 2002;17(2):242–249.
65. D'Alessandro R, Gamberini G, Granieri E, et al. Prevalence of Parkinson's disease in the Republic of San Marino. Neurology 1987;37(10):1679–1682.
66. de Rijk MC, Breteler MM, Graveland GA, et al. Prevalence of Parkinson's disease in the elderly: The Rotterdam Study. Neurology 1995;45(12):2143–2146.
67. de Rijk MC, Launer LJ, Berger K, et al. Prevalence of Parkinson's disease in Europe: A collaborative study of population-based cohorts. Neurologic Diseases in the Elderly Research Group. Neurology 2000;54(11 Suppl 5):S21–S23.
68. de Rijk MC, Tzourio C, Breteler MM, et al. Prevalence of parkinsonism and Parkinson's disease in Europe: The EUROPARKINSON Collaborative Study. European Community Concerted Action on the Epidemiology of Parkinson's disease. J Neurol Neurosurg Psychiatry 1997;62(1):10–15.
69. Dias JA, Felgueiras MM, Sanchez JP, Goncalves JM, Falcao JM, Pimenta ZP. The prevalence of Parkinson's disease in Portugal. A population approach. Eur J Epidemiol 1994;10(6):763–767.
70. Errea JM, Ara JR, Aibar C, et al. Prevalence of Parkinson's disease in lower Aragon, Spain. Mov Disord 1999;14(4):596–604.
71. Hobson P, Gallacher J, Meara J. Cross-sectional survey of Parkinson's disease and parkinsonism in a rural area of the United Kingdom. Mov Disord 2005;20(8):995–998.
72. Kis B, Schrag A, Ben-Shlomo Y, et al. Novel three-stage ascertainment method: Prevalence of PD and parkinsonism in South Tyrol, Italy. Neurology 2002;58(12):1820–1825.
73. Morgante L, Rocca WA, Di Rosa AE, et al. Prevalence of Parkinson's disease and other types of parkinsonism: A door-to-door survey in three Sicilian municipalities. The Sicilian Neuro-Epidemiologic Study (SNES) Group. Neurology 1992;42(10):1901–1907.
74. Porter B, Macfarlane R, Unwin N, et al. The prevalence of Parkinson's disease in an area of North Tyneside in the North-East of England. Neuroepidemiology 2006;26(3):156–161.
75. Schrag A, Ben-Shlomo Y, Quinn NP. Cross-sectional prevalence survey of idiopathic Parkinson's disease and Parkinsonism in London. BMJ 2000;321(7252):21–22.
76. Taba P, Asser T, Taba P, Asser T. Prevalence of Parkinson's disease in Estonia.[see comment]. Acta Neurol Scand2002;106(5):276–281.
77. Tison F, Dartigues JF, Dubes L, et al. Prevalence of Parkinson's disease in the elderly: A population study in Gironde, France. Acta Neurol Scand1994;90(2):111–115.
78. Totaro R, Marini C, Pistoia F, et al. Prevalence of Parkinson's disease in the L'Aquila district, central Italy. Acta Neurol Scand2005;112(1):24–28.
79. Trenkwalder C, Schwarz J, Gebhard J, et al. Starnberg trial on epidemiology of Parkinsonism and hypertension in the elderly. Prevalence of Parkinson's disease and related disorders assessed by a door-to-door survey of inhabitants older than 65 years. Arch Neurol 1995;52(10):1017–1022.
80. Harada H, Nishikawa S, Takahashi K. Epidemiology of Parkinson's disease in a Japanese city. Arch Neurol 1983;40(3):151–154.
81. Li SC, Schoenberg BS, Wang CC, et al. A prevalence survey of Parkinson's disease and other movement disorders in the People's Republic of China. Arch Neurol 1985;42(7):655–657.
82. Okada K, Kobayashi S, Tsunematsu T. Prevalence of Parkinson's disease in Izumo City, Japan. Gerontology 1990;36(5–6):340–344.
83. Tan LC, Venketasubramanian N, Hong CY, et al. Prevalence of Parkinson disease in Singapore: Chinese vs Malays vs Indians. Neurology 2004;62(11):1999–2004.
84. Wang SJ, Fuh JL, Liu CY, et al. Parkinson's disease in Kin-Hu, Kinmen: A community survey by neurologists. Neuroepidemiology 1994;13(1-2):69–74.
85. Wang SJ, Fuh JL, Teng EL, et al. A door-to-door survey of Parkinson's disease in a Chinese population in Kinmen. Arch Neurol 1996;53(1):66–71.
86. Zhang L, Nie ZY, Liu Y, et al. The prevalence of PD in a nutritionally deficient rural population in China. Acta Neurol Scand2005;112(1):29–35.
87. Zhang ZX, Anderson DW, Huang JB, et al. Prevalence of Parkinson's disease and related disorders in the elderly population of greater Beijing, China. Mov Disord 2003;18(7):764–772.

88. Zhang ZX, Roman GC, Hong Z, et al. Parkinson's disease in China: Prevalence in Beijing, Xian, and Shanghai. Lancet 2005;365(9459):595–597.
89. Barbosa MT, Caramelli P, Maia DP, et al. Parkinsonism and Parkinson's disease in the elderly:A community-based survey in Brazil (the Bambui study). Mov Disord 2006;21(6):800–808.
90. Chouza C, Ketzoian C, Caamano JL, et al. Prevalence of Parkinson's disease in a population of Uruguay. Preliminary results. Adv Neurol 1996;69:13–17.
91. Mayeux R, Denaro L, Hemenegildo N. A population-based investigation of Parkinson's disease with and without dementia: Relationships to age and gender. Arch Neurol 1992;42:492–497.
92. Melcon MO, Anderson DW, Vergara RH, Rocca WA. Prevalence of Parkinson's disease in Junin, Buenos Aires Province, Argentina. Mov Disord 1997;12(2):197–205.
93. Nicoletti A, Sofia V, Bartoloni A, et al. Prevalence of Parkinson's disease: A door-to-door survey in rural Bolivia. Parkinsonism Relat Disord 2003;10(1):19–21.
94. Svenson LW. Regional disparities in the annual prevalence rates of Parkinson's disease in Canada. Neuroepidemiology 1991;10(4):205–210.
95. Caradoc-Davies TH, Weatherall M, Dixon GS, et al. Is the prevalence of Parkinson's disease in New Zealand really changing? Acta Neurol Scand1992;86(1):40–44.
96. McCann SJ, LeCouteur DG, Green AC, et al. The epidemiology of Parkinson's disease in an Australian population. Neuroepidemiology 1998;17(6):310–317.
97. Guttman M, Slaughter PM, Theriault ME, et al. Parkinsonism in Ontario: Increased mortality compared with controls in a large cohort study. Neurology 2001;57(12): 2278–2282.
98. Wermuth L, Bech S, Petersen MS, et al. Prevalence and incidence of Parkinson's disease in The Faroe Islands. Acta Neurol Scand2008;118(2):126–131.
99. Beyer MK, Herlofson K, Arsland D, et al. Cause of death in a - study of Parkinson's disease. Acta Neurol Scand2001;103:7–11.
100. Imaizumi Y, Kaneko R. Rising mortality from Parkinson's disease in Japan, 1950–1992. Acta Neurol Scand1995;91(3):169–176.
101. Pressley JC, Tang MX, Marder K, et al. Disparities in the recording of Parkinson's disease on death certificates. Mov Disord 2005;20(3):315–321.
102. Bonifati V, Vanacore N, Bellatreccia A,et al. Mortality rates for parkinsonism in Italy (1969 to 1987). Acta Neurol Scand1993;87(1):9–13.
103. Chio A, Magnani C, Tolardo G, et al. Parkinson's disease mortality in Italy, 1951 through 1987. Analysis of an increasing trend. Arch Neurol 1993;50(2):149–153.
104. Clarke CE. Mortality from Parkinson's disease in England and Wales 1921–89. J Neurol Neurosurg Psychiatry 1993;56:690–693.
105. Kurtzke JF, Goldberg ID. Parkinsonism death rates by race, sex, and geography. Neurology 1988;38:1558–1561.
106. Lilienfeld DE, Chan E, Ehland J, et al. Two decades of increasing mortality from Parkinson's disease among the US elderly. Arch Neurol 1990;47(7):731–734.
107. Riggs JE. Longitudinal Gompertzian analysis of Parkinson's disease mortality in the U.S., 1955–1986: The dramatic increase in overall mortality since 1980 is the natural consequence of deterministic mortality dynamics. Mech Ageing Dev 1990;55(3):221–233.
108. Svenson LW. Geographic distribution of deaths due to Parkinson's disease in Canada: 1979–1986. Mov Disord 1990;5(4):322–324.
109. Treves TA, de Pedro-Cuesta J. Parkinsonism mortality in the US, 1. Time and space distribution. Acta Neurol Scand1991;84(5):389–397.
110. Vanacore N, Bonifati V, Bellatreccia A, et al. Mortality rates for Parkinson's disease and parkinsonism in Italy (1969–1987). Neuroepidemiology 1992;11(2):65–73.
111. Williams GR. Morbidity and mortality with parkinsonism. J Neurosurg1966;24:138–143.
112. Chandra V, Bharucha NE, Schoenberg BS. Mortality data for the US for deaths due to and related to twenty neurologic diseases. Neuroepidemiology 1984;3:149–168.
113. Griffiths C, Rooney C. Trends in mortality from Alzheimer's disease, Parkinson's disease and dementia, England and Wales, 1979–2004. Health Stat Q 2006;30:6–14.
114. Di Rocco A, Molinari SP, Kollmeier B, Yahr MD. Parkinson's disease: Progression and mortality in the L-DOPA era. Adv Neurol 1996;69:3–11.
115. Louis ED, Marder K, Cote L, et al. Mortality from Parkinson disease. Arch Neurol 1997;54(3):260–264.
116. Morgante L, Salemi G, Meneghini F, et al. Parkinson disease survival: A population-based study. Arch Neurol 2000;57(4):507–512.
117. D'Amelio M, Ragonese P, Morgante L, et al. Long-term survival of Parkinson's disease: A population-based study. J Neurol 2006;253(1):33–37.
118. de Lau LM, Schipper CM, Hofman A, et al. Prognosis of Parkinson disease: Risk of dementia and mortality: The Rotterdam Study. Arch Neurol 2005;62(8):1265–1269.
119. Herlofson K, Lie SA, Arsland D, et al. Mortality and Parkinson disease: A community based study. Neurology 2004;62(6):937–942.
120. Fall PA, Saleh A, Fredrickson M, et al. Survival time, mortality, and cause of death in elderly patients with Parkinson's disease: A 9-year follow-up. Mov Disord 2003;18(11):1312–1316.
121. Berger K, Breteler MM, Helmer C, et al. Prognosis with Parkinson's disease in Europe: A collaborative study of population-based cohorts. Neurologic Diseases in the Elderly Research Group. Neurology 2000;54(11 suppl 5).
122. Chen H, Zhang SM, Schwarzschild MA, Hernan MA, et al. Survival of Parkinson's disease patients in a large prospective cohort of male health professionals. Mov Disord 2006;21(7):1002–1007.
123. Hely MA, Reid WG, Adena MA, et al. The Sydney multicenter study of Parkinson's disease: The inevitability of dementia at 20 years. Mov Disord 2008;23(6): 837–844.
124. Driver JA, Kurth T, Buring JE, et al. Parkinson disease and risk of mortality: A prospective comorbidity-matched cohort study. Neurology 2008;70(16 Pt 2):1423–1430.
125. Marras C, McDermott MP, Rochon PA, et al. Survival in Parkinson's disease: Thirteen year follow-up of the DATATOP cohort. Neurology 2005;64:87–93.
126. Ishihara LS, Cheesbrough A, Brayne C, et al. Estimated life expectancy of Parkinson's patients compared

with the UK population. J Neurol Neurosurg Psychiatry 2007;78(12):1304–1309.
127. Lanska DJ. Comparison of utilization of Sinemet and Parkinson's disease mortality as surrogate indicators of Parkinson's disease in the United States. J Neurol Sci 1997;145(1):105–108.
128. Imaizumi Y. Geographical variations in mortality from Parkinson's disease in Japan, 1977–1985. Acta Neurol Scand1995;91(5):311–316.
129. Wooten GF, Currie LJ, Bovbjerg VE, et al. Are men at greater risk for Parkinson's disease than women? J Neurol Neurosurg Psychiatry 2004;75(4):637–639.
130. Kimura H, Kurimura M, Wada M, et al. Female preponderance of Parkinson's disease in Japan. Neuroepidemiology 2002;21(6):292–296.
131. Kessler II. Epidemiologic studies of Parkinson's disease. III. A - survey. Am J Epidemiol 1972;96(4):242–254.
132. Lombard A, Gelfand M. Parkinson's disease in the African. Centr Afr J Med 1978;24(1):5–8.
133. Paddison RM, Griffith RP. Occurrence of Parkinson's disease in black patients at Charity Hospital in New Orleans. Neurology 1974;24:688–690.
134. Reef HE. Prevalence of Parkinson's disease in a multiracial community. In Jage HWA, Bruyn GW, Heihstee APJ, eds. Eleventh World Congress of Neurology. Amsterdam: Excerpta Medica, 1977:125.
135. Schoenberg BS, Anderson DW, Haerer AF. Prevalence of Parkinson's disease in the biracial population of Copiah County, Mississippi. Neurology 1985;35(6): 841–845.
136. Dahodwala N, Siderowf A, Ming X, et al. Racial Differences in the Diagnosis of Parkinson's Disease. Mov Disord 2009;24(8):1200–1205.
137. Schoenberg BS, Osuntokun BO, Adeuja AO, et al. Comparison of the prevalence of Parkinson's disease in black populations in the rural United States and in rural Nigeria: Door-to-door community studies. Neurology 1988;38(4):645–646.
138. Ragothaman M, Murgod UA, Gururaj G, et al. Lower risk of Parkinson's disease in an admixed population of European and Indian origins. Mov Disord 2003;18(8): 912–914.
139. Milanov I, Kmetski TS, Lyons KE, et al. Prevalence of Parkinson's disease in Bulgarian Gypsies. Neuroepidemiology 2000;19(4):206–209.
140. Tanner CM, Thelen JA, Offord KP, et al. Parkinson's disease in Olmsted County, MN: 1935–1988. Neurology 1992;42:194.
141. Chan DK, Dunne M, Wong A, et al. Pilot study of prevalence of Parkinson's disease in Australia. Neuroepidemiology 2001;20(2):112–117.
142. Rocca WA, Bower JH, McDonnell SK, et al. Time trends in the incidence of parksinsonism in Olmsted County, Minnesota. Neurology 2001;57:462–467.
143. Zhang ZX, Roman GC. Worldwide occurrence of Parkinson's disease: An updated review. Neuroepidemiology 1993;12(4):195–208.
144. Wermuth L, von Weitzel-Mudersbach P, Jeune B. A two-fold difference in the age-adjusted prevalences of Parkinson's disease between the island of Als and the Faroe Islands. European J Neurol 2000;7(6):655–660.
145. Autere JM, Moilanen JS, Myllyla VV, et al. Familial aggregation of Parkinson's disease in a Finnish population. J Neurol Neurosurg Psychiatry 2000;69(1):107–109.
146. Bonifati V, Fabrizio E, Vanacore N, et al. Familial Parkinson's disease: A clinical genetic analysis. Can J Neurol Sci 1995;22:272–279.
147. De Michele G, Volpe G, Filla A, et al. Environmental and genetic risk factors in Parkinson's disease: A case-control study in Southern Italy. Mov Disord 1996;11(1): 17–23.
148. Morano A, Jimenez-Jimenez F, Molina J, et al. Risk factors for Parkinson's disease: Case-control study in the province of Caceres, Spain. Acta Neurol Scand 1994;89: 164–170.
149. Payami H, Larsen K, Bernard S, et al. Increased risk of Parkinson's disease in parents and siblings of patients. Ann Neurol 1994;36(4):659–661.
150. Preux PM, Condet A, Anglade C, et al. Parkinson's disease and enviromental factors. Matched case-control study in the Limousin region, France. Neuroepidemiology 2000;19:333–337.
151. Taylor CA, Saint-Hilaire MH, Cupples LA, et al. Environmental, medical, and family history risk factors for Parkinson's disease: A New England-based case control study. American Journal of Medical Genetics 1999;88:742–749.
152. Vieregge P, Heberlein I. Increased risk of Parkinson's disease in relatives of patients. Ann Neurol 1995;37:685.
153. Werneck AL, Alvarenga H. Genetics, drugs and environmental factors in Parkinson's disease. A case-control study. Arquivos de Neuro-Psiquiatria 1999;57:347–355.
154. Herishanu YO, Medvedovski M, Goldsmith JR, et al. A case-control study of Parkinson's disease in urban population of southern Israel. Can J Neurol Sci 2001;28(2): 144–147.
155. Zorzon M, Capus L, Pellegrino A, et al. Familial and environmental risk factors in Parkinson's disease: A case-control study in north-east Italy. Acta Neurol Scand2002;105(2):77–82.
156. Marder K, Levy G, Louis E. Familial aggregation of early- and late-onset Parkinson's disease. Ann Neurol 2003;54:507–513.
157. Korchounov A, Schipper HI, Preobrazhenskaya IS, et al. Differences in age at onset and familial aggregation between clinical types of idiopathic Parkinson's disease. Mov Disord 2004;19:1059–1064.
158. Spanaki C, Plaitakis A. Bilineal transmission of Parkinson disease on Crete suggests a complex inheritance. Neurology 2004;62:815–817.
159. Tan XH, Wang SM, Xue NQ, et al. Study on the risk factors and its interaction on Parkinson disease. Zhonghua Liu Xing Bing Xue Za Zhi 2004;25:527–530.
160. Elbaz A, Grigoletto F, Baldereschi M, et al. Familial aggregation of Parkinson's disease: A population-based case-control study in Europe. EUROPARKINSON Study Group. Neurology 1999;52:1876–1882.
161. Marder K, Tang MX, Mejia H, et al. Risk of Parkinson's disease among first-degree relatives: A community-based study. Neurology 1996;47(1):155–160.
162. Semchuk K, Love E, Lee R. Parkinson's disease: A test of the multifactorial etiologic hypothesis. Neurology 1993;43:1173–1180.

163. Kuopio AM, Marttila R, Helenius H, et al. Familian occurence of Parkinson's disease in a community-based case-control study. Parkinsonism Relat Disord 2001;7: 297–303.
164. Duzcan F, Zencir M, Ozdemir F, al. E. Familial influence on parkinsonism in a rural area of Turkey (Kizilcaboluk-Denizli): A case-control study. Mov Disord 2003;18: 799–804.
165. Kurz M, Alves G, Aarsland D, Larsen JP. Familial Parkinson's disease: A community-based study. European J Neurol 2003;10:159–163.
166. Rocca WA, McDonnell SK, Strain KJ, et al. Familial aggregation of Parkinson's disease: The Mayo Clinic family study. Ann Neurol 2004;56(4):495–502.
167. Sundquist K, Li X, Hemminki K, et al. Familial risks of hospitalization for Parkinson's disease in first-degree relatives: A nationwide follow-up study from Sweden. Neurogenetics 2006;7(4):231–237.
168. Thacker EL, Ascherio A, Thacker EL, et al. Familial aggregation of Parkinson's disease: A meta-analysis. Mov Disord 2008;23(8):1174–1183.
169. de Rijk MC, Breteler MM, Van der Meche FG, et al. The risk of Parkinson's disease among persons with a family history of Parkinson's disease or dementia: The Rotterdam study. Neurology 1997;48:A333.
170. Sveinbjornsdottir S, Hicks AA, Jonsson T, et al. Familial aggregation of Parkinson's disease in Iceland. N Engl J Med 2000;343:1765–1770.
171. Moilanen JS, Autere JM, Myllyla VV, et al. Complex segregation analysis of Parkinson's disease in the Finnish population. Hum Genet 2001;108:184–189.
172. Ozelius LJ, Senthil G, Saunders-Pullman R, et al. LRRK2 G2019S as a cause of Parkinson's disease in Ashkenazi Jews. N Engl J Med 2006;354(4):424–425.
173. Lesage S, Durr A, Tazir M, et al. LRRK2 G2019S as a cause of Parkinson's disease in North African Arabs. N Engl J Med 2006;354(4):422–423.
174. Marsden C. Parkinson's disease in twins. J Neurol Neurosurg Psychiatry 1987;50:105–106.
175. Marttila RJ, Kaprio J, Koskenvuo M, Rinne UK. Parkinson's disease in a nationwide twin cohort. Neurology 1988;38(8):1217–1219.
176. Tanner CM, Ottman R, Goldman SM, et al. Parkinson disease in twins. An etiologic study. JAMA 1999;281(4): 341–346.
177. Vieregge P, Schiffke KA, Friedrich HJ, et al. Parkinson's disease in twins. Neurology 1992;42:1453–1461.
178. Ward C, Duvoisin R, Ince S, et al. Parkinson's disease in 65 pairs of twins and in a set of quadruplets. Neurol 1983;33:815–824.
179. Zimmerman TR, Jr., Bhatt M, Calne DB, et al. Parkinson's disease in monozygotic twins: A follow-up study. Neurol Suppl 1991;41:255.
180. Wirdefeldt K, Gatz M, Schalling M, et al. No evidence for heritability of Parkinson disease in Swedish twins. Neurology 2004;63(2):305–311.
181. Burn D, Mark M, Playford E, et al. Parkinson's disease in twins studied with 18F-dopa and positron emission tomography. Neurology 1992;42:1894–1900.
182. Holthoff V, Vieregge P, Kessler J, et al. Discordant twins with Parkinson's disease: Positron emission tomography and early signs of impaired cognitive circuits. Ann Neurol 1994;36:176–182.
183. Langston J, Ballard P, Tetrud J, et al. Chronic parkinsonism in humans due to a product of meperidine-analog synthesis. Science 1983;219:979–980.
184. Davis GC, Williams AC, Markey SP, et al. Chronic parkinsonism secondary to intravenous injection of meperidine analogues. Psychiatry Res 1979;1:249–254.
185. Forno LS, Langston JW, DeLanney LE, et al. Locus ceruleus lesions and eosinophilic inclusions in MPTP-treated monkeys. Ann Neurol 1986;20:449–455.
186. Ricaurte GA, deLanney LE, Irwin I, et al. Older dopaminergic neurons do not recover from the effects of MPTP. Neuropharmacology 1987;26:97–99.
187. Betarbet R, Sherer TB, MacKenzie G, et al. Chronid systemic pesticide exposure reproduces feature of Parkinson's disease. Nat Neurosci 2000;3:1301–1306.
188. Barbeau A, Dallaire L, Buu NT, et al. Comparative behavioral, biochemical and pigmentary effects of MPTP, MPP+ and paraquat in Rana pipiens. Life Sciences 1985;37:1529–1538.
189. Priyadarshi A, Khuder SA, Schaub EA, et al. A meta-analysis of Parkinson's disease and exposure to pesticides. Neurotoxicology 2000;21(4):435–440.
190. Kamel F, Tanner C, Umbach D, et al. Pesticide exposure and self-reported Parkinson's disease in the agricultural health study. Am J Epidemiol 2007;165(4): 364–374.
191. Ritz B, Yu F. Parkinson's disease mortality and pesticide exposure in California 1984–1994. Int J Epidemiol 2000;29(2):323–329.
192. Nelson LM, Van Den Eeden SK, Tanner CM, et al. Home pesticide exposure and the risk of Parkinson's disease. Neurology 2000;54:A472–473.
193. Firestone JA, Smith-Weller T, Franklin G, et al. Pesticides and risk of Parkinson disease: A population based case-control study. Arch Neurol 2005;62(1):91–95.
194. Brown TP, Rumsby PC, Capleton AC, et al. Pesticides and Parkinson's disease--is there a link? Environ Health Perspect 2006;114(2):156–164.
195. Fleming L, Mann J, Bean J, et al. Parkinson's disease and brain levels of organochlorine pesticides. Ann Neurol 1994;36:100–103.
196. Smargiassi A, Mutti A, De Rosa A, et al. A case-control study of occupational and environmental risk factors for Parkinson's disease in the Emilia-Romagna region of Italy. Neurotoxicology 1998 Aug-Oct;19(4–5):709–712.
197. Rybicki BA, Johnson CC, Uman J, et al. Parkinson's disease mortality and the industrial use of heavy metals in Michigan. Mov Disord 1993;8(1):87–92.
198. Tanner CM. The role of environmental toxins in the etiology of Parkinson's disease. Trends Neurosci 1989;12: 49–54.
199. Seidler A, Hellenbrand W, Robra B, et al. Possible environmental, occupational, and other etiologic factors for Parkinson's disease: A case-control study in Germany. Neurology 1996;46:1275–1284.
200. Anthony JC, LeResche L, Niaz U, et al. Limits of the 'Mini-Mental State' as a screening test for dementia and delirium among hospital patients. Psychol Med 1982;12: 397–408.

201. Sofic E, Paulus W, Jellinger KA, et al. Selective increase of iron in substantia nigra zone compacta of Parkinsonian brains. J Neurochem 1991;56:978–982.
202. Gorell JM, Rybicki BA, Cole Johnson C, et al. Occupational metal exposures and the risk of Parkinson's disease. Neuroepidemiology 1999;18:303–308.
203. Coon S, Stark A, Peterson EL, et al. Whole-body lifetime occupational exposure and risk of Parkinson's disease. Environ Health Perspect 2006;114(12):1872–1876.
204. Kaiser J. Manganese: A high-octane dispute. Science 2003;300(5621):926–928.
205. Racette BA, McGee-Minnich L, Moerlein SM, et al. Welding-related parkinsonism: Clinical features, treatment, and pathophysiology. Neurology 2001;56(1):8–13.
206. Racette BA, Tabbal SD, Jennings D, et al. Prevalence of parkinsonism and relationship to exposure in a large sample of Alabama welders. Neurology 2005;64(2):230–235.
207. Frigerio R, Elbaz A, Sanft KR, et al. Education and occupations preceding Parkinson disease: A population-based case-control study. Neurology 2005;65(10):1575–1583.
208. Goldman SM, Tanner CM, Olanow CW, et al. Occupation and parkinsonism in three movement disorders clinics. Neurology 2005;65(9):1430–1435.
209. Dick S, Semple S, Dick F, Seaton A. Occupational titles as risk factors for Parkinson's disease. J Occup Med (London) 2007;57(1):50–56.
210. Marsh G, Gula MJ. Employment as a welder and Parkinson disease among heavy equipment manufacturing workers. J Occup Environ Med 2006;45(10):1031–1046.
211. Fored CM, Fryzek JP, Brandt L, et al. Parkinson's disease and other basal ganglia or movement disorders in a large nationwide cohort of Swedish welders. Occup Environ Med 2006;63(2):135–140.
212. Park J, Yoo CI, Sim CS, et al. A retrospective cohort study of Parkinson's disease in Korean shipbuilders. Neurotoxicology 2006;27(3):445–449.
213. Fryzek JP, Hansen J, Cohen S, et al. A cohort study of Parkinson's disease and other neurodegenerative disorders in Danish welders. J Occup Environ Med 2005;47(5): 466–472.
214. Park J, Yoo CI, Sim CS, et al. Occupations and Parkinson's disease: A multi-center case-control study in South Korea. Neurotoxicology 2005;26(1):99–105.
215. Gorell JM, Peterson EL, Rybicki BA, et al. Multiple risk factors for Parkinson's disease. J Neurol Sci 2004;217(2): 169–174.
216. Behari M, Srivastava AK, Das RR, et al. Risk factors of Parkinson's disease in Indian patients. J Neurol Sci 2001;190:49–55.
217. Chen H, Zhang SM, Hernan MA, et al. Diet and Parkinson's disease: A potential role of dairy products in men. Ann Neurol 2002;52:793–801.
218. Park M, Ross GW, Petrovitch H, et al. Consumption of milk and calcium in midlife and the future risk of Parkinson disease. Neurology 2005;64(6):1047–1051.
219. Chen H, O'Reilly EJ, McCullough ML, et al. Consumption of dairy products and risk of Parkinson's disease. Am J Epidemiol 2007;165:998–1006.
220. Johnson CC, Gorell JM, Rybicki BA, et al. Adult nutrient intake as a risk factor for Parkinson's disease. Int J Epidemiol 1999;28:1102–1109.
221. Logroscino G, Marder K, Cote L, et al. Dietary Lipids and Antioxidants in Parkinson's Disease: A Population-based, Case-Control Study. Ann Neurol 1996;39:89–94.
222. Anderson C, Checkoway H, Franklin G, et al. Dietary factors in Parkinson's disease: The role of food groups and specific foods. Mov Disord 1999;14(1):21–27.
223. Gaenslen A, Gasser T, Berg D. Nutrition and the risk for Parkinson's disease: Review of the literature. J Neural Transm 2008.
224. Abbott RD, Ross GW, White LR, et al. Midlife adiposity and the future risk of Parkinson's disease. Neurology 2002;59(7):1051–1057.
225. Chen H, Zhang SM, Schwarzschild MA, et al. Obesity and the risk of Parkinson's disease. Am J Epidemiol 2004;159:547–555.
226. Hu G, Jousilahti P, Nissinen A, et al. Body mass index and the risk of Parkinson's disease. Neurology 2006;67: 1955–1959.
227. Simon KC, Chen H, Schwarzschild M, et al. Hypertension, hypercholesterolemia, diabetes, and risk of Parkinson disease. Neurology 2007;69(17):1688–1695.
228. de Lau LM, Breteler MM, de Lau LML, et al. Epidemiology of Parkinson's disease. Lancet Neurol 2006;5(6):525–535.
229. Huang X, Chen H, Miller WC, et al. E. Lower low-density lipoprotein cholesterol levels are associated with Parkinson's disease. Mov Disord 2007;22(3):377–381.
230. Poskanzer DC, Schwab RS, Fraser DW. Further observations on the cohort phenomenon in Parkinson's syndrome. In Barbeau A, Brunette JR (eds). Progress in Neurogenetics. Amsterdam: Excerpta Medica Foundation, 1969, pp. 497–505.
231. Ehmeier KP, Mutch WJ, Calder SA, et al. Does idiopathic parkinsonism in Aberdeen follow intrauterine influenza? J Neurol Neurosurg Psychiatry 1989;52:911–913.
232. Elizan T, Casals J. The viral hypothesis in Parkinson's disease in Alzheimer's disease: A critique. In Kurstak E, Lipowski S, Morozov P (eds). Viruses, Immunity and Mental Disorders. New York: Plenum Press, 1987, pp. 47–59.
233. Fazzini E, Fleming J, Fahn S. Cerebrospinal fluid antibodies to coronaviruses in patients with Parkinson's disease. Neurology 1990;40(suppl 1):169.
234. Marttila R, Halonen P, Rinne U. Influenza virus antibodies in parkinsonism. Arch Neurol 1977;34:99–100.
235. Mattock C, Marmot M, Stern G. Could Parkinson's disease follow intra-uterine influenza?: A speculative hypothesis. J Neurol Neurosurg Psychiatry 1988;51(6):753–756.
236. Kohbata S, Beaman B. L-Dopa-Responsive movement disorder caused by Nocardia asteroides localized in the brains of mice. Infect Immun 1991;59(1):181–191.
237. Hubble J, Cao T, Kjelstrom J, et al. Nocardia species as an etiologic agent in Parkinson's disease: Serological testing in a case-control study. J Clin Microbiol 1995;33(10): 2768–2769.
238. Sasco AJ, Paffenbarger RS, Jr. Measles infection and Parkinson's disease. Am J Epidemiol 1985;122(6):1017–1031.
239. Snyder A, Stricker E, Zigmond M. Stress-induced neurological impairments in an animal model of parkinsonism. Ann Neurol 1985;18:544–551.
240. Spina M, Cohen G. Dopamine turnover and glutathione oxidation: Implications for Parkinson's disease. Proc Natnl Acad Sci U S A 1989;86:1398–1400.

241. Gibberd FB, Simmonds JP. Neurological disease in ex-far-east prisoners of war. Lancet 1980;ii:135–137.
242. Page WF, Tanner CM. Parkinson's disease and motor-neuron disease in former prisoners-of-war. Lancet 2000;355:843.
243. Treves TA, Rabey JM, Korczyn A. Case-control study, with use of temporal approach, for evaluation of risk factors for Parkinson's disease. Mov Disord 1990;5:11.
244. Kuopio AM, Marttila RJ, Helenius H, et al. Environmental risk factors in Parkinson's disease. Mov Disord 1999;14(6):928–939.
245. Lees AJ. Trauma and Parkinson disease. Revue Neurologique 1997;153:541–546.
246. Maher NE, Golbe LI, Lazzarini AM, et al. Epidemiologic study of 203 sibling pairs with Parkinson's disease: The GenePD study. Neurology 2002;58(1):79–84.
247. Goldman SM, Tanner CM, Oakes D, et al. Head injury and Parkinson's disease risk in twins. Ann Neurol 2006;60(1):65–72.
248. Bower JH, Maraganore DM, Peterson BJ, et al. Head trauma preceding PD: A case-control study. Neurology 2003;60(10):1610–1615.
249. Menza M. The personality associated with Parkinson's disease. Curr Psychiatry Rep 2000;2:421–426.
250. Liu B, Gao HM, Hong JS. Parkinson's disease and exposure to infections agents and pesticides and the occurrence of brain injuries: Role of neuroinflammation. Environ Health Perspect 2003;111:1065–1073.
251. Chen H, Zhang SM, Schwarzschild MA, Hernan MA, et al. Physical activity and the risk of Parkinson disease. Neurology 2005;64:664–669.
252. Hernan MA, Takkouche B, Caamano-Isorna F, et al. A meta-analysis of coffee drinking, cigarette smoking, and the risk of Parkinson's disease. Ann Neurol 2002;52(3):276–284.
253. Chade AR, Kasten M, Tanner CM. Nongenetic cause of Parkinson's disease. J Neural Transm Suppl 2006;70: 147–151.
254. Mellick GD, Gartner CE, Silburn PA, et al. Passive smoking and Parkinson's disease. Neurology 2006;67(1): 179–180.
255. Ritz B, Ascherio A, Checkoway H, et al. Pooled analysis of tobacco use and risk of Parkinson's disease. Arch Neurol 2007;64:990–997.
256. Menza M, Forman NE, Goldstein HS, et al. Parkinson's disease, personality, and dopamine. J Neuropsychiatry Clin Neurosci 1990;2:282–287.
257. Morens DM, Grandinetti A, Davis JW, et al. Evidence against the operation of selective mortality in explaining the association between cigarette smoking and reduced occurrence of idiopathic Parkinson disease. Am J Epidemiol 1996;144(4):400–404.
258. Morozova N, O'Reilly EJ, Ascherio A, et al. Variations in gender ratios support the connection between smoking and Parkinson's disease. Mov Disord 2008;23(10): 1414–1419.
259. Wirdefeldt K, Gatz M, Pawitan Y, et al. Risk and protective factors for Parkinson's disease: A study in Swedish twins. Ann Neurol 2005;57(1):27–33.
260. Quik M, O'Leary K, Tanner CM, et al. Nicotine and Parkinson's disease: Implications for therapy. Mov Disord 2008;23(12):1641–1652.
261. Kirch DG, Alho AM, Wyatt RJ. Hypothesis: A nicotine-dopamine interaction linking smoking with Parkinson's disease and tardive dyskinesia. Cell Mol Neurobiol 1988;8(3):285–291.
262. Soto-Otero R, Mendez-Alvarez E, Riguera-Vega R, et al. Studies on the interaction between 1,2,3,4-tetrahydro-beta-carboline and cigarette smoke: A potential mechanism of neuroprotection for Parkinson's disease. Brain Res 1998;802:155–162.
263. Hu G, Bidel S, Jousilahti P, et al. Coffee and tea consumption and the risk of Parkinson's disease. Mov Disord 2007;22:2242–2248.
264. Saaksjarvi K, Knekt P, Rissanen H, et al. Prospective study of coffee consumption and risk of Parkinson's disease. Eur J Clin Nutr 2008;62(7):908–915.
265. Ascherio A, Zhang SM, Hernan MA, et al. Prospective study of caffeine consumption and risk of Parkinson's disease in men and women. Ann Neurol 2001;50(1): 56–63.
266. Ross GW, Abbott RD, Petrovitch H, et al. Association of coffee and caffeine intake with the risk of Parkinson disease. JAMA 2000;283(20):2674–2679.
267. Chen J, Moratalla R, Impagnatiello F, et al. The role of the D(2) dopamine receptor (D(2)R) in A(2A) adenosine receptor (A(2A)R)-mediated behavioral and cellular responses as revealed by A(2A) and D(2) receptor knockout mice. Proc Natl Acad Sci U S A 2001;98(4):1970–1975.
268. Ulanowska K, Piosik J, Gwizdek-Wisniewska A, et al. Formation of stacking complexes between caffeine (1,2,3-trimethylxanthine) and 1-methyl-4-phenyl-1,2,3,-6-tetrahydropyridine may attenuate biological effects of this neurotoxin. Bioorg Chem 2005;33(5):402–413.
269. de Rijk MC, Breteler MB, den Breeijen JH, et al. Dietary antioxidants and Parkinson disease. Arch Neurol 1997;54:762–765.
270. Golbe L, Farrell T, Davis P. Case-control study of early life dietary factors in Parkinson's disease. Arch Neurol 1988;45:350–353.
271. Golbe L, Farrell T, Davis P. Follow-up study of early life protective and risk factors in Parkinson's disease. Mov Disord 1990;5:66–70.
272. Hellenbrand W, Boeing H, Robra B, et al. Diet and Parkinson's disease II: A possible role for the past intake of specific nutrients. Results from a self-administered food-frequency questionnaire in a case-control study. Neurology 1996;47:644–650.
273. Scheider WL, Hershey LA, Ven JE, et al. Dietary antioxidants and other dietary factors in etiology of Parkinson's disease. Mov Disord 1997;12:190–196.
274. Vieregge P, Maravic C, Friedrich HJ. Life-style and dietary factors early and late in Parkinson's disease. Can J Neurol Sci 1992;19:170–173.
275. Gao X, Chen H, Choi HK, et al. Diet, urate, and Parkinson's disease risk in men. Am J Epidemiol 2008;167(7): 831–838.
276. Davis JW, Grandinetti A, Waslien CI, et al. Observations on serum uric acid levels and the risk of idiopathic Parkinson's disease. Am J Epidemiol 1996;144(5):480–484.
277. de Lau LM, Koudstaal PJ, Hofman A, et al. Serum uric acid levels and the risk of Parkinson disease. Ann Neurol 2005;58(5):797–800.

278. Weisskopf MG, O'Reilly EJ, Chen H, et al. Plasma urate and risk of Parkinson's disease. Am J Epidemiol 2007;166:561–567.
279. Alonso A, Rodriguez LA, Logroscino G, et al. Gout and risk of Parkinson disease: A prospective study. Neurology 2007;69(17):1696–1700.
280. Schwarzschild MA, Schwid SR, Marek K, et al. Serum urate as a predictor of clinical and radiographic progression in Parkinson disease. Arch Neurol 2008;65(6):716–723.
281. Abbott RD, Ross GW, White LR, et al. Environmental, life-style, and physical precursors of clinical Parkinson's disease: Recent findings from the Honolulu-Asia Aging Study. J Neurol 2003;250 Suppl 3:III30–39.
282. Chen H, Zhang SM, Hernan MA, et al. Nonsteroidal anti-inflammatory drugs and the risk of Parkinson disease. Arch Neurol 2003;60:1059–1064.
283. Hernan MA, Logroscino G, Garcia Rodriguez LA, et al. Nonsteroidal anti-inflammatory drugs and the incidence of Parkinson disease. Neurology 2006;66(7):1097–1099.
284. Esposito E, Di Matteo V, Benigno A, et al. Non-steroidal anti-inflammatory drugs in Parkinson's disease. Exp Neurol2007;69(19):295–312.
285. Wahner AD, Bronstein JM, Bordelon YM, et al. Nonsteroidal anti-inflammatory drugs may protect against Parkinson disease. Neurology 2007;69(19):1836–1842.
286. Ton TG, Heckbert SR, Longstreth WT, Jr., et al. Nonsteroidal anti-inflammatory drugs and risk of Parkinson's disease. Mov Disord 2006;21(7):964–969.
287. Bornebroek M, de Lau LM, Haag MD, et al. Nonsteroidal anti-inflammatory drugs and the risk of Parkinson disease. Neuroepidemiology 2007;28(4):193–196.
288. Chen H, O'Reilly EJ, Schwarzschild MA, et al. Peripheral inflammatory biomarkers and risk of Parkinson's disease. Am J Epidemiol 2008;167(1):90–95.
289. Chan CS, Guzman JN, Ilijic E, et al. 'Rejuvenation' protects neurons in mouse models of Parkinson's disease. Nature 2007;447(7148):1081–1086.
290. Rodnitzky RL. Can calcium antagonists provide a neuroprotective effect in Parkinson's disease? Drugs 1999;57(6):845–849.
291. Ton TG, Heckbert SR, Longstreth WT, Jr., et al. Calcium channel blockers and beta-blockers in relation to Parkinson's disease. Parkinsonism Relat Disord 2007;13(3):165–169.
292. Becker C, Jick SS, Meier CR. Use of antihypertensives and the risk of Parkinson disease. Neurology 2008;DOI 10.1212/01.wnl.0000303818.38960.44.
293. Wolozin B, Wang SW, Li NC, et al. Simvastatin is associated with a reduced incidence of dementia and Parkinson's disease. BMC Medicine 2007;5:20.
294. Huang Y, Halliday GM, Vandebona H, et al. Prevalence and clinical features of common LRRK2 mutations in Australians with Parkinson's disease. Mov Disord 2007;22(7):982–989.
295. Thacker EL, Chen H, Patel A, et al. Recreational physical activity and risk of Parkinson's disease. Mov Disord 2007.
296. Logroscino G, Sesso HD, Paffenbarger RS, Jr., et al. Physical activity and risk of Parkinson's disease: A prospective cohort study. J Neurol Neurosurg Psychiatry 2006;77(12):1318–1322.
297. Dishman RK, Berthoud HR, Booth FW, al. E. Neurobiology of exercise. Obesity (Silver Spring) 2006;14(3):345–356.
298. Rocca WA, Bower JH, Maraganore DM, et al. Increased risk of parkinsonism in women who underwent oophorectomy before menopause. Neurology 2008;70(3):200–209.

CHAPTER 11

Neurochemistry and Neuropharmacology of Parkinson's Disease

Federico Micheli, Maria G. Cersosimo, and G. Frederick Wooten

▶ INTRODUCTION

Parkinsonism is a clinical syndrome characterized by tremor at rest, bradykinesia and hypokinesia and cogwheel rigidity. There are many causes or etiologies of parkinsonism, but the most common is Parkinson's disease (PD). PD has long been considered a clinical–pathologic entity defined clinically by parkinsonism and pathologically by depigmentation of the substantia nigra with the appearance of Lewy bodies: eosinophilic, intraneuronal, cytoplasmic inclusion bodies that contain high concentrations of ubiquitinated α-synuclein. Recent discoveries suggest, however, that the clinical phenotype of PD is much more heterogenous than originally conceived and strains the concept of a clinical entity. At the same time, doubt has been raised about the requirement for the presence of Lewy bodies in PD by the apparent absence of these inclusions from the brains of patients with some of the recently described autosomal dominant and recessive genetic mutations causing clinically typical PD. In addition, there is now an impressive body of evidence emerging that identifies a variety of clinical conditions that cluster in patients destined to develop PD before any of the classical features of parkinsonism are present. These include gastrointestinal dysfunction,[1] sleep disorders,[2] and anosmia.[3] Braak and colleagues have suggested that these "premonitory symptoms" are associated with Lewy body pathology in lower brain stem nuclei preceding the development of such pathology in dopaminergic neurons of the substantia nigra.[4] Further complicating the simplistic concept of a clinical–pathologic entity is the emerging evidence that many patients with the clinical features of PD will develop freezing and imbalance, depression, apathy, fatigue, psychosis, and dementia in the later clinical stages of their disease.[5] These typically late-emerging features are not particularly responsive to dopaminergic therapies and are unlikely to develop as a consequence of the death of dopamine neurons in the nigrostriatal pathway, per se.

Thus, according to the Braak hypothesis, one may identify three clinical phases of PD as the Lewy body pathology marches inexorably rostrally (see Fig. 11–1). (1) A predopamine phase would be characterized by some combination of gastrointestinal dysfunction, sleep disorders, anosmia, and restless leg syndrome; (2) a dopamine deficiency phase would be heralded by the onset of tremor, bradykinesia, and rigidity; and (3) a postdopamine deficiency phase would subsequently develop consisting of imbalance, freezing, falls, depression, apathy, fatigue, psychosis, and dementia. Although this is a useful structure for considering the various features associated with Lewy body pathology, experienced clinicians, however, recognize numerous exceptions to this "typical" sequence of symptom evolution. Recently, Burke and colleagues have critically reviewed the Braak staging scheme and raised a number of issues as to its validity.[6] Nevertheless, the defining clinical features of what we today call PD (tremor, bradykinesia, and rigidity) may now properly be viewed as merely a stage or phase of a more pervasive pathologic process with clinical features ranging from constipation to dementia.[7]

With the very concept of PD as a clinical pathologic entity eroding, with the rapid accumulation of knowledge regarding the role of disordered synuclein metabolism in the demise of central nervous system neurons, and with the lack of any clearly disease-modifying therapy for PD, the clinically oriented reader can take some solace in the remarkable progress reflected in the dopamine story. It may be "beating a dead horse"[8] and "so last century,"[9] but the development of dopaminergic therapy for PD over the past nearly 40 years has been associated with substantial improvement in the quality and duration of life for those affected with PD and remains the only pharmacotherapy with substantial

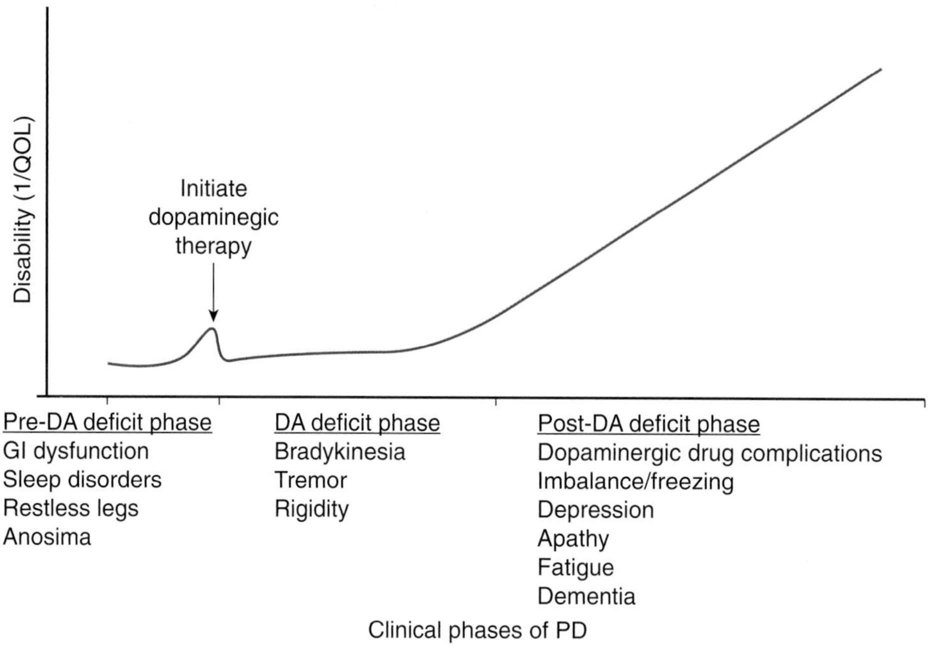

Figure 11–1. Clinical phases of Parkinson's disease and relationship to disability and decreased quality of life. DA, dopamine; QOL, quality of life.

clinical benefit in PD. It is at this point that we start with this chapter on the Neurochemistry and Neurophysiology of PD.

The defining motor signs and symptoms of what is called PD (tremor, bradykinesia, and rigidity) result primarily from dysfunction of the basal ganglia. The central mechanism for the physiologic dysfunction of the basal ganglia in PD is a progressive decline in the concentration of dopamine. In the past 40 years, much progress has been made in identifying the anatomic connections and in characterizing the regional neurochemistry of the basal ganglia. The major intrinsic and extrinsic connections of the several cell groups that comprise the basal ganglia and identified neurotransmitters for each pathway are summarized in Fig. 11–2. Probably the first findings to support the relationship between PD and the basal ganglia were the clinicopathologic correlations of Wilson,[10] coupled with the observations made by neuropathologists of neuronal loss and depigmentation of the substantia nigra in the brains of parkinsonian patients.[11] The subsequent discovery of profound reductions in the concentration of the monoamine neurotransmitter dopamine in the caudate nucleus and putamen of parkinsonian patients,[12] and the recognition that pigmented neurons of the substantia nigra project to the striatum and provide it with dopaminergic input, strengthened the evidence that the motor aspect of PD results from dysfunction of the basal ganglia.[13] Later observations that the neurotoxic opiate derivative 1-methyl-4-phenyl-1,2,3,6-tetrahydropyridine (MPTP) produced parkinsonism in humans and other primates, with resultant neuropathologic changes restricted primarily to the substantia nigra and large decrements in the striatal concentration of dopamine, provided further substantiation for the pathophysiologic basis of tremor, bradykinesia, and rigidity.[14]

The following structures are considered to comprise the basal ganglia: the putamen, caudate, globus pallidus (external and internal segments), subthalamic nucleus, and substantia nigra (pars reticulata, and pars compacta). The major sources of afferents to basal ganglia structures arising from extrinsic neuronal groups include the neocortex, which projects to the caudate and putamen (collectively referred to as the striatum), the intralaminar nuclei of the thalamus projection to the striatum, the locus ceruleus projection to the substantia nigra, and the raphe nuclei projecting to the substantia nigra and the striatum. The major efferent pathways from the basal ganglia structures to extrinsic neuronal groups include the projections from the substantia nigra pars reticulata and the globus pallidus internal segment to the thalamus, as well as the substantia nigra pars reticulata projection to the deep layers of the superior colliculus, the brain stem reticular formation, and the spinal cord. The various nuclear groups of the basal ganglia are intimately interconnected. The striatum and substantia nigra have prominent reciprocal connections. The striatum also projects to both segments of the globus pallidus. The subthalamic nucleus receives afferents from the external segment of the globus pallidus and projects to both the

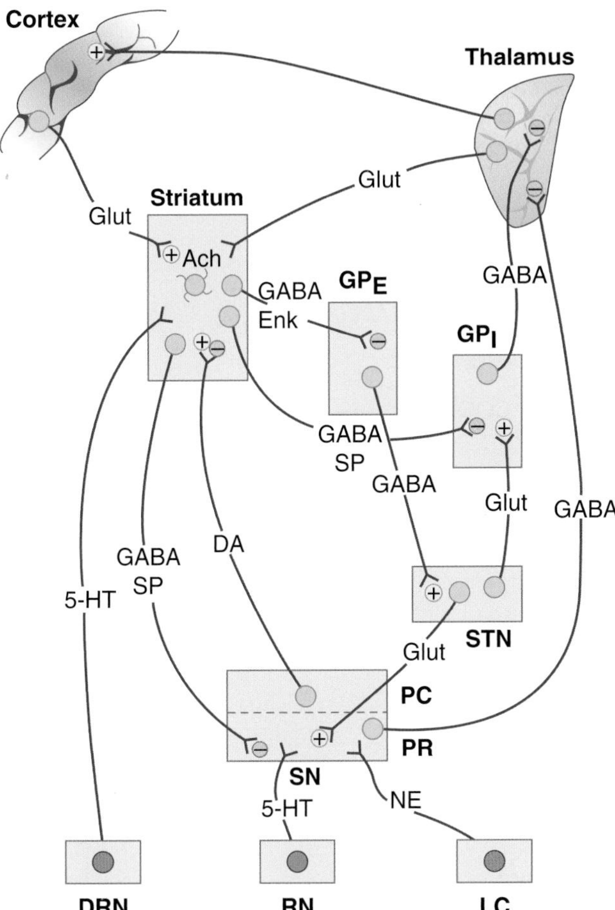

Figure 11–2. Simplified version of the major anatomic pathways within the basal ganglia, including identification of known neurotransmitters, when such information is available. Names and initials in large type identify anatomically distinct nuclear groups within the basal ganglia; abbreviations and contractions in small type denote neurotransmitters. 5-HT, serotonin; Ach, acetylcholine; DRN, dorsal raphe nucleus; Enk, enkephalin; GABA, gamma-aminobutyric acid; GPE, globus pallidus external segment; GPI, globus pallidus internal segment; Glut, glutamate; LC, locus ceruleus; NE, norepinephrine; SN, substantia nigra (PC, pars compacta; PR, pars reticulata); SP, substance P; STN, subthalamic nucleus; RN, raphe nuclei.

substantia nigra pars reticulata and the internal segment of the globus pallidus. In addition, the striatum contains numerous interneurons that do not project outside the striatum. (For an extensive review of basal ganglia anatomy, see Ref. 15.)

The neurotransmitters that have been identified for each projection pathway are depicted in Fig. 11–2, but the entirety of a particular projection may not be represented. For example, glutamate is used as a transmitter by neurons projecting from the neocortex to the stratum, but other as yet unidentified neurotransmitters may also be present in this extensive projection. The neurotransmitters used by many of the basal ganglia projection pathways are known; this provides the potential for selective modification of activity in specific basal ganglia circuits by drugs.

▶ DOPAMINE

GENERAL METABOLISM

Dopamine is synthesized in the brain from the amino acid L-tyrosine via the intermediate compound L-3,4-dihydroxyphenylalanine (L-dopa). Tyrosine hydroxylase (TH), the enzyme that catalyzes the conversion of L-tyrosine to L-dopa, is the rate-limiting step in dopamine synthesis. Because TH is highly localized in catecholamine neurons, it is often used by investigators as a specific marker for dopamine neurons. L-Aromatic amino acid decarboxylase (L-AAAD), the enzyme that catalyzes the conversion of L-dopa to dopamine, has a relatively low substrate specificity and is thought to be present not only in dopamine neurons but also in other cells not specialized to synthesize catecholamines. Once synthesized, dopamine is concentrated in storage vesicles; the membranes of these cytoplasmic organelles contain a high-affinity, energy-dependent, carrier-mediated transport system, the vesicular monoamine transporter ($VMAT_1$) that concentrates dopamine within the vesicle against a concentration gradient.

Under physiologic conditions, dopamine is released from dopaminergic neurons by a calcium-dependent mechanism. Dopamine thus released into the synaptic cleft is inactivated primarily by a high-affinity, stereospecific, carrier-mediated reuptake process mediated by the dopamine transporter (DAT). After reuptake, dopamine may be sequestered again in storage vesicles for rerelease. Released dopamine in the synaptic cleft may bind to specific cell-surface dopamine receptors on the same neuron from which it is released (autoreceptors) or on another neuron (postsynaptic receptors). Some dopamine receptors are linked positively to a dopamine-sensitive adenylate cyclase enzyme activity. When dopamine occupies this receptor, the rate of synthesis of cyclic adenosine monophosphate (cyclic AMP) is increased. Other cell-surface dopamine receptors appear to be linked negatively to adenylate cyclase. When these receptors are occupied by dopamine, there is a reduction in the rate of cyclic AMP synthesis.[16] At least five different dopamine receptors have been cloned and sequenced, each fitting into one of two large families, based on the nature of the linkage to adenylate cyclase (see Chapter 8).

Dopamine is inactivated enzymatically by the action of both monoamine oxidase (MAO), an enzyme

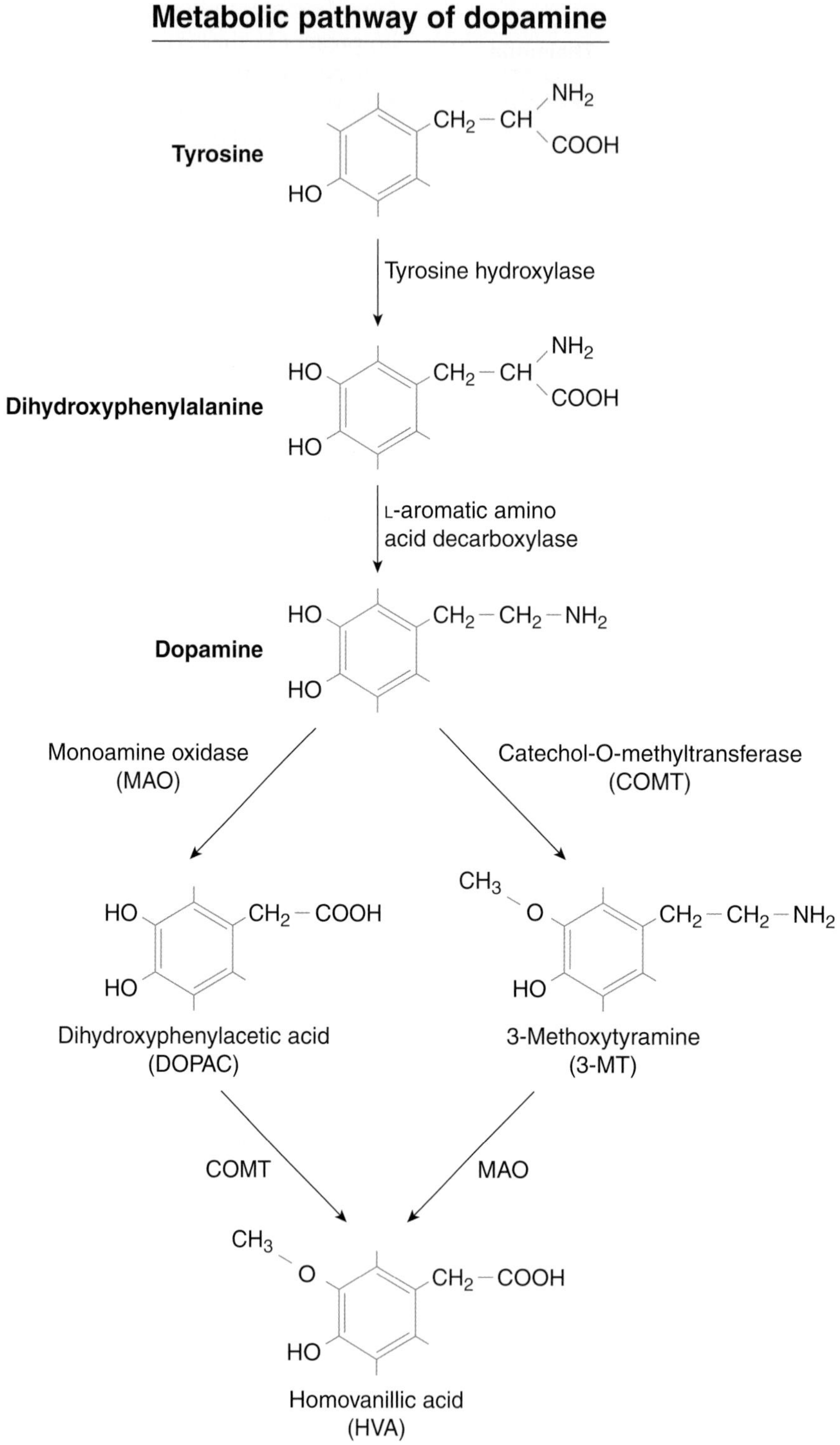

Metabolic pathway of dopamine

Tyrosine

HO – C_6H_4 – $CH_2-CH(NH_2)COOH$

Tyrosine hydroxylase

Dihydroxyphenylalanine

(HO)$_2$ – C_6H_3 – $CH_2-CH(NH_2)COOH$

L-aromatic amino acid decarboxylase

Dopamine

(HO)$_2$ – C_6H_3 – $CH_2-CH_2-NH_2$

Monoamine oxidase (MAO)

Catechol-O-methyltransferase (COMT)

Dihydroxyphenylacetic acid (DOPAC)

3-Methoxytyramine (3-MT)

COMT

MAO

Homovanillic acid (HVA)

Figure 11–3. Enzymatic synthesis and inactivation of dopamine.

associated with mitochondria and present in two forms (MAO-A and MAO-B), and catechol-*O*-methyltransferase (COMT), an enzyme localized primarily in glial cells in the brain. The resultant deamination and 3-*O*-methylation of dopamine produces homovanillic acid (HVA), the principal metabolite of dopamine (Fig. 11–3).

DISPOSITION OF DOPAMINE NEURONS IN BRAIN

Several dopaminergic neuronal cell groups have been identified in the central nervous system.[17] The most prominent group is the mesotelencephalic group. This group is composed of the nigrostriatal system, with cell bodies in the substantia nigra pars compacta that project primarily to the striatum; and the mesocortical system, with cell bodies in the ventral tegmental area that project to the mesial frontal, anterior cingulate, and entorhinal cortices, olfactory bulb, anterior olfactory nucleus, olfactory tubercle, piriform cortex, nucleus accumbens, and amygdaloid complex. The tuberohypophysial dopamine system projects from the arcuate and periventricular hypothalamic nuclei to the intermediate lobe of the pituitary gland and the median eminence. The incertohypothalamic dopamine system projects from the zona incerta and posterior hypothalamus to the dorsal hypothalamic area and septum. Finally, the periventricular dopamine system arises from cell bodies in the periventricular region of the medulla that project to the periventricular and periaqueductal gray, tegmentum, tectum, thalamus, and hypothalamus. The regional destruction of dopaminergic neurons in the substantia nigra of patients with PD appears to be rather specific and selective.[18] Loss of pigmented neurons is greatest in the lateral ventral tier, followed by the medial ventral tier and the dorsal tier. This contrasts dramatically with the pattern of pigmented neuron loss during normal aging in the substantia nigra. In normal aging, the lateral ventral tier is relatively spared, compared with the cell loss in other regions of the substantia nigra.

ROLE OF DOPAMINE IN PD

The first findings to suggest a role for dopamine in PD were the observations that the dopamine depleting drug reserpine (now known to act by inhibiting $VMAT_1$), reproduced both the clinical and pathophysiologic pictures of parkinsonism.[19] Subsequently, Carlsson and colleagues[19] showed that treatment with the dopamine precursor L-dopa reversed the behavioral effects of reserpine and partially restored brain dopamine levels in laboratory animals. These observations, coupled with early histofluorescence data showing very high concentrations of dopamine in the striatum, led Hornykiewicz to study the concentration of dopamine in postmortem brain material from patients who had died with PD.[12]

The discovery of marked reductions in the concentration of dopamine and HVA in the caudate, putamen, and substantia nigra of parkinsonian patients opened the door to a new era in the diagnosis and treatment of brain disease (Table 11–1).[12,20–22] Furthermore, there was a strong positive correlation between the severity of the premorbid parkinsonian clinical syndrome and the degree of dopamine depletion in the striatum. The data, which are summarized in Table 11–1, showed a reduction in dopamine concentration in all basal ganglia structures. A subsequent study of the postmortem striatal dopamine deficit in subregions of the parkinsonian basal ganglia found nearly complete depletion of dopamine in all segments of the putamen.[23] The greatest reduction was found in the caudal portion of the putamen, where dopamine levels were less than 1% of those in control postmortem brains.

Interestingly, the degree of reduction in dopamine concentration was much greater than the reduction in HVA concentration in brains of parkinsonian patients (see Table 11–1). Thus, the ratio of dopamine to HVA was much lower in these brains than in those of controls. Similar changes in the dopamine to HVA ratio have been noted following partial lesions of the nigrostriatal pathway in experimental animals, and as a consequence

▶ TABLE 11–1. DOPAMINE (DA) AND HVA CONCENTRATIONS IN DISCRETE BRAIN REGIONS FROM CONTROLS AND PD PATIENTS

Brain Region	DA (µg/g wet wt)	HVA (µg/g wet wt)	DA/HVA
Putamen*			
Control	5.06 ± 0.39(17)	4.92 ± 0.32(16)	1.03
Parkinsonian patient	0.14 ± 0.13(3)	0.54 ± 0.13(3)	0.26
Caudate nucleus*			
Control	4.06 ± 0.47(18)	2.92 ± 0.37(19)	1.39
Parkinsonian patient	0.20 ± 0.19(3)	1.19 ± 0.10(3)	0.17
Substantia nigra**,†			
Control	0.46(13)**	2.32(7)[c]	0.20
Parkinsonian patient	0.07(10)**	0.41(9)[c]	0.17
Nucleus accumbens‡			
Control	3.79 ± 0.82(8)	4.38 ± 0.64(8)	0.86
Parkinsonian patient	1.61 ± 0.28(4)	3.13 ± 0.13(3)	0.51

Results are expressed as mean ± SEM. Number in parentheses is number of cases.
*Ref. 20.
**Ref. 12.
†Ref. 21.
‡Ref. 22.

▶ **TABLE 11–2. ACTIVITIES OF TH, L-AAAD, COMT, AND MAO IN DISCRETE BRAIN REGIONS FROM CONTROLS AND PD PATIENTS**

Brain Region	TH (nmol CO_2/30 min /100 mg protein)	L-AAAD (nmol CO_2/ 2h/100 mg protein)	COMT (nmol NMN/h/100 mg protein)	MAO (nmol PPA/30 min/ 100 mg protein)
Putamen				
Control	17.4 ± 2.4(3)	432 ± 109(18)	24.1 ± 2.5(11)	1520 ± 127(11)
Parkinsonian patient	3.1 ± 1.2(3)*	32 ± 7(13)**	19.8 ± 3.7(9)	1648 ± 128(10)
Caudate nucleus				
Control	18.7 ± 2.0(3)	364 ± 95(19)	25.4 ± 2.8(10)	1726 ± 149(10)
Parkinsonian patient	3.2 ± 0.5(2)*	54 ± 14(13)**	17.8 ± 3.8(9)	1742 ± 197(10)
Substantia nigra				
Control	17.4(1)	549 ± 294(15)	26.4 ± 4.7(5)	1828 ± 200(5)
Parkinsonian patient	6.1 ± 1.5(3)	21 ± 6(10)	21.7 ± 10.2(9)	1477 ± 284(4)

Results are expressed as mean ± SEM. Number in parentheses is number of patients.
*Differs from control $p < 0.02$.
**Differs from control $p < 0.01$.
Source: Data from Ref. 20.

of treatment with dopamine antagonist drugs. These changes in the dopamine to HVA ratio may reflect both an increase in the metabolic activity of the few remaining dopamine neurons and a reduced capacity for reuptake and storage of released dopamine.[24]

Another postmortem study focused on enzymatic markers of dopamine neurons and dopamine metabolism (Table 11–2). This study revealed marked reductions in the activities of TH and L-AAAD in the caudate, putamen, and substantia nigra of patients with PD, but no changes were found in the levels of activity of MAO and COMT. These results reflect the high degree of localization of TH and L-AAAD in dopamine neurons in the striatum, compared with the more general distribution of MAO and nonneuronal distribution of COMT activities.

Radiolabeled cocaine has been used as a ligand marker for DAT, the neuronal membrane transport site responsible for the reuptake of catecholamines into catecholaminergic neurons. The binding of cocaine to striatal membranes in patients who died with PD was greatly reduced, compared to that of controls.[25] Similar findings have been obtained with ligands more selective for DAT, such as GBR-12935.[26] These results support previous evidence of a large reduction in all measurable neuronal markers for nigrostriatal dopaminergic neurons in the brains of patients with PD.

DOPAMINE RECEPTORS

The principal molecular site of action of dopamine in the brain is at dopamine receptors. Dopamine receptors are divided into two main families or categories: D1-like (positively linked to adenylate cyclase), and D2-like (negatively linked to adenylate cyclase).[16] Five different dopamine receptors have now been cloned and sequenced, but each falls into one of the two main "families." Thus, D1-like receptors include D1 and D5, whereas D2, D3, and D4 are D2-like receptors. The D1 and D2 types are expressed predominantly in the basal ganglia, whereas D3, D4, and D5 have a low level of expression in this structure (see Chapter 8).

D1 receptors in the basal ganglia appear to be expressed predominantly by striatonigral and striatopallidal (to medial pallidum) neurons that are GABAergic and also express substance P and dynorphin. In contrast, D2 receptors appear to be expressed primarily by striatopallidal neurons projecting to the lateral segment of the globus pallidus that are GABAergic and coexpress enkephalin, as well as substantia nigra dopaminergic neurons (autoreceptors), and cholinergic interneurons in the striatum (i.e., some large aspiny neurons). Physiologically, the striatonigral and striatomedial pallidal pathways appear to be activated by the action of dopamine, whereas the striatolateral pallidal pathway appears to be tonically inhibited by the action of dopamine. However, the capacity of dopamine to reverse optimally the bradykinesia, rigidity, and tremor caused by dopamine depletion appears to require the action of dopamine at both receptor types. (For a brief review of this subject, see Ref. 27.)

Numerous studies on dopamine receptor number and density have been carried out in the brains of patients with PD and in experimental animal models of the disease. So far, these studies have revealed overall modest or absent changes in dopamine receptor number, even in the face of large-scale depletion of dopamine. In addition, changes in dopamine receptor number have not proved to correlate well with the side-effects of L-dopa and dopamine agonists such as psychosis and dyskinesia. Collectively, these observations suggest that modifications in dopamine receptor number per se do not make a clinically meaningful contribution to the phenomenology of PD. More recently, some studies have suggested that there may be more important modulation of signaling pathways downstream of the dopamine receptors, such as that of the regulatory phosphoprotein DARRP-32. In addition, polymorphisms in dopamine receptor structure may be significant, as certain alleles of the short tandem repeat polymorphism of the dopamine receptor D2 gene have been found to reduce the risk of developing peak-of-dose dyskinesias and may contribute to decreased susceptibility to such induced dyskinesias.[28]

▶ NOREPINEPHRINE

The principal source of noradrenergic afferents to the forebrain is the locus ceruleus.[29] The locus ceruleus is one of the pigmented brain stem nuclei that is characteristically abnormal in the brains of parkinsonian patients. Specifically, these brains show depigmentation and loss of neurons, with Lewy bodies in the locus ceruleus. Several investigators have described reductions of norepinephrine concentration and dopamine-β-hydroxylase activity (a specific enzymatic marker of noradrenergic neurons) in forebrain regions.[30,31] Data are conflicting about whether norepinephrine levels are affected in the hypothalamus of patients with PD.[30,32] Studies of dopamine-β-hydroxylase activity in the A1 and A2 noradrenergic areas of the brain stem of parkinsonian patients did not reveal any changes, suggesting that these nuclear groups, which also have rostral projections, are spared in PD.[33] Because levels of norepinephrine were rarely below 50% of those of controls in the brains of parkinsonian patients, and, apparently, because certain noradrenergic cell groups of the lower brain stem were spared completely, it is unlikely that PD is associated with a generalized central catecholaminergic deficiency. The consequences of reduced norepinephrine levels in the adult brain are not clear, although evidence for both motor and cognitive functions of noradrenergic systems has been presented.[29]

▶ SEROTONIN

The principal locations of cell bodies of serotonergic neurons are the raphe nuclei of the brainstem. There is no neuropathologic evidence to suggest that these cell groups are specifically affected in PD. Nevertheless, serotonin levels were reduced throughout the forebrain in patients with PD, particularly in the striatum, substantia nigra, and hippocampus.[31,34] The mechanism and significance of the reduction in brain serotonin levels are not known; however, reduced serotonin levels may represent regulation of serotonergic neuronal activity in response to reduced activity of dopaminergic and/or noradrenergic neurons.

▶ GAMMA-AMINOBUTYRIC ACID

Gamma-aminobutyric acid (GABA) is a neurotransmitter found in several prominent basal ganglia projection pathways. There are probably GABA-releasing interneurons in the striatum, as well as GABAergic striatopallidal, striatonigral, nigrocollicular, and pallidothalamic projections.[15] No studies have suggested that these neurons are affected primarily by the pathologic process in PD. It is possible, however, that upregulation or downregulation of GABA activity might occur as a consequence of dopamine depletion in the striatum.

Two specific markers for GABAergic neurons have been studied in postmortem brain material from patients with PD. These include direct measurement of brain GABA levels and assay of the activity of glutamic acid decarboxylase (GAD), the enzyme that catalyzes the conversion of glutamic acid to GABA. Perry and colleagues found that GABA levels were elevated significantly in the putamen of parkinsonian patients,[35] whereas Laaksonen and colleagues found reduced GABA levels in cerebral and cerebellar cortices but no change in GABA levels in any other brain region.[36] Lloyd and Hornykiewicz found reduced GAD activity (approximately 50% of that of controls) in the striatum, globus pallidus, and substantia nigra,[37] a finding confirmed by Laaksonen.[36] Subsequently, Perry and colleagues reported, however, that GAD activity in the putamen of parkinsonian patients did not differ from that in controls.[35]

Thus, there is controversy about whether GAD activity is altered in the brains of patients with PD. Nevertheless, the critical issue is whether GABA turnover is altered and, if so, in which neuronal groups. The development of pharmacologic means to manipulate GABA neurotransmission is a potential avenue for new therapeutic strategies in the management of PD.

▶ ACETYLCHOLINE

The principal site of action of cholinergic neurons in basal ganglia circuitry is thought to be the numerous cholinergic interneurons identified in the striatum.[15] Measurement of the activity of choline acetyltransferase (ChAT), the enzyme that catalyzes the one-step synthesis of acetylcholine, is the most frequently used marker for the cholinergic neurons. Lloyd and colleagues reported a significant reduction in ChAT activity in the putamen, caudate nucleus, globus pallidus, and substantia nigra in the brains of parkinsonian patients.[38] These changes in activity, again, may reflect regulation in response to reduced dopamine levels rather than primary pathologic involvement. Ruberg and colleagues found reduced ChAT activity in cerebral cortex and hippocampus in brains of patients with PD, which perhaps relates to the dementing process in these patients.[39]

▶ NEUROPEPTIDES

Several of the neuropeptides regarded as neurotransmitters or neuromodulators are present in rather high concentrations in some nuclear groups of the basal ganglia. Their distribution has been mapped by immunocytochemical techniques, and radioimmunoassays have been used to quantify regional concentrations of various neuropeptides.

Motor signs of PD have been ascribed in part to overinhibition of the external globus pallidus secondary to hyperactivity of striatopallidal GABA or enkephalinergic neurons.[40]

Inhibition of pallidal GABA release following a dopamine-depleting lesion suggests that enkephalin may attenuate such release in the globus pallidus, specifically after striatal dopamine loss in PD animal models.[40]

Fernandez and colleagues measured the levels of the neuropeptides Met-enkephalin and Leu-enkephalin, substance P, and neurotensin by a combined high-performance liquid chromatography–radioimmunoassay method in autopsy samples of basal ganglia from PD patients, incidental Lewy body disease patients (presymptomatic PD) and matched controls. Dopamine levels were reduced in the caudate nucleus and putamen in PD, but were unaltered in incidental Lewy body disease, while Met-enkephalin values were reduced in the caudate nucleus, putamen, and substantia nigra in PD. Whereas Met-enkephalin levels were reduced in the caudate nucleus and in the putamen in incidental Lewy body disease, Leu-enkephalin levels were decreased in the putamen and undetectable in the substantia nigra in PD. Leu-enkephalin levels were unchanged in incidental Lewy body disease, although there was a trend to reduction in putamen. Substance P levels were reduced in the putamen in PD, but no significant changes were observed in incidental Lewy body disease. Neurotensin levels were increased in the substantia nigra in PD, but were not altered significantly in incidental Lewy body disease, tending to parallel the changes in PD. The changes in basal ganglia peptide levels in incidental Lewy body disease generally followed a trend similar to those seen in PD, but were less marked, suggesting that they are integral part of the disease pathology rather than secondary to dopaminergic neuronal loss or long-term drug therapy.

De Ceballos and Lopez-Lozano[42] assessed Met-enkephalin substance P, and TH immunostaining in caudate nucleus biopsies from 15 PD patients who underwent surgical procedures, and found that low Met-enkephalin immunostaining tended to correlate with disease severity. The different patterns of abnormalities found suggest that a variety of neurochemical phenotypes may exist among PD patients.

Changes in preproenkephalin gene expression in the caudate and putamen have been associated to striatal damage, but their role in the pathogenesis of L-DOPA-induced dyskinesias remains controversial.[43]

Functional interactions between somatostatinergic and dopaminergic transmitter systems have been well documented, supporting a role of somatostatin in several neuropsychiatric disorders, including PD.[44]

Some investigators have suggested that cholecystokinin-8 (CCK-8) coexists with dopamine in dopaminergic neurons.[45] However, using radioimmunoassay methods, Studler and colleagues found reduced CCK-8 levels in the substantia nigra but not in striatal or corticolimbic areas innervated by dopaminergic neurons.[46] These results from postmortem brains of parkinsonian patients cast doubt on the coexistence of dopamine and CCK-8 in nigral neurons.

Somatostatin levels in the basal ganglia of nondemented patients with PD failed to differ from those of controls.[47] However, somatostatin levels in the frontal cortex, hippocampus, and entorhinal cortex of demented parkinsonian patients were reduced, compared with levels in nondemented parkinsonian patients.[47]

As more information is accumulated about the cellular localization and physiologic function of neuropeptides, the significance of these various changes in PD may be elucidated.

▶ ENDOGENOUS FREE RADICAL SCAVENGERS AND GENERATORS

Oxidative stress may play a role in the pathogenesis of PD[48–50] (see Chapter 12). Studies aimed at elucidating the mechanism of MPTP- induced neuronal toxicity focused much attention on the possibility that oxidative MPTP metabolism generates cytotoxic free radical species. Cohen speculated that the generation of free radical species by MAO activity may contribute to dopaminergic neuronal death in PD.[51] In primates, the dopaminergic nigrostriatal neurons contain high concentrations of the pigment neuromelanin. Graham argued that PD may result from cytotoxicity of the products of catecholamine and melanin oxidation.[52] Furthermore, the concentration of iron is now known to be increased, and that of ferritin reduced, in the brains of patients with PD.[53] Iron catalyzes the production of hydroxyl radicals from hydrogen peroxide. Thus, the higher concentrations of free iron in the parkinsonian brain may predispose this disease state to a high rate of free radical production.[53]

Recently, disturbances in brain iron metabolism have been linked to synucleinopathies. Iron binding to α-synuclein accumulated in Lewy bodies was investigated by Golts and colleagues, who found that the conformation of α-synuclein may be modulated by metals, with iron stimulating aggregation and magnesium inhibiting.[54]

A similar study found that free radical generators such as dopamine and hydrogen peroxide also stimulate the production of intracellular aggregates of α-synuclein and ubiquitin.[55] Sangchot and colleagues documented that abnormal iron accumulation decreased cell viability, and increased lipid peroxidation. In addition, morphologic studies disclosed that iron altered mitochondrial morphology, disrupted the nuclear membrane, and translocated α-synuclein from perinuclear regions into the disrupted nucleus.[56] Borie and colleagues investigated the association between iron-related gene polymorphisms and PD and found a significantly higher frequency of G258S transferrin polymorphisms in PD patients, particularly in cases with onset after age 60 and negative family history. Such findings suggest that genetic variations in the control of iron metabolism may contribute to the pathogenesis of PD.[57]

Free radicals are generated constantly in all living tissue, and, when their intracellular concentrations become too high, damage to cellular elements (e.g., lipid, protein, DNA) may occur. Such damage is minimized by endogenous agents such as glutathione, ascorbate, β-carotene, and tocopherol,[58] which are free radical "scavengers." Also, enzymatic defenses exist that "scavenge" free radicals; these enzymes include superoxide dismutase, catalase, and glutathione peroxidase (which requires reduced glutathione).[58] Kunikowska and Jenner studied the regional distribution in rat basal ganglia of messenger ribonucleic acid (mRNA) for the antioxidant enzymes Cu-Zn superoxide dismutase (SOD), MnSOD, and glutathione peroxidase. mRNA levels were significantly higher in substantia nigra pars compacta than in other regions of the basal ganglia, suggesting that substantia nigra pars compacta would be vulnerable to oxidative stress without the high antioxidant capacity provided by these cytoprotective enzymes.[59]

Interestingly the substantia nigra of early PD patients has dramatically decreased levels of the thiol tripeptide glutathione.[49] Perry and colleagues reported that reduced glutathione levels were lower in the substantia nigra than in any other human brain region and that reduced glutathione levels were absent virtually from the substantia nigra of patients dying with PD.[60] Because reduced glutathione is an important endogenous antioxidant, as well as a cofactor for the free radical-scavenging enzyme glutathione peroxidase, it is interesting to speculate that the substantia nigra may be the region of the brain most susceptible to the toxic effects of free radicals. In vitro studies have demonstrated that the reduction in cellular glutathione is associated with a decrease in ubiquitin–protein conjugate levels, and such inhibition of the ubiquitin–proteosome protein degradation pathway may contribute to protein build-up and subsequent cell death.[61] Furthermore, it was shown that glutathione depletion results in selective inhibition of mitochondrial complex I activity.[48]

The activity of catalase has also been reported to be reduced in the brains of patients with PD.[62]

Increased products of lipid peroxidation have been found in the substantia nigra in the parkinsonian brain, and this was associated with a decrease in polyunsaturated fatty acids, which are the substrates for lipid peroxidation.[63] A 10-fold increase in lipid hydroperoxides in the parkinsonian brain has also been documented.[64]

Each of the above observations provides circumstantial evidence to support a role for excessive free radical production in the pathogenesis of PD.

▶ MITOCHONDRIAL FUNCTION

The mitochondrion has been regarded increasingly as the link for signaling pathways involved in degenerative processes. The mitochondrion seems to play a major role in the cellular decision-making that leads, irreversibly, toward the execution phase of cellular death processes[65] (see Chapters 5 and 13). Mitochondria are the major source of superoxide and are responsible for activating apoptosis and oxidative damage during acute neuronal cell death and neurodegenerative disorders such as Alzheimer's disease and PD.[65]

In 1989, Parker and colleagues reported a selective reduction in the activity of complex I of the mitochondrial electron transport chain in platelets of patients with PD,[66] a finding confirmed by several research teams (e.g., Benecke and colleagues,[67]). Subsequently, a selective reduction in NADH-coenzyme Q1 reductase activity (specific for complex I) was reported in the substantia nigra, but not in other areas of the brain, including the globus pallidum and cerebral cortex,[68] of patients with PD.[69] Furthermore, such abnormality was not found in postmortem material from patients with multisystem atrophy. It is thus a remarkable coincidence that MPP^+, the active toxic metabolite of MPTP, appears to exert its cytotoxic effects by inhibiting complex I of the mitochondrial electron transport chain.

Recently, a family of Sephardic Jews with progressive external ophthalmoparesis, skeletal muscle weakness, and parkinsonism with an autosomal-recessive inheritance suggesting a novel mitochondrial disorder of intergenomic communication has been reported.[70]

Experimental work with animal models chronically exposed to the pesticide rotenone, a complex I inhibitor that mimics the complex I deficit in PD, caused retrograde degeneration of the substantia nigra over several months.[71,72] In addition, recent studies showed that abnormal accumulation of α-synuclein could lead to mitochondrial alterations liable to result in oxidative stress and, eventually, cell death.[73]

Preliminary studies suggest that coenzyme Q10, an essential cofactor of the electron transport gene as well as a major antioxidant, which is particularly effective within mitochondria, may slow down the progressive deterioration of function in PD,[74] while blocking the apoptotic cascade has been proposed as a target of neuroprotective therapy.[75]

Again, whether these changes in complex I activity are primary or secondary and whether they are genetically transmitted or acquired remains to be shown. Hopefully, a deeper understanding of mitochondrial dysfunction in PD will afford clues to develop novel therapeutic efforts.

▶ IN VIVO NEUROCHEMISTRY: POSITRON EMISSION TOMOGRAPHY IN PD

Positron emission tomography (PET) techniques have provided the first reliable in vivo marker for neurochemical deficit in PD (see Chapter 3).

PET may be useful to assess disease progression and the efficacy of diverse neuroprotective therapies, as well as the impact of functional neurosurgery on PD patients.[76–78] More recently, PET techniques have been employed to assess subclinical dopaminergic dysfunction in asymptomatic (*parkin*) mutation carriers.[79,80]

Using ^{18}F-fluorodeoxyglucose and PET imaging techniques, it is possible to estimate in vivo the regional rate of glucose utilization in brains of parkinsonian patients.

Martin and colleagues found increased glucose utilization in the inferomedial portion of the basal ganglia, probably corresponding to the globus pallidus, in patients with PD.[81] Similar changes were also reported using ^{15}O imaging with PET techniques in parkinsonian patients.[82] Such an increase in glucose utilization in the globus pallidus was seen in experimental animals with lesions of the substantia nigra, and may represent increased physiologic activity in striatal efferents to the globus pallidus as a consequence of reduced dopamine neurotransmission in the striatum.[83]

Another advance in the field of in vivo neurochemistry using PET technology was the development of a method to image dopamine neurons, using radiolabeled L-dopa.[84] To date, ^{18}F-dopa has been the gold standard to measure presynaptic dopaminergic function. Striatal uptake of ^{18}F-dopa is markedly decreased in PD, more in putamen than in caudate nucleus, and inversely correlates with the severity of motor signs and disease duration.[85]

The uptake of this tracer depends not only on the density of dopaminergic terminals in the striatum but also on dopamine turnover, which in early-stage PD is increased as a result of compensatory mechanisms of surviving dopaminergic terminals. Therefore, ^{18}F-dopa uptake may be upregulated in early PD.[86,87] The density of dopaminergic terminals may be also assessed using new dopamine ligands such as ^{76}Br-Fe-CBT. Riveiro and colleagues compared the striatal uptake of ^{18}F-dopa and ^{76}Br-Fe-CBT in patients with early and advanced PD. They found that reduction in ^{76}Br-Fe-CBT uptake was more severe than reduction of ^{18}F-dopa uptake in early stages. Interestingly, no significant differences were found in the reduction of both tracers in advanced PD patients, suggesting that compensatory mechanisms are only present in early PD and that ^{18}F-dopa, but not ^{76}Br-Fe-CBT, is upregulated in early disease.[86]

Nurmi and colleagues, using ^{18}F-dopa PET scan, found that the disease process in PD first affects posterior putamen, followed by the anterior putamen, and caudate nucleus but, once started, the absolute rate of decline is the same.[76]

Finally, the use of PET for the differential diagnosis of movement disorders is gaining clinical relevance since new tracers are becoming available, as well as objective techniques for the interpretation of PET images to achieve an operator-independent analysis.[88] Unfortunately, these methods are extremely expensive and only available as a research tool.

▶ NEUROCHEMICAL ANALYSIS OF LEWY BODIES

These intraneuronal cytoplasmic inclusions were found first in neurons of the substantia innominata and dorsal motor nucleus of the vagus.[89] Subsequently, Lewy bodies were also detected in pigmented cells of the substantia nigra, as well as in the hypothalamus, locus ceruleus, raphe nuclei of the midbrain and rostral pons, sympathetic ganglia, and spinal cord.[90] The dense core of Lewy bodies is composed of tightly packed aggregates of filaments, vesicular profiles, and other granular material; at the periphery, filamentous structures emerge radially and are mixed with granular and vesicular material. Immunocytochemical studies using polyclonal antibodies to neurofilament polypeptides have demonstrated specific staining of Lewy bodies.[91]

Recently, intracytoplasmic inclusions consisting of α-synuclein, a brain presynaptic protein, have been shown to be characteristic of neurodegenerative Lewy body disorders, and an unprecedented and extensive burden of α-synuclein pathology in the striatum has been described.[92,93] α-Synuclein is a major component of Lewy bodies and Lewy neurites, intraneuronal inclusions that are regarded as neuropathologic hallmarks of PD.[94] These findings have provided important clues about the pathogenesis of PD.

Two missense mutations of the α-synuclein gene (A30P and A53T) have been described in several families with an autosomal dominant form of PD, but α-synuclein also constitutes one of the main components of Lewy bodies in sporadic cases of PD.[95] Moreover, it has been shown that glial cells, both astrocytes and oligodendrocytes, are also affected by α-synuclein pathology.[96] However, the pathogenic relationship between alterations in the biology of α-synuclein and PD-associated neurodegeneration remains speculative. Protein aggregation appears to be the common denominator in a series of distinct neurodegenerative diseases, although its role in the associated neuronal pathology in these various conditions is still elusive. The accumulation of α-synuclein, ubiquitin, and other proteins in Lewy bodies in degenerating dopaminergic neurons in substantia nigra in idiopathic PD suggests that inhibition of normal or abnormal protein degradation may contribute to neuronal death. However, although it appears likely that aggregation of α-synuclein may interfere with its normal function in the cell, this is not the primary cause of the related neurodegeneration.[97]

In support, in vitro models of proteasomal dysfunction that replicate the two cardinal pathologic features of Lewy body diseases (e.g., neuronal death, and the formation of cytoplasmic ubiquitinated inclusions) suggest that inclusion body formation and cell death may be dissociated from one another.[98]

Recent evidence that inhibition of the ubiquitin–proteasome pathway leads to altered protein handling and Lewy body formation suggests that this dysfunction may be responsible for degeneration of the nigrostriatal pathway in idiopathic PD.[99] Parkin mutations can also cause familial PD and parkin is also found in Lewy bodies. Interestingly, the absence of Lewy bodies in patients with parkin mutations suggests that parkin might be necessary for the formation of Lewy bodies.[100]

Recently, it has been shown that parkin interacts with and ubiquitinates the α-synuclein-interacting protein, synphilin-1, a novel protein that interacts with α-synuclein.[96,101] Coexpression of α-synuclein, synphilin-1, and parkin results in the formation of Lewy-body-like ubiquitin-positive cytosolic inclusions.[100]

Although little is known about its normal function, α-synuclein appears to interact with a variety of proteins and membrane phospholipids and may therefore participate in a number of signaling pathways. In particular, it may play a role in regulating cell differentiation, synaptic plasticity, cell survival, and dopaminergic neurotransmission.[20]

It should be noted, however, that Lewy bodies may simply represent a cellular response to some other primary insult (see also Chapter 19).

▶ POTENTIAL ROLE OF ION CHANNELS IN PD PATHOGENESIS

The cardinal motor symptoms and signs of PD result from the progressive death of dopaminergic neurons in the substantia nigra, which deprives the striatum of its dopaminergic innervation. Dopaminergic neurons in the substantia nigra pars compacta are autonomously active and maintain a rhythmic, pacemaking function. Surmeier and his colleagues have produced evidence that juvenile dopaminergic neurons use sodium channels to generate their rhythmic firing, but, as animals age, the sodium channels become latent and the rhythmic firing is taken over by calcium channels.[102,103]Surmeier and colleagues hypothesized that this reliance on calcium channels to maintain autonomous activity with age could, over a period of time, impose a sustained metabolic stress on mitochondria and activate cell death mechanisms. He and his colleagues have shown in experimental animals that administration of the calcium channel antagonist isradipine caused adult dopamine neurons to "revert" to the use of sodium channels to maintain their rhythmic firing function. In rodents this reversion to juvenile sodium channels confers protection against neurotoxins that are lethal for dopaminergic neurons employing calcium channels for their pacemaker function.[102,103] Clinical trials with isradipine in patients with PD will be initiated shortly to test whether this therapy delays the development or progression of symptoms of PD.

▶ SIGNIFICANCE AND FUTURE DIRECTIONS FOR NEUROCHEMICAL STUDIES OF PD

Selective degeneration of the dopaminergic nigrostriatal pathway is the most eloquent and characteristic consequence of the pathologic process in PD. The resulting reduction in striatal dopamine concentration is a sufficient condition for the emergence of tremor, bradykinesia and hypokinesia, and rigidity, the clinical hallmarks of PD. The development of L-dopa therapy and newer direct-acting dopamine agonists in the treatment of PD grew out of the recognition of this relationship between dopamine deficiency and parkinsonian symptoms.

There are numerous challenges and directions for future research in PD that are driven most importantly by the recognition that there are still no clearly disease-modifying therapies, and, despite numerous advances in therapy, PD still shortens life expectancy and decreases quality of life in those affected compared to age-matched controls.[104]

The role of the enigmatic Lewy body in PD pathology remains an important research challenge. Recognition of the pervasive nature of central and peripheral nervous system involvement in PD has appropriately broadened the focus of studying PD pathophysiology and pathogenesis beyond dopaminergic neurons of the nigrostriatal pathway. Many clues have emerged in recent years from elegant studies of rare autosomal dominant and recessive forms of parkinsonism. Two of the most prominent themes have focused on mishandling of proteins, particularly α-synuclein, by the ubiquitin–proteosome system and mitochondrial failure. Whatever the fundamental molecular and cellular pathologies turn out to be that result in PD, it is clear that dopaminergic neurons are specifically and characteristically susceptible.

REFERENCES

1. Abbott RD, Ross GW, White LR, et al. Environmental, lifestyle, and physical precursors of clinical Parkinson's disease: Recent findings from the Honolulu-Asia Aging Study. J Neurol 2003;250(suppl III):III30–III39.
2. Gagnon JF, Bedard MA, Fantini ML, et al. REM sleep behavior disorder and REM sleep without atonia in Parkinson's disease. Neurol 2002;59:585–589.
3. Muller A, Reichman H, Livermore A, Hummel T. Olfactory function in idiopathic Parkinson's disease (IPD): Results from cross-sectional studies in IPD patients and long-term follow-up of de-novo IPD patients. J Neural Transm 2002;109:805–811.
4. Braak H, Del Tredici K, Rub U, et al. Staging of brain pathology related to sporadic Parkinson's disease. Neurobiol Aging 2003;24:197–211.
5. Lang AE, Obeso JA. Challenges in Parkinson's disease: Restoration of the nigrostriatal dopamine system is not enough. Lancet Neurology 2004;3:309–316.
6. Burke RE, Dauer WT, Vonsattel JPG, et al. A critical evaluation of the Braak Staging Scheme for Parkinson's Disease. Ann Neurol 2008;64:485–491.
7. Langston JW. The Parkinson's complex: Parkinsonism just the tip of the iceberg. Ann Neurol 2006;59:591–596.
8. Ahlskog JE. Beating a dead horse: Dopamine and Parkinson Disease. Neurol 2007;69:1701–1711.
9. Shannon KM. Dopamine, so "last century". Neurol 2007;69:329–338.
10. Wilson SAK. Progressive lenticular degeneration: A familial nervous disease associated with cirrhosis of the liver. Brain 1912;34:295–489.
11. Hassler R. Zur Pathologie der Paralysis Agitans und des postenzephalitischen Parkinsonismus. J Psychol Neurol 1938;48:387–476.
12. Hornykiewicz O. Die topische Lokalisation und das Verhalten von Noradrenalin und Dopamin (3-Hydroxytyramin) in der Substantia Nigra des normalen und parkinsonkranken Menschen. Wien Klin Wochenschr 1963;75:309–312.
13. Hornykiewicz O. Dopamine (3-hydroxytyramine) and brain function. Pharmacol Rev 1966;18:925–962.
14. Langston JW, Ballard P, Tetrud JW, Irwin I. Chronic parkinsonism in humans due to a product of meperidine-analog synthesis. Science 1983;291:979–980.
15. Carpenter MB. Anatomy of the corpus striatum and brainstem integrating systems. In Brooks VB (ed.), Handbook of Physiology. Bethesda, MD: American Physiological Society, 1981, pp. 947–995.
16. Stoof JC, Kebabian JW. Two dopamine receptors: Biochemistry, physiology and pharmacology. Life Sci 1984;35:2281–2296.
17. Moore RY, Bloom FE. Central catecholamine neuron systems: Anatomy and physiology of the dopamine systems. Annu Rev Neurosci 1976;1:129–169.
18. Fearnley JM, Lees AJ. Aging and Parkinson's disease: Substantia nigra regional selectivity. Brain 1991;114: 2283–2301.
19. Carlsson A, Lindquist M, Magnusson T. 3,4-Dihydroxyphenylalanine and 5-hydroxytryptophan as reserpine antagonists. Nature 1957;180:1200–1201.
20. Lloyd KG, Davidson L, Hornykiewicz O. The neurochemistry of Parkinson's disease: Effect of L-dopa therapy. J Pharmacol Exp Ther 1975;195:453–464.
21. Bernheimer H, Hornykiewicz O. Herabgesetzte Konzentration der Homovanillinsäuure im Gehirn von parkinsonkranken Menschen als Ausdruck der Stöurung des zentralen Opaminstoffwechsels. Klin Wochenschr 1965;43:711–715.
22. Price KS, Farley IJ, Hornykiewicz O. Neurochemistry of Parkinson's disease: Relation between striatal and limbic dopamine. Adv Biochem Psychopharmacol 1978;19: 293–300.
23. Kish SJ, Shannak K, Hornykiewicz O. Uneven pattern of dopamine loss in the striatum of patients with idiopathic Parkinson's disease. N Engl J Med 1988;318:876–880.
24. Zigmond MJ, Stricker EM. Parkinson's disease: Studies with an animal model. Life Sci 1984;35:5–18.
25. Pimoule C, Schoemaker H, Javoy-Agid F, et al. Decrease in [^{3}H] cocaine binding to the dopamine transporter in Parkinson's disease. Eur J Pharmacol 1983;95:145–146.
26. Maloteaux J-M, Vanisberg M-A, Laterre C, et al. [^{3}H] GBR 12935 binding to dopamine uptake sites: Subcellular localization and reduction in Parkinson's disease and progressive supranuclear palsy. Eur J Pharmacol 1988;156:331–340.
27. Trugman JM, Leadbetter R, Zolis ME, et al. Treatment of severe axial tardive dystonia with clozapine: Case report and hypothesis. Mov Disord 1994;9:441–4464.
28. Oliveri RL, Annesi G, Zappia M, et al. Dopamine D2 receptor gene polymorphism and the risk of levodopa induced dyskinesias in PD. Neurology 1999;53:1425–1430.
29. Moore RY, Bloom FE. Central catecholamine neuron systems: Anatomy and physiology of the norepinephrine and epinephrine systems. Annu Rev Neurosci 1979;2: 113–168.
30. Farley IJ, Hornykiewicz O. Noradrenaline in subcortical brain regions of patients with Parkinson's disease and control subjects. In Birkmayer W, Hornykiewicz O (eds.), Advances in Parkinsonism. Basel: Editiones Roche, 1976, pp. 178–185.
31. Scatton B, Javoy-Agid F, Rouquier L, et al. Reduction of cortical dopamine, noradrenaline, serotonin, and their metabolites in Parkinson's disease. Brain Res 1983;275: 321–328.
32. Javoy-Agid F, Rubert M, Taquet H, et al. Biochemical neuropathology of Parkinson's disease. Adv Neurol 1984;40:189–198.
33. Kopp N, Denoroy L, Thomasi M, et al. Increase in noradrenaline-synthesizing enzyme activity in medulla oblongata in Parkinson's disease. Acta Neuropathol 1982;56:17–21.
34. Bernheimer H, Birkmayer W, Hornykiewicz O. Verteilung des 5-Hydroxytryptamin (Serotonin) in Gehirn des Menschen und sein Verhalten bei Patienten mit Parkinson-Syndrom. Klin Wochenschr 1961;39:1056–1059.
35. Perry TL, Javoy-Agid F, Agid Y, et al. Striatal GABAergic neuronal activity is not reduced in Parkinson's disease. J Neurochem 1983;40:1120–1123.
36. Laaksonen H, Rinne UK, Sonninen V, et al. Brain GABA neurons in Parkinson's disease. Acta Neurol Scand 1978;57(suppl 67):282–283.

37. Lloyd KG, Hornykiewicz O. L-Glutamic acid decarboxylase in Parkinson's disease: Effect of L-dopa therapy. Nature 1973;243: 521–523.
38. Lloyd KG, Möhler H, Hertz P, et al. Distribution of choline acetyltransferase and glutamate decarboxylase within the substantia nigra and in other brain regions from control and parkinsonian patients. J Neurochem 1975;25: 789–795.
39. Ruberg M, Ploska A, Javoy-Agid F, et al. Muscarinic binding and choline acetyltransferase activity in parkinsonian subjects with reference to dementia. Brain Res 1982;232: 129–139.
40. Schroeder JA, Schneider JS. GABA-opioid interactions in the globus pallidus: [D-Ala2]-Met-enkephalinamide attenuates potassium-evoked GABA release after nigrostriatal lesion. J Neurochem 2002;82:666–673.
41. Fernandez A, de Ceballos ML, Rose S, et al. Alterations in peptide levels in Parkinson's disease and incidental Lewy body disease. Brain 1996;119:823–830.
42. De Ceballos ML, Lopez-Lozano JJ. Subgroups of parkinsonian patients differentiated by peptidergic immunostaining of caudate nucleus biopsies. Peptides 1999;20:249–257.
43. Quik M, Police S, Langston JW, et al. Increases in striatal preproenkephalin gene expression are associated with nigrostriatal damage but not L-DOPA-induced dyskinesias in the squirrel monkey. Neuroscience 2002;113:213–220.
44. Lu JQ, Stoessl AJ. Somatostatin modulates the behavioral effects of dopamine receptor activation in parkinsonian rats. Neuroscience 2002;112:261–266.
45. Hökfelt T, Skirboll L, Rehfeld JF, et al. A subpopulation of mesencephalic dopamine neurons projecting to limbic areas contains a cholecystokinin-like peptide: Evidence from immunohistochemistry combined with retrograde tracing. Neuroscience 1980;5:2093–2124.
46. Studler JM, Javoy-Agid F, Cesselin F, et al. CCK-8-immunoreactivity distribution in human brain: Selective decrease in the substantia nigra from parkinsonian patients. Brain Res 1982;243:176–179.
47. Epelbaum J, Ruberg M, Moyse E, et al. Somatostatin and dementia in Parkinson's disease. Brain Res 1983;278: 376–379.
48. Jha N, Jurma O, Lalli G, et al. Glutathione depletion in PC12 results in selective inhibition of mitochondrial complex I activity. Implications in Parkinson's disease. J Biol Chem 2000;275:26096–26101.
49. Mytilineou C, Kramer BC, Yabut JA. Glutathione depletion and oxidative stress. Parkinsonism Relat Disord 2002;8:385–387.
50. Yoshioka M, Tanaka K, Miyazaki I, et al. The dopamine agonist cabergoline provides neuroprotection by activation of the glutathione system and scavenging free radicals. Neurosci Res 2002;43:259–267.
51. Cohen G. The pathobiology of Parkinson's disease: Biochemical aspects of dopamine neuron senescence. J Neural Trans 1983;19(suppl):89–103.
52. Graham DG. Catecholamine toxicity: A proposal for the molecular pathogenesis of manganese neurotoxicity and Parkinson's disease. Neurotoxicology 1984;5:83–96.
53. Fahn S, Cohen G. The oxidant stress hypothesis in Parkinson's disease: Evidence supporting it. Ann Neurol 1992;32:804–812.
54. Golts N, Snyder H, Frasier M, et al. Magnesium inhibits spontaneous and iron induced aggregation of alpha synuclein. J Biol Chem 2002;277:16116–16123.
55. Ostretova-Golts N, Petrucelli L, Hardy J, et al. The A53T alpha synuclein mutation increases iron dependent aggregation and toxicity. J Neurosci 2002;20:6048–6054.
56. Sangchot P, Sharma S, Chetsawang B, et al. Deferoxamine attenuates iron-induced oxidative stress and prevents mitochondrial aggregation and alpha-synuclein translocation in SK-N-SH cells in culture. Dev Neurosci 2002;24:143–153.
57. Borie C, Gasparini F, Verpillat P, et al. French Parkinson's Disease Genetic Study Group. Association study between iron-related genes polymorphisms and Parkinson's disease. J Neurol 2002;249:801–804.
58. Freeman BA, Crapo JD. Biology of disease: Free radicals and tissue injury. Lab Invest 1982;47:412–426.
59. Kunikowska G, Jenner P. The distribution of copper, zinc and manganese superoxide dismutase, and glutathione peroxidase messenger ribonucleic acid in rat basal ganglia. Biochem Pharmacol 2002;63:1159–1164.
60. Perry TL, Godin DV, Hansen S. Parkinson's disease: A disorder due to nigral glutathione deficiency? Neurosci Lett 1982;33:305–310.
61. Jha N, Kumar MJ, Boonplueang R, et al. Glutathione decreases in dopaminergic PC12 cells interfere with the ubiquitin protein degradation pathway: Relevance for Parkinson's disease? J Neurochem 2002;80:555–561.
62. Ambani LM, Van Woert MH, Murphy S. Brain peroxidase and catalase in Parkinson's disease. Arch Neurol 1975;32:114–118.
63. Dexter DT, Carter CJ, Wells FR. Basal lipid peroxidation in substantia nigra is increased in Parkinson's disease. J Neurochem 1989;52:381–389.
64. Jenner P. Oxidative stress as a cause of Parkinson's disease. Acta Neurol Scand 1991;84:6–15.
65. Tornero D, Ce a V, Gonzalez Garcia C, et al. The role of the mitochondrial permeability transition pore in neurodegenerative processes. Rev Neurol 2002;35:354–361.
66. Parker WD, Boyson SJ, Parks JK. Abnormalities of the electron transport chain in idiopathic Parkinson's disease. Ann Neurol 1989;26:719–723.
67. Benecke R, Strumper P, Weiss H. Electron transfer complexes I and IV of platelets are abnormal in Parkinson's disease but normal in Parkinson-plus syndromes. Brain 1993;116:1451–1463.
68. Ebadi M, Govitrapong P, Sharma S, et al. Ubiquinone (coenzyme Q10) and mitochondria in oxidative stress of Parkinson's disease. Biol Signals Recept 2001;10: 224–253.
69. Schapira AH, Mann VM, Cooper JM. Anatomic and disease specificity of NADH CoQ1 reductase (complex I) deficiency in Parkinson's disease. J Neurochem 1990;55: 2142–2145.
70. Casali C, Bonifati V, Santorelli FM, et al. Mitochondrial myopathy, parkinsonism, and multiple mtDNA deletions in a Sephardic Jewish family. Neurology 2001;56: 802–805.
71. Greenamyre JT, MacKenzie G, Peng TI, et al. Mitochondrial dysfunction in Parkinson's disease. Biochem Soc Symp 1999;66:85–97.

72. Greenamyre JT, Sherer TB, Betarbet R, et al. Complex I and Parkinson's disease. IUBMB Life 2001;52:135–141.
73. Hsu LJ, Sagara Y, Arroyo A, et al. Alpha-synuclein promotes mitochondrial deficit and oxidative stress. Am J Pathol 2000;157:401–410.
74. Lamensdorf I, Graeme E, Harvey-White J, et al. 3,4-Dihydroxyphenylacetaldehyde potentiates the toxic effects of metabolic stress in PC12 cells. Brain Res 2000;868:191–201.
75. Naoi M, Maruyama W, Akao Y, Yi H. Mitochondria determine the survival and death in apoptosis by an endogenous neurotoxin, N-methyl(R)salsolinol, and neuroprotection by propargylamines. J Neural Transm 2002;109:607–621.
76. Nurmi E, Ruottinen HM, Bergman J, et al. Rate of progression in Parkinson's disease: A 6-[18F]fluoro-L-dopa PET study. Mov Disord 2001;16:608–615.
77. Dagher A. Functional imaging in Parkinson's disease. Semin Neurol 2001;21:23–32.
78. Brooks DJ, Samuel M. The effects of surgical treatment of Parkinson's disease on brain function: PET findings. Neurology 2000;55:S52–59.
79. Khan NL, Valente EM, Bentivoglio AR, et al. Clinical and subclinical dopaminergic dysfunction in PARK6-linked parkinsonism: An 18F-dopa PET study. Ann Neurol 2002;52:849–853.
80. Khan NL, Brooks DJ, Pavese N, et al. Progression of nigrostriatal dysfunction in a parkin kindred: An [18F]dopa PET and clinical study. Brain 2002;125:2248–2256.
81. Martin WRW, Beckman JH, Calne DB, et al. Cerebral glucose metabolism in Parkinson's disease. Can J Neurol Sci 1984;11:169–173.
82. Leenders K, Wolfson L, Gibbs J, et al. Regional cerebral blood flow and oxygen metabolism in Parkinson's disease and their response to L-dopa. J Cereb Blood Flow Metab 1983;3:S488–S489.
83. Wooten GF, Collins RC. Metabolic effects of unilateral lesion of the substantia nigra. J Neurosci 1981;1:285–291.
84. Garnett ES, Firnau G, Nahmias C. Dopamine visualized in the basal ganglia of living man. Nature 1983;305: 137–138.
85. Thobois S, Guillouet S, Broussolle E. Contributions of PET and SPECT to the understanding of the pathophysiology of Parkinson's disease. Neurophysiol Clin 2001;31: 321–340.
86. Ribeiro MJ, Vidailhet M, Loc'h C, et al. Dopaminergic function and dopamine transporter binding assessed with positron emission tomography in Parkinson disease. Arch Neurol 2002;59:580–586.
87. Sossi V, de La Fuente-Fernandez R, Holden JE, et al. Increase in dopamine turnover occurs early in Parkinson's disease: Evidence from a new modeling approach to PET 18F-fluorodopa data. J Cereb Blood Flow Metab 2002;22:232–239.
88. Lucignani G, Gobbo C, Moresco RM, et al. The feasibility of statistical parametric mapping for the analysis of positron emission tomography studies using 11C-2-beta-carbomethoxy-3-beta-(4-fluorophenyl)-tropane in patients with movement disorders. Nucl Med Commun 2002;23:1047–1055.
89. Lewy FH. Paralysis agitans. I. Pathologische Anatomie, in Lewandowski M (ed), Handbuck der Neurologie. Berlin: Springer, 1912, pp. 920–933.
90. Greenfield JG, Bosanquet FD. The brainstem lesion in parkinsonism. J Neurol Neurosurg Psychiatry 1953;16: 213–226.
91. Goldman JE, Yen S-H, Chiu F-C, Peress NS. Lewy bodies of Parkinson's disease contain neurofilament antigens. Science 1983;221:1082–1084.
92. Duda JE, Giasson BI, Mabon ME, et al. Novel antibodies to synuclein show abundant striatal pathology in Lewy body diseases. Ann Neurol 2002;52:205–210.
93. Cole NB, Murphy DD. The cell biology of alpha-synuclein: A sticky problem? Neuromol Med 2002;1:95–109.
94. Lo Bianco C, Ridet JL, Schneider BL, et al: Alpha-synucleinopathy and selective dopaminergic neuron loss in a rat lentiviral-based model of Parkinson's disease. Proc Natl Acad Sci U S A 2002;99:10813–10818.
95. Lee MK, Stirling W, Xu Y, et al. Human alpha-synuclein-harboring familial Parkinson's disease-linked Ala-53–>Thr mutation causes neurodegenerative disease with alpha-synuclein aggregation in transgenic mice. Proc Natl Acad Sci U S A 2002;99:8968–8973.
96. Takahashi H, Wakabayashi K. The cellular pathology of Parkinson's disease. Neuropathology 2001;21:315–322.
97. Rajagopalan S, Andersen JK. Alpha synuclein aggregation: Is it the toxic gain of function responsible for neurodegeneration in Parkinson's disease? Mech Ageing Dev 2001;122:1499–1510.
98. Rideout HJ, Larsen KE, Sulzer D, et al. Proteasomal inhibition leads to formation of ubiquitin/alpha-synucleinimmunoreactive inclusions in PC12 cells. Neurochem 2001;78:899–908.
99. McNaught KS, Jenner P. Proteasomal function is impaired in substantia nigra in Parkinson's disease. Neurosci Lett 2001;297:191–194.
100. Chung KK, Zhang Y, Lim KL, et al. Parkin ubiquitinates the alpha-synuclein-interacting protein, synphilin-1: Implications for Lewy-body formation in Parkinson disease. Nat Med 2001;7:1144–1150.
101. Wakabayashi K, Engelender S, Yoshimoto M, et al. Synphilin-1 is present in Lewy bodies in Parkinson's disease. Ann Neurol 2000;47:521–523.
102. Chan CS, Guzman JN, Ilijic E, et al. "Rejuvenation" protects neurons in mouse models of Parkinson's disease. Nature 2007;447:1081–1086.
103. Surmeir DJ. Calcium, aging, and neuronal vulnerability in Parkinson's disease. Lancet Neurology 2007;6:933–938.
104. Ishihara LS, Cheesbrough A, Brayne C, et al. Estimated life expectancy of Parkinson's patients compared with UK population. J Neurol Neurosurg Psychiat 2007;78: 1304–1309.

CHAPTER 12

Etiology of Parkinson's Disease

Yoshikuni Mizuno, Nobutaka Hattori, and Hideki Mochizuki

▶ ETIOLOGY

HISTORICAL ASPECTS

The etiology of Parkinson's disease (PD) has long been discussed since the original description by James Parkinson.[1] Parkinson mentioned that chronic injury to the cervical cord might be the cause of this disease because the disease often started in the upper extremities. But he did not make any definite statement on the etiology and pathogenesis of the disease.

As parkinsonism was the frequent sequel of Von Economo's encephalitis, virus infection was once postulated as a cause of nigral degeneration in PD. Von Economo's encephalitis started with the epidemics in Vienna in 1916,[2] and resulted in worldwide pandemics until 1926, with a high morbidity of up to 80%.[3] The incidence of parkinsonism among recovered patients was up to 80%, or more by the tenth year after the acute episode of encephalitis.[4] The pathologic hallmark of postencephalitic parkinsonism is the presence of Alzheimer's neurofibrillary tangles in the remaining neurons in the substantia nigra (SN).[5] It is unlikely that Von Economo's encephalitis or other viral infections play any etiologic role in the pathogenesis of PD.[3]

Another possibility that was once postulated is chronic metal intoxication. Chronic manganese intoxication produces parkinsonism,[6,7] and the manganese and aluminum contents of water consumed by Guamanian people who developed parkinsonism–dementia complex were high.[8] However, the clinical pictures of chronic manganese intoxication are different from those of PD.[6] Pathologic changes are most prominent in the internal segment of the globus pallidus and subthalamic nucleus.[9] Furthermore, brain manganese level is not elevated in PD.[10]

Recently, high incidence of parkinsonism among welders was reported in the United States.[11] On the other hand, in a Swedish cohort study on welders did not prove higher incidence of parkinsonism and other movement disorders compared to general population.[12] It is unlikely that chronic manganese exposure represents one of the etiologic factors for PD.[13]

THE MODERN ERA

The modern era started with the discovery of the specific nigral neurotoxin 1-methyl-4-phenyl-1,2,3,6-tetrahydropyridine (MPTP). Since then, many PD specialists believe that nigral neuronal death is initiated by the interaction of environmental neurotoxins and genetic predisposition. Such interaction is likely to induce mitochondrial dysfunction and oxidative stress; furthermore, mitochondrial dysfunction and oxidative stress can induce dysfunctions of the 26S proteasome and the autophagy–lysosome system inducing accumulation of toxic, misfolded, and aggregated proteins, particularly of aggregated α-synuclein.

Today, many etiologic and pathogenetic factors are postulated in PD. Etiology denotes a cause of the disease, whatever the mechanism of neurodegeneration may be, and pathogenesis represents molecular mechanisms that lead neurons to death (Fig. 12–1). Studies on genetic forms of PD contributed a great deal to the understanding of etiology and pathogenesis of sporadic PD. Genetics of PD is discussed in Chapter 9 of this textbook. In this chapter, we mainly discuss etiologic factors of PD and discuss briefly pathogenetic mechanisms that connect the etiology and the nigral neuronal death. Readers who are interested in this subject are encouraged to read recent reviews as well.[14,15]

MPTP and Parkinsonism

In 1979, Davis and colleagues[16] reported a patient who developed severe parkinsonism after injecting a homemade illicit narcotic. This patient was examined by neurologists at the National Institutes of Health and the patient showed marked improvement after treatment with L-dopa and bromocriptine. However, 18 months later he was found dead. Postmortem examination revealed extensive degeneration and loss of pigmented neurons in the SN.[16] Then, in 1982, several young adults in northern California developed a parkinsonian syndrome after intravenous use of what was purported to be "synthetic heroin." Langston and colleagues[17] analyzed those drug samples and identified

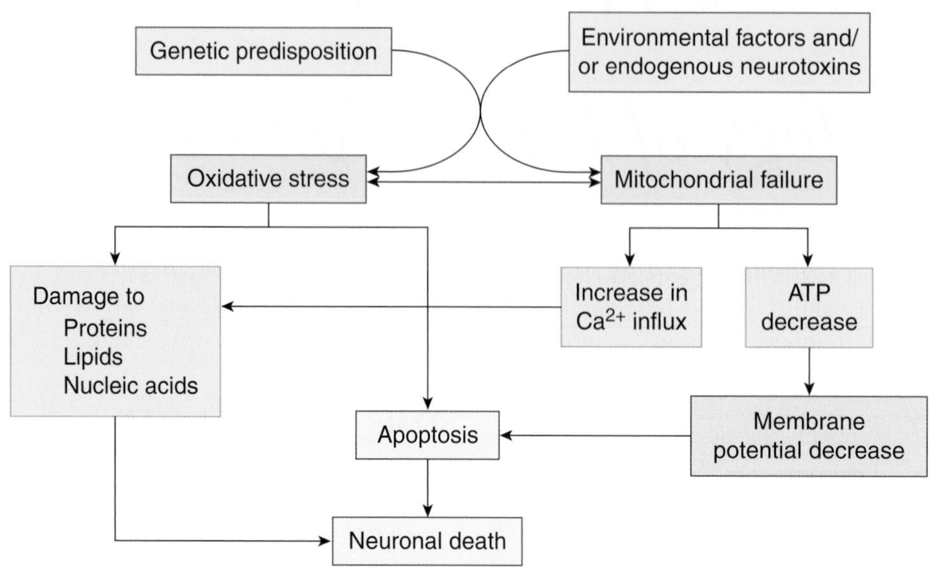

Figure 12–1. Etiology and pathogenesis of Parkinson's disease. Etiology means causes of the disease and pathogenesis represents abnormal molecular events that are induced by etiologic factors and are leading cells to death; in this case, the cells are nigral dopaminergic neurons.

MPTP as the probable toxin responsible for their parkinsonism.

The pathogenetic mechanism of nigral neuronal death in MPTP-induced parkinsonism has now been well elucidated. MPTP is taken up into astrocytes in the brain, and oxidized to MPP^+ (1-methyl-4-phenylpyridinium ion) by monoamine oxidase B.[18] Then MPP^+ is actively taken up into nigrostriatal neurons through dopamine transporters, with marked concentration within dopaminergic neurons.[19] MPP^+ is further concentrated within mitochondria by active uptake depending on the electrical potential gradient between the inside and the outside of the mitochondrial inner membrane.[20] Within the mitochondria, MPP^+ inhibits mitochondrial complex I and NADH-linked state 3 respiration.[21,22] The reason why MPP^+ can inhibit complex I is probably due to its structural similarity to NAD^+. The inhibition of mitochondrial respiration results in loss of oxidative phosphorylation and a rapid fall in the ATP level.[23] In addition to ATP depletion and energy crisis, MPP^+ induces apoptotic cell death at lower concentrations.[24,25] Although MPTP contributed a great deal to the understanding of etiology and pathogenesis of PD, it is not a cause of PD.

ENVIRONMENTAL NEUROTOXINS

Since the discovery of MPTP, environmental neurotoxins have emerged as a potential etiologic factor in PD. This subject is discussed in the Chapter 10 of this textbook, only pertinent points will be discussed briefly here.

Rural living and/or use of well water have been postulated as risk factors for PD; however, the results are conficting.[26,27] More recent case-controlled study in the Tuscany region of Italy did not find any difference in time spent in rural or industrial residence, in well water drinking, or in the exposure to herbicides and pesticides.[28]

Results on the exposure to pesticides and/or herbicides and a risk for PD are also conflicting.[29,30] A recent study on all subjects who developed PD in Olmsted County, Minnesota, from 1976 through 1995 revealed a risk of exposure to pesticides in PD only in men (149 cases; 129 controls and odds ratio (OR), 2.4; 95% confidence interval, 1.1–5.4; $P = 0.04$).[31] Also, exposure to pesticides was reported to increase a risk for PD in a Taiwanese cohort.[32] Thus, exposure to pesticides and herbicides may become a weak risk factor for PD depending on the country or gender. It is interesting to note that herbicides and pesticides, and some agricultural products, may contain substances that inhibit mitochondrial complex I.

Life Style (Smoking, Coffee Consumption, and NSAID Use)

It has been largely agreed that smoking is inversely associated with a risk of PD,[33–36] although some conflicting results were reported.[37,38] More recent studies on a large cohort also confirmed this inverse association.[35,36] But it is not known whether the nonsmoking life style is a cause of PD or a result of a premorbid personality from the disease.

Coffee drinking appears to be inversely associated with a risk for PD. In one of the studies, a positive association was found only in female patients.[39] More recent study on large cohorts of PD patients ($n = 356$) and family controls ($n = 317$) confirmed significant inverse association with coffee drinking and a risk for PD (test for trend $P = 0.05$).[36] Regarding NSAID use, conflicting results have been reported.[35,36,40] A recent study on large cohorts of PD patients ($n = 356$) and family controls ($n = 317$) failed to show association.[36] There is no association between alcohol consumption and a rise in PD.[35]

ENDOGENOUS NEUROTOXINS

The discovery of MPTP stimulated extensive studies on endogenous and exogenous neurotoxins that may accumulate in the SN and cause nigral neuronal death. Of these, tetrahydroisoquinolines (TIQs) and β-carbolines have been most extensively studied. TIQs are a group of compounds that are formed by condensation of aldehyde and phenylethylamine or its derivatives. β-Carbolines are derived from indolamines and aldehydes. These substances are structurally similar to MPTP or MPP^+. Isoquinoline derivatives are widely distributed in the environment, being present in many plants and foodstuffs, and readily cross the blood–brain barrier. Some are potent inhibitors of mitochondrial complex I and generate reactive oxygen species when oxidized by a monoamine oxidase.[41]

Nevertheless, even though these compounds were postulated to be candidate neurotoxins for nigral neuronal death in PD,[42–44] none of them has been explicitly proven to be accumulated in PD brains. Thus, it seems unlikely that endogenous compounds similar to MPTP play an important role in the etiology of PD.

Genetic Influence

There is no question about the genetic influence on the development of PD. Frequency of PD among first-degree relatives of the patients is 2–3 times higher than that in the control population.[45,46] Interestingly, conflicting results have been reported on twin studies. Concordance rates between monozygotic and dizygotic twins are low; 2.3% in monozygotic and 0% in dizygotic twins in one report.[47] Another study on a large veterans cohort showed high concordance rate in monozygotic twins with onset before age 50 (100%) and low in those with onset after age 50 (10.4%).[48] A more recent study on a large cohort of Swedish twins (154 twins) showed extremely low concordance rates for both zygosities, particularly no concordant affected with PD among 33 monozygotic twins.[49]

GENETIC ASSOCIATION STUDIES

As PD is believed to be caused by the interaction of genetic predisposition and environmental factors, many studies have attempted to find genetic risk factors for PD. Genetic risk is encoded in subtle differences in base sequences (polymorphism) in the gene. Such polymorphisms usually do not affect the function of encoded proteins. But at times, functions are modified by polymorphic mutations; in case of an enzyme, the activity of the variant type may be higher or lower than the wild type (functional polymorphism). The genetic association study usually compares the frequency of the wild type and the variant type of a candidate gene between PD patients and the controls (cohort study). Recent advances in the technologies allow genotyping of more than 100,000 genome wide polymorphisms in a large cohort of patients. But a lot of conflicting results have been reported in genetic association studies on PD. For instance, Maraganore and colleagues[50] reported 13 single-nucleotide polymorphisms (SNPs) significantly associated with PD in a genome-wide association study, whereas a subsequent study by Elbaz and colleagues[51] on these 13 SNPs using DNA samples from 5526 patients with PD and 6682 controls could not reproduce the association between any of the 13 SNPs and a risk for PD. Herein, we will review pertinent findings on genetic association studies on PD.

Familial PD-Related Genes

SNCA (α-Synuclein)

SNCA encodes α-synuclein. α-Synuclein is a brain-specific protein without a secondary structure aggregated in neurons of PD patients. Aggregation of α-synuclein is believed to be one of the most important pathogenetic mechanisms in PD. Therefore, its variants have been studied extensively for possible association with PD. *SNCA* has several SNPs in the coding region, introns, and also in the promoter region. The promoter region contains Rep1 polymorphism, which is a complex mixed dinucleotide repeats consisting of (TC)10-11TT(TC)8-11(TA)7-9(CA)10-11; the subscripts indicate usual numbers of dinucleotide repeats.[52] The length of the repeats varies considerably constituting Rep1 polymorphism. It is interesting to note that Rep1 polymorphism regulates expression of *SNCA* over threefold range.

Conflicting results have been reported on the genetic association between promoter polymorphisms and a risk for PD. Kruger and colleagues[53] first reported association between *SNCA* variants in the promoter region and a risk for PD. However, subsequent reports failed to reproduce their results.[54–56] More recently, some reports on larger cohorts indicated association between Rep1 polymorphism and PD.[57–63] For instance, Maraganore and colleagues[61] found association between genotypes defined by the 263 basepair allele of Rep1 polymorphism and PD (OR = 1.43, $n = 2692$ PD and 2652 controls). Overall trend is suggesting the presence of association between *SNCA* promoter variants and a risk for PD.

More consistent findings are the association between SNPs in the 3'-half of *SNCA* and PD. Mueller and colleagues[56] found two large linkage disequilibrium blocks spanning *SNCA* and several markers within the 3'-block around exons 5 and 6 with strong association with PD (p = 0.00009). Mizuta and colleagues[64] reported essentially similar results in that a SNP in *SNCA*, rs7684318, showed the strongest association with PD ($P = 5.0 \times 10^{-10}$); the entire *SNCA* lied within a single linkage disequilibrium. Winkler and colleagues[62] found a SNP in the 3'UTR (rs356165) of *SNCA* showing the greatest evidence for an association with PD ($p \leq 0.003$), with significant pairwise values for linkage disequilibrium. Thus, polymorphic variants in the 3'-half of *SNCA* appear to be strongly associated with a risk for PD. This is a few nonconflicting positive results among the many association studies on PD.

β-Synuclein may act as a natural negative regulator of alpha-synuclein aggregation and fibrillization; however, there is no evidence to suggest association between its variants and a risk for PD.[65]

PRKN (PARKIN)

PRKN is the disease gene for autosomal recessive young onset PD linked to *PARK2* locus. Conflicting results have been reported on the association of *PRKN* variants and PD. Earlier studies did not have a large number of patients to make a definite conclusion. Tan and colleagues[66] reported association between –258G variant in the promoter region and a risk for sporadic PD in a large cohort of the elderly ethnic Chinese population; however, a subsequent study failed to show association between *PRKN* and a risk for PD or for the age of onset.[67]

UCHLI (Ubiquitin Carboxyterminal Hydrolases L-1)

UCHL1 was reported as a rare cause of autosomal dominant familial PD. Conflicting results have been reported on the association between *UCHL1* variants and a risk for PD. The positive evidence came from a meta-analysis of small studies that reported the S18Y polymorphism as protective against PD.[68] Another study reported that the Y/Y genotype was protective only in young onset patients and the presence of this genotype delayed the onset of the disease.[69] Carmine Belin and colleagues[70] also reported positive association, whereas Healy and colleagues[71] found no protection against PD in the analysis of *S18Y* variant in a large white individual cohort (3023 subjects); furthermore, they conducted a meta-analysis on 6594 subjects and found no protective effect of *S18Y* variant. Subsequent studies in large cohorts also did not confirm this association.[72,73]

PINK1 (PTEN-Induced Kinase 1)

PINK1 encodes a mitochondrial protein with a kinase domain and is the disease gene for an autosomal recessive PD (PARK6-linked PD). Conflicting results have been reported on the association between *PINK1* variants and PD. Groen and colleagues[74] did not find any association between three *PINK1* variants (Leu63Leu, Ala340Thr, and Asn521Thr) and PD, whereas Wang and colleagues[75] reported association of *A340T* variant and with late-onset PD in Chinese. But the difference was too small to be an important risk factor for PD (The A-allele frequency was 6.2% in PD and 4.2% in controls, $p = 0.0404$.).

DJ-1

DJ-1 is the disease gene for PARK7-linked autosomal recessive familial PD. *DJ-1* encodes a protein that has a potent antioxidant property. DJ-1 appears to have a limited role in the etiology of PD. Morris and colleagues[76] analyzed a 18bp insertion/deletion variant in the promoter region of *DJ-1* and found no association with PD. Another study found no association between any of the four variants of *DJ-1* and PD, but SNP1 (position 4345 bp) and SNP3 (position 16,491 bp) were associated with PD in women (p = 0.03 and 0.002).[77]

LRRK2 (Leucin-Rich Repeat Kinase 2)

LRRK2 is the disease gene for PARK8-locus-linked autosomal dominant PD, which is the most frequent form of familial PD; more than 20 mutations are known. Conflicting results have reported on the association of *LRRK2* variants and the risk for PD. Skipper and colleagues[78] analyzed 25 SNPs of *LRRK2* and found that minor allele at rs10506151 (A) showed a significant association with a risk for PD, although Paisán-Ruíz and colleagues[79] found no association of 31 *LRRK2* variants and the risk for PD in European population.

The G2385R mutation of *LRRK2* is a genetic risk factor among orientals. Di Fonzo and colleagues[80] investigated *G2385R* variant in 608 Taiwanese PD cases and 373 ethnically matched controls and reported that heterozygosity for the *G2385R* variant was significantly more frequent among PD patients than controls (nominal p value = 0.004, gender- and age-adjusted OR = 2.24). Tan and colleagues[81] studied a large cohort of ethnically Chinese population living in Singapore (PD = 980, control = 980) and found essentially similar results, that is, a higher frequency of the heterozygous G2385R genotype in PD compared to controls (7.3 vs 3.6%, OR = 2.1, $P = 0.014$). They showed that under condition of oxidative stress, the *G2385R* variant was more toxic and associated with a higher rate of apoptosis, which may be related to hydrophilic arginine compared to hydrophobic glycine. Subsequent studies on Chinese and Japanese confirmed this association.[82,83] Thus,

G2385R variation appears to confer a risk for sporadic PD among Chinese and Japanese population.

NR4A2

NR4A2 encodes a member of nuclear receptor superfamily protein and is essential for the differentiation of the nigral dopaminergic neurons. *NR4A2* was once proposed as a candidate gene for an autosomal dominant form of PD.[84] Association between variants of *NR4A2* and PD seems unlikely.[85,86]

MAPT (Microtubule-Associated Protein Tau)

MAPT on chromosome 17q21 encodes microtubule-associated protein tau, which assembles microtubules into parallel arrays within axons. *MAPT* is the disease gene for chromosome 17-linked familial frontotemporal dementia and parkinsonism (FTD-17) as well as a susceptible gene for sporadic progressive supranuclear palsy (PSP). *MAPT* has H1/H2 polymorphism; H1 haplotype and its allelic counterpart, H2, are defined by eight SNPs and a 238-base pair deletion in intron 9 (*del-In9*); *del-In9* is found only on the H2 background.[87]

Conrad and colleagues[88] first reported association between a single allele (a0) and its genotype (a0/a0) of a TG dinucleotide repeat in intron 9 and a risk for PSP. Frequency of H1 varies 70% and 80% in Caucasian population, and in PSP this frequency is usually over 90%.[87,89] On the other hand, respect to PD, conflicting results have been reported. Several groups of investigators reported positive association between PD and A0 allele or H1 haplotype.[90–93] Additional studies reported a robust association between the H1/H1 diplotype and PD risk (OR for H1/H1 vs H1/H2 and H2/H2, 1.46, $p = 8 \times 10^{-7}$)[94] and an inverse association between the minor allele at SNP rs1800547 and a risk for PD;[95] whereas, other studies failed to prove association.[96,97] Zhang and colleagues[98] conducted a meta-analysis of 14 studies published before 2004 including 2093 PD cases and 2258 controls, after excluding two studies contributing to most of between-study heterogeneity, the pooled OR and 95% confidence intervals (CI) of PD were 1.42 (95% CI 1.23–1.65) for those with H1/H1 genotype compared with all others and 1.52 (95% CI 1.12–2.04) for all individuals carrying H1 haplotype versus all others.

There appears to be a racial difference in the frequency of H1 haplotype. Unlike Caucasians, the H1 haplotype are monomorphic in Japanese and no association was found between H1 haplotype and a risk for PD.[99] The issue of racial difference has to be studied further.

APOE (Apolipoprotein E)

APOE encodes apolipoprotein, and four variants are known (*APOE-1, APOE-2, APOE-3,* and *APOE-4*). *APOE-4* is associated with a risk for sporadic Alzheimer's disease and earlier age at onset in familial Alzheimer's disease, whereas *APOE-2* allele is protective. Conflicting results have been reported on the association of *APOE* variants and risk for PD. Huang and colleagues[100] reported association of *APOE-2* and a risk for PD (OR = 1.20, 95% CI 1.02–1.42), while Li and colleagues[101] found increased risk with *APOE-4* allele ($p = 0.015$) and decreased risk with *APOE-3* ($p = 0.019$) in a large cohort (282 multiplex and 376 singleton families). López and colleagues[102] also reported association of *APOE4* allele and *APOE4/3* genotype with a risk for PD (OR = 1.736, OR = 1.688, respectively) in a Mexican population ($n = 229$ PD and 229 controls).

Another question is whether dementia in PD is associated with *APOE* variants. Papapetropoulos and colleagues[103] found positive association between *APOE-4* allele and dementia in PD; whereas, Jasinska-Myga and colleagues[104] found no association between *APOE-4* and dementia in PD.

PGRN (Progranulin)

PGRN is the disease gene for ubiquitin-positive frontotemporal lobar degeneration linked to chromosome 17q21 (FTLDU-17).[105] No association was found between progranulin variants and PD.[106]

Synphiline 1

Synphiline 1 is an α-synuclein interacting protein expressed in the core of Lewy bodies; function of synphiline 1 is not well elucidated yet. It is an interesting protein; however, no association was found between *synphiline 1* variants and PD.[107]

Glucocerebrosidase Gene (GBA)

Glucocerebrosidase deficiency induces Gaucher disease, an autosomal recessive lipid storage disease. Recently, heterozygous carriers of *GBA* mutation have been reported among sporadic PD patients. Goker-Alpan and colleagues[108] reported 10 unrelated families of subjects with Gaucher disease, where obligate or confirmed carriers of *GBA* mutations developed parkinsonism. They indicated that mutant glucocerebrosidase, even in heterozygotes, might be a risk factor for the development of parkinsonism. In another study, five PD patients were found among 88 carriers and one PD among 122 controls, which was of marginal significance ($P = 0.048$).[109] De Marco and colleagues[110] studied large cohorts of sporadic PD patients (395) and controls (483) for the N370S and the L444P mutations in southern Italy; they found 11 patients (2.8%) carrying a heterozygous mutant *GBA* allele, whereas only one control subject (0.2%) had a heterozygous substitution ($P = 0.0018$).

Kono and colleagues[111] reported an interesting family, where the proband (38-year-old male) had Gaucher disease, who started to show parkinsonism at age 33; on the other hand, his father (an obligate carrier) developed parkinsonism at age 63; both of them showed marked reduction in [^{11}C]CFT binding in the striatum. Contrarily, Toft and colleagues[112] did not find any association with *GBA* variants and the risk for PD.

The reason why Gaucher carriers have increased risk for PD is not known. But it is interesting to note that glucocerebrosidase is a lysosomal enzyme regulating the metabolisms of glucocerebroside. In sporadic PD, lysosomal dysfunction has been implicated as a pathogenetic mechanism.[15] Decreased amount of glucocerebosidase in lysosomes might augment lysosomal dysfunction in PD brains.

Human Immunodeficiency Virus Enhancer-Binding Protein 3 Gene (HIVEP3)

HIVEP3 is one of the candidate genes for PARK10-locus (chromosome 1)-linked PD. Oliveira and colleagues[113] studied variants of *HIVEP3* in 267 multiplex and 361 singleton families with PD and found association between SNPs 13 and 19 of HIVEP3 and a risk for PD in the combined multiplex and singleton data set ($P = 0.006$ for SNP 13, $P = 0.002$ for SNP 19), whereas data set on singleton families alone did not reach the statistical significance.

Ubiquitin-Specific Protease 24 (USP24)

USP24 is another of the candidate genes for PARK10-linked PD. Li and colleagues[114] found strong linkages between SNPs of *USP24* and a risk for PD in age- and gender-matched case-control pairs ($n = 311$ pairs, most significant allelic p-value: 0.0006 for rs287235:C > G). Oliveira and colleagues[113] found no association; they found, however, association between SNP 227 of *USP24* and the age at onset of PD.

Ubiquitin-Specific Protease 40 (USP40)

USP40 is a candidate gene for chromosome 2-linked PD. Li and colleagues[114] found strong linkages between SNPs of *USP40* and a risk for PD in age- and gender-matched case-control pairs ($n = 311$ pairs, most significant allelic p-value: 0.005 for rs838552:T > C).

Genes Related to Catecholamines

Tyrosine Hydroxylase Gene (TH)

TH is the late-limiting enzyme for dopamine synthesis. No association between variants of TH and PD was found.[115]

Monoamine Oxidase A and B Genes (MAOA and MAOB)

MAOA and MAOB are mitochondrial enzymes involved in the metabolism of serotonin, dopamine, and norepinephrine. Both *MAOA* and *MAOB* have dinucleotide repeat (GT)n polymorphisms in intron 2 of *MAOA* and intron 2 of *MAOB*; *MAOB* also has a G-T substitution in intron 13. Results of early studies are conflicting, and the number of patients was not sufficiently large enough to make a definite conclusion.

Parsian and colleagues[116] reported strong association between the dinucleotide repeat polymorphism of *MAOA* and sporadic ($p < 0.00001$) as well as familial PD ($p < 0.00001$). But more recent studies are not so conclusive. Kang and colleagues[117] found association between intron 13 SNP of *MAOB* and a risk for PD only in the female subset ($P = 0.02$). The study by Dick and colleagues[118] on large cohorts of PD ($n = 959$) and controls ($n = 1989$) failed to show positive association between *MAOA* and a risk for PD; however, they found a modest association only in males.

There may be racial difference in the relationship between *MAO* variants and a risk for PD. Association between the length of (GT)n repeat sequence and the G-A genotype of *MAOB* and PD was reported in Australians, in which the (GT)n repeat alleles ≥188 base pairs were significantly associated with a risk for PD (OR = 4.60; $P < 0.00005$);[119] contrarily, a similar study in a Chinese cohort failed to show such association.[120] Thus, evidence is not sufficient to conclude that *MAO* variants are associated with a risk for PD. *MAO* variants may become a risk depending on the race.

Catechole-O-Methyl Transferase Gene (COMT)

COMT is regulating the metabolism of catecholamines by *O*-methylation of the OH residue of the catechol ring. An amino acid change at Val108Met determines the high-activity and low-activity forms of COMT (Val/Val = high, Met/Met = low).

Earlier studies suggested association of PD with *COMT* variants;[121,122] however, subsequent studies failed to show association.[123] More recently, Bialecka and colleagues[124] studied four SNPs of the *COMT*; a high-activity haplotype carriers were higher in late-onset PD patients ($P = 0.04$) compared with the controls, and they required higher amounts of L-Dopa for their treatment compared with low-activity haplotype carriers.

Dopamine Transporter (SLC6A3) and Vesicular Monoamine transporter 2 (VMA2)

SLC6A3 encodes plasma membrane dopamine transporter, which is responsible for active reuptake of dopamine released into the synaptic space. *VMAT2* encodes vesicular monoamine transporter protein, which is responsible for active uptake of cytoplasmic monoamine into synaptic vesicles. Not many studies have been reported on the association of these variants with PD.

Kelada and colleagues[125] reported a marginal association of *SLC6A3* SNPs and a risk for PD (OR = 1.58); for PD patients who had been exposed to pesticides, the odd ratio increased to 5.66, if they had two or more risk alleles. Contrarily, other studies did not find association between *SLC6A3* or *VMA2* and PD.[126–128]

Dopamine Receptor Genes (DRD1, DRD2, DRD3, DRD4, and DRD5)

D1 and D2 receptors are mainly expressed in the striatal neurons and other receptors in mesolimbic areas. *DRD2, DRD3*, and *DRD4* belong to the same family and *DRD1* and *DRD5* to another family. Conflicting results have been reported on the association between these receptor genes and PD.

Plante-Bordeneuve and colleagues[127] reported association between a *DRD2* variant and PD; individuals who were homozygous for allele 3 were 2.3 times more frequent in the sporadic PD than in controls. Ricketts and colleagues[129] reported a higher frequency of exon 3 alleles with 6 or more repeat units in PD (P = 0.039). More recently, Juyal and colleagues[130] also found association between *DRD4* variants and PD in an Indian population.

Nevertheless, no association was found between dopamine *DRD2, DRD3,* and *DRD4* variants and PD in a Japanese cohort,[126,131] no association between a *DRD2* variant and PD in Spanish PD,[132] no association between a *DRD4* variant and PD in Chinese patients in Hong Kong,[133] and no association between T978C variant of the *DRD5* and PD in a Chinese cohort.[134] Recent study by Dick and colleagues[118] on large cohort of PD (n = 959) and controls (n = 1989) failed to show positive association between *DRD2* polymorphisms and a risk for PD. It seems unlikely that *DRD* variants play a significant role in the etiology and pathogensis of PD. Readers who are interested in *DRD* variants in PD are encouraged to read the recent article by D'Souza and Craig.[135]

Serotonin 2A Receptor Gene (HTR2A)

Association with serotonin receptor genes have been extensively studied in psychiatric disorders such as schizophrenia.[135] Shadrina and colleagues[136] reported association between a *HTR2A* variant and the risk for PD (P = 0.043) in a Russian population.

Genes Related to Xenobiotic-Metabolizing Proteins

CYP2D6 (Debrisoquine hydroxylase gene)

As exogenous neurotoxins emerged as potential etiologic factors since the discovery of MPTP, hepatic cytochrome P450 enzyme-polymorphisms have been extensively studied as this enzyme system is responsible for detoxification of xenobiotic substances. Debrisoquine has a structure similar to that of TIQ, and is metabolized by one of the hepatic cytochrome P450 enzymes, CYP2D6 (debrisoquine hydroxylase). Extensive or poor debrisoquine metabolizers are determined by CYP2D6 polymorphisms. Conflicting results have been reported on the association between *CYP2D6* variants and a risk for PD.

Smith and colleagues[137] examined the frequency of mutant *CYP2D6* alleles in 229 patients with PD and 720 controls. Individuals with a metabolic defect in the *CYP2D6* gene with the poor metabolizer phenotype had a 2.54-fold (95% CI 1.51–4.28) increased risk for PD. The frequency of poor metabolizers among PD patients was 11.8%. Armstrong and colleagues made a similar observation.[138]

The age of onset of PD was not younger in CYP2D6 poor metabolizers and it was even older among them.[139] Christensen and colleagues[140] made a meta-analysis of case-control studies on *CYP2D6*. The overall OR for poor metabolizers was 1.48 (95% CI 1.10–1.99). This difference was caused by a single large study and they concluded that there was no convincing evidence of an association between debrisoquine/spartan polymorphism and PD.

Gene-environment interaction is an interesting subject; however, Dick and colleagues[118] found no significant association between PD and variants of the following genes, that is, *CYP2D6, PON1, GSTM1, GSTT1, GSTM3, GSTP1, NQO1, CYP1B1, MAO-A, MAO-B, SOD 2, EPHX, DAT1, DRD2,* and *NAP2* in a large cohort of PD patients (n = 959).

N-Acetyltransferase 2 (NAT2)

NAT2 is involved in the metabolism of drugs and environmental toxins. Variations in *NAT1* and *NAT2* are associated with slow or rapid acetylation. Conflicting results have been reported on *NAT2* variants and PD.[141,142] A recent meta-analysis on 10 studies that involved 1206 PD patients and 1619 control subjects revealed no association between slow acetylaters and a risk for PD.[143] It seems unlikely that *NAT2* variants play an role in the etiology of PD.

Paraoxonase 1 (PON1)

PON1 is involved in the metabolism and detoxification of insecticides and pesticides. Conflicting results have been reported on the association between *paraoxonase 1* variants and PD. Two polymorphisms, M54L and Q192R, affect the enzyme activity. Clarimon and colleagues[144] found no association between these variants and PD in a Finnish cohort; whereas, a meta-analysis by Zintzaras and colleagues[145] found an association of the *PON1*-55M allele and a risk for PD relative to the L allele (OR = 1.32, 95% CI 1.10–1.59).

Alcohol Dehydrogenase (ADH1C)

ADH1C plays multiple roles in detoxification pathways. Buervenich and colleagues[146] studied a large international cohort and found significant association between *ADH* Class IV variant as well as the G78stop mutation in *ADH1C* (P = 0.007, OR = 3.25). But only 2.0% of the PD patients and 0.6% of control subjects had this variant; thus, the etiological relevance of this variant appears to be small.

Genes Regulating the Metabolism of Free Radicals and Activated Oxygen Species

As oxidative stress has been implicated in the pathogenesis of PD for many years, studies on the possible association between PD and variants of oxidative stress-related genes are of interest.

SOD1 (Cu-Zn Superoxide Dismutase Gene) and SOD2 (Mn Superoxide Dismutase Gene)

SOD catalyzes superoxide anions into hydrogen peroxide. SOD1 is expressed in the cytoplasm and SOD2 within mitochondria. No association was found between *SOD1* variants and a risk for PD.[147]

Conflicting results have been reported on the association between *SOD2* variants and PD. Shimoda-Matsubayashi and colleagues[148] genotyped the –Val9Ala polymorphism in the mitochondrial targeting sequence of *SOD2*. The –9Ala allele was significantly more frequent in PD patients (12.1% vs 19.3%; $P < 0.05$); contrarily, subsequent studies could not find association.[134,147,149]

More recently, Fong and colleagues[150] failed to find positive association between a *SOD2* variant (–9T > C) and a risk for PD; however, for those PD patients who had been exposed to pesticide, this variant was a risk factor.

Glutathione Transferase Gene (GST)

GSTs are a family of enzymes protecting cells against oxidative stress; they conjugate reduced glutathione to a variety of compounds including pesticides and herbicides. Human glutathione transferases are subdivided into classes by substrate specificity such as GSTM1 and GSTP1. Conflicting results have been reported on the association between *GST* variants and a risk for PD.

Association between *GSTM1* null variant and a risk for PD[151,152] and association between *GSTP1* variant and a risk for PD[153] were reported; whereas, a recent study on large cohorts of PD (n = 959) and controls (n = 1989) failed to show positive association between PD and *GSTM1, GSTT1, GSTM3,* or *GSTP1* variants.[118]

Li and colleagues[154] analyzed relationship between *GST omega-1 (GSTO1)* variants and the age of onset of PD; the maximum average age at onset was delayed by 8.6 years (+/–5.71) in patients who carried A nucleotide at rs4825. Wilk and colleagues[155] found association between *GSTP1* variants and earlier onset by 8 years in men who had been occupationally exposed to pesticides. Wahner and colleagues[156] studied the relationship between smoking habit and polymorphism of *GST*. Those PD patients carrying at least one variant allele for *GSTO1* (OR = 0.68, 95% CI 0.47–0.98) and also *GSTO2* (OR = 0.64, 95% CI 0.44–0.93) were associated with a reduced risk for PD with smoking habit. Further studies are needed to see the role of *GST* in the etiology of PD.

Nitric Oxide Synthase Gene (NOS)

NOSs produce nitric oxide, a free radical serving as a messenger molecule. Overproduction of nitric oxide contributes to oxidative stress. Three isozymes are known, that is, inducible NOS (iNOS), neuronal NOS (nNOS), and endothelial NOS (eNOS). As iNOS produces high NO levels, the possible association between iNOS and PD has been studied recently. *NOS2A* encodes iNOS. Recent two studies failed to show association between variants of *iNOS, eNOS,* or *nNOS* and PD.[157,158] NOS2A potentially interacts with cigarette smoking. Hancock and colleagues[159] studied 13 *NOS2A* variants in 466 singleton families and in a validation set of 286 multiplex families; they found associations between *NOS2A* variants and a risk for PD as well as the age of onset.

8-Oxo-dGTPase Gene (MTH1)

8-Oxo-7,8-dihydrodeoxyguanosine triphosphatase (MTH1) is a key enzyme for preventing oxidative stress-induced DNA damage. However, no association between *NTH1* variants and PD was reported.[160]

Haptoglobin

The human haptoglobin (Hp) protein is a plasma α-2 glycoprotein that removes free hemoglobin from the circulation and tissues and is important in protection from oxidative stress; Costa-Mallen and colleagues[161] studied three polymorphisms of this gene and found that Hp 2-1 genotype was more frequent in PD (n = 312) compared to controls (n = 420) (56.4% vs 48.1%, P = 0.03).

Genes Encoding Mitochondrial Proteins

Mitochondrial dysfunction has been implicated as one of the most important mechanisms that leads nigral neurons to death. The activity and the protein level of mitochondrial complex I is significantly diminished in the SN of PD patients.

24-kDa Subunit of Mitochondrial Complex I Gene (NDUFV2)

Twenty-four-kilodalton subunit is one of the most important subunits of complex I. Hattori and colleagues[162] genotyped a polymorphism (Ala29Val) in the mitochondrial targeting sequence of NDUFV2 in 126 Japanese patients with PD and 113 controls. The frequency of homozygotes of the variant was significantly higher in PD (23.8%) than in controls (11.5%, OR = 2.40). On the other hand, Mellick and colleagues[163] did not find association between any of the variants of 70 potential SNPs in 31 nuclear complex I genes and PD in 306 patients and 321 controls.

NADH-Quinone: Quinone Oxidoreductase Gene (NQO1)

NQO1 encodes a component of complex I. No association between PD and *NQO1* was found; however, this polymorphisms became a risk factor in those PD patients who had been exposed to pesticide.[164]

Mitochondrial Transcription Factor A Gene (TFAM)

TFAM is regulating mtDNA copy number and is required for transcriptional initiation at mtDNA promoters; no association with PD was found.[165]

Mitochondrial Translation Initiation Factor 3 Gene (MTIF3)

MTIF3 affects the availability of mitochondrially encoded proteins, and its variant may lead to oxidative stress. Abahuni and colleagues[166] reported association between *MTIF3* variants and a risk for PD.

Mitochondrial DNA

Mitochondrial DNA encodes some of the subunits of the electron transport chain. Conflicting results have been reported on the association between mitochondrial DNA polymorphisms and PD. Early reports did not have enough numbers of patients to make a definite conclusion. More recently, Pyle and colleagues[167] found a reduction in a risk for PD by 22% in carriers of the UKJT haplogroup cluster. Huerta and colleagues[168] reported association of allele 4336C>T (a polymorphism in the tRNA gln gene) and PD (OR=4.45, 95% CI 1.23–15.96; p = 0.011). Recent article by Chen and colleagues[169] on large cohorts of PD (n = 416) and controls (n = 372) failed to show association of 9055G/A, 10398G/A, and 13708G/A polymorphisms and a risk for PD as a whole; however, those patients above 70 who carried 9055G-10398A-13708G demonstrated a significant decrease in a risk of developing PD.

Genes Related to Inflammation

IL (Interleukin Genes)

ILs are multifunctional cytokines released form glia cells in the brain, and they are involved in inflammatory processes in the central nervous system. Inflammatory process has been implicated as a contributing factor in the pathogenesis of PD. Håkansson and colleagues[170] investigated a G/C SNP at position 174 in the promoter of the *IL-6* and found a significantly increased frequency of the GG genotype in PD; when the GG genotype was combined with *the estrogen receptor beta (ERbeta)* G-1730A SNP, the combination was much more robustly associated with PD. Estrogen inhibits the production of IL-6 via action on estrogen receptors. Other reports did not find association between *IL-1beta* variants and a risk for PD.[171,172]

Tumor Necrosis Factor-Alpha Gene (TNF-α)

TNF-α is involved in inflammatory processes. Wu and colleagues[173] studied the genotype distribution at T-1031C and C-857T in PD (n = 326) and controls (n = 326) in Chinese in Taiwan and found association of the more frequent –1031 CC genotype and PD (P = 0.0085, OR = 2.96).

Heat-Shock Protein 70 Gene (HSP70)

HSP70 is a chaperone that is upregulated in stress responses and refolds protein. Wu and colleagues[174] analyzed five variants of *HSP70-1*, *HSP70-2*, and *HSP70-hom* gene in a large cohort of Taiwanese PD. The frequencies of the –110 CC and +190 CC genotypes of *HSP70-1* were significantly higher in PD than controls (P = 0.001 and 0.006, respectively), whereas there was no association between PD and *HSP70-2* or *HSP70*-hom variants.

Neurotrophic Factor Genes

Brain-Derived Neurotrophic Factor Gene (BDNF)

BDNF is a neurotrophic factor, deficiency of which has been implicated in the pathogenesis of PD. Conflicting results have been reported on the association of its variant with PD. Zintzaras and colleagues[175] conducted a meta-analysis of six reports and found no association between the G196A polymorphism and the risk for PD. More recent studies also reported no association.[176,177] Therefore, it seems unlikely that *BDNF* variants play an important role in the etiology of PD.

Fibroblast Growth Factor 20 Gene (FGF20)

FGF20 is a neurotrophic factor preferentially expressed in the SN in rat brain. Conflicting results have been reported on the association between *FGF20* variants and PD. Van der Walt and colleagues[178] reported a highly significant association between PD and one intronic SNP, rs1989754 (P = 0.0006), and two SNPs, rs1721100 (P = 0.02) and ss20399075 (P = 0.0008), located in the 3' regulatory region. Contrarily, Clarimon and colleagues[179] found no association between *FGF20* variants and PD. More recent study reported inverse association between haplotype 2 at rs1721100 and PD in a large cohort of Japanese patients.[180] Another group reported association between rs12720208 in the 3' untranslated region of *FGF20* and PD; the risk increased translation of *FGF20* and this increase was correlated with α-synuclein expression.[181]

Transforming Growth Factor β-2 Gene (TGFB2)

TGFB2 is regulating the immune system and promoting the survival of dopaminergic neurons. No association was reported between *TGFB2* variants and PD.[182]

Neural Precursor Cell Expressed, Developmentally Downregulated 9 (NEDD9)

NEDD9 is involved in the formation of neurite-like membrane extensions and neurite outgrowth. Li and colleagues[183] reported association of the major CC genotype of rs760768 SNP with the risk of developing AD and PD; later, Chaptus and colleagues[184] could not reproduce their results.

Genes Related to Intracellular Signaling Pathways

Embryonic Lethal, Abnormal Vision, Drosophila-Like 4 (ELAVL4)

ELAVL4 is implicated in neuronal differentiation and maintenance located on chromosome 1p in the PARK10 region. Two studies found association between SNP markers in *ELAVL4* and risk for PD in Irish and Caucasian population,[185,186] but not in Norwegian or US samples;[185] three additional studies found association between SNP markers of *ELAVL4* and the age of onset of PD.[186–188]

AKT 1

AKT1 encodes protein kinase B (PKB), an intracellular signaling molecule activated by phosphatidylinositol 3-kinase (PI3K); *AKT1* is related to cell survival, proliferation, growth, and is upregulated in many cancer cells. Xiromerisiou and colleagues[189] reported inverse association between *AKT 1* variants and a risk for PD.

Semaphorine 5A

Semaphorine protein plays an important role in nerurogenesis and in neuronal apoptosis. Maraganore and colleagues[50] reported association between a semaphrine 5A variant and a risk for PD.

ASCL1

ASCL1 protein is a transcription factor that coregulates catecholamine-synthesizing enzymes with *PHOX2B*, the gene for another transcription factor that plays important roles in the development of catecholaminergic neurons. Ide and colleagues[190] reported association between polyglutamine length variations of *ASCL1* and PD (P = 0.018).

Other Genes

α-Antichymotrypsin (ACT)

ACT is present in senile plaque and potentially associated with a risk for Alzheimer's disease. However, conflicting results have been reported on the association between *ACT* variants and PD. Yamamoto and colleagues[191] analyzed *ACT* in Japanese patients with PD. The number of individuals with two copies of the ACT-A allele (ACT-AA genotype) was increased significantly in PD compared to controls (19.9% vs 8.3%; $P < 0.02$), and the ACT-A allele frequency in PD was significantly higher than controls ($\chi^2 = 5.96$; $df = 1$; $P < 0.015$). The OR for developing PD in individuals with the ACT-AA genotype was 3.36 compared to other individuals. However, subsequent studies were unable to reproduce the above results in European nations.[192–194]

Calbindin 1 (CALB1)

CALB1 is a 28-kDa calcium-binding protein widely distributed in the brain; whereas in PD, CALB1-negative neurons in the SN are mainly involved and positive neurons are relatively spared.[195,196] Thus, CALB1 appears to be acting as a neuroprotective protein. Mizuta and colleagues[197] found significant association between *CALB1* SNP and a risk for PD; whereas, a previous study on Caucasian population failed to reveal association.[50]

Proopiomelanocortin

Proopiomelanocortin is a precursor of ACTH as well as a precursor of a number of other biologically active peptides, regulating steroidgenesis, feeding, and pigmentation. Shadrina and colleagues[136] reported association of the *proopiomelanocortin* (rs28930368, $P = 0.026$ and rs2071345, $P = 0.027$) and a risk for PD.

PATHOGENESIS

Mitochondrial and Oxidative Damage

There is ample evidence to indicate that there is a selective loss of complex I of the mitochondrial electron transport system in PD.[198–201] This decrease is specific for SN and is not seen in other brain regions, as well as being specific for PD. Conflicting results have been reported on the activity of complex I in platelets, lymphocytes, and skeletal muscle.[202–206] How complex I deficiency relates to nigral neuronal death has been extensively discussed. Readers who are interested in this subject are encouraged to read recent review articles.[207,208]

There is ample evidence to indicate the presence of oxidative damage to high molecular weight substances such as proteins, lipids, and nucleic acids in the SN of patients with PD. Generally, free radicals are highly reactive, oxidizing other substances by extracting electrons; they may oxidize various substances nonselectively by cross-linking sulfhydryl bonds of proteins, inactivating certain enzymes, and by inducing acquired DNA mutations.[209] Recently, aggregation of α-synuclein was proposed as a main pathogenetic mechanism for nigral neuronal death, and this aggregation is enhanced by oxidative stress.[210] Oxidative damage to mitochondrial proteins further deteriorates mitochondrial function and mitochondrial dysfunction further increases free radical formation. In this way, mitochondrial dysfunction and oxidative stress induce a vicious cycle within nigral neurons and further enhance the damage. Readers who are interested in oxidative damage in PD are encouraged to read recent review articles.[14,207]

Among the reactive oxygen species, hydroxyl radicals are most cytotoxic. These radicals are formed by Fenton reaction (Fig. 12–2) in the presence of ferrous iron. Increase in iron in the SN of PD has been reported by many groups.[211–213] Iron exists in two forms (i.e., Fe^{3+} and Fe^{2+}). Most of the tissue iron is in the ferric form (Fe^{3+}), although small amounts of ferrous iron (Fe^{2+}) may exist.[214] In the presence of reducing substance, Fe^{3+} can be reduced to Fe^{2+}; Fe^{2+} is highly reactive and may induce free radical reactions, Fe^{2+} catalyzes the Fenton reaction, and Fe^{3+} mediates iron-catalyzed Haber–Weiss reaction (Fig. 12–2); both reactions produce hydroxyl radicals from hydrogen peroxide. Neuromelanin has high-affinity binding sites for iron,[214,215] and, in the presence of neuromelanin, Fe^{3+} is believed to be reduced to Fe^{2+}.[216] The mechanism of iron accumulation in the SN in PD is not known.

$$
\begin{aligned}
&1.\ {}^3O_2 + e^- \longrightarrow O_2^-\\
&2.\ 2O_2^- + 2H^+ \longrightarrow H_2O_2 + {}^3O_2\\
&3.\ H_2O_2 + Fe^{2+} \longrightarrow HO\cdot + OH^- + Fe^{3+}\\
&4.\ O_2^- + H_2O_2 \longrightarrow HO\cdot + OH^- + {}^1O_2\\
&5.\ O_2^- + H_2O_2 \xrightarrow{(Fe^{3+})} HO\cdot + OH^- + {}^3O_2\\
&6.\ NO + O_2^- \longrightarrow ONOO^-\\
&7.\ ONOO^- + H^+ \longrightarrow HO\cdot + NO_2\cdot\\
&8.\ R\text{-}CH_2\text{-}NH_2 + O_2 + H_2O \longrightarrow RCHO + NH_3 + H_2O_2
\end{aligned}
$$

Figure 12–2. Reactive oxygen species and their formation. (1) Formation of superoxide anion, (2) reaction catalyzed by superoxide dismutase, (3) Fenton reaction, (4) Haber–Weiss reaction, (5) iron-catalyzed Haber–Weiss reaction, (6) formation of peroxinitrite, (7) formation of hydroxyl radical from peroxynitrite, (8) reaction catalyzed by monoamine oxidase, ${}^3O_2$: triplet oxygen, O^-_2: superoxide anion, H_2O_2: hydrogen peroxide, HO: hydroxyl radical, ${}^1O_2$: singlet oxygen, NO: nitric oxide, $ONOO^-$: peroxynitrite, NO_2: nitric dioxide.

Other evidence of oxidative damage in nigral neurons includes increase in lipid peroxidation as measured as increase in malondialdehyde,[217] decrease in reduced glutathione,[218,219] and oxidative damage to DNA; hydroxyl radicals interact with guanine molecules of DNA to yield 8-hydroxydeoxyguanine, which may be read as thymine at the time of DNA duplication; thus, a GC to AT pair mutation will be induced.[220] Interestingly, an increase in 8-hydroxydeoxyguanosine in the nigrostriatum of PD brain has been reported;[221–223] this would suggest that acquired mutation of nuclear DNA as well as mtDNA takes place under oxidative stress.

Proteins are also attacked by reactive oxygen species. An increase in hydroxynonenal-modified proteins has been reported in the nigral neurons;[224] 4-hydroxy-2-nonenal (HNE) is an unsaturated aldehyde released from fatty acids by lipid peroxidation. It reacts with proteins to form stable adducts, which represent a marker of oxidative stress-induced cellular damage. Protein carbonyl is another indicator of oxidative brain damage, and a twofold increase in the protein carbonyl has been reported in SN pars compacta of PD brains.[225] Protein nitration is another way of damaging normal protein functions, and nitration of aggregated α-synuclein proteins has been reported in PD brains.[226]

Protein Misfolding and Aggregation

Most of the newly synthesized proteins are folded into a three-dimensional structure (tertiary structure) and this folding process takes place within endoplasmic reticulum shortly after the synthesis of the protein with the aid of shaperons.[227] Misfolded proteins and toxic proteins are rapidly metabolized by 26S proteasome after polyubiquitilation of those proteins at lysine 48 residue of the ubiquitin molecule.[228,229] 26S Proteasome is an ATP-dependent proteolytic enzyme; thus, ATP deficiency from mitochondrial dysfunction will impair the function; furthermore, oxidative stress impairs its function as well. Therefore, proteasome function is believed to be impaired in the nigral neurons of PD. Loss of the α-subunit of the 26S proteasome was reported in the SN of PD.[230]

In PD brains, aggregates of α-synuclein are accumulating within Lewy bodies as well as in the cytoplasm, neurites, and axons.[231] Initially, oligomers of α-synuclein are formed; oligomers are more toxic than aggregated synuclein.[232] The exact mechanism of oligomer formation is not well understood; however, oxidative stress is one of the most important mechanisms of oligomer formation as it can oxidize sulfhydryl residues in proteins inducing disulfide bonds resulting in polymer formation. Once oligomers are formed, they can impair mitochondrial membranes, 26S proteasome, and the membranes of dopamine storage vesicles.[232] Release of dopamine into cytoplasm enhances oxidative stress as cytoplasmic dopamine is metabolized by monoamine oxidase to yield hydrogen peroxide. Thus, within nigral neurons vicious cycles are established aggravating the degenerative process.

Furthermore, recently autophagy–lysosome dysfunction has been implicated in the pathogenesis of PD. The autophagy–lysosome system is able to digest oligomers and aggregated proteins as well as intracellular organelles.[233] Oligomers and aggregated α-synuclein proteins are digested by the autophagy–lysosome system. An interesting observation is that Gaucher disease patients and its heterozygous carriers have a higher risk for PD.[108–111] Gaucher disease is an autosomal recessive lipid storage disease caused by mutations of *GBA* and glucocerebrosidase is a lysosomal enzyme. Even a carrier state of a *GBA* mutation predisposes to PD as the reduced amount of this enzyme may not be sufficient to keep the normal function of the autophagy–lysosome system.

Impairment of both proteolytic systems, that is, 26S proteasome and the autophagy–lysosome system would induce accumulation of toxic, unfolded, and oligomeric proteins leading to accumulation of aggregated proteins. Lewy bodies are full of aggregate proteins including α-synuclein. Aggregated proteins within axons and neurites may well impair axonal transport of important substances for the survival of neurons.

Inflammatory Changes

Inflammatory process has also been implicated as a pathogenetic mechanism of nigral degeneration in PD. Reactive astrocytes and microglia produce a number of cytokines, many of which are cytotoxic, although some are neurorestorative and neuroprotective. There are many studies on the content of cytokines in the nigrostriatal system in PD. Readers who are interested in this subject are encouraged to read recent review articles.[234–237]

Proinflammatory cytokines that were reported to be increased in the nigrostriatal system of PD brain includes TNF-α,[238] β-2-microglobulin,[238] and IL-2.[238] IL-6 was also reported to be increased in CSF;[239,240] whereas, conflicting results have been reported on peripheral blood IL-6.[241,242] TNF-α is released from activated astrocytes and induces β-2-microglobulin expression. IL-6 is a member of the neuropoietic cytokine family and has an essential role in the development, differentiation, regeneration, and degeneration of neurons in the peripheral and central nervous systems. It is expressed in both neurons and glial cells. IL-6 can exert completely opposite actions on neurons, triggering either neuronal survival after injury or causing neuronal degeneration and cell death in disorders such as Alzheimer's disease.[243]

Neuroprotective and neurorestorative cytokines that have been reported to be increased in the nigrostriatal system of PD brains include TGF-β[244] and EGF (epidermal growth factor).[245] TGF-β is expressed in both neurons and glial cells from early embryonic stages to adulthood. TGF-β is a potent antiapoptotic and neuroprotective agent and is significantly upregulated in response to lesions.

Neuropprotective or neurorestorative cytokines that have been reported to be decreased in the nigrostriatal system of PD brains include bFGF (basic fibroblast growth factor),[246] GDNF,[247,248] BDNF,[247,248] NGF,[247] and CNTF.[248] Glial cell line-derived neurotrophic factor (GDNF) is a potent neurotrophic factor for dopaminergic neurons.

Parkinson's Disease and Apoptosis

Apoptosis is a signal-mediated death of cells; it is frequently discussed in contrast to necrosis. Neurodegeneration is a chronic process; therefore, apoptotic neuronal death is more likely than necrotic cell death, which is a rather acute process triggered by life-threatening insult to cells. Apoptosis can be induced by mitochondrial respiratory failure as well as by oxidative stress. Thus, metabolic alterations in PD are likely to be able to induce apoptotic neuronal death. Indirect evidences suggesting apoptotic neuronal death in PD have been reported in the literature including TUNEL-positive neurons[249,250] and electron microscopic pictures of apoptotic neuronal death in the postmortem PD brains.[251] However, conflicting results have been reported on TUNEL-positive neurons in PD.[252–254]

Another evidence suggesting apoptotic neuronal death in PD includes increase in soluble FAS, an apoptosis-signaling receptor molecule on cell membranes, in the striatum,[255] increase in nuclear translocation of NF-κB in PD nigral neurons,[256] increase in caspase 3 in the SN,[257] and increase in bcl-2 in the nigrostriatal system.[258,259] However, conflicting results have been reported on the amount of bcl-2 and BAX in PD.[254,260] Also, decrease in caspase 3, an effector of apoptosis, and increase in caspase 8, a proximal effecter protein of the TNF receptor family death pathway, were reported in PD nigral neurons.[261,262] NF-κB is a transcription factor that is activated by oxidative stress-induced apoptosis, and its activation causes it to migrate from the cytoplasm to the nucleus. Bcl-2 is an antiapoptotic protein located in the mitochondrial membrane, regulating the opening of the permeability transition pore. Opening of the transition pore is associated with a proapoptotic molecule, cytochrome *c*. BAX is a proapoptotic member of the Bcl-2 family of proteins facilitating the release of cytochrome *c* from the mitochondrial intermembrane space into the cytosol, leading to caspase activation and cell death. Readers who are interested in apoptosis in PD are encouraged to read recent review articles.[263–265]

▶ SUMMARY AND CONCLUSION

Despite increase in our knowledge about the molecular biological abnormalities in PD, we still do not know the exact etiology of sporadic PD. Many experts believe that the interaction of environmental factors and genetic predisposition initiates the neurodegenerative process in the nigral neurons, leading to mitochondrial respiratory failure and oxidative stress. These two abnormalities are able to induce apoptotic cell death. However, no single environmental toxic molecule that has been explicitly proved to be able to causes PD has been identified; on the other hand, *SNCA* polymorphisms appear to be an important predisposing factor for the development of PD. Regarding polymorphisms of other genes, further studies are needed before conclusion. Studies on familial forms of PD are rapidly progressing field, and it is expected that molecular understanding of the pathogenesis of familial PD will greatly facilitate the elucidation of etiology and pathogenesis of more common sporadic PD.

▶ ACKNOWLEDGMENTS

This study was supported in part by Grant-in-Aid for Priority Areas and Grant-in-Aid for Neuroscience Research from the Ministry of Education and Science, Japan, Grant-in-Aid for Brain Science from the Ministry of Health and Labor, Japan, and a "Center of Excellence" project grant from the National Parkinson Foundation, Miami.

REFERENCES

1. Parkinson J. An Essay on the Shaking Palsy. London: Sherwood, Neely, and Jones, 1817.
2. Von Economo C. Encephalitis lethargica. Wien Klin Wochenschr 1917;30:581–585.
3. Duvoisin RC, Yahr MD. Encephalitis and parkinsonism. Arch Neurol 1965;12:227–239.
4. Holt WL Jr. Epidemic encephalitis. A follow-up study of two hundred and sixty-six cases. Arch Neurol Psychiatry 1937;38:1135–1144.
5. Hirano A, Zimmerman HM. Alzheimer's neurofibrillary changes: A topographic study. Arch Neurol 1962;7: 227–242.
6. Mena I, Marin O, Fuenzalida S, et al. Chronic manganese poisoning. Clinical picture and manganese turnover. Neurology 1967;17:128–136.
7. Cotzias GC. Metabolic modification of some neurologic disorders. JAMA 1969;210:1255–1262.
8. Yase Y. The pathogenesis of amyotrophic lateral sclerosis. Lancet 1972;ii:292–296.
9. Pentschew A, Ebner FF, Kovatch RM. Experimental manganese encephalopathy in monkeys. A preliminary report. J Neuropathol Exp Neurol 1963;22:488–499.
10. Larsen NA, Pakkenberg H, Damsgaard E, et al. Distribution of arsenic, manganese, and selenium in the human brain in chronic renal insufficiency, Parkinson's disease, and amyotrophic lateral sclerosis. J Neurol Sci 1981;51:437–446.
11. Racette BA, McGee-Minnich L, Moerlein SM, et al. Welding-related parkinsonism: Clinical features, treatment, and pathophysiology. Neurology 2005;64:2001–2003.
12. Fored CM, Fryzek JP, Brandt L, et al. Parkinson's disease and other basal ganglia or movement disorders in a large nationwide cohort of Swedish welders. Occup Environ Med 2006;63:135–140.
13. Santamaria AB, Cushing CA, Antonini JM, et al. State-of-the-science review: Does manganese exposure during welding pose a neurological risk? J Toxicol Environ Health B Crit Rev 2007;10:417–465,.
14. Mizuno Y, Hattori N, Kubo S, et al. Progress in the pathogenesis and genetics of Parkinson's disease. Philos Trans R Soc Lond B Biol Sci 2008;363:2215–2227.
15. Pan T, Kondo S, Le W, et al. The role of autophagy-lysosome pathway in neurodegeneration associated with Parkinson's disease. Brain 2008;131:1969–1978,.
16. Davis GC, Williams AC, Markey SP, et al. Chronic parkinsonism secondary to intravenous injection of meperidine analogues. Psychiatry Res 1979;1:249–254.

17. Langston JW, Ballard P, Tetrud JW, et al. Chronic parkinsonism in humans due to a product of meperidine-analog synthesis. Science 1983;219:979–980.
18. Chiba K, Trevor AJ, Castagnoli N Jr. Metabolism of the neurotoxic tertiary amine, MPTP, by brain monoamine oxidase. Biochem Biophys Res Commun 1984;120: 574–578.
19. Javitch JA, D'Amato RJ, Strittmatter SM, et al. Parkinsonism-inducing neurotoxin, N-methyl-4-phenyl-1,2,3,6-tetrahydropyridine: Uptake of the metabolite N-methyl-4-phenylpyridine by dopamine neurons explains selective toxicity. Proc Natl Acad Sci USA 1985;82:2173–2177.
20. Ramsay RR, Singer TP. Energy-dependent uptake of N-methyl-4-phenylpyridinium, the neurotoxic metabolite of 1-methyl-4-phenyl-1,2,3,6-tetrahydropyridine, by mitochondria. J Biol Chem 1986;261:7585–7587.
21. Nicklas WJ, Vyas I, Heikkila RE. Inhibition of NADH-linked oxidation in brain mitochondria by 1-methyl-4-phenylpyridine, a metabolite of the neurotoxin, 1-methyl-4-phenyl-1,2,5,6-tetrahydropyridine. Life Sci 1985;36:2503–2508.
22. Mizuno Y, Saitoh T, Sone N. Inhibition of mitochondrial NADH-ubiquinone oxidoreductase activity by 1-methyl-4-phenylpyridinium ion. Biochem Biophys Res Commun 1987;143:294–299.
23. Mizuno Y, Suzuki K, Sone N, et al. Inhibition of ATP synthesis by 1-methyl-4-phenylpyridinium ion (MPP+) in isolated mitochondria from mouse brains. Neurosci Lett 1987;81:204–208.
24. Dipasquale B, Marini M, Youl RJ. Apoptosis and DNA degradation by 1-methyl-4-phenylpyridinium in neurons. Biochem Biophys Res Commun 1991;181:1442–1448.
25. Mochizuki H, Nakamura N, Nishi K, et al. Apoptosis is induced by 1-methyl-4-phenylpyridinium ion (MPP+) in a ventral mesencephalic-striatal co-culture. Neurosci Lett 1994;170:191–194.
26. Rajput AH, Uitti RJ, Stern W, et al. Early onset Parkinson's disease in Saskatchewan: Environmental considerations for etiology. Can J Neurol Sci 1986;13:312–316.
27. Tanner CM, Langston JW. Do environmental toxins cause Parkinson's disease? A critical review. Neurology 1990;40(suppl 3):17–31.
28. Nuti A, Ceravolo R, Dell'Agnello G, Gambaccini Get al. Environmental factors and Parkinson's disease: A case-control study in the Tuscany region of Italy. Parkinsonism Relat Disord 2004;10:481–485.
29. Taylor CA, Saint-Hilaire MH, Cupples LA, et al. Environmental, medical, and family history risk factors for Parkinson's disease: A New England-based case control study. Am J Med Genet 1999;88:742–749.
30. Rajput AH, Uitti RJ, Stern W, et al. Geography, drinking water chemistry, pesticides and herbicides and the etiology of Parkinson's disease. Can J Neurol Sci 1987;14:414–418.
31. Frigerio R, Sanft KR, Grossardt BR, et al. Chemical exposures and Parkinson's disease: A population-based case-control study. Mov Disord 2006;21:1688–1692.
32. Fong CS, Cheng CW, Wu RM. Pesticides exposure and genetic polymorphism of paraoxonase in the susceptibility of Parkinson's disease. Acta Neurol Taiwan 2005;14:55–60.
33. Baron JA. Cigarette smoking and Parkinson's disease. Neurology 1986;36:1490–1496.
34. Hellenbrand W, Seidler A, Robra BP, et al. Smoking and Parkinson's disease: A case-control study in Germany. Int J Epidemiol 1997;26:328–339.
35. Wirdefeldt K, Gatz M, Pawitan Y, et al. Risk and protective factors for Parkinson's disease: A study in Swedish twins. Ann Neurol 2005;57:27–33.
36. Hancock DB, Martin ER, Stajich JM, et al. Smoking, caffeine, and nonsteroidal anti-inflammatory drugs in families with Parkinson disease. Arch Neurol 2007;64:576–580.
37. Tanner CM, Chen B, Wang W, et al. Environmental factors and Parkinson's disease: A case-control study in China. Neurology 1989;39:660–664.
38. Rajput AH, Offord KP, Beard CM, et al. A case-control study of smoking habits, dementia, and other illnesses in idiopathic Parkinson's disease. Neurology 1987;37:226–232.
39. Ascherio A, Zhang SM, Hernán MA, et al. Prospective study of caffeine consumption and risk of Parkinson's disease in men and women. Ann Neurol 2001;50: 56–63.
40. Chen H, Zhang SM, Hernán MA, et al. Nonsteroidal anti-inflammatory drugs and the risk of Parkinson disease. Arch Neurol 2003;60:1043–1044.
41. McNaught KS, Carrupt PA, Altomare C, et al. Isoquinoline derivatives as endogenous neurotoxins in the aetiology of Parkinson's disease. Biochem Pharmacol 1998;56:921–933.
42. Maruyama W, Strolin-Benedetti M, Naoi M. N-Methyl(R) salsolinol and a neutral N-methyltransferase as pathogenic factors in Parkinson's disease. Neurobiology 2000;8: 55–68.
43. Collins MA, Neafsey E. β-Carboline analogues of N-methyl-4-phenyl-1,2,5,6-tetrahydropyridine (MPTP): Endogenous factors underlying idiopathic parkinsonism? Neurosci Lett 1985;55:179–184.
44. Matsubara K, Gonda T, Sawada H, et al. Endogenously occurring beta-carboline induces parkinsonism in nonprimate animals: A possible causative protoxin in idiopathic Parkinson's disease. J Neurochem 1998;70:727–735.
45. Marder K, Tang M-X, Mejia H, et al. Risk of Parkinson's disease among first-degree relatives: A community-based study. Neurology 1996;47:155–160.
46. Elbaz A, Grigoletto F, Baldereschi M, et al. European Parkinson Study Group: Familial aggregation of Parkinson's disease. A population-based case-control study in Europe. Neurology 1999;52:1876–1882.
47. Ward CD, Duvoisin RC, Ince SE, et al. Parkinson's disease in 65 pairs of twins and in a set of quadruplets. Neurology 1983;33:815–824.
48 Tanner CM, Ottman R, Goldman SM, et al. Parkinson's disease in twins: An etiologic study. JAMA 1999;281:341–346.
49. Wirdefeldt K, Gatz M, Schalling M, et al. No evidence for heritability of Parkinson disease in Swedish twins. Neurology 2004;63;305–311.
50. Maraganore DM, de Andrade M, Lesnick TG, et al. High-resolution whole-genome association study of Parkinson disease. Am J Hum Genet 2005;77:685693.
51. Elbaz A, Nelson LM, Payami H, et al. Lack of replication of thirteen single-nucleotide polymorphisms implicated in Parkinson's disease: A large-scale international study Lancet Neurol 2006;5:917–923.
52. Farrer M, Marananore DM, Lackhart P, et al. Alpha-synuclein gene haplotypes are associated with Parkinson's disease. Hum Mol Genet 2001;10:1847–1851.

53. Kruger R, Vieira-Saecker AM, Kuhn W, et al. Increased susceptibility to sporadic Parkinson's disease by a certain combined alpha-synuclein/apolipoprotein E genotype. Ann Neurol 1999;45:611–617.
54. Khan N, Graham E, Dixon P, et al. Parkinson's disease is not associated with the combined alpha-synuclein/apolipoprotein E susceptibility genotype. Ann Neurol 2001;49:665–668.
55. Izumi Y, Morino H, Oda M, et al. Genetic studies in Parkinson's disease with an alpha-synuclein/NACP gene polymorphism in Japan. Neurosci Lett 2001;300:125–127.
56. Mueller JC, Fuchs J, Hofer A, et al. Multiple regions of a-synuclein are associated with Parkinson's disease. Ann Neurol 2005;57:535–41.
57. Tan EK, Chai A, Teo YY, et al. Alpha-synuclein haplotypes implicated in risk of Parkinson's disease. Neurology 2004;62:128–131.
58. Mellick GD, Maraganore DM, Silburn PA. Australian data and meta-analysis lend support for alpha-synuclein (NACP-Rep1) as a risk factor for Parkinson's disease. Neurosci Lett 2005;375:112–116.
59. Hadjigeorgiou GM, Xiromerisiou G, Gourbali V, et al. Association of alpha-synuclein Rep1 polymorphism and Parkinson's disease: Influence of Rep1 on age at onset. Mov Disord 2006;21:534–539.
60. Wang CK, Chen CM, Chang CY, et al. alpha-Synuclein promoter RsaI T-to-C polymorphism and the risk of Parkinson's disease. J Neural Transm 2006;113:1425–1433.
61. Maraganore DM, de Andrade M, Elbaz A, et al. Collaborative analysis of alpha-synuclein gene promoter variability and Parkinson disease. JAMA 2006;296:661–670.
62. Winkler S, Hagenah J, Lincoln S, et al. Alpha-Synuclein and Parkinson disease susceptibility. Neurology 2007;69:1745–1750.
63. Parsian AJ, Racette BA, Zhao JH, et al. Association of alpha-synuclein gene haplotypes with Parkinson's disease. Parkinsonism Relat Disord 2007;13:343–347.
64. Mizuta I, Satake W, Nakabayashi Y, et al. Multiple candidate gene analysis identifies alpha-synuclein as a susceptibility gene for sporadic Parkinson's disease. Hum Mol Genet 2006;15:1151–1158.
65. Brighina L, Okubadejo NU, Schneider NK, et al. Beta-synuclein gene variants and Parkinson's disease: A preliminary case-control study. Neurosci Lett 2007;420:229–234.
66. Tan EK, Puong KY, Chan DK, et al. Impaired transcriptional upregulation of Parkin promoter variant under oxidative stress and proteasomal inhibition: Clinical association. Hum Genet 2005;118:484–488.
67. Ross OA, Haugarvoll K, Stone JT, et al. Lack of evidence for association of Parkin promoter polymorphism (PRKN-258) with increased risk of Parkinson's disease. Parkinsonism Relat Disord 2007;13:386–388.
68. Maraganore DM, Lesnick TG, Elbaz A, et al. UCHL1 Global Genetics Consortium. UCHL1 is a Parkinson's disease susceptibility gene. Ann Neurol 2004;55:512–521.
69. Tan EK, Puong KY, Fook-Chong S, et al. Case-control study of UCHL1 S18Y variant in Parkinson's disease. Mov Disord 2006;21:1765–1768.
70. Carmine Belin A, Westerlund M, Bergman O, et al. S18Y in ubiquitin carboxy-terminal hydrolase L1 (UCH-L1) associated with decreased risk of Parkinson's disease in Sweden. Parkinsonism Relat Disord 2007;13:295–298.
71. Healy DG, Abou-Sleiman PM, Casas JP, et al. UCHL-1 is not a Parkinson's disease susceptibility gene. Ann Neurol 2006;59:627–633.
72. Hutter CM, Samii A, Factor SA, et al. Lack of evidence for an association between UCHL1 S18Y and Parkinson's disease. Eur J Neurol 2008;15:134–139.
73. Zhang ZJ, Burgunder JM, An XK, et al. Lack of evidence for association of a UCH-L1 S18Y polymorphism with Parkinson's disease in a Han-Chinese population. Neurosci Lett 2008;442:200–202.
74. Groen JL, Kawarai T, Toulina A, et al. Genetic association study of PINK1 coding polymorphisms in Parkinson's disease. Neurosci Lett 2004;372:226–229.
75. Wang F, Feng X, Ma J, et al. A common A340T variant in PINK1 gene associated with late-onset Parkinson's disease in Chinese. Neurosci Lett 2006;410:121–125.
76. Morris CM, O'Brien KK, Gibson AM, et al. Polymorphism in the human DJ-1 gene is not associated with sporadic dementia with Lewy bodies or Parkinson's disease. Neurosci Lett 2003;352:151–153.
77. Maraganore DM, Wilkes K, Lesnick TG, et al. A limited role for DJ1 in Parkinson disease susceptibility. Neurology 2004;63:550–553.
78. Skipper L, Li Y, Bonnard C, et al. Comprehensive evaluation of common genetic variation within LRRK2 reveals evidence for association with sporadic Parkinson's disease. Hum Mol Genet 2005;14:3549–3556.
79. Paisán-Ruíz C, Evans EW, Jain S, et al. Testing association between LRRK2 and Parkinson's disease and investigating linkage disequilibrium. J Med Genet 2006;43:e9.
80. Di Fonzo A, Wu-Chou YH, Lu CS, et al. A common missense variant in the LRRK2 gene, Gly2385Arg, associated with Parkinson's disease risk in Taiwan. Neurogenetics 2006;7:133–138.
81. Tan EK, Zhao Y, Skipper L, Tan MG, et al. The LRRK2 Gly2385Arg variant is associated with Parkinson's disease: Genetic and functional evidence. Hum Genet 2007;120:857–863.
82. Farrer MJ, Stone JT, Lin CH, et al. Lrrk2 G2385R is an ancestral risk factor for Parkinson's disease in Asia. Parkinsonism Relat Disord 2007;13:89–92.
83. Funayama M, Li Y, Tomiyama H, et al. Leucine-rich repeat kinase 2 G2385R variant is a risk factor for Parkinson disease in Asian population. Neuroreport 2007;18:273–275.
84. Wei-dong Le, Pingyi Xu, Jankovic J, et al. Mutations in NR4A2 associated with familial Parkinson disease. Nature Genetics 2002;33:85–89.
85. Nichols WC, Uniacke SK, Pankratz N, et al. Evaluation of the role of Nurr1 in a large sample of familial Parkinson's disease. Mov Disord 2004;649–655.
86. Healy DG, Abou-Sleiman PM, Ahmadi KR, et al. NR4A2 genetic variation in sporadic Parkinson's disease: A genewide approach. Mov Disord 2006;1960–1963.
87. Baker M, Litvan I, Houlden H, et al. Association of an extended haplotype in the tau gene with progressive supranuclear palsy. Hum Mol Genet 1999;8:711–715.

88. Conrad C, Andreadis A, Trojanowski JQ, et al. Genetic evidence for the involvement of tau in progressive supranuclear palsy. Ann Neurol 1998;44 707–708.
89. Pittman AM, Fung HC, de Silva R. Untangling the tau gene association with neurodegenerative disorders. Hum Mol Genet 2006;15 Spec No 2:R188–195.
90. Pastor P, Ezquerra M, Munoz E, et al. Significant association between the tau gene A0/A0 genotype and Parkinson's disease. Ann Neurol 2000;47:242–245.
91. Levecque C, Elbaz A, Clavel J, et al. Association of polymorphisms in the Tau and Saitohin genes with Parkinson's disease. J Neurol Neurosurg Psychiatry 2004;75:478–480.
92. Kwok JB, Teber ET, Loy C, et al. Tau haplotypes regulate transcription and are associated with Parkinson's disease. Ann Neurol 2004;55:329–334.
93. Skipper L, Wilkes K, Toft M, et al Linkage disequilibrium and association of MAPT H1 in Parkinson disease. Am J Hum Genet 2004;75:669–677.
94. Zabetian CP, Hutter CM, Factor SA, et al. Association analysis of MAPT H1 haplotype and subhaplotypes in Parkinson's disease. Ann Neurol 2007;62:137–144.
95. Tobin JE, Latourelle JC, Lew MF, et al. Haplotypes and gene expression implicate the MAPT region for Parkinson disease: The GenePD Study. Neurology 2008;71:28–34.
96. de Silva R, Hardy J, Crook J, et al. The tau locus is not significantly associated with pathologically confirmed sporadic Parkinson's disease. Neurosci Lett 2002;330:201–203.
97. Fung HC, Xiromerisiou G, Gibbs JR, et al. Association of tau haplotype-tagging polymorphisms with Parkinson's disease in diverse ethnic Parkinson's disease cohorts. Neurodegener Dis 2006;3:327–333.
98. Zhang J, Song Y, Chen H, et al. The tau gene haplotype h1 confers a susceptibility to Parkinson's disease. Eur Neurol 2005;53:15–21.
99. Kobayashi H, Ujike H, Hasegawa J, et al. Correlation of tau gene polymorphism with age at onset of Parkinson's disease. Neurosci Lett 2006;405:202–206.
100. Huang X, Chen PC, Poole C. APOE-[epsilon]2 allele associated with higher prevalence of sporadic Parkinson disease. Neurology 2004;62:2198–2202.
101. Li YJ, Hauser MA, Scott WK, et al. Apolipoprotein E controls the risk and age at onset of Parkinson disease. Neurology 2004;62:2005–2009.
102. López M, Guerrero J, Yescas P, et al. Apolipoprotein E epsilon4 allele is associated with Parkinson disease risk in a Mexican Mestizo population. Mov Disord 2007;22:417–420.
103. Papapetropoulos S, Farrer MJ, Stone JT, et al. Phenotypic associations of tau and ApoE in Parkinson's disease. Neurosci Lett 2007;414:141–144.
104. Jasinska-Myga B, Opala G, Goetz CG, et al. Apolipoprotein E gene polymorphism, total plasma cholesterol level, and Parkinson disease dementia. Arch Neurol 2007;64:261–265..
105. Baker M, Mackenzie IR, Pickering-Brown SM, et al. Mutations in progranulin cause tau-negative frontotemporal dementia linked to chromosome 17. Nature 2006;442: 916–919.
106. Nuytemans K, Pals P, Sleegers K, et al. Progranulin variability has no major role in Parkinson disease genetic etiology. Neurology 2008;71:1147–1151.
107. Myhre R, Klungland H, Farrer MJ, et al. Genetic association study of synphilin-1 in idiopathic Parkinson's disease. BMC Med Genet 2008;9:19.
108. Goker-Alpan O, Schiffmann R, LaMarca ME, et al. Parkinsonism among Gaucher disease carriers. J Med Genet 2004;41:937–940..
109. Sato C, Morgan A, Lang AE, et al. Analysis of the glucocerebrosidase gene in Parkinson's disease. Mov Disord 2005;20:367–370.
110. De Marco EV, Annesi G, Tarantino P, et al. Glucocerebrosidase gene mutations are associated with Parkinson's disease in southern Italy. Mov Disord 2008;23:460–463.
111. Kono S, Shirakawa K, Ouchi Y, et al. Dopaminergic neuronal dysfunction associated with parkinsonism in both a Gaucher disease patient and a carrier. J Neurol Sci 2007;252:181–184.
112. Toft M, Pielsticker L, Ross OA, et al. Glucocerebrosidase gene mutations and Parkinson disease in the Norwegian population. Neurology 2006;66:415–417.
113. Oliveira SA, Li YJ, Noureddine MA, et al. Identification of risk and age-at-onset genes on chromosome 1p in Parkinson disease. Am J Hum Genet 2005;77:252–264
114. Li Y, Schrodi S, Rowland C, T et al. Genetic evidence for ubiquitin-specific proteases USP24 and USP40 as candidate genes for late-onset Parkinson disease. Hum Mutation 2006;27:1017–1023
115 Plante-Bordeneuve V, Davis MB, Maraganore DM, et al. Tyrosine hydroxylase polymorphisms in familial and sporadic Parkinson's disease. Mov Disord 1994;9: 337–339.
116. Parsian A, Racette B, Zhang ZH, et al. Association of variations in monoamine oxidases A and B with Parkinson's disease subgroups. Genomics 2004;454–460.
117. Kang SJ, Scott WK, Li YJ, et al. Family-based case-control study of MAOA and MAOB polymorphisms in Parkinson disease. Mov Disord 2006;21:2175–2180.
118. Dick FD, De Palma G, Ahmadi A, et al. Geoparkinson Study Group. Gene-environment interactions in parkinsonism and Parkinson's disease: The Geoparkinson study. Occup Environ Med 2007;64:673–680.
119. Mellick GD, Buchanan DD, McCann SJ, et al. Variations in the monoamine oxidase B (MAOB) gene are associated with Parkinson's disease. Mov Disord 1999;14:219–224.
120. Mellick GD, Buchanan DD, Silburn PA, et al. The monoamine oxidase B gene GT repeat polymorphism and Parkinson's disease in a Chinese population. J Neurol 2000;247:52–55.
121. Kunugi H, Nanko S, Ueki A, et al. High and low activity alleles of catechol-O-methyltransferase gene: Ethnic difference and possible association with Parkinson's disease. Neurosci Lett 1997;221:202–204.
122. Yoritaka A, Hattori N, Yoshino H, et al. Catechol-O-methyltransferase genotype and susceptibility to Parkinson's disease in Japan. J Neural Transm 1997;104:1313–1317.
123. Hoda F, Nicholl D, Bennett P, et al. No association between Parkinson's disease and low-activity alleles of catechol-O-methyltransferase. Biochem Biophys Res Commun 1996;228:780–784.
124. Bialecka M, Kurzawski M, Klodowska-Duda G, et al. The association of functional catechol-O-methyltransferase haplotypes with risk of Parkinson's disease, levodopa

treatment response, and complications. Pharmacogenet Genomics 2008;18:815–821.

125. Kelada SN, Checkoway H, Kardia SL, et al. 5' and 3' region variability in the dopamine transporter gene (SLC6A3), pesticide exposure and Parkinson's disease risk: A hypothesis-generating study. Hum Mol Genet 2006;15:3055–3062.
126. Higuchi S, Muramatsu T, Arai H, et al. Polymorphisms of dopamine receptor and transporter genes and Parkinson's disease. J Neural Transm 1995;10:107–113.
127. Plante-Bordeneuve V, Taussig D, Thomas F, et al. Evaluation of four candidate genes encoding proteins of the dopamine pathway in familial and sporadic Parkinson's disease: Evidence for association of a DRD2 allele. Neurology 1997;48:1589–1593.
128. Kariya S, Hirano M, Takahashi N, et al. Lack of association between polymorphic microsatellites of the VMAT2 gene and Parkinson's disease in Japan. J Neurol Sci 2005;232:91–94.
129. Ricketts MH, Hamer RM, Manowitz P, et al. Association of long variants of the dopamine D4 receptor exon 3 repeat polymorphism with Parkinson's disease. Clin Genet 1998;54:33–38.
130. Jual RC, Das M, Punia S, et al. Genetic susceptibility to Parkinson's disease among South and North Indians: I. Role of polymorphisms in dopamine receptor and transporter genes and association of DRD4 120-bp duplication marker. Neurogenetics 2006;7:223–9.
131. Nanko S, Ueki A, Hattori M, et al. No allelic association between Parkinson's disease and dopamine D2, D3, and D4 receptor gene polymorphisms. Am J Med Genet 1994;54:361–364.
132. Pastor P, Munoz E, Obach V, et al. Dopamine receptor D2 intronic polymorphism in patients with Parkinson's disease. Neurosci Lett 1999;273:151–154.
133. Wan DC, Law LK, Ip DT, et al. Lack of allelic association of dopamine D4 receptor gene polymorphisms with Parkinson's disease in a Chinese population. Mov Disord 1999;14:225–229.
134. Wang J, Liu ZL, Chen B. Dopamine D5 receptor gene polymorphism and the risk of levodopa-induced motor fluctuations in patients with Parkinson's disease. Neurosci Lett 2001;308:21–24.
135. D'Souza UM, Craig IW. Functional polymorphisms in dopamine and serotonin pathway genes. Hum Mutat 2006;27:1–13
136. Shadrina M, Nikopensius T, Slominsky P, et al. Association study of sporadic Parkinson's disease genetic risk factors in patients from Russia by APEX technology. Neurosci Lett 2006;405:212–216.
137. Smith CA, Gough AC, Leigh PN, et al. Debrisoquine hydroxylase gene polymorphism and susceptibility to Parkinson's disease. Lancet 1992;339:1375–1377.
138. Armstrong M, Daly AK, Cholerton S, et al. Mutant debrisoquine hydroxylation genes in Parkinson's disease. Lancet 1992;339:1017–1018.
139. Payami H, Lee N, Zareparsi S, et al. Parkinson's disease, CYP2D6 polymorphism, and age. Neurology 2001;56: 1363–1370.
140. Christensen PM, Gotzsche PC, Brosen K. The sparteine/debrisoquine (CYP2D6) oxidation polymorphism and the risk of Parkinson's disease: A meta-analysis. Pharmacogenetics 1998;8:473–479.
141. Bandmann O, Vaughan J, Holmans P, et al. Association of slow acetylator genotype for N-acetyltransferase 2 with familial Parkinson's disease. Lancet 1997;350: 1136–1139.
142. Chaudhary S, Behari M, Dihana M, et al. Association of N-acetyl transferase 2 gene polymorphism and slow acetylator phenotype with young onset and late onset Parkinson's disease among Indians. Pharmacogenet Genomics 2005;15:731–735.
143. Borlak J, Reamon-Buettner SM. N-acetyltransferase 2 (NAT2) gene polymorphisms in Parkinson's disease. BMC Med Genet 2006;7:30.
144. Clarimon J, Eerola J, Hellström O, et al. Paraoxonase 1 (PON1) gene polymorphisms and Parkinson's disease in a Finnish population. Neurosci Lett 2004;367:168–170.
145. Zintzaras E, Hadjigeorgiou GM. Association of paraoxonase 1 gene polymorphisms with risk of Parkinson's disease: A meta-analysis. J Hum Genet 2004;49:474–481.
146. Buervenich S, Carmine A, Galter D, et al. A rare truncating mutation in ADH1C (G78Stop) shows significant association with Parkinson disease in a large international sample. Arch Neurol 2005;62:74–78.
147. Farin FM, Hitosis Y, Hallagan SE, et al. Genetic polymorphisms of superoxide dismutase in Parkinson's disease. Mov Disord 2001;16:705–707.
148. Shimoda-Matsubayashi S, Hattori T, Matsumine H, et al. Mn SOD activity and protein in a patient with chromosome 6-linked autosomal recessive parkinsonism in comparison with Parkinson's disease and control. Neurology 1997;49:1257–1262.
149. Grasbon-Frodl EM, Kosel S, Riess O, et al. Analysis of mitochondrial targeting sequence and coding region polymorphisms of the manganese superoxide dismutase gene in German Parkinson disease patients. Biochem Biophys Res Commun 1999;255:749–752.
150. Fong CS, Wu RM, Shieh JC, et al. Pesticide exposure on southwestern Taiwanese with MnSOD and NQO1 polymorphisms is associated with increased risk of Parkinson's disease. Clin Chim Acta 2007;378:136–141.
151. Stroombergen MCMJ, Waring RH, Bennett P, et al. Determination of the GSTM1 gene deletion frequency in Parkinson's disease by allele specific PCR. Parkinsonism Relat Disord 1996;2:151–154.
152. Perez-Pastene C, Graumann R, Díaz-Grez F, et al. Association of GST M1 null polymorphism with Parkinson's disease in a Chilean population with a strong Amerindian genetic component. Neurosci Lett 2007;418:181–185.
153. Vilar R, Coelho H, Rodrigues E, et al. Association of A313 G polymorphism (GSTP1*B) in the glutathione-S-transferase P1 gene with sporadic Parkinson's disease. Eur J Neurol 2007;14:156–161.
154. Li YJ, Scott WK, Zhang L, et al. Revealing the role of glutathione S-transferase omega in age-at-onset of Alzheimer and Parkinson diseases. Neurobiol Aging 2006;27:1087–1093.
155. Wilk JB, Tobin JE, Suchowersky O, et al. Herbicide exposure modifies GSTP1 haplotype association to Parkinson onset age: The GenePD Study. Neurology 2006;67: 2206–2210.

156. Wahner AD, Glatt CE, Bronstein JM, et al. Glutathione S-transferase mu, omega, pi, and theta class variants and smoking in Parkinson's disease. Neurosci Lett 2007;413:274–278.
157. Schulte C, Sharma M, Mueller JC, et al. Comprehensive association analysis of the NOS2A gene with Parkinson disease. Neurology 2006;67:2080–2082.
158. Huerta C, Sánchez-Ferrero E, Coto E, et al. No association between Parkinson's disease and three polymorphisms in the eNOS, nNOS, and iNOS genes. Neurosci Lett 2007;413:202–205.
159. Hancock DB, Martin ER, Fujiwara K, et al. NOS2A and the modulating effect of cigarette smoking in Parkinson's disease. Ann Neurol 2006;60:366–73.
160. Satoh J, Kuroda Y. A valine to methionine polymorphism at codon 83 in the 8-oxo-dGTPase gene MTH1 is not associated with sporadic Parkinson's disease. Eur J Neurol 2000;7:673–677.
161. Costa-Mallen P, Checkoway H, Zabeti A, et al. The functional polymorphism of the hemoglobin-binding protein haptoglobin influences susceptibility to idiopathic Parkinson's disease. Am J Med Genet B Neuropsychiatr Genet 2008;147B:216–222.
162. Hattori N, Yoshino H, Tanaka M, et al. Genotype in the 24-kDa subunit gene (NDUFV2) of mitochondrial complex I and susceptibility to Parkinson disease. Genomics 1998;49:52–58.
163. Mellick GD, Silburn PA, Prince JA, et al. A novel screen for nuclear mitochondrial gene associations with Parkinson's disease. J Neural Transm 2004;111:191–199.
164. Fong CS, Wu RM, Shieh JC, et al. Pesticide exposure on southwestern Taiwanese with MnSOD and NQO1 polymorphisms is associated with increased risk of Parkinson's disease. Clin Chim Acta 2007;378:136–141.
165. Belin AC, Björk BF, Westerlund M, et al. Association study of two genetic variants in mitochondrial transcription factor A (TFAM) in Alzheimer's and Parkinson's disease. Neurosci Lett 2007;420:257–262.
166. Abahuni N, Gispert S, Bauer P, et al. Mitochondrial translation initiation factor 3 gene polymorphism associated with Parkinson's disease. Neurosci Lett 2007;414: 126–129.
167. Pyle A, Foltynie T, Tiangyou W, et al. Mitochondrial DNA haplogroup cluster UKJT reduces the risk of PD. Ann Neurol 2005;57:564–567.
168. Huerta C, Castro MG, Coto E, et al. Mitochondrial DNA polymorphisms and risk of Parkinson's disease in Spanish population. J Neurol Sci 2005;236:49–54.
169. Chen CM, Kuan CC, Lee-Chen GJ, et al. Mitochondrial DNA polymorphisms and the risk of Parkinson's disease in Taiwan. J Neural Transm 2007;114: 1017–1021.
170. Håkansson A, Westberg L, Nilsson S, et al. Interaction of polymorphisms in the genes encoding interleukin-6 and estrogen receptor beta on the susceptibility to Parkinson's disease. Am J Med Genet B Neuropsychiatr Genet 2005;133B:88–92.
171. Nishimura M, Mizuta I, Mizuta E, et al. Influence of interleukin-1beta gene polymorphisms on age-at-onset of sporadic Parkinson's disease. Neurosci Lett 2000;284: 73–76.
172. Möller JC, Depboylu C, Kölsch H, et al. Lack of association between the interleukin-1 alpha (-889) polymorphism and early-onset Parkinson's disease. Neurosci Lett 2004;359:195–197.
173. Wu YR, Feng IH, Lyu RK, et al. Tumor necrosis factor-alpha promoter polymorphism is associated with the risk of Parkinson's disease. Am J Med Genet B Neuropsychiatr Genet 2007;144B:300–304.
174. Wu YR, Wang CK, Chen CM, et al. Analysis of heat-shock protein 70 gene polymorphisms and the risk of Parkinson's disease. Hum Genet 2004;114:236–241.
175. Zintzaras E, Hadjigeorgiou GM. The role of G196A polymorphism in the brain-derived neurotrophic factor gene in the cause of Parkinson's disease: A meta-analysis. J Hum Genet 2005;50:560–566.
176. Saarela MS, Lehtimaki T, Rinne JO, et al. No association between the brain-derived neurotrophic factor 196 G>A or 270 C>T polymorphisms and Alzheimer's or Parkinson's disease. Folia Neuropathol 2006;44:12–16.
177. Xiromerisiou G, Hadjigeorgiou GM, Eerola J, et al. BDNF tagging polymorphisms and haplotype analysis in sporadic Parkinson's disease in diverse ethnic groups. Neurosci Lett 2007;415:59–63.
178. van der Walt JM, Noureddine MA, Kittappa R, et al. Fibroblast growth factor 20 polymorphisms and haplotypes strongly influence risk of Parkinson disease. Am J Hum Genet 2004;74:1121–1127.
179. Clarimon J, Xiromerisiou G, Eerola J, et al. Lack of evidence for a genetic association between FGF20 and Parkinson's disease in Finnish and Greek patients. BMC Neurol 2005;5:11.
180. Satake W, Mizuta I, Suzuki S, et al. Fibroblast growth factor 20 gene and Parkinson's disease in the Japanese population. Neuroreport 2007;18:937–940.
181. Wang G, van der Walt JM, Mayhew G, et al. Variation in the miRNA-433 binding site of FGF20 confers risk for Parkinson disease by overexpression of alpha-synuclein. Am J Hum Genet 2008;82:283–289.
182. Goris A, Williams-Gray CH, Foltynie T, et al. Investigation of TGFB2 as a candidate gene in multiple sclerosis and Parkinson's disease. J Neurol 2007;254:846–848.
183. Li Y, Grupe A, Rowland C, et al. Evidence that common variation in NEDD9 is associated with susceptibility to late-onset Alzheimer's and Parkinson's disease. Hum Mol Genet 2008;17:759–767.
184. Chapuis J, Moisan F, Mellick G, et al. Association study of the NEDD9 gene with the risk of developing Alzheimer's and Parkinson's disease. Hum Mol Genet 2008;17: 2863–2867.
185. Haugarvoll K, Toft M, Ross OA, et al. ELAVL4, PARK10, and the Celts. Mov Disord 2007;22:585–587.
186. DeStefano AL, Latourelle J, Lew MF, et al. Replication of association between ELAVL4 and Parkinson disease: The GenePD study. Hum Genet 2008;124:85–99.
187. Li YJ, Scott WK, Hedges DJ, et al. Age at onset in two common neurodegenerative diseases is genetically controlled. Am J Hum Genet 2002;70:985–993.
188. Noureddine MA, Qin XJ, Oliveira SA, et al. Association between the neuron-specific RNA-binding protein ELAVL4 and Parkinson disease. Hum Genet 2005;117: 27–33.

189. Xiromerisiou G, Hadjigeorgiou GM, Papadimitriou A, et al. Association between AKT1 gene and Parkinson's disease: A protective haplotype. Neurosci Lett 2008;436:232–234.
190. Ide M, Yamada K, Toyota T, et al. Genetic association analyses of PHOX2B and ASCL1 in neuropsychiatric disorders: Evidence for association of ASCL1 with Parkinson's disease. Hum Genet 2005;117:520–527.
191. Yamamoto M, Kondo I, Ogawa N, et al. Genetic association between susceptibility to Parkinson's disease and alpha1-antichymotrypsin polymorphism. Brain Res 1997;759:153–155.
192. Grasbon-Frodl EM, Egensperger R, Kosel S, et al. The alpha1-antichymotrypsin A-allele in German Parkinson disease patients. J Neural Transm 1999;106:729–736.
193. Munoz E, Obach V, Oliva R, et al. Alpha1-antichymotrypsin gene polymorphism and susceptibility to Parkinson's disease. Neurology 1999;52:297–301.
194. Lin JJ, Yueh KC, Chang CY, et al. The homozygote AA genotype of the alpha1-antichymotrypsin gene may confer protection against early-onset Parkinson's disease in women. Parkinsonism Relat Disord 2004;10:469–473.
195. Yamada T, McGeer PL, Baimbridge KG, et al. Relative sparing in Parkinson's disease of substantia nigra dopamine neurons containing calbindin-D28K. Brain Res 1990;526:303–307.
196. Damier P, Hirsch EC, Agid Y, et al. The substantia nigra of the human brain. I. Nigrosomes and the nigral matrix, a compartmental organization based on calbindin D(28K) immunohistochemistry. Brain 1999;122:1421–1436.
197. Mizuta I, Tsunoda T, Satake W, et al. Calbindin 1, fibroblast growth factor 20, and alpha-synuclein in sporadic Parkinson's disease. Hum Genet 2008;124:89–94.
198. Schapira AHV, Cooper JM, Dexter D, et al. Mitochondrial complex I deficiency in Parkinson's disease. Lancet 1989;i:1269.
199. Schapira AHV, Cooper JM, Dexter D, et al. Mitochondrial complex I deficiency in Parkinson's disease. J Neurochem 1990;54:823–827.
200. Mizuno Y, Ohta S, Tanaka M, et al. Deficiencies in complex I subunits of the respiratory chain in Parkinson's disease. Biochem Biophys Res Commun 1989;163: 1450–1455.
201. Hattori N, Tanaka M, Ozawa T, et al. Immunohistochemical studies on complex I, II, III, and IV of mitochondria in Parkinson's disease. Ann Neurol 1991;30:563–571.
202. Parker WD Jr, Boyson SJ, Parks JK. Abnormalities of the electron transport chain in idiopathic Parkinson's disease. Ann Neurol 1989;26:719–723.
203. Kriege D, Carroll MT, Cooper JM, et al. Platelet mitochondrial function in Parkinson's disease. Ann Neurol 1992;32:782–788.
204. Mann VM, Cooper JM, Krige D, et al. Brain, skeletal muscle and platelet homogenate mitochondrial function in Parkinson's disease. Brain 1992;115:333–342.
205. Yoshino H, Nakagawa-Hattori Y, Kondo T, et al. Mitochondrial complex I and II activities of lymphocytes and platelets in Parkinson's disease. J Neural Transm 1992;4:27–34.
206. DiMauro S. Mitochondrial involvement in Parkinson's disease: The controversy continues. Neurology 1993;43: 2170–2178.
207. Fukui H, Moraes CT. The mitochondrial impairment, oxidative stress and neurodegeneration connection: Reality or just an attractive hypothesis? Trends Neurosci 31: 2008;251–256.
208. Schapira AHV. Mitochondria in the aetiology and pathogenesis of Parkinson's disease. Lancet Neurol 2008;7:97–109.
209. Halliwell B. Oxidants and the central nervous system: Some fundamental questions. Acta Neurol Scand 1989;126:23–33.
210. Galvin JE. Interaction of alpha-synuclein and dopamine metabolites in the pathogenesis of Parkinson's disease: A case for the selective vulnerability of the substantia nigra. Acta Neuropathol 2006;112:115–126.
211. Riederer P, Sofic E, Rausch WD, et al. Transition metals, ferritin, glutathione, and ascorbic acid in parkinsonian brains. J Neurochem 1989;52:515–520.
212. Youdim MBH, Ben-Shachar D, Riederer P. Is Parkinson's disease a progressive siderosis of substantia nigra resulting in ion and melanin induced neurodegeneration? Acta Neurol Scand 1989;126:47–54.
213. Dexter DT, Wells FR, Lees AJ, et al. Increased nigral iron content and alterations in other metal ions occurring in brain in Parkinson's disease. J Neurochem 1989;52: 1830–1836.
214. Gutteridge JNC. Iron and oxygen radicals in brain. Ann Neurol 1992;32:S16–S21.
215. Ben-Shachar D, Riederer P, Youdim MBH. Iron-melanin interaction and lipid peroxidation: Implications for Parkinson's disease. J Neurochem 1991;57:1609–1614.
216. Youdim MBH, Ben-Shachar, Riederer P. The possible role of iron in the etiopathology of Parkinson's disease. Mov Disord 1993;8:1–12.
217. Dexter DT, Carter CJ, Wells FR, et al. Basal lipid peroxidation in substantia nigra is increased in Parkinson's disease. J Neurochem 1989;52:381–389.
218. Perry TL, Yong VW: Idiopathic Parkinson's disease, progressive supranuclear palsy and glutathione metabolism in the substantia nigra of patients. Neurosci Lett 1986;67:269–274.
219. Jenner P, Dexter DT, Sian J, et al. Oxidative stress as a cause of nigral cell death in Parkinson's disease and incidental Lewy body disease. Ann Neurol 1992;32: S82–S87.
220. Cheng KC, Cahill DS, Kasai H, et al. 8-Hydroxyguanine, an abundant form of oxidative DNA damage, cause G→T and A→C substitutions. J Biol Chem 1992;267: 166–172.
221. Sanchez-Ramos JR, Övervik E, Ames BN. A marker of oxyradical-mediated DNA damage (8-hydroxy-2-deoxyguanosine) is increased in nigro-striatum of Parkinson's disease brain. Neurodegeneration 1994;3:197–204.
222. Alam ZI, Jenner A, Daniel SE, et al. Oxidative DNA damage in the parkinsonian brain: An apparent selective increase in 8-hydroxyguanine levels in substantia nigra. J Neurochem 1997;69:1196–1203.
223. Shimura H, Hattori N, Kang D, et al. Increase of 8-oxo-dGTPase in the mitochondria of substantia nigral neurons in Parkinson's disease. Ann Neurol 1999;46:920–924.
224. Yoritaka A, Hattori N, Uchida K, et al. Immunohistochemical detection of 4-hydroxynonenal protein adducts in Parkinson disease. Proc Natl Acad Sci USA 1996;93:2696–2701.

225. Floor E, Wetzel MG. Increased protein oxidation in human substantia nigra pars compacta in comparison with basal ganglia and prefrontal cortex measured with an improved dinitrophenylhydrazine assay. J Neurochem 1998;70:268–275.
226. Giasson BI, Duda JE, Murray IV, et al. Oxidative damage linked to neurodegeneration by selective alpha-synuclein nitration in synucleinopathy lesions. Science 2000;290:985–989.
227. Gregersen N. Protein misfolding disorders: Pathogenesis and intervention. J Inherit Metab Dis 2006;29: 456–470.
228. Tanaka K, Suzuki T, Hattori N, et al. Ubiquitin, proteasome and parkin. Biochim Biohys Acta 2004;1695: 235–247.
229. Rubinsztein RC. The role of intracellular protein-degradation pathways in neurodegeneration. Nature 2006;443:780–786.
230. McNaught KS, Belizaire R, Isacson O, et al. Altered proteasomal function in sporadic Parkinson's disease. Exp Neruol 2003;179:38–46.
231. Spillantini MG, Schmidt ML, Lee AMY, et al. alpha-Synuclein in Lewy bodies. Nature 1997;388:839–840.
232. Volles MJ, Lansbury PT Jr. Vesicle permeabilization by protofibrillar alpha-synuclein is sensitive to Parkinson's disease-linked mutations and occurs by a pore-like mechanism. Biochemistry 2002;41:4595–4602.
233. Yorimitsu T, Klionsky DJ. Autophagy: Molecular machinery for self-eating. Cell Death Differ 2005;12 (suppl 2):1542–1552.
234. Sawada M, Imamura K, Nagatsu T. Role of cytokines in inflammatory process in Parkinson's disease. J Neural Transm Suppl 2006;70:373–381.
235. Whitton PS. Inflammation as a causative factor in the aetiology of Parkinson's disease. Br J Pharmacol 2007;150:963–976.
236. Mrak RE, Griffin WS. Common inflammatory mechanisms in Lewy body disease and Alzheimer disease. J Neuropathol Exp Neurol 2007;66:683–686.
237. Tansey MG, Frank-Cannon TC, McCoy MK, et al. Neuroinflammation in Parkinson's disease: Is there sufficient evidence for mechanism-based interventional therapy? Front Biosci 2008;13:709–717.
238. Mogi M, Harada M, Kondo T, et al. Brain beta 2-microglobulin levels are elevated in the striatum in Parkinson's disease. J Neural Transm 1995;9:87–92.
239. Blum-Degen D, Muller T, Kuhn W, et al. Interleukin-1 beta and interleukin-6 are elevated in the cerebrospinal fluid of Alzheimer's and de novo Parkinson's disease patients. Neurosci Lett 1995;202:17–20.
240. Mogi M, Harada M, Narabayashi H, et al. Interleukin (IL)-1beta, IL-2, IL-4, IL-6 and transforming growth factor-alpha levels are elevated in ventricular cerebrospinal fluid in juvenile parkinsonism and Parkinson's disease. Neurosci Lett 1996;211:13–16.
241. Stypula G, Kunert-Radek J, Stepien H, et al. Evaluation of interleukins, ACTH, cortisol and prolactin concentrations in the blood of patients with Parkinson's disease. Neuroimmunomodulation 1996;3:131–134.
242. Wandinger KP, Hagenah JM, Kluter H, et al. Effects of amantadine treatment on in vitro production of interleukin-2 in de-novo patients with idiopathic Parkinson's disease. J Neuroimmunol 1999;98:214–220.
243. Gadient RA, Otten UH. Interleukin-6 (IL-6). A molecule with both beneficial and destructive potentials. Prog Neurobiol 1997;52:379–390.
244. Mogi M, Harada M, Kondo T, et al. Transforming growth factor-beta 1 levels are elevated in the striatum and in ventricular cerebrospinal fluid in Parkinson's disease. Neurosci Lett 1995;193:129–132.
245. Villares J, Faucheux B, Herrero MT, et al. [125I]EGF binding in basal ganglia of patients with Parkinson's disease and progressive supranuclear palsy and in MPTP-treated monkeys. Exp Neurol 1998;154:146–156.
246. Tooyama I, Kawamata T, Walker D, et al. Loss of basic fibro-blast growth factor in substantia nigra neurons in Parkinson's disease. Neurology 1993;43:372–376.
247. Mogi M, Togari A, Kondo T, et al. Brain-derived growth factor and nerve growth factor concentrations are decreased in the substantia nigra in Parkinson's disease. Neurosci Lett 1999;270:45–48.
248. Chauhan NB, Siegel GJ, Lee JM. Depletion of glial cell line-derived neurotrophic factor in substantia nigra neurons of Parkinson's disease brain. J Chem Neuroanat 2001;21:277–288.
249. Mochizuki H, Goto G, Mori H, Mizuno Y. Histochemical detection of apoptosis in Parkinson's disease. J Neurol Sci 1996;137:120–123.
250. Tompkins MM, Basgall EJ, Zamrini E, et al. Apoptotic-like changes in Lewy-body-associated disorders and normal aging in substantia nigral neurons. Am J Pathol 1997;150:119–131.
251. Anglade P, Vyas S, Javoy-Agid F, et al. Apoptosis and autophagy in nigral neurons of patients with Parkinson's disease. Histol Histopathol 1997;12:25–31.
252. Kosel S, Egensperger R, von Eitzen U, et al. On the question of apoptosis in the parkinsonian substantia nigra. Acta Neuropathol (Berl) 1997;93:105–108.
253. Banati RB, Daniel SE, Blunt SB. Glial pathology but absence of apoptotic nigral neurons in long-standing Parkinson's disease. Mov Disord 1998;13:221–227.
254. Wullner U, Kornhuber J, Weller M, et al. Cell death and apoptosis regulating proteins in Parkinson's disease: A cautionary note. Acta Neuropathol (Berl) 1999;97: 408–412.
255. Mogi M, Harada M, Kondo T, et al. The soluble form of Fas molecule is elevated in parkinsonian brain tissues. Neurosci Lett 1996;220:195–198.
256. Hunot S, Brugg B, Ricard D, et al. Nuclear translocation of NFkappaB is increased in dopaminergic neurons of patients with Parkinson disease. Proc Natl Acad Sci USA 1997;94:7531–7536.
257. Tatton NA. Increased caspase 3 and Bax immunoreactivity accompany nuclear GAPDH translocation and neuronal apoptosis in Parkinson's disease. Exp Neurol 2000;166:29–43.
258. Mogi M, Harada M, Kondo T, et al. Bcl-2 protein is increased in the brain from parkinsonian patients. Neurosci Lett 1996;215:137–139.
259. Marshall KA, Daniel SE, Cairns N, et al. Upregulation of the anti-apoptotic protein Bcl-2 may be an early event in neurode-generation: Studies on Parkinson's and

incidental Lewy body disease. Biochem Biophys Res Commun 1997;240:84–87.

260. Hartmann A, Michel PP, Troadec JD, et al. Is Bax a mitochondrial mediator in apoptotic death of dopaminergic neurons in Parkinson's disease? J Neurochem 2001;76:1785–1793.

261. Hartmann A, Hunot S, Michel PP, et al. Caspase-3: A vulnerability factor and final effector in apoptotic death of dopaminergic neurons in Parkinson's disease. Proc Natl Acad Sci USA 2000;97:2875–2880.

262. Hartmann A, Troadec JD, Hunot S, et al. Caspase-8 is an effector in apoptotic death of dopaminergic neurons in Parkinson's disease, but pathway inhibition results in neuronal necrosis. J Neurosci 2001;21:2247–2255.

263. Mattson MP. Neuronal life-and-death signaling, apoptosis, and neurodegenerative disorders. Antioxid Redox Signal 2006;8:1997–2006.

264. Loh KP, Huang SH, De Silva R, et al. Oxidative stress: Apoptosis in neuronal injury. Curr Alzheimer Res 2006;3:327–337.

265. Singh S, Dikshit M. Apoptotic neuronal death in Parkinson's disease: Involvement of nitric oxide. Brain Res Rev 2007;54:233–250.

CHAPTER 13

Clinical Manifestations of Parkinson's Disease

Jayne R. Wilkinson, Daniel Weintraub, and Matthew B. Stern

James Parkinson's original 1817 description of the "shaking palsy" remains a remarkably accurate account of the disease now bearing his name.[1] Although the cardinal manifestations of Parkinson's disease (PD) are no different today, our understanding of the full array of parkinsonian signs and symptoms continues to grow. In addition to motor symptoms, the nonmotor symptoms of PD are now recognized as a significant source of disability.[2] Given continuing advances in therapy, it is increasingly important that clinicians recognize PD in its earliest stages. Equally critical, PD must be distinguished from less common forms of parkinsonism because prognosis and treatment may differ. In this chapter, we discuss the motor and nonmotor clinical manifestations of PD, followed by a discussion of clinical signs that can distinguish PD from other parkinsonian syndromes.

▶ DEFINITIONS

In order to better recognize, understand, and distinguish PD, it is important to define and clarify the terminology used when assessing a patient with signs and/or symptoms of this hypokinetic movement disorder.

Parkinsonism is a clinical syndrome characterized by specific motor deficits, referred to as the *cardinal motor features* of PD: akinesia/bradykinesia, rigidity, tremor, and postural instability. A wide variety of unrelated disease states can result in parkinsonism. The common thread linking these disorders is an underlying disruption of the dopaminergic nigrostriatal pathways that play a central role in controlling voluntary movements. This disruption can take one of many forms, and depending on the etiology, other brain structures may be involved. For example, it may be chemical, as is seen with drugs that deplete dopamine from intraneuronal storage sites or block striatal dopamine receptors. Acute and chronic metabolic insults, structural causes, and some inherited neurodegenerative disorders can also cause parkinsonism by direct or indirect disruption of the substantia nigra or striatum and their respective connections. The many causes of parkinsonism can be grouped into primary (or idiopathic), secondary (or symptomatic), the parkinsonism-plus syndromes, and hereditary neurodegenerative diseases (Table 13–1). They are covered in detail in their respective chapters in this text.

In contrast to parkinsonism, idiopathic *Parkinson's disease* is a distinct clinical and pathological entity. It is the most common form of parkinsonism,[3] accounting for approximately 75% of all cases seen in a movement disorders clinic. The pathologic finding of PD includes massive loss of pigmented dopaminergic neurons in the substantia nigra and the presence of intracytoplasmic inclusions, or Lewy bodies.[4]

There is no definitive diagnostic test for PD. Therefore, a number of clinical diagnostic criteria have been put forth. The United Kingdom Parkinson's Disease Society Brain Bank (UKPDSBB) clinical criteria[5] for the diagnosis of probable PD and the National Institute of Neurological Disorders and Stroke (NINDS) diagnostic criteria for PD[6] are commonly used, with a diagnostic accuracy as high as 90%.[7] Most movement disorder specialists consider the presence of two of three cardinal motor signs (tremor, rigidity, and bradykinesia) and a consistent response to dopamine replacement (levodopa or dopamine agonist) indicative of clinical PD. The fourth clinical feature of parkinsonism, postural instability, is typically seen in advanced disease and is no longer a diagnostic criterion. Early or pronounced postural instability is more common in other forms of parkinsonism, such as multisystem atrophy (MSA) and progressive supranuclear palsy (PSP; Chapters 20 and 21). Because of the broad phenotypic variability in PD, and the lack of any one pathognomonic clinical feature, it is inevitable that a precise and rigid clinical definition is lacking.

An important part of diagnosis lies in excluding other potentials causes of parkinsonism. This is done so through a careful and systematic approach, incorporating

TABLE 13–1. CLASSIFICATION OF PARKINSONISM

Primary (idiopathic)
Parkinson's disease
Secondary (symptomatic)
Drug-induced (phenothiazines, butyrophenones, metoclopramide, reserpine, alpha-methyldopa)
Infectious/post-infectious (postencephalitic, syphilis)
Metabolic (hepatocerebral degeneration, hypoxia, parathyroid dysfunction)
Structural (brain tumor, hydrocephalus, trauma)
Toxin (carbon monoxide, carbon disulphide, cyanide, manganese, MPTP)
Vascular (stroke)
Parkinsonism-plus syndromes
Corticobasal degeneration
Hemiparkinsonism–hemiatrophy
Dementia syndromes
Alzheimer's disease with parkinsonism
Dementia with Lewy bodies
Multisystem atrophy
MSA-P
MSA-C
Parkinsonism-dementia-ALS complex of Guam
Progressive supranuclear palsy
Hereditary degenerative diseases
Genetic forms of PD
Autosomal dominant (PARK1,3,5,8: including alpha-synuclein and LRRK2 mutations)
Autosomal recessive (PARK2,6,7: including parkin mutations)
Spinocerebellar ataxias (especially Machado–Joseph disease, type 3)
Neurodegeneration with brain iron accumulation (PKAN; HSD)
Juvenile Huntington's disease
Mitochondrial disorders
Neuroacanthocytosis
Wilson's disease

MPTP, 1-methyl-4-phenyl-1,2,3,6-tetrahydropyridine; ALS, amyotrophic lateral sclerosis; PKAN, pantothenate kinase-associated neurodegeneration; HSD, Hallervorden–Spatz disease.

disease history and course, physical exam findings, past medical, family and medication histories, and dopaminergic treatment response.

To assist in organizing a disease with such wide clinical variability, some investigators have grouped PD into several subtypes,[8,9] including *juvenile* and *young-onset* forms, *tremor-predominant* versus *postural instability-dominant* forms, and *benign* versus *malignant* forms of PD. It is unknown whether these clinically defined subtypes correspond to differences at the biochemical or pathophysiological levels. Regardless, such distinctions can be useful, as some studies, for example, show that young-onset patients are more likely to display slower progression, increased dystonia, lower rate of dementia, and higher rate of levodopa-related dyskinesias.[10–12] Likewise, tremor-predominant PD tends to follow a slower, more benign course than postural instability-predominant disease.[8,9,13]

DISEASE ONSET/COURSE

PD is typically a disease of the middle to late years, beginning insidiously, and progressing slowly over a 10–20-year period.[3,14,15] PD is one of the most common causes of neurological disability, and prevalence increases with age. Average age of onset is about 65, with incidence of parkinsonism in age 0–29 at 0.8/100,000 increasing to 329/100,000 in those aged 80–99.[16] The overall age- and gender-adjusted incidence per 100,000 is 13.4.[17]

The underlying pathology of PD, the loss of nigral neurons, occurs slowly over the decades preceding the onset of symptoms. Up to 80% of dopaminergic neurons are lost before the cardinal signs and symptoms of PD first appear. It is not surprising, then, that PD begins insidiously and is heralded by a prodrome of nonspecific symptoms.[18,19] Motor signs typically present in subtle ways, such as subjective weakness, mild incoordination, or difficulty writing. Many will complain of pain or tension in a shoulder or arm, prompting a visit to an orthopedic surgeon before a neurologist.[20] Asymmetric onset is typical in PD and in the context of an insidious-onset, slowly progressive disease should raise clinical suspicion.

Easy fatigability, malaise, depression, sleep disorders, loss of smell, and constipation are examples of nonmotor symptoms that may appear years before the first motor signs.[19,21] These features represent a "premotor phase"[22] and have become increasingly important to recognize. However, given that many nonmotor sign/symptoms are nonspecific, their correlation to PD often goes unrecognized until motor symptoms evolve.

The signs and symptoms of early PD can be nonspecific, and therefore elicit a broad differential diagnosis. In addition to PD, this includes other neurodegenerative disease (parkinsonism-plus syndromes, Wilson's disease), myasthenia gravis, cerebrovascular disease, and other movement disorders. In many cases, the diagnosis will only become clear as motor signs develop. It is not uncommon that at the time of diagnosis, patients reflect back to subtle, yet progressive symptoms of PD that were present for months and even years. Understanding and recognizing the myriad of motor and nonmotor clinical manifestations of PD, and comparing/contrasting them with those of similar disorders, will give the clinician a high level of diagnostic accuracy.

▶ MOTOR MANIFESTATIONS

CARDINAL MOTOR FEATURES

Akinesia/Bradykinesia

Akinesia is the absence or failure of movement, while *bradykinesia* is slowness of movement. These terms are used to define the difficulty and slowness PD patients have in initiating and executing a motor plan. It is often the most disabling sign of PD, experienced by virtually all patients and manifested in a variety of ways (Table 13–2). It is considered by many to be the defining feature of PD, and is included in most diagnostic criteria.[6] As a general rule, the nature and severity of akinesia/bradykinesia worsen over the course of illness. Hypokinesia (falling short of the mark when executing a movement) is nearly always present early in the disease, later progressing to bradykinesia (slowed movements) and, finally, to akinesia, or absence of movement.

Often the patient's history and simple observation provide ample evidence of this PD symptom. Early signs may be confined to distal muscles (micrographia, decreased dexterity, and impaired sequential finger movements), and a general loss of spontaneous movements is usually noted. Sequential motor acts, such as alternating pronation–supination of the hand, and complex motor acts requiring fine motor control, such as buttoning a shirt, are difficult for patients. Quick repetitive movements, such as repeated opposition of the forefinger and thumb, will not only show slowness but also dampen the amplitude of the particular movement. In more advanced stages, patients have difficulty rising from a chair and display a generalized slowing of all voluntary movements. Facial and vocal manifestations of bradykinesia (hypomimia ["masked facies"], decreased blink rate, hypophonia, dysarthria, and sialorrhea) are often apparent to the clinician before the formal examination has even begun. The gait exam may show slow, short "shuffled" steps with reduced arm swing.

▶ TABLE 13–2. SIGNS OF AKINESIA IN PD

General
- Decreased dexterity
- Delayed motor initiation
- Difficulty executing sequential actions
- Diminution in voluntary movements (hypokinesia)
- Freezing/motor arrests (akinesia)
- Inability to perform simultaneous actions
- Rapid fatigue with repetitive movements; dampening of amplitude
- Slowed voluntary movements (bradykinesia)

Specific
- Decreased arm swing
- Decreased blink rate
- Difficulty rising from a chair
- Dysdiadochokinesia
- Hypokinetic dysarthria
- Hypometric saccades
- Hypophonia
- Masked facies (hypomimia)
- Micrographia
- Shuffling gait, short steps
- Sialorrhea (from decreased swallowing)

Freezing is a distinct form of akinesia, where a delay in initiating movements occurs. It is most common in advanced disease, and generally occurs during ambulation, called freezing of gait (FOG).[23] Patients have trouble initiating gait (start-hesitation), and experience hesitations while walking or attempting to turn, particularly when approaching a narrow or crowded space (doorways, corners, closets, and a sidewalk with heavy traffic). Also called "motor blocks," freezing may occur just before the patient reaches an intended target (e.g., a chair or bed). Sitting "en bloc" represents a special form of freezing in which a patient literally falls into a chair. Freezing is associated with an increased risk of falls.[24] Patients will also begin to experience "motor arrests," or pauses in movements; this can be observed during repetitive motor tasks (i.e., finger tapping).

The opposite of freezing can also occur in PD. *Kinesia paradoxica* is the term used to describe sudden short periods of relatively effortless mobility experienced by a few patients. These episodes are unrelated to medication and should not be confused with the "on-off" phenomenon that occurs in advanced patients on dopaminergic therapy.

Understanding the pathophysiology of motor control in PD is complex. Researchers generally agree that patients with PD have little or no trouble "planning" a motor task. The problem lies in initiating and executing the sequential motor acts that comprise a particular complex motor program.[25,26] When a simple movement at one joint is attempted, the initial burst of agonist activity is small, and the resulting movement is both too slow and inadequate in amplitude to generate the force to reach the target. This problem is exacerbated in complex motor tasks as it is compounded by the need to execute multiple motor programs simultaneously. Given that these types of "complex" movements are germane to performing activities of daily living, it is clear why bradykinesia is often the most disabling motor sign of PD. Dopamine plays a central role in modulating the striatal pathways that control motor initiation, execution, and adaptation.[27] Fortunately, dopaminergic replacement therapy is often quite effective in treating the manifestations of akinesia/bradykinesia.

Rigidity

Rigidity is the state of involuntary hypertonicity with unvarying resistance to passive movement. This stiffness can occur in all muscle groups: axial, limb, flexor, and extensor. The lack of velocity-dependency distinguishes rigidity from spasticity ("clasp-knife"). Spasticity is further distinguished from the rigidity of PD by its associated findings: pathological reflexes, weakness, and silent electromyogram (EMG) at rest. In PD, the EMG resembles the tonic voluntary muscle activity.[28] Likewise, rigidity can be distinguished from the Gegenhalten tone seen in a variety of encephalopathic conditions as Gegenhalten is intermittent and tends to increase in opposition to an applied force.

The rigidity of PD can be either smooth (lead pipe) or "ratchety" (cogwheel). Cogwheeling is thought to reflect the superimposition of tremor on existing rigidity. Both rigidity and cogwheeling can be accentuated by voluntary movement in the contralateral limb (Froment's maneuver[29]) or mental activation. These techniques are known as motor reinforcement. Rigidity frequently begins unilaterally, may vary during the course of the day, and is influenced by mood, stress, and medications.

Although the rigidity of PD limits the speed of voluntary movements, it is unclear to what degree it contributes to motor impairment. Some patients with prominent rigidity have relatively unimpeded motor function. Others, however, can develop postural and/or limb deformities as a result of increased muscle tone, called dystonia, which can be a source of significant disability. Rigidity also can effect posture and impair gait.

The pathophysiological basis of rigidity is not fully understood.[26] Afferent impulses must play a role because sectioning of dorsal roots or application of local anesthetic in the epidural or subarachnoid space decreases rigidity. There are competing theories explaining rigidity, which are not necessarily mutually exclusive. Increased activity in long-loop reflex pathways[30] and/or abnormalities in spinal interneuron function secondary to altered input from descending tracts are among these. There may be intrinsic changes in the muscle as well. The rigidity of PD usually responds to dopaminergic therapy.

Tremor

The rest tremor of PD, the "involuntary tremulous motion" first noted by Parkinson, remains the most recognized sign of disease. In about 75% of patients, it is the first motor manifestation. Typically it begins unilaterally in the distal limb, often an arm. The tremor may even be confined to a single finger before the appearance of other signs. The tremor often manifests as a rhythmic, alternating opposition of the forefinger and thumb, the classic, stereotypic "pill-rolling" tremor of PD. In others, it takes the form of a simple to-and-fro motion of the hand or arm. In all cases, the tremor oscillates with a characteristic slow frequency of 4–6 cycles/s (Hz). The tremor of PD is termed a "rest tremor" because it is present at rest and usually abates when the affected limb performs a motor task. When lower limbs are involved, tremor will be present in the legs when the patient is supine or sitting but disappears when the patient bears weight. The rest tremor of PD usually begins intermittently, and therefore careful examination is required. Tremor can be accentuated while walking, with contralateral limb activation and with mental activation. It disappears in sleep and worsens with stress or anxiety.

Occasionally, patients will complain that their tremor is felt internally, with only subtle external signs. Over several years, the tremor may spread proximally in the affected arm before involving the ipsilateral leg, and finally the contralateral limbs. Of the cardinal features of PD, however, tremor is the most slowly progressive.[31] Although tremor is bilateral in advanced disease, it often maintains asymmetry throughout the course. In later stages, an accompanying tremor of the face, lips, or chin is not uncommon.

It is important to note that patients with PD can demonstrate tremor during periods other than rest. With the arms outstretched, a re-emergent rest tremor can appear after a brief period of no tremor being observed. PD patients often also have a postural or kinetic component to their tremor, as well as an exaggerated physiological tremor. A moderate degree of action tremor is consistent with PD.[32,33] However, a pronounced action tremor at disease onset should suggest other diagnoses.

The pathophysiological basis of the parkinsonian tremor is uncertain.[26] Although several brain regions likely contribute to the tremor, the major source is thought to be a pathological central oscillator of 3–5 Hz. Cells of the ventral intermediate nucleus of the thalamus show oscillatory behavior correlating with the tremor, but it is unclear whether thalamic neurons are true pacemakers or simply oscillating as part of a long-loop reflex arc. Given that tremor can be affected by emotional state, motor activity, and general health, it is almost certain that modulation by other circuits in the nervous system occurs.

Postural Instability

Postural instability is typically the last of the four cardinal signs to appear and relates primarily to the loss of postural reflexes, leading to falls and problems with gait. It often proves to be the most disabling, largely due to the lack of therapeutic response to dopaminergic therapy.[34] This feature of PD is not a manifestation of any one single deficit. It not only represents the loss of postural ("righting") reflexes, but is compounded by the presence of rigidity and akinesia/bradykinesia. It represents the major contributing factor in progression from mild bilateral disease (Hoehn and Yahr stage 2) to wheelchair confinement (H&Y stage 5).[35]

Loss of postural reflexes often begins early, but is rarely disabling until years later. The patient adopts a stooped posture with flexion of the neck and trunk. The arms are held in an adducted position with elbows flexed. These signs are also related to rigidity, and to some extent, bradykinesia. Once a patient starts to lose the ability to make rapid postural corrections, a tendency to fall forward or backward becomes evident. The examiner can elicit this finding with the "pull test," standing behind the patient and pulling backward on the shoulders: patients with decreased righting reflexes will take more than two steps backwards before catching themselves (retropulsion), while others with more advanced disease would fall, unless caught.

The first sign of gait disturbance in PD is often decreased arm swing, but over time patients also begin to walk with a short, shuffling, uncertain step. Some patients feel that they are dragging one leg. Gait initiation and turning become particularly difficult. Festination occurs as a result of a tendency to lean/propulse forward, combined with an effort to retain balance. This is characterized by ineffective, short, rapid and accelerating steps, and the inability to stop. Often, stopping is only accomplished by grabbing onto an object or running into a wall. Although the gait is abnormal, the base is usually of normal width, and truncal ataxia is absent. Falls become increasingly common over time, in many cases resulting in fracture.[24] As mentioned previously, ambulation in later stages of PD is associated with freezing, often making walking even a short distance, very difficult.

The mechanisms that control normal locomotion and postural stability are complex, involving neural structures from cerebral cortex through the pedunculopontine nucleus, to proprioceptive sensory afferents. The pathophysiological basis of gait and postural abnormalities in PD is not well understood but is almost certainly multifactorial. This multifactorial origin may help explain why postural instability and gait disturbance are the least treatable signs of PD.

OTHER MOTOR FEATURES

Listing secondary motor manifestations of PD is common practice. However, most are simply special cases of one of the four cardinal motor signs. However, some motor features are distinct enough to merit separate discussion as they may not be immediately recognized as one of the cardinal manifestations (see Table 13–3).

Cranial Nerve Abnormalities

Oculomotor function is generally preserved in PD, in contrast to what is found in many parkinsonism-plus syndromes. Some patients will complain of blurred vision or difficulty reading, which may be a result of weakened convergence. Limited upgaze is common in PD patients but can also be seen in the asymptomatic elderly. Vertical gaze paresis downwards is not seen in PD. If it is present, one should consider the diagnosis of PSP or MSA. Although slow, hypometric saccades and jerky (saccadic) ocular pursuits are often seen in PD, ophthalmoparesis does not occur, and lid retraction is

TABLE 13–3. CLINICAL MANIFESTATIONS OF PD

Motor Features of PD
Cardinal manifestations
Akinesia/bradykinesia
Rigidity
Rest tremor
Postural instability
Cranial nerve abnormalities
Ocular:blurred vision, decreased blink rate, impaired upgaze, blepharospasm/eyelid apraxia
Glabellar reflex (Myerson's sign)
Dysarthria, hypokinetic; hypophonia
Dysphagia
Masked facies
Sialorrhea
Musculoskeletal
Dystonia
Hand and foot deformities (striatal hand/toe)
Compression neuropathies
Kyphoscoliosis
Peripheral edema
Nonmotor features of PD
Neuropsychiatric
Cognitive impairment and dementia; bradyphrenia
Depression
Anxiety
Psychosis
Impulse control disorder
Disorders of sleep and wakefulness
Autonomic
Gastrointestinal (constipation, nausea, ageusia)
Urinary dysfunction (frequency, hesitancy or urgency)
Sexual dysfunction (impotence, loss of libido)
Cardiovascular (orthostatic hypotension)
Hyperhydrosis
Seborrhea
Sensory
Cramps
Pain
Paresthesias
Restless leg syndrome/akathisia
Visual disturbances
Olfactory dysfunction

uncommon.[36] A typical feature of PD is persistent eye blinking when the forehead is repeatedly tapped; this is called the sustained glabellar reflex or Myerson's sign. This primitive reflex is intrinsic to the disease process and does not indicate dementia. Other primitive reflexes can also reappear in PD without associated dementia, most commonly the snout reflex.[37]

Facial bradykinesia leads to a mask-like, staring expression, with markedly decreased rate of spontaneous blinking. Some patients experience blepharospasm and/or apraxia of eyelid opening. The speech of PD is typically monotonal, hypophonic and can demonstrate a hypokinetic dysarthria. The first syllable may be repeated (pallilalia), and words and phrases may rush together. Excessive saliva with drooling occurs in up to 80% of patients and is a consequence of decreased transfer of saliva to the pharynx.[38] Dysphagia, a consequence of pharyngeal bradykinesia and rigidity, usually occurs later in disease and may prove life-threatening. Early and prominent dysphagia should suggest other forms of parkinsonism (PSP, MSA).

Dystonia and Musculoskeletal Changes

Dystonia and permanent deformities of the hands and feet can occur in PD. The parkinsonian hand displays ulnar deviation, flexion of the metacarpophalangeal and distal interphalangeal joints, and extension of the proximal interphalangeal joints ("striatal hand"). Likewise, the great toe can be tonically extended, with the remaining toes curled claw-like. Dystonic cramps, particularly of the feet, may be troublesome. These can occur as an "off" phenomenon, before medication, or as a side-effect of dopaminergic therapy.

As a result of rigidity, changes occur in the curvature of the spine resulting in abnormal postural. Early in the disease, mild scoliosis may be seen, resulting in a tilted gait. In advanced disease, kyphosis can become prominent and add greatly to posturally related disabling.

Many patients develop swelling in the lower extremities. Assuming it is not a medication side effect or of cardiac etiology, this can be a consequence of immobility and venous stasis. Measures taken to improve mobility will often reduce the swelling. Rarely, the profoundly immobile patient will develop compression neuropathies.

▶ NONMOTOR MANIFESTATIONS

The non-motor features of PD are increasingly recognized as a significant source of disability.[2,39,40] These symptoms occur throughout the disease, with some evident even years prior to the evolution of motor signs. Others, however, are a manifestation of later, more advanced disease. Non-motor symptoms are common, with at least one nonmotor symptoms being reported by 88% of PD patients in one study.[41] Many of these symptoms are likely mediated by non-dopaminergic neurotransmitters, instead are: serotonergic, cholinergic, adrenergic and/or peptidergic. In general, these non-motor symptoms can be divided into major categories: neuropsychiatric, disorders of sleep and wakefulness, automatic and sensory.

NEUROPSYCHIATRIC SYMPTOMS

Cognitive Impairment and Dementia

PD patients have a sixfold increased risk for becoming demented compared with non-PD elderly.[42] Most studies have reported PD dementia (PDD) prevalence rates of 20–30%,[43] but a recent long-term prospective study found an 8-year cumulative prevalence rate of 78%,[44] and longitudinal studies of non-demented PD patients have found that 20–30% of subjects develop dementia over a period of 2–5 years.[42,45–48]

Approximately half of non-demented PD patients have mild cognitive impairment,[49] and deficits are common even at disease onset or early in its course.[50] These include impairments in executive (i.e., impaired planning and working memory), visuospatial,[51] attentional,[52] and language functions.[53–56] Many patients report a "tip of the tongue" phenomenon. Early executive impairment and memory deficits are risk factors for the development of PDD.[48,57–60]

Clinical correlates or risk factors for PDD include increasing age, lower level of education, increased severity and longer duration of PD, and "atypical" parkinsonism.[42,43,55,61] Psychiatric correlates or risk factors include psychosis, apathy, and depression.[43,46,47] The cognitive deficits seen in PD depression may be quantitatively (i.e., an excess), but not qualitatively, different than that seen in nondepressed PD patients.[62,63]

Cognitive deficits in PD have traditionally been characterized as "subcortical" in nature, in contrast to the "cortical" deficits reported in Alzheimer's disease (AD).[64] A subcortical pattern is characterized by deficits in memory recall more than memory formation, by prominent psychomotor slowing and slowed thinking (i.e., bradyphrenia), and by amotivation (i.e., apathy).[65] At a group level, PD patients demonstrate more executive deficits and selective impairment in memory recall and benefit from cuing compared with AD patients, and less language deficits.[64,66,67] PDD is similar to AD, however, in that both commonly present with a variety of psychiatric disturbances, including psychosis, sleep disturbances, and agitation.[68]

PDD is associated with diffuse subcortical and cortical Lewy body disease pathology.[69–71] Impairment in the neural circuits connecting the basal ganglia and cortical regions, including the prefrontal cortex, are thought to contribute to cognitive impairment in PD.[54,72,73] There is significant acetylcholine depletion (i.e., neuronal degeneration and decreases in both neocortical acetylcholine transporters and choline acetyltransferase) that may contribute to the development of PDD.[74,75] Dopamine deficits in the prefrontal cortex likely contribute to attention impairment.[54] In addition to PD-related neuropathology, up to 40% of PD patients have AD-related neuropathological changes on autopsy,[69] and there is a positive correlation between the presence of AD pathology and severity of PD dementia.[76]

Affective Disorders

Depression

Prevalence estimates for depression in PD (dPD) are typically between 20–40%.[77–80] Recent studies using community samples and formal diagnostic criteria have reported that major depression may occur in 5–10% of patients, with an additional 10–30% experiencing non-major forms of depression (e.g., minor or subsyndromal depression).[79,81–84] Also, depressive symptoms can be specifically related to motor symptoms, as in patients who experience temporary dysphoria and anxiety during "off" periods.[85]

The presence of dPD is associated with excess disability,[2,84] worse quality of life,[86–88] increased caregiver distress,[89] more rapid progression of motor impairment and disability,[90] and the development of psychosis.[91] It may also be a risk factor for or a correlate of cognitive impairment[62,90,92] or dementia.[46,47]

Some studies have found that dPD is associated with female sex,[81] a personal history of depression,[77] early-onset PD (i.e., before age 55),[83,93] predominantly right-sided motor symptoms,[77] and "atypical" parkinsonism (e.g., prominent akinesia-rigidity or extensive vascular disease).[82,92] Most patients with dPD also meet criteria for an anxiety disorder, and vice versa.[94] Although apathy is a distinct psychiatric syndrome,[95] there is extensive overlap between depression and apathy in PD.[96]

Cognitive impairment and dPD adversely impact each other.[62,92,97] Executive impairment, which in particular has been associated with dPD,[63,98,99] may be due to the additive effects of PD and depression.[62]

Core non-somatic symptoms of depression (e.g., suicide thoughts, feelings of guilt, depressed mood, and anhedonia) discriminate highly between depressed and non-depressed patients, while somatic symptoms correlate variably with a diagnosis of depression.[100,101] Assessing dPD is challenging, partly as a result of symptom overlap with core PD symptoms (e.g., insomnia, psychomotor slowing, difficulty concentrating, and fatigue). Even the appearance of a non-depressed PD patient can be similar to that of someone with severe depression (i.e., bradykinetic movements and flat facies).

It has been suggested that the association between depression and early-onset PD reported in some studies[83,93] is due to the fact that younger patients experience more significant career, family, and financial disruptions.[102] However, dPD cannot be explained solely as a psychological process and likely results from a complex interaction of psychological and neurobiological factors. Interesting findings suggesting a biological basis for dPD come from studies reporting that PD patients have a higher lifetime prevalence of depressive disorders than non-PD controls,[103] and that non-PD patients with depression are at higher risk of subsequently developing PD than non-depressed controls.[104]

Biologically, the high frequency of dPD has been explained by dysfunction in (1) subcortical nuclei and the frontal lobes; (2) striatal–thalamic–frontal cortex circuits and the basotemporal limbic circuit; and (3) brainstem monoamine and indolamine systems (i.e., dopamine, serotonin, norepinephrine, and acetylcholine).

Neuroimaging studies have reported associations between depressive symptoms and either altered putaminal metabolism[105] or reduced basal limbic system echogenicity.[106] Likely as significant as the changes in subcortical structures are impairments in the pathways connecting this region and the frontal cortex.[107] Functional brain imaging studies have reported simultaneous pan-frontal cortex and caudate hypometabolism in dPD, changes that are presumed to reflect neurodegeneration of the cortical-striatal-thalamic-cortical circuits.[105,108]

Regarding neurotransmitters, disproportionate degeneration of dopamine neurons in the ventral tegmental area (VTA) has been reported in patients with a history of dPD.[109] In addition, imaging studies in dPD have found both a decrease in signal intensity from neural pathways originating in monoaminergic brainstem nuclei[106] and a negative correlation between depression scores and dorsal midbrain serotonin transporter (5-HTT) densities.[110]

Anxiety

Up to 40% of PD patients experience anxiety symptoms or disorders, including generalized anxiety disorder, panic attacks, and obsessive-compulsive disorder.[111,112] Anecdotal experience indicates that anxiety symptoms are often more upsetting and disabling than depressive symptoms in PD, perhaps due to their intensity, accompanying somatic complaints, and propensity to worsen parkinsonism. Similar to depression, studies have reported an increased prevalence of anxiety disorders up to 20 years prior to PD onset.[103,113]

Increasing anxiety and discrete anxiety attacks have been associated with motor complications, particularly the onset of "off" periods.[114] When it does occur, patients often describe a sensation of feeling "trapped" as they become increasingly immobilized, with symptoms resolving with improvement in motor symptoms.

Psychosis

Psychosis occurs in less than 10% of untreated PD patients,[115] but hallucinations or illusions occur in 15–40% of treated PD patients,[91,116–120] and approximately 5% of patients experience delusions in addition to hallucinations.[120,121] Persistent psychotic symptoms are associated with greater functional impairment, caregiver burden, and nursing home placement.[89,118,122]

Correlates of PD psychosis include exposure to PD medications,[123] older age,[119,120] greater cognitive impairment,[91,116–120] increasing severity[118,120] and duration of PD,[116,119] comorbid depression[91,116,118,120] or anxiety,[118] increasing daytime fatigue,[116] comorbid sleep disorder,[119] visual impairment,[124] polypharmacy,[123] and delirium.[118]

Psychotic syndromes can be roughly categorized into two phenomenological groups. One group experiences visual illusions or hallucinations only, though auditory and other hallucinations can also occur.[116,117,123] These patients typically retain insight into the hallucinations, do not find them troubling, and may not require treatment (i.e., "benign hallucinosis"). The other group experiences complex psychotic symptoms, typically hallucinations and persecutory delusions in the context of dementia. These patients typically do not have insight into their psychosis, may display behavioral changes (including "sundowning"), and typically require treatment.

Vivid perceptual changes and illogical thinking in PD can also occur as part of vivid dreaming or REM behavior disorder, and the overwhelming majority of psychotic PD patients also report sleep disturbances.[125–127] Clinically, it is difficult to distinguish nocturnal psychotic symptoms from sleep-related cognitive and perceptual changes.

Exposure to dopaminergic therapy has been implicated as the major cause of psychosis in PD.[128] Claims have been made that certain agents are less likely than others to induce psychosis, but evidence for this is anecdotal.[123] Despite the clear association between medication exposure and PD psychosis, some recent studies have reported that the dosage and duration of antiparkinsonian treatment are not correlated with psychosis,[119,120] indicating that PD psychosis likely results from a complex interaction of medication exposure, PD pathology, aberrant REM related phenomena, and comorbid vulnerabilities, particularly cognitive impairment and visual disturbances.

Dopaminergic medication exposure may lead to excessive stimulation or hypersensitivity of mesocorticolimbic D_2/D_3 receptors and induce psychosis.[129] However, the association between psychosis, cognitive impairment, and mood disorders suggests more widespread brain involvement involving other neurotransmitter systems or neural pathways. For instance, cholinergic deficits and a serotonergic/dopaminergic imbalance have also been implicated in the development of PD psychosis.[123,128–132]

Impulse Control Disorders

Impulse control disorders (ICDs), including problem or pathological gambling, compulsive buying, compulsive sexual behavior, and binge or compulsive eating, have been reported to occur in PD.[133,134] These psychiatric disorders, which have both impulsive and compulsive features, are commonly conceptualized as behavioral addictions.[135]

Preliminary cross-sectional prevalence estimates for ICDs in PD patients from formal assessment studies have ranged from 1.7–6.1% for problem or pathological gambling,[136–139] 2.0–4.0% for compulsive sexual behavior,[136,138,140] and 0.4–3.0% for compulsive buying;[136,138,140] there has been no formal prevalence estimate for eating disorders in PD.

Case reporting and cross-sectional studies have suggested an association between dopamine agonist (DA) treatment and ICDs in PD.[136–138,140–143] ICDs in PD have also been reported in the context of levodopa treatment[144] and after deep brain stimulation (DBS) surgery.[145]

Non-DA features have been associated with ICDs in PD, although not consistently across studies. ICD behaviors prior to PD onset, personal or familial histories of alcoholism, impulsive or novelty-seeking characteristics, young age, and early onset of PD onset have been associated with ICDs in PD.[146]

ICDs in PD may lead to significant impairments in psychosocial functioning, interpersonal relationships, and quality of life. Patients may not report such behaviors to a treating physician, perhaps due to embarrassment, not suspecting an association with PD treatment, or ambivalence regarding ceasing the behavior. Hence, there is evidence that ICDs are under-recognized in clinical practice.[136]

DISORDERS OF SLEEP AND WAKEFULNESS

Up to 90% of PD patients report insomnia, hypersomnia, sleep fragmentation, sleep terrors, nightmares, nocturnal movements, or REM behavior disorder (RBD),[123,127,147,148] the latter characterized by loss of normal skeletal muscle atonia during REM sleep, prominent motor activity, and dreams. RBD is another disorder that may be a prodrome of PD.[149,150]

Other sleep cycle-related disorders in PD are restless legs syndrome (RLS) and periodic leg movements in sleep (PLMS), which are overlapping but distinct disorders. In addition, patients with more advanced PD may have an increased frequency of obstructive or central apnea.[151]

RBD and other sleep disturbances have been attributed both to progressive degeneration of the cholinergic pedunculopontine nucleus[152] and reduced striatal dopaminergic activity.[153] Associated clinical factors that disrupt sleep are immobility due to nocturnal bradykinesia and rigidity, tremors and dyskinesias, cramps, micturition, pain, and excessive sweating.[148,151,154] Sleep disturbances also are correlated with psychosis,[155] depression,[148] and cognitive impairment.[154]

Excessive daytime sleepiness (EDS) or fatigue occurs in 15–50% of PD patients.[156–158] This clinical phenomenon has been attributed variably to impairments in the striatal-thalamic-frontal cortical system, exposure to dopaminergic medications (especially dopamine agonists), and nocturnal sleep disturbances.[151,154,158,159] In addition, advanced disease, depression, cognitive impairment, and psychosis are clinical correlates of EDS.[156,157,160] Daytime "sleep attacks" (i.e., sudden-onset REM sleep) have been reported rarely in this population, particularly in conjunction with dopamine agonist treatment, though it remains controversial whether this is a distinct clinical entity.[151,161]

AUTONOMIC DYSFUNCTION

Nearly all PD patients experience some degree of autonomic dysfunction during the course of illness.[162] However, prominent and/or early features may suggest MSA. Careful measurements of autonomic function in PD (QSART [quantitative sudomotor axon reflex test for sudomotor function], pulse variability, orthostatic blood pressure, responses to Valsalva maneuver, and cold pressor stimuli) indicate that the underlying disease does cause mild autonomic insufficiency.[163]

One of the most frequent autonomic complaints relates to gastrointestinal symptoms. Constipation is an exceedingly common problem that can become serious, occasionally leading to intestinal pseudo-obstruction or megacolon.[38] The basis of constipation is reduced colonic motility, possibly a direct consequence of PD as Lewy body neuropathology has been described within the myenteric plexus. Other factors exacerbate the problem, including poor diet, fluid depletion, and reduced physical activity. Weight loss often occurs as a result of reduced intake (dysphagia, gastroparesis, and oral difficulties) and increased energy expenditure (rigidity and/or dyskinesias). Urogenital involvement includes urinary difficulties such as: hesitancy, urgency, frequency, and even incontinence. Sexual dysfunction is a frequent complaint, often involving both loss of libido and impotence. The cause of sexual problems is multifactorial, with contributing factors including a depressed mood, chronic motor disability, and partial or complete loss of autonomic innervation.

Although more characteristic of MSA, cardiovascular autonomic dysfunction can cause orthostatic hypotension in some PD patients. More commonly in PD, however, postural hypotension occurs or is exacerbated, as a side-effect of dopaminergic therapy. Measures to treat orthostatic hypotension include: increased salt and fluid intake, fitted elastic stockings, fludrocortisone or other drugs to correct orthostatic hypotension, and rising slowly to the standing position. Thermoregulatory problems, such as hyperhydrosis and heat intolerance are also frequent nonmotor symptoms.

Chronic seborrhea is a common finding is PD. This leads to greasy skin, particularly on the face, which can be associated with erythema, and scaly patches in skin creases. The cause is not clear, as some research suggests it is related to sex hormone levels (testosterone/androgens), while others feel it mediated through the autonomic nervous system, with increased parasympathetic activity.[164] With respect to the visual systems, abnormal tear production is found as well,[165] which may be an autonomic symptom and result in dry eyes.

PAIN AND SENSORY SYMPTOMS

Although peripheral nerve disease is not associated with PD, pain and sensory complaints are surprisingly common. In a random group of parkinsonian patients, approximately 50% complained of pain directly related to their parkinsonism.[166,167] Estimates for prevalence of pain in PD range from 40–85%.[168,169] Pain is often proportional to the degree of motor dysfunction and may take the form of muscle cramps, stiffness, dystonia, radiculopathy or arthralgias. It is increasingly recognized as a complex and disabling aspect of the disease.

Sensory complaints are very common, and are not usually associated with signs of peripheral neuropathy. Numbness, burning, or tingling may occur at any stage of the disease, independent of medications and the degree of motor deficits, and, in some cases, even precedes motor manifestations. Paresthesias were noted in 40% of patients in one series, more commonly occurring on the affected side in hemiparkinsonism.[166] The basis of sensory disturbance in PD is unknown, but possibly reflects a role for the basal ganglia in sensory processing. One postulated mechanism is altered striatal input to sensory centers in the thalamus.

Patients with PD often report akathisia in the legs. This may be a sign of restless leg syndrome, which occurs more commonly in PD patients than in normal controls.[170,171] It can also occur when dopaminergic medications have worn off. Typically, symptoms of restless leg syndrome begin well after PD symptoms and may be associated with lower serum ferritin levels[171] (Chapter 46). Having restless leg syndrome earlier in life does not appear to be a predisposing factor for later development of PD.

The oculomotor aspects of vision impairment were previously discussed, but other nonmotor factors affect vision, as well. Abnormal tear function is also evident.[165] Impaired color discrimination and contrast sensitivity, as well as light sensitivity have been described. Decreased olfactory function is an early sign in PD.[172,173] Reduced ability to smell is not something patients complain about unless specifically asked; even then, only 25% will have noticed a change. However, testing indicates that decreased sense of smell is a significant and widespread manifestation, occurring early in disease and bilaterally. It neither correlates with motor signs nor progresses over the course of illness. Olfactory dysfunction may help distinguish PD from other forms of parkinsonism, and ultimately be helpful in identifying at-risk patient populations. Patient also often report ageusia, or loss of taste.

▶ ATYPICAL FEATURES AND DIFFERENTIAL DIAGNOSIS

Recognizing classic cases of PD should not be difficult. The 60-year old patient with insidious-onset, slowly progressive unilateral rest tremor, masked facies, hypokinetic dysarthria, generalized slowness and cogwheel rigidity, almost certainly has PD. A robust response to levodopa clinches the diagnosis. However, many cases are not straightforward, and have atypical clinical features, making the diagnosis more challenging. A complete history and thorough examination remain critical in establishing the correct diagnosis in cases with atypical features. The clinician must inquire thoroughly about medications, possible environmental exposures, family history of neurological disease, and the precise sequence and course of symptoms (insidious versus abrupt onset; rate of progression; age of onset). Atypical clinical features, particularly at the onset of symptoms, should raise suspicion of other forms of parkinsonism[174,175] (see Table 13–4) Nonetheless, despite a strong clinical acumen, there are cases of PD that will present atypically, and only be accurately diagnosed at autopsy.

There are a number of specific clinical features that should alert the clinician of a possible alternative diagnosis.[176] When these are present, additional testing is often required, such as MRI, genetic screening, neuropsychometric testing, or other laboratory studies.

▶ **TABLE 13–4. ATYPICAL FEATURES IN PARKINSONISM**

Early or Predominant Feature	Disease
Young-onset	Juvenile PD, WD, NBIA
Minimal or absent tremor	MSA-P (SND), PSP, vascular parkinsonism, hydrocephalic parkinsonism
Atypical tremor	CBD, MSA-C
Postural instability	PSP, MSA (all forms), vascular parkinsonism, hydrocephalic parkinsonism
Ataxia	MSA-C
Pyramidal signs	MSA-P, CBD, vascular or hydrocephalic parkinsonism
Neuropathy	MSA (particularly parkinsonism-amyotrophy)
Marked motor asymmetry	Hemiparkinsonism–hemiatrophy, CBD, stroke
Symmetric onset	MSA, vascular or hydrocephalic parkinsonism, medication-induced parkinsonism
Myoclonus	CBD, CJD
Dementia	DLB, AD, CJD, MID, PSP
Focal cortical signs	CBD
Alien limb sign	CBD
Oculomotor deficits	PSP, MSA-C, CBD
Dysautonomia	MSA
Rapid progression	MSA, CJD, NPH, secondary PD (medications)
Abrupt onset	Secondary PD (vascular, medications)

AD, Alzheimer's disease; CBD, corticobasal; CJD, Creutzfeldt–Jakob disease; DLB, dementia with Lewy bodies; MID, multi-infarct dementia; MSA, multisystem atrophy; NBIA neurodegenerative with brain iron accumulation; PSP, progressive supranuclear palsy; ccWD, Wilson's disease

YOUNG-ONSET PATIENT

Most movement disorder specialists define patients whose PD symptoms begin before age 40 as "young-onset PD."[177] This closely resembles older-onset PD, and probably represents the tail end (younger side) of the bell-shaped distribution for PD. "Juvenile-onset" is a separate term used by many authors to refer to patients whose parkinsonism begins in childhood (before age 20). Although resembling adult-onset PD in many ways,[178] it differs in that juvenile-onset patients are more likely to have a family history of PD and display dystonic features. It is important not to confuse dystonia in juvenile-onset Parkinsonism with dopa-responsive dystonia, another juvenile-onset disease.

Parkinsonism in the adolescent or young adult should only be diagnosed as idiopathic PD after all other potential causes have been ruled out. If clinical features seem otherwise typical for PD, and there is a strong family history, a genetic mutation[179] involving parkin, alpha-synuclein or ubiquitin, should be considered (Chapter 9). A strong family history of neurological disease should raise concern about trinucleotide repeat disorders, including Huntington's disease (Chapter 33) and some of the spinocerebellar ataxias (most notably, SCA-3; Chapter 41), both of which show anticipation and can present as juvenile parkinsonism. If the parkinsonism is accompanied by other, atypical clinical features, then other hereditary neurodegenerative diseases should be considered. Any young person with parkinsonism should be evaluated for Wilson's disease, although this is typically associated with significant neuropsychiatric symptoms, dystonia and manifestations of hepatic disease (Chapter 42). Wilson's disease would demonstrate Kayser-Fleisher rings on slit-lamp examination, elevated 24 hour urine copper and low serum ceruloplasmin. Signs of spasticity and retinal degeneration suggest neurodegeneration with brain iron accumulation (NBIA), also known as pantothenate kinase-associated neurodegeneration (PKAN), and formerly known as Hallervordan–Spatz disease. The diagnosis of NBIA is further supported by magnetic resonance imaging (MRI) evidence of symmetric signal abnormalities in the globus pallidus ("eye of the tiger" sign).[180]

ABSENT OR ATYPICAL TREMOR

The absence of rest tremor makes the diagnosis of PD difficult. If the patient also fails to respond to L-dopa, the diagnosis is unlikely. A careful search for symptomatic causes of parkinsonism must be undertaken. The patient should be examined with a close look for down-gaze paresis and facial dystonia (PSP), orthostatic hypotension and other autonomic signs (MSA), bulbar dysfunction with truncal ataxia (MSA-C, SCA) and pyramidal signs (cerebrovascular disease and hydrocephalus, among other disorders).

Parkinsonism-plus syndromes frequently present with minimal or no tremor. Of these, MSA-P, formerly termed striatonigral degeneration (SND; Chapter 20) most closely resembles PD and is often confused with it, especially when patients respond to L-dopa.[181,182] Some features helpful in distinguishing it from PD include early and significant gait disorder, symmetrical onset, severe dysarthria or dysphonia, respiratory stridor, rapid progression, and pyramidal signs. A poor or transient response to L-dopa can occur as well.[183]

A markedly asymmetric tremor with myoclonic features suggests corticobasal degeneration (CBD; Chapter 22). Initially described by Rebeiz et al.[184] this disorder is characterized by progressive asymmetric motor impairment and both cortical and basal ganglionic dysfunction.[185,186] Typical features include asymmetric parkinsonism with dystonia, myoclonus, apraxia, cortical sensory loss, the alien-limb phenomenon, ocular motility disturbance, and late-onset dementia. The tremor of CBD often begins as an action tremor in one arm, and over time, the arm becomes increasingly rigid and contracted. By late stages of disease, stimulus-induced myoclonus in the affected arm is often apparent. Although stimulus-induced myoclonus is also seen in CJD disease and occasionally in MSA, the combination of focal cortical and extrapyramidal signs usually distinguishes CBD from these two diseases.

In the patient without tremor, risk factors for cerebrovascular disease should raise concern of vascular parkinsonism. In rare cases, the vascular Parkinsonian will fulfill clinical criteria for PD, but most patients will have minimal tremor, poor response to L-dopa and pyramidal signs. Vascular parkinsonism can have a stepwise progression. Brain MRI supports the diagnosis, demonstrating widespread subcortical small-vessel ischemic changes. The MRI is frequently helpful in other forms of Parkinsonism as well: symmetric abnormal signal in the basal ganglia suggests manganese or iron deposition, and atrophy within the brainstem, cerebellum, or striatum suggests several different parkinsonism-plus conditions. Medication-induced (secondary) parkinsonism may also present symmetrically and without tremor.

A coarse kinetic tremor originating proximally in the limb (rubral tremor) is not typical of PD. Degenerative and vascular diseases affecting the cerebellum and its outflow tracts can cause this type of tremor and are associated with other cerebellar signs.

Essential tremor can be mistaken for the tremor of PD (Chapter 25). The patient with pronounced kinetic or postural tremor, minimal or no signs of rigidity and bradykinesia, and a strong family history of tremor is more likely to have essential tremor. However, it is important to remember that many patients with PD have, as part of their disease, a superimposed kinetic tremor that may resemble essential tremor. PD patients rarely display the tremulous voice that is characteristic of familial essential tremor. It is important to remember that cogwheeling is not pathognomonic for PD; essential tremor can also cause ratcheting during passive movement of the limb, but without rigidity. Because both PD and essential tremor are common disorders, a small number of PD patients will inherit the trait for familial tremor as well.

PROMINENT POSTURAL INSTABILITY

Although postural instability is one of the cardinal features of PD, it is not prominent early in disease. When initial signs include pronounced postural instability, the clinician should consider several parkinsonism-plus syndromes, including PSP (Chapter 21), MSA (Chapter 20), NPH (Chapter 24), and some forms of SCA.

PSP[187,188] may be the most common parkinsonism-plus syndrome, accounting for 7.5% of cases of parkinsonism in one series.[175] In early PSP, pronounced postural instability is a clue to the diagnosis because the disease otherwise can resemble PD. Instead of the stooped, shuffling gait of PD, patients with PSP may walk stiffly with extended trunk and knees. Additional features include axial and nuchal rigidity with opisthotonic neck posturing, and a fixed facial expression with dystonic features such as blepharospasm. It is important to note that in early stages of PSP the most characteristic feature, vertical and (later) horizontal ophthalmoparesis, may be absent or manifested only by abnormal vertical optokinetic nystagmus. The vestibulo-ocular reflex remains intact, even in advanced disease, hence the designation supranuclear. Other early clues distinguishing PSP from PD include less prominent or absent tremor, prominent cognitive deficits, and a poor or transient response to L-dopa. The cognitive disturbance of PSP tends to have more frontal lobe features than that of PD.[189]

MSA also frequently presents with marked postural instability. MSA represents a spectrum of related clinical syndromes characterized by deficits in the extrapyramidal and pyramidal systems, cerebellum, and autonomic nervous system. Particular forms of MSA are now identified based on the predominant motor system involved: the cerebellum in MSA-C (sporadic olivopontocerebellar degeneration [OPCD]), the extrapyramidal and pyramidal systems in MSA-P (striatonigral degeneration, parkinsonism-amyotrophy). Autonomic dysfunction, including orthostatic hypotension, sexual dysfunction, urinary urgency or frequency, sexual dysfunction and anhydrosis,[190] is common in MSA. Despite this, there remains considerable overlap between PD and MSA. In addition to postural instability, the parkinsonism of MSA typically shows features of an akinetic rigid form of disease. Clues to the diagnosis of MSA-C include progressive truncal and gait ataxia, ophthalmoparesis, and bulbar dysfunction. If a strong family history is present, the patient may instead have one of the hereditary cerebellar ataxias.

Parkinsonism with marked postural instability also occurs in normal pressure hydrocephalus (NPH), and is usually accompanied by urinary incontinence and dementia. These patients may find it difficult to raise their leg from the floor (magnetic gait) while walking. The gait is slow, apraxic, and characterized by short mincing, irregular steps ("march à petits pas"). Leg function usually improves markedly in the recumbent position. Hydrocephalic parkinsonism is not limited to normal pressure hydrocephalus as noncommunicating hydrocephalus has also been reported with parkinsonian features. Associated clinical features suggesting hydrocephalic parkinsonism include a history of head trauma, subarachnoid hemorrhage, or meningitis, symmetrical onset involving the lower extremities, prominent gait disturbance, early cognitive or urinary symptoms, minimal or absent tremor, position-dependent bradykinesia (less when lying down), and brisk leg reflexes. A similar clinical picture may be seen in multi-infarct dementia. MRI can distinguish between hydrocephalus and multi-infarct dementia as the former typically shows prominent dilated ventricles and an aqueductal void on MRI. Additionally, the course would likely be more rapid than that of idiopathic PD.

Finally, it is important to remember that the differential diagnosis of early postural instability includes PD itself. Early postural instability in PD is of prognostic importance because evidence suggests that postural instability-predominant disease tends to progress more rapidly and show a less effective response to medication than tremor-predominant PD.[8]

PROMINENT AUTONOMIC DYSFUNCTION

Although autonomic dysfunction is found in PD, even in the earliest stages, it is typically not significant. If significant autonomic signs are found early in disease, MSA must be strongly considered in the differential diagnosis. Detailed signs/symptoms were previously reviewed.

EARLY DEMENTIA

Dementia at the onset of illness argues against PD, suggesting instead primary dementia with parkinsonian features. Forms of dementia with parkinsonian features include dementia with Lewy body disease (DLB), CJD, PSP, and AD. Although parkinsonism is not a classic feature of AD, some patients will have subtle bradykinesia and rigidity. DLB accounts for up to 20% of all dementia in the elderly.[191] Early psychiatric disturbance is said to be more common in DLB, with fluctuating mental status, hallucinations and significant RBD. Early on the dementia of DLB may resemble that of AD, except that the latter often displays parkinsonian features and fluctuating levels of consciousness. CJD typically progresses rapidly, over months instead of years, and usually can be identified by the presence of startle myoclonus and periodic complexes on the electroencephalogram; 5–10% of CJD patients will have a long-duration variant in which disease may last for more than 2 years. There is considerable overlap in the clinical and pathological features of the various dementia syndromes, and in some patients, definitive diagnosis cannot be made until autopsy.

It is important to recognize that PD can exist concurrently with depression, masquerading as dementia, so-called pseudodementia. Compared to PD patients who are not depressed, those with depression show greater cognitive deficits and are more likely to show a rapid decline in global function.[47,192,193] Formal neuropsychological testing may distinguish bona fide dementia from PD associated with depression, as well as outline that cognitive domains are most effected. This can also help provide evidence for one diagnosis over another.

PERSISTENT UNILATERAL MOTOR FEATURES

Although usually unilateral in onset, PD typically becomes bilateral within several years. A patient whose disease persists in a markedly asymmetric manner may have CBD, discussed earlier, or hemiparkinsonism-hemiatrophy (HPHA). The latter is a rare condition characterized by unilateral body atrophy (face, arm, or leg), ipsilateral parkinsonism often accompanied by dystonia, and poor response to L-dopa.[194] Parkinsonism in this condition may represent a late manifestation of hypoxic-ischemic injury during brain development. Although imaging studies in CBD and HPHA may demonstrate similar focal brain metabolic abnormalities, the two are distinguishable by the younger-onset, slower progression and focal body atrophy in HPHA, and by the prominence of cortical signs in CBD.

Equally atypical is symmetrical onset of disease. It is more common in forms of parkinsonism: secondary (medication-induced, toxic-metabolic causes), vascular, hydrocephalic, several parkinsonism-plus syndromes. Table 14–4 outlines a complete list of atypical features and possible diagnoses.

▶ CLINICAL RATING SCALES

In order to most effectively mange patients with PD, it is crucial to have standardized methods to quantify disease severity, motor manifestations, and quality of life. Clinical rating scales have proved useful in evaluating an individual patient's response to medication changes, and in assessing the contribution of treatment-related fluctuations and dyskinesias to a patient's disability. For these reasons, a variety of PD rating scales have been developed, three of which are discussed here. Other ways of assessing manifestations of PD are available, including videotape analysis (routinely used in movement disorders centers), patient diaries to assess on-off status, and simple timed maneuvers such as walking a defined distance.

Investigators created the Unified Parkinson's Disease Rating Scale (UPDRS) in the 1980s, in response to the need for standardized assessment of PD. This widely used scale has undergone several revisions. Most recently, it was revised (MDS-UPDRS) in an effort to capture more nonmotor features and enable better distinction of mild disabilities, which is critical to clinical trial designs that focus on early disease.[195] The UPDRS contains four sections. Part I concerns "nonmotor experiences of daily living," Part II concerns "motor experiences of daily living," Part III is the "motor examination," and Part IV concerns "motor complication." It provides a detailed and accurate assessment of PD by evaluating 64 items on a 5-point range: normal [0], slight [1], mild [2], moderate [3], and severe [4]. Another important addition includes details instructions that will serve to maintain good interrater consistency. The detail and thoroughness of the UPDRS may be its greatest weakness because completing the entire scale can prove somewhat cumbersome in a routine clinic practice.

The Hoehn and Yahr Staging Scale[13] is a widely adopted and useful scale designed to give a rough estimate of disease severity. Its developers designed five stages of disease severity:

1. Unilateral disease only
2. Bilateral mild disease, with or without axial involvement
3. Mild-to-moderate bilateral disease, with first signs of deteriorating balance
4. Severe disease requiring considerable assistance
5. Confinement to wheelchair or bed unless aided

Stage 3 is distinguished from stage 2 by the appearance of postural instability. The stage 3 patient remains fully independent, whereas the stage 4 patient is unable to live alone without assistance. Interrater correlation with the Hoehn and Yahr Staging Scale is excellent. It was not designed for use in therapeutic trials and is clearly inadequate for such purposes when used in isolation. However, it is a useful measure of disease milestones, and is often incorporated into several rating scales, including the UPDRS. Two additional stages, 1.5 and 2.5, were later added.

The Schwab and England Capacity for Daily Living Scale[196] is a widely used scale to assess patient disability in performing activities of daily living. It has a 10-point scoring system, with 100% representing completely normal function and 0% total helplessness. The Schwab and England Capacity for Daily Living Scale has also been incorporated as an arm of patient assessment, along with the Hoehn and Yahr and UPDRS.

REFERENCES

1. Parkinson J. An essay on the shaking palsy. 1817. J Neuropsychiatry Clin Neurosci 2002;14:223.
2. Weintraub D, Moberg PJ, Duda JE, et al. Effect of psychiatric and other non-motor symptoms on disability in Parkinson's disease. J Am Geriatr Soc 2004;52:784. PMCID: PMC15086662.
3. Rajput AH, Offord KP, Beard CM, et al. Epidemiology of parkinsonism: Incidence, classification, and mortality. Ann Neurol 1984;16:278.
4. Gibb WR. Neuropathology of Parkinson's disease and related syndromes. Neurol Clin 1992;10:361.
5. Gibb WR, Lees AJ. The relevance of the Lewy body to the pathogenesis of idiopathic Parkinson's disease. J Neurol Neurosurg Psychiatry 1988;51:745.
6. Gelb DJ, Oliver E, Gilman S. Diagnostic criteria for Parkinson disease. Arch Neurol 1999;56:33.

7. Hughes AJ, Daniel SE, Lees AJ. Improved accuracy of clinical diagnosis of Lewy body Parkinson's disease. Neurology 2001;57:1497.
8. Jankovic J, McDermott M, Carter J, et al. Variable expression of Parkinson's disease. A base-line analysis of the DATATOP cohort. The Parkinson Study Group. Neurology 1990;40:1529.
9. Zetusky WJ, Jankovic J, Pirozzolo FJ. The heterogeneity of Parkinson's disease: Clinical and prognostic implications. Neurology 1985;35:522.
10. Gibb,WR, Lees AJ. A comparison of clinical and pathological features of young- and old-onset Parkinson's disease. Neurology 1988;38:1402.
11. Kostic V, Przedborski S, Flaster E, et al. Early development of levodopa-induced dyskinesias and response fluctuations in young-onset Parkinson's disease. Neurology 1991;41:202.
12. Wickremaratchi MM, Ben Shlomo Y, Morris HR. The effect of onset age on the clinical features of Parkinson's disease. Eur J Neurol 2009. Apr;16(4):450–456.
13. Elbaz A, Bower JH, Peterson BJ, et al. Survival study of Parkinson disease in Olmsted County, Minnesota. Arch Neurol 2003;60:91.
14. Hoehn MM, Yahr MD. Parkinsonism: Onset, progression and mortality. Neurology 1967;17:427.
15. Hoehn MM. The natural history of Parkinson's disease in the pre-levodopa and post-levodopa eras. Neurol Clin 1992;10:331.
16. Bower JH, Maraganore DM, McDonnell SK, et al. Incidence and distribution of parkinsonism in Olmsted County, Minnesota, 1976-1990. Neurology 1999; 52:1214.
17. Van Den Eeden SK, Tanner CM, Bernstein AL, et al. Incidence of Parkinson's disease: Variation by age, gender, and race/ethnicity. Am J Epidemiol 2003;157:1015.
18. Koller WC. When does Parkinson's disease begin? Neurology 199242:27.
19. Langston JW. The Parkinson's complex: Parkinsonism is just the tip of the iceberg. Ann Neurol 2006;59:591.
20. Riley D, Lang AE, Blair RD, et al. Frozen shoulder and other shoulder disturbances in Parkinson's disease. J Neurol Neurosurg Psychiatry 1989;52:63.
21. Siderowf A, Stern MB. Preclinical diagnosis of Parkinson's disease: are we there yet? Curr Neurol Neurosci Rep 2006;6:295.
22. Tolosa E, Gaig C, Santamaria J, et al. Diagnosis and the premotor phase of Parkinson disease. Neurology 2009;72:S12-S20.
23. Giladi N, McMahon D, Przedborski S, et al. Motor blocks in Parkinson's disease. Neurology 1992;42:333.
24. Hely, MA, Morris JG, Reid WG, et al. Sydney Multicenter Study of Parkinson's disease: Non-L-dopa-responsive problems dominate at 15 years. Mov Disord 2005; 20:190.
25. Bloxham, CA, Mindel TA, Frith CD. Initiation and execution of predictable and unpredictable movements in Parkinson's disease. Brain 1984;107(Pt 2):371.
26. Hallett, M. Parkinson revisited: pathophysiology of motor signs. Adv Neurol 2003;91:19.
27. Graybiel, AM, Aosaki T, Flaherty AW, et al. The basal ganglia and adaptive motor control. Science 1994;265:1826.
28. Cantello R, Gianelli M, Civardi C, et al. Parkinson's disease rigidity: EMG in a small hand muscle at "rest". Electroencephalogr Clin Neurophysiol 1995;97:215.
29. Broussolle E, Krack P, Thobois S, et al. Contribution of Jules Froment to the study of parkinsonian rigidity. Mov Disord 2007;22:909.
30. Tatton WG, Lee RG. Evidence for abnormal long-loop reflexes in rigid Parkinsonian patients. Brain Res 1975;100:671.
31. Louis ED, Tang MX, Cote L, et al. Progression of parkinsonian signs in Parkinson disease. Arch Neurol 1999;56:334.
32. Lance JW, Schwab RS, Peterson EA. Action tremor and the cogwheel phenomenon in Parkinson's disease. Brain 1963;86:95.
33. Louis ED, Levy G, Cote LJ, et al. Clinical correlates of action tremor in Parkinson disease. Arch Neurol 2001; 58:1630.
34. Sethi K. Levodopa unresponsive symptoms in Parkinson disease. Mov Disord 2008;23(suppl 3):S521–S533.
35. Klawans HL. Individual manifestations of Parkinson's disease after ten or more years of levodopa. Mov Disord 1986;1:187.
36. Pelak VS, Hall DA. Neuro-ophthalmic manifestations of neurodegenerative disease. Ophthalmol Clin North Am 2004;17:311, v.
37. Vreeling FW, Verhey FR, Houx PJ, et al. Primitive reflexes in Parkinson's disease. J Neurol Neurosurg Psychiatry 1993;56:1323.
38. Edwards LL, Quigley EM, Pfeiffer RF. Gastrointestinal dysfunction in Parkinson's disease: Frequency and pathophysiology. Neurology 1992;42:726.
39. Chaudhuri KR, Healy DG, Schapira AH. Non-motor symptoms of Parkinson's disease: diagnosis and management. Lancet Neurol 2006;5:235.
40. Poewe W. Non-motor symptoms in Parkinson's disease. Eur J Neurol 2008;15(suppl 1):14.
41. Shulman LM, Taback RL, Bean J, et al. Comorbidity of the nonmotor symptoms of Parkinson's disease. Mov Disord 2001;16:507.
42. Aarsland D, Andersen K, Larsen JP, et al. Risk of dementia in Parkinson's disease: A community-based, prospective study. Neurology 2001;56:730.
43. Aarsland D, Tandberg E, Larsen JP, et al. Frequency of dementia in Parkinson's disease. Arch Neurol 1996; 53:538.
44. Aarsland D, Andersen K, Larsen JP, et al. Prevalence and characteristics of dementia in Parkinson disease: An 8-year prospective study. Arch Neurol 2003;60:387.
45. Levy G, Schupf N, Tang M-X, et al. Combined effect of age and severity on the risk of dementia in Parkinson's disease. Ann Neurol 2002;51:722.
46. Marder K, Tang M-X, Cote L, et al. The frequency and associated risk factors for dementia in patients with Parkinson's disease. Arch Neurol 1995;52:695.
47. Stern Y, Marder K, Tang M-X, et al. Antecedent clinical features associated with dementia in Parkinson's disease. Neurology. 1993;43:1690.
48. Mahieux F, Fenelon G, Flahault A, et al. Neuropsychological prediction of dementia in Parkinson's disease. J of Neurol, Neurosurgery and Psychiatry. 1998;64:178.

49. Janvin C, Aarsland D, Larsen JP, et al. Neuropsychological profile of patients with Parkinson's disease without dementia. Dement Geriatr Cogn Disord 2003;15:126.
50. Muslimovic D, Post B, Speelman JD, et al. Cognitive profile of patients with newly diagnosed Parkinson disease. Neurology 2005;65:1239.
51. Cronin-Golomb A, Braun AE. Visuospatial dysfunction and problem solving in Parkinson's disease. Neuropsychology 1997;11:44.
52. Dujardin K, Degreef JF, Rogelet P, et al. Impairment of the supervisory attentional system in early untreated patients with Parkinson's disease. J Neurol 1999;246:783.
53. Levin BE, Katzen HL. Early cognitive changes and nondementing behavioral abnormalities in Parkinson's disease. In: Weiner WJ, Lang AE, eds. Behavioral Neurology of Movement Disorders. New York, NY: Raven Press, Ltd.; 1995:85–95.
54. Dubois B, Pillon B. Cognitive deficits in Parkinson's disease. J Neurol 1997;244:2.
55. Green J, McDonald WM, Vitek JL, et al. Cognitive impairments in advanced PD without dementia. Neurology 2002;59:1320.
56. Lewis SJG, Cools R, Robbins TW, et al. Using executive heterogeneity to explore the nature of working memory deficits in Parkinson's disease. Neuropsychologia 2003;41:645.
57. Azuma T, Cruz RF, Bayles KA, et al. A longitudinal study of neuropsychological change in individuals with Parkinson's disease. Int J Geriatr Psychiatry 2003;18:1043.
58. Levy G, Jacobs DM, Tang M-X, et al. Memory and executive function impairment predict dementia in Parkinson's disease. Mov Disord 2002;17:1221.
59. Woods SP, Tröster AI. Prodromal frontal / executive dysfunction predicts incident dementia in Parkinson's disease. J Int Neuropsychol Soc 2003;9:17.
60. Jacobs DM, Marder K, Côté LJ, et al. Neuropsychological characteristics of preclinical dementia in Parkinson's disease. Neurology 1995;45:1691.
61. Tomer R, Levin BE, Weiner WJ. Side of onset of motor symptoms influences cognition in Parkinson's disease. Ann Neurol 1993;34:579.
62. Tröster AI, Stalp LD, Paolo AM, et al. Neuropsychological impairment in Parkinson's Disease with and without depression. Arch Neurol 1995;52:1164.
63. Kuzis G, Sabe L, Tiberti C, et al. Cognitive functions in major depression and Parkinson disease. Arch Neurol 1997;54:982.
64. Pillon B, Deweer B, Agid Y, et al. Explicit memory in Alzheimer's, Huntington's, and Parkinson's diseases. Arch Neurol 1993;50:374.
65. Turner MA, Moran NF, Kopelman MD. Subcortical dementia. Br J Psychiatry 2002;180:148.
66. Helkala E-L, Laulumaa V, Soininen H, et al. Recall and recognition memory in patients with Alzheimer's and Parkinson's diseases. Ann Neurol 1988;24:214.
67. Cahn-Weiner DA, Grace J, Ott BR, et al. Cognitive and behavioral features discriminate between Alzheimer's and Parkinson's disease. Neuropsychiatry Neuropsychol Behav Neurol 2002;15:79.
68. Bliwise DL, Watts RL, Watts N, et al. Disruptive nocturnal behavior in Parkinson's disease and Alzheimer's disease. J Geriatr Psychiatry Neurol 1995;8:107.
69. Lieberman AN. Point of view: Dementia in Parkinson's disease. Parkinsonism Relat Disord 1997;3:151.
70. Hurtig HI, Trojanowski JQ, Galvin J, et al. Alpha-synuclein cortical Lewy bodies correlate with dementia in Parkinson's disease. Neurology 2000;54:1916.
71. Kovari E, Gold G, Herrmann FR, et al. Lewy body densities in the entorhinal and anterior cingulate cortex predict cognitive deficits in Parkinson's disease. Acta Neuropathol 2003;106:83.
72. Burn DJ, O'Brien JT. Use of functional imaging in parkinsonism and dementia. Mov Disord 2003;18(suppl 6): S88-S95.
73. Carbon M, Ma Y, Barnes A, et al. Caudate nucleus: Influence of dopaminergic input on sequence learning and brain activation in Parkinsonism. NeuroImage 2003;21:1497.
74. Perry EK, Curtis M, Dick DJ, et al. Cholinergic correlates of cognitive impairment in Parkinson's disease: Comparisons with Alzheimer's disease. J Neurol Neurosurg Psychiatry 1985;48:413.
75. Kuhl DE, Minoshima S, Fessler JA, et al. In vivo mapping of cholinergic terminals in normal aging, Alzheimer's disease, and Parkinson's disease. Ann Neurol 1996;40:399.
76. Jellinger KA, Seppi K, Wenning GK, et al. Impact of coexistent Alzheimer pathology on the natural history of Parkinson's disease. J Neural Transm 2002;109:329.
77. Starkstein SE, Preziosi TJ, Bolduc PL, et al. Depression in Parkinson's disease. J Nerv Ment Dis 1990;178:27.
78. Allain H, Schuck S, Manduit N. Depression in Parkinson's disease. Br Med J 2000;320:1287.
79. Hantz P, Caradoc-Davies G, Caradoc-Davies T, et al. Depression in Parkinson's disease. Am J Psychiatry 1994;151:1010.
80. Cummings JL. Depression and Parkinson's disease: A review. Am J Psychiatry 1992;149:443.
81. Tandberg E, Larsen JP, Aarsland D, et al. The occurrence of depression in Parkinson's disease. A community-based study. Arch Neurol 1996;53:175.
82. Starkstein SE, Petracca G, Chemerinski E, et al. Depression in classic versus akinetic-rigid Parkinson's disease. Mov Disord 1998;13:29.
83. Cole SA, Woodard JL, Juncos JL, et al. Depression and disability in Parkinson's disease. J Neuropsychiatry Clin Neurosci. 1996;8:20.
84. Liu CY, Wang SJ, Fuh JL, et al. The correlation of depression with functional activity in Parkinson's disease. J Neurol 1997;244:493.
85. Menza MA, Sage J, Marshall E, et al. Mood changes and "on-off" phenomena in Parkinson's disease. Mov Disord 1990;5:148.
86. Kuopio A-M, Marttila RJ, Helenius H, et al. The quality of life in Parkinson's disease. Mov Disord 2000;15:4216.
87. Karlsen KH, Larsen JP, Tandberg E, et al. Influence of clinical and demographic variables on quality of life in patients with Parkinson's disease. J Neurol Neurosurg Psychiatry 1999;66:431.
88. Caap-Ahlgren M, Dehlin O. Insomnia and depressive symptoms in patients with Parkinson's disease. Relationship to health-related quality of life. An interview of patients living at home. Arch Gerontol Geriatr 2001;32:23.

89. Aarsland D, Larsen JP, Tandberg E, et al. Predictors of nursing home placement in Parkinson's disease: A population-based, prospective study. J Am Geriatr Soc 2000;48:938.
90. Starkstein SE, Mayberg HS, Leiguarda R, et al. A prospective longitudinal study of depression, cognitive decline, and physical impairments in patients with Parkinson's disease. J Neurol Neurosurg Psychiatry 1992;55:377.
91. Giladi N, Treves TA, Paleacu D, et al. Risk factors for dementia, depression and psychosis in long-standing Parkinson's disease. J Neural Transm 2000;107:59.
92. Tandberg E, Larsen JP, Aarsland D, et al. Risk factors for depression in Parkinson disease. Arch Neurol 1997;54:625.
93. Kostic VS, Filipovic SR, Lecic D, et al. Effect of age at onset of frequency of depression in Parkinson's disease. J Neurol Neurosurg Psychiatry 1994;57:1265.
94. Menza MA, Robertson-Hoffman DE, Bonapace AS. Parkinson's disease and anxiety: Comorbidity with depression. Biol Psychiatry 1993;34:465.
95. Pluck GC, Brown RG: Apathy in Parkinson's disease. J Neurol Neurosurg Psychiatry 2002;73:636.
96. Starkstein SE, Mayberg HS, Preziosi TJ, et al. Reliability, validity, and clinical correlates of apathy in Parkinson's disease. J Neuropsychiatry Clin Neurosci 1992;4:134.
97. Norman S, Tröster AI, Fields JA, et al. Effects of depression and Parkinson's disease on cognitive functioning. J Neuropsychiatry Clin Neurosci 2002;14:31.
98. Wertman E, Speedie L, Shemesh Z, et al. Cognitive disturbances in Parkinsonian patients with depression. J Neuropsychiatry Neuropsychol Behav Neurol 1993;6:31.
99. Anguenot A, Loll PY, Neau JP, et al. Depression and Parkinson's disease: Study of a series of 135 Parkinson's patients. Can J Neurol Sci 2002;29:139.
100. Leentjens AF, Marinus J, Van Hilten JJ, et al. The contribution of somatic symptoms to the diagnosis of depression in Parkinson's disease: A discriminant analytic approach. J Neuropsychiatry Clin Neurosci 2003;15:74.
101. Starkstein SE, Preziosi TJ, Forrester AW, et al. Specificity of affective and autonomic symptoms of depression in Parkinson's disease. J Neurol Neurosurg Psychiatry 1990;53:869.
102. Brown RG, Maccarthy B, Gotham A-M, et al. Depression and disability in Parkinson's disease: A follow-up of 132 cases. Psychol Med 1988;18:49.
103. Shiba M, Bower JH, Maraganore DM, et al. Anxiety disorders and depressive disorders preceding Parkinson's Disease: A case-control study. Mov Disord 2000;15:669.
104. Schuurman AG, van den Akker, M, et al. Increased risk of Parkinson's disease after depression. Neurology 2002;58:1501.
105. Mentis MJ, McIntosh AR, Perrine K, et al. Relationships among the metabolic patterns that correlate with mnemonic, visuospatial, and mood symptoms in Parkinson's disease. Am J Psychiatry 2002;159:746.
106. Berg D, Supprian T, Hofmann E, et al Depression in Parkinson's disease: Brainstem midline alteration on transcranial sonography and magnetic imaging. J Neurol 1999;246:1186.
107. Mayberg HS. Modulating dysfunctional limbic-cortical circuits in depression: Towards development of brain-based algorith.ms for diagnosis and optimised treatment. Br Med Bull 2003;65:193.
108. Mayberg HS, Starkstein SE, Sadzot B, et al. Selective hypometabolism in the inferior frontal lobe in depressed patients with Parkinson's disease. Ann Neurol 1990;28:57.
109. Brown AS, Gershon S. Dopamine and depression. J Neural Transm Gen Sect 1993;91:75.
110. Murai T, Muller U, Werheid K, et al. In vivo evidence for differential association of striatal dopamine and midbrain serotonin systems with neuropsychiatric symptoms in Parkinson's disease. J Neuropsychiatry Clin Neurosci. 2001;13:222.
111. Richard IH, Schiffer RB, Kurlan R. Anxiety and Parkinson's disease. J Neuropsychiatry Clin Neurosci. 1996;8:383.
112. Walsh K, Bennett G. Parkinson's disease and anxiety. Postgrad Med J 2001;77:89.
113. Gonera EG, van't Hof M, Berger HJC, et al. Symptoms and duration of the prodromal phase in Parkinson's disease. Mov Disord 1997;12:871.
114. Richard IH, Justus AW, Kurlan R. Relationship between mood and motor fluctuations in Parkinson's disease. J Neuropsychiatry Clin Neurosci. 2001;13:35.
115. Cummings JL. Neuropsychiatric complications of drug treatment in Parkinson's disease. In Huber SJ, Cummings JL, eds. Parkinson's disease. Neurobehavioral aspects. New York: Oxford University Press; 1992. p. 313–327.
116. Fénelon G, Mahieux F, Huon R, et al. Hallucinations in Parkinson's disease: Prevalence, phenomenology, and risk factors. Brain 2000;123:733.
117. Inzelberg R, Kipervasser S, Korczyn AD. Auditory hallucinations in Parkinson's disease. J Neurol Neurosurg Psychiatry 1998;64:533.
118. Marsh L, Williams JR, Rocco M, et al. Psychiatric comorbidities in patients with Parkinson disease and psychosis. Neurology 2004;63:293.
119. Sanchez-Ramos JR, Ortoll R, Paulson GW. Visual hallucinations associated with Parkinson disease. Arch Neurol 1996;53:1265.
120. Aarsland D, Larsen JP, Cummings JL, et al. Prevalence and clinical correlates of psychotic symptoms in Parkinson disease: A community-based study. Arch Neurol 1999;56:595.
121. Wint DP, Okun MS, Fernandez HH. Psychosis in Parkinson's disease. J Geriatr Psychiatry Neurol 2004;17:127.
122. Goetz CG, Stebbins GT. Risk factors for nursing home placement in advanced Parkinson's disease. Neurology 1993;43:2227.
123. Henderson MJ, Mellers JDC. Psychosis in Parkinson's disease: 'Between a rock and a hard place'. Int Rev Psychiatry 2000;12:319.
124. Diederich N, Goetz C, Raman R, et al. Primary deficits in visual discrimination is a risk factor for visual hallucinations in Parkinson's disease. Neurology 1997;48(3, suppl 2):A181.
125. Moskovitz C, Moses H, Klawans HL. Levodopa-induced psychosis: A kindling phenomenon. Am J Psychiatry 1978;135:669.
126. Pappert E, Goetz C, Niederman F. Hallucinations, sleep fragmentation and altered dream phenomena in Parkinson's disease. Mov Disord 1999;14:117.

127. Arnulf I, Bonnet AM, Damier P, et al. Hallucinations, REM sleep, and Parkinson's disease: A medical hypothesis. Neurology 2000;55:281.
128. Wolters ECh. Intrinsic and extrinsic psychosis in Parkinson's disease. J Neurol 2001;248(suppl 3):22.
129. Wolters ECh. Dopaminomimetic psychosis in Parkinson's disease patients: Diagnosis and treatment. Neurology 1999;52(suppl 3):S10-S13.
130. Cheng A, Ferrier I, Morris C, et al. Cortical serotonin S-2 receptor-binding in Lewy body dementia, Alzheimer's and Parkinson's diseases. J Neurol Sci 1991;106:50.
131. Perry E, Marshall E, Kerwin J. Evidence of monoaminergic-cholinergic imbalance related to visual hallucinations in Lewy body dementia. J Neurochem 1990;55:1454.
132. Birkmayer W, Danielczyk W, Neumayer E, et al. Nucleus ruber and L-dopa psychosis: Biochemical and postmortem findings. J Neural Transm 1974;35:93.
133. Galpern W, Stacy M. Management of impulse control disorders in Parkinson's disease. Curr Opin Neurol 2007;9:189.
134. Voon V, Fox SH. Medication-related impulse control and repetitive behaviors in Parkinson disease. Arch Neurol 2007;64:1089.
135. Holden C. 'Behavioral' addictions: Do they exist? Science 2001;294:980.
136. Weintraub D, Siderowf AD, Potenza MN, et al. Association of dopamine agonist use with impulse control disorders in Parkinson disease. Arch Neurol 2006;63:969.
137. Voon V, Hassan K, Zurowski M, et al Prospective prevalence of pathological gambling and medication association in Parkinson disease. Neurology 2006;66:1750.
138. Pontone G, Williams JR, Bassett SS, et al. Clinical features associated with impulse control disorders in Parkinson disease. Neurology 2006;67:1258.
139. Avanzi M, Baratti M, Cabrini S, et al. Prevalence of pathological gambling in patients with Parkinson's disease. Mov Disord 2006;21:2068.
140. Voon V, Hassan K, Zurowski M, et al. Prevalence of repetitive and reward-seeking behaviors in Parkinson disease. Neurology 2006;67:1254.
141. Ondo W, Lai D. Predictors of impulsivity and reward seeking behavior with dopamine agonists. Parkinsonism Relat Disord 2008;14:28.
142. Singh A, Kandimala G, Dewey RB, et al. Risk factors for pathological gambling and other compulsions among Parkinson's disease patients taking dopamine agonists. J Clin Neurosci 2007;14:1178.
143. Grosset KA, Macphee G, Pal G, et al. Problematic gambling on dopamine agonists: Not such a rarity. Mov Disord 2006;21:2206.
144. Molina JA, Sáinz-Artiga MJ, Fraile A, et al. Pathologic gambling in Parkinson's disease: A behavioral manifestation of pharmacologic treatment? Mov Disord 2000;15:869.
145. Smeding HMM, Goudriaan AE, Foncke EMJ, et al. Pathological gambling after bilateral subthalamic nucleus stimulation in Parkinson disease. J Neurol Neurosurg Psychiatry 2007;78:517.
146. Potenza MN, Voon V, Weintraub D. Drug insight: Impulse control disorders and dopamine therapies in Parkinson's disease. Nature Clin Pract Neurol 2007;3:664. PMCID: PMC18046439.
147. Aarsland D, Larsen JP, Lim NG, et al. Range of neuropsychiatric disturbances in patients with Parkinson's disease. J Neurol Neurosurg Psychiatry 1999;67:492.
148. Smith MC, Ellgring H, Oertel WH. Sleep disturbances in Parkinson's disease patients and spouses. J Am Geriatr Soc 1997;45:194.
149. Schenck CH, Bundlie SR, Mahowald MW. Delayed emergence of a parkinsonian disorder in 38% of 29 older men initially diagnosed with idiopathic rapid eye movement sleep behaviour disorder. Neurology 1996; 46:388.
150. Tan A, Salgado M, Fahn S. Rapid eye movement sleep behavior disorder preceding Parkinson's disease with therapeutic response to levodopa. Mov Disord 1996;1996:214.
151. Stacy M. Sleep disorders in Parkinson's disease. Drugs Aging 2002;19:733.
152. Jellinger K. The pedunculopontine nucleus in Parkinson's disease. J Neurol, Neurosurg Psychiatry 1988;51:540.
153. Eisensehr I, Linke R, Noachtar S, et al. Reduced striatal dopamine transporters in idiopathic rapid eye movement sleep behavior disorder. Comparison with Parkinson's disease and controls. Brain 2000;123:1155.
154. Phillips B. Movement disorders: A sleep specialist's perspective. Neurol 2004;62(suppl 2):S9–S16.
155. Comella CL, Tanner CM, Ristanovic RK. Polysomnographic sleep measures in Parkinson's disease patients with treatment-induced hallucinations. Ann Neurol 1993;34:710.
156. Tandberg E, Larsen JP, Karlsen K. Excessive daytime sleepiness and sleep benefit in Parkinson's disease: A community-based study. Mov Disord 1999;14:922.
157. Friedman J, Friedman H. Fatigue in Parkinson's disease. Neurology 1993;43:2016.
158. Hitten JJ, van Hoogland G, van der Velde EA, et al. Diurnal effects of motor activity and fatigue in Parkinson's disease. J Neurol Neurosurg Psychiatry 1993;56:874.
159. Chaudhuri A, Behan PO. Fatigue and basal ganglia. J Neurolog Sci 2000;179:34.
160. Karlsen K, Larsen JP, Tandberg E, et al. Fatigue in patients with Parkinson's disease. Mov Disord 1999;14:237.
161. Olanow CW, Schapira AH, Roth T. Waking up to sleep episodes in Parkinson's disease. Mov Disord 2000;15:212.
162. Appenzeller O, Goss JE. Autonomic deficits in Parkinson's syndrome. Arch Neurol 1971;24:50.
163. Goetz CG, Lutge W, Tanner CM. Autonomic dysfunction in Parkinson's disease. Neurology 1986;36:73.
164. Martignoni E, Godi L, Pacchetti C, et al. Is seborrhea a sign of autonomic impairment in Parkinson's disease? J Neural Transm 1997;104:1295.
165. Tamer C, Melek IM, Duman T, et al. Tear film tests in Parkinson's disease patients. Ophthalmology 2005;112:1795.
166. Koller WC. Sensory symptoms in Parkinson's disease. Neurology 1984;34:957.
167. Snider SR, Fahn S, Isgreen WP, et al. Primary sensory symptoms in parkinsonism. Neurology 1976;26:423.
168. Buzas,B, Max MB. Pain in Parkinson disease. Neurology 2004;62:2156.
169. Defazio G, Berardelli A, Fabbrini G, et al. Pain as a nonmotor symptom of Parkinson disease: Evidence from a case-control study. Arch Neurol 2008;65:1191.

170. Krishnan,PR, Bhatia M, Behari M. Restless legs syndrome in Parkinson's disease: A case-controlled study. Mov Disord 2003;18:181.
171. Ondo WG, Vuong KD, Jankovic J. Exploring the relationship between Parkinson disease and restless legs syndrome. Arch Neurol. 2002;59:421.
172. Doty RL, Golbe LI, McKeown DA, et al. Olfactory testing differentiates between progressive supranuclear palsy and idiopathic Parkinson's disease. Neurology 1993;43:962.
173. Stern MB, Doty RL, Dotti M, et al. Olfactory function in Parkinson's disease subtypes. Neurology 1994;44:266.
174. Facca AG, Koller WC. Differential diagnosis of parkinsonism. Adv Neurol 2003;91:383.
175. Stacy M, Jankovic J. Differential diagnosis of Parkinson's disease and the parkinsonism plus syndromes. Neurol Clin 1992;10:341.
176. Suchowersky O, Reich S, Perlmutter J, et al. Practice parameter: Diagnosis and prognosis of new onset Parkinson disease (an evidence-based review). Report of the Quality Standards Subcommittee of the American Academy of Neurology 2006 Apr 11;66(7):976–982.
177. Quinn N, Critchley P, Marsden CD. Young onset Parkinson's disease. Mov Disord 1987;2:73.
178. Muthane UB, Swamy HS, Satishchandra P, et al. Early onset Parkinson's disease: Are juvenile- and young-onset different? Mov Disord 1994;9:539.
179. Gasser T. Update on the genetics of Parkinson's disease. Mov Disord 2007;22:S343-S350.
180. Hayflick SJ, Westaway SK, Levinson B, et al. Genetic, clinical, and radiographic delineation of Hallervorden-Spatz syndrome. N Eng J Med 2003;348:33.
181. Fearnley JM, Lees AJ. Striatonigral degeneration. A clinicopathological study. Brain 1990;113 (Pt 6):1823.
182. Gilman S, Wenning GK, Low PA, et al. Second consensus statement on the diagnosis of multiple system atrophy. Neurology 2008;71:670.
183. Gouider-Khouja N, Vidailhet M, Bonnet AM, et al. "Pure" striatonigral degeneration and Parkinson's disease: A comparative clinical study. Mov Disord 1995;10:288.
184. Rebeiz JJ, Kolodny EH, Richardson EP Jr. Corticodentatonigral degeneration with neuronal achromasia. Arch Neurol 1968;18:20.
185. Brunt ER, van Weerden TW, Pruim J, et al. Unique myoclonic pattern in corticobasal degeneration. Mov Disord 1995;10:132.
186. Riley DE, Lang AE, Lewis A, et al. Cortical-basal ganglionic degeneration. Neurology 1990;40:1203.
187. Gearing M, Olson DA, Watts RL, et al. Progressive supranuclear palsy: Neuropathologic and clinical heterogeneity. Neurology 1994;44:1015.
188. Steele JC, Richardson JC, Olazewski J. Progressive supranuclear palsy. A heterogeneous degeneration involving the brain stem, basal ganglia and cerebellum with vertical gaze and pseudobulbar palsy, nuchal dystonia and dementia. Arch Neurol 1964;10:333.
189. Pillon B, Dubois B, Ploska A, et al. Severity and specificity of cognitive impairment in Alzheimer's, Huntington's, and Parkinson's diseases and progressive supranuclear palsy. Neurology 1991;41:634.
190. Shy GM, Drager GA. A neurological syndrome associated with orthostatic hypotension: A clinical-pathologic study. Arch Neurol. 1960;2:511.
191. McKeith IG. Spectrum of Parkinson's disease, Parkinson's dementia, and Lewy body dementia. Neurol Clin 2000;18:865.
192. Slaughter JR, Slaughter KA, Nichols D, et al. Prevalence, clinical manifestations, etiology, and treatment of depression in Parkinson's disease. J Neuropsychiatry Clin Neurosci 2001;13:187.
193. Troster AI, Paolo AM, Lyons KE, et al. The influence of depression on cognition in Parkinson's disease: A pattern of impairment distinguishable from Alzheimer's disease. Neurology 1995;45:672.
194. Giladi N, Burke RE, Kostic V, et al. Hemiparkinsonism-hemiatrophy syndrome: Clinical and neuroradiologic features. Neurology 1990;40:1731.
195. Goetz,CG, Tilley BC, Shaftman SR, et al. Movement disorder society-sponsored revision of the Unified Parkinson's Disease Rating Scale (MDS-UPDRS): Scale presentation and clinimetric testing results. Mov Disord 2008; 23:2129.
196. Schwab RS, Chafetz ME. Kemadrin in the treatment of parkinsonism. Neurology 1955;5:273.

CHAPTER 14

Neuroprotective Therapies for Parkinson's Disease

Talene A. Yacoubian and David G. Standaert

▶ INTRODUCTION: THE NEED FOR NEUROPROTECTIVE THERAPY

Parkinson's disease (PD) is a relentlessly progressive disorder. The symptoms are usually mild at onset, most frequently a resting tremor of a hand, but worsen steadily over years to cause severe disability in most cases. Indeed, much evidence suggests that the onset of the neurodegenerative process precedes the appearance of clinical symptoms by as much as a decade, and that the neurodegenerative process is well established by the time the disease is clinically apparent.

The motor deficits—tremor, rigidity, bradykinesia, and gait impairment—are the most obvious features of the disorder, and have been mainly attributed to the progressive loss of dopaminergic neurons in the substantia nigra (SN). Consequently, the focus of PD therapy has been on the replacement of dopamine. This approach has, in some respects, been remarkably effective and has led to treatments, which can substantially improve both the duration and quality of life of patients affected by PD. Ultimately, however, the success of this approach is limited by the development of motor complications that are difficult to control with currently available treatments (see Chapter 16). In addition, patients develop a variety of nonmotor symptoms, including anosmia, sleep disorders, autonomic impairment, and cognitive impairment (see Chapter 14). These nonmotor symptoms are refractory to most current treatments, and frequently become the most significant source of disability.

Recent pathological studies have revealed a spectrum of degeneration that corresponds with this broader range of symptomatology. Dopaminergic degeneration is only a part of a much broader process of PD-related neurodegeneration that may begin with pathology in the brainstem and then progress beyond the SN to cortical and subcortical regions (see Chapter 20).[1] Given the complexity of these late-stage complications and the widespread neurodegenerative changes that underlie them, it is unlikely that it will be possible to control all of these symptoms with pharmacological replacement therapies and preventative strategies are required.

It is important to recognize that the long, slow course of neurologic impairment in PD offers an important opportunity: if treatments that delay or prevent the neurodegenerative process are developed, they could be employed at an early stage of the disease to prevent the severely debilitating complications of advanced PD. Such a therapy, although not a cure, could convert PD into a disorder that is readily treatable and not a source of long-term disability. Indeed, it is likely technologies that can detect the disease process before the onset of visible symptoms will become practical in the near future. The main barrier to progress against PD is the lack of a meaningful neuroprotective treatment that can be applied after the disease is identified.

▶ WHAT IS NEUROPROTECTION?

A DEFINITION OF NEUROPROTECTION

In this chapter, we define "neuroprotective" therapies as those that slow or prevent further neurodegeneration of cell populations, both dopaminergic and nondopaminergic, which are affected in PD. This is a mechanistic definition, which focuses on the fundamental processes of brain degeneration in PD. It is a useful framework for approaching experimental studies, but it should be recognized that it may be difficult to translate these ideas directly to more patient-centered measures, such as life span and accumulation of disability. Indeed, the inability at present to directly observe the neurodegenerative process of PD in living patients, and thereby measure the rate of neurodegeneration, is one of the main challenges in the field; these issues are discussed in detail later. We define neuroprotective therapies as different from "neurorestorative" approaches, which seek to reconstruct the circuitry of the brain through transplantation of fetal

▶ TABLE 14–1. MECHANISMS OF PD PATHOGENESIS AND TARGETS FOR THERAPY

PD Pathogenic Mechanism	Targets for Neuroprotection
Oxidative stress and mitochondrial dysfunction	Inhibitors of dopamine metabolism (e.g., MAO inhibitors, dopamine receptor agonists) Electron transport enhancers (e.g., CoQ10) Other antioxidants (e.g., vitamin E, uric acid) Glutathione promoters (e.g., selenium)
Protein aggregation and misfolding	Inhibitors of α-syn aggregation Agents that reduce α-syn protein levels Enhancers of parkin function Enhancers of UCH-L1 function Other enhancers of proteosomal or lysosomal pathways
Neuroinflammation	Anti-inflammatory agents (e.g., NSAIDs, statins, minocycline)
Excitotoxicity	NMDA receptor antagonists Calcium channel antagonists
Apoptosis and cell death pathways	Antiapoptotic agents
Loss of trophic factors	Neurotrophic factors (e.g., GDNF, neurturin)

tissue or stem cells or other methods. Neurorestorative approaches are discussed in Chapter 17.

MECHANISMS FOR PD PATHOGENESIS AND TARGETS FOR NEUROPROTECTION

An understanding of the mechanisms underlying the development and progression of PD pathology is critical for the development of neuroprotective therapies. A complex interplay of multiple environmental and genetic factors has been implicated in PD, suggesting that PD likely represents a syndrome instead of a single disorder with the same primary cause in all cases. Several mechanisms have been implicated as crucial to PD pathogenesis: oxidative stress, mitochondrial dysfunction, protein aggregation and misfolding, inflammation, excitotoxicity, apoptosis and other cell death pathways, and loss of trophic support (Table 14–1). No one mechanism appears to be primary in all cases of PD, and these pathogenic mechanisms likely act synergistically through complex interactions to promote neurodegeneration. Discussion of these mechanisms is briefly reviewed here in reference to their implications for the development of neuroprotective therapies. The reader is referred to Chapter 13, which addresses PD pathogenesis in more detail.

Oxidative Stress and Mitochondrial Dysfunction

Oxidative stress results from an overabundance of reactive free radicals secondary to either an overproduction of reactive species or a failure of cell buffering mechanisms that normally limit their accumulation. Excess reactive species can react with cellular macromolecules and thereby disrupt their normal functions. Oxidative damage to proteins, lipids, and nucleic acids has been found in the SN of patients with PD.[2–4] Both overproduction of reactive species and failure of cellular protective mechanisms appear to be operative in PD.

Dopamine metabolism promotes oxidative stress through the production of quinones, peroxides, and other reactive oxygen species (ROS).[5,6] Mitochondrial dysfunction is another source for the production of ROS, which can then further damage mitochondria. Complex I activity is diminished in the SN of PD patients,[7] while inhibitors of complex I, such as 1-methyl-4-phenylpyridinium (MPP^+) and rotenone, cause a Parkinsonian syndrome in animal models.[8–10] The mechanisms responsible for mitochondrial dysfunction in PD are not well understood, but inherited or acquired mutations in mitochondrial DNA may contribute.[11–13] Increased iron levels seen in the SN of PD patients[14,15] also promote free radical damage, particularly in the presence of neuromelanin.

There is also evidence of impairment of endogenous protective mechanisms in PD. The antioxidant protein glutathione is reduced in postmortem PD nigra.[16–18] Several of the genes linked to familial forms of PD appear to be involved in protection against oxidative stress, including PTEN-induced putative kinase (*PINK1*) and *DJ-1*.[19–22]

Several different strategies have been proposed to limit oxidative stress in PD. These strategies include inhibitors of monoamine oxidase, a key enzyme involved in dopamine catabolism; enhancers of mitochondrial electron transport, such as Coenzyme Q10; compounds that can directly quench free radicals, such as vitamin E; and molecules that can promote endogenous mechanisms to buffer free radicals, such as selenium. The advantage of many of these agents is that they are well tolerated with few adverse effects, although convincing clinical evidence for the effectiveness of this approach is still lacking.

Protein Aggregation and Misfolding

Protein aggregation and misfolding have emerged as important mechanisms in many neurodegenerative disorders, including PD, Alzheimer's disease, and Huntington's disease. Although the proteins involved in these disorders are different, each is associated with characteristic aggregates of misfolded protein, and these abnormal aggregates appear to acquire toxic properties.

In PD, the primary aggregating protein is alpha-synuclein (α-syn), whose link to PD was first identified through rare families with autosomal dominant PD caused by mutations in this protein.[23–26] Although mutations in α-syn are found in a very small number of inherited PD cases, α-syn is the major component of Lewy bodies and Lewy neurites found in sporadic PD.[27,28] Gene multiplication of the *α-syn* locus also causes PD, further supporting the central role of this protein in PD pathogenesis.[29] Point mutations,[30–33] overexpression,[34] and oxidative damage of α-syn[35] have all been postulated to promote self-aggregation.

Abundant evidence links α-syn to PD, but the mechanism by which overabundance or aggregation of α-syn causes neuronal injury is not understood. Likewise, it is unclear which molecular form of α-syn is toxic. Hypotheses include toxic effects of oligomers on cell membranes or proteosomal function, effects of α-syn on gene transcription or regulation, interactions of α-syn with cell signaling and cell death cascades, alterations in dopamine storage and release, and α-syn-mediated activation of inflammatory mechanisms.[36–46]

Recent studies implicating *parkin* and *ubiquitin carboxyl-terminal hydrolase L1 (UCH-L1)* in genetic forms of PD reinforce the connection between protein aggregation and PD pathogenesis.[47,48] Parkin is an E3 ubiquitin ligase involved in targeting misfolded proteins for degradation, and mutations of parkin found in genetic forms of PD disrupt its E3 ubiquitin ligase activity.[49–51] Interestingly, native α-syn does not appear to be a substrate for parkin, although modified forms may be,[52,53] and brains from patients with parkin-associated PD do not usually contain Lewy bodies.[54–57] Parkin does appear to have a variety of other substrates that may play a role in protein turnover and degradation, including HSP70, which is known to modulate α-syn toxicity.[58,59] UCH-L1 serves as an ubiquitin recycling enzyme in neurons, and its dysfunction promotes aggregation of damaged proteins, including α-syn.[60–62] Although UCH-L1 has a plausible role in regulating misfolded proteins, it should be noted that UCH-L1 has been linked to PD in only a single family, and thus evidence of involvement in PD is not as strong as the other factors discussed.

The misfolding of α-syn can be placed in the broader context of the ability of cells to clear proteins with abnormal conformations, termed "proteostasis." This recently developed concept emphasizes that the capacity of cells to clear misfolded proteins is limited.[63–65] Clearance requires the coordinated activity of chaperones, proteosomal degradation and lysosomal mechanisms, and these mechanisms may become overwhelmed if a large number of aberrant proteins are present. Experimental evidence suggests that these mechanisms are shared among the total pool of proteins present in a cell, so that overabundance of any single protein may lead to the accumulation of a variety of unwanted other proteins with abnormal conformations. In the case of PD, overabundance of α-syn may lead to the accumulation of other proteins, and similarly other proteins may perturb cellular proteostasis and promote the accumulation of α-syn.

Strategies to prevent protein aggregation or to enhance the clearance of misfolded proteins are the subject of intensive study at present. Inhibitors of α-syn aggregation could serve as potential neuroprotective therapies, although a clearer understanding of the toxic form of α-syn is important. Viewed from the broader perspective of proteostasis, molecules that promote clearance of abnormally folded proteins could also have therapeutic potential, even if they do not directly target α-syn. Promoters of protein clearance could include enhancers of parkin or UCH-L1 function, or molecules that promote proteosomal or lysosomal degradation pathways.

Neuroinflammation

Neuroinflammation has been increasingly recognized as a primary mechanism involved in PD pathogenesis.[66–68] Activation of microglia is a constant feature of postmortem human PD as well as PD animal models.[69–73] Proinflammatory cytokines, such as IL-1β, IL-6, and TNF-α, are elevated in the CSF and basal ganglia in PD patients.[74,75] The complement system is also implicated in PD pathogenesis, as elevated serum levels of complement proteins and the presence of complement proteins in Lewy bodies have been detected in PD.[76,77] There is also infiltration of T cells into the SN in PD.[69]

A central issue is how the inflammatory process is related to neurodegeneration. Until recently, inflammation was viewed primarily as a secondary consequence of cell death, with macrophages playing a role in removing cellular debris. Recent work, however, has pointed to a much earlier and active role of inflammation and has suggested that inflammation may promote progression of neural injury. α-Syn may be one trigger for the activation of inflammation in PD. In vitro, both aggregated and nitrated forms of α-syn can directly trigger a microglial response and release of cytotoxic factors.[78–80] In vivo, α-syn or modified forms of the protein can trigger both microglial and humoral responses,[45,81] and inhibition of NF-KB signaling is neuroprotective.[82]

Given the evidence for neuroinflammation in PD, agents with anti-inflammatory effects have been investigated for their neuroprotective potential. Many of these anti-inflammatory drugs are already in common use for other indications. Nonsteroidal anti-inflammatory agents (NSAIDs) reduce dopaminergic cell death in animal and culture PD models,[67] and epidemiological studies have suggested that certain NSAIDs and statin drugs may reduce PD risk.[83–89] Minocycline is another agent with anti-inflammatory capabilities that is currently being investigated in human trials.[90] None of these approaches, however, has been specifically designed to the inflammatory process in PD, and considerable additional work is needed to define these mechanisms.

Excitotoxicity

Excitotoxicity has been implicated as a pathogenic mechanism in several neurodegenerative disorders, including PD. Glutamate is the primary excitatory transmitter in the mammalian central nervous system and a primary driver of the excitotoxic process. Dopaminergic neurons in the SN have high levels of glutamate receptors and receive glutamatergic innervation from the subthalamic nucleus and cortex. Excessive NMDA receptor activation by glutamate could increase intracellular calcium levels that then activate cell death pathways.[91] Calcium influx produced by excessive glutamate receptor activation can also promote peroxynitrite production through the activation of nitric oxide synthase.[92] Levels of 3-nitrotyrosine, a marker of peroxynitrite formation, are increased in postmortem SN from PD patients.[93] NMDA receptor antagonists protect against dopaminergic cell loss in MPTP models,[94,95] but a major limitation to clinical application is the low potency and poor tolerability of currently available agents. Riluzole has glutamate antagonist properties, but a small clinical trial failed to show any neuroprotective effect.[96] Neuroprotective effects have also been attributed to amantadine, which has modest NMDA antagonist properties as well as other actions.[97]

Another approach to modifying excitotoxicity is to address the downstream processes, which include intracellular calcium and related signaling systems. An important recent development is the discovery of the calcium-dependent pacemaking properties of nigral dopaminergic neurons, which expose the cells to high levels of intracellular calcium in the course of normal physiological activity.[98] This reliance on calcium channels results in a large energetic burden for these neurons, as intracellular calcium has to be sequestered regularly into the endoplasmic reticulum and mitochondria to prevent the activation of cell death pathways. The consequence is nigral cell aging through the production of free radicals and ROS. Blockade of L-type Cav1.3 calcium channels leads to a reversion of the cells to a "juvenile" Na^+-dependent form of pacemaking and resistance to MPTP and 6-OHDA toxicity.[99] Epidemiological studies have suggested that patients treated with dihydropyridines for hypertension have a lower incidence of PD.[100] The dihydropyridine isradipine is currently being investigated as a potential neuroprotective agent.

Apoptosis

Apoptosis, or programmed cell death, is a mechanism that has been demonstrated to participate in neural development and to play a role in some forms of neural injury. There has been controversy as to whether apoptosis is directly involved in PD. Several pathological studies have revealed signs of both apoptotic and autophagic cell death in the SN of PD brains,[101–105] although the extent is limited, perhaps because of the slow process of cell death which underlies PD. Apoptotic cell death has also been observed in animal PD models.[106–108] Alterations in cell death pathways are unlikely to be the primary cause for PD, but both apoptotic and autophagic cell death pathways are hypothesized to become activated in PD through oxidative stress, protein aggregation, excitotoxicity, or inflammatory processes. Activation of these cell death pathways most likely represents end-stage processes in PD neurodegeneration. Therefore, inhibitors of these cell death pathways have been proposed as potential neuroprotective agents regardless of the initial cause for neurodegeneration in PD. Two different compounds that inhibit apoptotic signaling have been recently tested in human PD trials (see later;[109,110]).

Loss of Trophic Factors

The loss of neurotrophic factors has been implicated as a potential contributor to cell death observed in PD. The neurotrophic factors brain-derived neurotrophic factor (BDNF), glial-derived neurotrophic factor (GDNF), and nerve growth factor (NGF) have all been demonstrated to be reduced in the nigra in PD.[111–113] As a result, treatment with growth factors has been proposed as a potential neuroprotective therapy in PD. Indeed, the potent ability of these agents to stimulate growth and arborization of dopaminergic neurons suggests that they may be useful treatments, even if deficiency of the factors is not the primary cause of the disease process. These trophic factors and others are discussed in detail in Chapter 6.

▶ CURRENT STATE OF NEUROPROTECTION IN CLINICAL STUDIES

Many drugs have shown promise in animal PD models, but this promise has not yet translated into therapies that are clearly neuroprotective in human PD. A recent practice parameter from the American Academy of Neurology concluded that "no treatment has been shown to be neuroprotective."[114] The barriers to establishing a neuroprotective therapy stem from the complexity of the disease process as well as the limits of the clinical tools available to monitor the progression of the disease and to observe the effects of an intervention. Recent studies seeking a neuroprotective effect illustrate the importance of both of these factors (Table 14–2).

LEVODOPA AS A NEUROPROTECTIVE AGENT: THE ELLDOPA TRIAL

Levodopa (L-dopa) is one of the oldest and most effective therapies for the symptoms of PD. Although widely used, until recently there was little data on the impact of L-dopa therapy on the long-term progression of PD. Because dopamine catabolism produces free radicals, there has been concern that treatment of PD patients with the precursor L-dopa could potentially promote neurodegeneration in PD.[115,116] On the other hand, a variety of preclinical data have suggested a neuroprotective effect.[117,118]

The Earlier versus Later L-Dopa (ELLDOPA) trial was a placebo-controlled, double-blind study designed to evaluate whether treatment of PD patients with L-dopa-modified disease progression compared with those treated with placebo.[119] In all, 361 patients were treated with placebo or L-dopa at 150 mg/day, 300 mg/day, or 600 mg/day for 40 weeks, followed by a two-week washout period. The primary outcome measure was change in Unified Parkinson's Disease Rating Scale (UPDRS) score from baseline. Patients on L-dopa, particularly those on the highest dose, showed a smaller change in UPDRS score from baseline than those on placebo (Fig. 14–1). This result suggests that L-dopa does not have a deleterious effect, but instead is neuroprotective. This interpretation has been controversial, as the findings could be explained by the possibility that the effects of L-dopa outlasted the two-week washout period. In addition, a secondary outcome measure of the trial, β-CIT neuroimaging, suggested the opposite conclusion, with patients on the highest dose of L-dopa showing the greatest decline in the uptake of β-CIT, a dopamine transporter ligand.

The ELLDOPA trial illustrates some of the most confounding issues in studies of PD neuroprotection. The potent effect of many dopaminergic agents on the symptoms of the disease can make assessment of the rate of progression difficult. Neuroimaging techniques are a more direct measure of the physiology of brain dopamine systems, but the reliability of these techniques as measures for PD progression remains uncertain.[120,121] At this time, it is not clear whether L-dopa is neuroprotective, but fears of its potential toxicity have been somewhat allayed by the ELLDOPA trial.

NEUROPROTECTIVE EFFECTS OF DOPAMINE RECEPTOR AGONISTS

Dopamine receptor agonists have been hypothesized as potentially neuroprotective by acting at D_2 autoreceptors found on dopaminergic SN terminals to suppress dopamine release and thus reduce oxidative stress. Indeed, in vitro and animal studies have shown that dopamine receptor agonists can reduce dopaminergic cell death.[122–129] Certain agonists, such as pramipexole, may also act as direct antioxidants because of their hydroxylated benzyl ring structure.[122,130]

Two large-scale clinical trials—comparison of the agonist pramipexole with levodopa on motor complications of Parkinson's disease (CALM–PD) and requip as early therapy versus L-dopa – PET (REAL–PET)—have attempted to assess the neuroprotective properties of dopamine agonist drugs using neuroimaging strategies. The CALM–PD trial compared pramipexole with L-dopa treatment in patients with early PD.[131] In this study, all patients received an active treatment: 301 patients were randomized to pramipexole or L-dopa. In a subset of 82 patients, the uptake of radiolabeled β-CIT was assessed. Patients treated with pramipexole did show less of a decline in β-CIT uptake compared with those treated with L-dopa alone (Fig. 14–2). The imaging data suggest that pramipexole may slow neurodegeneration, but no difference in UPDRS score was found between the two treatment groups at 46 months. In addition, since the pramipexole group was compared with patients on L-dopa and not a placebo control group, an alternative interpretation is that the imaging difference could be secondary to L-dopa promoting dopaminergic cell loss. Of note, no extended washout was incorporated into the trial design.

A similar result was obtained in the REAL–PET trial, which compared patients with early PD treated with ropinirole with those treated with L-dopa.[132] 162 patients had fluorodopa (^{18}F-dopa) PET imaging to assess ^{18}F-dopa uptake in the putamen at four weeks and at 24 months after initiating drug treatment. Patients on ropinirole showed less of a decrease in putaminal ^{18}F-dopa uptake. Clinically, the L-dopa-treated group showed a greater decline

▶ **TABLE 14–2. KEY NEUROPROTECTIVE CLINICAL TRIALS IN PARKINSON'S DISEASE**

Drug/Therapy	Name of Trial	Mechanism	Number of Subjects	Duration	Primary Outcome	Finding	Reference
CEP-1347	PRECEPT	Mixed lineage kinase inhibitor	806	21.4 mo	Time to need for dopaminergic therapy	Terminated early secondary to futility	(110)
Coenzyme Q10	QE2	Cofactor in mitochondrial electron transport chain	80	16 mo	Change in total UPDRS score	Trend toward reduced change in UPDRS in CoQ10 group	(147)
Coenzyme Q10		Cofactor in mitochondrial electron transport chain	213	1 yr	Change in total UPDRS score	Nonfutility of CoQ10	(148)
Creatine		Promoter of mitochondrial ATP production	60	2 yr	β-CIT SPECT	No difference in β-CIT uptake but small difference in UPDRS Part I subscore between creatine and placebo groups	(153)
Creatine		Promoter of mitochondrial ATP production	200	1 yr	Change in total UPDRS score	Non-futility of creatine	(90)
GDNF		Neurotrophic factor	50	8 mo	Change in motor UPDRS score	No difference between GDNF and placebo groups	(Nutt et al. 2003. Neurology 60:69–73)
GDNF		Neurotrophic factor	34	6 mo	Change in motor UPDRS score	No difference between GDNF and placebo groups	(Lang et al. 2006. Ann Neurol 59:459–466)
L-dopa	ELLDOPA	Dopamine precursor	361	40 wk	Change in total UPDRS score	Less change in UPDRS score in L-dopa group vs. placebo group	(119)
Minocycline		Anti-inflammatory	200	1 yr	Change in total UPDRS score	Nonfutility of minocycline	(90)
Neurturin		Neurotrophic factor	12	1 yr	Safety monitoring	Reduction in off-medication UPDRS motor subscore from baseline (no placebo group)	(Marks et al. 2008. Lancet Neurol 7:400–408)
Pramipexole	CALM-PD	Dopamine receptor agonist	82	46 mo	β-CIT SPECT	Less decline in β-CIT SPECT uptake in pramipexole group vs. L-dopa group	(131)

Rasagiline	TEMPO	MAO-B antagonist	404	1 yr	Change in total UPDRS score	Less change in UPDRS score in early rasagiline group vs. early placebo group	(144)
Rasagiline	ADAGIO	MAO-B antagonist	1176	72 wk	(1) superiority of slopes between weeks 12–36; (2) superiority in change from baseline to week 72; and (3) noninferiority of slopes during weeks 48–72	Early 1 mg/day rasagiline group met all 3 end points	(145)
Riluzole		Glutamate antagonist	20	6 mo	Change in UPDRS (Part II and III) score	No difference between riluzole and placebo groups	(96)
Ropinirole	REAL–PET	Dopamine receptor agonist	186	2 yr	^{18}F-dopa PET	Less decline in ^{18}F-dopa PET uptake in ropinirole group vs. L-dopa group	(132)
Selegiline	DATATOP	MAO-B antagonist	800	Mean 14 mo	Time to need for L-dopa therapy	Delay in need for L-dopa in selegiline group vs. placebo group	(133,134)
TCH346		GAPDH inhibitor	301	12 to 18 mo	Time to need for dopaminergic therapy	No difference between TCH346 and placebo groups	(109)
Vitamin E	DATATOP	Antioxidant	800	Mean 14 mo	Time to need for L-dopa therapy	No difference between vitamin E and placebo groups	(133,134)

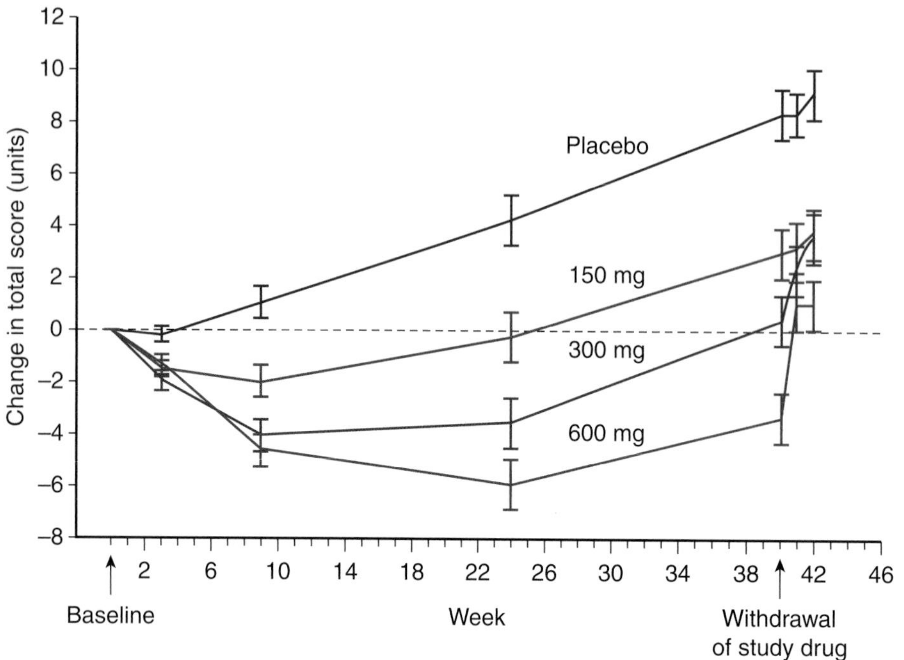

Figure 14–1. Change in UPDRS scores in the ELLDOPA trial. Subjects with PD were treated with placebo or L-dopa at 150 mg/day, 300 mg/day, or 600 mg/day for 40 weeks, followed by a two-week washout period. Total UPDRS score was measured at baseline, during interim visits (weeks 3, 9, 24, and 40), and during the washout phase. Patients treated with L-dopa had smaller changes in total UPDRS score from baseline compared with those treated with placebo, with those on 600 mg of L-dopa showing the least change. (Reproduced with permission from Ref. 119. Copyright © Massachusetts Medical Society. All rights reserved.)

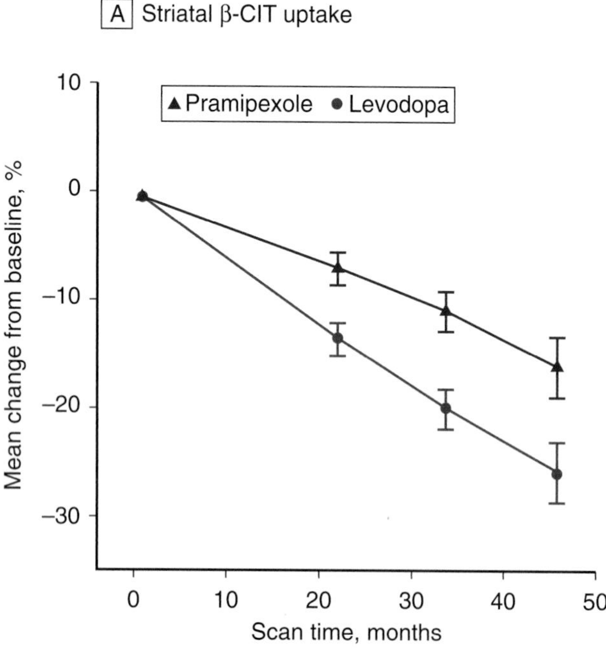

Figure 14–2. β-CIT uptake in the CALM-PD trial. Patients with early PD were randomized to pramipexole or L-dopa. Striatal uptake of [I123]β-CIT was assessed in a subset of 82 patients at 22, 34, and 46 months after initiation of treatment. Subjects treated with pramipexole showed less decline in striatal [I123] β-CIT uptake compared with patients treated with L-dopa. (Reproduced with permission from Ref. 131. Copyright © American Medical Association. All rights reserved.)

in UPDRS, but as UPDRS assessment was performed on-treatment, this likely reflects L-dopa's more potent symptomatic effect. Although the REAL–PET results also suggest a neuroprotective effect of dopamine agonists, this study suffers from similar limitations as the CALM–PD study, including lack of a placebo control and lack of an extended washout of the medications. The most substantial limitation of these studies is the difficulty of establishing that the neuroimaging measures reflect long-term neuroprotection of dopamine systems and not short-term pharmacological modification of the uptake of the radiotracers.[120,121]

ANTIOXIDANT THERAPIES

Given the role of oxidative stress in PD pathogenesis, several agents with antioxidant properties have been studied in clinical trials, including selegiline, vitamin E, and rasagiline. Whereas none of these clinical studies has yet provided irrefutable evidence that antioxidant therapies can slow disease progression, the results are intriguing and suggest that this approach does have promise. In addition, all of the antioxidant approaches have had a good safety record, a desirable property in a neuroprotective therapy that may need to be administered to a large number of patients for many years. The clinical experience with these agents is briefly summarized later.

Selegiline and the DATATOP Trial

Selegiline reduces dopamine oxidation by inhibiting monoamine oxidase B (MAO-B) and is the antioxidant drug most studied in clinical trials. The deprenyl and tocopher-

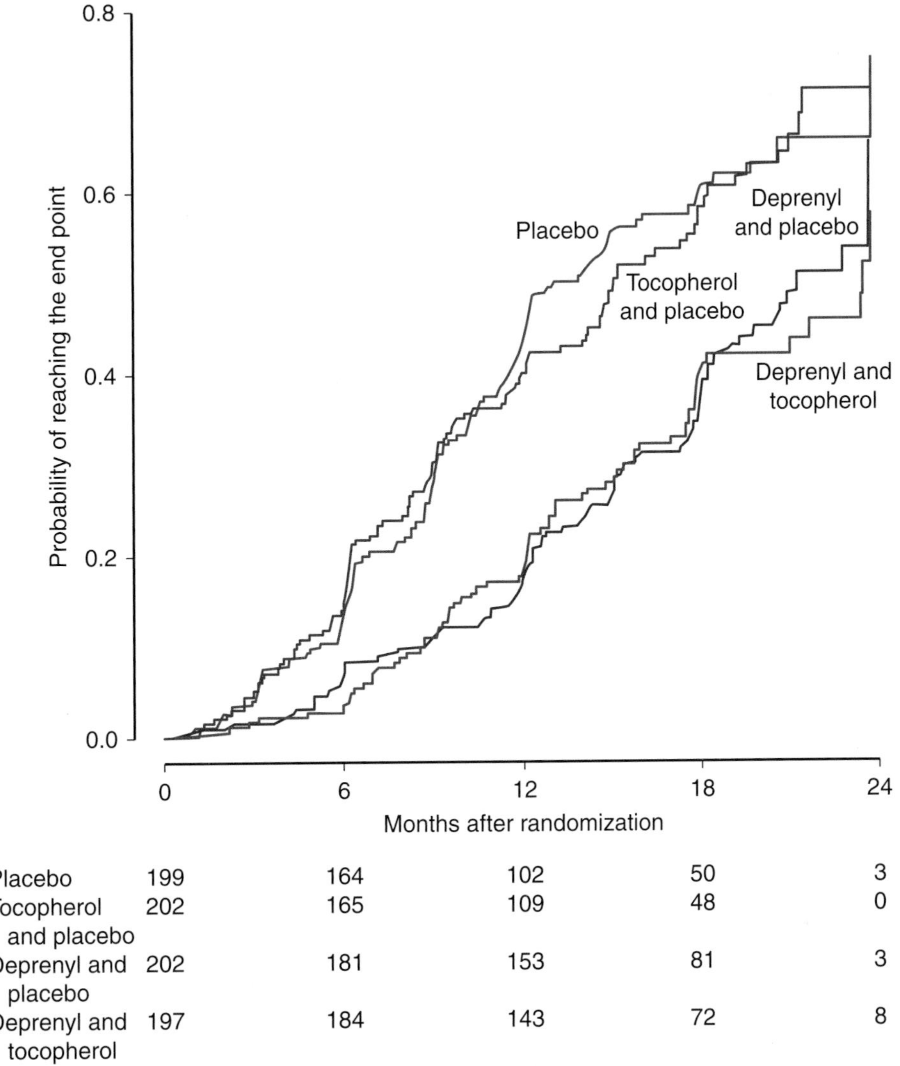

Figure 14–3. Kaplan–Meier estimate of the cumulative probability of requiring L-dopa in the DATATOP trial. Untreated patients with early PD were randomized to placebo, vitamin E, selegiline, or the combination of vitamin E and selegiline. The primary outcome measure was the time to clinical decision to treat with L-dopa. Those subjects treated with selegiline required L-dopa at a later time than those treated with placebo. Those treated with vitamin E showed no difference compared with placebo-treated patients. The number of patients evaluated at each time point is illustrated later. (Reproduced with permission from Ref. 134. Copyright © Massachusetts Medical Society. All rights reserved.)

ol antioxidative therapy of Parkinsonism (DATATOP) trial was the largest clinical trial to investigate the neuroprotective potential of selegiline, along with vitamin E, in patients with early PD.[133,134] In all, 800 patients were randomized to placebo, vitamin E, selegiline, or the combination of vitamin E and selegiline, and evaluated every three months up to a maximum of 24 months. The primary outcome measure was the time to clinical decision to treat with L-dopa. Secondary measures included the UPDRS score, Hoehn and Yahr staging, and Schwab and England Activities of Daily Living Scale. Selegiline did significantly delay the time of onset of L-dopa treatment; the initial difference of an 11-month delay was so striking that the interim analysis was published in 1989 prior to completion of the trial,[133] and the protocol was modified to switch patients who had not reached the end point to open-label selegiline (with patient consent) after a washout period.

The DATATOP trial was continued in this open-label fashion and has produced a number of additional observations. With longer follow-up, more patients reached the end point of need for L-dopa therapy, and by the conclusion of the study, the median delay was slightly reduced to 9 months (Fig. 14–3).[134] The secondary measures showed that patients treated with selegiline did better in terms of motor disability. Those treated with vitamin E showed no difference compared with that of placebo-treated patients, and vitamin E did not appear to add any benefit to selegiline's effects.[134]

The DATATOP trial was a landmark in studies of neuroprotection because of its size and novel approach to clinical outcomes, but the authors' conclusion that selegiline may delay disease progression spawned much controversy and discussion.[135–138] At the core of the controversy is the issue of whether selegiline had a direct effect on the symptoms of PD (comparable to the effect of L-dopa or other dopaminergic drugs) and how this effect may have confounded the outcome. Studies of selegiline prior to DATATOP had suggested that this drug does not have symptomatic effects,[139] and the trial design did not take symptomatic effects into account. The evidence from DATATOP shows quite clearly that selegiline does have symptomatic effects, as illustrated both by the early improvement in UPDRS score within three months from start of treatment (so-called wash-in effects) and by worsening in UPDRS score in patients reexamined two months after stopping treatment (so-called washout effects).[134] Despite a symptomatic benefit of selegiline, the data analysis could still suggest neuroprotection if the rates of reaching the primary outcome remained divergent.[136,137] However, the Kaplan–Meier curves became parallel at 18 months of follow-up (Fig. 14–3),[134] whereas follow-up of patients in the open-label phase showed no significant difference between the group originally treated with selegiline and the group initially treated with placebo.[140] Viewed with the benefit of the many years that have passed since the initiation of the DATATOP study, it is clear that this effort taught investigators many lessons about the difficulties of clinical trials in search of neuroprotection, but in the end, the study did not resolve the question of whether or not selegiline has neuroprotective effects. This issue remains under study, with long-term follow-up of additional clinical cohorts.

Rasagiline

Rasagiline is a newer MAO-B inhibitor that is both more potent than selegiline and has distinct metabolites with potential antioxidant properties. It has efficacy in cellular and animal models of PD.[141–143] Clinical data supporting a neuroprotective effect of rasagiline were first obtained in the TEMPO study, a trial with a delayed-start design (Fig. 14–4) intended to reduce the confounding effect of symptomatic efficacy. In this trial, 404 patients with early, untreated PD were treated with either placebo or rasagiline for six months and then all were placed on rasagiline for another six months.[144] The primary outcome was change in UPDRS score from baseline at 12 months. Those treated initially with rasagiline had a smaller increase in UPDRS scores compared with those first started on placebo (Fig. 14–5). Because all patients were on rasagiline at the end of the study, the assumption is that symptomatic effects of rasagiline were similar between the two groups. This study does suggest that early treatment confers a long-lasting improvement, but the overall duration of this study was relatively short, and the group sizes were modest.

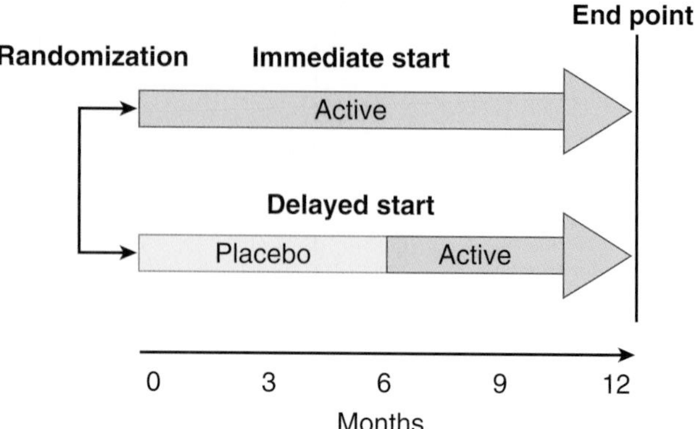

Figure 14–4. Delayed-start design. Subjects are randomized to either immediate or delayed initiation of the therapeutic agent. Patients in the immediate group start active therapy at the onset of the study and stay on active therapy for the duration of the trial. Those randomized to delayed initiation take placebo initially for a predetermined time period and then are switched to active therapy.

The attenuation of disease progression with azilect given once-daily (ADAGIO) study is a larger study designed specifically to address whether rasagiline can alter the rate of disease progression.[145] Compared with TVP-1012 in early monotherapy for parkinson's disease outpatients (TEMPO) in which there was no time limit on duration since PD diagnosis, patients enrolled in ADAGIO were required to have been diagnosed with PD within 1.5 years. This study was designed prospectively as a delayed-start clinical trial to follow more patients for a longer period compared with that of TEMPO. In this study, 1176 patients with early PD were initiated with placebo, 1 mg/day rasagiline, or 2 mg/day rasagiline for 36 weeks and then all patients were switched to rasagiline at 1 or 2 mg/day. A hierarchical set of end points for this study were based on the UPDRS score: (1) superiority of slopes between weeks 12–36; (2) superiority in change from baseline to week 72, and (3) noninferiority of slopes during weeks 48–72. Patients who were on the 1-mg rasagiline dose from the onset met all three end points. At the end of the study, patients started early on rasagiline had a significantly lower UPDRS score than those initiated 36 weeks later, and the curves were parallel, suggesting a lasting benefit.[145] At the higher dose of 2 mg, the end points were not met, perhaps because this dose produced a stronger symptomatic effect, which may have obscured an underlying neuroprotective effect. This trial shows that early treatment with rasagiline provides a benefit that cannot be matched with the later addition of the same treatment and is the strongest evidence to date for a disease-modifying effect of a medication in PD. Whether

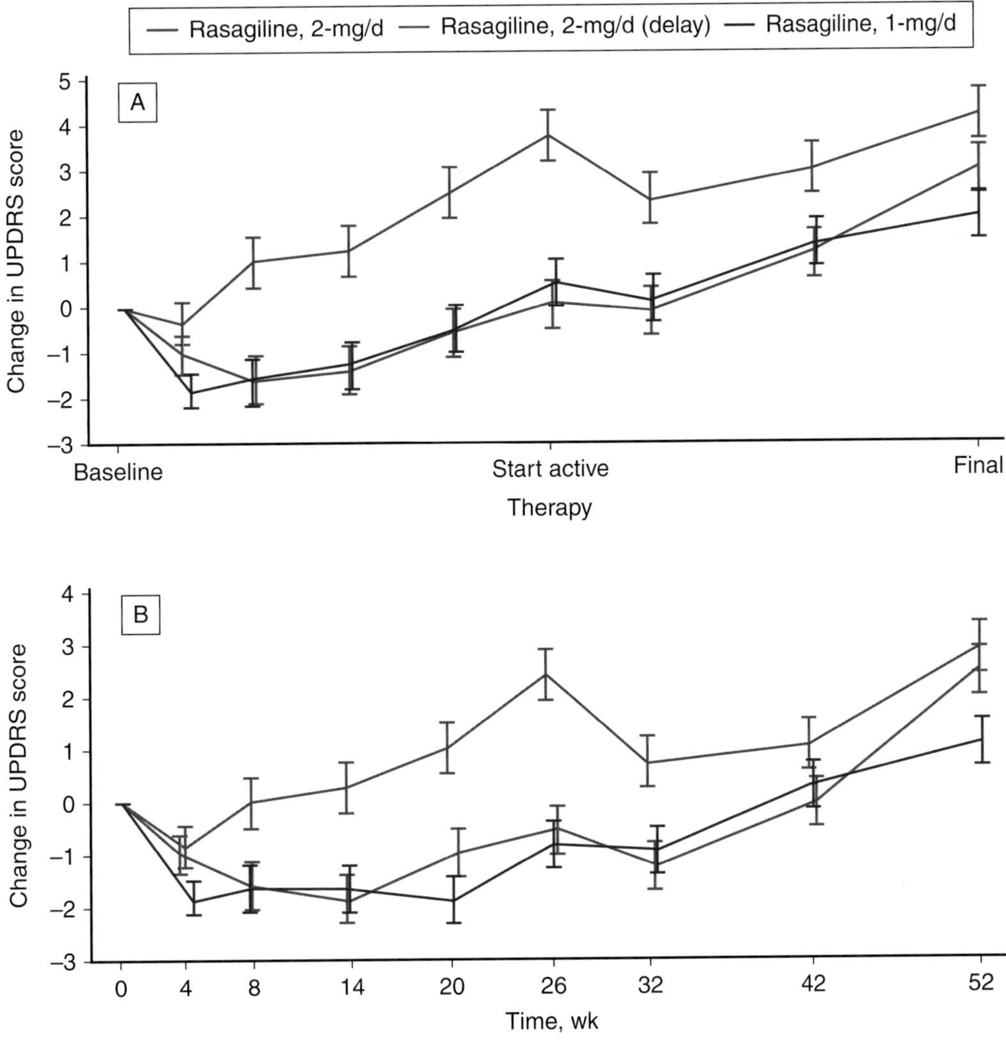

Figure 14-5. Change in UPDRS scores in the TEMPO trial. Subjects with early, untreated PD were randomized to either placebo or rasagiline for six months and then all were placed on rasagiline for another six months. Total UPDRS score was measured at baseline and at 4, 8, 14, 20, 26, 32, 42, and 52 weeks after randomization. Those treated initially with rasagiline had a smaller increase in UPDRS score compared to those first started on placebo. **A.** Total UPDRS score for all subjects in the efficacy cohort (371 subjects). **B.** Total UPDRS score for subgroup of subjects that did not require additional therapy by the end of the trial (249 subjects). (Reproduced with permission from Ref. 144). Copyright © American Medical Association. All rights reserved.)

it is the result of MAO-B inhibition or the effects of some of the metabolites of rasagiline that have other properties is not clear at present. Whether the difference is secondary to a true neuroprotective effect is also not clear. Longer treatment with rasagiline could result in increased sensitivity to the drug such that symptomatic effects may be more prominent in the early treatment group.

Coenzyme Q10

Coenzyme Q10 (CoQ10) is a cofactor in the electron transport chain in mitochondria and has been shown to reduce dopaminergic neurodegeneration in mouse PD models.[146] A small pilot study of 80 patients compared patients treated with CoQ10 at 300 mg/day, 600 mg/day, or 1200 mg/day to patients treated with placebo.[147] Patients were followed for 16 months or until they required L-dopa treatment. The primary outcome was change in total UPDRS compared to baseline. There was a trend toward reduction in UPDRS score change in patients treated with CoQ10 compared with those treated with placebo ($p = 0.09$), and secondary analysis suggested that most of the benefit was in the group treated with 1200 mg/day of CoQ10 (Fig. 14–6). More recently, CoQ10 has been examined using a "futility study."[148] This design employs small group sizes and is intended to identify treatments that clearly do not have a significant effect on disease progression and, therefore, should be excluded from further study.[149–151] In this para-

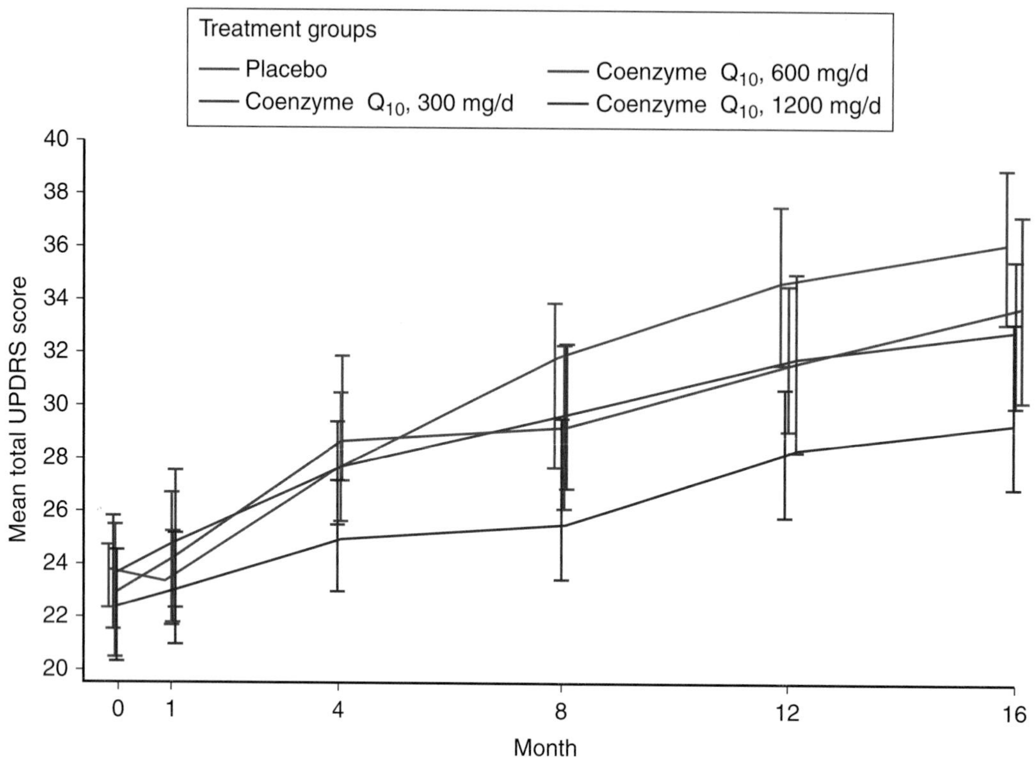

Figure 14–6. Change in UPDRS scores in subjects treated with CoEnzyme Q10. Eighty patients with early PD were randomized to treatment with placebo or with CoQ10 at 300 mg/day, 600 mg/day, or 1200 mg/day. Total UPDRS score was measured at baseline and at 1, 4, 8, 12, and 16 months. UPDRS score was significantly lower in subjects treated with 1200 mg/day CoQ10 compared with placebo-treated subjects. (Reproduced with permission from Ref. 147).

digm, CoQ10 did not meet the criteria for futility, and a larger, long-term study comparing high doses of CoQ10 with that of placebo has recently been initiated.

Creatine

Creatine promotes mitochondrial ATP production and has been shown to be neuroprotective in animal models.[152] A pilot study compared 60 patients with early PD treated with either creatine or placebo for two years.[153] No difference was seen in the UPDRS score or in the β-CIT uptake between the control and creatine groups. Subanalysis of the individual UPDRS subscales showed a difference in the "mentation, behavior, and mood" section. Creatine has also been examined in a futility study paradigm and could not be rejected as futile.[90] A large phase III trial examining creatine's effect on disease progression in a diverse population of patients with different stages of PD is in progress.

ANTIAPOPTOTIC AGENTS

Several antiapoptotic agents have been examined in controlled clinical trials. The propargylamine TCH346 is an antiapoptotic factor that inhibits the glycolytic enzyme glyceraldehyde-3-phosphate dehydrogenase (GAPDH), which can initiate apoptosis. Although TCH346 was shown in both 6-OHDA and MPTP animal models to reduce dopaminergic cell loss,[154,155] a double-blind, randomized trial involving 301 patients over 12 to 18 months failed to show a significant difference in clinical outcome.[109] CEP-1347, an inhibitor of mixed lineage kinases that can activate the c-Jun *N*-terminal kinase (JNK) pathway involved in cell death, is another antiapoptotic agent that showed promise in preclinical studies.[156–158] The PRECEPT trial involved 806 patients with early PD randomized to placebo or CEP-1347, and the primary outcome was time to need for dopaminergic therapy.[110] This study was terminated early when an interim analysis revealed futility of the experimental treatment.

The failure of these two antiapoptotic drugs has raised a number of important questions. Both were very effective in commonly used neurotoxin-based animal models of PD, raising the question of the predictive validity of these models. These failures have also raised the question of whether antiapoptotic strategies are an effective approach when applied at the relatively late stage of the disease when symptoms are clinically evident.

If activation of cell death pathways is the end stage of PD pathogenesis, then interference at this end stage may not be sufficient as "saved" neurons may remain dysfunctional. Combination of antiapoptotic therapies with trophic support or other treatments may be required.[159] It is also possible that multiple cell death pathways need to be blocked in concert to prevent neurodegeneration, as inhibition of single apoptotic pathways may just result in a shift from one cell death pathway to another.

▶ CHALLENGES FOR THE DEVELOPMENT OF NEUROPROTECTIVE THERAPY

Despite the promise of many different neuroprotective strategies, treatments that can stop the progression of PD and prevent later complications remain elusive. This is despite exploration of a wide range of potential pathogenic mechanisms and many different trial designs. What are some of the limitations of testing for neuroprotection that may have lead to these "failures"?

LIMITATIONS OF CLINICAL MEASURES OF DISEASE

One of the major challenges is the difficulty of testing a potential neuroprotective treatment in a living patient. Traditionally, clinical measures based on neurological exam have been used to assess progression (or lack of progression) of PD. Many different PD scales have been developed and employed for clinical studies over the years, including the Webster, Columbia University Rating Scale, Northwestern University Disability Scale, King's College, New York University PD Scale, UCLA Rating Scale, and the UPDRS.

The UPDRS Scale

The UPDRS scale is the most widely used and accepted scale since its development in the 1980s.[160] This scale is divided into four parts that involve clinical examination of motor function combined with scales rating patient's subjective view of function in daily activities. This scale has been investigated thoroughly in terms of clinimetrics, and overall has been demonstrated to have good reliability and validity.[161] Although interrater consistency is excellent overall, some studies have shown low interrater reliability for certain items, including speech, facial masking, posture, global bradykinesia, tremor, and rigidity.[162,163] There are several other limitations to this scale, particularly toward its usefulness for testing neuroprotection.[160,161] First, available symptomatic treatments have a large effect on the UPDRS scale, which may obscure evidence of neuroprotection. Second, the scale is also heavily weighted toward motor dysfunction, particularly bradykinesia and tremor-related symptoms. Much of the disability associated with PD is not considered in the scale, such as that related to autonomic dysfunction. Third, the current scale emphasizes signs and symptoms of moderate to severe disease and is not designed to assess adequately very mild symptoms and signs seen in early PD.[161] As trials investigating the potential neuroprotective effects of tested therapies typically enroll patients in the early stages of PD to maximize the potential for neuroprotection, "floor" effects of the UPDRS could limit the ability of this scale to detect neuroprotection. A new version of the UPDRS is currently under development to address some of these limitations.[164]

Symptomatic Effects and the Delayed-Start Design

To overcome the potentially confounding symptomatic effects of a treatment, many trials have incorporated a washout period before assessing the primary outcome measure. However, these symptomatic drug effects may be longstanding and outlast the washout period.[165,166] Another concern with the washout approach is that patients with severe PD may not tolerate stopping of PD medications so that they may withdraw from the study. The consequence would be skewing of the study population toward those patients with less severe disease.

An alternative approach used in several recent trials has been to use a delayed-start design where one group of patients is started on the therapy several months before the comparative group (Fig. 14–4).[165] This approach is based on the assumption that the symptomatic effects would be similar across the groups at the end of the study. However, there are still some potential problems with this approach.[144] The delayed-start paradigm is very sensitive to distortion from different rates of dropout between groups; patients randomized to placebo start are more likely to discontinue the study than those assigned to an effective therapy.[144,167] Longer treatment could result in increased sensitivity to drug such that symptomatic effects may be more prominent in patients in the early treatment group.[144] Finally, delaying any form of treatment may lead to worsened long-term disability, because failure to treat PD early may lead to orthopedic and musculoskeletal limitations. Despite these problems, many investigators regard the delayed-start design as the best currently available approach for evaluating neuroprotection.

NEUROIMAGING STRATEGIES

In laboratory studies the "gold standard" for evaluating neuroprotection is direct counts of surviving dopamine neurons, an approach not currently feasible in living patients. SPECT and PET imaging have been used as default measures of dopamine cell numbers, yet these imaging techniques, which are based on dopamine neurochemistry, have their limitations.[120,121] β-CIT SPECT imaging measures the binding of the radioactive tracer to the dopamine transporter on dopaminergic terminals in the striatum, while [18F]fluorodopa PET imaging measures the conversion of the radioactive tracer into fluorodopamine within the terminals. Although they rely on different aspects of dopamine neurochemistry, a concern with both approaches is that the underlying chemistry may be altered by the pharmacological effects of the treatments under investigation such that imaging changes may not necessarily reflect changes in dopaminergic neuron counts.[120] In addition, the amount of dopamine transporter per neuron or the ability of neurons to convert L-dopa into dopamine may not be stable over the course of the disease. Several clinical trials, including ELLDOPA and CALM–PD, have demonstrated a discrepancy between clinical and imaging outcome measures. None of these imaging techniques have yet been validated as appropriate surrogate measures of neuroprotection through correlation with neuropathology and/or clinical symptoms,[121,168,169] and considerably more long-term data with these methods are required.

LIMITATIONS OF ANIMAL MODELS

Most neuroprotective therapies are developed through the use of animal models of PD. The apparent "failure" of so many potential neuroprotective therapies may reflect the limitations of these animal models. Currently, there is no one animal model for PD that mimics the full pathology and clinical symptomology of the illness. Traditionally, preclinical studies have focused on toxin-based models using 6-OHDA or MPTP. Both of these models show degeneration of SN neurons, but the time course and pathological features of these models are different from human disease.[170,171] These toxins induce an acute neurodegeneration which may not be relevant to the slow progression seen in human PD. Both of these toxin models show nigral neurodegeneration, but neither leads to the formation of Lewy bodies, a hallmark of the human disease. These toxin models also fail to mimic the loss of other, nondopaminergic cell populations seen in human PD. Other toxins, such as rotenone and paraquat, cause a more chronic nigral neurodegeneration, yet these pesticides show considerable variability in their effects, limiting their utility in preclinical studies.[8,170,172]

With the discovery of α-syn, parkin, and other proteins identified through genetic PD studies, genetic-based models have been developed as alternatives to toxin-based models. These models incorporate some additional features of the disease but still fall short of an authentic re-creation. For example, transgenic mice that either express mutant α-syn (A30P or A53T) or overexpress wild type α-syn show variable motor deficits, α-syn inclusions, and dopaminergic terminal loss, but none of these transgenic animals show actual loss of dopaminergic neurons.[173,174] Some of these transgenic α-syn mice have pathology involving nervous system areas not typically involved in human PD.[175] Viral vector-mediated overexpression of wild type or mutant α-syn in rats and monkeys has resulted in neuronal loss and could serve as alternative animal models for examining neuroprotection.[176–178] However, while vector-mediated models allow for site-specific targeting of α-syn, it is not possible to target all areas affected in PD with these models.

The predictive power of animal models of PD will be confirmed only if there is some success in demonstrating neuroprotection in humans. In the meantime, most in the field rely on examining effectiveness of potential treatments in several different animal models, with the hope that treatments exhibiting a broad effect in these diverse models are the ones mostly likely to exhibit effectiveness against human disease.

HETEROGENEITY AND TIME COURSE OF THE DISEASE

The discovery of genes that cause PD has emphasized the diversity of the disorder: not only does it involve anatomical sites outside the dopaminergic system but it likely also has many interrelated causes. Most of the single-gene mutations discovered so far are rare and unlikely to play a significant role in broad-based clinical trials. However, *parkin* mutations are relatively frequent in young-onset patients,[48,179,180] and *LRRK2* mutations may account for 2% of a general clinical population of PD.[181–184] A more problematic issue is that there are likely a number of genetic risk factors for PD, which could alter the response to putative neuroprotective strategies. Therefore, defining subgroups of PD may be essential in order to establish neuroprotective efficacy. In addition, as PD involves many different pathogenic mechanisms, several agents may need to be combined to block multiple pathways in order to achieve neuroprotection.

For a potential neuroprotective agent to be most effective, patients need to be treated early, before much cell loss has occurred. By the time most patients develop the typical clinical symptoms of PD, it is estimated that at least 60% of nigral dopaminergic neurons have degenerated.[185–187] They may already have a variety of nonmotor symptoms, including sleep disturbance and autonomic dysfunction.[188] Such earlier symptoms are guiding the ongoing search for methods to detect "presymptomatic" PD, ranging from simple tests of olfaction to sophisticated neuroimaging studies.

Finally, since PD is a chronic, slowly progressive disorder, the ability to detect modest effects on progression using clinical scales is affected by sample size and length of follow-up. For example, in the ADAGIO trial, the largest neuroprotective study conducted to date, 1.7 was the difference in the total UPDRS score, a scale with

168 possible points. This difference arises from a difference of treatment duration of nearly 9 months and was detectable only with a very large sample size. Testing every potential neuroprotective agent in such a large and expensive trial is not feasible. Resolution of this bottleneck to development will require the development of reliable laboratory methods for studying PD progression ("biomarkers"), most likely using either neuroimaging or biochemical methods.

▶ NEUROPROTECTIVE THERAPIES OF THE FUTURE

In 2003, the NIH-appointed Committee to Identify Neuroprotective Agents in Parkinson's (CINAPS) published an assessment of potential neuroprotective compounds and prioritized 12 compounds to be studied further in clinical trials.[189] Since then, the list of potential therapies has grown longer, but a convincing success in human trials is still awaited. Of those strategies still under active study, several of the most promising are described later. The wealth of information regarding PD pathogenesis from genetic studies is leading to novel approaches to neuroprotection based on the biology of α-syn, *LRRK2*, and others. Although much more research is needed before translating such theoretical therapies into clinical trials, these approaches may lead to therapies that protect not only against dopaminergic cell loss but also against the loss of other neuronal populations at risk in PD and related disorders.

ADENOSINE RECEPTOR ANTAGONISTS

Epidemiological studies have indicated that caffeine may reduce the incidence of PD, at least in men.[190,191] As caffeine mediates its action by antagonizing adenosine receptors, this finding has led to interest in evaluating adenosine receptor antagonists as potential neuroprotective agents.[192] In the striatum, the A_{2A} receptor can heterodimerize with the D_2 receptor to inhibit dopamine signaling,[193,194] while inhibition of the A_{2A} receptor can promote dopamine function. Two small clinical trials of the A_{2A} antagonist istradefylline (KW-6002) has demonstrated potential symptomatic effects in advanced PD.[195,196] More recent research has suggested that A_{2A} antagonists may also be neuroprotective. Caffeine and istradefylline are both neuroprotective in the MPTP model,[197,198] and caffeine (and related A_{2A} antagonists) has been identified by CINAPS as a priority agent to be evaluated for neuroprotection in clinical trials.[189] A potential advantage of A_{2A} antagonists is that they have also been shown to be neuroprotective in nondopaminergic brain areas[199–201] so that they may protect against PD neurodegeneration found in regions besides the SN.

ANTI-INFLAMMATORY AGENTS

The role of inflammation in PD has become increasingly clear. As a means to slow disease progression, anti-inflammatory agents, including NSAIDs and minocycline, have been pursued as potential disease-modifying treatments for PD. Several studies in culture and in animal models have shown that certain NSAIDs have neuroprotective qualities, although there are conflicting data regarding which NSAIDs, what dosing, and what timing provides the best neuroprotection.[67] Epidemiological studies examining the association of regular NSAID use with the risk of PD have provided conflicting results. An initial study by Chen and colleagues showed that NSAID use lowers the risk of PD by 45%,[85] and a follow-up study by the same group showed that only ibuprofen had this neuroprotective effect.[84] Other epidemiological studies examining this association have shown nonsignificant trends or have shown this association only in men.[83,86,87] At this time, it is unclear that any of the currently available NSAIDs have genuine neuroprotective properties in PD, but the more general strategy of targeting the mechanisms of neuroinflammation seems very promising.

An example of an alternative approach to targeting neuroinflammation may be the use of statins (3-hydroxy-3-methylglutaryl-coenzyme A reductase inhibitors). In addition to lowering cholesterol, these drugs have anti-inflammatory effects, including reduction of TNFα, nitric oxide, and superoxide production by microglia.[202] Statins may also act to scavenge free radicals.[203] Simvastatin has been shown to reduce dopamine loss in MPTP animal models.[202] Recent epidemiological studies showed that statin use, particularly simvastatin, is associated with reduced PD incidence.[88,89] A limitation of these studies is that they were retrospective, and the use of statins was not randomized. Other studies have suggested low LDL cholesterol levels increased PD risk,[204,205] so that the increased use of statins among controls may just reflect high LDL levels that would be protective against PD. These issues need to be explored in a prospective, randomized study.

Minocycline, a second-generation tetracycline long used as an antimicrobial agent, has anti-inflammatory effects independent of its antimicrobial activity. Minocycline blocks microglial activation and may also have antiapoptotic activity.[206,207] It protects against dopaminergic cell loss in both the MPTP and 6-OHDA animal models.[208–210] A recent futility study showed that minocycline was well tolerated and could not be rejected as futile, setting the stage for larger phase III trials.[90]

OTHER ANTIOXIDANTS

Epidemiological studies have pointed to uric acid as a potential neuroprotective agent in PD. Uric acid acts as an antioxidant by scavenging reactive oxygen and nitrogen species.[211] Studies have shown a decreased incidence of PD among subjects with high serum urate levels[212–214] and among subjects with gout.[215] In patients with early PD, higher plasma urate levels correlate with slower disease progression.[216] Uric acid can reduce dopaminergic cell death in response to rotenone and homocysteine in culture.[217] A recent study showed that subjects on diets that promote high urate levels have a reduced risk of developing PD.[218] Such a urate-rich diet could serve as a neuroprotective therapy in PD. However, the potential benefits of a urate-rich diet have to be weighed against the risk of developing gout and cardiovascular disease. A large-scale clinical trial of the effectiveness of elevating urate in patients with PD is in the planning stages.

ALPHA-SYNUCLEIN-DIRECTED THERAPIES

Although its mechanism for inducing neurotoxicity is not well understood, α-syn appears to be an important mediator of toxicity in PD. Reduction of α-syn protein levels and disruption of α-syn aggregation have been the focus of research to develop novel therapies against PD. Potential methods to reduce α-syn protein production include small-molecule modifiers of transcription and RNAi-based methods to knock down translation. α-Syn clearance could become enhanced by activation of proteosomal or lysosomal pathways. Augmentation of parkin or UCH-L1 activity could promote the clearance of α-syn and other aggregated proteins. Indeed, parkin overexpression can rescue cells from α-syn pathology in animal models.[219–221] Activation of lysosomal degradation could also induce α-syn clearance; the lysosomal enzyme cathepsin D reduces α-syn aggregation and toxicity.[222] In addition, vaccine-based therapies have been pursued as potential strategies for increasing α-syn clearance. α-Syn transgenic mice vaccinated with antibodies against α-syn showed decreased α-syn accumulation secondary to increased degradation via lysosomal pathways.[223] Direct blockers of α-syn aggregation could also be developed into therapeutic strategies for PD. Peptide-based inhibitors have been developed that can block α-syn self-association and aggregation.[224–226] All of these strategies are at a relatively early stage of development and await further study before proceeding to human intervention trials.

KINASE INHIBITORS

The most common genetic cause of PD to date is mutation in the gene *LRRK2*, which causes about 2% of all cases of PD[181–183] and up to 40% in historically isolated populations.[227–230] The *LRRK2* gene codes for a large protein, also known as dardarin, which contains a serine/threonine kinase domain and a GTPase domain. The native function of this protein is currently poorly understood. The most common pathogenic mutation of *LRRK2* is associated with increased kinase activity.[231–233] Evidence that pathogenic mutations increase this activity makes the kinase activity of LRRK2 an important target for neuroprotective therapy. Kinases are generally good targets for small molecule therapies, and indeed certain therapies in other diseases are based on inhibition of kinase activity. At this time, however, the endogenous substrates of LRRK2 are unknown, making it difficult to devise the development of LRRK2 kinase inhibitors. As the function of LRRK2 is further characterized, a clearer therapeutic strategy based on LRRK2 biology should become more apparent.

▶ CONCLUSIONS

Neuroprotection in PD remains an important but elusive goal. A successful neuroprotective treatment could transform PD from a relentlessly progressive and disabling disease to a problem that can be managed with only a modest effect on quality of life. Current barriers include a lack of knowledge of the basic mechanisms of PD, and the insensitivity of the methodologies used to study disease progression. Overall, however, the activity aimed at understanding and treating PD has grown exponentially and should ultimately result in better therapies for PD.

REFERENCES

1. Braak, H, Del Tredici K, Rub U, et al. Staging of brain pathology related to sporadic Parkinson's disease. Neurobiol Aging 2003;24:197–211.
2. Alam, ZI, Jenner A, Daniel SE, et al. Oxidative DNA damage in the parkinsonian brain: An apparent selective increase in 8-hydroxyguanine levels in substantia nigra. J Neurochem 1997;69:1196–1203.
3. Dexter, DT, Holley AE, Flitter WD, et al. Increased levels of lipid hydroperoxides in the parkinsonian substantia nigra: An HPLC and ESR study. Mov Disord 1994;9:92–97.
4. Dexter, DT, Sian J, Rose S, et al. Indices of oxidative stress and mitochondrial function in individuals with incidental Lewy body disease. Ann Neurol 1994;35:38–44.
5. Hastings, TG, Lewis DA, Zigmond MJ. Reactive dopamine metabolites and neurotoxicity: Implications for Parkinson's disease. Adv Exp Med Biol 1996;387:97–106.
6. Sulzer, D, Zecca L. Intraneuronal dopamine-quinone synthesis: A review. Neurotox Res 2000;1:181–195.
7. Schapira, AH, Cooper JM, Dexter D, et al. Mitochondrial complex I deficiency in Parkinson's disease. Lancet 1989;1:1269.
8. Betarbet, R, Sherer TB, MacKenzie G, et al. Chronic systemic pesticide exposure reproduces features of Parkinson's disease. Nat Neurosci 2000;3:1301–1306.
9. Langston, JW, Ballard P, Tetrud JW, et al. Chronic Parkinsonism in humans due to a product of meperidine-analog synthesis. Science 1983;219:979–980.

10. Langston, JW, Forno LS, Rebert CS, et al. Selective nigral toxicity after systemic administration of 1-methyl-4-phenyl-1,2,5,6-tetrahydropyrine (MPTP) in the squirrel monkey. Brain Res 1984;292:390–394.
11. Wooten, GF, Currie LJ, Bennett JP, et al. Maternal inheritance in Parkinson's disease. Ann Neurol 1997;41: 265–268.
12. Schapira, AH. Mitochondria in the aetiology and pathogenesis of Parkinson's disease. Lancet Neurol 2008; 7:97–109.
13. Cantuti-Castelvetri, I, Lin MT, Zheng K, et al. Somatic mitochondrial DNA mutations in single neurons and glia. Neurobiol Aging 2005;26:1343–1355.
14. Dexter, DT, Wells FR, Lees AJ, et al. Increased nigral iron content and alterations in other metal ions occurring in brain in Parkinson's disease. J Neurochem 1989;52: 1830–1836.
15. Riederer, P, Sofic E, Rausch WD, et al. Transition metals, ferritin, glutathione, and ascorbic acid in parkinsonian brains. J Neurochem 1989;52:515–520.
16. Perry, TL, Yong VW. Idiopathic Parkinson's disease, progressive supranuclear palsy and glutathione metabolism in the substantia nigra of patients. Neurosci Lett 1986;67:269–274.
17. Sian, J, Dexter DT, Lees AJ, et al. Alterations in glutathione levels in Parkinson's disease and other neurodegenerative disorders affecting basal ganglia. Ann Neurol 1994;36:348–355.
18. Sofic, E, Lange KW, Jellinger K, et al. Reduced and oxidized glutathione in the substantia nigra of patients with Parkinson's disease. Neurosci Lett 1992;142:128–130.
19. Clark, IE, Dodson MW, Jiang C, et al. Drosophila pink1 is required for mitochondrial function and interacts genetically with parkin. Nature 2006;441:1162–1166.
20. Kim, RH, Smith PD, Aleyasin H, et al. Hypersensitivity of DJ-1-deficient mice to 1-methyl-4-phenyl-1,2,3,6-tetrahydropyrindine (MPTP) and oxidative stress. Proc Natl Acad Sci U S A. 2005;102:5215–5220.
21. Park, J, Lee SB, Lee S, et al. Mitochondrial dysfunction in Drosophila PINK1 mutants is complemented by parkin. Nature 2006;441:1157–1161.
22. Yokota, T, Sugawara K, Ito K, et al. Down regulation of DJ-1 enhances cell death by oxidative stress, ER stress, and proteasome inhibition. Biochem Biophys Res Commun 2003;312:1342–1348.
23. Athanassiadou, A, Voutsinas G, Psiouri L, et al. Genetic analysis of families with Parkinson disease that carry the Ala53Thr mutation in the gene encoding alpha-synuclein. Am J Hum Genet 1999;65:555–558.
24. Kruger, R, Kuhn W, Muller T, et al. Ala30Pro mutation in the gene encoding alpha-synuclein in Parkinson's disease. Nat Genet 1998;18:106–108.
25. Polymeropoulos, MH, Lavedan C, Leroy E, et al. Mutation in the alpha-synuclein gene identified in families with Parkinson's disease. Science 1997;276:2045–2047.
26. Zarranz, JJ, Alegre J, Gomez-Esteban JC, et al. The new mutation, E46K, of alpha-synuclein causes Parkinson and Lewy body dementia. Ann Neurol 2004;55:164–173.
27. Irizarry, MC, Growdon W, Gomez-Isla T, et al. Nigral and cortical Lewy bodies and dystrophic nigral neurites in Parkinson's disease and cortical Lewy body disease contain alpha-synuclein immunoreactivity. J Neuropathol Exp Neurol 1998;57:334–337.
28. Spillantini, MG, Schmidt ML, Lee VM, et al. Alpha-synuclein in Lewy bodies. Nature 1997;388:839–840.
29. Singleton, AB, Farrer M, Johnson J, et al. alpha-Synuclein locus triplication causes Parkinson's disease. Science 2003;302:841.
30. El-Agnaf, OM, Jakes R, Curran MD, et al. Effects of the mutations Ala30 to Pro and Ala53 to Thr on the physical and morphological properties of alpha-synuclein protein implicated in Parkinson's disease. FEBS Lett 1998; 440:67–70.
31. Narhi, L, Wood SJ, Steavenson S, et al. Both familial Parkinson's disease mutations accelerate alpha-synuclein aggregation. J Biol Chem 1999;274:9843–9846.
32. Conway, KA, Harper JD, Lansbury PT. Accelerated in vitro fibril formation by a mutant alpha-synuclein linked to early-onset Parkinson disease. Nat Med 1998;4: 1318–1320.
33. Conway, KA, Lee SJ, Rochet JC, et al. Acceleration of oligomerization, not fibrillization, is a shared property of both alpha-synuclein mutations linked to early-onset Parkinson's disease: Implications for pathogenesis and therapy. Proc Natl Acad Sci U S A 2000;97:571–576.
34. Masliah, E, Rockenstein E, Veinbergs I, et al. Dopaminergic loss and inclusion body formation in alpha-synuclein mice: Implications for neurodegenerative disorders. Science 2000;287:1265–1269.
35. Souza, JM, Giasson BI, Chen Q, et al. Dityrosine cross-linking promotes formation of stable alpha-synuclein polymers. Implication of nitrative and oxidative stress in the pathogenesis of neurodegenerative synucleinopathies. J Biol Chem 2000;275:18344–18349.
36. Abeliovich, A, Schmitz Y, Farinas I, et al. Mice lacking alpha-synuclein display functional deficits in the nigrostriatal dopamine system. Neuron 2000;25:239–252.
37. Murphy, DD, Rueter SM, Trojanowski JQ, et al. Synucleins are developmentally expressed, and alpha-synuclein regulates the size of the presynaptic vesicular pool in primary hippocampal neurons. J Neurosci 2000;20:3214–3220.
38. Flower, TR, Chesnokova LS, Froelich CA, et al. Heat shock prevents alpha-synuclein-induced apoptosis in a yeast model of Parkinson's disease. J Mol Biol 2005;351: 1081–1100.
39. Saha, AR, Ninkina NN, Hanger DP, et al. Induction of neuronal death by alpha-synuclein. Eur J Neurosci 2000;12:3073–3077.
40. Smith, WW, Jiang H, Pei Z, et al. Endoplasmic reticulum stress and mitochondrial cell death pathways mediate A53T mutant alpha-synuclein-induced toxicity. Hum Mol Genet 2005;14:3801–3811.
41. Volles, MJ, Lansbury PT, Jr. Zeroing in on the pathogenic form of alpha-synuclein and its mechanism of neurotoxicity in Parkinson's disease. Biochemistry 2003;42: 7871–7878.
42. Cookson, MR, van der Brug M. Cell systems and the toxic mechanism(s) of alpha-synuclein. Exp Neurol 2008; 209:5–11.
43. Kontopoulos, E, Parvin JD, Feany MB. Alpha-synuclein acts in the nucleus to inhibit histone acetylation and promote neurotoxicity. Hum Mol Genet 2006;15:3012–3023.

44. Yacoubian, TA, Cantuti-Castelvetri I, Bouzou B, et al. Transcriptional dysregulation in a transgenic model of Parkinson disease. Neurobiol Dis 2008;29:515–528.
45. Benner, EJ, Banerjee R, Reynolds AD, et al. Nitrated alpha-synuclein immunity accelerates degeneration of nigral dopaminergic neurons. PLoS ONE 2008;3:e1376.
46. Theodore, S, McLean PJ, Standaert DG. Microglial activation following targeted over-expression of human alpha-synuclein in the mouse substantia nigra. Soc Neurosci Abstract Viewer/Itinerary Planner. Program #50.3/M162007.
47. Leroy, E, Boyer R, Auburger G, et al. The ubiquitin pathway in Parkinson's disease. Nature 1998;395:451–452.
48. Kitada, T, Asakawa S, Hattori N, et al. Mutations in the parkin gene cause autosomal recessive juvenile parkinsonism. Nature 1998;392:605–608.
49. Imai, Y, Soda M, Takahashi R. Parkin suppresses unfolded protein stress-induced cell death through its E3 ubiquitin-protein ligase activity. J Biol Chem 2000;275: 35661–35664.
50. Shimura, H, Hattori N, Kubo S, et al. Familial Parkinson disease gene product, parkin, is a ubiquitin-protein ligase. Nat Genet 2000;25:302–305.
51. Zhang, Y, Gao J, Chung KK, et al. Parkin functions as an E2-dependent ubiquitin- protein ligase and promotes the degradation of the synaptic vesicle-associated protein, CDCrel-1. Proc Natl Acad Sci U S A 2000;97: 13354–13359.
52. Chung, KK, Zhang Y, Lim KL, et al. Parkin ubiquitinates the alpha-synuclein-interacting protein, synphilin-1: Implications for Lewy-body formation in Parkinson disease. Nat Med 2001;7:1144–1150.
53. Shimura, H, Schlossmacher MG, Hattori N, et al. Ubiquitination of a new form of alpha-synuclein by parkin from human brain: Implications for Parkinson's disease. Science 2001;293:263–269.
54. Mori, H, Kondo T, Yokochi M, et al. Pathologic and biochemical studies of juvenile parkinsonism linked to chromosome 6q. Neurology 1998;51:890–892.
55. Takahashi, H, Ohama E, Suzuki S, et al. Familial juvenile parkinsonism: Clinical and pathologic study in a family. Neurology 1994;44:437–441.
56. Hayashi, S, Wakabayashi K, Ishikawa A, et al. An autopsy case of autosomal-recessive juvenile parkinsonism with a homozygous exon 4 deletion in the parkin gene. Mov Disord 2000;15:884–888.
57. Farrer, M, Chan P, Chen R, et al. Lewy bodies and parkinsonism in families with parkin mutations. Ann Neurol 2001;50:293–300.
58. Klucken, J, Shin Y, Masliah E, et al. Hsp70 Reduces alpha-Synuclein Aggregation and Toxicity. J Biol Chem 2004;279:25497–25502.
59. Moore, DJ, West AB, Dikeman DA, et al. Parkin mediates the degradation-independent ubiquitination of Hsp70. J Neurochem 2008;105:1806–1819.
60. McNaught, KS, Mytilineou C, Jnobaptiste R, et al. Impairment of the ubiquitin-proteasome system causes dopaminergic cell death and inclusion body formation in ventral mesencephalic cultures. J Neurochem 2002;81:301–306.
61. Chung, KK, Dawson VL, Dawson TM. The role of the ubiquitin-proteasomal pathway in Parkinson's disease and other neurodegenerative disorders. Trends Neurosci 2001;24:S7–S14.
62. Nishikawa, K, Li H, Kawamura R, et al. Alterations of structure and hydrolase activity of parkinsonism-associated human ubiquitin carboxyl-terminal hydrolase L1 variants. Biochem Biophys Res Commun 2003;304:176–183.
63. Balch, WE, Morimoto RI, Dillin A, et al. Adapting proteostasis for disease intervention. Science 2008;319: 916–919.
64. Morimoto, RI. Proteotoxic stress and inducible chaperone networks in neurodegenerative disease and aging. Genes Dev 2008;22:1427–1438.
65. Prahlad, V, Morimoto RI. Integrating the stress response: Lessons for neurodegenerative diseases from *C. elegans*. Trends Cell Biol 2009;19:52–61.
66. Tansey, MG, McCoy MK, Frank-Cannon TC. Neuroinflammatory mechanisms in Parkinson's disease: Potential environmental triggers, pathways, and targets for early therapeutic intervention. Exp Neurol 2007;208:1–25.
67. Esposito, E, Di Matteo V, Benigno A, et al. Non-steroidal anti-inflammatory drugs in Parkinson's disease. Exp Neurol 2007;205:295–312.
68. McGeer, EG, McGeer PL. The role of anti-inflammatory agents in Parkinson's disease. CNS Drugs 2007;21: 789–797.
69. McGeer, PL, Itagaki S, Boyes BE, et al. Reactive microglia are positive for HLA-DR in the substantia nigra of Parkinson's and Alzheimer's disease brains. Neurology 1988;38:1285–1291.
70. McGeer, PL, Schwab C, Parent A, et al. Presence of reactive microglia in monkey substantia nigra years after 1-methyl-4-phenyl-1,2,3,6-tetrahydropyridine administration. Ann Neurol 2003;54:599–604.
71. Orr, CF, Rowe DB, Mizuno Y, et al. A possible role for humoral immunity in the pathogenesis of Parkinson's disease. Brain 2005;128:2665–2674.
72. Cicchetti, F, Brownell AL, Williams K, et al. Neuroinflammation of the nigrostriatal pathway during progressive 6-OHDA dopamine degeneration in rats monitored by immunohistochemistry and PET imaging. Eur J Neurosci 2002;15:991–998.
73. Sherer, TB, Betarbet R, Kim JH, et al. Selective microglial activation in the rat rotenone model of Parkinson's disease. Neurosci Lett 2003;341:87–90.
74. Mogi, M, Harada M, Kondo T, et al. Interleukin-1 beta, interleukin-6, epidermal growth factor and transforming growth factor-alpha are elevated in the brain from parkinsonian patients. Neurosci Lett 1994;180:147–150.
75. Mogi, M, Harada M, Riederer P, et al. Tumor necrosis factor-alpha (TNF-alpha) increases both in the brain and in the cerebrospinal fluid from parkinsonian patients. Neurosci Lett 1994;165:208–210.
76. Yamada, T, McGeer PL, McGeer EG. Lewy bodies in Parkinson's disease are recognized by antibodies to complement proteins. Acta Neuropathol 1992;84:100–104.
77. Goldknopf, IL, Sheta EA, Bryson J, et al. Complement C3c and related protein biomarkers in amyotrophic lateral sclerosis and Parkinson's disease. Biochem Biophys Res Commun 2006;342:1034–1039.
78. Zhang, W, Wang T, Pei Z, et al. Aggregated alpha-synuclein activates microglia: a process leading to disease

progression in Parkinson's disease. FASEB J 2005;19: 533–542.

79. Reynolds, AD, Glanzer JG, Kadiu I, et al. Nitrated alpha-synuclein-activated microglial profiling for Parkinson's disease. J Neurochem 2008;104:1504–1525.
80. Reynolds, AD, Kadiu I, Garg SK, et al. Nitrated alpha-synuclein and microglial neuroregulatory activities. J Neuroimmune Pharmacol 2008;3:59–74.
81. Theodore, S, Cao S, McLean PJ, et al. Targeted overexpression of human alpha-synuclein triggers microglial activation and an adaptive immune response in a mouse model of Parkinson disease. J Neuropathol Exp Neurol 2008;67:1149–1158.
82. Ghosh, A, Roy A, Liu X, et al. Selective inhibition of NF-kappaB activation prevents dopaminergic neuronal loss in a mouse model of Parkinson's disease. Proc Natl Acad Sci U S A 2007;104:18754–18759.
83. Bower, JH, Maraganore DM, Peterson BJ, et al. Immunologic diseases, anti-inflammatory drugs, and Parkinson disease: A case-control study. Neurology 2006;67: 494–496.
84. Chen, H, Jacobs E, Schwarzschild MA, et al. Nonsteroidal antiinflammatory drug use and the risk for Parkinson's disease. Ann Neurol 2005;58:963–967.
85. Chen, H, Zhang SM, Hernan MA, et al. Nonsteroidal anti-inflammatory drugs and the risk of Parkinson disease. Arch Neurol 2003;60:1059–1064.
86. Hernan, MA, Logroscino G, Garcia Rodriguez LA. Nonsteroidal anti-inflammatory drugs and the incidence of Parkinson disease. Neurology 2006;66:1097–1099.
87. Ton, TG, Heckbert SR, Longstreth WT, Jr., et al. Nonsteroidal anti-inflammatory drugs and risk of Parkinson's disease. Mov Disord 2006;21:964–969.
88. Wolozin, B, Wang SW, Li NC, et al. Simvastatin is associated with a reduced incidence of dementia and Parkinson's disease. BMC Med 2007;5:20.
89. Wahner, AD, Bronstein JM, Bordelon YM, et al. Statin use and the risk of Parkinson disease. Neurology 2008;70:1418–1422.
90. A randomized, double-blind, futility clinical trial of creatine and minocycline in early Parkinson disease. Neurology 2006;66:664–671.
91. Mody, I, MacDonald JF. NMDA receptor-dependent excitotoxicity: the role of intracellular Ca2+ release. Trends Pharmacol Sci 1995;16:356–359.
92. Dawson, VL, Dawson TM. Nitric oxide neurotoxicity. J Chem Neuroanat 1996;10:179–190.
93. Good, PF, Hsu A, Werner P, et al. Protein nitration in Parkinson's disease. J Neuropathol Exp Neurol 1998;57:338–342.
94. Turski, L, Bressler K, Rettig KJ, et al. Protection of substantia nigra from MPP+ neurotoxicity by N-methyl-D-aspartate antagonists. Nature 1991;349:414–418.
95. Brouillet, E, Beal MF. NMDA antagonists partially protect against MPTP induced neurotoxicity in mice. Neuroreport 1993;4:387–390.
96. Jankovic, J, Hunter C. A double-blind, placebo-controlled and longitudinal study of riluzole in early Parkinson's disease. Parkinsonism Relat Disord 2002;8:271–276.
97. Kornhuber, J, Weller M, Schoppmeyer K, et al. Amantadine and memantine are NMDA receptor antagonists with neuroprotective properties. J Neural Transm Suppl 1994;43:91–104.
98. Surmeier, DJ. Calcium, ageing, and neuronal vulnerability in Parkinson's disease. Lancet Neurol 2007;6:933–938.
99. Chan, CS, Guzman JN, Ilijic E, et al. 'Rejuvenation' protects neurons in mouse models of Parkinson's disease. Nature 2007;447:1081–1086.
100. Rodnitzky, RL. Can calcium antagonists provide a neuroprotective effect in Parkinson's disease? Drugs 1999;57:845–849.
101. Anglade, P, Vyas S, Javoy-Agid F, et al. Apoptosis and autophagy in nigral neurons of patients with Parkinson's disease. Histol Histopathol 1997;12:25–31.
102. Tompkins, MM, Basgall EJ, Zamrini E, et al. Apoptotic-like changes in Lewy-body-associated disorders and normal aging in substantia nigral neurons. Am J Pathol 1997;150:119–131.
103. Hirsch, EC, Hunot S, Faucheux B, et al. Dopaminergic neurons degenerate by apoptosis in Parkinson's disease. Mov Disord 1999;14:383–385.
104. Tatton, NA. Increased caspase 3 and Bax immunoreactivity accompany nuclear GAPDH translocation and neuronal apoptosis in Parkinson's disease. Exp Neurol 2000;166:29–43.
105. Tatton, WG, Chalmers-Redman R, Brown D, et al. Apoptosis in Parkinson's disease: Signals for neuronal degradation. Ann Neurol 2003;53(suppl 3):S61–S70; discussion S70–S62.
106. Blum, D, Torch S, Lambeng N, et al. Molecular pathways involved in the neurotoxicity of 6-OHDA, dopamine and MPTP: Contribution to the apoptotic theory in Parkinson's disease. Prog Neurobiol 2001;65:135–172.
107. Jellinger, KA. Cell death mechanisms in neurodegeneration. J Cell Mol Med 2001;5:1–17.
108. Mattson, MP. Neuronal life-and-death signaling, apoptosis, and neurodegenerative disorders. Antioxid Redox Signal 2006;8:1997–2006.
109. Olanow, CW, Schapira AH, LeWitt PA, et al. TCH346 as a neuroprotective drug in Parkinson's disease: A double-blind, randomised, controlled trial. Lancet Neurol 2006;5:1013–1020.
110. Mixed lineage kinase inhibitor CEP-1347 fails to delay disability in early Parkinson disease. Neurology 2007;69:1480–1490.
111. Howells, DW, Porritt MJ, Wong JY, et al. Reduced BDNF mRNA expression in the Parkinson's disease substantia nigra. Exp Neurol 2000;166:127–135.
112. Chauhan, NB, Siegel GJ, Lee JM. Depletion of glial cell line-derived neurotrophic factor in substantia nigra neurons of Parkinson's disease brain. J Chem Neuroanat 2001;21:277–288.
113. Mogi, M, Togari A, Kondo T, et al. Brain-derived growth factor and nerve growth factor concentrations are decreased in the substantia nigra in Parkinson's disease. Neurosci Lett 1999;270:45–48.
114. Suchowersky, O, Gronseth G, Perlmutter J, et al. Practice Parameter: Neuroprotective strategies and alternative therapies for Parkinson disease (an evidence-based review): Report of the Quality Standards Subcommittee of the American Academy of Neurology. Neurology 2006;66:976–982.

115. Fahn, S. Is levodopa toxic? Neurology 1996;47: S184–S195.
116. Barzilai, A, Melamed E, Shirvan A. Is there a rationale for neuroprotection against dopamine toxicity in Parkinson's disease? Cell Mol Neurobiol 2001;21:215–235.
117. Murer, MG, Dziewczapolski G, Menalled LB, et al. Chronic levodopa is not toxic for remaining dopamine neurons, but instead promotes their recovery, in rats with moderate nigrostriatal lesions. Ann Neurol 1998;43:561–575.
118. Datla, KP, Blunt SB, Dexter DT. Chronic L-DOPA administration is not toxic to the remaining dopaminergic nigrostriatal neurons, but instead may promote their functional recovery, in rats with partial 6-OHDA or FeCl(3) nigrostriatal lesions. Mov Disord 2001;16:424–434.
119. Fahn, S, Oakes D, Shoulson I, et al. Levodopa and the progression of Parkinson's disease. N Engl J Med 2004;351:2498–2508.
120. Ravina, B, Eidelberg D, Ahlskog JE, et al. The role of radiotracer imaging in Parkinson disease. Neurology 2005;64:208–215.
121. Allain, H, Bentue-Ferrer D, Akwa Y. Disease-modifying drugs and Parkinson's disease. Prog Neurobiol 2008;84:25–39.
122. Ogawa, N, Tanaka K, Asanuma M, et al. Bromocriptine protects mice against 6-hydroxydopamine and scavenges hydroxyl free radicals in vitro. Brain Res 1994;657: 207–213.
123. Carvey, PM, Pieri S, Ling ZD. Attenuation of levodopa-induced toxicity in mesencephalic cultures by pramipexole. J Neural Transm 1997;104:209–228.
124. Kitamura, Y, Kosaka T, Kakimura JI, et al. Protective effects of the antiparkinsonian drugs talipexole and pramipexole against 1-methyl-4-phenylpyridinium-induced apoptotic death in human neuroblastoma SH-SY5Y cells. Mol Pharmacol 1998;54:1046–1054.
125. Iida, M, Miyazaki I, Tanaka K, et al. Dopamine D2 receptor-mediated antioxidant and neuroprotective effects of ropinirole, a dopamine agonist. Brain Res 1999;838:51–59.
126. Vu, TQ, Ling ZD, Ma SY, et al. Pramipexole attenuates the dopaminergic cell loss induced by intraventricular 6-hydroxydopamine. J Neural Transm 2000;107:159–176.
127. Zou, L, Xu J, Jankovic J, et al. Pramipexole inhibits lipid peroxidation and reduces injury in the substantia nigra induced by the dopaminergic neurotoxin 1-methyl-4-phenyl-1,2,3,6-tetrahydropyridine in C57BL/6 mice. Neurosci Lett 2000;281:167–170.
128. Iravani, MM, Haddon CO, Cooper JM, et al. Pramipexole protects against MPTP toxicity in non-human primates. J Neurochem 2006;96:1315–1321.
129. Olanow, CW, Jenner P, Brooks D. Dopamine agonists and neuroprotection in Parkinson's disease. Ann Neurol 1998;44:S167–S174.
130. Cassarino, DS, Fall CP, Smith TS, et al. Pramipexole reduces reactive oxygen species production in vivo and in vitro and inhibits the mitochondrial permeability transition produced by the parkinsonian neurotoxin methylpyridinium ion. J Neurochem 1998;71:295–301.
131. Dopamine transporter brain imaging to assess the effects of pramipexole vs levodopa on Parkinson disease progression. The Parkinson Study Group. JAMA 2002;287:1653–1661.
132. Whone, AL, Watts RL, Stoessl AJ, et al. Slower progression of Parkinson's disease with ropinirole versus levodopa: The REAL-PET study. Ann Neurol 2003;54:93–101.
133. Effect of deprenyl on the progression of disability in early Parkinson's disease. The Parkinson Study Group. N Engl J Med 1989;321:1364–1371.
134. Effects of tocopherol and deprenyl on the progression of disability in early Parkinson's disease. The Parkinson Study Group. N Engl J Med 1993;328:176–183.
135. Landau, WM. Clinical neuromythology IX. Pyramid sale in the bucket shop: DATATOP bottoms out. Neurology 1990;40:1337–1339.
136. Schulzer, M, Mak E, Calne DB. The antiparkinson efficacy of deprenyl derives from transient improvement that is likely to be symptomatic. Ann Neurol 1992;32:795–798.
137. Ward, CD. Does selegiline delay progression of Parkinson's disease? A critical re-evaluation of the DATATOP study. J Neurol Neurosurg Psychiatry 1994;57:217–220.
138. Maki-Ikola, O, Heinonen E. Study design problems of DATATOP study analysis. Ann Neurol 1996;40:946–948.
139. Eisler, T, Teravainen H, Nelson R, et al.: Deprenyl in Parkinson disease. Neurology 1981;31:19–23.
140. Impact of deprenyl and tocopherol treatment on Parkinson's disease in DATATOP subjects not requiring levodopa. Parkinson Study Group. Ann Neurol 1996;39: 29–36.
141. Akao, Y, Maruyama W, Yi H, et al. An anti-Parkinson's disease drug, N-propargyl-1(R)-aminoindan (rasagiline), enhances expression of anti-apoptotic bcl-2 in human dopaminergic SH-SY5Y cells. Neurosci Lett 2002;326:105–108.
142. Heikkila, RE, Duvoisin RC, Finberg JP, et al. Prevention of MPTP-induced neurotoxicity by AGN-1133 and AGN-1135, selective inhibitors of monoamine oxidase-B. Eur J Pharmacol 1985;116:313–317.
143. Maruyama, W, Akao Y, Carrillo MC, et al. Neuroprotection by propargylamines in Parkinson's disease: Suppression of apoptosis and induction of prosurvival genes. Neurotoxicol Teratol 2002;24:675–682.
144. A controlled, randomized, delayed-start study of rasagiline in early Parkinson disease. Arch Neurol 2004;61: 561–566.
145. Olanow CW, Rascol O, Hauser R, et al. A double-blind, delayed-start trial of rasagiline in Parkinson's disease for the ADAGIO Study Investigators. N Engl J Med 2009;361:1268–1278.
146. Beal, MF, Matthews RT, Tieleman A, et al. Coenzyme Q10 attenuates the 1-methyl-4-phenyl-1,2,3,tetrahydropyridine (MPTP) induced loss of striatal dopamine and dopaminergic axons in aged mice. Brain Res 1998;783: 109–114.
147. Shults, CW, Oakes D, Kieburtz K, et al. Effects of coenzyme Q10 in early Parkinson disease: Evidence of slowing of the functional decline. Arch Neurol 2002;59:1541–1550.
148. A randomized clinical trial of coenzyme Q10 and GPI-1485 in early Parkinson disease. The NINDS NET-PD Investigators. Neurology 2007;68:20–28.
149. Elm, JJ, Goetz CG, Ravina B, et al. A responsive outcome for Parkinson's disease neuroprotection futility studies. Ann Neurol 2005;57:197–203.
150. Schwid, SR, Cutter GR. Futility studies: Spending a little to save a lot. Neurology 2006;66:626–627.

151. Tilley, BC, Palesch YY, Kieburtz K, et al. Optimizing the ongoing search for new treatments for Parkinson disease: Using futility designs. Neurology 2006;66:628–633.
152. Matthews, RT, Ferrante RJ, Klivenyi P, et al. Creatine and cyclocreatine attenuate MPTP neurotoxicity. Exp Neurol 1999;157:142–149.
153. Bender, A, Koch W, Elstner M, et al. Creatine supplementation in Parkinson disease: A placebo-controlled randomized pilot trial. Neurology 2006;67:1262–1264.
154. Andringa, G, Eshuis S, Perentes E, et al. TCH346 prevents motor symptoms and loss of striatal FDOPA uptake in bilaterally MPTP-treated primates. Neurobiol Dis 2003;14:205–217.
155. Andringa, G, van Oosten RV, Unger W, et al. Systemic administration of the propargylamine CGP 3466B prevents behavioural and morphological deficits in rats with 6-hydroxydopamine-induced lesions in the substantia nigra. Eur J Neurosci 2000;12:3033–3043.
156. Saporito, MS, Brown EM, Miller MS, et al. CEP-1347/KT-7515, an inhibitor of c-jun N-terminal kinase activation, attenuates the 1-methyl-4-phenyl tetrahydropyridine-mediated loss of nigrostriatal dopaminergic neurons In vivo. J Pharmacol Exp Ther 1999;288:421–427.
157. Mathiasen, JR, McKenna BA, Saporito MS, et al. Inhibition of mixed lineage kinase 3 attenuates MPP+-induced neurotoxicity in SH-SY5Y cells. Brain Res 2004;1003: 86–97.
158. Lotharius, J, Falsig J, van Beek J, et al. Progressive degeneration of human mesencephalic neuron-derived cells triggered by dopamine-dependent oxidative stress is dependent on the mixed-lineage kinase pathway. J Neurosci 2005;25:6329–6342.
159. Wang, LH, Johnson EM, Jr. Mixed lineage kinase inhibitor cep- 1347 fails to delay disability in early Parkinson disease. Neurology 2008;71:462; author reply 462–463.
160. Ramaker, C, Marinus J, Stiggelbout AM, et al. Systematic evaluation of rating scales for impairment and disability in Parkinson's disease. Mov Disord 2002;17:867–876.
161. The Unified Parkinson's Disease Rating Scale (UPDRS). Status and recommendations. Mov Disord 2003;18: 738–750.
162. Martinez-Martin, P, Gil-Nagel A, Gracia LM, et al. Unified Parkinson's Disease Rating Scale characteristics and structure. The Cooperative Multicentric Group. Mov Disord 1994;9:76–83.
163. Richards, M, Marder K, Cote L, et al. Interrater reliability of the Unified Parkinson's Disease Rating Scale motor examination. Mov Disord 1994;9:89–91.
164. Goetz, CG, Fahn S, Martinez-Martin P, et al. Movement Disorder Society-sponsored revision of the Unified Parkinson's Disease Rating Scale (MDS-UPDRS): Process, format, and clinimetric testing plan. Mov Disord 2007; 22:41–47.
165. Kieburtz, K. Issues in neuroprotection clinical trials in Parkinson's disease. Neurology 2006;66:S50–S57.
166. Hauser, RA, Zesiewicz TA. Clinical trials aimed at detecting neuroprotection in Parkinson's disease. Neurology 2006;66:S58–S68.
167. Siderowf, A, Stern M. Clinical trials with rasagiline: evidence for short-term and long-term effects. Neurology 2006;66:S80–S88.
168. Morrish, PK, Rakshi JS, Bailey DL, et al. Measuring the rate of progression and estimating the preclinical period of Parkinson's disease with [18F]dopa PET. J Neurol Neurosurg Psychiatry 1998;64:314–319.
169. Marek, K, Innis R, van Dyck C, et al. [123I]beta-CIT SPECT imaging assessment of the rate of Parkinson's disease progression. Neurology 2001;57:2089–2094
170. Betarbet, R, Sherer TB, Greenamyre JT. Animal models of Parkinson's disease. Bioessays 2002;24:308–318.
171. Hung, AY, Schwarzschild MA. Clinical trials for neuroprotection in Parkinson's disease: Overcoming angst and futility? Curr Opin Neurol 2007;20:477–483.
172. Brooks, AI, Chadwick CA, Gelbard HA, et al. Paraquat elicited neurobehavioral syndrome caused by dopaminergic neuron loss. Brain Res 1999;823:1–10.
173. Hashimoto, M, Rockenstein E, Masliah E. Transgenic models of alpha-synuclein pathology: Past, present, and future. Ann N Y Acad Sci 2003;991:171–188.
174. Maries, E, Dass B, Collier TJ, et al. The role of alpha-synuclein in Parkinson's disease: insights from animal models. Nat Rev Neurosci 2003;4:727–738.
175. van der Putten, H, Wiederhold KH, Probst A, et al. Neuropathology in mice expressing human alpha-synuclein. J Neurosci 2000;20:6021–6029.
176. Kirik, D, Annett LE, Burger C, et al. Nigrostriatal alpha-synucleinopathy induced by viral vector-mediated overexpression of human alpha-synuclein: a new primate model of Parkinson's disease. Proc Natl Acad Sci U S A 2003;100:2884–2889.
177. Kirik, D, Rosenblad C, Burger C, et al. Parkinson-like neurodegeneration induced by targeted overexpression of alpha-synuclein in the nigrostriatal system. J Neurosci 2002;22:2780–2791.
178. Lo Bianco, C, Ridet JL, Schneider BL, et al. Alpha-Synucleinopathy and selective dopaminergic neuron loss in a rat lentiviral-based model of Parkinson's disease. Proc Natl Acad Sci U S A 2002;99:10813–10818.
179. Lohmann, E, Periquet M, Bonifati V, et al. How much phenotypic variation can be attributed to parkin genotype? Ann Neurol 2003;54:176–185.
180. Lucking, CB, Durr A, Bonifati V, et al. Association between early-onset Parkinson's disease and mutations in the parkin gene. N Engl J Med 2000;342:1560–1567.
181. Deng, H, Le W, Guo Y, et al. Genetic and clinical identification of Parkinson's disease patients with LRRK2 G2019S mutation. Ann Neurol 2005;57:933–934.
182. Gilks, WP, Abou-Sleiman PM, Gandhi S, et al. A common LRRK2 mutation in idiopathic Parkinson's disease. Lancet 2005;365:415–416.
183. Kachergus, J, Mata IF, Hulihan M, et al. Identification of a novel LRRK2 mutation linked to autosomal dominant parkinsonism: Evidence of a common founder across European populations. Am J Hum Genet 2005;76:672–680.
184. Healy, DG, Falchi M, O'Sullivan SS, et al. Phenotype, genotype, and worldwide genetic penetrance of LRRK2-associated Parkinson's disease: a case-control study. Lancet Neurol 2008;7:583–590.
185. Riederer, P, Wuketich S. Time course of nigrostriatal degeneration in parkinson's disease. A detailed study of influential factors in human brain amine analysis. J Neural Transm 1976;38:277–301.

186. Tissingh, G, Bergmans P, Booij J, et al. Drug-naive patients with Parkinson's disease in Hoehn and Yahr stages I and II show a bilateral decrease in striatal dopamine transporters as revealed by [123I]beta-CIT SPECT. J Neurol 1998;245:14–20.
187. Tissingh, G, Booij J, Bergmans P, et al. Iodine-123-N-omega-fluoropropyl-2beta-carbomethoxy-3beta-(4-iod ophenyl)tropane SPECT in healthy controls and early-stage, drug-naive Parkinson's disease. J Nucl Med 1998;39:1143–1148.
188. Tolosa, E, Compta Y, Gaig C. The premotor phase of Parkinson's disease. Parkinsonism Relat Disord 2007;13(suppl):S2–S7.
189. Ravina, BM, Fagan SC, Hart RG, et al. Neuroprotective agents for clinical trials in Parkinson's disease: A systematic assessment. Neurology 2003;60:1234–1240.
190. Ross, GW, Abbott RD, Petrovitch H, et al. Association of coffee and caffeine intake with the risk of Parkinson disease. JAMA 2000;283:2674–2679.
191. Ascherio, A, Zhang SM, Hernan MA, et al. Prospective study of caffeine consumption and risk of Parkinson's disease in men and women. Ann Neurol 2001;50:56–63.
192. Schwarzschild, MA, Agnati L, Fuxe K, et al. Targeting adenosine A2A receptors in Parkinson's disease. Trends Neurosci 2006;29:647–654.
193. Ferre, S, Fuxe K. Dopamine denervation leads to an increase in the intramembrane interaction between adenosine A2 and dopamine D2 receptors in the neostriatum. Brain Res 1992;594:124–130.
194. Ferre, S, O'Connor WT, Fuxe K, et al. The striopallidal neuron: A main locus for adenosine-dopamine interactions in the brain. J Neurosci 1993;13:5402–5406.
195. Bara-Jimenez, W, Sherzai A, Dimitrova T, et al. Adenosine A(2A) receptor antagonist treatment of Parkinson's disease. Neurology 2003;61:293–296.
196. Hauser, RA, Hubble JP, Truong DD. Randomized trial of the adenosine A(2A) receptor antagonist istradefylline in advanced PD. Neurology 2003;61:297–303.
197. Chen, JF, Xu K, Petzer JP, et al. Neuroprotection by caffeine and A(2A) .adenosine receptor inactivation in a model of Parkinson's disease. J Neurosci 2001;21: RC143.
198. Ikeda, K, Kurokawa M, Aoyama S, et al. Neuroprotection by adenosine A2A receptor blockade in experimental models of Parkinson's disease. J Neurochem 2002;80: 262–270.
199. Phillis, JW. The effects of selective A1 and A2a adenosine receptor antagonists on cerebral ischemic injury in the gerbil. Brain Res 1995;705:79–84.
200. Jones, PA, Smith RA, Stone TW. Protection against hippocampal kainate excitotoxicity by intracerebral administration of an adenosine A2A receptor antagonist. Brain Res 1998;800:328–335.
201. Monopoli, A, Lozza G, Forlani A, et al. Blockade of adenosine A2A receptors by SCH 58261 results in neuroprotective effects in cerebral ischaemia in rats. Neuroreport 1998;9:3955–3959.
202. Selley, ML. Simvastatin prevents 1-methyl-4-phenyl-1,2,3,6-tetrahydropyridine-induced striatal dopamine depletion and protein tyrosine nitration in mice. Brain Res 2005;1037:1–6.
203. Di Napoli, P, Taccardi AA, Oliver M, et al. Statins and stroke: evidence for cholesterol-independent effects. Eur Heart J 2002;23:1908–1921.
204. de Lau, LM, Koudstaal PJ, Hofman A, et al. Serum cholesterol levels and the risk of Parkinson's disease. Am J Epidemiol 2006;164:998–1002.
205. Huang, X, Chen H, Miller WC, et al. Lower low-density lipoprotein cholesterol levels are associated with Parkinson's disease. Mov Disord 2007;22:377–381.
206. Tikka, T, Fiebich BL, Goldsteins G, et al. Minocycline, a tetracycline derivative, is neuroprotective against excitotoxicity by inhibiting activation and proliferation of microglia. J Neurosci 2001;21:2580–2588.
207. Tikka, TM, Koistinaho JE. Minocycline provides neuroprotection against N-methyl-D-aspartate neurotoxicity by inhibiting microglia. J Immunol 2001;166:7527–7533.
208. Du, Y, Ma Z, Lin S, et al. Minocycline prevents nigrostriatal dopaminergic neurodegeneration in the MPTP model of Parkinson's disease. Proc Natl Acad Sci U S A 2001;98:14669–14674.
209. Wu, DC, Jackson-Lewis V, Vila M, et al. Blockade of microglial activation is neuroprotective in the 1-methyl-4-phenyl-1,2,3,6-tetrahydropyridine mouse model of Parkinson disease. J Neurosci 2002;22:1763–1771.
210. He, Y, Appel S, Le W. Minocycline inhibits microglial activation and protects nigral cells after 6-hydroxydopamine injection into mouse striatum. Brain Res 2001;909: 187–193.
211. Ames, BN, Cathcart R, Schwiers E, et al. Uric acid provides an antioxidant defense in humans against oxidant- and radical-caused aging and cancer: a hypothesis. Proc Natl Acad Sci U S A 1981;78:6858–6862.
212. Davis, JW, Grandinetti A, Waslien CI, et al. Observations on serum uric acid levels and the risk of idiopathic Parkinson's disease. Am J Epidemiol 1996;144:480–484.
213. de Lau, LM, Koudstaal PJ, Hofman A, et al. Serum uric acid levels and the risk of Parkinson disease. Ann Neurol 2005;58:797–800.
214. Weisskopf, MG, O'Reilly E, Chen H, et al. Plasma urate and risk of Parkinson's disease. Am J Epidemiol 2007;166:561–567.
215. Alonso, A, Rodriguez LA, Logroscino G, et al. Gout and risk of Parkinson disease: a prospective study. Neurology 2007;69:1696–1700.
216. Schwarzschild, MA, Schwid SR, Marek K, et al. Serum urate as a predictor of clinical and radiographic progression in Parkinson disease. Arch Neurol 2008;65:716–723.
217. Duan, W, Ladenheim B, Cutler RG, et al. Dietary folate deficiency and elevated homocysteine levels endanger dopaminergic neurons in models of Parkinson's disease. J Neurochem 2002;80:101–110.
218. Gao, X, Chen H, Choi HK, et al. Diet, urate, and Parkinson's disease risk in men. Am J Epidemiol 2008;167: 831–838.
219. Haywood, AF, Staveley BE. Parkin counteracts symptoms in a Drosophila model of Parkinson's disease. BMC Neurosci 2004;5:14.
220. Lo Bianco, C, Schneider BL, Bauer M, et al. Lentiviral vector delivery of parkin prevents dopaminergic degeneration in an alpha-synuclein rat model of Parkinson's disease. Proc Natl Acad Sci U S A 2004;101:17510–17515.

221. Yamada, M, Mizuno Y, Mochizuki H. Parkin gene therapy for alpha-synucleinopathy: A rat model of Parkinson's disease. Hum Gene Ther 2005;16:262–270.
222. Qiao, L, Hamamichi S, Caldwell KA, et al. A neuroprotective role of lysosomal enzyme cathepsin D against a-synuclein pathogenesis. Movement Disorders 2008;23:S8.
223. Masliah, E, Rockenstein E, Adame A, et al. Effects of alpha-synuclein immunization in a mouse model of Parkinson's disease. Neuron 2005;46:857–868.
224. Bodles, AM, El-Agnaf OM, Greer B, et al. Inhibition of fibril formation and toxicity of a fragment of alpha-synuclein by an N-methylated peptide analogue. Neurosci Lett 2004;359:89–93.
225. El-Agnaf, OM, Paleologou KE, Greer B, et al. A strategy for designing inhibitors of alpha-synuclein aggregation and toxicity as a novel treatment for Parkinson's disease and related disorders. FASEB J 2004;18:1315–1317.
226. Amer, DA, Irvine GB, El-Agnaf OM. Inhibitors of alpha-synuclein oligomerization and toxicity: A future therapeutic strategy for Parkinson's disease and related disorders. Exp Brain Res 2006;173:223–233.
227. Lesage, S, Durr A, Tazir M, et al. LRRK2 G2019S as a cause of Parkinson's disease in North African Arabs. N Engl J Med 2006;354:422–423.
228. Lesage, S, Ibanez P, Lohmann E, et al. G2019S LRRK2 mutation in French and North African families with Parkinson's disease. Ann Neurol 2005;58:784–787.
229. Ozelius, LJ, Senthil G, Saunders-Pullman R, et al. LRRK2 G2019S as a cause of Parkinson's disease in Ashkenazi Jews. N Engl J Med 2006;354:424–425.
230. Hulihan, MM, Ishihara-Paul L, Kachergus J, et al. LRRK2 Gly2019Ser penetrance in Arab-Berber patients from Tunisia: A case-control genetic study. Lancet Neurol 2008;7:591–594.
231. West, AB, Moore DJ, Biskup S, et al. Parkinson's disease-associated mutations in leucine-rich repeat kinase 2 augment kinase activity. Proc Natl Acad Sci U S A 2005;102:16842–16847.
232. Greggio, E, Jain S, Kingsbury A, et al. Kinase activity is required for the toxic effects of mutant LRRK2/dardarin. Neurobiol Dis 2006;23:329–341.
233. West, AB, Moore DJ, Choi C, et al. Parkinson's disease-associated mutations in LRRK2 link enhanced GTP-binding and kinase activities to neuronal toxicity. Hum Mol Genet 2007;16:223–232.

CHAPTER 15

Pharmacological Treatment of Parkinson's Disease

Werner Poewe and Cht P Mahlkne

▶ INTRODUCTION

The first empirical attempts of a pharmacological treatment of Parkinson's disease (PD) were made in the 1860s by Ordenstein and Charcot in Paris by using extracts from *Hyscyamus niger*, *Atropia belladonna,* and *Datura stramonium* containing the anticholinergic compounds hyoscine and scopolamine.[1,2] With the development of synthetic anticholinergic drugs in the 1940s[3] these agents became the mainstay of antiparkinsonian drug treatment. However, while improving tremor and rigidity, they had little effect on akinesia.[4]

The classical experiments on reserpinized animals by Carlsson in 1957, which showed that the akinesia of catecholamine-depleted animals could be reversed by levodopa (L-dopa) administration,[5] led to the hypothesis of a dopaminergic disorder as the pathophysiological basis of PD. Shortly afterwards, the finding in postmortem studies of dopamine deficiency in the striatum of PD patients, by Ehringer and Hornykiewicz in Vienna in 1960,[6] and the observation of reduced dopamine excretion in the urine of PD patients, by Barbeau and colleagues,[7] marked the beginning of a new "era" in the treatment of PD. In 1961, two groups in Vienna and Montreal independently reported positive results of open-label small-scale clinical trials with L-dopa in parkinsonian patients.[8,9] Five years later, Cotzias and colleagues demonstrated striking efficacy of high-dose oral L-dopa,[10] the potentiation of its effects and the improvement of side effects with coadministration of peripheral dopa decarboxylase inhibitors (DCIs),[11] as well as the long-term side effects of L-dopa treatment.[12]

Until today L-dopa substitution has remained the gold standard of antiparkinsonian drug therapy, although important advances have been made, including the introduction of directly acting dopamine agonists and MAO-B inhibitors. L-dopa treatment of PD, however, has also introduced new therapeutic challenges such as response fluctuations and drug-induced dyskinesias, which have not only prompted the continuing development of novel pharmacokinetic formulations and delivery systems for L-dopa itself but also focussed drug development efforts on nondopaminergic systems. Finally, the progression of PD is associated with a plethora of nonmotor symptoms, which can make advanced PD one of the most complex therapeutic scenarios in neurology.

This chapter first summarizes medical treatment options to control motor symptoms both in early and in advanced disease and will then move on to describe the pharmacological management of the most common nonmotor problems of this illness.

▶ SECTION 1: MEDICAL MANAGEMENT OF THE MOTOR SYMPTOMS OF PD

This section reviews the most commonly used drugs to treat the motor symptoms of PD both for initial monotherapy in early PD and for the management of L-dopa-related motor complications in advanced PD. For each stage, drugs are reviewed by class of agents. For each drug, a brief synopsis of its pharmacology and mechanism of action is followed by a summary of the available evidence for efficacy from controlled clinical trials, a review of safety data, closing with recommendations for clinical use by North American and European guidelines.

PHARMACOLOGICAL TREATMENT OF EARLY PD

The decision when and how to initiate pharmacotherapy in early PD is very much an individualized decision, taking into account factors of drug efficacy, safety, and ease of use, but also patient needs and perceptions. In the past, many physicians have adopted a strategy to withhold pharmacotherapy until symptoms had become sufficiently severe to impact significantly on a patient's daily performance. There is increasing evidence,

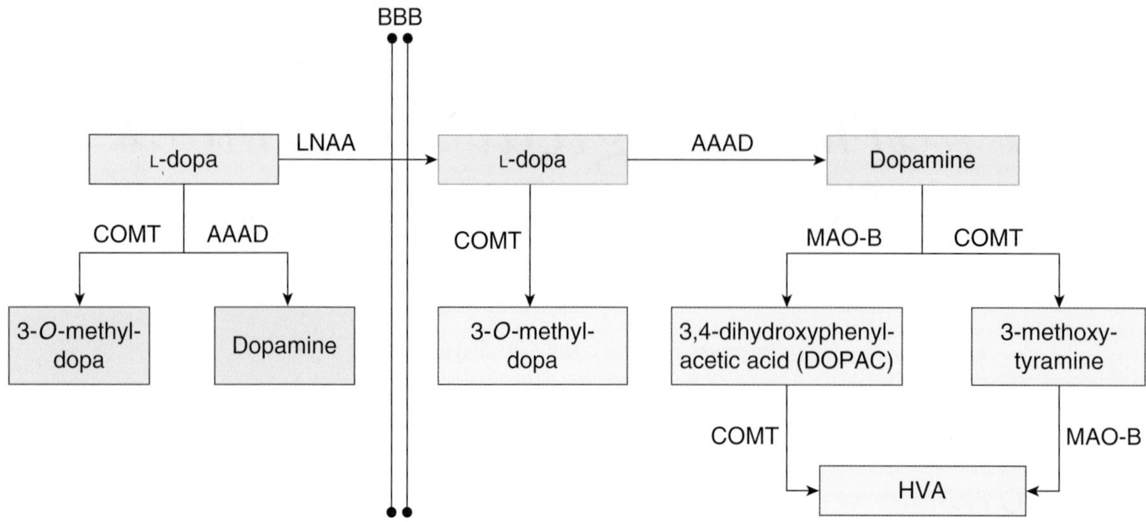

Figure 15–1. Schematic diagram of the two major avenues of enzymatic handling of L-dopa. *Abbreviations:* AAAD, aromatic amino acid decarboxylase; BBB, blood–brain barrier; COMT, catechol-*O*-methyltransferase; HVA, homovanillic acid; LNAA, large neutral amino acid transport system; MAO, monoamine oxidase.

however, that early initiation of drug treatment may be beneficial as compared with delayed therapy. Which agent to choose again depends on data on efficacy and safety as well as patient needs and preferences. For most drugs, there is sufficient evidence from clinical trials and many years of clinical use to give physicians a sound basis for making rational choices.

L-Dopa

Basic Pharmacology and Mechanisms of Action

L-dopa is absorbed in the gastrointestinal tract at the level of the small bowel, utilizing the large neutral amino acid (LNAA) transport system. L-dopa is then rapidly distributed into other tissues, mainly muscle, with a half-life of 5–10 minutes. It crosses the blood–brain barrier via LNAA, competing with the normal concentration of plasma amino acids. Peripherally, L-dopa is rapidly catabolized by aromatic amino acid decarboxylase (AADC) and catechol-*O*-methyltransferase (COMT) (Fig. 15–1) and eliminated from plasma with a half-life of approximately 60–90 minutes (Table 15–1). The amount of L-dopa that eventually reaches the brain following ingestion of an oral dose is dependent on a number of variables that may interfere with absorption and transport of the drug.[13,14] The speed of gastric emptying is crucial for the time interval to reach plasma levels as absorption sites for L-dopa are in the intestinal wall. Food may delay gastric transit time, and in case of protein-rich meals, competition between L-dopa and dietary LNAA for transmucosal transport further contributes to erratic intestinal absorption. L-dopa versus LNAA transport competition may also significantly reduce the amount of plasma L-dopa crossing the endothelial blood–brain barrier.[15,16] The stomach mucosa, as well as the bowel and the liver, is rich in AADC and COMT. Those enzymes convert L-dopa into dopamine and *O*-methyldopa, reducing the bioavailability of L-dopa.[17,18] For this reason commonly used L-dopa preparations contain

TABLE 15–1. L-DOPA PHARMACOKINETIC PARAMETERS: SUMMARY OF HUMAN STUDIES

Study	Apparent Volume of Distribution	Plasma Clearance	$T_{1/2}\alpha$	$T_{1/2}\beta$
Hardie et al. 1986	83.1 L	36.2 L/hr	5.5 min	1.6 hr
Sasahara et al. 1980	87.8 L	96.6 L/hr	–	0.6 hr
Fabbrini et al. 1987	0.26 L/kg	0.13 L/hr	–	1.4 hr
Nutt et al. 1985	0.67 L/kg	0.3 L/hr	–	1.4 hr
Poewe et al. (unpublished data)	3 L/kg	1.4 L/hr	5.4 min	1.5 hr

▶ TABLE 15–2. RESULTS OF THE MAIN TRIALS OF LEVODOPA VERSUS DOPAMINE AGONISTS IN EARLY PD

Results of the Main Trials of Levodopa versus Dopamine Agonists in Early Parkinson's DiseaseTrial [Ref]	Duration (Years)	Number On		ΔUPDRS Part III Score or % of Baseline		Dyskinesia (% of Patients)		Wearing-Off (% of Patients)	
		L-Dopa	Agonist	L-Dopa	Agonist	L-Dopa	Agonist	L-Dopa	Agonist
L-Dopa vs Ropinirole [27]	5	89	179	−4.8 ± 8.3	−0.8 ± 10.1	45	20	34	23
L-Dopa vs Pramipexole [28]	2	151	150	−7.3 ± 8.6	−3.4 ± 8.6	30.7	9.9	38.0	23.8
L-Dopa vs Pergolide [30]	3	146	148	−2.8 ± 7.8	2.8 ± 9.8	26.0	8.2	43.8*	30.6*
L-Dopa vs Cabergoline [26]	4	204	208	−30.0%	−22.5%	13.7	5.8	18.6	12.0

ΔUPDRS = Change in Unified Parkinson's Disease Rating Scale.
* Frequency of motor complications (fluctuations plus dyskinesia).

inhibitors of the peripheral AADC (benserazide or carbidopa),.[19,20] and more recently, inhibitors of COMT have been introduced into clinical practice.

Coadministration of peripherally acting AADC inhibitors doubles the bioavailability of L-dopa without significant effects on elimination half-life.[18] Consequently, therapeutically effective L-dopa doses are much lower when admininistered in combination with DCI and the incidence of peripheral side effects such as nausea, vomiting, and hypotension is markedly reduced. Inhibition of COMT is associated with an increase in the plasma half-life of L-dopa and an increase in bioavailability without significant changes in maximal plasma concentrations following a dose (C_{max}) or the time to peak plasma levels (T_{max}).[21,22]

The exact central mechanisms of L-dopa action are disputed. The classical hypothesis assumes that L-dopa is taken up by residual dopaminergic neurons, decarboxylated by AADC in these surviving cells, and finally synaptically released.[23] According to this hypothesis, there should be a continuous loss of L-dopa efficacy with disease duration, which is clearly not observed in most PD patients. This suggests alternative mechanisms of presynaptic handling of L-dopa, but the exact site of decarboxylation of exogenous L-dopa to dopamine remains unknown.[24]

Evidence for Efficacy from Clinical Trials

The clinical efficacy of L-dopa in reducing the motor symptoms of PD is established by more than 40 years of clinical use. Curiously, the first large placebo-controlled randomized trial of L-dopa monotherapy was only performed recently and confirmed the pronounced potential of L-dopa to reduce motor scores on the UPDRS in a dose-dependent fashion.[25] In addition, several randomized controlled trials have compared the efficacy of various ergolinic and nonergolinic dopamine agonists (see "Dopamine Agonists") with L-dopa as initial monotherapy for PD. (See Refs. Cabergoline,[26] Ropinirole,[27] Pramipexole,[28,29] Pergolide[30].) These trials have consistently shown superior symptomatic efficacy of L-dopa compared with dopamine agonists (Table 15–2).

Tolerability and Safety

Despite coadministration of AADC some patients initially experience nausea and vomiting when L-dopa treatment is started. Most patients, however, develop tolerance to these side effects within days. In severe cases, they may be controlled outside the United States by coadministration of domperidone (10–20 mg) 1 hour before dosing. The same is true for postural hypotension induced by L-dopa.[31] Sedation and daytime sleepiness is another common and occasionally dose-limiting side effect of L-dopa. Although randomized controlled comparative trials of L-dopa versus various dopamine agonists suggest a decreased incidence of this side effect with L-dopa compared with dopamine agonists, attacks of irresistible sleep following L-dopa doses have been occasionally described.[32] In addition, L-dopa is known to trigger a variety of psychiatric symptoms, including illusions, hallucinations, and paranoid psychosis. Rarely, high-dose L-dopa treatment—particularly in patients with young-onset PD—may cause behavioral abnormalities including compulsive medication overuse, drug hoarding, associated with marked neglect of occupational and social responsibilities and relations (dopamine dysregulation syndrome).[33] Affected patients may perform continuous, purposeless, non-goal-oriented repetitive behaviors, frequently related to a patients' premorbid occupational habits or interests and hobbies ("PUNDING").[34] Impulse control disorders such as pathological gambling, hypersexuality, or binge eating are rare with L-dopa monotherapy as opposed to treatment with dopamine agonists.[35]

There have been concerns that L-dopa via its oxidative metabolism might further induce oxidative stress in nigral neurons, thereby enhancing neuronal cell death and ultimately progression of PD.[36] However, evidence from in vitro and in vivo studies of potential L-dopa toxicity has been conflicting showing both neurotoxicity and neuroprotection.[37] Likewise, after more than 30 years of extensive use in PD, there is no clinical indication of deleterious effects of L-dopa treatment on the progression of PD. A recent placebo-controlled 9 months trial of early L-dopa monotherapy, on the contrary, has found sustained beneficial effects on symptomatic scores even after prolonged washout.[25]

A majority of patients eventually develop a variety of motor complications in response to sustained treatment with oral L-dopa . These include oscillations in motor performance and drug-induced dyskinesias affecting about one-third of patients of nearly 2 years of exposure,[28] increasing to more than 50% after 5–6 years[38,39] (see Medical Management of the Nonmotor Symptoms of PD).

Practical Recommendations

Despite of all recent developments L-dopa continues to be the gold standard of symptomatic efficacy in the treatment of PD. Still, there is consensus through most international guidelines[40–42] to initiate dopaminergic monotherapy in early PD with dopamine agonists or in cases with mild symptoms also with a MAO-B-inhibitor to delay the occurrence of L-dopa-related motor complications. This is particularly the case for patients with younger age at onset because of their increased risks to develop L-dopa-induced dyskinesias. Most patients initiated on MAO-B-inhibitors or dopamine agonists monotherapy will, however, require adjunct L-dopa to maintain symptomatic control with disease progression. Patients older than 70 years continue to be candidates for first-line L-dopa monotherapy because of their reduced risk of developing disabling motor complications. L-dopa should also be used in those patients started on dopamine agonists who develop serious side effects, in particular sleep attacks and impulse dyscontrol, regardless of their age.

Dopamine Agonists

Dopamine agonists were first introduced in the 1970s, when Cahne and colleagues reported on the efficacy of bromocryptine as adjunct to L-dopa.[43,44] Over the past decades multiple new agents of this class have entered in clinical practice.

Basic Pharmacology and Mechanisms of Action

Dopamine agonists share the capacity to directly stimulate brain dopamine receptors. The first generation of dopamine agonists were all ergot derivatives, including bromocryptine, cabergoline, dihydroergocriptine, lisuride, and pergolide. Although more than 50 years have passed since the nonergot agonist apomorphine was first reported to exert strong antiparkinsonian effects,[3,45] most of the currently used nonergot dopamine agonists have entered the clinic more recently and include pramipexole, ropinirole, rotigotine, and piribedil. The pharmacological profiles of all dopamine agonists differ from that of L-dopa in many ways, offering several theoretical advantages. First, dietary amino acids do not compete with dopamine agonists for absorption from the gut and for crossing of the blood–brain barrier. Second, they do not require metabolic conversion to an active product to exert their pharmacologic effect; therefore, they do not undergo oxidation and do not generate free radicals. Third, all of them have in part a substantial longer half-life than L-dopa, the only exception being apomorphine. Finally, dopamine agonists have differential affinities within the D_1 and D_2 families of dopamine receptors (see Table 15–3).

Some agonists can also be administered via nonoral routes, providing the possibility of continuous delivery: Rotigotine is available as a once-daily transdermal patch formulation;[46,47] apomorphine is used as subcutaneous infusion treatment for patients with refractory response oscillations (see "Dopamine Agonists" below, pages 14–16)[48] or as rescue medication for sudden unpredictable off periods.[49] Orally active extended-release formulations have recently become available for ropinirole[50] and pramipexole.[51,52]

Evidence for Efficacy from Clinical Trials

There is robust evidence for the efficacy of dopamine agonists as monotherapies to control the motor symptoms of early PD patients. Well-designed randomized placebo-controlled trials have established the efficacy of the ergot compounds pergolide,[53] dihydroergocryptine,[54] as well as the nonergolinic agonists pramipexole,[55,56] ropinirole,[57] rotigotine,[46,47] and piribedil.[58] There is weaker evidence for the efficacy of bromocryptine, lisuride, and cabergoline, which have not been tested in placebo-controlled trials in early PD and apomorphine has not been studied as initial monotherapy.[59]

Several randomized controlled trials of dopamine agonists have also tested their comparative efficacy and

▶ **TABLE 15-3. PHARMACOLOGY OF DOPAMINE AGONISTS**

Substance	Dopamine Receptor Interaction**		Interaction with Other Receptors		T/2 (h)	Average Daily Dose (mg)		References
	D_2/D_3	D1	NA	5-HT		Monotherapy	Adjunct to L-Dopa	
Bromocryptine	D_2	–	+	+/–	3–6	25–45	15–25	[321–323]
Lisuride	D_2	–	+	Antag.	2–3	0.8–1.6	0.6–1.2	[324–326]
Pergolide	$D_3 > D_2$	+	+	+	15–24	1.5–5.0	0.75–5	[327–329]
Cabergoline	$D_3 > D_2$	–	+	+	65	2–6	2–4	[26,60]
Dihydroergocryptine*	D_2	+/–	+	+	12–16	60–80	40	[54,330]
Apomorphine*	$D_3 > D_2$	+	–		0.5	–	1.5–6 (s.c. bolus)	[331–333]
Pramipexole	$D_3 > D_2$	–	+/–	–	9–12	0.375–4.5	0.375–4.5	[55,56,195]
Ropinirole	$D_3 > D_2$	–	–	–	6	6–18	6–12	[27,334]
Piribedil	$D_3 > D_2$	–	+/–	–	20	150–300	150	[58,335]
Rotigotine	$D_3 > D_2$	+		–	5–7	4–8	4–16	[46,47,195]

*not available in the United States.
**within D_2 family all agonists have D_3–D_2 affinity ratio of >1 except for lisuride, bromocriptine, and dihydroergocryptine.

tolerability versus L-dopa and consistently found smaller effect sizes on the UPDRS for pergolide, cabergoline, ropinirole, and pramipexole. The primary outcome of these trials, however, was the incidence of motor complications, where pergolid,[30] cabergoline,[26,60] ropinirole,[27] and pramipexole,[28,29] were all superior to L-dopa in reducing the risk for dyskinesias and response oscillations over follow-up periods of 2–5 years (Table 15–2). Longer-term, open-label follow-up in L-dopa controlled studies of pramipexole over 6 years[61] and ropinirole over 10 years[62] have shown maintained reductions in overall dyskinesia rates despite adjunct L-dopa, and similar results have been reported over 14 years in the UK-Parkinson's Disease Research Group (PDRG) bromocriptine trial.[63]

Tolerability and Safety

The acute side effects of dopamine agonists are similar to those observed with L-dopa and include nausea, vomiting, and postural hypotension. These adverse events tend to occur with the initiation of treatment, can be overridden by treatment with domperidone, and tend to abate as tolerance to the drug develops.[64] Discontinuation rates associated with adverse events do not differ between different dopamine agonists and L-dopa in randomized double-blind trials.[59,65] However, compared with L-dopa, dopamine agonists are associated with a higher rate of some central dopaminergic side effects, including hallucinations or paranoid psychosis, excess daytime sleepiness (EDS), and sudden-onset sleep (SOS).[66]

SOS was first reported as a side effect of treatment with pramipexole and ropinirole,[67] but has since been established as a class effect common to all dopamine agonists.[68] In a questionnaire-based survey of a large cohort of patients with PD SOS occurred in 3% of patients on L-dopa monotherapy, in 5% of patients on dopamine agonist monotherapy, and in 7% of patients on combined treatment with L-dopa plus a dopamine agonist, regardless of its type,[69] while the incidence of excessive daytime sleepiness with or without SOS has been between 16 and 51% in different series.[68]

Whereas dopamine dysregulation syndrome and punding have been primarily associated with high-dose L-dopa or continuous subcutaneous apomorphine treatment, impulse control disorders (ICD) seem to be mainly associated with dopamine agonists. ICDs are characterized by a failure to resist an impulse, drive, or temptation to carry out an act that is harmful to oneself or to others.[35] In PD, typical ICD include hypersexuality, gambling, compulsive shopping, and compulsive eating. The lifetime prevalence of impulse dyscontrol is 6% in all patients with PD, and increases to 14–17% in patients on dopamine agonists.[70] Data suggest that risk factors for an ICD may include male sex, younger age, history of substance abuse, and a personality style characterized by impulsiveness or novelty seeking.[71]

Peripheral edema can be induced by all types of dopamine agonists, but data on the incidence in clinical practice are lacking. In a 4-year follow-up survey of a pramipexole-study incidence of leg edema was 45% in patients who were initially randomized to active treatment,[72] but severity was usually mild and discontinuation rates of agonist therapy because of leg edema have been low in clinical trials.[28,61]

The ergolinic agonists pergolide and cabergoline have recently become associated with cardiac valvular fibrosis. In a meta-analysis of heart valve abnormalities in patients with PD treated with dopamine agonists,[73] moderate to severe valvular changes were detected in a quarter of patients treated with pergolide and cabergoline. In contrast, patients treated with nonergot agonists had the same rate of valvular changes as control patients of only 10%. Overall, the severity of ergot-induced vavulopathies tends to correlate with cumulative doses.[74] The mechanisms underlying cardiac valvulopathy induced by cabergoline or pergolide are likely to involve agonism of these two drugs at the 5-HT2B receptor subtype, which is expressed on heart valve leaflets.[75] Consistently no link has been found between lisuride, a 5-HT2B receptor antagonist, and fibrotic cardiac valvulopathy.[76] However, fibrotic reactions are not exclusively related to the heart, but may also include pleuropulmonary fibrosis. On the basis of such findings, the European Medicines Agency has added new warnings and contraindications to the product information of cabergoline and pergolide to reduce the risk of fibrosis.

General Practical Recommendations

Initial monotherapy with a dopamine agonist is an established first-line therapy for early PD by many international guidelines.[40,41] Advantages include good efficacy in controlling motor symptomes and the reduced risk to induce motor complications as compared with L-dopa. In addition, some agonists offer the convenience of once-daily dosing, either via transdermal patches for rotigotine or once-daily extended-release tablets for ropinirole or pramipexole. Disadvantages include the somewhat smaller effects size versus L-dopa and a greater risk for EDS/SOS, ICDs, hallucinosis, and leg edema. The use of ergolinic dopaminergic agonists such as pergolide or cabergoline in early PD monotherapy is no longer recommended because of their poor overall benefit to risk ratio when compared with initial L-dopa monotherapy, based on their additional risk of potentially life-threatening pleuropulmonary or cardiac valvular fibrosis. Whether or not a dopamine agonist should be used as early monotherapy will largely depend on the overall balance of level of symptomatic control required, perceived risk of dyskinesias(for which younger age is a major determinant), and also patient perceptions related to a risk of developing ICDs.

MAO-B Inhibitors

Early attempts to enhance dopaminergic neurotransmission through inhibition of one of dopamine's major metabolizing enzyme—monoamine oxidase (MAO)—were made soon after the discovery of the striatal dopaminergic deficit and the efficacy of L-dopa.[79] However, side effects ("cheese effect") associated with the nonselective type A plus B MAO inhibitors used in those days prevented further use. Meanwhile, selective MAO-B inhibitors such as selegiline and rasagiline have been introduced into clinical practice and a third one, safinamide, is in clinical development.

Basic Pharmacology and Mechanisms of Action

Both selegeline and rasagiline are propargylamine drugs and irreversibly inhibit the MAO-B, an enzyme that oxidatively deaminates dopamine primarily in neuronal glial cells. At the dose commonly given in PD (2 × 5 mg/day for selegiline and 1 × 1 mg/day for rasagiline) they effect a complete and irreversible inhibition of MAO-B, with only minimal effects on MAO-A, an enzyme that deaminates serotonin, noradrenaline, and thyramine mainly in the gut. Inhibition of MAO-B activity remains significant for a week and returns to baseline after 2 weeks.[80,81] Selegiline is metabolized to methamphetamine and to a lesser extent, to amphetamine,[82] which blocks dopamine reuptake and releases dopamine and may account for some of the dopaminergic effects. Rasagiline is even highly potent and does not give rise to amphetamine-like metabolites, but degrades to aminoindan.[83] There is evidence to suggest that selegeline and both rasagiline and aminoindan have neuroprotective properties, whereas methamphetamine may block this effect.[84] Neuroprotection does not occur due to MAO-B inhibition,[85] which is responsible for the symptomatic effect of these substances, but seems to be related to activation of anti-apoptotic *Bcl-2* and protein kinase C (PKC), and down-regulating proapoptotic FAS and Bax.[86]

A new once-daily sublingual formulation of selegeline named zydis selegiline (Zelapar) avoids the first-pass mechanism by being absorbed via the buccal mucosa. Therefore, levels of metabolites (and attributed side effects) are decreased and higher serum and brain concentrations of selegeline are attained.[87]

The new reversible MAO-B inhibitor safinamide has additional effects as an inhibitor of dopamine uptake and glutamate release and is currently studied in a phase III clinical trial program.[88]

Evidence for Efficacy from Clinical Trials

When given as monotherapy to de novo patients with PD selegiline has a small but definitive symptomatic effect according to several placebo-controlled trials—usually with doses of 10 mg/day.[89–92] The majority of these randomized controlled trials conducted with selegiline were designed to assess the potential of selegiline to modify PD progression. Delayed need for L-dopa was mostly demonstrated, but such results are insufficient to prove neuroprotective properties because of selegiline's symptomatic efficacy as evident from "wash-in" effects.[89,92] One study found improved scores after 12 months of selegiline versus placebo treatment added to L-dopa or bromocriptine in de novo patients after an extended 2 months washout period and argued that such effects were more readily explained by neuroprotective than symptomatic properties of selegiline.[93] Overall the evidence available indicates that selegiline delays the progression of the signs and symptoms of PD, but is insufficient to demonstrate neuroprotection through selegiline.[94]

Rasagiline was only recently introduced into clinical practice, and its symptomatic effect in early PD as monotherapy was described in two large randomized placebo-controlled trials. The TEMPO study[95] showed a clear symptomatic "wash-in" effect of rasagiline that persisted over the trial duration. At the 6-month analysis, the effect size for the total UPDRS score was—4 points in favor of the rasagiline group as compared with placebo. Similar results have been recently obserevd for 1 mg of rasagiline after 9 months of treatment in the large, placebo-controlled delayed-start ADAGIO trial.[96] While these effect sizes are smaller than those reported in most placebo-controlled trials of dopamine agonists or L-dopa, around 50% of patients from the TEMPO trial were successfully maintained on rasagiline monotherapy for 2 years.[97]

The TEMPO trial was the first PD study to employ the delayed-start design in order to test for potential disease-modifying efficacy of rasagiline,[95] where after first 6-month study period placebo-treated patients were switched to rasagiline for another 6 months in a double-blind fashion. Differences in the UPDRS outcome after phase II, where all patients received identical treatment with rasagiline, would not be explicable by a pure symptomatic effect and suggest additional disease-modifying effects.[98] TEMPO was positive on this outcome and the recent ADAGIO trial provided additional support for a disease-modifiying effect of rasagiline, with an extended 9 plus 9 months delayed-start trial in a total of more than 1100 patients using a rigorous and sophisticated hierarchical statistical analysis, which included slope analyses of rates of UPDRS decline in both phases of the trial.[96]

Tolerability and Safety

Rasagiline is generally well tolerated. The most frequent adverse events seen during monotherapy with selegiline have been insomnia, nausea, benign cardiac arrhythmias, dizziness, and headache.[99] Insomnia has been linked to selegiline's metabolism via methamphetamine and may occur particularly if doses are given late in the day. Selegiline does not potentiate tyramine-induced hypertension (the cheese effect) at the doses used for the treatment of PD, but coadministration with unselective MAO inhibitors such as moclobemide should be avoided.[99]

Rasagiline was shown to be generally safe and well tolerated,[83] in pivotal trials that found similar incidences of adverse reactions between active treatment and placebo. Like selegiline, rasagiline is free of the cheese-effect, and dietary tyramine restriction is generally not deemed necessary. Only in the United States, patients must still be advised to restrict consumption of foods rich in tyramine such as cheese and red wine. It is not metabolized to amphetamine-like substances, and its major metabolite is aminoindan, which has shown neuroprotective effects in some experimental models.[100] There have been concerns of using MAO-B inhibitors in combination with selective serotonin reuptake inhibitors (SSRIs) because of a risk to induce a serotonine syndrome. Such reactions have been reported for selegiline administered in combination with fluvoxamine and fluoxetine,[101] but were found in only 0.04% of patients receiving combined selegiline and TCAs or SSRIs in a large survey.[102] Clinical trials with rasagiline have included patients on SSRIs (except fluoxetine) and AE rates have not been different from those patients not receiving SSRIs.[103] Nevertheless, physicians should remain vigilant for serotonine syndromelike reactions in patients on combined therapy, since this appears to be a class effect with either MAO-B inhibitor or SSRIs.[104]

Practical Recommendations

Both MAO-B inhibitors are considered first-line options for initial monotherapy of early PD by international guidelines.[40,41,105] Effect sizes are smaller than those reported for dopamine agonists or L-dopa, but a recent long-term follow-up observation of patients entered into the TEMPO trial has shown that around 50% of patients could be sufficiently managed on rasagiline monotherapy for 2 years.[106] Both currently used inhibitors are well tolerated, and rasagiline has the additional benefit of a once-daily drug not requiring titration. Selegiline or rasagiline are therefore perfectly reasonable choices in patients with early disease and mild symptoms.

Although early claims for additional neuroprotective efficacy of selegiline could not be substantiated by clinical trials because of confounding symptomatic effects,[89] there is recent evidence for the disease-modifying potential of rasagiline on the basis of two positive delayed-start trials.[95,96] Although these results have been interpreted with caution, they add another consideration to the use of rasagiline as initial monotherapy.

Amantadine

According to current models of basal ganglia function increased glutamatergic neurotransmission contributes to parkinsonian motor dysfunction at multiple levels. Increased glutamatergic drive from the subthalamic nucleus to the internal pallidum contributes to increased inhibitory pallidal input to the motor thalamus and is therefore involved in the pathophysiology of akinesia.[107] It has also been shown that specific stimulation of either NMDA or non-NMDA glutamate receptors by stereotactic injection in different subcortical targets induces parkinsonian features in rodents in a regionally specific manner.[108] Glutamate antagonists might therefore be expected to reduce parkinsonism. The antiparkinsonian efficacy of the antiviral agent amantadine was first reported in 1969 by Schwab and colleagues.[109]

Basic Pharmacology and Mechanisms of Action

Although amantadine's exact mechanism of action remains uncertain, its NMDA receptor–blocking activity is generally believed to play a major role in producing its antiparkinsonian effcts.[110] In addition, amantadine has been shown to enhance the release of catecholamines from intact dopaminergic terminals and also inhibit catecholamine reuptake.[111] Other studies have suggested effects on dopamine receptors as well as anticholinergic activity.[112] Amantadine hydrochloride produces peak plasma levels 1–4 hours after an oral dose with a clinical duration of action of up to 8 hours.

Evidence for Efficacy from Clinical Trials

Virtually all trials studying symptomatic efficacy of amantadine have been formed in the 1970s and generally do not meet modern standards of trial methodology in PD. Oral treatment with 200–300 mg per day of amantadine has consistently been shown to produce mild to moderate antiparkinsonian effects on all cardinal symptoms in at least two-thirds of patients both as monotherapy or as adjunct to L-dopa in open-label observations.[111] The clinical benefit from amantadine has often been described as transient with about a third of patients showing slight to moderate loss of improvement within the first months of treatment, but some studies have reported sustained benefit for more than a year.[113–116]

Tolerability and Safety

Doses of 100 to 300 mg amantadine per day, given in two or three divided doses, are usually well tolerated. The major route of elimination is via renal clearance of the unmetabolized drug; such patients with renal impairment should receive lower doses, and renal function should be monitored carefully. Most of adverse reactions can be attributed to central effects and are generally mild but may be more severe in elderly patients with cognitive impairment. They include dizziness, nausea and vomiting, anxiety, insomnia, and nervousness. Less than 5% of the patients report headaches, nightmares, depression, ataxia, confusion, somnolence/drowsiness, agitation, and hallucinations. Amantadine is best avoided in patients with cognitive impairment and PD dementia.[111] Occasionally amantadine may cause ankle edema and livedo reticularis for which the underlying mechanism is unclear. Occasional urinary retention and constipation have been related to anticholinergic properties of the drug; combination with anticholinergics should be avoided. Before starting treatment with amantadine, a long QT-interval and bradycardic arrhythmias should be excluded.

Practical Recommendations

Amantadine is a second-line drug for initial monotherapy, but in countries with limited access to more modern and costly PD therapies, it is still commonly used in the routine management of early PD. Amantadine is best used as short-term monotherapy in early patients with mild functional impairment. In most countries, the drug is available as amantadine hydrochloride 100-mg capsules or coated tablets, and in several European countries, amantadine is also available as a liquid formulation of 50 mg/mL as well as a parenteral form for infusions (200 mg/500 mL). The recommended daily oral dose is 200–400 mg.

Anticholinergics

In the 1860s Ordenstein and Charcot were the first to treat (PD) by using extracts from *Hyscyamus niger*, *Atropa belladonna*, and *Datura stramonium*, but without recognizing the principle of cholinergic antagonism underlying their effects. With the development of synthetic anticholinergic drugs anticholinergics became the gold standard for treating PD in the 1940s, followed by a sharp decline after the advent of L-dopa in the 1960s.[117]

Basic Pharmacology and Mechanisms of Action

The precise mechanism of action of anticholinergic drugs in PD is not completely understood. Acetylcholine is released from cholinergic interneurons in the striatum and is a powerful modulator of excitability of striatal projection neurons.[118] Since cholinergic drugs worsen PD symptoms, a disbalance between acetylcholine and dopamine-related striatal neurotransmission with relative cholinergic muscarinic overactivity has been postulated to exist in the parkinsonian striatum. D_2 dopamine receptor stimulation inhibits striatal release of acetylcholine,[119,120] whereas D_1 dopamine receptor stimulation has the opposite effect.[121,122] Cholinergic modulation of striatal neurotransmission involves both muscarinic-[118] and nicotinic receptor-subtypes.[123] Table 15–4 summarizes the most commonly available compounds of this class.

Evidence for Efficacy from Clinical Trials

Similar as for amantadine there are no randomized controlled trials of modern standard available to document the efficacy and safety of anticholinergics as a treatment

TABLE 15-4. COMMONLY AVAILABLE ANTICHOLINERGIC DRUGS

Substance	Recommended Daily Dose
Benzatropine-mesylate	3–6 mg
Biperiden-HCl/lactate	4–8 mg
Trihexyphenidyl-HCl	4–8 mg
Orphenadrine-HCl	150–300 mg
Procyclidine-HCl	10–15 mg

for PD.[124] Overall randomized clinical trials[125] suggest that anticholinergic drugs improve parkinsonian tremor and rigidity, but have little effect on bradykinesia. One small, single-dose L-dopa and apomorphine controlled study has found similar effects on rest tremor amplitude for biperidin as compared with dopaminergic pulses.[126]

Tolerability and Safety

Because of their peripheral antimuscarinic action anticholinergics are contraindicated in narrow-angle glaucoma, tachycardia, prostate hypertrophy, gastrointestinal obstruction, and megacolon. They may cause blurred vision, urinary retention, nausea, constipation, and rarely paralytic ileus. Reduced sweating may interfere with temperature regulation and central anticholinergic activity impairs short-term memory and may interfere with mental function, such that the use of anticholinergics is contraindicated in patients with cognitive decline and dementia.[40] Particularly in the elderly anticholinergics may induce acute confusion and hallucinations. Some reports suggest that anticholinergic treatment has the potential to induce dyskinesias either by itself[127] or exacerbate them in combination with L-dopa.[128,129] The abrupt withdrawal of anticholinergic drugs may induce marked worsening of parkinsonism so that these agents should be discontinued gradually.[130,131]

Practical Recommendations

Although anticholinergics are now only rarely used, they may still be occasionally considered for patients presenting with predominant rest tremor and age below 60, if there is otherwise no need for dopamine replacement. Likewise, there are occasional patients, in whom dopamine replacement, while improving bradykinesia and rigidity, fails to control rest tremor, who will profit from a trial of adjunct anticholinergic treatment. Generally, patients over 60 years of age or those exhibiting clinical signs of cognitive impairment should be excluded from this class of agents. Clinically there is little difference between the various available anticholinergic agents but trihexyphenidyle and benztropine are the two most widely used candidates worldwide. As mentioned earlier, discontinuation should be carried out gradually to avoid a withdrawal syndrome.

Initiating Drug Treatment in Newly Diagnosed PD—Pragmatic Approach

Initiating medical treatment in newly diagnosed patients with PD requires careful counseling and weighing of multiple disease- and patient-related factors that impact when and how to start. The two main themes that generally feature foremost in patients' needs and expectations in this situation are related to symptom control and prevention of emerging or progressive disability—the latter often dominating in those in whom symptoms are still mild and without major consequence on professional or other activities of daily living. Particularly in these latter patients, a common strategy has been to withhold symptomatic therapies until increasing symptom severity begins to have functional impact. This 'wait-and-see' approach was mainly driven by concerns about side effects of medications—such as L-dopa-related motor complications or issues such as somnolence or impulse dyscontrol with dopamine agonists—and the absence of drugs that would unequivocally retard disease progression.

Recently, there is growing belief that initiating symptomatic drug treatment early—as soon as patients have been diagnosed—may offer benefits via correction or prevention of maladaptive functional or neuroplastic responses in the parkinsonian brain.[132] Although this has not been proven scientifically, the recent ADAGIO trial showing potential disease-modifying efficacy of early treatment with the MAO-B inhibitor rasagiline[96] has added another piece of evidence in favor of initiating drug therapy early rather than later in the course of disease. In any case, patients will have to be informed about these emerging developments and the final decision about when to start will be emerging from the interplay between the patient's and the treating physician's beliefs and expectations.

Which drugs to use once a decision to treat has been made will likewise very much depend on individual factors of symptom type and severity, age, as well as cognitive and social (professionally active versus retired) status of the patient, comorbidities, and the risk profile for drug-specific side effect profiles resulting from all these factors. Counseling by the experienced neurologist will be assisted by a growing body of evidence regarding efficacy and safety from well-designed clinical trials and long-term post-marketing data on most agents coming into consideration (see earlier sections—L-Dopa, Dopamine Agonists, MAO Inhibitor).

Table 15–5 presents a summarize of the differential profile of available drug classes for early monotherapy along the pragmatic dimensions of efficacy, safety, and tolerability, long-term complication rates, ease of use, and convenience.

▶ **TABLE 15–5. THE DIFFERENTIAL PROFILES OF THE AVAILABLE DRUG CLASSES FOR EARLY MONOTHERAPY**

Substance Class	L-Dopa	DA-Agonists	MAO-B Inhibitors	Other Medication
Symptomatic efficacy	+++	++	+	E.g., amantadine and anticholinergics:
Acute dopaminergic side effects	++	+	+++	Overall lower level of evidence: slightly efficacious.
Prevention of motor complications		++	+	To be avoided in patients with cognitive decline (and in patients older than 65 years for anticholinergics).
Neuroprotection	+/–	+/–	+	
Convenience	+	++	+++	
Risk profile				
Somnolence	+	++	–	
Hallucinosis	+	++	+/–	
Impulse dyscontrol	+/–	++	–	
Leg edema	–	+	–	
Fibrotic reactions	–	+*	–	

Advantage level: + mild; + + moderate; + + + marked; +/- uncertain.
*For ergolinic DA-agonists with agonism at the 5-HT2B receptor subtype.
(Data from Antonini et al. 2009 and Olanow et al. 2009 [Refs. 70, 42])

PHARMACOLOGICAL TREATMENT OF MOTOR COMPLICATIONS IN ADVANCED DISEASE

Although L-dopa continues to be the single-most effective drug to control the motor symptoms of PD[36] and marked clinical responsiveness to oral L-dopa is one of the diagnostic hallmarks of this disease,[133] its chronic use is associated with the emergence of drug-induced motor complications in a majority of cases.[117] These include motor response oscillations and drug-induced dyskinesias, which may affect more than 10% of patients already during the first year of therapy, around 30 % after 2 years, and 50% or more after treatment duration of more than 5 years.[39,134–137] Risk factors for the development of drug-induced dyskinesias include younger age, treatment duration, and dose and the latter also determine the onset of motor response oscillations.[39] More than 50% of patients with L-dopa-related motor complications develop fluctuations before or simultaneous with dyskinesias.[138] Both types of complications can cause significant disability.

Management of Motor Fluctuations

Initially motor response oscillations are usually related to dose intervals and are characterized by re-emergence of parkinsonian symptoms some 3–4 hours post dosing ("wearing-off-phenomenon"). In addition, patients may begin to experience "delayed-on" phenomena consisting of lag times of more than 30 minutes from oral drug intake until onset of clinical effect.[139] While wearing-off fluctuations are related to L-dopa half-life, delayed-on or complete dose failure ("No-on") has been shown to best correlate with erratic gastric emptying.[140]

A minority of patients progress to develop more malignant and unpredictable "on–off" swings with sudden releases of parkinsonian symptoms without apparent relation to their L-dopa dosing schedule. This latter type of response oscillation has been linked to postsynaptic changes in receptor pharmacodynamics induced by long-term pulsatile stimulation[141] Table 15–6 summarizes the different types of motor response oscillations by their underlying pathophysiology.

L-Dopa-Based Approaches

Adjusting the dosing frequency and interdose intervals of L-dopa to smooth out motor response oscillations is a commonly used approach when wearing-off fluctuations first appear, for example by introducing a fourth daily dose in patients on a t.i.d. regimen. In addition, altering the pharmacokinetics via extended-release preparations

▶ **TABLE 15–6. CLASSIFICATION OF L-DOPA-RELATED MOTOR FLUCTUATIONS IN PD**

Clinical Pattern	Pathophysiology
Wearing-off	L-Dopa–$t_{1/2}$ Presynaptic storage
"Delayed-on"	Gastric emptying Intestinal absorption
Dose failures ("No-on")	Gastric emptying Intestinal absorption BBB-transport
Complex on-off	Striatal pharmacodynamic changes

or the addition of COMT inhibitors has also been shown to reduce off time in such patients. More recently, intrajejunal infusions of L-dopa have become available in the European Union.

L-Dopa Extended-Release Formulations

L-dopa slow-release preparations have been introduced in an attempt to produce prolonged clinical effects from each individual dose and thereby smooth out response oscillations. Two formulations are currently available worldwide (Sinemet CR® [Merck & Co., Inc., Whitehouse station, NJ, USA] and Madopar CR® [Roche Products Ltd., Hertfordshire, UK.]).

Basic Pharmacology and Mechanisms of Action

Sinemet CR is a combination of 200 mg L-dopa and 50 mg carbidopa, imbedded in a slow-eroding matrix.[142,143] A rate-controlled erosion and dissolution take place as the preparation passes along the duodenal–jejunal mucosa. Madopar CR contains 100 mg of L-dopa and 25 mg of benserazide, which upon gastric contact are transformed into a gelatinous diffusion body that floats upon the fluid contents of the stomach.[144] Both these controlled-release preparations cause a delayed onset of peak L-dopa concentrations (T_{max}), a prolonged decline of plasma levels as compared with conventional preparations. Further pharmacokinetic features of L-dopa slow-release preparations include reduced peak plasma levels and decreased bioavailability of about 25% compared with conventional L-dopa formulations.[145]

Evidence for Efficacy from Clinical Trials

There are 10 randomized controlled trials available that have compared L-dopa standard versus slow-release formulations with control motor fluctuations in advanced PD. Results have been inconsistent, not showing significant effects on off time reduction in the slow-release arm in several of them.[146] One trial specifically addressed the effect of Madopar HBS versus standard L-dopa to control nocturnal problems and failed to find significant differences in favor of the slow-release compound.[147]

Three randomized controlled long-term trials have compared standard versus slow-release L-dopa as initial treatment in de novo patients[148–150] with the rate of occurrence of motor fluctuations and dyskinesias after 5 years as their primary endpoint. All three trials failed to detect significant differences in the rate of motor complications observed with either type of initial treatment, thereby failing to show efficacy of slow-release L-dopa regarding prevention of motor complications.

Tolerability and Safety

The side-effect profile of available L-dopa slow-release formulations does not differ from that of standard formulations (see "L-Dopa").

Practical Recommendations

Overall, the use of L-dopa CR formulations is of limited value in reducing motor response fluctuations, often yielding transient and inconsistent improvement.[151,152] The main reasons for failure are lack of predictability of onset of clinical effects and increased peak dose or prolonged biphasic dyskinesias.[153] The delay in T_{max} causes delayed "on" effects particularly after the first morning dose, which may be overcome by combined use of slow-release plus standard L-dopa formulations. The decreased bioavailability of slow-release L-dopa requires greater total daily doses compared with standard preparations.

Alternative L-Dopa Preparations

While L-dopa slow-release preparations and add-on treatment with COMT-inhibitors (see later) are aimed at increasing the half-life of L-dopa, a number of strategies have been used to improve gastrointestinal absorption of L-dopa to overcome onset of dose difficulties. Such formulations include dispersible L-dopa-preparations that have been shown to produce shorter T_{max} and more rapid onset of clinical effects as compared with standard formulations.[154] Dispersible L-dopa is marketed as Madopar LT in several European countries.

Recently a novel dual-release preparation of L-dopa consisting of a three-layer tablet combining immediate-release and slow-release properties has been developed and small-scale open-label studies have reported significantly shorter times to switch on compared with slow-release formulations and a trend to longer on duration.[155] This formulation is currently marketed in some countries in Europe.

COMT Inhibitors

Following continued administration of L-dopa with dopamine-decarboxylase inhibitors the major catabolism of the drug is shifted to conversion to 3-OMD by the action of COMT (Fig. 15–1). Because of its long half-life of approximately 15 hours, 3-OMD accumulates during chronic L-dopa treatment and competes with L-dopa for intestinal absorption and active transport through the blood–brain barrier. COMT inhibition is associated with a significant prolongation of L-dopa terminal half-life of up to 75%, increase in AUC (bioavailability), and avoidance of deep trough levels with multiple daily dosing.[156]

Basic Pharmacology and Mechanisms of Action

Two COMT-inhibitors, tolcapone and entacapone, have been introduced into clinical practice. *Entacapone* acts as a reversible inhibitor of peripheral COMT.[157] with a half-life of approximately 1.5 hours[158] and inhibits erythrocyte COMT activity in a dose-dependent fashion.[159] Clinical pharmacokinetic studies have shown that coadministration of 200 mg of entacapone prolongs the elimination half-life and approximately doubles the bioavailability of L-dopa due to significantly reduced metabolic loss of L-dopa into 3-OMD.[21,22,160–162] Plasma 3-OMD levels from a given dose of L-dopa are reduced by 40–60%. [^{18}F]fluoro-L-dopa PET studies have shown significant increase in striatal signal following coadministration of entacapone.[163,164] With repeated dosing L-dopa peak plasma concentration (C_{max}) is increased over standard L-dopa and average trough levels are also higher, while time to C_{max} (T_{max}) is unchanged.[156] Recently, a triple combination of L-dopa with carbidopa and entacapone (Stalevo) has become available offering the advantage of decreased pill burden when combining L-dopa treatment with entacapone.

Tolcapone has a similar pharmacological profile to entacapone. However, half-life is longer (approximately 3–4 hours), allowing for t.i.d. dosing. High doses of tolcapone may pass the blood–brain barrier in humans and also block central COMT in addition to peripheral blocking effects.

Evidence for Efficacy from Clinical Trials

Both tolcapone and entacapone have been shown to reduce off time and increase on time in L-dopa-treated patients with motor fluctuations. Randomized placebo-controlled trials in patients with wearing-off type of response oscillations have consistently shown increases in on time by between 1 and 2 hours with tolcapone and close to 1 hour with entacapone.[165] Entacapone has also been shown to improve symptomatic control of parkinsonism by enhancing on motor functions in patients with fluctuating PD.[166,167] In addition, both COMT-inhibitors are able to improve symptomatic control in PD patients with a stable response to L-dopa.[168,169] Comparative trials of entacapone and tolcapone have yielded evidence for somewhat greater clinical efficacy of tolcapone in reducing off time in patients with fluctuating PD.[165]

Recently, two large trials have assessed efficacy and safety of the L-dopa/carbidopa/entacapone triple combination in de novo patients with PD. One of these found superior efficacy in reducing UPDRS motor scores when giving 300 mg/t.i.d. of L-dopa with entacapone as compared with the same dose of standard L-dopa/carbidopa. Secondary outcomes included the emergence of wearing-off fluctuations and dyskinesias after 9 months of treatment that were overall very low and not different between the two treatments.[59,97] The large Stalevo reduction in dyskinesia evaluation (STRIDE-PD) trial was designed to specifically address the risk of developing dyskinesia when using L-dopa/carbidopa/entacapone versus L-dopa/carbidopa in either de novo patients or those already on dopamine agonists requiring for the first time adjunct L-dopa. This study has recently been completed and failed to detect benefits in terms of delaying the onset of dyskinesias when prolonging L-dopa half-life by using entacapone. On the contrary, patients in the triple combination arm, particularly those on previous dopamine agonist therapy, had short delays to and greater incidences of dyskinesias compared with L-dopa/carbidopa–presumably reflecting the higher total dopaminergic load due to increasing L-dopa bioavailability.[170]

Tolerability and Safety

Worsening of preexisting L-dopa-induced dyskinesias and nausea are the most common dopaminergic adverse reactions when COMT-inhibitors are added to L-dopa. They are usually transient and can be relieved by reducing the L-dopa dose. Newly emergent dyskinesias or hallucinations are rare. Diarrhea is the most common nondopaminergic side effect of both tolcapone and entacapone, but diarrhea-related withdrawal was somewhat rarer in studies with entacapone compared with tolcapone. Urine discoloration in up to 40% of patients taking entacapone is a clinically irrelevant side effect related to the formulation.

Tolcapone exposure has been associated with liver toxicity, and following published reports on three fatal cases of fulminant liver failure on treatment with tolcapone, the drug was withdrawn from the market in the European Union and labeling was changed in the United States restricting its use to patients for whom there is no alternative treatment and requiring regular monitoring of liver enzymes (every 2–4 weeks for the first 6 months, then by physician judgment with a requirement to stop treatment when transaminase levels exceed the twofold upper limit of normal). Recently, tolcapone has been reintroduced in the European Union as well with still stricter monitoring requirements. No such monitoring is required for entacapone, and to date there have been no cases of fatal liver injury associated with entacapone in postmarketing surveillance. The exact mechanism of liver toxicity of tolcapone is not clear.[171,172]

Practical Recommendations

Adding entacapone to L-dopa or switching from standard L-dopa to Stalevo are first-line options for the drug treatment of motor fluctuations of the wearing-off type. Tolcapone can be used as a second-line option in patients failing entacapone. When adding COMT-inhibitors the total daily dose of L-dopa may have to be reduced, and preemptive dose reductions of approximately 10–20% may be considered in fluctuating patients with bothersome dyskinesias at baseline. The reported dose reductions of L-dopa were generally above 100 mg/day in clinical trials with tolcapone and somewhat lower in studies with entacapone.

Although the use of Stalevo in patients with early PD has been shown to provide greater symptomatic control compared with standard L-dopa, this approach may increase dyskinesia risk, particularly in patients with previous monotherapy with dopamine agonists. In addition, this approach is associated with increased incidence of gastrointestinal side effects such that the use of entacapone is not recommended in patients without motor fluctuations.

L-Dopa Infusions

The efficacy of constant-rate intravenous infusions in reducing motor fluctuations was first shown more than 25 years ago.[173]

Following this, proof-of-concept studies of subsequent trials showed similar effects using intrajejunal delivery of L-dopa via nasogastric tubes.[174,175] Long-term open-label observation in small numbers of patients receiving intraintestinal L-dopa infusions provided additional evidence for reductions in preexisting dyskinesias following a continuous L-dopa delivery.[176] The major limitation of this approach was the poor solubility of L-dopa of approximately 2 mg/mL, whereby requiring the delivery of large fluid volumes in order to meet daily dosing requirements. Recently a new formulation for intraintestinal infusion continuous infusion of L-dopa has been introduced into clinical routine in the European Union (Duodopa).

Basic Pharmacology

The duodopa principle is based on a novel L-dopa formulation insisting of a carboxymethylcellulose gel containing a concentrated suspension of L-dopa/carbidopa (20 mg of L-dopa per mL). A cassette of 100 mL containing 2 g/0.5 g of L-dopa/carbidopa can therefore comfortably cover daily dosing requirements over a wide range. The suspension, commercially delivered as a PVC bag of 100 mL in a protective cassette, can be stored at refrigerator temperature for about 15 weeks and will remain stable for 16 hours after opening. Delivery is achieved via percutaneous gastrostomy tubes with the catheter tip located in the proximal jejunum (below Treitz fold) using portable programmable pumps that can achieve delivery rates between 10 and 2000 mg of L-dopa per hour for up to 24 hours. In addition, there is a bolus function to rapidly induce on periods or counteract intervening of periods.

Evidence from Clinical Trials

There are no randomized placebo-controlled trials to demonstrate the efficacy of this approach to smooth out motor oscillations as compared with standard oral L-dopa treatment. Available studies have all been open-label so far with one trial using a randomized cross-over design between conventional oral treatment and infusion therapy.[177] This study and other open-label approaches[178] have consistently shown reductions of daily off-time when switching patients from oral therapy to continuous intrajejunal infusions of more than 17%.[178,179] In addition, these studies have also provided evidence for reductions in dyskinesia severity using continuous enteral L-dopa delivery.[180]

Tolerability and Safety

To date there have been no reports of tolerability or safety issues related to the carboxymethylcellulose gel formulation itself. The main side effects and complications of duodopa therapy are related to either technical problems with the delivery system or the invasiveness of the approach using percutaneous endoscopic gastrostomy and permanent enteral catheters. The biggest long-term follow-up series reported so far covered a total of 58 patients observed for a mean of 3.7 years of which 52 had used duodopa infusions for at least 1 year. The incidence of pump-related technical problems was 24%. Almost all patients experienced some problem associated with the intestinal tube over the follow-up period (dislocation, kinking, erosion, or occlusion). Of the patients, 60% had episodes of pain, secretion, infection, or granulation at the gastrostomy site during follow-up.[179] A more recent series[180] with shorter mean follow-up had reported lesser percentages but a similar side-effect/complication spectrum.

Practical Recommendations

Enteral L-dopa infusions using the duodopa principle are an option for patients failing noninvasive pharmacotherapy for disabling motor fluctuations with or without dyskinesias. Results in terms of off-time reduction and also reduction of preexisting dyskinesias seem to be similar to those achievable with subcutaneous apomorphine infusions (see "Dopamine Agonists") or deep brain stimulation (see Chapter 17). Enteral L-dopa infusion approaches may be particularly considered for patients with certain contraindications for STN/DBS, including issues with cognitive decline and dementia or those with significant depression at baseline as well as patients with nonneurological comorbidity that would raise concern about DBS procedure. Major limitations are related to the relatively high drug cost as well as the size and weight of the pump (approximately 400 g) plus the need for permanent PEG tubing.

MAO-B Inhibitors

Selegiline and rasagiline are both irreversible inhibitors of MAO-B producing dopaminergic effects that are independent of their half-life. Both drugs are therefore candidates for use as adjunct therapies to L-dopa and fluctuating PD in an attempt to smooth out motor fluctuations.

Basic Pharmacology

See earlier mention of basic pharmacology of MAO-B inhibitors (page 6).

Available Trials

Three randomized placebo-controlled studies have assessed the efficacy of selegiline to improve motor fluctuations.[181–183] All have had short durations of up to 8 weeks and have included less than 100 patients. Results have been inconsistent with a trend to increase daily on-time and decrease wearing-off symptoms. More recently, the rapidly sublingual dissolving formulation of selegiline (zydes selegiline) has been tested for efficacy to reduce motor fluctuations in a large placebo-controlled trial showing significant greater reductions in off-time compared with placebo.[184]

In contrast to selegiline, there is robust and consistent evidence for efficacy to treat motor fluctuations for rasagiline from well-designed large-scale placebo-controlled trials.[185,186] Both randomized placebo-controlled trials showed off-time reductions in patients with L-dopa-related motor fluctuations receiving adjunct rasagiline (1 mg/day) of close to one hour per day. In addition, the lasting effect in adjunct therapy with rasagiline given once daily (LARGO) trial[186] included an active comparator arm where patients received double-blind adjunct treatment with the COMT-inhibitor entacapone. Effect sizes with both adjunct rasagiline or adjunct entacapone regarding reduction in off-time were similar, and the trial provided some indication for longer duration of the dopaminergic enhancement with rasagiline in a substudy assessing early morning motor function.

Tolerability and Safety

Using selegiline or rasagiline as adjunct therapies to L-dopa in patients with motor fluctuations is associated with similar tolerability as when these drugs are used as early monotherapy (see MAO Inhibitors, pages 6–7). However, there is a risk for increasing the existing L-dopa dyskinesias.

Practical Recommendations

The use of adjunct rasagiline is a first-line option for the treatment of wearing-off type motor fluctuations in L-dopa-treated Parkinson patients. Rasagiline and entacapone are the only drugs with a level A recommendation for this indication in a recent parameter by the American Academy of Neurology.[187] Similar recommendations exist from a guideline report by the EFNS,[188] while NICE recommendations from the UK comprise MAO-B inhibitors as a class (including selegiline) for a level A recommendation in this situation (see http://guidance.nice.org.uk/CG35).[105]

Dopamine Agonists

Dopamine agonists were originally introduced as adjunct therapies for L-dopa-treated patients in the 1970s when bromocriptine was shown to enhance efficacy of L-dopa in patients with advanced PD.[189] Since then most available dopamine agonists have been shown to extend on-time when given as adjunct therapy to patients with L-dopa-related motor fluctuations.[65]

Basic Pharmacology

The efficacy of dopamine agonists to reduce motor fluctuations likely reflects their longer half-lives as compared with L-dopa (see Table 15–3). Apomorphine is an exception and its use in treating motor fluctuations is related to possibility of subcutaneous delivery.

Apomorphine is a potent mixed D_1-type and D_2-type dopamine agonist receptor agonist with L-dopa-like antiparkinsonian effects. It has a poor bioavailability when administered orally because of extensive first-pass metabolism, but is readily absorbed via sublingual, intranasal, or rectal routes. With subcutaneous or intravenous injections, it has a half-life of about 30 minutes[190] corresponding to a 45- to 60-minute duration of clinical effect. Following a subcutaneous bolus injection maximal plasma concentrations are reached in about 8 minutes and clinical effects have a latency of 10–20 minutes. Latencies are longer for the various transmucosal routes.[191–193]

Evidence for Efficacy from Clinical Trials

The efficacy of several dopamine agonists in reducing off-time in patients with fluctuating PD has been demonstrated in well-designed randomized controlled trials for apomorphine, pergolide, pramipexole, ropinirole, and rotigotine, while there is less robust evidence for bromocriptine, piribedil, dihydroergocriptine, cabergoline, and lisuride[59,194,195] (see Table 15–7). Placebo-adjusted effect sizes are usually somewhat less than 2 hours with the exception of continuous subcutaneous

▶ TABLE 15–7. EFFICACY OF DOPAMINE AGONISTS TO REDUCE MOTOR FLUCTUATIONS BY STRENGTH OF EVIDENCE FROM RCTS

Agent	Efficacious	Likely Efficacious	Insufficient Evidence
Ergolinic Drugs			
– bromocriptine		✓	
– lisuride			✓
– pergolide	✓		
– cabergoline		✓	
– dihydroergocriptine			✓
Nonergolinic Drugs			
– apomorphine	✓		
– pramipexole	✓		
– ropinirole	✓		
– rotigotine	✓		
– piribedil			✓

(Data from Goetz et al. 2002–2005 and Poewe et al. 2007 [59,195])

infusions of apomorphine (available only outside the United States). This approach has not been tested in placebo-controlled trials, but there is a consistent body of evidence from open-label studies showing greater than 50% off-time reduction.[196,197] In addition, small open-label studies have found improvements in preexisting dyskinesias with continuous subcutaneous apomorphine therapy.[198]

Intermittent subcutaneous apomorphine injections are able to reverse off-periods within 10–15 minutes ("rescue-injections") at single doses between 2 mg and 7 mg. These effects have recently been confirmed in a double-blind placebo-controlled trial.[199]

Tolerability and Safety

Tolerability and safety of oral dopamine agonists or transdermal rotigotine in patients with advanced PD and motor fluctuations is generally similar to their use in early disease (see Dopamine Agonists, pages 5–6). In addition, adjunct dopamine agonist therapy in L-dopa-treated patients may induce or exacerbate preexisting dyskinesias.

Subcutaneous injections or infusions of apomorphine frequently cause nausea and vomiting upon initiation of therapy, which can be largely prevented by coadministration of domperidone (10–20 mg t.i.d.). Red itching nodules at injection sites are also common, but are usually well tolerated and transient. More severe application site reactions with large areas of inflammation or subcutaneous abscesses or necrosis can occur and lead to discontinuation in a minority of cases.[200,201] Apomorphine-induced autoimmune hemolytic anemia is a rare complication, requiring monthly blood counts in patients on subcutaneous continuous infusions.[202]

Practical Recommendations

Adjunct treatment with dopamine agonists is a first-line approach in the management of L-dopa-related motor response oscillations. Nonergolinic drugs such as ropinirole, pramipexole, or rotigotine have been best studied in this indication and are three of the added safety concerns of fibrotic reactions reported for ergolinic agents such as pergolide or cabergoline. Ropinirole and pramipexole are now available as once-daily extended-release formulations offering additional ease of use. This also applies to transdermal rotigotine, however, at the cost of possible application side reactions. Efficacious dose ranges for these agents are summarized in Table 15–3. Switching from one agent to another can usually be achieved overnight using equivalent daily doses. In patients with refractory response oscillations, subcutaneous rescue injections of apomorphine using a self-injection pen device is usually efficacious and sufficient for patients who will need less than 3–5 injections per day. In patients with more frequent refractory periods, continuous subcutaneous apomorphine infusions should be considered.

Treating Motor Fluctuations in Advanced PD—Pragmatic Approach

Management of L-dopa-related motor response oscillations is aimed at various aspects of the underlying pathophysiology and includes measures to enhance absorption and transport of L-dopa, stabilizing L-dopa plasma levels via changes of drug delivery and L-dopa pharmacokinetics and finally also through non-L-dopa-related strategies of continuous dopaminergic receptor stimulation (see Table 15–8). Which of the different

▶ TABLE 15–8. PHARMACOLOGICAL MANAGEMENT OF MOTOR FLUCTUATIONS

1. **Improve L-Dopa Absorption and Transport**
   - Avoid dosing with protein-rich food.
   - Enhance gastric motility (avoid anticholinergics or dosing with meals).
   - Soluble L-dopa preparations (Madopar dispersible*).
2. **Revise L-Dopa Regimen**
   - Increase dosing frequency (decrease time interval between doses to <4 hr).
   - Introduce sustained-release formulations for nocturnal or early morning offs.
3. **Provide Prolonged Striatal DA-ergic Stimulation**
   - Add COMT inhibitors.
   - Add MAO-B-inhibitors.
   - Add orally active DA-agonists, preferably ER-formulations (ropinirole and pramipexole).
   - Add transdermal DA-agonist delivery (rotigotine).
4. **Consider Invasive Therapies (If Available)**
   - Introduce s.c. apomorphine "rescue" injections up to 3–5/day.
   - Introduce s.c. apomorphine infusions.
   - Duodenal L-dopa infusions.*

*Not available in the United States.

options listed in Table 15–8 is used will depend on the type of drug regimen the patient is on when motor fluctuations begin, patient factors such as age and comorbidity, as well as ease of use and complexity of motor response swings.

Patients with wearing-off-type motor fluctuations will profit from multiple approaches including increased dosing frequency with shortened interdose intervals (particularly for those on four or less daily doses of L-dopa), the addition of COMT-inhibitors such as entacapone (first-line) or tolcapone (second-line), adjunct rasagiline or selegiline, as well as oral dopamine agonists. Frequently patients with motor fluctuations will require combinations of several of these approaches. Once-daily drugs, such as pramipexole or ropinirole extended-release, rasagiline, or transdermal rotigotine, offer benefits in terms of convenience, but the more continuous plasma level profiles of these drugs are not mirrored by greater efficacy in terms of reducing motor fluctuations as compared with t.i.d. dosing of pramipexole or ropinirole.

Patients with refractory and disabling motor response oscillations will be considered for invasive approaches, including subcutaneous apomorphine rescue injections, continuous infusions, or enteral L-dopa infusions, where available. Both continuous infusion approaches impose significant demand on day-to-day technical handling of the patient and caregiver and a supportive caring environment is usually required before considering such regimens in the elderly PD patient. Table 15–8 summarizes the flow of pragmatic treatment decisions for patients with motor fluctuations.

Management of Dyskinesias

The emergence of response oscillations is usually associated with the appearance of L-dopa induced abnormal involuntary movements. These may occur in 30% of patients already after 2 years of L-dopa exposure[28] or even earlier in patients with young-onset PD .[203]

L-dopa-induced dyskinesias most often consist of choreic movements involving the trunk and extremities at times of peak effect (on-period dyskinesia), while in some patients involuntary movements is linked to the phases of onset or waning of a motor response to an individual dose of L-dopa.[204,205] Some 30% of patients additionally suffer from painful dystonic cramps, particularly involving the foot and leg at times of wearing-off of L-dopa effects (off-period dystonia)[31] (see Table 15–9).

The exact pathophysiology of L-dopa-induced dyskinesias (LIDs) is not fully understood, but they are probably related to the short half-life of L-dopa leading to discontinuous or pulsatile stimulation of striatal dopamine receptors, which over time induces altered gene expression and firing patterns in basal ganglia output neurons of the indirect pathway.[170] One approach to the medical management of LIDs, therefore, is focussed on providing more continuous dopminergic stimulation, while a second area of ongoing development is to target nondopaminergic receptors involved in the expression of dyskinesias via corticostriatal and striatopallidal signaling.[206]

▶ TABLE 15–9. DRUG-INDUCED DYSKINESIAS IN PD

On-Period Dyskinesias ("Interdose")
- phasic (choreic) limb movements
- dystonic craniocervical movements
- more pronounced on side initially affected by PD

Biphasic Dyskinesias
- at onset or wearing-off of clinical benefit from a dose of L-dopa (or both)
- mix of phasic and dystonic movements ("mobile dystonia")

Off-Period Dystonia
- most often distal limb (feet)
- painful

L-Dopa Based Approaches

Continuous delivery of L-dopa itself has been shown to reduce levels of preexisting dyskinesias in studies of enteral L-dopa infusions.[176,177,207] Duodopa is currently marketed in the European Union as an enteral infusion system for patients with refractory L-dopa-related motor complications (see section on motor fluctuations); antidyskinetic responses of this approach are not immediate and may take several weeks of continuous infusion before they become apparent.

Altering pharmacokinetics of L-dopa through slow-release formulations or, more recently, the use of COMT-inhibitors has not been successful in reducing dyskinesia risk of oral L-dopa treatment.[208,209]

Dopamine Agonists

Dopamine agonists are able to provide more continuous dopaminergic receptor stimulation either through their longer half-life in comparison to L-dopa (pramipexole, ropinirole, pergolide, cabergoline) or via continuous delivery options (subcutaneous infusions for apomorphine, transdermal delivery for rotigotine). More continuous dopaminergic stimulation via prolonged half-life is the most popular hypothesis to explain the decreased dyskinesia risk when initiating PD monotherapy with a dopamine agonist as compared with L-dopa. Substituting L-dopa with high-dose or oral dopamine agonist monotherapy as a treatment for L-dopa-induced dyskinesias, however, is only exceptionally successful.[210] A majority of chronically L-dopa-treated patients will not obtain sufficient symptomatic control with dopamine agonist monotherapy.

The only exception to this rule is with apomorphine, which has been shown to produce equivalent motor benefits to L-dopa and single-dose experiments.[211] Continuous subcutaneous infusions of apomorphine have been shown to reduce dyskinesias in small open-label studies.[198,212]

Glutamate Antagonists

Altered glutamate receptor–mediated signaling is believed to play an important role in pathogenesis of direct striatal pallidal pathway hyperactivity (which mediates L-dopa-induced dyskinesias via disinhibition of thalamocortical motor outputs).[213] The NMDA-glutamate receptor antagonist amantadine remains the only drug to date with proven antidyskinetic efficacy. Placebo-controlled trials assessing the antidyskinetic potential of amantadine[214–217] have consistently shown that adjunct treatment with oral amantadine at 300–400 mg/day significantly reduces the intensity of preexisting L-dopa-induced dyskinesias. Such benefit may be maintained for at least 12 months.

The novel mGluR5 antagonist AFQ506 has recently been found to also reduce LIDs in a small double-blind placebo-controlled proof-of-concept study.[218]

Novel Non-Dopaminergic Approaches

Other than cortical striatal glutamate receptors several additional nondopaminergic receptors expressed on striatal medium spiny neurons have been implicated in the pathological basal ganglia signaling underlying L-dopa-induced dyskinesias.[206] These include adenosine A_{2A} receptors that are preferentially expressed on striatal medium spiny neuron dendrites of the indirect pathway and may increase excitability of these neurons. The A_{2A} antagonist istradefylline failed clinical trials testing its efficacy to treat motor fluctuations,[219,220] and there are currently no human data showing modulation of dyskinesias through A_{2A} antagonism. Adrenergic α-2A receptors are believed to modulate striatopallidal transmission via the indirect pathway and antagonism on this side may help to counteract the direct striatal pathway overactivity in L-dopa-induced dyskinesias. The A_{2A} receptor antagonist fipamazole has been shown to reduce dyskinesias in a phase IIA study.

Finally, there is experimental evidence also for a role of striatal 5-HT2 receptors in mediating erratic motor signaling in dyskinetic MPTP monkeys. Clinical trials with a 5-HT1A agonist sarizotane have not been successful, however.[221,222]

Medical Treatment of LID - Pragmatic Approach

In many patients, L-dopa-induced dyskinesias are nondisabling and may not necessarily require changes in medical treatment. If bothersome to the patient, simple measures such as reductions of daily L-dopa dose may be tried, but this usually requires concomitant and up-titration of dopamine agonists to counterbalance loss of efficacy. Sometimes patients may profit from receiving lower L-dopa single doses at shorter time intervals, but this approach may enhance motor fluctuations. A switch from L-dopa treatment to high-dose monotherapy with dopamine agonists has the potential of reducing intensity of preexisting dyskinesias but is not often possible because of the reduced efficacy of dopamine agonists versus L-dopa.

Adding amantadine, on the other hand, has the advantage of both being simple and usually successful leading to reductions in the order of 40–60% of dyskinesia intensity at daily doses of 200–400 mg.

Disabling refractory dyskinesias often require more invasive approaches. For pharmacotherapy, this includes the use of continuous subcutaneous infusions of apomorphine or continuous intrajejunal L-dopa infusions,

▶ TABLE 15–10. PHARMACOLOGICAL MANAGEMENT OF L-DOPA-INDUCED DYSKINESIAS

- Revise L-dopa regimen (reduce individual doses, use more frequent dosing).
- Add/increase dopamine agonists (ER-formulations).
- Consider parenteral dopamine agonist (transdermal rotigotine).
- Add amantadine.
- Use continuous drug delivery (duodenal L-dopa, s.c. apomorphine).
- Add low-dose clozapine (recommended by EFNS-[188], but not by AAN-guideline [187]).
- Consider bilateral STN-DBS.

where available. All of these approaches have been shown to reduce preexisting dyskinesias in many open-label case series, but a substantial portion of patients with disabling L-dopa-induced dyskinesias will require deep brain surgery to control them. Table 15–10 summarizes the most commonly used drug options to treat L-dopa-induced dyskinesias.

▶ SECTION 2: MEDICAL MANAGEMENT OF THE NON MOTOR SYMPTOMS OF PD

Although idiopathic PD is generally considered a paradigmatic movement disorder, nonmotor symptoms (NMS) are increasingly recognized as important elements in the clinical spectrum of PD (for overview see Table 15–11). They are assumed to reflect α-synuclein pathology and cell loss in multiple areas of the nervous system including nondopaminergic brain stem nuclei such as the locus coeruleus, cholinergic nucleus basalis of the forebrain, the olfactory tubercle, neocortical and limbic brain areas, as well as peripheral sympathetic ganglia and sympathetic or parasympathetic efferents. For many of these pathologies, which are regularly found in the parkinsonian nervous system, the exact clinical pathological correlations have not been clearly established.[223] While some of these extranigral sites may show α-synuclein pathology prior to the occurrence of Lewy body formation and cell loss in the substantia nigra itself, disabling NMS are related to advanced disease stages[224] and may include disturbances of the sleep–wake cycle regulation, cognitive dysfunction, depression and psychosis, as well as autonomic dysfunction. In line with the motor response oscillations to dopaminergic stimulation, some NMS may likewise fluctuate and can therefore respond to dopaminergic treatment.[225] However, rarely NMS are relieved satisfactorily by such treatment and therefore various NMS-combinations may become the foremost therapeutic challenge in advanced stages of PD.

▶ TABLE 15–11. NONMOTOR SYMPTOMS (NMS) IN PD

Neuropsychiatric Dysfunction	Mood disorders Apathy and anhedonia Frontal executive dysfunction Dementia Psychosis Dopamine dysregulation syndrome (DDS) Impulse control disorders (ICD)
Sleep Disorders	Sleep fragmentation and insomnia RBD Restless legs syndrome (+/–PLMS) Excess daytime sleepiness (EDS) Sudden-onset sleep (SOS)
Autonomic Dysfunction	Orthostatic hypotension Urogenital dysfunction Constipation
Sensory Symptoms and Pain	Olfactory dysfunction Abnormal sensations Pain

DEPRESSION

Depressive symptoms are relatively common in PD, affecting 40–50% of patients,[226,227] and in many cases, anxiety and depression precede the onset of classical motor symptoms by years or even decades.[228] However, only less than half of affected PD patients will meet DSM IV criteria for major depression.[227,229] Depression was described to be more common in PD with prominent bradykinesia and gait instability than in tremor-dominant syndromes;[229] other studies failed to demonstrate a correlation between depression severity and duration of the illness.[227,230] With its core features loss of interest and anhedonia, depression in PD could be overdiagnosed, because the physical appearance of a nondepressed PD patient can easily mimic that of depression due to hypomimia, hypophonia, and psychomotor retardation, but in fact remains often under-recognized and undertreated.[231] Anxiety, insomnia, fatigue, and loss of appetite are also commonly present,[231] whereas other depressive features, such as feelings of self-blame, guilt, sense of failure, and self-destructive thoughts, often encountered in major depression are rare in PD.[232] Whether depression in PD is exogenous or endogenous or both is unclear and causes may vary from patient to patient. It is likely that the diagnosis of a chronic disease contributes to depressed mood as an exogenous cause,[230] but PD patients are even more likely to be depressed than patients with other chronic disabling diseases.[233] In fact, there are many clinicopathological correlation studies that suggest dopaminergic and noradrenergic denervation due to cell loss in mesocorticolimbic projections and the locus ceruleus, respectively, to underlie depressive symptoms.[234] Moreover, the serotonergic systems seem to be involved in the pathophysiology of depression in PD.[235]

Evidence for Efficacy from Clinical Trials

According to a questionnaire-based survey of Parkinson Study Group investigators, SSRIs are the most—and tricyclic antidepressants (TCAs) the second most commonly used drugs to treat PD depression.[236] A paucity of controlled trials in PD-depression has assessed these classical antidepressants in terms of ameliorating depressed mood.

The largest and most recent RCT compared nortryptiline versus paroxetin versus placebo.[237] As assessed by the Hamilton depression scale (HADS), significantly more patients responded to nortryptiline than to placebo and paroxetin (53% versus 24% and 10%, respectively). Amitriptyline was more efficacious than fluoxetine in one randomized comparator trial.[238] In another single-blind clinical trial, amitriptyline and sertraline were shown to have comparable antidepressant effects, although only sertraline was associated with enhanced quality of life.[239] However, in two relatively small RCT the SSRIs sertraline and citaloprame failed to be superior to placebo,[240,241] but both active treatment and placebo led to a significant reduction of depression scores.

In some patients mood troughs are related to the motor off-state and this may well mirror the role of dopaminergic deficiency in PD depression.[225] Therefore, the antidepressant potential of dopaminergic drugs used to treat the motor symptoms of PD has been assessed in randomized open-label studies. One study demonstrated the antidepressant effect of pramipexole in fluctuating PD patients.[242] In another study in nonfluctuating patients pramipexole had an even greater number of patient responders compared with sertraline.[243] Furthermore, data of a pilot study suggest that also adjunctive ropinirole may be effective in treatment-resistant depression.[244] All three studies produced positive results for dopaminergic treatment but are limited by a lack of a placebo-control arm. Recently a large placebo-controlled study on the effects of pramipexole on depressive symptoms in PD has been completed and positive results have been published in abstract form.[245]

In terms of nonpharmacological treatment, two trials addressed the antidepressant potential of repetitive transcranial magnetic stimulation (rTMS). There was no difference between sham and effective stimulation with respect to depression and PD measures in one study,[246] and the other study found rTMS as effective as fluoxetine in improving depression.[247]

Practical Recommendations

All available guidelines regarding PD depression have been published before 2007[105,188,248] and do not consider results of the most recent published trials. There is a general consensus that antiparkinsonian drug treatment should be optimized first in patients displaying depressive symptoms. Particularly off-period-related depressive episodes should be managed by measures that will smooth out motor fluctuations (see Table 15–8), also including the use of pramipexole, for which there are a number of studies demonstrating improvement of depressive symptoms.

Many patients, particular those with depressive symptoms not related to off-periods, will require adjunct therapy with antidepressants. Although SSRIs are still the most commonly used class of agents in clinical routine, data from recent studies suggest that TCAs may be more effective in PD depression. SSRIs may occasionally worsen tremor in PD but this is a rare cause for discontinuation. Concomitant use of SSRIs in patients receiving MAO-B-inhibitors such as selegiline or rasagiline requires special attention regarding the potential but rare development of a serotonin-like syndrome. TCAs have a potential to produce anticholinergic side effects and their use in cognitively impaired patients is usually not recommended. Because of their sedating properties TCAs can be beneficial in depressed patients with insomnia and their anticholinergic component may excerpt some benefit on tremor as well. Medical antidepressant treatment options are summarized in Table 15–12.

TABLE 15–12. MEDICAL ANTIDEPRESSANT TREATMENT OPTIONS IN PD

1. **Revise DA-ergic Therapy**
   - Optimize DA-ergic therapy in case of insufficient motor control.
   - Smooth out motor fluctuations especially in case of off period–related depressive symptoms (see Table 15–8).
2. **Add Classical Antidepressant Depending on Major Symptom(s)**
   - Depression and anxiety: Consider SSRI or TCA (e.g., sertraline 50 mg/day, paroxetine 20–40 mg/day, fluvoxamine 100 mg/day, fluoxetine 20 mg/day).
   - Caveat when combining with MAO-B inhibitor (serotonine syndrome, see "MAO-B Inhibitors") (e.g., amitriptyline 25–75 mg/day, nortriptyline up to 150 mg/day (Caveat: anticholinergic activity).
   - Anhedonia and apathy: Consider SSRI/SNRI (e.g., venlafaxin 75–150 mg/day, nefazodone 100–300 mg/day, reboxetine up to 12 mg/day).
   - Agitation or insomnia: Consider sedating TCAs or mirtazapine (e.g., amitriptyline 25–75 mg/day; mirtazapine 15–30 mg/day).

COGNITIVE DYSFUNCTION AND DEMENTIA

Cognitive decline and hallucinosis are key milestones in the progression of nonmotor disability of PD and important risk factors for nursing home care and mortality[249] (see also Chap. 18). A recent meta-analysis of cross-sectional studies has found a point prevalence of PD-Dementia (PD-D) of about 30%.[250] Patients with early hallucinations and akinetic-dominant PD have a higher risk of dementia. PD-D is characterized by impairment in attention, memory, and visuospatial and executive function, frequently accompanied by behavioral symptoms such as affective changes, hallucinations, and apathy.[251] Once dementia in PD becomes clinically significant, median survival time is 5 years.[252] The pathophysiology of cognitive decline and dementia in PD is complex and may include Alzheimer-type changes as well as subcortical vascular lesions. The hallmark neuropathological and neurochemical findings, however, are limbic and neocortical Lewy-bodies in combination with cholinergic deficiency of the nucleus basalis Meynert in the basal forebrain.[253,254]

Evidence for Efficacy from Clinical Trials

Several RCTs have assessed the efficacy of cholinesterase inhibitors to treat PD-D. In two small studies, treatment with donepezil over 10 weeks was associated with a significant improvement in MMSE scores of 2 points.[255,256] A large-scale study with 541 patients demonstrated a small, but significant benefit in patients randomized to rivastigmine compared with controls as assessed by different Alzheimer rating scales (Alzheimer's Disease Assessment Scale—cognitive subscale and Alzheimer's Disease Cooperative Study—Clinicians Global Impression of Change).[257] Benefit was greatest after a period of 16 weeks, and after the whole study period of 24 weeks, there was a significant difference of 1 score point in the MMSE in favor of the active comparator arm. A subanalysis revealed greater response in patients experiencing visual hallucinations at baseline,[258] and an open-label extension of the trial demonstrated sustained efficacy over the period of 12 months.[259] Finally galantamine, a cholinesterase inhibitor with additional modulating activity on nicotinic cholinergic receptors has been assessed in an open controlled trial reporting improvement in the clock drawing test, in the neuropsychiatric inventory, the MMSE, and the frontal assessment battery.[260] Worsening of tremor occurred in some patients.

Most recently memantine, a glutamatergic antagonist at NMDA receptors with a similar pharmacodynamic profile as amantadine (see Chapter 13), was tested in a relatively large RCT.[261] The authors of this study observed significant improvement in clinical global impression of change after a trial duration of 24 weeks and concluded that treatment with memantine is well tolerated and might be beneficial to patients with PD-D.

Practical Recommendations

Management of PD-D should always include discontinuation of potential aggravators of central cholinergic dysfunctions such as anticholinergic drugs, amantadine, and TCAs. Orthostatic hypotension may be another potential aggravator of attentional dysfunction[262] and should be approximately treated as well. A MMSE score of less than 24 points represents the indication to start treatment with a cholinesterase inhibitor. To date, the best-studied drug in this class of agents and the only approved in this indication in the United State and European is rivastigmine.[105,188,248] Data on donepezil, galantamine, and memantine are few but do support their use. They should be used as second-line drugs for PD-D. The results to be expected from antidementive therapy are improvement of memory, attention, concentration, as well as the fluctuation in these tasks. Hallucinosis and erratic behavior may also respond to such treatment, and the overall caregiver burden should be reduced. However, the overall responder rates are not very high and benefit may be temporary due to ongoing Lewy-body degeneration. Once started, discontinuation of treatment in such cases may be associated with further worsening and should therefore be omitted.

PSYCHOSIS

Drug trials clearly suggest that PD-Psychosis (PDPsy) is a common and significant problem in around 20% of patients with PD and may affect up to 40% in hospital-based series.[263] A case-control study[264] identified hallucinosis as a primary risk factor for nursing home placements.[265] "Psychosis" is often used as an umbrella term for illusions, delusions, hallucinations, confusion, and paranoid ideation.[266] Illusions, false sense of presence, and hallucinations are the most common manifestations in PD, mostly visual in nature, and other sensory modalities such as acoustic and tactile may be present only in combination with visual misperceptions.[263] Initially, patients often retain insight into their hallucinations and are not bothered by them, but as the disease progresses, hallucinations become frightening and sometimes accompanied by paranoid delusions and delirium. The major risk factors for psychotic symptoms in PD include cognitive impairment, severity, and duration of PD as well as depression and anxiety. All major antiparkinsonian drugs can contribute to psychosis in at-risk patients: anticholinergics, amantadine, dopamine agonists, MAO-B, and COMT inhibitors in combination with L-dopa and finally L-dopa itself (in order of relative risk to induce psychosis).[188] However, hallucinations are associated with Lewy-body pathology in the visuoperceptual system including the basolateral nucleus of the amygdala and parahyppocampus[267] and imbalances of monoaminergic neurotransmitters.[266]

Evidence for Efficacy from Clinical Trials

Several trials have assessed the antipsychotic potency of mainly atypical neuroleptics in PDPsy. The best-studied drug in this setting is clozapine, and there are two RCTs firmly proving efficacy of this substance.[268,269] In both trials, 60 patients were treated for 4 weeks with a mean clozapine dose of 25 and 36 mg/day, respectively, and improved significantly in the clinical global impression scale, while psychotic symptoms diminished. Overall in 1 of 120 patients clozapine was discontinued because of leukopenia.[269] Both studies were followed by an open-label period of 12 weeks, throughout which treatment benefit from clozapine was maintained.[270,271] There are inconsistent findings from different trials addressing the antipsychotic potency of quetiapine in PDPsy. Two of these trials failed to demonstrate superiority of quetiapine over placebo,[272,273] whereas two other trials showed similar efficacy of quetiapine when compared with clozapine.[274,275] In open-label studies, this substance was generally associated with an improvement of psychosis in 70–80% of patients,[263,276] but in the long term in one-third of patients minor worsening of motor function was noted.[276] In small studies, other substances of this class such as risperidone or olanzapine either failed to exhibit antipsychotic effect or were associated with marked worsening of motor function and are therefore not recommended for their use in PDPsy.[188,248] There is some evidence from small-scale open studies for rivastigmine,[277,278] donepezil,[279,280] and galantamine[281] that cholinesterase inhibitors may improve PDPsy when accompanied by cognitive dysfunction.

Practical Recommendations

Similar to the management of PDD, the occurrence of confusion and hallucinosis in a parkinsonian patient should initially prompt search for intercurrent illnesses, particularly infections, metabolic disturbances, or structural lesions. After excluding those conditions, patients on polypharmacotherapy should be discontinued first from anticholinergics, TCAs and/or amantadine, second from dopamine agonists, third from MAO-B and/or COMT inhibitors, and finally the L-dopa should be adjusted to the minimum dose sufficient to control the motor symptoms of disease. Those patients continuing to hallucinate despite antiparkinsonian drug reductions should receive antipsychotic treatment.[105,188,248] Although not formally established as efficacious in RCTs, quetiapine is usually the pragmatic first choice because of its improved safety profile as compared with clozapine. Treatment should start with 25 mg bedtime and can gradually be increased to 200 mg/day. Clozapine is the only antipsychotic agent with proven efficacy based on RCTs and should be used in all cases failing treatment with quetiapine but can also be considered as first-line option in severe cases of psychosis. It should be started at a very low dose (6.25 mg) at bedtime and increased gradually until psychosis remits or adverse events occur. Because of the small but definite risk of leukopenia associated with clozapine treatment (1–2% of patients not dose related), weekly blood monitoring for the first 6 months of treatment and biweekly monitoring thereafter are needed. In patients with concomitant dementia, treatment with cholinesterase-inhibitors should be considered. Table 15–13 hierarchically summarizes treatment options for psychosis in PD.

TABLE 15–13. PHARMACOLOGICAL MANAGEMENT OF PSYCHOSIS IN PD

1. **Control Nondrug Triggers and Aggravators**
   - Treat infection.
   - Rectify fluid/electrolyte balance.
   - Exclude acute organic brain disease (stroke, encephalitis), if reasonable.
2. **Reduce Polypharmacy**
   - Discontinue tricyclic antidepressants.
   - Discontinue anticholinergics and/or amantadine.
   - Reduce/discontinue DA-agonists before L-dopa.
   - Discontinue MAO-B inhibitor before L-dopa.
   - Discontinue COMT-inhibitors before L-dopa.
3. **Add Antipsychotics**
   - Clozapine (start with 6,25–12,5 mg at bedtime, monitor blood counts).
   - Quetiapine (start with 50–75 mg/day).

   Caveat: Olanzapine and risperidone have failed efficacy in controlled trials of PD and may induce motor worsening.
4. **Add Cholinesterase Inhibitors in Patients with Cognitive Impairment**
   - Rivastigmine 4.5–9 mg/day (or donepezil 5–10 mg/day, galantamine 8–24 mg/day).

DISORDERS OF SLEEP AND WAKEFULNESS

Generally, sleep disorders are among the most frequent NMS in PD affecting 70–90% of patients,[282] although two thirds of patients rate sleep quality as acceptable or good[283] (see also Chapter 47). Subjective complaints about sleep in patients with IPD include difficulties falling asleep, frequent awakenings, discomfort and pain in the legs, difficulties turning in bed, nycturia, nocturnal confusion, and hallucinosis as well as daytime sleepiness. Difficulty with the initiation and maintenance of sleep in PD may occur because of a primary sleep disorder or secondary to advancing PD with sleep-interfering motor complications, especially motor offs, painful off-period dystonia, and early morning akinesia, as well as NMS such as nycturia, dementia, and psychosis. Primary reasons for sleep disturbances range from REM-sleep behavior disorder (RBD) and excessive daytime sleepiness (EDS) in around 50% of patients[284,285] to comorbidities such as restless legs syndrome (RLS) and obstructive sleep apnea syndrome (OSAS) in around 20% of patients.[286,287] Disturbances of sleep architecture such as sleep fragmentation, reduced sleep efficiency, reduced REM-sleep, and particularly RBD seems to be closely related to Lewy-body pathology in lower brain stem nuclei.[288] Because of this plethora of possible contributing factors, diagnosis and treatment of sleep disturbance and daytime sleepiness in PD are usually complex. It is essential, to perform a careful history taking including additional information from spouses or caregivers to identify the treatment target. Optimizing treatment of nocturnal PD features, counseling about "sleep hygiene," as well as treatment of interfering NMS such as nycturia, mental dysfunction, and hallucinosis may be first important targets. EDS may in part derive from primary sleep disorders, but might be exacerbated by dopaminergic drugs (see Chapter 11). New-onset EDS following changes in dopaminergic medication should raise suspicion of drug-induced EDS and therefore lead to dose reduction or change of treatment regimen. If this is not feasible, the addition of a wake-promoting drug such as modafinile should be considered.[105] Table 15–14 summarizes general principles of sleep management in PD.

▶ TABLE 15–14. MANAGEMENT OF SLEEP DISORDERS IN PD

Treatment of Underlying Causes
- Nocturnal motor problems (tremor, nocturnal akinesia, off-period dystonia): Bedtime doses of CR L-dopa, and/or transdermal or ER dopamine agonists (see Table 15–8; management of motor fluctuations).
- RLS/PLMS: Bedtime doses of CR L-dopa or DA-agonists.
- Sleep-disordered breathing: CPAP if necessary.
- REM sleep behavior disorder: Bedtime clonazepam 0.5–2 mg (and/or bedtime melatonin 3–12 mg).
- Nocturia: Consider desmopressin spray (also trospiumchloride, oxybutinin, tolterodine; see Table 15–15).
- Nocturnal hallucinosis/confusion (see Table 15–11).

Symptomatic Treatment
- Sleep hygiene (establishment of a regular pattern of sleep, comfortable bedding and temperature, restriction of daytime siestas).
- Provision of assistive devices, such as a bed lever or rails to aid with moving and turning, allowing the person to get more comfortable.
- Avoid substances that might interfere with sleep (e.g., caffeine, alcohol).
- Short-acting benzodiazepines (e.g., triazolam).
- Low-dose, sedating antidepressants (e.g., amitriptyline, mirtazapin).

REM Sleep Behavior Disorder (RBD)

RBD is a parasomnia characterized by lack of atonia during REM-sleep, resulting in dream-enacting behavior, occasionally associated with violent motor activity.[289] Significantly increased risk factors for clinical PD have been reported in individuals with idiopathic REM sleep behavior disorder.[290] RBD is frequently associated with poor sleep quality and daytime somnolence and sleep-related injuries; complaints may often be voiced by bed partners of patients.

Standard treatment recommendations of RBD lack evidence based on RCT. Before starting patients on active treatment, potentially aggravating factors should be identified (e.g., TCAs) and removed. Several open-label case series demonstrated clonazepam completely suppressing dream-enacting behavior with overall high responder rates,[291–293] and clonazepam given as a single bedtime dose of 0.5–2 mg is considered first-line treatment of RBD. The endogenous hormone melatonin, either given as sole agent or in combination with clonazepam, was consistently reported as beneficial in three open-label studies in RBD patients[294–296] and is therefore regarded as second-line option in a dose of 3–12 mg to be given also as single bedtime dose.

AUTONOMIC DYSFUNCTION

Autonomic dysfunction is a common treatment problem in PD and may include orthostatic hypotension (OH), urinary dysfunction (urinary frequency, urgency, and urge incontinence), erectile dysfunction and impotence, gastrointestinal motility problems, and constipation (see also Chapter 13). Retrospective chart reviews in a large series of pathologically confirmed PD cases found an overall prevalence of autonomic dysfunction of three-quarters.[297] 30% were affected from symptomatic OH, 32% from bladder dysfunction, and 36% from constipation. It usually occurs in advanced disease compared with atypical parkinsonism such as multiple system atrophy (MSA). The pathophysiology and clinicopathological correlations of dysautonomia in PD are not entirely understood. Lewy-body-related neurodegeneration affecting lower brain stem nuclei such as the dorsal vagal nucleus, the nucleus ambiguous, and some medullary centers as well as peripheral sympathetic ganglia and efferents of the gastrointestinal and cardiovascular system[224,297–299] is supposed to play a crucial role.

TABLE 15–15. PRACTICAL MANAGEMENT OF DYSAUTONOMIC FUNCTION IN PD

Pharmacotherapy

1. For orthostatic hypotension
   - Head-up tilt of bed at night, elastic stockings or tights, increased salt and fluid intake.
   - Midodrine 2.5–10 mg/day.
   - Fludrocortisone 0.1–0.4 mg/day.
   - Etilefrine 7.5–15 mg/day.
   - DOPS 200–400 mg/day.
2. For postprandial hypotension
   - Octreotide 25–50 μg s.c.30 minutes before a meal.
3. For bladder symptoms
   - Check for bladder infections, antibiotic treatment if positive.
   - Add anticholinergics: trospiumchloride 20–40 mg/day (or oxybutynin 5–15 mg, tolterodine 2–4 mg).
   - Intermittent self-catheterization for retention or residual volume—100 mL.
   - If unmanageable, use long-term urethral catheter.
4. For erectile failure
   - PDE-5 inhibitors: sidenafil 50 mg (vardenafil 10 mg, tadalafil 20 mg)—Caveat: OH.
   - Sublingual apomorphine 3mg.
   - Penis implant.
5. For gastrointestinal motility problems
   - Domperidone up to 150 mg/day.
   - Tegaserod 6–12 mg, mosaprde 15–45 mg, cisapride 2.5–20 mg (Caveat: arrhythmias)
6. For constipation
   - Adequate fiber and water intake.
   - Lactulose 20–60 g/day.
   - Macrogol-water solution to increase intraluminal fluid.

Other therapies

- Physiotherapy
- Occupational therapy

Unfortunately, there is no casual therapy of autonomic dysfunction available and symptomatic management is largely based on pragmatic recommendations[105,188] rather than firm evidence from RCT. Table 15–15 provides a summarization.

Orthostatic Hypotension (OH)

OH is clinically defined as a decrease of at least 20 mmHg in systolic and/or 10 mmHg in diastolic blood pressure within 3 minutes in upright position, with or without postural symptoms.[300] Symptoms from OH include blurred vision, postural instability, light-headedness and dizziness, coat hanger pain, and syncope.[301] OH can be caused or triggered by large and heavy meals.

Data from controlled trials on OH in PD derive mostly from studies performed in patients with mixed neurogenic causes for hypotension. Guidelines consistently recommend to adopt general nonpharmacological measures before starting active treatment: firstly it is important to avoid aggravating factors such as large meals, alcohol, exposure to a warm environment, and drugs known to cause orthostatic hypotension such as diuretics or antihypertensive drugs (L-dopa and dopamine agonists may also aggravate orthostatic hypotension); and second, it is recommended to increase salt intake, keep the head-up tilt of the bed at night, wear elastic stockings, and take frequent but small meals. If these nonpharmacological measures are insufficient, active treatment should be started.

The postsynaptically acting α_1-adrenergic agonist midodrine was shown as efficacious in two RCTs in improving OH[302,303] and is regarded as first-line therapy in OH in the EFNS guideline on treatment of late PD.[188] Smaller open-label studies established beneficial effects on OH of the unselective adrenergic agonist etilefrine and the mineralocorticoid fludrocortisone,[300,304] and fludrocortisone is preferred by NICE guideline on treatment of PD[105] and EFNS guideline on diagnosis and treatment of OH[300] as first-line treatment. The prodrug dihydroxyphenylserine (DOPS), which is converted to the endogenous catecholamine norepinephrine, was shown to decrease blood pressure falls during orthostatism[305] with only minor side effects, and received a level A recommendation from the EFNS guidelines on diagnosis and treatment of OH.[300] Further studies are ongoing to assess the potential benefit from DOPS treatment in OH.

Bladder Dysfunction

Urinary dysfunction is a common feature of advanced PD and includes urinary urgency, frequency. and urge incontinence as well as incomplete bladder emptying.[306,307] Urodynamic studies in PD patients demonstrated that the most common urdynamic abnormality is detrusor hyperreflexia, whereas detrusor hypoactivity seems to be less prominent.

The anticholinergic agents oxybutinin, tolteridone, and trospium chloride were found to be efficacious in treating detrusor overactivity-related urgency and urge incontinence in non-PD patients with neurogenic bladder syndromes.[188,304,306,307] In a small open-label study, desmopressin given intranasally has shown reductions in frequency of nocturnal voids.[308] Novel approaches include the intravesical instillation of botulinum toxin, and so far results are promising in non-PD patients.[309]

Patients with persistent urinary dysfunction should have a detailed urological evaluation including urodynamic studies and measurement of postmicturial residual volume. Urinary dysfunction because of secondary cases should carefully be excluded (e.g., drug side effects, infections, benign prostatic hyperplasia). If nycturia is the problem, it may be helped by curtailing the fluid intake (especially coffee) after evening meals. Refractory nycturia may respond to nighttime doses of intranasal desmopressin. In cases in which this is not effective, anticholinergic should be tried to treat detrusor hyperreflexia. Since trospium-chloride acts more locally in the urinary tract and largely lacks systemic anticholinergic properties, it is preferred to oxybutinine and tolteridone, which may worsen cognitive dysfunction.[306] When urge and frequency are unmanageable, a long-term urethral catheter may be required, possibly restoring a degree of independency. Urinary tract infections should be treated immediately, and if they are recurrent, a suprapubic catheter is preferable to a urethral catheter for chronic use.[306,307]

Constipation

Constipation is another common autonomic symptom of PD and may even precede the onset of motor symptoms in PD.[310] This symptom can cause large discomfort to patients and end in a rare but severe complication, the toxic megacolon.[311]

The treatment of constipation consists of dietary changes, exercise, and pharmacotherapy.[105,188] Dietary modification is primarily aimed at increasing the bulk as well as softening the stools and consists in raising the fiber (e.g., raw vegetables or bran) and total fluid intake. If stool remains hard, despite dietary modifications and adequate exercise, stool softeners such as lactulose may be used. Laxatives such as bisacodyl, picosulfate, or macrogol may be further therapeutic options. Open-label trials with macrogol, a polyethylene glycol electrolyte solution working on an osmotic basis, and also dietary herb extracts have reported an improvement of constipation in small PD cohorts.[312,313] Prokinetic drugs including cisapride and mosapride were found to be effective in small-scale studies;[314,315] an RCT of the prokinetic tegaserod found a trend toward improvement of constipation measures.[316] However, these drugs have been withdrawn from the market in several countries worldwide because of their risk of fatal arrhythmia. Domperidone may also be considered, since it blocks peripheral dopamine receptors, thus increasing gastric emptying, and reduces dopaminergic drug-related gastrointestinal symptoms in patients with PD.[188]

Erectile Dysfunction

Erectile dysfunction (ED) typically affects men several years after onset, and relative risk increases as the disease progresses.[317]

Management of ED involves identifying and correcting underlying treatable causes such as drug side effects (e.g., propranolol), depression, prostate disorders, or diabetes. Symptomatic treatment is mostly carried out with orally active inhibitors of the type 5 cGMP-specific phosphodiesterase (PDE). Among the oral PDE-5 inhibitors, sildenafil is the only one with evidence from clinical trials for ED in PD patients.[318] In non-PD patients all PDE-5 inhibitors seem to share the same efficacy and safety profile,[319] and may therefore all be applicable for ED treatment in PD. Cautious use is advised in patients with symptomatic OH, and PDE-5 inhibitors are contraindicated in patients with nitrate medication for coronary artery disease.[319] Sublingual apomorphine may represent an alternative, but has been less effective in non-PD populations.[320]

REFERENCES

1. Ordenstein L. [Sur la paralysie agitante et la sclérose en plaque generalisèe]. Martinet 1867.
2. Charcot J. Lecons sur les maladies du systeme nerveux. A Delahaye 1872.
3. Schwab RS, Mador LV, and Lettvin JY. Apomorphine in Parkinson's disease. Trans Am Neurol Assoc 1951;56: 251–253.
4. Corbin KB. Trihexyphenidyl; evaluation of the new agent in the treatment of Parkinsonism. J Am Med Assoc 1949 Oct 8;141(6):377–382.
5. Carlsson A, Lindqvist M, and Magnusson T. 3,4-Dihydroxyphenylalanine and 5-hydroxytryptophan as reserpine antagonists. Nature 1957 Nov 30;180(4596):1200.
6. Ehringer H, Hornykiewicz O. [Distribution of noradrenaline and dopamine (3-hydroxytyramine) in the human brain and their behavior in diseases of the extrapyramidal system.]. Klin Wochenschr 1960 Dec 15;38: 1236–1239.
7. Barbeau A, Murphy GF, and Sourkes TL. Excretion of dopamine in diseases of basal ganglia. Science 1961 May 26;133:1706–1707.
8. Barbeau A, Sourkes TL, and Murphy C. [Les catecholamines dans la maladie de Parkinson. In de Ajuriaguerra J (ed). Monoamines et System Nerveaux Central. Geneva: Georg, 1962, p. 247–262.
9. Birkmayer W and Hornykiewicz O. [The L-3,4-dioxyphenylalanine (DOPA)-effect in Parkinson-akinesia.]. Wien Klin Wochenschr 1961 Nov 10;73:787–788.
10. Cotzias GC, Van Woert MH, and Schiffer LM. Aromatic amino acids and modification of parkinsonism. N Engl J Med 1967 Feb 16;276(7):374–379.
11. Papavasiliou PS, Cotzias GC, Duby SE, et al. Levodopa in Parkinsonism: Potentiation of central effects with a peripheral inhibitor. N Engl J Med 1972 Jan 6;286(1):8–14.
12. Cotzias GC, Papavasiliou PS, and Gellene R. Modification of Parkinsonism—chronic treatment with L-dopa. N Engl J Med 1969 Feb 13;280(7):337–345.
13. Nutt JG and Fellman JH. Pharmacokinetics of levodopa. Clin Neuropharmacol 1984;7(1):35–49.
14. Rivera-Calimlim L, Dujovne CA, Morgan JP, et al. Absorption and metabolism of L-dopa by the human stomach. Eur J Clin Invest 1971 May;1(5):313–320.
15. Leenders KL, Poewe WH, Palmer AJ, et al. Inhibition of L-[18F]fluorodopa uptake into human brain by amino acids demonstrated by positron emission tomography. Ann Neurol 1986 Aug;20(2):258–262.

16. Nutt JG, Woodward WR, Hammerstad JP, et al. The "on-off" phenomenon in Parkinson's disease. Relation to levodopa absorption and transport. N Engl J Med 1984 Feb 23;310(8):483–488.
17. Schultz E. Catechol-O-methyltransferase and aromatic L-amino acid decarboxylase activities in human gastrointestinal tissues. Life Sci 1991;49(10):721–725.
18. Nutt JG, Woodward WR, Anderson JL. The effect of carbidopa on the pharmacokinetics of intravenously administered levodopa: The mechanism of action in the treatment of parkinsonism. Ann Neurol 1985 Nov;18(5):537–543.
19. Barbeau A, Gillo-Joffroy L, and Mars H. Treatment of Parkinson's disease with levodopa and Ro 4-4602. Clin Pharmacol Ther 1971 Mar;12(2):353–359.
20. Calne DB, Reid JL, Vakil SD, et al. Idiopathic Parkinsonism treated with an extracerebral decarboxylase inhibitor in combination with levodopa. Br Med J 1971 Sep 25;3(5777):729–732.
21. Kaakkola S, Teravainen H, Ahtila S, et al. Effect of entacapone, a COMT inhibitor, on clinical disability and levodopa metabolism in parkinsonian patients. Neurology 1994 Jan;44(1):77–80.
22. Merello M, Lees AJ, Webster R, Bovingdon M, et al. Effect of entacapone, a peripherally acting catechol-O-methyltransferase inhibitor, on the motor response to acute treatment with levodopa in patients with Parkinson's disease. J Neurol Neurosurg Psychiatry 1994 Feb;57(2):186–189.
23. Hefti F, Melamed E, and Wurtman RJ. The site of dopamine formation in rat striatum after L-dopa administration. J Pharmacol Exp Ther 1981 Apr;217(1):189–197.
24. Poewe W, Wenning G. L-dopa in Parkinson's disease: Mechanisms of action and pathophysiology of late failure. In Jankovic P and Tolosa, E (eds). Parkinson's disease and movement disorders. 4th edn. Baltimore: Williams&Wilkins; 2002, p. 104–115.
25. Fahn S, Oakes D, Shoulson I, et al. Levodopa and the progression of Parkinson's disease. N Engl J Med 2004 Dec 9;351(24):2498–2508.
26. Rinne UK, Bracco F, Chouza C, et al. Early treatment of Parkinson's disease with cabergoline delays the onset of motor complications. Results of a double-blind levodopa controlled trial. The PKDS009 Study Group. Drugs 1998;55(suppl 1):23–30.
27. Rascol O, Brooks DJ, Korczyn AD, et al. A five-year study of the incidence of dyskinesia in patients with early Parkinson's disease who were treated with ropinirole or levodopa. 056 Study Group. N Engl J Med 2000 May 18;342(20):1484–1491.
28. Pramipexole vs levodopa as initial treatment for Parkinson disease: A randomized controlled trial. Parkinson Study Group. JAMA 2000 Oct 18;284(15):1931–1938.
29. Holloway RG, Shoulson I, Fahn S, et al. Pramipexole vs levodopa as initial treatment for Parkinson disease: A 4-year randomized controlled trial. Arch Neurol 2004 Jul;61(7):1044–1053.
30. Oertel WH, Wolters E, Sampaio C, et al. Pergolide versus levodopa monotherapy in early Parkinson's disease patients: The PELMOPET study. Mov Disord 2006 Mar;21(3):343–353.
31. Quinn NP. Anti-parkinsonian drugs today. Drugs 1984 Sep;28(3):236–262.
32. Hogl B, Seppi K, Brandauer E, et al. Increased daytime sleepiness in Parkinson's disease: A questionnaire survey. Mov Disord 2003 Mar;18(3):319–323.
33. Giovannoni G, O'Sullivan JD, Turner K, et al. Hedonistic homeostatic dysregulation in patients with Parkinson's disease on dopamine replacement therapies. J Neurol Neurosurg Psychiatry 2000 Apr;68(4):423–428.
34. Evans AH, Katzenschlager R, Paviour D, et al. Punding in Parkinson's disease: Its relation to the dopamine dysregulation syndrome. Mov Disord 2004 Apr;19(4):397–405.
35. Voon V and Fox SH. Medication-related impulse control and repetitive behaviors in Parkinson disease. Arch Neurol 2007 Aug;64(8):1089–1096.
36. Olanow CW, Agid Y, Mizuno Y, et al. Levodopa in the treatment of Parkinson's disease: Current controversies. Mov Disord 2004 Sep;19(9):997–1005.
37. Schapira AH. The clinical relevance of levodopa toxicity in the treatment of Parkinson's disease. Mov Disord 2008;23(suppl 3):S515–S520.
38. Poewe WH, Lees AJ, and Stern GM. Low-dose L-dopa therapy in Parkinson's disease: A 6-year follow-up study. Neurology 1986 Nov;36(11):1528–1530.
39. Schrag A and Quinn N. Dyskinesias and motor fluctuations in Parkinson's disease. A community-based study. Brain 2000 Nov;123 (pt 11):2297–2305.
40. Horstink M, Tolosa E, Bonuccelli U, et al. Review of the therapeutic management of Parkinson's disease. Report of a joint task force of the European Federation of Neurological Societies and the Movement Disorder Society-European Section. Part I: Early (uncomplicated) Parkinson's disease. Eur J Neurol 2006 Nov;13(11):1170–1185.
41. Miyasaki JM, Martin W, Suchowersky O, et al. Practice parameter: Initiation of treatment for Parkinson's disease: An evidence-based review: Report of the Quality Standards Subcommittee of the American Academy of Neurology. Neurology 2002 Jan 8;58(1):11–17.
42. Olanow CW, Stern MB, and Sethi K. The scientific and clinical basis for the treatment of Parkinson disease (2009). Neurology 2009 May 26;72(21 suppl 4):S1–S136.
43. Calne DB, Teychenne PF, Claveria LE, et al. Bromocriptine in Parkinsonism. Br Med J 1974 Nov 23;4(5942): 442–444.
44. Calne DB, Teychenne PF, Leigh PN, et al. Treatment of parkinsonism with bromocriptine. Lancet 1974 Dec 7;2(7893):1355–1356.
45. Struppler A and von Uexkull T. [Studies of mechanism of action of apormorphine on Parkinson's tremor.] Z Klin Med 1953;152(1–2):46–57.
46. Giladi N, Boroojerdi B, Korczyn AD, et al. Rotigotine transdermal patch in early Parkinson's disease: A randomized, double-blind, controlled study versus placebo and ropinirole. Mov Disord 2007 Dec;22(16):2398–2404.
47. Watts RL, Jankovic J, Waters C, et al. Randomized, blind, controlled trial of transdermal rotigotine in early Parkinson disease. Neurology 2007 Jan 23;68(4):272–276.
48. Stibe CM, Lees AJ, Kempster PA, et al. Subcutaneous apomorphine in parkinsonian on-off oscillations. Lancet 1988 Feb 20;1(8582):403–406.
49. Frankel JP, Lees AJ, Kempster PA, et al. Subcutaneous apomorphine in the treatment of Parkinson's disease. J Neurol Neurosurg Psychiatry 1990 Feb;53(2):96–101.

50. Stocchi F, Hersh BP, Scott BL, et al. Ropinirole 24-hour prolonged release and ropinirole immediate release in early Parkinson's disease: A randomized, double-blind, non-inferiority crossover study. Curr Med Res Opin 2008 Oct;24(10):2883–2895.
51. Poewe W, Barone P, Hauser R, et al. Pramipexole extended-release is effective in early Parkinson's disease. Mov Disord 24(suppl 1):S273. 2009.
52. Schapira A, Barone P, Hauser R, et al. Efficacy and safety of pramipexole extended-release for advanced Parkinson's Disease. Mov Disord 24(suppl 1): S277–S273. 2009.
53. Barone P, Bravi D, Bermejo-Pareja F, et al. Pergolide monotherapy in the treatment of early PD: A randomized, controlled study. Pergolide Monotherapy Study Group. Neurology 1999 Aug 11;53(3):573–579.
54. Bergamasco B, Frattola L, Muratorio A, et al. Alpha-dihydroergocryptine in the treatment of de novo parkinsonian patients: Results of a multicentre, randomized, double-blind, placebo-controlled study. Acta Neurol Scand 2000 Jun;101(6):372–380.
55. Safety and efficacy of pramipexole in early Parkinson disease. A randomized dose-ranging study. Parkinson Study Group. JAMA 1997 Jul 9;278(2):125–130.
56. Shannon KM, Bennett JP, Jr., Friedman JH. Efficacy of pramipexole, a novel dopamine agonist, as monotherapy in mild to moderate Parkinson's disease. The Pramipexole Study Group. Neurology 1997 Sep;49(3):724–728.
57. Adler CH, Sethi KD, Hauser RA, Davis TL, et al. Ropinirole for the treatment of early Parkinson's disease. The Ropinirole Study Group. Neurology 1997 Aug;49(2): 393–399.
58. Rascol O, Dubois B, Caldas AC, et al. Early piribedil monotherapy of Parkinson's disease: A planned seven-month report of the REGAIN study. Mov Disord 2006 Dec;21(12):2110–2115.
59. Goetz CG, Poewe W, Rascol O, et al. Evidence-based medical review update: Pharmacological and surgical treatments of Parkinson's disease: 2001 to 2004. Mov Disord 2005 May;20(5):523–539.
60. Rinne UK, Bracco F, Chouza C, et al. Cabergoline in the treatment of early Parkinson's disease: Results of the first year of treatment in a double-blind comparison of cabergoline and levodopa. The PKDS009 Collaborative Study Group. Neurology 1997 Feb;48(2):363–368.
61. Long-term Effect of Initiating Pramipexole vs Levodopa in Early Parkinson Disease. Arch Neurol 2009 Mar 9.
62. Hauser RA, Rascol O, Korczyn AD, et al. Ten-year follow-up of Parkinson's disease patients randomized to initial therapy with ropinirole or levodopa. Mov Disord 2007 Dec;22(16):2409–2417.
63. Katzenschlager R, Head J, Schrag A, et al. Fourteen-year final report of the randomized PDRG-UK trial comparing three initial treatments in PD. Neurology 2008 Aug 12;71(7):474–480.
64. Yamamoto M, Schapira AH. Dopamine agonists in Parkinson's disease. Expert Rev Neurother 2008 Apr;8(4): 671–677.
65. Rascol O, Goetz C, Koller W, et al. Treatment interventions for Parkinson's disease: An evidence based assessment. Lancet 2002 May 4;359(9317):1589–1598.
66. Hubble JP. Long-term studies of dopamine agonists. Neurology 2002 Feb 26;58(4 suppl 1):S42–S50.
67. Frucht S, Rogers JD, Greene PE, et al. Falling asleep at the wheel: Motor vehicle mishaps in persons taking pramipexole and ropinirole. Neurology 1999 Jun 10;52(9):1908–1910.
68. Frauscher B, Poewe W. Excessive daytime sleepiness in Parkinson's disease. In Chaudhuri K, Tolosa E, Schapira A and Poewe W (eds). Non-motor symptoms of Parkinson's Disease.Oxford: Oxford University Press, 2009, p. 205–213.
69. Paus S, Brecht HM, Koster J, et al. Sleep attacks, daytime sleepiness, and dopamine agonists in Parkinson's disease. Mov Disord 2003 Jun;18(6):659–667.
70. Antonini A, Tolosa E, Mizuno Y, et al. A reassessment of risks and benefits of dopamine agonists in Parkinson's disease. Lancet Neurol 2009 Aug 24.
71. Weintraub D. Dopamine and impulse control disorders in Parkinson's disease. Ann Neurol 2008 Dec;64(suppl 2):S93–S100.
72. Biglan KM, Holloway RG, Jr., McDermott MP, et al. Risk factors for somnolence, edema, and hallucinations in early Parkinson disease. Neurology 2007 Jul 10;69(2): 187–195.
73. Simonis G, Fuhrmann JT, Strasser RH. Meta-analysis of heart valve abnormalities in Parkinson's disease patients treated with dopamine agonists. Mov Disord 2007 Oct 15;22(13):1936–1942.
74. Zanettini R, Antonini A, Gatto G, et al. Valvular heart disease and the use of dopamine agonists for Parkinson's disease. N Engl J Med 2007 Jan 4;356(1):39–46.
75. Roth BL. Drugs and valvular heart disease. N Engl J Med 2007 Jan 4;356(1):6–9.
76. Hofmann C, Penner U, Dorow R, et al. Lisuride, a dopamine receptor agonist with 5-HT2B receptor antagonist properties: Absence of cardiac valvulopathy adverse drug reaction reports supports the concept of a crucial role for 5-HT2B receptor agonism in cardiac valvular fibrosis. Clin Neuropharmacol 2006 Mar;29(2):80–86.
77. Tintner R, Manian P, Gauthier P, Jankovic J. Pleuropulmonary fibrosis after long-term treatment with the dopamine agonist pergolide for Parkinson Disease. Arch Neurol 2005 Aug;62(8):1290–1295.
78. Townsend M, MacIver DH. Constrictive pericarditis and pleuropulmonary fibrosis secondary to cabergoline treatment for Parkinson's disease. Heart 2004 Aug;90(8):e47.
79. Gerstenbrand F, Prosenz P. [On the treatment of Parkinson's syndrome with monoamine oxidase inhibitors alone and in combination with L-dopa]. Praxis 1965 Nov 18;54(46):1373–1377.
80. Thebault JJ, Guillaume M, Levy R. Tolerability, safety, pharmacodynamics, and pharmacokinetics of rasagiline: A potent, selective, and irreversible monoamine oxidase type B inhibitor. Pharmacotherapy 2004 Oct;24(10): 1295–1305.
81. Turkish S, Yu PH, Greenshaw AJ. Monoamine oxidase-B inhibition: A comparison of in vivo and ex vivo measures of reversible effects. J Neural Transm 1988;74(3):141–148.
82. Reynolds GP, Elsworth JD, Blau K, et al. Deprenyl is metabolized to methamphetamine and amphetamine in man. Br J Clin Pharmacol 1978 Dec;6(6):542–544.

83. Chen JJ, Swope DM. Clinical pharmacology of rasagiline: A novel, second-generation propargylamine for the treatment of Parkinson disease. J Clin Pharmacol 2005 Aug;45(8):878–894.
84. Bar AO, Amit T, Youdim MB. Contrasting neuroprotective and neurotoxic actions of respective metabolites of anti-Parkinson drugs rasagiline and selegiline. Neurosci Lett 2004 Jan 30;355(3):169–172.
85. Youdim MB, Wadia A, Tatton W, et al. The anti-Parkinson drug rasagiline and its cholinesterase inhibitor derivatives exert neuroprotection unrelated to MAO inhibition in cell culture and in vivo. Ann N Y Acad Sci 2001 Jun;939:450–458.
86. Mandel S, Weinreb O, Amit T, et al. Mechanism of neuroprotective action of the anti-Parkinson drug rasagiline and its derivatives. Brain Res Brain Res Rev 2005 Apr;48(2):379–387.
87. Clarke A, Johnson ES, Mallard N, et al. A new low-dose formulation of selegiline: Clinical efficacy, patient preference and selectivity for MAO-B inhibition. J Neural Transm 2003 Nov;110(11):1257–1271.
88. Onofrj M, Bonanni L, and Thomas A. An expert opinion on safinamide in Parkinson's disease. Expert Opin Investig Drugs 2008 Jul;17(7):1115–1125.
89. Effects of tocopherol and deprenyl on the progression of disability in early Parkinson's disease. The Parkinson Study Group. N Engl J Med 1993 Jan 21;328(3):176–183.
90. Myllyla VV, Sotaniemi KA, Vuorinen JA, et al. Selegiline as initial treatment in de novo parkinsonian patients. Neurology 1992 Feb;42(2):339–343.
91. Mally J, Kovacs AB, and Stone TW. Delayed development of symptomatic improvement by (--)-deprenyl in Parkinson's disease. J Neurol Sci 1995 Dec;134(1–2):143–145.
92. Palhagen S, Heinonen EH, Hagglund J, et al. Selegiline delays the onset of disability in de novo parkinsonian patients. Swedish Parkinson Study Group. Neurology 1998 Aug;51(2):520–525.
93. Olanow CW, Hauser RA, Gauger L, et al. The effect of deprenyl and levodopa on the progression of Parkinson's disease. Ann Neurol 1995 Nov;38(5):771–777.
94. Palhagen S, Heinonen E, Hagglund J, et al. Selegiline slows the progression of the symptoms of Parkinson disease. Neurology 2006 Apr 25;66(8):1200–1206.
95. A controlled, randomized, delayed-start study of rasagiline in early Parkinson disease. Arch Neurol 2004 Apr;61(4):561–566.
96. Olanow CW, Rascol O, Hauser R, et al. A double-blind, delayed-start trial of rasagiline in Parkinson's disease. N Engl J Med 2009 Sep 24;361(13):1268–1278.
97. Hauser RA, Panisset M, Abbruzzese G, et al. Double-blind trial of levodopa/carbidopa/entacapone versus levodopa/carbidopa in early Parkinson's disease. Mov Disord 2009 Mar 15;24(4):541–550.
98. D'Agostino RB, Sr. The delayed-start study design. N Engl J Med 2009 Sep 24;361(13):1304–1306.
99. Heinonen EH, Myllyla V. Safety of selegiline (deprenyl) in the treatment of Parkinson's disease. Drug Saf 1998 Jul;19(1):11–22.
100. Schapira AH. Molecular and clinical pathways to neuroprotection of dopaminergic drugs in Parkinson disease. Neurology 2009 Feb 17;72(7 suppl):S44–S50.
101. Ritter JL, Alexander B. Retrospective study of selegiline-antidepressant drug interactions and a review of the literature. Ann Clin Psychiatry 1997 Mar;9(1):7–13.
102. Richard IH, Kurlan R, Tanner C, et al. Serotonin syndrome and the combined use of deprenyl and an antidepressant in Parkinson's disease. Parkinson Study Group. Neurology 1997 Apr;48(4):1070–1077.
103. Hauser RA, Lew MF, Hurtig HI, et al. Long-term outcome of early versus delayed rasagiline treatment in early Parkinson's disease. Mov Disord 2009 Mar 15;24(4):564–573.
104. Boyer EW, Shannon M. The serotonin syndrome. N Engl J Med 2005 Mar 17;352(11):1112–1120.
105. Stewart DA. NICE guideline for Parkinson's disease. Age Ageing 2007 May;36(3):240–242.
106. Hauser RA, Lew MF, Hurtig HI, et al. Long-term outcome of early versus delayed rasagiline treatment in early Parkinson's disease. Mov Disord 2009 Mar 15;24(4):564–573.
107. Obeso JA, Marin C, Rodriguez-Oroz C, et al. The basal ganglia in Parkinson's disease: Current concepts and unexplained observations. Ann Neurol 2008 Dec;64(suppl 2):S30–S46.
108. Klockgether T, Turski L. Toward an understanding of the role of glutamate in experimental parkinsonism: Agonist-sensitive sites in the basal ganglia. Ann Neurol 1993 Oct;34(4):585–593.
109. Schwab RS, England AC, Jr., Poskanzer DC, Young RR. Amantadine in the treatment of Parkinson's disease. JAMA 1969 May 19;208(7):1168–1170.
110. Stoof JC, Booij J, and Drukarch B. Amantadine as N-methyl-D-aspartic acid receptor antagonist: New possibilities for therapeutic applications? Clin Neurol Neurosurg 1992;94(suppl):S4–S6.
111. Amantadine and other antiglutamate agents: Management of Parkinson's disease. Mov Disord 2002;17(suppl 4):S13–S22.
112. Pimentel L and Hughes B. Amantadine toxicity presenting with complex ventricular ectopy and hallucinations. Pediatr Emerg Care 1991 Apr;7(2):89–92.
113. Butzer JF, Silver DE, and Sahs AL. Amantadine in Parkinson's disease. A double-blind, placebo-controlled, crossover study with long-term follow-up. Neurology 1975 Jul;25(7):603–606.
114. Cox B, Danta G, Schnieden H, et al. Interactions of L-dopa and amantadine in patients with Parkinsonism. J Neurol Neurosurg Psychiatry 1973 Jun;36(3):354–361.
115. Parkes JD, Baxter RC, Curzon G, et al. Treatment of Parkinson's disease with amantadine and levodopa. A one-year study. Lancet 1971 May 29;1(7709):1083–1086.
116. Parkes JD, Baxter RC, Marsden CD, et al. Comparative trial of benzhexol, amantadine, and levodopa in the treatment of Parkinson's disease. J Neurol Neurosurg Psychiatry 1974 Apr;37(4):422–426.
117. Poewe W. Treatments for Parkinson disease—past achievements and current clinical needs. Neurology 2009 Feb 17;72(7 suppl):S65–S73.
118. Galarraga E, Hernandez-Lopez S, Reyes A, et al. Cholinergic modulation of neostriatal output: A functional antagonism between different types of muscarinic receptors. J Neurosci 1999 May 1;19(9):3629–3638.

119. Friedman E, Wang HY, and Butkerait P. Decreased striatal release of acetylcholine following withdrawal from long-term treatment with haloperidol: Modulation by cholinergic, dopamine-D1 and -D2 mechanisms. Neuropharmacology 1990 Jun;29(6):537–544.
120. Stoof JC and Kebabian JW. Independent in vitro regulation by the D-2 dopamine receptor of dopamine-stimulated efflux of cyclic AMP and K+-stimulated release of acetylcholine from rat neostriatum. Brain Res 1982 Nov 4;250(2):263–270.
121. Abercrombie ED, DeBoer P. Substantia nigra D1 receptors and stimulation of striatal cholinergic interneurons by dopamine: A proposed circuit mechanism. J Neurosci 1997 Nov 1;17(21):8498–8505.
122. Damsma G, Tham CS, Robertson GS, et al. Dopamine D1 receptor stimulation increases striatal acetylcholine release in the rat. Eur J Pharmacol 1990 Sep 21;186 (2–3):335–338.
123. Zhou FM, Liang Y, Dani JA. Endogenous nicotinic cholinergic activity regulates dopamine release in the striatum. Nat Neurosci 2001 Dec;4(12):1224–1229.
124. Katzenschlager R, Sampaio C, Costa J, et al. Anticholinergics for symptomatic management of Parkinson's disease. Cochrane Database Syst Rev 2003;(2):CD003735.
125. Anticholinergic therapies in the treatment of Parkinson's disease. Mov Disord 2002;17(suppl 4):S7–S12.
126. Schrag A, Schelosky L, Scholz U, et al. Reduction of Parkinsonian signs in patients with Parkinson's disease by dopaminergic versus anticholinergic single-dose challenges. Mov Disord 1999 Mar;14(2):252–255.
127. Birket-Smith E. Abnormal involuntary movements induced by anticholinergic therapy. Acta Neurol Scand 1974;50(6):801–811.
128. Birket-Smith E. Abnormal involuntary movements in relation to anticholinergics and levodopa therapy. Acta Neurol Scand 1975 Aug;52(2):158–160.
129. Linazasoro G. Anticholinergics and dyskinesia. Mov Disord 1994 Nov;9(6):689.
130. Horrocks PM, Vicary DJ, Rees JE, et al. Anticholinergic withdrawal and benzhexol treatment in Parkinson's disease. J Neurol Neurosurg Psychiatry 1973 Dec;36(6): 936–941.
131. Hughes RC, Polgar JG, Weightman D, et al. Levodopa in Parkinsonism: The effects of withdrawal of anticholinergic drugs. Br Med J 1971 May 29;2(5760):487–491.
132. Schapira AH, Obeso J. Timing of treatment initiation in Parkinson's disease: A need for reappraisal? Ann Neurol 2006 Mar;59(3):559–562.
133. Clarke CE, Davies P. Systematic review of acute levodopa and apomorphine challenge tests in the diagnosis of idiopathic Parkinson's disease. J Neurol Neurosurg Psychiatry 2000 Nov;69(5):590–594.
134. A randomized controlled trial comparing pramipexole with levodopa in early Parkinson's disease: Design and methods of the CALM-PD Study. Parkinson Study Group. Clin Neuropharmacol 2000 Jan;23(1):34–44.
135. Fahn S. Parkinson disease, the effect of levodopa, and the ELLDOPA trial. Earlier vs Later L-DOPA. Archives of neurology 1999 May;56(5):529–535.
136. Fahn S. A new look at levodopa based on the ELLDOPA study. J Neural Transm Suppl 2006;(70):419–426.
137. Rascol O, Brooks DJ, Korczyn AD, et al. A five-year study of the incidence of dyskinesia in patients with early Parkinson's disease who were treated with ropinirole or levodopa. 056 Study Group. N Engl J Med 2000 May 18;342(20):1484–1491.
138. Hauser RA, McDermott MP, Messing S. Factors associated with the development of motor fluctuations and dyskinesias in Parkinson disease. Arch Neurol 2006 Dec;63(12):1756–1760.
139. Djaldetti R, Ziv I, Melamed E. Impaired absorption of oral levodopa: A major cause for response fluctuations in Parkinson's disease. Isr J Med Sci 1996 Dec;32(12): 1224–1227.
140. Djaldetti R, Baron J, Ziv I, et al. Gastric emptying in Parkinson's disease: Patients with and without response fluctuations. Neurology 1996 Apr;46(4):1051–1054.
141. Mouradian MM, Juncos JL, Fabbrini G, et al. Motor fluctuations in Parkinson's disease: Central pathophysiological mechanisms, Part II. Ann Neurol 1988 Sep;24(3):372–378.
142. Yeh KC, August TF, Bush DF, et al. Pharmacokinetics and bioavailability of Sinemet CR: A summary of human studies. Neurology 1989 Nov;39(11 Suppl 2):25–38.
143. LeWitt PA, Nelson MV, Berchou RC, et al. Controlled-release carbidopa/levodopa (Sinemet 50/200 CR4): Clinical and pharmacokinetic studies. Neurology 1989 Nov;39(11 suppl 2):45–53.
144. Erni W, Held K. The hydrodynamically balanced system: A novel principle of controlled drug release. Eur Neurol 1987;27(suppl 1):21–27.
145. Koller WC, Pahwa R. Treating motor fluctuations with controlled-release levodopa preparations. Neurology 1994 Jul;44(7 suppl 6):S23–S28.
146. Levodopa: Management of Parkinson's disease. Mov Disord 2002;17 Suppl 4:S23–S37.
147. A comparison of Madopar CR and standard Madopar in the treatment of nocturnal and early-morning disability in Parkinson's disease. The U.K. Madopar CR Study Group. Clin Neuropharmacol 1989 Dec;12(6):498–505.
148. Block G, Liss C, Reines S, et al. Comparison of immediate-release and controlled release carbidopa/levodopa in Parkinson's disease. A multicenter 5-year study. The CR First Study Group. Eur Neurol 1997;37(1):23–27.
149. Dupont E, Andersen A, Boas J, et al. Sustained-release Madopar HBS compared with standard Madopar in the long-term treatment of de novo parkinsonian patients. Acta Neurol Scand 1996 Jan;93(1):14–20.
150. Koller WC, Hutton JT, Tolosa E, et al. Immediate-release and controlled-release carbidopa/levodopa in PD: A 5-year randomized multicenter study. Carbidopa/Levodopa Study Group. Neurology 1999 Sep 22;53(5):1012–1019.
151. Kleedorfer B, Poewe W. Comparative efficacy of two oral sustained-release preparations of L-dopa in fluctuating Parkinson's disease. Preliminary findings in 20 patients. J Neural Transm Park Dis Dement Sect 1992;4(2):173–178.
152. Poewe WH, Lees AJ, Stern GM. Treatment of motor fluctuations in Parkinson's disease with an oral sustained-release preparation of L-dopa: Clinical and pharmacokinetic observations. Clin Neuropharmacol 1986;9(5):430–439.
153. LeWitt PA. Clinical studies with and pharmacokinetic considerations of sustained-release levodopa. Neurology 1992 Jan;42(1 suppl 1):29–32.

154. Contin M, Riva R, Martinelli P, et al. Concentration-effect relationship of levodopa-benserazide dispersible formulation versus standard form in the treatment of complicated motor response fluctuations in Parkinson's disease. Clin Neuropharmacol 1999 Nov;22(6):351–355.
155. Descombes S, Bonnet AM, Gasser UE, et al. Dual-release formulation, a novel principle in L-dopa treatment of Parkinson's disease. Neurology 2001 May 8;56(9): 1239–1242.
156. Kuoppamaki M, Korpela K, Marttila R, et al. Comparison of pharmacokinetic profile of levodopa throughout the day between levodopa/carbidopa/entacapone and levodopa/carbidopa when administered four or five times daily. Eur J Clin Pharmacol 2009 May;65(5):443–455.
157. Kaakkola S, Wurtman RJ. Effects of COMT inhibitors on striatal dopamine metabolism: A microdialysis study. Brain Res 1992 Aug 7;587(2):241-9.
158. Keranen T, Gordin A, Karlsson M, et al. Inhibition of soluble catechol-O-methyltransferase and single-dose pharmacokinetics after oral and intravenous administration of entacapone. Eur J Clin Pharmacol 1994;46(2):151–157.
159. Nissinen E, Linden IB, Schultz E, et al. Biochemical and pharmacological properties of a peripherally acting catechol-O-methyltransferase inhibitor entacapone. Naunyn Schmiedebergs Arch Pharmacol 1992 Sep;346(3): 262–266.
160. Sawle GV, Burn DJ, Morrish PK, et al. The effect of entacapone (OR-611) on brain [18F]-6-L-fluorodopa metabolism: Implications for levodopa therapy of Parkinson's disease. Neurology 1994 Jul;44(7):1292–1297.
161. Myllyla VV, Sotaniemi KA, Illi A, et al. Effect of entacapone, a COMT inhibitor, on the pharmacokinetics of levodopa and on cardiovascular responses in patients with Parkinson's disease. Eur J Clin Pharmacol 1993;45(5):419–423.
162. Keranen T, Gordin A, Harjola VP, et al. The effect of catechol-O-methyl transferase inhibition by entacapone on the pharmacokinetics and metabolism of levodopa in healthy volunteers. Clin Neuropharmacol 1993 Apr;16(2):145–156.
163. Nutt JG, Woodward WR, Beckner RM, et al. Effect of peripheral catechol-O-methyltransferase inhibition on the pharmacokinetics and pharmacodynamics of levodopa in parkinsonian patients. Neurology 1994 May;44(5): 913–919.
164. Limousin P, Pollak P, Gervason-Tournier CL, et al. Ro 40-7592, a COMT inhibitor, plus levodopa in Parkinson's disease. Lancet 1993 Jun 19;341(8860):1605.
165. Lees AJ. Evidence-based efficacy comparison of tolcapone and entacapone as adjunctive therapy in Parkinson's disease. CNS Neurosci Ther 2008;14(1):83–93.
166. Safety and efficacy of pramipexole in early Parkinson disease. A randomized dose-ranging study. Parkinson Study Group. JAMA 1997;278(2):125–130.
167. Rinne UK, Larsen JP, Siden A, Worm Petersen J. Entacapone enhances the response to levodopa in parkinsonian patients with motor fluctuations. Nomecomt Study Group. Neurology 1998;51(5):1309–1314.
168. Poewe WH, Deuschl G, Gordin A, et al. Efficacy and safety of entacapone in Parkinson's disease patients with suboptimal levodopa response: A 6-month randomized placebo-controlled double-blind study in Germany and Austria (Celomen study). Acta Neurol Scand 2002 Apr;105(4):245–255.
169. Waters CH, Kurth M, Bailey P, , et al. Tolcapone in stable Parkinson's disease: Efficacy and safety of long-term treatment. The Tolcapone Stable Study Group. Neurology 1997;49(3):665–671.
170. Olanow CW, Obeso JA, Stocchi F. Continuous dopamine-receptor treatment of Parkinson's disease: Scientific rationale and clinical implications. Lancet Neurol 2006 Aug;5(8):677–687.
171. Assal F, Spahr L, Hadengue A, et al. Tolcapone and fulminant hepatitis. Lancet 1998 Sep 19;352(9132):958.
172. Colosimo C. The rise and fall of tolcapone. J Neurol 1999 Oct;246(10):880–882.
173. Quinn N, Parkes JD, Marsden CD. Control of on/off phenomenon by continuous intravenous infusion of levodopa. Neurology 1984 Sep;34(9):1131–1136.
174. Kurlan R, Rubin AJ, Miller C, et al. Duodenal delivery of levodopa for on-off fluctuations in parkinsonism: Preliminary observations. Ann Neurol 1986;20(2):262–265.
175. Kurth MC, Adler CH. COMT inhibition: A new treatment strategy for Parkinson's disease. Neurology 1998 May;50(5 suppl 5):S3–S14.
176. Syed N, Murphy J, Zimmerman T, Jr., et al. Ten years' experience with enteral levodopa infusions for motor fluctuations in Parkinson's disease. Mov Disord 1998 Mar;13(2):336–338.
177. Nyholm D, Nilsson Remahl AI, Dizdar N, et al. Duodenal levodopa infusion monotherapy vs oral polypharmacy in advanced Parkinson disease. Neurology 2005 Jan 25;64(2):216–223.
178. Antonini A, Isaias IU, Canesi M, et al. Duodenal levodopa infusion for advanced Parkinson's disease: 12-month treatment outcome. Mov Disord 2007 Jun 15;22(8): 1145–1149.
179. Nyholm D, Lewander T, Johansson A, et al. Enteral levodopa/carbidopa infusion in advanced Parkinson disease: Long-term exposure. Clin Neuropharmacol 2008 Mar;31(2):63–73.
180. Devos D. Patient profile, indications, efficacy and safety of duodenal levodopa infusion in advanced Parkinson's disease. Mov Disord 2009 May 15;24(7):993–1000.
181. Golbe LI. Deprenyl as symptomatic therapy in Parkinson's disease. Clin Neuropharmacol 1988;11:387–400.
182. Lees AJ, Frankel J, Eatough V, et al. New approaches in the use of selegiline for the treatment of Parkinson's disease. Acta Neurol Scand Suppl 1989;126:139–145.
183. Lieberman AN, Neophytides A, Leibowitz M, et al. Comparative efficacy of pergolide and bromocriptine in patients with advanced Parkinson's disease. Adv Neurol 1983;37:95–108.
184. Waters CH, Sethi KD, Hauser RA, et al. Zydis selegiline reduces off time in Parkinson's disease patients with motor fluctuations: A 3-month, randomized, placebo-controlled study. Mov Disord 2004 Apr;19(4):426–432.
185. A randomized placebo-controlled trial of rasagiline in levodopa-treated patients with Parkinson disease and motor fluctuations: The PRESTO study. Arch Neurol 2005 Feb;62(2):241–248.
186. Rascol O, Brooks DJ, Melamed E, et al. Rasagiline as an adjunct to levodopa in patients with Parkinson's disease

and motor fluctuations (LARGO, Lasting effect in Adjunct therapy with Rasagiline Given Once daily, study): A randomized, double-blind, parallel-group trial. Lancet 2005 Mar 12;365(9463):947–954.

187. Pahwa R, Factor SA, Lyons KE, et al. Practice Parameter: Treatment of Parkinson disease with motor fluctuations and dyskinesia (an evidence-based review): Report of the Quality Standards Subcommittee of the American Academy of Neurology. Neurology 2006 Apr 11;66(7):983–995.
188. Horstink M, Tolosa E, Bonuccelli U, et al. Review of the therapeutic management of Parkinson's disease. Report of a joint task force of the European Federation of Neurological Societies (EFNS) and the Movement Disorder Society-European Section (MDS-ES). Part II: Late (complicated) Parkinson's disease. Eur J Neurol 2006 Nov;13(11):1186–1202.
189. Calne DB, Plotkin C, Williams AC, et al. Long-term treatment of parkinsonism with bromocriptine. Lancet 1978 Apr 8;1(8067):735–738.
190. Gancher ST, Woodward WR, Boucher B, et al. Peripheral pharmacokinetics of apomorphine in humans. Ann Neurol 1989 Aug;26(2):232–238.
191. Durif F, Lemaire JJ, Debilly B, et al. Acute and chronic effects of anteromedial globus pallidus stimulation in Parkinson's disease. J Neurol Neurosurg Psychiatry 1999 Sep;67(3):315–322.
192. Kapoor R, Turjanski N, Frankel J, et al. Intranasal apomorphine: A new treatment in Parkinson's disease. J Neurol Neurosurg Psychiatry 1990 Nov;53(11):1015.
193. Van Laar T, Jansen EN, Essink AW, et al. Rectal apomorphine: A new treatment modality in Parkinson's disease [letter]. J Neurol Neurosurg Psychiatry 1992;55:737–8X.
194. Goetz CG, Leurgans S, Raman R. Placebo-associated improvements in motor function: Comparison of subjective and objective sections of the UPDRS in early Parkinson's disease. Mov Disord 2002 Mar;17(2):283–288.
195. Poewe WH, Rascol O, Quinn N, et al. Efficacy of pramipexole and transdermal rotigotine in advanced Parkinson's disease: A double-blind, double-dummy, randomized controlled trial. Lancet Neurol 2007 Jun;6(6):513–520.
196. Poewe W, Wenning GK. Apomorphine: An underutilized therapy for Parkinson's disease. Mov Disord 2000 Sep;15(5):789–794.
197. Garcia Ruiz PJ, Sesar IA, Ares PB, et al. Efficacy of long-term continuous subcutaneous apomorphine infusion in advanced Parkinson's disease with motor fluctuations: A multicenter study. Mov Disord 2008 Jun 15;23(8):1130–1136.
198. Katzenschlager R, Hughes A, Evans A, et al. Continuous subcutaneous apomorphine therapy improves dyskinesias in Parkinson's disease: A prospective study using single-dose challenges. Mov Disord 2005 Feb;20(2):151–157.
199. Dewey RB, Jr., Hutton JT, Lewitt PA, et al. A randomized, double-blind, placebo-controlled trial of subcutaneously injected apomorphine for parkinsonian off-state events. Archives of neurology 2001 Sep;58(9):1385–1392.
200. Poewe W, Kleedorfer B, Wagner M, et al. Continuous subcutaneous apomorphine infusions for fluctuating Parkinson's disease. Long-term follow-up in 18 patients. Adv Neurol 1993;60:656–659.
201. Hughes AJ, Bishop S, Kleedorfer B, et al. Subcutaneous apomorphine in Parkinson's disease: Response to chronic administration for up to five years. Mov Disord 1993 Apr;8(2):165–170.
202. Poewe W, Kleedorfer B, Gerstenbrand F, et al. Subcutaneous apomorphine in Parkinson's disease. Lancet 1988 Apr 23;1(8591):943.
203. Schrag A, Ben-Shlomo Y, Brown R, et al. Young-onset Parkinson's disease revisited—clinical features, natural history, and mortality. Mov Disord 1998 Nov;13(6):885–894.
204. Muenter MD, Sharpless NS, Tyce GM, et al. Patterns of dystonia ("I-D-I" and "D-I-D-") in response to l-dopa therapy for Parkinson's disease. Mayo Clin Proc 1977 Mar;52(3):163–174.
205. Nutt JG. Levodopa-induced dyskinesia: Review, observations, and speculations. Neurology 1990 Feb;40(2): 340–345.
206. Fox SH, Brotchie JM, Lang AE. Non-dopaminergic treatments in development for Parkinson's disease. Lancet Neurol 2008 Oct;7(10):927–938.
207. Stocchi F, Vacca L, Ruggieri S, et al. Intermittent vs continuous levodopa administration in patients with advanced Parkinson disease: A clinical and pharmacokinetic study. Arch Neurol 2005 Jun;62(6):905–910.
208. Koller WC. Management of motor fluctuations in Parkinson's disease. Eur Neurol 1996;36(suppl 1):43-48.
209. Olanow CW, Hauser RA, Jankovic J, et al. A randomized, double-blind, placebo-controlled, delayed start study to assess rasagiline as a disease modifying therapy in Parkinson's disease (the ADAGIO study): Rationale, design, and baseline characteristics. Mov Disord 2008 Nov 15;23(15):2194–2201.
210. Facca A, Sanchez-Ramos J. High-dose pergolide monotherapy in the treatment of severe levodopa-induced dyskinesias. Mov Disord 1996 May;11(3):327–329.
211. Kempster PA, Frankel JP, Bovingdon M, et al. Levodopa peripheral pharmacokinetics and duration of motor response in Parkinson's disease. J Neurol Neurosurg Psychiatry 1989;52(6):718–723.
212. Colzi A, Turner K, Lees AJ. Continuous subcutaneous waking day apomorphine in the long term treatment of levodopa induced interdose dyskinesias in Parkinson's disease. J Neurol Neurosurg Psychiatry 1998;64(5): 573–576.
213. Cenci MA. Dopamine dysregulation of movement control in L-DOPA-induced dyskinesia. Trends Neurosci 2007 May;30(5):236–243.
214. Lemstra AW, Verhagen ML, Lee JI, et al. Tremor-frequency (3-6 Hz) activity in the sensorimotor arm representation of the internal segment of the globus pallidus in patients with Parkinson's disease. Neurosci Lett 1999 May 28;267(2):129–132.
215. Luginger E, Wenning GK, Bosch S, et al. Beneficial effects of amantadine on L-dopa-induced dyskinesias in Parkinson's disease. Mov Disord 2000 Sep;15(5):873–878.
216. Snow BJ, Macdonald L, Mcauley D, et al. The effect of amantadine on levodopa-induced dyskinesias in Parkinson's disease: A double-blind, placebo-controlled study. Clin Neuropharmacol 2000 Mar;23(2):82–85.
217. Verhagen Metman L, Del Dotto P, van den Munckhof P, et al. Amantadine as treatment for dyskinesias and motor fluctuations in Parkinson's disease [see comments]. Neurology 1998;50(5):1323–1326.

218. Gasparini F, Bilbe G, Gomez-Mancilla B, et al. mGluR5 antagonists: Discovery, characterization and drug development. Curr Opin Drug Discov Devel 2008 Sep;11(5): 655–665.
219. Hauser RA, Shulman LM, Trugman JM, et al. Study of istradefylline in patients with Parkinson's disease on levodopa with motor fluctuations. Mov Disord 2008 Nov 15;23(15):2177–2185.
220. Stacy M, Silver D, Mendis T, et al. A 12-week, placebo-controlled study (6002-US-006) of istradefylline in Parkinson disease. Neurology 2008 Jun 3;70(23):2233–2240.
221. Bara-Jimenez W, Bibbiani F, Morris MJ, et al. Effects of serotonin 5-HT1A agonist in advanced Parkinson's disease. Mov Disord 2005 Aug;20(8):932–936.
222. Goetz CG, Damier P, Hicking C, et al. Sarizotan as a treatment for dyskinesias in Parkinson's disease: A double-blind placebo-controlled trial. Mov Disord 2007 Jan 15;22(2):179–186.
223. Lees AJ. The Parkinson chimera. Neurology 2009 Feb 17;72(7 suppl):S2–S11.
224. Braak H, Del TK, Rub U, et al. Staging of brain pathology related to sporadic Parkinson's disease. Neurobiol Aging 2003 Mar;24(2):197–211.
225. Witjas T, Kaphan E, Azulay JP, et al. Nonmotor fluctuations in Parkinson's disease: Frequent and disabling. Neurology 2002 Aug 13;59(3):408–413.
226. Tandberg E, Larsen JP, Aarsland D, et al. The occurrence of depression in Parkinson's disease. A community-based study. Arch Neurol 1996 Feb;53(2):175–179.
227. Starkstein SE, Preziosi TJ, Bolduc PL, et al. Depression in Parkinson's disease. J Nerv Ment Dis 1990 Jan;178(1): 27–31.
228. Shiba M, Bower JH, Maraganore DM, et al. Anxiety disorders and depressive disorders preceding Parkinson's disease: A case-control study. Mov Disord 2000 Jul;15(4):669–677.
229. Cummings JL. Depression and Parkinson's disease: A review. Am J Psychiatry 1992 Apr;149(4):443–454.
230. Brown R, Jahanshahi M. Depression in Parkinson's disease: A psychosocial viewpoint. Adv Neurol 1995;65: 61–84.
231. Shulman LM, Taback RL, Rabinstein AA, et al. Non-recognition of depression and other non-motor symptoms in Parkinson's disease. Parkinsonism Relat Disord 2002 Jan;8(3):193–197.
232. Mayeux R. Depression in the patient with Parkinson's disease. J Clin Psychiatry 1990 Jul;51(suppl):20–23.
233. Ehmann TS, Beninger RJ, Gawel MJ, et al. Depressive symptoms in Parkinson's disease: A comparison with disabled control subjects. J Geriatr Psychiatry Neurol 1990 Jan;3(1):3–9.
234. Remy P, Doder M, Lees A, et al. Depression in Parkinson's disease: Loss of dopamine and noradrenaline innervation in the limbic system. Brain 2005 Jun;128(Pt 6): 1314–1322.
235. Frisina PG, Haroutunian V, Libow LS. The neuropathological basis for depression in Parkinson's disease. Parkinsonism Relat Disord 2009 Feb;15(2):144–148.
236. Richard IH, Kurlan R. A survey of antidepressant drug use in Parkinson's disease. Parkinson Study Group. Neurology 1997 Oct;49(4):1168–1170.
237. Menza M, Dobkin RD, Marin H, et al. A controlled trial of antidepressants in patients with Parkinson disease and depression. Neurology 2009 Mar 10;72(10): 886–892.
238. Serrano-Duenas M. [A comparison between low doses of amitriptyline and low doses of fluoxetin used in the control of depression in patients suffering from Parkinson's disease]. Rev Neurol 2002 Dec 1;35(11):1010–1014.
239. Antonini A, Tesei S, Zecchinelli A, et al. Randomized study of sertraline and low-dose amitriptyline in patients with Parkinson's disease and depression: Effect on quality of life. Mov Disord 2006 Aug;21(8):1119–1122.
240. Leentjens AF, Vreeling FW, Luijckx GJ, et al. SSRIs in the treatment of depression in Parkinson's disease. Int J Geriatr Psychiatry 2003 Jun;18(6):552–554.
241. Wermuth L, Sorensen P, Timm S. Depression in diopathic Parkinson's Disease treated with citalopram. A placebo-controlled trial. Nord J Psychiatry 1998;52:163–169.
242. Rektorova I, Rektor I, Bares M, et al. Pramipexole and pergolide in the treatment of depression in Parkinson's disease: A national multicentre prospective randomized study. Eur J Neurol 2003 Jul;10(4):399–406.
243. Barone P, Scarzella L, Marconi R, et al. Pramipexole versus sertraline in the treatment of depression in Parkinson's disease: A national multicenter parallel-group randomized study. J Neurol 2006 May;253(5):601–607.
244. Cassano P, Lattanzi L, Fava M, et al. Ropinirole in treatment-resistant depression: A 16-week pilot study. Can J Psychiatry 2005 May;50(6):357–360.
245. Barone P, Poewe W, Tolosa E, et al. Efficacy of double-blind, placebo-controlled pramipexole against depression in Parkinson's disease. Mov Disord 2009;24(suppl 1): 27–25.
246. Okabe S, Ugawa Y, Kanazawa I. 0.2-Hz repetitive transcranial magnetic stimulation has no add-on effects as compared to a realistic sham stimulation in Parkinson's disease. Mov Disord 2003 Apr;18(4):382–328.
247. Fregni F, Santos CM, Myczkowski ML, et al. Repetitive transcranial magnetic stimulation is as effective as fluoxetine in the treatment of depression in patients with Parkinson's disease. J Neurol Neurosurg Psychiatry 2004 Aug;75(8):1171–1174.
248. Miyasaki JM, Shannon K, Voon V, et al. Practice Parameter: Evaluation and treatment of depression, psychosis, and dementia in Parkinson disease (an evidence-based review): Report of the Quality Standards Subcommittee of the American Academy of Neurology. Neurology 2006 Apr 11;66(7):996–1002.
249. Factor SA, Feustel PJ, Friedman JH, et al. Longitudinal outcome of Parkinson's disease patients with psychosis. Neurology 2003 Jun 10;60(11):1756–1761.
250. Aarsland D, Zaccai J, Brayne C. A systematic review of prevalence studies of dementia in Parkinson's disease. Mov Disord 2005 Oct;20(10):1255–1263.
251. Emre M, Aarsland D, Brown R, et al. Clinical diagnostic criteria for dementia associated with Parkinson's disease. Mov Disord 2007 Sep 15;22(12):1689–1707.
252. Hely MA, Reid WG, Adena MA, et al. The Sydney multicenter study of Parkinson's disease: The inevitability of dementia at 20 years. Mov Disord 2008 Apr 30;23(6): 837–844.

253. Aarsland D, Perry R, Brown A, et al. Neuropathology of dementia in Parkinson's disease: A prospective, community-based study. Ann Neurol 2005 Nov;58(5):773–776.
254. Perry EK, Irving D, Kerwin JM, et al. Cholinergic transmitter and neurotrophic activities in Lewy body dementia: Similarity to Parkinson's and distinction from Alzheimer disease. Alzheimer Dis Assoc Disord 1993;7(2):69–79.
255. Aarsland D, Laake K, Larsen JP, et al. Donepezil for cognitive impairment in Parkinson's disease: A randomised controlled study. J Neurol Neurosurg Psychiatry 2002 Jun;72(6):708–712.
256. Ravina B, Putt M, Siderowf A, et al. Donepezil for dementia in Parkinson's disease: A randomised, double blind, placebo controlled, crossover study. J Neurol Neurosurg Psychiatry 2005 Jul;76(7):934–939.
257. Emre M, Aarsland D, Albanese A, et al. Rivastigmine for dementia associated with Parkinson's disease. N Engl J Med 2004 Dec 9;351(24):2509–2518.
258. Burn D, Emre M, McKeith I, et al. Effects of rivastigmine in patients with and without visual hallucinations in dementia associated with Parkinson's disease. Mov Disord 2006 Nov;21(11):1899–1907.
259. Poewe W, Wolters E, Emre M, et al. Long-term benefits of rivastigmine in dementia associated with Parkinson's disease: An active treatment extension study. Mov Disord 2006 Apr;21(4):456–461.
260. Litvinenko IV, Odinak MM, Mogil'naya VI, et al. Efficacy and safety of galantamine (reminyl) for dementia in patients with Parkinson's disease (an open controlled trial). Neurosci Behav Physiol 2008 Nov;38(9):937–945.
261. Aarsland D, Ballard C, Walker Z, et al. Memantine in patients with Parkinson's disease dementia or dementia with Lewy bodies: A double-blind, placebo-controlled, multicentre trial. Lancet Neurol 2009 Jul;8(7):613–618.
262. Peralta C, Stampfer-Kountchev M, Karner E, et al. Orthostatic hypotension and attention in Parkinson's disease with and without dementia. J Neural Transm 2007;114(5):585–588.
263. Poewe W. Psychosis in Parkinson's disease. Mov Disord 2003 Sep;18(suppl 6):S80–S87.
264. Goetz CG and Stebbins GT. Risk factors for nursing home placement in advanced Parkinson's disease. Neurology 1993 Nov;43(11):2227–2229.
265. Goetz CG and Stebbins GT. Mortality and hallucinations in nursing home patients with advanced Parkinson's disease. Neurology 1995 Apr;45(4):669–671.
266. Ravina B, Marder K, Fernandez HH, et al. Diagnostic criteria for psychosis in Parkinson's disease: Report of an NINDS, NIMH work group. Mov Disord 2007 Jun 15;22(8):1061–1068.
267. Williams DR and Lees AJ. Visual hallucinations in the diagnosis of idiopathic Parkinson's disease: A retrospective autopsy study. Lancet Neurol 2005 Oct;4(10):605–610.
268. Clozapine in drug-induced psychosis in Parkinson's disease. The French Clozapine Parkinson Study Group. Lancet 1999 Jun 12;353(9169):2041–2042.
269. Low-dose clozapine for the treatment of drug-induced psychosis in Parkinson's disease. The Parkinson Study Group. N Engl J Med 1999 Mar 11;340(10):757–763.
270. Factor SA, Friedman JH, Lannon MC, et al. Clozapine for the treatment of drug-induced psychosis in Parkinson's disease: Results of the 12 week open label extension in the PSYCLOPS trial. Mov Disord 2001 Jan;16(1):135–139.
271. Pollak P, Tison F, Rascol O, et al. Clozapine in drug induced psychosis in Parkinson's disease: A randomized, placebo controlled study with open follow up. J Neurol Neurosurg Psychiatry 2004 May;75(5):689–695.
272. Ondo WG, Tintner R, Voung KD, et al. Double-blind, placebo-controlled, unforced titration parallel trial of quetiapine for dopaminergic-induced hallucinations in Parkinson's disease. Mov Disord 2005 Aug;20(8):958–963.
273. Rabey JM, Prokhorov T, Miniovitz A, et al. Effect of quetiapine in psychotic Parkinson's disease patients: A double-blind labeled study of 3 months' duration. Mov Disord 2007 Feb 15;22(3):313–318.
274. Morgante L, Epifanio A, Spina E, et al. Quetiapine and clozapine in parkinsonian patients with dopaminergic psychosis. Clin Neuropharmacol 2004 Jul;27(4):153–156.
275. Merims D, Balas M, Peretz C, et al. Rater-blinded, prospective comparison: qQuetiapine versus clozapine for Parkinson's disease psychosis. Clin Neuropharmacol 2006 Nov;29(6):331–337.
276. Fernandez HH, Trieschmann ME, Burke MA, et al. Long-term outcome of quetiapine use for psychosis among Parkinsonian patients. Mov Disord 2003 May;18(5):510–514.
277. Reading PJ, Luce AK, and McKeith IG. Rivastigmine in the treatment of parkinsonian psychosis and cognitive impairment: Preliminary findings from an open trial. Mov Disord 2001 Nov;16(6):1171–1174.
278. Bullock R and Cameron A. Rivastigmine for the treatment of dementia and visual hallucinations associated with Parkinson's disease: A case series. Curr Med Res Opin 2002;18(5):258–264.
279. Fabbrini G, Barbanti P, and Aurilia C, et al. Donepezil in the treatment of hallucinations and delusions in Parkinson's disease. Neurol Sci 2002 Apr;23(1):41–43.
280. Bergman J and Lerner V. Successful use of donepezil for the treatment of psychotic symptoms in patients with Parkinson's disease. Clin Neuropharmacol 2002 Mar;25(2):107–110.
281. Aarsland D, Hutchinson M, and Larsen JP. Cognitive, psychiatric and motor response to galantamine in Parkinson's disease with dementia. Int J Geriatr Psychiatry 2003 Oct;18(10):937–941.
282. Tandberg E, Larsen JP, and Karlsen K. A community-based study of sleep disorders in patients with Parkinson's disease. Mov Disord 1998 Nov;13(6):895–899.
283. Lees AJ, Blackburn NA, and Campbell VL. The nighttime problems of Parkinson's disease. Clin Neuropharmacol 1988 Dec;11(6):512–519.
284. Gagnon JF, Bedard MA, Fantini ML, et al. REM sleep behavior disorder and REM sleep without atonia in Parkinson's disease. Neurology 2002 Aug 27;59(4):585–589.
285. Hobson DE, Lang AE, Martin WR, et al. Excessive daytime sleepiness and sudden-onset sleep in Parkinson disease: A survey by the Canadian Movement Disorders Group. JAMA 2002 Jan 23;287(4):455–463.
286. Ondo WG, Vuong KD, and Jankovic J. Exploring the relationship between Parkinson disease and restless legs syndrome. Arch Neurol 2002 Mar;59(3):421–424.

287. Arnulf I, Konofal E, Merino-Andreu M, et al. Parkinson's disease and sleepiness: An integral part of PD. Neurology 2002 Apr 9;58(7):1019–1024.
288. Boeve BF, Silber MH, Saper CB, et al. Pathophysiology of REM sleep behaviour disorder and relevance to neurodegenerative disease. Brain 2007 Nov;130(Pt 11):2770–2788.
289. Mahowald MW, Schenck CH, and Bornemann MA. Pathophysiologic mechanisms in REM sleep behavior disorder. Curr Neurol Neurosci Rep 2007 Mar;7(2):167–172.
290. Iranzo A, Molinuevo JL, Santamaria J, et al. Rapid-eye-movement sleep behaviour disorder as an early marker for a neurodegenerative disorder: A descriptive study. Lancet Neurol 2006 Jul;5(7):572–577.
291. Schenck CH, Bundlie SR, Patterson AL, et al. Rapid eye movement sleep behavior disorder. A treatable parasomnia affecting older adults. JAMA 1987 Apr 3;257(13): 1786–1789.
292. Ozekmekci S, Apaydin H, and Kilic E. Clinical features of 35 patients with Parkinson's disease displaying REM behavior disorder. Clin Neurol Neurosurg 2005 Jun;107(4):306–309.
293. Schenck CH and Mahowald MW. Long-term, nightly benzodiazepine treatment of injurious parasomnias and other disorders of disrupted nocturnal sleep in 170 adults. Am J Med 1996 Mar;100(3):333–337.
294. Boeve BF, Silber MH, and Ferman TJ. Melatonin for treatment of REM sleep behavior disorder in neurologic disorders: Results in 14 patients. Sleep Med 2003 Jul;4(4):281–284.
295. Kunz D, and Bes F. Melatonin as a therapy in REM sleep behavior disorder patients: An open-labeled pilot study on the possible influence of melatonin on REM-sleep regulation. Mov Disord 1999 May;14(3):507–511.
296. Takeuchi N, Uchimura N, Hashizume Y, et al. Melatonin therapy for REM sleep behavior disorder. Psychiatry Clin Neurosci 2001 Jun;55(3):267–269.
297. Magalhaes M, Wenning GK, Daniel SE, et al. Autonomic dysfunction in pathologically confirmed multiple system atrophy and idiopathic Parkinson's disease—a retrospective comparison. Acta Neurol Scand 1995 Feb;91(2):98–102.
298. Braak H, de Vos RA, Bohl J, et al. Gastric alpha-synuclein immunoreactive inclusions in Meissner's and Auerbach's plexuses in cases staged for Parkinson's disease-related brain pathology. Neurosci Lett 2006 Mar 20;396(1):67–72.
299. Braak H, Muller CM, Rub U, et al. Pathology associated with sporadic Parkinson's disease—where does it end? J Neural Transm Suppl 2006;(70):89–97.
300. Lahrmann H, Cortelli P, Hilz M, et al. EFNS guidelines on the diagnosis and management of orthostatic hypotension. Eur J Neurol 2006 Sep;13(9):930–936.
301. Pathak A and Senard JM. Blood pressure disorders during Parkinson's disease: Epidemiology, pathophysiology and management. Expert Rev Neurother 2006 Aug;6(8): 1173–1180.
302. Low PA, Gilden JL, Freeman R, et al. Efficacy of midodrine vs placebo in neurogenic orthostatic hypotension. A randomized, double-blind multicenter study. Midodrine Study Group. JAMA 1997 Apr 2;277(13):1046–1051.
303. Jankovic J, Gilden JL, Hiner BC, et al. Neurogenic orthostatic hypotension: A double-blind, placebo-controlled study with midodrine. Am J Med 1993 Jul;95(1):38–48.
304. Drugs to treat autonomic dysfunction in Parkinson's disease. Mov Disord 2002;17(suppl 4):S103–S111.
305. Mathias CJ. L-dihydroxyphenylserine (Droxidopa) in the treatment of orthostatic hypotension: The European experience. Clin Auton Res 2008 Mar;18(suppl 1):25–29.
306. Fowler CJ and O'Malley KJ. Investigation and management of neurogenic bladder dysfunction. J Neurol Neurosurg Psychiatry 2003 Dec;74(suppl 4):iv27–iv31.
307. Winge K and Fowler CJ. Bladder dysfunction in Parkinsonism: Mechanisms, prevalence, symptoms, and management. Mov Disord 2006 Jun;21(6):737–745.
308. Suchowersky O, Furtado S, and Rohs G. Beneficial effect of intranasal desmopressin for nocturnal polyuria in Parkinson's disease. Mov Disord 1995 May;10(3):337–340.
309. Giannantoni A, Mearini E, Del ZM, et al. Botulinum A toxin in the treatment of neurogenic detrusor overactivity: A consolidated field of application. BJU Int 2008 Jul 25;102(suppl 1):2–6.
310. Abbott RD, Petrovitch H, White LR, et al. Frequency of bowel movements and the future risk of Parkinson's disease. Neurology 2001 Aug 14;57(3):456–462.
311. Kaufmann H and Biaggioni I. Autonomic failure in neurodegenerative disorders. Semin Neurol 2003 Dec;23(4):351–363.
312. Eichhorn TE and Oertel WH. Macrogol 3350/electrolyte improves constipation in Parkinson's disease and multiple system atrophy. Mov Disord 2001 Nov;16(6):1176–1177.
313. Sakakibara R, Odaka T, Lui Z, et al. Dietary herb extract dai-kenchu-to ameliorates constipation in parkinsonian patients (Parkinson's disease and multiple system atrophy). Mov Disord 2005 Feb;20(2):261–262.
314. Liu Z, Sakakibara R, Odaka T, et al. Mosapride citrate, a novel 5-HT4 agonist and partial 5-HT3 antagonist, ameliorates constipation in parkinsonian patients. Mov Disord 2005 Jun;20(6):680–686.
315. Jost WH and Schimrigk K. Cisapride treatment of constipation in Parkinson's disease. Mov Disord 1993 Jul;8(3):339–343.
316. Sullivan KL, Staffetti JF, Hauser RA, et al. Tegaserod (Zelnorm) for the treatment of constipation in Parkinson's disease. Mov Disord 2006 Jan;21(1):115–116.
317. Papatsoris AG, Deliveliotis C, Singer C, et al. Erectile dysfunction in Parkinson's disease. Urology 2006 Mar;67(3):447–451.
318. Hussain IF, Brady CM, Swinn MJ, et al. Treatment of erectile dysfunction with sildenafil citrate (Viagra) in parkinsonism due to Parkinson's disease or multiple system atrophy with observations on orthostatic hypotension. J Neurol Neurosurg Psychiatry 2001 Sep;71(3): 371–374.
319. Briganti A, Salonia A, Gallina A, et al. Drug Insight: Oral phosphodiesterase type 5 inhibitors for erectile dysfunction. Nat Clin Pract Urol 2005 May;2(5):239–247.
320. Porst H, Behre HM, Jungwirth A, et al. Comparative trial of treatment satisfaction, efficacy and tolerability of sildenafil versus apomorphine in erectile dysfunction—an open, randomized cross-over study with flexible dosing. Eur J Med Res 2007 Feb 26;12(2):61–67.
321. Rinne UK. Early combination of bromocriptine and levodopa in the treatment of Parkinson's disease: A 5-year follow-up. Neurology 1987 May;37(5):826–828.

322. Nakanishi T, Iwata M, Goto I, et al. Nation-wide collaborative study on the long-term effects of bromocriptine in the treatment of parkinsonian patients. Final report. Eur Neurol 1992;32(suppl 1):9–22.
323. Montastruc JL, Rascol O, Senard JM, et al. A randomized controlled study comparing bromocriptine to which levodopa was later added, with levodopa alone in previously untreated patients with Parkinson's disease: A five year follow up. J Neurol Neurosurg Psychiatry 1994 Sep;57(9):1034–1038.
324. Rinne UK. Lisuride, a dopamine agonist in the treatment of early Parkinson's disease. Neurology 1989 Mar;39(3):336–339.
325. Gopinathan G, Teravainen H, Dambrosia JM, et al. Lisuride in parkinsonism. Neurology 1981 Apr;31(4):371–376.
326. Giovannini P, Scigliano G, Piccolo I, et al. Lisuride in Parkinson's disease. 4-year follow-up. Clin Neuropharmacol 1988 Jun;11(3):201–211.
327. Lieberman AN, Goldstein M, Gopinathan G, et al. Further studies with pergolide in Parkinson disease. Neurology 1982 Oct;32(10):1181–1184.
328. Olanow CW, Fahn S, Muenter M, et al. A multicenter double-blind placebo-controlled trial of pergolide as an adjunct to Sinemet in Parkinson's disease. Mov Disord 1994 Jan;9(1):40–47.
329. Goetz CG, Tanner CM, Glantz R, et al. Pergolide in Parkinson's disease. Arch Neurol 1983 Dec;40(13):785–787.
330. Martignoni E, Pacchetti C, Sibilla L, et al. Dihydroergocryptine in the treatment of Parkinson's disease: A six months' double-blind clinical trial. Clin Neuropharmacol 1991 Feb;14(1):78–83.
331. Baas H, Harder S, Burklin F, et al. Pharmacodynamics of levodopa coadministered with apomorphine in parkinsonian patients with end-of-dose motor fluctuations. Clin Neuropharmacol 1998;21(2):86–92.
332. Ostergaard L, Werdelin L, Odin P, et al. Pen injected apomorphine against off phenomena in late Parkinson's disease: A double blind, placebo controlled study. J Neurol Neurosurg Psychiatry 1995;58(6):681–687.
333. Pietz K, Hagell P, and Odin P. Subcutaneous apomorphine in late stage Parkinson's disease: A long term follow up. J Neurol Neurosurg Psychiatry 1998;65(5):709–716.
334. Lieberman A, Olanow CW, Sethi K, et al. A multicenter trial of ropinirole as adjunct treatment for Parkinson's disease. Ropinirole Study Group. Neurology 1998 Oct;51(4):1057–1062.
335. Ziegler M, Castro-Caldas A, Del SS, . Efficacy of piribedil as early combination to levodopa in patients with stable Parkinson's disease: A 6-month, randomized, placebo-controlled study. Mov Disord 2003 Apr;18(4):418–425.

CHAPTER 16

Restorative Therapies for Parkinson's Disease

Olle Lindvall

▶ INTRODUCTION

The main pathology underlying the motor symptoms in Parkinson's disease (PD) is a rather selective degeneration of the nigrostriatal dopamine (DA) neuron system. The experimental strategies to restore brain function in PD patients have all been based on a very simple principle, namely, to replace the dead dopaminergic neurons by new, transplanted DA-producing cells. The interest in cell replacement dates back to the late 1970s when it was demonstrated that intrastriatal grafts of embryonic mesencephalic tissue, rich in DA neuroblasts, induced functional recovery in rats with neurotoxin-induced lesions of the nigrostriatal DA system. There is now a solid experimental basis showing functional efficacy of such transplantation to the striatum in animal models of PD, and a biological mechanism underlying the observed improvement, that is, restoration of striatal DA transmission.[1,2] Extensive animal studies have shown that the grafted DA neurons display many of the morphological and functional characteristics of the intrinsic mesencephalic DA neurons: they reinnervate the denervated striatum and form synaptic contacts with host neurons, are spontaneously active and release DA, and receive afferent inputs from the host. Reinnervation by the grafts ameliorates several aspects of the DA deficiency syndrome in rodents and monkeys.

Based on these animal experimental data, clinical trials with transplantation of human embryonic mesencephalic tissue to the striatum in patients with PD were started in 1987. At that time, it was unknown whether cell replacement could work at all in the human brain. Therefore, the first phase of clinical transplantation research aimed at answering several basic scientific questions: first, can the grafted DA neurons survive and form connections? Second, can the patient's brain integrate and use the grafted DA neurons? Third, can the grafts induce a measurable clinical improvement in PD patients? So far, 300–400 patients with PD have been grafted with human embryonic mesencephalic tissue. The results have provided proof-of-principle that cell replacement can work in the PD patient's brain.

Besides transplantation of embryonic mesencephalic tissue, several other sources of cells secreting catecholamines have been tested clinically in PD patients. Intrastriatal implantation of tissue from the patient's own adrenal medulla was pioneered by Backlund and coworkers already in the early 1980s.[3] These trials were the first attempts to apply the cell transplantation strategy to the human brain. The main interest in this approach arose in 1987, when dramatic improvements were described after adrenal medulla transplantation in PD patients using a new surgical technique.[4] This report led to a large number of clinical trials. When the outcome in these studies had been evaluated, it was concluded that adrenal medulla transplantation can lead to modest improvement but with a serious level of mortality and morbidity[5] and poor graft survival.[6] Another approach has used autotransplantation of dopaminergic glomus cells from carotid body into the striatum of PD patients. An open-label trial showed modest mean improvement in operated patients and no direct positron emission tomography (PET) evidence for graft survival.[7] Finally, based on their ability to produce L-dopa, human retinal pigment epithelial cells, attached to gelatine microcarriers, have been implanted into the striatum in PD patients. However, whereas an open-label study indicated substantial improvement,[8] a recent placebo-controlled Phase II trial revealed no significant clinical benefit.

Cell therapy research in PD now enters a new phase, the main objective being to develop this approach into a clinically competitive treatment. There is a lot of hope that stem cells could become a source of virtually unlimited numbers of DA neuroblasts for transplantation. However, several new therapeutic options for the PD patient have been added over the past decades. Most importantly, deep brain stimulation (DBS) in the subthalamic nucleus has been shown to substantially improve motor deficits in advanced PD.[9] Therefore, in order to become clinically useful, stem cell therapy has to give rise to long-lasting, major improvement of mobility, suppression of dyskinesias, amelioration of symptoms resistant to other treatments, or counteraction of disease progression. In this chapter, I will summarize the experiences from the clinical trials with embryonic mesencephalic grafts. I will also describe how far stem cells have reached toward the clinic in PD, and what are the major scientific and clinical problems to be solved for successful application in patients.

▶ CLINICAL TRIALS WITH TRANSPLANTATION OF HUMAN EMBRYONIC MESENCEPHALIC TISSUE

Dopaminergic neuroblasts, obtained from the ventral mesencephalon of 6- to 9-week-old human embryos, can survive transplantation into the brain of PD patients (Fig. 16–1). PET has detected increases of ^{18}F-dopa uptake in the grafted striatum,[10–24] and histopathological studies have shown long-term, extensive synaptic reinnervation of the patient's striatum.[24–31] The grafts are able to restore DA release in the denervated striatum. One patient with major clinical improvement, in whom ^{18}F-dopa uptake was normalized in the grafted putamen from 3 to 10 years post-surgery (Figs. 16–2A and 16–2B), showed normal basal and drug-induced DA release, as assessed using ^{11}C-raclopride binding, at 10 years after transplantation.[32] No evidence has been obtained for abnormal DA release from the terminals of grafted neurons in PD patients (Fig. 16–3A).[33] The grafts also become functionally integrated into the neural circuitries in the PD patient's brain.[34] The supplementary motor area and the dorsolateral prefrontal cortex are influenced by the basal ganglia–thalamo-cortical neural circuitries, and their impaired activation is believed to underlie parkinsonian akinesia. With a time course which paralleled that of the clinical improvement, bilateral striatal grafts restituted the movement-related activation of these frontal cortical areas (Fig. 16–2C).[34]

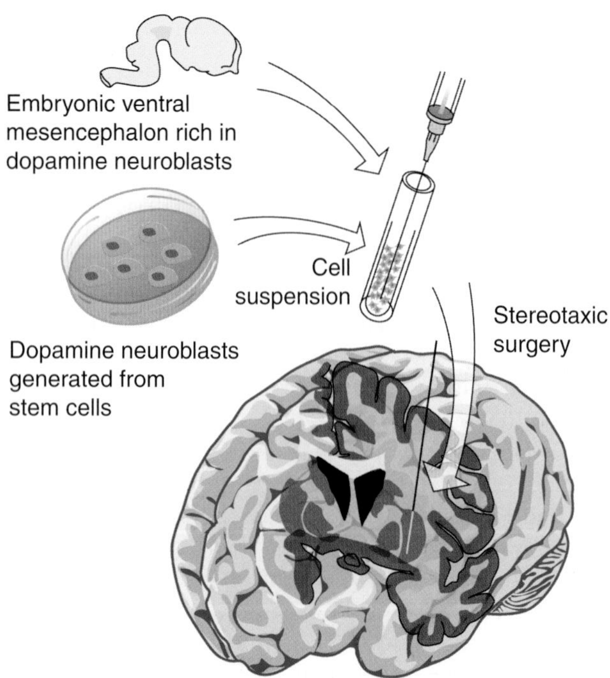

Figure 16–1. Schematic representation of procedure for cell transplantation in PD patients using either embryonic ventral mesencephalon, rich in dopamine neuroblasts, or dopamine neuroblasts generated from stem cells.

Clear clinical benefits associated with survival of the human embryonic mesencephalic grafts have been reported from open-label trials.[10–19,24,35–37] The most successful cases have been able to withdraw L-dopa treatment and have exhibited major clinical improvement during several years after transplantation.[16,17,19,32] In four open-label trials, the Unified Parkinson's Disease Rating Scale (UPDRS) motor score during practically defined "off" (i.e., in the morning, at least 12 hours after the last dose of antiparkinsonian medication) revealed 30–50% symptomatic relief at 1–3 years after bilateral transplantation into putamen (Table 16–1).[17–19,24] Patients showed significant increases of ^{18}F-dopa uptake in the operated putamen indicating graft survival. However, in three of these studies, the uptake after transplantation was still only about 50% of the normal mean. This probably explains, at least to some extent, the incomplete functional recovery and indicates that there is room for improvement. Some support for this idea is provided by the more pronounced reduction of UPDRS motor score observed in the patients of Mendez and colleagues,[24] in whom 72% of the normal ^{18}F-dopa uptake was restored.

The functional improvement in two sham surgery–controlled clinical trials was only modest and clearly less than that in the open-label trials. It is now well established that surgical interventions in PD are associated with substantial placebo responses,[38] which could hypothetically explain the discrepancy in outcome between the open-label and sham surgery–controlled studies. Arguing against such an interpretation, improvements of motor function after unilateral grafts have been predominantly on the contralateral side of the body. In several patients, their "worst" side has switched after transplantation. Functional recovery has developed gradually, from about 3 months and up to 1–2 years after grafting. Objective neurophysiological methods measuring arm and hand movements have confirmed the improvements. Some patients have recovered to the extent that they have returned to work and withdrawn L-dopa treatment for many years. Finally, changes in motor function have broadly corresponded to the degree of graft survival and restoration of movement-related cortical activation.

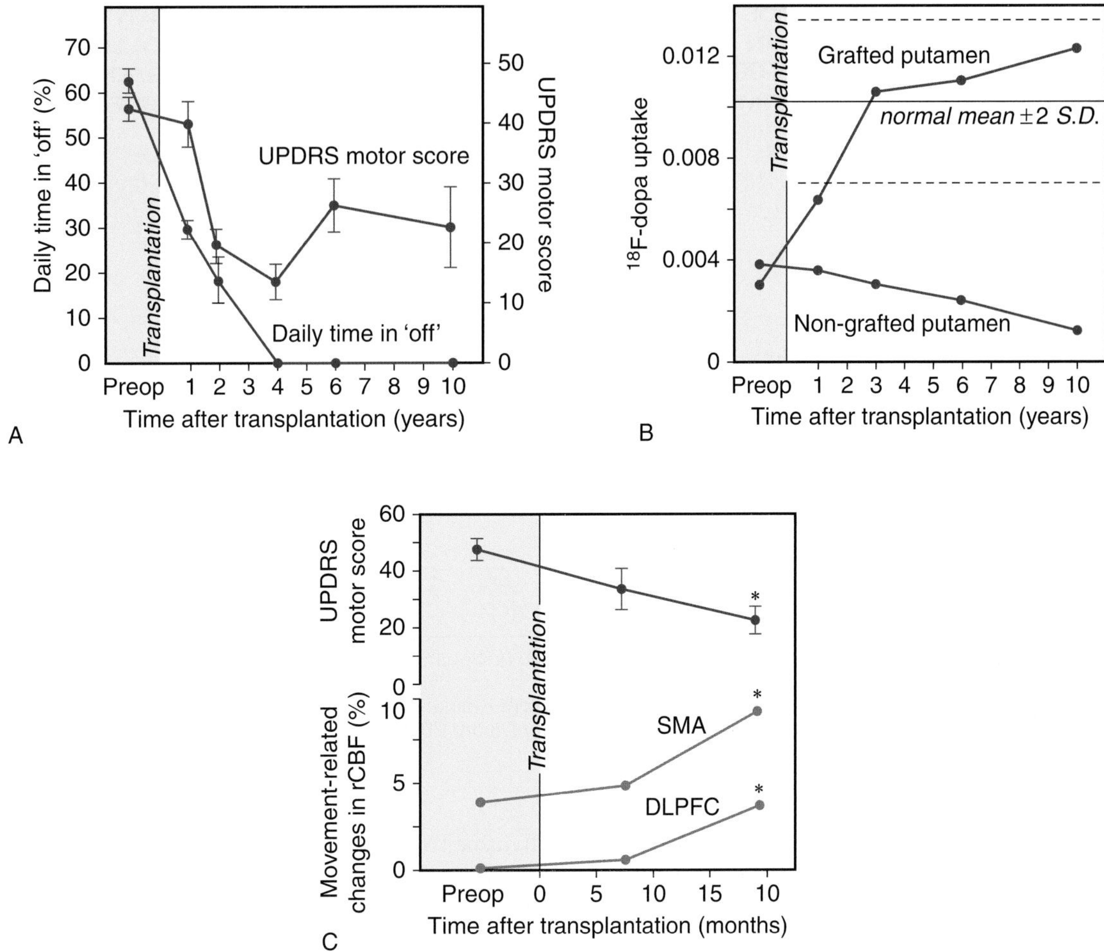

Figure 16–2. Grafts of embryonic mesencephalic dopaminergic neurons can become functionally integrated in the PD patient's brain, restore striatal DA synthesis and release to normal levels, and give rise to major long-lasting improvements in some patients. (A) Percentage of the day spent in the off-phase and Unified Parkinson's Disease Rating Scale (UPDRS) motor score in off preoperatively and at various time points after transplantation to the right putamen in a PD patient. Mean ± 95% confidence interval. (B) ^{18}F-Dopa uptake in grafted and non-grafted putamen of the same patient with comparative values from a group of 16 healthy volunteers. (C) UPDRS motor score and percentage of movement-related levels of regional cerebral blood flow in comparison to rest in the supplementary area (SMA) and dorsolateral prefrontal cortex (DLPFC) before surgery and at 6.5 and 18.3 months after bilateral implantation of embryonic mesencephalic tissue in the caudate and putamen of four PD patients. *, $p < 0.001$ compared to preoperative value, Student's t-test. (Data from Piccini P, Brooks DJ, Björklund A, et al. Dopamine release from nigral transplants visualized *in vivo* in a Parkinson's patient. Nat Neurosci 1999;2:1137–1140 and Piccini P, Lindvall O, Björklund A, et al. Delayed recovery of movement-related cortical function in Parkinson's disease after striatal dopaminergic grafts. Ann Neurol 2000;48:689–695.)

The first sham surgery–controlled study (Fig. 16–4 and Table 16–1)[20] demonstrated modest clinical response with 18% reduction of the UPDRS motor score in off-phase at 12 months after bilateral putaminal grafts, but no improvement in the sham-operated group. In patients younger than 60 years, the improvement of the UPDRS was 34%. Two patients who died after grafting had only between 7000 and 40,000 grafted dopaminergic neurons in each putamen,[20] which was much lower than that found in two patients in one of the open-label trials (80,000–135,000).[25–27] The low numbers of surviving DA neurons could be due to that less tissue was implanted as compared to the open-label trials, tissue was stored in cell culture for up to 4 weeks, or there was lack of immunosuppressive treatment leading to compromised graft survival. Several open-label trials reporting clear clinical benefits used strictly controlled immunosuppressive regimens for 1–2 years after transplantation.

In the second sham surgery–controlled clinical trial,[23] the tissue was implanted in the putamen and cyclosporine was given for 6 months thereafter. The trial showed no group difference in the change in UPDRS

▶ **TABLE 16–1. MAGNITUDE OF POSTOPERATIVE CHANGES OF SYMPTOMATOLOGY AND PUTAMINAL ^{18}F-DOPA UPTAKE IN OPEN-LABEL AND SHAM SURGERY–CONTROLLED TRIALS WITH EMBRYONIC MESENCEPHALIC TISSUE TRANSPLANTATION, AS COMPARED TO SUBTHALAMIC DEEP BRAIN STIMULATION IN PATIENTS WITH PARKINSON'S DISEASE**

	Hauser et al. (1999; *n* = 6)	Hagell et al. (1999; *n* = 4)	Brundin et al. (2000; *n* = 5)	Freed et al. (2001; *n* = 19)	Olanow et al. (2003; *n* = 11/12)*	Mendez et al. (2005; *n* = 2)	DBS-STN (22 studies)
UPDRS motor score in "off" (Δ)	−30%	−30%	−40%	−18%	+3.5%/ −0.72%	−51%	−52%
Daily time in "off" (Δ)	−43%	−59%	−43%	n.r.	+7.8%/ −0.9%	−50%	−68%
Daily L-dopa dose (Δ)	−16%	−37%	−45%	n.r.	−20%/ −11%	±0/−30%	−56%
^{18}F-dopa uptake (putamen; % of normal mean)							
Preop	34%	31%	31%	39%	n.r.**	28%	
Postop	55%	52%	48%	55%	n.r.**	72%	

n, number of patients; DBS-STN, deep brain stimulation in subthalamic nucleus; UPDRS, Unified Parkinson's Disease Rating Scale.
*One-/four-donor groups, respectively.
**Only change in uptake from baseline reported. DBS-STN data are from Kleiner-Fisman G, Herzog J, Fisman DN, et al. Subthalamic deep brain stimulation: Summary and meta-analysis of outcomes. Mov Disord 2006;21:(suppl.14) S290–S304.

motor score at 24 months compared to baseline. However, similar to the time course of improvement in the open-label trials, patients showed progressive symptomatic relief up to between 6 and 9 months after surgery (but deteriorated thereafter) (Fig. 16–4). Putaminal ^{18}F-dopa uptake was significantly increased in grafted patients at 1 and 2 years after transplantation. Possible explanations for the lack of efficacy include the fact that the patients of Olanow and colleagues[23] were more severely disabled and required higher doses of antiparkinsonian medication as compared to, for example, the patients described by Wenning and colleagues,[16] Hagell and colleagues,[17] and Brundin and colleagues.[19] In support, Olanow and colleagues[23] showed significant improvement compared to sham-operated group at 2 years in their less severely disabled patients. This finding agrees well with the observation[33] that the extent of degeneration of dopaminergic and non-dopaminergic neurons in the patient's brain prior to transplantation influences the magnitude of functional recovery induced by a dopaminergic graft. Although the grafts survived in the study of Olanow and colleagues,[23] their function may have been compromised due to an immune reaction. The improvement up to between 6 and 9 months and the deterioration thereafter (Fig. 16–4) are consistent with an immune reaction after withdrawal of immunosuppression at 6 months. Autopsies in two patients demonstrated that the grafts were surrounded by activated microglia suggesting a delayed immune response.[23] In contrast, in two patients who had been subjected to 6-month immunosuppressive treatment in the study of Mendez and colleagues[24] and showed clinical improvement, only few macrophages and activated microglia were found in grafted regions at 3–4 years after surgery.

The most troublesome complication caused by transplantation of embryonic mesencephalic tissue in PD patients has been the occurrence of dyskinesias in the off-phase.[39] In the study of Freed and colleagues,[20] 15% of the grafted patients developed severe dyskinesias. Hagell and colleagues[40] found that among 14 grafted PD patients, 8 displayed mild off-phase dyskinesias. The remaining six patients exhibited dyskinesias of moderate severity, which in one patient constituted a clinical therapeutic problem. Olanow and colleagues[23] reported that 56.5% of the grafted patients developed off-phase dyskinesias. Severity of dyskinesias appeared to be generally mild, but they were disabling and required surgery in three cases. The off-phase dyskinesias in grafted patients have been effectively treated with DBS of the globus pallidus internus.[41,42]

The off-phase dyskinesias are most likely not caused by dopaminergic overgrowth or excessive DA release from the grafts.[23,33,40,43] No correlation was found between the magnitude of dyskinesias and that of the antiparkinsonian response.[23,40] Dyskinesias and functional improvements showed different time course following transplantation.[20,23,40] Moreover, off-phase dyskinesias were not associated with high postoperative striatal ^{18}F-dopa uptake or the most pronounced graft-induced increases in striatal ^{18}F-dopa uptake.[23,40] Ma and colleagues[43]

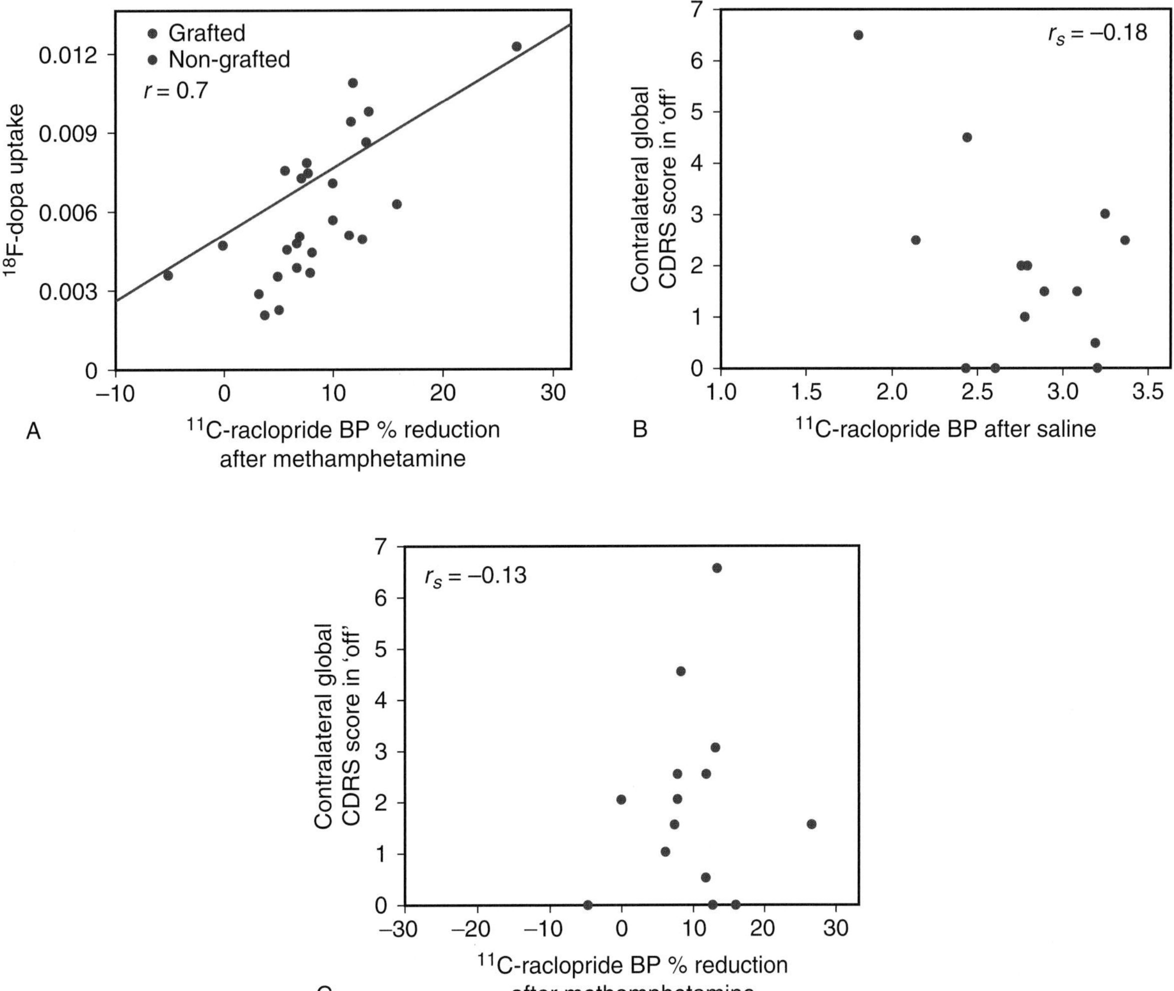

Figure 16–3. Transmitter release from grafted embryonic dopaminergic neurons resembles that of intrinsic neurons, and off-phase dyskinesias are not due to excessive DA release. (A) Correlation between ^{18}F-dopa uptake and percentage reduction of ^{11}C-raclopride binding potential after methamphetamine in the grafted putamen (filled circles and line; data from the two sides are pooled). For comparison, values from the left and right putamen in a group of non-grafted PD patients are given (open circles). (B) and (C) Correlation between ^{11}C-raclopride binding potential in the putamen after saline (B) or its percentage reduction after methamphetamine (C) and the global dyskinesia (CDRS) score in the off-phase in the contralateral side of the body. Data from six PD patients with bilateral and two patients with unilateral grafts. (Data from Piccini P, Pavese N, Hagell P, et al. Factors affecting the clinical outcome after neural transplantation in Parkinson's disease. Brain 2005;128:2977–2986.)

found evidence of an imbalance between the dopaminergic innervation (regional putaminal ^{18}F-dopa uptake) in the ventral and that in the dorsal putamen in dyskinetic grafted patients. However, no differences were observed in either regional or global levels of striatal FD uptake between patients with and without off-phase dyskinesias by Olanow and colleagues.[23] Piccini and colleagues[33] found no correlation between ^{11}C-raclopride binding (as a measure of DA release) in the putamen and dyskinesia severity scores (Figs. 16–3B and 16–3C). Finally, off-phase dyskinesias have resembled biphasic dyskinesias,[23,39,43] suggesting intermediate (not excess) DA levels.

Whether off-phase dyskinesias only develop in patients with already-established L-dopa-induced dyskinesias is unclear. Three main hypotheses regarding the mechanisms underlying off-phase dyskinesias can be proposed: first, they may be due to small grafts giving rise to islands of reinnervation, "hot spots," surrounded by supersensitive, denervated striatal areas.[44] The dyskinesias could also be due to an unfavorable cellular composition in the graft with a relative predominance of serotonergic neurons, from which L-dopa-derived DA is released as a "false transmitter."[45] Carlsson and colleagues[46,47] reported that serotonin neurons caused a worsening of L-dopa-induced dyskinesias in grafts with few but not with large

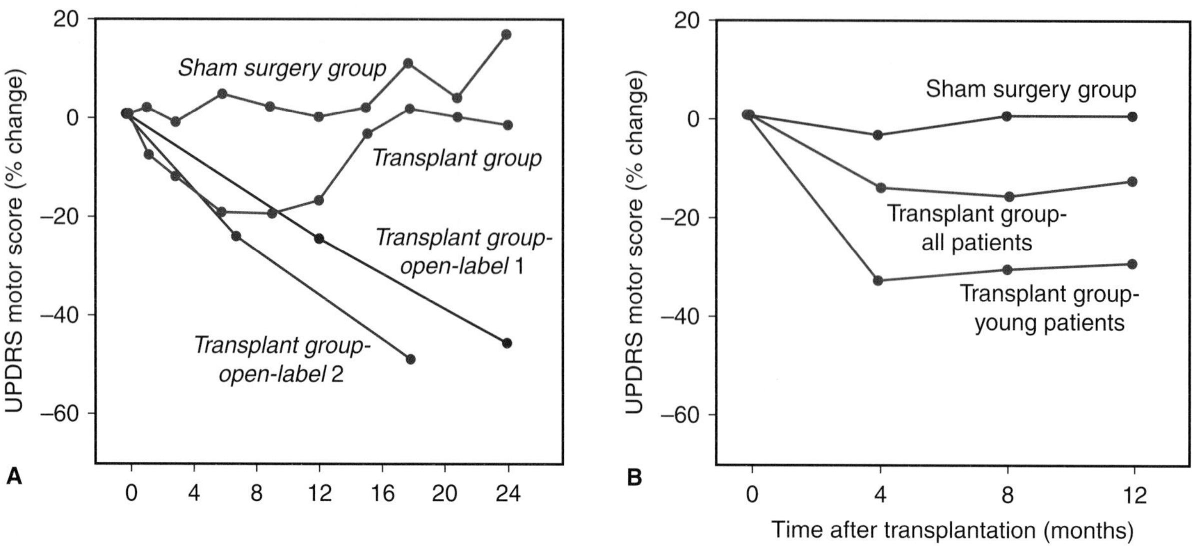

Figure 16–4. Time course of symptomatic improvement following transplantation of embryonic mesencephalic tissue in two sham surgery–controlled trials (A, Olanow et al.[23]; B, Freed et al.[20]) as compared to two open-label trials (1, Wenning et al.[16]; 2, Piccini et al.[34]). The magnitude of symptomatic improvement was similar over the first 4–6 months. However, in contrast to the patients in the controlled studies (Freed et al.,[20] Olanow et al.[23]), those in the open-label trials (Wenning et al.,[16] Piccini et al.[34]) continued to improve over the subsequent 12–18 months. This difference may be explained by the differences in immunosuppressive treatment: in the controlled studies, patients were treated with cyclosporine only for the first 6 months (Olanow et al.[23]) or no immunosuppression was given (Freed et al.[20]). The patients in the open-label trials were subjected to triple-drug immunosuppressive regimen for at least 12 months (Wenning et al.,[16] Piccini et al.[34]). Young patients in B $\leq$ 60 years old.

numbers of dopaminergic neurons and with a density of striatal DA innervation below a critical threshold (about 10–20% of normal). Blockade of serotonin neuron activity by administration of a combination of 5-HT_{1A} and 5-HT_{1B} agonists markedly ameliorated L-dopa-induced dyskinesias in nonhuman primates.[48] It remains to be shown, although, whether this treatment strategy is effective also against off-phase dyskinesias evoked by grafts. Finally, off-phase dyskinesias may be dependent on chronic inflammatory and immune responses around the graft. Off-phase dyskinesias did not develop until after withdrawal of immunosuppression at 6 months,[23] and at later autopsies, inflammation and activated microglia were observed around the graft. Piccini and colleagues[33] found that withdrawal of immunosuppression at 29 months after transplantation was accompanied by increased dyskinesia severity (Fig. 16–5). Animal studies have reported both increased and unchanged dyskinesia-like behavior in grafted rats with elevated immune response and inflammation.[49,50]

▶ DOPAMINERGIC GRAFTS AND THE DISEASE PROCESS

For the clinical usefulness of a cell-based therapy in PD, it is of major importance whether the grafts at some stage will be affected by the disease process. Three recent reports on patients transplanted with human embryonic mesencephalic tissue provide evidence that PD pathology may indeed propagate from the host to the graft.[28–30] In four patients, who died 11–16 years after surgery, a fraction (1–4%; Li and colleagues, unpublished observations) of the grafted DA neurons contained α-synuclein-rich Lewy bodies (LBs) and Lewy neurites (LNs). These pathological features are observed in affected brain regions, including the substantia nigra, of patients with PD. One study reported no LBs in a patient 14 years after transplantation.[31] Interestingly, four patients who had survived 4 or 9 years following transplantation showed no α-synuclein pathology in the grafts,[28,31] suggesting that at least one decade is required for the development of LBs. The pathological changes are probably progressive because LBs were more frequent in the grafts implanted 16 years prior to death than in those transplanted in the contralateral hemisphere 4 years later in one PD patient (Li and colleagues, unpublished observations).

Potential mechanisms that may underlie the pathological changes include inflammation, oxidative stress, excitotoxicity, reduced levels of trophic factors, or a prion-like mechanism.[51] What are the consequences of these findings for the further development of the DA cell replacement strategy in PD? Imaging studies have shown that embryonic mesencephalic grafts can synthesize and

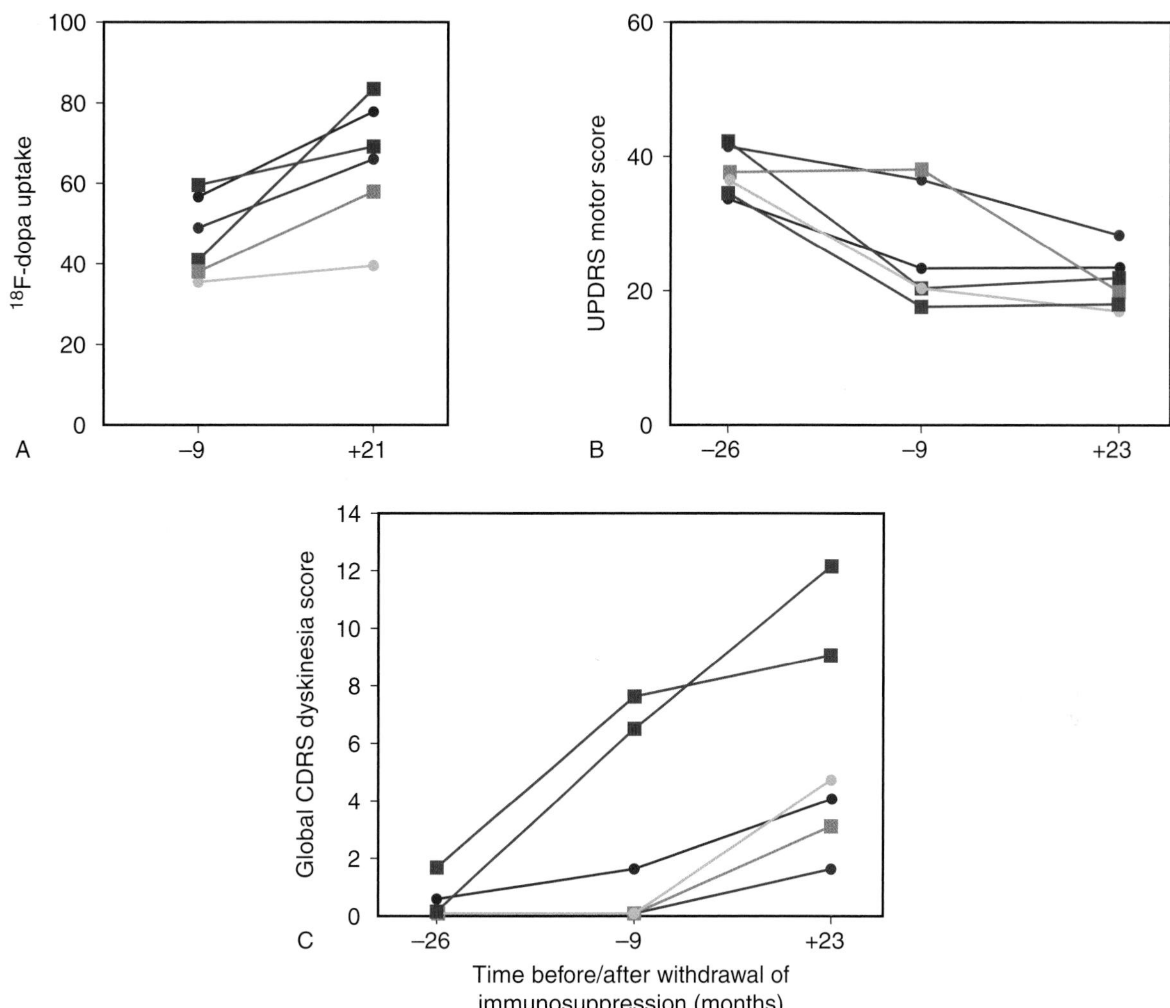

Figure 16–5. Withdrawal of immunosuppression late after transplantation of embryonic mesencephalic tissue does not compromise survival or antiparkinsonian action of the grafts but may contribute to worsening of off-phase dyskinesias. (A–C) Effects of withdrawal of immunosuppression in six PD patients on (A) ^{18}F-dopa uptake in grafted putamen (expressed as percentage of normal mean), and (B) UPDRS motor score and (C) global dyskinesia (CDRS) score in the off-phase. Immunosuppression was completely withdrawn at a mean of 29 months after the last transplantation and time points given on x-axis depict when in relation to withdrawal respective data were collected. (Data from Piccini P, Pavese N, Hagell P, et al. Factors affecting the clinical outcome after neural transplantation in Parkinson's disease. Brain 2005;128:2977–2986.)

release normal DA levels 10 years after transplantation associated with major clinical improvement.[32] This indicates that the majority of the grafted cells are not functionally impaired after one decade. It should be mentioned, although, that in two patients who died 14 years after transplantation, immunostaining for the DA transporter (DAT) was very light or absent in the grafts, despite robust staining for tyrosine hydroxylase (TH).[28,29] These patients experienced progressive worsening of PD from 11 and 12 years after surgery. The reduced DAT staining combined with TH and vesicular monoamine transporter (VMAT) staining may indicate an early compensatory response to graft failure.[28,29] In summary, cell replacement is still a viable therapeutic option because (i) the process is slow, (ii) the majority of grafted neurons are unaffected after a decade, and (iii) the patients experience long-term symptomatic relief.

▶ GENERATION OF DOPAMINE NEURONS FOR TRANSPLANTATION FROM STEM CELLS

It is unlikely that transplantation of human embryonic mesencephalic tissue will become routine treatment for PD due to problems with tissue availability and standardization of the grafts, leading to much variation in

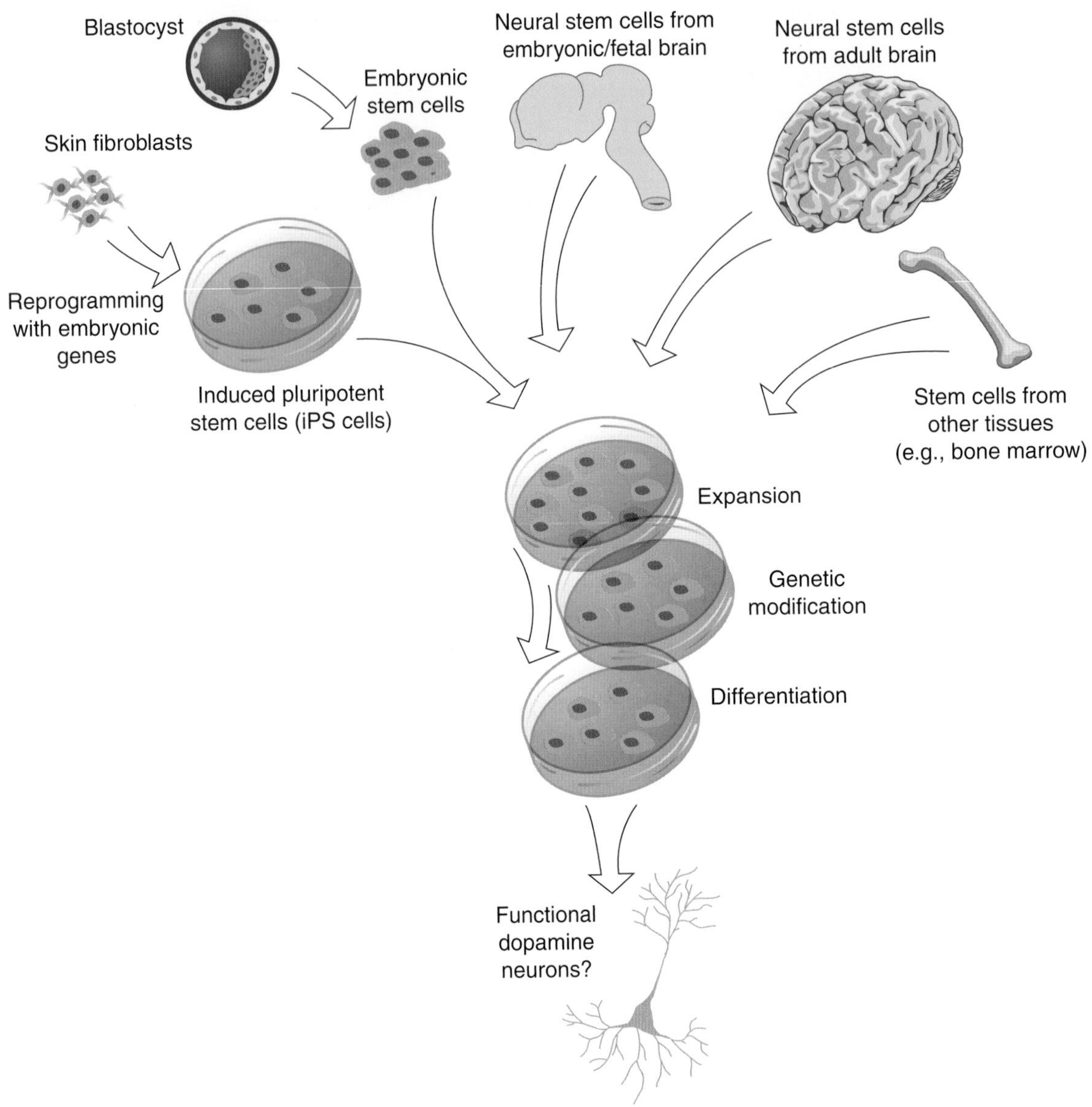

Figure 16–6. Potential sources of stem cells for the in vitro generation of functional DA neurons for restorative therapy in PD.

functional outcome. The main interest is now focused on the production of DA neuroblasts for transplantation from stem cells. It should be emphasized, although, that after maturation, these neurons have to work at least as well as those in the embryonic mesencephalic grafts. Conceivably, the stem cell–derived cells have to fulfil the following requirements in order to induce marked clinical improvement after transplantation: (1) release DA in a regulated manner, and exhibit the molecular, morphological, and electrophysiological properties of substantia nigra neurons[24,52]; (2) reverse motor deficits in animal models resembling the symptoms in patients; (3) allow for 100,000 or more grafted DA neurons to survive long term in each human putamen[53]; (4) reestablish a dense terminal network throughout the striatum; and (5) become functionally integrated into host neural circuitries.[34]

In a clinical setting, the stem cell–derived DA neuroblasts used for transplantation most likely have to be of human origin. Cells exhibiting at least some characteristics of mesencephalic DA neurons have been produced from stem cells of different sources, that is, embryonic stem cells, embryonic/fetal brain, adult brain, and other tissues, obtained from rodents, nonhuman primates, and humans (Fig. 16–6). The differentiation to DA neuroblasts has followed different culture protocols in the presence of various combinations of growth factors and signaling molecules. Based on the identification of transcription factors that determine mesencephalic DA neuron specification or maturation during normal development, it has

▶ TABLE 16–2. **CLINICALLY IMPORTANT PROPERTIES OF DOPAMINERGIC STEM/PRECURSOR CELL GRAFTS IN ANIMAL MODELS OF PARKINSON'S DISEASE**

Cell Source	Striatal Reinnervation	In Vivo Dopamine Release	Improvement of Parkinson-like Symptoms
Mouse ES cells	Partial	Significant	Significant
Mouse ES cells (therapeutically cloned)	N.D.	N.D.	Significant
Monkey ES cells	Partial	N.D.	Partial
Human ES cells	N.D.	N.D.	Partial
Rat embryonic VM-derived NSCs	Partial	N.D.	N.D.
Human embryonic VM-derived NSCs	Fibers	N.D.	N.D.
Rat adult SVZ-derived NSCs	N.D.	N.D.	N.D.
Rat bone marrow stem cells	Fibers	N.D.	Partial
Mouse fibroblasts (iPS cells)	Fibers	N.D.	N.D.

ES cells, embryonic stem cells; iPS cells, induced pluripotent stem cells; N.D., not demonstrated; NSCs, neural stem cells; SVZ, subventricular zone; VM, ventral mes-encephalon. Based on data from Björklund LM, Sánchez-Pernaute R, Chung S, et al. Embryonic cells develop into functional dopaminergic neurons after transplantation in a Parkinson rat model. Proc Natl Acad Sci USA 2002;99:2344–2349; Cho MS, Lee Y-E, Kim JY, et al. Highly efficient and large-scale generation of functional dopamine neurons from human embryonic stem cells. Proc Natl Acad Sci USA 2008;105:3392–3397; Dezawa M, Kanno H, Hoshino M, et al. Specific induction of neuronal cells from bone marrow stromal cells and application for autologous transplantation. J Clin Invest 2004;113:1701–1710; Kawasaki H, Mizuseki K, Nishikawa S, et al. Induction of midbrain dopaminergic neurons from ES cells by stromal cell-derived inducing activity. Neuron 2000;28:31–40; Kawasaki H, Suemori H, Mizuseki K, et al. Generation of dopaminergic neurons and pigmented epithelia from primate ES cells by stromal cell-derived inducing activity. Proc Natl Acad Sci USA 2002;99:1580–1585; Kim JH, Auerbach JM, Rodriguez-Gomez JA, et al. Dopamine neurons derived from embryonic stem cells function in an animal model of Parkinson's disease. Nature 2002;418:50–56; O'Keeffe FE, Scott SA, Tyers P, et al. Induction of A9 dopaminergic neurons from neural stem cells improves motor function in an animal model of Parkinson's disease. Brain 2008;131:630–641; Parish CL, Castelo-Branco G, Rawal N, et al. Wnt5a-treated midbrain neural stem cells improve dopamine cell replacement therapy in parkinsonian mice. J Clin Invest 2008;118:149–160; Rodriguez-Gomez JA, Lu J-Q, Velasco I, et al. Persistent dopamine functions of neurons derived from embryonic stem cells in a rodent model of Parkinson disease. Stem Cells 2007;25:918–928; Roy NS, Cleren C, Singh SK, et al. Functional engraftment of human ES cell-derived dopaminergic neurons enriched by coculture with telomerase-immortalized midbrain astrocytes. Nat Med 2006;12:1259–1268; Sanchez-Pernaute R, Studer L, Bankiewicz KS, et al. In vitro generation and transplantation of precursor-derived human dopamine neurons. J Neurosci Res 2001;65:284–288; Sanchez-Pernaute R, Lee H, Patterson M, et al. Parthenogenetic dopamine neurons from primate embryonic stem cells restore function in experimental Parkinson's disease. Brain 2008;131:2127–2139; Shim J-W, Park C-H, Bae Y-C, et al. Generation of functional dopamine neurons from neural precursor cells isolated from the subventricular zone and white matter of the adult rat brain using Nurr1 overexpression. Stem Cells 2007;25:1252–1262; Studer L, Tabar V, McKay RDG. Transplantation of expanded mesencephalic precursors leads to recovery in parkinsonian rats. Nat Neurosci 1998;1:290–295; Tabar V, Tomishima M, Panagiotakos G, et al. Therapeutic cloning in individual parkinsonian mice. Nat Med 2008;14:379–381; Takagi Y, Takahashi J, Saiki H, et al. Dopaminergic neurons generated from monkey embryonic stem cells function in a Parkinson primate model. J Clin Invest 2005;115:102–109; Wernig M, Zhao J-P, Pruszak J, et al. Neurons derived from reprogrammed fibroblasts functionally integrate into the fetal brain and improve symptoms of rats with Parkinson's disease. Proc Natl Acad Sci USA 2008;105, 5856–5861.

been possible to increase the yield of DA neurons with correct phenotype from stem cells by overexpressing the corresponding genes, for example, *Nurr1*,[54] *Pitx3*,[55,56] and *Lmx1a*.[57] In most cases, however, the improved efficiency in DA neuron generation has been shown only for animal and not for human stem cells. Moreover, it is unclear if this genetic modification of the stem cells would be acceptable in a clinical protocol.

Table 16–2 summarizes reported data when stem cell–derived DA neurons have been tested in animal models of PD with focus on properties of particular importance for the decision whether the cells are suitable for clinical application. In most cases, it has not been demonstrated that the stem cell–derived cells can substantially reinnervate the striatum, restore DA release, and markedly improve deficits resembling the PD patient's symptoms (Table 16–2). Thus, much experimental work remains before any stem cell–derived DA neuroblast can be selected as a clinical candidate cell for transplantation in a PD patient. A major concern, even when transplanting embryonic stem cell–derived DA neuroblasts, which have been pre-differentiated in culture, is the risk for tumor growth.[65] These tumors are most likely formed from residual proliferating embryonic stem cells or precursors. Because life expectancy is virtually normal in PD patients, it is unacceptable even with a minor risk of tumor formation associated with stem cell therapy in this disorder.

One of the most exciting, recent developments is the demonstration that somatic cells such as skin cells can be reprogrammed to a pluripotent state (Fig. 16–6).

Wernig and colleagues[72] recently reported that DA neurons can be generated from such induced pluripotent stem (iPS) cells, derived from mouse fibroblasts, and ameliorate behavioral deficit after transplantation in a rodent PD model. The major potential advantage with this approach is that patient-specific DA neuroblasts suitable for transplantation, avoiding immune reactions, can be produced without the use of human embryonic stem cells. However, several problems have to be solved before transplantation of DA neurons derived from iPS cells could be considered in a clinical setting. First, the risk for tumor formation, which resembles that with embryonic stem cells, has to be eliminated. The development of small molecules for reprogramming and cell sorting to separate the tumorigenic cells[72] could be the solution to this problem. Much work also remains to determine the survival, growth capacity, and functionality of the DA neurons generated from iPS cells (Table 16–2). A specific problem could be envisaged if the DA neurons are produced by iPS cells derived from the PD patient's skin cells. These human PD-specific iPS cells could be ideal for studies on disease pathophysiology and for drug development.[73] However, it seems possible that the use of the patient's own cells could be associated with increased susceptibility to the degenerative process, making the neurons more vulnerable to be affected by the disease. Consistent with this idea, increased α-synuclein expression was recently reported in PD patient fibroblasts.[74]

Therapeutic cloning provides another possibility to avoid immune reactions after DA neuron transplantation. Genetically identical embryonic stem cell–derived DA neurons, generated by transfer of autologous nuclei from fibroblasts, ameliorate functional deficits without immune reaction in PD mice.[70] However, to produce cells using therapeutic cloning for clinical application would be a logistical challenge. It has to be shown that therapeutic cloning leading to the generation of DA neurons also works with human cells and that substantial recovery can be obtained. Tumor formation has to be eliminated. The patient may exhibit a gene profile that would make the cells particularly susceptible to pathological changes. Finally, it can be questioned whether all the efforts to produce patient-specific DA neurons for transplantation in PD are justified. Immune reactions to brain allografts are moderate, and survival can be obtained even without immunosuppression,[20] although most investigators favor immunosuppression for 6–12 months after transplantation.[19,23,24]

▶ MAKING CELL THERAPY WORK IN PATIENTS WITH PARKINSON'S DISEASE

If DA cell replacement should become a clinically competitive therapy in PD, it has to provide advantages over currently available, rather effective treatments for alleviation of motor symptoms in PD patients. So far, the improvements after intrastriatal transplantation of DA neurons in patients[17–20,23,24] have not exceeded those found with DBS in the subthalamic nucleus (Table 16–1),[9] and there is no convincing evidence that drug-resistant symptoms are reversed by these grafts.[75] Even if it will be possible to produce virtually unlimited numbers of DA neuroblasts in standardized and quality-controlled preparations from stem cells, also other scientific advancements will be necessary for the development of a clinically competitive DA cell replacement therapy in PD (Fig. 16–1).

IMPROVED PATIENT SELECTION

Better criteria for how to select the most suitable patients for cell transplantation with respect to stage and type of PD have to be defined, and the preoperative degeneration pattern has to be determined using imaging techniques such as PET. Dopaminergic cell therapy will most likely be successful only in those patients who exhibit marked symptomatic (albeit too short-lasting) improvement of motor symptoms in response to L-dopa, and in whom the main pathology is a loss of DA neurons. Debilitating symptoms in PD and related disorders are also caused by pathological changes in non-dopaminergic systems leading to postural dysfunction, dementia, and autonomic disturbances. Until it is known how to repair these systems, patients in whom such symptoms are predominant should not undergo cell transplantation.

IMPROVED FUNCTIONAL EFFICACY OF GRAFTS

The transplantation procedure needs to be tailor-made with respect to the dose and site of implantation of the DA cells based on preoperative imaging so that the repair of the DA system in striatum and extra-striatal areas is as complete as possible in each patient's brain. Piccini and colleagues[33] have shown that the occurrence of dopaminergic denervation in areas not reached by intraputaminal grafts, before or after surgery, exerts a marked influence on the overall outcome following transplantation of human embryonic mesencephalic tissue. Statistical parametric mapping (SPM) of ^{18}F-dopa uptake, comparing each patient vs. appropriate control across the whole brain, was used to show the pattern of dopaminergic denervations outside the grafted areas and also to explore whether these changes were present already prior to transplantation or if they developed during the postoperative assessment period. Out of eight patients, all having surviving grafts bilaterally in the putamen, three patients showed no reduction of ^{18}F-dopa uptake outside the grafted areas either before or after transplantation, indicating that the dopaminergic denervation remained confined to the caudate-putamen throughout the period of assessment. Three patients showed denervation outside the areas to be grafted already prior to transplantation. Two patients developed such denervation during the first 2 years after surgery. Remarkably, the three patients with denervation confined to grafted areas exhibited major improvements, whereas those that had widespread denervation already prior to transplantation showed no overall benefit or even deteriorated. The two patients who developed denervation outside the grafted areas in the postoperative course showed modest overall benefit. These findings indicate that the occurrence of dopaminergic denervation in non-grafted areas before or after transplantation exerts a marked negative influence on the overall outcome. In contrast, long-lasting successful outcome in PD patients with more widespread denervations including, for example, ventral striatum and cerebral cortex will require that grafts are placed also in areas outside the caudate-putamen.

STRATEGIES TO AVOID ADVERSE EFFECTS

The risk of off-phase dyskinesias following cell transplantation has to be minimized. Available data indicate that this could be achieved by excluding serotonergic neurons from the graft material, by carefully monitored immunosuppressive treatment for at least 6–12 months, and by using a surgical procedure that gives rise to optimum distribution of cells over the putamen, and complete and even reinnervation without "hot-spots." The risk for tumor formation when the grafted DA neurons have been derived from pluripotent stem cells, and the consequences of the introduction of new genes in stem cell–derived neurons, should be carefully evaluated after transplantation in animal models prior to clinical application. However, some evidence suggests that embryonic stem cells are more prone to generate tumors when implanted into the same species from which they were derived.[76] Absence of tumors after xenotransplantation, as with human cells implanted into rodent PD model, may therefore not exclude their occurrence in the PD patient's brain. To improve safety, it may be necessary to engineer the stem cells with regulatable suicide genes or to use cell sorting to eliminate those cells that could give rise to tumors.

▶ PERSPECTIVES

Parkinson's disease is progressive and also affects areas outside the putamen, where most grafts have been placed, and non-dopaminergic systems, which are not replaced by embryonic mesencephalic tissue or stem cell–derived dopaminergic neurons. Moreover, it has not yet been possible to reconstruct the nigrostriatal pathway and; therefore, the dopaminergic grafts have, in virtually all cases, been placed in an ectopic location, that is, the striatum. Several arguments support that cell replacement research, despite these problems, should continue with the aim to develop a clinically useful transplantation treatment for PD patients. Dopaminergic cell therapy leads to replacement, specifically of those neurons that have died because of the disease process, and thereby targets the impaired biological mechanism underlying a substantial part of the patient's symptoms. In successful cases, dopaminergic cell therapy has induced major, long-lasting clinical improvements and allowed PD patients to stop medication for several years. Moreover, imaging techniques, in particular PET, have improved to the extent that it is now possible, with high resolution, to monitor the extent and pattern of innervation as well as the function of different neural systems, for example, the nigrostriatal DA system. Finally, in the future, it may be possible to implant also neurons with other phenotypes as well as to reconstruct the nigrostriatal pathway by transplantation into substantia nigra and subsequent suppression of axonal growth inhibitory mechanisms.

Stem cell–based approaches for the first time open up the possibility for the development of a restorative treatment for large numbers of PD patients. Based on the available experimental and clinical data, it should now be possible to define a road map including the six main steps toward clinical application of stem cells in PD: (1) production of DA-releasing cells, expressing markers and electrophysiological properties of substantia nigra neurons, under GMP conditions in vitro without the use of animal components; (2) demonstration of survival, effective reinnervation of striatum, in vivo DA release, and efficacy in reversing clinically relevant behavioral deficits after transplantation in rodent PD model; (3) assessment of scaling up, cell migration, and graft effects on complex behaviors in large animals; (4) assessment of risks and toxicity (e.g., tumorigenicity and dyskinesias) in rodents and large animals, and development of clinical plan for treatment of toxicity; (5) selection of patients with dopaminergic denervation restricted to striatal areas and without predominating dementia, depression, and autonomic symptoms; and (6) Phase 1 clinical trials: bilateral implants in putamen, evenly distributed, 100,000 surviving DA neurons per putamen, low numbers of serotonin neurons, immunosuppression for 12 months.

Besides the scientific and clinical advancements, it is important that the relevant ethical, regulatory, societal, and economical issues are also addressed in this translation of stem cells to patient application. It should be emphasized that, with respect to efficacy and risk of adverse effects, the requirements for stem cell therapy to become a clinically competitive treatment in PD are high. Moreover, permanent symptomatic relief in PD patients will most likely require that the DA cell replacement by stem cells is combined with strategies to hinder disease progression.

▶ ACKNOWLEDGMENTS

Our own research was supported by the Swedish Research Council, and the Söderberg, Crafoord, and Kock Foundations. The Lund Stem Cell Center is supported by a Center of Excellence grant in Life Sciences from the Swedish Foundation for Strategic Research.

REFERENCES

1. Brundin P, Duan W-M, Sauer H. Functional effects of mesencephalic dopamine neurons and adrenal chromaffin cells grafted to the rodent striatum. In Dunnett SB, Björklund A (eds). Functional Neural Transplantation. New York: Raven Press, 1994, pp. 9–46.
2. Winkler C, Kirik D, Björklund A, et al. Transplantation in the rat model of Parkinson's disease: Ectopic versus homotopic graft placement. Prog Brain Res 2000;127:233–265.
3. Backlund E-O, Granberg P-O, Hamberger B, et al. Transplantation of adrenal medullary tissue to striatum in parkinsonism: First clinical trials. J Neurosurg 1985;62: 169–173.
4. Madrazo I, Drucker-Colin R, Diaz V, et al. Open microsurgical autograft of adrenal medulla to the right caudate nucleus in two patients with intractable Parkinson's disease. N Engl J Med 1987;316:831–834.
5. Goetz CG, Stebbins GT 3rd, Klawans HL, et al. United Parkinson Foundation Neurotransplantation Registry on adrenal medullary transplants: Presurgical, and 1- and 2-year follow-up. Neurology 1991;41:1719–1722.
6. Kompoliti K, Chu Y, Shannon KM, et al. Neuropathological study 16 years after autologous adrenal medullary transplantation in a Parkinson's disease patient. Mov Disord 2007;22:1630–1633.
7. Minguez-Castellanos A, Escamilla-Sevilla F, Hotton GR, et al. Carotid body autotransplantation in Parkinson disease. A clinical and positron emission tomography study. J Neurol Neurosurg Psychiatry 2007;78:825–831.
8. Stover NP, Bakay RAE, Subramanian T, et al. Intrastriatal implantation of human retinal pigment epithelial cells attached to microcarriers in advanced Parkinson's disease. Arch Neurol 2005;62:1833–1837.
9. Kleiner-Fisman G, Herzog J, Fisman DN, et al. Subthalamic deep brain stimulation: Summary and meta-analysis of outcomes. Mov Disord 2006;21:(suppl.14) S290–S304.
10. Lindvall O, Brundin P, Widner H, et al. Grafts of fetal dopamine neurons survive and improve motor function in Parkinson's disease. Science 1990;247:574–577.
11. Sawle GV, Bloomfield PM, Björklund A, et al. Transplantation of fetal dopamine neurons in Parkinson's disease: PET [^{18}F]6-L-fluorodopa studies in two patients with putaminal implants. Ann Neurol 1992;31:166–173.
12. Lindvall O, Sawle G, Widner H, et al. Evidence for long-term survival and function of dopaminergic grafts in progressive Parkinson's disease. Ann Neurol 1994;35: 172–180.
13. Peschanski M, Defer G, N'Guyen JP, et al. Bilateral motor improvement and alteration of L-dopa effect in two patients with Parkinson's disease following intrastriatal transplantation of foetal ventral mesencephalon. Brain 1994;117:487–499.
14. Freeman TB, Olanow CW, Hauser RA, et al. Bilateral fetal nigral transplantation into the postcommissural putamen in Parkinson's disease. Ann Neurol 1995;38:379–388.
15. Remy P, Samson Y, Hantraye P, et al. Clinical correlates of [^{18}F]fluorodopa uptake in five grafted parkinsonian patients. Ann Neurol 1995;38:580–588.
16. Wenning GK, Odin P, Morrish P, et al. Short- and long-term survival and function of unilateral intrastriatal dopaminergic grafts in Parkinson's disease. Ann Neurol 1997;42:95–107.
17. Hagell P, Schrag A, Piccini P, et al. Sequential bilateral transplantation in Parkinson's disease: Effects of the second graft. Brain 1999;122:1121–1132.
18. Hauser RA, Freeman TB, Snow BJ, et al. Long-term evaluation of bilateral fetal nigral transplantation in Parkinson disease. Arch Neurol 1999;56:179–187.
19. Brundin P, Pogarell O, Hagell P, et al. Bilateral caudate and putamen grafts of embryonic mesencephalic tissue treated with lazaroids in Parkinson's disease. Brain 2000;123:1380–1390.
20. Freed CR, Greene PE, Breeze RE, et al. Transplantation of embryonic dopamine neurons for severe Parkinson's disease. N Engl J Med 2001;344:710–719.
21. Mendez I, Dagher A, Hong M, et al. Simultaneous intrastriatal and intranigral fetal dopaminergic grafts in patients with Parkinson disease: A pilot study. Report of three cases. J Neurosurg 2002;96:589–596.
22. Cochen V, Ribeiro MJ, Nguyen JP, et al. Transplantation in Parkinson's disease: PET changes correlate with the amount of grafted tissue. Mov Disord 2003;18:928–932.
23. Olanow CW, Goetz CG, Kordower JH, et al. A double-blind controlled trial of bilateral fetal nigral transplantation in Parkinson's disease. Ann Neurol 2003;54:403–414.
24. Mendez I, Sanchez-Pernaute R, Cooper O, et al. Cell type analysis of functional fetal dopamine cell suspension transplants in the striatum and substantia nigra of patients with Parkinson's disease. Brain 2005;128:1498–1510.
25. Kordower JH, Freeman TB, Snow BJ, et al. Neuropathological evidence of graft survival and striatal reinnervation after the transplantation of fetal mesencephalic tissue in a patient with Parkinson's disease. New Engl J Med 1995;332:1118–1124.
26. Kordower JH, Rosenstein JM, Collier TJ, et al. Functional fetal nigral grafts in a patient with Parkinson's disease: Chemoanatomic, ultrastructural, and metabolic studies. J Comp Neurol 1996;370:203–230,
27. Kordower JH, Freeman TB, Chen EY, et al. Fetal nigral grafts survive and mediate clinical benefit in a patient with Parkinson's disease. Mov Disord 1998;13:383–393.
28. Kordower JH, Chu Y, Hauser RA, et al. Lewy body-like pathology in long-term embryonic nigral transplants in Parkinson's disease. Nat Med 2008;14:504–506.
29. Kordower JH, Chu Y, Hauser RA, et al. Transplanted dopaminergic neurons develop PD pathologic changes: A second case report. Mov Disord 2008;23:2303–2306.
30. Li J-Y, Englund E, Holton JL, et al. Lewy bodies in grafted neurons in subjects with Parkinson's disease suggest host-to-graft disease propagation. Nat Med 2008;14: 501–503.

31. Mendez I, Vinuela A, Astradsson A, et al. Dopamine neurons implanted into people with Parkinson's disease survive without pathology for 14 years. Nat Med 2008;14:507–509.
32. Piccini P, Brooks DJ, Björklund A, et al. Dopamine release from nigral transplants visualized in vivo in a Parkinson's patient. Nat Neurosci 1999;2:1137–1140.
33. Piccini P, Pavese N, Hagell P, et al. Factors affecting the clinical outcome after neural transplantation in Parkinson's disease. Brain 2005;128:2977–2986.
34. Piccini P, Lindvall O, Björklund A, et al. Delayed recovery of movement-related cortical function in Parkinson's disease after striatal dopaminergic grafts. Ann Neurol 2000;48:689–695.
35. Lindvall O, Widner H, Rehncrona S, et al. Transplantation of fetal dopamine neurons in Parkinson's disease: 1-year clinical and neurophysiological observations in two patients with putaminal implants. Ann Neurol 1992;31: 155–165.
36. Defer GL, Geny C, Ricolfi F, et al. Long-term outcome of unilaterally transplanted parkinsonian patients: I. Clinical approach. Brain 1996;119:41–50.
37. Mendez I, Dagher A, Hong M, et al. Enhancement of survival of stored dopaminergic cells and promotion of graft survival by exposure of human fetal nigral tissue to glial cell line-derived neurotrophic factor in patients with Parkinson's disease. J Neurosurg 2000;92:863–869.
38. Goetz CG, Wuu J, McDermott MP, et al. Placebo response in Parkinson's disease: Comparisons among 11 trials covering medical and surgical interventions. Mov Disord 2008;23:690–699.
39. Hagell P, Cenci MA. Dyskinesias and dopamine cell replacement in Parkinson's disease: A clinical perspective. Brain Res Bull 2005;68:4–15.
40. Hagell P, Piccini P, Björklund A, et al. Dyskinesias following neural transplantation in Parkinson's disease. Nat Neurosci 2002;5:627–628.
41. Graff-Radford J, Foote KD, Rodriguez RL, et al. Deep brain stimulation of the internal segment of the globus pallidus in delayed runaway dyskinesia. Arch Neurol 2006;63:1181–1184.
42. Herzog J, Pogarell O, Pinsker MO, et al. Deep brain stimulation in Parkinson's disease following fetal nigral transplantation. Mov Disord 2008;23:1293–1296.
43. Ma Y, Feigin A, Dhawan V, et al. Dyskinesia after fetal cell transplantation for parkinsonism: A PET study. Ann Neurol 2002;52:628–634.
44. Maries E, Kordower JH, Chu Y, et al. Focal not widespread grafts induce novel dyskinetic behavior in parkinsonian rats. Neurobiol Dis 2006;21:165–180.
45. Carta M, Carlsson T, Kirik D, Bjorklund A. Dopamine released from 5-HT terminals is the cause of L-DOPA-induced dyskinesia in parkinsonian rats. Brain 2007;130: 1819–1833.
46. Carlsson T, Carta M, Winkler C, et al. Serotonin neuron transplants exacerbate L-DOPA-induced dyskinesias in a rat model of Parkinson's disease. J Neurosci 2007;27: 8011–8022.
47. Carlsson T, Carta M, Munoz A, et al. Impact of grafted serotonin and dopamine neurons on development of L-DOPA-induced dyskinesias in parkinsonian rats is determined by the extent of dopamine neuron degeneration. Brain 2009;132(2):319–335.
48. Munoz A, Li Q, Gardoni F, et al. Combined 5-HT_{1A} and 5-HT_{1B} receptor agonists for the treatment of L-DOPA-induced dyskinesia. Brain. 2008 Dec;131(Pt 12):3380–3394.
49. Lane EL, Soulet D, Vercammen L, et al. Neuroinflammation in the generation of post-transplantation dyskinesia in Parkinson's disease. Neurobiol Dis 2008;32:220–228.
50. Soderstrom KE, Meredith G, Freeman TB, et al. The synaptic impact of the host immune response in a parkinsonian allograft rat model: Influence on graft-derived aberrant behaviors. Neurobiol Dis. 2008 Nov;32(2):229–242.
51. Brundin P, Li J-Y, Holton JL, et al. Research in motion: The enigma of Parkinson's disease pathology spread. Nat Rev Neurosci 2008;9:741–745.
52. Isacson O, Bjorklund LM, Schumacher JM. Toward full restoration of synaptic and terminal function of the dopaminergic system in Parkinson's disease by stem cells. Ann Neurol 2003;53:(suppl 3):S135–S146.
53. Hagell P, Brundin P. Cell survival and clinical outcome following intrastriatal transplantation in Parkinson's disease. J Neuropathol Exp Neurol 2001;60:741–752.
54. Kim JH, Auerbach JM, Rodriguez-Gomez JA, et al. Dopamine neurons derived from embryonic stem cells function in an animal model of Parkinson's disease. Nature 2002;418:50–56.
55. Chung S, Hedlund E, Hwang M, et al. The homeodomain transcription factor Pitx3 facilitates differentiation of mouse embryonic stem cells into AHD2-expressing dopaminergic neurons. Mol Cell Neurosci 2005;28:241–252.
56. O'Keeffe FE, Scott SA, Tyers P, et al. Induction of A9 dopaminergic neurons from neural stem cells improves motor function in an animal model of Parkinson's disease. Brain 2008;131:630–641.
57. Andersson E, Tryggvason U, Deng Q, et al. Identification of intrinsic determinants of midbrain dopamine neurons. Cell 2006;124:393–405.
58. Björklund LM, Sánchez-Pernaute R, Chung S, et al. Embryonic cells develop into functional dopaminergic neurons after transplantation in a Parkinson rat model. Proc Natl Acad Sci USA 2002;99:2344–2349.
59. Cho MS, Lee Y-E, Kim JY, et al. Highly efficient and large-scale generation of functional dopamine neurons from human embryonic stem cells. Proc Natl Acad Sci USA 2008;105:3392–3397.
60. Dezawa M, Kanno H, Hoshino M, et al. Specific induction of neuronal cells from bone marrow stromal cells and application for autologous transplantation. J Clin Invest 2004;113:1701–1710.
61. Kawasaki H, Mizuseki K, Nishikawa S, et al. Induction of midbrain dopaminergic neurons from ES cells by stromal cell-derived inducing activity. Neuron 2000;28: 31–40.
62. Kawasaki H, Suemori H, Mizuseki K, et al. Generation of dopaminergic neurons and pigmented epithelia from primate ES cells by stromal cell-derived inducing activity. Proc Natl Acad Sci USA 2002;99:1580–1585.
63. Parish CL, Castelo-Branco G, Rawal N, et al. Wnt5a-treated midbrain neural stem cells improve dopamine cell replacement therapy in parkinsonian mice. J Clin Invest 2008;118:149–160.

64. Rodriguez-Gomez JA, Lu J-Q, Velasco I, et al. Persistent dopamine functions of neurons derived from embryonic stem cells in a rodent model of Parkinson disease. Stem Cells 2007;25:918–928.
65. Roy NS, Cleren C, Singh SK, et al. Functional engraftment of human ES cell-derived dopaminergic neurons enriched by coculture with telomerase-immortalized midbrain astrocytes. Nat Med 2006;12:1259–1268.
66. Sanchez-Pernaute R, Studer L, Bankiewicz KS, et al. In vitro generation and transplantation of precursor-derived human dopamine neurons. J Neurosci Res 2001;65:284–288.
67. Sanchez-Pernaute R, Lee H, Patterson M, et al. Parthenogenetic dopamine neurons from primate embryonic stem cells restore function in experimental Parkinson's disease. Brain. 2008 Aug;131(Pt 8):2127–2139.
68. Shim J-W, Park C-H, Bae Y-C, et al. Generation of functional dopamine neurons from neural precursor cells isolated from the subventricular zone and white matter of the adult rat brain using Nurr1 overexpression. Stem Cells 2007;25:1252–1262.
69. Studer L, Tabar V, McKay RDG. Transplantation of expanded mesencephalic precursors leads to recovery in parkinsonian rats. Nat Neurosci 1998;1:290–295.
70. Tabar V, Tomishima M, Panagiotakos G, et al. Therapeutic cloning in individual parkinsonian mice. Nat Med 2008;14:379–381.
71. Takagi Y, Takahashi J, Saiki H, et al. Dopaminergic neurons generated from monkey embryonic stem cells function in a Parkinson primate model. J Clin Invest 2005;115: 102–109.
72. Wernig M, Zhao J-P, Pruszak J, et al. Neurons derived from reprogrammed fibroblasts functionally integrate into the fetal brain and improve symptoms of rats with Parkinson's disease. Proc Natl Acad Sci USA 2008;105, 5856–5861.
73. Park I-H, Arora N, Huo H, et al. Disease-specific induced pluripotent stem cells. Cell 2008;134:1–10.
74. Hoepken H-H, Gispert S, Azizov M, et al. Parkinson patient fibroblasts show increased alpha-synuclein expression. Exp Neurol 2008;212:307–313.
75. Lindvall O, Hagell P. Clinical observations after neural transplantation in Parkinson's disease. Prog Brain Res 2000;127:299–320.
76. Erdö F, Bührle C, Blunk J, et al. Host-dependent tumorigenesis of embryonic stem cell transplantation in experimental stroke. J Cereb Blood Flow Metab 2003;23: 780–785.

CHAPTER 17

Stereotaxic Surgery and Deep Brain Stimulation for Parkinson's Disease and Movement Disorders

Milind Deogonkar, Andre Machado, and Jerrold L. Vitek

▶ INTRODUCTION

Functional surgery for movement disorders can significantly alleviate the motor symptoms associated with these disorders and improve the quality of life for patients with disabling diseases such as Parkinson's disease (PD), essential tremor (ET), and dystonia in appropriately selected patients. The surgical approach to movement disorders has evolved dramatically from the pre-L-dopa era to the development of modern magnetic resonance imaging (MRI)-based stereotaxic and neurophysiologic guided targeting. Current stereotactic approaches have benefited from the concurrent growth in our understanding of the functional organization of target structures and the pathophysiological basis underlying the development of these disorders. The resurgence of ablative therapy in the 1990s has given way to the development of chronic electrical stimulation of deep brain structures, that is, deep brain stimulation (DBS). DBS has given us the ability to explore surgical therapies for neurological disorders not previously approachable through ablative therapy, given the reversibility of side effects and the ability to modify stimulation parameters to optimize results.

Although an effective treatment for the motor symptoms associated with PD, over time medical treatment with L-dopa leads to motor fluctuations and drug-induced dyskinesias, side effects that compromise efficacy and diminish quality of life. Even with advances in molecular- and genetic-based therapies on the horizon, it seems likely that there will be, for the foreseeable future, a large population of patients significantly burdened by these neurodegenerative diseases who are candidates for DBS.

While many patients with ET have mild symptoms that may be controlled with medication, others are refractory to or develop a tolerance to medication, have significant disability as the tremor becomes more severe, and are often unable to perform simple activities of daily living or maintain employment.

Dystonia is a particularly disabling condition that is difficult to treat with medical therapy requiring large doses of anticholinergic medications alone or in combination with other medications such as baclofen, clonazepam, or the dopamine-depleting drug tetrabenazine. While some patients may get adequate benefit from this combination of medications alone or in conjunction with botulinum toxin injections, many require such large doses that side effects compromise the patient's quality of life. Although many patients with focal dystonias may respond to botulinum toxin alone, some of these patients will develop antibodies to the toxin and lose benefit, while others with more diffuse involvement or involvement of larger muscle groups are not candidates for botulinum therapy.

Thus there is a need for a therapy that can provide relief from the symptoms of these disorders when medical therapy is no longer effective. With the advent of DBS, a therapy is now available for these patients. As data from larger controlled clinical trials become available, neurologists and neurosurgeons will be better able to tailor therapy for individual patients through the appropriate choice of target site and mode of treatment (ablative or stimulation) that best fits the patient's disease characteristics.

▶ HISTORY OF STEREOTAXIC SURGERY FOR MOVEMENT DISORDERS

The history of stereotaxic surgery for the treatment of movement disorders is replete with a multitude of approaches to different targets in an attempt to ameliorate a variety of movement disorders. Reports of remarkable successes are mixed with complete failures after the same stereotaxic intervention.[1,2] The earliest approaches were generally not based on sound scientific principles but were empirically driven or based on simplistic rationales that led to what often appears as a desperate search for an effective target. The first known attempts to treat PD surgically were based on the presumed relationship between the motor symptoms and the foci of infection in patients with encephalitis lethargica. These consisted of removing the various organs suspected of harboring the infection evolving to sympathetic ramisectomies and cervical ganglionectomies. In 1930, Pollack and Davis,[3] in a failed attempt to relieve parkinsonian tremor, sectioned the dorsal roots of a patient. Although the rigidity was lessened, the tremor remained. Subsequent attempts included anterolateral cordotomies,[4,5] dentatectomy,[6] and extirpation of the precentral cortex.[7] These were generally unsuccessful and were associated with considerable morbidity. Meyers[8] subsequently reported improvements in some patients in which various parts of the basal ganglia, including the caudate, putamen, and globus pallidus (GP) or its outflow tracts, the ansa lenticularis or fascicularis lenticularis, were removed or sectioned, respectively. However, there remained significant morbidity and mortality associated with these procedures. In 1952, Cooper observed alleviation of parkinsonian motor signs after accidental ligation of the anterior choroidal artery, which led to a number of unpredictable outcomes after subsequent ligations in other PD patients.[9] A variety of approaches were subsequently used to interrupt the pallidofugal pathways, including heating, freezing, and injections of procaine oil into the pallidum. Results, however, were inconsistent. Was it a problem of appropriate target selection, or an inability to consistently reach the chosen target that led to such a wide variation in the results for patients with similar movement disorders? With the development of stereotaxis by Spiegel and Wycis,[10] there was an opportunity to improve target localization. Yet results, although somewhat improved, were still quite variable. This led to the report by Svennilson and colleagues, who described the effect of pallidotomy on 81 patients operated on by Lars Leksell.[11] Leksell, varying the lesion site within the globus pallidus pars interna (GPi), observed a clear difference in outcome that was correlated with lesion location. In the last 20 patients with lesions placed in the posteroventral portion of GPi, 19 were substantially improved. These early successes led to the further development of stereotaxy and to a variety of lesioning procedures of the basal ganglia and the thalamus for the treatment of rigidity and tremor in the 1950s and 1960s. Various surgical techniques, lesion locations, lesion sizes, and outcomes were reported.[12–15] The motor thalamus and the pallidal targets lying in the ventral and posterior portions of the GPi as well as the pallidal projections were considered to be the most effective targets. With the advent of L-dopa, however, surgical treatment of PD became less frequent. Subsequent approaches were focused on thalamotomy for parkinsonian tremor, because most surgeons, at that time, felt that this was a better target for tremor alleviation.[11,16] Although Svennilson and colleagues had reported more than 80% of patients experienced complete tremor alleviation after pallidotomy, the target site was moved to the thalamus. This was likely due in part to the immediate and oftentimes dramatic cessation of tremor following the thalamic lesion compared to pallidotomy where the tremor may more often than not wane over time following the lesion. For the next 20 years, surgery for movement disorders was predominantly limited to thalamotomy[17–25] for the treatment of tremor and pallidotomy and thalamotomy for dystonia.[26–29] PD surgery was rarely performed during this time. It was not until the late 1980s that interest in the neurosurgical treatment for PD underwent resurgence due to the increasing realization of the limitations and side effects of L-dopa. Lauri Laitien[30,31] and others repopularized the use of pallidotomy for the treatment of PD during this time.

Thalamotomy, although effective for tremor, rigidity, and L-dopa-induced dyskinesia, was ineffective for akinesia, and often worsened gait or speech. It remained the target of choice; however, until the early 1990s when pallidotomy was favorably reexplored by Laitinen and colleagues.[31] Laitinen's report of significant improvement in parkinsonian motor signs, and drug-induced dyskinesias after posteroventral pallidotomy, together with separate reports of improvement of parkinsonian motor signs after ablation or inactivation of the subthalamic nucleus (STN) and GPi in animal models of PD, led to a resurgence of stereotaxic pallidotomy for PD. Several centers corroborated earlier reports[11,31] of amelioration of parkinsonian motor signs after stereotaxic pallidotomy.[32–36] Results, however, were not uniformly successful across centers, with some reporting minimal improvement,[37] whereas others, such as Svennilson and colleagues and Laitinen, reported significant improvement across the vast majority of patients.[32–36] Short- and long-term benefits of pallidotomy for PD have now been confirmed in two blinded randomized trials versus best medical therapy.[37–39] Inconsistencies in results of earlier studies were likely due to a variety of clinical variables, including lesion location and size, the patient's age and cognitive state, and other, as yet unidentified variables, such as the presence of cerebral atrophy, response to medication, associated medical problems, and varied brain pathology. These variables, of which lesion location, age, and etiology of the movement disorder likely played a central role, may also account, in part, for the variable success rates of stereotaxic intervention in other movement disorders.

DBS evolved from experience with thalamotomies for PD in the 1950s and 1960s. Hassler and others noted that intraoperative high-frequency stimulation (>100 Hz) in Vim temporarily arrested parkinsonian tremor.[40,41] Chronic Vim stimulation was soon employed as an alternative to thalamotomy for parkinsonian tremor and ET.[42,43] As the revival of pallidotomy for parkinsonism was meeting renewed success with modern techniques, investigators started applying chronic stimulation successfully in Vim,[42–47] GPi,[48–50] and STN.[51] It was not long before DBS was applied to these targets for other movement disorders, including hemiballism[52] and dystonia.[53–55] Over the past 20 years DBS, with its inherent features of reversibility and adjustability and ability to perform bilateral procedures without the high incidence of side effects associated with ablative therapies, has gained in popularity and emerged as the neurosurgical standard of care for movement disorders such as PD, dystonia, and essential tremor.[25,42,56–75] Since its inception, more than 50,000 DBS implants have been performed in over 500 centers worldwide.[76] In addition to the widespread use of DBS for movement disorders, a number of clinical investigations using DBS are underway exploring its safety and efficacy for conditions such as Tourette's syndrome,[77–85] chronic pain,[85–90] addiction, epilepsy, disorders of consciousness, and psychiatric disorders such as depression[91–95] and obsessive compulsive disorder (OCD).[96–101]

▶ PATHOPHYSIOLOGICAL BASIS OF HYPO- AND HYPERKINETIC MOVEMENT DISORDERS

ORGANIZATION OF BASAL GANGLIA AND THALAMOCORTICAL CIRCUITS

Based on our understanding of the anatomy and physiology of the basal ganglia and related structures, a scheme for the functional organization of the basal ganglia has been developed. This scheme views the basal ganglia as a family of segregated circuits involving specific portions of the thalamus and cerebral cortex. These circuits take origin from different cortical areas and project to separate portions of the basal ganglia, which in turn project to separate portions of the thalamus, returning to the same areas of the frontal cortex from which they took origin. One of these circuits, the "motor" circuit, plays an important role in the pathogenesis of hypo and hyperkinetic movement disorders, including PD, dystonia, hemiballismus, and Huntington's chorea.[102] Parkinsonian tremor, although implicated in this circuit, may have a more diverse etiology,[103,104] whereas ET and intention tremor are most likely the result of alterations in cerebellothalamic pathways.[105–107]

The motor circuit takes origin from precentral motor and postcentral somatosensory cortical areas and projects to motor areas of the basal ganglia and thalamus en route to its return to motor and premotor cortical areas (Fig. 17–1). This circuit is somatotopically organized throughout the different cortical and subcortical motor areas. Cortical input to subcortical portions of the motor circuit occurs via their projections to the putamen. Putaminal output arrives at the two major output routes from the basal ganglia, the internal segment of the globus pallidus (GPi) and the substantia nigra pars reticulata (SNr), via two pathways, termed the "direct" and the "indirect" pathways (see Fig. 17–1). The direct pathway takes origin from medium spiny neurons with presumed dopaminergic excitatory responses and monosynaptic projections to GPi and SNr. The indirect pathway takes origin from medium spiny neurons with presumed dopaminergic inhibitory responses that project, via globus pallidus pars externa (GPe) and STN, to the GPi and SNr. In addition, there are return projections from the STN to GPe as well as direct projections from GPe to GPi, SNr, and the reticularis nucleus of the thalamus.[108] More recently a hyperdirect pathway has been described with cortical projections directly to the STN.

Based on this organizational scheme of the basal ganglia, two putative roles for the pallidothalamocortical motor circuit have been proposed: (1) scaling movement and (2) focusing motor activity. Scaling of movement could occur through the opposing effects of inhibitory striatal neurons in the direct pathways and excitatory effect of indirect pathway neurons from the STN on output neurons from GPi/SNr. Thus, movement can be scaled by facilitation of movement through increasing direct pathway activity and inhibition of movement through increased indirect pathway activity converging on these same inhibitory output neurons. Similarly, focusing of movement may occur when neurons controlling agonist activity are facilitated through the direct pathway, while at the same time neurons controlling antagonist activity are inhibited through the indirect pathway.[109]

The primary projection site from GPi is to the "motor" thalamus, ventralis lateralis pars oralis (VLo), and ventralis anterior (VA).[110–114] These areas project predominantly to the supplementary motor area (SMA) and premotor areas, respectively, but also have projections to the primary motor and arcuate premotor areas.[115–117] The SNr projects predominantly to ventralis anterior magnocellularis (VAmc), which projects to the prefrontal[110] cortex. GPi and SNr also have smaller projections to the midbrain tegmentum and the superior colliculus.[118,119] All intrinsic and output projections from the basal ganglia

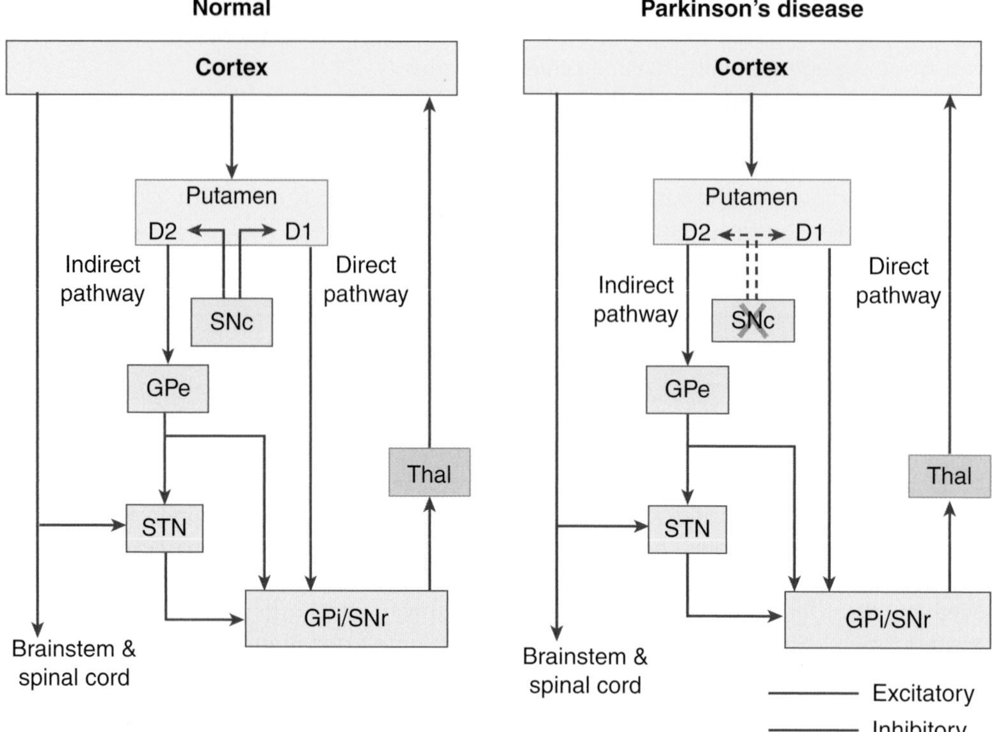

Figure 17–1. Schematic illustration of the basal ganglia–thalamocortical "motor" circuit and its neurotransmitters in the normal and parkinsonian state. "Indirect" and "direct" pathways from the striatum to basal ganglia output nuclei are shown by the arrows. GPe, globus pallidus par externa; GPi, globus pallidus pars interna; STN, subthalamic nucleus; SNr, substantia nigra pars reticulata; SNc, substantia nigra pars compacta; Thal, thalamus; D_1, D_2, dopamine receptor subtypes 1 and 2. Wider lines represent an increase in neuronal activity, and thinner lines represent a decrease.

are GABAergic and inhibitory, with the exception of the STN, which is glutaminergic and excitatory. Projections from the cortex to the putamen and from the thalamus to the cortex are excitatory.

Through the use of retrograde transynaptic tracers, it has been discovered that within the motor circuit there may be a series of segregated subcircuits, each taking origin in different motor and premotor cortical areas (motor cortex, supplementary and arcuate premotor cortex), and involving different portions of the basal ganglia and thalamus.[120,121] It has been proposed that these subcircuits may subserve different motor functions and may contribute differentially to the motor symptoms of PD. The proposal that these subcircuits may differentially affect movement receives some support from the differential role these cortical areas are proposed to play in motor control,[122–125] as well as from observations that neurons in different portions of GPi, electrophysiologically identified to project to different thalamic and cortical motor areas, have characteristic patterns of activity related to different components of the behavioral task.[121] Thus, it appears likely that these subcircuits may indeed be differentially involved in motor control and, when altered in a particular fashion, may lead to the development of specific motor signs (i.e., rigidity, tremor, akinesia, dystonia, and dyskinesias).

▶ PATHOPHYSIOLOGY UNDERLYING HYPO- AND HYPERKINETIC MOVEMENT DISORDERS

PARKINSON'S DISEASE (PD)

The Rate Model

Based on our understanding of the pathophysiological changes that occur in the basal ganglia thalamocortical circuit in the parkinsonian monkey, a rate model for PD was developed (Fig. 17–1). In this model, loss of dopamine in the substantia nigra pars compacta (SNc) was proposed to lead to differential changes in neuronal activity of striatal cells in the direct and indirect pathways. In the direct pathway, loss of dopamine at striatal excitatory D_1 receptors leads to a decrease of inhibitory activity from the putamen to GPi. In the indirect pathway, there is loss of dopamine at inhibitory D_2 receptors leading to increased activity of inhibitory putaminal neurons projecting to GPe, causing a reduction of GPe activity. The decrease in inhibitory output from GPe to STN leads to excessive excitation from the STN to the GPi. Thus, there is an increase in inhibitory activity from the GPi to the thalamus and brain stem, which occurs via both the direct and indirect pathways.

In this model, inhibition of thalamocortical and midbrain projections in the motor circuit has been proposed as the primary cause for the development of parkinsonian motor signs and the hypokinetic features associated with PD.[102] Similarly, the model predicts that a loss or lowering of inhibitory input from GPi to the thalamus may result in the hyperkinetic movements associated with drug-induced dyskinesias.[16,126] Changes in mean firing rates of neurons in GPe, GPi, STN, and VLo in the 1-methyl-4-phenyl-1,2,3,6-tetrahydropyridine (MPTP) monkey model of PD, and in STN, GPe, and GPi in patients with idiopathic PD, are consistent with those predicted by the model, that is, a decrease in mean discharge rates in GPe and VLo and an increase in mean discharge rates in STN and GPi.[102,127–132] Furthermore, positron emission tomography (PET) studies in PD patients have shown increased activity in cortical motor areas after pallidotomy, consistent with disinhibition of thalamocortical pathways.[133]

Problems with the Rate Model

Patient and experimental animal responses to surgical interventions, however, contradict the prediction of the rate model. Lesions within the motor thalamus do not exacerbate or induce parkinsonian motor signs but, instead, are reported to improve or abolish parkinsonian tremor, rigidity, and drug-induced dyskinesias.[126,134,135] This suggests that a decrease in activity of thalamic neurons cannot by itself account for the development of parkinsonian motor signs. Furthermore, the rate model would predict that pallidotomy would produce excessive involuntary movements or dyskinesias by disinhibiting the thalamus. It does not, and, in fact, pallidotomy is very effective in alleviating drug-induced dyskinesias. These contradictions of the rate model and subsequent observations of altered patterns of neuronal activity in the parkinsonian state have led to the development of an alternative, pattern model.[132,136–138]

The Pattern Model

Increased bursting, broadened receptive fields, and increased incidence of synchronized oscillations have been described in animal models of PD and in humans with idiopathic PD. Furthermore, improvement in the motor signs associated with PD have been associated with a reduction in synchronized oscillations, a reduction in bursting, and a narrowing of receptive fields in pallidal neurons.[139,140] Incorporation of these findings

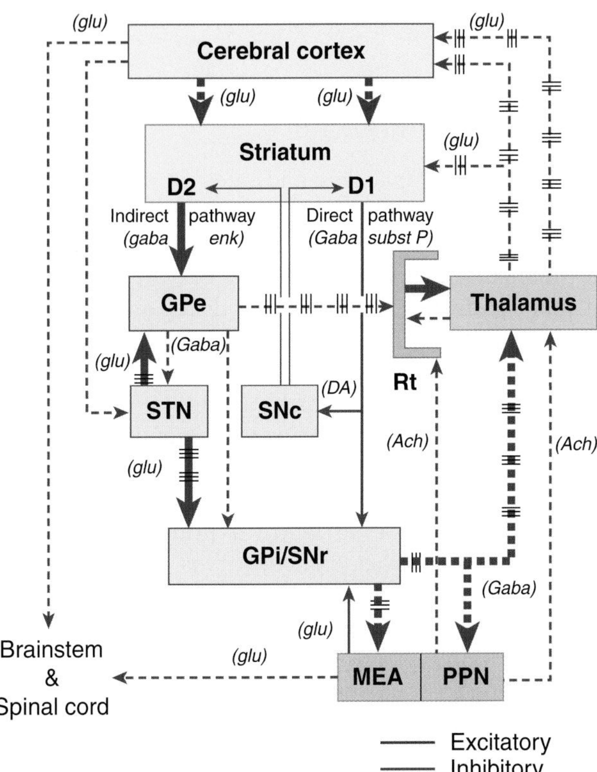

Figure 17–2. Schematic illustration of the basal ganglia thalamocortical "motor" circuit incorporating changes in pattern of neuronal activity and alternative pathways from the external segment of the globus pallidus (GPe) and pedunculopontine nucleus (PPN). Interrupted arrows represent an alternation in the pattern of neuronal activity. The grouped lines crossing the projections from the subthalamic nucleus (STN), the internal segment of the globus pallidus (GPi), and thalamus represent the presence of bursting activity. SNc, substantia nigra pars compacta; SNr, substantia nigra pars reticulata; D_1, D_2, dopamine receptor 1 and 2 subtypes; glu, glutamate; GABA, gamma-aminobutyric acid; enk, enkephalin; DA, dopamine; Rt, nucleus reticularis of the thalamus; Ach, acetylcholine; MEA, midbrain extrapyramidal area; PPN, pedunculopontine nucleus; subst P; substance P.

have led to the proposed "pattern" model of PD, which predicts that pattern rather than rate plays a predominant role in the development of parkinsonian motor signs (Fig. 17–2). These altered patterns of neuronal activity permeate throughout the pallidothalamocortical circuit and disrupt the normal operation of corticocortical circuits involved in motor control. Reports of increased bursting and rhythmic oscillatory patterns of activity within the thalamus in parkinsonian monkeys, together with the clear improvement in most parkinsonian motor signs after thalamotomy, lend further support to this hypothesis.[132,141,142] Based on this model, pallidotomy or thalamotomy or DBS in these regions is effective in PD because they remove disorganized output from the basal ganglia that is interrupting the motor circuit.

Additional Pathways

Although altered patterns and rates of neuronal activity within the pallidothalamocortical motor circuit likely provide a significant contribution to the development of the motor signs associated with PD, the contribution of other pathways should not be disregarded, either in terms of their role in the underlying pathophysiology or in our approach to treatment. Perhaps the best example of the role of alternative pathways in the development of parkinsonian motor signs is the potential role of the cerebellothalamocortical pathway in the development of parkinsonian tremor. In previous animal models of parkinsonian tremor, in which a portion of the midbrain tegmentum was ablated, it was necessary to include cerebellothalamic projections in order for tremor to develop.[143] Furthermore, whereas lesions in the sensorimotor portion of GPi are effective in improving or ameliorating parkinsonian tremor, lesions within the pallidal receiving area of the thalamus (Vop and Voa) have not generally been reported to be as effective as those within the cerebellar receiving area (Vim).[134,144–146] Although Hassler and colleagues reported that lesions within Vop were effective for parkinsonian tremor, he considered Vop to be a cerebellar receiving area not associated with pallidothalamic input.[16,147] The importance of interrupting the cerebellothalamic pathway in alleviating tremor was emphasized in his report of postmortem material obtained after thalamotomy. In patients with complete tremor arrest, he reported "coagulations either in the Vop or in the dentatothalamic fibers, which end in the Vop." The discrepancy between the observations of Hassler and colleagues and others concerning the most effective site in the thalamus for alleviation of parkinsonian tremor may be no more than a difference in nomenclature, or may be the result of a difference in interpretation of the cytoarchitectonic boundaries of thalamic subnuclei. Both groups, however, argue that the most effective lesions for relief of parkinsonian tremor lie in the cerebellar receiving area of the motor thalamus.

Additional support for a role of the cerebellothalamic pathway in the pathogenesis of parkinsonian tremor are the observations of rhythmic activity of neurons in Vim strongly correlated with tremor, as well as reports that the optimal location for lesions to alleviate such tremor appears to be within or includes significant portions of this region within Vim.[148–151]

Another potentially significant pathway in the development of parkinsonian motor signs is the projection from GPe to the nucleus reticularis of the thalamus (NRT).[112,152] Other than through its effect on the STN, the role of GPe in the development of the motor signs associated with PD has been largely disregarded. Given the significant decrease in mean firing rates and altered patterns of activity in GPe in PD, and the diffuse projections of reticularis neurons within and across thalamic subnuclei, the projection from GPe to NRT may serve an important role in the underlying pathophysiology of PD. Other potentially important pathways in PD involve the role of brain stem regions, including the pedunculopontine nucleus (PPN) and midbrain extrapyramidal area (MEA), which receive input from GPi and SNr and project to the thalamus, as well as the locus ceruleus (LC). The LC has widespread projections to the thalamus, cerebellum, and brain stem and may suffer significant cellular loss in PD (see Fig. 17–2). The MEA sends projections back to the GPi and SNr, as well as to the brain stem and spinal cord, whereas the PPN has extensive projections to the thalamus.[153–156] Cholinergic projections from the PPN have a differential effect on thalamic relay and reticular neurons, depolarizing relay neurons and hyperpolarizing reticular neurons.[157–160] Thus, cholinergic brain stem projections from the PPN are generally excitatory to thalamic relay neurons and inhibitory to reticular neurons. Therefore, in addition to the direct effect of GPi and PPN projections on thalamic relay cells, there are likely indirect effects on these cells from GPe and PPN projections to the NRT. The extensive projections from NRT and PPN throughout the motor thalamus may explain the observed changes in neuronal activity reported in both pallidal and cerebellar receiving areas in animal models of PD.[132,153–155,161] Such a diffuse change in both the rate and pattern of neuronal activity in the motor thalamus is hard to account for without considering the potential role of GPe and/or brain stem thalamic projections in mediating them (Fig. 17–2).

Recent studies also suggest that GPi, in addition to the role played in motor circuits, also plays a major role in information processing in nonmotor cognitive circuits.[162–165] Whether these functions operate in parallel via functionally segregated pathways or through integrated circuits has been a point of contention, given the apparent functional segregation as demonstrated by lesioning and other studies versus anatomical studies that suggest significant interplay between motor and nonmotor circuits.[166,171] {Alexander, 1990 #3414; Alexander, 1986 #3147}. Whether operating in parallel or utilizing integration of motor and nonmotor pathways, it is clear that the information carried along the corticostriatopallidal pathway is critical for proper motor execution and that it also plays an integrative role in cognitive information processing.[162–165,172] {Fukuda, 2001 #2215}. Alterations in neuronal activity in the final output pathway of this circuit, the GPi, have been associated with both hypokinetic and hyperkinetic movement disorders, while lesioning this region to remove or stimulation to modify this output has been associated with improvement in motor function, making GPi a prime target for the treatment of these disorders.[133,173–177]{Okun, 2004 #11; Vitek, 2003 #14; Vitek, 1998 #22}

DYSTONIA

Dystonia is a movement disorder characterized by sustained muscle contractions, leading to twisting, repetitive movements, and abnormal postures. Clinicopathological studies in patients with dystonia indicate that the most common site in which a lesion can be identified is in the basal ganglia (i.e., caudate, putamen, or pallidum). Thalamic lesions, although less common, have also been observed in patients with dystonia[178,179] (see also Chapter 32).

In mapping the receptive fields of thalamic neurons in patients with dystonia undergoing microelectrode-guided thalamotomy, an increased area of representation of the affected body part in the motor thalamus has been reported when compared to that in patients without dystonia (i.e., patients with ET or intention tremor).[180,181] The incidence of somatosensory responses in Vop and Vim was significantly greater than that in a control group comprising chronic pain or tremor (non-PD) patients.[182,183] In this study, the percentage of sensory cells in the motor thalamus (22%) was significantly greater than that observed in control patients (9.5%). Notably, the number of sensory cells responding to movement of more than one joint was significantly higher in dystonic patients (23%) than in control patients (9%), an observation similar to that made in the MPTP monkey model of parkinsonism.[184] In addition, microstimulation in and around Vim produced simultaneous contraction of multiple muscles in the forearm of dystonic patients, with the activity of many neurons in Vop and Vim showing peaks of activity at the frequency of the dystonic movements, which were significantly correlated with electromyogram (EMG) activity in the affected limb segment.[182,183] A small lesion, presumably involving Vop and part of Vim, produced an immediate and dramatic decrease in the involuntary movements of these dystonic patients. These observations provide compelling evidence that pallidal (Vop) and cerebellar (Vim) receiving areas of the motor thalamus are both involved in the pathogenesis of some types of dystonia.

Recordings of pallidal neuronal activity in patients with primary dystonia have also revealed broadened receptive fields, an increase on low-frequency oscillatory activity in the 4- to 10-Hz range and reduced mean discharge rates. Neurons in both Gpi and GPe show irregularly group discharges similar in pattern to one another, making discernment of GPe from GPi a challenge in mapping these patients. [ref- vitek original paper- see others for osc activity, etc.]

Pathophysiologically, dystonia may be a presenting symptom in parkinsonian patients who are not taking antiparkinsonian medications, or alternatively may appear as a consequence of L-dopa treatment (peak-dose dystonia). Whether this reflects etiologically different "types" of dystonia or merely represents a variation along the same general pathophysiological scheme is unclear. Although both types of dystonia likely reflect an alteration in the neural activity in the pallidothalamocortical and, probably, the cerebellothalamocortical circuit, the exact relationship between changes in neural activity in these regions and the development of dystonia remains unclear. In addition, pallidal projections to the brain stem are also likely to contribute to the pathogenesis of some "types" of dystonia. As with the pallido- and cerebellothalamic pathways, the particular changes in neural activity in these areas and their relationship to the development of dystonia is unclear.

Essential and Action Tremor

Cerebellothalamic pathways, although likely contributing to the development of parkinsonian tremor, may also play a significant role in the development of ET and intention tremor. In both disorders, tremor-related activity has been identified in Vim, and lesions within this area can significantly reduce or abolish both benign essential and cerebellar outflow tremors.

The physiological basis for the development of these tremors has been a much-debated issue. Neurons in the "cerebellar" thalamus in patients with either ET or cerebellar tremor have rhythmic bursting activity at tremor frequency.[185,186] Whether this occurs as a result of inherent neuronal rhythmicity expressed secondarily to conditions particular to these disorders and results in tremor, or occurs secondarily to or coincident with the development of these tremors, remains unclear. Thus, although the central mechanisms underlying the development of these tremors are not well defined, they clearly appear to involve thalamic neurons, given the resolution of such tremors after thalamotomy.

The contribution of peripheral afferent mechanisms to the development of these tremors is also debated. Some investigators have argued that the contribution of peripheral afferent mechanisms could be assessed by determining the degree of phase resetting of bursting neuronal activity in the thalamus after unexpected perturbations to the tremulous limb, and they termed this the resetting index.[178] An index of 0 suggested that there was no resetting, whereas an index of 1 implied complete resetting. The resetting index for ET was high, suggesting a significant peripheral contribution. It can be argued, however, that the index simply describes the degree to which tremor-related activity may be altered by peripheral input and not necessarily whether it underlies tremor genesis. Support implicating peripheral afferent mechanisms in the genesis of cerebellar tremor was provided by Vilis and Hore, who cooled the deep cerebellar nuclei and examined the change in response of motor cortical neurons, as well as the change in timing and duration of agonist and antagonist EMG responses to torque pulses applied to the upper limb.[107,187] They concluded that cerebellar tremor occurred secondary to disordered reflex loops involving the motor cortex, because the delay in the response of motor cortex cells related to agonist–antagonist EMG activity was correlated with the delay observed in these EMG responses to controlled perturbation.[107,187] These data, although suggestive of a peripheral contribution to the pathogenesis of cerebellar tremor, however, do not address the role of inherent oscillatory mechanisms in the development of cerebellar tremor. Given the reports of rhythmically bursting neuronal activity in the motor thalamus in patients with cerebellar tremor who undergo thalamotomy, there is likely a significant central component underlying the genesis of this tremor.[134,188] One explanation for the development of cerebellar tremor lies in the inherent tendency for hyperpolarized thalamic neurons to burst after a depolarizing pulse.[160,161,189] Interruption of excitatory cerebellar projections to thalamic neurons could put these neurons into a hyperpolarized "burst-promoting" state. With initiation of movement, depolarizing corticothalamic projections may produce synchronous bursting activity of a population of thalamic neurons. When a critical population of thalamic neurons bursts synchronously, it may lead to the development of rhythmic bursting activity which, when transmitted to a critical number of alpha-motoneurons via the motor cortex, induces an action tremor. Thus, although both peripheral and central tremorgenic mechanisms likely contribute to the development of cerebellar tremor, the relative contribution remains unclear.

HEMIBALLISMUS

Hemiballism consists of involuntary, often violent, movements of the limbs. These movements are most closely associated with inactivation or destruction of the STN or its efferent pathway and occur contralateral to the side of the lesion.[190] Hemiballismus has been observed in humans after vascular lesions restricted to the STN, as well as in monkeys after selective lesioning of the STN with ibotenic acid, and is thought to occur predominantly as a result of disinhibition of the thalamus.[191]

This model receives support from both experimental studies in the monkey and studies of patients with intractable hemiballismus,[142,190,–194] who have undergone microelectrode-guided pallidotomy.[142] In both humans and monkeys, there is a significant reduction in the tonic discharge rate in GPi after an STN lesion and the development of hemiballismus. Consistent with this observation, monkeys with hemiballismus after inactivation of STN show decreased metabolic activity in both the GPi and the ventral lateral thalamus.[195] However, the reduced rate in GPi would suggest that thalamotomy and not pallidotomy would effectively treat hemiballism, yet both alleviate hemiballism.[33,35,136,196] {Vitek, 1997 #13836; Suarez, 1997 #3991} This lends further support to the hypothesis that altered patterns of activity in the pallidothalamic motor circuit underlie the abnormal movement found in both hypokinetic and hyperkinetic movement disorders.

SUMMARY PATHOPHYSIOLOGICAL FINDINGS

Our understanding of the pathophysiological basis of hypo- and hyperkinetic movement disorders has increased significantly over the last decade (see Chapter 5). Altered patterns of neuronal activity are now considered to play a predominant role in the genesis of both hypo- and hyperkinetic movement disorders. The contribution of altered receptive fields, development of oscillatory activity, and changes in synchrony are just now being fully appreciated for their contribution to the pathophysiological basis underlying the development of movement disorders. Although not drawing much attention at this time, it is also highly likely that alternative pathways are involved in the genesis of these disorders with alterations in different motor and nonmotor subcircuits mediating different motor symptoms.

RADIOGRAPHIC LOCALIZATION AND MICROELECTRODE MAPPING TECHNIQUES FOR TARGET LOCALIZATION

Radiographic Techniques

Initial target coordinates are obtained by conventional radiographic techniques using computed tomography (CT), MRI, and/or ventriculography. The location of the anterior (AC) and the posterior commissure (PC) relative to fiducial markers on the stereotaxic frame is used to calculate the x-, y-, and z-coordinates of the target.

Guiot[197,198] defined the position of various deep nuclei based on the distance between the AC and the PC and the height of the thalamus, obtained from ventriculography. This method was used for decades and is still used in several centers worldwide. However, modern imaging has replaced ventriculography with CT and MRI scans.

A thin cut stereotactic CT (1- or 2-mm slices with no gap and no gantry tilt) can be easily obtained to localize the AC and PC and can be fused with the MRI on a stereotactic planning station. CT is free from image distortions sometimes seen in MRI and allows the stereotactic space to be defined with a higher degree of accuracy.

MRI is the imaging modality of choice in stereotactic targeting and planning due to excellent visualization of deeper subcortical structure, sulci, and vasculature, which is important in trajectory planning. Various sequences are used based on the target nucleus. T_1-weighted volumetric acquisition of the whole brain with gadolinium enhancement, a T_2-weighted axial and coronal acquisition, and inversion recovery (IR) sequences are some of the most commonly used. The T_2 and IR sequences delineate the STN and the GPi relatively well. The thalamic nuclei, however, are not readily visualized on MRI imaging. 3 Tesla (3T) MRI and diffusion tensor imaging (DTI) improve the visualization of thalamic nuclei.[199] However, few centers employ these techniques for targeting the thalamus.

Anatomical Targeting

Anatomical targeting is the initial method for localizing the nucleus of interest. Different centers use various combinations of imaging sources for anatomical targeting strategies. In general, these strategies of indirect targeting employing reformatted anatomical atlases and formulas of known distances and direct targeting based on visualization are complimentary.

Indirect Targeting Formulas and Brain Atlas Approaches

Indirect targeting techniques utilize the stereotactic coordinates of the AC and the PC as determined by the imaging (Fig. 17–3). The location of the subcortical nuclei such as STN, GPi, and Vim can be subsequently determined based on their average anatomical distance with respect to the AC, PC, and the midcommissural point (MCP). Typical anatomical coordinates for the sensorimotor components of these nuclei can be calculated. This includes the STN (11–13 mm lateral to the midline, 4–5 mm ventral to

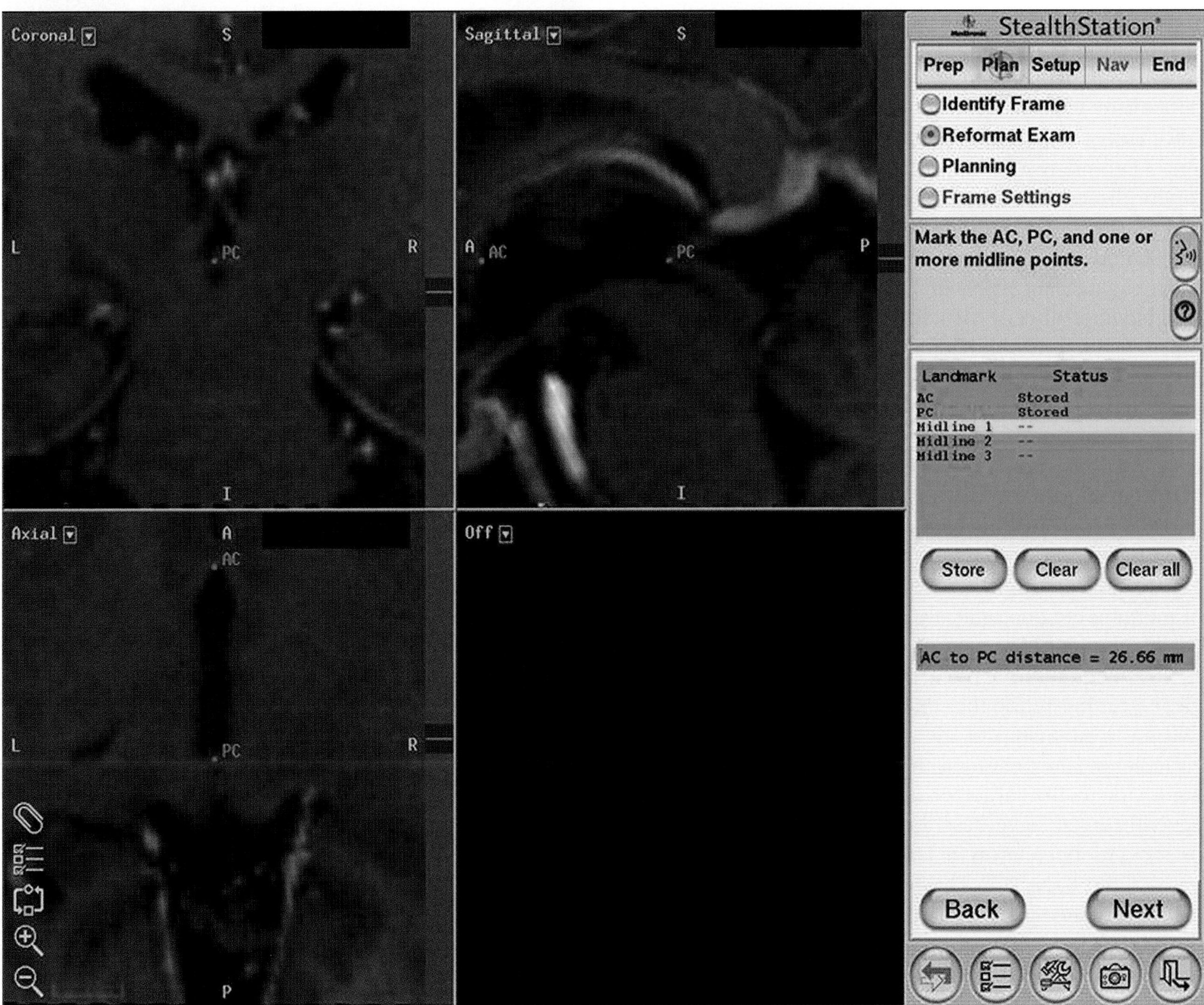

Figure 17–3. A snap shot of Stealth station showing the anterior commissure (AC) and posterior commissure (PC) location on axial, sagittal, and coronal planes.

the AC-PC plane, and 3–4 mm posterior to the MCP), the GPi (19–21 mm lateral to the midline, 2–3 mm anterior to the MCP, and 4–5 mm ventral to AC-PC plane), and the Vim upper extremity target (11–12 mm lateral to the wall of the third ventricle, at the level of the AC-PC plane, and the AP location located between 2/12 and 3/12 of the AC-PC distance anterior to the PC).

A standardized brain atlas can be used to locate the x-, y-, and z-coordinates of the STN, GPi, and Vim in relation to the MCP.[200] The stereotactic atlas can be stretched and morphed using surgical navigation software to better fit each patient's anatomy. However, despite these technological advances, it is important to realize the limitations of the stereotactic atlases. Most atlases are based on a small number of patients. The Schaltenbrand and Wahren atlas[200] uses one brain for the frontal series and one brain for the axial and sagittal series.

Direct Targeting

With the advances in neuroimaging technology, direct visualization of the various nuclei has become possible. While CT has excellent stereotactic precision, it can be difficult to visualize various targets and periventricular landmarks. MRI has the advantage of providing excellent anatomic resolution in multiple planes. This allows for localization of the AC and the PC on T_1-weighted images (Fig. 17–3), and the visualization of the pallidum on IR and T_2 sequences (Fig. 17–4) and the STN on axial, sagittal, and coronal T_2 images (Fig. 17–5).[201] The advantage of directly visualizing deep targets is implicit, given the patient's individual anatomical variation rather than relying on a fixed brain from one or two patients sectioned several decades ago. Some centers currently rely entirely on MR images to calculate anatomical targets.[201] The accuracy of MR as a sole targeting tool has been questioned due to magnetic warping and distortion. A fusion of CT images with MR images is supposed to improve the accuracy. To reduce the possibility of MRI-related inaccuracies, several centers use a protocol of merging the anatomically superior MRI to a stereotactically acquired CT.

Several authors have described additional strategies to further refine the image-based targeting. Arguing that the relationship of the AC-PC and the STN may be variable and inconsistent, the use of a physically closer landmark to the target of interest has been proposed. Several centers have described using the anterior border of the red nucleus as a landmark for the AP coordinate of the STN.[203–205] The axial and coronal T_2 images are particularly important for adequate visualization of the STN, as a sharp contrast can often be seen between the nucleus and the surrounding white matter. The red nucleus and the STN can be clearly visualized. The STN lies anterior and lateral to the red nucleus, and in this regard, the anterior border of the red nucleus can be used as a landmark for the STN target. The possibility of directly visualizing and targeting the STN and GPi has brought forth innovative imaging application possibilities for DBS surgery. The use of intraoperative MRI to perform DBS surgery is being investigated.

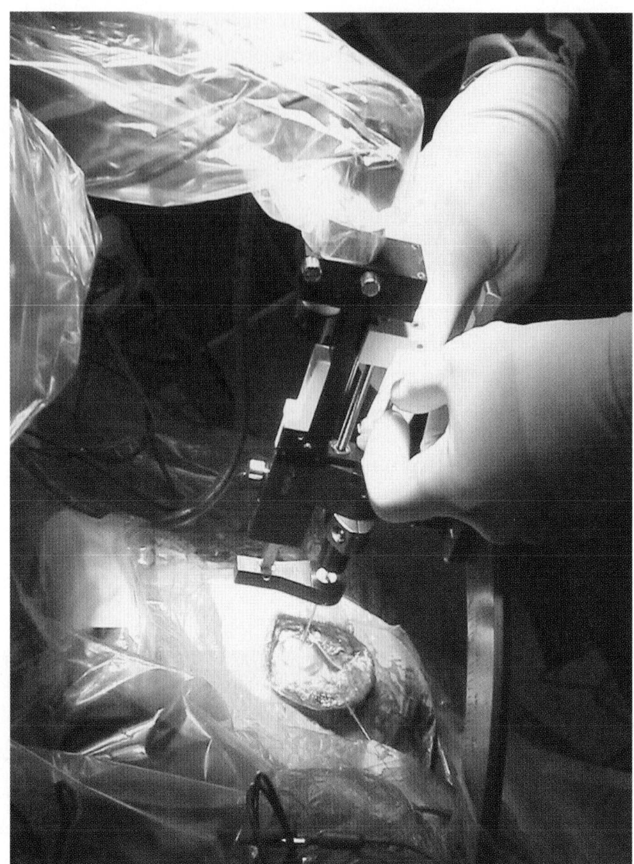

Figure 17–4. Assembly and placement of the microdrive on the arc of Leksell stereotaxic frame with a canula entering the burrhole.

For Vim thalamus, a good starting point is approximately 3 mm anterior to the PC at 15 mm lateral to the AC-PC line. These coordinates should allow the first pass with the recording electrode to penetrate portions of the sensory thalamus which, combined with determination of the receptive fields of neurons in the adjacent motor thalamus, provides a highly reliable landmark for subsequent penetrations.

For the GPi, the coordinates are 21 mm lateral, 3 mm anterior, and 3–6 mm ventral to the midcommissural line. Based on physiological data gathered during microelectrode-guided pallidotomies, these coordinates target the sensorimotor portion of GPi.[128]

For the STN, initial targeting coordinates are 2–3 mm posterior to the MCP, 11–13 mm lateral, and 4–6 mm inferior to the AC-PC line.

The final target selection should be based on the type of movement disorder being treated. Other factors

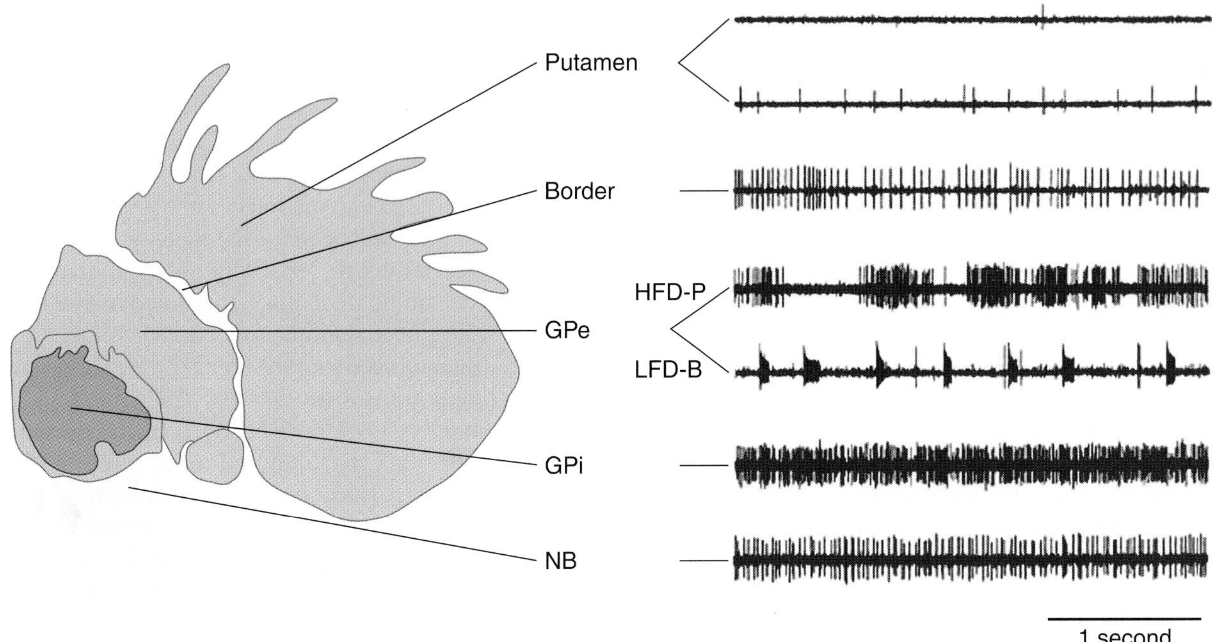

Figure 17–5. Microelectrode physiology encountered when targeting GPi. Typical neural activity is shown for striatum (putamen and caudate), GPe (globus pallidus externa), GPi (globus pallidus interna), and NB (nucleus basalis). Populations of high-frequency discharge pausing cells (HFD-P) and low-frequency discharge bursting cells (LFD-B) are found in GPe. The line drawing shows a parasagittal representation of these structures from the Schaltenbrand and Bailey Atlas. (Reproduced with permission from Vitek JL, et al. Microelectrode-guided pallidotomy: Technical approach and its application in medically intractable Parkinson's disease. J Neurosurg 1998;**88**(6):1027–1043. Fig. 4.)

that can and should be taken into consideration include the somatotopic organization of the structure, the portion of the body involved, and the relative location of nearby critical structures to be avoided. This information is readily obtained with the use of electrophysiological mapping techniques. Some reports suggest that errors in radiographic targeting are greater than 3 mm in 43% of GPi cases and 45% of STN cases. Assuming a 3- to 4-mm-diameter spread of current with DBS, with a 3-mm inaccuracy, there would be significantly less than an optimal amount of target effected by the DBS lead in these cases.[206]

Because of individual variation in the length of the AC-PC line, size of the third ventricle, and radiographic distortion inherent in these techniques, these coordinates should serve only as a starting point. MRI is prone to error due to magnetic susceptibility artifact in the direction of frequency encoding (usually the anterior–posterior direction),[207] whereas CT does not provide sufficient contrast of subcortical structures. Some advocate use of combined techniques fusing MR and CT images to minimize these errors while still providing high resolution.[208–210] There is also a significant degree of anatomical variation from patient to patient. Some of this variation may be accounted for by variation in the width of the third ventricle, and one approach advocated is to normalize the lateral coordinate to the width of the third ventricle.[211,212] Another approach is to use direct targeting based on the boundaries of the target.[212] This approach has been shown to be more accurate than reliance on coordinates based on AC-PC dimensions. Microelectrode mapping can define the borders of structures with much better accuracy than current imaging techniques. Thus, despite improvements in MRI- and CT-based targeting techniques, electrophysiological mapping provides information for target delineation not available by other means.

MICROELECTRODE MAPPING TECHNIQUE FOR PHYSIOLOGICAL LOCALIZATION OF THE TARGET SITE

Microelectrode recording techniques used in conjunction with radiographic methods and macrostimulation techniques facilitate identification and localization of the target structure. This approach enhances the ability of the surgeon to locate and place the stimulator or lesion within the identified target while avoiding adjacent structures. A variety of electrodes can be used for electrophysiologic recording; however, platinum–iridium glass-coated microelectrodes with an impedance of 0.5–2.0 MΩ (at 1000 Hz) provide excellent recording characteristics that do not deteriorate after microstimulation.

Electrophysiology of the Thalamus

The thalamus contains 50–60 different subnuclei. The targeted subnuclei lie adjacent to regions which, when interrupted, may lead to significant cognitive, language, or sensory impairment. It is important, therefore, to map precisely the boundaries of the region(s) to be included within the target area to obtain the maximal benefit while minimizing potential complications as a result of encroachment on adjacent subnuclei.

The thalamus is generally mapped in a parasagittal plane to allow one to cross subnuclei as the electrode is advanced. An angle of approximately 30–35° from the vertical is taken, except for cases in which one wants to include Vop or portions of Voa, in which case one may choose an angle of 45°. A sharper angle allows one microelectrode penetration to cross a greater portion of adjacent thalamic subnuclei and provides a better approximation of the borders between thalamic subnuclei. However, placement of a DBS lead at this angle means that contacts located more dorsally are also significantly more anterior and may lie outside of the Vim as well as away from the targeted body part. As such different approaches and angles may be taken based upon the ultimate goal of surgery and how that may vary with individual patients. To avoid the ventricle, many centers will also plan the trajectory to also take a lateral-to-medial approach.

Using the parasagittal approach just after entering the thalamus, one encounters neurons with broad receptive fields responding to passive or active movement, confrontational hand gestures, or changes in attention. These types of responses are typical of neurons in the NRT. This nucleus is only a few hundred micrometers thick and is followed by a thin lamina of similar diameter before the characteristic rhythmic discharge of thalamic neurons is encountered. At this point, single units are discriminated throughout the track. In patients with tremor, "tremor cells" may be identified in pallidal and cerebellar receiving areas (Vim, Voa, or Vop), where neurons have bursting discharges synchronous with the patient's tremor.

Neuronal responses to passive and active movement of individual body parts are sought, and microstimulation is carried out at 5–100 μA, with trains of symmetric biphasic pulse pairs at a frequency of 300–400 Hz. The patient is instructed to report any change in sensation that occurs with microstimulation, describing its location, quality, and intensity. At each stimulation site, when changes in sensation occur with stimulation, sensory thresholds are determined by decreasing the current intensity progressively, until the stimulus no longer elicits a sensory response. For each microelectrode penetration, response to microstimulation, sensory thresholds, spontaneous activity patterns, and the response of each isolated cell to sensorimotor examination are plotted on plastic overlays, then fitted to computer-generated maps of the human thalamus taken from the Schaltenbrand and Bailey atlas,[213] and scaled to the patient's AC-PC coordinates.

Lateral, anterior, and ventral boundaries of the motor (Voa, Vop, and Vim) and sensory (Vc) thalamus are determined based on microstimulation effects, the presence or absence of neuronal activity, and neuronal response properties to sensorimotor examination. The lateral border of the thalamus is bounded by the internal capsule where microstimulation results in evoked movements, allowing this region to be easily identified. Along the anterior border of the sensory thalamus is the ventrocaudal nucleus (Vc). It is identified by the presence of neurons with small, well-defined fields receptive to tactile sensation in a body region in which low-threshold (5- to 10-μA) stimulation-induced paresthesias occur. The relative distance of the recording electrode from the anterior border of Vc can be approximated by the sensory threshold at which microstimulation induces paresthesias. Sites sufficiently anterior to Vc are characterized by a lack of microstimulation-induced paresthesias, even at current intensities of 40–50 μA or greater. The sensorimotor thalamus is somatotopically organized with areas representing leg, arm, jaw, face, and intraoral structures arrayed in a lateral-to-medial direction in onion skin–like lamellae. Thus, penetrations near the lateral border of the sensory thalamus are characterized by microstimulation-induced paresthesias of somatosensory responses predominantly restricted to the leg. Penetrations made progressively more medially will have responses largely restricted to the arm and the face, respectively. As one moves rostrally from Vc to Vim, Vop, and Voa, there is a gradation of cell responses to sensorimotor examination: cells in Vc predominantly respond to tactile stimuli, while the most rostral "shell" portion of Vc has proprioceptive responses. Cells in Vim, Vop, and Voa do not respond to tactile stimulation; however, cells in Vim readily respond to passive manipulations of the limbs and orofacial structures. Cells in Vop and Voa tend to respond more selectively to voluntary movement and less to passive manipulations, which is similar to that described in the monkey for homologous subnuclei.[214,215]

Electrophysiology of the Globus Pallidus Pars Interna

Microelectrode penetrations are generally made in the parasagittal plane, proceeding from the anterodorsal to posteroventral direction at an angle of approximately 30–35° from the vertical. As the microelectrode is advanced, patterns of neural activity are noted throughout the track. The major structures that are identified using this plane of approach are striatum (caudate and putamen), followed by GPe, GPi, and more ventrally the internal capsule and/or optic tract. The nucleus basalis may be encountered with anteriorly placed penetrations.

Each cellular region has a characteristic pattern of neural activity similar to that described in the monkey[216] (Fig. 17–5). Low spontaneous discharge rates (<1 Hz) that increase transiently up to 4–6 Hz as the electrode is advanced typify neural activity from the striatum. As the electrode enters GPe, two distinct cell types can be identified: (1) units with high-frequency discharges (50 ± 21 Hz) separated by pauses (HFD-P) and (2) units that are active in bursts separated by periods of single-spike discharges at low frequency at 18 ± 12 Hz (LFD-B). Next, in GPi, high-frequency (82 ± 24 Hz) tonic activity characterizes the majority of neural activity, although a variety of other patterns may be present, including bursts with little pause between them, emitting a "chugging" sound, or lower-frequency bursting in the range of 4–6 Hz that may correspond to the patient's tremor frequency ("tremor cells"). Within the laminae of the pallidum (i.e., between the GPe and the GPi, as well as laminae within GPi), neurons with slower rates of tonic neural activity ("border" cells) may be encountered. These cells help identify border regions of the pallidal segments.[128]

Once through the pallidum, the optic tract or the internal capsule can be identified by microstimulation. In the optic tract, microstimulation at 5–40 μA typically results in brief flashes of light (phosphenes). In the internal capsule, microstimulation induces movement of the limbs or orofacial structures. The relative proximity of these structures (i.e., optic tract and internal capsule) can be ascertained by the stimulation threshold at which these phosphenes are noted or muscle contraction occurs. The optic tract can also be identified by flashing a light in the patient's eyes and listening for high-frequency modulation of the background audio signal coincident with the light stimulus.

The target region within GPi is determined by identifying neurons with responses to passive manipulations and active movement of the extremities and orofacial structures of the patient. The presence of bursting activity and its relationship to tremor, if present, is noted, along with each type of neural activity. The presence and the somatotopic location of neuronal responses in the GPi to passive or active movement, as well as the relative location of the optic tract and internal capsule (noting the thresholds), are used to generate a topographic map of this subcortical region. This topographic map is, in turn, used to determine the location within GPi and guide stimulator or lesion placement.

There is somatotopic organization within the sensorimotor region of GPi, with a preponderance of leg cells found medially, arm cells laterally, and face ventrally (Fig. 17–6).[214] Neurons in this area are characterized by

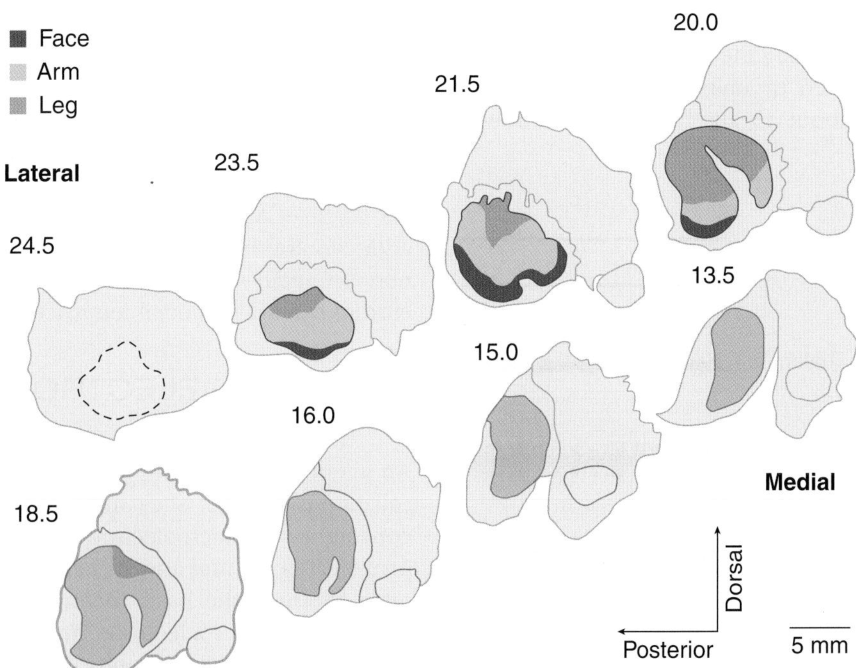

Figure 17–6. Somatotopic organization of GPi. Drawing representing a composite of 10 patients showing the somatotopic organization of receptive fields in GPi. The numbers represent the distance in millimeters from the midline of each parasagittal plane. (Reproduced with permission from Vitek JL, et al. Microelectrode-guided pallidotomy: technical approach and its application in medically intractable Parkinson's disease. J Neurosurg 1998;**88**(6):1027–1043. Fig. 6.)

increased activity to deep-muscle palpation, passive joint movement, or active movement of the somatotopically related body parts. These responses are predominantly contralateral and specific to a single joint, although neurons with responses to multiple joints or limbs or even the ipsilateral limb are commonly encountered in patients with PD and dystonia may be encountered.[136] {Vitek, 1998 #4054}

Sensorimotor responses are found predominantly in the posterolateral portions of GPi, whereas neurons in regions more anterior and medial are not as likely to respond to active or passive manipulations of the limbs or orofacial structures. Based on anatomical studies, these neurons are likely related to nonmotor "associative" functions.[217] Stimulation or lesions in this region alone will likely result in no or partial improvement in the motor symptoms of PD. Targeting this region of GPi produces similar results for dystonia and hemiballismus.[31,218]

Electrophysiology of the Subthalamic Nucleus

When targeting STN, depending upon the depth at which recording begins, the microelectrode may pass through the striatum (usually caudate) before coursing through the anterior thalamus. Here the reticular thalamus may be identified with its characteristic units that respond to broad receptive field with active and passive movement.[219] Figure 17–7 shows examples of characteristic electrophysiological recordings in structures encountered when targeting the STN. Anterior thalamic nuclei may be identified by units with a characteristic bursting pattern at about 15 Hz.[219] If the electrode is more anteriorly located, it may pass through the internal capsule with low background noise and a paucity of cellular activity. Just below the thalamus there is a quiet region, likely the thalamic fasciculus (H1 fields of Forel), followed by a narrow strip of cells with large-amplitude neurons or bursting neurons at 25–45 Hz characteristic of zona incerta.[220] These neurons may not be encountered, and this quiet region may continue into another quiet region corresponding to the lenticular fasciculus (H2 fields of Forel). As the STN is approached further inferiorly, there is a striking increase in background activity, reflecting increased cellular density. STN neurons are then found with a discharge rate of about 35 Hz; however, they may range from 20 to 70 Hz.[220] Two patterns of units can sometimes be discerned: (1) a mixed pattern with tonic activity, irregular discharges, and occasional bursts and (2) a burst pattern with periodic oscillating bursts that may or may not be synchronous with the patient's tremor when present.[220,221] Below the inferior border of STN, there is another short quit area followed by the SNr, which has units with a regular firing pattern at 71 ± 23.2 Hz, similar to those present in GPi.[220]

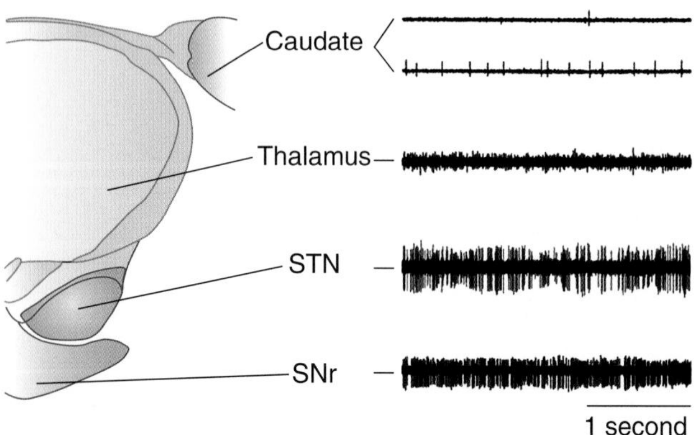

Figure 17-7. Microelectrode physiology encountered when targeting STN. Typical neural activity is shown for striatum (putamen and caudate), thalamus, subthalamic nucleus (STN), and substantia nigra pars reticulata (SNr). The line drawing shows a parasagittal representation of these structures from the Schaltenbrand and Bailey atlas.

Careful somatotopic mapping of the STN in the African green monkey shows that the dorsorostral STN contains most of the cells responding to somatosensory input, with the face represented dorsomedially, the leg ventrolateral to this, and the arm at the most lateral extent of the nucleus (see Fig. 17–8).[222] Our knowledge of the somatotopic organization in the human is incomplete, but existing studies seem to correlate roughly with the monkey data.[223,224]

Micro- and macrostimulation in STN can be used to help identify its borders and proximity to adjacent structures (Fig. 17–9). Stimulation lateral to the STN causes muscle contractions identifying its proximity to the internal capsule. Medially, stimulation may cause ipsilateral adduction of the eye from stimulation of the oculomotor nerve. Caudal stimulation may cause paresthesias from current spread to medial lemniscus.

SEMIMICROELECTRODE TECHNIQUE

An alternative recording technique for physiological localization of target sites involves the use of a bipolar concentric semimicroelectrode with a tip diameter of approximately 0.6 mm and an interpole distance of 0.3–0.6 mm. Although the basic technique is the same as that used for the microelectrode, the type of information it provides differs significantly. The semimicroelectrode gives a broader, more integrated sampling of multicellular activity, whereas the microelectrode allows characterization of the response properties of single units. Basically, the semimicroelectrode is better suited to locate and differentiate individual subnuclei, or to identify

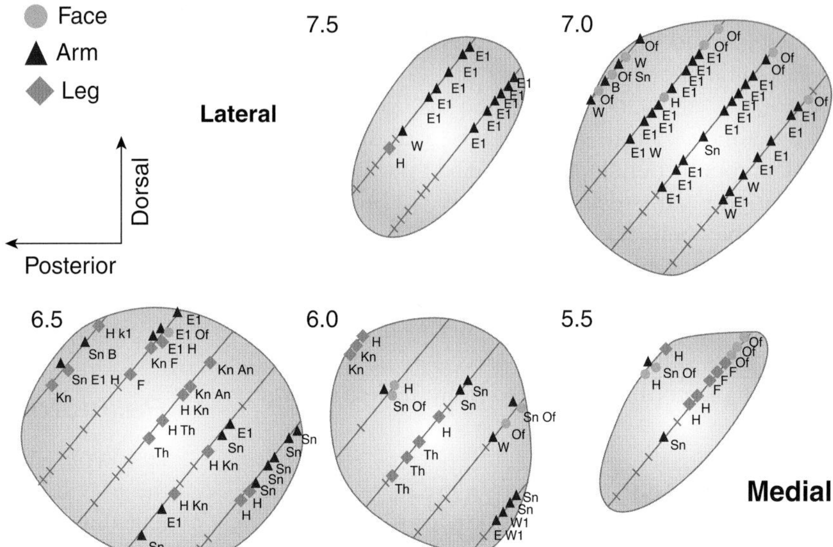

Figure 17–8. Somatotopic organization of STN. Monkey data showing distribution of cells responding to somatosensory input in subthalamic nucleus (STN). The numbers represent the distance in millimeters from the midline of each parasagittal plane. (Modified from Wichmann T, Bergman H, DeLong MR. The primate subthalamic nucleus. I. Functional properties in intact animals. J Neurophysiol 1994;72(2):494–506, with permission.)

the borders of the targeted nucleus, whereas the microelectrode is more precise, allowing for the determination of spontaneous activity patterns and sensorimotor response properties of single neurons.

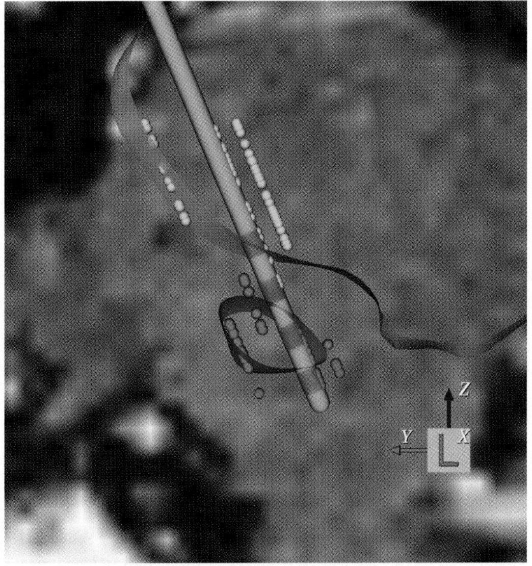

Figure 17–9. Anatomical modeling using microelectrode mapping for STN implant. Preoperative imaging data with fiducial markers from the stereotactic frame were imported into the Cicerone software system. A 2-D brain atlas with representations of the thalamus (yellow outline) and subthalamic nucleus (green outline) were warped to match the MRI of the patient. The stereotactic coordinates of the 3387 DBS electrode (blue shaft, pink contacts) and microelectrode recordings of neural activity representative of the thalamus (yellow dots), STN (green dots), and substantia nigra (red dots) are depicted within the context of the MRI and 3-D brain atlas.

▶ ABLATIVE SURGERY TECHNIQUE

Lesions or ablation of the pallidum (pallidotomy) or thalamus (thalamotomy) is commonly performed with a radiofrequency lesioning electrode. Once the target is determined by imaging and electrophysiological mapping, the lesioning electrode is advanced into the target. Macrostimulation through the lesioning electrode can help confirm the location of the lesioning probe in the target region and allow one to assess side effects. We have previously determined that when making 75°C lesions, thresholds of >0.5 mA at 300 Hz are safe for avoiding encroachment into the internal capsule, while thresholds of >1.0 mA are safe for avoiding the optic tract. It should be noted that these thresholds may vary depending on the equipment and how it is configured. During macrostimulation and lesioning, the patient is serially examined for side effects. We generally made our initial lesions at 60°C for 60 sec. Subsequent lesions can be made at temperatures up to 80–90°C. There is a linear relationship between temperature and lesion diameter; while 60°C lesions are approximately 1 mm in diameter, 90°C lesions are roughly 5 mm.[128]

▶ DEEP BRAIN STIMULATION SURGICAL TECHNIQUE

After the target nucleus is identified by preoperative radiologic techniques and intraoperative electrophysiology, the stimulator lead is implanted in the chosen target. The FDA-approved Medtronic system has two lead configurations that are commonly used. Both are platinum–iridium quadripolar leads approximately 1.3 mm in diameter. The 3387 lead has four 1.5-mm contacts separated by 1.5 mm, and the 3389 has 1.5-mm contacts separated by 0.5 mm. The device is capable of bipolar stimulation between any of the four contacts or monopolar stimulation using the pulse generator casing as the anode. Before securing the lead, one can assess the therapeutic benefit and side-effect profile of different simulation parameters using an external pulse generator that can be connected to the lead to pass current into the target region. Once satisfactory placement is achieved, the lead is secured and connected to a programmable pulse generator located in the subclavicular region. This can be done during the same procedure or at a later date once the patient has recovered from the initial surgery.

▶ SURGICAL APPROACH TO SPECIFIC MOVEMENT DISORDERS

PARKINSON'S DISEASE

Patient Selection

Patients with medically intractable idiopathic PD are considered candidates for surgery. In addition to tremor, rigidity, bradykinesia, and gait disorder motor fluctuations, on–off phenomenon, dystonia (off or on), and drug-induced dyskinesia also respond to surgical intervention and may be the predominant feature in some patients for which they are undergoing surgery. Patients should have demonstrated a clear and historically a long-lasting benefit from antiparkinsonian medication. Patients with multiple-system atrophy, striatonigral degeneration, progressive supranuclear palsy, or olivopontocerebellar atrophy are not candidates. Medical management of patients with idiopathic PD should be optimized before surgery, depression should be treated, and the cognitive state of patients should be thoroughly assessed. Patients with significant cognitive impairment are less likely to have long-lasting improvement and may be unable to cooperate with motor and visual field testing during the procedure.[128] {Vitek, 1998 #4054} These patients also tend to have a more complicated and prolonged postoperative recovery period.

Ablative Therapy

Thalamotomy

The thalamus has been targeted predominantly for its benefit on tremor. Lesions within Vim are highly effective in alleviating parkinsonian tremor in more than 85% of patients,[22,76,133,144] and if extended anteriorly to include Vop, and possibly portions of Voa, they may also improve rigidity and dopa-induced dyskinesia.[126] Thalamic lesions generally have not been reported to improve bradykinesia or akinesia and have been reported to exacerbate speech and gait disorders in some patients.[225,226] Studies showing exception to this are sparse; Hassler reported that bradykinesia did improve following lesions that included more anterior portions of the motor thalamus (i.e., Voa).[16] While thalamotomy has similar benefit on parkinsonian tremor as pallidotomy (see below), its efficacy on other symptoms is more limited. As PD progresses, akinesia, rigidity, and gait problems invariably become problematic. Given the success of other procedures in improving all of these symptoms, thalamotomy is usually not recommended for PD patients.

Pallidotomy

Lesions in either the sensorimotor portion of the GPi or the STN have been reported effective in reducing or alleviating the motor signs associated with PD. Lesions that lie outside or involve only a portion of the sensorimotor territory are likely to result in no or only a partial benefit.[227] Optimal benefit is most likely to occur with lesions that most completely interrupt the motor circuit by encompassing a significant portion of the sensorimotor territory of the targeted nucleus.[214] {Vitek, 1994 #4056} The optimal location and size of the lesion within the GPi, although not fully defined, should in theory involve as much of the sensorimotor portion of GPi as possible without infringing on nearby critical structures (i.e., GPe, nucleus basalis, internal capsule, and the optic tract). Modern techniques using MRI-guided stereotaxic targeting and electrophysiological mapping techniques to identify the target structure and its borders, together with an improved understanding of the pathophysiological basis underlying the development of parkinsonian motor signs, have lead to improved and more reliable outcomes.

A prospective single-blind trial randomizing 36 patients to unilateral pallidotomy or best medical therapy was conducted at our center. Results at 6 months showed unilateral pallidotomy improved the total UPDRS (Unified Parkinson's Disease Rating Scale) score by 32% over the presurgical baseline while, at the same time, patients with medical therapy alone worsened by 5%. The UPDRS "off" motor subscore in the surgical arm improved by 33%; there was no significant improvement in the "on"-period motor subscore. There was significant improvement in contralateral tremor, rigidity, bradykinesia, and dyskinesias. Gait and "off"-period freezing were also significantly improved.[38] Significant improvement in ipsilateral rigidity, bradykinesia, and drug-induced dyskinesia was also observed.

After meeting the primary outcome criteria at 6 months, control patients were offered pallidotomy and a total of 20 patients were followed for 2 years. Over this time, the patients continued to have a significant (25%) benefit in their off-medicine motor UPDRS subscore. Dyskinesias, rigidity, and bradykinesia continued to show bilateral improvement, and tremor maintained contralateral improvement. Although there was loss of benefit in midline symptoms, including postural stability, gait, and freezing, 50% of patients still maintained an average of 38% improvement.[38] Some of the worsening gait and balance problems were likely due to progression of the underlying disease, particularly since only unilateral procedures were performed.

One other randomized study showed similar results with the UPDRS "off" motor score improving 31% from baseline in the surgical arm at 6 months.[228] On average, other nonrandomized series showed similar benefit with a roughly 30% improvement in the motor "off" score at 6 months postoperatively.[33,35,229–238] {Ondo, 1998 #11157}

Results of long-term studies are more divergent. Most studies show loss of gait and postural benefit beyond 1 year;[38,239–243] however, a few show persistent benefit beyond 2 years.[11,31,244]

Improvement of ipsilateral "off" rigidity often does not last beyond 1 year,[239,242,243] {Lang, 1997 #3701} although our recent randomized single-blinded study showed a persistent 55% reduction at 2 years. Improvement of ipsilateral bradykinesia[38] and dyskinesia[240,242] {Vitek, 2003 #4053} is usually more robust than other ipsilateral symptomatology and has been shown to persist for as long as 2 years in several studies. Studies of patients followed for up to 4 years showed significant reductions of contralateral tremor and dyskinesia and a milder reduction of contralateral rigidity and bradykinesia that was not always significant.[240,245,246] Much of the variability in outcomes may be due in part to the varying lesion size and location reported across studies.

The current use of pallidotomy for PD is mostly restricted to unilateral procedures due to the finding of significant hypophonia, dysarthria, and worsening cognitive and neuropsychiatric function with bilateral pallidotomy.[247–250] With unilateral pallidotomy, cognitive side effects are mild and often transient. Detailed neuropsychological evaluation of patients randomized to unilateral pallidotomy or medical management found a mild defect in phonemic fluency, with left pallidotomy surgeries producing a slightly higher risk. There was no overall change in mood; however, patients with a history of depression were at risk for recurrence.[251] A detailed analysis of lesion location and outcome showed that anteromedially placed lesions lead to impairment in memory and cognition, whereas posterolateral lesions improved cognition as well as motor performance.[252]

Weight gain was common after pallidotomy.[253] More serious but rare complications of pallidotomy include delayed infarction of the internal capsule causing hemiparesis or dysarthria,[33,236,239,254] and compromise of the optic tract from a poorly placed lesion causing visual field defects.[255] Delayed infarctions, although rare, have occurred in patients 2 weeks to 3–4 months after surgery. Patients with delayed infarctions often have a history of prior stroke, suggesting that patients with cerebrovascular disease may be at risk for this complication.[254] Most complications of pallidotomy are avoidable by appropriate screening and patient selection, and precise targeting. With careful targeting, lesions can be limited to the motor territory and spare more anterior areas that are more likely to be associated with cognitive and neuropsychological changes.

Subthalamotomy

The STN is another potential target in the treatment of parkinsonian motor signs. Although STN lesions in monkeys have been highly successful in ameliorating parkinsonian motor signs,[256–258] there has been reluctance to use this technique in humans because of the association of such lesions with the development of hemiballismus.[133,190,191,193,194] Although transient in most cases, intractable hemiballismus may occur after subcortical lesions involving the STN.[259] In addition, although the intensity of hemiballism has been reported to decrease over time, in animal experiments it has been reported to persist to some degree for the duration of the experiments (8 months) and is difficult to control pharmacologically.[256,257] Monkeys in which these observations were made, however, had not been on chronic L-dopa therapy, and the effect of subthalamotomy on dopa-induced dyskinesia in patients with long-term dopaminergic drug use is unclear. These observations and the location of the STN near the internal capsule, together with its rich blood supply, have made this a less popular target for an ablative lesion in the treatment of PD.

With modern neurosurgical techniques, including the use of MRI and neurophysiology for target localization, some groups have reexplored the use of subthalamic lesions for control of parkinsonian symptoms.[260–263] {Su, 2002 #3989} Alvarez and colleagues performed unilateral subthalamotomies in 10 patients, resulting in a 50% decrease in the off-medicine UPDRS motor score, and stable benefit in contralateral symptoms in patients followed up to 2 years. There was a less robust ipsilateral benefit that disappeared at 1 year. "On" time was improved from 53% at baseline to 94% at 12 months. Hemichorea was common but usually transient, occurring in 6 of 11 patients, and lasted from a few hours to 5 days. One additional patient had a thalamic infarct and developed disabling hemichorea at 7 days, which continued until an ipsilateral pallidotomy was performed.[171,263] Su and colleagues performed unilateral subthalamotomy in 13 patients with a 30% and 32% improvement in off-medicine UPDRS scores at 6 months and 1 year, respectively.[264] Three patients (23%) developed hemichorea, two of which resolved spontaneously without treatment. The third patient developed intractable chorea at 1 month postoperatively and died at 5 months from aspiration pneumonia.

Alvarez and colleagues performed bilateral subthalamotomy in 18 patients. One patient dropped out due to ataxia and cognitive decline; the remaining 17 patients were followed for 2 years. Three patients had postoperative chorea and dysarthria. They had a 58% reduction in the "off" UPDRS motor subscore. There was also a significant improvement in the "on" subscore of 63%. There was an average decrease of L-dopa by 72% with five patients stopping L-dopa therapy altogether. At the same time, dopamine dyskinesias were reduced by 50%.[265]

These promising results show that subthalamotomy can be performed safely and with efficacy and that the risk of hemichorea may not be as high as previously thought. Like pallidotomy, this approach is particularly attractive when stimulation therapy is considered too costly or when the associated need for close follow-up and periodic surgery for battery changes and follow-up visits for programming adjustments are not acceptable or feasible.

Deep Brain Stimulation

Vim DBS

The Vim nucleus of the thalamus, although initially pursued aggressively as a target for stimulation therapy for parkinsonian tremor, has fallen out of favor due to its lack of efficacy on akinesia, rigidity, and L-dopa-induced dyskinesias. Early reports from the Grenoble group showed that, of 80 parkinsonian patients undergoing Vim DBS, 88% showed improvement in their tremor;[74] several smaller series from other groups showed similar results ranging from 64% to 100% of patients having improvement of their contralateral tremor.[44,48,75,266] However, 65% of the Grenoble patients eventually required further surgery due to progression of akinetic-rigid symptoms or dyskinesias for which the Vim DBS was ineffective.[221] Although most studies of Vim DBS have not found improvement of dyskinesia or rigidity, one group has shown some improvement in dyskinesia with a more anterior electrode placement.[43,44] At 8 mm anterior to the PC, they were likely affecting Voa and Vop. Consistent with these observations, others have targeted more anterior portions of the motor thalamus for relief of L-dopa-induced dyskinesias[127] and rigidity.[216,267–269]

The most common complication of Vim stimulation for PD tremor is worsening dysarthria, which has been reported to occur in approximately 20% of patients. It is more common with bilateral stimulation and can often be reduced with reduction of the amplitude of stimulation.[45] In patients who have a contralateral thalamotomy, the incidence of dysarthria following Vim DBS on the intact side is higher, at approximately 27–30%.[48,74] This compares to a higher (30–50%) incidence of speech difficulties in patients with bilateral thalamotomies. The major advantage to Vim stimulation over lesioning is that the side effects associated with stimulation are reversible, whereas those that occur as a result of lesioning are not.[270]

Although very effective for tremor, the lack of reliable efficacy on the other cardinal parkinsonian symptoms has limited the use of Vim DBS for PD.[221] Even in patients with tremor-predominant disease, other features manifest over time that would have potentially been controlled if another target had been selected.[271] Perhaps, with stimulation of Vim and Voa/Vop, tremor, rigidity, and dyskinesia could be controlled; however, this has not been possible with stimulation, as current spread is not sufficient to cover such a broad territory with a single DBS lead. Using two DBS leads in the thalamus to control symptoms that could be controlled with one DBS lead in another target has led to little interest by physicians in using this approach.

GPi DBS

After initial successes with modern pallidotomy for PD and Vim stimulation to relieve parkinsonian and essential tremor, GPi DBS appeared as an attractive intervention, one which may match or supercede the efficacy of pallidotomy with less risk of irreversible disability. Furthermore, bilateral GPi DBS does not have the risk of speech disturbances seen with anteriorly placed bilateral pallidotomy and can therefore be used more safely to obtain better bilateral benefit.

In the largest prospective double-blind multicenter study to date, bilateral GPi DBS showed a 37% improvement in the off-medicine UPDRS motor subscore in 38 patients at 3 months.[272] Results from other studies have been consistently positive, and long-term studies of bilateral GPi DBS up to 3–4 years have shown stable benefit.[273] Two series of 6 patients showed 53% and 36% improvement at 6 months, and 50% and 38% at 2 years.[274,275] In the DBS for Parkinson's study, patients followed for 3–4 years demonstrated an increase in "on" time without dyskinesia from 29% to 69% and the "off" medication "on" stimulation UPDRS III motor subscore remained improved at 39%.[273]

Unlike thalamotomy or Vim DBS, GPi DBS has reliably alleviated not only tremor but all the cardinal motor symptoms of PD including akinesia/bradykinesia, rigidity, and gait.[177,272–283] {Krack, 1998 #3676; Loher, 2002 #3744} "Off" dystonia is improved,[283,284] and like pallidotomy, GPi DBS has a potent direct suppressing effect on L-dopa-induced dyskinesias.[49,275,278,285,286]

In gait kinematic studies, GPi DBS has been shown to improve both postural instability and gait, albeit less so than L-dopa. Defebvre and colleagues found that gait velocity increased with GPi DBS. This was considered to occur as a result of an increased stride length along with a compensatory increase in cadence.[287] Other studies have shown similar improvement along with an approximately 50% improvement in the UPDRS gait subscore.[50,277,288] {Krack, 1998 #3676} These changes tended to be more dramatic in patients with bilateral rather than unilateral stimulation.

Complications directly due to GPi DBS are minimal and are usually eliminated with adjustment of the stimulation parameters. There are fewer reports of adverse effects on speech, mood, and cognition reported with GPi DBS than have been reported for stimulation in STN (see below).[289] There are, however, case reports of mania,[290] apathy,[291] and mild decline in lexical verbal memory with GPi DBS.[274] Of the studies that have performed detailed neuropsychological testing, most have shown minimal subclinical changes in some patients, and overall no significant change.[292,293]

STN DBS

Like GPi stimulation, bilateral STN stimulation has been shown to improve all of the cardinal motor symptoms of PD. A multicenter double-blinded crossover study showed 49% improvement in the off-medicine UPDRS motor subscore in 96 patients after bilateral STN stimulation.[272] These results and those of other studies have been consistently robust, with most studies showing 45–55% improvement and some showing as high as 60–70% improvement in the off-medicine motor subscore (Table 17–1). Like GPi DBS, improvement appears to be relatively stable with several studies showing significant improvement out 24–36 months,[294,295] and one showing sustained improvement out 5 years following implanation[296] (see Table 17–1). "On" time was also increased: the 96 patients in the DBS for Parkinson's study improved from spending 27% at baseline to 74% at 3 months of the day in an "on" state.[272]

Bilateral STN stimulation may produce dramatic beneficial effects on midline symptoms such as gait, posture, and balance.[279,297] Unlike GPi DBS, it has been reported to increase walking velocity to a degree that is comparable to that of L-dopa.[298,299] Most studies of patients with bilateral STN DBS attribute this increase in velocity to an increase in stride length and thus more closely approximating normal gait.[297–302]

STN DBS has an additive effect to L-dopa on dyskinesias and, if stimulation parameters are titrated too quickly, dyskinesia can become significantly worse unless antiparkinsonian medications are reduced.[303] With STN DBS postoperative dopamine and dopamine-agonist therapy can (and usually must) be decreased.[51,295,304] If done properly, patients tolerate this well, and postoperative UPDRS scores in most studies demonstrate significant benefit despite lower doses of dopaminergic therapy.[51] In turn, by treating patients with less L-dopa, particularly if done early in their disease course, the long-term side effect of inducing motor fluctuations and dyskinesia may be minimized.

The results of STN DBS originally reported by Benabid and his group;[51,279,297,303–308] {Krack, 1998 #118} resulted in a large number of studies that have further validated the safety and efficacy of this procedure.[309–335] {Zhang, 2006 #225} A meta-analysis of the literature published in 2006 shows mean reduction in UPDRS part III scores among the 34 articles included in the study was 52% (range 82–17%). The mean reduction in UPDRS part II scores was 49.9% (range 72–29.5%). The correlation between levodopa response and positive outcomes following STN-DBS was confirmed by this meta-analysis as well as other studies.[327] A few prospective, controlled studies have since been published. In 2001, the DBS for PD Study Group reported on the outcomes of 96 patients undergoing STN DBS. The improvements in UPDRS part III motor subscores at 3-month follow-up (assessed with double-blinded evaluations after randomly assigning patients to stimulation on or off) were 49%. A continuation of this study was reported in 2005 with 3-year or greater follow-up of 69 patients from the initial study. The 3-year or greater follow-up data demonstrated that the effects of DBS for PD are long lasting. The long-term benefits of DBS were later substantiated by Krack and colleagues.[296] Forty-nine consecutive patients treated with bilateral STN-DBS were assessed at 1, 3, and 5 years postimplantation. The mean reductions in UPDRS part III at these time points were 66%, 59%, and 54%, respectively. Activities of daily living were also improved. A significant drop in efficacy was observed when comparing the 1st and 5th years after surgery. Nevertheless, most of these patients were dependent upon others before surgery and continued to enjoy independence throughout the entire follow-up period. Similar 5-year follow-up results were reported by Schüpbach and colleagues with 54% reductions in UPDRS part III scores, and 40% maintained reduction in UPDRS part II scores. Additional long-term outcome studies with follow-up ranging from 2 to 4 years reported on mean UPDRS part III reductions of 48% in 25 patients,[336] 43% in 20 patients,[337] 55% in 22 patients,[318] 57% in 29 patients,[338] and 45% in 20 patients.[295] The latter study also reported on complete withdrawal of medication (replaced by stimulation) in 10 of 20 patients. Such a dramatic and early reduction of medication intake may have accounted for some of the complications observed by the authors, such as dysarthria and cognitive problems.[339]

In addition to stimulation-induced dyskinesias, there are more reports of mood, behavioral, and cognitive side effects associated with STN compared to GPi stimulation. This may be due to the fact that more centers perform STN stimulation and, therefore, there are more reports of side effects; however, the STN also has unique anatomical characteristics that may make stimulation in this site more likely to be associated with such side effects. These include (1) its small size, requiring implantation of the DBS lead in regions near nonmotor

▶ **TABLE 17–1. COMPARISON OF RESULTS FROM STUDIES WITH BILATERAL STN OR GPi DBS**

Study	3 Months	6 Months	9 Months	12 Months	24 Months	36 Months	48 Months	60 Months
Bilateral STN DBS								
Krack 1998[279]		71 (8)						
Burchiel 1999[278]				44 (5)				
Scotto di Luzio 2001[280]	44 (9)	54 (9)		57 (9)				
DBS Study Group 2001[272]	49 (96)							
Volkmann 2001[281]		67 (16)		60 (16)				
Limousin 1998[306]				60 (20)				
Brown 1999[340]	57 (6)							
Moro 1999[341]	34 (7)	36 (6)		41 (5)				
Pinter 1999[342]	54 (9)			55 (8)				
Bejjani 2000[205]		62 (10)						
Fraix 2000[343]	17 (24)			9 (24)				
Molinuevo 2000[344]		66 (15)						
Alegret 2001[345]	57 (15)							
Capus 2001[346]		56 (7)						
Lopiano 2001[347]	57 (16)							
Figueiras-Mendez 2002[348]				63 (22)	49 (9)			
Iansek 2002[332]								
Ostergaard 2002[318]	57 (26)			64 (26)				
Romito 2002[294]					49 (10)	49 (7)		
Simuni 2002[349]				47 (12)				
Thobois 2002[350]		55 (18)		62 (14)				
Vingerhoets 2002[295]	46 (19)	49 (19)		49 (19)	63 (10)			
Average	47 (227)	58 (108)		49 (180)	50 (29)	49 (7)		
Bilateral GPi DBS								
Krack 1998[279]		39 (5)						
Burchiel 1999[278]				39 (4)				
Scotto di Luzio 2001[280]	49 (5)	44 (5)		42 (5)				
DBS Study Group 2001[272]	37 (38)							
Volkmann 2001[281]		56 (11)		51 (11)		43		24
Ghika 1998[274]		53 (6)	52 (6)	55 (6)	50			
Volkmann 1998[276]	44 (9)							
Kumar 2000[177]		31 (17)						
Durif 2002[275]		36 (6)		26 (6)	38			
Loher 2002[282]	36 (10)			41 (10)				
Krack 2003[296]				66 (43)		59 (42)		54 (42)
Average	39 (62)	42 (50)	52 (6)	43 (42)	44	43	46	24

Data are presented as percent improvement from preoperative off-medication UPDRS motor score, by postoperative months. The numbers of patients are given in parentheses.

portions of the STN and (2) its close proximity to important neighboring structures such as the median forebrain bundle and lateral hypothalamus. Because of its small size and location to nonmotor structures, inadvertent current spread into nonmotor STN or adjacent structures may affect cognition and behavior by modulating frontal and limbic function. Indeed, reprogramming these patients to reduce current spread into these nonmotor areas may reduce the cognitive deficits while maintaining motor improvement.[351,352]

Worsening cognitive function has been reported in some patients with subthalamic stimulation, more commonly in older patients and patients who demonstrate preoperative cognitive decline. In contrast, as a whole, young and non-demented patients show no significant cognitive change. Several reports show worsening of frontal lobe function as demonstrated on the Stroop test. PET studies done during evaluation of patients taking the Stroop test implicate changes in striatoanterior cingulate cortex circuits as potentially having a role in this disturbance. Whereas such findings are subclinical to routine examination, modulation of these important frontal circuits may become more important in older or demented patients with less cognitive reserve.

Limbic circuits have strong connections with medial STN, and not surprisingly, STN stimulation has been reported to cause apathy, depression, or mania. Depression and apathy may also occur in part due to a reduction or sudden withdrawal of L-dopa, as such patients may show improvement with increasing dopaminergic treatment. Depression has also been reported to occur in some patients, particularly with left STN stimulation. Right-sided STN DBS may produce laughter. One patient appeared to have a pseudobulbar depression with uncontrollable crying associated only with left STN stimulation, while having no change in the Geriatric Depression Scale.[353] She also had an exaggerated gag reflex that was present only when stimulation was turned on. The most common cognitive side effect in the immediate postoperative period following STN DBS is transient confusion with an incidence between 1% and 36%.[273,296,314,324,345,354–366] Neuropsychological deficits prior to surgery are significantly associated with increased confusion following surgery.[367] The most frequently observed long-term neuropsychological change following STN DBS is a decline in word fluency.[314] There is also decline in measures assessing executive function, verbal learning, and memory.[359,364] However, it is critical to understand that the majority of available neuropsychological outcome studies have not included control groups, are biased, and consist of small groups. The incidence of dementia in PD patients who underwent STN DBS over a 3-year follow-up was similar to the incidence reported in medically treated patients.[365] Whereas speech can improve with STN stimulation, current spread in the neighboring corticobulbar fibers may cause worsening speech. Subthalamic stimulation can also induce conjugate horizontal or vertical eye deviation that is usually contraversive to the stimulation side. This is most common with a laterally placed lead and may involve the oculomotor loop. Ipsilateral deviation of the homolateral eye, on the other hand, is common with medially placed leads and is likely due to direct stimulation of the oculomotor nerve. Many of the side effects of STN stimulation can be ameliorated by changing the stimulation contact or parameter; however, mood and cognitive changes can be more occult, may not be noticed immediately, and can persist once stimulation is turned off.[368]

In addition to its size and location, the rapid medication adjustments necessitated by the prodyskinetic effect may also lead to induction of side effects associated with too rapid a reduction in dopaminergic medications. STN stimulation also provides for more difficult postoperative management of dopamine agonist therapy in patients with dyskinesias; however, the benefits are very rewarding in properly selected patients when managed closely in the postoperative period.

Comparison of STN to GPi DBS

Multiple retrospective and prospective studies have compared the outcomes of GPi and STN DBS in PD.[290,369,370] Both targets have shown to be beneficial.[296,369] It is often argued based on these studies that STN DBS is more effective and allows for a greater reduction in postoperative medication.[273,371,372] The only three prospective randomized double-blind studies comparing these two targets, however, fail to authenticate any of these arguments. Burchiel and colleagues[278] randomized 10 patients with idiopathic PD, dyskinesia, and motor fluctuations to implantation of bilateral GPi or STN stimulators. Patients and evaluating clinicians were blinded to the stimulation site throughout the study period. After analysis of 12-month follow-up data, they reported 39% and 44% improvement in "off" UPDRS scores in the GPi and STN groups, respectively. Rigidity, tremor, and bradykinesia improved equally in both groups. "On" UPDRS scores were improved more by GPi than by STN stimulation. Reduction in dyskinesia was equally seen by DBS at either site, although the medication requirement was reduced only in the STN group. An extension of this randomized, blinded pilot study was carried out and enrolled 23 patients with idiopathic PD, dyskinesia, and motor fluctuations.[373] They were randomized to implantation of bilateral GPi or STN stimulators. Patients and evaluating clinicians were blinded to stimulation site. At 1-year follow-up, "off" UPDRS motor subscores were improved in both GPi and STN groups (39% vs. 48%). Medication reduction was more marked in the STN group but was not statistically significant from the GPi group (P = .08). Dyskinesias were reduced in both GPi and STN groups (89% vs. 62%). Cognitive and behavioral complications were observed only in combination with STN stimulation. Anderson and colleagues also found increased frequency of postoperative delirium and confusion in STN stimulation patients.[373] A third prospective, randomized, blinded study assessed the effects of unilateral DBS in the STN versus GPi on fine motor skills in 33 patients with advanced PD.[374] Stimulation of either the STN (18 subjects) or the GPi (15 subjects) in the off-medication state significantly improved movement time and dexterity with no significant difference between the two targets. A recent study that systematically examined the long-term effects of unilateral GPi or STN DBS on the force-producing capabilities of both limbs under unimanual and bimanual motor conditions has found persistent improvements in the control and coordination of grasping forces during maximal efforts and functional dexterous actions.[375] Overall, the results indicate that unilateral GPi or STN DBS is effective in improving overall motor function, maximum force production, and the control and specification of grasping forces in both limbs.[375] Stimulation produced greater clinical gains in motor function and strength for the contralateral limb; however, significant improvements were also observed in the ipsilateral limb.[375] In general there appears to be little difference in the motor scores of patients receiving either STN or GPi DBS in trials where patients were randomized and assessments were blinded. On the other hand, these studies suggest that DBS in the STN may result in greater cognitive and neurobehavioral changes than GPi DBS in patients with PD.[273,373,376] Two large blinded randomized trials currently completed but not yet published should help to further address this question.

Target/Procedure Selection

STN and GPi DBS are the most common neurosurgical procedures performed today for PD. Although most studies of STN stimulation have shown greater improvement in off-medicine motor subscores than those of GPi stimulation (Table 17–1), two large randomized comparisons of these two targets recently completed enrollment, but results are not yet published. Several smaller studies, however, did not demonstrate a significant difference in motor outcome.[296,369] One small study of 10 patients randomized to GPi or STN showed no significant difference between the two targets, with STN showing a slightly higher improvement of 44% as compared to 39% with GPi stimulation.[278] The errors in taking these data at face value without proper comparison are numerous. Average improvement is inextricably linked to targeting accuracy. There is a great degree of center-to-center variability in targeting techniques used, ranging from combined stereotaxic MRI-guided initial targeting with microelectrode and macroelectrode neurophysiologic characterization of the target structure to those relying predominately on CT-guided targeting with minimal or no neurophysiology. If there is a difference in the ability to accurately target these different structures (as may be suggested by their differing size and proximity to neighboring structures with adverse stimulatory effects), then a bias in targeting accuracy is likely, which in turn will lead to different degrees of improvement based purely on targeting accuracy. We must also be reminded that different centers target different areas within these structures, and there is no clear consensus on the site of optimal lead placement, nor has the relationship between lead location and clinical outcome been defined. Furthermore, most STN leads are placed bilaterally, whereas more GPi leads are unilateral; thus although these patient group should not be directly compared, several studies that have reported superiority of STN over Gpi include a combination of unilateral and bilateral GPi cases and compare them to predominately bilaterally operated STN patients. The side-effect profile differs between the two targets, with STN stimulation having more reports of mood, cognitive, and speech effects, and may be more difficult to manage postoperatively. As more data are collected directly comparing these procedures, it may be determined that there is a select patient population better suited for each procedure. At present, however, the data by which we could make these decisions do not exist.

In PD, bilateral pallidotomies are now generally felt to have unjustifiable side effects of hypophonia and dysarthria. Unilateral pallidotomy, however, is safe, has proven efficacy, and still exists as a good alternative to DBS for some patients. It has clear advantages when cost is an issue, when patients do not want repeated procedures for battery replacement, or when programming along with the risk of infection of the implanted hardware. If the patient has bilateral disease, a different procedure may eventually be necessary for the unoperated side. Subthalamotomy, although studied less, may provide a safe alternative.[262,265] More studies regarding the use of this approach for the treatment of PD are clearly needed.

ESSENTIAL TREMOR (ET) AND OTHER TREMORS

Patient Selection

ET is the most common movement disorder. It is often mild and controlled symptomatically with oral medications. However, approximately 10% of patients have severe disabling tremor that is refractory to medical therapy.[377] Patients with medically intractable ET who are functionally compromised in performing activities of daily living are considered candidates for surgical intervention. Maximal doses of propranolol and primidone alone and in combination should be tried before recommending surgical intervention. Deuschl and Bain also recommend a trial of gabapentin and a test dose of 12.5 mg of clozapine (if significant hand and head tremor is present) or a trial of botulinum toxin (if significant head and voice tremor is present) before declaring patients medically refractory.[377]

Patients with predominantly distal limb postural tremor are most likely to benefit from surgery. There may be a physiological explanation for this observation. The thalamus has a somatotopic lamellar organization with leg, trunk, proximal arm, distal arm, and face arranged in sequential lamellae toward the center of the nuclei.[378,379] Due to this somatotopic organization, proximal tremors are more difficult to treat surgically and require a larger lesion or larger area of current spread to affect more proximal limb segments. Improvement following surgery is contralateral to the side of the lesion, with little or no improvement in the ipsilateral side.

Those patients with bilateral tremor should have the side operated on, which, in the patient's and physician's view, will give the most functional benefit.

Midline symptoms such as head and voice tremor may improve with unilateral procedure; however, these symptoms generally require bilateral procedures to achieve maximal improvement. When bilateral procedures are needed, DBS is the method of choice over thalamotomy for at least one side due to the significantly high risk of dysarthria after bilateral thalamotomy.

Patients with other non-Parkinson tremor etiologies can sometime benefit from surgery as well. Patients with cerebellar outflow tremors, multiple sclerosis, or posttraumatic brain injury may be considered for surgery as these tremors rarely respond well to medical therapy. However, success among this group of patients has been highly variable, with many undergoing several procedures, only to have their tremor return. Larger lesions or greater areas of current spread are required for these tremors and should involve as much of the affected limb region within Vim, and possibly Vop, as possible. These patients usually have extensive and diffuse brain pathology and thus may have less functional reserve, raising the risk of adverse outcomes with surgery. Thus, the risk-versus-benefit ratio must be carefully weighed for these patients before recommending surgical intervention.

Results: Thalamotomy versus Vim DBS

Both thalamic stimulation and thalamotomy have been shown to be effective in the relief of postural tremor in patients with ET. Most studies show approximately 90% of patients having marked improvement or complete elimination of tremor with either thalamotomy[380–383] or Vim stimulation.[42,73,384–389] Long-term follow-up of patients with thalamotomies shows that nearly 80% of patients continue to have significant improvement.[390]

Voice tremor is less responsive to unilateral thalamotomy but has been reported to improve in some series.[391,392] Several studies have noted improvement of voice and head tremors with thalamic DBS most consistently when performed bilaterally.[391,392] However, there is some evidence that unilateral stimulation can be efficacious in treating voice and head tremor. Koller and colleagues reported that 71% of patients had improvement in head tremor with unilateral Vim DBS and maintained this benefit when reexamined 1 year later.[393] There was also improvement in voice tremor in 57% of patients. Others have also seen similar improvement in both head and voice tremor[394] with unilateral stimulation.

Complications of unilateral thalamotomy are often mild and transient, lasting only a few days to weeks postoperatively. Two percent to 9% of patients may experience some permanent neurological deficit. These deficits include numbness, weakness, dysarthria, ataxia, and cognitive problems. There are few data on adverse outcome with bilateral thalamotomy in ET patients in the modern era. Most do not recommend bilateral thalamotomy, because of the high incidence of speech and cognitive dysfunction found in PD patients undergoing bilateral procedures for parkinsonian tremor.[390,395,396] No recent study of thalamotomy for ET has operated on more than three patients bilaterally for ET.[384,389,390] One such study showed that two of the three patients with ET had dysarthria after bilateral thalamotomy.[397]

Vim DBS has a comparatively lower incidence of permanent neurological complications but does carry all the common risks of implantation of stimulation hardware, including infection and device failure, which may necessitate repeated surgical procedures. One major advantage of Vim DBS over thalamotomy is the ability to perform bilateral surgeries without the high incidence of side effects associated with bilateral thalamotomy. Alternatively, unilateral thalamotomy can be combined with contralateral Vim stimulation safely and, at the same time, reduces the number of battery replacements required for patients undergoing bilateral Vim DBS.

In summary, DBS, initially considered an alternative to stereotactic thalamotomies, has become the surgical procedure of choice for the treatment of essential tremor, as it demonstrated similar efficacy rates and lower risks.[24,25,386,398] A direct comparison between thalamotomy and thalamic stimulation was reported by Schuurman and colleagues.[398] Seventy patients with PD, ET, or tremor from multiple sclerosis (MS) were randomized to stimulation or ablative surgery. Patients with unilateral symptoms underwent a single intervention contralateral to the symptoms. Patients with bilateral tremors underwent either bilateral thalamic stimulation or a unilateral thalamotomy with contralateral stimulation. Patients with PD and ET who had undergone thalamic stimulation performed significantly better in activities of daily living (ADL) than those undergoing ablation. Sixteen adverse effects occurred among the patients randomized to thalamotomy. In comparison, only six patients with thalamic stimulation experienced adverse effects, which were successfully resolved with stimulation cessation. Pahwa and colleagues[24] reported similar results when comparing outcomes of 17 patients undergoing thalamic stimulation to the outcomes of 17 patients who had previously undergone thalamotomy. Although the effects in tremor suppression were very similar between both groups, complications were more common among patients with thalamotomies, particularly intracerebral hemorrhages (35% vs. 0%). Likewise, cognitive deterioration and hemiparesis occurred, respectively, in 29% and 12% of patients who had undergone thalamotomies but in none of those with thalamic stimulation. Although thalamic stimulation is chronically effective for most patients,[42,66,385,398–402] reductions in efficacy during longer-term follow-ups have been reported.[74,403]

DYSTONIA

Patient Selection

Patients with generalized or focal dystonia have been considered candidates for stereotaxic functional surgery. Although all groups of patients have been reported to benefit from ablative and stimulation procedures in both the thalamus and pallidum, results vary considerable across studies and etiology, with primary dystonia doing significantly better than those with secondary dystonia, the one exception being tardive dystonia. No randomized trials comparing the site (pallidum or thalamus), technique (ablation versus stimulation), or etiology have been conducted.

Interpretation of results is also difficult due to the fact that dystonia is not a single disease, but rather a syndrome that has been traditionally divided into subcategories based on etiologic and phenomenologic criteria. Some processes that cause dystonia also cause more diffuse brain pathology and may lead to a higher risk of neuropsychological or other complications. It is also important to consider whether the disease process is progressive, raising the risk of worsening symptoms due to progression of the underlying disease process. As our understanding of the molecular and genetic basis of these diseases and the circuitry involved improves, we will be better able to categorize patients so that subsequent studies of surgical therapy will be able to provide the necessary information to better predict which patients are most likely to respond to surgery.

Such studies will be critically dependent on the use of validated, standardized rating scales to allow comparisons across investigations. In contemporary studies, patients are usually assessed by one of three commonly used scales: the Burke–Fahn–Marsden Dystonia Rating Scale (BFMDRS), the Unified Dystonia Rating Scale (UDRS), and the Physicians Global Dystonia Rating Scale (PGDS). Although all three have been compared in a multicenter trial and show excellent internal consistency, interrater reliability, and high correlation ($r = 0.977-0.983$),[404] the majority of reports of DBS for dystonia have used the BFMDRS. Additionally, the Toronto Western Spasmodic Torticollis Rating Scale (TWSTRS) has been used in several studies for cervical dystonia.[404–406]

Ablative Therapy

Thalamotomy

The thalamus was initially the preferred target for surgical therapy for dystonia. In 1976, Cooper published long-term follow-up results on 226 dystonia patients (followed on average for 7.9 years) showing that, overall, 70% of patients had mild-to-marked improvement following thalamotomy.[407] Cardoso and colleagues showed that 47% of patients improved in his series.[408] Andrew and colleagues found that 64% of patients with generalized dystonia improved with thalamotomy (most of which were bilateral);[409] however, 1 year after surgery, only 35% retained benefit and by 3 years only 19% were still improved. In contrast, Cardoso found in his series that 80% of patients with generalized dystonia had moderate-to-marked improvement, and did better than other subgroups.[408] Other major studies also reported positive results, which varied depending on the disease characteristics.[408–410]

Patients with hemidystonia had dramatic initial postoperative improvement in Andrew's series, with 100% showing improvement—91% were rated as good to excellent and 9% as fair. However, after 3 years, the benefit was greatly diminished with only 17% continuing to show improvement. In contrast, Cardoso found that only 33% of patients with hemidystonia had a moderate or better response to thalamotomy.[408] He also found that one of three patients with segmental dystonia improved.

For spasmodic torticollis, four major studies of thalamotomy showed that, on average, 63% of patients had good-to-excellent improvement.[409,411–414] Complications ranged from 63% of patients showing significant complications to 11%, with 54–82% of patients demonstrating good results.[409,413,414]

Forty-five percent of patients with primary dystonia had greater than 25% improvement in Tasker and colleagues' series.[415] Cooper also found significant improvement and noted that Jewish patients with a significant family history of dystonia did better than others, with 85% of those with a family history of dystonia improving significantly. Although this series preceded the discovery of the DYT1 gene, it is likely that many of these patients may have been DYT1-positive. In contrast, non-Jewish patients with familial dystonia only improved in 56% of cases in his series.

Broggi's group performed thalamic lesions in patients with cerebral palsy and dystonia and achieved a good benefit in 46% of patients, and a fair benefit in 18%. Others have reported only transient benefit in patients with secondary dystonia, not lasting longer than a year.

The reported lesion location and size vary dramatically from study to study, making direct comparisons difficult. Having performed a large number of thalamotomies in varied locations, Cooper suggested that the best target for dystonia is the posterior half of the ventrolateral thalamus extending into VPL, VPM, and centromedian thalamus. Targets chosen by others vary greatly, and included Vim, Voa, Vop, Vce, Vci, CeM, and pulvinar. Given the imaging capabilities of the day, the actual location of these lesions remain speculative.

Complications varied significantly by series. Cooper reported a 0.7% mortality rate per operation and 2% per patient.[416] Similarly, Tasker had a 1.8% mortality rate per patient.[416] Dysarthria or dysphonia occured in 18–25%

of all dystonia patients after thalamotomy. There was a greater incidence of dysarthria, ranging from 56% to 73% after bilateral thalamotomies compared with only 8–11% of patients after unilateral thalamotomy. Additionally, Tasker reported that 6% of patients undergoing thalamotomy for secondary dystonia developed permanent dysphagia. Overall, Tasker noted a 21% incidence of major complications in patients with secondary dystonia and 25% in primary dystonia patients undergoing surgery.[416]

In summary, thalamotomy can have dramatic benefit in carefully selected patients. Side effects are not trivial, particularly when bilateral procedures are required, as is the case with axial-predominant symptoms. In these instances, given the reports of improvement in patients following alternative approaches not associated with such a high incidence of side effect, one must consider whether the underlying disability is significant enough to warrant the risk of surgery and then consider which approach may provide the greatest benefit with the least risk. These alternative procedures are described below.

Pallidotomy

Early surgeries for dystonia were principally thalamotomies. After witnessing the beneficial effect of pallidotomy on dystonia in patients undergoing surgery for PD, several groups pursued the use of pallidotomy for other dystonic syndromes. Our group, as well as Iacono and Lozano, reported individual cases of primary generalized dystonia with dramatic improvement, which was soon followed by several case series.[27,29,417–420]

In all of the series reported to date, the vast majority of idiopathic generalized dystonia patients have improved following pallidotomy. Although many of the secondary dystonia patients have improved as well, their response has generally been less dramatic and less consistent.[27,29,233,418,420] {Vitek, 1997 #830; Ondo, 1998 #926; Vitek, 1997 #951} In primary dystonia, the BFMDRS has been reported to improve 67–80%,[27,418,420] {Vitek, 1997 #830; Ondo, 1998 #926; Vitek, 1997 #951} whereas improvement in secondary dystonia is approximately 18%. This has ranged from transient benefit that was lost by 3 months in a patient reported by Teive and colleagues,[421] to 13% benefit found in 18 patients reported by Lin and colleagues,[422] to 59% average improvement in four patients reported by Ondo and colleagues.[423] Even in Ondo's series, in which the results in secondary dystonia were comparatively better than others, primary dystonia still had a better response. All case series reported have been retrospective, and many consist of patients who have had unilateral or bilateral pallidotomies with variable length of follow-up. In most cases, improvement is gradual, and patients continue to improve for 3–6 months or more after surgery.

Most complications reported in unilateral or bilateral pallidotomy for dystonia are mild and transient, ranging from 0 to 38% of patients.[29,233,418,,420,424] {Vitek, 1997 #830; Ondo, 1998 #926; Vitek, 1997 #951} Of note, unlike cases with PD, dystonia patients have not been reported to develop incapacitating hypophonia following bilateral pallidotomy.

To date, there has been no randomized prospective trial comparing surgical targets for dystonia. One group has retrospectively compared thalamotomy and pallidotomy and suggests that pallidotomy is more effective in primary dystonia, whereas thalamotomy may be better in focal secondary dystonia.[423] However, this study was limited not only because it was retrospective but also because unilateral or bilateral surgeries were performed and some patients underwent both pallidotomy and thalamotomy. Palliodotomy has been shown to be useful in some cases of tardive dystonia.[28] Future studies with careful characterization of patients into focal, segmental, hemi-, and generalized dystonia will be needed to document carefully which patient populations respond best to the various therapies.

Deep Brain Stimulation

Thalamic DBS

Data from pallidotomy and thalamotomy studies have suggested that pallidotomy may be more effective and safer and allow for bilateral procedures in patients without the high incidence of side effects seen with bilateral thalamotomy; however, it is important to note that there have been no randomized controlled clinical trials that have compared the two procedures. It is unlikely that such a trial will be done, given the fact that DBS now plays such a predominate role in the surgical treatment of these patients together with the previously reported high incidence of side effects following bilateral thalamotomy. At present most studies of DBS for dystonia have chosen GPi as the target. This is due primarily to the success of GPi as a target site for PD and the associated improvement in dystonic symptoms in these patients, which led to targeting GPi for patients with primary dystonia. The marked success of this procedure for these patients has kept physicians from exploring alternative targets. Nevertheless, some studies have investigated thalamic stimulation in patients with primary and secondary dystonia, and more recently, several centers have implanted or lesioned the STN for the treatment of dystonia.[425–430]

Vercueil has the largest series of thalamic stimulation patients, and implanted 12 patients (4 primary, 8 secondary) in VLp thalamus.[431,432] Five of these patients had moderate-to-marked improvement of their dystonia and three of the remaining seven were reimplanted in GPi with good benefit in two. Three of the four primary dystonia patients had good improvement with VLp stimulation, and the fourth patient had benefit in her dystonic tremor but no other dystonic movements until her thalamic leads were removed and GPi was implanted. This study shows one group's clinical experience with DBS for dystonia suggesting that GPi may be a superior target; however, it is limited by its retrospective design, variable follow-up, and study of a mixed population of primary and secondary dystonia. There is also limited support from individual case reports also suggesting that thalamic stimulation is not as good as GPi.

Trottenburg and colleagues implanted bilateral leads each with contacts in Vim and GPi in a single patient with tardive dystonia.[433] There was no benefit with Vim stimulation but 73% improvement in the BMFDS with bilateral GPi stimulation. They reported another patient with dystonia-myoclonus with Vim stimulation who had improvement of the myoclonus but not dystonia.[434] In contrast, Ghika reported a case of postanoxic dystonia who failed to improve from bilateral pallidal DBS but subsequently improved after explanting and reimplanting in bilateral Voa thalamus.[435] This is an interesting finding. The patient had MRI evidence of bilateral pallidal anoxic damage, possibly rendering it a poor target due to lack of functional brain to stimulate. However, by stimulating Voa thalamus, a pallidal receiving area, they may have disrupted the abnormal pallidal output responsible for the patient's symptoms. Thus, theoretically, the motor thalamus is a sound target for the treatment of dystonia. Experimentally, it has been demonstrated that lesions or stimulation in Voa and Vop can be effective in treating the symptoms of dystonia. Lest we make the mistakes of the past, we should not dismiss the motor thalamus as a viable target for the treatment of dystonia. Without clear documentation of lesion or lead location and standardized modes of assessment at selective intervals, negative outcomes are hard to interpret. Is it the failure of the procedure to help the patient or the failure of the physician to perform the procedure?

GPi DBS

Pallidal stimulation has also been successful for the treatment of primary dystonia and is presently the surgical procedure of choice for such patients. Similar to the experience with pallidotomy, the experience with GPi DBS is predominately in patients with primary dystonia. One of the first reports of GPi DBS for dystonia was that of Coubes and colleagues who reported seven patients with DYT1-positive dystonia. All patients had a dramatic response to bilateral pallidal stimulation with an average improvement in the BFMDRS of 90.3% (range 60–100%). Results were stable for over 1 year.[54,436] {Coubes, 2000 #3442} They also reported a larger series, including the 7 DYT1 patients as well as 9 DYT1-negative primary generalized dystonia patients with an average improvement in the BFMDRS of 80.3%.[54,436] {Coubes, 2000 #3442} A subsequent study included 1 patient with DYT1-positive generalized dystonia with 86% improvement in the BMFDRS and 3 patients with DYT1-negative primary generalized or multifocal dystonia with an average improvement of 59%. Additionally, 1 secondary posttraumatic patient with hemidystonia had 72 percent improvement. Other studies have also shown significant improvement in patients with segmental and cervical dystonia.[54,436] {Coubes, 2000 #3442}

Pallidal stimulation for dystonia has been formally assessed in prospective, controlled, multicenter studies. Results from a series of 22 patients with primary generalized dystonia (7 DYT1-positive) were described by Vidailhet and the French stimulation du pallidum interne dans la dystonie study group.[437] At 3-month follow-up, investigators blinded to the status of stimulation assessed dystonia severity through video recordings. At 12-month follow-up, the dystonia movement scores had dropped to a mean of 21, compared to a baseline preoperative mean score of 46.3. Similar blinding methodologies were used by Kupsch, and DBS was used by dystonia study groups[438] to assess patients with primary generalized or segmental dystonia. Greater reductions in the dystonia movement scores were evident in the stimulation group (15.8 points/39.3%) than in the sham stimulation group (1.4 points/4.9%). Surprisingly, there were no significant differences in the degree of amelioration of patients who were positive for the DYT1 mutation versus those who were negative for the mutation. Nor were significant differences apparent when the outcomes of patients with generalized dystonia were compared to those with segmental dystonia.

It is important to note that the literature has a selective bias against reporting negative results, and there have been a few DYT1-positive patients with reportedly good placement and poor outcome that have been described in unpublished abstracts. The reasons for this, while unclear, remain important and require further study. It is also important to note that there have been no randomized trials comparing pallidal DBS to other therapies, either medical or surgical. It is important to keep in mind that the recommendations we make today are based largely on nonrandomized series with only two randomized controlled studies for comparison. Given the difficult in characterizing lead location, there is little data demonstrating with reasonable accuracy the location of the lead within the targeted structure for any of these studies. This is not a criticism of the studies performed as much as a statement of the shortcoming of current technology and one that needs to be addressed if we are to move the field forward.

Target/Procedure Selection

Despite the lack of careful controlled prospective trials, given the dramatic benefit, relative safety, and reversibility of GPi DBS, most physicians consider GPi DBS the preferred surgical approach to dystonia. Thalamic DBS may still have a role, and has not been thoroughly evaluated. Some have suggested that Vim thalamic DBS may be particularly beneficial in patients with secondary dystonia or in patients with dystonia and tremor or other hyperkinetic movements. Others have suggested that Vim is the wrong thalamic target for dystonia, and instead, the pallidal receiving areas Voa and Vop should be targeted. Just as we should not dismiss the thalamus as a potential target for dystonia, we should not disregard pallidotomy for the treatment of dystonia. Although there has been no randomized evaluation of pallidotomy versus GPi DBS, they appear to have roughly similar efficacy in improving the symptoms of primary dystonia as measured by the BFMRS. Unlike patients with PD, patients with dystonia appear to tolerate bilateral pallidotomy and do not appear to develop hypophonia. Pallidotomy may also have some advantages over pallidal DBS for dystonia since many dystonia patients require high voltages with DBS, thus leading to frequent battery changes. The associated risks of surgery for battery replacements, although small, are ever present and should not be dismissed, particularly in young patients in whom battery replacements could be required every couple of years. Given the associated issues of safety and efficacy, it will be important that these techniques are compared in a randomized clinical study to assess their relative efficacy, complications, and economic implications. In future, the STN could be a target with some advantages such as lower current requirements, capturing a greater target volume, and since it is in younger patients, we may not see the same incidence of cognitive issues as with PD.[60] {Zhang, 2006 #15951}

HEMIBALLISMUS

Patient Selection

Hemiballism is most often secondary to acute stroke but may also be due to trauma or other insult involving the subthalamic region. Medical therapies include haloperidol, diazepam, and clozapine. Many patients (56%) fully recover spontaneously or with medical therapy alone within 15 days of the event.[439] There is a high rate of death after post-stroke hemiballism, but the vast majority of deaths are due to cerebrovascular or cardiac etiologies. A small percentage of patients have such severe hemiballism that physical exhaustion due to uncontrolled muscle activity eventually leads to death.

Patients in whom medical therapy has been unsuccessful and/or whose health is at risk, secondary to continuous excessive hemiballistic movements should be considered candidates for surgery.

Target/Procedure Selection

Both thalamotomy and pallidotomy have been reported to be effective in the surgical treatment of intractable hemiballismus.[196,440–443] Although there are few cases with histological confirmation of lesion location, the effective lesions in GPi are reported to lie in the posterior pallidum. Those in the thalamus are placed in the ventrolateral thalamus and would appear to include portions of what is now termed Vop and Vim. These lesions, however, likely involve surrounding subnuclei and, in some histologically verified cases, involve portions of the zona incerta and reticular nucleus of the thalamus.[441] DBS in Vim thalamus has also been reported to be successful in isolated cases of hemiballism.[52] As GPi DBS is effective in hyperkinetic movement disorders,[444,445] it would also likely be effective for hemiballism.

▶ PUTATIVE MECHANISMS OF ACTION OF DBS AND ABLATIVE THERAPY

As the surgical treatment of PD and other movement disorders has evolved from ablative techniques such as pallidotomy and thalamotomy to DBS, the traditional models of hypo- and hyperkinetic movement disorders have been challenged and revised. Alternative models of basal ganglia function were developed that focused attention on the pattern of neural discharges and the content of information that it represents. Subsequent studies of DBS supported and reinforced these alternative models. This transition from the rate model to models focusing on altered patterns and uncontrolled synchrony of neuronal activity remains in a dynamic state with modifications occurring with each new piece of data supplied through experimental studies.

Based on the rate model, one might assume that pallidal or subthalamic stimulation must be inhibitory, thus explaining the similar effect of stimulation to ablation on tremor and PD motor signs. However, there is an evolving consensus based on neurophysiologic data from primate animal models and functional imaging of patients that DBS is likely *excitatory* and causes an increased output from its target nuclei.

The mechanisms proposed by which DBS may paradoxically ameliorate symptoms of PD with comparable efficacy to ablation at the same sites are numerous, and include (1) activation of inhibitory presynaptic axons terminating in the target structure, (2) depolarization blockade, (3) block of ion channels, (4) synaptic depletion and failed transmission, (5) jamming of pathological neuronal signals, and (6) activation of output from the stimulated structure or nearby adjacent fiber pathways.[446–450] Theories (1)–(4) would require stimulation to have an inhibitory effect on target nucleus activity, which is not supported by the majority of data available to us today. Our group and others are now proposing that DBS causes an alteration of the pattern of neural activity possibly by altering abnormal neural signals responsible for many of the symptoms of PD, leading either to what some refer to as an informational lesion[451,452] or alternatively to an improvement in information processing.[446–450,453]

Hashimoto and colleagues showed that chronic stimulation of the STN in parkinsonian monkeys causes an increased mean discharge rate of neurons in GPi during stimulation, suggesting activation of glutamatergic subthalamic neuron projections to GPi.[450] There appeared to be a dose–response relationship between STN stimulation and the response observed in GPi activity: with subtherapeutic stimulation parameters, there were nearly equal numbers of neurons with increased, decreased, or unchanged activity. At stimulation parameters that improved bradykinesia and rigidity (i.e., therapeutic stimulation), there was a dramatic shift in the percentage of neurons with increased mean discharge rates in GPi. More important than the rate change, however, was the observation that the pattern of neural activity in GPi locked to the stimulus in STN leading to an increased regularity. As the mean discharge rate increased, parkinsonian symptoms paradoxically improved. Thus, the rate model could not explain the mechanism by which pallidal DBS was improving PD. What is often ignored in this study, however, is the fact that the pattern of GPi neuronal activity was significantly modified by therapeutic stimulation. Thus, the change in pattern that occurred and was correlated with improvement in parkinsonian motor signs provided support for the etiology of hypo- and hyperkinetic movement disorders and their relationship to altered patterns of neuronal activity.

Support for activation of the output from the site of stimulation has also been supported by studies in normal monkeys. Anderson and colleagues demonstrated that GPi stimulation inhibited thalamic neuronal activity consistent with activation of GABAergic GPi projections.[454] In further support of these data, microdialysis performed in GPi and SNr during STN stimulation in the rat showed increased extracellular levels of glutamate, consistent with increased activity of STN efferent projections during STN stimulation.[455]

Functional MRI (fMRI) studies of patients with deep brain stimulators implanted in STN are also consistent with stimulation-induced neuronal activation. In a study by Jech and colleagues, increased BOLD (blood oxygenation level-dependent) signal changes were seen in ipsilateral GPi in two of three patients, and in ipsilateral thalamus in all three patients with STN stimulation.[456] Interestingly, the only patient that did not have GPi activation lost benefit of stimulation within 4 weeks of surgery and required reimplantation inferiorly before gaining benefit. In a recent report, these authors extended the work to eight patients with STN DBS, all of which had ipsilateral GPi and thalamic BOLD signal changes with stimulation parameters giving the patient clinical benefit.[457] A PET study of six patients with GPi stimulation showed increased cerebral blood flow in ipsilateral thalamus.[173] With Vim thalamic stimulation, both PET and fMRI studies have shown ipsilateral thalamic activation and ipsilateral SMA activation—an efferent target of Vim.[173] Further clues to our understanding of how DBS works may be gained from functional imaging during motor tasks. Parkinson patients have abnormal hyperactivation of SM1 and SMA. With STN or Vim stimulation, Jech and colleagues found that contralateral hand movement caused less activity in these areas when stimulation was turned on. Thus, there seems to be a normalization of cortical activity with stimulation.[457]

Although experimental support for activation of the site of stimulation is substantial, there remains disagreement as to whether DBS activates or inhibits neurons. Early reports that STN stimulation caused a subsequent decreased activity of neurons in the SNr and the enteropeduncular nucleus (analogous to GPi), as well as VL thalamus in the anesthetized rat, led many to believe that stimulation may have a net inhibitory effect.[446–448] However, this conflicts with primate studies mentioned above.[455–457] One major difference in these studies is that in both primate studies data were collected during the stimulus train by using a spike sorter, whereas in the rat experiments data were collected after the stimulus and may not reflect the true concurrent effects of the electrical stimulation. Additionally, the anesthesia used in the rat model could have affected firing rates. Dostrovsky and colleagues used low current stimulation in GPi in order to record close to the stimulating electrode and found inhibition, and suggested that pallidal DBS causes excitation of inhibitory subthalamic axon terminals synapsing in GPi.[458] However, their stimulation was at a much lower intensity and frequency than that of DBS, and may not be comparable. In evidence of this, our data did not show net stimulation of GPi until stimulation reached therapeutic parameters.[453]

In summary, there is substantial evidence that DBS causes activation of fibers exiting the targeted structures (GPi, STN, or thalamus). More importantly, however, is that the pattern of activity in these pathways has been changed, replacing what may have been abnormal feedback loops with a less-disruptive, more regular pattern of activation. Therefore, the clinical effect of DBS may be similar to ablative therapy in that an abnormal pattern of activity is removed, allowing the cortex to process information in a more normal manner. For a review of this topic, see Johnson and colleagues.[459]

REFERENCES

1. Cooper IS. A review of surgical approaches to the treatment of parkinsonism. In Cooper IS (ed). Parkinsonism: Its Medical and Surgical Therapy. Springfield, IL: Charles C. Thomas, 1961, pp. 14–128.

2. Meyers R. Surgical interruption of the pallidofugal fibres: Its effect on the syndrome paralysis agitans and technical considerations in its application. N Y State J Med 1942;42:317–325.
3. Pollack LT, Davis L. Muscle tone in parkinsonian states. Arch Neurol Psychiat 1930;23:303–319.
4. Putnam TJ. Treatment of unilateral paralysis agitans by section of the lateral pyramidal tract. Arch Neurol Psychiatry 1940;44.
5. Foerster O, Gagel O. Die Vorderseitenstrangdurchschneidung beim Menschen. Ztschr ges Neurol u Psychiat 1932;138:1.
6. Delmas-Marsalat P, Van Bogaert L. Sur un cas de myoclonies rhythmique continues par une intervention chirurgicale sur le tronc cerebral. Rev Neurol 1935;64:728–740.
7. Bucy JC. Cortical extirpation in the treatment of involuntary movement. Arch Neurol Psychiatry 1942;21.
8. Meyers R. Surgical interruption of pallidofugal fibres: Its effect on the syndrome parlysis agitans and technical considerations in its application. N Y State J Med 1942;42:317–325.
9. Cooper IS. Ligation of the anterior choroidal artery for involuntary movements; parkinsonism. Psychiatr Q 1953;27(2):317–319.
10. Spiegel EA, et al. Stereotaxic apparatus for operations on the human brain. Science 1946;106:349–350.
11. Svennilson E, Torvik A, Lowe R, et al. Treatment of Parkinsonism by stereotactic thermolesions in the pallidal region: A clinical evaluation of 81 cases. Acta Psychiatr Neurol Scand 1960;35:358–377.
12. Crevier PH. [Various considerations on pallidotomy for relief of abnormal movements]. Union Med Can 1957;86(7):734–750.
13. Spiegel EA, Wycis HT, Baird HW, 3rd. Pallidotomy and pallido-amygdalotomy in certain types of convulsive disorders. Trans Am Neurol Assoc 1957;82nd Meeting:51–52; discussion 52–54.
14. Wycis HT,. Baird HW, Spiegel EA. Pallidotomy and pallido-amygdalotomy in certain types of convulsive disorders. Confin Neurol 1957;17(1):67–68.
15. Narabayashi H, et al. Procaine-oil-wax pallidotomy for double athetosis and spastic states in infantile cerebral palsy: Report of 80 cases. Neurology 1960;10:61–69.
16. Hassler R, Mundinger F, Reichert T. Stereotaxis in Parkinsonian Syndromes. Berlin: Springer-Verlag, 1979.
17. Alterman RL, et al. Stereotactic ventrolateral thalamotomy: Is ventriculography necessary? Neurosurgery 1995;37(4):717–721; discussion 721–722.
18. Goldman MS, Ahlskog JE, Kelly PJ. The symptomatic and functional outcome of stereotactic thalamotomy for medically intractable essential tremor. J Neurosurg 1992;76(6):924–928.
19. Goldman MS, Kelly PJ. Symptomatic and functional outcome of stereotactic ventralis lateralis thalamotomy for intention tremor. J Neurosurg 1992;77(2):223–229.
20. Goldman MS, Kelly PJ. Stereotactic thalamotomy for medically intractable essential tremor. Stereotact Funct Neurosurg 1992;58(1–4):22–25.
21. Hitchcock E, Flint GA, Gutowski NJ. Thalamotomy for movement disorders: A critical appraisal. Acta Neurochir Suppl (Wien) 1987;39:61–65.
22. Kelly PJ, et al. Computer-assisted stereotactic ventralis lateralis thalamotomy with microelectrode recording control in patients with Parkinson's disease. Mayo Clin Proc 1987;62(8):655–664.
23. Narabayashi H, Maeda T, Yokochi F. Long-term follow-up study of nucleus ventralis intermedius and ventrolateralis thalamotomy using a microelectrode technique in parkinsonism. Appl Neurophysiol 1987;50(1–6):330–337.
24. Pahwa R, Lyons KE, Wilkinson SB, et al. Comparison of thalamotomy to deep brain stimulation of the thalamus in essential tremor. Mov Disord 2001;16(1):140–143.
25. Tasker RR, Munz M, Junn FS, et al. Deep brain stimulation and thalamotomy for tremor compared. Acta Neurochir Suppl 1997;68:49–53.
26. Tasker RR. Deep brain stimulation is preferable to thalamotomy for tremor suppression. Surg Neurol 1998;49(2):145–153; discussion 153–154.
27. Lozano AM, Kumar R, Gross RE, et al. Globus pallidus internus pallidotomy for generalized dystonia. Mov Disord 1997;12(6):865–870.
28. Weetman J, Anderson IM, Gregory RP, Gill SS. Bilateral posteroventral pallidotomy for severe antipsychotic induced tardive dyskinesia and dystonia. J Neurol Neurosurg Psychiatry 1997;63(4):554–556.
29. Vitek JL, Bakay RA. The role of pallidotomy in Parkinson's disease and dystonia. Curr Opin Neurol 1997;10(4):332–339.
30. Laitinen LV, Bergenheim AT, Hariz MI. Ventroposterolateral pallidotomy can abolish all parkinsonian symptoms. Stereotact Funct Neurosurg 1992;58(1–4):14–21.
31. Laitinen LV, Bergenheim AT, Hariz MI. Leksell's posteroventral pallidotomy in the treatment of Parkinson's disease. J Neurosurg 1992;76(1):53–61.
32. Vitek JL, Bakay RA, DeLong MR. Microelectrode-guided pallidotomy for medically intractable Parkinson's disease. Adv Neurol 1997;74:183–198.
33. Baron MS, Vitek JL, Bakay RA, et al. Treatment of advanced Parkinson's disease by posterior GPi pallidotomy: 1-year results of a pilot study. Ann Neurol 1996;40(3):355–366.
34. Dogali M, Fazzini E, Kolodny E, et al. Stereotactic ventral pallidotomy for Parkinson's disease. Neurology 1995;45(4):753–761.
35. Lozano AM, Lang AE, Galvez-Jimenez N, et al. Effect of GPi pallidotomy on motor function in Parkinson's disease. Lancet 1995;346:1383–1387.
36. Vitek JL, Bakay RA, DeLong MR. Microelectrode-guided pallidotomy is an effective treatment for medically intractable Parkinson's disease. Neurology 1994;44(4):P703 (Abstract).
37. Sutton JP, Couldwell W, Lew MF, et al. Ventroposterior medial pallidotomy in patients with advanced Parkinson's disease. Neurosurgery 1995;36(6):1112–1116; discussion 1116–1117.
38. Vitek JL, Bakay RA, Freeman A, et al. Randomized trial of pallidotomy versus medical therapy for Parkinson's disease. Ann Neurol 2003;53(5):558–569.
39. de Bie RM, Schuurman PR, Bosch DA, et al. Outcome of unilateral pallidotomy in advanced Parkinson's disease: Cohort study of 32 patients. J Neurol Neurosurg Psychiatry 2001;71(3):375–382.

40. Hassler R, Riechert T, Mundinger F, et al. Physiological observations in stereotaxic operations in extrapyramidal motor disturbances. Brain 1960;83:337–349.
41. Ohye C, Kubota K, and Hooper HE Ventrolateral and subventrolateral thalamic stimulation. Arch Neurol 1964;11:427–434.
42. Benabid AL, Pollak P, Seigneuret E, et al. Chronic VIM thalamic stimulation in Parkinson's disease, essential tremor and extra-pyramidal dyskinesias. Acta Neurochir Suppl (Wien) 1993;58: 39–44.
43. Caparros-Lefebvre D, Blond S, Vermersch P, et al. Chronic thalamic stimulation improves tremor and levodopa induced dyskinesias in Parkinson's disease. J Neurol Neurosurg Psychiatry 1993;56(3):268–273.
44. Blond S, Caparros-Lefebvre D, Parker F, et al. Control of tremor and involuntary movement disorders by chronic stereotactic stimulation of the ventral intermediate thalamic nucleus. J Neurosurg 1992;77(1):62–68.
45. Benabid AL, Pollak P, Gervason C, et al. Long-term suppression of tremor by chronic stimulation of the ventral intermediate thalamic nucleus. Lancet 1991;337(8738): 403–406.
46. Blond S. and J. Siegfried. Thalamic stimulation for the treatment of tremor and other movement disorders. Acta Neurochir Suppl (Wien) 1991;52:109–111.
47. Benabid AL, Pollak P, Louveau A, et al. Combined (thalamotomy and stimulation) stereotactic surgery of the VIM thalamic nucleus for bilateral Parkinson disease. Appl Neurophysiol 1987;50(1–6):344–346.
48. Siegfried J, Lippitz B. Chronic electrical stimulation of the VL-VPL complex and of the pallidum in the treatment of movement disorders: Personal experience since 1982. Stereotact Funct Neurosurg 1994;62(1–4):71–75.
49. Gross C, Rougier A, Guehl D, et al. High-frequency stimulation of the globus pallidus internalis in Parkinson's disease: A study of seven cases. J Neurosurg 1997;87: 491–498.
50. Pahwa R, Wilkinson S, Smith D, et al. High-frequency stimulation of the globus pallidus for the treatment of Parkinson's disease. Neurology 1997;49(1):249–253.
51. Limousin P, Krack P, Pollak P, et al. Electrical stimulation of the subthalamic nucleus in advanced Parkinson's disease. N Engl J Med 1998;339(16):1105–1111.
52. Tsubokawa T, Katayama Y, Yamamoto T. Control of persistent hemiballismus by chronic thalamic stimulation. Report of two cases. J Neurosurg 1995;82(3): 501–505.
53. Islekel S, Zileli M Zileli B. Unilateral pallidal stimulation in cervical dystonia. Stereotact Funct Neurosurg 1999;72 (2–4):248–252.
54. Coubes P, Roubertie A, Vayssiere N, et al. Treatment of DYT1-generalised dystonia by stimulation of the internal globus pallidus. Lancet 2000;355(9222):2220–2221.
55. Coubes P, et al. Early onset generalised dystonia: Neurosurgical treatment by continuous bilateral stimulation of the internal globus pallidus in sixteen patients. Mov Disord 2000;15(suppl 3):S154.
56. Tisch S, Zrinzo L, Limousin P, et al. Effect of electrode contact location on clinical efficacy of pallidal deep brain stimulation in primary generalised dystonia. J Neurol Neurosurg Psychiatry. 2007;78(12):1314–1319.
57. Parr JR, Green AL, Joint C, et al. Deep brain stimulation in childhood: an effective treatment for early onset idiopathic generalised dystonia. Arch Dis Child. 2007;92(8): 708–711.
58. Cohen OS, Hassin-Baer S, Spiegelmann R. Deep brain stimulation of the internal globus pallidus for refractory tardive dystonia. Parkinsonism Relat Disord. 2007; 13(8):541–544.
59. Alterman RL, Shils JL, Miravite J, Tagliati M. Lower stimulation frequency can enhance tolerability and efficacy of pallidal deep brain stimulation for dystonia. Mov Disord 2007;22(3):366–368.
60. Zhang JG, Zhang K, Ma Y, Hu WH, et al. Follow-up of bilateral subthalamic deep brain stimulation for Parkinson's disease. Acta Neurochir Suppl 2006;99:43–47.
61. Krauss JK, Yianni J, Loher TJ, Aziz TZ. Deep brain stimulation for dystonia. J Clin Neurophysiol 2004;21(1): 18–30.
62. Lee JY, Deogaonkar M, Rezai A. Deep brain stimulation of globus pallidus internus for dystonia. Parkinsonism Relat Disord 2007;13(5):261–265.
63. Pahwa R, Lyons KE, Wilkinson SB, et al. Long-term evaluation of deep brain stimulation of the thalamus. J Neurosurg 2006;104(4):506–512.
64. Ondo WG. Essential tremor: Treatment options. Curr Treat Options Neurol 2006;8(3):256–267.
65. Lee JY, Kondziolka D. Thalamic deep brain stimulation for management of essential tremor. J Neurosurg 2005;103(3):400–403.
66. Putzke JD, Uitti RJ, Obwegeser AA, et al. Bilateral thalamic deep brain stimulation: Midline tremor control. J Neurol Neurosurg Psychiatry 2005;76(5):684–690.
67. Foote KD, Okun MS. Ventralis intermedius plus ventralis oralis anterior and posterior deep brain stimulation for posttraumatic Holmes tremor: Two leads may be better than one: Technical note. Neurosurgery 2005;56(2 suppl):E445; discussion E445.
68. Ushe M, Mink JW, Revilla FJ, et al. Effect of stimulation frequency on tremor suppression in essential tremor. Mov Disord 2004;19(10):1163–1168.
69. Putzke JD, Wharen RE Jr, et al. Thalamic deep brain stimulation for essential tremor: Recommendations for long-term outcome analysis. Can J Neurol Sci 2004;31(3):333–342.
70. Lyons KE, Pahwa R. Deep brain stimulation in Parkinson's disease. Curr Neurol Neurosci Rep 2004;4(4):290–295.
71. Kumar R, Lozano AM, Sime E, Lang AE. Long-term follow-up of thalamic deep brain stimulation for essential and parkinsonian tremor. Neurology 2003;61(11):1601–1604.
72. Murata J, Kitagawa M, Uesugi H, et al. Electrical stimulation of the posterior subthalamic area for the treatment of intractable proximal tremor. J Neurosurg 2003;99(4): 708–715.
73. Benabid AL, Benazzouz A, Hoffmann D, et al. Long-term electrical inhibition of deep brain targets in movement disorders. Mov Disord 1998;13(suppl 3):119–125.
74. Benabid AL, Pollak P, Gao D, et al. Chronic electrical stimulation of the ventralis intermedius nucleus of the thalamus as a treatment of movement disorders. J Neurosurg 1996;84(2):203–214.
75. Alesch F, Pinter MM, Helscher RJ, et al. Stimulation of the ventral intermediate thalamic nucleus in tremor domi-

nated Parkinson's disease and essential tremor. Acta Neurochir (Wien) 1995;136(1–2):75–81.

76. Benabid AL, Deuschl G, Lang AE, et al. Deep brain stimulation for Parkinson's disease. Mov Disord 2006;21(suppl 14): S168–S170.
77. Diallo R, Welter ML Mallet L [Therapeutic management of tics in Tourette's syndrome]. Rev Neurol (Paris) 2007;163(3):375–386.
78. Okun MS, Rodriguez RL, Mikos A, et al. Deep brain stimulation and the role of the neuropsychologist. Clin Neuropsychol 2007;21(1):162–189.
79. Mink JW, Walkup J, Frey KA, Como P, et al. Patient selection and assessment recommendations for deep brain stimulation in Tourette syndrome. Mov Disord 2006; 21(11):1831–1838.
80. Anderson TR, Hu B, Iremonger K, Kiss ZH. Selective attenuation of afferent synaptic transmission as a mechanism of thalamic deep brain stimulation-induced tremor arrest. J Neurosci 2006;26(3):841–850.
81. Skidmore FM, Rodriguez RL, Fernandez HH, et al. Lessons learned in deep brain stimulation for movement and neuropsychiatric disorders. CNS Spectr 2006;11(7): 521–536.
82. Visser-Vandewalle V, Ackermans L, van der Linden C. Deep brain stimulation in Gilles de la Tourette's syndrome. Neurosurgery 2006;58(3):E590.
83. Houeto JL, Karachi C, Mallet L, Pillon B, et al. Tourette's syndrome and deep brain stimulation. J Neurol Neurosurg Psychiatry 2005;76(7):992–995.
84. Gilbert DL, Lipps TD. Tourette's syndrome. Curr Treat Options Neurol 2005;7(3):211–219.
85. Kringelbach ML, Jenkinson N, Green AL, et al. Deep brain stimulation for chronic pain investigated with magnetoencephalography. Neuroreport 2007; 18(3): 223–228.
86. Rasche D, Rinaldi PC, Young RF, Tronnier VM. Deep brain stimulation for the treatment of various chronic pain syndromes. Neurosurg Focus 2006; 21(6):E8.
87. Coffey RJ, Lozano AM. Neurostimulation for chronic noncancer pain: An evaluation of the clinical evidence and recommendations for future trial designs. J Neurosurg 2006; 105(2):175–189.
88. Green AL, Nandi D, Armstrong G, Carter H, Aziz T. Postherpetic trigeminal neuralgia treated with deep brain stimulation. J Clin Neurosci 2003; 10(4):512–514.
89. Levy RM. Deep brain stimulation for the treatment of intractable pain. Neurosurg Clin N Am 2003; 14(3): 389–399, vi.
90. Bittar RG, Kar-Purkayastha I, Owen SL, et al. Deep brain stimulation for pain relief: A meta-analysis. J Clin Neurosci 2005; 12(5):515–519.
91. Sartorius A, Henn FA. Deep brain stimulation of the lateral habenula in treatment resistant major depression. Med Hypotheses. 2007;69(6):1305–1308.
92. Schlaepfer TE, Cohen MX, Frick C, et al. Deep brain stimulation to reward circuitry alleviates anhedonia in refractory major depression. Neuropsychopharmacology. 2008;33(2):368–377.
93. George MS, Nahas Z, Borckardt JJ, et al. Brain stimulation for the treatment of psychiatric disorders. Curr Opin Psychiatry 2007; 20(3):250–254; discussion 247–249.
94. Carpenter LL. Neurostimulation in resistant depression. J Psychopharmacol 2006;20(suppl 3):35–40.
95. Mayberg HS, Lozano AM, Voon V, et al. Deep brain stimulation for treatment-resistant depression. Neuron 2005; 45(5):651–660.
96. Greenberg BD, Malone DA, Friehs GM, et al. Three-year outcomes in deep brain stimulation for highly resistant obsessive-compulsive disorder. Neuropsychopharmacology 2006; 31(11):2384–2393.
97. Greenberg BD, Rezai AR. Mechanisms and the current state of deep brain stimulation in neuropsychiatry. CNS Spectr 2003;8(7):522–526.
98. Cosyns P, Gabriels L, Nuttin B. Deep brain stimulation in treatment refractory obsessive compulsive disorder. Verh K Acad Geneeskd Belg 2003;65(6):385–399; discussion 399–400.
99. Millet B, Jaafari N. [Treatment of obsessive-compulsive disorder]. Rev Prat 2007;57(1):53–57.
100. Kuhn J, Lenartz D, Mai JK, Huff W, et al. Deep brain stimulation of the nucleus accumbens and the internal capsule in therapeutically refractory Tourette-syndrome. J Neurol. 2007;254(7):963–965.
101. Wichmann T, Delong MR. Deep brain stimulation for neurologic and neuropsychiatric disorders. Neuron 2006;52(1):197–204.
102. DeLong MR. Primate models of movement disorders of basal ganglia origin. Trends Neurosci 1990;13:281–285.
103. Vitek JL, Wichmann T, DeLong MR. Current concepts of basal ganglia neurophysiology with respect to tremorgenesis. In Findley LJ, Koller W (eds). Handbook of Tremor Disorders. New York: Marcel Dekker, Inc., 1994, pp. 37–50.
104. Lamarre Y, Joffroy, AJ. Experimental tremor in monkey: Activity of thalamic and precentral cortical neurons in the absence of peripherial feedback. Adv Neurol 1979;24: 109–122.
105. Lamarre Y. Tremorogenic mechanisms in primates. Adv Neurol 1975;10:23–34.
106. Llinas RR. Rebound excitation as the physiological basis for tremor: A biophysical study of the oscillatory properties of mamalian central neurones in vitro. In Findley LJ, Capildeo R (eds). Movement Disorders: Tremor. New York: Oxford University Press, 1984.
107. Vilis T, Hore J. Central neural mechanisms contributing to cerebellar tremor produced by limb perturbations. J Neurophysiol 1980;43:279–291.
108. Hazrati LN, Parent A. Projection from the external pallidum to the reticular thalamic nucleus in the squirrel monkey. Brain Res 1991;550(1):142–146.
109. Vitek JL, Giroux M. Physiology of hypokinetic and hyperkinetic movement disorders: Model for dyskinesia. Ann Neurol 2000;47(4 suppl 1):S131–S140.
110. Ilinsky IA, Jouandet ML, Goldman-Rakic PS. Organization of the nigrothalamocortical system in the rhesus monkey. J Comp Neurol 1985;236:315–330.
111. Asanuma C, Thach WT, Jones EG. Distribution of cerebellar terminations and their relation to other afferent terminations in the ventral lateral thalamic region of the monkey. Brain Res 1983;286(3):237–265.
112. Asanuma C, Thach WR, Jones EG. Anatomical evidence for segregated focal groupings of efferent cells and their

terminal ramifications in the cerebellothalamic pathway of the monkey. Brain Res 1983;286(3):267–297.
113. Asanuma C, Thach WT, Jones EG. Cytoarchitectonic delineation of the ventral lateral thalamic region in the monkey. Brain Res Rev 1983;5:219–235.
114. DeVito JL, Anderson ME. An autoradiographic study of efferent connections of the globus pallidus in Macaca mulatta. Exp Brain Res 1982;46(1):107–117.
115. Schell GR, Strick PL. The origin of thalamic inputs to the arcuate premotor and supplementary motor areas. J Neurosci 1984;4:539–560.
116. Jones EG, Coulter JD, Burton H, Porter R. Cells of origin and terminal distribution of corticostriatal fibers arising in the sensory-motor cortex of monkeys. J Comp Neurol 1977;173:53–80.
117. Darian-Smith C, Darian-Smith I, Cheema SS. Thalamic projections to sensorimotor cortex in the macaque monkey: Use of multiple retrograde fluorescent tracers. J Comp Neurol 1990;299:17–46.
118. Harnois C, Filion M. Pallidofugal projections to thalamus and midbrain: A quantitative antidromic activation study in monkeys and cats. Exp Brain Res 1982;47(2):277–285.
119. Parent A, De Bellefeuille L. Organization of efferent projections from the internal segment of globus pallidus in primate as revealed by fluorescence retrograde labeling method. Brain Res 1982;245(2):201–213.
120. Hoover JE, Strick P L. Multiple output channels in the basal ganglia. Science 1993;259:819–821.
121. Jinnai K, Nambu A, Yoshida S, et al. The two separate neuron circuits through the basal ganglia concerning the preparatory or execution processes of motor control. In Mano N, Hamada I, DeLong MR (eds). Role of the Cerebellum and Basal Ganglia in Voluntary Movement. New York: Elsevier Science Publishers, 1985, pp. 153–161.
122. Tanji J. Comparison of neuronal activities in the monkey supplementary and precentral motor areas. Behav Brain Res 1985;18:137–142.
123. Tanji J, Kurata K. Contrasting neuronal activity in supplementary and precentral motor cortex of monkeys. I. Responses to instructions determining motor responses to forthcoming modalities. J Neurophysiol 1985;53:129–141.
124. Tanji J, Okano K Sato KC. Relation of neurons in the nonprimary motor cortex to bilateral hand movement. Nature 1987;327:618–620.
125. Wise SP, Godschalk M. Functional fractionation of frontal fields. Trends in Neuroscience 1987;10:449–450.
126. Narabayashi H, Yokochi F, Nakajima Y. Levodopa-induced dyskinesia and thalamotomy. J Neurol Neurosurg Psychiatry 1984;47:831–839.
127. Ohye, 1982C. Ohye, Depth microelectrode studies. In: G. Schaltenbrand and A.E. Walker, Editors, Stereotaxy of the Human Brain, Thieme, Stuttgart (1982) pp. 372–389.
128. Vitek JL, Bakay RA, Hashimoto T, et al. Microelectrode-guided pallidotomy: Technical approach and its application in medically intractable Parkinson's disease. J Neurosurg 1998;88(6):1027–1043.
129. Miller WC, DeLong MR. Altered tonic activity of neurons in the globus pallidus and subthalamic nucleus in the primate MPTP model of parkinsonism. In Carpenter MB, Jayaraman A (eds). The Basal Ganglia II. New York: Plenum Press, 1987, pp. 415–427.
130. Filion M, Tremblay L. Abnormal spontaneous activity of globus pallidus neurons in monkeys with MPTP-induced parkinsonism. Brain Res 1991;547:142–151.
131. Vitek JL, Kaneoke Y, Turner R. Neuronal activity in the internal (GPi) and external (GPe) segments of the globus pallidus (GP) of parkinsonian patients is similar to that in the MPTP-treated primate model of parkinsonism. Soc Neurosci 1993;19:561.
132. Vitek JL, Ashe J, Kaneoke Y. Spontaneous neuronal activity in the motor thalamus: Alteration in pattern and rate in parkinsonism. Neuroscience 1994;20(Pt 1):561 (#237.4).
133. Ceballos-Baumann AO, et al. Restoration of thalamocortical activity after posteroventral pallidotomy in Parkinson's disease. Lancet 1994;344(8925):814.
134. Narabayashi H. Tremor mechanisms. In Schaltenbrand G, Walker AE (eds). Stereotaxy of the Human Brain. Stuttgart: Thieme, 1982, pp. 510–514.
135. Hassler R, Dieckmann G. Stereotactic treatment of different kinds of spasmodic torticollis. Confinia Neurologica 1970;32:135–143.
136. Vitek JL, Chockkan V, Zhang JY, et al. Neuronal activity in the basal ganglia in patients with generalized dystonia and hemiballismus. Ann Neurol 1999;46(1):22–35.
137. Vitek JL, Zhang J, Evatt M, et al. GPi pallidotomy for dystonia: Clinical outcome and neuronal activity. Adv Neurol 1998;78:211–219.
138. Wichmann T, DeLong MR. Functional and pathophysiological models of the basal ganglia. Curr Opin Neurobiol 1996;6(6):751–758.
139. Levy R, Dostrovsky JO, Lang AE, et al. Effects of apomorphine on subthalamic nucleus and globus pallidus internus neurons in patients with Parkinson's disease. J Neurophysiol 2001;86(1):249–260.
140. Brown P. Oscillatory nature of human basal ganglia activity: Relationship to the pathophysiology of Parkinson's disease. Mov Disord 2003;18(4):357–363.
141. Tasker RR, Yamashiro K, Lenz F, Dostrovsky JO. Thalamotomy in Parkinson's disease: Microelectrode techniques. In Lundsford D (ed). Modern Stereotactic Surgery. Norwell, MA: Academic Press, 1988, pp. 297–313.
142. Kaneoke Y, Vitek JL. The motor thalamus in the parkinsonian primate: Enhanced burst and oscillatory activities. Neuroscience 1995;21(Pt 2):1428 (#560.5).
143. Nakaoka T. Experimental tremor produced by ventromedial tegmental lesion in monkeys. Neuroanatomical study. Appl Neurophysiol 1983;46(1–4):92–106.
144. Narabayashi H. Surgical approach to tremor. In Marsden CD (ed). Neurology 2: Movement Disorders. England: London, Butterworths and Company, 1982.
145. Ohye C, Nakamura R, Fukamachi A, et al. Recording and stimulation of the ventralis intermedius nucleus of the human thalamus. Conf Neurol 1975;37:258.
146. Ohye C, Narabayashi H. Physiological study of presumed ventralis intermedius neurons in the human thalamus. J Neurosurg 1979;50:290–297.
147. Hassler R, Mundinger F, Riechert T. Correlations between clinical and autoptic findings in stereotaxic operations of parkinsonism. Confin Neurol 1965;26(3): 282–290.
148. Hirai T, Miyazaki M, Nakajima H, et al. The correlation between tremor characteristics and the predicted volume

of effective lesions in stereotaxic nucleus ventralis intermedius thalamotomy. Brain 1983;106:1001–1018.
149. Lenz FA, Schnider S, Tasker RR, et al. The role of feedback in the tremor frequency activity of tremor cells in the ventral nuclear group of human thalamus. Acta Neurochir Suppl (Wien) 1987;39:54–56.
150. Narabayashi H. Tremor: Its generation mechanism and treatment. Handbook Clin Neurol 1986;5:597–607.
151. Lenz FA, Kwan HC, Martin RL, et al. Single unit analysis of the human ventral thalamic nuclear group Tremor-related activity in functionally identified cells. Brain 1994;117:531–543.
152. Asanuma C. Organization of the external pallidal projection upon the thalamic reticular nucleus in squirrel monkeys. Soc Neurosci 1994;20:332.
153. Hallanger AE, Levey AI, Lee HJ, et al. The origins of cholinergic and other subcortical afferents to the thalamus in the rat. J Comp Neurol 1987;262:105–124.
154. Levey AI, Hallanger AE and Wainer BH. Cholinergic nucleus basalis neurons may influence the cortex via the thalamus. Neurosci Lett 1987;b–74:7–13.
155. Paré D, Smith Y, Parent A, Steriade M. Projections of brainstem core cholinergic and non-cholinergic neurons of cat to intralaminar and reticular thalamic nuclei. Neuroscience 1988;25:69–86.
156. Steriade M, Paré D, Parent A, Smith Y. Projections of cholinergic and non-cholinergic neurons of the brainstem core to relay and associational thalamic nuclei in the cat and macaque monkey. Neuroscience 1988;25:47–67.
157. McCormick DA, Prince DA. Acetylcholine induces burst firing in thalamic reticular neurones by activating a potassium conductance. Nature 1986;a–319:402–405.
158. McCormick DA, Prince DA. Actions of acetylcholine in the guinea-pig and cat medial and lateral geniculate nuclei, in vitro. J Physiol 1987;392:147–165.
159. McCormick DA, Pape HC. Acetylcholine inhibits identified interneurons in the cat lateral geniculate nucleus. Nature 1988;334(6179):246–248.
160. McCormick DA. Cholinergic and noradrenergic modulation of thalamocortical processing. Trends Neurosci 1989;12(6):215–221.
161. Steriade M, Jones EG, Llinas RR. Thalamic Oscillations and Signaling. New York: Wiley Interscience, 1990.
162. Chan CS, Surmeier DJ, Yung WH. Striatal information signaling and integration in globus pallidus: Timing matters. Neurosignals 2005;14(6):281–289.
163. Morris G, Hershkovitz Y, Raz A, et al. Physiological studies of information processing in the normal and Parkinsonian basal ganglia: Pallidal activity in Go/No-Go task and following MPTP treatment. Prog Brain Res 2005;147: 285–293.
164. Rektor I, Bares M, Brázdil M, et al. Cognitive- and movement-related potentials recorded in the human basal ganglia. Mov Disord 2005;20(5):562–568.
165. Romanelli P, Esposito V, Schaal DW, Heit G. Somatotopy in the basal ganglia: Experimental and clinical evidence for segregated sensorimotor channels. Brain Res Brain Res Rev 2005;48(1):112–128.
166. Alexander GE, Crutcher MD. Functional architecture of basal ganglia circuits: Neural substrates of parallel processing. Trends Neurosci 1990;13(7):266–271.
167. Alexander GE, Crutcher MD, DeLong MR. Basal ganglia-thalamocortical circuits: Parallel substrates for motor, oculomotor, "prefrontal" and "limbic" functions. Prog Brain Res 1990;85:119–146.
168. Alexander GE, DeLong MR, Strick PL. Parallel organization of functionally segregated circuits linking basal ganglia and cortex. Annu Rev Neurosci 1986;9:357–381.
169. Parent A, Hazrati LN. Anatomical aspects of information processing in primate basal ganglia. Trends Neurosci 1993;16(3):111–116.
170. Parent A, Hazrati LN. Functional anatomy of the basal ganglia. I. The cortico-basal ganglia-thalamo-cortical loop. Brain Res Brain Res Rev 1995;20(1):91–127.
171. Parent A, Sato F, Wu Y, et al. Organization of the basal ganglia: The importance of axonal collateralization. Trends Neurosci 2000;23(10 suppl):S20–S27.
172. Fukuda M, Mentis MJ, Ma Y, Dhawan V, et al. Networks mediating the clinical effects of pallidal brain stimulation for Parkinson's disease: A PET study of resting-state glucose metabolism. Brain 2001;124(Pt 8):1601–1609.
173. Fukuda M, Mentis M, Ghilardi MF, et al. Functional correlates of pallidal stimulation for Parkinson's disease. Ann Neurol 2001;49(2):155–164.
174. Davis KD, Taub E, Houle S, et al. Globus pallidus stimulation activates the cortical motor system during alleviation of parkinsonian symptoms. Nat Med 1997;3(6): 671–674.
175. Okun MS, Vitek JL. Lesion therapy for Parkinson's disease and other movement disorders: Update and controversies. Mov Disord 2004;19(4):375–389.
176. Bakay RA, Starr PA, Vitek JL, DeLong MR. Posterior ventral pallidotomy: Techniques and theoretical considerations. Clin Neurosurg 1997;44:197–210.
177. Kumar R, Lang AE, Rodriguez-Oroz MC, et al. Deep brain stimulation of the globus pallidus pars interna in advanced Parkinson's disease. Neurology 2000;55(12 suppl 6):S34–S39.
178. Lee MS, Marsden CD. Movement disorders following lesions of the thalamus or subthalamic region. Mov Disord 1994;9:493–507.
179. Marsden CD, Obeso JA, Zarranz JJ, Lang AE. The anatomical basis of symptomatic hemidystonia. Brain 1985; 108:463–483.
180. Lenz F, Byl N, Garonzik I, Lee J, Hua S. Microelectrode studies of basal ganglia and VA, VL and VP thalamus in patients with dystonia: Dystonia-related activity and sensory reorganization. In Kultas-Ilinsky K, Ilinsky I (eds). Basal Ganlia and Thalamus in Health and Movement Disorders. New York: Kluwer Academic/Plenum Publishers, 2001, pp. 225–237.
181. Lenz FA, Jaeger CJ, Seike MS, et al. Thalamic single neuron activity in patients with dystonia: Dystonia-related activity and somatic sensory reorganization. J Neurophysiol 1999;82(5):2372–2392.
182. Lenz FA, Tasker RR, Kwan HC, et al. Cross-correlation analysis of thalamic neurons and EMG activity in parkinsonian tremor. Appl Neurophysiol 1985;48:305–308.
183. Lenz FA, Jaeger CJ, Seike MS, et al. Single-neuron analysis of human thalamus in patients with intention tremor and other clinical signs of cerebellar disease. J Neurophysiol 2002;87(4):2084–2094.

184. Vitek, JL, Ashe L, DeLong MR, Alexander GE. Altered somatosensory response properties of neurons in the 'motor' thalamus of MPTP treated parkinsonian monkeys. Soc Neurosci 1989;16:425.
185. Narabayashi H, Ohye C. Importance of microstereoencephalotomy for tremor alleviation. Appl Neurophysiol 1980;43:222–227.
186. Vilis T,. Hore J. Effects of changes in mechanical state of limb on cerebellar intention tremor. J Neurophysiol 1977;40:1214–1224.
187. Hore J, Flament D. Changes in motor cortex neural discharge associated with the development of cerebellar limb ataxia. J Neurophysiol 1988;60:1285–1302.
188. Narabayashi H. A consideration of intention tremor. In Ito M.(ed). Integrative Control Function of the Brain. Tokyo: Kodansha, 1979, pp. 185–187.
189. Llinas RR. The intrinsic electrophysiological properties of mammalian neurons: Insights into central nervous system function. Science 1988;242:1654–1664.
190. Carpenter MB, Whittier JR, Mettler FA. Analysis of choreoid hyperkinesia in the rhesus monkey: Surgical and pharmacological analysis of hyperkinesia resulting from lesions in the subthalamic nucleus of Luys. J Comp Neurol 1950;92:293–332.
191. Hamada I, DeLong MR. Excitotoxic acid lesions of the primate subthalamic nucleus result in reduced pallidal neuronal activity during active holding. J Neurophysiol 1992;68:1859–1866.
192. Hamada I, DeLong MR. Excitotoxic acid lesions of the primate subthalamic nucleus result in transient dyskinesias of the contralateral limbs. J Neurophysiol 1992;68:1850–1858.
193. Whittier JR, Mettler FA. Studies of subthalamus of the rhesus monkey. II. Hyperkinesia and other physiologic effects of subthalamic lesions with special reference to the subthalamic nucleus of Luys. J Comp Neurol 1949;90:319–372.
194. Martin JP. Hemichorea (hemiballismus) without lesions in the corpus luysii. Brain 1957;80:1–10.
195. Crossman AR, Mitchell IJ, Sambrook MA. Regional brain uptake of 2-deoxyglucose in N-methyl-4-phenyl-1,2,3,6-tetrahydropyridine (MPTP)-induced parkinsonism in the macaque monkey. Neuropharmacology 1985;24: 587–591.
196. Suarez JI, Metman LV, Reich SG, et al. Pallidotomy for hemiballismus: Efficacy and characteristics of neuronal activity. Ann Neurol 1997;42(5):807–811.
197. Guiot G. Le treatement des syndromes parkinsoniens par la destruction du pallidum interne. Neurochirurgie 1958;1:94–98.
198. Guiot G, Brion S. Traitement des mouvements anormaux par la coagulation pallidale. Technique et resultats. Rev Neurol (Paris) 1953;89:578–580.
199. Wiegell MR, Tuch DS, Larsson HB, Wedeen VJ. Automatic segmentation of thalamic nuclei from diffusion tensor magnetic resonance imaging. Neuroimage 2003;19(2 Pt 1):391–401.
200. Schaltenbrand G, Wahren W. Atlas for Stereotaxy of the Human Brain. Stuttgart: Thieme, 1977.
201. Rezai AR, Machado AG, Deogaonkar M, et al. Surgery for movement disorders. Neurosurgery 2008;62(suppl 2):809–838; discussion 838–839.
202. Rezai AR, Kopell BH, Gross RE, et al. Deep brain stimulation for Parkinson's disease: Surgical issues. Mov Disord 2006;21(suppl 14):S197–S218.
203. Andrade-Souza YM, Schwalb JM, Hamani C, et al. Comparison of three methods of targeting the subthalamic nucleus for chronic stimulation in Parkinson's disease. Neurosurgery 2005;56(2 suppl):360–368; discussion 360–368.
204. Starr PA, Christine CW, Theodosopoulos PV, et al. Implantation of deep brain stimulators into the subthalamic nucleus: Technical approach and magnetic resonance imaging-verified lead locations. J Neurosurg 2002;97(2): 370–387.
205. Bejjani BP, Dormont D, Pidoux B, Yelnik J, et al. Bilateral subthalamic stimulation for Parkinson's disease by using three-dimensional stereotactic magnetic resonance imaging and electrophysiological guidance. J Neurosurg 2000;92(4):615–625.
206. Guridi J, Rodriguez-Oroz MC, Lozano AM, et al. Targeting the basal ganglia for deep brain stimulation in Parkinson's disease. Neurology 2000;55(12 suppl 6):S21–S28.
207. Burchiel KJ, Nguyen TT, Coombs BD, Szumoski J. MRI distortion and stereotactic neurosurgery using the Cosman-Roberts-Wells and Leksell frames. Stereotact Funct Neurosurg 1996;66(1–3):123–136.
208. Liu X, Rowe J, Nandi D, et al. Localisation of the subthalamic nucleus using Radionics Image Fusion and Stereoplan combined with field potential recording. A technical note. Stereotact Funct Neurosurg 2001;76(2):63–73.
209. Duffner F, Schiffbauer H, Breit S, et al. Relevance of image fusion for target point determination in functional neurosurgery. Acta Neurochirurgica 2002;144(5):445–451.
210. Egidi M, Rampini P, Locatelli M, et al. Visualisation of the subthalamic nucleus: A multiple sequential image fusion (MuSIF) technique for direct stereotaxic localisation and postoperative control. Neurological Sciences 2002;23(suppl 2):S71–S72.
211. Kelly PJ, Derome P, Guiot G. Thalamic spatial variability and the surgical end results of lesions placed with neurophysiologic control. Surg Neurol 1978;9:307–315.
212. Starr PA, Vitek JL, DeLong M, Bakay RA. Magnetic resonance imaging-based stereotactic localization of the globus pallidus and subthalamic nucleus. Neurosurgery 1999;44(2):303–313; discussion 313–314.
213. Schaltenbrand G, Bailey P. Introduction to Stereotaxis with an Atlas of the Human Brain. New York: Grune & Stratton, Inc., 1959, Vol. II.
214. Vitek JL, Ashe J, DeLong MR, Alexander GE. Physiologic properties and somatotopic organization of the primate motor thalamus. J Neurophysiol 1994;71(4): 1498–513.
215. Hirai T, Jones EG. A new parcellation of the human thalamus on the basis of histochemical staining. Brain Res Rev 1989;14:1–34.
216. DeLong MR. Activity of pallidal neurons during movement. J Neurophysiol 1971;34:414–427.
217. DeLong MR, Alexander GE, Miller WC, Crutcher MD. Anatomical and functional aspects of basal ganglia-thalamocortical circuits. In Winslow W (ed). Studies in Neuroscience 1989; Manchester University Press: Manchester.
218. Bronte-Stewart H, et al. Lesion location predicts clinical outcome of pallidotomy. Mov Disord 1998;13(2):300.

219. Hutchison WD, Allan RJ, Opitz H, et al. Neurophysiological identification of the subthalamic nucleus in surgery for Parkinson's disease. Ann Neurol 1998;44(4): 622–628.
220. Sterio D, Zonenshayn M, Mogilner AY, et al. Neurophysiological refinement of subthalamic nucleus targeting. Neurosurgery 2002;50(1):58–67; discussion 67–69.
221. Benazzouz A, Breit S, Koudsie A, et al. Intraoperative microrecordings of the subthalamic nucleus in Parkinson's disease. Mov Disord 2002;17(suppl 3):S145–S149.
222. Wichmann T, Bergman H, DeLong MR. The primate subthalamic nucleus. I. Functional properties in intact animals. J Neurophysiol 1994;72(2):494–506.
223. Abosch A, Hutchison WD, Saint-Cyr JA, et al. Movement-related neurons of the subthalamic nucleus in patients with Parkinson disease. J Neurosurg 2002;97(5):1167–1172.
224. Rodriguez-Oroz MC, Rodriguez M, Guridi J, et al. The subthalamic nucleus in Parkinson's disease: Somatotopic organization and physiological characteristics. Brain 2001;124(Pt 9):1777–1790.
225. Selby G. Stereotactic surgery for the relief of Parkinson's disease. 1. A critical review. J Neurol Sci 1967;5(2): 315–342.
226. Speelman JD. Parkinson's Disease and Stereotaxic Surgery. Amsterdam: Rodorpi, 1991.
227. Vitek JL, Hashimoto T, Baron M. Lesion location related to outcome in microelectrode-guided pallidotomy. Ann Neurol 1994;36(2):279.
228. de Bie RM, Schuurman PR, de Haan PS, et al. Unilateral pallidotomy in Parkinson's disease: A randomised, single-blind, multicentre trial. Lancet 1999;354(9191):1665–1669.
229. Uitti RJ, Wharen RE Jr, Turk MF, et al. Unilateral pallidotomy for Parkinson's disease: Comparison of outcome in younger versus elderly patients. Neurology 1997;49(4):1072–1077.
230. Shannon KM, Penn RD, Kroin JS, et al. Stereotactic pallidotomy for the treatment of Parkinson's disease. Efficacy and adverse effects at 6 months in 26 patients. Neurology 1998;50(2):434–438.
231. Scott R, Gregory R, Hines N, Carroll C, et al. Neuropsychological, neurological and functional outcome following pallidotomy for Parkinson's disease. A consecutive series of eight simultaneous bilateral and twelve unilateral procedures. Brain 1998;121(Pt 4):659–675.
232. Samuel M, Caputo E, Brooks DJ, Schrag A, et al. A study of medial pallidotomy for Parkinson's disease: Clinical outcome, MRI location and complications. Brain 1998;121 (Pt 1):59–75.
233. Ondo WG, Jankovic J, Lai EC, Sankhla C, et al. Assessment of motor function after stereotactic pallidotomy. Neurology 1998;50(1):266–270.
234. Lang AE. Pallidal surgery: Pallidotomy vs. pallidal stimulaiton: Which to choose? In Teaching Courses of the American Academy Meeting. Saint Paul, MN: American Academy of Neurology, 1999.
235. Kopyov O, Jacques D, Duma C, Buckwalter G, et al. Microelectrode-guided posteroventral medial radiofrequency pallidotomy for Parkinson's disease. J Neurosurg 1997;87(1):52–59.
236. Giller CA, Dewey RB, Ginsburg MI, et al. Stereotactic pallidotomy and thalamotomy using individual variations of anatomic landmarks for localization. Neurosurgery 1998;42(1):56–62; discussion 62–65.
237. Kishore A, Turnbull IM, Snow BJ, de la Fuente-Fernandez R, et al. Efficacy, stability and predictors of outcome of pallidotomy for Parkinson's disease. Six-month follow-up with additional 1-year observations. Brain 1997;120(Pt 5):729–737.
238. Krack P, Poepping M, Weinert D, et al. Thalamic, pallidal, or subthalamic surgery for Parkinson's disease? J Neurol 2000;247(suppl 2):II122–II134.
239. Lang AE, Lozano AM, Montgomery E, et al. Posteroventral medial pallidotomy in advanced Parkinson's disease. N Engl J Med 1997;337(15):1036–1042.
240. Baron MS, Vitek JL, Bakay RA, Green J, et al. Treatment of advanced Parkinson's disease by unilateral posterior GPi pallidotomy: 4-year results of a pilot study. Mov Disord 2000;15(2):230–237.
241. Pal PK, Samii A, Kishore A, Schulzer M, et al. Long term outcome of unilateral pallidotomy: Follow up of 15 patients for 3 years. J Neurol Neurosurg Psychiatry 2000;69(3):337–344.
242. Lai EC, Jankovic J, Krauss JK, et al. Long-term efficacy of posteroventral pallidotomy in the treatment of Parkinson's disease. Neurology 2000;55(8):1218–1222.
243. Kondziolka D, Bonaroti E, Baser S, et al. Outcomes after stereotactically guided pallidotomy for advanced Parkinson's disease. J Neurosurg 1999;90(2):197–202.
244. Fazzini E, Dogali M, Sterio D, Eidelberg D, Berić A. Stereotactic pallidotomy for Parkinson's disease: A long-term follow-up of unilateral pallidotomy. Neurology 1997;48(5):1273–1277.
245. Samii A, Turnbull IM, Kishore A, et al. Reassessment of unilateral pallidotomy in Parkinson's disease. A 2-year follow-up study. Brain 1999;122(Pt 3):417–425.
246. Fine J, Duff J, Chen R, Chir B, et al. Long-term follow-up of unilateral pallidotomy in advanced Parkinson's disease. N Eng J Med 2000;342(23):1708–1714.
247. De Bie RM, Schuurman PR, Esselink RA, et al. Bilateral pallidotomy in Parkinson's disease: A retrospective study. Mov Disord 2002;17(3):533–538.
248. Favre J, Burchiel KJ, Taha JM, Hammerstad J. Outcome of unilateral and bilateral pallidotomy for Parkinson's disease: Patient assessment. Neurosurgery 2000;46(2): 344–353; discussion 353–355.
249. Intemann PM, Masterman D, Subramanian I, et al. Staged bilateral pallidotomy for treatment of Parkinson disease. J Neurosurg 2001;94(3):437–444.
250. Merello M, Starkstein S, Nouzeilles MI, et al. Bilateral pallidotomy for treatment of Parkinson's disease induced corticobulbar syndrome and psychic akinesia avoidable by globus pallidus lesion combined with contralateral stimulation. J Neurol Neurosurg Psychiatry 2001;71(5):611–614.
251. Green J, McDonald WM, Vitek JL, Haber M, et al. Neuropsychological and psychiatric sequelae of pallidotomy for PD: Clinical trial findings. Neurology 2002;58(6): 858–865.
252. Lombardi WJ, Gross RE, Trepanier LL, et al. Relationship of lesion location to cognitive outcome following microelectrode-guided pallidotomy for Parkinson's disease: Support for the existence of cognitive circuits in the human pallidum. Brain 2000;123(Pt 4):746–758.

253. Lang AE, Lozano A, Tasker R, et al. Neuropsychological and behavioral changes and weight gain after medial pallidotomy. Ann Neurol 1997;41(6):834–836.
254. Lim JY, De Salles AA, Bronstein J, Masterman DL, Saver JL. Delayed internal capsule infarctions following radiofrequency pallidotomy. Report of three cases. J Neurosurg 1997;87(6):955–960.
255. Biousse V, Newman NJ, Carroll C, et al. Visual fields in patients with posterior GPi pallidotomy. Neurology 1998; 50(1):258–265.
256. Bergman H, Wichmann T, DeLong MR. Reversal of experimental parkinsonism by lesions of the subthalamic nucleus. Science 1990;249:1436–1438.
257. Guridi J, Luquin MR, Herrero MT, Obeso JA. The subthalamic nucleus: a possible target for stereotaxic surgery in Parkinson's disease. Mov Disord. 1993;8(4):421–429.
258. Aziz TZ, Peggs D, Sambrook MA, Crossman AR. Lesion of the subthalamic nucleus for the alleviation of 1-methyl-4-phenyl-1,2,3,6-tetrahydropyridine (MPTP)-induced parkinsonism in the primate. Mov Disord 1991;6: 288–292.
259. Lang AE. Persistent hemiballismus with lesions outside the subthalamic nucleus. Can J Neurol Sci 1985;12:125–128.
260. Su PC, Tseng HT. Subthalamotomy for end-stage severe Parkinson's disease. Mov Disord 2002;17(3):625–627; author reply 627.
261. Su PC, Tseng HM, Liu HM, Yen RF, Liou HH. Subthalamotomy for advanced Parkinson disease. J Neurosurg 2002;97(3):598–606.
262. Alvarez L, Macias R, Guridi J, Lopez G, et al. Dorsal subthalamotomy for Parkinson's disease. Mov Disord 2001;16(1):72–78.
263. Gill SS, Heywood P. Bilateral dorsolateral subthalamotomy for advanced Parkinson's disease. Lancet 1997;350(9086):1224.
264. Su PC, Tseng HM, Liu HM, Yen RF, Liou HH. Treatment of advanced Parkinson's disease by subthalamotomy: One-year results. Mov Disord 2003;18(5):531–538.
265. Alvarez L, Macias R, Guridi J, et al. Bilateral dorsal subthalamotomy in Parkinson's disease (PD): Initial response and evolution after 2 years. Mov Disord 2002;17(suppl 5):S95.
266. Hubble JP, Busenbark KL, Wilkinson S, et al. Effects of thalamic deep brain stimulation based on tremor type and diagnosis. Mov Disord 1997;12(3):337–341.
267. Smith MC. Location of stereotatic lesions confirmed at necropsy. Br Med J. 1962;1(5282):900–906.
268. Ohye C. Functional organization of the human thalamus: Stereotactic interventions. In Steriade M, Jones EG, McCormick DA (eds). Thalamus Amsterdam: Elsevier, 1997, pp. 517–542.
269. Wester K, Hauglie-Hanssen E. Stereotaxic thalamotomy-experiences from the levodopa era. J Neurol Neurosurg Psychiatry 1990;53(5):427–430.
270. Matsumoto K, Shichijo F, Fukami T. Long-term follow-up review of cases of Parkinson's disease after unilateral or bilateral thalamotomy. J Neurosurg 1984;60(5): 1033–1044.
271. Krack P, Pollak P, Limousin P, Benazzouz A, Benabid AL. Stimulation of subthalamic nucleus alleviates tremor in Parkinson's disease. Lancet 1997;350(9092):1675.
272. Deep-Brain Stimulation for Parkinson's Disease Study Group. Deep-brain stimulation of the subthalamic nucleus or the pars interna of the globus pallidus in Parkinson's disease. N Engl J Med 2001;345(13):956–963.
273. Rodriguez-Oroz MC, Obeso JA, Lang AE, et al. Bilateral deep brain stimulation in Parkinson's disease: A multicentre study with 4 years follow-up. Brain 2005;128(Pt 10):2240–2249.
274. Ghika J, Villemure JG, Fankhauser H, et al. Efficiency and safety of bilateral contemporaneous pallidal stimulation (deep brain stimulation) in levodopa-responsive patients with Parkinson's disease with severe motor fluctuations: A 2-year follow-up review. J Neurosurg 1998;89(5):713–8.
275. Durif F, Lemaire JJ, Debilly B, Dordain G. Long-term follow-up of globus pallidus chronic stimulation in advanced Parkinson's disease. Mov Disord 2002;17(4): 803–807.
276. Volkmann J, Sturm V, Weiss P, et al. Bilateral high-frequency stimulation of the internal globus pallidus in advanced Parkinson's disease. Ann Neurol 1998;44(6): 953–961.
277. Krack P, Pollak P, Limousin P, Hoffmann D, et al. Opposite motor effects of pallidal stimulation in Parkinson's disease. Ann Neurol 1998;43(2):180–192.
278. Burchiel KJ, Anderson VC, Favre J, Hammerstad JP. Comparison of pallidal and subthalamic nucleus deep brain stimulation for advanced Parkinson's disease: Results of a randomized, blinded pilot study. Neurosurgery 1999;45(6):1375–1382; discussion 1382–1384.
279. Krack P, Pollak P, Limousin P, Hoffmann D, et al. Subthalamic nucleus or internal pallidal stimulation in young onset Parkinson's disease. Brain 1998;121(Pt 3):451–457.
280. Scotto di Luzio AE, Ammannati F, Marini P, et al. Which target for DBS in Parkinson's disease? Subthalamic nucleus versus globus pallidus internus. Neurological Sciences 2001;22(1):87–88.
281. Volkmann J, Allert N, Voges J, Weiss PH, et al. Safety and efficacy of pallidal or subthalamic nucleus stimulation in advanced PD. Neurology 2001;56(4):548–551.
282. Loher TJ, Burgunder JM, Pohle T, et al. Long-term pallidal deep brain stimulation in patients with advanced Parkinson disease: 1-year follow-up study. J Neurosurg 2002;96(5):844–853.
283. Loher TJ, Burgunder JM, Weber S, et al. Effect of chronic pallidal deep brain stimulation on off period dystonia and sensory symptoms in advanced Parkinson's disease. J Neurol Neurosurg Psychiatry 2002;73(4):395–399.
284. Sugiyama K, Yokoyama T, Namba H. Neurosurgical treatment for dopamine-induced dyskinesias in Parkinson's disease patients. Nippon Rinsho – Jap J Clin Med 2000;58(10):2115–2119.
285. Nutt JG, Rufener SL, Carter JH, et al. Interactions between deep brain stimulation and levodopa in Parkinson's disease. Neurology 2001;57(10):1835–1842.
286. Katayama Y. Deep brain stimulation(DBS) therapy for parkkinson,s disease. Nippon Rinsho – Jap J Clin Med 2000;58(10):2078–2083.
287. Defebvre LJ, Krystkowiak P, Blatt JL, et al. Influence of pallidal stimulation and levodopa on gait and preparatory postural adjustments in Parkinson's disease. Mov Disord 2002;17(1):76–83.

288. Krystkowiak P, Blatt JL, Bourriez JL, Duhamel A, et al. Chronic bilateral pallidal stimulation and levodopa do not improve gait in the same way in Parkinson's disease: A study using a video motion analysis system. J Neurol 2001;248(11):944–949.
289. Vitek JL. Deep brain stimulation for Parkinson's disease: A critical re-evaluation of STN versus GPi DBS. Stereotact Funct Neurosurg 2002;78:119–131.
290. Miyawaki E, Perlmutter JS, Tröster AI, et al. The behavioral complications of pallidal stimulation: A case report. Brain Cogn 2000;42(3):417–434.
291. Dujardin K, Krystkowiak P, Defebvre L, et al. A case of severe dysexecutive syndrome consecutive to chronic bilateral pallidal stimulation. Neuropsychologia 2000; 38(9):1305–1315.
292. Tröster AI, Fields JA, Wilkinson SB, et al. Unilateral pallidal stimulation for Parkinson's disease: Neurobehavioral functioning before and 3 months after electrode implantation. Neurology 1997;49(4):1078–1083.
293. Vingerhoets G, van der Linden C, Lannoo E, et al. Cognitive outcome after unilateral pallidal stimulation in Parkinson's Disease. J Neurol Neurosurg Psychiatry 1999; 66:297–304.
294. Romito LM, Scerrati M, Contarino MF, et al. Long-term follow up of subthalamic nucleus stimulation in Parkinson's disease. Neurology 2002;58(10):1546–1550.
295. Vingerhoets FJ, Villemure JG, Temperli P, et al. Subthalamic DBS replaces levodopa in Parkinson's disease: Two-year follow-up. Neurology 2002;58(3):396–401.
296. Krack P, Batir A, Van Blercom N, et al. Five-year follow-up of bilateral stimulation of the subthalamic nucleus in advanced Parkinson's disease. N Engl J Med 2003;349(20):1925–1934.
297. Limousin P, Pollak P, Benazzouz A, et al. Effect of parkinsonian signs and symptoms of bilateral subthalamic nucleus stimulation. Lancet 1995;345(8942):91–95.
298. Faist M, Xie J, Kurz D, Berger W, et al. Effect of bilateral subthalamic nucleus stimulation on gait in Parkinson's disease. Brain 2001;124(Pt 8):1590–1600.
299. Yokoyama T, Sugiyama K, Nishizawa S, et al. Subthalamic nucleus stimulation for gait disturbance in Parkinson's disease. Neurosurgery 1999;45(1):41–47; discussion 47–49.
300. Rizzone M, Ferrarin M, Pedotti A, et al. High-frequency electrical stimulation of the subthalamic nucleus in Parkinson's disease: Kinetic and kinematic gait analysis. Neurol Sci 2002;23 (suppl 2):S103–S104.
301. Allert N, Volkmann J, Sturm V, et al. Improvement of gait in Parkinson patients treated by bilateral stimulation of subthalamic nucleus or internal pallidum. [abstract]. Mov Disord 2000;15(suppl 3):51.
302. Krystkowiak P, Defebvre L, Blatt JL, et al. Influence of subthalamic nucleus stimulation on gait in Parkinson's disease: A study using the optoelectronic VICON system [abstract]. Mov Disord 2000;15(suppl 3):48.
303. Benabid AL, Benazzouz A, Limousin P, et al. Dyskinesias and the subthalamic nucleus. Ann Neurol 2000;47(4 suppl 1):S189–S192.
304. Albanese A, Nordera GP, Caraceni T, Moro E. Long-term ventralis intermedius thalamic stimulation for parkinsonian tremor. Italian Registry for Neuromodulation in Movement Disorders. Adv Neurol 1999;80:631–634.
305. Pollak P, Benabid AL, Gross C, et al. [Effects of the stimulation of the subthalamic nucleus in Parkinson disease]. Rev Neurol (Paris) 1993;149(3):175–176.
306. Limousin P, Pollak P, Benazzouz A, et al. Bilateral subthalamic nucleus stimulation for severe Parkinson's disease. Mov Disord 1995;10(5):672–674.
307. Krack P, Limousin P, Benabid AL, Pollak P. Chronic stimulation of subthalamic nucleus improves levodopa-induced dyskinesias in Parkinson's disease. Lancet 1997;350(9092):1676.
308. Benabid AL, Krack PP, Benazzouz A, et al. Deep brain stimulation of the subthalamic nucleus for Parkinson's disease: Methodologic aspects and clinical criteria. Neurology 2000;55(12 suppl 6):S40–S44.
309. Lyons KE, Davis JT, Pahwa R. Subthalamic Nucleus Stimulation in Parkinson's Disease Patients Intolerant to Levodopa. Stereotact Funct Neurosurg 2007;85(4): 169–174.
310. Vergani F, Landi A, Antonini A, Sganzerla EP. Bilateral subthalamic deep brain stimulation in a patient with Parkinson's disease who had previously undergone thalamotomy and autologous adrenal grafting in the caudate nucleus: Case report. Neurosurgery 2006;59(5):E1140; discussion E1140.
311. Hertel F, Züchner M, Weimar I, et al. Implantation of electrodes for deep brain stimulation of the subthalamic nucleus in advanced Parkinson's disease with the aid of intraoperative microrecording under general anesthesia. Neurosurgery 2006;59(5):E1138; discussion E1138.
312. Liang GS, Chou KL, Baltuch GH, et al. Long-term outcomes of bilateral subthalamic nucleus stimulation in patients with advanced Parkinson's disease. Stereotact Funct Neurosurg 2006;84(5–6):221–227.
313. Katayama Y, Oshima H, Kano T, et al. Direct effect of subthalamic nucleus stimulation on levodopa-induced peak-dose dyskinesia in patients with Parkinson's disease. Stereotact Funct Neurosurg 2006;84(4):176–179.
314. Parsons TD, Rogers SA, Braaten AJ, et al. Cognitive sequelae of subthalamic nucleus deep brain stimulation in Parkinson's disease: A meta-analysis. Lancet Neurol 2006;5(7):578–588.
315. Siderowf A, Jaggi JL, Xie SX, et al. Long-term effects of bilateral subthalamic nucleus stimulation on health-related quality of life in advanced Parkinson's disease. Mov Disord 2006;21(6):746–753.
316. Schüpbach WM, Chastan N, Welter ML, et al. Stimulation of the subthalamic nucleus in Parkinson's disease: A 5 year follow up. J Neurol Neurosurg Psychiatry 2005;76(12):1640–1644.
317. Erola T, Heikkinen ER, Haapaniemi T, et al. Efficacy of bilateral subthalamic nucleus (STN) stimulation in Parkinson's disease. Acta Neurochir (Wien) 2006;148(4):389–394.
318. Ostergaard K, Aa Sunde N. Evolution of Parkinson's disease during 4 years of bilateral deep brain stimulation of the subthalamic nucleus. Mov Disord 2006;21(5):624–631.
319. Pahwa R, Wilkinson SB, Overman J, Lyons KE. Preoperative clinical predictors of response to bilateral subthalamic stimulation in patients with Parkinson's disease. Stereotact Funct Neurosurg 2005;83(2–3):80–83.
320. Hamani C, Richter E, Schwalb JM, Lozano AM. Bilateral subthalamic nucleus stimulation for Parkinson's disease:

A systematic review of the clinical literature. Neurosurgery 2005;56(6):1313–1321; discussion 1321–1324.
321. Nilsson MH, Tornqvist AL, Rehncrona S. Deep-brain stimulation in the subthalamic nuclei improves balance performance in patients with Parkinson's disease, when tested without anti-parkinsonian medication. Acta Neurol Scand 2005;111(5):301–308.
322. Rodriguez-Oroz MC, Zamarbide I, Guridi J, et al. Efficacy of deep brain stimulation of the subthalamic nucleus in Parkinson's disease 4 years after surgery: Double blind and open label evaluation. J Neurol Neurosurg Psychiatry 2004;75(10):1382–1385.
323. Ford B, Winfield L, Pullman SL, Frucht SJ, et al. Subthalamic nucleus stimulation in advanced Parkinson's disease: Blinded assessments at one year follow up. J Neurol Neurosurg Psychiatry 2004;75(9):1255–1259.
324. Funkiewiez A, Ardouin C, Caputo E, et al. Long term effects of bilateral subthalamic nucleus stimulation on cognitive function, mood, and behaviour in Parkinson's disease. J Neurol Neurosurg Psychiatry 2004;75(6):834–839.
325. Cintas P, Simonetta-Moreau M, Ory F, et al. Deep brain stimulation for parkinson's disease: Correlation between intraoperative subthalamic nucleus neurophysiology and most effective contacts. Stereotact Funct Neurosurg 2003;80(1–4):108–113.
326. Romito LM, Scerrati M, Contarino MF, et al. Bilateral high frequency subthalamic stimulation in Parkinson's disease: Long-term neurological follow-up. J Neurosurg Sci 2003;47(3):119–128.
327. Welter ML, Houeto JL, Tezenas du Montcel S, et al. Clinical predictive factors of subthalamic stimulation in Parkinson's disease. Brain 2002;125(Pt 3):575–583.
328. Eriksen SK, Tuite PJ, Maxwell RE, et al. Bilateral subthalamic nucleus stimulation for the treatment of Parkinson's disease: Results of six patients. J Neurosci Nurs 2003;35(4):223–231.
329. Tavella A, Bergamasco B, Bosticco E, et al. Deep brain stimulation of the subthalamic nucleus in Parkinson's disease: Long-term follow-up. Neurol Sci 2002;23 (suppl 2):S111–S112.
330. Daniele A, Albanese A, Contarino MF, et al. Cognitive and behavioural effects of chronic stimulation of the subthalamic nucleus in patients with Parkinson's disease. J Neurol Neurosurg Psychiatry 2003;74(2):175–182.
331. Varma TR, Fox SH, Eldridge PR, et al. Deep brain stimulation of the subthalamic nucleus: Effectiveness in advanced Parkinson's disease patients previously reliant on apomorphine. J Neurol Neurosurg Psychiatry 2003;74(2):170–174.
332. Iansek R, Rosenfeld JV, Huxham FE, Deep brain stimulation of the subthalamic nucleus in Parkinson's disease. Med J Aust 2002. 177(3):142–146.
333. Vesper J, Klostermann F, Stockhammer F, et al. Results of chronic subthalamic nucleus stimulation for Parkinson's disease: A 1-year follow-up study. Surg Neurol 2002;57(5):306–311; discussion 311–313.
334. Schüpbach WM, Chastan N, Welter ML, et al. Deep-Brain Stimulation for Parkinson's Disease Study Group. Deep-brain stimulation of the subthalamic nucleus or the pars interna of the globus pallidus in Parkinson's disease. N Engl J Med 2001;345(13):956–963.
335. Lévesque MF, Taylor S, Rogers R, et al. Subthalamic stimulation in Parkinson's disease. Preliminary results. Stereotact Funct Neurosurg 1999;72(2–4):170–173.
336. Kleiner-Fisman G, Fisman DN, Sime E, et al. Long-term follow up of bilateral deep brain stimulation of the subthalamic nucleus in patients with advanced Parkinson disease. J Neurosurg 2003;99(3):489–495.
337. Visser-Vandewalle V, van der Linden C, Temel Y, et al. Long-term effects of bilateral subthalamic nucleus stimulation in advanced Parkinson disease: A four year follow-up study. Parkinsonism Relat Disord 2005;11(3):157–165.
338. Herzog J, Volkmann J, Krack P, et al. Two-year follow-up of subthalamic deep brain stimulation in Parkinson's disease. Mov Disord 2003;18(11):1332–1337.
339. Lang AE, Kleiner-Fisman G, Saint-Cyr JA, et al. Subthalamic DBS replaces levodopa in Parkinson's disease: Two-year follow-up. Neurology 2003;60(1):154–155; author reply 154–155.
340. Brown RG, Dowsey PL, Brown P, et al. Impact of deep brain stimulation on upper limb akinesia in Parkinson's disease. Ann Neurol 1999; 45(4):473–488.
341. Moro E, Scerrati M, Romito LM, Roselli R, et al. Chronic subthalamic nucleus stimulation reduces medication requirements in Prakinson's disease. Neurology 1999:53(1): 85–90.
342. Pinter MM, Alesch F, Murg M, et al. Deep brain stimulation of the subthalamic nucleus for control of extrapiramidal features in advnaced idiopathic parkinson's disease: One year follow-up. J Neural Transm 1999;106(7–8):693–709.
343. Fraix V, Pollak P, Van Blercom N, et al. Effect of subthalamic nucleus stimulation on levodopa-induced dyskinesia in Parkinson's disease. Neurology 2000;55(12):1921–1923.
344. Molinuevo JL, Valldeoriola F, Tolosa E, et al. Levodopa withdrawal alter bilateral subthalamic nucleus stimulation in advanced Parkinson disease. Arch Neurol 2000; 57(7):983–988.
345. Alegret M, Junqué C, Valldeoriola F, et al. Effects of bilateral subthalamic stimulation on cognitive function in Parkinson disease. Arch Neurol 2001;58(8):1223–1227.
346. Capus L, Melatini A, Zorzon M, Torre P, et al. Chronic bilateral electrical stimulation of the subthalamic nucleus for the treatment of advanced Parkinosn's disease. Neurol Sci 2001;22(1):57–58.
347. Lopiano L, Rizzone M, Bergamasco B, Tavella A, et al. Deep brain stimulation of the subthalamic nucleus: Clinical effectiveness and safety. Neurology 2001; 56(4):552–554.
348. Figueiras-Mendez R, Regidor I, Riva-Meana C, Magariños-Ascone CM. Further supporting evidence of beneficial subthalamic stimulation in Parkinson's patients. Neurology 2002;58(3):469–470.
349. Simuni T, Jaggi JL, Mulholland H, Hurtig HI, Colcher A, et al. Bilateral stimulation of the subthalamic nucleus in patients with Parkinson disease: A study of efficacy and safety. J Neurosurg 2002; 96(4):666–672.
350. Thobois S, Mertens P, Guenot M, Hermier M, et al. Subthalamic nucleus stimulation in Parkinson's disease: clinical evaluation of 18 patients. J Neurol 2002;249(5):529–534.
351. Alberts JL, Voelcker-Rehage C, Hallahan K, et al. Bilateral subthalamic stimulation impairs cognitive-motor performance in Parkinson's disease patients. Brain 2008;131(Pt 12):3348–3360.

352. Alberts JL, Hass CJ, Vitek JL, Okun MS. Are two leads always better than one: An emerging case for unilateral subthalamic deep brain stimulation in Parkinson's disease. Exp Neurol 2008.
353. Okun MS, Raju DV, Walter BL, et al. Pseudobulbar crying induced by stimulation in the region of the subthalamic nucleus. J Neurol Neurosurg Psychiatry 2004;75(6): 921–923.
354. Fields JA, Troster AI. Cognitive outcomes after deep brain stimulation for Parkinson's disease: A review of initial studies and recommendations for future research. Brain Cogn 2000;42(2):268–293.
355. Pillon B, Ardouin C, Damier P, Krack P, et al. Neuropsychological changes between "off" and "on" STN or GPi stimulation in Parkinson's disease. Neurology 2000;55(3):411–418.
356. Trépanier LL, Kumar R, Lozano AM, et al. Neuropsychological outcome of GPi pallidotomy and GPi or STN deep brain stimulation in Parkinson's disease. Brain Cogn 2000;42(3):324–347.
357. Woods SP, Fields JA, Lyons KE, et al. Neuropsychological and quality of life changes following unilateral thalamic deep brain stimulation in Parkinson's disease: A one-year follow-up. Acta Neurochir (Wien) 2001;143(12):1273–1277; discussion 1278.
358. Hariz MI. Complications of deep brain stimulation surgery. Mov Disord 2002;17 (suppl 3):S162–S166.
359. Woods SP, Fields JA, Troster AI. Neuropsychological sequelae of subthalamic nucleus deep brain stimulation in Parkinson's disease: A critical review. Neuropsychol Rev 2002;12(2):111–126.
360. Morrison CE, Borod JC, Perrine K, et al. Neuropsychological functioning following bilateral subthalamic nucleus stimulation in Parkinson's disease. Arch Clin Neuropsychol 2004;19(2):165–181.
361. Halbig D, Gruber U, Kopp G, et al. Pallidal stimulation in dystonia: Effects on cognition, mood, and quality of life. J Neurol Neurosurg Psychiatry 2005;76(12):1713–1716.
362. Castelli L, Perozzo P, Zibetti M, et al. Chronic deep brain stimulation of the subthalamic nucleus for Parkinson's disease: Effects on cognition, mood, anxiety and personality traits. Eur Neurol 2006;55(3):136–144.
363. Pillon B, Ardouin C, Dujardin K, et al. Preservation of cognitive function in dystonia treated by pallidal stimulation. Neurology 2006;66(10):1556–1558.
364. Voon V, Kubu C, Krack P, et al. Deep brain stimulation: Neuropsychological and neuropsychiatric issues. Mov Disord 2006;21 (suppl 14):S305–S327.
365. Aybek S, Gronchi-Perrin A, Berney A, et al. Long-term cognitive profile and incidence of dementia after STN-DBS in Parkinson's disease. Mov Disord. 2007;22(7):974–981.
366. Contarino MF, Daniele A, Sibilia AH, et al. Cognitive outcome 5 years after bilateral chronic stimulation of subthalamic nucleus in patients with Parkinson's disease. J Neurol Neurosurg Psychiatry 2007;78(3):248–252.
367. Pilitsis JG, Rezai AR, Boulis NM, et al. A preliminary study of transient confusional states following bilateral subthalamic stimulation for Parkinson's disease. Stereotact Funct Neurosurg 2005;83(2–3):67–70.
368. Okun MS, Green J, Saben R, et al. Mood changes with deep brain stimulation of STN and GPi: Results of a pilot study. J Neurol Neurosurg Psychiatry 2003;74(11): 1584–1586.
369. Krause M, Fogel W, Heck A, et al. Deep brain stimulation for the treatment of Parkinson's disease: Subthalamic nucleus versus globus pallidus internus. J Neurol Neurosurg Psychiatry 2001;70(4):464–470.
370. Mazzone P. Deep brain stimulation in Parkinson's disease: Bilateral implantation of globus pallidus and subthalamic nucleus. J Neurosurg Sci 2003;47(1):47–51.
371. Deuschl G, Fogel W, Hahne M, et al. Deep-brain stimulation for Parkinson's disease. J Neurol 2002;249 (suppl 3):III/36–39.
372. Peppe A, Pierantozzi M, Bassi A, et al. Stimulation of the subthalamic nucleus compared with the globus pallidus internus in patients with Parkinson disease. J Neurosurg 2004;101(2):195–200.
373. Anderson VC, Burchiel KJ, Hogarth P, et al. Pallidal vs subthalamic nucleus deep brain stimulation in Parkinson disease. Arch Neurol 2005. 62(4):554–560.
374. Nakamura K, Christine CW, Starr PA, Marks WJ Jr. Effects of unilateral subthalamic and pallidal deep brain stimulation on fine motor functions in Parkinson's disease. Mov Disord 2007. 22(5):619–626.
375. Alberts JL, Okun MS and Vitek JL. The persistent effects of unilateral pallidal and subthalamic deep brain stimulation on force control in advanced Parkinson's patients. Parkinsonism Relat Disord. 2008;14(6):481–488.
376. Volkmann J, Allert N, Voges J, et al. Long-term results of bilateral pallidal stimulation in Parkinson's disease. Ann Neurol 2004;55(6):871–875.
377. Deuschl G, Bain P. Deep brain stimulation for tremor [correction of trauma]: Patient selection and evaluation. Mov Disord 2002;17 (suppl 3):S102–S111.
378. Vitek JL, Ashe J, DeLong MR, Alexander GE. Physiologic properties and somatotopic organization of the primate motor thalamus. J Neurophysiol 1994;71:1498–1513.
379. Vitek JL, Ashe J, DeLong MR, Kaneoke Yl. Microstimulation of primate motor thalamus: Somatotopic organization and differential distribution of evoked motor responses among subnuclei [published erratum appears in J Neurophysiol 1997 Mar;77(3):1049]. J Neurophysiol 1996;75(6):2486–2495.
380. Lenz F, Dougherty P, Reich S. The effectiveness of thalamotomy for treatment of tremor and dystonia. Mov Disord 1996;11:18.
381. Bakay RAE, Vitek JL, DeLong MR. Thalamotomy for tremor. In Rengachary S, Wilkins R (eds). Neurosurgical Operative Atlas. Baltimore: Williams & Wilkins, 1992, pp. 299–312.
382. Miyamoto T, Bekku H, Moriyama E, Tsuchida S. Present role of stereotactic thalamotomy for parkinsonism: Retrospective analysis of operative results and thalamic lesions in computed tomograms. Appl Neurophysiol 1985;48:294–304.
383. Tasker RR. Tremor of parkinsonism and stereotactic thalamotomy. Mayo Clin Proc 1987;62:736–739.
384. Vaillancourt DE, Sturman MM, Verhagen Metman L, et al. Deep brain stimulation of the VIM thalamic nucleus modifies several features of essential tremor. Neurology 2003;61(7):919–925.
385. Lozano AM. Vim thalamic stimulation for tremor. Arch Med Res 2000;31(3):266–269.

386. Koller WC, Pahwa PR, Lyons KE, Wilkinson SB. Deep brain stimulation of the Vim nucleus of the thalamus for the treatment of tremor. Neurology 2000;55(12 suppl 6):S29–S33.
387. Kumar K, Kelly M, Toth C. Deep brain stimulation of the ventral intermediate nucleus of the thalamus for control of tremors in Parkinson's disease and essential tremor. Stereotact Funct Neurosurg 1999;72(1):47–61.
388. Koller WC, Lyons KE, Wilkinson SB, Pahwa R. Efficacy of unilateral deep brain stimulation of the VIM nucleus of the thalamus for essential head tremor. Mov Disord 1999;14(5):847–850.
389. Pfann KD, Penn RD, Shannon KM, et al. Effect of stimulation in the ventral intermediate nucleus of the thalamus on limb control in Parkinson's disease: A case study. Mov Disord 1996;11(3):311–316.
390. Shahzadi S, Tasker RR, Lozano A. Thalamotomy for essential and cerebellar tremor. Stereotact Funct Neurosurg 1995;65(1–4):11–17.
391. Obwegeser AA, Uitti RJ, Turk MF, et al. Thalamic stimulation for the treatment of midline tremors in essential tremor patients. Neurology 2000;54(12):2342–2344.
392. Pahwa R, Lyons KL, Wilkinson SB, et al. Bilateral thalamic stimulation for the treatment of essential tremor. Neurology 1999;53(7):1447–1450.
393. Koller W, Pahwa R, Busenbark K, et al. High-frequency unilateral thalamic stimulation in the treatment of essential and parkinsonian tremor. Ann Neurol 1997;42(3): 292–299.
394. Carpenter MA, Pahwa R, Miyawaki KL, et al. Reduction in voice tremor under thalamic stimulation. Neurology 1998;50(3):796–798.
395. Nagaseki Y, Shibazaki T, Hirai T, et al. Long-term follow-up results of selective VIM-thalamotomy. J Neurosurg 1986;65(3):296–302.
396. Ohye C, Hirai T, Miyazaki M, et al. Vim thalamotomy for the treatment of various kinds of tremor. Appl Neurophysiol 1982;45(3):275–280.
397. Zirh A, Reich SG, Dougherty PM, Lenz FA. Stereotactic thalamotomy in the treatment of essential tremor of the upper extremity: Reassessment including a blinded measure of outcome. J Neurol Neurosurg Psychiatry 1999;66(6):772–775.
398. Schuurman PR, Bosch DA, Bossuyt PM, et al. A comparison of continuous thalamic stimulation and thalamotomy for suppression of severe tremor. N Engl J Med 2000;342(7):461–468.
399. Bryant JA, De Salles A, Cabatan C, et al. The impact of thalamic stimulation on activities of daily living for essential tremor. Surg Neurol 2003;59(6):479–484; discussion 484–485.
400. Krauss JK, Simpson RK Jr, Ondo WG, et al. Concepts and methods in chronic thalamic stimulation for treatment of tremor: Technique and application. Neurosurgery 2001;48(3):535–541; discussion 541–543.
401. Limousin-Dowsey P. Thalamic stimulation in essential tremor. Lancet Neurol 2004;3(2):80.
402. Lyons KE, Pahwa R. Long-term benefits in quality of life provided by bilateral subthalamic stimulation in patients with Parkinson disease. J Neurosurg 2005;103(2): 252–255.
403. Koller WC, Lyons KE, Wilkinson SB, et al. Long-term safety and efficacy of unilateral deep brain stimulation of the thalamus in essential tremor. Mov Disord 2001;16(3):464–468.
404. Comella CL, Leurgans S, Wuu J, et al. Rating scales for dystonia: A multicenter assessment. Mov Disord 2003; 18(3):303–312.
405. Lindeboom R, Brans JW, Aramideh M, et al. Treatment of cervical dystonia: A comparison of measures for outcome assessment. Mov Disord 1998;13(4):706–712.
406. Tarsy D. Comparison of clinical rating scales in treatment of cervical dystonia with botulinum toxin. Mov Disord 1997; 12(1):100–102.
407. Cooper IS. 20-year followup study of the neurosurgical treatment of dystonia musculorum deformans. In Eldridge R, Fahn S (eds). Advances in Neurology. New York: Raven Press, 1976, pp. 423–452.
408. Cardoso F, Jankovic J, Grossman RG, Hamilton WJ. Outcome after stereotactic thalamotomy for dystonia and hemiballismus. Neurosurgery 1995;36(3):501–508.
409. Andrew J, Fowler CJ, Harrison MJ. Stereotaxic thalamotomy in 55 cases of dystonia. Brain 1983;106(Pt 4):981–1000.
410. Evatt M, Hashimoto T, Triche S, et al. Thalamotomy for dystonia using electrophysiolgic mapping. Third International dystonia Symposium, Abstracts, 1996.
411. von Essen C, Augustinsson LE, Lindqvist G. VOI thalamotomy in spasmodic torticollis. Appl Neurophysiol 1980;43(3–5):159–163.
412. Bertrand C, Molina-Negro P, Martinez SN Combined stereotactic and peripheral surgical approach for spasmodic torticollis. Appl Neurophysiol 1978;41(1–4):122–133.
413. Laitinen LV. CT-guided ablative stereotaxis without ventriculography. Appl Neurophysiol 1985;48(1–6):18–21.
414. Colbassani HJ, Jr, Wood JH, Management of spasmodic torticollis. Surg Neurol 1986;25(2):153–158.
415. Tasker RR, Doorly T, Yamashiro K. Thalamotomy in generalized dystonia. Adv Neurol 1988;50:615–631.
416. Tasker RR, Doorly T, Yamashiro K. Thalamotomy in generalized dystonia. In Fahn S, Marsden C, Calne D (eds). Advances in Neurology: Dystonia 2. New York: Raven Press, 1988, pp. 615–631.
417. Ondo WG, Desaloms JM, Jankovic J, et al. Pallidotomy for dystonia. Ann Neurol 1997;42:446 (abstract).
418. Vitek JL, Evatt ML, Zhang J, et al. Pallidotomy as a treatment for medically intractable dystonia. Ann Neurol 1997; 42(3):409.
419. Ondo WG, Desaloms JM, Jankovic J, Grossman RG. Pallidotomy for generalized dystonia. Mov Disord 1998;13(4): 693–698.
420. Blount J, Kondoh T, Ebner T, et al. Pallidotomy for the treatment of dystonia. Third International Dystonia Symposium Abstracts, October 9–11, 1996, p. 190.
421. Teive HA, Sá DS, Grande CV, et al. Bilateral pallidotomy for generalized dystonia. Arq Neuropsiquiatr 2001;59 (2–B):353–357.
422. Lin JJ, Lin SN, Chang DC. Pallidotomy and generalized dystonia. Mov Disord 1999;14(6):1057–1059.
423. Ondo WG, Desaloms JM. Pallidotomy and thalamotomy for dystonia. In Krauss JK, Jankovic J, Grossman RG (eds). Surgery for Parkinson's Disease and Movement Disorders. Philadelphia, PA: Lippincott Williams & Wilkins, 2001, pp. 299–306.

424. Iacono RP , Lonser RR , Ulloth JE , et al. Posteroventral pallidotomy in the treatment of primary and secondary dystonia. Third International Dystonia Symposium Abstracts, Miami, Florida, 1996, p. 37.
425. Pastor-Gómez J, Hernando-Requejo V, Luengo-Dos Santos A, et al. [Treatment of a case of generalised dystonia using subthalamic stimulation]. Rev Neurol 2003;37(6): 529–531.
426. Novak KE, Nenonene EK, Bernstein LP, et al. Successful bilateral subthalamic nucleus stimulation for segmental dystonia after unilateral pallidotomy. Stereotact Funct Neurosurg 2008;86(2):80–86.
427. Sun B, Chen S, Zhan S, Le W, Krahl SE. Subthalamic nucleus stimulation for primary dystonia and tardive dystonia. Acta Neurochir Suppl 2007;97(Pt 2):207–214.
428. Kleiner-Fisman G, Liang GS, Moberg PJ, et al. Subthalamic nucleus deep brain stimulation for severe idiopathic dystonia: Impact on severity, neuropsychological status, and quality of life. J Neurosurg 2007;107(1):29–36.
429. Zhang JG, Zhang K, Wang ZC, Ge M, Ma Y. Deep brain stimulation in the treatment of secondary dystonia. Chin Med J (Engl) 2006;119(24):2069–2074.
430. Zhang JG, Zhang K, Wang ZC. Deep brain stimulation in the treatment of tardive dystonia. Chin Med J (Engl) 2006;119(9):789–792.
431. Vercueil L, Pollak P, Fraix V, et al. Deep brain stimulation in the treatment of severe dystonia. J Neurol 2001; 248(8):695–700.
432. Vercueil L, Krack P, Pollak P. Results of deep brain stimulation for dystonia: A critical reappraisal. Mov Disord 2002;17 (suppl 3):S89–S93.
433. Trottenberg T, Volkmann J, Deuschl G, et al. Treatment of severe tardive dystonia with pallidal deep brain stimulation. Neurology 2005;64(2):344–346.
434. Trottenberg T, Paul G, Meissner W, et al. Pallidal and thalamic neurostimulation in severe tardive dystonia. J Neurol Neurosurg Psychiatry 2001;70(4):557–559.
435. Ghika J, Villemure JG, Miklossy J, et al. Postanoxic generalized dystonia improved by bilateral Voa thalamic deep brain stimulation. Neurology 2002;58(2):311–313.
436. Coubes P, Echenne B, Roubertie A, et al. Bilateral chronic electrical stimulation of the internal globus pallidus as a treatment of idiopathic dystonia in musculorum deformans: Case report. Stereotact Funct Neurosurg 1997;67:70.
437. Vidailhet M, Vercueil L, Houeto JL, et al. Bilateral deep-brain stimulation of the globus pallidus in primary generalized dystonia. N Engl J Med 2005;352(5):459–467.
438. Kupsch A, Benecke R, Müller J, et al. Pallidal deep-brain stimulation in primary generalized or segmental dystonia. N Engl J Med 2006;355(19):1978–1990.
439. Ristic A, Marinkovic J, Dragasevic N, et al. Long-term prognosis of vascular hemiballismus. Stroke 2002;33(8): 2109–2111.
440. Guridi J, Obeso J. The subthalamic nucleus, hemiballismus and Parkinson's disease: Reappraisal of a neurosurgical dogma. Brain 2001;124:5–19.
441. Suarez JI, Metman LV, Reich SG, et al. Pallidotomy for hemiballismus: Efficacy and characteristics of neuronal activity. Ann Neurol 1997;42(5):807–811.
442. Vitek JL, Kaneoke Y, Hashimoto T, et al. Neuronal activity in the pallidum of a patient with hemiballismus. American Neurological Association Abstract, Washington, DC, 1995, 120th Annual Meeting, pp. 38–39.
443. Jallo GI, Dogali M. Ventral intermediate thalamotomy for hemiballismus. Stereotactic Func Neurosurg 1995;65 (1–4):23–25.
444. Vidailhet M, Yelnik J, Lagrange C, et al. Bilateral pallidal deep brain stimulation for the treatment of patients with dystonia-choreoathetosis cerebral palsy: A prospective pilot study. Lancet Neurol 2009;8(8):709–717.
445. Sato K, Nakagawa E, Saito Y, et al. Hyperkinetic movement disorder in a child treated by globus pallidus stimulation. Brain Dev 2009;31(6):452–455.
446. Benabid A, Benazzous A, Pollak P. Mechanisms of deep brain stimulation. Mov Disord 2002;17(suppl 3):S73–S74.
447. Benazzouz A, Gao DM, Ni ZG, et al. Effect of high-frequency stimulation of the subthalamic nucleus on the neuronal activities of the substantia nigra pars reticulata and ventrolateral nucleus of the thalamus in the rat. Neuroscience 2000;99(2):289–295.
448. Benazzouz A, Hallett M. Mechanism of action of deep brain stimulation. Neurology 2000;55(12 suppl 6): S13–S16.
449. Xu W, Russo GS, Hashimoto T, et al. STN DBS differentially modulates neuronal activity in the pallidal and cerebellar receiving areas of the motor thalamus. In Movement Disorders Society Meeting. Chicago, IL: The Movement Disorders Society, 2008.
450. Hashimoto T, Elder CM, Okun MS, et al. Stimulation of the Subthalamic Nucleus Changes the Firing Pattern of Pallidal Neurons. J Neurosci 2003;23(5):1916–1923.
451. Grill WM, Snyder AN, Miocinovic S. Deep brain stimulation creates an informational lesion of the stimulated nucleus. Neuroreport 2004;15(7):1137–1140.
452. Grill W. Mechanisms of deep brain stimulation. In Neuromodulation: Defining the Future. Cleveland, OH: The Cleveland Clinic Foundation, 2001.
453. Vitek JL. Mechanisms of deep brain stimulation: Excitation or inhibition. Mov Disord 2002;17(suppl 3):S69–S72.
454. Anderson ME, Postupna N, Ruffo M. Effects of high-frequency stimulation in the internal globus pallidus on the activity of thalamic neurons in the awake monkey. J Neurophysiol 2003;89(2):1150–1160.
455. Windels F, Bruet N, Poupard A, et al. Influence of the frequency parameter on extracellular glutamate and gamma-aminobutyric acid in substantia nigra and globus pallidus during electrical stimulation of subthalamic nucleus in rats. J Neurosci Res 2003;72(2):259–267.
456. Jech R, Urgosík D, Tintera J, et al. Functional magnetic resonance imaging during deep brain stimulation: A pilot study in four patients with Parkinson's disease. Mov Disord 2001;16(6):1126–1132.
457. Jech R. Effects of deep brain stimulation of the STN and Vim nuclei in the resting state and during simple movement task. A functional MRI study at 1.5 Tesla. Mov Disord 2002;17(suppl 5):S173.
458. Dostrovsky JO, Levy R, Wu JP, et al. Microstimulation-induced inhibition of neuronal firing in human globus pallidus. J Neurophysiol 2000;84(1):570–574.
459. Johnson MD, Miocinovic S, McIntyre CC, Vitek JL. Mechanisms and targets of deep brain stimulation in movement disorders. Neurotherapeutics 2008;5(2):294–308.

CHAPTER 18

Parkinson's Disease Dementia: Features and Management

Murat Emre, Haşmet A. Hanağası, and David J. Burn

▶ INTRODUCTION

Cognitive changes and dementia in Parkinson's disease (PD) were largely ignored in early descriptions of the condition. These aspects, however, have become increasingly more recognized and highly relevant, as the life expectancy of patients has increased with modern treatments for motor problems, and better healthcare in general. Consequently, disorders of cognition, which tend to emerge in advanced age, have become more apparent. Over the past decade in particular, there has been greater attention to mental aspects of PD, with increasing research devoted to the epidemiology, clinical characteristics, underlying pathophysiology, and treatment of dementia in PD (PD-D). This chapter summarizes the features and management of dementia associated with PD.

▶ EPIDEMIOLOGY

Cognitive impairment can be detected at the time of diagnosis in PD if appropriate neuropsychological tests are administered, even though patients may not have subjective complaints. The presence of dementia at the onset of disease would preclude the diagnosis of PD by current definitions and would qualify the patient as having dementia with Lewy Bodies (DLB). In a community-based study in the United Kingdom, 36% of newly diagnosed patients were found to have cognitive impairment, [1] while 57% of this cohort developed cognitive deficits (described as frontostriatal or posterior cortical in type) within 3.5 (±0.7) years from disease onset. [2] In the Netherlands, 24% of newly presenting cases were reported to have varying degrees of cognitive impairment.[3]

Both prevalence and incidence of dementia are substantially increased in PD compared with age-matched controls. A meta-analysis of 27 earlier studies found a prevalence rate of 40%.[4] A more recent systematic review of 12 selected studies reported a point prevalence of 24–31%, it estimated that 3–4% of all dementias in the general population would be due to PD.[5]

Prevalence studies may not accurately reflect the true frequency of PD-D, as demented patients are unlikely to survive as long as nondemented PD cases. Incidence rates are thus more reliable, as they are prospective and relatively free of survival bias. The incidence rate of dementia was reported to be six times higher in PD compared with controls.[6] In the Sydney cohort 48% of surviving patients had developed dementia 15 years after the diagnosis,[7] the cumulative incidence had risen to 83% 20 years after the diagnosis.[8] Similarly, in a UK-based study, the cumulative incidence of dementia was 53% after 14 years.([9] Another study conducted in Norway reported that 78% of the patients had dementia at the 8-year follow-up, 26% of cases being demented already at baseline.[10] The 12-year cumulative incidence of dementia was also reported for this cohort: by the end of the follow-up period 60% of patients had developed dementia, the cumulative incidence steadily increasing with age and duration of PD.[11]

▶ RISK FACTORS

Old age at disease onset or at the time of evaluation, long disease duration, and atypical neurological features such as early autonomic failure, symmetrical disease presentation, and unsatisfactory response to dopaminergic treatment are associated with increased risk of developing PD-D.[12–14] Other studies indicate severe motor disability, low cognitive scores at baseline, early development of confusion, hallucinations or psychosis on dopaminergic medication, axial involvement including speech impairment and postural imbalance, presence of depression, smoking, and excessive daytime sleepiness as additional risk factors.[6,9,15–22] Rapid eye movement (REM), sleep behavior disorder (RBD) is frequently seen in PD and may be more frequent in patients who eventually develop dementia. In one study, the frequency of RBD was significantly higher in PD-D compared with a nondemented PD group; PD patients with RBD had a sixfold higher occurrence of dementia than those without RBD.[23]

Although a number of risk factors have been reported, three of them are consistently found across almost all studies: advanced age, motor phenotype, and baseline mental performance. Advanced age is the single most significant risk factor, both in cross-sectional and prospective studies: In a population-based cross-sectional survey the prevalence was zero in patients younger than 50 years as opposed to 69% older than 80 years.[13] Old age and severe motor symptoms are synergistic in predicting a poor prognosis: Patients with old age and severe disease had a 12-fold increased risk for incident dementia as compared with young patients with mild disease.[20] As younger patients with greater disease severity and older patients with less severe motor symptoms did not show a significantly increased risk, a combined effect of age and disease severity was assumed. A nontremor-dominant motor phenotype also predicts a greater risk for incident dementia in PD. In one prospective study of 40 PD patients, 25% of the 16 so-called postural instability-gait difficulty (PIGD) subtype developed dementia over 2 years, compared with none of the 18 tremor-dominant or six indeterminate phenotype cases.[24] Of note is that conversion from a tremor-dominant to a PIGD subtype is also a risk factor for a more rapid rate of cognitive decline and dementia.[25] Poor verbal fluency at baseline is significantly and independently associated with incident dementia,[26] as well as poor performance on verbal memory,[27] and the presence of subtle impairment in executive functions.[28] A prospective community-based study of incident PD cases determined that neuropsychological tasks with a more "posterior cortical" basis, including semantic fluency and ability to copy an intersecting pentagons figure, as well as a nontremor-dominant motor phenotype at baseline assessment were highly predictive of PD-D.[2]

▶ GENETICS OF PD-D

Carrying an apolipoprotein (Apo)E4 allele is the most frequent genetic risk factor for Alzheimer's disease (AD). In a meta-analysis of 22 eligible case-control studies, the ApoE2, but not the ApoE4 allele, was positively associated with sporadic PD.[29] The same association was also noted in a population-based study, the presence of at least one ApoE2 allele significantly increasing the risk of PD. In this study both ApoE2 and ApoE4 alleles appeared to increase the risk of PD-D; the risk of dementia for ApoE4 carriers was, however, not significantly different for subjects with or without PD, whereas ApoE2 strongly increased the risk of dementia in patients with PD.[30] No excess of AD was found among the relatives of patients with PD,[31] the risk of cognitive impairment or dementia was, however, higher in first-degree relatives of patients with PD compared with first-degree relatives of controls; the risk was notably greater in relatives of patients with onset of PD under age 67 years.[32]

Inherited genetic variation in the tau (*MAPT*) gene may influence rate of cognitive decline and the development of dementia in PD. The *MAPT* H1/H1 genotype has been associated with a greater rate of cognitive decline in 109 incident PD patients prospectively followed up over a 3.5-year period: 15% of H1/H1 homozygotes, but none of the H2 carriers developed dementia within the follow-up period.[33]

A significantly higher heterozygote frequency for mutations in the glucocerebrosidase (*GBA*) gene has been reported in PD and dementia with Lewy bodies (DLB) compared with control subjects. *GBA* mutations may exert a large effect on susceptibility for Lewy body disorders at the individual level, but they are associated with a modest (approximately 3%) population-attributable risk in individuals of European ancestry.[34] Up to half of the PD patients heterozygous for *GBA* mutations developed cognitive impairment later in their disease in one series.[35]

Familial forms of dementia associated with PD are rare. Such cases have mostly been associated with mutations in, or multiplication of, the α-synuclein (*SNCA*) gene, the protein product of which is a major component of LB. Altered expression of, or missense mutations in, the α-synuclein gene have been linked to early-onset familial PD, sometimes associated with dementia.[36–38] It seems that the age of onset of PD and the likelihood of dementia increase as the additional copies of the gene increase: dementia is rare in families with duplication of the gene, whereas triplication is frequently associated with dementia.[36,38–40] The additional copies of the gene result in an excess of wild-type α-synuclein protein, triplication leading to a doubling of α-synuclein expression.[38] Studies of monogenic forms of PD have not systematically reported the frequency of nonmotor symptoms, including dementia: for series of cases with *SNCA*, *LRRK-2*, *PINK-1*, or parkin mutations, the respective percentages of reports including nonmotor features are 18%, 31%, 40%, and 24% (Meike Kasten and Christine Klein, personal communication). In these, dementia has been reported in 5–26% of patients, with the highest frequency in *SNCA* mutations and multiplications (Meike Kasten and Christine Klein, personal communication). Clearly, these reports may be subject to significant bias, and currently the most parsimonious explanation is that the frequency of dementia in monogenic forms of PD does not appear to be higher, and indeed may be lower than in sporadic PD. Relatively younger age of patients, especially in recessive forms may be one reason for this observation.

▶ TABLE 18–1. **CLINICAL FEATURES OF DEMENTIA ASSOCIATED WITH PD**

I Core Features

1. Diagnosis of Parkinson's disease according to Queen Square Brain Bank criteria
2. A dementia syndrome with insidious onset and slow progression, developing within the context of established Parkinson's disease and diagnosed by history, clinical, and mental examination, defined as:
   - Impairment in more than one cognitive domain
   - Representing a decline from premorbid level
   - Deficits severe enough to impair daily life (social, occupational, or personal care), independent of the impairment ascribable to motor or autonomic symptoms

II Associated Clinical Features

1. **Cognitive features:**
   - Attention: Impaired. Impairment in spontaneous and focused attention, poor performance in attentional tasks; performance may fluctuate during the day and from day to day
   - Executive functions: Impaired. Impairment in tasks requiring initiation, planning, concept formation, rule finding, set shifting or set maintenance; impaired mental speed (bradyphrenia)
   - Visuospatial functions: Impaired. Impairment in tasks requiring visual-spatial orientation, perception, or construction
   - Memory: Impaired. Impairment in free recall of recent events or in tasks requiring learning new material, memory usually improves with cueing, recognition is usually better than free recall
   - Language: Core functions largely preserved. Word finding difficulties and impaired comprehension of complex sentences may be present
2. **Behavioral features:**
   - Apathy: decreased spontaneity; loss of motivation, interest, and effortful behavior
   - Changes in personality and mood including depressive features and anxiety
   - Hallucinations: mostly visual, usually complex, formed visions of people, animals or objects
   - Delusions: usually paranoid, such as infidelity, or phantom boarder (unwelcome guests living in the home) delusions
   - Excessive daytime sleepiness

III Features Which Do Not Exclude PD-D But Make the Diagnosis Uncertain

- Coexistence of any other abnormality which may by itself cause cognitive impairment, but judged not to be the cause of dementia, e.g. presence of relevant vascular disease in imaging
- Time interval between the development of motor and cognitive symptoms not known

IV Features Suggesting Other Conditions or Diseases as Cause of Mental Impairment, Which, When Present Make It Impossible to Reliably Diagnose PD-D

- Cognitive and behavioral symptoms appearing solely in the context of other conditions such as:
  Acute confusion due to
    a) systemic diseases or abnormalities
    b) drug intoxication
  Major Depression according to DSM IV
- Features compatible with "Probable Vascular dementia" criteria according to NINDS-AIREN (dementia in the context of cerebrovascular disease as indicated by focal signs in neurological exam such as hemiparesis, sensory deficits, and evidence of relevant cerebrovascular disease by brain imaging AND a relationship between the two as indicated by the presence of one or more of the following: onset of dementia within 3 months after a recognized stroke, abrupt deterioration in cognitive functions, and fluctuating, stepwise progression of cognitive deficits)

(Reproduced with permission from Emre et al., 2007)[42]

▶ CLINICAL FEATURES

In typical cases, dementia associated with PD can be best described as a dysexecutive syndrome with prominent impairment of attention and visuospatial functions, moderately impaired memory and a high neuropsychiatric symptom burden including apathy and psychosis.[41,42] Cognitive, behavioral, and other associated clinical features are summarized in Table 18–1 and are described in detail later.

COGNITIVE FEATURES

Cognitive impairment in nondemented PD patients has a similar profile to those fulfilling criteria for dementia, with quantitative rather than qualitative differences.

Most deficits are in executive functions, visuospatial functions, memory, and attention.[1,3,43] Transition from cognitive impairment to dementia is gradual, in terms of both symptom severity and temporal course. A diagnosis of dementia becomes justified once mental dysfunction is severe enough to impair daily life.

Impairment of attentional functions is an early and prominent feature of patients with PD-D.[44] Reaction time and vigilance are impaired, fluctuating attention is similar to those seen in patients with DLB.[45] PD-D patients are more apathetic and have more prominent cognitive slowing, compared with those with AD.[46] The magnitude of cognitive slowing is disproportionately higher as compared with the general level of cognitive performance.[47] Impaired attention is an important determinant of activities of daily living (ADL) in PD-D: the measure of vigilance and focused attention was the single strongest cognitive predictor of ADL status, matching the strength of the effect of motor function on ADL.[48]

Executive functions span a broad spectrum of abilities including the ability to plan, organize, and perform goal-directed behavior, insight, and foresight. Impairment in executive functions is one of the core features of PD-D. Deficits in executive functions have been demonstrated in diverse tasks assessing rule finding, problem solving, planning, set elaboration, set shifting, and set maintenance.[49] Using the Mattis Dementia Rating Scale, which is more sensitive for executive functions, PD-D patients have lower initiation, perseverance, and construction, but higher memory subscores.[50] Internally cued behavior is more impaired, hence patients have more difficulties when they have to develop their own pace and mental strategies, performance improves when external cues are provided. Deficits in executive functions occur early in the course of PD-D and are prominent throughout the disease course.[44,46,49,51] One particular aspect is insight, which is usually preserved in PD-D, in contrast to patients with AD, where deficits are usually denied.[22]

Working memory, explicit memory, involving both verbal and visual modalities, and implicit memory such as procedural learning can all be impaired in PD-D. Deficits in working memory are found early in the disease course.[52] The relative severity of memory impairment as compared with general level of cognitive deficits, and the profile of impairment differ from that seen in AD. Patients with PD-D have difficulties learning new material in tests of explicit memory, but these deficits are less severe than in AD.[16,53,54] In typical cases, the memory impairment is characterized by a deficit in free recall with preserved recognition, indicating that information is stored, but not readily accessed; when structured cues or multiple choices are provided, retrieval improves.[55–57] Memory scores in patients with PD-D were found to correlate with performance in executive function tests.[56] On the basis of this observation, it was suggested that impairment of memory in PD-D, at least to some extent, may be due to difficulties in internally built search strategies.[49] This contrasts with the limbic type of amnesia in AD, where both free recall as well as recognition are impaired, because of lack of storage of new information.

Impairment in visuospatial functions occurs early and is prominent in PD-D,[16,51,58]and is more severe that seen in AD patients with similar global dementia severity.[16,51] Patients with PD-D perform worse in all perceptual tests compared with AD, those with visual hallucinations tend to have worse visual perception than those without.[59] Visuospatial abilities such as abstraction and reasoning are more impaired in PD-D, whereas visuospatial memory tasks are worse in AD.[60] Deficits in visuospatial functions become more evident in more complex tasks, which require planning and sequencing of response or self-generation of strategies. These deficits may thus be, at least partly, because of problems in sequential organization of behavior[61] or in executive functions.[62,63]

Main language functions are largely preserved in PD-D as compared with AD,[51,64] and deficits usually consist of mild anomia. As a consequence, verbal fluency is impaired and may constitute the main deficit in the language domain in a given patient; it is usually more severe than that seen in AD.[16,51] In nondemented PD patients, verb generation is more impaired than generation of nouns, suggesting that deficits may affect representation of actions more than they do grammatical representation.[65] Ideomotor apraxia is not common in PD-D.[51]

Cognitive profiles in patients with PD-D, DLB, and AD have been directly compared in several studies, where gross similarities between PD-D and DLB were found, as opposed to consistent differences between these Lewy body dementias and AD. Key differences between PD-D and AD are a retrieval deficit type memory abnormality in PD-D as compared with storage type amnesia in AD, relative lack of language abnormalities, predominance of executive and visuospatial deficits, preserved insight, and more prominent fluctuations in PD-D as compared with AD.[22,46,50,57,59] Patients with PD-D and DLB perform significantly worse on attentional tasks, but better on memory tests than patients with AD. A comparison of 488 PDD patients with the same number of AD patients, recruited independently for clinical trials of rivastigmine, revealed that diagnosis was predicted from the cognitive profile with an overall accuracy of 75%. The main discriminating factors were poor performance of AD patients on tests of orientation and poor performance of PDD patients on the attentional tasks.[66]

BEHAVIORAL FEATURES

Prominent behavioral symptoms and changes in personality are characteristic of PD-D. In a recent large multicenter trial of rivastigmine, patients with PD-D were assessed at baseline for the presence of behavioral symptoms using the 10-item Neuropsychiatric Inventory

(NPI). At least one neuropsychiatric symptom was present in 89% of the patients, while 77% had two or more symptoms. With regard to severity, 64% had at least one symptom with a score of 4 or more, 60% of the caregivers reported at least one symptom to be of moderate to severe distress. The most common symptoms were depression (58%), apathy (54%), anxiety (49%), and hallucinations (44%).[67] Hallucinations and delusions may follow treatment with dopaminergic agents, but occur more frequently in PD patients with dementia.[68] When minor forms such as feeling of presence are included, hallucinations occur in 70% of patients with PD-D, as opposed to 25% of those with AD.[69] Delusional misidentification syndromes are found in 17% of PD-D patients, and are associated with hallucinations, and more severe memory and language deficits.[70] Depressive features are more common in PD-D than AD.[44,51] Subthreshold depression was found in 21% of 538 patients with PD-D and was associated with younger age, age at onset, and female gender, but not with severity of parkinsonism, cognition, or ADL functions.[71] In PD-D, apathy is common in the earlier stages while delusions increase with more severe motor and cognitive dysfunction.[68] In a longitudinal study, patients with PD-D were discriminated by the presence of cognitive fluctuations, visual and auditory hallucinations, depression, and sleep disturbance compared with patients with AD; these features were identical to those observed in DLB patients.[22]

MOTOR, AUTONOMIC, AND OTHER ASSOCIATED FEATURES

In PD-D patients, motor symptoms are frequently described as being more symmetrical with predominance of bradykinesia, rigidity, and postural instability. Such features are also correlated with more rapid cognitive decline,[72–75] whereas tremor dominance has been associated with relative preservation of mental status.[75] In a cross-sectional study, a "postural imbalance gait difficulty" subtype was overrepresented with 88% in patients with PD-D in contrast to 38% in nondemented patients.[76] PD patients with falls are more likely to have lower MMSE scores than those without falls and also more likely to have frank dementia.[77] L-dopa-responsiveness may diminish as cognitive impairment emerges, although this assertion is largely based on retrospective clinical data.[78,79] Mechanisms for relative loss of L-dopa response may include development of α-synuclein pathology in striatum,[80] and loss of striatal dopamine D_2 and D_3 receptors.[79,81] Alternatively, this might simply reflect the development or predominance of nondopaminergic features, such as postural instability.[19,76] Life-threatening neuroleptic sensitivity, similar to that seen in DLB, has also been reported in PD-D.[82]

Signs of autonomic dysregulation such as orthostatic and postprandial hypotension resulting in syncope and falls, bowel, and bladder dysfunction such as urinary incontinence and constipation, reduced heart rate variability predisposing to ventricular arrhythmias, and sexual dysfunction are frequent and may significantly contribute to disability in patients with PD-D.[83] In a comparative study, cardiovascular autonomic dysfunction was most frequent in patients with PD-D as compared with those with DLB, vascular dementia, and AD, with PD-D patients demonstrating consistent impairment of both parasympathetic and sympathetic function tests as compared with controls.[84]

RBD is common in PD-D. In some patients it can be an early indicator of incipient dementia and may antedate the onset of dementia for many years.[85,86] In nondemented patients with PD, only those with concomitant RBD had impaired performance on neuropsychological tests, specifically on measures of episodic verbal memory, executive function, and visuospatial and visuoperceptual processing.[87] Excessive daytime somnolence (EDS) and poor sleep quality are more common in patients with PD, PDD, and DLB as compared with AD. A PIGD phenotype predicts more frequent and severe EDS in PD-D patients, although this association may be lost during the course of the disease.[88]

▶ NEUROPATHOLOGICAL AND BIOCHEMICAL CORRELATES OF PD-D

The neuropathology of PD is covered extensively elsewhere in this book (see Chapter 19); hence, it will only be briefly mentioned here in the context of dementia. In general, PD-D may be characterized by variable combinations of degeneration in subcortical nuclei, the involvement of AD-type pathology and LB-type degeneration.[89] A key outstanding issue is the correlation of these pathological features with antemortem clinical data, with some studies suggesting a close correlation between dementia and synuclein pathology,[78,90–92] while others[93–96] have determined a closer association with Alzheimer-like changes. Ultimately, it is probably the topographic and temporal cell sequence of neuronal loss rather than protein aggregations that determine the clinical phenotype. Indeed, protein aggregation (i.e., accumulation of α-synuclein, β-amyloid) may be synergistic, with one protein promoting the aggregation of another,[78] although what these accumulations actually mean in terms of cellular function is unknown. Recent studies in which α-synuclein immunohistochemistry was used (a more sensitive method to detect LB) with concomitant assessment of AD-type changes revealed that dementia better correlates with LB, although AD-type pathology of variable extent (more plaques than tangles) is usually coexistent. Evidence from studies in families with α-synuclein gene duplications or triplications also supports a primary role for "dose-dependent" synuclein-based pathology in development of PD-D.

Subcortical cell loss may affect neurons projecting to areas involved in cognition,[97] or damage to subcortical structures involved in neuronal loops connecting with cortical areas, such as thalamic components of the limbic loop.[98] Dementia in PD usually develops later in the disease course and may be related to an ascending order of pathological changes, as suggested by Braak and colleagues.[99,100] Some support for this "bottom–up" is also provided by other studies.[101] PD patients with relatively long disease duration prior to dementia onset had lower levels of cortical choline acetyltransferase than those with a short disease duration before dementia onset, implying greater loss of ascending cholinergic projections. In contrast, a more "top–down" pathological process, with greater burden of cortical pathology in PD patients with a more malignant disease course and short time before dementia supervenes has also been described.[100,101] In a clinicopathological study, approximately 25% of the cases with dementia had severe neocortical Lewy body disease, more consistent with a "DLB-like" phenotype, but also with a high amyloid burden.[100] It is currently unknown which factors determine this clinical and pathological variability. Furthermore, a recent study found that around 55% of subjects with widespread α-synuclein pathology (Braak PD stages 5–6) lacked clinical signs of dementia or extrapyramidal signs antemortem.[102] It is unclear why these subjects appear to "tolerate" high levels of synuclein deposition without developing symptoms.

Biochemically, PD-D is associated with a profound cholinergic deficit. Although deficits in other ascending monoaminergic pathways (dopaminergic, serotoninergic, noradrenergic) have been reported, and they may all contribute to some aspects of mental dysfunction,[49] their association with dementia has not been as consistent as that found with changes in cholinergic markers. Loss of cholinergic cells in the nucleus basalis of Meynert (nbM) greater than that observed in AD occurs in patients with PD-D,[103,104] cholinacetyltransfarase (ChAT) activity is markedly decreased in the frontal cortex and nbM.[105] In a comparative study of AD, DLB, and PD, mean midfrontal ChAT activity was markedly reduced in PD and DLB when compared with normal controls and AD.[106] In contrast to AD, PD-D is also associated with neuronal loss in the pedunculopontine cholinergic nuclei that project to structures such as thalamus.[98] Using vesicular acetylcholine transporter as a marker of cholinergic integrity, [^{123}I] iodobenzovesamicol (IBVM) SPECT demonstrated reduction in IBVM binding in parietal and occipital cortices in nondemented PD patients, while demented PD cases have a more extensive decrease in cortical binding, similar to patients with early-onset AD.[107] Functional imaging studies with PET demonstrated that compared with controls mean cortical AChE activity was lowest in patients with PD-D, followed by patients with PD without dementia and AD patients with equal severity of dementia.[108] A subsequent study revealed that the degree of cortical cholinergic deficits correlated particularly well with typical cognitive deficits found in PD-D, for example, impaired performance on tests of attention and executive functions.[109]

CORRELATES IN NEUROIMAGING

Structural imaging with MRI can determine the pattern and rate of cerebral atrophy using voxel-based morphometry. There is frontal gray matter loss in PD[110] compared with control subjects and a nearly fourfold increased rate of whole-brain atrophy in PD-D compared with nondemented PD and controls.[111] Furthermore, rates of cerebral atrophy in PD correlate with global measures of cognitive decline in some,[112] but not all studies,[111] implying that MRI may be a useful technique in predicting preclinical onset of dementia in PD. In general, temporal lobe atrophy, including the hippocampus and parahippocampal gyrus may be more severe in AD patients, with more severe atrophy of the thalamus and occipital lobe in patients with PD-D.[110]

A review of SPECT studies performed in PD described that in PD-D, rCBF assessments often demonstrate frontal hypoperfusion or bilateral temporoparietal deficits.[113] Perfusion deficits in precuneus and inferior lateral parietal regions, areas associated with visual processing, have also been described in PD-D, compared with AD where perfusion deficits are found in a more anterior and inferior location.[114] Reduced metabolism in temporoparietal regions of patients with PD-D compared with PD is also observed in FDG-PET studies,[115] while PD-D and DLB patients demonstrate similar patterns of decreased metabolism in bilateral inferior and medial frontal lobes, and right parietal lobe.[116]

^{123}I meta-iodobenzylguanidine (^{123}I-MIBG) is an analogue of noradrenaline and may be used in conjunction with SPECT imaging to quantify postganglionic sympathetic cardiac innervation. The heart to mediastinum ratio (H:M ratio) is lower in PD compared with normal controls and also lower than in other akinetic-rigid syndromes such as multiple system atrophy and progressive supranuclear palsy.[117] This ratio is also lower in patients with DLB. Since in AD tracer uptake is expected to be normal, cardiac ^{123}I-MIBG can be used to distinguish between the Lewy body dementias and AD.[118]

The integrity of nigrostriatal dopaminergic terminals can be visualized using markers of dopamine transporter, such as ^{123}I-FP-CIT SPECT. Significant reductions were found in ^{123}I-FP-CIT binding in the caudate, anterior, and posterior putamens in subjects with DLB compared with those with AD and controls. Transporter loss in DLB was of similar magnitude to that seen in PD, the greatest loss in all three areas was seen in patients with PD-D.[119]

Thus, this method can be used to differentiate patients with DLB or PD-D from AD patients with extrapyramidal symptoms.[119]

In PET studies with the Pittsburgh B compound (11C-PIB), which binds to amyloid, mean cortical levels of amyloid were increased twofold in AD.[120] and by 60% in DLB.[121] In PD-D mean cortical amyloid load was not significantly elevated, although 20% of individuals showed an Alzheimer pattern of increased 11C-PIB uptake.[122] Whether cortical deposition of amyloid protein is a time-dependent process hence different in DLB and PD-D is, however, not known. Amyloid may play a greater role the shorter the time of onset of dementia in PD-D, a hypothesis supported by recent clinicopathological studies.[100,101]

▶ DIAGNOSIS OF PD-D

Until recently, a formal diagnosis of dementia in PD was based on *DSM IV* criteria, which are descriptive and fail to capture several of the core features of PD-D. The need for more specific criteria was recognized by the Movement Disorder Society, leading to an International Task Force, which published clinical diagnostic criteria for PD-D,[42] along with practical recommendations for diagnostic procedures.[123] Clinical features of PD-D are described in Table 18–1, diagnostic requirements for Probable and Possible PD-D, representing two levels of diagnostic certainity, are given in Table 18–2.

The diagnosis of PD-D is not always easy as there are several confounding factors, such as motor and speech dysfunction, which can make it difficult to judge if impairment in function is due primarily to cognitive deficits. Comorbidities such as depression, systemic disorders, and adverse events of drugs may also mimic dementia and need to be considered. The onset, course and pattern of behavioral and neuropsychological impairment and the clinical context within which these symptoms occur can be helpful in identifying dementia. In certain situations, for example, a new referral where the temporal sequence of events is unclear, presence of significant comorbid illness, or when the clinical course is atypical (e.g., a rapid onset of confusion) the differential may include vascular parkinsonism, AD with or without drug-induced parkinsonism, confusion, depression, and DLB. Use of appropriate neuropsychological tests, including those that assess attention, visuospatial, and executive functions as well as memory, a detailed history including a deliberate screening for features known to be associated with PD-D and a review of current medication, are the essential diagnostic tools.

Simple cognitive screening test batteries and scales specifically developed for PD have been published, including the Parkinson Neuropsychometric Dementia Assessment,[124] and Mini Mental Parkinson.[125] Among the more generic scales, the Montreal Cognitive Assessment (MoCA) is probably more suited to PD than MMSE, because executive functions are better represented in the former instrument. More elaborate assessments can be achieved using the SCOPA-COG,[126] PD-CRS,[127,] or Mattis Dementia Rating Scale, which is more time consuming.

▶ TABLE 18–2. DIAGNOSTIC CRITERIA FOR PD-D

Probable PD-D

A. Core features: Both must be present
B. Associated clinical features:
   - Typical profile of cognitive deficits including impairment in at least two of the four core cognitive domains (impaired attention which may fluctuate, impaired executive functions, impairment in visuospatial functions, and impaired free recall memory which usually improves with cueing)
   - The presence of at least one behavioral symptom (apathy, depressed or anxious mood, hallucinations, delusions, excessive daytime sleepiness) supports the diagnosis of Probable PD-D, lack of behavioral symptoms, however, does not exclude the diagnosis
C. None of the group III features present
D. None of the group IV features present

Possible PD-D

A. Core features: Both must be present
B. Associated clinical features:
   - Atypical profile of cognitive impairment in one or more domains, such as prominent or receptive-type (fluent) aphasia, or pure storage-failure type amnesia (memory does not improve with cueing or in recognition tasks) with preserved attention
   - Behavioral symptoms may or may not be present

OR

C. One or more of the group III features present
D. None of the group IV features present

(Reproduced with permission from Emre et al., 2007)[42]

▶ RELATION TO DLB

The clinical and pathological features of DLB and PD-D grossly overlap; clinically, the time course of the symptoms and presenting features differentiate these two disorders. The clinical and pathological overlap between these two conditions led to the assumption that they represent two disorders on the spectrum of LB-related dementias, with different temporal and spatial sequence of events, and hence different chronology of clinical symptoms.[128]

In research studies in which distinction is made between DLB and PD-D, it is proposed that a "12-month rule" between the onset of dementia and parkinsonism should be maintained .[129] There is, however, no solid clinical or pathological basis to stipulate a fixed time interval between the development of motor symptoms versus onset of dementia symptoms in differentiating PD-D from DLB. In fact, it is often difficult to determine retrospectively when in the course of the disease cognitive or behavioral changes emerged. Therefore, on the basis of an empirical and practical approach, it is suggested that the diagnosis of PD-D should be entertained when dementia develops following the diagnosis of idiopathic PD, whereas the diagnosis of DLB is warranted when the symptoms of dementia precedes or coincides with the development of motor symptoms.

TABLE 18–3. MANAGEMENT OF PD PATIENTS WITH DEMENTIA

1. Exclude other causes for mental dysfunction such as depression, systemic disorders, and adverse effects of medication
2. Specific treatment
   - Cholinesterase inhibitors such as rivastigmine, possibly donepezil
3. Nonspecific treatment
   - Evaluate the need for treatment
   - Atypical antipsychotics such as clozapine, or possibly quetiapine for psychosis
   - Antidepressants other than tricyclics for depressive features or sleep disturbances
   - Consider modafinil for excessive daytime sleepiness

▶ MANAGEMENT OF PATIENTS WITH PD-D

The management of patients with PD-D involves both pharmacological and nonpharmacolocigal interventions. The main nonpharmacological measures include education of the patient and the family about the disease, sufficient mental and physical activation, avoidance of aggravating factors such as undue sensory stimuli and inappropriate environmental factors. As a general rule, before a pharmacological intervention for dementia is implemented, other conditions that can trigger or aggravate mental dysfunction should be investigated. These include systemic abnormalities and diseases, depression, adverse events of antiparkinson medication and treatment for concomitant diseases. Those agents that can potentially cause mental dysfunction, such as anticholinergics, tricyclic antidepressants, and benzodiazepines should be discontinued. Once these are excluded or optimized, the need for pharmacological treatment, especially of behavioral symptoms, should be determined, on the basis of symptom frequency, severity, and burden. In principal, one drug should be introduced at a time with low doses and titrated up as needed. One should attempt to discontinue nonspecific treatment for behavioral symptoms, once sufficient symptom control is attained. The basic approach to management of patients with PD-D is described in Table 18–3.

SPECIFIC TREATMENT

Cholinesterase Inhibitors (ChE-I)

ChE-I inhibit the enzyme acetylcholinesterase, which breaks down acetylcholine released to the synaptic cleft from presynaptic terminals, thus terminating its postsynaptic action. This prolongs the synaptic residency time of acetylcholine and enhances cholinergic transmission. After becoming available for the treatment of AD and establishment of cholinergic deficits in PD-D, all available ChE-Is have been tested in this population. The earlier trials were mostly in the form of open-label or small randomized, placebo-controlled studies. A review of these studies demonstrated that, although not having sufficient power, there was a consistent pattern, suggesting benefits on cognitive and behavioral symptoms, worsening of motor symptoms such as increased tremor occurred only in a small proportion of cases.[130] These preliminary findings prompted the initiation of large-scale studies, one with rivastigmine and the other with donepezil.

Rivastigmine

The first large, randomized, placebo-controlled, double-blind study in patients with PD-D was performed with rivastigmine, which inhibits both acetyl-cholinesterase as well as butyryl-cholinesterase.[131] In this multicenter study (EXPRESS), 541 patients with mild to moderate PD-D received either rivastigmine up to 12 mg day or placebo over 24 weeks. Primary efficacy parameters included Alzheimer Disease Assessment Scale-cognitive part (ADAS-cog) as a composite measure of cognitive function, and Alzheimer Disease Collaborative Study-Clinical Global Impression of Change scale (ADCS-CGIC) to assess global change from baseline. Both primary end points showed statistically significant improvements in favor of rivastigmine. On the ADAS-cog, patients on rivastigmine showed a 2.1 improvement at week 24, whereas patients on placebo deteriorated by 0.7 points ($p < 0.001$). On the ADCS-CGIC, more patients on rivastigmine showed any degree of improvement (40.8% versus 29.7% on placebo) and more patients on placebo had deteriorated (42.5% on placebo versus33.7% on rivastigmine) ($p = 0.007$). Likewise, all secondary efficacy measures demonstrated statistically significant differences in favor of rivastigmine, including neuropsychiatric symptoms as assessed by NPI, Ten-Point Clock Drawing test, verbal fluency, computerized attention tests, and MMSE. The ADL scores showed a minimal worsening in patients on rivastigmine, whereas those on placebo did significantly more so. Adverse events were more frequent in the rivastigmine group, mainly related to gastrointestinal system (29.0% versus 11.2% nausea, and 16.6% versus 1.7% vomiting on rivastigmine and placebo, respectively). Worsening of parkinsonian symptoms was also more frequently reported as an adverse event on rivastigmine (27.3% versus 15.6% on placebo), basically driven by worsening of tremor (10.2% on rivastigmine versus 3.9% on placebo), whereas the change in UPDRS motor score from baseline did not reveal any significant differences between the two treatments. Premature discontinuations due to adverse events were more frequent under rivastigmine (17.1% versus 7.8% under placebo). During a 6-month extension phase, where all patients received rivastigmine, the beneficial effects seen during the first 6 months were largely preserved, although there was some decline from the initial improvement, but no evidence of worsening motor function over the course of one year treatment.[132] A comparison of patients who had visual hallucinations at baseline with those who did not showed that hallucinators did derive greater benefits in cognitive outcomes, although this was mainly driven by a more rapid decline from baseline in the hallucinating group.[133] An analysis of rivastigmine's effects on various aspects of attention as assessed by a computerized test battery revealed that all aspects of attention (including focused attention, sustained attention, consistence of responding, and central processing speed) improved with rivastigmine treatment.[134]

On the basis of the EXPRESS study, rivastigmine was granted a marketing approval for treatment of patients with mild to moderate PD-D, both in the European Union and the United States, becoming the first specific treatment for this condition. A patch form of rivastigmine has also become available, and this has been approved for PD-D in several countries.

Donepezil

An initial small placebo-controlled, crossover study in patients with PD-D[135] suggested beneficial effects of donepezil on mental functions. Subsequently a randomized, double-blind, placebo-controlled study was conducted in a large PD-D population[136] This was a 24-week study, which recruited 550 patients with mild to moderate PD-D (MMSE range 10–26), and randomized into three groups to receive either placebo, donepezil 5 mg, or donepezil 10 mg. The primary efficacy parameters were ADAS-cog and an overall measure of change from baseline, the Clinician Interview-Based Impression of Change-plus (CIBIC-plus). At week 24, there was a 0.3 point improvement in ADAS-cog with placebo, 2.45 point improvement with 5 mg, and 3.72 point improvement with 10 mg of donepezil. The difference between placebo and donepezil groups did not reach statistical significance in the primary analysis of efficacy, although a type II weighted analysis and omission of country interaction did result in significance ($p < 0.001$). The CIBIC-plus showed statistically significant superiority for the 10 mg, but the 5 mg dose of donepezil. Significant differences in favor of donepezil were also found on a number of secondary end points, the MMSE, Brief Test of Attention and Verbal Fluency Test, whereas there were no significant differences from placebo on activities of daily living (using the Disability Assessment for Dementia scale) or NPI score. UPDRS III scores did not indicate significant worsening of motor function on donepezil. In an open-label study, the effects of donepezil on central processing speed and other attentional measures have been evaluated over 20 weeks of treatment. As compared with baseline, power of attention, continuity of attention, and reaction time variability all improved with donepezil.[137]

Galantamine

Open-label studies have suggested that galantamine has beneficial effects in patients with PD-D.[130] In a placebo-controlled, randomized, double-blind trial of galantamine 16–24 mg, in 69 nondemented PD patients over 16 weeks, there were no beneficial effects on any of the cognitive functions assessed, while there was a high and significant drop-out rate in the galantamine group due to gastrointestinal side effects and self reported worsening of PD symptoms.[138]

In summary, ChE-Is are efficacious in PD-D in randomized trials, although questions remain regarding clinical significance of the benefits in a given patient, which patients might derive greatest benefit, and cost-effectiveness. In a Cochrane meta-analysis evaluating the efficacy of ChE-Is, 5.3% of PD-D patients showed benefits on outcome scales, whereas 10.1% patients on placebo demonstrated worsening, suggesting that the clinically meaningful effect size for treatment of PD-D with these agents approaches 15%.[139]

Other Neurotransmitter-Based Treatments

The effects of dopaminergic treatment on mental functions have mostly been studied in nondemented patients. In one of the few studies that specifically included demented patients, subjects with PD, PD-D and DLB were tested for cognitive functions and behavioral symptoms after acute L-dopa challenge and followed for 3 months on treatment. Following acute challenge patients reported improvement in subjective alertness, but fluctuations increased; reaction time and accuracy remained unchanged in those with PD-D. After 3 months, neuropsychiatric scores improved both in PD and PD-D, mean global cognitive score was better, but attention and memory scores were worse in PD patients without dementia, reaction time became slower in those with PD-D, but no patient demonstrated marked deterioration.[140] In a study of 19 patients with DLB, motor benefit (defined as >10% improvement over baseline UPDRS Part III score) occurred in only one-third of subjects, whereas worsened hallucinations or psychosis developed in one-third. Considering motor benefit without exacerbation of psychosis was the therapeutic objective in this study, only four DLB subjects (22%) achieved this goal.[141]

In an 8-week open-label study, the norepinephrine reuptake inhibitor atomoxetine was tested in 12 patients with PD and disabling executive dysfunction. Executive dysfunction improved, on the basis of global change scores, behavioral measures of executive function, and a measure of recognition memory.[142] Further randomized trials are required to determine whether norepinephrinergic agents have a role in PD-D.

There is only scarce data on the effects of the *N*-methly-D-aspartate (NMDA) antagonist memantine in PD-D. In a small case series, good tolerability and possible benefits have been suggested.[143] A large, randomized, controlled trial with memantine in patients with PD-D and DLB is currently being conducted. Interestingly, the related NMDA antagonist amantadine has been reported to delay the onset of dementia in PD and to attenuate its severity,[144] although given the retrospective nonrandomized nature of the study these results should be interpreted with caution.

NONSPECIFIC TREATMENT OF BEHAVIORAL SYMPTOMS

Neuropsychiatric symptoms such as psychosis, depression, and sleep–wake cycle disturbances are frequent in patients with PD-D, at times they may constitute a more significant problem than cognitive impairment. Visual hallucinations may improve with ChE-I drugs, and these agents should therefore probably be considered first in PD-D patients with hallucinations. Neuroleptic treatment, however, may sometimes become necessary, especially in patients with florid psychosis or severe agitation. Classical neuroleptics are contraindicated as they worsen motor function and may result in life-threatening neuroleptic hypersensitivity. Specific studies of new generation ("atypical") neuroleptics in PD-D patients are few, most of those mentioned later were performed in PD patients with hallucinations or psychosis, without indicating the presence or absence of dementia. In a systematic review of atypical neuroleptics for the treatment of psychosis in PD, clozapine was concluded to be the only drug with proven efficacy and acceptable tolerability provided appropriate safety monitoring is performed.[145] Olanzapine does not improve psychosis and may worsen motor function,[146] while risperidone is also associated with worsening extrapyramidal symptoms.[147] In two studies that included patients with PD-D, one open label[148] and the other placebo–controlled,[149] quetiapine did not show significant benefits in treating agitation or psychosis, although it did not worsen motor function. In a retrospective analysis of all PD patients receiving quetiapine, more quetiapine nonresponders were demented and motor worsening also tended to occur more frequently in demented patients.[150]

There have been no randomized, controlled studies of antidepressants in patients with PD-D. In a meta-analysis of antidepressants in PD patients with depression, large effect sizes were seen both under active treatment and placebo, but no statistically significant differences were found between them; increasing age and major depression predicted better response.[151] In another systematic review, amitriptyline was reported to be the only compound with evidence of efficacy in PD depression.[152] Tricyclic antidepressants such as amitriptyline, however, should not be administered in patients with PD-D, because of their anticholinergic effects and their potential to worsen cognition. Selective serotonin, or mixed serotonin and noradrenalin reuptake inhibitors should therefore be the preferred choice in PD-D, taking into account their adverse effects and potential interaction with other medication such as MAO-B inhibitors. Antidepressants with sedating properties can also be considered to treat nighttime sleep disturbances. In case RBD is a source of significant distress very low doses of clonazepam may be used, induction of daytime sedation, however, should be monitored.

Disturbances of sleep–wake cycle are common in patients with PD-D. Excessive daytime sleepiness (EDS) is frequent, it occurs more frequently than in nondemented PD patients. Modafinil, an agent that promotes wakefulness, was significantly better than placebo in treating EDS in nondemented PD patients in two small randomized, placebo-controlled and one open-label study,[153–155] although no difference was found in another small, placebo-controlled trial.[156] The drug was well tolerated in all studies. Modafinil has not been tested in PD-D.

▶ CONCLUSIONS

Cognitive impairment and dementia are an integral part of the disease spectrum in PD. Dementia affects approximately one-third of patients in cross-sectional studies, it develops in up to 85% of patients 20 years after diagnosis and has a major impact on quality of life. The typical profile of dementia in PD is a dysexecutive syndrome with prominent impairment of attention and visuospatial functions, relatively milder impairment of memory and frequent association of behavioral symptoms such as apathy, psychosis, and depressive features. Currently there is no treatment capable of halting or reversing the disease pathology, and symptomatic treatment approaches are based on rectifying neurotransmitter deficits. The most prominent biochemical deficits are cholinergic, and treatment with ChE-I drugs can provide mild to moderate benefits in cognitive and behavioral symptoms without undue worsening in motor functions. There remains an urgent need to evaluate and develop new symptomatic drug treatments in PD dementia, while the "holy grail" remains the introduction of disease modifying therapies.

REFERENCES

1. Foltynie T, Brayne CEG, Robbins TW, et al. The cognitive ability of an incident cohort of Parkinson's patients in the UK. The CamPaIGN study. Brain 2004;127: 1–11.
2. Williams-Gray CH, Foltynie T, Brayne CE, et al. Evolution of cognitive dysfunction in an incident Parkinson's disease cohort. Brain 2007;130:1787–1798.
3. Muslimovic D, Post B, Speelman JD, Cognitive profile of patients with newly diagnosed Parkinson disease. Neurology 2005;65:1239–1245.
4. Cummings JL. Intellectual impairment in Parkinson's disease: clinical, pathologic, and biochemical correlates. J Geriatr Psychiatry Neurol 1988;1:24–36.
5. Aarsland D, Zaccai J, and Brayne C. A systematic review of prevalence studies of dementia in Parkinson's disease. Mov Disord 2005;20:1255–1263.
6. Aarsland D, Andersen K, Larsen JP, et al. Risk of dementia in Parkinson's disease: A community-based, prospective study. Neurology 2001;56:730–736.
7. Hely MA, Morris JG, Reid WG, et al. Sydney Multicenter Study of Parkinson's disease: Non-L-dopa-responsive problems dominate at 15 years. Mov Disord 2005;20: 190–199.
8. Hely MA, Reid WG, Adena MA, et al. The Sydney multicenter study of Parkinson's disease: the inevitability of dementia at 20 years. Mov Disord 2008;23:837–844.
9. Read N, Hughes TA, Dunn EM, et al. Dementia in Parkinson's disease: incidence and associated factors at 14-years of follow up. Parkinsonism and Related Disord 2001;7(suppl):S109.
10. Aarsland D, Andersen K, Larsen JP, et al. Prevalence and characteristics of dementia in Parkinson disease: An 8-year prospective study. Arch Neurol 2003;60:387–392.
11. Buter TC, van den Hout A, Matthews FE, et al. Dementia and survival in Parkinson disease. A 12-year population study. Neurology 2008;70:1017–1022.
12. Mayeux R, Stern Y, Rosenstein R, et al. An estimate of the prevalence of dementia in idiopathic Parkinson's disease. Arch Neurol 1988;45:260–262.
13. Mayeux R, Denaro J, Hemenegildo N, et al. A population-based investigation of Parkinson's disease with and without dementia. Relationship to age and gender. Arch Neurol 1992;49:492–497.
14. Aarsland D, Tandberg E, Larsen JP, et al. Frequency of dementia in Parkinson disease. Arch Neurol 1996;53: 538–542.
15. Starkstein SE, Mayberg HS, Leiguarda R, et al. A prospective longitudinal study of depression, cognitive decline, and physical impairments in patients with Parkinson's disease. J Neurol Neurosurg Psychiatry 1992;55:377–382.
16. Stern Y, Marder K, Tang MX, et al. Antecedent clinical features associated with dementia in Parkinson's disease. Neurology 1993;43:1690–1692.
17. Marder K, Tang MX, Cote L, et al. The frequency and associated risk factors for dementia in patients with Parkinson's disease. Arch Neurol 1995;52:695–701.
18. Goetz CG, Vogel C, Tanner CM, et al. Early dopaminergic drug-induced hallucinations in parkinsonian patients. Neurology 1998;51:811–814.
19. Levy G, Tang MX, Cote LJ, et al. Motor impairment in PD: relationship to incident dementia and age. Neurology 2000;55:539–544.
20. Levy G, Schupf N, Tang MX, et al. Combined effect of age and severity on the risk of dementia in Parkinson's disease. Ann Neurol 2002;51:722–729.
21. Gjerstad MD, Aarsland D, and Larsen JP. Development of daytime somnolence over time in Parkinson's disease. Neurology 2002;58:1544–1546.
22. Galvin JE, Pollack J, and Morris JC. Clinical phenotype of Parkinson disease dementia. Neurology 2006;67: 1605–1611.
23. Marion MH, Qurashi M, Marshall G, et al. Is REM sleep behaviour disorder (RBD) a risk factor of dementia in idiopathic Parkinson's disease? J Neurol 2008;255:192–196.
24. Burn DJ, Rowan EN, Allan LM, et al. Motor subtype and cognitive decline in Lewy body disease. A two-year longitudinal study J Neurol Neurosurg Psychiatry 2006;77: 585–589.
25. Alves G, Larsen JP, Emre M, et al. Changes in motor subtype and risk for incident dementia in Parkinson's disease. Mov Disord 2006;21:1123–1130.
26. Jacobs DM, Marder K, Cote LJ, et al. Neuropsychological characteristics of preclinical dementia in Parkinson's disease. Neurology 1995;45:1691–1696.
27. Levy G, Tang MX, Cote LJ, et al. Do risk factors for Alzheimer's disease predict dementia in Parkinson's disease? An exploratory study. Mov Disord 2002;17: 250–257.
28. Woods SP and Troster AI. Prodromal frontal/executive dysfunction predicts incident dementia in Parkinson's disease. J Int Neuropsychol Soc 2003;9:17–24.
29. Huang X, Chen PC, and Poole C. APOE-epsilon2 allele associated with higher prevalence of sporadic Parkinson disease. Neurology 2004;62:2198–2202.
30. Harhangi BS, de Rijk MC, van Duijn CM et al. APOE and the risk of PD with or without dementia in a population-based study. Neurology 2000;54:1272–1276.
31. Levy G, Louis ED, Mejia-Santana H, et al. Lack of familial aggregation of Parkinson disease and Alzheimer disease. Arch Neurol 2004;61:1033–1039.
32. Rocca WA, Bower JH, Ahlskog JE, et al. Risk of cognitive impairment or dementia in relatives of patients with Parkinson disease. Arch Neurol 2007;64:458–1464.
33. Goris A, Williams-Gray CH, Clark GR, et al. Common variation in tau and alpha synuclein genes influences risk of developing idiopathic Parkinson disease and related cognitive impairment. Ann Neurol 2007;62:145–153.

34. Mata IF, Samii A, Schneer SH, et al. Glucocerebrosidase gene mutations: a risk factor for Lewy body disorders. Arch Neurol 2008;65:379–382.
35. Goker-Alpan O, Lopez G, Vithayathil J, et al. The spectrum of parkinsonian manifestations associated with glucocerebrosidase mutations. Arch Neurol 2008;65: 1353–1357.
36. Singleton AB, Farrer M, Johnson J, et al. Alpha-Synuclein locus triplication causes Parkinson's disease. Science 2003;302:841.
37. Singleton A and Gwinn-Hardy K. Parkinson's disease and dementia with Lewy bodies: A difference in dose? Lancet 2004;364:1105–1107.
38. Farrer M, Kachergus J, Forno L, et al. Comparison of kindreds with parkinsonism and alpha-synuclein genomic multiplications. Ann Neurol 2004;55:174–179.
39. Chartier-Harlin MC, Kachergus J, Roumier C, et al. Alpha-synuclein locus duplication as a cause of familial Parkinson's disease. Lancet 2004;364:1167–1169.
40. Ibanez P, Bonnet AM, Debarges B, et al. Causal relation between alpha-synuclein gene duplication and familial Parkinson's disease. Lancet 2004;364:1169–1171.
41. Emre M. Dementia associated with Parkinson's disease. Lancet Neurology 2003;2:229–237.
42. Emre M, Aarsland D, Brown R, et al. Clinical diagnostic criteria for Dementia associated with Parkinson's Disease. Mov Disord 2007;22:1689–1707.
43. Caviness JN, Driver-Dunckley E, Connor DJ, et al. Defining mild cognitive impairment in Parkinson's disease. Mov Disord 2007;22:1272–1277.
44. Litvan I, Mohr E, Williams J, et al. Differential memory and executive functions in demented patients with Parkinson's and Alzheimer's disease. J Neurol Neurosurg Psychiatry 1991;54:25–29.
45. Ballard CG, Aarsland D, McKeith I, et al. Fluctuations in attention: PD dementia vs DLB with parkinsonism. Neurology 2002;59:1714–1720.
46. Cahn-Weiner DA, Grace J, Ott BR, et al. Cognitive and behavioral features discriminate between Alzheimer's and Parkinson's disease. Neuropsychiatry Neuropsychol Behav Neurol 2002;15:79–87.
47. Pate DS and Margolin DI. Cognitive slowing in Parkinson's and Alzheimer's patients: distinguishing bradyphrenia from dementia. Neurology 1994;44:669–674.
48. Bronnick K, Ehrt U, Emre M, et al. Attentional deficits affect activities of daily living in dementia-associated with Parkinson's disease. J Neurol Neurosurg Psychiatry 2006;77:1136–1142.
49. Pillon B, Boller F, Levy R, et al. Cognitive deficits and dementia in Parkinson's disease, In Boller F and Cappa S (eds). Handbook of Neuropsychology, 2nd. Ed., Amsterdam: Elsevier Sciences B.V., 2001, pp. 311–371.
50. Aarsland D, Litvan I, Salmon D, et al. Performance on the dementia rating scale in Parkinson's disease with dementia and dementia with Lewy bodies: comparison with progressive supranuclear palsy and Alzheimer's disease. J Neurol Neurosurg Psychiatry 2003;74:1215–1220.
51. Huber SJ, Shuttleworth EC, Freidenberg DL. Neuropsychological differences between the dementias of Alzheimer's and Parkinson's diseases. Arch Neurol 1989;46: 1287–1291.
52. Kensinger EA, Shearer DK, Locascio JJ, et al. Working memory in mild Alzheimer's disease and early Parkinson's disease. Neuropsychology 2003;17:230–239.
53. Helkala EL, Laulumaa V, Soininen H, et al. Different error pattern of episodic and semantic memory in Alzheimer's disease and Parkinson's disease with dementia. Neuropsychologia 1989;27:1241–1248.
54. Pillon B, Dubois B, Ploska A, et al. Severity and specificity of cognitive impairment in Alzheimer's, Huntington's, and Parkinson's diseases and progressive supranuclear palsy. Neurology 1991;41:634–643.
55. Helkala EL, Laulumaa V, Soininen H, et al. Recall and recognition memory in patients with Alzheimer's and Parkinson's diseases. Ann Neurol 1988;24:214–217.
56. Pillon B, Deweer B, Agid Y, et al. Explicit memory in Alzheimer's, Huntington's, and Parkinson's diseases. Arch Neurol 1993;50:374–379.
57. Noe E, Marder K, Bell KL, et al. Comparison of dementia with Lewy bodies to Alzheimer's disease and Parkinson's disease with dementia. Mov Disord 2004;19:60–67.
58. Girotti F, Soliveri P, Carella F, et al. Dementia and cognitive impairment in Parkinson's disease. J Neurol Neurosurg Psychiatry 1988;51:1498–1502.
59. Mosimann UP, Mather G, Wesnes KA, et al. Visual perception in Parkinson disease dementia and dementia with Lewy bodies. Neurology 2004;63:2091–2096.
60. Mohr E, Litvan I, Williams J, et al. Selective deficits in Alzheimer and parkinsonian dementia: visuospatial function. Can J Neurol Sci 1990;17:292–297.
61. Stern Y, Mayeux R, Rosen J, et al. Perceptual motor dysfunction in Parkinson's disease: a deficit in sequential and predictive voluntary movement. J Neurol Neurosurg Psychiatry 1983;46:145–151.
62. Bondi MW, Kaszniak AW, Bayles KA, et al. Contribution of frontal system dysfunction to memory and perceptual abilities in Parkinson's disease. Neuropsychology 1993;7:89–102.
63. Crucian GP and Okun MS. Visual-spatial ability in Parkinson's disease. Front Biosci 2003;8:992–997.
64. Cummings JL, Darkins A, Mendez M, et al. Alzheimer's disease and Parkinson's disease: comparison of speech and language alterations. Neurology 1988;38: 680–684.
65. Peran P, Rascol O, Demonet JF, et al. Deficit of verb generation in nondemented patients with Parkinson's disease. Mov Disord 2003;18:150–156.
66. Bronnick K, Emre M, Lane R, et al. Profile of cognitive impairment in dementia associated with Parkinson's disease compared with Alzheimer's disease. J Neurol Neurosurg Psychiatry 2007;78:1064–1068.
67. Aarsland D, Brønnick K, Ehrt U, et al. Neuropsychiatric symptoms in patients with Parkinson's disease and dementia: Frequency, profile and associated care giver stress. J Neurol Neurosurg Psychiatry 2007;78:36–42.
68. Aarsland D, Cummings JL, and Larsen JP. Neuropsychiatric differences between Parkinson's disease with dementia and Alzheimer's disease. Int J Geriatr Psychiatry 2001;16:184–191.
69. Fenelon G, Mahieux F, Huon R, et al. Hallucinations in Parkinson's disease: prevalence, phenomenology and risk factors. Brain 2000;123:733–745.

70. Pagonabarraga J, Llebaria G, García-Sánchez C, et al. A prospective study of delusional misidentification syndromes in Parkinson's disease with dementia. Mov Disord 2008;23:443–448.
71. Ehrt U, Brønnick K, De Deyn PP, et al. Subthreshold depression in patients with Parkinson's disease and dementia: Clinical and demographic correlates. Int J Geriatr Psychiatry 2007;22:980–985.
72. Pillon B, Dubois B, Cusimano G, et al. Does cognitive impairment in Pakinson's disease result from non-dopaminergic lesions? J Neurol Neurosurg Psychiatry 1989;52:201–206.
73. Ebmeier KP, Calder SA, Crawford JR, et al. Clinical features predicting dementia in idiopathic Parkinson's disease: A follow-up study. Neurology 1990;40:1222–1224.
74. Hershey LA, Feldman BJ, Kim KY, et al. Tremor at onset: predictor of cognitive and motor outcome in Parkinson's disease? Arch Neurol 1991;48:1049–1051.
75. Foltynie T, Brayne C, and Barker RA. The heterogeneity of idiopathic Parkinson's disease. J Neurol 2002;249:138–145.
76. Burn DJ, Rowan EN, Minett T, et al. Extrapyramidal features in Parkinson's disease with and without dementia and dementia with Lewy bodies: a cross-sectional comparative study. Mov Disord 2003;218:884–889.
77. Wood BH, Bilclough JA, Bowron A, et al. Incidence and prediction of falls in Parkinson's disease: A prospective multidisciplinary study. J Neurol Neurosurg Psychiatry 2002;72:721–725.
78. Apaydin H, Ahlskog JE, Parisi JE, et al. Parkinson disease neuropathology: Later-developing dementia and loss of the levodopa response. Arch Neurol 2002;59:102–112.
79. Joyce JN, Ryoo HL, Beach TB, et al. Loss of response to levodopa in Parkinson's disease and co-occurrence with dementia: Role of D3 and not D2 receptors. Brain Res 2002;1955:138–152.
80. Duda JE, Giasson BI, Mabon ME, et al. Novel antibodies to synuclein show abundant striatal pathology in Lewy body diseases. Ann Neurol 2002;52:205–210.
81. Piggott MA, Marshall EF, Thomas N, et al. Striatal dopaminergic markers in dementia with Lewy bodies, Alzheimer's and Parkinson's diseases. Rostrocaudal distribution. Brain 1999;122:1449–1468.
82. Aarsland D, Ballard CG, Larsen JP, et al. Marked neuroleptic sensitivity in dementia with Lewy bodies and Parkinson's disease. Nord J Psychiatry, 2003;57:94.
83. Kaufmann H and Biaggioni I. Autonomic failure in neurodegenerative disorders. Semin Neurol 2003;23:351–363.
84. Allan LM, Ballard CG, Allen J, et al. Autonomic dysfunction in dementia. J Neurol Neurosurg Psychiatry 2007;78: 671–677.
85. Iranzo A, Molinuevo JL, Santamaría J, et al. Rapid-eye-movement sleep behaviour disorder as an early marker for a neurodegenerative disorder: a descriptive study. Lancet Neurology 2006;5:572–577.
86. Boeve BF, Silber MH, Saper CB, et al. Pathophysiology of REM sleep behaviour disorder and relevance to neurodegenerative disease. Brain 2007;130:2770–2788.
87. Vendette M, Gagnon JF, Decary A, et al. REM sleep behavior disorder predicts cognitive impairment in Parkinson disease without dementia. Neurology 2007;69: 1843–1849.
88. Boddy F, Rowan EN, Lett D, et al. Subjectively reported sleep quality and excessive daytime somnolence in Parkinson's disease with and without dementia, dementia with Lewy bodies and Alzheimer's disease. Int J Geriatr Psychiatry 2007;22:529–535.
89. Emre M. What causes mental dysfunction in Parkinson's disease? Mov Disord 2003;18(suppl. 6): S63–S71.
90. Hurtig HI, Trojanowski JQ, Galvin J, et al. Alpha-synuclein cortical Lewy bodies correlate with dementia in Parkinson's disease. Neurology 2000;54:1916–1921.
91. Mattila PM, Rinne JO, Helenius H, et al. Alpha-synuclein-immunoreactive cortical Lewy bodies are associated with cognitive impairment in Parkinson's disease. Acta Neuropathol (Berl) 2000;100:285–290.
92. Kovari E, Gold G, Herrmann FR, et al. Lewy body densities in the entorhinal and anterior cingulate cortex predict cognitive deficits in Parkinson's disease. Acta Neuropathol (Berl) 2003;106:83–88.
93. Boller F, Mizutani T, Roessmann U, et al. Parkinson disease, dementia, and Alzheimer disease: Clinicopathological correlations. Ann Neurol 1980;7:329–335.
94. Mann DM and Jones D. Deposition of amyloid (A4) protein within the brains of persons with dementing disorders other than Alzheimer's disease and Down's syndrome. Neurosci Lett 1990;109:68–75.
95. de Vos RA, Jansen EN, Stam FC, et al. 'Lewy body disease': clinico-pathological correlations in 18 consecutive cases of Parkinson's disease with and without dementia. Clin Neurol Neurosurg 1995;97:13–22.
96. Jellinger KA, Seppi K, Wenning GK, et al. Impact of coexistent Alzheimer pathology on the natural history of Parkinson's disease. J Neural Transm 2002;109:329–339.
97. Rinne JO, Rummukainen J, Paljarvi L, et al. Dementia in Parkinson's disease is related to neuronal loss in the medial substantia nigra. Ann Neurol 1989;26:47–50.
98. Rub U, Del Tredici K, Schultz C, et al. Parkinson's disease: the thalamic components of the limbic loop are severely impaired by alpha-synuclein immunopositive inclusion body pathology. Neurobiol Aging 2002;23:245–254.
99. Braak H, Del Tredici K, Rub U, et al. Staging of brain pathology related to sporadic Parkinson's disease. Neurobiol Aging 2003;24:197–211.
100. Halliday G, Hely M, Reid W, et al. The progression of pathology in longitudinally followed patients with Parkinson's disease. Acta Neuropathol 2008;115:409–415.
101. Ballard C, Ziabreva I, Perry R, et al. Differences in neuropathologic characteristics across the Lewy body dementia spectrum. Neurology 2006;67:1931–1934.
102. Parkkinen L, Pirttilä T, and Alafuzoff I. Applicability of current staging/categorization of alpha-synuclein pathology and their clinical relevance. Acta Neuropathol 2008;115:399–407.
103. Candy JM, Perry RH, Perry EK, et al. Pathological changes in the nucleus of Meynert in Alzheimer's and Parkinson's diseases. J Neurol Sci 1983;59:277–289.
104. Whitehouse PJ, Hedreen JC, White CL 3rd, et al. Basal forebrain neurons in the dementia of Parkinson disease. Ann Neurol 1983;13:243–248.
105. Dubois B, Ruberg M, Javoy-Agid F, et al. A subcortico-cortical cholinergic system is affected in Parkinson's disease. Brain Res 1983;288:213–218.

106. Tiraboschi P, Hansen LA, Alford M, et al. Cholinergic dysfunction in diseases with Lewy bodies. Neurology 2000;54:407–411.
107. Kuhl DE, Koeppe RA, Minoshima S, et al. In vivo mapping of cholinergic terminals in normal aging, Alzheimer's disease, and Parkinson's disease. Ann Neurol 1996;40: 399–410.
108. Bohnen NI, Kaufer DI, Ivanco LS, et al: Cortical cholinergic function is more severely affected in parkinsonian dementia than in Alzheimer disease: An in vivo positron emission tomographic study. Arch Neurol 2003;60: 1745–1748.
109. Bohnen NI, Kaufer DI, Hendrickson R, et al. Cognitive correlates of cortical cholinergic denervation in Parkinson's disease and parkinsonian dementia. J Neurol 2006;253:242–247.
110. Burton EJ, McKeith IG, Burn DJ, et al. Cerebral atrophy in Parkinson's disease with and without dementia: A comparison with Alzheimer's disease, dementia with Lewy bodies amnd controls. Brain 2004;127:791–800.
111. Burton EJ, McKeith IG, Burn DJ, et al. Brain atrophy rates in Parkinson's disease with and without dementia using serial magnetic resonance imaging. Mov Disord 2005;20:1571–1576.
112. Hu MTM, White SJ, Chaudhuri KR, et al. Correlating rates of cerebral atrophy in Parkinson's disease with measures of cognitive decline. J Neural Transm 2001;108: 571–580.
113. Bissessur S, Tissingh G, Wolters EC, et al. rCBF SPECT in Parkinson's disease patients with mental dysfunction. J Neural Transm Suppl 1997;50:25–30.
114. Firbank MJ, Colloby SJ, Burn DJ, et al. Regional cerebral blood flow in Parkinson's disease with and without dementia. Neuroimage 2003;20:1309–1319.
115. Peppard RF, Martin WR, Carr GD, et al. Cerebral glucose metabolism in Parkinson's disease with and without dementia. Arch Neurol 1992;49:1262–1268.
116. Yong SW, Yoon JK, An YS, et al. A comparison of cerebral glucose metabolism in Parkinson's disease, Parkinson's disease dementia and dementia with Lewy bodies. Eur J Neurol 2007;14:1357–1362.
117. Yoshita M. Differentiation of idiopathic Parkinson's disease from striatonigral degeneration and progressive supranuclear palsy using iodine-123 metaiodobenzylguanidine myocardial scintigraphy. J Neurol Sci 1998;155:60–67.
118. Yoshita M, Taki J, and Yamada M. A clinical role for [(123)I]MIBG myocardial scintigraphy in the distinction between dementia of the Alzheimer's type and dementia with Lewy bodies. J Neurol Neurosurg Psychiatry 2001;71:583–588.
119. O'Brien JT, Colloby S, Fenwick J, et al. Dopamine transporter loss visualized with FP-CIT SPECT in the differential diagnosis of dementia with Lewy bodies. Arch Neurol 2004;61: 919–925.
120. Edison P, Archer HA, Hinz R, et al. Amyloid, hypometabolism, and cognition in Alzheimer disease. An [11C]PIB and [18F]FDG PET study. Neurology 2007;68:501–508.
121. Rowe CC, Ng S, Ackermann U, et al: Imaging β-amyloid burden in aging and dementia. Neurology 2007;68: 1718–1725.
122. Edison P, Rowe CC, Rinne JO, et al. Amyloid load in Parkinson's disease dementia and Lewy Body dementia measured with [11C]PIB-PET. J Neurol Neurosurg Psychiatry 2008;79:1331–1338.
123. Dubois B, Burn D, Goetz C, et al. Diagnostic procedures for Parkinson's disease dementia: Recommendations from the movement disorder society task force. Mov Disord 2007;22:2314–2324.
124. Kalbe E, Calabrese P, Kohn N, et al. Screening for cognitive deficits in Parkinson's disease with the Parkinson neuropsychometric dementia assessment (PANDA) instrument. Parkinsonism Relat Disord 2008;14:93–101.
125. Mahieux F, Michelet D, Manifacier MJ, et al. Mini-mental Parkinson: first validation study of a new bedside test constructed for Parkinson's disease. Behav Neurol 1995;8:15–22.
126. Marinus J, Visser M, Verwey NA, et al. Assessment of cognition in Parkinson's disease. Neurology 2003;61: 1222–1228.
127. Pagonabarraga J, Kulisevsky J, Llebaria G, et al. Parkinson's disease-cognitive rating scale: a new cognitive scale specific for Parkinson's disease. Mov Disord 2008;23: 998–1005.
128. Lippa CF, Duda JE, Grossman M, et al. DLB and PDD boundary issues: diagnosis, treatment, molecular pathology, and biomarkers. Neurology 2007;68:812–819.
129. McKeith IG, Dickson DW, Lowe J, et al. Diagnosis and management of dementia with Lewy bodies: Third report of the DLB Consortium. Neurology 2005;65: 1863–1872.
130. Aarsland D, Mosimann UP, and McKeith IG. Role of Cholinesterase Inhibitors in Parkinson's Disease and dementia with Lewy Bodies. J Geriatr Psychiatry Neurol 2004;17:164–171.
131. Emre M, Aarsland D, Albanese A, et al. Rivastigmine for dementia associated with Parkinson's disease. N Engl J Med 2004;351:2509–2518.
132. Poewe W, Wolters E, Emre M, et al. Long-term benefits of rivastigmine in dementia associated with Parkinson's disease: An active treatment extension study. Mov Disord 2005;21:456–461.
133. Burn D, Emre M, McKeith I, et al. Effects of rivastigmine in patients with and without visual hallucinations in dementia associated with Parkinson's disease. Mov Disord 2006;21:1899–1907.
134. Wesnes KA, McKeith I, Edgar C, et al: Benefits of rivastigmine on attention in dementia associated with Parkinson disease. Neurology 2005;65:1654–1656.
135. Ravina B, Putt M, Siderowf A, et al. Donepezil for dementia in Parkinson's disease: A randomised, double blind, placebo controlled, crossover study. J Neurol Neurosurg Psychiatry 2005;76:934–939.
136. Dubois B, Tolosa E, Kulisevsky J, et al. Efficacy and safety of donepezil in the treatment of Parkinson's disease patients with dementia. Poster presented at AD-PD, March 14th–18th 2007, Salzburg.
137. Rowan E, McKeith IG, Saxby BK, et al. Effects of donepezil on central processing speed and attentional measures in Parkinson's disease with dementia and dementia with Lewy Bodies. Dement Geriatr Cogn Disord 2007; 23:161–167.

138. Grace J, Amick MM, and Friedman JH. A Double Blind Comparison of Galantamine Hydrobromide ER and Placebo in Parkinson's Disease. J Neurol Neurosurg Psychiatry 2008 Oct 17. [Epub ahead of print].
139. Maidment I, Fox C, and Boustani M. Cholinesterase inhibitors for Parkinson's disease dementia. Cochrane Database Syst Rev 2006;1:CD004747.
140. Molloy SA, Rowan EN, O`Brien JT, et al. Effect of levodopa on cognitive function in Parkinson`s disease with and without dementia and dementia with Lewy bodies. J Neurol Neurosurg Psychiatry 2006;77:1323–1328.
141. Goldman JG, Goetz CG, Brandabur M, et al. Effects of dopaminergic medications on psychosis and motor function in dementia with Lewy bodies. Mov Disord 2008 Sep 29 [Epub ahead of print].
142. Marsch L, Biglan K, Gerstenhaber M, et al. Atomoxetine for the treatment of executive dysfunction in Parkinson's disease: A pilot open-label study. Mov Disord. 2009 Jan 30;24(2):277–282.
143. Fox CG, Umoh G, Samuel M, et al. Memantine in Parkinson's disease dementia: clinical experience. Mov Disord 2005;20(suppl. 10):P418.
144. Inzelberg R, Chapman J, Treves TA, et al. Apolipoprotein E4 in Parkinson disease and dementia: New data and meta-analysis of published studies. Alzheimer Dis Assoc Disord 1998;12:45–48.
145. Goetz CG, Koller WC, Poewe W, et al. Drugs to treat dementia and psychosis. Mov Disord 2002;17(suppl 4): 120–127.
146. Ondo WG, Levy JK, Vuong KD, et al. Olanzapine treatment for dopaminergic-induced hallucinations. Mov Disord 2002;17:1031–1035.
147. Ellis T, Cudkowicz ME, Sexton PM, et al. Clozapine and risperidone treatment of psychosis in Parkinson's disease. J Neuropsychiatry Clin Neurosci 2000;12:364–369.
148. Prohorov T, Klein C, Miniovitz A, et al. The effect of quetiapine in psychotic Parkinsonian patients with and without dementia. An open-labeled study utilizing a structured interview. J Neurol 2006;253:171–175.
149. Kurlan R, Cummings J, Raman R, et al. Alzheimer`s Disease Cooperative Study Group: Quetiapine for agitation or psychosis in patients with dementia and parkinsonism. Neurology 2007;68:1356–1363.
150. Fernandez HH, Trieschamann ME, Burke MA, et al. Long-term outcome of quetiapine use for psychosis among Parkinsonian patients. Mov Disord 2003;18:510–514.
151. Weintraub D, Morales KH, Moberg PJ, et al. Antidepressant studies in Parkinsons's disease: A review and meta-analysis. Mov Disord 2005;20:161–169.
152. Miyasaki JM, Shannon K, Voon V, et al. Practice Parameter: evaluation and treatment of depression, psychosis, and dementia in Parkinson disease (an evidence-based review): Report of the Quality Standards Subcommittee of the American Academy of Neurology. Neurology 2006;66:996–1002.
153. Hogl B, Saletu M, Brandauer E, et al. Modafinil for the treatment of daytime sleepiness in Parkinson's disease: A double-blind, randomized, cross-over, placebo-controlled, polygraphic trial. Sleep 2002;25:905–909.
154. Nieves AV and Lang AE. Treatment of excessive daytime sleepiness in patients with Parkinson's disease with modafinil. Clin Neuropharmacol , 2002;25:111–114.
155. Adler CH, Caviness JN, Hentz JG, et al. Randomized trial of modafinil for treating subjective daytime sleepiness in patients with Parkinson's disease. Mov Disord 2003;18:287–293.
156. Ondo WG, Fayle R, Atassi F, et al. Modafinil for daytime somnolence in Parkinson's disease: Double blind, placebo controlled parallel trial. J Neurol Neurosurg Psychiatry 2005;76:1636–1639.

CHAPTER 19

Parkinson's Disease: Neuropathology

John E. Duda

▶ INTRODUCTION

From the recognition of 1-methyl-4-phenyl-1,2,3,6-tetrahydropyridine (MPTP)-induced parkinsonism to the discovery of numerous genes responsible for rare Mendelian forms of parkinsonism, our understanding of the mechanisms involved in rare causes of parkinsonism has exploded in the past 25 years. It was hoped that further understanding of the pathophysiologic mechanisms involved in these conditions would lead to novel therapeutic interventions for people afflicted with what is by far the most common form of parkinsonism, Lewy body Parkinson's disease (hereafter referred to as PD). As clues to the pathophysiology of these other forms of parkinsonism arose, cellular and animal models designed to recapitulate these mechanisms were developed. These models have enhanced our understanding of nigrostriatal degeneration and basal ganglionic circuitry.

These advancements have also laid the framework for the development of several novel therapies to alleviate the symptoms of nigrostriatal degeneration, including dopamine agonists and deep brain stimulation. In contrast, these models have also led to the development of neuroprotective strategies that have been far less successfully translated to clinical use and have led to questions about the validity of their use for this purpose.[1,2] While the reason for these failures of translation is highly debatable, at least one potential problem that must be considered is the possibility that the pathophysiologic underpinnings of these genetic and acute intoxication forms of parkinsonism may play little if any role in the pathophysiology of PD. Indeed, there are likely myriad ways to cause degeneration of what appear to be highly vulnerable dopaminergic midbrain neurons and understanding one mechanism may in no way lead to a better understanding of the others. Alternatively, while a component of a particular mechanism may be relevant in various etiologies at a downstream level, critically important upstream components may differ, and truly neuroprotective therapies may depend on modifying these essential components in the neurodegenerative cascade. For example, while inhibition of mitochondrial complex 1 may be a critical factor in some toxin-induced causes of parkinsonism, it may be present only as an effect of an upstream pathophysiologic process in PD. Similarly, it seems entirely likely that while some of the genetic causes of parkinsonism have led to important discoveries regarding the pathophysiology of PD, most notably the recognition that α-synuclein is the primary component of Lewy bodies (LBs), nonmutated forms of some of the genes implicated in Mendelian parkinsonism may play no role in the pathophysiology of PD. This seems particularly likely for causes of parkinsonism that do not share one of the two essential neuropathological hallmarks of PD, LB accumulation, which include MPTP intoxication, mutations in Parkin and potentially several other genetic causes of parkinsonism that have as yet undetermined neuropathology. An extensive review of the known neuropathology of Mendelian parkinsonism has been recently reported.[3]

These assumptions highlight the need to gain a better understanding of the neuropathology of PD so that improved cellular and animal models that recapitulate essential components of the pathophysiology of PD may be developed. Fortunately, concurrent with advances in our understanding of rare causes of parkinsonism, great strides have been made in our understanding of the neuropathology of PD. The highlights of those advances will be the focus of this chapter.

▶ MACROSCOPIC PATHOLOGY

Grossly, the PD brain has so little specific pathology that the eminent neurologist and neuropathologist Charcot, considered PD a névrose, a term he used to describe neurological conditions with no identifiable neuropathological lesions.[4] As late as 1910, Wilhelm Erb commented, "We must still admit that we do not know the positive and constant pathologico-anatomical foundation of paralysis agitans."[5] However, later investigations did reveal subtle changes that are apparent on gross examination of the vast majority of brains from patients with PD. Although the external surfaces of the brain remain essentially unremarkable in the PD brain, sectioning of the brain stem reveals depigmentation of the

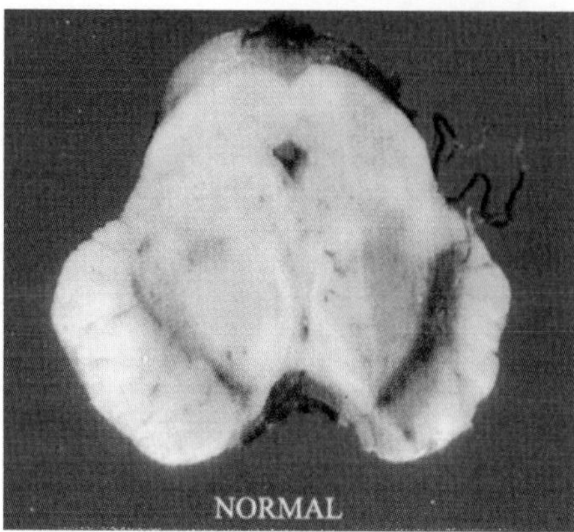

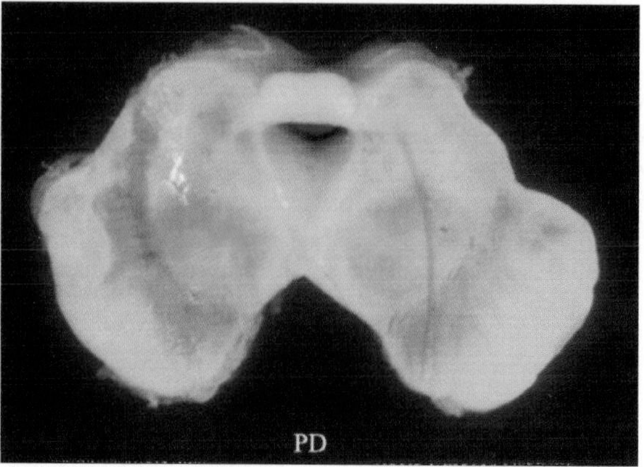

Figure 19–1. Macroscopic pathology of Substantia nigra. Gross photograph of a coronal section through the midbrain from a normal brain (*left*) and from a case of PD (*right*). Note the normal pigmentation pattern of the substantia nigra in the normal specimen, and the loss of pigmentation in the case of PD.

pars compacta of the substantia nigra in the midbrain (Fig. 19–1) and the locus coeruleus in the ventral pons. Caused by decreased numbers of melanized neurons, this depigmentation often leads to a smearing of the borders of the substantia nigra compared with control brains. In contrast to the previous conceptions of early neuropathologists,[6] the basal ganglia are now accepted to appear grossly normal in PD.

▶ MICROSCOPIC PATHOLOGY

Although the substantia nigra pars compacta (SNpc) has been the focus of investigation ever since Greenfield solidified neuronal loss and the LBs therein as the essential pathology of PD,[7] one of the most important findings of the past decade has been the recognition that the pathology of PD occurs throughout the brain and brain stem and that our traditional focus on the SNpc may have been artificially enhanced by its role in the generation of motor symptoms. Nonetheless, the SNpc remains one of the most thoroughly examined areas in the PD brain and a thorough discussion of the neuropathology described therein is warranted.

▶ PATHOLOGY OF THE SUBSTANTIA NIGRA

TRADITIONAL FINDINGS

The sine qua non of neurodegenerative disease has been neuronal loss, and the SNpc is one area of the PD brain where this is readily demonstrable, even at the earliest stages of motor symptom development. Neuronal loss and depigmentation is not homogenous throughout the SNpc but predominates in areas that might be predicted on the basis of the resulting symptomatology. In normal aging, there is a controversy over whether there is age-associated neuronal loss[8,9] that occurs primarily in the dorsal tier,[10] or whether there is merely highly variable neuronal loss at all ages with no correlation with age.[11,12] In the PD brain, neuronal loss predominates in the SNpc ventrolateral tier neurons (Fig. 19–2), which project to the motor aspect of the striatum.[11] Neuronal loss can also occur in the medial SNpc in PD and increasing severity has been associated with the development of dementia.[11,13]

In addition to the absence of melanin-containing SNpc neurons, other indications of ongoing neuronal dysfunction and demise are readily identifiable in the PD SNpc. It is not unusual to see deposits of extracellular neuromelanin, melanophagia or phagocytosed neuromelanin, and occasionally neuronophagia of pigmented neurons (Fig. 19–2). In addition, with immunostaining to tyrosine hydroxylase (TH), the enzyme responsible for catalyzing the conversion of the amino acid L-tyrosine to dihydroxyphenylalanine in the synthesis of dopamine, it is possible to identify melanized neurons in the SNpc that are not expressing TH (Fig. 19–2). It is probable that these TH-negative melanized SNpc neurons are not producing dopamine, which can be considered a 'luxury' function for these neurons, and therefore, are probably 'sick' neurons. The frequency of these TH-negative neurons is increased in the SNpc of patients with PD compared with age-matched controls and 82% of SNpc neurons with aggregates of α-synuclein do not express TH.[14] Although their significance has traditionally been thought to reflect a benign marker of normal aging, spherical eosinophilic nuclear inclusions known as Marinesco bodies (Fig. 19–2) were recently examined as another possible marker of neuronal dysfunction in PD and related disorders.[15] Another rarely discussed aberration observed in the SNpc of PD brains is the

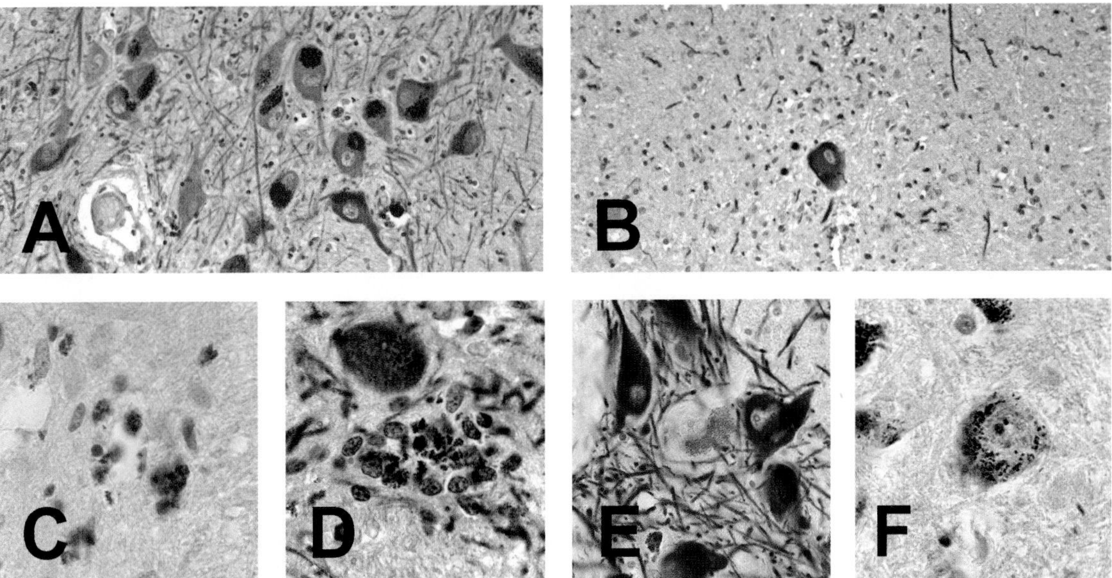

Figure 19–2. Pathological alterations of the substantia nigra in PD. Compared to the normal substantia nigra (A), there are numerous pathological alterations visible in the substantia nigra of patients with PD including depletion of pigmented neurons (B), extracellular neuromelanin (C), melanophagia and neuronophagia (D), tyrosine hydroxylase pigmented neurons (in center of panel E), and Marinesco bodies (aggregate in nucleus of panel F). Panels were immunostained with antibodies against tyrosine hydroxylase (A,B,C,D,E) and ubiquitin (F). Original magnification 200× (A,B) and 600× (C-F).

presence of grumose degeneration that entails 'foamy' appearing spheroids, which were originally described by Tretiakoff.[16,17] A recent study also suggests that SNpc neurons in early PD have a higher density of neuromelanin pigment that is associated with α-synuclein and may be a clue to their selective vulnerability.[11]

Finally, the second essential feature for the pathologic diagnosis of PD is the accumulation of LBs in the SNpc. The SNpc is one of the few areas of the brains wherein classical LBs form, characterized ultrastructurally by a dense fibrillar core surrounded by a clearly defined corona of radially projecting fibrils. By standard immunohistochemistry, classical LBs may appear as a solid, round inclusion, or with the core being unlabeled with only the corona staining (Fig. 19–3). However, our ability to demonstrate LBs sensitively and specifically dramatically changed when hematoxylin and eosin histostaining was replaced originally by neurofilament and ubiquitin immunohistochemistry, and more recently by α-synuclein immunohistochemistry. In addition to classical LBs, it is typical to visualize several other forms of Lewy pathology in the SNpc with α-synuclein immunostaining, which with LBs are collectively referred to as Lewy pathology. These include inclusions within the neuronal soma including pale bodies (pale staining of softly defined inclusion within the neuromelanin), somatodendritic staining of the cell soma, punctuate staining within the cell soma and multilobular LBs (Fig. 19–3). In addition numerous forms of Lewy pathology may be observed in the neuronal processes, including intraneuritic LBs (LB-like structures located within processes), spheroids (long tubular inclusions within processes), and Lewy neurites (small curvilinear or punctuate staining within processes) (Fig. 19–4). In addition, occasional inclusions within glia are present (Fig. 19–4). While first described with ubiquitin immunochemistry,[18,19] Lewy neurites have been established as the predominate form of Lewy pathology with α-synuclein immunochemistry.[20–23] Recently, novel antibodies raised against oxidized α-synuclein provided an even more sensitive method for recognizing Lewy neurites, including a burden of neuritic dystrophy within the striatum of the LB disorders[21] that may contribute to the parkinsonism in these disorders. These studies, in combination with the recognition that Lewy neurites appear to form prior to LBs[24,25] and that α-synuclein transgenic mice undergo axonal degeneration due to the formation of Lewy neurites and resultant disruption of axonal transport[26] has led to a hypothesis that neuritic dystrophy is an early and important component in the Lewy neurodegenerative cascade[27] (Fig. 19–5).

Recently, variability in the sensitivity and specificity of α-synuclein immunohistochemical protocols was assessed in several studies.[28–30] One study of protocols thought to be selective for Lewy pathology, with blinded comparison of identical cases for all protocols, revealed that some protocols, particularly those with aggressive antigen-retrieval protocols, were more sensitive and specific than others.[29] In another study comparing only commercially available

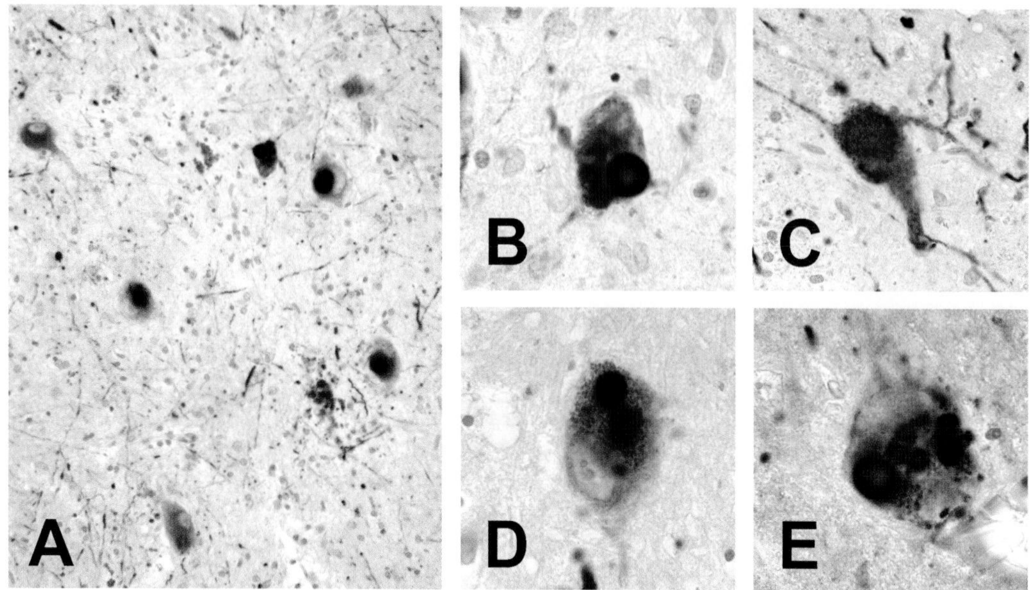

Figure 19-3. Lewy pathology of the substantia nigra. α-Synuclein immunostaining reveals Lewy pathology of many different forms in the substantia nigra pars compacta. Lower power magnification reveals LBs in many remaining pigmented neurons, somatodendritic staining in others, and diffuse Lewy neurites in the neuropil (A). Higher power magnification in individual pigmented neurons reveals a classical LB (B), somatodendritic staining with punctuate inclusions and a pale body (C), LBs in various stages of development in the same neuron (D) and multilobular LBs (E). All panels were immunostained with antibodies against α-synuclein. Original magnification 200× (A) and 600× (B-E).

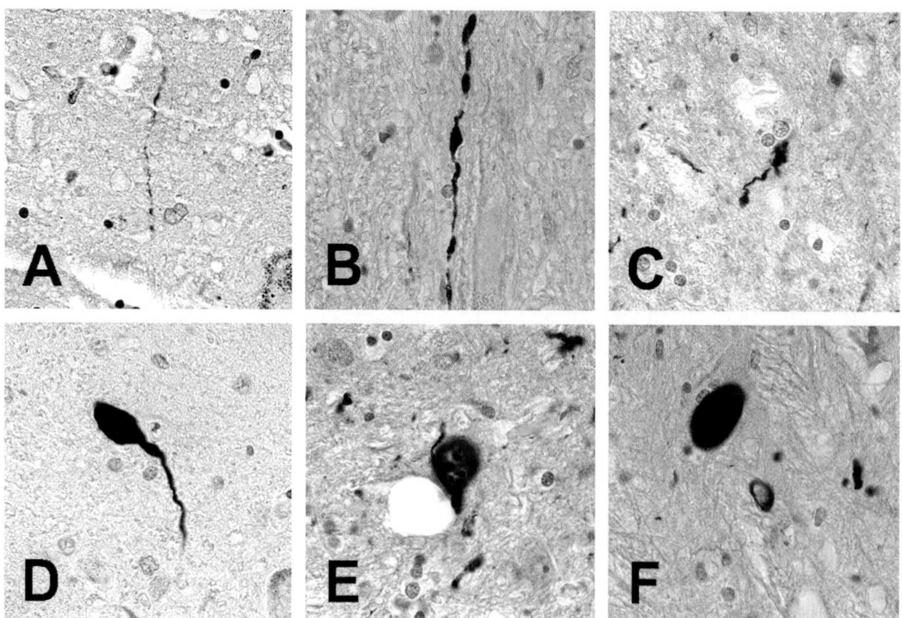

Figure 19-4. Lewy pathology within neuronal processes and glia. Alpha-synuclein immunostaining also reveals Lewy pathology of many different forms in neuronal processes and glia. The finest or filiform inclusions involve one neuronal process without significant dilatation of the process (A), while other inclusions dilate the process in a repeated fusiform pattern (B). Occasionally filiform or fusiform neurites will develop a tangled or knotted appearance (C), and further dilatation of the process will lead to the formation of axonal spheroids (D). Rarely, these spheroids will have a foamy appearance described as 'grumose degeneration' (E) but will more commonly have homogenous staining of the entire axonal compartment (upper inclusion in F). In addition, alpha-synuclein immunostaining will occasionally identify cytoplasmic inclusions within glial cells (central inclusion in F). All panels immunostained with antibodies against alpha-synuclein. Original magnification 600× (A-F).

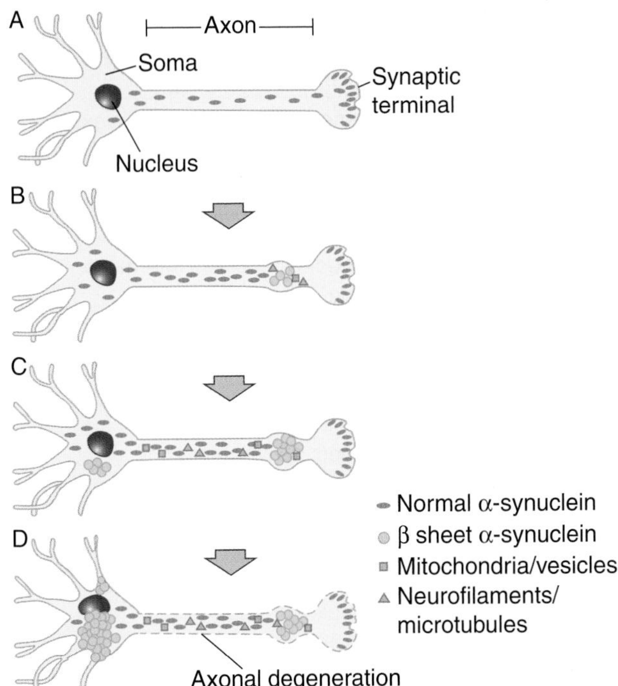

Figure 19–5. Neuritic dystrophy hypothesis of Lewy neurodegeneration. α-synuclein is produced in the cell soma, transported down the axon and located at the synaptic terminal (A). In this model, the aggregation of α-synuclein begins as Lewy neurites are formed within axons of neurons (B). These axonal aggregates enlarge by the sequestration of additional α-synuclein, other proteins and subcellular elements, until interruption of axonal transport occurs (B/C). The axonal transport blockade causes an accumulation of anterogradely transported subcellular elements proximal to the occlusion and a supersaturation of the cell soma with α-synuclein (C). The supersaturation of α-synuclein predisposes the neuron to the formation of somatic α-synuclein aggregates, known as Lewy bodies (LBs) (C). LB growth continues until the normal somatic architecture is disrupted, with nuclear displacement, and α-synuclein aggregates form within proximal dendrites as Lewy neurites (D). Finally, continued axonal transport blockade prohibits distal axonal viability, leading to axonal degeneration (D) with the possibility of resultant neuronal degeneration. (Reproduced from Ref. 27 with permission from S. Karger AG, Basel.)

α-synuclein antibodies, Croisier and colleagues reported that antibodies directed against amino acids 116–131 and 15–123 of the α-synuclein molecule had the best sensitivity and specificity for detecting Lewy pathology.[30]

COMPONENTS OF LBS

Although previously considered a "trash can" in the neurons of PD patients with little consequence, LBs slowly became a primary focus of research efforts in pathophysiologic studies as well as in the development of cellular and animal model systems. Early immunohistochemical studies revealed that two of the primary components were ubiquitin and neurofilament subunits.[31,32] Early purification studies of LBs confirmed these findings and identified other unidentified components.[33–35] Since that time, there has been an explosion of proteins identified as components of LBs, some with questionable significance, as they are present in only a small subset of LBs. There are currently more than 70 proteins identified and a recent review[36] suggests that they may be divided into several categories, including (1) structural elements of the LB fibril; (2) α-synuclein-binding proteins; (3) synphilin-1-binding proteins; (4) components of the ubiquitin-proteasome system; (5) proteins implicated in cellular responses; (6) proteins associated with phosphorylation and signal transduction; (7) cytoskeletal proteins; (8) cell cycle proteins; and (9) cytosolic proteins that passively diffuse into LBs. To date, however, there have been no proteins shown to immunolabel a higher percentage of LBs than antibodies to α-synuclein.[23]

▶ NON-NIGRAL LEWY PATHOLOGY

SYNUCLEIN PATHOLOGY

In addition to the SNpc, nigral pathology has been known to involve numerous other regions of the brain ever since the first description of LBs by Frederick Henry Lewy in 1912 who observed these aggregates in the dorsal vagal nucleus, nucleus accumbens, locus coeruleus and other areas, but not the SNpc, which, in his defense, was not known to be involved with the generation of parkinsonian symptoms.[37] Since that time, areas selectively vulnerable to Lewy pathology have been described throughout the brain stem, diencephalon, and cortex that are highlighted in Table 19–1 and reviewed thoroughly elsewhere.[38] In fact, in cases with severe Lewy neurodegeneration, at least traces of Lewy pathology are present in nearly every area of the brain in selectively vulnerable neurons. However, that is not to say that all neurons are vulnerable to Lewy neurodegeneration. There are clearly neuronal subtypes that are selectively vulnerable to Lewy neurodegeneration and others that are rarely if ever affected. Braak and colleagues have identified common features of neurons that are selectively vulnerable, which are summarized in Table 19–2.[38] Patients with long disease duration and greater severity typically have higher burdens of Lewy pathology throughout the neuraxis although there are exceptions. In the case of the SNpc, it has been recognized that patients with long duration PD typically have lower densities of Lewy pathology than patients with DLB with shorter durations, which has been thought to

TABLE 19–1. NERVOUS SYSTEM REGIONS SELECTIVELY VULNERABLE TO LEWY NEURODEGENERATION

Spinal Cord and Peripheral Nervous Tissues	Meissner's and Auerbach's plexus of the enteric nervous system Postganglionic sympathetic neurons and celiac ganglion Vagal nerve Intermediolateral and intermediomedial nuclei of the spinal cord Lamina 1 of the spinal cord Olfactory bulb and anterior olfactory nucleus
Medulla Oblongata	Dorsal motor nucleus Intermediate reticular zone Lower raphe nuclei Gigantocellular nucleus of reticular formation
Pons	Locus coeruleus–subcoeruleus complex
Midbrain	Substantia nigra pars compacta Pedunculopontine tegmental nucleus Ventral tegmental area
Diencephalon	Hypothalamic tuberomamillary nucleus Median forebrain bundle Magnocellular nuclei of the basal forebrain Intralaminar thalamic nuclei Interstitial nucleus of the stria terminalis Ventral striatum and ventral claustrum
Telencephalon	Central subnucleus and basal complex of the amygdala Hippocampal CA2/3 sector Cingulate, insular, and subgenual cortices Temporal mesocortex Frontal, temporal ,and parietal association cortices Prefrontal cortex

TABLE 19–2. CHARACTERISTICS COMMON TO MOST SELECTIVELY VULNERABLE NEURONS

Projection neurons with long axons relative to cell soma
Unmyelinated or thinly myelinated axons
Lipofuscin or neuromelanin accumulations
High metabolic demand

be an artifact of the long disease course in PD that allows more neurons with Lewy pathology to be completely phagocytosed after dying, giving the SNpc a "burnt out" appearance with rare remaining pigmented neurons. However, another more dramatic exception to the clinicopathologic correlation of Lewy pathology has been the recognition of numerous patients who have little if any evidence of neurodegenerative disease during life and at autopsy have large burdens of Lewy pathology.[39–42] What the mechanisms are that allow these patients to tolerate large burdens of Lewy pathology without symptoms are yet unidentified, but a promising area of ongoing research. Better characterization of these patients as well as patients who have the earliest stages of Lewy neurodegeneration will lead to better understanding of the pathophysiological mechanisms involved. To date, careful characterization of the Lewy pathology present in patients with low levels of pathology have led to surprising insights into selective vulnerability that are detailed in the following sections.

UNDERSTANDING THE PATTERN OF PROGRESSION OF LEWY BODY PATHOLOGY THROUGH THE BRAIN

Until very recently, there was very little insight into the progression of Lewy body formation through the brain. It was known that there were selectively vulnerable neuronal populations throughout the brain,[43–54] but it was not clear if they were all affected concurrently or if there was sequential involvement through these vulnerable populations. This was due in large part to the limitations of human neuropathological assessment as a 'snapshot' in time, without the ability to observe more than one time point in a single brain, and the reliance on examination of brains in the later stages of disease, when most patients come to autopsy.

BRAAK STAGES

A landmark body of work was carried out by Kelly Del Tredici and Heiko Braak who completed the first large-scale attempt to develop a staging system of Lewy neurodegeneration in the human brain that included patients without symptoms.[55–59] Largely, the traditional limitations of human neuropathological assessment were circumvented by the use of large numbers of brains representing the breath of human Lewy neurodegeneration, especially many cases defined as incidental Lewy body disease in which there was no obvious evidence of clinical parkinsonism and yet the brains from these patients had at least mild Lewy neurodegeneration. The study included a large-scale assessment of autopsied brains, including 413 patients over the age of 40 with no known history of psychiatric or neurological disorders that identified 30 cases of incidental Lewy pathology.[55] In these cases, 26 of which had no Lewy pathology in the SNpc, it became clear that the earliest predilection sites of those examined were in the dorsal motor nucleus of the vagal/glossopharangeal nuclei, the intermediate reticular nucleus and the olfactory bulb and anterior olfactory nucleus. This was supported by the presence of several cases that had mild Lewy pathology in these areas but not in the other areas examined, and the fact that there were no cases with pathology in the other areas that did not have pathology in most of these early predilection sites.

With these cases as the starting point, the authors then endeavored to determine the progression of Lewy pathology throughout the central nervous system by including other cases with more advanced pathology and concomitant clinical symptoms.[56] In a comprehensive assay of Lewy pathology in the brains of 110 patients, including 41 with clinical PD and 69 with incidental LBs, Braak and colleagues developed a staging system of the progression of Lewy pathology. This staging system was similarly determined by comparing the regional distribution of pathology throughout the brain and brain stem and assuming that if the pathology progresses in a stepwise fashion, brains with less pathology in more restricted distributions would represent earlier pathological stages. In this system, six stages are delineated, with stages 1 and 2 representing "preclinical" stages, stages 3 and 4 representing early "clinical" stages when typical motor features of PD are expected to arise and stage 5 and 6 representing later stages with widespread pathology and frequently characterized by the development of dementia and other late nonmotor symptoms (Fig. 19–6).

In what has become known as the 'Braak LB staging system' each stage includes additional areas wherein Lewy pathology may be found and increasing burdens of pathology in the areas wherein pathology was present in previous stages. Stage 1 is characterized by involvement of the olfactory system including the olfactory bulb and anterior olfactory nucleus (AON), which extends into the olfactory tract and select areas of the medulla including the dorsal visceromotor nucleus of vagus and the intermediate reticular zone. In stage 2, pathology extends to the 'gain-setting nuclei' of the medulla and pons, including the caudal raphe nuclei, the gigantocellular reticular nucleus, and the coeruleus/subcoeruleus complex. Stage 3 is the first stage wherein pathology is present in the SNpc as well as in the tegmental pedunculopontine nucleus and in the prosencephalon with involvement of the central subnucleus and basal complex of the amygdala, the magnocellular nuclei of the basal forebrain and the hypothalamic tuberomamillary nucleus. The cerebral cortex is involved for the first time in stage 4, with involvement of the anteromedial temporal mesocortex, as well as CA2 of Ammon's horn (Fig. 19–7), the interstitial nucleus of

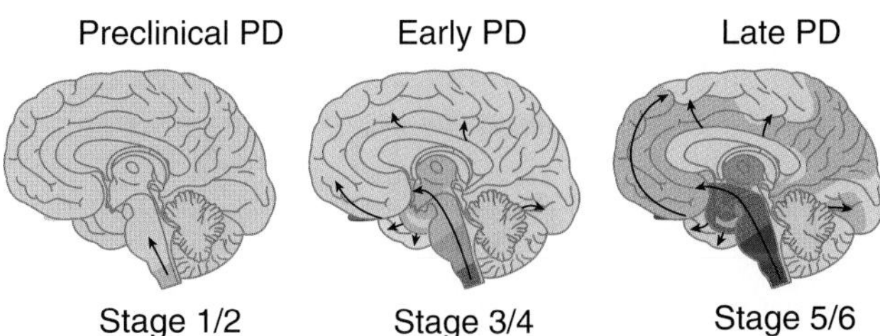

Figure 19–6. Stages in the evolution of Parkinson-related LB pathology. The first LBs occur in the dorsal motor nucleus of the vagal nerve and olfactory bulb (stage 1). From these induction sites, LB pathology makes inroads, first into additional brain stem nuclei, such as the locus coeruleus (stage 2) and SNpc (stage 3), then into the amygdala (stage 3), and finally into the cerebral cortex (stages 4 to 6). (Modified with permission from Kelly Del Tredici, MD and Heiko Braak, MD.)

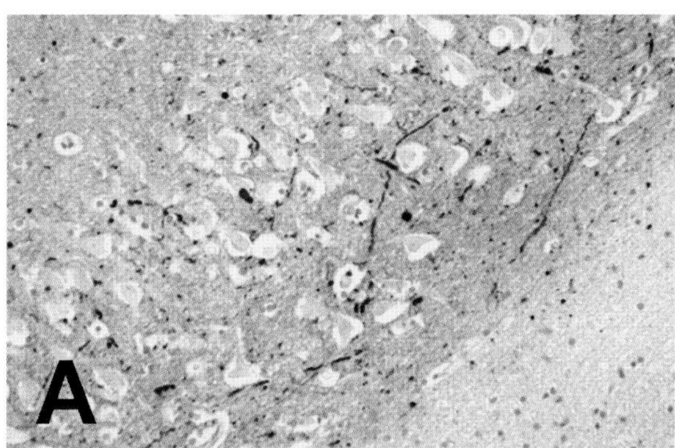

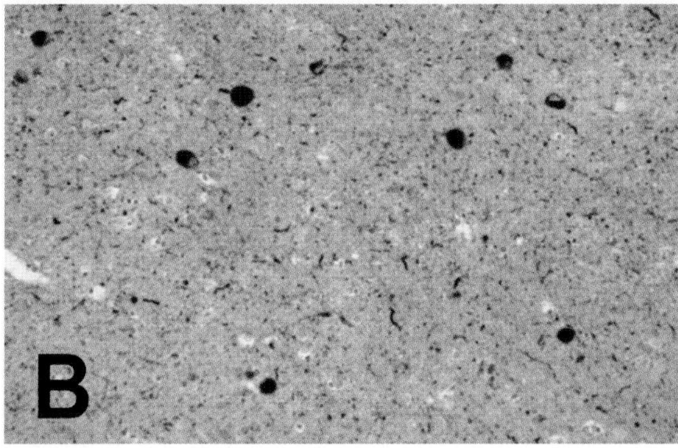

Figure 19–7. Lewy pathology develops typical patterns in several brain regions. Typical patterns of Lewy pathology predominate in several other areas of the brain including sectors 2 of Ammon's horn in the hippocampus that often form a network of long filamentous Lewy neurites (A) and limbic cortex that is subject to the formation of numerous cortical LBs in the pyramidal cells of layers IV–V as well as dense accumulations of Lewy neurites (B). Both panels immunostained with antibodies against alpha-synuclein. Original magnification 100× (A-B).

the stria terminalis and the midline and intralaminar thalamic nuclei. Stage 5 heralds a more diffuse involvement of the cerebral cortex, including many limbic cortical areas (Fig. 19–7) including the anterior cingulate cortex, the insular and subgenual cortices as well as higher-order sensory association cortices and prefrontal cortex. Also in stage 5, the striatum becomes involved for the first time with pathology found in the ventral striatum and ventral claustrum. Finally, in stage 6, the progression of involvement of cortical areas culminates with involvement of the first-order sensory association cortices and premotor fields followed ultimately by the primary sensory and motor cortices in extreme cases.

For the sake of simplicity, Braak and his colleagues have recently devised an alternative system for LB staging that retains the essential components of the original staging system while employing the necessity of only assessing five different sections of tissue, namely the medulla at the level of the dorsal motor nucleus of the vagus, the pons at the level of the locus coeruleus, the midbrain with the SNpc, the uncal portion of the hippocampal formation including the entorhinal cortex and the anteromedial temporal mesocortex, and the first temporal gyrus.[60] These tissue sections are then assessed for pathology in eight different anatomical locations and based on the presence or absence of pathology a stage of 0 through 6 is given. This protocol was designed for everyday use in routine neuropathological assessment and when assessed in a blinded fashion by six different raters, showed high interrater and intrarater reliability.

LIMITATIONS OF THE BRAAK LEWY BODY STAGING SYSTEM

It should be recognized that there are several limitations of the methodologies utilized in devising the Braak LB staging system, including the absence of investigation of spinal cord or peripheral autonomic nervous system tissues, the practice of screening patients with only immunostaining of the medulla oblongata and the exclusion of cases with significant Alzheimer's pathology.

Given the LB predilection sites in stage 1 and the topographical progression of pathology throughout the brain stem and spinal cord, it is very tempting to assume that the Braak LB staging system delineated LB induction sites within the brain stem and olfactory system because of a lack of investigation of more peripheral nervous system tissues, including spinal cord and peripheral autonomic nervous system tissues. The presence of Lewy pathology in the spinal cord[61–63] and peripheral autonomic nervous system tissues[64–68] has been well documented in patients with PD. Indeed, Braak and colleagues, suggested that this pathology might be the real induction sites for LB pathology in a separate report.[69] They presented the evidence for involvement of enteric nervous system tissues in idiopathic PD and a scheme by which each succeeding stage of Lewy pathology predilection sites connects axonally to nuclear areas involved in the previous stage. They also presented a hypothesis for the retrograde transport of a neurotropic pathogen all the way from the mucosal layer of the gastrointestinal tract, through postganglionic enteric neurons and into the central nervous system via unmyelinated preganglionic fibers of the vagus nerve. However, no previous studies had rigorously examined the spinal cord and peripheral autonomic nervous tissues for the presence of Lewy pathology in normal patients and these tissues were not included in the landmark studies of Braak and colleagues. Recently, several groups have completed this task to varying degrees and added supporting evidence to the Braak induction hypothesis by demonstrating that spinal cord and the peripheral autonomic nervous system tissues are susceptible to the formation of Lewy pathology in apparently normal elderly.[70,71]

In a study that examined the spinal cord for the presence of Lewy pathology in 106 neurologically normal patients who had been followed longitudinally and examined within the last year of life, Klos and colleagues reported the presence of Lewy pathology within the thoracic spinal cord of nine patients (8% of the patients examined).[71] Lewy pathology was most commonly observed in the intermediolateral cell column of the spinal cord but was also occasionally seen in other areas, including the lateral aspects of the anterior and posterior horns. Not surprisingly, all nine cases also demonstrated pathology within the dorsal motor nucleus of the vagus, the locus coeruleus, and the central raphe nuclei. Interestingly, in addition, the authors also identified four cases with Lewy pathology in the higher predilection sites, including the dorsal motor nucleus of the vagus, locus coeruleus, dorsal raphe nuclei, SNpc, nucleus basalis of Meynert and/or the amygdala, without any Lewy pathology in the spinal cord. Because of this, the authors suggested that spinal cord involvement occurs early in the Braak staging system, but probably after involvement of the lower brain stem, consistent with at least Braak LB stage 2. However, it is important to recognize that these authors did not sample the sacral spinal cord for evidence of Lewy pathology in the parasympathetic neurons found therein.

In a similar study by Bloch and colleagues,[70] 98 brains of patients with no reference of PD-associated symptoms on retrospective review of clinical records were examined for evidence of Lewy pathology. This study was somewhat limited because of restricted information concerning the thoroughness of the clinical records and premortem evaluations, but was superior to the previous study by the inclusion of sampling in the sacral spinal cord and peripheral autonomic nervous system tissues including the esophagus, the paravertebral sympathetic chain, and the vagus nerve. In this study, the authors identified 17 brains (17.3%) with Lewy pathology somewhere in the neuraxis. Of these cases, classified as incidental LB cases, the authors observed Lewy pathology in 82% of the esophageal samples, usually in the myenteric plexus, in 82% of the paravertebral sympathetic chains examined and in 75% of the vagal nerves examined. In all of the 17 brains, Lewy pathology was demonstrated at both the sacral parasympathetic cell column of the spinal cord and the intermediolateral and intermediomedial nuclei of the thoracic spinal cord. Interestingly, they described one case of Lewy pathology with the highest density in the olfactory bulb and some pathology in the association cortices with little or no pathology in the lower brain stem predilection sites. This case of what appears to be an olfactory bulbcentric progression of Lewy pathology is important as an example of a possible alternate pathway of Lewy progression through the brain. The authors conclude that the high incidence of Lewy pathology in the spinal cord and peripheral autonomic nervous system suggests that these structures are involved very early on in the progression of Lewy pathology at least at the same time as the dorsal motor nucleus, locus coeruleus, and olfactory bulb. However, the relatively lower density found in these areas compared to the lower brain stem areas suggests that the pathology may start in the lower brain stem and progress both caudally into higher levels of the brain stem and rostrally into the spinal cord and peripheral autonomic nervous system.

In a recent contribution of their own to this literature, Braak and colleagues examined five patients, three with clinical PD (Braak Lewy body stage 4–5) and two with some Lewy pathology but no evidence of parkinsonism (Braak Lewy body stage 2 and 3), and five control patients with no evidence of Lewy pathology.[72] All cases underwent α-synuclein immunohistochemical examination of the stomach and esophagus. In this study, they were able to demonstrate Lewy pathology in both the Auerbach's and Meissner's plexuses throughout the gastric enteric nervous system in all five cases. It is important to note that there have been no cases of incidental Lewy body disease with Lewy pathology limited to the spinal cord or peripheral autonomic nervous system. However, in addition to these investigations of elderly individuals with no clear history of symptoms relevant to their Lewy pathology, there have been several cases reported of patients with early stages of Lewy pathology and autonomic symptoms relevant to their underlying pathology. Polvikoski and colleagues reported a case of an 82-year-old patient with carotid sinus hypersensitivity and no other evidence of parkinsonism who exhibited mild Lewy pathology in her dorsal motor nucleus of the vagus and solitary tract and marked pathology in her stellate ganglion.[73] Similarly, in a postmortem examination of patients with achalasia but no overt parkinsonism before the advent of α-synuclein immunohistochemistry, Lewy pathology was demonstrated in the esophageal myenteric plexus in several cases.[74] Finally, in several different case reports, Lewy pathology has been observed throughout the autonomic nervous system, both centrally in the spinal cord and peripherally in autonomic neurons, in cases of pure autonomic failure, or Bradbury–Eggleston syndrome.[75–77]

Certainly, one of the greatest difficulties in this area is the rarity with which investigators obtain the brains of patients at the earliest stages of Lewy neurodegeneration and are confident that any relevant symptoms were documented during the last years of the patient's lives. Whether these cases with incidental Lewy pathology are truly patients who would have gone on to develop PD or DLB had they lived long enough is still a matter of some debate. In support of this hypothesis, there have been several studies that demonstrate that patients with incidental Lewy pathology have evidence of subclinical degeneration of the dopaminergic nigrostriatal system.[78–80] In addition, in a study with a novel design that deserves further follow-up and replication, Minguez-Castellanos and colleagues conducted α-synuclein immunohistochemical examination of abdominopelvic tissues from patients who had surgical resections with no history of neurodegenerative disease.[81] They found that 9% contained Lewy pathology in the autonomic plexus of these tissues. Interestingly, after 16 months of follow-up, all four patients with Lewy pathology who underwent cardiac MIBG scintigraphy, a measure of sympathetic innervation of the heart, had abnormal scans while none of three patients without Lewy pathology had abnormal scans. Similarly, 1 out of 3 patients with Lewy pathology had an abnormal SPECT examination of cerebral dopamine with FP-CIT, while none of five patients without Lewy pathology had abnormal scans. Taken together, these studies suggest that patients with incidental Lewy pathology are indeed at risk for developing PD or DLB. However, further studies of clinically well-characterized patients will help to identify more brains with truly incidental Lewy pathology at the earliest stages and determine whether there is a clear progression of pathology between the peripheral autonomic nervous system neurons and spinal cord and the lower brain stem susceptibility areas.

The second major area of concern with the methodologies employed in developing the Braak Lewy body staging is the exclusion of all brains with significant burdens of Alzheimer's pathology from consideration. It has been recognized for some time that patients with dementia, and particularly those with concomitant Alzheimer's pathology, are highly susceptible to develop LBs that are predominant in the amygdala.[82–84] How these patients fit into the Braak Lewy body staging system is not at all clear, as they often do not have pathology in many sites of higher predilection than the amygdala, which is not involved until Braak LB stage 3. In addition, previous studies of the distribution of Lewy pathology in the brains of patients with DLB have recognized the possibility that some patients with this condition have pathology predominantly in the neocortex[25,85] and have even gone so far as to suggest the Lewy body pathology in DLB patients progresses from the cerebrum descending to the brain stem.[86] Limitations of some of these studies include a reliance on late-stage brains, a lack of sampling in many of the lower brain stem areas and utilizing less sensitive methodologies for detecting Lewy pathology. However, a reexamination of 35 DLB brains, including examination throughout the brain stem and diencephalon with α-synuclein immunohistochemistry, revealed consistent results with three patterns of Lewy pathology, a brain stem predominant form, a form with equal burdens in the brain stem and cerebral cortex and a cerebral cortex predominant form.[87] The presence or absence of Alzheimer's pathology varied with the Lewy pathology forms with patients exhibiting little or no Alzheimer's pathology being primarily of the brain stem predominant type and patients with more Alzheimer's pathology comprising the cases in the other two Lewy pathology forms. The authors suggest that this is further evidence that the majority of patients with DLB develop Lewy pathology in the cerebrum with later progression to the brain stem although this remains controversial.

Finally, the last limitation of the Braak LB staging system involves the inability to stage a variable proportion of brains in any given autopsy series because they do not conform to the prescribed distribution pattern. Several studies have attempted to determine what proportion can be appropriately staged according to the Braak staging system and the percentage that do not seem to fit the pattern ranges from 53–83%.[88–92] The reasons for the high variability in the proportion of brains with Lewy pathology that conform to the Braak LB staging system are undoubtedly numerous, but include technical variations in the way that brains were assayed for Lewy pathology and how brains were determined to conform, or not conform, to the staging system. In addition, inclusion of large numbers of brains with other concomitant neurodegenerative diseases such as progressive supranuclear palsy or Alzheimer's disease has contributed to some of the discrepancy. In fact, it has become clear that patients with Alzheimer's disease commonly do not conform to the Braak staging system and the relationship between Lewy pathology and Alzheimer's pathologies is discussed further in the next section.

▶ PATHOLOGY OF PARKINSON'S DISEASE DEMENTIA AND DEMENTIA WITH LEWY BODIES

While a comprehensive discussion of the neuropathology of DLB and PD with dementia (PDD) is beyond the scope of this chapter, there are several concepts that have developed in the past decade that should be recognized. In particular, the significance and relationship between the two most commonly cited correlates of dementia in PD and DLB, namely diffuse Lewy body pathology and Alzheimer's pathology, are beginning to be elucidated. While LBs in the brain stem have been associated with PD for almost a century, the relevance of LBs to dementia has only been fully recognized for the past 2 decades.[85,93,94] The presence of Lewy pathology is considered the pathological hallmark of DLB and PDD just as senile (amyloid) plaques (SP) and neurofibrillary tangles (NFT) are the hallmarks of AD. However, Lewy pathology, SPs and NFTs frequently coexist in patients with dementia, and in some cases, make it difficult to discern the pathologic source of the dementia.[95–98] In fact, the frequency of concurrent pathology in these diseases suggests that there may be a common underlying etiology.[99] In addition, several studies have shown that the burden of concomitant AD pathology alters the DLB phenotype,[98,100–112] which certainly contributed to the low sensitivity of prior diagnostic criteria. The most recent modifications to the consensus criteria for the clinicopathologic diagnosis of DLB attempt to address this complex interaction by providing guidelines for assessing both Lewy pathology and AD pathology and then assigning probability statements of the likelihood that a specific combination is likely to manifest the DLB phenotype.[103]

Recently, several studies have been conducted to investigate further the role of Lewy pathology in the generation of dementia in DLB and PDD and many demonstrated a correlation between Lewy pathology and dementia in DLB[96,104–106] and PD.[107–111] There may be a synergistic effect between Lewy pathology and AD pathology as Samuel and colleagues found that patients with AD who had concomitant Lewy pathology, which they referred to as the Lewy body variant of AD, were more severely demented than DLB patients with the same cortical LB count.[112] Similarly, Serby and colleagues found that dementia is more severe and LBs are more frequent when AD and Lewy pathology coexist.[113] Several recent reports have examined the presence of Alzheimer's pathology in the striatum and have suggested that amyloid pathology in the striatum of patients with PD correlates with dementia[114] and may even differentiate patients with DLB from those with PDD.[115]

In addition, several recent studies suggest that concomitant AD pathology can modify the presentation of PDD so that patients with more AD pathology will develop dementia earlier in the course of PD and will possibly have worse dementia.[94,116,117] Another common observation is that the AD pathology in DLB and PDD may be different from typical AD pathology in that it primarily involves the diffuse type of senile plaques, and there is a relative paucity of NFTs.[118–120] Interestingly, Lashley and colleagues recently found that diffuse plaque burden correlated strongly with the cortical Lewy pathology burden in an assessment of 40 PD patients and 20 age-matched controls, stregthening the argument that amyloid pathology may contribute to the development of dementia in PD.[121] While a detailed discussion of the pathological relathionship between PDD and DLB is beyond the scope of this chapter, this topic has been recently reviewed elsewhere.[122]

In summary, while the pendulum of consensus had previously swung towards the notion that diffuse Lewy pathology, rather than Alzheimer's pathology, was the main contributor towards the development of dementia in PD, recent studies have suggested that both pathologies probably play important roles in this process.[123]

▶ SUMMARY AND CONCLUSIONS

The past decade has seen remarkable advancements in our understanding of the pathology of PD and other forms of parkinsonism. Recognition that α-synuclein is the primary component of Lewy pathology, that Lewy neurites are more prevalent than previously accepted, that Lewy pathology often follows a predictable pattern of progression through the neuraxis and that Lewy pathology and Alzheimer's pathology both contribute to the development of dementia in PD are all significant advancements that provide targets for the development of novel therapeutics in the near future. Recently, consensus criteria for the neuropathologic diagnosis of PD were drafted and will be published shortly (D.W. Dickson personal communication). It is hoped that these and other advancements from the continuing exploration of the neuropathology of PD will lead to better model systems for the development of truly effective neuroprotective therapies leading to a paradigm shift away from merely symptomatic therapies for PD.

REFERENCES

1. Ahlskog, JE. I can't get no satisfaction: Still no neuroprotection for Parkinson disease. Neurology 2007;69:1476.
2. Waldmeier, P, Bozyczko-Coyne D, Williams M, et al. Recent clinical failures in Parkinson's disease with apoptosis inhibitors underline the need for a paradigm shift in drug discovery for neurodegenerative diseases. Biochem. Pharmacol 2006;72:1197.
3. Cookson, MR, Hardy J, and Lewis PA. Genetic neuropathology of Parkinson's disease. Int J Clin Exp Pathol 2008;1:217.
4. Goetz CG. Charcot, the Clinician: The Tuesday lessons. New York: Ravens Press, 1987, p. 139.
5. Erb WH. Paralysis agitans (Parkinson's disease). In A Church (ed). Diseases of the nervous system. New York: D. Appleton and Company, 1910, p. 880.
6. Greenfield JG. The pathology of Parkinson's disease. In M Critchley (ed). James Parkinson (1755-1824), London: MacMillan and Company Limited, 1955, p. 219.
7. Greenfield JG, Bosanquet FD: The brain-stem lesions in Parkinsonism. J Neurol Neurosurg Psychiatry 1953;16:213.
8. McGeer PL, McGeer EG, and Suzuki JS. Aging and extrapyramidal function. Arch Neurol 1977;34:33.
9. Rudow G, O'Brien R, Savonenko AV, et al. Morphometry of the human substantia nigra in ageing and Parkinson's disease. Acta Neuropathol 2008;115:461.
10. Gibb WR and Lees AJ. Anatomy, pigmentation, ventral and dorsal subpopulations of the substantia nigra, and differential cell death in Parkinson's disease. J Neurol Neurosurg Psychiatry 1991:54:388.
11. Halliday GM, McRitchie DA, Cartwright H, et al. Midbrain neuropathology in idiopathic Parkinson's disease and diffuse Lewy body disease. J Clin Neurosci 1996;3:52.
12. Pakkenberg B, Moller A, Gundersen HJ, et al. The absolute number of nerve cells in substantia nigra in normal subjects and in patients with Parkinson's disease estimated with an unbiased stereological method. J Neurol Neurosurg Psychiatry 1991;54:30.
13. Rinne JO, Rummukainen J, Paljarvi L, et al. Dementia in Parkinson's disease is related to neuronal loss in the medial substantia nigra. Ann Neurol 1989;26:47.
14. Mori F, Nishie M, Kakita A, et al. Relationship among alpha-synuclein accumulation, dopamine synthesis, and neurodegeneration in Parkinson disease substantia nigra. J Neuropathol Exp Neurol 2006;65:808.
15. Beach TG, Walker DG, Sue LI, et al. Substantia nigra Marinesco bodies are associated with decreased striatal expression of dopaminergic markers. J Neuropathol Exp Neurol 2004;63:329.
16. Arai N, Yagishita S, Amano N, et al. "Grumose degeneration" of Tretiakoff. J Neurol Sci 1989;94:319.
17. Lees AJ, Selikhova M, Andrade LA, et al. The black stuff and Konstantin Nikolaevich Tretiakoff. Mov Disord 2008;23:777.
18. Dickson DW, Ruan D, Crystal H, et al. Hippocampal degeneration differentiates diffuse Lewy body disease (DLBD) from Alzheimer's disease: Light and electron microscopic immunocytochemistry of CA2-3 neurites specific to DLBD. Neurology 1991;41:1402.
19. Gai WP, Blessing WW, Blumbergs PC: Ubiquitin-positive degenerating neurites in the brainstem in Parkinson's disease. Brain 1995;118 (pt 6):1447.
20. Braak H, Sandmann-Keil D, Gai W, et al. Extensive axonal Lewy neurites in Parkinson's disease: A novel pathological feature revealed by alpha-synuclein immunocytochemistry. Neurosci Lett 1999;265:67.
21. Duda JE, Giasson BI, Mabon ME, et al. Novel antibodies to synuclein show abundant striatal pathology in Lewy body diseases. Ann Neurol 2002;52:205.
22. Gomez-Tortosa E, Newell K, Irizarry MC, et al. Alpha-Synuclein immunoreactivity in dementia with Lewy bodies: morphological staging and comparison with ubiquitin immunostaining. Acta Neuropathol (Berl) 2000;99:352.
23. Irizarry MC, Growdon W, Gomez-Isla T, et al. Nigral and cortical Lewy bodies and dystrophic nigral neurites in Parkinson's disease and cortical Lewy body disease contain alpha-synuclein immunoreactivity. J Neuropathol Exp Neurol 1998;57:334.

24. Braak H, Del Tredici K, Rub U, et al. Staging of brain pathology related to sporadic Parkinson's disease. Neurobiol Aging 2003;24:197.
25. Marui W, Iseki E, Nakai T, et al. Progression and staging of Lewy pathology in brains from patients with dementia with Lewy bodies. J Neurol Sci 2002;195:153.
26. Giasson BI, Duda JE, Quinn SM, et al. Neuronal alpha-synucleinopathy with severe movement disorder in mice expressing A53T human alpha-synuclein. Neuron 2002;34:521.
27. Duda JE: Pathology and neurotransmitter abnormalities of dementia with Lewy bodies. Dement Geriatr Cogn Disord. ,200417(suppl 1):3.
28. Alafuzoff I, Parkkinen L, Al Sarraj S, et al. Assessment of alpha-synuclein pathology: A study of the BrainNet Europe Consortium. J Neuropathol Exp Neurol 2008;67:125.
29. Beach TG, White CL, Hamilton RL, et al. Evaluation of alpha-synuclein immunohistochemical methods used by invited experts. Acta Neuropathol 2008;116:277.
30. Croisier E, MRes DE, Deprez M, et al. Comparative study of commercially available anti-alpha-synuclein antibodies. Neuropathol Appl Neurobiol 2006;32:351.
31. Galvin JE, Lee VM, Baba M, et al. Monoclonal antibodies to purified cortical Lewy bodies recognize the mid-size neurofilament subunit. Ann Neurol 1997;42:595.
32. Goldman JE, Yen SH, Chiu FC, et al. Lewy bodies of Parkinson's disease contain neurofilament antigens. Science 1983;221:1082.
33. Hirsch E, Ruberg M, Portier MM, et al. Characterization of two antigens in parkinsonian Lewy bodies. Brain Res 1988;441:139.
34. Iwatsubo T, Yamaguchi H, Fujimuro M, et al. Lewy bodies: Purification from diffuse Lewy body disease brains. Ann N Y Acad Sci 1996;786:195.
35. Pollanen MS, Bergeron C, and Weyer L. Deposition of detergent-resistant neurofilaments into Lewy body fibrils. Brain Res 1993;603:121.
36. Wakabayashi K, Tanji K, Mori F, et al. The Lewy body in Parkinson's disease: Molecules implicated in the formation and degradation of alpha-synuclein aggregates. Neuropathology 2007;27:494.
37. Lewy FH. Zur Pathologischen Anatomie der Paralysis agitans. Dtsch Z Nervenheilk 1914;1:50.
38. Braak H and Del Tredici K. Neuroanatomy and pathology of sporadic Parkinson's disease. Adv. Anat. Embryol. Cell Biol. 201:1,2009.
39. Aho L, Parkkinen L, Pirttila T, et al. Systematic appraisal using immunohistochemistry of brain pathology in aged and demented subjects. Dement Geriatr Cogn Disord 2008;25:423.
40. Parkkinen L, Pirttila T, Tervahauta M, et al. Widespread and abundant alpha-synuclein pathology in a neurologically unimpaired subject. Neuropathology 2005; 25:304.
41. Parkkinen L, Kauppinen T, Pirttila T, et al. Alpha-synuclein pathology does not predict extrapyramidal symptoms or dementia. Ann Neurol 2005;57:82.
42. Parkkinen L, Pirttila T, and Alafuzoff I. Applicability of current staging/categorization of alpha-synuclein pathology and their clinical relevance. Acta Neuropathol 2008;115:399.
43. Braak E, Sandmann-Keil D, Rub U, et al. Alpha-synuclein immunopositive Parkinson's disease-related inclusion bodies in lower brain stem nuclei. Acta Neuropathol (Berl) 2001;101:195.
44. Braak, H, Braak E, Yilmazer D, et al. Amygdala pathology in Parkinson's disease. Acta Neuropathol. (Berl). 88:493,1994.
45. Braak H and Braak E. Pathoanatomy of Parkinson's disease. J Neurol 2000;247(suppl 2):II3.
46. Braak H, Rub U, Sandmann-Keil D, et al. Parkinson's disease: affection of brain stem nuclei controlling premotor and motor neurons of the somatomotor system. Acta Neuropathol (Berl)2000;99:489.
47. Hirsch EC, Graybiel AM, Duyckaerts C, et al. Neuronal loss in the pedunculopontine tegmental nucleus in Parkinson disease and in progressive supranuclear palsy. Proc Natl Acad Sci U S A 1987;84:5976.
48. Gai WP, Blumbergs PC, Geffen LB, et al. Age-related loss of dorsal vagal neurons in Parkinson's disease. Neurology 1992;42:2106.
49. Goto S and Hirano A. Catecholaminergic neurons in the parabrachial nucleus of normal individuals and patients with idiopathic Parkinson's disease. Ann Neurol 1991;30:192.
50. Hawkes CH, Shephard BC, and Daniel SE. Olfactory dysfunction in Parkinson's disease. J Neurol Neurosurg Psychiatry 1997;62:436.
51. Pearce RK, Hawkes CH, and Daniel SE. The anterior olfactory nucleus in Parkinson's disease. Mov Disord 1995;10:283.
52. Jellinger KA. Pathology of Parkinson's disease. Changes other than the nigrostriatal pathway. Mol Chem Neuropathol 1991;14:153.
53. Langston JW and Forno LS. The hypothalamus in Parkinson disease. Ann Neurol 1978;3:129.
54. Pahapill PA and Lozano AM. The pedunculopontine nucleus and Parkinson's disease. Brain 2000;123 (pt 9):1767.
55. Del Tredici K, Rub U, de Vos RA, et al. Where does Parkinson disease pathology begin in the brain? J Neuropathol Exp Neurol 2002;61:413.
56. Braak H, Del Tredici K, Bratzke H, et al. Staging of the intracerebral inclusion body pathology associated with idiopathic Parkinson's disease (preclinical and clinical stages). J Neurol 2002;249(suppl 3:III/1–III/5.
57. Braak H, Rub U, Gai WP, et al. Idiopathic Parkinson's disease: possible routes by which vulnerable neuronal types may be subject to neuroinvasion by an unknown pathogen. J Neural Transm 2003;110:517.
58. Braak H, Del Tredici K, Rub U, et al. Staging of brain pathology related to sporadic Parkinson's disease. Neurobiol Aging 2003;24:197.
59. Braak H, Ghebremedhin E, Rub U, et al. Stages in the development of Parkinson's disease-related pathology. Cell Tissue Res 2004;318:121.
60. Muller CM, de Vos RA, Maurage CA, et al. Staging of sporadic Parkinson disease-related alpha-synuclein pathology: inter- and intra-rater reliability. J Neuropathol Exp Neurol 2005;64:623.
61. Hishikawa N, Hashizume Y, Yoshida M, et al. Clinical and neuropathological correlates of Lewy body disease. Acta Neuropathol (Berl) 2003;105:341.

62. Oyanagi K, Wakabayashi K, Ohama E, et al. Lewy bodies in the lower sacral parasympathetic neurons of a patient with Parkinson's disease. Acta Neuropathol (Berl) 1990;80:558.
63. Wakabayashi K and Takahashi H. The intermediolateral nucleus and Clarke's column in Parkinson's disease. Acta Neuropathol (Berl) 1997;94:287.
64. Forno LS, Norville RL: Ultrastructure of Lewy bodies in the stellate ganglion. Acta Neuropathol (Berl) 1976; 34:183.
65. Wakabayashi K and Takahashi H. Neuropathology of autonomic nervous system in Parkinson's disease. Eur Neurol 1997;38(suppl 2):2.
66. Wakabayashi K, Takahashi H, Ohama E, et al. Lewy bodies in the visceral autonomic nervous system in Parkinson's disease. Adv Neurol 1993;60:609.
67. Wakabayashi K, Takahashi H, Takeda S, et al. Parkinson's disease: The presence of Lewy bodies in Auerbach's and Meissner's plexuses. Acta Neuropathol (Berl) 1988;76:217.
68. Takeda S, Yamazaki K, Miyakawa T, et al. Parkinson's disease with involvement of the parasympathetic ganglia. Acta Neuropathol (Berl)1993;86:397.
69. Braak H, Rub U, Gai WP, et al. Idiopathic Parkinson's disease: Possible routes by which vulnerable neuronal types may be subject to neuroinvasion by an unknown pathogen. J Neural Transm 2003;110:517.
70. Bloch A, Probst A, Bissig H, et al. Alpha-synuclein pathology of the spinal and peripheral autonomic nervous system in neurologically unimpaired elderly subjects. Neuropathol Appl Neurobiol 2006;32:284.
71. Klos KJ, Ahlskog JE, Josephs KA, et al. Alpha-synuclein pathology in the spinal cords of neurologically asymptomatic aged individuals. Neurology 2006;66:1100.
72. Braak H, de Vos RA, Bohl J, et al. Gastric alpha-synuclein immunoreactive inclusions in Meissner's and Auerbach's plexuses in cases staged for Parkinson's disease-related brain pathology. Neurosci Lett 2006;396:67.
73. Polvikoski T, Kalaria RN, Perry R, et al. Carotid sinus hypersensitivity associated with focal alpha-synucleinopathy of the autonomic nervous system. J Neurol Neurosurg Psychiatry 2006;77:1064.
74. Qualman SJ, Haupt HM, Yang P, et al. Esophageal Lewy bodies associated with ganglion cell loss in achalasia. Similarity to Parkinson's disease. Gastroenterology 1984;87:848.
75. Arai K, Kato N, Kashiwado K, et al. Pure autonomic failure in association with human alpha-synucleinopathy. Neurosci Lett 2000;296:171.
76. Hague K, Lento P, Morgello S, et al. The distribution of Lewy bodies in pure autonomic failure: Autopsy findings and review of the literature. Acta Neuropathol (Berl) 1997;94:192.
77. van Ingelghem E, van Zandijcke M, and Lammens M. Pure autonomic failure: a new case with clinical, biochemical, and necropsy data. J Neurol Neurosurg Psychiatry 1994;57:745.
78. Beach TG, Adler CH, Sue LI, et al. Reduced striatal tyrosine hydroxylase in incidental Lewy body disease. Acta Neuropathol 2008;115:445.
79. DelleDonne A, Klos KJ, Fujishiro H, et al. Incidental Lewy body disease and preclinical Parkinson disease. Arch Neurol 2008;65:1074.
80. Dickson DW, Fujishiro H, DelleDonne A, et al. Evidence that incidental Lewy body disease is pre-symptomatic Parkinson's disease. Acta Neuropathol 2008;115:437.
81. Minguez-Castellanos A, Chamorro CE, Escamilla-Sevilla F, et al. Do alpha-synuclein aggregates in autonomic plexuses predate Lewy body disorders? A cohort study. Neurology 2007;68:2012.
82. Hamilton RL. Lewy bodies in Alzheimer's disease: A neuropathological review of 145 cases using alpha-synuclein immunohistochemistry. Brain Pathol 2000;10:378.
83. Lippa CF, Fujiwara H, Mann DM, et al. Lewy bodies contain altered alpha-synuclein in brains of many familial Alzheimer's disease patients with mutations in presenilin and amyloid precursor protein genes. Am J Pathol 1998;153:1365.
84. Lippa CF, Schmidt ML, Lee VM, et al. Antibodies to alpha-synuclein detect Lewy bodies in many Down's syndrome brains with Alzheimer's disease. Ann Neurol 1999;45:353.
85. McKeith IG, Galasko D, Kosaka K, et al. Consensus guidelines for the clinical and pathologic diagnosis of dementia with Lewy bodies (DLB): Report of the consortium on DLB international workshop. Neurology 1996;47:1113.
86. Marui W, Iseki E, Kato M, et al. Pathological entity of dementia with Lewy bodies and its differentiation from Alzheimer's disease. Acta Neuropathol (Berl) 2004;108:121.
87. Yamamoto R, Iseki E, Marui W, et al. Non-uniformity in the regional pattern of Lewy pathology in brains of dementia with Lewy bodies. Neuropathology 2005;25:188.
88. Ballard C, Ziabreva I, Perry R, et al. Differences in neuropathologic characteristics across the Lewy body dementia spectrum. Neurology 2006;67:1931.
89. Halliday GM and McCann H. Human-based studies on alpha-synuclein deposition and relationship to Parkinson's disease symptoms. Exp Neurol 2008;209:12.
90. Kalaitzakis ME, Graeber MB, Gentleman SM, et al. The dorsal motor nucleus of the vagus is not an obligatory trigger site of Parkinson's disease: A critical analysis of alpha-synuclein staging. Neuropathol Appl Neurobiol 2008;34:284.
91. Uchikado H, DelleDonne A, Ahmed Z, et al. Lewy bodies in progressive supranuclear palsy represent an independent disease process. J Neuropathol Exp Neurol 2006;65:387.
92. Zaccai J, Brayne C, McKeith I, et al. Patterns and stages of alpha-synucleinopathy: Relevance in a population-based cohort. Neurology ,2008;70:1042.
93. Kosaka K, Yoshimura M, Ikeda K, et al. Diffuse type of Lewy body disease: progressive dementia with abundant cortical Lewy bodies and senile changes of varying degree--a new disease? Clin Neuropathol 1984;3:185.
94. Perry RH, Irving D, Blessed G, et al. Senile dementia of Lewy body type. A clinically and neuropathologically distinct form of Lewy body dementia in the elderly. J Neurol Sci 1990;95:119.
95. Galasko D, Hansen LA, Katzman R, et al. Clinical-neuropathological correlations in Alzheimer's disease and related dementias. Arch Neurol 1994;51:888.
96. Samuel W, Crowder R, Hofstetter CR, et al. Neuritic plaques in the Lewy body variant of Alzheimer disease lack paired helical filaments. Neurosci Lett 1997;223:73.

97. Szpak GM, Lewandowska E, Lechowicz W, et al. Lewy body variant of Alzheimer's disease and Alzheimer's disease: A comparative immunohistochemical study. Folia Neuropathol 2001;39:63.
98. Merdes AR, Hansen LA, Jeste DV, et al. Influence of Alzheimer pathology on clinical diagnostic accuracy in dementia with Lewy bodies. Neurology 2003;60:1586.
99. Pompeu F and Growdon JH. Diagnosing dementia with Lewy bodies. Arch Neurol 2002;59:29.
100. Del Ser T, Hachinski V, Merskey H, et al. Clinical and pathologic features of two groups of patients with dementia with Lewy bodies: Effect of coexisting Alzheimer-type lesion load. Alzheimer Dis Assoc Disord 2001;15:31.
101. Lopez OL, Becker JT, Kaufer DI, et al. Research evaluation and prospective diagnosis of dementia with Lewy bodies. Arch Neurol 2002;59:43.
102. Weisman D, Cho M, Taylor C, et al. In dementia with Lewy bodies, Braak stage determines phenotype, not Lewy body distribution. Neurology 2007;69:356.
103. McKeith IG, Dickson DW, Lowe J, et al. Diagnosis and management of dementia with Lewy bodies: Third report of the DLB Consortium. Neurology 2005;65:1863.
104. Haroutunian V, Serby M, Purohit DP, et al. Contribution of Lewy body inclusions to dementia in patients with and without Alzheimer disease neuropathological conditions. Arch Neurol 2000;57:1145.
105. Lennox G, Lowe J, Morrell K, et al. Anti-ubiquitin immunocytochemistry is more sensitive than conventional techniques in the detection of diffuse Lewy body disease. J Neurol Neurosurg Psychiatry 1989;52:67.
106. Samuel W, Galasko D, Masliah E, et al. Neocortical lewy body counts correlate with dementia in the Lewy body variant of Alzheimer's disease. J Neuropathol Exp Neurol 1996;55:44.
107. Apaydin H, Ahlskog JE, Parisi JE, et al. Parkinson disease neuropathology: later-developing dementia and loss of the levodopa response. Arch Neurol 2002;59:102.
108. Hurtig, HI, Trojanowski JQ, Galvin J, et al): Alpha-synuclein cortical Lewy bodies correlate with dementia in Parkinson's disease. Neurology 2000;54:1916.
109. Kovari, E, Gold G, Herrmann FR, et al. Lewy body densities in the entorhinal and anterior cingulate cortex predict cognitive deficits in Parkinson's disease. Acta Neuropathol (Berl) 2003;106:83.
110. Mattila PM, Roytta M, Torikka H, et al. Cortical Lewy bodies and Alzheimer-type changes in patients with Parkinson's disease. Acta Neuropathol (Berl) 1998;95:576.
111. Mattila PM, Rinne JO, Helenius H, et al. Alpha-synuclein-immunoreactive cortical Lewy bodies are associated with cognitive impairment in Parkinson's disease. Acta Neuropathol (Berl) 2000;100:285.
112. Samuel W, Alford M, Hofstetter CR, et al. Dementia with Lewy bodies versus pure Alzheimer disease: differences in cognition, neuropathology, cholinergic dysfunction, and synapse density. J Neuropathol Exp Neurol,1997; 56:499.
113. Serby M, Brickman AM, Haroutunian V, et al. Cognitive burden and excess Lewy-body pathology in the Lewy-body variant of Alzheimer disease. Am J Geriatr Psychiatry 2003;11:371.
114. Kalaitzakis ME, Graeber MB, Gentleman SM, et al. Striatal beta-amyloid deposition in Parkinson disease with dementia. J Neuropathol Exp Neurol 2008;67:155.
115. Jellinger KA and Attems J. Does striatal pathology distinguish Parkinson disease with dementia and dementia with Lewy bodies? Acta Neuropathol 2006; 112:253.
116. Jellinger KA. Morphological substrates of parkinsonism with and without dementia: a retrospective clinico-pathological study. J Neural Transm 2007;Suppl 91.
117. Galvin JE, Pollack J, and Morris JC. Clinical phenotype of Parkinson disease dementia. Neurology 2006;67:1605.
118. Hansen LA, Masliah E, Galasko D, et al): Plaque-only Alzheimer disease is usually the lewy body variant, and vice versa. J. Neuropathol. Exp. Neurol. 52:648,1993.
119. Mann DM, Brown SM, Owen F, et al. Amyloid beta protein (A beta) deposition in dementia with Lewy bodies: predominance of A beta 42(43) and paucity of A beta 40 compared with sporadic Alzheimer's disease. Neuropathol Appl Neurobiol 1998;24:187.
120. Samuel W, Alford M, Hofstetter CR, et al. Dementia with Lewy bodies versus pure Alzheimer disease: Differences in cognition, neuropathology, cholinergic dysfunction, and synapse density. J Neuropathol Exp Neurol 1997;56:499.
121. Lashley T, Holton JL, Gray E, et al. Cortical alpha-synuclein load is associated with amyloid-beta plaque burden in a subset of Parkinson's disease patients. Acta Neuropathol 2008;115:417.
122. Duda JE, and McKeith I. Cortical Lewy body disease: dementia with Lewy bodies and Parkinson's disease with dementia. In Cappa SF, Abutalebi J, Demonet J-F, et al (eds), Cognitive Neurology: a Clinical Textbook. Oxford, Oxford University Press, 2008, p. 293.
123. Thal DR, Del Tredici K, and Braak H. Neurodegeneration in normal brain aging and disease. Sci. Aging Knowledge. Environ. 2004;2004:e26.

OTHER PARKINSONIAN SYNDROMES

CHAPTER 20

Multiple-System Atrophy

Bradley J. Robottom, Lisa M. Shulman, and William J. Weiner

The topic multiple-system atrophy (MSA) alerts the reader that a description of a neurodegenerative disorder characterized by predominant involvement of the basal ganglia, cerebellar, and autonomic pathways follows. The uninitiated may be understandably misled by the broad inference of the term MSA. We describe the historical derivation of this appellation, although perhaps we should not dismiss the impulse to reexamine the congruity of this diagnostic subset with the range of patients seen in the clinical setting. The sharp distinction of MSA from the other neurodegenerative processes, as depicted in discrete chapters of this book, belies the challenge facing the clinician when diagnosing the individual patient. Despite the prodigious advances in medicine, MSA and neurodegenerative disorders as a group remain clinical diagnoses, and the heterogeneity of our patients defies simple classification.

▶ HISTORICAL BACKGROUND AND NOSOLOGY

The conceptualization of the diagnosis of MSA emerged from a series of publications that each described fragments of a larger picture. Dejerine and Thomas[1] first coined the term olivopontocerebellar atrophy (OPCA) in 1900 to describe two sporadic cases of progressive cerebellar degeneration with parkinsonism. Sixty years later, Shy and Drager[2] published the first clinicopathological study of a patient with idiopathic orthostatic hypotension (OH). They recognized the association of OH with a primary degenerative disorder of the nervous system involving the intermediolateral cell column of the spinal cord, medulla, pons, midbrain, cerebellum, and basal ganglia. The full clinical syndrome comprised "orthostatic hypotension, urinary and rectal incontinence, loss of sweating, iris atrophy, external ocular palsies, rigidity, tremor, loss of associated movement, impotence, the findings of an atonic bladder and loss of the rectal sphincter tone, fasciculations, wasting of distal muscles, and evidence of a neuropathic lesion."[2]

Also in 1960, van der Eecken et al.[3] described a unique pathological subgroup among a large number of patients with paralysis agitans. Striatopallidonigral degeneration was identified with "virtual disappearance of the small cells of the caudate nucleus and putamen" in a few patients with rigidity but minimal tremor. The full clinicopathological study was published the following year.[4] In addition to parkinsonism, brisk reflexes, extensor plantar responses, ataxia, dysarthria, syncope, incontinence, and impotence were described among the three patients reported. Neurodegeneration was also identified in the cerebellum, olivary nuclei, and pons.

The conceptual threads of the three disorders, OPCA, Shy–Drager syndrome (SDS), and striatonigral degeneration (SND), were tied together in a seminal paper by Graham and Oppenheimer[5] in 1969:

> What is needed is a general term to cover this collection of overlapping progressive presenile multisystem degenerations. As the causes of this group of conditions are still unknown, such a general term would merely be a temporary practical convenience... What we wish to avoid is the multiplication of names for 'disease entities' which in fact are merely the expressions of neuronal atrophy in a variety of overlapping combinations. We therefore propose to use the term multiple system atrophy to cover the whole group.

Graham and Oppenheimer also identified two subgroups of patients with idiopathic OH: those with Lewy body pathology and those without. This latter group comprised the patients with MSA. Bannister and Oppenheimer[6] again highlighted this distinction in their clinicopathological review of 16 patients in 1972. Although parkinsonian features and lesions of the pigmented nuclei were common to both groups, MSA was distinguished by an earlier mean age of onset than idiopathic paralysis agitans (49 years, as compared to 65), and a worsened prognosis.

Although the terms SND, OPCA, and SDS confer additional information about the predominant clinical presentation, they are no longer regularly used. Instead, MSA is designated MSA-P if parkinsonism is the predominant motor symptom at presentation and MSA-C if a cerebellar syndrome predominates.[7] Autonomic dysfunction is present with both MSA-P and MSA-C. While parkinsonism, autonomic failure, or cerebellar dysfunction may mark the beginning of the disease, the emergence of the other two syndromes can be predicted when the patient survives long enough.

Familial associations of MSA are rarely observed. Historically, there was considerable debate regarding MSA-C (OPCA) and heredity. Older descriptions of autosomal dominant OPCA likely represent spinocerebellar ataxias (SCA), which are discussed in a different chapter. MSA-C may present with a predominant cerebellar syndrome. Penney pointed out that there is a growing body of evidence from positron emission tomography (PET) studies and pathology to indicate that sporadic cerebellar degeneration of the Dejerine and Thomas type is MSA and is distinct from the dominantly inherited cerebellar degenerations.[8] While an autosomal dominant pattern of inheritance should call into doubt the diagnosis of MSA, recent reports indicate that some cases of MSA may be autosomal recessive.[9]

We use the term MSA to refer to a gradually progressive, idiopathic neurodegenerative process of adult onset characterized by varying proportions of cerebellar dysfunction, autonomic failure, and parkinsonism that is poorly responsive to L-dopa therapy. The clinical syndrome is dominated but not confined to these features. Familial presentations will be excluded from the discussion. It is understood that these lines are currently drawn more to conform with precedent and practicality than to reflect genuine and fundamental attributes of pathophysiology.

▶ EPIDEMIOLOGY

MSA affects both sexes equally. The exact prevalence of MSA is unknown because of limited epidemiologic data. However, one cross-sectional study in a primary care service reported a prevalence of 4.4 per 100,000 in the UK.[10] Estimates from France based on data from specialty clinics reveals a prevalence of 1.9 per 100,000.[11] Vanacore et al.[12] reported the annual incidence of new cases as about 0.6 per 100,000 population. Ben-Shlomo et al., in a meta-analysis of published cases of pathologically proven MSA, calculated a mean age at onset of 54.2 years and a median survival of 6.2 years.[13] MSA usually begins in middle age and advances over a period of 1–18 years.[14,15] Estimated survival rates at 5 and 10 years after clinical onset are 83.5% and 39.9%, respectively.[16]

▶ CLINICAL DIAGNOSIS

The initial evaluation of a patient with MSA is simply a "snapshot" of the evolving neurodegenerative process. Although the initial presentation may suggest the diagnosis, often the full picture will remain obscured for some time. In fact, the akinetic-rigid patient who is poorly responsive to L-dopa therapy has a broad differential diagnosis. The impression will be later refined by the emerging signs: a vertical supranuclear ophthalmoparesis suggests progressive supranuclear palsy (PSP), whereas prominent OH suggests MSA. Ironically, an initial evaluation of a patient with an advanced neurodegenerative disorder may also be difficult to sort out, particularly when historical data regarding the order and time frame of the symptoms are lacking. For example, cerebellar signs may be difficult to appreciate in the wheelchair-bound patient with profound rigidity and bradykinesia. Therefore, diagnostic accuracy requires either long-term follow-up of the individual patient or the good fortune to be confronted by the patient when all the diagnostic pieces of the puzzle are in place. Even then, confidence in our diagnostic impression is tempered by the inability to confirm our clinical intuition.

Although MSA patients can manifest any combination of basal ganglia, autonomic, and cerebellar features, movement disorders of basal ganglia origin (i.e., parkinsonism) are the most common. Quinn[17] reported that parkinsonism was present in 89% of MSA case reports at some point in the course of their illness. Autonomic failure occurred in 78% and cerebellar signs in 55%. Pyramidal involvement is also very common, occurring in 61%. Twenty-eight percent of MSA patients developed the full clinical spectrum (i.e., parkinsonism, autonomic failure, cerebellar signs, and pyramidal signs) before death.

Quinn[18] first proposed a set of clinical diagnostic criteria for MSA in 1989. A consensus conference on diagnosis of MSA was convened in 1998 and a statement on the diagnosis of MSA published.[19] These guidelines were updated in 2008 to reflect advances in neuroimaging techniques.[7] The guidelines for diagnosis of MSA are presented in Table 20–1. Application of either the Quinn or the 1998 consensus criteria is far superior to actual clinical diagnosis made early in the disease.[20] The second consensus criteria have not yet been validated, but the changes from the first consensus criteria are not expected to reduce diagnostic accuracy. As with previous criteria, the term definite MSA is reserved for cases with autopsy findings of typical pathological features.[21] Probable MSA is the term used for patients with autonomic failure plus parkinsonism or cerebellar ataxia. Possible MSA is the diagnosis in patients with clinical findings that are suggestive of the disease but do not clearly represent MSA.[7] Clinical features that do not support a diagnosis of MSA include a classic, pill-rolling rest tremor, clinically significant neuropathy, hallucinations in absence of dopaminergic medications, age of onset >75 years, dementia, family history of ataxia or parkinsonism, and abnormal brain MRI suggestive of multiple sclerosis. Additional features that should lead one to consider a diagnosis of

TABLE 20-1. CRITERIA FOR THE DIAGNOSIS OF MSA

Probable MSA	Possible MSA
• Autonomic failure: Involving urinary incontinence (with erectile dysfunction in men) *or* An orthostatic decrease of blood pressure within 3 min of standing by at least 30 mm Hg systolic or 15 mm Hg diastolic	• Parkinsonism (bradykinesia with rigidity, tremor, sor postural instability) *or* • A cerebellar syndrome (gait ataxia with cerebellar dysarthria, limb ataxia, or cerebellar oculomotor dysfunction)
and	*and*
• Poorly levodopa–responsive parkinsonism (bradykinesia with rigidity, tremor, or postural instability) *or* • A cerebellar syndrome (gait ataxia with cerebellar dysarthria, limb ataxia, or cerebellar oculomotor dysfunction)	• At least one feature suggesting autonomic dysfunction: Otherwise unexplained urinary urgency, frequency, or incomplete bladder emptying Erectile dysfunction in males Significant orthostatic blood pressure decline that does not meet the level required in probable MSA
	and
	• One of the following features: Babinski sign with hyperreflexia Stridor Rapidly progressive parkinsonism Poor response to levodopa Postural instability within 3 years of motor onset A combination of a cerebellar syndrome and parkinsonism Dysphagia within 5 years of motor onset Atrophy on MRI of putamen, middle cerebellar peduncle, pons, or cerebellum Hypometabolism on FDG-PET in putamen, brain stem, or cerebellum Atrophy on MRI of putamen, middle cerebellar peduncle, or pons Hypometabolism on FDG-PET in putamen Presynaptic nigrostriatal dopaminergic denervation on SPECT or PET

Data adapted from Gilman S, Wenning GK, Low PA, et al. Second consensus statement on the diagnosis of multiple system atrophy. Neurology 2008;71:670–676.

MSA but are not part of the diagnostic criteria include the following:

- Orofacial dystonia
- Disproportionate anterocollis
- Camptocormia and/or Pisa syndrome
- Inspiratory sighs
- Severe dysphonia
- Severe dysarthria
- New or increased snoring
- Contractures of hands or feet
- Cold hands and feet
- Pathologic laughter or crying
- Jerky, myoclonic postural or action tremor

PARKINSONIAN FEATURES

Progressive akinesia, rigidity, and postural instability are common features of MSA. Tremor may occur, although it is less frequent than in Parkinson's disease (PD). Bilateral onset of symptoms favors MSA over PD, although unilateral presentations do occur.[22] Hypomimia, micrographia, and a narrow-based, shuffling gait with flexion posture appear. Extreme anterior (camptocormia) or lateral flexion (Pisa syndrome) of the trunk is more suggestive of MSA than PD. The primary distinguishing factors between PD and MSA presenting with isolated parkinsonian signs are early postural instability, rapid progression, and a poor or atypical response to dopaminergic therapy.[23]

In practice, MSA is most frequently confused with PD or PSP. Mild limitation of upward gaze alone is nonspecific, whereas a prominent (>50%) limitation of upward gaze or any limitation of downward gaze suggests PSP. Before the onset of vertical gaze limitation, a clinically obvious slowing of voluntary vertical saccades may be detectable in PSP and assists in the differentiation of these two disorders. Loss of optokinetic nystagmus also differentiates PSP from MSA.

An adequate trial of L-dopa assumes a central role in identifying patients with MSA, although one can be misled. One-third of early MSA patients reported by Rajput et al.[24] experienced a moderate-to-marked improvement with L-dopa therapy, and Quinn[18] similarly observed a moderate-to-good response in one-third. Hughes et al.[25] reported that 65% of pathologically confirmed MSA patients had an initial response to L-dopa, and 35% remained partially responsive until death. The benefits are generally less impressive than those observed in PD and tend to decline over 1–2 years of treatment. L-Dopa-induced dyskinesias occur in MSA. They may appear unusually early and with an atypical predilection for the face and neck. Dyskinesias may be observed without concomitant symptomatic improvement. It is uncommon to obtain symptomatic relief from other antiparkinsonian agents in the absence of a response to L-dopa. Although the benefits are less gratifying than in PD, this should not discourage the clinician from attempting an adequate trial of high-dose L-dopa (1000 mg/day) in MSA patients with parkinsonism.

▶ AUTONOMIC FAILURE

Practically all patients with MSA develop some degree of clinically apparent autonomic failure. For example, postural hypotension ranging from mild symptoms of "dizziness" to frank syncope manifests in 88% of patients.[2,26,27] From the perspective of a neurological clinic, where the neurological history and examination are more intensive than the autonomic evaluation, the prevalence, severity, and time frame of the dysautonomia may be underestimated. Although orthostasis and genitourinary difficulties are most likely to be brought to the attention of the physician, problems of thermoregulation and gastrointestinal and respiratory function are not uncommon.

Autonomic dysfunction may also occur in PD; therefore, this array of symptoms and signs in a patient with an akinetic-rigid syndrome does not immediately imply a diagnosis of MSA. Magalhaes et al.,[26] in a retrospective review of autonomic dysfunction in pathologically confirmed cases of MSA and PD, identified certain distinctions regarding prevalence and severity that may prove useful in differentiating MSA and PD when autonomic signs and symptoms are present. All patients with MSA had some autonomic involvement, whereas 24% of PD had none. Autonomic dysfunction in MSA involved more autonomic functions and was more severe than that seen in PD, particularly with regard to inspiratory stridor. Although this investigation concluded that autonomic disturbance alone does not distinguish among MSA and PD in individual patients, the presence of severe autonomic dysfunction, autonomic dysfunction that precedes parkinsonism, and inspiratory stridor are all suggestive of MSA.

On initial evaluation of the patient with autonomic signs, the distinction between the primary autonomic failure of MSA and secondary autonomic dysfunction should be considered. ...Common medical disorders, including diabetes mellitus, autoimmune disease, neoplasia, and renal failure, may give rise to autonomic dysfunction. A variety of medications, including antihypertensives, cardiovascular agents, diuretics, tricyclic antidepressants, and antiparkinsonian drugs, may contribute to postural hypotension.

OH is the most commonly recognized symptom of autonomic dysfunction and develops in nearly all patients with autonomic failure. A strict definition of OH is used in the diagnosis of probable MSA, requiring blood pressure to fall greater than 30-mmHg systolic blood pressure or 15-mmHg diastolic blood pressure within 3 minutes of standing from a seated position. Not infrequently, significant orthostasis is documented in asymptomatic patients, as gradually progressive and chronic autonomic failure promotes compensatory adjustments of cerebral autoregulation. The symptoms related to postural hypotension are variable, ranging from vague descriptions of lethargy or weakness to full syncope. Other complaints include dizziness, visual disturbances, and craniocervical discomfort, although patients rarely relate their symptoms to changes of position without direct questioning. Craniocervical pain has been referred to as "coat-hanger" pain, and may represent hypoperfusion of contracted muscles.[28]

Postural hypotension is exacerbated after prolonged recumbency, mealtime, and physical exertion. Other contributory factors are heat, alcohol, coughing, and defecation.[29,30] Management of OH involves a number of prophylactic measures. As nocturnal diuresis in the elderly contributes to inadequate blood volume and OH upon arising, recommendations are designed to improve intravascular volume and diminish peripheral edema. Liberalizing salt and water intake, the application of elastic stockings before arising, elevation of the legs periodically during the day, and elevation of the head at night may be helpful. Physical exertion should be delayed until the afternoon and should not closely follow mealtime. Pharmacological therapies for the treatment of OH include fludrocortisone and midodrine.[31,32]

Genitourinary dysfunction in MSA is very common. Beck et al.[33] studied urological features of 62 patients clinically diagnosed with MSA. All patients had abnormal urethral or anal sphincter electromyograms, a finding the authors considered diagnostic in the appropriate clinical setting. Impotence was the presenting symptom in 37% of men and occurred in 96% with progression of the illness. Frequent spontaneous penile erections may antedate erectile failure. The absence of penile erection upon awakening in the morning favors a neurogenic rather than a functional etiology for impotence. Urinary symptoms resulted from a combination of detrusor hyperreflexia, urethral sphincter weakness, and, finally, failure of detrusor contraction. The urinary symptoms simulated outflow obstruction in men, and 43 percent underwent prostatic or bladder neck surgery. Fifty-seven percent of the women had stress incontinence, and one-half had undergone surgical bladder repair. The results of operative procedures in both sexes were poor. Nonsurgical treatment with intermittent catheterization, anti-cholinergic medication, and desmopressin spray improved continence in over one-half of the patients. Anticholinergic medication may result in urinary retention, and intermittent catheterization may result in recurrent infection.

Sakakibara et al. also studied micturitional disturbance in 86 patients with clinically diagnosed MSA.[34] The authors subdivided their MSA patients into those with SDS, SND, and OPCA to further classify urinary dysfunction. Micturitional symptoms were found in more than 90 percent of patients, regardless of MSA subdivision. Urinary symptoms appeared earlier and were more severe in SDS than in SND or OPCA. Urinary symptoms progressed with disease progression. In men with MSA, a careful history will reveal that erectile dysfunction often precedes bladder dysfunction.[35] Preserved erectile function should call into question a diagnosis of MSA.[7]

Constipation is the most common gastrointestinal symptom and affects 57 percent of patients.[36] Straining during evacuation or micturition elevates intrathoracic pressure and may result in symptomatic hypotension. Daily use of dietary fiber, adequate liquid intake, and laxatives is helpful. Fecal incontinence occasionally occurs, although it is less common than urinary incontinence. Dysphagia is not uncommon in more advanced stages of the disorder. Laryngeal stridor is another serious manifestation of MSA, which may be due to the loss of motor neurons of the nucleus ambiguus innervating the laryngeal abductor muscles.[37] A study by Benarroch et al. of the number of cholinergic neurons in the nucleus ambiguus of patients with MSA and PD failed to confirm neuronal loss as the sole cause of stridor in patients with MSA.[38] Bilateral abductor vocal fold paresis, a life-threatening condition, has also been reported in patients with MSA.[39] The advisability of either gastrostomy or tracheostomy should be approached on an individual basis with a realistic appraisal of the patient's quality of life.

A mild, normocytic, normochromic anemia may exist due to loss of sympathetic stimulation of renal erythropoietin production.[40] It is rarely severe enough to be clinically significant.

▶ CEREBELLAR DYSFUNCTION

Whereas the majority of MSA patients present with parkinsonism, in others a cerebellar syndrome heralds the development of multisystem involvement. The initial manifestations are gait ataxia accompanied by ataxia of speech and cerebellar oculomotor abnormalities.[7] Limb ataxia may develop as the disease progresses.[41] Dysarthria is nearly universal, although its nature may vary. Speech may be scanning, bulbar, pseudobulbar, monotone, slow, or hypophonic. Kinetic tremor with dysmetria may occur. Other cerebellar features include hypotonia and exaggerated rebound with loss of checking response. Myoclonus may be seen. Nystagmus, jerky pursuit, ocular dysmetria, square wave jerks, and slowing of saccades are common in MSA patients.[42] Mild limitations of gaze are also common. Supranuclear vertical gaze palsy or severe slowing of saccades is not consistent with a diagnosis of MSA.[7]

Therapeutics for cerebellar signs remains a disappointing and frustrating area for the clinician. When tremor or myoclonus is prominent, trials of clonazepam or valproate may prove worthwhile. Patients with isolated cerebellar dysfunction are frequently diagnosed with cerebellar degeneration. The later emergence of autonomic, basal ganglia, and pyramidal signs is often overlooked, delaying both appropriate diagnosis as well as therapeutic opportunities for parkinsonian or autonomic symptoms. While no specific pharmacologic therapies are available for the cerebellar features of MSA, physical therapy may be useful for gait ataxia.

▶ PYRAMIDAL SIGNS

Exaggerated deep tendon reflexes, extensor plantar responses, pseudobulbar palsy, and spasticity are present in the majority of MSA patients, often early in the disorder. The presence of prominent rigidity and bradykinesia often masks both pyramidal spasticity and cerebellar incoordination.

▶ COGNITIVE FUNCTION AND BEHAVIOR

Although progressive dementia is not a feature of MSA, cognitive deficits and alterations of personality and mood are common. When the cognitive performance of 16 patients with probable MSA of the striatonigral type (mean Hoehn and Yahr stage 3.7) was studied and compared to that of normal controls, the MSA group showed significant deficits on tests of frontal lobe function.[43] Specifically, attentional set shifting and speed of thinking were impaired, although there was no consistent evidence of intellectual deterioration, as measured by the Wechsler Adult Intelligence Scale. Cognitive deficits were not correlated with either the duration or the severity of disease. The pattern of deficits was distinctive, markedly in contrast to Alzheimer's dementia, but similar to that of non-demented PD patients. Personality alterations include apathy, passivity, emotional lability, and depression. This confluence of impaired executive functions, apathy, and impulsivity is characteristic of frontal subcortical circuit dysfunction.[44] The presence of significant dementia or psychosis should signal to the clinician that the diagnosis of MSA may not be correct.

▶ DIAGNOSTIC INVESTIGATIONS

Neuroradiological evaluation is routinely performed in the investigation of a patient with progressive neurological deficits. Cranial computed tomography (CT) may reveal infratentorial atrophy. When CT images of 33 MSA patients and 40 age-matched controls were blindly analyzed by neuroradiologists, atrophy of the cerebellar hemispheres, vermis, pons, midbrain, and cerebral hemispheres, as well as enlargement of the basilar cisterns and fourth ventricle, were differentially discriminated between the two groups.[45] However, in no case did CT imaging confirm cerebellar or brain stem involvement that was not clinically evident. Wenning et al.[46] concluded that CT is of limited diagnostic use in MSA.

Magnetic resonance imaging (MRI) of the brain can differentiate MSA from multi-infarct conditions or normal pressure hydrocephalus as a cause of dopa-unresponsive parkinsonism. MRI may also show putaminal, pontine, and middle cerebellar peduncle atrophy.[47] MRI findings such as the "putaminal slit" and the "cross sign" or "hot cross bun sign" (Figs. 20–1 to 20–3) are characteristic of MSA-P and MSA-C, respectively, but may take years after the onset of clinical symptoms to appear.[48] MRI with diffusion-weighted imaging may be used to discriminate MSA-P from PD on the basis of increased putaminal and middle cerebellar peduncle diffusivity.[49] The "putaminal slit" is thought to be due to iron deposition, which manifests as hypointense signals on T_2-weighted images as well as gliosis presenting as slit-like hyperintense signals on T_2-weighted images at the posterolateral border of the putamen occur.[50,51] These findings are supportive, but not diagnostic of MSA.[10,52]

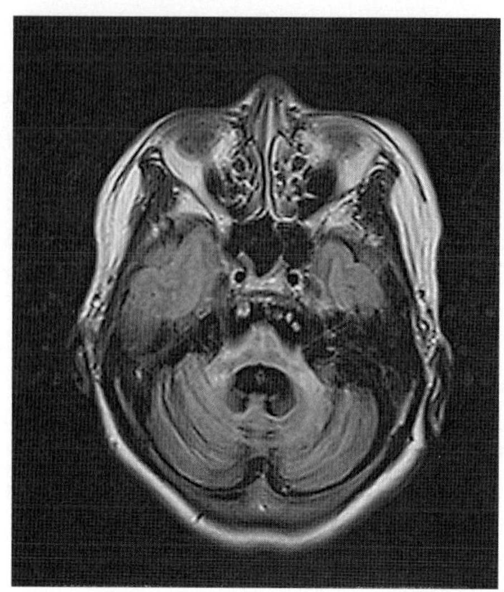

Figure 20–2. MSA-C. Increased signal on MRI in the middle cerebellar peduncles.

PET studies have been performed with ^{18}F-6-fluorodopa (FD), ^{11}C-raclopride (RAC), and ^{11}C-diprenorphine in order to examine both the pre- and postsynaptic segments of the dopaminergic pathway. Reduced putaminal

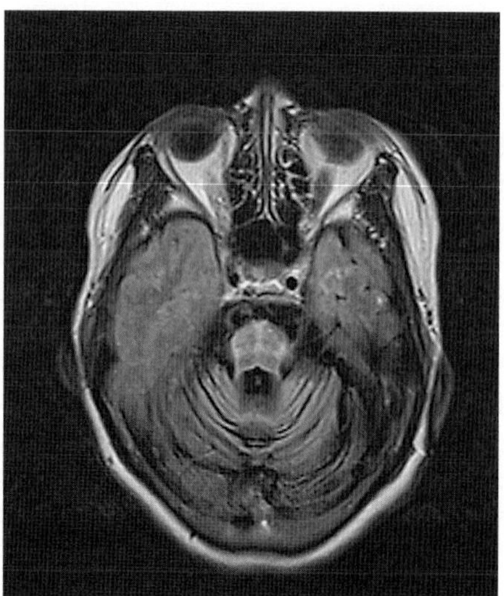

Figure 20–1. MRI FLAIR image demonstrating increased signal in the brain stem involving the midline raphe and transverse pontine fibers and sparing the tegmentum, pyramidal tracts, and superior cerebellar peduncles. This image demonstrates the "hot cross bun sign."

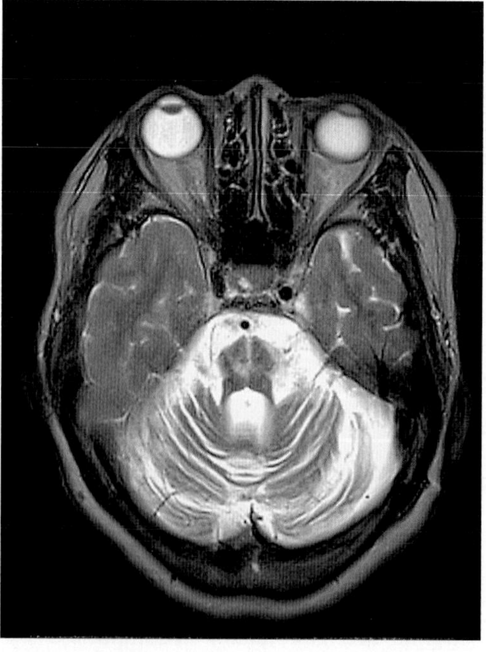

Figure 20–3. MSA-C. MRI T_2-weighted axial image showing the brain stem and cerebellar atrophy.

uptake of FD has been reported in MSA, as well as reduced striatal binding of diprenorphine and RAC.[53–55] Abnormalities of striatal glucose metabolism have also been demonstrated with ^{18}F-fluorodeoxyglucose PET studies.[56–58] These results suggest that selective metabolic reduction in the putamen and cerebellum may be a marker for MSA. In addition, PET studies have contributed to the evidence that sporadic OPCA is MSA, whereas dominantly inherited OPCA is a separate entity. ^{123}I-iodobenzamide single-photon emission CT scanning may be useful in assessing the integrity of striatal dopamine receptors in early parkinsonism.[59] While functional imaging techniques show promise in the diagnosis of MSA, they are not routinely used in clinical practice. Brain parenchyma sonography has also been reported to differentiate PD from atypical parkinsonian syndromes including MSA.[60]

Nerve conduction and electromyographic (EMG) studies may reveal subclinical polyneuropathy in MSA. EMG of external urethral sphincter demonstrates denervation in almost all patients with MSA.[61] However, the capability of this test to differentiate patients with MSA from those with PD has been challenged.[62] Electroencephalographic studies are normal in MSA, and evoked responses yield widely varying results.

Although autonomic failure is commonly diagnosed with an appropriate history and the demonstration of a significant drop in blood pressure upon arising, there are a number of sophisticated investigations of autonomic function available.[30] Postural hypotension is best evaluated with the use of a tilt table. Plasma norepinephrine responses to postural change may provide a quantitative biochemical assessment of the sympathetic nervous system. In individual patients, barium swallowing studies for dysphagia, urodynamic studies for urinary difficulties, and laryngoscopy or sleep studies for respiratory stridor may be useful for both diagnosis and management.

In summary, although diagnostic investigations are routinely pursued, their major contribution is the exclusion of diagnoses that are more amenable to therapy than MSA. The accumulated data may add to the clinical impression; however, no diagnostic study alone can reliably distinguish the autonomic failure, electrophysiology, or neuroradiology of MSA from the other possible etiologies in this setting. Certain features on MRI, FDG-PET, or SPECT may be used as supportive features in possible MSA.[7]

▶ NEUROPATHOLOGY

Postmortem brains of MSA patients demonstrate selective neuronal loss and gliosis in the following regions: striatum, substantia nigra, locus ceruleus, Edinger–Westphal nucleus, dorsal motor nucleus of the vagus, middle cerebellar peduncles, cerebellar Purkinje cells, inferior olives, intermediolateral cell columns, and Onuf's nucleus.[18,63,64] Gross specimens show severe pontine atrophy (Fig. 20–4). Characteristic neuropathological features of

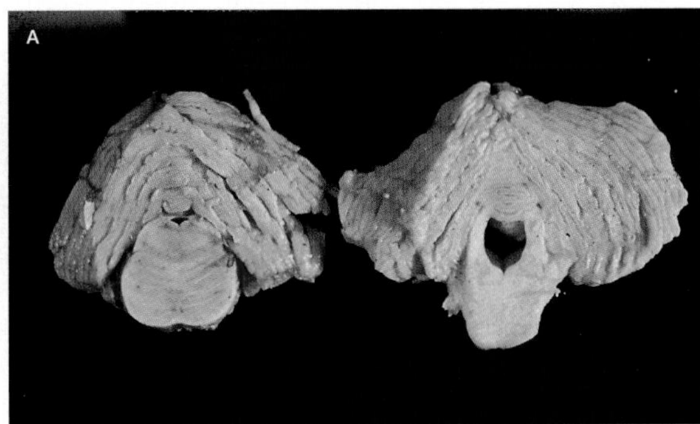

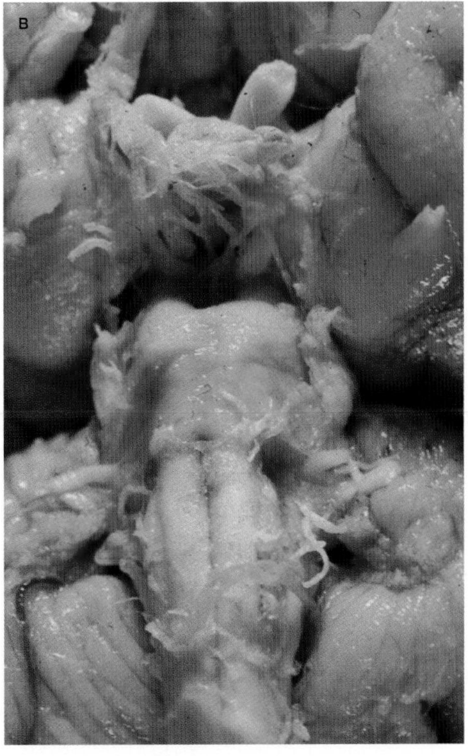

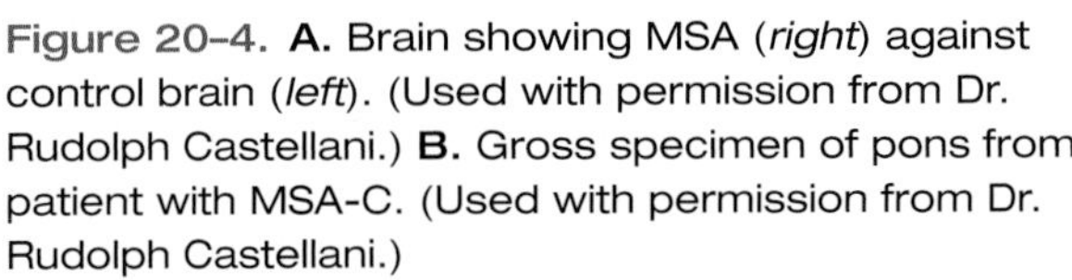

Figure 20–4. **A.** Brain showing MSA (*right*) against control brain (*left*). (Used with permission from Dr. Rudolph Castellani.) **B.** Gross specimen of pons from patient with MSA-C. (Used with permission from Dr. Rudolph Castellani.)

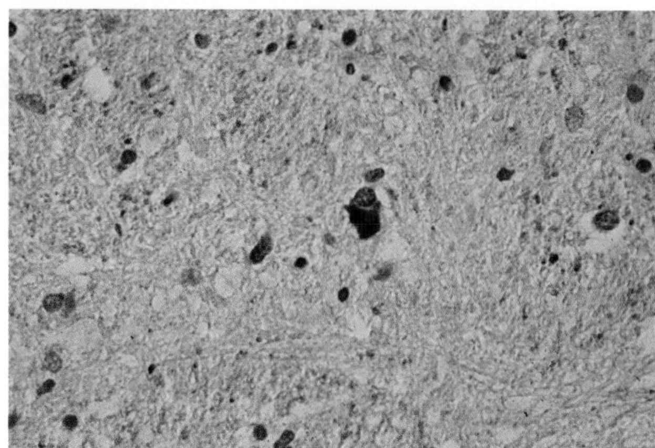

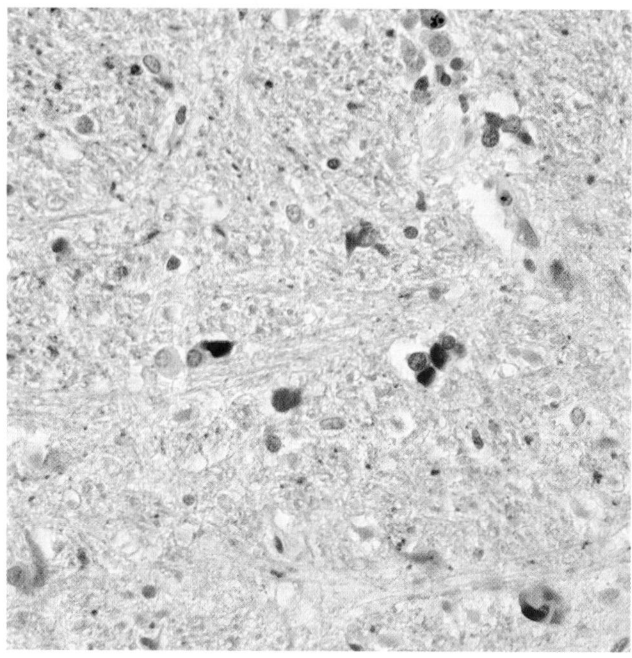

Figures 20–5 and 20-6. *Left.* Glial cytoplasmic inclusions in a patient with MSA. *Right.* Alpha-synuclein stain. (Used with permission from Dr. Rudolph Castellani.)

MSA include glial cytoplasmic inclusions (GCIs), neuronal cytoplasmic inclusions, neuronal nuclear inclusions, glial nuclear inclusions, and neuropil threads. GCIs (also known as Papp-Lantos inclusions) are the most significant neuropathological feature of MSA[21,65,66] (Figs. 20–5 and 20–6). GCIs surround the nuclei of oligodendroglia with a crescent- or flame-shaped morphology. They are found in large numbers in many regions of the central nervous system, with a particular predilection for the white matter tracts. The clinicopathological correlation of MSA is not high in the early stages of the disorder. As the disease progresses GCI lesion burden correlates with striatonigral and olivopontocerebellar degeneration.[67,68] In the gray matter, there is no clear correlation between lesion burden and disease severity.[69] The GCIs demonstrate variable immunoreactivity for tau protein,[70] ubiquitin, tubulin, microtubule-binding protein, and alpha B-crystallin. The most abundant protein found in GCI is alpha-synuclein.[71] Ultrastructural examination of GCIs has shown inclusions composed of randomly arranged tubules or filaments with a diameter of 20–40 nm associated with granular material.[66] The filaments appear in two forms: twisted and straight filaments.[71] Neuronal cytoplasmic inclusions may be located in neurons of pontine nuclei, putamen, subthalamic nucleus, arcuate nucleus, subiculum, amygdala, inferior olivary nucleus, and the reticular formation of brain stem. These neuronal inclusions are argentophilic and show immunoreactivity with anti-alpha-synuclein. Argentophilic inclusions are both alpha-synuclein- and ubiquitin-positive, and may be observed in both neuronal and glial nuclei. The mechanism(s) of cell loss in MSA remains unknown; however, the oligodendroglial GCIs stain heavily for alpha-synuclein.[72–74] Mounting evidence of extensive oligodendroglial involvement has led recently to a theory proposing that MSA is actually a primary oligodendrogliopathy with secondary neurodegeneration.[75]

▶ DIFFERENTIAL DIAGNOSIS

The most instrumental tool currently available to the clinician to make the diagnosis of MSA is the passage of time. Indeed, we all have congratulated ourselves for diagnosing MSA in patients with previous misdiagnoses of PD or cerebellar ataxia, when we simply have been the beneficiary of information unavailable to our predecessors. There is considerable similarity between the neurological signs that appear in the various neurodegenerative disorders (Table 20–2). The particular vulnerability of the substantia nigra and striatum to neuronal injury is borne out by the presence of moderate-to-severe parkinsonism in the full range of disorders. Autonomic failure, cognitive dysfunction, oculomotor impairment, dysarthria, dysphagia, and involuntary movements are also pervasive. The clinical impression is formed by the relative proportions of a similar array of neurological signs, tempered by knowledge of the natural history of the individual disorders. Nonetheless, the astute clinician

▶ TABLE 20–2. NEUROLOGICAL SIGNS IN THE NEURODEGENERATIVE DISORDERS

	MSA-P	MSA-C	PSP	PD	DLB	CBD	AD
Parkinsonism	++++	++	++++	++++	++++	++++	++
Cerebellar signs	++	++++	+	0	0	+	+
Autonomic failure	+++	+++	+	++	++	+	+
Pyramidal signs	++	++	++	0	+	++	++++
Cognitive dysfunction	++	++	+++	++	++++	++	++++
Oculomotor impairment	++	++	++++	++	++	++	+
Dysarthria	+++	+++	+++	++	++	+++	++
Dysphagia	++	++	+++	+	++	+	++
Peripheral neuropathy	+	+	+	0	0	++	+
Involuntary movements	+	+	+	+++	+++	++	+

0, none; +, uncommon or unusual; ++, common or moderate; +++, frequent or marked; ++++, present in nearly all cases or severe. DLB, dementia with Lewy body; CBD, corticobasal degeneration; AD, Alzheimer's disease.

can be sensitized to clues or idiosyncrasies that suggest the presence of one disorder over another.

MSA is most commonly confused with PD, although PSP often bears the greatest similarity. Corticobasal degeneration (CBD) also deserves consideration in the differential diagnosis of atypical parkinsonism, especially in the early years before the fully developed clinical picture emerges. In a prospective clinical pathological study of diagnostic accuracy in parkinsonism, the initial diagnosis of PD was correct in 65% of cases, and improved to 76% with follow-up.[24] The diagnostic accuracy for MSA with at least 5 years of follow-up was 69%. MSA was misdiagnosed as PD in 31%. Higher accuracy was reported in a retrospective analysis of patients with neuropathological correlation who were diagnosed at a movement disorders specialty clinic.[76] When followed at a movement disorders specialty clinic, final clinical diagnosis had a sensitivity of 88.2% and specificity of 95.4%.[76]

The major clinical features that raise suspicion about a diagnosis of MSA are a poor response to L-dopa; the presence of pyramidal, cerebellar, or autonomic signs; early postural instability; and rapid clinical deterioration. Questions are also raised by the absence of rest tremor, the presence of a symmetrical onset of signs, a severe dysarthria, disproportionate antecollis, and respiratory stridor. Recently, a "red flag" checklist was proposed to assist in the diagnosis of MSA.[77] The checklist is composed of six clinical categories (early instability, rapid progression, abnormal postures, bulbar dysfunction, respiratory dysfunction, emotional incontinence). If features are present in two or more of the six categories, the diagnosis of MSA should be considered. When administered to a group of patients who did not yet meet criteria for probable MSA but were followed over time, the red flag checklist resulted in a positive predictive value of 96% and a negative predictive value of 92.7%.[77]

PSP is most frequently distinguished from MSA by the appearance of a prominent supranuclear vertical ophthalmoparesis with associated visual impairment. Hyperextension of the head or unusually erect posture, lid retraction associated with a surprised facial expression, disproportionate nuchal and axial rigidity, and apraxia of eyelid opening also suggest the presence of PSP. CBD is most frequently distinguished from MSA by the presence of early signs of cortical dysfunction (especially apraxia, and cortical sensory loss), prominent myoclonus, and asymmetric perirolandic frontoparietal cortical atrophy on CT or MRI. Vascular parkinsonism may be confused with MSA; however, history, the association of hypertension or other stroke risk factors, and neuroimaging help the clinician distinguish between them.

Our current knowledge of MSA and other neurodegenerative disorders that have similar presentations is fragmentary, and the conundrum of where to draw the lines that define and compartmentalize "unique" disorders remains an ongoing challenge. Clinical description, diagnostic investigations, and neuropathology are helpful but ultimately insufficient due to the great degree of overlap. Perhaps advances in cellular biochemistry and molecular biology will ultimately help to identify fundamental, distinguishing attributes of these disorders.

▶ TREATMENT

There is great variability of therapeutic results from L-dopa in patients win MSA. L-Dopa may improve rigidity, bradykinesia, and postural instability in possible and probable MSA patients.[25,78] L-Dopa therapy can be started with (carbidopa/L-dopa 25/100 0.5–1 tablet twice daily). The dosage can be increased until patients show toxicity or response. Compared with patients with

PD, MSA patients may need far larger doses of L-dopa. Approximately 30% of patients with MSA will show a clinically significant response, although it is often short-lived.[25]

Dopamine agonists have been used in treatment of MSA, although less successfully than L-dopa. Bromocriptine (10–80 mg daily) and lisuride (up to 2.4 mg daily) have been used. No formal efficacy trials of pramipexole or ropinirole are available. However, use of dopamine agonists has been linked to pathological hypersexuality and other compulsive behaviors in MSA.[79,80] Apomorphine, an injectable dopamine agonist, has been used in a clinical trial involving 28 patients with MSA. In the trial, apomorphine had some positive effects on these patients with an average improvement in motor scores of 11.9%, 14.3%, and 13.3% at doses of 1.5, 3, and 4.5 mg daily.[81] In general, L-Dopa is better tolerated than dopamine agonists with fewer side effects and should be considered the drug of choice in the treatment of the motor symptoms of MSA.

Symptomatic orthostatic hypotension can be managed with sodium and volume replacement, unless there are contraindications such as congestive heart failure or renal failure. Even without sodium supplementation, oral ingestion of water increases standing blood pressure in patients with MSA, although the effect may not be clinically significant.[82] Physical maneuvers such as crossing the legs or squatting may be helpful to transiently improve the symptoms of orthostatic hypotension.[83] Elastic stockings are an effective adjunct to volume replacement and pharmacologic therapies.[84] The mineralocorticoid fludrocortisone, used in doses of 0.1–0.3 mg per day, expands body fluid volume and improves alpha-adrenergic sensitivity.[85] The most serious potential adverse effect is supine hypertension. Midodrine, an alpha-adrenergic agonist, is a suitable alternative. Treatment starts with 2.5 mg three times a day, increasing to 10 mg three times a day. Midodrine, a selective aplha1-adrenoceptor agonist, increases blood pressure through arterial and venous vasoconstriction.[85] Care must be taken in the use of midodrine due to the potential serious side effect of supine hypertension, which has been reported in up to 25% of patients undergoing treatment and may be more common in patients with orthostatic hypotension due to autonomic failure.[86] Pyridostigmine is also beneficial for the symptoms of orthostatic hypotension.[87] Pyridostigmine may be used in combination with midodrine and does not lead to or aggravate supine hypertension.[87] While clinical experience is limited, a small follow-up survey suggests that pyridostigmine has continued efficacy and an acceptable side effect profile.[88]

In patients with MSA, urinary symptoms such as frequency or incontinence may result from a combination of detrusor hyperreflexia and urethral sphincter weakness. Urinary frequency may be managed with anticholinergic agents such as oxybutynin 5–10 mg or tolterodine 2 mg at bedtime or propantheline 15–30 mg at bedtime. The use of alpha1 blockers such as prazosin, tamsulosin, and moxisylyte improve bladder symptoms and decrease residual urine volume, but these agents may worsen orthostatic hypotension.[89,90] Intermittent catheterization is utilized in patients with significant urinary retention (>100 mL).[90] Recently, sildenafil citrate has been used for treatment of erectile dysfunction in patients with MSA. Despite its efficacy, sildenafil often worsens the orthostatic hypotension.[91] This is likely a class effect, and a similar problem is anticipated with vardenafil or tadalafil.

REFERENCES

1. Dejerine J, Thomas A. L'atrophie olivo-ponto-cerebelleuse. Nouv Iconogr Salpet 1900;13:330–370.
2. Shy GM, Drager GA. A neurological syndrome associated with orthostatic hypotension. Arch Neurol 1960;2: 511–527.
3. van der Eecken H, Adams RD, van Bogaert L. Striopallidal-nigral degeneration: A hitherto undescribed lesion in paralysis agitans. J Neuropathol Exp Neurol 1960;19:159–161.
4. Adams RD, von Bogaert L, van der Eecken H. Degeneres cences nigro-striees et cerebello-nigro-striees. Psychiatr Neurol 1961;142:219–259.
5. Graham JG, Oppenheimer DR. Orthostatic hypotension and nicotine sensitivity in a case of multiple system atrophy. J Neurol Neurosurg Psychiatry 1969;32:28–34.
6. Bannister R, Oppenheimer DR. Degenerative diseases of the nervous system associated with autonomic failure. Brain 1972;95:457–474.
7. Gilman S, Wenning GK, Low PA, et al. Second consensus statement on the diagnosis of multiple system atrophy. Neurology 2008;71:670–676.
8. Penney JB. Multiple systems atrophy and nonfamilial olivopontocerebellar atrophy are the same disease. Ann Neurol 1995;37:553–554.
9. Hara K, Momose Y, Tokiguchi S, et al. Multiplex families with multiple system atrophy. Arch Neurol 2007;64: 545–551.
10. Schrag A, Ben-Shlomo Y, Quinn NP. Prevalence of progressive supranuclear palsy and multiple system atrophy: A cross-sectional study. Lancet 1999;354:1771–1775.
11. Chrysostome V, Tison F, Yekhlef F, et al. Epidemiology of multiple system atrophy: A prevalence and pilot risk factor study in Aquitaine, France. Neuroepidemiology 2004;23:201–208.
12. Vanacore N, Bonifati V, Colosimo C, et al. Epidemiology of progressive supranuclear palsy. ESGAP Consortium. European Study Group on Atypical Parkinsonisms. Neurol Sci 2001;22:101–103.
13. Ben-Shlomo Y, Wenning GK, Tison F, et al. Survival of patients with pathologically proven multiple system atrophy: A meta-analysis. Neurology 1997;48:384–393.
14. Wenning GK, Ben Shlomo Y, Magalhaes M, et al. Clinical features and natural history of multiple system atrophy: An analysis of 100 cases. Brain 1994;117:835–845.

15. Klockgether T, Ludtke R, Kramer B, et al. The natural history of degenerative ataxia: A retrospective study in 466 patients. Brain 1998;121:589–600.
16. Watanabe H, Saito Y, Terao S, et al. Progression and prognosis in multiple system atrophy. An analysis of 230 Japanese patients. Brain 2002;125:1070–1083.
17. Quinn NP. Multiple system atrophy. In Marsden CD, Fahn S (eds). Movement Disorders 3. Oxford: Butterworth-Heinemann, 1994, pp. 262–281.
18. Quinn N. Multiple system atrophy: The nature of the beast. J Neurol Neurosurg Psychiatry 1989;52(suppl):78–89.
19. Gilman S, Low P, Quinn N, et al. Consensus statement on the diagnosis of multiple system atrophy. American Autonomic Society and American Academy of Neurology. Clin Auton Res 1998;8:359–362.
20. Osaki Y, Wenning GK, Daniel SE, et al. Do published criteria improve clinical diagnostic accuracy in multiple system atrophy? Neurology 2002;59:1486–1491.
21. Trojanowski JQ, Revesz T. Proposed neuropathological criteria for the post mortem diagnosis of multiple system atrophy. Neuropahtol Appl Neurobiol 2007;33:615–620.
22. Adams RD, Salam-Adams M. Striatonigral degeneration. In Vinken PJ, Bruyn GW, Klawans HL (eds). Extrapyramidal Disorders. Amsterdam: Elsevier Science Publishers, 1986, pp 205–212.
23. Gouider-Khouja N, Vidailhef M, Bonnef AM, et al. "Pure" striatonigral degeneration and Parkinson's disease: A comparative clinical study. Mov Disord 1995;10:288–294.
24. Rajput AH, Rodzilsky B, Rajput A. Accuracy of clinical diagnosis in parkinsonism: A prospective study. Can J Neurol Sci 1991;18:275–278.
25. Hughes AJ, Colosimo C, Kleedorfen B, et al. The dopaminergic response in multiple system atrophy. J Neurol Neurosurg Psychiatry 1992;55:1009–1013.
26. Magalhaes M, Wenning GK, Daniel SE, et al. Autonomic dysfunction in pathologically confirmed multiple system atrophy and idiopathic Parkinson's disease: A retrospective comparison. Acta Neurol Scand 1995;91:98–102.
27. Mathias CJ. Autonomic disorders and their recognition. N Engl J Med 1997;336:721–724.
28. Mathias CJ, Mallipeddi R, Bleasdale-Barr K. Symptoms associated with orthostatic hypotension in pure autonomic failure and multiple system atrophy. J Neurol 1999;246: 893–898.
29. Mathias CJ. Orthostatic hypotension: Causes, mechanisms and influencing factors. Neurology 1995;45:S6–S11.
30. Robertson D, Davis TL. Recent advances in the treatment of orthostatic hypotension. Neurology 1995;45:S26–S32.
31. Colosimo C ,and Pezzella FR. The symptomatic treatment of multiple system atrophy. Eur J Neurol 2002; 9:195–199.
32. Mathias CJ, Williams AC. The Shy-Drager syndrome and multiple system atrophy. In Calne DB (ed). Neurodegenerative Diseases. Philadelphia: WB Saunders, 1994, pp. 743–767.
33. Beck RO, Betts CD, Fowler CJ. Genitourinary dysfunction in multiple system atrophy: Clinical features and treatment in 62 cases. J Urol 1994;151:1336–1341.
34. Sakakibara R, Hattori T, Tojo M, et al. Micturitional disturbance in multiple system atrophy. Jpn J Psychiatry Neurol 1993;47:591–598.
35. Kirchhol K, Apostolidis AN, Mathias CJ, et al. Erectile and urinary dysfunction may be the presenting features in patients with multiple system atrophy: A retrospective study. Int J Impot Res 2003;15:293–298.
36. Stocchi F, Badiali D, Vacca L, et al. Anorectal function in multiple system atrophy and Parkinson's disease. Mov Disord 2000;15:71–76.
37. Isozaki E, Matsubara S, Hayashida T, et al. Morphometric study of nucleus ambiguus in multiple system atrophy presenting with vocal cord abductor paralysis. Clin Neuropathol 2000;19:213–220.
38. Benarroch EE, Schmeichel AM, Parisi JE. Preservation of branchimotor neurons of the nucleus ambiguus in multiple system atrophy. Neurology 2003;60:115–117.
39. Blumin JH, Berke GS. Bilateral vocal fold paresis and multiple system atrophy. Arch Otolaryngol Head Neck Surg 2002;128:1404–1407.
40. Winkler AS, Marsden J, Parton M, et al. Erythropoietin deficiency and anaemia in multiple system atrophy. Mov Disord 2001;16:233–239.
41. Berciano J. Olivopontocerebellar atrophy. In Jankovic J, Tolosa E (eds). Parkinson's Disease and Movement Disorders. Baltimore: Williams & Wilkins, 1993, pp. 163–189.
42. Duvoisin RC. The olivopontocerebellar atrophies. In Marsden CD, Fahn S (eds). Movement Disorders 2. London: Butterworth, 1987, pp. 249–271.
43. Robbins TW, James M, Lange KW, et al. Cognitive performance in multiple system atrophy. Brain 1992; 115:271–291.
44. Cummings JL. Frontal-subcortical circuits and human behavior. Arch Neurol 1993;50:873–880.
45. Wenning GK, Jager K, Kendall B, et al. Is cranial computerized tomography useful in the diagnosis of multiple system atrophy? Mov Disord 1994;9:333–336.
46. Wenning GK, Ben-Shlomo Y, Magalhaes M, et al. Clinicopathological study of 35 cases of multiple system atrophy. J Neurol Neurosurg Psychiatry 1995;58:160–166.
47. Seppi K, Schocke MF, Wenning GK, et al. How to diagnose MSA early: The role of magnetic resonance imaging. J Neural Transm 2005;112:1625–1634.
48. Horimoto Y, Aiba I, Yasuda T, et al. Longitudinal MRI study of multiple system atrophy – when do the findings appear, and what is the course? J Neurol 2002;249:847–854.
49. Nicoletti G, Lodi R, Condino F, et al. Apparent diffusion coefficient measurements of the middle cerebellar peduncle differentiate the Parkinson variant of MSA from Parkinson's disease and progressive supranuclear palsy. Brain 2006;129:2679–2687.
50. Konagaya M, Konagaya Y, Iida M. Clinical and magnetic resonance imaging study of extrapyramidal symptoms in multiple system atrophy. J Neurol Neurosurg Psychiatry 1994;57:1528–1531.
51. Macia F, Yekhlef F, Ballan G, et al. T2-hyperintense lateral rim and hypointense putamen are typical but not exclusive of multiple system atrophy. Arch Neurol 2001;58: 1024–1026.
52. Kraft E, Schwarz J, Trenkwalder C, et al. The combination of hypointense and hyperintense signal changes on T2-weighted magnetic resonance imaging sequences: A specific marker of multiple system atrophy? Arch Neurol 1999;56:225–228.
53. Brooks DJ, Ibanez V, Sawle GV, et al. Differing patterns of striatal 18F-dopa uptake in Parkinson's disease, multiple

system atrophy, and progressive supranuclear palsy. Ann Neurol 1990;28:547–555.
54. Sawle GV, Playford ED, Brooks DJ, et al. Asymmetrical pre-synaptic and post-synaptic changes to the striatal dopamine projection in dopa naive parkinsonism: Diagnostic implications of the D2 receptor status. Brain 1993;116: 853–867.
55. Rinne JO, Burn DJ, Mathias CJ, et al. Positron emission tomography studies on the dopaminergic system and striatal opioid binding in the olivopontocerebellar atrophy variant of multiple system atrophy. Ann Neurol 1995;37:568–573.
56. Eidelberg D, Takikawa S, Moeller JR, et al. Striatal hypometabolism distinguishes striatonigral degeneration from Parkinson's disease. Ann Neurol 1993;33:518–527.
57. Perani D, Bressi S, Testa D, et al. Clinical/metabolic correlations in multiple system atrophy: A fluorodeoxyglucose F18 positron emission tomographic study. Arch Neurol 1995;52:179–185.
58. Gilman S, Koeppe RA, Junck L, et al. Patterns of cerebral glucose metabolism detected with positron emission tomography differ in multiple system atrophy and olivopontocerebellar atrophy. Ann Neurol 1994;36:166–175.
59. Schwarz J, Taksen K, Arnold G, et al. 123I-iodobenzamide SPECT predicts dopaminergic responsiveness in patients with de novo parkinsonism. Neurology 1992;42:556–561.
60. Walter U, Niehaus L, Probst T, et al. Brain parenchyma sonography discriminates Parkinson's disease and atypical parkinsonian syndromes. Neurology 2003;60:74–77.
61. Wenning GK, Kraft E, Beck R, et al. Cerebellar presentation of multiple system atrophy. Mov Disord 1997;12:115–117.
62. Giladi N, Simon ES, Korczyn AD, et al. Anal sphincter EMG does not distinguish between multiple system atrophy and Parkinson's disease. Muscle Nerve 2000;23:731–734.
63. Wenning GK, Ebersbach G, Verny M, et al. Progression of falls in postmortem-confirmed parkinsonism disorders. Mov Disord 1999;14:947–950.
64. Ozawa T. Morphological substrate of autonomic failure and neurohormonal dysfunction in multiple system atrophy: Impact of on -determining phenotype spectrum. Acta Neuropathol 2007;114:201–211.
65. Papp MI, Kahn JE, Lantos PL. Glial cytoplasmic inclusions in the CNS of patients with multiple system atrophy (striatonigral degeneration, olivopontocerebellar atrophy and Shy-Drager syndrome). J Neurol Sci 1989;94:79–100.
66. Papp MI, Lantos PL. Accumulation of tubular structures in oligodendroglial and neuronal cells as the basic alteration in multiple system atrophy. J Neurol Sci 1992;107:172–182.
67. Ozawa T, Paviour D, Quinn NP, et al. The spectrum of pathological involvement of the striatonigral and olivopontocerebellar systems in multiple system atrophy: Clinicopathological correlations. Brain 2004;127:2657–2671.
68. Jellinger KA, Seppi K, Wenning GK. Grading of neuropathology in multiple system atrophy: Proposal for a new scale. Mov Disord 2005;20(suppl 12):S29–S36.
69. Ishizawa K, Komori T, Arai N, et al. Glial cytoplasmic inclusions and tissue injury in multiple system atrophy: A quantitative study in white matter (olivopontocerebellar system) and gray matter (nigrostriatal system). Neuropathology 2008;28;249–257.
70. Piao YS, Hayashi S, Hasegawa M, et al. Co-localization of alpha-synuclein and phosphorylated tau in neuronal and glial cytoplasmic inclusions in a patient with multiple system atrophy of long duration. Acta Neuropathol (Berl) 2001;101:285–293.
71. Spillantini MG, Crowther RA, Jakes R, et al. Filamentous alpha-synuclein inclusions link multiple system atrophy with Parkinson's disease and dementia with Lewy bodies. Neurosci Lett 1998;251:205–208.
72. Arima K, Ueda K, Sunohara N, et al. NACP/alpha-synuclein immunoreactivity in fibrillary components of neuronal and oligodendroglial cytoplasmic inclusions in the pontine nuclei in multiple system atrophy. Acta Neuropathol (Berl) 1998;96:439–444.
73. Gai WP, Power JH, Blumbergs PC, et al. Multiple system atrophy: A new alpha-synuclein disease? Lancet 1998;352:547–548.
74. Duda JE, Giasson BI, Gur TL, et al. Immunohistochemical and biochemical studies demonstrate a distinct profile of alpha-synuclein permutations in multiple system atrophy. J Neuropathol Exp Neurol 2000;59:830–841.
75. Wenning GK, Stefanova N, Jellinger KA, et al. Multiple system atrophy: A primary oligodendrogliopathy. Ann Neurol 2008;64:239–246.
76. Hughes AJ, Daniel SE, Ben-Shlomo Y, et al. The accuracy of diagnosis of parkinsonian syndromes in a specialist movement disorder service. Brain 2002;125:861–870.
77. Kollensperger M, Geser M, Seppi K, et al. Red flags for multiple system atrophy. Mov Disord 2008;23:1093–1099.
78. Parati EA, Fetoni V, Geminiani GC, et al. Response to L-DOPA in multiple system atrophy. Clin Neuropharmacol 1993;16:139–144.
79. Klos KJ, Bower JH, Josephs KA, et al. Pathological hypersexuality linked to adjuvant dopamine agonist therapy in Parkinson's disease and multiple system atrophy. Parkinsonism Relat Disord 2005;11:381–386.
80. McKeon A, Josephs KA, Klos KJ, et al. Unusual compulsive behaviors primarily related to dopamine agonist therapy in Parkinson's disease and multiple system atrophy. Parkinsonism Relat Disord 2007;13:516–519.
81. Rossi P, Colosimo C, Moro E, et al. Acute challenge with apomorphine and levodopa in Parkinsonism. Eur Neurol 2000;43:95–101.
82. Young TM, Mathias CJ. The effects of water ingestion on orthostatic hypotension in two groups of chronic autonomic failure: Multiple system atrophy and pure autonomic failure. J Neurol Neurosurg Psychiatry 2004;75: 1737–1741.
83. Wieling W, van Lieshout JJ, van Leeuwen AM. Physical manuoeuvres that reduce postural hypotension in autonomic failure. Clin Auton Res 1993;3:57–65.
84. Henry R, Rowe J, O'Mahony D. Haemodynamic analysis of efficacy of compression hosiery in elderly fallers with orthostatic hypotension. Lancet 1999;354:45–46.
85. Maule S, Papotti G, Naso D, et al. Orthostatic hypotension: Evaluation and treatment. Cardiovasc Hematol Disord Drug Targets 2007;7:63–70.
86. Sandroni P, Benarroch EE, Wijdicks EFM. Caudate hemorrhage as a possible complication of midodrine-induced supine hypertension. Mayo Clin Proc 2001;76:1275.
87. Singer W, Sandromi P, Opfer-Gehrking TL, et al. Pyridostigmine treatment trial in neurogenic orthostatic hypotension. Arch Neurol 2006;63:513–518.

88. Sandroni P, Opfer-Gehrking TL, Singer W, et al. Pyridostigmine for treatment of neurogenic orthostatic hypertension: A follow-up survey study. Clin Auton Res 2005;15:51–53.
89. Sakakibara R, Hattori T, Uchiyama T, et al. Are alpha-blockers involved in the lower urinary tract dysfunction in multiple system atrophy? A comparison of prazosin and moxisylyte. J Auton Nerv Syst 2000;79:191–195.
90. Ito T, Sakakibara R, Yasuda K, et al. Incomplete emptying and urinary retention in multiple-system atrophy: When does it occur and how do we manage it? Mov Disord 2006;21:816–823.
91. Hussain IF, Brady CM, Swinn MJ, et al. Treatment of erectile dysfunction with sildenafil citrate (Viagra) in parkinsonism due to Parkinson's disease or multiple system atrophy with observations on orthostatic hypotension. J Neurol Neurosurg Psychiatry 2001;71:371–374.

II. PARKINSONIAN STATES: AKINETIC-RIGID SYNDROMES

CHAPTER 21

Progressive Supranuclear Palsy

Lawrence I. Golbe

The first clinicopathologic descriptions of progressive supranuclear palsy (PSP) to draw widespread attention were published in 1963 and 1964.[1–3] The full-blown, typical case is at once unusually complex in its combination of motor and behavioral features and so distinctive that the diagnosis is unmistakable at a glance. Lack of objective diagnostic markers and poor response to treatment make PSP a challenge for the clinician and a trial for the patient and family. But recent progress in understanding its genetic, molecular, and cellular pathology offer hope that PSP will become more easily diagnosed and treated in the near future.

▶ CLINICAL SUMMARY

PRESENTING FEATURES AND CLINICAL COURSE

Three retrospective studies found gait disturbance, often unheralded falls, to be a presenting feature in 90%, 62%, and 61%, respectively.[4–6] In contrast, Parkinson's disease (PD) presents with gait disturbance in only 11% of cases.[7] The falls may prompt a workup for vestibulopathy, myelopathy, basilar artery ischemia, cardiac syncope, or epilepsy. However, in most cases, the gait disturbance is accompanied by enough bradykinesia and/or rigidity to prompt an initial diagnosis of PD.

The next most common presenting feature is a nonspecific mental and physical slowness, irritability, social withdrawal, or fatigability[8] that is usually interpreted by the patient as normal aging. If medical attention is sought at this point, a diagnosis of primary depression or Alzheimer's disease (AD) is common.

In the minority of cases that present with gaze palsy, dysarthria or dysphagia, the initial workup may embark on a search for myasthenia gravis, progressive bulbar palsy, or local causes of esophageal dysmotility. Cataract extraction may be performed in a futile effort to correct the nonrefractible visual deficit of early, unrecognized supranuclear gaze fixation instability. Gaze palsy is often absent until the middle of the illness and is only rarely the presenting symptom (Table 21–1). In one series of autopsy-confirmed patients, gaze palsy failed to appear during life in half of cases.[9] Yet many physicians fail to consider the diagnosis of PSP until vertical gaze restriction occurs.

In its full-blown clinical state, PSP will not be confused with other illnesses. There can be little diagnostic doubt in a patient with a progressive syndrome of gait instability with early falls, bradykinesia, disproportionately nuchal rigidity with unexpectedly upright or even retrocollis posture,[10] predominantly vertical supranuclear gaze abnormality, spastic dysarthria, dangerous

▶ **TABLE 21–1. SYMPTOMS AT ONSET OF PSP**

Symptom	Percentage of Cases (N = 187)
Gait	
Unsteadiness	61
Slow/weak gait	6
Behavior	
Memory difficulty	7
Personality change	4
Depression/anxiety/apathy	3
Wordfinding difficulty	1
Bulbar/speech/language	
Dysarthria/dysphagia	9
Reduced speech output	3
Palilalia/echolalia	1
Dysphonia	1
Vision	
Blurring or diplopia	10
Other visual symptom	3
Other	
Tremor	13
Dizziness	3
Localized pain	3

Data adapted from Nath U, Ben-Shlomo Y, Thomson RG, et al. Clinical features and natural history of PSP: A clinical cohort study. Neurology 2003;60:910–916.

dysphagia, and behavioral abnormalities referrable disproportionately to frontal lobe dysfunction.

The illness progresses to an immobile state over less than a decade in most cases,[4,5] but the order of appearance of the cardinal deficits is highly variable. On average, the gait difficulty appears first, followed by dysarthria, visual symptoms, and dysphagia in that order.[4] Symptoms present at the onset are also highly variable and are described in Table 21–1. A clinical disability rating scale, the PSP Rating Scale, has been published,[11] and is available via www.curepsp.org. It requires about 10 minutes to administer and can be performed by a neurologist with no specialized familiarity with PSP. The scores span 0 (normal) to 100 and progress at an average of 10–12 points per year. Its utility as a clinical prognostic tool is discussed below.

PSP VERSUS PD

The most important competing diagnostic consideration, PD, may often be discarded by a glance at the patient's tonically contracted facial muscles, unmoving gaze with coarse square-wave jerks and unexpectedly erect posture for the degree of bradykinesia. More careful clinical inquiry and examination are likely to reveal a history of poor response to dopaminergic treatment (a common reason for the patient's referral), pseudobulbar affect, slow or hypometric saccades in the upward or downward directions, dysarthria that is too spastic or cerebellar in quality for PD, unexpected mildness of rigidity in the wrists and elbows, and postural instability as the most disabling feature of all.

One pathologically based series using logistic regression analysis found gait instability, paucity of tremor and poor L-dopa response to be the features that best differentiated PSP from PD.[12] The same series found that falls in the first year of illness had high sensitivity and positive predictive value in distinguishing PSP from PD, multiple-system atrophy (MSA), dementia with Lewy bodies, and corticobasal degeneration (CBD).[13] While PD may display restrictions of vertical gaze and early PSP may not, a sign that is highly sensitive and specific for PSP is slowing of downward saccades.[14] Another that is quite sensitive for PSP but shared with other conditions involving the cerebellum is square-wave jerks.[15]

ATYPICAL FEATURES

Cases departing from this typical picture are common. Some patients with PSP have prominent dementia suggestive of AD.[16] Others have asymmetric apraxia or dystonia suggestive of CBD,[1] and others resemble PD or MSA of the parkinsonian type (formerly called striatonigral degeneration) until late in the illness, when marked vertical supranuclear gaze abnormalities finally appear. Even such findings as moderate asymmetry and mild rest tremor,[17,18] claimed by earlier authors to virtually exclude PSP, occurred in 2 of 12 pathologically confirmed cases in a recent series.[19] Another autopsy series[20] found asymmetric onset in 3 of 16 cases.

Atypical clinical features tend to cluster in patients with atypical pathological and molecular features that occur in AD.[21] This suggests that there may be two or more disease entities presently lumped as "PSP."

Indeed, the notion of "PSP" as a category comprising multiple disorders has been advanced by the recent observation of Williams and colleagues[22] that approximately one-third of patients with pathologically confirmed PSP had presented with a syndrome more suggestive of PD. Dubbed "PSP-parkinsonism," this entity, relative to classic PSP, features a better levodopa response, more motor asymmetry, more tremor, longer survival, and an even sex ratio.[23] The classic form has been called "Richardson's syndrome" to honor the senior member of the team that first described PSP. A third variant comprising only 1% of cases starts with "pure akinesia with gait freezing," which remains its only prominent finding for years in some cases. It has received the name "PSP-PAGF."[24]

DIAGNOSTIC CRITERIA

A set of diagnostic criteria formulated by Golbe and colleagues[4] for use in settings that permit detailed examination of patients are shown in Table 21–2. This set is suitable for drug trials or for small epidemiologic studies in which an experienced neurologist examines each patient. Under such conditions, its specificity is 98% and its positive predictive value 92%.[25] It would not be suitable when only retrospective examination data by nonneurologists are available. Likewise, its sensitivity, 50%, is insufficient for prevalence or incidence surveys.

Litvan and colleagues[25] formulated a now widely accepted set of "probable" clinical criteria (Table 21–3) that achieve 100% specificity and positive predictive value while sacrificing sensitivity (50%). They reviewed clinical records of 24 patients with autopsy-proven PSP and approximately three times that number with other conditions in the differential diagnosis of PSP. The same project also formulated a set of "possible" criteria with the higher sensitivity, 83%, necessary to a prevalence or incidence study. The "possible" criteria sacrifice only little specificity (93%) and positive predictive value (83%) in achieving this goal. The likely source of the suboptimal sensitivity of the "probable" criteria is the insistence on falls within the first year. These criteria have been named the National Institute of Neurological Disorders and Stroke/Society for Progressive Supranuclear Palsy (NINDS-SPSP) Criteria in honor of the cosponsors of the project and are the most commonly used set of criteria worldwide.

TABLE 21–2. DIAGNOSTIC CRITERIA FOR PSP

All 4 of these
- Onset at age 40 or later
- Progressive course
- Bradykinesia
- Supranuclear gaze palsy, per criteria below

Plus any 3 of these
- Dysarthria or dysphagia
- Neck rigidity (to flexion/extension) greater than limb rigidity
- Neck in a posture of extension
- Minimal or absent tremor
- Frequent falls or gait disturbance early in course

Without any of these
- Early or prominent cerebellar signs
- Unexplained polyneuropathy
- Prominent noniatrogenic dysautonomia other than isolated postural hypotension

Criteria for supranuclear gaze palsy

Either both of these
- Voluntary downgaze less than 15 degrees (tested by instructing patient to "look down" without presenting a specific target; accept the best result after several attempts)
- Preserved horizontal oculocephalic reflexes (except in very advanced stages)

Or all 3 of these
- Slowed downward saccades (defined as slow enough for the examiner to perceive the movement itself)
- Impaired opticokinetic nystagmus with the stimulus moving downward
- Poor voluntary suppression of vertical vestibulo-ocular reflex

Data proposed by Golbe LI, Davis PH, Schoenberg BS, et al. Prevalence and natural history of PSP. Neurology 1988;38:1031–1034.

TABLE 21–3. NINDS-SPSP CRITERIA FOR THE DIAGNOSIS OF PSP

"Possible" PSP

All 3 of these:
1. Gradually progressive disorder
2. Onset at age 40 or later
3. No evidence for competing diagnostic possibilities

Plus either of these:

4. Vertical gaze palsy

   Or

5. Slowing of vertical saccades *and* prominent postural instability with falls in the first year

"Probable" PSP

All 5 of these:
1. Gradually progressive disorder
2. Onset at age 40 or later
3. No evidence for competing diagnostic possibilities
4. Vertical gaze palsy
5. Slowing of vertical saccades *and* prominent postural instability with falls in the first year

Criteria that would exclude PSP from consideration
1. Recent encephalitis
2. Alien limb syndrome, cortical sensory defects or temporoparietal atrophy
3. Psychosis unrelated to dopaminergic treatment
4. Important cerebellar signs
5. Important unexplained dysautonomia
6. Severe, asymmetric parkinsonian signs
7. Relevant structural abnormality of basal ganglia on neuroimaging
8. Whipple's disease on CSF PCR, if indicated

PCR, polymerase chain reaction.
Data proposed by Litvan I, Agid Y, Calne D, et al. Clinical research criteria for the diagnosis of PSP: Report of the NINDS-SPSP International Workshop. Neurology 1996;47:1–9.

DIFFERENTIAL DIAGNOSIS

For a neuropathologist with access to the full range of modern, but routine, histopathologic techniques, the principal entities competing with PSP are only corticobasal degeneration (CBD), postencephalitic parkinsonism (PEP), and the Parkinson–dementia complex of Guam (PDC) (Table 21–4). The clinician must contend with a longer list that includes some cases of PD, CBD, MSA (principally striatonigral degeneration but also olivopontocerebellar atrophy),[26] progressive subcortical gliosis,[27] Creutzfeldt–Jakob disease,[28] AD with parkinsonism, diffuse Lewy body disease,[29] Pick's disease, and the primary pallidal atrophies, including dentatorubropallidoluysian atrophy.[30] The mitochondrial encephalomyopathies, which are protean in their presentations, can rarely resemble PSP.[31]

Some clinical points by which PSP can be differentiated from some of the most common of these entities are listed in Table 21–4. Perhaps the most difficult differentiation of PSP is from MSA. One study[20] found that certain clinical features could distinguish MSA from PD with acceptable certainty, but that they could not distinguish MSA from PSP in the absence of specific signs such as downgaze palsy or extensor axial dystonia.

CLINICAL EVALUATION

A thorough clinical examination and history will generally reveal PEP, PDC, myasthenia gravis (as a cause of gaze palsy, dysarthria, and dysphagia), mitochondrial myopathy (as a cause of gaze palsy), and bulbar amyotrophic lateral sclerosis. Magnetic resonance imaging (MRI) or X-ray computed tomography (CT) will reveal, although not necessarily incriminate, mimics such as

▶ TABLE 21–4. CLINICAL POINTS DIFFERENTIATING PSP FROM SOME OTHER PARKINSONIAN DISORDERS

Clinical Points	PSP	PD	MSA (SND)	CBD
Symmetry of deficit	+++	+	+++	–
Axial rigidity	+++	++	++	++
Limb dystonia	+	+	+	+++
Postural instability	+++	++	++	+
Vertical supranuclear gaze restriction	+++	+	++	++
Frontal behavior	+++	+	+	++
Dysautonomia	–	+	++	–
L-Dopa response early in course	+	+++	+	–
L-Dopa response late in course	–	++	+	–
Asymmetric cortical atrophy on MRI	–	–	–	++

SND, striatonigral degeneration.

hydrocephalus,[32] midbrain tumors, and a multi-infarct state. The last is the most common nondegenerative PSP mimic. In fact, lacunar states can reproduce virtually the full range of clinical features of PSP, as they can reproduce the clinical features of AD and PD.[33–35] It may be suspected in the patient with stepwise progression, marked pyramidal signs, focal weakness, and, as mentioned, ischemic changes on MRI or CT.

RADIOLOGIC EVALUATION

Positron emission tomography using ^{18}F-dopa distinguished 90% of patients with clinically diagnosed PSP from a group with PD.[36] Similar results are produced by use of ^{18}F-glucose as a marker of cortical and subcortical metabolic rate,[36–39] and by calculating the relative deficiencies of caudate and putamen with regard to uptake of a dopamine transporter marker.[40]

Although ^{18}F-dopa and ^{18}FDG (fluorodeoxyglucose) positron emission tomography (PET) can identify presymptomatic members of families with PSP,[41] the sensitivity and specificity of PET in distinguishing patients with clinically equivocal or early PSP from other conditions has not been assessed. For this reason, PET is not yet considered a standard diagnostic tool in PSP. The cost of that technology is a separate problem that would limit the use of PET in PSP to research settings for the foreseeable future.

MRI and CT imaging are nonspecific in most cases of PSP (Table 21–5). In the moderate-to-advanced stages, they may reveal thinning of the anteroposterior diameter of the midbrain tectum and tegmentum with atrophy of the colliculi and disproportionate enlargement of the sylvian fissures and posterior third ventricle.[42–47] MRI may show high signal in the periaqueductal gray compatible with gliotic change, a nonspecific finding in the parkinsonisms. The MRI features that are most likely to permit a differentiation of PSP from MSA are the absence (in PSP) of abnormal signal and/or atrophy in the cerebellum, middle cerebellar peduncle, pons and inferior olive, and of the hyperintense putaminal rim caused by iron deposition.[47] The MRI features most helpful in distinguishing PSP from CBD are the absence of asymmetric frontal atrophy and the presence of midbrain atrophy.As is the case with PET imaging, the value of MRI and CT in the early, diagnostically doubtful case is not established, except to rule out nondegenerative pathology or to rule out cerebellar atrophy that would direct suspicion toward olivopontocerebellar atrophy as the diagnosis.

A similar challenge faces the use of single photon emission computed tomography (SPECT) using markers of cerebral blood flow and/or metabolism. Such

▶ TABLE 21–5. MRI FEATURES OF PSP AND SOME OTHER CONDITIONS

MRI Features	PSP	PD	MSA (OPCA)	MSA (SND)	CBD	AD
Cortical atrophy	++	+	+/–	+	++/–	++
Putaminal atrophy	–	–	–	++	–	–
Pontine atrophy	+	–	+++	–	+/–	–
Midbrain atrophy	++	–	+	–	+/–	–
Cerebellar atrophy	–	–	++/–	–	–	–
High putaminal iron	–	–	+/–	+/–	–	–
Lateral putaminal "gliotic slit"	+	-	+	+	-	-
Pontine "hot cross bun sign"	-	-	+	+	-	-

–, absent or rare; +, occasional, mild, or late; ++, usual, moderate; +++, usual, severe, or early; OPCA, olivopontocerebellar atrophy; SND, striatonigral degeneration.

studies show bifrontal hypometabolism in established PSP[50–52] and have yet to be evaluated in equivocal cases. However, SPECT imaging of D_2 receptor sites using ^{123}I-iodobenzamide is promising as a means of differentiating PSP, where there is often detectable striatal D_2 loss, from PD, where there is not.[53,54]

Magnetic resonance spectroscopy is starting to show promise as a means of differentiating PSP from PD or other states.[55–57] The diagnostic finding is a reduction in the ratio of *N*-acetylaspartate to creatine in the region of the putamen and/or pallidum. However, as for PET, the ability of this modality to distinguish the conditions during their early, clinically equivocal phases is unproven.

Transcranial sonography (TCS) in PSP[58] shows hyperechogenicity of the lenticular nucleus and widening of the third ventricle, unlike in PD, where the sole finding is hyperechogenicity of the substantia nigra. However, TCS cannot reliably distinguish PSP from MSA and the distinction from PD is robust only for younger-onset PD. TCS has not yet proven useful in documenting PSP progression. The modality requires extensive operator training and experience but is inexpensive and safe.

MRI modalities that are showing promise in monitoring disease progression include diffusion-weighted imaging, diffusion-tensor imaging, and voxel-based morphometry.[59,60]

CEREBROSPINAL FLUID (CSF) STUDIES

CSF tau levels are elevated in CBD but not in PSP[61,62] or AD.[62] The CSF level of neurofilament protein has been found in one small series to distinguish PSP from PD and controls but not from MSA.[63] Protein, glucose, and cell counts are uniformly normal in PSP.

One recent study found that the ratio of truncated (33kD) to extended (55kD) tau protein in CSF distinguished PSP from competing diagnostic possibilities with no overlap.[64] Confirmation, particularly in early, diagnostically uncertain, cases is awaited.

▶ NEUROPATHOLOGY, NEUROCHEMISTRY, AND THEIR CLINICAL CORRELATES

OVERVIEW

PSP is one of the neurofibrillary tangle (NFT) diseases. This group also includes AD, corticobasal degeneration, dementia pugilistica, Down's syndrome, frontotemporal dementia, Guadelouopean tauopathy, PDC, Pick's disease, and PEP.

Dopaminergic damage in the nigrostriatal pathway and cholinergic damage in many areas are the most consistent, severe neurotransmitter-related changes in PSP.[65–68] GABAergic function of the basal ganglia (in striatum, globus pallidus interna, GPi, and globus pallidus externa, GPe) is moderately but widely impaired.[69] Unlike the case in PD, the peptidergic systems and the mesolimbic and mesocortical dopaminergic systems are intact. Serotonergic receptor sites are reduced in the cortex, but unlike in PD, are normal in basal ganglia.[70] The loss of adrenoceptors is widespread,[71] reflecting the wide projections of the severely damaged locus ceruleus.

NEUROFIBRILLARY TANGLES (NFTS)

While neuronal loss and gliosis are the most prominent microanatomic features of PSP[72] and their characteristic anatomic distribution can produce suspicion of PSP, the diagnosis cannot be made in the absence of NFTs. While most of the NFTs of most brains with PSP have a rounded ("globose") shape, a few are "flame-shaped." This situation is reversed in AD and seems to relate more closely to the structure of the neuron containing the tangle than to the disease producing the damage.[73]

The filaments composing the NFTs of PSP are unpaired straight filaments 15–18 nm in diameter, comprising at least 6 protofilaments 2–5 nm in diameter.[74–77] Filaments of AD, by contrast, are mostly paired helical filaments 22 nm in diameter with a minor component of straight filaments similar to those of PSP.[78] A few cortical areas in PSP, or even subcortical nuclei, may display paired helical filaments of the Alzheimer type.[79–84] Paired straight filaments and unpaired twisted filaments, which may be a more advanced stage of filament formation, also occur occasionally in PSP.[80]

The immunostaining and ultrastructural properties of the filaments of PSP tangles are nearly identical to those of CBD.[80,81] However, the white matter tangles of CBD occur in oligodendroglia rather than in astrocytes, as in most[82] cases of PSP. Furthermore, "pretangles" are far more frequent in CBD than in PSP.[83]

The recently described "PSP-parkinsonism" variant develops milder and more anatomically restricted NFTs and other tau pathology than the classic "Richardson's syndrome" or "PSP-PAGF" forms of PSP described above.[24,84,85]

TAU PROTEIN

Cortical NFTs of PSP appear to be antigenically identical to those of AD, most notably with regard to the presence of abnormally phosphorylated tau protein.[86–89] Tau is a low molecular weight component of microtubule-associated protein (MAP). The latter is involved in axonal transport of vesicles. PSP tau exhibits bands of 64 and 69 kDa on Western blot, while AD and Down's syndrome tau has those two bands plus one of 55 kDa.[91,92]

Staining with anti-tau antibody greatly aids the identification of NFTs in PSP and has largely replaced silver stains and hematoxylin and eosin for this purpose, at least in the research setting. Anti-tau staining has revealed the existence of neuropil threads, also known as curly fibers, in the same neurons that include NFTs and in oligodendroglia of white matter tracts connecting affected areas of subcortical gray matter.[93–95] Most neuropil threads of AD, on the other hand, occur in neurons, sparing glia. Staining for ubiquitin, a peptide involved in proteolysis and occurring in NFTs of AD and Lewy bodies of PD, is weak or variable in the NFTs of PSP.[96]

A transgenic mouse[97,98] is the most widely used animal model for PSP. It expresses one of the mutant forms of tau that causes frontotemporal dementia, but the distribution of lesions is closely analogous to that of human PSP. *Drosophila*[99] and zebrafish[100] transgenic models of a generic tauopathy have also been reported.

The molecular biology of tau abnormalities in PSP is discussed in more detail in the section on genetics below.

OTHER CHANGES

Grumose degeneration, in which eosinophilic material surrounds degenerating neurons, accompanied by spherical argentophilic components, occurs in a significant minority of cases with PSP, particularly in the cerebellar dentate nucleus.[2,101] It appears to comprise abnormally regenerated synaptic terminal material of Purkinje cells. Grumose degeneration of the dentate occurs also in dentatorubropallidoluysian atrophy, a condition with more obvious ataxia than occurs in PSP.

While amyloid or senile plaques do not occur in PSP, another hallmark of AD, granulovacuolar degeneration, does occur to a mild extent. In addition, swollen, achromatic neurons characteristic of CBD or Pick's disease occur in a few cases of otherwise typical PSP, generally in tegmental and inferior temporal areas.[102]

The overlap of PSP with AD is illustrated by a recent series of 13 autopsies with the full pathologic picture of PSP,[103] of which 4 also exhibited pathologic changes of "definite AD" and 2 had "probable AD." A primary clinical diagnosis of AD with memory loss as the first neurologic symptom was present in 2 of these 6 and in 3 of the 7 without AD pathology.

Microglial activation, another pathologic change that occurs in some neurodegenerative disorders, is common in PSP.[104,105] In the brain stem in PSP, microglial activation does not correlate well with the presence of NFTs. This suggests that neither is the direct cause of the other and that microglia may help produce the neuronal loss of PSP.

Anatomic Distribution of Degeneration

The major areas of primary involvement in PSP, together with an oversimplified but convenient scheme of their clinical correlates, are the cerebral cortex, producing cognitive and behavioral changes; the nigrostriatalpallidal area, producing rigidity, bradykinesia, and postural instability; the cholinergic pontomesencephalic nuclei area, producing gaze palsies, sleep disturbances, and axial motor abnormalities; and the hindbrain area, producing dysarthria and dysphagia. The daunting complexity of this syndrome, the interactions of its parts, and its tremendous interpatient variability may be the principal reason for the continuing resistance of PSP to pathophysiologic understanding and pharmacologic intervention.

▶ CEREBRAL CORTEX

PATHOANATOMY

The marked central and cortical atrophy of cerebrum seen on gross postmortem examination in AD is only mild in PSP.[106] Early studies of PSP found scant microscopical pathology in cerebral cortex, but the advent of tau immunostaining has permitted identification of the motor strip (area 4) and a partly ocular motor association area (area 39) as the most important sites of pathology.[107–109] Many other cortical areas are affected, but much less severely. The least affected area appears to be the primary visual cortex (area 17), as is the case in AD.[110] The affection of the motor area of cortex may be secondary to the severe degeneration of subcortical areas, such as the subthalamic nucleus, that have projections to cortex.[111] Overlap with the topography of the pathology of corticobasal degeneration can produce in some cases of PSP cortical signs such as apraxia.[112] PSP affects the large pyramidal and small neurons of layers V and VI, while AD affects the medium-sized neurons of layers III and V.[112]

Cortical involvement in PSP therefore differs importantly from that in AD at the gyral, laminar, cytologic, ultrastructural, and biochemical levels.

FRONTAL LOBES

Behavioral changes were the initial symptom of PSP in 22% of patients in one series[4] that used family interview data, and in 2 of 24 (8%) in a series with autopsy confirmation and good clinical records (I Litvan, personal communication). Disabling mental changes eventually occur in 80% or more of cases.[5,113]

ANATOMIC AND NEUROCHEMICAL CHANGES

The prefrontal areas, which are the most obviously affected by behavioral testing and by measures of cerebral blood flow,[50–52,114–117] display relatively little neurofibrillary pathology or neuronal loss in PSP.[99,102] This suggests that, in PSP, secondary cortical dysfunction is caused by subcortical pathology, as in the cholinergic nucleus basalis of Meynert and the cholinergic pedunculopontine nucleus (PPN), both important and relatively constant sites of involvement.[118–120] The situation is not so simple, however, because, in PSP, unlike in PD, dementia does not correlate with the degree of reduction in choline acetyltransferase activity.[66,121] Frontal cortical degeneration in PSP correlates well with the atrophy of the anterior corpus callosum, which presumably is its result[122] and with disproportionate frontal EEG slowing.[123]

Damage to the striatopallidal complex may also contribute to dementia via reduction in its output to the frontal lobes.[111,124] However, in PSP, unlike in PD, damage to noncholinergic subcorticocortical projections via dopaminergic, noradrenergic, and serotonergic pathways is minimal.

CLINICAL CORRELATES

Clinically, the frontal lobe dysfunction in PSP is often striking and rapidly progressing.[125] Apathy, intellectual slowing, and impairment of "executive" functions are the consistent findings. These are partly related to slowed central sensory processing.[126,127] Tests of reaction time that control for motor slowing show that the cognitive component of such tasks is greatly prolonged in PSP, approximately 50% longer than in PD.[128] It is a common clinical observation that the patient with PSP can supply correct answers to complex questions after a delay of several minutes.

The executive dysfunction[129] is illustrated by difficulty in shifting mental set, as in following an alternating numerical/alphabetical trail with a pencil.[130] Other defects are poor performance of sorting, problem-solving, abstract thinking, and lexical fluency (as when given 1 minute to name as many items as possible from a given category such as words starting with "m").[131,132] Other examining room tasks that can reveal a frontal defect are the ability to perform task A (e.g., tapping once) when the examiner performs task B (e.g., tapping twice) and vice versa, and the ability, when confronted by the examiner's widely separated hands, to direct horizontal gaze toward the hand that does not wave the "antisaccade task." Disinhibition in other forms occurs in a significant minority.

Prominent frontal deficits of this sort with little agitation, irritability, or abnormal motor behaviors help distinguish the dementia of PSP from that of AD.[133]

Spontaneous frontal motor behaviors can also be dramatic in some patients with PSP.[130,134] Most obvious are forced grasping (either with the hand or gaze), imitative behavior (such as mimicking the examiner's hand movements), and motor perseveration (as when unable to cease clapping after being asked to imitate the examiner's three handclaps—the "applause sign"). These signs in the presence of parkinsonism are a useful alert to the possibility of PSP, but the combination also occurs in PD and SND.[26] Arm levitation[135] and other forms of apraxia[136] have been described. Palilalia is a common and, at times, disabling problem in PSP.[131]

HIPPOCAMPUS

The hippocampus, a primary site of pathology in AD, is involved in only half of cases of PSP.[137] This probably explains the relative preservation of memory in PSP, at least until late in the course.[16] The qualitative pattern of involvement of the hippocampus in PSP, however, is similar to that in AD and PD.[109] Memory tasks that require goal-directed searching of memory are, as one would expect given the frontal lobe function, an early area of impairment in PSP.[138] The pattern of memory impairment is similar to that of PD and Huntington's disease and different from that in AD, where forgetting is more rapid.[139]

▶ NIGROSTRIATAL SYSTEM

DISTRIBUTION OF PATHOLOGY

Damage to the pigmented neurons of the zona compacta of the substantia nigra, the most consistent abnormality in PSP, occurs in a distribution different from that in PD.[140] In PSP, the damage is relatively uniform except for relative sparing of a small, extreme lateral portion, while, in PD, both the dorsal and extreme lateral portions are relatively spared. A similar pattern occurs in striatonigral degeneration.[140] The dorsal portion projects principally to the caudate, the ventral to the putamen. This probably explains the relative sparing of presynaptic caudate dopamine reuptake in PD and its involvement in PSP, as measured by ^{18}F-fluorodopa PET.[36,141]

In the striatum, there is also severe loss of acetylcholinergic activity,[67] although the majority of affected striatal cells appear to be astrocytes rather than neurons ("tufted" astrocytes).[89] They include tau-positive, argyrophilic tangles and neuropil threads similar to those in affected neurons. Such astrocytic pathology may be unique to PSP. Most of the few affected striatal neurons are probably cholinergic interneurons.[68,142,143]

It is unclear whether the poor response of the parkinsonian components of PSP to dopamine replacement therapy and the relative resistance of PSP to the hyperkinetic side effects of such therapy are the result of pathology in the striatum or further downstream in the striatal system. It is also unclear whether the loss of the cholinergic striatal interneurons explains the failure of anticholinergic treatment (relative to its success in PD) and the hints of improvement from cholinergic treatment.[144]

As predicted from the paucity of striatal neuronal damage, there is no loss of postsynaptic dopamine D_1 receptors, as measured by binding studies, and by D_1

receptor mRNA levels.[65] Density of D_2 receptors is probably normal or only slightly decreased.[65,137,138]

CLINICAL COURSE

Postural instability is the initial symptom in approximately two-thirds of patients with PSP and for the remainder, frank falls typically start within the first year.[4–6] The falls are often unheralded in that the patient had had no concomitant gait difficulty and typically complains of having "tripped over nothing." This has prompted the term "paroxysmal dysequilibrium." Patients often have a normal neurological examination at this point and are investigated for vestibulopathy, syncope, epilepsy, myelopathy, or posterior fossa ischemia. The initial or only gait abnormality occasionally takes the form of severe gait "freezing" or "apraxia"[84,137–150] with no rigidity. In PD, by contrast, gait difficulty or postural instability is a presenting feature in only 11%.[7]

The postural instability is usually the most disabling feature of later PSP. The median intervals from initial symptom, corrected by the Kaplan-Meier lifetable method, are 3.1 years until assistance is required, and 8.2 years until wheelchair confinement.[4]

Contrary to widespread impression, rest tremor is not unknown in PSP, occurring in about 5–10% of patients, usually early in the course.[151,152] Action or postural tremor occurs in about 25%. The limb rigidity and distal bradykinesia are mild relative to axial rigidity and bradykinesia. The rigidity tends to increase from wrist to elbow to shoulder and is far greater in the neck than in the trunk.[10] The retrocollis that many neurologists consider a hallmark of PSP is specific but not sensitive, occurring in only about 10%, although a neck posture that is unexpectedly erect for a parkinsonian disorder is far more common.

▶ OTHER BASAL GANGLIA

SUBTHALAMIC NUCLEUS

Damage to the subthalamic nucleus ranks beside that of the substantia nigra as a constant in PSP and is far more specific to PSP. Subthalamic neuronal depletion is so severe that the posteroinferior portion of the third ventricle may be disproportionately dilated on CT or magnetic resonance MRI.[42] This can give the third ventricle the shape of a bowling pin on axial imaging, contrasting with the cigar-shaped characteristic of AD.

GLOBUS PALLIDUS INTERNA

The basal ganglia damage that is furthest "downstream" and therefore perhaps the most relevant with regard to therapeutic intervention in PSP is in the GPi. This structure acts as the common outflow pathway from the basal ganglia to the thalamus. This lesion is not quite as constant as that of the substantia nigra or subthalamic nucleus, but it probably explains the failure of stereotactic GPi lesions to ameliorate PSP despite their efficacy against PD. Similarly, the outflow function of the GPi probably explains the therapeutic failure of fetal mesencephalic implants into the striatum in PSP.

GLOBUS PALLIDUS EXTERNA

A careful comparison of PSP with PD and controls with regard to neuronal counts in the GPe showed an important loss in PSP but not in PD.[153] This offers the possibility that GPe dysfunction provides the most direct source of the hypokinesis of PSP by increasing thalamic inhibition, particularly in patients lacking the excitatory input from the subthalamic nucleus.

PEDUNCULOPONTINE NUCLEUS

Despite the status of the GABAergic GPi (and the partly GABAergic substantia nigra reticulata, SNr) as the final outflow from the basal ganglia, and despite low GABAergic activity in many parts of the basal ganglia, efforts to treat PSP with the GABAergic drug valproic acid have failed, at least on informal assessment at the symptomatic level.[154] Part of the explanation may be that the GPi projects not only to the thalamus, which is nearly intact in PSP, but also to the cholinergic PPN, which is severely affected.[119,120,155] There is evidence that lesions of the PPN alone can cause severe postural instability.[156] Nevertheless, GABA agonists more selective for basal ganglia function should be tested in PSP. At the same time, preliminary studies of PPN stimulation in PSP are under way.[157]

THALAMUS

Although the thalamus is not classically considered a major center of pathology in PSP, Steele and colleagues[1–3] did mention the presence of tangles in the glutamatergic caudal intralaminar nuclei, which regulate caudate and putamen, and more recent studies have confirmed this quantitatively.[158] PET using a cholinergic marker has documented loss of those thalamic neurons, producing a picture different from that of the cholinergic loss in PD.[159]

OTHERS

The GPe, ventral tegmental area, red nucleus, intralaminar nuclei of the thalamus, and locus ceruleus are also involved in PSP, although not as constantly or as severely as the foregoing areas.

Experimental lesions of the interstitial nucleus of Cajal in monkeys produce extensor rigidity at the neck and postural instability,[160] and this nucleus is characteristically affected in PSP.[161] However, the severe damage in the striatopallidal pathway could also help explain the unusual extensor tone of PSP.[162]

▶ MESENCEPHALIC AND PONTINE OCULAR MOTOR AREAS

PATHOANATOMY

The supranuclear, predominantly vertical, eye movement abnormality for which PSP was named presumably originates in the rostral midbrain, where there is variable involvement of the interstitial nucleus of Cajal, the nucleus of Darkschewitsch, the rostral interstitial nucleus of the medial longitudinal fasciculus, and the mesencephalic reticular formation.[111,119,161,163] The relative contributions of these nuclei have not been sorted out.

There have been cases of damage to some of these areas in patients without clinical supranuclear gaze abnormality.[164–167] Conversely, there is one report of idiopathic calcification of basal ganglia sparing dorsal midbrain with PSP-like gaze palsy.[168] One quantitative study of neuronal loss in the SNr[169] found a correlation of damage there with gaze palsy in patients with PSP. This may be explained by the projection of the SNr to the superior colliculus.

Some of the vertical paresis may result from subselective involvement of these nuclei themselves, followed by nuclear ocular paresis at the endstage of PSP in some cases. The horizontal gaze palsy that appears eventually in most cases is attributable to degeneration of nuclei of the pontine base.[170]

CLINICAL PHENOMENOLOGY

Symptomatic eye movement difficulty does not begin until a median of 3.9 years after disease onset, nearly half the clinical course.[4] Before that time, however, most patients with otherwise diagnosable PSP will exhibit slowing of vertical saccades, saccadic pursuit, breakdown of opticokinetic nystagmus in the vertical plane, disordered Bell's phenomenon, poor convergence, and subtle square-wave jerks.[171–173] The last finding has perhaps the greatest sensitivity for PSP, occurring in all or nearly all patients with the condition.[173,174] Square-wave jerks occur in very few patients with PD, but are sufficiently common in MSA and other conditions that they cannot be used to differentiate them from PSP.[174] Of great specificity for PSP is a delay in saccade initiation, at times so prolonged as to give the appearance of the patient's not having heard or attended to the examiner's command. Such delays may constitute visual prehension, also called perseveration of gaze, a result of frontal lobe damage.[175]

The frontal dysfunction is also expressed via such ocular motor phenomena as poor performance on the antisaccade task. Here, the patient quickly directs the gaze to the examiner's hand that does *not* move. An altitudinal visual attentional deficit[176] arising from damaged tectal centers may contribute to overloading the fork, poor aim of the urinary stream, and poor attention to dress out of proportion to dementia. In addition, patients with PSP seem less aware of their postural instability than patients with the same degree of instability of other causes.

Later in the course, the patient loses range of vertical gaze, with downgaze usually, but far from always, worse than upgaze. Voluntary gaze without a specific target (i.e., "look down") is usually worse than command gaze to a target, which is worse than pursuit, and reflex gaze is by far the least affected. Some patients with autopsy-confirmed PSP never display gaze paresis during life, even on careful prospective examination.[9]

REFLEX GAZE

From the earliest stages, most patients also lose the ability to voluntarily suppress the vestibulo-ocular reflex.[177] This may be tested by seating the patient in a swivel chair or wheelchair and asking him to extend the arms at the level of the eyes, clasp his hands, and fixate on one thumbnail as the examiner slowly rotates the chair and patient en bloc. Patients with PSP (and many other basal ganglia disorders) are unable to suppress the opticokinetic nystagmus produced by relative movement of the environment. Performing this maneuver in the vertical plane, if the patient's axial rigidity permits, reveals an abnormality which, when out of proportion to concomitant poor horizontal vestibulo-ocular reflex suppression, may be a valuable clue to the presence of very early PSP.

EYELID MOVEMENT

Eyelid movement abnormalities, particularly apraxia of eyelid opening (perhaps better termed "lid levator inhibition"[178]), and blepharospasm, occur in about one-third of patients and can cause functional blindness.[179–181] Apraxia of lid closing and the very slow blink rate of PSP, often less than 5/minute, can allow conjunctival drying with annoying reactive inflammation and lacrimation. The electrical blink reflex is severely impaired, unlike in PD, CBD, or MSA,[182,183] testament to the profound brain stem pathology in PSP.

BRAIN STEM CENTERS CONTROLLING SLEEP AND AROUSAL

Sleep disturbance is a prominent abnormality in PSP. It is presumably related principally to damage to the (serotonergic) raphe nuclei, the (cholinergic) PPN and others, the (noradrenergic) locus ceruleus, and the periaqueductal gray. The most important clinical component is a severe reduction in rapid eye movement (REM) sleep.[184] There is a loss of sleep spindles and K-complexes. During what REM sleep remains, there are abnormal slow waves and absence of normal sawtooth waves.[185] The diagnostic value of the REM abnormalities prompted Agid and colleagues[137] to advocate polysomnography in all patients with a suspicion of PSP.

Daytime hypersomnolence, probably related to damage of dopaminergic systems that maintain wakefulness, is a disabling problem in PSP. There is a fragmentation of sleep–wake periods that culminate, at the endstage of PSP, in a constant sleep-like or stuporous state from which the patient can be roused but briefly. The auditory startle and auditory blink reflexes are absent or severely impaired in PSP[186] despite normal auditory evoked potentials.[187] Startle is mediated via the lower pontine reticular formation, in particular the nucleus reticularis pontis caudalis, which degenerates in PSP.

BRAIN STEM CENTERS CONTROLLING SPEECH AND SWALLOWING

Dysarthria

Steele and colleagues[3] were referring to the lower brain stem functions as much as to the eye movements in applying the term "supra-nuclear palsy." Indeed, degeneration of the cranial nerve nuclei in PSP is mild except in the oculomotor nucleus.[188] Likewise, the dysarthria of PSP reveals no lower motoneuron features. Rather, it is a variable combination of, in descending order of importance, spasticity, hypophonia, and ataxia.[189] The combination is unique among the competing diagnostic considerations, at least from a statistical standpoint (Table 21–6). The slow rate of speech with a strained and strangled quality and some hyperkinetic, ataxic components is highly specific for PSP.

Dysarthria can be an early symptom that often brings the patient to a physician.[5] Within 2 years after disease onset, 41% of patients or their families have detected dysarthria. By the fifth year, the figure is 68%.[4]

Dysphagia

Relative to the morbidity it causes, the dysphagia of PSP has received only little and belated research attention. Aspiration pneumonia is a major risk in advanced PSP, but only 18% of patients report symptomatic dysphagia within 2 years after PSP onset and 46% do so by 5 years.[4] Dysphagia occurred in 26 of 27 patients in one study in which the mean disease duration was 52 months.[190,191] The median latency to onset of dysarthria was 48 months in one study[4] and 42 in another.[192]

In a study[193] that performed videofluoroscopy in 22 patients with mild-to-moderate PSP with symptomatic dysphagia, at least 80% of patients exhibited abnormalities attributable to parkinsonian rigidity of the oral and pharyngeal muscles. Esophageal problems occurred in fewer than half of patients and nasal reflux occurred in none. Only 4.5% (1 patient) aspirated contrast material, but 27% coughed or choked. The dysphagia of PSP, while arising from many levels of the oropharyngeal axis,[191] emphasizes oral rather than pharyngeal abnormalities, distinguishing it from the dysphagia of PD.[194]

It is common for patients with PSP, but not with PD, to exacerbate the effects of dysphagia by overloading the fork, probably through a combination of poor downgaze, frontal disinhibition, and vertical visual inattention.[195] The neck hyperextension that occurs eventually in some patients with PSP may decrease the ability of the epiglottis to protect the airway. However, relative to patients with PD, those with PSP appear more aware of their dysphagia and have less rigidity and tremor of the tongue, major causes of dysphagia in PD.[193]

SPINAL AND AUTONOMIC CENTERS

PSP includes less dysautonomia than PD,[197] a point useful in its clinical differentiation from MSA. Nevertheless, there can be disabling bladder dysfunction,[198] which is probably the result of the severe degeneration of brain stem autonomic nuclei,[199] and of some white matter tracts in the spinal cord.[200] The latter occurs mainly in the motor area (lamina IX) and the intermediolateral column. There is also mild gray matter tract degeneration in the spinal cord.[111] In one series,[86] urinary incontinence occurred in 42% of patients, beginning a mean of 3.5 years into the disease course.

▶ TABLE 21–6. COMPONENTS OF DYSARTHRIA IN PSP AND SOME RELATED CONDITIONS[190,193]

Components of Dysarthria	Hypokinesia	Ataxia	Spasticity
PSP	++	+	+++
PD	+++	–	–
MSA (striatonigral degeneration)	+++	++	+
MSA (olivopontocerebellar atrophy)	+	+++	++

TABLE 21-7. SURVIVAL ESTIMATES AND 95% CI FOR PATIENTS WITH TOTAL PSPRS SCORES IN THE SPECIFIED RANGES*

PSPRS Score	Subsequent Survival Percentage and 95% CI						
	6 months	12 months	24 months	36 months	48 months	60 months	72 months
20–29	97.1 91.9–100	94.2 86.8–100	83.8 71.8–97.7	64.1 48.7–84.5	40.1 25.4–63.1	18.0 8.1–40.2	9.0 2.5–32.0
30–39	96.4 91.7–100	92.6 86.0–99.7	76.4 65.7–88.8	57.7 45.3–73.6	25.3 15.1–42.3	12.6 5.6–28.5	6.3 1.8–22.6
40–49	91.5 85.2–98.1	86.9 79.4–95.2	58.9 47.9–72.5	41.9 31.0–56.6	17.9 10.2–31.5	13.0 6.5–26.2	5.2 1.5–18.5
50–59	88.0 80.6–96.0	76.9 67.4–87.6	54.9 44.0–68.6	26.0 16.8–40.2	16.2 8.7–30.2	**	**
60–69	83.7 74.1–94.4	70.2 58.5–84.3	28.5 17.8–45.4	11.4 4.7–27.6	7.6*** 2.5–22.8	7.6*** 2.5–22.8	3.8*** 0.9–16.6
>70	69.2 54.9–87.2	47.4 33.0–68.0	16.4*** 7.5–30.4	16.4*** 7.5–30.4	**	**	**

*Survival times are calculated as the interval between initial entry into the PSPRS score range and death.
**Not estimable because there were no survivors.
***These are the same because there were no observed deaths between the two successive time points.

EPIDEMIOLOGY AND ETIOLOGY

DESCRIPTIVE EPIDEMIOLOGY

Onset Age

In most series, PSP begins, on average, in the late fifties to mid-sixties, as is the case for PD. Approximately a third of cases begin before age 60.[4] The standard deviation of the onset age is typically between 6 and 7 years,[4] far less than the 11 years typical for PD. For a late-life-onset condition, such raw onset age data are less useful to the epidemiologist than age-specific incidence figures, which do not exist for PSP. That is, we do not know whether there is an age of maximal risk for PSP or whether the incidence of new cases in a given age group relative to the number of people alive in that age group declines after a certain age. This would have implications for etiology and pathogenesis.

Survival

Death occurred at an actuarially corrected median of 9.7, 7.0, and 5.9 years in three studies.[4,5,201] Ten-year survival is typically approximately 30%.[201] In a study based on complete ascertainment of a well-documented community, Olmsted County, Minnesota, median survival was only 5.3 years.[202] The onset age distribution was older in that study than in many others that were based on referred cases. Therefore, the median survival in that study may be a more valid measure of the natural history of PSP in general.

The PSP Rating Scale[11] score provides a useful prognostic guide to expected survival. Table 21–7 shows the subsequent expected survival given the PSPRS score on examination.

Death is usually related to pneumonia and other inevitable complications of immobility, but frank aspiration, head trauma due to falls, and complications of hip fracture are important preventable causes of death in PSP.

Prevalence

The prevalence ratio of previously diagnosed PSP was found by one study in three counties in central New Jersey[4] to be 1.4 per 100,000, and by another in the UK[203] to be 1.0 per 100,000. This figure would be useful in determining the demand for PSP-specific services or treatment.

In an attempt to count undiagnosed cases, two studies, one in London[204] and the other in the north of England,[203] examined patients in defined geographical areas whose medical records suggested any sort of parkinsonism. Most of the patients thereby identified as having PSP had not previously received that diagnosis. The age-adjusted prevalence ratios were 6.4[204] and 5.0[203] per 100,000. The 4–5-fold difference between these prevalence ratios and those based only on previously diagnosed cases is a measure of the difficulty in accurately diagnosing PSP when the index of suspicion is low.

Incidence

For a chronic disease, incidence (the number of new cases in a defined population per year) gives a more valid measure than prevalence of the intensity of the etiologic agent in the population or environment. The incidence of PSP has been measured directly in Rochester, Minnesota (population 50,000) by two separate studies. The first used patients previously diagnosed over the interval 1967–1979, giving an incidence of 0.3 per 100,000 per year.[205] The second, which covered the years 1976–1990 and used a more thorough method that captured patients with inobvious clinical presentations, gave an annual incidence of 1.1 per 100,000 per year.[202] This compares with approximately 20 per 100,000 per year for PD.[206]

Sex Ratio

Published cases of PSP reveal a sex ratio (M/F) of approximately 2:1, similar to that reported for PD but different from most other neurodegenerative disorders. While gender-related referral bias may be a contributor, the magnitude and the specificity of the effect point to underlying biological differences in susceptibility or possibly differences in environmental exposures, such as an occupational toxin.

ANALYTIC EPIDEMIOLOGY

The first case-control study of risk factors in PSP was an 85-item questionnaire administered to 50 tertiary referral patients and 100 matched controls in New Jersey.[207] Patients, relative to controls, reported more years of schooling and were more likely to have lived in a small town. Suspecting that this may have been the result of using widely referred outpatient affected cases and locally ascertained inpatient controls, the authors performed a second study[208] using controls who, like the PSP subjects, were referred outpatients. This yielded the opposite result, where those with PSP were less likely to have completed 12 years' schooling (odds ratio = 0.35, 95% CI = 0.12–0.95, p = 0.022).

Neither study[207,208] gave statistically significant results concerned living overseas, occupations implicated in other neurologic illnesses, potential exposure to occupational toxins or pesticides, smoking, alcohol, caffeine, contact sports, head trauma, type A personality, early menopause, estrogen supplementation, multiparity, various medical conditions, surgical history, psychiatric history, animal exposure, maternal age, birth order, and family neurologic history.

Anecdotal reports from one investigator in Canada suggest greater than expected exposure to hydrocarbons in a small series of patients with PSP.[209,210] This may help explain the asymmetric sex ratio, but has not yet been specifically examined in a controlled study. Smoking, which is negatively correlated with PD and MSA, has no relation to PSP.[211]

A TRANSMISSIBLE AGENT?

The pathologic and clinical similarity between PSP and PDC aroused suspicion that a slow virus may be their cause, as it is in Kuru, another neurodegenerative disease of the western Pacific. However, after a mean of 9.1 (range 3–24) years' observation of 29 chimpanzees receiving intracerebral inoculation of brain tissue from 10 patients with PSP results were negative.[212] A search for prion protein in PSP and other parkinsonian disorders, despite the pathologic similarities between PSP and Creutzfeldt–Jakob disease, was also negative.[213]

In PD and AD, but not in PSP,[214] there is a deficit in the sense of smell, the function of which involves dopaminergic transmission. This is evidence against the hypothesis that, at least in PSP, an etiologic agent gains entry to the CNS via the olfactory epithelium.

A HEREDITARY COMPONENT?

In reviewing the records of 104 patients with PSP, Jankovic and colleagues[215] found no allegations of secondary cases of PSP among their 409 relatives, and the frequency of PD, tremor, and dementia among the relatives was only that expected in the population. A retrospectively controlled survey from the same clinic[216] found a family history of tremor in relatives of patients with (nonfamilial) PSP (2.6%) to be similar to that among relatives of controls (2.2%).

However, in a formal case-control study,[207] the question inquiring into the presence of "Parkinson's disease" among parents, siblings, grandparents, aunts, uncles, and first cousins elicited a positive answer 5.0 times as frequently in those with PSP as in controls. For "Alzheimer's or dementia," the ratio was 3.6. These results were not statistically significant but suggest more sensitive studies.[217] Another intriguing observation of deficits in reaction time in 39% of 23 asymptomatic close relatives of patients with PSP but in no controls.[218]

Recent reports of families with more than one member with PSP give additional reason to reconsider the issue of a genetic factor in the cause of PSP. Eight such reports with autopsy confirmation in at least one member have appeared, all most compatible with autosomal-dominant transmission.[219–223] Paternal transmission was a component of the mechanism in most of these families, a strong point against a mitochondrial gene as the sole culprit. In fact, point mutations in the MAPT (tau) gene have been found in some of these families.[224]

It is intriguing that some of these families, including a Spanish family that is by far the largest, include additional members with reports of typical PD or essential tremor.[225] Some asymptomatic members of such families show caudate and putaminal abnormalities in ^{18}F-fluorodopa uptake on PET.[227,228]

GEOGRAPHIC CLUSTERS

Two geographic clusters of PSP-like tauopathies are known. Lytigo-bodig, or the amyotrophic lateral sclerosis–parkinsonism–dementia complex of Guam (PDC), has resisted multiple careful etiologic investigations, but its markedly declining incidence since the westernization of Guam after World War II suggests an environmental cause.[229,230] The anatomic pathology of PDC has been called both easily distinguishable[83] and indistinguishable[231] from PSP. At the biochemical level, however, the predominance of 4-repeat tau in PSP tangles is absent in PDC, where the 4-repeat/3-repeat ratio is unity, as in controls and AD.[83]

An unusual concentration of a PSP-like tauopathy on the Caribbean island of Guadeloupe was described in 1999 by Caparros-Lefebvre and colleagues[232] Their case-control survey found that illness to be associated with dietary or medicinal use of two indigenous plants, soursop, and sweetsop (*Annona muricata* and *A. squamosa*). These species contain reticuline and corexime, which are dopaminergic toxins.[233] Discontinuing the use of these products resulted in marked and prolonged clinical improvement in some of the younger patients on Guadeloupe. Relative to PSP, patients with the Guadeloupean PSP have greater prevalence of rest tremor, dysautonomia, and hallucinations.[233] The active toxin in sweetsop and soursop, annonacin, is a mitochondrial complex I inhibitor that can produce a tauopathy in rats.[230]

A MITOCHONDRIAL OR OXIDATIVE MECHANISM?

Molecular genetic study of PSP has been advancing in recent years. One candidate locus, the apolipoprotein E (ApoE) locus, which exhibits a disproportionate prevalence of the ε4 allele in AD, exhibits only the normal distribution of alleles in PSP.[234–236] Other candidate genes could be subjected to similar allelic association studies in PSP, but there are as yet too few multiplex families or affected sibling pairs to perform linkage analysis.

A more promising lead arises from the finding[237] that skeletal muscle mitochondrial respiratory function, assessed at the biochemical level, is reduced by about 30% in PSP. In brain tissue, activity levels of superoxide dismutase 1 and/or 2,[238] malondialdehyde,[239] and lipid peroxidation products[240] are markedly increased specifically in areas that degenerate in PSP as a result of oxidative stress.

Evidence that deficiency of complex I of mitochondrial genetic origin contributes to the cause of typical PSP is provided by the observation of low complex I activity and mitochondrial dysfunction in cultured neuronal cells in which native mitochondria were replaced by mitochondria from patients with PSP.[241,242]

An area of recent inquiry is the role of transglutaminases in PSP.[243] Enzymes normally important in stabilizing protein structure, they are aberrantly activated in PSP and other neurodegenerative disorders by oxidative stress. The resulting crosslinking of tau protein could help explain the formation of NFTs or the dysfunction of other proteins.

Another promising molecular hypothesis concerns abnormal phosphorylation of tau protein. First reported in the 1980's, tau hyperphosphorylation via aberrant kinases or cell signaling pathways differs from that in Alzheimer's disease and offers attractive treatment targets.[244] Trials of neuroprotection by lithium and valproic acid, each of which inhibits tau phosphorylation by glycogen synthase kinase-3β, are under way.

A NUCLEAR GENETIC MECHANISM?

Tau Isoforms

In normal human brain, tau occurs in approximately equal proportions of isoforms: with either 3 or 4 repeats of the microtubule-binding peptide domain.[245] The isoform is determined by whether the transcript of the tau gene's exon 10 is spliced in or out of the final tau protein product. In PSP, the ratio is at least 3:1 in favor of 4-repeat tau.[91] In some other tauopathies such as Pick's disease, 3-repeat tau predominates; in others, such as AD, the normal 1:1 ratio occurs. Disordered regulation of exon 10 splicing may therefore explain tau aggregation into NFTs in PSP and other tauopathies.

The PSP-like illness highly prevalent on Guadeloupe, at least in the three cases autopsied so far,[246] is biochemically identical to PSP itself. That is, the NFTs in both conditions present a major doublet at 64 and 69 kDa and a minor 74 kDa band, and the tau is predominantly 4-repeat. This contrasts with the Guamanian disease, where there is a triplet at 60, 64 and 69 kDa, and the tau occurs equally in 3-repeat and 4-repeat forms.[247] The Guamanian biochemical signature is therefore closer to that of AD than PSP.[229]

A CLUE FROM FTD

A valuable clue to PSP, a sporadically occurring tauopathy, arises from frontotemporal dementia (FTD), a dominantly inherited tauopathy.[248] Several mutations in and near the 5′ splice site downstream of exon 10 have been described in FTD families. Here, the 3-repeat/4-repeat skew is similar to that of PSP.[249] The pathogenic mechanism of these mutations is probably disruption of a stem-loop structure in the RNA transcribed at the downstream end of exon 10. This stem-loop regulates splicing of the exon 10 transcript. Its dysfunction in FTD produces predominantly 4-repeat tau. One etiologic factor, then, in PSP and other sporadic tauopathies may be dysfunction of the same RNA stem-loop, but of nongenetic or nonmendelian genetic cause. This prospect has been strengthened by the description[250] of a family with inherited, autopsy-typical PSP and a mutation at the downstream end of exon 10 close to those described in FTD. This single nucleotide substitution does not alter the tau amino acid sequence but would disrupt the RNA stem-loop.

A TAU ALLELIC VARIANT

Following the lead of the FTD story, Conrad and colleagues[251] found an association between sporadic PSP and a genetic marker, the A0 allele, located in the intron upstream of exon 10. Subsequently, A0 was found to be part of a haplotype, H1, extending across the tau (MAPT) gene.[252,253] Homozygosity for H1 is present in 92% of patients with PSP but in only 60% of controls.[254] This suggests that a genetic variation necessary but not sufficient to cause PSP is located in or near the tau gene at chromosome 17q21. The precise causative mutation and its pathogenic mechanism are not known, but may involve overexpression of tau.[255–258]

The occurrence of PSP in sporadic rather than familial fashion must then require an additional exogenous or genetic factor. It is sobering in this regard to note that corticobasal degeneration shares the haplotype that characterizes PSP,[259,260] as does PD to a lesser degree.[261] It is equally sobering that the presence or absence of this H1 haplotype or the H1/H1 genotype has no effect on the age of onset, clinical progression,[262,263] or on the biochemical features of the abnormal tau protein.[264] However, the overrepresentation of H1 in PSP appears to be driven primarily by the Richardson syndrome clinical form.[22]

Variants in apoE that are associated with AD and variants in α-synuclein and synphilin that are associated with PD are absent in PSP.[265] However, a whole-genome analysis using pooled autopsy-proven samples revealed an association of PSP with a region at chromosome 11p12-p11 along with several areas of weaker value.[266] A more sensitive whole-genome analysis using individual autopsy-proven samples is under way and will report results in 2009.

▶ TREATMENT

PHARMACOTHERAPY

As is the case for most other degenerative disorders, neurotransmitter replacement or receptor stimulation in PSP encounters little or none of the success it has with PD (Table 21–8).[154,267] The multiplicity of neurotransmitter defects in PSP has prompted trials of many synaptic drugs.

Dopaminergics

The extent and nature of the benefit of L-dopa in PSP has not been adequately studied in double-blind fashion, but any benefit is nearly always mild and/or brief. In two retrospective, uncontrolled studies, 51%[268] and 38%[154] of patients responded, most of them minimally. (The placebo response rate in PD drug trials is generally about 30%.) Only the rigidity and bradykinesia, including those components of dysarthria and dysphagia attributable to them, may respond more than would be expected from placebo. Therefore, there is no reason to prescribe dopaminergic treatment for patients whose activities are not impaired by those specific abnormalities.

While hyperkinetic side effects and response fluctuations of L-dopa are very rare in PSP (0 of 82 patients in one survey[154]), agitation, confusion, and/or hallucinations are less rare (5 of 82, 6%). Still, it is the author's practice to prescribe for PSP approximately twice the L-dopa/carbidopa dosages used for PD with the equivalent degree of parkinsonism. Dopamine receptor agonists give similar benefit with additional risks.[154,269] This impression has been confirmed by a multicenter double-blind trial of pramipexole as well as by anecdotal experience with that drug.[270]

Cholinergics and Anticholinergics

It is perhaps symptomatic of our state of knowledge of PSP therapy that opposite directions in cholinergic intervention have been advocated. Anticholinergics have been used by analogy with PD, but are far less efficacious than L-dopa.[154,268,271] An exception may be amantadine, which has dopaminergic and antiglutamatergic properties as well, and is a close second to L-dopa in

▶ TABLE 21–8. **DRUGS MOST LIKELY TO RELIEVE SYMPTOMS IN PSP**

Drug	Starting dosage	MaxiNumber of dosage in PSP
L-Dopa* (with carbidopa)	100 mg per day	2000 mg per day
Amantadine	100 mg once daily	100 mg twice daily
Amitriptyline	10 mg at bedtime	20 mg in the morning, 20 mg at bedtime

*L-Dopa as a rule will only relieve limb rigidity and bradykinesia.

risk/benefit ratio.[154] Amantadine starting at 100 mg daily and increasing to a maximum of 100 mg twice daily is worthwhile as a trial for most patients with PSP. It should be tapered and discontinued if symptomatic benefit is not apparent within a month.

Trials of cholinergics have been inspired by the severe and widespread degeneration of acetylcholinergic systems in PSP. The cholinesterase inhibitor physostigmine was reported to improve PET evidence of prefrontal dysfunction, long-term verbal memory, and visuospatial attention, all very slightly,[127,144] but a subsequent trial by one of these groups gave negative results, with worsening of gait.[272] Donepezil, a commercially available cholinesterase inhibitor minimally effective in AD, has no benefit against PSP.[273] The benefits of RS-86, another cholinergic agent, were limited to some aspects of sleep.[274]

OTHER CATEGORIES OF SYNAPTIC DRUGS

Antidepressants

In a double-blind trial,[275] amitriptyline improved gait and rigidity in 3 of 4 patients, and desipramine improved "apraxia" of eyelid opening in both of 2 patients. In a retrospective series,[154] amitriptyline gave a risk/benefit ratio that was slightly less favorable than those of L-dopa and amantadine. Amitriptyline is generally safest started at 10 mg at bedtime, increasing by that amount each week, given in two divided doses. If 20 mg twice daily proves ineffective, higher dosages are unlikely do otherwise. Amitriptyline may paradoxically worsen postural instability in PSP and its anticholinergic effect may worsen the cognitive impairment of the illness. Imipramine confers a slightly less favorable risk/benefit ratio than amitriptyline,[154] and desipramine a quite unfavorable ratio.

Antiserotonergics

The antiserotonergic drug methysergide was found moderately efficacious in a controlled trial published in 1981,[195] but subsequent informal experience has not confirmed this benefit.[154,276]

GABAergics

Zolpidem, a commonly prescribed bedtime sedative, has been reported to ameliorate overall parkinsonian scores and some eye movement problems in PSP,[277] but the benefit lasts only a few hours at best and has not been confirmed. Sedation is common.

Antiglutamatergics

Riluzole, as an antiglutamatergic that modestly prolongs survival in amyotrophic lateral sclerosis and offers multiple other mechanisms of action that in theory could do the same for PSP. However, in a 44-center double-blind trial of 362 patients followed for approximately 3 years, the drug failed to provide benefit in slowing clinical progression or delaying death.[278]

Adrenergics

Idazoxan, a nonselective drug with a predominantly alpha-2 antagonistic action, gave favorable results in one controlled trial in PSP.[279] This was refuted, however, by observations that the adverse effects of that drug make a truly blinded trial difficult and by the negative results in a large trial of efaroxan, a more selective alpha-2 antagonist.[280]

Botulinum Toxin

Blepharospasm in PSP responds well to botulinum A injections.[281] Even "apraxia" of lid opening may respond to botulinum A.[282] Torticollis or retrocollis in PSP may also respond, but the occasional occurrence of mild dysphagia after botulinum injection for idiopathic spasmodic torticollis dictates caution in the case of PSP, where slight exacerbation of dysphagia could allow aspiration. Botulinum toxin may also be useful in focal dystonia of PSP.[283]

Coenzyme Q-10

Coenzyme Q-10 is a component of mitochondrial complex I that is available as a nutritional supplement. It has shown modest success in a small trial[284] in PSP, improving the PSP Rating Scale score by 1.6 points relative to placebo ($p = 0.008$), approximately 3.5% of the baseline score. The drug was administered as a highly bioavailable nanoparticulate emulsion at 5 mg/kg/day over 6 weeks. Magnetic resonance spectroscopic measures of basal ganglia energy metabolism improved modestly as well. A larger trial is being organized.

NONPHARMACOLOGIC THERAPY

Gaze and Lid Pareses

Blepharospasm or lid levator inhibition may be overcome if a family member presents a finger-counting task. Some patients can overcome the voluntary downgaze palsy that impairs eating by using their remaining pursuit downgaze ability to follow the fork down to the plate. If downgaze palsy or inattention to the lower half of space is present, low-lying objects such as children's toys, loose rugs, and coffee tables should be removed from the patient's path. While prisms are not usually useful in correcting the patient's inability to attend to the lower half of space, they may help diplopia related to dysconjugate gaze.

The chronic conjunctivitis and reactive lacrimation caused by the low blink rate may be treated by instillation of methyl-cellulose or polyvinyl alcohol drops when awake, and a petrolatum-based ointment or mineral oil at bedtime.

PHYSICAL, SPEECH, AND SWALLOWING THERAPY

Physical therapy seems to be of little or no benefit against the postural instability of PSP, but instruction for the family in the physical care of the poorly ambulatory patient may be useful, and regular exercise has a clear psychological benefit.[285] Similarly, speech therapy has proved of little benefit in most patients, but the speech pathologist may be able to arrange adjunctive means of communication such as electronic typing devices or simple pointing boards.

Dysphagia in PSP is also unlikely to respond to therapy. However, the family may be instructed in the preparation of foods of proper consistency, using a blender or cornstarch-based thickeners as necessary. A barium swallow radiograph using boluses of varying consistency will guide this advice. The speech pathologist can teach the patient safer swallowing techniques and can monitor the patient for the need for a feeding gastrostomy. The high morbidity and mortality related to aspiration in advanced PSP has led the author to recommend endoscopic placement of a feeding gastrostomy after the first episode of aspiration pneumonitis, if the patient requires more time to finish a meal than the family can practically provide, if there is significant weight loss because of reduced intake, or if a minor degree of aspiration occurs with every mouthful (K Kluin, personal communication).

SURGICAL IMPLANTS

Fetal or porcine nigral cell striatal allografts have not been attempted in PSP, but the advanced state of degeneration of centers downstream from the striatum, contrasting with the situation in PD, suggests that such procedure is unlikely to be of benefit. This prediction is supported by the unfavorable results of a trial of adrenal medullary tissue autografts to striatum.[286]

A similar rationale predicts that deep brain stimulation would not help PSP. PD, a condition in which the subthalamic nucleus and GPi do not degenerate, responds to stimulation of those areas, possibly via suppression of disinhibited activity there. In PSP, however, both areas are among the most severely affected by the degenerative process, and reduction in activity there could be expected only to exacerbate the functional abnormality.

Interest in stimulation of the PPN in PSP has recently arisen.[287] Very small, preliminary trials of the procedure for PD with drug-refractory gait difficulty have been modestly favorable. This suggests a similar approach for PSP, where the PPN partly degenerates. Early trials are in progress.

ELECTROCONVULSIVE THERAPY (ECT)

Two personal cases and one from the literature[288] have markedly worsened with ECT with regard to both motor and cognitive functioning. All 3 patients improved nearly to baseline over subsequent weeks. Another trial gave results that were mixed at best.[289] This contrasts with the benefit of ECT in PD.[290]

▶ PATIENT RESOURCES

CurePSP (the Society for Progressive Supranuclear Palsy) is headquartered in Maryland and serves North America. The Progressive Supranuclear Palsy Association is based in the UK and serves all of Europe. Smaller organizations have recently been founded in other countries. These patient service and advocacy organizations offer support meetings and lay-language literature. The two listed below also offer research funding to scientists in all countries. Just as important as these formal activities is these organizations' message to patients that having an "orphan disease" does not mean neglect by the medical world.

REFERENCES

1. Richardson JC, Steele J, Olszewski J. Supranuclear ophthalmoplegia, pseudobulbar palsy, nuchal dystonia and dementia: A clinical report on eight cases of "heterogeneous system degeneration." Trans Am Neurol Assoc 1963;88: 25–29.
2. Olszewski J, Steele J, Richardson JC. Pathological report on six cases of heterogeneous system degeneration. J Neuropathol Exp Neurol 1963;23:187–188.
3. Steele JC, Richardson JC, Olszewski J. PSP: A heterogeneous degeneration involving the brain stem, basal ganglia and cerebellum, with vertical gaze and pseudobulbar palsy, nuchal dystonia and dementia. Arch Neurol 1964;10:333–359.
4. Golbe LI, Davis PH, Schoenberg BS, et al. Prevalence and natural history of PSP. Neurology 1988;38:1031–1034.
5. Maher ER, Lees AJ. The clinical features and natural history of the Steele-Richardson-Olszewski syndrome (PSP). Neurology 1986;36:1005–1008.
6. Nath U, Ben-Shlomo Y, Thomson RG, et al. Clinical features and natural history of PSP: A clinical cohort study. Neurology 2003;60:910–916.
7. Hoehn MM, Yahr MD. Parkinsonism: Onset, progression, and mortality. Neurology 1967;17:427–442.
8. Duvoisin RC. Clinical diagnosis. In Litvan I, Agid Y (eds). PSP: Clinical and Research Approaches. New York: Oxford University Press, 1992, pp. 15–33.

9. Birdi S, Rajput AH, Fenton M, et al. PSP diagnosis and confounding features: Report on 16 autopsied cases. Mov Disord 2002;17:1255–1267.
10. Tanigawa A, Komiyama A, Hasegawa O. Truncal muscle tonus in PSP. J Neurol Neurosurg Psychiatry 1998;64:190–196.
11. Golbe LI, Ohman-Strickland PA. A clinical disability rating scale for PSP. Brain 2007;130:1552–1565.
12. Litvan I, Campbell G, Mangone CA, et al. Which clinical features differentiate PSP from related disorders? A clinicopathological study. Brain 1997;120:65–74.
13. Wenning GK, Ebersbach G, Verny M, et al. Progression of falls in postmortem-confirmed parkinsonian disorders. Mov Disord 1999;14:947–950.
14. Leigh RJ, Riley DE. Eye movements in parkinsonism: It's saccadic speed that counts. Neurology 2000;54:1018–1019.
15. Rivaud-Péchoux S, Vidailhet M, Gallouedec G, et al. Longitudinal ocular motor study in corticobasal degeneration and PSP. Neurology 2000;54:1029–1032.
16. Milberg W, Albert M. Cognitive differences between patients with PSP and Alzheimer's disease. J Clin Exp Neuropsychol 1989;11:605–611.
17. Rivest J, Quinn N, Marsden CD. Dystonia in Parkinson's disease, multiple system atrophy, and PSP. Neurology 1990;40:1571–1578.
18. Gibb WRG, Luthert PJ, Marsden CD. Corticobasal degeneration. Brain 1989;112:1171–1192.
19. Collins SJ, Ahlskog JE, Parisi JE, et al. PSP: Neuropathologically based diagnostic clinical criteria. J Neurol Neurosurg Psychiatry 1995;58:167–173.
20. Colosimo C, Albanese A, Hughes AJ, et al. Some specific clinical features differentiate multiple system atrophy (striatonigral variety) from Parkinson's disease. Arch Neurol 1995;52:294–298.
21. Morris HR, Gibb G, Katzenschlager R, et al. Pathological, clinical and genetic heterogeneity in PSP. Brain 2002;125:969–975.
22. Williams DR, de Silva R, Paviour DC, et al. Characteristics of two distinct clinical phenotypes in pathologically proven PSP: Richardson's syndrome and PSP-parkinsonism. Brain 2005;128:1247–1258.
23. O'Sullivan SS, Massey LA, Williams DR, et al. Clinical outcomes of PSP and multiple system atrophy. Brain 2008;131:1362–1372.
24. Williams DR, Holton JL, Strand K, et al. Pure akinesia with gait freezing: A third clinical phenotype of PSP. Mov Disord 2007;22:2235–2241.
25. Litvan I, Agid Y, Calne D, et al. Clinical research criteria for the diagnosis of PSP: Report of the NINDS-SPSP International Workshop. Neurology 1996;47:1–9.
26. Robbins TW, James M, Owen AM, et al. Cognitive deficits in PSP, Parkinson's disease, and multiple system atrophy in tests sensitive to frontal lobe dysfunction. J Neurol Neurosurg Psychiatry 1994;57:79–88.
27. Will RG, Lees AJ, Gibb W, et al. A case of progressive subcortical gliosis presenting clinically as Steele-Richardson-Olszewski syndrome. J Neurol Neurosurg Psychiatry 1988;51:1224–1227.
28. Bertoni JN, Label LS, Sackellares C, et al. Supranuclear gaze palsy in familial Creutzfeldt-Jakob disease. Arch Neurol 1983;40:618–622.
29. Fearnley JM, Revesz T, Brooks DJ, et al. Diffuse Lewy body disease presenting with a supranuclear gaze palsy. J Neurol Neurosurg Psychiatry 1991;54:159–161.
30. Pahwa R, Koller WC, Stern MB. Primary pallidal atrophy. In Stern MB, Koller WC (eds). Parkinsonian Syndromes. New York: Marcel Dekker, 1993, pp. 433–440.
31. Truong DD, Harding AE, Scaravilli F, et al. Movement disorders in mitochondrial myopathies: A study of nine cases with two autopsy studies. Mov Disord 1990;5:109–117.
32. Curran T, Lang AE. Parkinsonian syndromes associated with hydrocephalus: Case reports, a review of the literature, and pathophysiological hypotheses. Mov Disord 1994;9:508–520.
33. Tanner CM, Goetz CG, Klawans HL. Multi-infarct PSP. Neurology 1987;37:1819.
34. Winikates J, Jankovic J. Vascular PSP. J Neural Transm Suppl 1994;42:189–201.
35. Dubinsky RM, Jankovic J. PSP and a multi-infarct state. Neurology 1987;37:570–576.
36. Burn DJ, Sawle GV, Brooks DJ. Differential diagnosis of Parkinson's disease, multiple system atrophy, and Steele-Richardson-Olszewski syndrome: Discriminant analysis of striatal ^{18}F-dopa PET data. J Neurol Neurosurg Psychiatry 1994;57:278–284.
37. Foster NL, Gilman S, Berent S, et al. Cerebral hypometabolism in PSP studied with PET. Ann Neurol 1988;24:399–406.
38. D'Antona R, Baron JC, Samson Y, et al. Subcortical dementia: Frontal cortex hypometabolism detected by PET in patients with PSP. Brain 1985;108:785–799.
39. Nagahama Y, Fukuyama H, Turjanski N, et al. Cerebral glucose metabolism in corticobasal degeneration: Comparison with PSP and normal controls. Mov Disord 1997;12:691–696.
40. Ilgin N, Zubieta J, Reich SG, et al. PET imaging of the dopamine transporter in PSP and PD. Neurology 1999;52:1221–1226.
41. Piccini P, Lees AJ, de Yébenes JG, et al. ^{18}F-dopa and ^{18}FDG studies in 3 kindreds with familial PSP. Neurology 1998;50:A429.
42. Schonfeld SM, Golbe LI, Safer J, et al. Computed tomographic findings in PSP: Correlation with clinical grade. Mov Disord 1987;2:263–278.
43. Drayer BP, Olanow W, Burger P, et al. Parkinson plus syndrome: Diagnosis using high field MR imaging of brain iron. Radiology 1986;159:493–498.
44. Savoiardo M, Strada L, Girotti F, et al. MR imaging in PSP and Shy-Drager syndrome. J Comput Assist Tomogr 1989;13:555–560.
45. Saitoh H, Yoshii F, Shinohara Y. Computed tomographic findings in PSP. Neuroradiology 1987;29:168–171.
46. Yuki N, Sato S, Yuasa T, et al. Computed tomographic findings of PSP compared with Parkinson's disease. Jpn J Med 1990;29:506–511.
47. Stern MB, Braffman BH, Skolnick BE, et al. Magnetic resonance imaging in Parkinson's disease and parkinsonian syndromes. Neurology 1989;39:1524–1526.
48. Schrag A, Good CD, Miszkiel K, et al. Differentiation of atypical parkinsonian syndromes with routine MRI. Neurology 2000;54:697–702.
49. Wenning GK, Ebersbach G, Verny M, et al. Progression of falls in postmortem-confirmed parkinsonian disorders. Mov Disord 1999;14:947–950.

50. Timmons JH, Bonikowski FW, Harshorne MF. Iodoamphetamine-123 brain imaging demonstrating cortical deactivation in a patient with PSP. Clin Nucl Med 1989;14:841–842.
51. Habert MO, Spampinato U, Mas JL, et al. A comparative technetium 99m hexamethylpropylene amine oxime SPECT study in different types of dementia. Eur J Nucl Med 1991;18:3–11.
52. Neary D, Snowdon JS, Shields RA, et al. Single photon emission tomography using[99] mTc-HM-PAO in the investigation of dementia. J Neurol Neurosurg Psychiatry 1987;50:1101–1109.
53. van Royen E, Verhoeff NF, Speelman JD, et al. Multiple system atrophy and PSP: Diminished striatal D2 dopamine receptor activity demonstrated by[123] I-IBZM single photon emission computed tomography. Arch Neurol 1993;50:513–516.
54. Schwarz J, Tatsch K, Arnold G, et al.[123] I-Iodobenzamide-SPECT predicts dopaminergic responsiveness in patients with de novo parkinsonism. Neurology 1992;42: 556–561.
55. Davie CA, Barker GJ, Machado C, et al. Proton magnetic resonance spectroscopy in Steele-Richardson-Olszewski syndrome. Mov Disord 1997;12:767–771.
56. Abe K, Terakawa H, Takanashi M, et al. Proton magnetic resonance spectroscopy of patients with parkinsonism. Brain Res Bull 2000;52:589–595.
57. Paviour DC, Thornton JS, Lees AJ, et al. Diffusion-weighted magnetic resonance imaging differentiates Parkinsonian variant of multiple-system atrophy from PSP. Mov Disord 2007;22:68–74.
58. Walter U, Dressler D, Probst T, et al. Transcranial brain sonography findings in discriminating between parkinsonism and idiopathic Parkinson disease. Arch Neurol 2007;64:1635–1640.
59. Clarke CE, Lowry M. Systematic review of proton magnetic resonance spectroscopy of the striatum in parkinsonian syndromes. Eur J Neurol 2001;8:573–577.
60. Padovani A, Borroni B, Brambati SM, et al. Diffusion tensor imaging and voxel based morphometry study in early PSP. J Neurol Neurosurg Psychiat 2006;77:457–463.
61. Urakami K, Mori M, Wada K, et al. A comparison of tau protein in CSF between CBD and PSP. Neurosci Lett 259: 1999;127–129.
62. Arai H, Morikawa Y, Higuchi M, et al. Cerebrospinal fluid tau levels in neurodegenerative diseases with distinct tau-related pathology. Biochem Biophys Res Commun 1997;236:262–264.
63. Holmberg B, Rosengren L, Karlsson J-E, et al. Increased cerebrospinal fluid levels of neurofilament protein in PSP and MSA compared with PD. Mov Disord 1998;13:70–77.
64. Borroni B, Malinverno M, Gardoni F, et al. Tau forms in CSF as a reliable biomarker for PSP. Neurology 2008;71:1796–1803.
65. Jellinger K, Riederer P, Tomonaga M. PSP: Clinicopathological and biochemical studies. J Neural Transm Suppl 1980;16:111–128.
66. Kish SJ, Chang LJ, Mirchandani L, et al. PSP: Relationship between extrapyramidal disturbances, dementia and brain neurotransmitter markers. Ann Neurol 1985;18: 530–536.
67. Ruberg M, Javoy-Agid F, Hirsch E, et al. Dopaminergic and cholinergic lesions in PSP. Ann Neurol 1985;18:523–529.
68. Young AB. PSP: Postmortem chemical analysis. Neurology 1985;18:521–522.
69. Levy R, Ruberg M, Herrero MT, et al. Alterations of GABAergic neurons in the basal ganglia of patients with PSP: An in situ hybridization study of GAD_{67} messenger RNA. Neurology 1995;45:127–134.
70. Landwehrmeyer B, Palacios JM. Neurotransmitter receptors in PSP. J Neural Transm Suppl 1994;42:229–246.
71. Pascual J, Berciano J, Gonzalez AM, et al. Autoradiographic demonstration of loss of alpha-2-adrenoceptors in PSP: Preliminary report. J Neurol Sci 1993;114:165–169.
72. Hauw J-J, Daniel SE, Dickson D, et al. Preliminary NINDS neuropathologic criteria for Steele-Richardson-Olszewski syndrome (PSP). Neurology 1994;44:2015–2019.
73. Ishino H, Otsuki S. Frequency of Alzheimer's neurofibrillary tangles in the cerebral cortex in PSP. J Neurol Sci 1976;28:309–316.
74. Powell HC, London GW, Lampert PW. Neurofibrillary tangles in PSP. J Neuropathol Exp Neurol 1974;33:98–106.
75. Tellez-Nagel I, Wisniewski HM. Ultrastructure of neurofibrillary tangles in Steele-Richardson-Olszewski syndrome. Arch Neurol 1973;29:324–327.
76. Tomonaga M. Ultrastructure of neurofibrillary tangles in PSP. Acta Neuropathol (Berl) 1977;37:1771–1781.
77. Montpetit V, Clapin DR, Guberman A. Substructure of 20 nm filaments of PSP. Acta Neuropathol 1985;68:311–318.
78. Dickson DW, Kress Y, Crowe A, et al. Monoclonal antibodies to Alzheimer neurofibrillary tangles (ANT): 2. Demonstration of a common antigenic determinant between ANT and neurofibrillary degeneration in PSP. Am J Pathol 1985;120:292–303.
79. Ghatak NR, Nochlin D, Hadfield MG. Neurofibrillary pathology in PSP. Acta Neuropathol (Berl) 1980;52:73–76.
80. Ikeda K, Akiyama H, Haga C, et al. Argyrophilic thread-like structure in corticobasal degeneration and supranuclear palsy. Neurosci Lett 1994;174:157–159.
81. Mori H, Nishimura M, Namba Y, et al. Corticobasal degeneration: A disease with widespread appearance of abnormal tau and neurofibrillary tangles, and its relation to PSP. Acta Neuropathol 1994;88:113–121.
82. Wakabayashi K, Oyanagi K, Makifuchi T, et al. Corticobasal degeneration: Etiopathological significance of the cytoskeletal alterations. Acta Neuropathol 1994;87:545–553.
83. Oyanagi K, Tsuchiya K, Yamazaki M, et al. Substantia nigra in PSP, corticobasal degeneration and parkinsonism-dementia complex of Guam: Specific pathological features. J Neuropathol Exp Neurol 2001;60:393–402.
84. Williams DR, Holton JL, Strand C, et al. Pathological tau burden and distribution distinguishes PSP-parkinsonism from Richardson's syndrome. Brain 2007;130:1566–1576.
85. Jellinger KA. Different tau pathology pattern in two clinical phenotypes of PSP. Neurodegener Dis 2008;5: 339–346.
86. Pollock NJ, Mirra SS, Binder LI, et al. Filamentous aggregates in Pick's disease, PSP, and Alzheimer's disease share antigenic determinants with microtubule-associated protein, tau. Lancet 1986;ii:1211.
87. Love S, Saitoh T, Quijada S, et al. Alz-50, ubiquitin and tau immunoreactivity of neurofibrillary tangles, Pick

bodies and Lewy bodies. J Neuropathol Exp Neurol 1988;47:393–405.

88. Tabaton M, Whitehouse PJ, Perry G, et al. Alz 50 recognized abnormal filaments in Alzheimer's disease and PSP. Ann Neurol 1988;24:407–413.

89. Yamada T, Calne DB, Akiyama H, et al. Further observations on tau-positive glia in the brains with PSP. Acta Neuropathol 1993;85:308–315.

90. Schmidt ML, Huang R, Martin J A, et al. Neurofibrillary tangles in PSP contain the same tau epitopes identified in Alzheimer's disease PHFtau. J Neuropathol Exp Neurol 1996;55:534–539.

91. Flament S, Delacourte A, Verny M, et al. Abnormal tau proteins in PSP. Acta Neuropathol (Berl) 1991;81: 591–596.

92. Vermersch P, Robitaille Y, Bernier L, et al. Biochemical mapping of neurofibrillary degeneration in a case of PSP: Evidence for general cortical involvement. Acta Neuropathol 1994;87:572–577.

93. Probst A, Langui D, Lautenschlager C, et al. PSP: Extensive neuropil threads in addition to neurofibrillary tangles. Acta Neuropathol (Berl) 1988;77:61–68.

94. Nelson SJ, Yen S-H, Davies P, et al. Basal ganglia neuropil threads in PSP. J Neuropathol Exp Neurol 1989;48:324.

95. Iwatsubo T, Hasegawa M, Ihara Y. Neuronal and glial tau-positive inclusions in diverse neurologic diseases share common phosphorylation characteristics. Acta Neuropathol (Berl) 1994;88:129–136.

96. Lennox G, Lowe J, Morrell K, et al. Ubiquitin is a component of neurofibrillary tangles in a variety of neurodegenerative diseases. Neurosci Lett 1988;94:211–217.

97. Lewis J, McGowan E, Rockwood J, et al. Neurofibrillary tangles, amyotrophy and progressive motor disturbance in mice expressing mutant (P301L) tau protein. Nat Genet 2000;25:402–405.

98. Wittmann CW, Wszolek MF, Shulman JM, et al. Tauopathy in Drosophila: Neurodegeneration without neurofibrillary tangles. Science 2001;293:711–714.

99. Bai Q, Garver JA, Hukriede NA, et al. Generation of a transgenic zebrafish model of Tauopathy using a novel promoter element derived from the zebrafish eno2 gene. Nucleic Acids Res 2007;35:6501–6516.

100. Lewis J, Dickson KW, Lin W-L, et al. Enhanced neurofibrillary degeneration in transgenic mice expressing mutant tau and APP. Science 2001;293:1487–1491.

101. Arai N. "Grumose degeneration" of the dentate nucleus: A light and electron microscopic study in PSP and dentatorubropallidoluysian atrophy. J Neurol Sci 1987;90:131–145.

102. Giaccone G, Tagliavini F, Street JS, et al. PSP with hypertrophy of the olives: An immunohistochemical study of artyrophilic neurons. Acta Neuropathol (Berl) 1988;77:14–20.

103. Gearing M, Olson DA, Watts RL, et al. PSP: Neuropathologic and clinical heterogeneity. Neurology 1994;44: 1015–1024.

104. Ishizawa K, Dickson DW. Microglial activation parallels system degeneration in PSP and corticobasal degeneration. J Neuropathol Exp Neurol 2001;60:647–657.

105. Gerhard A, Trender-Gerhard I, Turkheimer F, et al. In vivo imaging of microglial activation with [11C](R)-PK11195 PET in PSP. Mov Disord 2006;21:89–93.

106. Cordato NJ, Halliday GM, Harding AJ, et al. Regional brain atrophy in PSP and Lewy body disease. Ann Neurol 2000;47:718–728.

107. Hauw J-J, Verny M, Delaere P, et al. Constant neurofibrillary changes in the neocortex in PSP. Basic differences with Alzheimer's disease and aging. Neurosci Lett 1990;119:182–186.

108. Hof PR, Delacourte A, Bouras C. Distribution of cortical neurofibrillary tangles in PSP: A quantitative analysis of six cases. Acta Neuropathol (Berl) 1992;84:45–51.

109. Braak H, Jellinger K, Braak E, et al. Allocortical neurofibrillary changes in PSP. Acta Neuropathol 1992;84:478–483.

110. Verny M, Duyckaerts C, Delaére P, et al. Cortical tangles in PSP. J Neural Transm Suppl 1994;42:179–188.

111. Jellinger KA, Bancher C. Neuropathology. In Litvan I, Agid Y (eds). PSP: Clinical and Research Approaches. New York: Oxford University Press, 1992, pp. 44–88.

112. Bergeron C, Pollanen MS, Weyer L, et al. Cortical degeneration in PSP: A comparison with cortical-basal ganglionic degeneration. J Neuropathol Exp Neurol 1997;56:726–734.

113. Jankovic J, Van der Linden C. PSP. In Chokroverty S (ed). Movement Disorders. New York: PMA Publishing, 1990, pp. 267–286.

114. D'Antona R, Baron JC, Sanson Y, et al. Subcortical dementia: Frontal cortex hypometabolism detected by positron tomography in patients with PSP. Brain 1985;108:785–799.

115. Foster NL, Gilman S, Berent S, et al. Cerebral hypometabolism in PSP studied with positron emission tomography. Ann Neurol 1988;24:399–406.

116. Leenders KL, Frackowiak RSJ, Lees AJ. Steele-Richardson-Olszewski syndrome: Brain energy metabolism, blood flow and fluorodopa uptake measured by positron emission tomography. Brain 1988;111:615–630.

117. Goffinet AM, De Volder AG, Guillain C, et al. Positron tomography demonstrates frontal lobe hypometabolism in PSP. Ann Neurol 1989;25:131–139.

118. Tagliavini F, Pilleri G, Bouras C, et al. The basal nucleus of Meynert in patients with PSP. Neurosci Lett 1984;44: 37–42.

119. Zweig RM, Whitehouse PJ, Casanova MF, et al. Loss of pedunculopontine neurons in PSP. Ann Neurol 1987;22:18–25.

120. Jellinger K. The pedunculopontine nucleus in Parkinson's disease, PSP and Alzheimer's disease. J Neurol Neurosurg Psychiatry 1988;52:540–543.

121. Perry RH, Tomlinson BE, Candy JM, et al. Cortical cholinergic deficit in mentally impaired parkinsonian patients. Lancet ii: 1983;789–790.

122. Yamauchi H, Fukuyama H, Nagahama Y, et al. Atrophy of the corpus callosum, cognitive impairment, and cortical hypometabolism in PSP. Ann Neurol 1997;41:606–614.

123. Montplaisir J, Petit D, Decary A, et al. Sleep and quantitative EEG in patients with PSP. Neurology 1997;49:999–1003.

124. Agid Y, Graybiel AM, Ruberg M, et al. The efficacy of levodopa treatment declines in the course of Parkinson disease: Do nondopaminergic lesions play a role? Adv Neurol 1990;53:83–100.

125. Soliveri P, Monza D, Paridi D, et al. Neuropsychological follow up in patients with PD, SND-type MSA, and PSP. J Neurol Neurosurg Psychiatry 2000;69:313–318.

126. Johnson R, Litvan I, Grafman J. PSP: Altered sensory processing leads to degraded cognition. Neurology 1991;41:1257–1262.
127. Kertzman C, Robinson DL, Litvan I. Effects of physostigmine on spatial attention in patients with PSP. Arch Neurol 1990;47:1346–1350.
128. Dubois B, Pillon B, Legault F, et al. Slowing of cognitive processing in PSP. Arch Neurol 1988;45:1194–1199.
129. Pillon B, Gouider-Khouja N, Deweer B, et al. Neuropsychological pattern of striatonigral degeneration: Comparison with Parkinson's disease and PSP. J Neurol Neurosurg Psychiatry 1995;58:174–179.
130. Grafman J, Litvan I, Gomez C, et al. Frontal lobe function in PSP. Arch Neurol 1990;47:553–558.
131. Podoll K, Schwarz M, Noth J. Language functions in PSP. Brain 1991;114:1457–1472.
132. Rosser A, Hodges JR. Initial letter and semantic category fluency in Alzheimer's disease, Huntington's disease, and PSP. J Neurol Neurosurg Psychiatry 1994;57:1389–1394.
133. Litvan I, Mega MS, Cummings JL, et al. Neuropsychiatric aspects of PSP. Neurology 1996;47:1184–1189.
134. Cambier J, Masson M, Viader F, et al. Le syndrome frontal de paralysie supranucleaire progressive. Rev Neurol (Paris) 1985;141:528–536.
135. Barclay CL, Bergeron C, Lang AE. Arm levitation in PSP. Neurology 1999;52:879–882.
136. Leiguarda RC, Pramstaller PP, Merello M, et al. Apraxia in PD, PSP, MSA and neuroleptic-induced parkinsonism. Brain 1997;120:75–90.
137. Agid Y, Javoy-Agid F, Ruberg M, et al. PSP: Anatomoclinical and biochemical considerations. Adv Neurol 1987;45:191–206.
138. Pillon B, Dubois B. Cognitive and behavioral impairments. In Litvan I, Agid Y (eds). PSP: Clinical and Research Approaches. New York: Oxford University Press, 1992, pp. 223–239.
139. Pillon B, Deweer B, Michon A, et al. Are explicit memory disorders of PSP related to damage to striatofrontal circuits? Comparison with Alzheimer's, Parkinson's and Huntington's diseases. Neurology 1994;44:1264–1270.
140. Fearnley JM, Lees AJ. Ageing and Parkinson's disease: Substantia nigra regional selectivity. Brain 1991;114:2283–2301.
141. Brooks DJ, Ibanez V, Sawle GV, et al. Differing patterns of striatal ^{18}F-dopa uptake in Parkinson's disease, multiple system atrophy, and PSP. Ann Neurol 1990;28:547–555.
142. Villares J, Strada O, Faucheux B, et al. Loss of striatal high affinity NGF binding sites in PSP but not in Parkinson's disease. Neurosci Lett 1994;182:59–62.
143. Oyanaki K, Takahashi H, Wakabayashi K, et al. Large neurons in the neostriatum in Alzheimer's disease and PSP: A topographic, histologic and ultrastructural investigation. Brain Res 1991;544:221–226.
144. Litvan I, Gomez C, Atack JR, et al. Physostigmine treatment of PSP. Ann Neurol 1989;26:404–407.
145. Baron JC, Mazière B, Loc'h C, et al. Loss of striatal [^{76}Br] bromospiperone binding sites demonstrated by positron emission tomography in PSP. J Cereb Blood Flow Metab 1986;6:131–136.
146. Brooks DJ, Ibanez V, Sawle GV, et al. Striatal D_2 receptor status in patients with Parkinson's disease, striatonigral degeneration, and PSP, measured with[11] C-raclopride and positron emission tomography. Ann Neurol 1992;31:184–192.
147. Matsuo H, Takashima H, Kishikawa M, et al. Pure akinesia: An atypical manifestation of PSP. J Neurol Neurosurg Psychiatry 1991;54:397.
148. Imai H, Nakamura T, Kondo T, et al. Dopa-unresponsive pure akinesia or freezing: A condition with a wide spectrum of PSP? Adv Neurol 1993;60:622–625.
149. Mizusawa H, Mochizuki A, Ohkoshi N, et al. PSP presenting with pure akinesia. Adv Neurol 1993;60:618–621.
150. Riley DE, Fogt N, Leigh RJ. The syndrome of "pure akinesia" and its relationship to PSP. Neurology 1994;44:1025–1029.
151. Masucci EF, Kurtzke JF. Tremor in PSP. Acta Neurol Scand 1989;80:296–300.
152. Jankovic J, Van der Linden C. PSP (Steele-Richardson-Olszewski syndrome). In Chokroverty S (ed). Movement Disorders. New York: PMA Publishing, 1990, pp 267–286.
153. Hardman CD, Halliday GM. The external globus pallidus in patients with PD and PSP. Mov Disord 1999;14:626–633.
154. Nieforth KA, Golbe LI. Retrospective study of drug response in 87 patients with PSP. Clin Neuropharmacol 1993;16:338–346.
155. Moriizumi T, Hattori T. Separate neuronal populations of the rat globus pallidus projecting to the subthalamic nucleus, auditory cortex and pedunculopontine tegmental area. Neuroscience 1992;46:701–710.
156. Masdeu JC, Alampur U, Cavaliere R, et al. Astasia and gait failure with damage of the pontomesencephalic locomotor region. Ann Neurol 1994;35:619–621.
157. Weinberger M, Hamani C, Hutchison WD, et al. Pedunculopontine nucleus microelectrode recordings in movement disorder patients. Exp Brain Res 2008;188:165–174.
158. Henderson JM, Carpenter K, Cartwright H, et al. Loss of thalamic intralaminar nuclei in PSP and PD: Clinical and therapeutic implications. Brain 2000;123:1410–1421.
159. Shinotoh H, Namba H, Yamaguchi M, et al. PET measurement of acetylcholinesterase activity reveals differential loss of ascending cholinergic systems in PD and PSP. Ann Neurol 1999;46:62–69.
160. Carpenter MB, Harbison JW, Peter P. Accessory oculomotor nuclei in the monkey: Projections and effects of discrete lesions. J Comp Neurol 1970;140:131–147.
161. Fukushima-Kudo J, Fukushima K, Tahiro K. Rigidity and dorsiflexion of the neck in PSP and the interstitial nucleus of Cajal. J Neurol Neurosurg Psychiatry 1987;50:1197–1203.
162. Lees AJ. The Steele-Richardson-Olszewski syndrome (PSP). Mov Disord 1987;2:272–287.
163. Juncos JL, Hirsch EC, Malessa S, et al. Mesencephalic cholinergic nuclei in PSP. Neurology 1991;41:25–30.
164. Davis PH, Bergeron C, McLachlan DR. Atypical presentation of PSP. Ann Neurol 1985;17:337–343.
165. Dubas F, Gray F, Escourolle R. Maladie de steele-Richardson-Olszewski sans ophthalmoplégie: 6 cas anatomo-cliniques. Rev Neurol (Paris) 1992;139:407–416.
166. Nuwer MR. PSP despite normal eye movements. Arch Neurol 1981;38:784.
167. Kida E, Barcikowska M, Niemszewska M. Immunohistochemical study of a case with PSP without ophthalmoplegia. Acta Neuropathol 1992;83:328–332.
168. Saver, Liu GT, Charness ME. Idiopathic striopallidodentate calcification with prominent supranuclear abnormality of eye movement. J Neuroophthalmol 1994;14:29–33.

169. Halliday GM, Hardman CD, Cordato NJ, et al. A role for the substantia nigra pars reticulata in the gaze palsy of PSP. Brain 2000;123:724–732.
170. Malessa S, Gaymard B, Rivaud S, et al. Role of pontine nuclei damage in smooth pursuit impairment of PSP: A clinical-pathologic study. Neurology 1994;44:716–721.
171. Pfaffenbach DD, Layton DD, Kearns TP. Ocular manifestations in PSP. Am J Ophthalmol 1972;74:1179–1184.
172. Chu FC, Reingold DB, Cogan DG, et al. The eye movement disorders of PSP. Ophthalmology 1979;86:422–428.
173. Troost BT, Daroff RB. The ocular motor defects in PSP. Ann Neurol 1977;2:397–403.
174. Rascol O, Sabatini U, Simonetta-Moreau M, et al. Square wave jerks in parkinsonian syndromes. J Neurol Neurosurg Psychiatry 1991;54:599–602.
175. Pierrot-Deseilligny C, Rivaud S, Pillon B, et al. Lateral visually-guided saccades in PSP. Brain 1989;112:471–487.
176. Rafal RD, Posner MI, Friedman JH, et al. Orienting of visual attention in PSP. Brain 1988;111:267–280.
177. Rascol OJ, Clanet M, Senard JM, et al. Vestibulo-ocular reflex in Parkinson's disease and multiple system atrophy. Adv Neurol 1993;60:395–397.
178. Lepore FE, Duvoisin RC. "Apraxia" of eyelid opening: An involuntary levator inhibition. Neurology 1985;35:423–427.
179. Dehaene I. Apraxia of eyelid opening in PSP. Neurology 1984;15:115–116.
180. Jankovic J. Apraxia of eyelid opening in PSP: Reply. Neurology 1984;15:116.
181. Golbe LI, Davis PH, Lepore FE. Eyelid movement abnormalities in PSP. Mov Disord 1989;4:297–302.
182. Valls-Solé J, Valldeoriola F, Tolosa E, et al. Distinctive abnormalities of facial reflexes in patients with PSP. Brain 1997;120:1877–1883.
183. Bologna M, Agostino R, Gregori B, et al. Voluntary, spontaneous and reflex blinking in patients with clinically probable PSP. Brain 2008.
184. Aldrich MS, Foster NL, White RF, et al. Sleep abnormalities in PSP. Ann Neurol 1989;25:577–581.
185. Leygonie F, Thomas J, Degos JD, et al. Troubles du sommeil dans la maladie de Steele-Richardson: Étude polygraphique de 3 cas. Rev Neurol (Paris) 1976;132: 125–136.
186. Vidailhet M, Rothwell JC, Thompson PD, et al. The auditory startle response in the Steele-Richardson-Olszewski syndrome and Parkinson's disease. Brain 1992;115: 1181–1192.
187. Tolosa ES, Zeese JA. Brainstem auditory evoked responses in PSP. Ann Neurol 1979;6:369.
188. De Bruin VMS, Lees AJ. Subcortical neurofibrillary degeneration presenting as Steele-Richardson-Olszewski and other related syndromes. A review of 90 pathologically verified cases. Mov Disord 1994;9:381–389.
189. Kluin KJ, Foster NL, Berent S, et al. Perceptual analysis of speech disorders in PSP. Neurology 1993;43:563–566.
190. Litvan I, Sastry N, Sonies BC. Characterizing swallowing abnormalities in PSP. Neurology 1997;48:1654–1662.
191. Leopold NA, Kagel MC. Dysphagia in PSP: Radiologic features. Dysphagia 1997;12:140–143.
192. Muller J, Wenning GK, Verny M, et al. Progression of dysarthria and dysphagia in postmortem-confirmed parkinsonian disorders. Arch Neurol 2001;58:259–264.
193. Sonies BC. Swallowing and speech disturbances. In Litvan I, Agid Y (eds). PSP: Clinical and Research Approaches. New York: Oxford University Press, 1992, pp. 240–254.
194. Johnston BT, Castell JA, Stumacher S, et al. Comparison of swallowing function in PD and PSP. Mov Disord 1997;12:322–327.
195. Rafal RD, Grimm RJ. PSP. Functional analysis of the response to methysergide and antiparkinsonian agents. Neurology 1981;31:1507–1518.
196. Gert van Dijk J, Haan J, Koenderink M, et al. Autonomic nervous function of PSP. Arch Neurol 1991;48:1083–1084.
197. Kimber J, Mathias CJ, Lees AJ, et al. Physiological, pharmacological and neurohormonal assessment of autonomic function in PSP. Brain 2000;123:1422–1430.
198. Sakakibara R, Hattori T, Tojo M, et al. Micturitional disturbance in PSP. J Auton Nerv Syst 1993;45:101–106.
199. Rub U, Del Tredici K, Schultz C, et al. PSP: Neuronal and glial cytoskeletal pathology in the higher order processing autonomic nuclei of the lower brainstem. Neuropathol Appl Neurobiol 2002;28:12–22.
200. Vitaliani R, Scaravilli T, Egarter-Vigl E, et al. The pathology of the spinal cord in PSP. J Neuropathol Appl Neurol 2002;61:268–274.
201. Testa D, Monza D, Ferrarini M, et al. Comparison of natural histories of PSP and multiple system atrophy. Neurol Sci 2001;22:247–251.
202. Bower JH, Maraganore DM, McDonnell SK, et al. Incidence of PSP and multiple system atrophy in Olmsted County, Minnesota, 1976 to 1990. Neurology 1997;49:1284–1288.
203. Nath U, Ben-Shlomo Y, Thomson RG, et al. The prevalence of PSP (Steele-Richardson-Olszewski syndrome) in the UK. Brain 2001;124:1438–1449.
204. Schrag A, Ben-Shlomo Y, Quinn N. Prevalence of PSP and MSA: A cross-sectional study. Lancet 1999;354:1771–1772.
205. Rajput AH, Offord KP, Beard CM, et al. Epidemiology of parkinsonism: Incidence, classification, and mortality. Ann Neurol 1984;16:278–282.
206. Kurtzke JF, Kurland LT. Neuroepidemiology: A Summation. In Kurland LT, Kurtzke JF, Goldberg ID (eds). Epidemiology of Neurologic and Sense Organ Disorders. Cambridge: Harvard University Press, 1973, pp. 305–332.
207. Davis PH, Golbe LI, Duvoisin RC, et al. Risk factors for PSP. Neurology 1988;38:1546–1552.
208. Golbe LI, Rubin RS, Cody RP, et al. Follow-up study of risk factors in PSP. Neurology 1996;47:148–154.
209. McCrank E. PSP risk factors. Neurology 1990;40:1637.
210. McCrank E, Rabheru K. Four cases of PSP in patients exposed to organic solvents. Can J Psychiatry 1989;34:934–935.
211. Vanacore N, Bonifati V, Fabbrini G, et al. Smoking habits in multiple system atrophy and PSP. Neurology 2000;54:114–119.
212. Brown P, Gibbs CJ, Rodgers-Johnson P, et al. Human spongi-form encephalopathy: The National Institutes of Health series of 300 cases of experimentally transmitted disease. Ann Neurol 1994;35:513–529.
213. Jendroska K, Hoffmann O, Schelosky L, et al. Absence of disease related prion protein in neurodegenerative disorders presenting with Parkinson's syndrome. J Neurol Neurosurg Psychiatry 1994;57:1249–1251.
214. Doty RL, Golbe LI, McKeown DA, et al. Olfactory testing differentiates between PSP and Parkinson's disease. Neurology 1993;43:962–965.

215. Jankovic J, Friedman DI, Pirozzolo FJ, et al. PSP: Motor, neurobehavioral, and neuro-ophthalmic findings. Adv Neurol 1990;53:293–304.
216. Jankovic J, Beach J, Schwartz K, et al. Tremor and longevity in relatives of patients with Parkinson's disease, essential tremor, and control subjects. Neurology 1995;45:645–648.
217. Golbe LI. The epidemiology of PSP. Adv Neurol 1996;69:25–31.
218. Baker KB, Montgomery EB Jr. Performance on the PD test battery by relatives of patients with PSP. Neurology 2001;56:25–30.
219. Brown J, Lantos P, Stratton M, et al. Familial PSP. J Neurol Neurosurg Psychiatry 1993;56:473–476.
220. Ohara S, Kondo K, Morita H, et al. PSP-like syndrome in two siblings of a consanguineous marriage. Neurology 1992;42:1009–1014.
221. Golbe LI, Dickson DW. Familial autopsy-proven PSP. Neurology 1995;45(suppl 4):A255.
222. Tetrud JW, Golbe LI, Farmer PM, et al. Autopsy-proven PSP in two siblings. Neurology 1996;46:931–934.
223. Gazely S, Maguire J. Familial PSP. Brain Pathol 1994;4:534.
224. Ros R, Thobois S, Streichenberger N, et al A new mutation of the tau gene, G303V, in early-onset familial PSP. Arch Neurol 2005;62:1444–1450.
225. García de Yébenes J, Sarasa JL, Daniel SE, et al. Familial PSP: description of a pedigree and review of the literature. Brain 1995;118:1095–1103.
226. Uitti R, Evidente VGH, Dickson DW, et al. A kindred with familial PSP. Neurology 1999;52:A227.
227. Rojo A, Pernaute S, Fontán A, et al. Clinical genetics of familial PSP. Brain 1999;122:1233–1245.
228. Piccini P, de Yebenes, Lees AJ, et al. Familial PSP: Detection of subclinical cases using 18F-dopa and 18-fluorodeoxyglucose positron emission tomography. Arch Neurol 2001;58:1846–1851.
229. Lannuzel A, Höglinger GU, Verhaeghe S, et al. Atypical parkinsonism in Guadeloupe: A common risk factor for two closely related phenotypes. Brain; 2007;130:816–827.
230. Champy P, Höglinger GU, Féger J, et al. Annonacin, a lipophilic inhibitor of mitochondrial complex I, induces nigral and striatal neurodegeneration in rats: possible relevance for atypical parkinsonism in Guadeloupe. J Neurochem 2004;88:63–69.
231. Geddes JF, Hughes AJ, Lees AJ, et al. Pathological overlap in cases of parkinsonism associated with neurofibrillary tangles: A study of recent cases of postencephalitic parkinsonism and comparison with PSP and Guamanian parkinsonism-dementia complex. Brain 1993;116:281–302.
232. Caparros-Lefebvre D, Elbaz A and the Caribbean Parkinsonism Study Group: Possible relation of atypical parkinsonism in the French West Indies with consumption of tropical plants: A case-control study. Lancet 1999;354:281–286.
233. Lannuzel A, Michel PP, Caparros-Lefebvre D, et al. Toxicity of Annonaceae for dopaminergic neurons: Potential role in atypical parkinsonism in Guadeloupe. Mov Disord 2002;17:84–90.
234. Anouti A, Schmidt K, Lyons KE, et al. Normal distribution of apolipoprotein E alleles in PSP. Neurology 1996;46:1156–1157.
235. Morris HR, Schrag A, Nath U, et al. Effect of ApoE and tau on age of onset of PSP and multiple system atrophy. Neurosci Lett 2001;312:118–120.
236. Schneider JA, Gearing M, Robbins RS, et al. Apolipoprotein E genotype in diverse neurodegenerative disorders. Ann Neurol 1995;38:131–135.
237. Di Monte CA, Harati Y, Jankovic J, et al. Muscle mitochondrial ATP production in PSP. J Neurochem 1994;62: 1631–1634.
238. Cantuti-Castelvetri I, Standaert DG, Albers DS, et al. Antioxidant enzymes in the PSP brain. Mov Disord 2000;15:1045.
239. Albers DS, Augood SJ, Martin DM, et al. Evidence for oxidative stress in the subthalamic nucleus in PSP. J Neurochem 1999;73:881–884.
240. Odetti P, Garibaldi S, Norese R, et al. Lipoperoxidation is selectively involved in PSP. J Neuropathol Exp Neurol 2000;59:393–397.
241. Swerdlow RH, Golbe LI, Parks JK, et al. Mitochondrial dysfunction in cybrid lines expressing mitochondrial genes from patients with PSP. J Neurochem 2000;75:1681–1684.
242. Chirichigno J, Manfredi G, Beal M, et al. Stress-induced mitochondrial depolarization and oxidative damage in PSP cybrids. Brain Res 2002;95:31–35.
243. Kim SY, Jeiter TM, Steinert PM. Transglutaminases in disease. Neurochem Int 2002;40:85–103.
244. Guillozet-Bongaarts AL, Glajch KE, Libson EG, et al. Phosphorylation and cleavage of tau in non-AD tauopathies. Acta Neuropathol 2007;113:513–520.
245. Dickson DW. Neurodegenerative diseases with cytoskeletal pathology: A biochemical classification. Ann Neurol 1997;42:541–544.
246. Caparros-Lefebvre D, Sergeant N, Lees A, et al. Guadeloupean parkinsonism: A cluster of PSP-like tauopathy. Brain 2002;125:801–811.
247. Bueé-Scherrer V, Bueé L, Hof PR, et al. Neurofibrillary degeneration in amyotrophic lateral sclerosis/parkinsonism-dementia complex of Guam. Immunochemical characterisation of tau proteins. Am J Pathol 1995;146:924–932.
248. Hutton M, Lendon CL, Rizzu P, et al. Association of missense and 5 -splice-site mutation in tau with the inherited dementia FTDP-17. Nature 1998;393:702–705.
249. Spillantini MG, Murrell JR, Goedert M, et al. Mutation in the tau gene in familial multiple system tauopathy with presenile dementia. Proc Natl Acad Sci USA 1998;95:7737–7741.
250. Stanford PM, Halliday GM, Brooks WS, et al. PSP pathology caused by a novel silent mutation in exon 10 of the tau gene. Brain 2000;123:880–893.
251. Conrad C, Andreadis A, Trojanowski JQ, et al. Genetic evidence for the involvement of tau in PSP. Ann Neurol 1997;41:277–281.
252. Baker M, Litvan I, Houlden H, et al. Association of an extended haplotype in the tau gene with PSP. Hum Mol Genet 1999;8:711–715.
253. Higgins JJ, Adler RL, Loveless JM. Mutational analysis of the tau gene in PSP. Neurology 1999;53:1421–1424.
254. Webb A, Miller B, Bonasera S, et al. Role of the tau gene region chromosome inversion in PSP, corticobasal degeneration, and related disorders. Arch Neurol 2008;65:1473–1478.
255. Ezquerra M, Pastor P, Valldeoriola F, et al. Identification of a novel polymorphism in the promoter region of the

tau gene highly associated to PSP in humans. Neurosci Lett 1999;275:183–186.
256. de Silva R, Weiler M, Morris HR, et al. Strong association of a novel tau promoter haplotype in PSP. Neurosci Lett 2001;311:145–148.
257. Pastor P, Ezquerra M, Tolosa E, et al. Further extension of the H1 haplotype associated with PSP. Mov Disord 2002;17:550–556.
258. Ingelsson M, Ramasamy K, Russ C, et al. Increase in the relative expression of tau with four microtubule binding repeat regions in frontotemporal lobar degeneration and PSP brains. Acta Neuropathol 2007;114:471–479.
259. Di Maria E, Tabaton M, Vigo T, et al. Corticobasal degeneration shares a common genetic background with PSP. Ann Neurol 2000;47:374–377.
260. Houlden H, Baker M, Morris HR, et al. Corticobasal degeneration and PSP share a common tau haplotype. Neurology 2001;56:1702–1706.
261. Golbe LI, Lazzarini AM, Spychala JR, et al. The tau A0 allele in Parkinson's disease. Mov Disord 2001;16:442–447.
262. Morris HR, Schrag A, Nath U, et al. Effect of ApoE and tau on age of onset of PSP and multiple system atrophy. Neurosci Lett 2001;312:118–120.
263. Litvan I, Baker M, Hutton M. Tau genotype: No effect on onset, symptom severity, or survival in PSP. Neurology 2001;57:138–140.
264. Liu WK, Le TV, Adamson J, et al. Relationship of the extended tau haplotype to tau biochemistry and neuropathology in PSP. Ann Neurol 2001;50:494–502.
265. Morris HR, Vaughan JR, Datta SR, et al. Multiple system atrophy/PSP: α-Synuclein, synphilin, tau, and APOE. Neurology 2000;55:1918–1920.
266. Melquist S, Craig DW, Huentelman MJ, et al. Identification of a novel risk locus for PSP by a pooled genome-wide scan of 500,288 SNP's. Am J Hum Genet 2007;80:769–778.
267. Kompoliti K, Goetz CG, Litvan I, et al. Pharmacological therapy in PSP. Arch Neurol 1998;55:1099–1102.
268. Jankovic J. PSP: Clinical and pharmacologic update. Neurol Clin 1984;2:473–486.
269. Jankovic J. Controlled trial of pergolide mesylate in Parkinson's disease and PSP. Neurology 1983;33:505–507.
270. Weiner WJ, Minagar A, Shulman LM. Pramipexole in PSP. Neurology 1999;52:873–874.
271. Jackson JA, Jankovic J, Ford J. PSP: Clinical features and response to treatment in 16 patients. Ann Neurol 1983;13:273–278.
272. Litvan I, Blesa R, Clark K, et al. Pharmacological evaluation of the cholinergic system in PSP. Ann Neurol 1994;36:55–61.
273. Litvan I, Phipps M, Pharr VL, et al. Randomized placebo-controlled trial of donepezil in patients with PSP. Neurology 2001;57:467–473.
274. Foster NL, Aldrich MS, Bluemlein L, et al. Failure of cholinergic agonist RS-86 to improve cognition and movement in PSP despite effects on sleep. Neurology 1989;39:257–261.
275. Newman GC. Treatment of PSP with tricyclic antidepressants. Neurology 1985;35:1189–1193.
276. Gaudet RJ, Kessler II. Transparently blinded trials of methysergide. N Engl J Med 1987;316:279–280.
277. Daniele A, Moro E, Bentivoglio AR. Zolpidem in PSP. N Engl J Med 1999;341:543–544.
278. Bensimon G, Ludolph A, Agid Y, Vidailhet M, Payan C, Leigh PN; for the NNIPPS Study Group. Riluzole treatment, survival and diagnostic criteria in Parkinson plus disorders: The NNIPPS Study. Brain (in press).
279. Ghika J, Tennis M, Hoffman E, et al. Idazoxan treatment in PSP. Neurology 1991;41:986–991.
280. Rascol O, Sieradzan K, Peyro-Saint-Paul H, et al. Efaroxan, an alpha-2 antagonist, in the treatment of PSP. Mov Disord 1998;13:673–676.
281. Müller J, Wenning GK, Wissel J, et al. Botulinum toxin treatment in atypical parkinsonian disorders associated with disabling focal dystonia. J Neurol 2002;249:300–304.
282. Piccione F, Mancini E, Tonin P, et al. Botulinum toxin treatment of apraxia of eyelid opening in PSP: Report of two cases. Arch Phys Med Rehab 1997;78:525–529.
283. Polo KB, Jabbari B. Botulinum toxin-A improves the rigidity of progressive supranculear palsy. Ann Neurol 1994;35:237–239.
284. Stamelou M, Reuss A, Pilatus U, et al. Short-term effects of coenzyme Q-10 in PSP: A randomized, placebo-controlled trial. Mov Disord 2008;23:942–949.
285. Sosner J, Wall GC, Sznajder J. PSP: Clinical presentation and rehabilitation of two patients. Arch Phys Med Rehab 1993;74:537–539.
286. Koller WC, Morantz R, Vetere-Overfield B, et al. Autologous adrenal medullary transplant in PSP. Neurology 1989;39:1066–1068.
287. Lozano AM, Snyder BJ. Deep brain stimulation for parkinsonian gait disorders. J Neurol 2008;255(suppl 4):30–31.
288. Hauser RA, Trehan R. Initial experience with electroconvulsive therapy for PSP. Mov Disord 1994;9:466–468.
289. Barclay CL, Duff J, Sandor P, et al. Limited usefulness of electroconvulsive therapy in PSP. Neurology 1996;46:1284–1286.
290. Rasmussen K, Abrams R. Treatment of Parkinson's disease with electroconvulsive therapy. Psychiatr Clin North Am 1991;14:925–933.

CHAPTER 22

Corticobasal Degeneration

Natividad P. Stover and Ray L. Watts

▶ HISTORY AND DESCRIPTION OF THE INITIAL CASES

Corticobasal degeneration (CBD) is a neurodegenerative disorder that has gained interest of neurologists, neuropathologists, and other neuroscientists in the last four to five decades. Over the past years, there has been a tendency to consider CBD as a syndrome more than a nosologic entity because of the heterogeneity of clinical presentations and overlap of the clinical and pathological features with other neurodegenerative diseases. The patients with the classical motor presentation may be still very characteristic, and currently most of the pathologically confirmed cases of CBD can be divided into two distinct groups: (1) patients that present mainly with a movement disorder and (2) patients that develop cognitive problems. As the disease progresses, most of the patients may manifest both types of symptoms. The lack of biomarkers for the diagnosis of the different neurodegenerative processes makes the premortem diagnosis of these disorders even more inaccurate and difficult to differentiate in a clinical setting. CBD was originally called corticodentatonigral degeneration with neuronal achromasia, based in the pathological findings of three original cases described by Rebeiz and colleagues in 1967.[1] The term "CBD" was initially used by Gibb and colleagues in 1989,[2] and in 2000, the term CBD Syndrome was proposed by Kertesz.[3] Other names used to describe the cases of CBD included corticonigral degeneration with neuronal achromasia,[4] corticodentatonigral degeneration,[5] cortical-basal ganglionic degeneration,[6] and myoclonic dystonia.[7] In the nineteenth century, Jean-Martin Charcot, Alfred Vulpian, and their disciples described cases of atypical Parkinson's disease (PD) with jerking movements and abnormal posture of the limbs, called originally "hemiplegic parkinsonism."[8,9] Many of these clinical cases lack a complete description, since the characterization of many neurologic signs and symptoms such as apraxia, dystonia, cortical sensory deficits, and myoclonus were not a regular part of the neurological examination performed at that time. The description of some of Charcot's atypical parkinsonian cases has some of the distinctive features that we consider today associated with CBD. Jacques Lhermitte in 1925 described a clinical case to the French Neurological Society that is suggestive of CBD.[10] "A 67-year-old carpenter with progressive right hand clumsiness, unable to ambulate independently at age of 72, with the right arm flexed and an involuntary right arm movement 'like a foreign body,' unable to recognize objects in his right hand, in spite of normal primary sensation."

In this chapter, we describe our current understanding of CBD and its place in the spectrum of neurodegenerative disorders. However, before we embark on a formal delineation of current concepts, we will review the original reported cases. Rebeiz and colleagues described three patients in 1967 at the Massachusetts General Hospital with a unique pattern of progressive motor impairment in later mid-life. The clinical symptoms were characterized by slow, awkward involuntary limb movements accompanied by tremor and dystonic posturing. In all three cases, dysfunction began and remained most prominent in the left limbs. Stiffness, slowness, lack of dexterity or clumsiness, and "numbness" or "deadness" were the initial symptoms. The leg was affected first in two of the three patients and gait impairment was an early manifestation, with particular difficulty initiating steps. The cases had marked limbs rigidity, impaired sensory function of the limbs, as well as interference of attempted voluntary movements with involuntary synkinesias of the contralateral limb. All the cases had some tremulous movements of the limbs even if this was not a predominant feature. Motor disability progressed in the affected limbs without motor weakness, except late in the disease. Two of the cases had cortical sensory changes with impaired position sense and tactile localization, difficulties with two-point discrimination exam and recognizing objects by touch. All of the cases had finger contractures and increased tendon reflexes. As the disease progressed, all of the patients developed problems with speech and dysphagia. Although motor impairment progressed, intellectual function was said to remain relatively preserved. Motor disability progressed, and the illness terminated in death six to eight years after the onset of the disease. General physical examination and laboratory studies, including cerebrospinal fluid analysis, were normal. The radiological studies showed asymmetrical cerebral atrophy in the three patients, most evident in the opposite side of the brain from where the symptoms initiated. Seizures and myoclonic phenomena were not described in any of the patients. Electroencephalogram showed asymmetrical slow and sharp activity without specific changes. Pneumoencephalograms studies showed cerebral atrophy greater on the right side of the brain in two of the patients.

The pathological findings in all three patients were distinctive, with an unusual pattern of asymmetric frontoparietal cortical atrophy contralateral to the side of the body where the symptoms presented. The cerebral arteries showed little or no atherosclerosis, with no evidence of vascular occlusion. The microscopic examination of the atrophic cortex showed extensive neuronal loss mainly in the outer three cortical layers with associated astrocytic gliosis and minimal microglial activation. These changes co-localized with the appearance of pale and swollen cell bodies frequently with accompanied vacuolization of the pyramidal neurons mainly in the third and fifth cortical layers and presented an eosinophilic hyaline appearance with hematoxylin–eosin staining. The swollen neurons often had eccentric displacement of the nucleus, as reminiscent of the axonal reaction described in cases of pellagra, but the cases lacked Nissl substance in the cytoplasm, thus prompting the use of the terms "achromatic" and "ballooned neurons." These abnormal neurons were situated in the areas of cortical neuronal loss in the cortex, mostly in the frontal, Rolandic, and parietal regions. The hippocampal formation, occipital cortex, and inferior and medial temporal cortex were spared in the original cases. Considerable loss of pigmented neurons in the substantia nigra (SN) was observed in the three patients. These striking pathological findings were not accompanied by microscopic features typical of any other neurodegenerative condition, such as Lewy bodies, senile plaques, or Pick's bodies. The subcortical nuclei were relatively intact except for some old lacunar infarcts in one of the patients. The medial portion of the subthalamic nucleus also showed gliosis and swollen neurons. In two patients, there were similar neuronal changes in the dentate and deep nuclei of the cerebellum with retrograde atrophy of the superior cerebellar peduncles with an intact appearance of the cerebellar cortex. The cases also showed gliosis of the red nuclei and ventrolateral portion of the thalamus. In one of the patients, there were a few swollen neurons in the oculomotor nucleus. There were no significant neuronal abnormalities in the spinal cord. The white matter areas showed considerable demyelination and gliosis, as corresponding with areas of secondary cortical degeneration and without evidence of an independent white matter disease process. In each case, the general autopsy gave no clues concerning the pathogenesis of the intriguing neuropathological findings.

In later years, Obeso and colleagues described a case of "myoclonic dystonia" with akinetic rigid syndrome, focal dystonia, and myoclonus of the arm with alien hand phenomenon that developed supranuclear gaze palsy, parkinsonism, and mild cerebellar signs. The pathological exam revealed frontoparietal atrophy with cortical cell loss, Pick-like cells, and gliosis in the basal ganglia, midbrain tegmentun, SN, and locus ceruleus. The inclusions in the SN were similar to the neurofibrillary tangles (NFT) seen in progressive supranuclear palsy (PSP) and Pick's disease (PiD) cases and they were called "corticobasal inclusions."[7] Watts and colleagues described in 1985 a patient who presented with stiffness and severe dystonic posturing of the right arm and leg with rapid, irregular action tremor and impairment of balance that progressed to inability to walk independently. The patient lost the ability to perform motor tasks previously learned with the right arm. He also developed blepharospasm and saccadic breakdown of smooth pursuit eye movements and progressed to be dysarthric and have poor language content in a short period. Fasciculations were described in several muscle groups of the extremities. The patient did not have a family history of neurologic disease and the imaging studies showed cortical atrophy in the peri-Rolandic area. The neuropathological examination showed asymmetrical neuronal loss with reactive gliosis in all layers of the premotor, anterior cingulate, inferior parietal, insular, and anterior temporal regions with extensive loss of myelinated axons and gliosis in the white matter. The cortical areas that were not so severely affected were populated with swollen neurons with achromasia. There was neuronal loss in the SN bilaterally, but there were no Lewy bodies. There were no abnormalities in the globus pallidus, striatum, amygdala, hypothalamus, cerebellum, brain stem, and spinal cord. The peripheral nerves showed demyelination and there were denervation changes in skeletal muscles. The treatment of the patient with multiple medications was not effective.[11]

Over the past decades, many other authors have described a wide spectrum of clinical phenotypes with characteristic pathologic findings of CBD. Many patients with atypical parkinsonian syndromes and a predominance of cognitive dysfunction have turned out to have the classical pathologic picture of CBD.[12] The literature has also reported cases presenting with clinical features of CBD that lack the specific pathological findings.[13]

With this historical backdrop, we now address current knowledge of epidemiology, clinical features, diagnosis, neuropathological findings, and differential diagnosis of CBD. Finally, the treatment of CBD constitutes one of the greatest challenges facing basic and clinical neuroscientists as we seek to understand the molecular mechanisms and develop effective disease-modifying strategies.[14,15]

▶ EPIDEMIOLOGY

The general incidence and prevalence of CBD are unknown and most likely underestimated.[16] Studies with neuropathological confirmed CBD cases showed very low sensitivity in the clinical diagnosis based on medical records only, reflecting that the disorder is likely underdiagnosed, especially after an intitial visit. Most of the CBD cases are manifested in middle to late adult life with a mean onset of symptoms at 63 (±7.7) years.[17,18] Clinical cases diagnosed as CBD have been reported as early as age 34 and 40 years, and the youngest case with pathological confirmation was 45 years old.[19] Some authors have observed predominance in women and two of the three original cases were women.[1,5] No clear ethnic preponderance has been observed and most of the cases are described in Caucasians. Current knowledge suggests that it is mainly a sporadic disease with negative family history of affected patients in most of the cases, although a small series reported family history of a parkinsonian disorder.[20] It is becoming more evident that certain genetic backgrounds may be a risk factor,[21] and there are described several families with clinical and pathological correlation of CBD.[22,23] Many cases that were originally reported as familial CBD were later identified as frontal temporal dementia and parkinsonism linked to chromosome 17 (FTDP-17).[24,25] Some authors consider CBD and PSP as different phenotypes of the same disorder, on the basis of clinocopathological and genetic overlap.[26] Other risk factors such as toxic exposures or infectious agents have not been implicated in the pathogenesis of CBD, but we lack large epidemiological, occupational, or toxicological studies of CBD cases.

▶ CLINICAL PRESENTATION AND FEATURES

There have been several attempts to establish diagnostic criteria for CBD. Among movement disorder specialists most cases present with predominantly motor symptoms, but the pathological examination of cases from brain banks showed dementia as the most frequent initial symptom in patients with pathological confirmation of CBD.[27,28] The early presentation of subcortical and cortical symptoms is usually a clue to consider the diagnosis of CBD. The motor symptoms respond poorly or not at all to dopaminergic and other medications, and this represents an early important characteristic clue that suggests an atypical parkinsonian syndrome.[29,30] The most frequent initial motor symptom reported by patients is limb clumsiness with or without increased tone, and in some studies, it is observed in half of the patients at the first visit.[31,32] Overall, bradykinesia, rigidity, and apraxia were reported in over 90% of cases within the first 3 years of illness.[33,34] An asymmetrical, insidiously progressive parkinsonism usually of the akinetic-rigid type, limb dystonia, apraxia, with or without tremulous movements, is also typical. Signs of cortical impairment develop within 1–3 years of onset in most of the reported cases, but in studies done with both dementia and movement disorder referrals, cognitive, or language disturbances were the most frequent presenting features and, at times, the sole manifestation in patients with pathologic confirmation of CBD.[12]

Riley and Lang[35] tried to establish practical inclusion and exclusion criteria for the clinical diagnosis of CBD with manifestations reflecting dysfunction of basal ganglia (akinesia, rigidity, postural and action tremor, limb dystonia, myoclonus, postural instability, falls and disequilibrium, and other dyskinesias) and cerebral cortex dysfunction (cortical sensory loss, apraxia, alien limb phenomenon, frontal lobe release signs, dementia, and dysphasia). Other findings did not localize specifically to either of these regions: oculomotor dysfunction, eyelid motor dysfunction, dysarthria, dysphagia, cerebellar signs, and autonomic symptomatology. The inclusion criteria included the presence of rigidity plus one cortical sign or asymmetric rigidity, dystonia, and focal reflex myoclonus. Exclusion criteria initially were defined as early dementia, early vertical gaze palsy, typical rest tremor, severe autonomic dysfunction, sustained improvement with dopaminergic medications, or imaging studies that offer an alternative diagnosis.[36] Watts and colleagues proposed major and minor criteria for the diagnosis of CBD.[18] The major criteria included a strong degree of asymmetry with rigidity, bradykinesia/akinesia, gait disorder, action or postural tremor, alien limb phenomenon, dystonia, myoclonus, and cortical signs. Among the minor criteria they described choreoathetosis, dementia, cerebellar signs, supranuclear gaze palsy, frontal release signs, and blepharospasm. Rinne and colleagues[37] analyzed the clinical features of 36 patients with clinical diagnosis of CBD of which six patients had pathological confirmation. Of the 36 patients, 20 presented with symptoms of a useless arm related to jerky movements, stiffness, or clumsiness and 10 patients began with the symptom of difficulty walking with clumsiness and loss of motor control of one leg due to disequilibrium, apraxia, or both. Other less common presentations included combined arm and leg involvement with motor dysfunction, isolated sensory syndromes, unilateral painful paresthesias, myoclonus, dysarthria, orofacial dyspraxia, and behavioral symptoms.[38] Most of the patients presented and maintained an asymmetric distribution of the symptoms but they extended gradually over the next years to the contralateral side, with worsening of the postural instability, dysphagia, dysarthria, and hypomimic facial expression.[39]

Litvan and colleagues[40] published the statistical analysis of 105 clinical cases with known neuropathologic diagnosis of different neurodegenerative diseases presented to a group of neurologists trained in movement disorders to determine the accuracy of the clinical diagnosis. The specialists then provided clinical diagnoses that were subsequently correlated with the pathologic findings. The results of the 10 patients with CBD with pathologic confirmation showed high specificity and low sensitivity, mainly during the first 3 years of symptoms. In this study, the best predictors for the diagnosis of CBD during the first visit of the patient included limb dystonia, asymmetric akinetic-rigid parkinsonian syndrome, ideomotor apraxia, myoclonus, and problems with balance or gait disturbances. There are, however, cases of limb dystonia with a pathological diagnosis of PSP.[41–43]The absence of a gait disturbance may be a key feature for differentiating CBD from PSP and striatonigral degeneration (SND) if some of the other characteristic clinical symptoms are present. Other clinical features commonly seen were an irregular, jerky postural/action tremor and focal stimulus-sensitive myoclonus, choreoathetoid movements, cortical sensory loss, the alien limb phenomenon, abnormal eye movements, blepharospasm, neuropsychological and cognitive symptoms, language disturbances, and speech and swallowing problems[44–47] (Table 22–1).

TABLE 22–1. CLINICAL FEATURES OF CBD

Nature of Symptoms:
Motor and cognitive symptoms
Insidious onset, progressive, may be asymmetric
Atypical parkinsonism
Unresponsive to dopaminergic medication
Motor Dysfunction:
Bradykinesia-akinesia, limb clumsiness
Rigidity
Dystonia
Atypical tremor (mainly postural and action)
Focal, reflex myoclonus
Oculomotor symptoms: slowed saccadic pursuit and hypometric saccades
Blepharospasm
Speech problems: dysarthria, hypophonia
Dysphagia
Alien limb phenomenon
Gait disorder and postural instability
Involuntary synkinesias and athetosis/pseudoathetosis
Facial dyskinesias
Corticospinal signs and upper motor neuron syndrome
Cortical Dysfunction:
Apraxia (limb kinetic, ideomotor, ideational)
Cortical sensory abnormalities: agraphestesia, astereognosis, extinction to double simultaneous somatosensory stimulation.
Cognitive impairment/dementia
Progressive aphasia
Neuropsychiatric Dysfunction:
Frontal lobe behavior disorder: disinhibition, irritability
Depression and anxiety
Obsessive compulsive behavior
Apathy
Other symptoms:
Sleep disorders
Urinary dysfunction
Constipation
Pain syndromes

MOTOR SYMPTOMS

The tremor in CBD differs from the typical pill-rolling rest tremor seen in PD. It is a faster tremor with postural and action components, more irregular and jerky and affects mainly the upper extremities.[48]

Myoclonus has been traditionally considered a distinctive clinical finding in patients with CBD and frequently appears during the first year.[49–51] Myoclonus may happen in other neurodegenerative diseases and some recent clinicopathologic correlation studies have found myoclonus to be more frequent in patients diagnosed clinically as CBD but with pathologic findings of Alzheimer's disease (AD).[52] Myoclonus may also be seen early in the course of Creutzfeldt–Jakob disease (CJD), and later in the course of multiple system atrophy (MSA), Huntington's disease, and cerebellar degeneration. The myoclonus in CBD is unilateral, focal, and reflex stimulus-sensitive or triggered by action. It may coexist with tremor and usually precedes or accompanies the development of dystonic posturing and it tends to be present, at least initially, to a greater extent in the most affected limbs.[53,54] The myoclonus, like the tremor, is better observed during action or maintenance of a posture; it may be elicited by cutaneous or auditory stimulation; and it may be in part attenuated by the presence of severely increased muscle tone.[55,56] Spontaneous myoclonus may also appear but is less common and difficult to evaluate in the setting of tremor and limb rigidity.[57]

The presence of asymmetric limb dystonia is very suggestive of the diagnosis of CBD in the setting of atypical parkinsonism cases without benefit from medical treatment.[35,40,58] Asymmetric dystonia of the upper extremity is the most frequent presentation with flexion of the hand and forearm, adduction of the shoulder, flexion of the fingers at the metacarpophalangeal joints, extension or flexion of the fingers at the proximal and distal interphalangeal joints, and variable degrees of dystonic postures with or without associated contractures. Involvement of the arm and leg by dystonia may happen but predominantly lower extremity dystonia is less frequent.[59] Orofacial, head, neck, and trunk dystonia are less common in the course of the disease, and the axial distribution of the dystonia may be manifested as retrocollis, anterocollis, or torticollis. Blepharospasm can be present in CBD as well as in PSP and other parkinsonian syndromes. Dystonia is often associated with myoclonus, tremor, apraxia, alien limb phenomenon, and cortical sensory abnormality in the affected limb and, as dystonia progresses, patients may develop rigid postures. Pain accompanying dystonia is described frequently, and it may be very intense, resembling cases of complex regional pain syndrome, usually associated with contractures.[60] Pathology and imaging studies have failed to identify a distinctive marker for CBD patients with dystonia, but in general, cases with dystonia tend to have more generalized cortical and subcortical brain atrophy.

Oculomotor dysfunction is frequent in CBD and evaluation of these symptoms can provide useful clues to improve the diagnostic accuracy in the early stages of the disease and to differenciate it from PSP (mainly) and other parkinsonian syndromes.[61,62] In most patients with CBD, horizontal and vertical eye movements may be equally affected compared with PSP patients that have vertical saccades more affected in upward and downward directions than horizontal saccades. Initiation of horizontal saccades in patients with CBD have increased latency bilaterally and higher frequency of eye blinking to perform voluntary saccades compared with controls and PSP patients, with the latter group manifesting a sustained decreased velocity of eye movements. Vertical saccadic eye movements may be slightly impaired in patients with CBD. In contrast, PSP patients usually have slow and hypometric saccades early in the disease and need to perform multiple steps to reach a target with frequent downward saccade paralysis.[63,64] Smooth pursuit eye movements in early stages of CBD may be slow and exhibit saccadic breakdown, but the range of movements is generally full (except for upgaze in elderly patients). As the illness progresses, patients with CBD gradually lose the ability to make rapid saccades to verbal commands, and frequently retain spontaneous saccades with optokinetic nystagmus, but after years they can reach the level of abnormalities observed in PSP patients.[65,66]

Speech problems and difficulties swallowing are frequently reported in CBD cases, mainly as the disease progresses and cortical and subcortical areas are affected. These deficits are not clearly distinguishable from those found in other parkinsonian syndromes. The speech changes include dysarthria, slowness of speech production, monotonous voice, dysphonia, echolalia, or palilalia. The difficulties may evolve to include aphonia and patients may become anarthric in advanced stages. Dysarthria may be present even in early phases of the disease, is usually mild in severity, and may include reduced loudness of voice, slow rate of performance, and difficulties with sound articulation. Spastic dysarthria has been described inconsistently in cases of CBD, as well as the presence of vocal tremor and stridor.[67] Dysarthria and pathological laughter or crying have been also described as the presenting symptoms of CBD cases.[68–70] Swallowing disorders are very common, especially in later phases of the disease. Dysphagia is reported more frequently with liquids than with solids and confirmed by modified barium swallow studies. The dysphagia is characterized by delay in initiation of swallowing and pooling of the food bolus in valleculae and may affect the oral, pharyngeal, and esophageal phases of swallowing in different grades.[71]

The alien limb phenomenon is a failure to recognize ownership of one's extremity in the absence of visual cues.[72–75] It is frequently associated with autonomous activity or personification of the affected limb, which may be perceived by the subject as foreign, outside his or her control. This interesting sign is probably one of the most frequently associated with typical cases of CBD, although it is not an exclusive element of this disease and it is usually rare on initial presentation.[76–78] The alien limb phenomenon in cases of CBD often coexists with dystonia, myoclonus, apraxia, and cortical sensory loss. Alien arm is the most frequent location in cases of suspected and confirmed CBD, but alien leg has been reported also as a presentation of the disease. The complete manifestation of the alien limb phenomenon with posturing and levitation of the affected extremity is associated with CBD more commonly than with other etiologies.[79,80] Alien face syndrome has been reported also in association with probable CBD.[81] The anatomical localization of lesions associated with the alien hand syndrome is in the corpus callosum, the parietal cortex, or the frontal cortical regions.

Postural instability and gait disorders with shuffling, start hesitation, freezing episodes, leg bradykinesia or akinesia, and falls may occur early in the disease if the legs are initially involved or may be seen as the disease progresses with the combination of cortical, subcortical, and cognitive symptoms producing marked disequilibrium and the inability to walk.

Spontaneous onset of dyskinesias, mainly athetosis or pseudoathetotic movements involving the limbs or facial muscles, may develop occasionally in the course of CBD but they are not frequent at presentation. The presence of synkinesias with the urgency to use the less affected limb when instructed to use the opposite extremity is also described in CBD.

As the disease advances, most of the patients exhibit signs of corticospinal dysfunction with an upper motor neuron syndrome, Babinski sign and spasticity, and the involvement of the primary motor and sensory cortex has been confirmed with the corresponding pathological findings.[82] Increased tone in the affected limbs may be difficult to differentiate whether it is related to rigidity or spasticity, but most likely, it is the result of cortical and subcortical involvement. In more advanced stages, frontal release signs such as grasp, glabellar, and exaggerated facial and palmomental reflexes, may become prominent.

Symptoms associated with shorter survival in CBD patients are early onset of bilateral parkinsonism and the presence of a frontal lobe syndrome. The motor symptoms usually progresses to a state of bilateral rigid immobility, and death related to secondary causes may occur after 5–10 years after disease onset.

CORTICAL SYMPTOMS

Apraxia is considered the hallmark of CBD and raises the possibility of this diagnosis if seen as part of the additional characteristic symptoms on presentation. Limb apraxia includes a wide spectrum of cognitive and motor disorders affecting the performance of learned movements that cannot be accounted for by simple sensory or motor deficits.[83] Different types of apraxia have been described in suspected and confirmed cases of CBD, depending not only on the initial cortical area affected but also in the time frame of disease progression in which the symptom is evaluated.[84] Initial reports of cases with CBD considered ideomotor apraxia to be the most frequent type but new studies suggests that limb-kinetic apraxia is predominant in CBD, while idomotor apraxia can be seen most frequently in more advanced disease or PSP cases.[85,86] In limb kinetic apraxia the manipulative behavior is affected by a decrease in dexterity and fine movements in the affected limb, and it may be difficult to evaluate properly when the rigidity, bradykinesia, dystonia, or other motor symptoms are present in the affected extremity.[87–89] Limb kinetic apraxia is a dysfunction of the "praxis conceptual system" where the fingers and hand movements are affected with awkward movements unnecessary to perform a task. The evaluation is done by asking the patient to perform a fine movement with the fingers, usually manipulating an object. This type of apraxia is mainly seen with lesions of the premotor cortex with or without associated parietal cortex or basal ganglia involvement. Ideomotor apraxia constitutes a problem at the level of the "praxis production system" and it is manifested by impairment of timing, sequencing, spatial organization, and mimicking of movements.[90] Patients with ideomotor apraxia commit mainly temporal (irregular speed and sequencing) and spatial errors (abnormal amplitude, orientation of objects and movements), and they demonstrate abnormal use of body parts as objects. The evaluation of ideomotor apraxia is done asking the patient to pretend to manipulate an object in order to perform a task. This type of apraxia is associated with damage to the parietal association areas, premotor cortex and intrahemispheric white matter bundles that connect them, as well as basal ganglia and thalamus. Patients with CBD may also demonstrate ideational apraxia, considered also a dysfunction of the "praxis conceptual system."[91,92] The performance of the movement in ideational apraxia is abnormal in the content and tool selection, and it may include the presence of perseverations and pantomime-related errors. The patients with ideational apraxia cannot sequence correctly different movements needed to perform a specific task. This type of apraxia has been observed in later stages of the disease and in patients mainly with cognitive problems and language dysfunction at presentation.[93,94]

Apraxia of speech has been described in CBD and Rosenfield and colleagues described two patients (one with pathological confirmation of CBD) with speech apraxia as a presenting sign in the evolution of the classical clinical motor syndrome.[95] Apraxia of speech and nonfluent aphasia are strongly associated with a diagnosis of CBD, PSP, or both.[96,97] Orofacial apraxia with dysarthria was also reported in a series of ten patients, and patients, with facial apraxia may have impaired ability to voluntarily generate facial expressions with relatively spared ability to generate spontaneous emotional faces.[98,99] Truncal apraxia has also been described in patients with a clinical diagnosis of CBD.[100]

Cortical sensory abnormalities, mainly loss of two point discrimination and somatosensory extinction to double simultaneous stimulation, agraphesthesia and astereognosis may precede the development of apraxia and other cortical symptoms in CBD. Patients with parkinsonian syndromes usually do not have major sensory complaints, and this finding may raise the suspicion of CBD. It is important to note that cortical sensory symptoms may be present several years before apraxia and some of the other symptoms become evident.[88]

Cognitive and language problems in CBD patients are frequently associated with motor and praxis disorders. Cases mainly with motor symptoms may have preservation of the cognitive function in the early stages of the disease, and varying degrees of cognitive dysfunction and language impairment may develop overtime. Cognitive impairment and dementia may be the presenting or even sole feature in some cases.[12,101] One of our studies, with 11 cases of neuropathologically confirmed CBD, showed that all patients eventually developed cognitive deficits but the onset, nature, and severity of the impairment varied widely. Cognitive disorder preceded or accompanied the onset of the movement disorder in four patients and an additional three patients developed memory loss, progressing to more global dementia, within 2–3 years of the onset of the symptoms. Another patient displayed mild early memory impairment, and in three individuals, dementia was a late feature.[47] In another study with 15 patients with pathologic confirmation of CBD, the authors found a specific pattern of impaired cognition with persistent impairment of praxis and executive function, worsening of language performance, and preserved memory in many cases.[102] The cognitive dysfunction in CBD fits mainly a subcortical pattern with pronounced impairment in executive function, resembling that of PSP, except for the presence of apraxia that is usually worse in CBD cases. The origin of the cognitive dysfunction in these patients without significant pathology in the hippocampus and temporal regions is explained by the disruption of subcortical circuits, and the deficits can be evaluated assessing word fluency and difficulties switching between different activities, requiring a sequence of movements. The patients may have problems with motor programming, temporal organization of the different movements as well as problems with bimanual coordination, and inhibition of interfering movements that are not necessary to perform a specific task.[103] Temporospatial orientation and recent and remote memories are usually preserved in early stages of the disease. In a study comparing clinically diagnosed CBD and AD patients with extrapyramidal features, CBD patients displayed better performance on tests of immediate recall and attention, whereas they performed significantly worse on tests of praxis, digit span, and uni- and bimanual motor series examinations.[104,105] Naming may be impaired in CBD patients, although their naming ability often benefits from phonemic cuing, unlike that of AD patients. Recognition memory may be preserved, but encoding and recall strategies could be dysfunctional. Impairment mainly with handling large numbers despite the present of minimal aphasia has been described as a characteristic of CBD.[106] The initial speech difficulties may progress to include language problems that include paraphasic errors with aphasia. Also, an impairment of syntactic knowledge was only found in patients with CBD syndrome, even in the absence of aphasia when compared with frontotemporal dementia (FTD) cases[107] but progressive nonfluent aphasia is often a precursor of CBD and PSP patients.[108] Cases with primary progressive conduction aphasia as the presenting symptom of CBD have been described.[109–111] A frontosubcortical pattern of cognitive impairment with the presence of abnormal gesture in one extremity may be very suggestive of CBD as well.

OTHER SYMPTOMS

Neuropsychiatric features have been described in many cases of probable and confirmed CBD. In the past, depression and irritability were found more frequently, whereas apathy was less frequent in CBD compared with PSP.[112,113] Most recently, three behavioral syndromes have been shown to be associated more specifically with CBD: a frontal lobe type behavioral disorder, depression and obsessive compulsive behavior.[114] Over the last years, this group of symptoms was confirmed in 36 pathologically confirmed cases of CBD.[115] In this study, 8 out of the 36 patients had well-documented neuropsychiatric disorders and only two of the patients were diagnosed with typical motor symptoms of CBD during life: depression refractory to treatment was present in one patient and obsessive compulsive behavior in the other. The rest of the patients were diagnosed initially with progressive aphasia and FTD, which developed compulsive behavior disorders, including excessive eating and new onset of excessive alcohol drinking, socially inappropriate and disinhibited behaviors, agressiveness, impaired judgment, and irritability. Previous studies found that at least half of patients with CBD had neuropsychiatric symptoms. Depression and anxiety were the most common disorders, followed by apathy and sleep disturbances. Manifestations of obsessive–compulsive disorder, including recurrent thoughts, repetitive acts, indecisiveness, checking behaviors, and preoccupation with perfectionism, are frequently included in the neuropsychological profile of CBD patients.[116,117] Compared with AD, patients with CBD have less apathy, agitation, anxiety, and delusions.[118–120] Patients diagnosed with FTD are said to manifest more disinhibition and euphoria but many of those studies have no pathologic confirmation. CBD patients usually manifest rates of depression similar to PD but lower rates of anxiety.

The presence of prominent or severe autonomic dysfunction is not characteristic of CBD, although different grades of postural hypotension and dizziness, urinary and bowel dysfunction, sexual dysfunction, sweating episodes, esophageal reflux, and sleep problems have been described. Sleep disorders with the presence of insomnia, periodic leg movements during the sleep, and sleep-related respiratory disorders also have been described in a minority of patients with CBD.[121] Rapid eye movement (REM) sleep behavior disorder, although more frequently described in the synucleinopathies, has also been reported in cases of CBD.[122] Although visual hallucinations have been described, they are not systematically reported in CBD patients with neuropathological confirmation of the disease.[123] Urinary dysfunction, manifested mainly as frequency and overactive bladder are a common feature in patients with CBD.[124] Constipation to the point of repeated stool impactions is a frequently reported symptom in most of the neurodegenerative diseases. Olfactory dysfunction has not been reported in CBD.[125,126]

▶ DIAGNOSIS

Debate continues as to whether CBD is a distinct nosologic entity or contained in the spectrum of tauopathies (such as PSP and Pick's Disease). When fully developed and observed over time, the motoric presentation is sufficiently characteristic to allow correct diagnosis during life with a relatively high accuracy. Although not diagnostic, additional studies, summarized below, can provide supportive data, including laboratory, imaging, and electrophysiologic studies. Neuropsychological testing and evaluation of praxis may be helpful when patients do not have the typical motor presentation. The ultimate

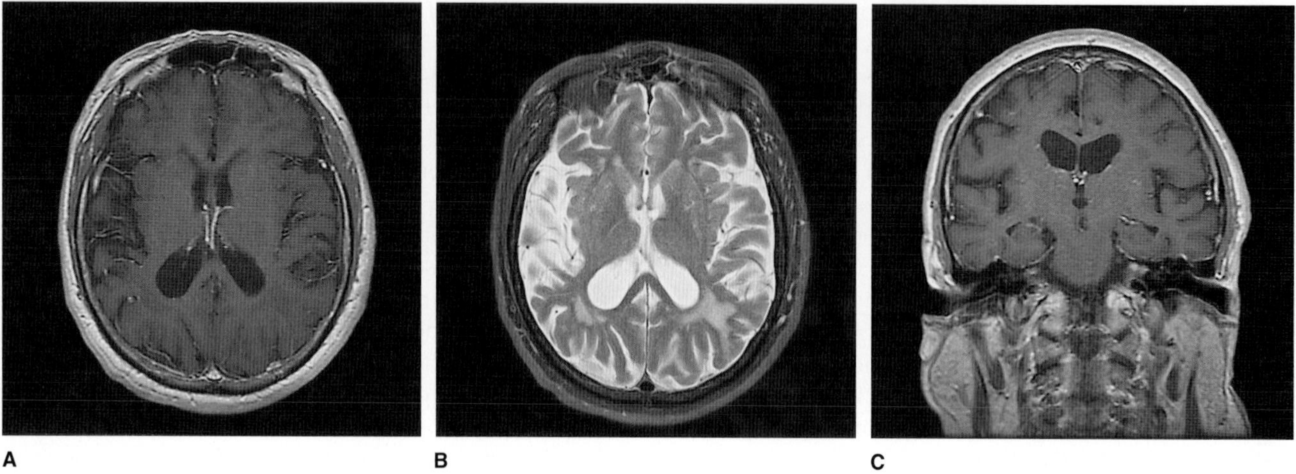

Figure 22–1. **(A,B)** Axial T_1 and T_2-weighted 1.5 T MRI of a patient with clinical CBD with atrophy in the right posterior frontal, parietal and temporal regions. **(C)** Coronal T_1-weighted 1.5 T MRI image with asymmetric right frontal atrophy in a patient with CBD.

confirmation, however, still depends on the neuropathological findings in concert with the clinical picture.

LABORATORY STUDIES

Routine laboratory studies of blood, urine, and cerebrospinal fluid (CSF) are normal. Serum copper and ceruloplasmin levels are normal. Heavy metal toxic screens of urine have been negative. Watts and colleagues found that CSF levels of somatostatin were significantly decreased in all three patients assayed, two of whom had autopsy confirmation of CBD.[127] A tendency towards decreased serum folate concentration was found in CBD patients, compared with other neurodegenerative diseases.[128] The levels of the protein tau are elevated in CSF of AD patients but its diagnostic value was found to be inadequate for the differential diagnosis of the different types of dementia syndromes.[129,130]

NEUROIMAGING STUDIES

A distinctive feature that needs to be considered when evaluating brain images of patients with suspected CBD is the presence of asymmetric brain atrophy. In this regard, serial radiographic evaluations with brain computed tomography (CT) scans or magnetic resonance imaging (MRI) are usually more useful than an isolated study to observe the progression of the atrophy. The studies may be normal in the early stages of the disease, but as the disease progresses, a pattern of asymmetric frontoparietal cortical atrophy (greater contralateral to the most severely affected limbs) is frequently observed, mainly in the cases with motor symptoms.[131] The less characteristic cases usually show a pattern of diffuse generalized atrophy. The areas most affected are usually the posterior frontal and parietal regions. The cortex may appear thin and frequently with slight increase in signal intensity in proton density images. Abnormalities of the cortex are more easily detectable with fluid-attenuated inversion recovery (FLAIR: T_2-weighted images but with suppression of the signal of the spinal fluid) sequences in the MRI.[132,133] As the cortical atrophy becomes more prominent, abnormal signal attenuation with hyperintensity is seen in the underlying subcortical white matter of the Rolandic region, together with the asymmetric atrophy[134] (Fig. 22–1A,B,C).

Atrophy of the corpus callosum has been described in cases of CBD, PSP, and FTD (Fig. 22–2). Atrophy and abnormal signal in the corpus callosum are frequently described because of the cortical degeneration, as can be dilatation of the ventricle opposite to the most affected body side in cases with marked asymmetry. Neither cortical nor corpus callosum atrophy or subcortical and periventricular white matter signal changes on MRI are specific to CBD.[135] However, MRI can provide strong support for the diagnosis of CBD, and it may be helpful in distinguishing CBD from other neurodegenerative disorders. The corpus callosum has been described smaller in cases of AD, compared with normal controls, and was not atrophic in PD and PD with dementia (PDD) patients.[136] The degree of cognitive impairment shows a strong correlation with the severity of callosal atrophy and ventricular dilatation in some studies.[137] Savoiardo and colleagues addressed the role of MRI in various parkinsonian syndromes:[138,139] Compared with CBD, MRI abnormalities in patients with typical PSP are easy to differentiate and demonstrate atrophy in the midbrain and tectum without asymmetrical cortical atrophy.[140,141] AD cases may be differentiated from CBD by observing in AD diffuse atrophy in the hippocampal and adjacent

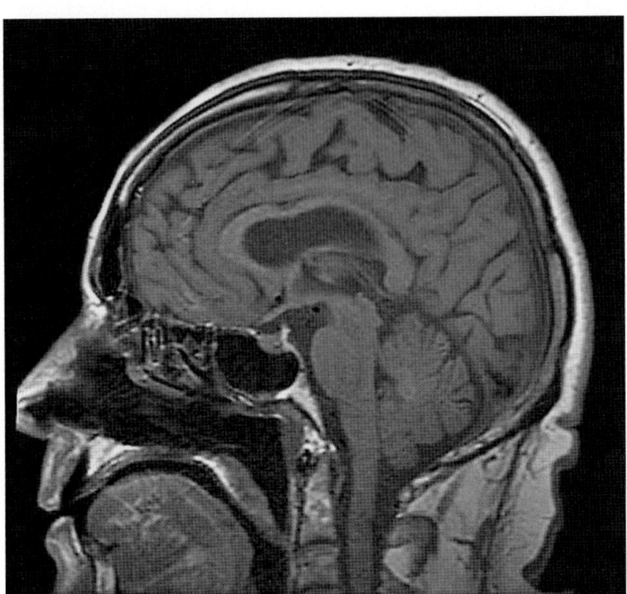

Figure 22-2. Sagital T_1-weighted 1.5 MRI images that show the atrophy of the corpus callosum and the frontoparietal atrophy in a patient with CBD.

mesial temporal structures in the MRI with enlarged temporal horns, suprasellar cisterns and sylvian fissures. In patients with MSA, the MRI may show changes in the basal ganglia, infratentorial structures and intermediolateral columns of the spinal cord. MRI in patients with SND type of MSA often demonstrates T_2 hypointensities in the posterior lateral putamen. In patients with MSA of the olivopontocerebellar atrophy (OPCA) type, the atrophy is more evident in the pons and cerebellar areas. Cases of clinically diagnosed FTD and PiD have MRI findings consistent with marked brain atrophy in the frontal and temporal regions, with enlarged supratentorial ventricles.[142]

Other techniques such as MRI voxel-based morphometry has been used to quantify structural neuroanatomical differences on MRI and manifest the distinct patterns of brain atrophy that help distinguish between CBD and other neurodegenerative diseases. In cases of PSP, the technique has focused on cortical and brain stem areas related to ocular motor control.[143] This technique of neuroimaging analysis uses statistical parametric mapping and compares every evaluated brain to a template, considered as normal.[144,145] MRI voxed-based morphometry and diffusion tensor images were able to associate limb apraxia with parietofrontal fractional anisotropy reduction in cases with CBD.[146,147]

Functional imaging with positron emission tomography (PET), single-photon emission computed tomography (SPECT) and proton magnetic resonance spectroscopy (PMRS) have been used in suspected CBD cases to study changes in regional cerebral blood flow (CBF), cerebral metabolism of oxygen or glucose, dopamine receptor binding, and neuronal composition and status.[148–150] CBD patients show an asymmetrical global reduction of cortical oxygen metabolism and side-to-side regional glucose metabolism (fluorodeoxyglucose, FDG) under resting metabolic studies done with PET, most prominent in the cerebral hemisphere contralateral to the most affected limbs and more evident in the inferior parietal, posterior frontal and superior temporal cortex, compared with primary visual cortex, an area that is spared in CBD. There is a relative asymmetrical reduction of CBF and oxygen metabolism in the superior prefrontal cortex, lateral and mesial premotor cortex, and sensorimotor cortex regions.[151–155] Eidelberg and colleagues corroborated the asymmetric regional cerebral glucose reduction in the same areas when compared with PD and normal controls: FDG was not asymmetric in PD cases, although they had asymmetrical parkinsonism and the levels of striatal metabolism were consistently preserved.[156] In functional imaging studies, the most significantly affected subcortical area in CBD cases is the thalamus, where glucose metabolism can be significantly reduced asymmetrically and the caudate and lenticular nuclei may be affected to a lesser degree. Changes in regional CBF can also be studied with technetium-99m hexamethylpropyleneamineoxine (^{99m}Tc-HMPAO) and N-isopropyl-p-(iodine-123) iodoamphetamine (^{123}I-IMP) SPECT. Markus and colleagues[157] found significant asymmetric changes in contralateral parietal cortex in seven out of eight patients with clinically diagnosed CBD, even though the asymmetry was reported in MRI studies in only one patient. Other authors have agreed with this finding, confirming that SPECT may be useful in the study of cases presented as probable CBD.[158,159] Magnetic resonance spectroscopy studies can be used to study regional cerebral metabolism and blood flow in cases of CBD, and these studies suggest neuronal loss or degeneration in the parietal cortex, lentiform nucleus and centrum semiovale, as revealed by significant reduction of *N*-acetylaspartate/choline (NA/Cho) and creatine (NA/Cre) ratios, compared with PD patients. There was also a trend in these studies to reduce the NA/Cho ratio in the frontal cortex as well as brain stem. The significant reduction in the centrum semiovale suggests the degeneration of the axons interconnecting subcortical nuclei with cortical areas. This asymmetry was significant in the parietal cortex, a result that confirms the pathological findings frequently described in CBD cases.[160,161]

Dysfunction of the nigrostriatal dopaminergic system has been demonstrated by decreased PET tracer ^{18}F-6-fluorodopa (^{18}F-dopa) uptake in the caudate and putamen, and moderately reduced postsynaptic mean striatal dopamine receptor 2 (D_2) binding of ^{123}I-iodobenzamide (^{123}I-IBZM) on SPECT scanning, both in an asymmetric fashion.[162] This reduction of the postsynaptic D_2 receptors is not a constant finding, since other studies have found relatively preserved D_2 receptors in cases of CBD.[163] SPECT labeling of the dopamine transporter by 2β-carboxymethoxy-3β(4-iodophenyl)-tropane (^{123}I-β-CIT) and ^{123}I-fluoropropyl (FP)-CIT has demonstrated homogeneous reduction in caudate and putamen to as low as 25% of normal values in clinically diagnosed CBD, PSP, and MSA cases, compared with an asymmetric reduction in PD patients, where binding is selectively reduced in the putamen.[164–168] The characteristic pattern of asymmetrically reduced frontoparietal cerebral cortical metabolism and/or CBF coupled with equal reduction of FP uptake in the caudate and putamen provides strong supportive evidence in a patient with a clinical diagnosis of possible CBD. Decreased presynaptic dopamine D_2 transporter (DAT) binding was found in all CBD cases studied while D_2 receptor binding was reduced in only one patient in a study of eight clinically diagnosed CBD cases.[169–173]

It is not clear the roll that microglia may play in the neurodegenerative disorders so far. Evidence for microglial activation in CBD cases was found with PET studies using a marker of peripheral benzodiazepine-binding sites. Expression of this marker was found to be increased significantly in the frontal lobe, pre and postcentral gyrus, caudate, putamen, SN, and pons of patients with CBD, compared with normal controls.[174,175]

Brain parenchyma sonography is another neuroimaging technique relatively new that uses ultrasound to display the echogenicity of the different tissues and nuclei. Ultrasonography[176] as well as transcranial magnetic stimulation[177] are not fully developed for the diagnosis of neurodegenerative diseases but could represent noninvasive ways to help with the characterization, diagnosis, and study of CBD. Patients diagnosed clinically with CBD were found to have hyperechogenicity in the SN, a finding that is also seen in PD patients but not in cases of PSP and MSA. The neuroimaging studies support the diagnosis of CBD, but there are cases with pathological confirmation of CBD that have normal functional imaging studies years after the beginning of the symptoms.[178]

ELECTROPHYSIOLOGIC STUDIES

Electrophysiologic studies can be useful in the evaluation of patients with CBD to further support the diagnosis. The electroencephalogram (EEG) is usually normal in early stages of the disease. As the disease progresses, the EEG may reveal asymmetric slowing without spike discharges, most prominent over the cerebral hemisphere contralateral to the most affected limb.[179] In later stages, the EEG may show nonspecific bilateral slowing, so the time reference of the EEG in the evaluation of an individual patient can be important. This finding further supports the diagnosis when it correlates with asymmetric radiographic changes in a similar distribution and a typical clinical picture of CBD is present. EEG analysis is important because it may be very characteristic in cases of prion disease, which can mimic a CBD motor clinical presentation.[180]

Electrophysiologic studies of the tremor with accelerometric and electromyographic (EMG) recording techniques demonstrate that the tremor present in CBD clearly differs from the classic parkinsonian tremor: it is mainly an action and postural tremor with higher frequency (6–8 Hz) and more irregular amplitude, with a myoclonic component frequently superimposed.

Study of the myoclonus with electrophysiologic techniques in CBD patients demonstrates action or stimulus sensitive reflex myoclonus. The myoclonus is best recorded using provocative maneuvers: voluntary movement of the affected extremity or auditory or tactile stimulation of the affected limb(s). The myoclonus is originated by brief muscle discharges of 2–3 Hz with simultaneous activation of agonists and antagonist muscles. The activation continues during the period of voluntary muscle movement in the case of action myoclonus. Cortical activity preceding myoclonus can be detected on back-averaged magnetoencephalography but is not consistently evident on EEG recordings of clinically probable CBD cases. The pattern of motor activation of the myoclonus is consistent frequently with a cortical origin, although a subcortical origin cannot always be ruled out.[181,182] Pathophysiologically, reflex myoclonus in CBD may be caused by enhancement of the response to direct sensory input or by exaggeration of inputs/outputs in motor cortical areas due to increased cortical excitability.[54,55] Routine EMG of the extremities is usually normal in early stages or confirms the presence of dystonia or tremor in the affected limb. Nerve conduction studies may show occasional focal or generalized neuropathies that are usually subclinical in the context of the other symptoms.

Somatosensory-evoked potentials (SEP) have minimal utility in evaluating patients with suspected CBD and the results have not been conclusive. The N30 frontal component has been reported absent in symmetrical and asymmetrical way, as well as with increased latency in some patients with clinical diagnosis of CBD. Thalamocortical potentials of the SEP and motor evoked potentials are occasionally reported to be prolonged. Abnormalities on electro-oculography may be evident early in the disease and may help to improve the diagnostic accuracy.[40,183,184] Brain stem auditory evoked potentials and visual evoked potentials are usually of no help for the diagnosis of CBD.[185]

▶ NEUROPATHOLOGY

The neuropathologic diagnosis of CBD requires careful macroscopic, microscopic, histochemical, immunologic and at times biochemical and molecular genetic examination of the tissue. The criteria for the diagnosis are

▶ TABLE 22-2. **PATHOLOGICAL FEATURES OF CBD**

Macroscopic Findings:
- Cerebral cortical atrophy: frontoparietal and perirolandic (may be asymmetric)
- Hydrocephalus ex-vacuo
- Corpus callosum atrophy
- Subcortical atrophy
- Pallor of substantia nigra
- White matter atrophy at the level of internal capsules, cerebral peduncles, and spinal cord

Microscopic Findings:
- Cortical areas: neuronal loss and gliosis
- Balloned achromatic neurons, originating a vacuolar or spongiosis appearance of the cerebral cortex
- Loss of pigmented cells and gliosis in the substantia nigra
- Neurofibrillary tangles in neuronal and glial cells
- Astrocytic plaques
- Neuropil thread-like lesions
- Subcortical areas: neuronal loss and gliosis (globus pallidus, putamen and ventrolateral nucleus of thalamus and subthalamus)
- White matter pathology with swollen axons and demyelination

Tau Pathology:
- Tau positive structures in glial and neuronal cells of cortex, subcortical regions, brain stem, and spinal cord
- Astrocytic plaques
- Tufted astrocytes
- Thorn-shaped astrocytes
- Oligodendroglial coiled bodies
- Pretangles and neurofibrillary tangles (caudate, putamen, SN)
- White matter tau pathology with neuronal inclusions and threads

focused on the presence of neuronal loss and gliosis as well as confirmation of tau positive immunoreactive lesions affecting glial and neuronal processes at cortical and subcortical levels. Use of appropriate stains identifies the underlying tau pathology and rules out other neurodegenerative processes (Table 22–2).

MACROSCOPIC FINDINGS

The typical macroscopic finding is atrophy, mainly of the frontoparietal cortex, that can be asymmetric in the cases of typical motor presentation and correlates with the laterality of the clinical manifestations.[186] Detailed study of the atrophy shows that it is usually most marked in the medial perirolandic superior frontal gyrus, the parasagittal pre- and postcentral gyri, and the superior parietal lobule.[187,188] The distribution of the atrophy may be more generalized, also involving the inferior frontal and temporal lobes in cases presenting with cognitive or language problems as well as in advanced cases. Cingulate and insular cortical regions exhibit variable involvement and the occipital lobe, hippocampus, and parahippocampal gyrus are usually spared.[189] Secondary to the cortical atrophy, hydrocephalus exvacuo and dilatation of the cerebral aqueduct may be seen. Atrophy of subcortical nuclei varies widely from case to case in both severity and topography. The thalamus tends to be smaller than normal, and the head of the caudate may have a flattened appearance. Transverse sections of the brain stem show severe loss of neuromelanin pigment in the SN; however, neuromelanin within the locus ceruleus is usually preserved. Some of these findings may also be seen in PD and other dementia syndromes, but in cases of AD, the locus ceruleus is usually pale and the SN is preserved.[190] Significant atrophy of the pons, inferior olivary nuclei, and cerebellar dentate nuclei suggests an alternative diagnosis such as MSA.

Atrophy of the white matter was not remarkable in the initial cases, but further studies reveal that it can be severe, particularly in regions underlying extensively affected cortex and it is related, at least partially, to retrograde cortical axonal degeneration. The myelin appears pale and the corpus callosum is frequently thin. The anterior limb of the internal capsule may show attenuation, but other white matter pathways are usually unaffected, such as the optic tract, anterior commissure, and fornix. The cerebral peduncles may show atrophy of sections containing corticospinal (middle) and frontopontine (medial) tracts. There may also be atrophy of corticospinal fascicles within the base of the pons and the medullary pyramids.

MICROSCOPIC FINDINGS

Microscopic examination of cortical sections stained with hematoxylin–eosin show a variable amount of neuronal loss and astrogliosis. Specific cholinergic neuronal loss has also been described in cases of CBD and PSP.[191] The cerebral white matter shows mild loss of myelin and gliosis, following the cortical, corticostriatal, and corticobulbar fibers distribution of the atrophy.[192,193]

Ballooned neurons (BN) or swollen achromatic cells represent an important pathologic finding for the diagnosis of CBD. The BN frequently have swollen perikarya and eccentric nuclei, indicative of central chromatolysis and reactive changes to neuronal and axonal damage. The BN lack Nissl substance in the cytoplasm when studied with cresyl violet stain, creating a pale appearance. Due to the presence of BN, the upper cortical layers, mainly laminae 2 and 3, have a vacuolar appearance or spongiosis, a characteristic finding in CBD. This spongiosis of the neocortical and limbic areas is not specific for CBD, and it may be seen in other neurodegenerative

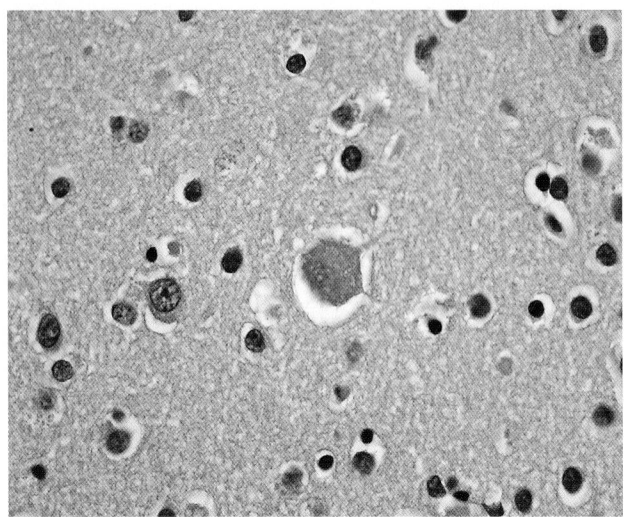

Figure 22–3. Ballooned neuron. 40× (50 bar) in the middle frontal gyrus. (Used with permission from Dr. SL Carrol, UAB Neuropathology.)

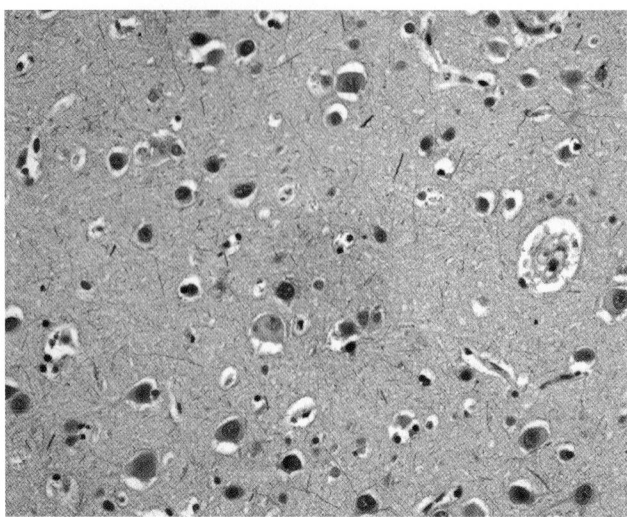

Figure 22–4. A lower-power image of a Bielschowsky stain. 20× (100 bar). This image shows that there are no Alzheimer's type plaques and tangles in an area of dense tau pathology. (Used with permission from Dr. SL Carrol, UAB Neuropathology.)

diseases such as AD, CJD,[194] PSP,[195] and amyotrophic lateral sclerosis (ALS),[196,197] as well as aging, but the presence of BN in the perirolandic region strongly suggests the diagnosis of CBD. The BN are eosinophilic to amphophilic and weakly argyrophilic. Further microscopic studies of the cell organelles has revealed fragmentation of the neuronal Golgi apparatus in CBD as well as in other neurodegenerative diseases such as ALS, CJD, and spinal cerebellar ataxias[198,199] (Fig. 22–3).

Preparations with argyrophilic stains reveal the presence of neurofibrillary tangles (NFT) in neuronal and glial cells. The morphology of the NFT varies from delicate threadlike structures to compact globoid[186,200,201] morphologies, but the typical flame-like appearance of AD tangles is not frequent. Astrocytic plaques are considered the most specific histopathologic feature of CBD and they have glial origin as demonstrated by immunoreactivity to astrocytic glial fibrillary acidic protein and other astrocytic markers.[187] Astrocytic plaques are located mainly in the neocortex and have the appearance of an annular cluster of short processes, resembling the neuritic plaque from AD pathology. Neuropil threads, indicative of dystrophic axonal and glial processes in gray and white matter areas, may also be present in CBD, but neuronal threads are less frequent than in AD pathology. The neuropil thread described in AD is considered to be of neuronal origin, as can be confirmed by immunoelectron microscopy. The remaining neurons of the SN in cases of CBD contain also NFT that are similar to globose NFT of PSP or AD and this pathology is usually mild at the level of the locus ceruleus (Fig. 22–4).

The subcortical nuclei, mainly the globus pallidus and putamen, show variable neuronal loss with gliosis and NFT. The ventrolateral nucleus of the thalamus, subthalamic nuclei, raphe nuclei, and tegmental gray matter may have similar lesions but are usually less severely involved. The fibrillary gliosis typical of PSP in the subthalamic nucleus is not seen consistently in CBD. Cell loss and gliosis in the SN is almost uniformly severe in CBD, with extraneuronal neuromelanin in phagocytes (melanophagia), and without the presence of Lewy bodies, except in elderly cases with associated pathology. The cerebellar dentate nuclei, inferior olivary nuclei, red nucleus, oculomotor complex, and colliculi are relatively spared, but may show a variable degree of neuronal loss and gliosis. The cerebellar cortex may also show different grades of focal or diffuse Purkinje cell axonal torpedoes and Bergmann gliosis.

TAU-ASSOCIATED PATHOLOGY

Tau is a microtubule-associated phosphoprotein expressed in neurons and glial cells that promotes tubulin polymerization and stabilization of microtubules, playing a fundamental role in promoting the integrity of neuronal processes as well as maintaining axoplasmic transport.[202–204] Abnormal deposits of tau positive structures are the major component of the filamentous deposits that are indicative of the tauopathies. It was not clear initially if the dysfunctional tau was the product of the disease or whether the abnormal tau was a byproduct of the neurodegeneration. This was resolved when several tau mutations were described that produced the inability of tau to interact with microtubules and thus promoting aggregation of the protein.[203–208] Tau is normally found in axons, but in the tauopathies the

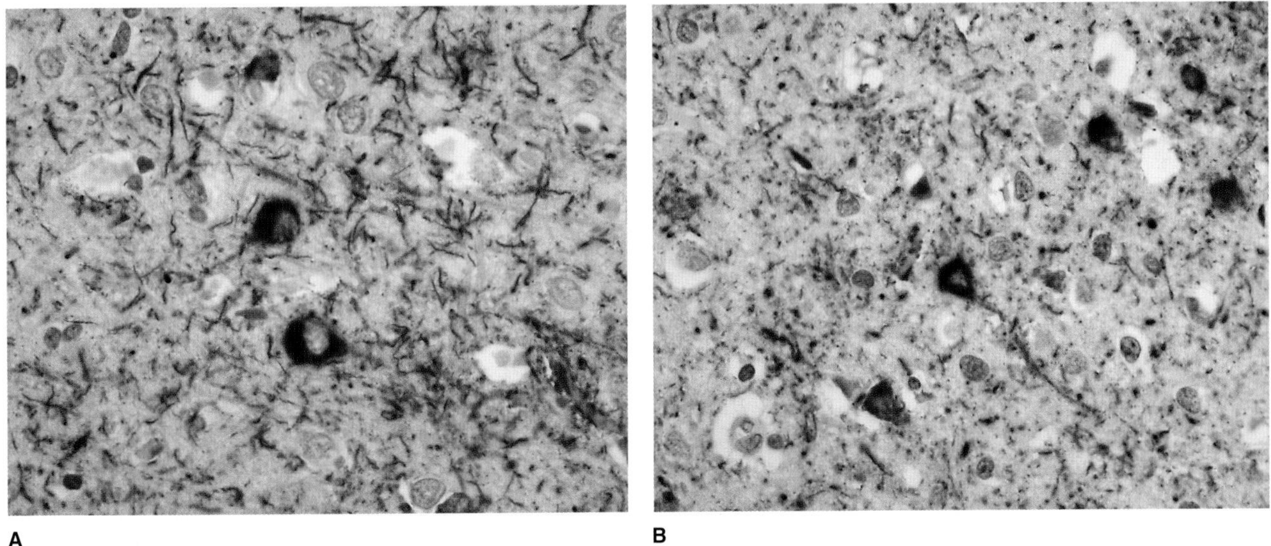

Figure 22–5. **(A,B)** Neurofibrillary tangles (NFT) 40× (50 bar). These images show paired helical filaments (PHF) tau positive antibodies in NFT within neurons in the middle frontal gyrus. These NFTs are set against a background of numerous PHF tau positive astrocytic threads. (Used with permission from Dr. SL Carrol, UAB Neuropathology.)

lesions with aggregation of proteins appear distributed in the cell body and dendrites. Tau protein undergoes selective phosphorylation, which controls its functional state. Normal tau is soluble and heat-stable, but it forms aggregates and becomes insoluble under pathological conditions. Tau pathology may originate from abnormal phosphorylation and selective reduction, or from loss or alteration of the different isoforms.[209–212] The presence of tau pathology may be demonstrated with specific immunohistochemical methods, using different monoclonal antibodies specific to tau protein, as well as with Gallyas silver stain preparations.[205]

Abnormal deposits of tau positive structures are the most important diagnostic finding in CBD and the other tauopathies.[206] The tau pathology in CBD is more extensive that the macroscopic findings and involves neuronal and glial cells in the cortex, subcortical nuclei, brain stem, and spinal cord. The distribution of tau positive immunoreactivity in most affected cells is pleomorphic, presented as diffuse or granular cytoplasmic deposits, called pretangles and more frequently located in cell bodies and proximal cell structures of neurons and glia. The tau lesions of the NFT are highly organized in deposits that appear similar to the threadlike structures of AD or globoid inclusions typical of PSP. The ultrastructure of the tangle in CBD consists of a 15 nm straight and paired helical or twisted stranded filaments with wider diameter than the filaments found in AD.[201,207] The tangles found in PSP cases have more straight and uniform filaments with compact and globoid configuration.[208,209] The immunocytochemical staining of BN is weakly positive for tau protein and immunoreactive for phosphorylated neurofilaments, αB-crystallin, heat-shock proteins and sometimes ubiquitin, but it is negative for amyloid (Fig. 22–5A,B).

The tau positive immunoreactive glial inclusions in the astrocytic plaques are probably the most characteristic lesion of CBD, although it can be present in other tauopathies[210] (Fig. 22–6A,B). Astrocytic plaques may resemble the neuritic plaque of AD, but they do not contain amyloid and are mainly found in proximity to astrocytic processes, instead of dystrophic neurons. The astrocytic plaques are located mainly in the neocortex, although they may be detected in the striatum as well.[211] Another lesion similar to the astrocytic plaque is the so called tufted astrocyte, which consists of fibrillary accumulations of tau within cell bodies and processes, and is believed to be more characteristic of PSP than of CBD.[212,213] Thorn shape astrocytes are also tau positive lesions, located at subpial and perivascular spaces that can be found in CBD, normal aging and other pathologies. Tau positive threads in CBD are believed to be present mainly in glial processes and are derived from astrocytes, while in AD the threads are localized mainly to neuronal processes and considered of neuronal origin. Coiled bodies are tau-positive inclusions in oligodendroglia, frequently present in CBD as well as in other tauopathies. The appearance of the coiled bodies is of a fine bundle of filaments coiled around a core located at cortical and subcortical preparations. These inclusions are distinct from the oligodendroglial inclusions that are the hallmark of MSA, called glial cytoplasmic inclusions, which are immunoreactively positive for alpha-synuclein and ubiquitin but negative for tau protein[214] (Fig. 22–7A,B).

In the subcortical structures, the caudate and putamen, as well as the SN and the nucleus basalis of Meynert

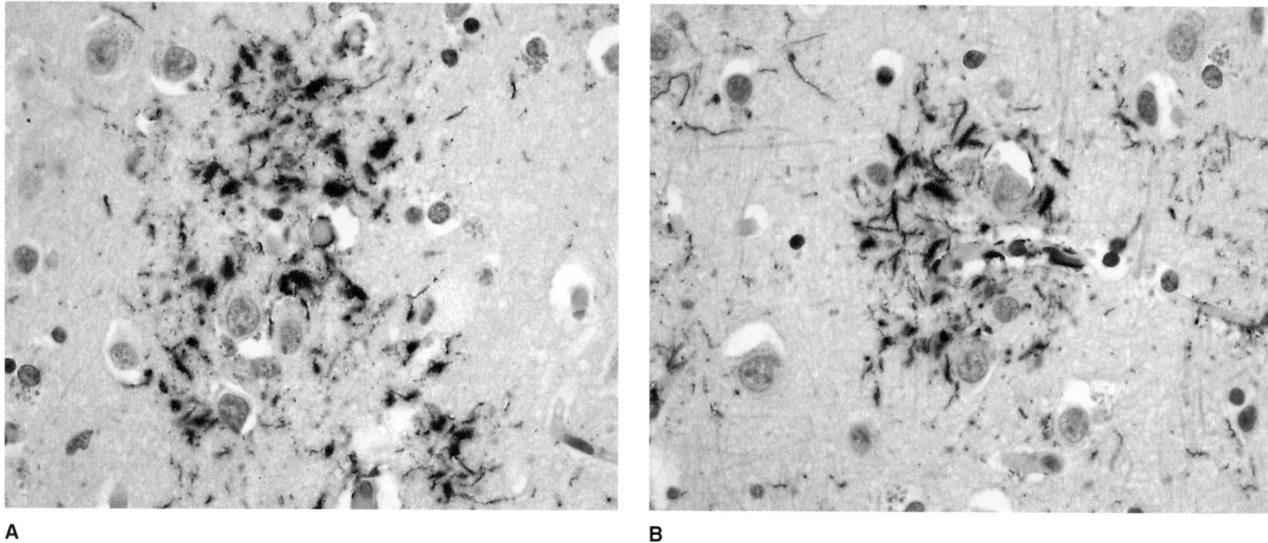

Figure 22-6. **(A,B)** Astrocytic plaques 40× (50 bar). Images of astrocytic plaques in the superficial white matter of the middle frontal gyrus. (Used with permission from Dr. SL Carrol, UAB Neuropathology.)

contain tau-immunoreactive lesions, most numerous in the form of pretangles, and less frequently as NFT. White matter areas not contiguous to cortical atrophy in CBD may also contain tau-immunoreactive threadlike lesions and coiled bodies. Some studies found white matter pathology to be more abundant in PSP cases than in CBD by immunohistochemical analysis, although the internal capsule and thalamic fasciculus often have many threadlike processes in CBD.[215,216] Involvement also of the spinal cord with tau positive neuronal inclusions and threads, mainly at the level of the cervical intermediate gray matter, has been described in CBD and PSP cases.[217–219]

TAU BIOCHEMISTRY AND GENETIC ANALYSIS

The tauopathies have a fundamental abnormality in tau processing that causes the abnormal isoform composition, hyperphosphorylation and finally aggregation of the protein. The abnormal protein aggregates can be

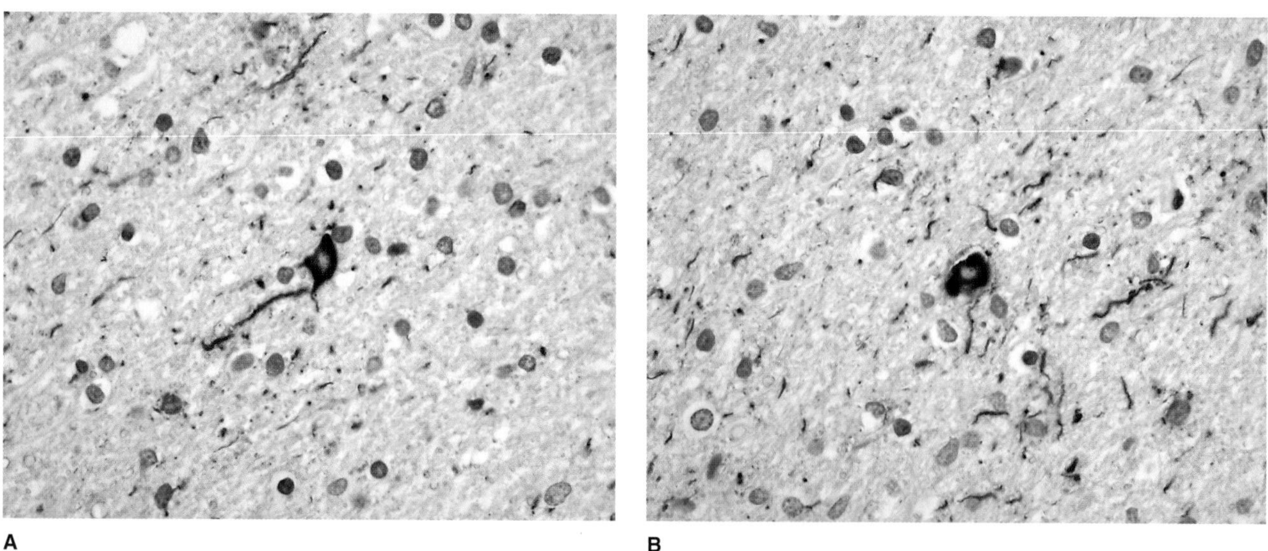

Figure 22-7. **(A,B)** Coiled Bodies 40× (50 bar). The images show PHF tau-positive coiled bodies (tau-positive oligodendroglial inclusions) in the white matter underlying the middle frontal gyrus. (Used with permission from Dr. SL Carrol, UAB Neuropathology.)

isolated from brain tissue as detergent-insoluble tau fractions, and analyzed for isoform composition and phosphorylation state.[220–224]

The tau gene is located on chromosome 17 and has 16 exons. The major tau protein in the human brain is encoded by 11 exons. The variable tau mRNA splicing of exons 2, 3, and 10 results in 6 different tau isoforms that are phosphorylated at specific serine and threonine residues.[225–226] Three of these isoforms carry the segment specified by exon 10 (E10) and when this is included, the result is a protein with 4 microtubule-binding repeats (4-repeat, 4R tau) and when E10 is excluded, the result is a protein with 3 microtubule–binding repeats (3-repeat, 3R tau).[227] The binding domains are located in the carboxy-terminus of the protein, and under normal circumstances, there are the same concentrations of 4R and 3R tau. Phosphorylation of tau is regulated by a group of kinases, but hyperphosphorylation and exon splitting may alter the affinity of tau filaments and can result in self-assembly of tangles with helical and straight filaments and microtubules and these may cause protein aggregates that constitute the pathologic changes of the tauopathies. The 4R isoforms are better at stabilizing microtubules than those with 3R binding domains.[228] The insoluble tau from CBD, PSP and argyriphilic grain disease (AGD) cases have elevated 4R/3R ratios, compared with AD and normal aging controls. Studies of the tau aggregates found in CBD and PSP revealed similar epitopes to each other but distinct from that of AD. Despite clinical and pathologic heterogeneity, a unifying genetic etiology appears likely between PSP and CBD.[229–231] In PiD cases, the insoluble tau consists of elevated levels of 3R tau. In contrast, the insoluble tau of AD shows ratios of 4R/3R that are similar to normal control brains, but the tau is abnormally phosphorylated and hyperphosphorylated. The tau pathology in AD is thought to be mediated, at least in part, by the amyloid cascade, causing the hyperphosphorylation at the level of the neuritic plaques.[232]

Dysfunction of the tau protein was initially found to cause neurodegeneration and dementia in cases of FTDP-17. The morphology of the filaments and isoform composition vary among the different tauopathies but it is the repeat region with the amino and carboxy terminal region that forms the core of the filaments. In the cases of FTDP-17, two main types of mutations (missense and splite site) originate an abnormal tau protein that alters the 4R/3R ratios and could trigger neurodegeneration.[233–240]

A selective loss or reduction in the levels of all six tau isoforms has been also described in sporadic cases of FTD and are classified as tau deficient tauopathies.[241–244] The variability of the different tauopathies is probably related to the presence of other genes and essential factors that may influence the neurodegenerative process.[240] These factors affecting the abnormal processing of tau are not well understood, however, a detailed genetic analysis of the tau gene and haplotype structure has revealed two ancestral haplotypes, called H1 and H2. In cases of CBD and PSP, H1 homozygosity (H1/H1) is overexpressed in close to 90% of patients, compared with 60% of normal controls.[245,246] These findings suggest that genetic polymorphisms of the tau gene may influence the risk of developing the sporadic 4R tau diseases.[247] The H1 and H1/H1 haplotype cases displayed lower regional gray matter volume in MRI studies, compared with healthy subjects. These data may suggest that H1 haplotype is associated with a particular cerebral morphology that may increase the susceptibility of the healthy carriers to develop neurodegenerative diseases such as sporadic tauopathies. One of these mutations, seen only in astrocytic plaques in cases of CBD, include the DJ-1 gene that is associated with autosomal recessive PD and both 3R and 4R tau isoforms.[248–250] Other mutations originating TAR-DNA-binding protein 43 (TDP-43) were mainly found in a glial distribution and in 15% of cases with CBD. Additional modifying factors and mutations may ultimately contribute to the development of abnormal tau protein composition and tau aggregation.[251]

▶ HETEROGENEITY AND OVERLAP IN NEURODEGENERATIVE DISEASES

The clinical phenotype and the pathological findings overlap significantly between the neurodegenerative disorders. Most recently LRRK2 mutations have been associated with pleomorphic pathology leading to speculation on an upstream role of the mutations in the cascade of events triggering both tauopathies and alpha-synucleinopathies.[15,252] In this regard we can identify several general types of pathological diagnostic situations that may be encountered. First, there are situations where two different diseases may be present concomitantly. A common example is PD and AD and the explanation of a coincidence for both diseases looks unlikely based on the results of several studies that suggested the development of dementia in PD patients to more likely result from progression of Lewy body pathology to the cortex than from coexistent AD pathology.[253–257] The study of Lewy body presence and distribution in cases of AD showed the presence of this pathology in 20–40% with a higher frequency in limbic areas.[253,258–261] These findings suggest that amyloid and perhaps tau pathology may trigger abnormalities in α-synuclein processing. Experimental support for this hypothesis was provided by Masliah and colleagues when beta-amyloid pathology was shown to facilitate α-synuclein accumulation and neuronal deficits in a transgenic mouse model of AD and PD.[262] There are cases where related diseases have overlapping pathology.

This is particularly relevant to CBD where there may be overlapping or coexisting features with other forms of tauopathies and/or synucleinopathies. In these cases the predominant pathological phenotype is reported, along with other changes.

The pathology underlying sporadic frontotemporal lobar degeneration syndrome (FTLD) that includes frontotemporal dementia, primary progressive aphasia and semantic dementia is heterogeneous and not predictable.[263,264] This syndrome may show cortical atrophy, spongiosis, and gliosis, and BN may be present.[265,266] One finding that may be present in this disorder is ubiquitin-positive/tau-negative inclusions. This lack of visible tau pathology should help with differentiation from CBD, but clinical phenotypes with pathological findings of CBD have been described. These patients may also have concomitant motor neuron disease with the same inclusions identified in familial FTDP-17.[267] The pathological differentiation between CBD and FTDP-17 was not possible in the study reported by Dickson and colleagues[186] Both disorders have widespread cortical and subcortical tau pathology and BN, and family history with genetic studies was crucial in making the diagnosis in these cases.

There is substantial neuropathological overlap between CBD and PiD, and the "Pick's complex" cases. BN, variable degeneration of the SN and basal ganglia, and tau-positive inclusions occur in both disorders. However, Pick bodies, a characteristic feature of PiD, are rarely observed in CBD. Although both disorders exhibit cortical atrophy, in PiD the temporal cortex and the hippocampus are usually involved and the perirolandic sensorimotor cortex is often spared. CBD and PiD can also have overlapping clinical features, and CBD patients may manifest behavioral changes and language disturbances, at times as the initial presentation. The main features to determine the pathological diagnosis in PiD are related to the presence of Pick bodies and involvement of the limbic and neocortices with less subcortical involvement, and usually in a symmetric distribution. The SN and brain stem nuclei are only mildly affected in PiD, and tau-positive immunoreactive lesions are located mainly in the neurons. PiD and CBD may have numerous BN in cortex but, in the CBD cases, this pathology usually extends outside the limbic cortices.

AGD is a newly recognized tauopathy with neuronal and glial tau-positive lesions and BN.[268,269] AGD pathology is mainly restricted to the medial temporal lobe and hypothalamus and includes elevated 4R tau isoforms.[270–273]

Links among these disorders may occur also at a genetic level. The apolipoprotein E4 allele is recognized as a major risk factor for familial and sporadic AD.[274,275] However, some studies observed an increased frequency of the E4 allele in CBD, PiD, and PSP, compared to that of control populations. Finally, tau mutations are found in only 25% of sporadic cases without familial history of neurodegenerative disease.[276] This broad heterogeneity in phenotype, pathology, different age of presentation of symptoms, and duration of disease suggests that mutations may be influenced also by multiple other modifiers.[277]

▶ CLINICAL DIFFERENTIAL DIAGNOSIS

The different phenotypes of CBD reflect the variability of distribution and severity of neuronal loss and pathological changes. A broad view is that CBD should be considered in the differential diagnosis of a parkinsonian or a cognitive disorder with atypical features[37,47] Table 22–3. The typical pattern of CBD presenting mainly with motor deficits, and cortical signs such as apraxia and/or cortical sensory loss, is usually sufficiently distinctive such that, when fully developed, it would allow a confident clinical diagnosis and not be confused with PD. The best early clues that can help to distinguish CBD from idiopathic PD are the lack of beneficial response to dopaminergic medication and the signs of cortical dysfunction, most notably apraxia and/or cortical sensory impairment. Many other neurodegenerative diseases can mimic CBD. The differential diagnosis list of the motoric presentation of CBD includes PSP[278] and MSA, either the parkinsonian or cerebellar phenotype.[279–282] Primary dementing and behavioral disorders should also be included in the differential diagnosis: atypical PiD,[283–285] Lewy body dementia (LBD), PD with dementia, AD with extrapyramidal features,[286] AGD,[287] the parkinsonism-dementia-ALS complex,[288–290] and the FTD syndromes, including primary progressive aphasia and semantic dementia pictures. Other diagnoses described as mimickers of CBD are widespread cerebrovascular disease, multi-infarct disorders and variants of the Binswanger's disease,[291] progressive multifocal leukodystrophies and hereditary diffuse leukoencephalopathy with spheroids, [292–296] Wilson's disease,[297] Huntington's disease,[298] hemiatrophy-hemiparkinson syndrome,[299] variants of Azorean disease and SCA 8,[300–303] late-onset Hallervorden–Spatz disease,[304,305] and adult neuronal ceroid lipofuscinosis,[306] all of which typically differ in several clinical and pathological features. CBD has been also presented as a Balint's syndrome[307] and a case of neuropsyphilis resembling CBD has been described.[308]

PSP is the atypical parkinsonian disorder most likely to be confused with CBD. PSP classically presents with prominent axial rigidity, postural instability with frequent early falls, and abnormal vertical eye movements. Several cases of "atypical PSP" have been reported, with clinical features similar to those of CBD. Atypical features such

▶ **TABLE 22-3. CLINICAL DIFFERENTIAL DIAGNOSIS OF NEURODEGENERATIVE DISEASES**

Diagnosis	Clinical Features	Features Suggesting an Alternative Diagnosis
CBD	Asymmetric parkinsonism with lack of response to medications. Apraxia. Dystonia, myoclonus, action tremor cortical sensory loss, alien limb phenomenon. Cognitive dysfunction, language problems.	Typical resting tremor, good response to medications. Early severe gait disorder/falls. Severe axial dystonia. Prominent autonomic symptoms. Early vertical gaze palsy.
PSP	Supranuclear ophthalmoplegia, symmetric symptoms. Severe gait disorder and falls. Pseudobulbar palsy and axial dystonia. Dysarthria, dysphagia. Executive dysfunction.	Asymmetric symptoms. Lack of eye movements abnormalities. Apraxia, alien limb phenomenon, cortical sensory loss. Prominent cognitive dysfunction.
MSA	Symmetric symptoms. Lack of typical resting tremor. Cerebellar and pyramidal symptoms. Autonomic dysfunction. Suboptimal response to medication.	Apraxia, cortical sensory symptoms. Early or prominent ocular dysfunction. Prominent cognitive dysfunction.
FTD/Pick's Syndromes	Behavioral dysfunction, frontal lobe syndrome, personality changes, desinhibition. Speech and language problems. Cognitive dysfunction.	Gait disorder, ocular symptoms. Asymmetric parkinsonism, motor cortical symptoms, cerebellar symptoms. Severe autonomic dysfunction. Response to medications
PD-Dementia/ DLBD	Asymmetric parkinsonism, early memory problems, fluctuating symptoms, gait disorder. Mild response to medications and dopaminergic-induced psychosis.	Symmetric parkinsonian syndrome or asymmetric dystonia, apraxia, or alien limb phenomenon. Prominent gait disorder and ophtalmoplegia. Frontal lobe syndrome. Autonomic dysfunction
AD with Parkinsonism	Early memory problems. Visuospatial and language changes. Mild parkinsonian syndrome with modest response to medications. Insidious progression.	Initial parkinsonian syndrome with minimal cognitive disorder. Frontal syndrome. Severe gait disorder and ophtalmoplegia. Apraxia and cortical sensory symptoms. Cerebellar syndrome and profound autonomic disorder.
CJD	Rapid course of dementia, personality changes. Apraxia, myoclonus. Pyramidal, extrapyramidal symptoms. Prominent gait apraxia/cerebellar syndrome.	Asymmetric, typical parkinsonism or cortical symptoms. Lack of cognitive dysfunction. Symptoms present for long time. Response to medications.

Abbreviations: CBD, corticobasal degeneration; CJD, Creutzfeldt–Jakob disease; DLBD, dementia with Lewy bodies; FTD, frontotemporal dementia; PD, Parkinson's disease; PSP, progressive supranuclear palsy; MSA, multisystem atrophy.

as asymmetric onset, mild oculomotor impairment, focal dystonia, and involuntary limb levitation resembling the alien limb phenomenon are the most frequent features that may cause confusion with CBD.[309]

Asymmetric cortical degenerations including PiD, primary progressive aphasia, and FTDP-17 may present with features resembling early CBD, such as focal myoclonus, apraxia, alien limb phenomenon, and asymmetric rigidity.[310] In FTDP-17 there are usually several family members affected. These syndromes, in general, lack the prominent and progressive extrapyramidal dysfunction characteristic of the typical motoric presentation of CBD. Cases with either a motoric or cognitive presentation with a rapidly progressive picture should raise the possible diagnosis of prion-related diseases.[311–313]

There is significant overlap of these disorders with CBD, not only at the clinical level but also at pathological and molecular levels as discussed earlier. The delineation of specific molecular and genetic markers for each disorder or the factors that modify the initial neurodegenerative event will help to further characterize the different diseases.

▶ THERAPY

Pharmacotherapy for CBD cases is ineffective or produced limited benefit in most of the cases. Currently pharmacological treatment is mainly symptomatic and oriented to modify the abnormal motor manifestations (such as myoclonus, dystonia, and/ or tremor) and ameliorate the neuropsychological problems. There is little or no beneficial response to dopaminergic medication; indeed, this is an initial characteristic feature and probably related to the widespread pathological involvement of cortical and subcortical neuronal systems.

The future treatment of CBD and the tauopathies must be directed to better understanding the molecular mechanisms that mediate tau neurotoxicity and develop options to alter the process. We know that the pathological hyperphosphorylation and aggregation of the tau protein plays a central role in the neuronal dysfunction and neurodegeneration. The hyperphosphorylation of tau results in an imbalance between the activities of tau kinases and tau phosphatases. Some of the experimental therapeutic options that are being considered for the treatment of the tauopathies include decreasing the activity of the protein phosphatases that promote abnormal hyperphosphorylation, as well as the use of specific protein kinases that will change the abnormal tau conformation and interactions.[314–316]

TREATMENT OF MOTOR SYMPTOMS

Mild improvement of the parkinsonian features in CBD with the treatment of carbidopa/levodopa was only reported in one quarter of patients clinically diagnosed with CBD in retrospective studies.[317–319] The rest of the dopaminergic agents (dopamine agonists, amantadine, MAO-B and COMT inhibitors) may produce more side effects with less clinical benefits and they are usually not indicted. Clonazepam or the other benzodiazepines, usually in small doses, have been the most beneficial agents for the treatment of myoclonus and action tremor. Baclofen, tizanidine, dantrolene, and cyclobenzaprine or methocarbamol may improve rigidity and tremor also but to a lesser degree. Anticholinergics are usually poorly tolerated in this group of patients, especially if cognitive problems are present, and are overall not recommended. Botulinum toxin injections may be useful in the treatment of painful focal dystonias as well as for blepharospasm. If the blepharospasm does not respond to the treatment with botulinum toxin, it may indicate eyelid opening apraxia. Stereotactic surgeries with lesions or deep brain stimulation have shown little or no benefit in atypical parkinsonian disorders.[320]

TREATMENT OF COGNITIVE AND NEUROPSYCHIATRIC SYMPTOMS

Treatments of cognitive dysfunction with medications that enhance cholinergic neurotransmitters have not been studied well but probably have limited benefit. Depression, apathy, and obsessive–compulsive symptomatology may be treated with some efficacy with serotonin reuptake inhibitors, but cautious tritation and low doses are recommended because these medications can exacerbate agitation. Antidepressants with anticholinergic side-effects, including tricyclic compounds, may also exacerbate confusion. More severe obsessive compulsive symptoms as well as paranoid delusions, psychotic behavior, severe agitation, and irritability may be treated with small doses of atypical neuroleptic medications such as quetiapine, olanzapine, or clozapine. The use of typical antipsychotic medications such as haloperidol may worsen parkinsonian motor symptoms and are not recommended. The use of transcranial magnetic stimulation for treatment of depression and other psychiatric symptoms is still investigational.[321]

TREATMENT OF OTHER SYMPTOMS

Gastrointestinal symptoms described in cases of CBD include dysphagia, hypersalivation, nausea, esophageal reflux, and constipation. The goal of treatment of the dysphagia is to maintain safe and efficient nutrition and hydration. Evaluation of the dysphagia with a barium swallow study may be necessary to further determine the place and level of the abnormality. Treatment includes dietary modifications, postural changes, swallowing maneuvers and exercises, and surgical interventions in some specific cases. Selection of foods with a consistency that facilitates swallowing is a critical aspect and some patients may require thickened liquids. If they are not able to ingest enough food to meet nutritional requirements, placement of a percutaneous feeding gastrostomy tube may be needed, although the decision to place a gastrostomy in a patient with a chronically progressive neurodegenerative disease must be handled on an individual basis. Excessive salivation may respond to small doses of anticholinergic therapy, but side-effects are a limiting factor in most cases. The use of antiemetics should be oriented to short periods of treatment and dopamine blocking antiemetic medications should be avoided. The use of histamine-2 blocker medications is helpful for gastroesophageal reflux problems in this group of patients. Constipation in parkinsonism is very frequently reported by patients and can be the result of gastrointestinal outlet dysfunction, colonic hypomotility, or both. Constipation also has been associated with pelvic floor dystonia and the incidence of obstructions is overall increased in the parkinsonian syndromes. The appropriate intake of fluids is usually one of the most important preventive therapies, but the use of stool softeners, foods rich in fiber, and laxatives may be beneficial and necessary. Polyethylene glycol or similar compounds are another alternative for severe constipation. The urinary symptoms in CBD patients are mainly urgency and frequency, and they may improve with the use of hyoscyamine, tolterodine, or oxybutynin. Close observation for central and peripheral anticholinergic side-effects is warranted when using these or related medications.

Sleep problems, mainly insomnia and fragmented sleep, may be treated with small doses of sedative hypnotics or atypical neuroleptic agents. They may be helpful to decrease sleep latency and increase total sleep time but one must keep in mind that they may exacerbate confusion and agitation. Benzodiacepines and agents such as diphenhydramine, chloral hydrate, and zolpidem may have a relative role. Symptomatic orthosthatic hypotension, although more frequently seen in MSA, may be treated with fludrocortisone, midodrine, or droxidopa. Pain related to severe dystonic contraction can be lessened by maintenance of good range of motion, and occasionally splinting can be helpful. Gabapentin and other modifiers of the pain threshold have been tried in the dystonias and pain syndromes without much success. The painful dystonias may be resistant even to the use of narcotic medications. Speech therapy may offer practical suggestions and exercises to optimize speech function and guard against aspiration secondary to swallowing difficulty. Good home care assistance may help prolong the time a patient can remain at home before requiring nursing home placement. Prevention and aggressive treatment of dehydration, infection, and other metabolic abnormalities are necessary in CBD patients to avoid toxic encephalopathy, which can worse motor and cognitive function.

Other aspects of patient care, not involving pharmacotherapy, can be of special importance for these patients and their families, although a small number of patients have been studied. Physical therapy interventions to maintain mobility and prevent contractures may have some general benefit.[322,323] Occupational therapy can help patients maintain some degree of functional independence by providing specially made devices such as eating utensils with large handles. Patients with severe cognitive symptoms and their families require similar treatments and support measures as are used in AD patients.

▶ ACKNOWLEDGEMENT

We would like to thank Bruce Wainer, MD, PhD, for his contributions to this chapter in the second edition, some of which has been carried over to this chapter in the third edition. Suzanne S. Mirra, MD, Randal P. Brewer, MD, and Julie A. Schhneider, MD, contributed to this chapter in the first edition. This work was supported in part by The UAB Parkinson Research Fund, the Sartain Lanier Family Foundation, the Mary Louise Morris Brown Foundation, and the American Parkinson Disease Association.

REFERENCES

1. Rebeiz JJ, Kolodny EH, and Richardson EP. Corticodentatonigral degeneration with neuronal achromasia: A progressive disorder of late adult life. Trans Am Neurol Assoc 1967;92:23–26.
2. Gibb WRG, Luthert PJ, and Marsden CD. Corticobasal degeneration. Brain 1989;112:1171–1192.
3. Kertesz A, Martinez-Lage P, Davidson W, et al. The corticobasal degeneration syndrome overlaps progressive aphasia and frontotemporal dementia. *Neurology* 2000;55:1368–1375.
4. Case Records of the Massachusetts General Hospital (Case 38-1985) (Case of corticonigral degeneration with neuronal achromasia). N Engl J Med 1985;313:739–748.
5. Rebeiz JJ, Kolodny EH, and Richardson EP. Corticodentatonigral degeneration with neuronal achromasia. Arch Neurol 1968;18:20–33.
6. Riley DE and Lang AE. Cortical-basal ganglionic degeneration. In Appel SH (ed). Current Neurology (12). St. Louis: Mosby, 1992, pp.155–171.
7. Obeso JA, Rothwell JC, and Lang AE, et al. Myoclonic dystonia. Neurology 1983;33:825–830.
8. Charcot JM. Leçons du mardi: Policlinique de la Salpêtrière. Paris: Bureaux du Progrès Médical 1887–1888.
9. Charcot JM and Vulpian A. De la paralysie agitante. Gazette Hebdomadaire de Médecine et de Chirurgie 1861–1862:8:765–767; 8: 616–820; 9:54–59;
10. Ballan G and Tison F. A historical case of probable corticobasal degeneration? Mov Disord 1997;12(6):1073–1074.
11. Watts RL, William RS, Growdon JH, et al. Corticobasal ganglionic degeneration. Neurology 1985;35(1):178.
12. Grimes DA, Lang AE, and Bergeron CB. Dementia as the most common presentation of cortical-basal ganglionic degeneration. Neurology 1999;53:1969–1974.
13. Kurz AF. Uncommon neurodegenerative causes of dementia. Int Psychogeriatr 2005;17 (1):S35–S49.
14. Galpern WR and Lang AE. Interface between tauopathies and synucleionopathies: A tale of two proteins. Ann Neurol 2006;59(3):449–458.
15. Newman J, Rissman RA, Sarsoza F, et al. Caspase-cleaved tau accumulation in neurodegenerative diseases associated with tau and α-synuclein pathology. J Acta Neuropathologica 2005;10(2)135–144.
16. Tanner CM. Epidemiologic approaches to cortical-basal ganglionic degeneration. Mov Disord 1996;11:346–357.
17. Wenning GK, Litvan I, Jankovic J, et al. Natural history and survival of 14 patients with corticobasal degeneration confirmed at postmortem examination. J Neurol Neurosurg Psychiatry 1998;64:184–189.

18. Watts RL, Mirra SS, and Richardson EP. Corticobasal ganglionic degeneration. In Marsden CD, Fahn S (eds). Movement Disorders 3. London: Butterworths, 1994, pp. 282–299.
19. DePold Hohler A, Ranson BR, Chun MR, et al. The youngest reported case of corticobasal degeneration. Parkinsonism Relat Disord 2003;10(1): 47–50.
20. Brown J, Lantos PL, and Rossor MN. Familial dementia lacking specific pathological features presenting with clinical features of corticobasal degeneration. J Neurol Neurosurg Psychiatry 1998;65:600–603.
21. Di Maria E, Tabaton M, Vigo T, et al. Corticobasal degeneration shares a common genetic background with progressive supranuclear palsy. Ann Neurol 2000;47:374–377.
22. Tuite PJ, Clark HB, Bergeron C, et al. Clinical and pathological evidence of corticobasal degeneration and progressive supranuclear palsy in familial tauopathy. Arch Neurol 2005;62(9):1453–1457.
23. Uchihara T and Nakayama H. Familial tauopathy mimicking corticobasal degeneration and autopsy study on three siblings. J Neurol Sci 2006;15;246(1–2):45–51.
24. Verin M, Rancurel G, De Marco O, et al. First familial cases of corticobasal degeneration. Mov Disord 1997;12:55.
25. Brown J, Lantos PL, Roques P, et al. Familial dementia with swollen achromatic neurons and corticobasal inclusion bodies: A clinical and pathological study. J Neurol Sci 1996;135:21–30.
26. Scaravilli T, Tolosa E, and Ferrer I. Progressive supranuclear palsy and corticobasal degeneration: lumping versus splitting. Mov Disord 2005;20(l)12:S21–S28.
27. Bergeron C, Davis A, and Lang AE. Corticobasal ganglionic degeneration and progressive supranuclear palsy presenting with cognitive decline. Brain Pathology 1998;8(2):355–365.
28. Beatty WW, Scott JG, Wilson DA, et al. Memory deficits in a demented patient with probable corticobasal degeneration. J Geriatr Psychiatry Neurol 1995;8:132–136.
29. Riley DE and Lang AE. Cortical-basal ganglionic degeneration. In Stern MB, Koller WC (eds). Parkinsonian Syndromes. New York: Marcel Dekker, 1993, pp. 379–392.
30. Caselli RJ. Asymmetric cortical degeneration syndromes. Curr Opin Neurol 1996;9:276–280.
31. Riley DE and Lang AE. Cortical-basal ganglionic degeneration in Appel SH (ed): Current Neurology (12). St. Louis: Mosby, 1992, pp. 155–171.
32. Case records of the Massachusetts General Hospital. Case16. N Engl J Med 1986;314:1101–1111.
33. Greene PE, Fahn S, Lang AE, et al. Progressive unilateral rigidity, bradykinesia, tremulousness, and apraxia, leading to fixed postural deformity of the involved limb. Mov Disord 1990;5:341–351.
34. Lang AE. Parkinsonism in corticobasal degeneration. Adv Neurol 2000;82:83–89.
35. Riley DE, Lang AE, Lewis A, et al. Cortical-basal ganglionic degeneration. Neurology 1990;40:1203–1212.
36. Litvan I, Bhatia KP, Burn DJ, et al. Movement Disorders Society Scientific Issues Committee report: SIC Task Force appraisal of clinical diagnostic criteria for Parkinsonian disorders. Mov Disord 2003;18(5):467–486.
37. Rinne JO, Lee MS, Thompson PD, et al. Corticobasal degeneration: A clinical study of 36 cases. Brain 1994;117:1183–1196.
38. Lang AE. Corticobasal ganglionic degeneration presenting with "progressive loss of speech output and orofacial dyspraxia". J Neurol Neurosurg Psychiatry 1992;55:1101.
39. Maraganore DM, Ahlskog JE, and Petersen RC. Progressive asymmetric rigidity with apraxia: A distinctive clinical entity. Mov Disord 1992;7:80.
40. Litvan I, Agid Y, Goetz CG, et al. Accuracy of the clinical diagnosis of corticobasal degeneration: A clinicopathologic study. Neurology 1997;48:119–125.
41. Litvan I, Agid Y, Jankovic J, et al. Accuracy of clinical criteria for the diagnosis of progressive supranuclear palsy (Steele-Richardson-Olszewski syndrome). Neurology 1996;46:922–930.
42. Rivest J, Quinn N, and Marsden CD. Dystonia in Parkinson's disease, multiple system atrophy, and progressive supranuclear palsy. Neurology 1990;40:1571–1578.
43. Collins SJ, Ahlskog JE, Parisi JE, et al. Progressive supranuclear palsy: Neuropathologically based diagnostic clinical criteria. J Neurol Neurosurg Psychiatry 1995;58: 167–173.
44. Gibb WRG, Luther PJ, and Marsden CD. Corticobasal degeneration. Brain 1989;112:1171–1192.
45. Graham NL, Bak T, and Hodges JR. Corticobasal degeneration as a cognitive disorder. Mov Disord 2003;18(11):1224–1232.
46. Lang AE, Riley DE, and Bergeron C. Cortical-basal ganglionic degeneration in Calne DB (ed): Neurodegenerative Diseases. Philadelphia: WB Saunders, 1994, pp. 877–894.
47. Schneider JA, Watts RL, Gearing M, et al. Corticobasal degeneration: Neuropathological and clinical heterogeneity. Neurology 1994;48:959–989.
48. Stover NP and Watts RL. Corticobasal degeneration. Semin Neurol 2001;21:49–58.
49. Brunt ERP, Van Weerden TW, Pruim J, et al. Unique myoclonic pattern in corticobasal degeneration. Mov Disord 1995;10:132–142.
50. Thompson PD and Shibasaki H. Myoclonus in corticobasal degeneration and other neurodegenerations. Adv Neurol 2000;82:69–81.
51. Shibasaki H. Myoclonus. Curr Opin Neurology 1995;8(4):331–334.
52. Hu WT, Rippon GW, Boeve BF, et al. Alzheimer's disease and corticobasal degeneration presenting as corticobasal syndrome. Mov Disord 2009;15;24(9):1375–1379.
53. Carella F, Scaioli V, Franceschetti S, et al. Focal reflex myoclonus in corticobasal degeneration. Funct Neurol 1991;6:165–170.
54. Chen R, Ashby P, and Lang AE. Stimulus sensitive myoclonus in akinetic-rigid syndromes. Brain 1992;115: 1875–1888.
55. Thompson PD, Day BL, Rothwell JC, et al. The myoclonus of corticobasal degeneration: Evidence of two forms of corticobasal reflex myoclonus. Brain 1994;117:1197–1207.
56. Piccione F, Meneghello F, Priftis K, et al. Masked myoclonus in corticobasal degeneration: Neurophysiological study of a case. Electromyogr Clin Neurophysiol 2002;42:57–63.
57. Grosse P, Kuhn A, Cordivani C, et al. Coherence analysis in the myoclonus of corticobasal degeneration. Mov Disords 2003;(18)11:1345–1350.

58. Godeiro-Junior C, Felício AC, Barsottini OG, et al. Clinical features of dystonia in atypical parkinsonism. Arq Neuropsiquiatr 2008;66(4):800–804.
59. Vanek ZF and Jankovic J. Dystonia in corticobasal degeneration. Adv Neurol 2000;82:61–67.
60. Gatto EM, Garretto NS, Etcheverry JL, et al. Corticobasal degeneration presenting as complex regional pain syndrome. Mov Disord 2009;30;24(6):947–948.
61. Vidailhet M and Rivaud-Pechoux S. Eye movement disorders in corticobasal degeneration. Adv Neurol 2000;82:161–167.
62. Garbutt S, Matlin A, Hellmuth J, et al. Oculomotor function in frontotemporal lobar degeneration, related disorders and Alzheimer's disease. Brain 2008;131: 1268–1281.
63. Rivaud-Pechoux S, Vidailhet M, Gallouedec G, et al. Longitudinal ocular motor study in corticobasal degeneration and progressive supranuclear palsy. Neurology 2000;54:1029–1032.
64. Vidailhet M, Rivaud S, Gouider-Khouja N, et al. Eye movements in parkinsonian syndromes. Ann Neurol 1994;35:420–426.
65. Rottach KG, Riley DE, Di Scenna AO, et al. Dynamic properties of horizontal and vertical eye movements in parkinsonian syndromes. Ann Neurol 1996;39: 368–377.
66. Pierrot-Deseilligny C, Rivaud S, Pillon B, et al. Lateral visually-guided saccades in progressive supranuclear palsy. Brain 1989;112:471–487.
67. Ozsancak C, Auzou P, Jan M, et al. The place of perceptual analysis of dysarthria in the differential diagnosis of corticobasal degeneration and Parkinson's disease. J Neurol 2005;253(1):92–97.
68. Thumler BH, Urban PP, Davids E, et al. Dysarthria and pathological laughter/crying as presenting symptoms of corticobasal-ganglionic degeneration syndrome. J Neurol 2003;250(9):1107–1108.
69. Darley FL, Aronson AE, and Brown JR. Motor Speech Disorders. Philadelphia: W.B. Saunders, 1975.
70. Duffy JR. Motor Speech Disorders: Substrates, Differential Diagnosis, and Management. St. Louis: Mosby, 1995.
71. Frattali CM and Sonies BC. Speech and swallowing disturbances in corticobasal degeneration. Adv Neurol 2000;82:153–160.
72. Doody RS and Jankovic J. The alien hand and related signs. J Neurol Neurosurg Psychiatry 1992;55:806–810.
73. Bogen JE. The callosal syndromes. In Heilman KM, Valenstein E (eds). Clinical Neuropsychology, 3rd ed. New York: Oxford University Press, 1993, pp. 337–407.
74. Kikkert MA, Ribbers GM, and Koudstaal PJ. Alien hand syndrome in stroke: a report of 2 cases and review of the literature. Arch Phys Med Rehabil 2006;87(5):728–732.
75. Ay H, Buonanno FS, Price BH, et al. Sensory alien hand syndrome: Case report and review of the literature. J Neurol Neurosurg Psychiatry 1998;65:366–369.
76. Ball JA, Lantos PL, Jackson M, et al. Alien hand sign in association with Alzheimer's histopathology. J Neurol Neurosurg Psychiatry 1993;56:1020–1023.
77. Tiwari D and Amar K. A case of corticobasal degeneration presenting with alien limb syndrome. Age and Ageing 2008;37(5):600–601.
78. Hu Wt, Josephs KA, and Ashskog JE. MRI correlates of alien leg-like phenomenon in corticobasal degeneration. Mov Disords 2005;20(7):870–873.
79. Banks G, Short P, Martinez J, et al. The alien hand syndrome. Clinical and postmortem findings. Arch Neurol 1989;46:456–459.
80. Goldberg G and Bloom KK. The alien hand sign. Localization, lateralization and recovery. Am J Physical Med Rehab 1990;69:228–238.
81. Borroni B, Agosti C, Alberici A, et al."Alien face" in corticobasal degeneration syndrome: extending clinical features. International Psychogeriatrics 2007;19: 1175–1177.
82. Mitani K. Constant and severe involvement of Betz cells in corticobasal degeneration is not consistent with pyramidal signs: a clinicopathological study of ten autopsy cases. Acta Neuropathologica 2005;109(4):353–366.
83. Gross RG and Grossman M. Update on apraxia. Curr Neurol Neurosci Rep 2008;8(6):490–496.
84. Jacobs DH, Boston MA, Adair JC, et al. Apraxia in corticobasal degeneration. Neurology 1995;45:A266–A267.
85. Soliveri P, Piacentini S, and Girotti F. Limb apraxia in corticobasal degeneration and progressive supranuclear palsy. Neurology 2005;64:448–453.
86. Zafikoff C and Lang A. Apraxia in movement disorders. Brain 2005;128:1480–1497.
87. Rothi LJ and Heilman KM. Introduction to limb apraxia. In LJ Rothi and KM Heilman (eds). Apraxia: The Neuropsychology of action. Psychology Press, Hove UK, 1997, pp. 1–6.
88. Otsuki M, Soma Y, Yoshimura N, et al. Slowly progressive limb-kinetic apraxia. Eur Neurol 1997;37:100–103.
89. Okuda B, Tachibana H, Kawabata K, et al. Slowly progressive limb-kinetic apraxia with a decrease in unilateral cerebral blood flow. Acta Neurol Scand 1992;86:76–81.
90. Rothi LJG, Mack L, Verfaellie M, et al. Ideomotor apraxia: Error pattern analysis. Aphasiology 1988;2:381–388.
91. De Renzi E and Lucchelli F. Ideational apraxia. Brain 1988;111:1173–1185.
92. Poeck K. Ideational apraxia. J Neurol 1983;230:1–5.
93. Okuda B and Tachibana H. The nature of apraxia in corticobasal degeneration. J Neurol Neurosurg Psychiatry 1994;57:(12):1548–1549.
94. Leiguarda R, Lees AJ, Merello M, et al. The nature of apraxia in corticobasal degeneration. J Neurol Neurosurg Psychiatry 1994;57:455–459.
95. Rosenfield DB, Bogatka CJ, Viswanath NS, et al. Speech apraxia in corticobasal ganglionic degeneration. Ann Neurol 1991;30:296–297.
96. Josephs KA and Duffy JR. Apraxia of speech and nonfluent aphasia: a new clinical marker for corticobasal degeneration and progressive supranuclear palsy. Curr Opin Neurol 2008;21(6):1410–1414.
97. Duffy JR. Apraxia of speech in degenerative neurologic disease. Aphasiology 2006;20(6) 511–527.
98. Kluger BM and Heilman KM. Dysfunctional facial emotional expression and comprehension in a patient with corticobasal degeneration. Neurocase 2007;13(3):165–168.
99. Ozsancak C, Auzou P, and Hannequin D. Dysarthria and orofacial apraxia in corticobasal degeneration. Mov Disord 2000;15:905–910.

100. Okuda B, Tanaka H, Kawabata K, et al. Truncal and limb apraxia in corticobasal degeneration. Mov Disord 2001;16:760–762.
101. Lerner A, Friedland R, Riley D, et al. Dementia with pathological findings of corticobasal ganglionic degeneration. Ann Neurol 1992;32:271.
102. Murray R, Neumann M, Forman MS, et al. Cognitive and motor assessment in autopsy-proven corticobasal degeneration. Neurology 2007;17;68(16):1274–1278.
103. Green J. Neuropsychological profiles in corticobasal degeneration. In Green J (ed). Neuropsychological Evaluation of the Older Adult. New York: Academic Press, 2000, pp. 142–143.
104. Massman PJ, Kreiter KT, Jankovic J, et al. Neuropsychological distinction between corticobasal ganglionic degeneration and Alzheimer's disease with extrapyramidal signs. Neurology 1994;44:194–195.
105. Massman PJ, Kreiter KT, Jankovic J, et al. Neuropsychological functioning in cortical-basal ganglionic degeneration: Differentiation from Alzheimer's disease. Neurology 1996;46:720–726.
106. Halpern C, Clark R, Moore P, et al. Verbal mediation of number knowledge: evidence from semantic dementia and corticobasal degeneration. Brain Cogn 2004;56(1):107–115.
107. Cotelli M, Borroni B, Manenti R, et al. Universal grammar in the frontotemporal dementia spectrum: Evidence of a selective disorder in the corticobasal degeneration syndrome. Neuropsychologia 2007;45(13): 3015–3023.
108. Sha S, Hou C, Viskontas IV, et al. Are frontotemporal lobar degeneration, progressive supranuclear palsy and corticobasal degeneration distinct diseases? Nat Clin Pract Neurol 2006;2(12):658–665.
109. Ioannides P, Karacostas D, Hatzipantazi M, et al. Primary progressive aphasia as the initial manifestation of corticobasal degeneration. A "three in one" syndrome? Funct Neurol 2005;20(3):135–137.
110. Kimura N, Kumamoto T, Hanaoka T, et al. Corticobasal degeneration presenting with progressive conduction aphasia. J Neurol Sci 2008;15;269(1–2):163–168.
111. McMonagle P, Blair M, and Kertesz A. Corticobasal degeneration and progressive aphasia. Neurology 2006;24;67(8):1444–1451.
112. Borroni B, Turla M, Bertasi V, et al. Cognitive and behavioral assessment in the early stages of neurodegenerative extrapyramidal syndromes. Arch Gerontol Geriatr, 2008;47(1):53–61.
113. Borroni B, Alberici A, Agosti C, et al. Pattern of behavioral disturbances in corticobasal degeneration syndrome and progressive supranuclear palsy. Int Psychogeriatr 2009;21(3):463–468.
114. Litvan I, Cummings JL, and Mega M. Neuropsychiatric features of corticobasal degeneration. J Neurol Neurosurg Psychiatry 1998;65:717–721.
115. Geda YE, Boeve BF, Negash S, et al. Neuropsychiatric features in 36 pathologically confirmed cases of corticobasal degeneration. J Neuropsychiatry Clin Neurosci 2007;19:1.
116. Cummings JL and Litvan I. Neuropsychiatric aspects of corticobasal degeneration. Adv Neurol 2000;82:147–152.
117. Pillon B, Blin J, Vidailhet M, et al. The neuropsychological pattern of corticobasal degeneration: Comparison with progressive supranuclear palsy and Alzheimer's disease. Neurology 1995;45:1477–1483.
118. Mega MS, Cummings JL, Fiorello T, et al. The spectrum of behavioral changes in Alzheimer's disease. Neurology 1996;46:130–135.
119. Levy ML, Miller BL, Cummings JL, et al. Alzheimer disease and frontotemporal dementias. Behavioral distinctions. Arch Neurol 1996;53:687–690.
120. Cummings JL, Mega M, Gray K, et al. The Neuropsychiatric Inventory: Comprehensive assessment of psychopathology in dementia. Neurology 1994;44:2308–2314.
121. Roche S, Jacquesson JM, Destee A, et al. Sleep and vigilance in corticobasal degeneration: a descriptive study. Neurophysiol Clin 2007;37(4): 261–264.
122. Kimura K, Tachibana N, Aso T, et al. Subclinical REM sleep behavior disorder in a patient with corticobasal degeneration. Sleep 1997;(20):10, 891–894.
123. Diederich NJ, Leurgans S, Fan W, et al. Visual hallucinations and symptoms of REM sleep behavior disorder in Parkinsonian tauopathies. Int J Geriatr Psychiatry 2008;23(6):598–603.
124. Sakakibara R, Uchiyama T, Yamanishi T et al. Urinary function in patients with corticobasal degeneration; comparison with normal subjects. Neurourol Urodyn 2004;23(2):154–158.
125. Muller A, Reichmann H, Livermore A, et al. Olfatory function in idiopathic Parkinson's disease: results from cross-sectional studies in idiopathic Parkinson's disease patients and long term follow up of de novo idiopathic Parkinson's disease. J Neural Transmi 2002;109(5–6): 805–811.
126. Hawkes CH. Olfaction in neurodegenerative disorders. Mov Disord 2003;18(4):364–372.
127. Watts RL, William RS, Growdon JH, et al. Corticobasal ganglionic degeneration. Neurology 1985;35:178.
128. Lovati C, Galimberti D, and Pomati S. Serum folate concentrations in patients with cortical and subcortical dementias. Neuroscience Letters 2007;40(3):213–216.
129. Noguchi M, Yoshita M, MatsumotoY, et al. Decreased beta-amyloid peptide 42 in cerebrospinal fluid of patients with progressive supranuclear palsy and corticobasal degeneration. J Neurol Sci 2005;15;237(1–2):61–65.
130. Paraskevas GP, Kapaki E, Liappas I, et al. The diagnostic value of cerebrospinal fluid tau protein in dementing and nondementing neuropsychiatric disorders. J Geriatr Psychiatry Neurol 2005;8(3):163–173.
131. Vitali P, Migliaccio R, Agosta F, et al. Neuroimaging in dementia. Semin Neurol 2008;28(4):467–483.
132. Savoiardo M, Grisoli M, and Girotti F. Magnetic resonance imaging in corticobasal degeneration, related atypical parkinsonian disorders, and dementias. Adv Neurol 2000;82:197–208.
133. Schrag A, Good CD, Miszkiel K, et al. Differentiation of atypical parkinsonian syndromes with routine MRI. Neurology 2000;54:697–702.
134. Rizzo G, Martinelli P, Manners D, et al. Diffusion-weighted brain imaging study of patients with clinical diagnosis of corticobasal degeneration, progressive supranuclear palsy and Parkinson's disease. Brain 2008;131(10):2690–2700.

135. Josephs KA, Tang-Wai DF, Edland SD, et al. Correlation between antemortem magnetic resonance imaging findings and pathologically confirmed corticobasal degeneration. Arch Neurol 2004;61:1881–1884.
136. Wiltshire K, Foster, S, Kaye, et al. Corpus callosum in neurodegenerative diseases: findings in Parkinson's disease. Dement Geriatric Cogn Disorder 2005;20(6):345–351.
137. Yamauchi H, Fukuyama H, Nagahama Y, et al. Atrophy of the corpus callosum, cortical hypometabolism, and cognitive impairment in corticobasal degeneration. Arch Neurol 1998;55:609–614.
138. Savoiardo M, Girotti F, Strada L, et al. Magnetic resonance imaging in progressive supranuclear palsy and other parkinsonian disorders. J Neural Transm 1994;42:93–110.
139. Savoiardo M, Strada L, Girotti F, et al. MR imaging in progressive supranuclear palsy and Shy-Drager syndrome. J Comput Assist Tomogr 1989;13:555–560.
140. Schonfeld SM, Golbe LI, Sage JI, et al. Computed tomographic findings in progressive supranuclear palsy: Correlation with clinical grade. Mov Disord 1987;2:263–278.
141. Boxer AL, Geschwind MD, Belfor N, et al. Patterns of brain atrophy that differentiate corticobasal degeneration syndrome from progressive supranuclear palsy. Arch Neurol 2006;63(1):81–6.
142. Whitwell JL and Jack CR. Rates of cerebral atrophy differ in different degenerative pathologies. Brain 2007;130(4):1148–1158.
143. Josephs KA, Whitwell JL, Dickson DW, et al. Voxel-based morphometry in autopsy proven progressive supranuclear palsy and corticobasal degeneration. Neurobiol Aging 2006;29(2):280–289.
144. Hosaka K, Ishii K, Sakamoto S, et al. Voxel-based comparison of regional cerebral glucosa metabolism between PSP and corticobasal degeneration. J Neurol Sci 2002;199(1–2):67–71.
145. Bozzali M, Cercignani M, Baglioo F, et al. Voxel-wise analysis of diffusion tensor MRI improves the confidence of diagnosis of corticobasal degeneration non-invasively. Parkinsonism and Rel Disords 2008;14(5):436–439.
146. Borroni B, Garibotto V, Agosti C, et al. White matter changes in corticobasal degeneration syndrome and correlation with limb apraxia. Arch Neurol 2008;65(6): 796–801.
147. Bozzali M and Cherubini A. Diffusion tensor MRI to investigate dementias: a brief review. Magnetic resonance imaging 2007;(25) 6:969–977.
148. Brooks DJ. Functional imaging studies in corticobasal degeneration. Adv Neurol 2000;82:209–215.
149. Juh R, Pae CU, Kim TS, et al. Cerebral glucose metabolism in corticobasal degeneration comparison with progressive supranuclear palsy using statistical mapping analysis. Neurosci Lett 2005;22–29; 383(1–2):22–27.
150. Eckert T, Barnes A, Dhawan V, et al. FDG PET in the differential diagnosis of parkinsonian disorders. Neuroimage 2005;1; 26(3):912–921.
151. Nagahama Y, Fukuyama H, Turjanski N, et al. Cerebral glucose metabolism in corticobasal degeneration: Comparison with progressive supranuclear palsy and normal controls. Mov Disord 1997;12:691–696.
152. Sawle GV, Brooks DJ, Marsden CD, et al. Corticobasal degeneration. A unique pattern of regional cortical oxygen hypometabolism and striatal fluorodopa uptake demonstrated by positron emission tomography. Brain 1991;114:541–556.
153. Okuda B, Tachibana H, Kawabata K, et al. Cerebral blood flow correlates of higher brain dysfunctions in corticobasal degeneration. J Geriatr Psychiatry Neurol 1999;12:189–193.
154. Laureys S, Salmon E, Garraux G, et al. Fluorodopa uptake and glucose metabolism in early stages of corticobasal degeneration. J Neurol 1999;246:1151–1158.
155. Brooks DJ. Functional imaging in relation to parkinsonian syndromes. J Neurol Sci 1993;115:1–17.
156. Eidelberg D, Takikawa S, Dhawa V, et al. Striatal 18-Fdopa uptake: absence of an aging effect. J cerebral flow and metabolism 1993;13(5):881–888.
157. Markus HS, Lees AJ, Lennox G, et al. Patterns of regional cerebral blood flow in corticobasal degeneration studied using HMPAO SPECT; comparison with Parkinson's disease and normal controls. Mov Disords 2004;10(2): 179–187.
158. Storey E, Lichtenstein M, Desmond MS, et al. Clinical features and SPECT scanning in presumed cortico-basal ganglionic degeneration. J of Clinical Neuroscience 1995;2(4):321–328.
159. Okuda B, Tachibama H, Takeda M, et al. Focal cortical hypoperfusion in corticobasal degeneration demostrated by three-dimensional surface display with 123I-IMP: a possible cause of apraxia. Neuroradiology 1995;37(8): 642–644.
160. Seritan AL, Mendez MF, Silverman DHS, et al. Functional imaging as a window to dementia: corticobasal degeneration. J Neuropsychiatry Clin Neurosci 2004;12:393–399.
161. Blin J, Vidailhet MJ, Pillon B, et al. Corticobasal degeneration: Decreased and asymmetrical glucose consumption as studied with PET. Mov Disord 1992;7:348–354.
162. Nagasawa H, Tanji H, Nomura H, et al. PET study of cerebral glucose metabolism and fluorodopa uptake in patients with corticobasal degeneration. J Neurol Sci 1996;139:210–217.
163. Klaffke S, Kuhn AA, Plotkin M, et al. Dopamine transporters, D2 receptors, and glucose metabolism in corticobasal degeneration. Mov Disord 2006;21(10):1724–1727.
164. Schwarz J, Tatsch K, Gasser T, et al. 123I-IBZM binding compared with long-term clinical follow up in patients with de novo parkinsonism. Mov Disord 1998;13:16–19.
165. Sawle GV, Brooks DJ, Thompson PD, et al. PET studies on the dopaminergic system and regional cortical metabolism in corticobasal degeneration. Neurology 1989;39:163.
166. Eidelberg D, Moeller JR, Sidtis JJ, et al. Corticodentatonigral degeneration: Metabolic asymmetries studied with 18F-fluorodeoxyglucose and positron emission tomography. Neurology 1989;39:164.
167. Eidelberg D, Dhawan V, Moeller JR, et al. The metabolic landscape of corticobasal ganglionic degeneration: Regional asymmetries studied with positron emission tomography. J Neurol Neurosurg Psychiatry 1991;54:856–862.
168. Blin J, Vidailhet M, Bonnet AM, et al. PET study in corticobasal degeneration. Mov Disord 1990;5:19.
169. Brooks DJ: PET studies on the early and differential diagnosis of Parkinson's disease. Neurology 1993;43:S6–S16.

170. Marek K, Seibyl J, Fussell B, et al. Dopamine transporter imaging in Parkinson disease and Parkinson plus syndromes. Mov Disord 1995;10:3.
171. Frisoni GB, Pizzolato G, Zanetti O, et al. Corticobasal degeneration: Neuropsychological assessment and dopamine D2 receptor SPECT analysis. Eur Neurol 1995;35:50–54.
172. Turjanski N, Lees AJ, and Brooks DJ. In vivo studies on striatal dopamine D1 and D2 site binding in l-dopa-treated Parkinson's disease patients with and without dyskinesias. Neurology 1997;49:717–723.
173. Kish SJ, Shannak K, and Hornykiewicz O. Uneven pattern of dopamine loss in the striatum of patients with idiopathic Parkinson's disease. Pathophysiologic and clinical implications. N Engl J Med 1988;318:876–880.
174. Gerhard A, Watts J, Trender-Gerhard I, et al. In vivo imaging of microglial activation with [11C] (R)-PK11195 PET in corticobasal degeneration. Mov Disord 2004;19(10): 1221–1226.
175. Henkel K, Karitzky J, Schmid M, et al. Imaging of activated microglia with PET and [11C]PK 11195 in corticobasal degeneration. Mov Disord 2004;19(7):817–821.
176. Walter U, Dressler D, Wolters A, et al. Sonographic discrimination of corticobasal degeneration vs progressive supranuclear palsy. Neurology 2004;10; 63(3):504–509.
177. Alberici A, Bonato C, Calabria M, et al. The contribution of TMS to frontotemporal dementia variants. Acta Neurol Scand 2008;118(4):275–280.
178. O'Sullivan SS, Burn DJ, Holton JL, et al. Normal dopamine transporter single photon-emission CT scan in corticobasal degeneration. Mov Disord 2008;15; 23(16):2424–2426.
179. Tashiro K, Ogata K, Goto Y, et al. EEG findings in early-stage corticobasal degeneration and progressive supranuclear palsy: a retrospective study and literature review. Clin Neurophysiol 2006;117(10):2236–2242.
180. Wieser HG, Schwarz U, Blattler T, et al. Serial EEG findings in sporadic and iatrogenic Creutzfeldt-Jakob disease. Clin Neurophysiol 2004;115(11):2467–2478.
181. Defebvre L. Myoclonus and extrapyramidal diseases. Clinical Neurophysiol 2006;(36) 319–325.
182. Tyvaert L, Cassim F, Derambue P, et al. Neurophysiology of corticobasal degeneration. Rev Neurol 2007;163 (8–9):779–791.
183. Takeda M, Tachibana H, Okuda B, et al. Electrophysiological comparison between corticobasal degeneration and progressive supranuclear palsy. Clin Neurol Neurosurg 1998;100:94–98.
184. Okuda B, Tachibana H, Takeda M, et al. Asymmetric changes in somatosensory evoked potentials correlate with limb apraxia in corticobasal degeneration. Acta Neurol Scand 1998;97:409–412.
185. Homma A, Harayama H, Kondo H, et al. P300 findings in patients with corticobasal degeneration. Brain Nerve 1996;48:925–929.
186. Dickson DW, Bergeron C, Chin SS, et al. Office of rare diseases of the national institutes of health, office of rare diseases neuropathologic criteria for corticobasal degeneration. J Neuropathol Exp Neurol 2002;61:935–946.
187. Dickson DW and Litvan I. Corticobasal degeneration. In Dickson DW (ed). Neurodegeneration: The Molecular Pathology of Dementia and Movement Disorder. Neuropath Press, 2003, pp. 115–123.
188. Lowe J and Leigh N. Disorders of movement and system degenerations in Graham D, Lantos P (eds): Greenfield's Neuropathology. New York: Gray Publishing, 2002, pp. 325–430.
189. Ikeda K, Akiyama H, Iritani S, et al. Corticobasal degeneration with primary progressive aphasia and accentuated cortical lesion in superior temporal gyrus: Case report and review. Act Neuropathol 1996;92:534–539.
190. Kaida K, Takuda K, Nagata N, et al. Alzheimer's disease with asymmetrical parietal lobe atrophy: A case report. J Neurologi Sci 1998;160(1):96–99.
191. Karashima S and Oda Y. Cholinergic ineuronal loss in the basal forebrain and mesopontine tegmentum of progressive supranuclear palsy and corticobasal degeneration. Acta Neuropathol 2003;105:117–124.
192. Feany MB and Dickson DW. Widespread cytoskeletal pathology characterizes corticobasal degeneration. Am J Pathol 1995;146:1388–1396.
193. Dickson DW, Feany MB, Yen SH, et al. Cytoskeletal pathology in non-Alzheimer degenerative dementia: new lesions in diffuse Lewy body disease, Pick's disease, and corticobasal degeneration. J Neural Trans 1996;47: 31–46.
194. Nakazato Y, Hirato J, Ishida Y, et al. Swollen cortical neurons in Creutzfeldt-Jakob disease contain a phosphorylated neurofilament epitope. J Neuropathol Exp Neurol 1990;49:197–205.
195. Mackenzie IRA and Hudson LP. Achromatic neurons in the cortex of progressive supranuclear palsy. Acta Neuropathol 1995;90:615–619.
196. Manetto V, Sternberger NH, Perry G, et al. Phosphorylation of neurofilaments is altered in amyotrophic lateral sclerosis. J Neuropathol Exp Neurol 1988;47:642–653.
197. Fujino Y, Delucia MW, Davies P, et al. Balloned neurons in the limbic lobe are associated with Alzheimer type pathology and lack diagnostic specificity. Neuropathol Appl Neurobiol 2004;30(6):676–682.
198. Gonatas NK, Stieber A, and Gonatas JO. Fragmentation of the Golgi apparatus in neurodegenerative disease and cell death. J Neural Sci 2006;15:246(1-2):21–30.
199. Sakurai A, Okamoto K, Fujita Y, et al. Fragmentation of the Golgi apparatus of the ballooned neurons in patients with corticobasal degeneration and Creutzfeldt-Jakob disease. Acta Neuropathol 2000;100:270–274.
200. Dickson DW. Neuropathology of Parkinsonism in Pahwa R, Lyons KE, Koller WC (eds): Handbook of Parkinson's Disease. New York: Marcel Dekker, 2003, pp. 203–220.
201. Ksiezak-Reding H, Morgan K, Mattiace LA, et al. Ultrastructure and biochemical composition of paired helical filaments in corticobasal degeneration. Am J Pathol 1994;145:1496–1508.
202. Delacourte A and Buee L. Normal and pathological tau proteins as factors for microtubule assembly. Int Rev Cytol 1997;171:167–224.
203. Buee L and Delacourte A. Comparative biochemistry of tau in progressive supranuclear palsy, corticobasal degeneration, FTDP-17 and Pick's disease. Brain Pathol 1999;9:681–693.
204. Arvanitakis Z and Wszolek ZK. Recent advances in the understanding of tau protein and movement disorders. Curr Opin Neurol 2001;14:491–497.

205. Tolnay M and Probst A. The neuropathological spectrum of neurodegenerative tauopathies. IUBMB Life 2003;55(6):299–305.
206. Dickson DW. Tau and synuclein and their role in neuropathology. Brain Pathol 1999;9:657–661.
207. Bancher C, Brunner C, Lassmann H, et al. Accumulation of abnormally phosphorylated tau precedes the formation of neurofibrillary tangles in Alzheimer's disease. Brain Res 1989;477:90–99.
208. Tellez-Nagel I and Wisniewski H. Ultrastructure of neurofibrillary tangles in Steele Richardson-Olszewski syndrome. Arch Neurol 1973;29:324–327.
209. Dickson DW. Neuropathologic differentiation of progressive supranuclear palsy and corticobasal degeneration. J Neurol 1999;246:II6–15.
210. Matsusaka H, Ikeda K, Akiyama H, et al. Astrocytic pathology in progressive supranuclear palsy: Significance for neuropathological diagnosis. Acta Neuropathol 1998;96:248–252.
211. Wakabayashi K, Mori F, Hasegawa M, et al. Co-localization of beta-peptide and phosphorylated tau in astrocytes in a patient with corticobasal degeneration. Neuropath 2006;26(1):66–71.
212. Hattori M, Hashizume Y, Yoshida M, et al. Distribution of astrocytic plaques in the corticobasal degeneration brain and comparison with tuft-shaped astrocytes in the progressive supranuclear palsy brain. Acta Neuropathol 2003;106:143–149.
213. Komori T. Tau-positive glial inclusions in progressive supranuclear palsy, corticobasal degeneration and Pick's disease. Brain Pathol 1999;9:663–679.
214. Wakabayashi K, Yoshimoto M, Tsuji S, et al. Alpha-synuclein immunoreactivity in glial cytoplasmic inclusions in multiple system atrophy. Neurosci Lett 1998;249:180–182.
215. Sakai K, Piao YS, Kikugawa K, et al. Corticobasal degeneration with focal massive tau accumulation in the subcortical white matter astrocytes. Acta Neuropathol 2006;112(3):341–348.
216. Zhukareva V, Joyce S, Schuck T, et al. Unexpected abundance of pathological tau in progressive supranuclear palsy white matter. Ann Neurol 2006;60(1):335–345.
217. Iwasaki Y, Yoshida M, Hattori M, et al. Widespread spinal cord involvement in corticobasal degeneration. Acta Neuropathol 2005;109:632–638.
218. Kikuchi H, Doh-ura K, Kira J, et al. Preferential neurodegeneration in the cervical spinal cord of progressive supranuclear palsy. Acta Neuropathol 1999; 97(6):577–584.
219. Josephs KA, Katsuse O, Beccano-Kelly DA, et al. Atypical progressive supranuclear palsy with corticospinal tract degeneration. J Neuropathol Exp Neuro 2006;65(4):396–405.
220. Yoshida M. Cellular tau pathology and immunohistochemical study of tau isoforms in sporadic tauopathies. Neuropathol 2006;26(5):457–470.
221. Arima K. Ultrastructural characteristics of tau filaments in tauopathies: immuno – electron microscopic demonstration of tau filaments in tauopathies. Neuropathol 2006;26(5):475–483.
222. Pittman AM, Fung HC, and de Silva R. Untangling the tau gene association with neurodegenerative disorders. Hum Mol Genet 2006;15(2:R)188–195.
223. D'Souza I and Schellenberg GD. Regulation of tau isoform expression and dementia. Biochimica et biophysica Acta 2005;1739:104–115.
224. Goedert M. Tau gene mutations and their effects. Mov Disord 2005;20(12):S45–S52.
225. Terada S, Ishizu H, Ishiguro K, et al. Exon 3 insert of tau protein in neurodegenerative diseases. Acta Neuropathol 2005;110(1):12–8.
226. Ferrer I, Gomez-Isla T, Puig B, et al. Current advances on different kinases involved in tau phosphorylation, and implications in Alzheimer's disease and tauopathies. Curr Alzheimer Res 2005;2(1):3-18.
227. Caffrey TM, Joachim C, Paracchini S, et al. Haplotype-specific expression of exon 10 at the human MAPT locus. Hum Mol Genet 2006;15(24):3529–3537.
228. Togo T, Sahara N, Yen SH, et al. Argyrophilic grain disease is a sporadic 4-repeat tauopathy. J Neuropathol Exp Neurol 2002;61:547–556.
229. Berry RW, Sweet AP, Clark FA, et al. Tau epitope display in progressive supranuclear palsy and corticobasal degeneration. J Neurocytol 2004;33(3):287–295.
230. Tuite PJ, Clark HB, Bergeron C, et al. Clinical and pathologic evidence of corticobasal degeneration and progressive supranuclear palsy in familial tauopathy. Arch Neurol 2005;62(9):14531457.
231. Pittman AM, Myers AJ, Abou-Sleiman P, et al. Linkage disequilibrium fine mapping and haplotype association analysis of the tau gene in progressive supranuclear palsy and corticobasal degeneration. J Med Genet 2005;42(11):837–846.
232. Webb A, Miller B, Bonasera S, et al. Role of the tau gene region chromosome inversion in progressive supranuclear palsy, corticobasal degeneration and related disorders. Arch Neurol 2008;65(11):1473-8.
233. Rosso SM and van Swieten JC. New developments in frontotemporal dementia and parkinsonism linked to chromosome 17. Curr Opin Neurol 2002;15:423–428.
234. Kertesz A, McMonagle P, Blair M, et al. The evolution and pathology of frontotemporal dementia. Brain 2005;128(9):1996–2005.
235. Kertesz A and Munoz DG. Relationship between frontotemporal dementia and corticobasal degeneration/ progressive supranuclear palsy. Dement Geriatr Cogn Disord 2004;17(4):282–286.
236. Godbolt AK, Josephs KA, Revesz T, et al. Sporadic and familial dementia with ubiquitin-positive tau-negative inclusions: clinical features of one histopathological abnormality underlying frontotemporal lobar degeneration. Arch Neurol 2005;62(7): 1097–1101.
237. Wray S, Saxton M, Anderton BH, et al. Direct analysis of tau from PSP brain identifies new phosphorylation sites and a major fragment of N-terminally cleaved tau containing four microtubule-binding repeats. J Neurochem 2008;105(6):2343–2352.
238. Ksiezak-Reding H, Yang G, Simon M, et al. Assembled tau filaments differ from native paired helical filaments as determined by scanning transmission electron microscopy (STEM). Brain Res 1998;814(1–2): 86–98.
239. Grinberg LT and Heinsen H. Argyrophilic grain disease. Dementia and Neuropsychol 2009;3(1):2–7.

240. Boeve BF. Links between frontotemporal lobar degeneration, corticobasal degeneration, progressive supranuclear palsy, and amyotrophic lateral sclerosis. Alzheimer Dis Assoc Disord 2007:21(4).
241. Zhukareva V, Vogelsberg-Ragaglia V, Van Deerlin VMD, et al. Loss of brain tau defines novel sporadic and familial tauopathies with frontotemporal dementia. Ann. Neurol 2001;49:165–175.
242. Zhukareva V, Sundarraj S, Mann D, et al. Selective reduction of soluble tau proteins in sporadic and familial frontotemporal dementias: an international follow up study. Acta Neuropathol 2003;105:469-476.
243. Rademakers R, Cruts M, and van Broeckhoven C. The role of tau (MAPT) in frontotemporal dementia and related tauopathies. Hum Mut 2004;24:277–295.
244. Kawasaki K, Iwanaga K, Wakabayashi K et al. Corticobasal degeneration with neither argyrophilic inclusions nor tau abnormalities: a new subgroup? Acta Neuropathol 1996;91(2):140–144.
245. Baker M, Litvan I, Houlden H, et al. Association of an extended haplotype in the tau gene with progressive supranuclear palsy. Hum Mol Genet 1999;8:711–715.
246. Houlden H, Baker M, Morris HR, et al. Corticobasal degeneration and progressive supranuclear palsy share a common tau haplotype. Neurology 2001;56:1702–1706.
247. Myers AJ, Pittman AM, Zhao AS, et al. The MAPT H1c risk haplotype is associated with increased expression of tau and especially of 4 repeat containing transcripts. Neurobiol Dis 2007;25(3):561–570.
248. Kumaran R, Kingsbury A, Coulter I, et al. DJ-1 (PARK7) is associated with 3R and 4R tau neuronal and glial inclusions in neurodegenerative disorders. Neurobiol Dis 2007;28 (1):122–132.
249. Neumann M, Müller V, Görner K, et al. Pathological properties of the Parkinson's disease-associated protein DJ-1 in synucleinopathies and tauopathies: relevance for multiple system atrophy and Pick's disease. Acta neuropathol 2004;107(6):489–496.
250. Canu E, Boccardi M, Ghidoni R, et al. H1 haplotype of the MAPT gene is associated with lower regional gray matter volume in healthy carriers. Eur J Hum Genet 2009;17(3):287–294.
251. Uryu K, Nakashima-Yasuda H, Forman MS, et al. Concomitant TAR-DNA-binding protein 43 pathology is present in Alzheimer disease and corticobasal degeneration but not in other tauopathies. J Neuropathol Exp Neurol 2008;67(6):555–564.
252. Gaig C, Ezquerra M, Martí M, et al. Screening for the LRRK2 G2019S and codon-1441 mutations in a pathological series of parkinsonian syndromes and frontotemporal lobar degeneration. J Neurol Sci 2008;270(1):94–98.
253. Pollanen MS, Dickson DW, and Bergeron C. Pathology and biology of the Lewy body. J Neuropathol Exp Neurol 1993;52:183–191.
254. Mattila PM, Rinne JO, Helenius H, et al. Alpha-synuclein-immunoreactive cortical Lewy bodies are associated with cognitive impairment in Parkinson's disease. Acta Neuropathol 2000;100:285–290.
255. Hurtig HI, Trojanowski JQ, Galvin J, et al. Alpha-synuclein cortical Lewy bodies correlate with dementia in Parkinson's disease. Neurology 2000;54:1916–1921.
256. Haroutunian V, Serby M, Purohit DP, et al. Contribution of Lewy body inclusions to dementia in patients with and without Alzheimer disease neuropathological conditions. Arch Neurol 2000;57:1145–1150.
257. Dickson DW. Alzheimer-Parkinson disease overlap: Neuropathology in Clark CM, Trojanowski JQ (eds). Neurodegenerative Dementias: Clinical Features and Pathological Mechanism. New York: McGraw-Hill, 2000, pp. 247–259.
258. Hamilton RL. Lewy bodies in Alzheimer's disease: A neuropathological review of 145 cases using alpha-synuclein immunohistochemistry. Brain Pathol 2000;10:378–384.
259. Dickson DW, Corral A, and Lin W. Alzheimer's disease with amygdaloid Lewy bodies: A form of Lewy body disease distinct from AD and diffuse Lewy body disease. Neurology 2000;54:A451.
260. Arai Y, Yamazaki M, Mori O, et al. Alpha-synuclein-positive structures in cases with sporadic Alzheimer's disease: Morphology and its relationship to tau aggregation. Brain Res 2001;888:287–296.
261. Marui W, Iseki E, Ueda K, et al. Occurrence of human alpha-synuclein immunoreactive neurons with neurofibrillary tangle formation in the limbic areas of patients with Alzheimer's disease. J Neurol Sci 2000;174:81–84.
262. Masliah E, Rockenstein E, Veinbergs I, et al. Beta-amyloid peptides enhance alpha-synuclein accumulation and neuronal deficits in a transgenic mouse model linking Alzheimer's disease and Parkinson's disease. Proc Natl Acad Sci U S A 2001;98:12245–12250.
263. LLado A, Sanchez-Valle R, Rey MJ, et al. Clinicopathological and genetic correlates of frontotemporal lobar degeneration and corticobasal degeneration. J Neurol 2008;255(4):488–494.
264. Murray B, Lynch T, and Farrell M. Clinicopathological features of the tauopathies. Biochemical Society Transactions 2005;33:595–599.
265. Trojanowski JQ and Dickson D. Update on the neuropathological diagnosis of frontotemporal dementias. J Neuropathol Exp Neurol 2001;60:1123–1126.
266. Giannakopoulos P, Hof PR, and Bouras C. Dementia lacking distinctive histopathology: Clinicopathological evaluation of 32 cases. Act Neuropathol 1995;89:346–355.
267. Bugiani O. The many ways to frontotemporal degeneration and beyond. Neurol Sci; 2007;28:241–244.
268. Braak H and Braak E. Cortical and subcortical argyrophilic grains characterize a disease associated with adult onset dementia. Neuropathol Appl Neurobiol 1989;15:13–26.
269. Jellinger KA. Dementia with grains (argyrophilic grain disease). Brain Pathol 1998;8:377–386.
270. Ferrer I, Santpere G, and van Leeuwen FW. Argyrophilic grain disease. Brain 2008;131(6):1416–1432.
271. Masellis M, Momeni P, Meschino W, et al. Novel splicing mutation in the progranulin gene causing familial corticobasal syndrome. Brain 2006;129(11):3115–3123.
272. Le Ber I, Camuzat A, Hannequin D, et al. Phenotype variability in progranulin mutation carriers: A clinical, neuropsychological imaging and genetic study. Brain 2008;131(Pt 3):732–746.
273. Kelley BJ, Haidar W, Boeve BF, et al. Prominent phenotypic variability associated with mutations in Progranulin. Neurobiol Aging 2009;30(5):739–751.

274. Strittmatter WJ, Saunders AM, Schmechel D, et al. Apolipoprotein E: High avidity binding to beta-amyloid and increased frequency of type 4 allele in late onset familial Alzheimer's disease. Proc Natl Acad Sci U S A 1993;90:1977–1981.
275. Corder EH, Saunders AM, Strittmatter WJ, et al. Gene dose of apolipoprotein E type 4 allele and the risk of Alzheimer's disease in late onset families. Science 1993;261:921–923.
276. Stanford PM, Brooks WS, Teber ET, et al. Frequency of tau mutations in familial and sporadic frontotemporal dementia and other tauopathies. J Neurol 2004;251(9):1098–1104.
277. Skoglund L, Viitanen M, Kalimo H, et al. The tau S305S mutation causes frontotemporal dementia with parkinsonism. Eur J Neurol 2008;15(2):156–161.
278. Steele JC, Richardson JC, and Olszewski J. Progressive supranuclear palsy. Arch Neurol 1964;10:333–358.
279. Adams RD, Van Bogaert L, and Vander Eecken H. Striatonigral degeneration. J Neuropathol Exp Neurol 1964;23:584–608.
280. Takei Y and Mirra SS. Striatonigral degeneration: A form of multiple system atrophy with clinical parkinsonism. Prog Neuropathol 1973;2:217–251.
281. Spokes EGS, Bannister R, and Oppenheimer DR. Multiple system atrophy with autonomic failure. J Neurol Sci 1979;43:59–82.
282. Wenning GK, Ben Shlomo Y, Magalhaes M, et al. Clinical features and natural history of multiple system atrophy. An analysis of 100 cases. Brain 1994;117:835–845.
283. Jendroska K, Rossor MN, Mathias CJ, et al. Daniel SE: Morphological overlap between corticobasal degeneration and Pick's disease: A clinicopathological report. Mov Disord 1995;10:111–114.
284. Lang AE, Bergeron C, Pollanen MS, et al. Parietal Pick's disease mimicking cortical-basal ganglionic degeneration. Neurology 1994;44:1436–1440.
285. Cole M, Wright D, and Banker BQ. Familial aphasia due to Pick's disease. Ann Neurol 1979;6:158.
286. Molsa PK, Marttila RJ, and Rinne UK. Extrapyramidal signs in Alzheimer's disease. Neurology 1984;34:1114–1116.
287. Chui HC, Teng EL, Henderson VW, et al. Clinical subtypes of dementia of the Alzheimer type. Neurology 1985;35:1544–1550.
288. Hirano A, Kurland LT, Krooth RS, et al. Parkinsonism-dementia complex, an endemic disease on the Island of Guam. I. Clinical features. Brain 1961;84:642–661.
289. Hirano A, Malamud M, and Kurland LT. Parkinsonism-dementia complex on the Island of Guam. II. Pathological features. Brain 1961;84:662–679.
290. Yamazaki M, Hasegawa M, Mori O, et al. Tau-positive fine granules in the cerebral white matter: a novel finding among the tauopathies exclusive to Parkinsonism-Dementia Complex of Guam. J Neuropathol and Exp Neurol 2005;64(10):839–846.
291. Kreisler A, Mastain B, Tison F, et al. Multi-infart disorder presenting as corticobasal degeneration (DCB): Vascular pseudocorticobasal. Rev Neurol 2007;163(12):1191–1199.
292. Baba Y, Ghetti B, Baker MC, et al. Hereditary diffuse leukoencephalopathy with spheroids: Clinical, pathologic and genetic studies of a new kindred. Acta Neuropathol 2006;111(4):300–311.
293. Okeda R, Matsuo T, Kawahara Y, et al. Adult pigment type (Pfeiffer) of sudanophilic leukodystrophy. Pathological and morphometrical studies on two autopsy cases of siblings. Acta Neuropathol 1989;78:533–542.
294. Gray F, Destee A, Bourre JM, et al. Pigmentary type of orthochromatic leukodystrophy (OLD): A new case with ultra-structural and biochemical study. J Neuropathol Exp Neurol 1987;46:585–596.
295. Pietrini V, Tagliavini F, Pilleri G, et al. Orthochromatic leukodystrophy with pigmented glial cells. An adult case with clinical-anatomical study. Acta Neurol Scand 1979;59:140–147.
296. Bhatia KP, Morris JH, and Frackowiak RS. Primary progressive multifocal leukoencephalopathy presenting as an extrapyramidal syndrome. J Neurol 1996;243:91–95.
297. Wilson SAK. Progressive lenticular degeneration: a familial nervous disease associated with cirrhosis of the liver. Brain 1912;34:295–309.
298. Bruyn GW. The Westphal variant and juvenile type of Huntington's chorea in Barbeau A, Brunette JR (eds): Progress in Neurogenetics. Amsterdam: Excerpta Medica, 1967, pp. 666–673.
299. Giladi N and Fahn S. Hemiparkinsonism-hemiatrophy syndrome may mimic early-stage cortical-basal ganglionic degeneration. Mov Disord 1992;7:384–385.
300. Baba Y, Uitti RJ, Farrer MJ, et al. Sporadic SCA8 mutation resembling corticobasal degeneration. Parkinsonism Relat Disord 2005;11(3):147–150.
301. Nakano KK, Dawson DM, and Spence A. Machado disease: A hereditary ataxia in Portuguese emigrants to Massachusetts. Neurology 1972;22:49–55.
302. Romanul FCA, Fowler HL, Radvany J, et al. Azorean disease of the nervous system. N Engl J Med 1977;296: 1505–1508.
303. Sachdev HS, Forno LS, and Kane CA. Joseph disease: A multisystem degenerative disorder of the nervous system. Neurology 1982;32:192–195.
304. Jankovic J, Kirkpatrick JB, Blonquist KA, et al. Late onset Halloverden-Spatz disease presenting as familial parkinsonism. Neurology 1985;35:227–234.
305. Kritchevsky N, Hansen LA, Deteresa R, et al. Slowly progressive ideomotor apraxia: A presentation of adult onset Hallervorden Spatz disease. Neurology 1989;39:237.
306. Martin JJ. Adult type of neuronal ceroid lipofuscinosis. Dev Neurosci 1991;13:331–338.
307. Mendez M. Corticobasal ganglionic degeneration with Balint's syndrome. J Neuropsychiatry Cli Neurosci 2000;12:273–275.
308. Benito-Leon J, Alvarez Linera J, and Louis ED. Neurosyphilis masquerading as corticobasal degeneration. Mov Disord 2004;19(11):1367–1370.
309. Mizuno T, Shiga K, Nakata Y, et al. Discrepancy between clinical and pathological diagnoses of CBD and PSP. J Neurol 2005;252(6):687–697.
310. Bugiani O. The many ways to frontotemporal degeneration and beyond. Neurological Sciences 2007;28(5) 241–244.
311. Avanzino L, Marinelli L, Buccolieri A, et al. Creutzfeldt-Jakob disease presenting as corticobasal degeneration: a neurophysiological study. Neurol Sci 2006;27(2): 118–121.

312. Moreaud O, Monavon A, Brutti-Mairesse MP, et al. Creutzfeldt-Jakob disease mimicking corticobasal degeneration: Clinical and MRI data of a case. J Neurol 2005;252(10):1283–1284.
313. Cannard KR, Galvez-Jimenez N, and Watts RL. Creutzfeldt-Jakob disease presenting and evolving as rapidly progressive corticobasal degeneration. Neurology 1998;50:A95.
314. Rankin CA and Gamblin TC. Assessing toxicity of tau aggregation. J Alzheimer's Dis 2008;14(4):411–416.
315. Schneider A and Mandelkow E. Tau-based treatment strategies in neurodegenerative diseases. Neurotherapeutics 2008;5(3):443–457.
316. Reich SG and Grill SE. Corticobasal degeneration. Curr Treat Options Neurol 2009;11(3):179–185.
317. Kompoliti K, Goetz CG, Boeve BF, et al. Clinical presentation and pharmacological therapy in corticobasal degeneration. Arch Neurol 1998;55:957–961.
318. Parati EA, Fetoni V, Geminiani GC, et al. Response to L-DOPA in multiple system atrophy. Clin Neuropharmacol 1993;16:139–144.
319. Hughes AJ, Colosimo C, Kleedorfer B, et al. The dopaminergic response in multiple system atrophy. J Neurol Neurosurg Psychiatry 1992;55:1009–1013.
320. Fazzini E, Dogali M, Beric A, et al. The effects of unilateral ventral posterior medial pallidotomy in patients with Parkinson's disease and Parkinson's plus syndromes In Koller WC, Paulson G (eds). Therapy of Parkinson's Disease. New York: Marcel Dekker, 1995, pp. 353–379.
321. Cantello R. Applications of transcranial magnetic stimulation in movement disorders. J Clin Neurophysiol 2002;19:272–293.
322. Steffen TM, Boeve BF, Mollinger-Riemann LA, et al. Long-term locomotor training for gait and balance in a patient with mixed progressive supranuclear palsy and corticobasal degeneration. Phys Ther 2007;87(8):1078–1087.
323. Kawahira K, Noma T, Iiyama J, et al. Improvements in limb kinetic apraxia by repetition of a newly designed facilitation exercise in a patient with corticobasal degeneration. Int J Rehabil Res 2009;32(2):178–183.

CHAPTER 23

Infectious, Postinfectious, Toxin-Induced, and Drug-Induced Parkinsonism

Rajesh Pahwa and Kelly E. Lyons

Parkinsonism is defined by the presence of the cardinal symptoms of bradykinesia, rigidity, tremor, and postural instability. The most common cause of parkinsonism is idiopathic Parkinson's disease (PD) but a number of cases are due to secondary parkinsonism for which there are multiple causes. This chapter will review parkinsonism resulting from infectious causes[1] and exposure to various toxins and drugs.[2]

▶ INFECTIOUS CAUSES OF PARKINSONISM

There are several potential infectious causes of parkinsonism (Table 23–1).[3–9] This chapter reviews postencephalitic parkinsonism as well as other infectious causes of parkinsonism, including acquired immune deficiency syndrome (AIDS), syphilis, fungal and parasitic infections, and Creutzfeldt–Jakob disease.

▶ TABLE 23–1. POTENTIAL INFECTIOUS CAUSES OF PARKINSONISM

Acquired immune deficiency syndrome (AIDS)
Coxsackie B types 2 and 4
Creutzfeldt–Jakob disease (CJD)
Epstein–Barr virus
Fungal and parasitic infections
Herpes simplex
Japanese encephalitis
Measles
Mycoplasma pneumoniae
Poliomyelitis
Postencephalitic parkinsonism
Syphilis
West Nile virus
Western equine encephalitis
Whipple's disease

POSTENCEPHALITIC PARKINSONISM

"Postencephalitic parkinsonism," "von Economo's disease," and "encephalitis lethargica" are multiple terms used to describe a form of parkinsonism, which occurs after a bout of encephalitis. In 1917, von Economo[9] described this condition, which became an epidemic during World War I. Postencephalitic parkinsonism accounted for the majority of the cases of parkinsonism from 1920 to 1930 and for one-half of the cases seen during the 1930s.[10] The incidence of postencephalitic parkinsonism was significantly reduced over time, and by the late 1960s, it represented less than 1% of the cases of parkinsonism. There have been no new cases in the recent literature.

Clinical Features

Initial symptoms were consistent with a viral infection, including influenza and pharyngeal symptoms with fever followed by a variety of neurological symptoms.[11] The majority of patients had ophthalmoplegia in combination with a persistent pathological somnolence lasting for days to weeks in which arousal was brief and often required vigorous stimulation.[12] Signs of cortical dysfunction, like aphasia, convulsions, psychosis, and sensory disturbances were rare. Clinical, laboratory, and pathological features were consistent with a viral infection. Elevated cerebrospinal fluid protein with lymphocytic pleocytosis was seen in about one-half of patients. No specific virus was ever identified and the encephalitis was not contagious.[13–15]

The initial symptoms generally lasted for several weeks, and mortality was as high as 40%. A large percentage of patients who survived had delayed symptoms with the most common including central respiratory irregularities, oculogyric crises, and parkinsonism.[16,17] Oculogyric crisis consisted most commonly of upward deviation of the eyes although downward deviations and convergence rarely occurred.[18] Most attacks lasted minutes to hours and disappeared during sleep. Oculogyric crisis occurred in approximately 20% of parkinsonian patients.[19] In some patients with oculogyric crisis, symptoms similar to Meige's syndrome or other forms of dystonia also occurred. Patients frequently complained of fear, anxiety, depression, or suicidal ideation, which preceded or accompanied oculogyric crisis.

Parkinsonian or extrapyramidal features generally included rigidity, masked facies, bradykinesia, impaired gait, and dysarthria. Rigidity was more common than tremor, which did not occur in all patients.[20,21] The majority of patients had catatonic akinesia and akathisia was occasionally seen. In addition to features reported in idiopathic PD, signs such as myoclonus, chorea, tics or spasms, oculogyric crisis, respiratory disturbances, pupillary dysfunction, ocular palsies, and behavioral disorders were also present.[12] Vertical gaze paresis and eyelid opening apraxia also occurred, making the distinction from progressive supranuclear palsy important.[22] The progression of parkinsonian features was variable although generally a slow worsening of motor features was observed.[23,24] Dementia was rare, in contrast to its relatively high prevalence in PD.[25]

Pathology

The characteristic pathological feature of postencephalitic parkinsonism was a loss of pigmentation in the substantia nigra and also to some degree in the locus ceruleus.[26,27] This loss of pigmented nigral neurons could be as high as 90%, which is significantly higher than seen in most PD brains.[28] In contrast to PD, Lewy bodies were not reported in postencephalitic parkinsonism but neurofibrillary tangles were typically present in the substantia nigra, locus ceruleus, reticular formation, hippocampus, nucleus basalis of Meynert, and in some cases in the neocortex and spinal cord.[29]

Treatment

Belladonna alkaloids were the initial treatment for postencephalitic parkinsonism and synthetic anticholinergics continued to be a beneficial treatment option.[30] These drugs were well-tolerated compared with levodopa and in addition to the parkinsonian symptoms, also provided some benefit for oculogyric crisis, tics, and behavioral issues. Amphetamines were often used in the treatment of postencephalitic oculogyric crisis and were also shown to improve parkinsonian motor symptoms by approximately 20% in some patients.[31] Another treatment option was levodopa; however, at that time, a decarboxylase inhibitor was not used, and many patients could not tolerate levodopa alone. In a double-blind, 6-week study of 20 institutionalized postencephalitic parkinsonism patients, the maximum tolerated dose of levodopa was determined to be 2.5 g daily, which was much less than doses used at that time for PD.[32] In this study, 50% improved, 25% withdrew due to intolerable side effects and 25% had no benefit. The primary benefit was seen in walking, but oculogyric crises and drooling were also improved. The most common side effects included dyskinesia and restlessness.[32] In a long-term open-label study of levodopa in 50 patients, 32% had continued benefit, 32% did not benefit, and 36% did not tolerate levodopa.[33] Side effects included respiratory problems, tics, and worsening of oculogyric crisis.

ACQUIRED IMMUNE DEFICIENCY SYNDROME (AIDS)

Clinical Features

Approximately 70% of AIDS patients have neurological symptoms and neurological abnormalities are observed in more than 90% of autopsied cases.[34] Movement disorders have been identified in 3% of patients with HIV infection seen at tertiary referral centers and 50% of patients with AIDS develop tremor, parkinsonism, or other extrapyramidal features.[35] Hemiballism, chorea, and tremor are the most common movement disorders seen in patients who are HIV positive, but dystonia, myoclonus, tics, paroxysmal dyskinesia, and parkinsonism have also been reported. In a study of 2460 HIV-positive patients neurological symptoms were reported in 43%, movement disorders in 3%, and parkinsonism in only 0.6%.[36,37] The mean onset of parkinsonism after HIV diagnosis was 5 months. In the majority of patients, these movement disorders occur from lesions caused by opportunistic infections, particularly toxoplasmosis. However, parkinsonism can result from dopaminergic dysfunction resulting from HIV or from the use of dopamine-blocking drugs.

Many patients with HIV or AIDS have a sensitivity to dopamine-blocking drugs resulting in parkinsonism.[38] In a study of 31 men with AIDS compared with 32 men of similar demographics without AIDS or HIV risk factors, the development of neuroleptic-induced extrapyramidal signs as measured by chlorpromazine equivalents was 2.4 times greater in the AIDS group. In fact, 50% of AIDS patients taking less than 4 mg/kg of chlorpromazine equivalents and 80% receiving greater than 4 mg/kg per day developed parkinsonism.[39] This may be a result of neuronal loss in the substantia nigra[40] and the globus pallidus[41] possibly due to the toxicity of the virus.[42–44] HIV-1 DNA has been identified in macrophages and microglia, as well as in basal ganglia astrocytes and neurons contributing to HIV toxicity in the brain.[45] In HIV-positive patients, positron emission tomography (PET) studies have shown hypermetabolism of the basal ganglia, which changed to hypometabolism as extrapyramidal signs developed.[46]

Treatment

The management of HIV positive patients with movement disorders involves recognition and treatment of opportunistic infections, symptomatic treatment of the movement disorder, and the use of highly active antiretroviral therapy (HAART).[35] Symptomatic treatment of the parkinsonian features and the movement disorder is often disappointing. Mild to no improvement has been reported with levodopa.[37,47] However, in a study of HIV-positive children with parkinsonism, levodopa was reported to improve extrapyramidal symptoms.[48] In some cases, treatment of opportunistic infections has also been shown to improve parkinsonism.[47,49]

MYCOPLASMA PNEUMONIAE

Mycoplasma pneumoniae, a nonviral infection, has been reported to cause parkinsonism. In one report, a 7-year-old boy with flu symptoms resulting from *M. pneumoniae* developed parkinsonism including hypophonia, hypomimia, bradykinesia, and dystonia.[50] In addition, imaging studies showed abnormalities in the basal ganglia. After treatment, the parkinsonian symptoms and basal ganglia abnormalities on imaging resolved.

SYPHILIS

Rare cases of meningovascular syphilis as a cause for parkinsonism have been reported. In one report, a 43-year-old patient with active neurosyphilis developed parkinsonism, which improved with penicillin.[51]

FUNGAL AND PARASITIC INFECTIONS

The development of parkinsonism after cryptococcal meningoencephalitis or cryptococcal granulomata is rare.[52–54] In one case, a patient developed parkinsonian features before meningoencephalitic symptoms, which continued to worsen and eventually improved with anticryptococcal therapy. Imaging studies indicated no basal ganglia abnormalities in this patient.[54] In another case, an intravenous drug user developed severe parkinsonism with bilateral striatal lesions. On biopsy, septate hyphae consistent with either aspergillosis or mucormycosis was identified.[55] Systemic amphotericin B therapy improved the parkinsonism and the striatal lesions were gradually reduced.

In one report neurocysticercosis led to the development of parkinsonism. In this case, midbrain encephalitis resulting from cysticercosis was treated with praziquantel. The patient developed asymmetric parkinsonism related to midbrain cysticercus cysts. The parkinsonian symptoms resolved after treatment.[56]

CREUTZFELDT–JAKOB DISEASE (CJD)

CJD is potentially transmissible and therefore is often classified as an infectious cause of parkinsonism.[57,58] The characteristic pathology involves spongiform changes, which are generally in the cortex and basal ganglia. The primary symptoms are cognitive dysfunction, personality changes, anxiety, depression, cerebellar ataxia, and involuntary and uncoordinated movements. Rigidity is uncommon at diagnosis but frequently occurs as the disease progresses. In one study, 56% of sporadic CJD patients developed extrapyramidal signs at some point during the disease course; however, they were present in only 9% at diagnosis.[59]

▶ TOXIN-INDUCED PARKINSONISM

A variety of toxins can induce parkinsonism (Table 23–2). Manganese was the first toxin reported to cause parkinsonism in 1837.[60] However, the discovery of the neurotoxin MPTP (1-methyl-4-phenyl-1,2,3,6-tetrahydropyridine) as a cause of parkinsonism has benefited almost every aspect of PD research.[61] MPTP-induced parkinsonism in animal models has become a standard and powerful tool in the laboratory investigation of parkinsonism.[61] Multiple other toxins such as carbon monoxide, carbon disulfide, cyanide, and methanol can cause symptoms of parkinsonism.

MPTP-INDUCED PARKINSONISM

In 1947, Ziering and colleagues[62] synthesized the compound 1-methyl-4-phenyl-4-propionoxypiperdine (MPPP). This compound underwent testing as a possible antiparkinsonian drug.[63] Primates who received this

▶ **TABLE 23-2. VARIOUS TOXINS THAT CAN INDUCE PARKINSONISM**

1-Methyl-4-phenyl-1,2,3,6-tetrahydropyridine (MPTP)
Manganese
Carbon monoxide
Carbon disulfide
Cyanide
Methanol

compound became rigid and immobile, and two humans died during or shortly after the study; this agent was therefore abandoned as a possible therapeutic agent.[63] In 1979, Davis and colleagues [64] reported a 23-year-old college student who became parkinsonian after injecting a compound that he had synthesized. It is believed that the offending agent was a mixture of MPPP and MPTP.[65] The parkinsonian symptoms responded to levodopa and bromocriptine, and at autopsy there was neuronal loss in the substantia nigra.[64]

In 1982, a chemist in northern California synthesized and distributed MPPP as a heroin substitute.[66] because of shortcuts in the synthesis, he produced a mixture of MPPP and MPTP that resulted in a number of young addicts being admitted with acute parkinsonism. Samples of the substance used by the addicts were analyzed and MPPP and MPTP were identified in the samples, and in one batch MPTP was the only compound identified.[67] Subsequent animal studies confirmed that MPTP was the neurotoxin that caused selective and irreversible damage to the substantia nigra and produced clinical characteristics similar to those of PD.[68]

Clinical Features

Although the majority of the 400 intravenous drug users estimated to be exposed to MPTP[69] have remained asymptomatic, there are reports of addicts who developed parkinsonism.[70–72] In seven patients reported to have developed moderate-to-severe parkinsonism, the acute reactions associated with intravenous use of MPTP included a burning sensation at the injection site followed by a high sensation and visual changes with hallucinations.[70] The majority of these patients experienced generalized jerking movements and one patient reported twisting postures of the arms, legs, and neck. Within a few days, patients developed drooling, oily face, slow generalized movements, low-volume speech, and tremor. All seven patients developed rapidly progressive parkinsonian features within 2 weeks. The patients had the cardinal signs of PD, namely resting tremor, bradykinesia, rigidity, and postural instability. Other features of PD, including flexed posture, shuffling gait, micrographia, loss of associated movements, masked facies, freezing, and akinesia paradoxica, were also present. None of the patients had dementia[(73)] or associated corticospinal tract, cerebellar, or sensory findings.[70] These patients had a dramatic response to levodopa. Long-term complications of levodopa therapy, namely dyskinesia, motor fluctuations, and psychiatric disturbances, occurred within weeks to months and continued to worsen over time.[61,74] This is in contrast to PD, where it usually takes years for these adverse effects to occur.

Tetrud and Langston[61] reported a series of 22 individuals who developed mild parkinsonism after exposure to MPTP. These individuals demonstrated parkinsonian features similar to early PD, which progressively worsened. Two surveys carried out in a group of MPTP-exposed individuals supported the findings of symptom progression.[69,75] One survey was a retrospective chart review of individuals who complained of typical PD symptoms,[75] the second was a survey of 83 individuals exposed to MPTP who developed parkinsonian symptoms about 1 year after exposure.[69] Although these surveys suggest symptom progression, they cannot be considered definitive as they relied on patient reports.

Snow and colleagues[76] used PET to examine the distribution of striatal dopaminergic function in MPTP-induced parkinsonian patients. They scanned nine patients with MPTP-induced parkinsonism and compared them with 10 patients with PD and 6 normal subjects. In the MPTP group there was an equal reduction of dopaminergic function in the caudate and putamen, in contrast to PD where there was a greater putaminal than caudate loss.

Pathology

Brains of three subjects with MPTP-induced parkinsonism have undergone detailed neuropathological evaluations.[64,77] Gross examination of the brain indicated a pale to almost completely depigmented substantia nigra. Microscopically there was moderate-to-severe depletion of pigmented nerve cells of the substantia nigra, along with gliosis and clustering of microglia around nerve cells. Lewy bodies or other inclusions were not present. One of the cases had large amounts of extraneuronal melanin.

Mechanism of Toxicity

MPTP is a protoxin converted to MPP^+, which is the toxin responsible for cell damage in the substantia nigra.[78,79] MPTP is metabolized by extraneuronal monoamine oxidase type B (MAO-B), located in the glial cells,[80] to 1-methyl-4-phenyl-2,3-dihydropyridinium ($MPDP^+$), which is converted to MPP^+.[81] Pretreatment of animals with an MAO-B inhibitor blocks the toxicity of MPTP.[82,83]

MPP^+ enters the neurons through the dopamine uptake systems.[84] It is unclear why the toxicity is limited to the dopaminergic neurons in the substantia nigra. However, Langston and Irwin[85] proposed that if the presence of a dopamine uptake system is a prerequisite for MPTP toxicity, there are three primary dopaminergic projection systems in the brain: the hypothalamic dopaminergic system, ventral tegmental system, and nigrostriatal system. The hypothalamic dopaminergic system is more resistant to the toxicity of MPTP.[86] The glia surrounding the substantia nigra but not the ventral tegmental area is rich in MAO-B,[85] and, hence, only the substantia nigra has all the requirements for the generation of toxic MPP^+.

Once MPP^+ enters the neuron, it was postulated to destroy cells through a process of free radical generation. Once within the cell, MPP^+ is accumulated by the mitochondria.[87] This process is dependent on the mitochondrial membrane gradient and appears to be driven by the mitochondrial membrane potential. In the mitochondria, MPP^+ appears to act by interfering with the mitochondrial energy metabolism, inhibiting nicotinamide adenine dinucleotide (NAD^+)-linked oxidation in complex J,[88,89] thereby interrupting the process of cellular energy production. In spite of the lack of definitive evidence, most investigators believe that this energy depletion is the ultimate cause of cell death.[87]

Treatment

Patients with MPTP-induced parkinsonism have a dramatic and unequivocal response to levodopa and dopamine agonists.[67,70,74] Unfortunately, long-term complications of levodopa therapy, such as end-of-dose "wearing-off," peak-dose dyskinesia, on–off phenomenon, and psychiatric complications, including hallucinations and agitation develop.[74] Interestingly, these complications occur much more rapidly than seen in PD.

In 1992, Widner and colleagues[90] reported the outcome of grafting human fetal tissue bilaterally to the caudate and putamen in two immunosuppressed patients with MPTP-induced parkinsonism. The patients were assessed during the 18 months before surgery and the 22–24 months after the surgery. Both patients had substantial, sustained improvement in motor function. Striatal uptake of fluorodopa as measured by PET showed a marked increase in uptake on both sides, paralleling the patients' clinical improvement. However, this surgical technique is investigational and not widely used. There was also a report of a patient with MPTP-induced parkinsonism who underwent deep brain stimulation of the subthalamic nucleus with marked improvement in parkinsonian symptoms.[91]

MANGANESE

Manganese is the twelfth most common element in the earth's crust and the fourth most widely used metal in the world.[92] Its main application is in the manufacture of steel. Manganese dioxide is used in the manufacture of dry batteries and methylcyclopentadienyl manganese tricarbonyl is used as an antiknock agent in gasoline. Potassium permanganate is used industrially for bleaching resins and fabrics, printing fabrics, dying wood, tanning leather, and for water purification, and these can also be sources of manganese intoxication.[60,93] Maneb, a fungicide, also contains manganese. Recently there have been reports of manganese poisoning following use of ephedrone. "Ephedrone" is a slang term for the street drug that contains manganese to produce an amphetamine-like euphoria. The desired chemical product, phenylpropanoneamine (also called methcathinone), is synthesized from ephedrine or pseudoephedrine using permanganate as the catalyst. Manganese is the by-product in the ephedrone mixture, and when addicts inject the compound, they develop manganese poisoning.[94,95] Manganese plays an important role as a cofactor in many enzymatic reactions in humans, but excess amounts can cause irreversible damage to the central nervous system (CNS).

Clinical Features

Couper[96] was the first to describe the effects of chronic manganese intoxication in 1837. He described five patients who worked in a manganese ore-crushing plant and developed features of parkinsonism. The clinical syndrome has since been reported in miners, smelters, industrial and agricultural workers, patients on long-term parenteral nutrition, and after ingestion of Chinese herbal pills.[97–100] The clinical syndrome of manganese intoxication can be divided into three stages: behavioral and psychiatric manifestations, parkinsonian features, and dystonia with severe gait disturbances.[60] The initial symptoms are nonspecific, such as fatigue, headache, muscle cramps, anorexia, insomnia, memory problems, and impotence. Psychiatric and behavioral manifestations ("manganese madness" or "locura manganesa") are generally seen in miners but are not present in industrial workers.[101,102] Psychiatric disturbances include nervousness, irritability, emotional instability, illusions, and hallucinations, which usually last for 1–3 months.[101,102] Parkinsonian features include seborrhea, increased sweating, soft speech, clumsiness with impaired dexterity, dystonic reactions, balance difficulties, and gait problems.[103] Bradykinesia and rigidity are the predominant signs. Tremor is infrequently observed and is usually upper extremity postural tremor. The patients often have a peculiar gait ("cock walk"), in which the trunk is extended, arms are flexed, and patients swagger on their toes. Limb and truncal dystonia is often present, resulting in painful cramps.[104,105] Other neurologic signs include corticospinal signs, dementia, cranial nerve palsies, sensory deficits, muscle weakness, and cerebellar dysfunction.[60] There may be progression of signs and symptoms even after withdrawal from the exposure.[103]

Manganese-induced parkinsonism should be suspected in patients with dystonic parkinsonism. Tremor is usually absent, and dystonia along with postural impairment occur early in the course of the illness. In addition, there is failure to have a sustained response to dopaminomimetic agents.[92] A history of occupational exposure to manganese is helpful. The value of testing biological specimens (blood, hair) for diagnosing manganese-induced parkinsonism is controversial. Blood manganese levels have been reported to be higher in healthy individuals exposed to manganese and lower in manganese-induced parkinsonian patients if they have been removed from exposure.[101] Manganese can be estimated in hair but the concentrations increase with the degree of pigmentation.[60] Electroencephalography, cerebrospinal fluid, and evoked potentials are generally normal.[103,106] Magnetic resonance imaging (MRI) of the brain usually shows high signal intensity on T_1-weighted images in the globus pallidus.[107] These hyperintense signals on T_1-weighted images gradually disappear after cessation of exposure.[98,107] In patients with manganese-induced parkinsonism, PET studies with ^{18}F-6-fluorodopa are normal, and ^{11}C-raclopride (RAC) studies show that RAC binding is mildly reduced in the caudate and normal in the putamen; cerebral glucose metabolism studies show widespread decline in cortical glucose metabolism.[108,109]

Pathology

Pathological changes with manganese intoxication result in neuronal loss and gliosis in the globus pallidus.[110,111] The changes are more extensive in the medial segment of the globus pallidus compared with the lateral segment. There is also some degeneration of the caudate nucleus and the substantia nigra reticulata. The areas of the brain that are affected inconsistently include the substantia nigra pars compacta, the pons, cerebral cortex, the thalamus, the hypothalamus, the red nucleus, and the cerebellum. Histologically, there is a prominent reduction of the myelinated fibers and astrocyte proliferation.[111,112]

Mechanism of Toxicity

Normally, manganese functions in carbohydrate metabolism and gluconeogenesis. However, overexposure to manganese will result in neurotoxicity, possibly due to increased auto-oxidation of dopamine by a higher valence manganese (Mn^{3+}) ion causing increased generation of free radicals.[113,114] However, manganese in its Mn^{2+} form or in complexes such as superoxide dismutase is normally a scavenger of free radicals.[115,116] Barbeau[104] proposed that brain regions with high concentrations of oxidative enzymes, such as nuclei of the basal ganglia, promote the oxidation of Mn^{2+} to Mn^{3+}, which causes increased auto-oxidation of dopamine to toxic quinones and hydroxyl radicals. However, manganese toxicity also results in degeneration of nondopaminergic neurons in the pallidum, caudate, and putamen. It is postulated that the rich dopaminergic innervation of the striatum results in high extracellular concentrations of dopamine, which in the presence of Mn^{3+} are sufficient to injure the adjacent neurons.[102,117] Other possible theories include mitochondrial damage, leading to excitotoxic cell death, and enhanced iron and aluminum in the brain.[60] Manganese accumulates within the mitochondria[118] and can inhibit both the sodium-dependent and sodium-independent calcium efflux in the brain.[119] It can produce a bioenergetic defect by impairing oxidative phosphorylation and reducing ATP synthesis.[120] This can lead to calcium-dependent enzyme activation and cell death.

Treatment

Administration of the chelating agent ethylenediaminetetraacetic acid (EDTA) has not resulted in significant clinical improvement.[121] Open-label studies with levodopa have reported some response.[105,122] Mena and colleagues[105] reported a dramatic improvement with levodopa in rigidity, hypokinesia, postural reflexes, and balance in five patients, and dystonia in two patients; however, no other studies have been able to duplicate these results. There is another report of improvement in cognition and bradykinesia but not dystonia in one patient after levodopa therapy.[122] Cook and colleagues [121] and Greenhouse[123] reported minimal to no benefit with levodopa. Similarly, in a placebo-controlled study with levodopa in six patients there were no changes in motor scores, finger tapping, gait, or dystonia.[124] There is, however, one report of para-aminosalicylic acid improving two patients with chronic manganese poisoning.[125]

CARBON MONOXIDE

Carbon monoxide is a colorless, odorless, nonirritating gas that can cause CNS damage. Approximately 2–26% of affected individuals die due to acute intoxication of carbon monoxide,[125–129] and 2–49% of the survivors develop sequelae.[125,129–132] The recovery in patients with sequelae is 53–75%; the morbidity is 17–21%, and mortality is 8–25%.[125,130]

Clinical Features

The sequelae of carbon monoxide intoxication are either progressive or delayed relapsing.[133] In the progressive-type, acute encephalopathy progresses directly into the vegetative state, whereas, in the delayed relapsing-type, neurological deficits develop after a period of recovery from the acute poisoning. Lee and Marsden[133] described eight patients with progressive sequelae. The patients opened their eyes spontaneously 2–15 days after recovery from coma, but remained in a mute vegetative state. The patients were nonresponsive, rigid, spastic, bed-bound, and exhibited little or no spontaneous movement. In patients with delayed relapsing carbon monoxide intoxication, after the initial coma they recovered completely after a period of days to weeks.[130,134] The delayed symptoms may be parkinsonian or akinetic-mute. The parkinsonian patients have a slow shuffling gait, loss of armswing, retropulsion, bradykinesia, rigidity, masked facies, and occasionally resting tremor.[135] There may also be fixed dystonia of the hands and feet.[133] Emotional change, confusion, memory disturbances, anxiety, and depression may occur.[125,130,133,136] In the akinetic-mute patients, initial mental changes progress to apathy and mutism along with motor deterioration. Incontinence, rigidity, and primitive responses to painful stimuli may be present.[133] The delayed deterioration may progress, stop at any time, or eventually improve.[133,137]

Rare patients develop tremor,[133,138] chorea,[139,140] myoclonus,[131,141] and Tourette syndrome[142] after carbon monoxide intoxication. Choi and Cheon[143] examined 242 patients with carbon monoxide poisoning and reported movement disorders in 32 (13.2%). These included parkinsonism in 23 patients, dystonia in 5, chorea in 3, and myoclonus in 1. Median latency after exposure for the onset of parkinsonism and chorea was four weeks, dystonia was 51 weeks, and myoclonus was 8 weeks.

Patients with carbon monoxide intoxication may have a normal CT scan, white matter low-density lesions, bilateral globus pallidus lesions, or both white matter and globus pallidus lesions.[133,144–146] Mimura and colleagues[147] performed MRIs in 129 of their 156 patients. They reported abnormal findings of cerebral atrophy (72%), pallidum lesions (38%), lacunar and cerebral infarctions (53%), and hippocampal atrophy (19%). Among the patients with extrapyramidal symptoms, pallidum lesions occurred in 59% of the cases. Follow-up CT scans may show new lesions or progression of white matter and globus pallidus lesions.[133,148–150]

Pathology

The most prominent pathological changes with carbon monoxide poisoning are white matter changes and necrosis of the globus pallidus.[151–153] If death occurs a few hours after acute intoxication the pathological changes are similar to those seen with asphyxia. The brain appears swollen, with congestion of the capillaries and veins, along with petechial hemorrhages.[154] Three types of white matter damage have been reported: small multifocal necrotic lesions with fragmentation of axis cylinders, extensive diffuse necrotic lesions with severe axis cylinder damage, and diffuse demyelination with sparing of axis cylinders.[153,155] These changes may be due to differences in the severity of poisoning.[156] Unilateral or bilateral necrosis of the globus pallidus is the most striking finding.[154,157] The hemorrhage or necrosis of the globus pallidus is limited to the anterior and superior part of the inner pallidum.[151,153,154] Rarely, the pallidum may be spared in cases of carbon monoxide encephalopathy, where the predominant finding is white matter lesions.[154,158]

Mechanism of Toxicity

Carbon monoxide is an asphyxiant that has a much greater affinity for hemoglobin oxygen-binding sites compared with oxygen. It enters the blood, where it binds with the ferrous ion complex of protoporphyrin IX in hemoglobin and hence blocks the binding of oxygen.[93] This results in anoxia, leading to tissue damage. The globus pallidus is vulnerable to anoxic injury, which could be due to intrinsic metabolic susceptibility[159] such as high oxygen consumption[160] and high iron content.[161] Carbon monoxide also blocks ATP production by binding to the cytochrome oxidase of the mitochondrial chain[93] and potentiates the injury due to anoxia.

Treatment

There have been some reports that levodopa and anticholingerics have been helpful in a few patients.[162,163] Lee and Marsden[133] used anticholinergic drugs and carbidopa/levodopa (375–750 mg/day) in 23 patients. Because of spontaneous improvement of symptoms, they found it difficult to evaluate the benefits of these medications. None of their patients had a dramatic response, nor was there any deterioration after the medications were discontinued. Hyperbaric oxygen therapy is the most efficient method of reversing the effects of acute carbon monoxide poisoning and prevents the development of delayed neurological sequelae.

CARBON DISULFIDE

Carbon disulfide is a clear, colorless, and highly volatile liquid used in various industries, such as the production of cellophane and viscose rayon; as a solvent for resins, fats, and rubber; and the manufacture of carbon tetrachloride. It is also used as a fumigant, in combination with carbon tetrachloride, to treat corn, wheat, rye, and other grains.

Clinical Features

The three principal manifestations of carbon disulfide neurotoxicity are acute and chronic encephalopathy, peripheral and cranial neuropathies, and movement disorders. Nervousness, irritability, confusion, disorientation, insomnia, memory problems, and hallucinations are mental changes that can be seen with carbon disulfide intoxication.[164] Neurological findings associated with carbon disulfide exposure include peripheral sensorimotor neuropathy, cranial nerve, and abnormalities, pyramidal, and extrapyramidal dysfunction, cerebellar dysfunction, and rarely dystonia and choreoathetosis.[164–167] Resting tremor, gait abnormalities, decreased associated movements, and rigidity are the common parkinsonian features.[168,169] MRI may be normal or show a pattern consistent with central demyelination or lesions of the basal ganglia and corona radiata.[167,170]

Pathology

There have been very few reports of pathological findings after chronic carbon disulfide intoxication. The available data indicate that the pathological changes in the brain include diffuse neuronal degeneration over the cerebral cortex, globus pallidus, and putamen, and a decrease in Purkinje cells in the cerebellar cortex.[171,172]

Mechanism of Toxicity

Carbon disulfide may induce neurotoxicity by the formation of dithiocarbamate metabolites.[173] Dithiocarbamate complexes are capable of chelating metal ions such as copper and zinc, which are of physiological importance.[174] It is also possible that carbon disulfide inhibits cytochrome oxidase and brain tissue respiration,[175] which induces lesions of the striatopallidum.

Treatment

The treatment of carbon disulfide poisoning is limited. There are no reports of dramatic improvement in parkinsonian features with levodopa.

CYANIDE

Clinical Features

Cyanide poisoning may result from exposure through ingestion, injection, or asphyxiation with hydrocyanic fumes. A dose of 50 mg[176] or 0.5 mg per kg of body weight[177] has been estimated as the minimum lethal dose. Acute intoxication results in dizziness, headaches, confusion, restlessness, coma, and convulsions; death usually occurs within seconds to minutes.[102,178] The clinical picture also includes cardiac arrhythmias and hypotension.[178] The mortality rate with acute cyanide poisoning is 95%.[179] Although survival following acute intoxication is rare, in those who recover consciousness parkinsonian features develop over a period of days.[179–181] Gait abnormalities, masked facies, infrequent blinking, rigidity, and weak hypophonic voice are the common parkinsonian features.[179–181] Mild postural and resting tremor has been reported.[179,181] Dystonia and dementia are other features that may occur.[179,180,182]

Immediately following acute intoxication, neuroimaging studies are unremarkable; however, after 3–6 months, bilateral symmetric lesions in the globus pallidus and posterior putamen are reported.[180–182] 6-Fluorodopa PET has revealed diffuse decreased activity in the posterior regions of the basal ganglia, similar to that in patients with PD.[181]

Pathology

Pathologic changes after acute cyanide intoxication have demonstrated selective destruction of the striatum, especially the globus pallidus and pathological findings in a patient with cyanide-induced parkinsonism demonstrated destruction of the putamen and globus pallidus.[179] There was also atrophy of the cerebellum, subthalamic nucleus, and complete nerve cell loss, along with marked fibrous gliosis in the zona reticularis of the substantia nigra.[179]

Mechanism of Toxicity

Similar to the other neurotoxins discussed in this chapter, cyanide radicals inactivate cytochrome oxidase and other oxidative enzymes, leading to cell death due to tissue anoxia.[183]

Treatment

Amantadine, anticholinergics and carbidopa/levodopa have been used in patients with cyanide-induced parkinsonism.[179–181] None of the patients had a dramatic response to these medications.

METHANOL

Methanol is a common industrial solvent. It is a colorless, clear, volatile liquid with a weak odor and is slightly sweeter than ethanol.[184] Methanol poisoning commonly occurs from illegal adulteration of ethanol with methanol.[185,186] Suicidal or accidental poisoning can also occur from ingestion of industrial or household products that contain methanol (e.g., windshield wiper fluid).[187,188]

Clinical Features

Acute intoxication with methanol results in severe acidosis, confusion, and coma.[189] Blindness due to retinal degeneration and subsequent optic atrophy is the most common deficit in patients who survive the acute intoxication.[189,190] There are multiple reports of parkinsonism developing a few days after acute intoxication with methanol.[189–193] Soft voice, masked facies, drooling, tremor, rigidity, bradykinesia, and slow shuffling gait are the common parkinsonian features. Limb and foot dystonia has also been reported.[191] CT and MRI demonstrate bilateral putaminal abnormalities, localized areas of cerebral edema, with necrosis and hemorrhage in the cortex, subcortical white matter, cerebellum, and optic nerve.[189,191,193]

Pathology

Bilateral necrosis of the putamen along with optic atrophy and widespread lesions in the cerebral cortex, anterior horn, and other gray matter nuclei are often induced by methanol intoxication.[154,189,193]Although the duration of survival after methanol ingestion determines the severity of the lesions, bilateral putaminal necrosis has been reported after survival of at least 24 hours.[192]

Mechanism of Toxicity

The exact pathogenesis of methanol intoxication is controversial. Methanol is metabolized to formaldehyde and formic acid by liver alcohol dehydrogenase.[194] Formic acid is believed to be largely responsible for the severe systemic acidosis.[195,196] Since formaldehyde and formic acid achieve high concentrations within the putamen, it is believed to have selective toxicity to the putamen.

Treatment

There are reports of levodopa and bromocriptine having dramatic improvement in rigidity, tremor, and hypokinesia in patients with methanol-induced parkinsonism;[190,191] however, other reports have not confirmed this finding.[189]

OTHER SOLVENTS

Various other solvents have also been reported to cause parkinsonism. Uitti and colleagues [197] described a case of parkinsonism after sniffing lacquer thinner daily for 9 months. The constituents of lacquer thinner are toluene, methanol, ethyl acetate, xylene, n-hexane, isopropyl alcohol, isobutyl acetate, and isobutyl isobutyrate. Although methanol and n-hexane[198] have been reported to cause parkinsonism, the authors believed that toluene was the most likely toxin that produced parkinsonism in their patient. Hageman and colleagues [199] described three patients who developed a variety of neurological features, including parkinsonism, after exposure to a variety of organic solvents, including toluene, xylene, methyl ethyl ketone, and resins. It is possible that mixtures of organic solvents may have a synergistic effect or an antagonistic effect, depending on the solvents in the mixture. Studies of long-term exposure to solvents may lead to identification of other specific neurotoxins that can cause parkinsonism.

SUMMARY

Parkinsonism, particularly rigidity and bradykinesia, following exposure to toxins is rare but can occur. MPTP-induced parkinsonism has clinical characteristics similar to those of PD (Tables 23–3 and 23–4). Unlike parkinsonism induced by MPTP, the other toxins usually cause rigidity and bradykinesia and usually do not respond to levodopa (Table 23–5). These cases have lesions primarily in the pallidostriatum.

▶ DRUG-INDUCED PARKINSONISM

Drug-induced parkinsonism is the most common cause of secondary parkinsonism. Although many drugs can produce parkinsonism, antipsychotic drugs or neuroleptics are the leading cause of drug-induced parkinsonism.[2] Chlorpromazine was one of the first neuroleptics reported to cause parkinsonism in the early 1950s.[200,201] The reported incidence of drug-induced parkinsonism varies from 15–60%.[202,203] Drug-induced parkinsonism tends to be more common in women and the elderly.[202–204]

NEUROLEPTICS

Parkinsonism can result from the use of numerous drugs; however, neuroleptics are the most recognized cause of drug-induced parkinsonism (Table 23–6). Some reports suggest that certain neuroleptics such as piperazine phenothiazines and butyrophenones are more likely to cause parkinsonism.[204] However, controlled studies comparing the risk of parkinsonism between different neuroleptics are lacking. In one series of 125 patients, haloperidol was the most common cause of drug-induced movement disorders followed by amitriptyline-perphenazine and thioridazine.[202]

Higher doses of neuroleptics are thought to increase the risk of parkinsonism; however, studies have failed to show a correlation between the incidence of parkinsonism and total neuroleptic dosage.[205] Depot preparations of neuroleptics are more likely to cause parkinsonism.[206] Other risk factors for neuroleptic-induced parkinsonism include advanced age, female gender, coexisting brain damage, genetic predisposition, and individual susceptibility.[203,207–209]

Neuroleptic-induced parkinsonism is generally reversible and patients usually recover within several months after the offending agent is discontinued; however, in some patients symptoms may persist for more

▶ TABLE 23–3. CLINICAL FEATURES COMMON TO MPTP-INDUCED PARKINSONISM AND PD

Resting tremor
Bradykinesia
Rigidity
Dramatic response of motor disabilities to levodopa
Development of motor fluctuations, and dyskinesia
Progression of symptoms over time

▶ TABLE 23–4. CLINICAL FEATURES MORE COMMON TO MPTP-INDUCED PARKINSONISM THAN TO PD

Young age of onset (<40 yr)
History of intravenous drug abuse
Rapidly progressive symptoms and complications of levodopa therapy

▶ **TABLE 23-5. CLINICAL FEATURES ASSOCIATED WITH PD AND TOXIN-INDUCED PARKINSONISM**

Clinical Features	PD	MPTP	Mn	CO	CS	CN	Methanol
Tremor	++	++	±	±	+	±	+
Bradykinesia	++	++	++	++	++	++	++
Rigidity	++	++	++	++	++	++	++
Gait abnormality	++	++	++	++	++	++	++
Dystonia	±	±	++	+	±	±	±
Mental changes	+	±	++	+	–	+	–
L-Dopa response	++	++	±	±	–	±	+
Motor fluctuations	++	++	–	–	–	–	–

–, not present; ±, may be present; +, rarely present; ++, commonly present.
CN, cyanide-induced parkinsonism; CO, carbon monoxide-induced parkinsonism; CS, carbon disulfide-induced parkinsonism; Methanol, methanol-induced parkinsonism; MN, manganese-induced parkinsonism; MPTP, 1-methyl-4-phenyl-1,2,3,6-tetrahydropyridine-induced parkinsonism; PD, Parkinson's disease.

▶ **TABLE 23-6. NEUROLEPTICS AND RELATED AGENTS REPORTED TO CAUSE PARKINSONISM**

Trade Name	Generic Name
Abilify	Aripiprazole
Compazine	Prochlorperazine
Etrafon (Triavil)	Perphenazine and amitripyline
Fentanyl	Droperidol
Geodon	Ziprasidone
Haldol	Haloperidol
Levoprome	Methotrimeprazine
Loxitane	Loxapine
Mellaril	Thioridazine
Moban	Molindone
Navane	Thiothixene
Norzine	Thiethylperazine
Phenergan	Promethazine
Proketazine	Carphenazine maleate
Prolixin	Fluphenazine
Reglan	Metoclopramide
Risperdal	Risperadone
Serentil	Mesoridazine
Seroquel	Quetiapine
Sparine	Promaxine
Stelazine	Trifluoperazine
Taractan	Chlorprothixene
Thorazine	Chlorpromazine
Torecan	Thiethylperazine
Trilafon	Perphenazine
Vesprin	Triflupromazine hydrochloride
Zyprexa	Olanzapine

than a year.[207] In some patients signs of parkinsonism do not resolve after the offending drug is discontinued and these patients may develop signs of idiopathic PD.[207,209] In one report, two patients who had complete recovery of parkinsonism following discontinuation of a neuroleptic underwent brain autopsy and had mild–to-moderate nigral dopaminergic cell loss and Lewy bodies suggesting preclinical PD.

Although neuroleptics are used primarily as antipsychotic agents, they are sometimes prescribed for depression, anxiety, and insomnia. Typically used to control nausea and vomiting, the neuroleptic prochlorperazine and related agents can cause parkinsonism.[210] Similarly, metoclopramide, an atypical neuroleptic belonging to the benzamide class, is used as an antiemetic and to ameliorate gastric stasis and can cause parkinsonism.[211–213] In a series of 2,557 metoclopramide-treated patients, only 5 (<0.2%) patients, all over the age of 40, developed parkinsonism.[214]

Clinical Features

Clinical features of neuroleptic-induced parkinsonism are similar to PD and include bradykinesia, rigidity, and tremor.[215] Bradykinesia is the most common symptom, generally the initial symptom and often the only symptom of neuroleptic-induced parkinsonism. It results in masked facies, slowed, or reduced movement and speech difficulties. Rigidity may also occur and generally affects the limbs, neck, or trunk. Although the resting tremor of PD may be present, postural tremor resembling essential tremor may also be seen.[216,217] Gait abnormalities and postural instability can also occur with neuroleptic-induced parkinsonism.[218]

Differentiating neuroleptic-induced parkinsonism from PD can be challenging; however, there are several characteristics that can help to distinguish the two

TABLE 23–7. CLINICAL FEATURES THAT MAY DISTINGUISH DRUG-INDUCED PARKINSONISM FROM PARKINSON'S DISEASE (PD)[2]

	Drug-Induced Parkinsonism	PD
Symptom at onset	Bilateral and symmetric	Unilateral or asymmetrical
Course	Acute or subacute	Insidious, chronic
Tremor type	Bilateral or symmetric postural or rest tremor	Unilateral or asymmetric rest tremor
Anticholinergic drug response	May be pronounced	Usually moderate
Withdrawal of suspected offending drug	Remittance typically within weeks to months	Symptoms and signs slowly progress

disorders (Table 23–7).[219] PD is slowly progressive and is generally initially unilateral, affecting the other side as the disease progresses. In contrast, drug-induced parkinsonism is generally bilateral and symmetric with an acute onset. In one series, the signs of parkinsonism emerged within a few days of neuroleptic treatment with a gradual increase in incidence, so that 50–70% of cases appeared by 1 month and 90% of cases within 3 months.[215] It has been suggested that tolerance to neuroleptic-induced parkinsonism develops; however, this has not been confirmed. The only clinical basis for this assumption is the observation that withdrawal of anticholinergic drugs, co-administered for several months with neuroleptics, is followed by the appearance of relatively few cases of drug-induced parkinsonism.

After discontinuation of neuroleptics, in the majority of patients parkinsonian signs resolve within a few weeks. However, the effects may last longer, even several years in some cases.[219] Metoclopramide-induced parkinsonism has been reported to take several months to resolve completely.[220,221] Drug-induced parkinsonism will usually slowly improve after the reduction or discontinuation of the offending drug, whereas the signs and symptoms of PD progressively worsen.

Neuroleptic-induced movement disorders, including parkinsonism, are frequently not initially recognized.[220] In a review of metoclopramide-induced movement disorders, it was reported that the offending drug was continued for an average of 6 months after the onset of extrapyramidal symptoms.[212] Hansen and colleagues reported that psychiatry residents diagnosed drug-induced parkinsonism in 11% of neuroleptic-treated patients, whereas researchers determined the prevalence to be 26% in this study population.[222]

Pathogenesis

The primary neurochemical abnormality of PD is striatal dopamine depletion. Therefore, since neuroleptics are dopamine-blocking drugs, it follows that the clinical features of parkinsonism may result from their use. However, the mechanism of action is not this simple as the incidence and severity of neuroleptic-induced parkinsonism has not been shown to correlate with drug dosage;[205] furthermore, plasma neuroleptic drug levels do not usually correlate with the severity of parkinsonism.[223] Parkinsonism appearing within several days of treatment with relatively small drug doses is a common clinical experience; yet, other patients are successfully maintained on relatively high doses for several years without developing parkinsonism. It had been suggested that neuroleptic-induced parkinsonism is simply PD occurring by chance in neuroleptic-treated individuals. The reported prevalence of neuroleptic-induced parkinsonism varies, but clinically significant parkinsonism reportedly occurs in 10–15% of treated individuals, which is likely an underestimate.[224–226] Therefore, coincidental PD could not account for all cases of neuroleptic-induced parkinsonism because the incidence of parkinsonism in neuroleptic-treated patients is much greater than the incidence of PD in the general population.

The mechanisms determining susceptibility to neuroleptic-induced parkinsonism are unclear. It has been suggested that women may be at a greater risk due to estrogen-related dopamine receptor blockade.[203,224,227] However, others have not found differences related to gender.[228,229] These inconsistencies could be related to differences in the ascertainment of the subjects studied and also to differences in medication prescription and usage based on gender. In one report, low urinary levels of free dopamine were associated with the subsequent development of phenothiazine-induced parkinsonism, suggesting that an inherent metabolic defect may be causative.[230] Human leukocyte antigen B44 (HLA-B44) has been reported in persons with drug-induced parkinsonism, suggesting a genetic influence.[231] In one study of 16 patients with metoclopramide-induced movement disorders, 31% had a family history of parkinsonism, tremor, or chorea.[212] However, the potential genetic influences in drug-induced parkinsonism are unclear.

Treatment

The first treatment option is to discontinue the offending agent; however, it is important to consider the risks and benefits of discontinuation of the drug. This is a particular issue in the instance of neuroleptics used for psychosis associated with schizophrenia. If the psychosis is under good control and the parkinsonism is mild, discontinuation may not be the best option. Another consideration for persons with more severe parkinsonism is to switch to an atypical antipsychotic such as quetiapine or clozapine with less potential to cause parkinsonism. Similarly, domperidone, a peripherally acting dopamine antagonist, may be considered to replace the antiemetics metoclopramide or chlorpromazine.[232] Although it has less potential to cause parkinsonism due to low central nervous system (CNS) penetration, parkinsonian symptoms have been reported with domperidone.[233] Another option is to try an antiemetic such as ondansetron or benzquinamide hydrochloride not associated with dopamine blockade.

Antiparkinsonian medications can be used to treat neuroleptic-induced parkinsonism. Treatment with anticholinergics is common, and they can also be used as prophylactic therapy along with a neuroleptic. Anticholinergics have been reported to be more beneficial for neuroleptic-induced parkinsonism than for PD. It has been suggested that anticholinergics could be used to differentiate between drug-induced parkinsonism and PD; however, this has not been confirmed.[234] Dopaminergic drugs, including levodopa, can improve neuroleptic-induced parkinsonism; however, they may also worsen the symptoms for which the neuroleptic was prescribed, such as nausea and hallucinations.[235]

DOPAMINE STORAGE AND TRANSPORT INHIBITORS

Reserpine, an antihypertensive, depletes brain dopamine and other biogenic amines by interfering with presynaptic vesicular storage mechanisms and can cause parkinsonism.[236] Currently, it is rarely used to control blood pressure but may be prescribed for tardive dyskinesia.[237,238] Individuals with tardive dyskinesia may have an increased risk for the development of drug-induced parkinsonism, so close monitoring is warranted if reserpine is used. Tetrabenazine is a synthetic analogue of reserpine that also depletes amines and may block postsynaptic dopamine receptors.[239] Tetrabenazine, like reserpine, is useful in the treatment of hyperkinetic disorders.[240,241] In a study of 217 patients receiving tetrabenazine for hyperkinesia, parkinsonism was the most common side effect, affecting 24% of patients.[241] Although several cases of parkinsonism have been reported with α-methyldopa,[242,243] it is believed to act as a "false" neurotransmitter and has been used in the treatment of PD.[244] Therefore, the significance of the few reported cases of α-methyldopa-induced parkinsonism is unclear.

CALCIUM CHANNEL BLOCKERS

Available in Europe and Latin America, the piperazine derivatives, flunarizine, and cinnarizine, act as calcium-entry blockers and have been prescribed for various disorders, including vertigo, migraine, and tinnitus. Extrapyramidal reactions, including drug-induced parkinsonism and worsening of PD, have been associated with their use.[245,246] Parkinsonism is thought to be a result of the antidopaminergic effects of these compounds that may be presynaptic or postsynaptic.[247,248] In a 15-year follow-up of 74 patients with cinnarizine-induced parkinsonism, the majority of patients recovered within 16 months of discontinuation of the drug. Interestingly, 15% of the patients later developed PD.[249] Calcium-channel blockers are widely available in the United States and have not been associated with parkinsonism except for isolated case reports with diltiazem.[250]

OTHER MEDICATIONS

Various other drugs have occasionally been reported to be associated with the development of parkinsonism (Table 23–8). The cardiac anti-arrhythmic agent, amiodarone, may cause tremor that is typically postural, resembling essential tremor; however, other parkinsonian signs and symptoms have also been described with this drug.[251–253] Lithium often causes postural tremor and in a small percentage of patients, rigidity.[254] Two patients were reported to develop parkinsonism with lithium, but both had prior exposure to neuroleptics.[255]

Cholinergic drugs like bethanechol and the cholinesterase inhibitor pyridostigmine have been reported to cause parkinsonism.[256,257] This side effect is theorized to be a result of drug-induced cholinergic overactivity,

▶ TABLE 23–8. MISCELLANEOUS DRUGS ASSOCIATED WITH PARKINSONISM

α-Methyldopa
Amiodarone
Amphotericin B
Bethanechol
Calcium-channel blockers (cinnarizine, flunarizine)
Cephaloridine
Diazepam
Doxorubicin hydrochloride
5-Fluorouracil
Fluoxetine
Lithium
Meperidine
Phenelzine
Procaine
Pyridostigmine
Reserpine
Tetrabenazine

which is an imbalance of striatal acetylcholinedopamine activity. In one instance of bethanechol-induced parkinsonism, post-mortem analysis demonstrated pathological changes consistent with PD, suggesting that the drug may clinically manifest the underlying nigrostriatal pathology.[256]

Drug-induced parkinsonism was reported in 4 patients on high dose (≥100 mg/day) diazepam for schizophrenia.[258] Fluoxetine has also been associated with parkinsonism.[259–261] Isolated reports of drug-induced parkinsonism have involved various drugs including phenelzine,[262] procaine,[263] meperidine,[264] amphotericin B,[53] cephaloridine,[265] 5-fluorouracil,[266] and vincristine combined with doxorubicin hydrochloride.[267]

SUMMARY

Drug-induced parkinsonism is the most common cause of secondary parkinsonism. It is most often caused by neuroleptics and other dopamine receptor blockers, used primarily as antipsychotics and antiemetics. Other types of medications can less commonly lead to symptoms of parkinsonism. The susceptibility to the development of drug-induced parkinsonism has not been established, but in some cases, may represent latent PD or a heritable trait. Further scrutiny of the occurrence and characteristics of drug-induced parkinsonism would yield a better understanding of this phenomenon and may also provide greater insight into the cause and pathogenesis of PD.

REFERENCES

1. Nisipeanu P, Paleacu D, and Korczyn AD. Infectious and postinfectious parkinsonism. In Watts RL and Koller WC (eds). Movement Disorders: Neurologic Principles & Practice, 2nd ed. New York: McGraw Hill, 2004, pp. 373–382.
2. Hubble JP. Drug-induced parkinsonism. In Watts RL and Koller WC (eds). Movement Disorders: Neurologic Principles & Practice, 2nd ed. New York: McGraw Hill, 2004, pp. 395–402.
3. Poser CM, Huntley CJ, and Poland JD. Para-encephalitic parkinsonism. Report of an acute case due to coxsackie virus type B 2 and re-examination of the etiologic concepts of postencephalitic parkinsonism. Acta Neurol Scand 1969;45:199–215.
4. Cree BC, Bernardini GL, Hays AP, et al. A fatal case of coxsackievirus B4 meningoencephalitis. Arch Neurol 2003;60:107–112.
5. Yazaki M, Yamazaki M, Urasawa N, et al. Successful treatment with alpha-interferon of a patient with chronic measles infection of the brain and parkinsonism. Eur Neurol 2000;44:184–186.
6. Solbrig MV and Nashef L. Acute parkinsonism in suspected herpes simplex encephalitis. Mov Disord 1993;8:233–234.
7. Hsieh JC, Lue KH, and Lee YL. Parkinson-like syndrome as the major presenting symptom of Epstein-Barr virus encephalitis. Arch Dis Child 2002;87:358.
8. Solomon T, Ooi MH, Beasley DW, et al. West Nile encephalitis. BMJ 2003;326:865–869.
9. von Economo C. Encephalitis lethargica. Wien Klin Wochnschr 1917;30:581–585.
10. Dimsdale H. Changes in Parkinson syndrome in the 20th century. Q J Med 1946;15:155–170.
11. von Economo C. Encephalitis Lethargica: Its sequelae and Treatment. New York: Oxford University Press, 1931.
12. Wilson S, ed. Epidemic encephalitis. London: Arnold, 1940.
13. Elizan TS, Madden DL, Noble GR, et al. Viral antibodies in serum and CSF of Parkinsonian patients and controls. Arch Neurol 1979;36:529–534.
14. Esiri MM and Swash M. Absence of herpes simplex virus antigen in brain in encephalitis lethargica. J Neurol Neurosurg Psychiatry 1984;47:1049–1050.
15. Martilla RJ, Halonen P, and Rinne UK. Influenza virus antibodies in parkinsonism: Comparison of postencephalitic and idiopathic Parkinson patients and matched controls. Arch Neurol 1977;34:99–100.
16. Grinker RR and Bucy PC. Epidemic Encephalitis in Neurology, 4th ed. Oxford: Blackwell Scientific, 1949.
17. Krusz JC, Koller WC, and Ziegler DK. Historical review: abnormal movements associated with epidemic encephalitis lethargica. Mov Disord 1987;2:137–141.
18. Oeckinghaus W. Encephalitis epidemica und Wilsonsches Krankleithbild. Dtsch Z Nervenkr 1921;72:294–309.
19. McCowan PK and Cook LC. Oculogyric crises in chronic epidemic encephalitis. Brain 1928;51:285–309.
20. Litvan II, Jankovic J, Goetz CG, et al. Accuracy of the clinical diagnosis of postencephalitic parkinsonism: A clinicopathologic study. Eur J Neurol 1998;5:451–457.
21. Duvoisin RC and Yahr MD. Encephalitis and Parkinsonism. Arch Neurol 1965;12:227–239.
22. Wenning GK, Jellinger K, and Litvan I. Supranuclear gaze palsy and eyelid apraxia in postencephalitic parkinsonism. J Neural Transm 1997;104:845–865.
23. Geddes JF, Hughes AJ, Lees AJ, et al. Pathological overlap in cases of parkinsonism associated with neurofibrillary tangles. A study of recent cases of postencephalitic parkinsonism and comparison with progressive supranuclear palsy and Guamanian parkinsonism-dementia complex. Brain 1993;116 (Pt 1):281–302.
24. Calne DB and Lees AJ. Late progression of post-encephalitic Parkinson's syndrome. Can J Neurol Sci 1988;15:135–138.
25. Korczyn AD. Dementia in Parkinson's disease. J Neurol 2001;248 Suppl 3:III1–4.
26. Forno L. Pathology of parkinsonism. A preliminary report of 24 cases. J Neurosurg 1966;1:266–271.
27. Greenfield JG and Bosanquet FD. The brain-stem lesions in Parkinsonism. J Neurol Neurosurg Psychiatry 1953;16:213–226.
28. Gibb WR and Lees AJ. The progression of idiopathic Parkinson's disease is not explained by age-related changes. Clinical and pathological comparisons with post-encephalitic parkinsonian syndrome. Acta Neuropathol 1987;73:195–201.

29. Yen SH, Houroupian DS, and Terry RD. Immunocytochemical comparison of neurofibrillary tangles in Alzheimer type dementia, progressive supranuclear palsy and postencephalitic parkinsonism. Ann Neurol 1982;13:175.
30. Mark MH and Duvoisin RC. The history of the medical therapy of Parkinson's disease. In Koller WC and Paulson G (eds). Therapy of Parkinson's Disease, 2nd ed. New York: Marcel Dekker, 1995: 1–20.
31. Parkes JD, Tarsy D, Marsden CD, et al. Amphetamines in the treatment of Parkinson's disease. J Neurol Neurosurg Psychiatry 1975;38:232–237.
32. Calne DB, Stern GM, Laurence DR, et al. L-dopa in postencephalitic parkinsonism. Lancet 1969;1:744–746.
33. Hunter KR, Stern GM, and Sharkey J. Levodopa in postencephalitic parkinsonism. Lancet 1970;2:1366–1367.
34. Holloway RG and Kieburtz KD. Neurologic manifestations of human immunodeficiency virus infection. In Mandell GL, Bennett JE, and Polin R (eds). Mandell, Douglas and Bennett's Principles and Practice of Infectious Diseases, 5 ed. Philadelphia: Churchill-Livingstone, 2000: 1432–1439.
35. Cardoso F. HIV-related movement disorders: Epidemiology, pathogenesis and management. CNS Drugs 2002;16:663–668.
36. De Mattos JP, Rosso AL, Correa RB, et al. Involuntary movements and AIDS: Report of seven cases and review of the literature. Arq Neuropsiquiatr 1993;51:491–497.
37. Mattos JP, Rosso AL, Correa RB, et al. Movement disorders in 28 HIV-infected patients. Arq Neuropsiquiatr 2002;60:525–530.
38. Berger JR and Arendt G. HIV dementia: The role of the basal ganglia and dopaminergic systems. J Psychopharmacol 2000;14:214–221.
39. Hriso E, Kuhn T, Masdeu JC, et al. Extrapyramidal symptoms due to agents in patients with AIDS encephalopathy. Am J Psychiatry 1991;148:1558–1561.
40. Reyes MG, Faraldi F, Senseng CS, et al. Nigral degeneration in acquired immune deficiency syndrome (AIDS). Acta Neuropathol 1991;82:39–44.
41. Factor SA, Podskalny GD, and Barron KD. Persistent neuroleptic-induced rigidity and dystonia in AIDS dementia complex: A clinico-pathological case report. J Neurol Sci 1994;127:114–120.
42. Itoh K, Mehraein P, and Weis S. Neuronal damage of the substantia nigra in HIV-1 infected brains. Acta Neuropathol 2000;99:376–384.
43. Koutsilieri E, Sopper S, Scheller C, et al. Parkinsonism in HIV dementia. J Neural Transm 2002;109:767–775.
44. Nath A, Anderson C, Jones M, et al. Neurotoxicity and dysfunction of dopaminergic systems associated with AIDS dementia. J Psychopharmacol 2000;14:222–227.
45. Trillo-Pazos G, Diamanturos A, Rislove L, et al. Detection of HIV-1 DNA in microglia/macrophages, astrocytes and neurons isolated from brain tissue with HIV-1 encephalitis by laser capture microdissection. Brain Pathol 2003;13:144–154.
46. von Giesen HJ, Antke C, Hefter H, et al. Potential time course of human immunodeficiency virus type 1-associated minor motor deficits: Electrophysiologic and positron emission tomography findings. Arch Neurol 2000;57:1601–1607.
47. Maggi P, de Mari M, Moramarco A, et al. Parkinsonism in a patient with AIDS and cerebral opportunistic granulomatous lesions. Neurol Sci 2000;21:173–176.
48. Mintz M, Tardieu M, Hoyt L, et al. E. Levodopa therapy improves motor function in HIV-children with extrapyramidal syndromes. Neurology 1995;47:278–279.
49. Murakami T, Nakajima M, Nakamura T, et al. Parkinsonian symptoms as an initial manifestation in a Japanese patient with acquired immunodeficiency syndrome and Toxoplasma infection. Intern Med 2000;39:1111–1114.
50. Kim JS, Choi IS, and Lee MC. Reversible parkinsonism and dystonia following probable mycoplasma pneumoniae infection. Mov Disord 1995;10:510–512.
51. Neill KG. An unusual case of syphilitic parkinsonism. Br Med J 1953;2:320–322.
52. Balakrishnau J, Becker PS, Jumar AY, et al. E. Acquired immune deficiency syndrome: Correlation of radiologic and pathologic findings in the brain. Radiographics 1990;10:201–216.
53. Fisher JF and Dewald J. Parkinsonism associated with intraventricular amphotericin B. J Antimicrob Chemother 1983;12:97–99.
54. Wszolek Z, Monsour H, Smith P, et al. Cryptococcal meningoencephalitis with parkinsonian features. Mov Disord 1988;3:271–273.
55. Adler CH, Stern MB, and Brooks ML. Parkinsonism secondary to bilateral striatal fungal abscesses. Mov Disord 1989;4:333–337.
56. Verma A, Berger JR, Bowen BC, et al. Reversible parkinsonian syndrome complicating cysticercus midbrain encephalitis. Mov Disord 1995;10:215–219.
57. Brown P, Gibbs CJ, Jr., Rodgers-Johnson P, et al. Human spongiform encephalopathy: The National Institutes of Health series of 300 cases of experimentally transmitted disease. Ann Neurol 1994;35:513–529.
58. Chapman J, Brown P, Rabey JM, et al. Transmission of spongiform encephalopathy from a familial Creutzfeldt-Jakob disease patient of Jewish Libyan origin carrying the PRNP codon 200 mutation. Neurology 1992;42:1249–1250.
59. Chapman J and Korczyn AD. Genetic and environmental factors determining the development of Creutzfeldt-Jakob disease in Libyan Jews. Neuroepidemiology 1991;10: 228–231.
60. Pal PK, Samii A, and Calne DB. Manganese neurotoxicity: A review of clinical features, imaging and pathology. Neurotoxicology 1999;20:227–238.
61. Tetrud JW and Langston JW. MPTP and Parkinson's disease: One decade later. In Stern MB and Koller WC (eds). Parkinsonian Syndromes. New York: Marcel Dekker, 1993: 173–193.
62. Ziering A, Berger L, et al. Piperidine derivatives; 4-arylpiperidines. J Org Chem 1947;12:894–903.
63. Langston JW, Langston EB, and Irwin I. MPTP-induced parkinsonism in human and non-human primates: Clinical and experimental aspects. Acta Neurol Scand Suppl 1984;100:49–54.
64. Davis GC, Williams AC, Markey SP, et al. Chronic Parkinsonism secondary to intravenous injection of meperidine analogues. Psychiatry Res 1979;1:249–254.

65. Markey SP. MPTP: A new tool to understand Parkinson's disease. Discuss Neurosci 1986;3:11–51.
66. Langston JW. MPTP: The promise of a new neurotoxin. In Marsden CD and Fahn S (eds). Movement Disorders 2. London: Butterworths, 1987: 73–90.
67. Langston JW, Ballard P, Tetrud JW, et al. Chronic Parkinsonism in humans due to a product of meperidine-analog synthesis. Science 1983;219:979–980.
68. Langston JW, Forno LS, Rebert CS, et al. Selective nigral toxicity after systemic administration of 1-methyl-4-phenyl-1,2,5,6-tetrahydropyrine (MPTP) in the squirrel monkey. Brain Res 1984;292:390–394.
69. Ruttenber AJ, Garbe PL, Kalter HD, et al. Meperdine analog exposure in California narcotics abusers: Initial epidemiologic findings. In Markey SP, Castagnoli NJ, Trevor AJ, et al. (eds). MPTP: A Neurotoxin Producing Parkinsonian Syndrome. New York: Academic Press, 1986: 339–353.
70. Ballard PA, Tetrud JW, and Langston JW. Permanent human parkinsonism due to 1-methyl-4-phenyl-1,2,3, 6-tetrahydropyridine (MPTP): Seven cases. Neurology 1985;35:949–956.
71. Tetrud JW, Langston JW, Garbe PL, et al. Mild parkinsonism in persons exposed to 1-methyl-4-phenyl-1,2,3,6-tetrahydropyridine (MPTP). Neurology 1989;39: 1483–1487.
72. Tetrud JW, Langston JW, Redmond DEJ, et al. MPTP-induced tremor in human and non-human primates. Neurology 1986;36:308.
73. Stern Y and Langston JW. Intellectual changes in patients with MPTP-induced parkinsonism. Neurology 1985;35:1506–1509.
74. Langston JW and Ballard P. Parkinsonism induced by 1-methyl-4-phenyl-1,2,3,6-tetrahydropyridine (MPTP): Implications for treatment and the pathogenesis of Parkinson's disease. Can J Neurol Sci 1984;11:160–165.
75. Langston JW. MPTP-induced parkinsonism: How good a model is it? In Fahn S, Marsden CD, Teychenne P, and Jenner P (eds). Recent Advances in Parkinson's Disease. New York: Raven Press, 1986: 119–126.
76. Snow BJ, Vingerhoets FJ, Langston JW, et al. Pattern of dopaminergic loss in the striatum of humans with MPTP induced parkinsonism. J Neurol Neurosurg Psychiatry 2000;68:313–316.
77. Langston JW, Forno LS, Tetrud J, et al. Evidence of active nerve cell degeneration in the substantia nigra of humans years after 1-methyl-4-phenyl-1,2,3,6-tetrahydropyridine exposure. Ann Neurol 1999;46:598–605.
78. Langston JW, Irwin I, Langston EB, et al. 1-Methyl-4-phenylpyridinium ion (MPP+): Identification of a metabolite of MPTP, a toxin selective to the substantia nigra. Neurosci Lett 1984;48:87–92.
79. Sanchez-Ramos J, Barrett JN, Goldstein M, et al. 1-Methyl-4-phenylpyridinium (MPP+) but not 1-methyl-4-phenyl-1,2,3,6-tetrahydropyridine (MPTP) selectively destroys dopaminergic neurons in cultures of dissociated rat mesencephalic neurons. Neurosci Lett 1986;72:215–220.
80. Uhl GR, Javitch JA, and Snyder SH. Normal MPTP binding in parkinsonian substantial nigra: Evidence for extraneuronal toxin conversion in human brain. Lancet 1985;1:956–957.
81. Chiba K, Trevor A, and Castagnoli N, Jr. Metabolism of the neurotoxic tertiary amine, MPTP, by brain monoamine oxidase. Biochem Biophys Res Commun 1984;120:574–578.
82. Cohen G, Pasik P, Cohen B, et al. Pargyline and deprenyl prevent the neurotoxicity of 1-methyl-4-phenyl-1,2,3,6-tetrahydropryidine (MPTP) in monkeys. Eur J Pharmacol 1985;106:209–210.
83. Langston JW, Irwin I, Langston EB, et al. Pargyline prevents MPTP-induced parkinsonism in primates. Science 1984;225:1480–1482.
84. Javitch JA, D'Amato RJ, Strittmatter SM, et al. Parkinsonism-inducing neurotoxin, N-methyl-4-phenyl-1,2,3,6-tetrahydropyridine: Uptake of the metabolite N-methyl-4-phenylpyridine by dopamine neurons explains selective toxicity. Proc Natl Acad Sci U S A 1985;82:2173–2177.
85. Langston JW and Irwin I. MPTP: Current concepts and controversies. Clin Neuropharmacol 1986;9:485–507.
86. Demarest KT and Moore KE. Lack of a high affinity transport system for dopamine in the median eminence and posterior pituitary. Brain Res 1979;171:545–551.
87. Di Monte DA. Mitochondrial DNA and Parkinson's disease. Neurology 1991;41:38–42; discussion 42–33.
88. Nicklas WJ, Vyas I, and Heikkila RE. Inhibition of NADH-linked oxidation in brain mitochondria by 1-methyl-4-phenyl-pyridine, a metabolite of the neurotoxin, 1-methyl-4-phenyl-1,2,5,6-tetrahydropyridine. Life Sci 1985;36:2503–2508.
89. Poirier J and Barbeau A. 1-Methyl-4-phenyl-pyridinium-induced inhibition of nicotinamide adenosine dinucleotide cytochrome c reductase. Neurosci Lett 1985; 62:7–11.
90. Widner H, Tetrud J, Rehncrona S, et al. Bilateral fetal mesencephalic grafting in two patients with parkinsonism induced by 1-methyl-4-phenyl-1,2,3,6-tetrahydropyridine (MPTP). N Engl J Med 1992;327:1556–1563.
91. Christine CW, Langston JW, Turner RS, et al. The neurophysiology and effect of deep brain stimulation in a patient with 1-methyl-4-phenyl-1,2,3,6-tetrahydropyridine-induced parkinsonism. J Neurosurg 2009;110:234–238.
92. Calne DB, Chu NS, Huang CC, et al. Manganism and idiopathic parkinsonism: Similarities and differences. Neurology 1994;44:1583–1586.
93. Spencer PS and Butterfield PG. Environmental agents and Parkinson's disease. In Ellenberg JH, Koller WC, and Langston JW (eds). Etiology of Parkinson's Disease. New York Marcel Dekker, 1995: 319–365.
94. Sanotsky Y, Lesyk R, Fedoryshyn L, et al. Manganic encephalopathy due to "ephedrone" abuse. Mov Disord 2007;22:1337–1343.
95. Stepens A, Logina I, Liguts V, et al. A Parkinsonian syndrome in methcathinone users and the role of manganese. N Engl J Med 2008;358:1009–1017.
96. Couper J. On the effects of black oxide of manganese when inhaled into the lungs. Br Ann Med Pharm 1987;1:41–42.
97. Canavan MM, Cobb S, and Drinker CK. Chronic manganese poisoning. Arch Neurol Psychiatry 1934;32: 501–512.
98. Ejima A, Imamura T, Nakamura S, et al. Manganese intoxication during total parenteral nutrition. Lancet 1992;339:426.

99. Emara AM, el-Ghawabi SH, Madkour OI, et al. Chronic manganese poisoning in the dry battery industry. Br J Ind Med 1971;28:78–82.
100. Flinn RH, Neal PA, and Fulton WB. Industrial manganese poisoning. J Ind Hyg Toxicol 1941;23:374–387.
101. Mena I, Marin O, Fuenzalida S, et al. Chronic manganese poisoning. Clinical picture and manganese turnover. Neurology 1967;17:128–136.
102. Sanchez-Ramos JR. Toxin-induced parkinsonism. In Stern MB and Koller WC (eds). Parkinsonian Syndromes. New York: Marcel Dekker, 1993: 155–172.
103. Huang CC, Chu NS, Lu CS, et al. Chronic manganese intoxication. Arch Neurol 1989;46:1104–1106.
104. Barbeau A. Manganese and extrapyramidal disorders (a critical review and tribute to Dr. George C. Cotzias). Neurotoxicology 1984;5:13–35.
105. Mena I, Court J, Fuenzalida S, et al. Modification of chronic manganese poisoning. Treatment with L-dopa or 5-OH tryptophane. N Engl J Med 1970;282:5–10.
106. Mena I. Manganese poisoning. In Vinken PJ, Bruyn EW, Cohen MM, et al. (eds). Intoxications of the Nervous System, Part I. Handbook of Clinical Neurology. Amsterdam: North-Holland, 1979: 217–237.
107. Nelson K, Golnick J, Korn T, et al. Manganese encephalopathy: Utility of early magnetic resonance imaging. Br J Ind Med 1993;50:510–513.
108. Shinotoh H, Snow BJ, Chu NS, et al. Presynaptic and postsynaptic striatal dopaminergic function in patients with manganese intoxication: A positron emission tomography study. Neurology 1997;48:1053–1056.
109. Wolters EC, Huang CC, Clark C, et al. Positron emission tomography in manganese intoxication. Ann Neurol 1989;26:647–651.
110. Canavan M, Cobb S, and Drinker CK. Chronic manganese poisoning: Report of a case with autopsy. Arch Neurol Psychiatry 1934;32:500–505.
111. Yamada M, Ohno S, Okayasu I, et al. Chronic manganese poisoning: A neuropathological study with determination of manganese distribution in the brain. Acta Neuropathol 1986;70:273–278.
112. Banta RG and Markesbery WR. Elevated manganese levels associated with dementia and extrapyramidal signs. Neurology 1977;27:213–216.
113. Donaldson J. The pathophysiology of trace metal: Neurotransmitter interaction in the CNS. Trends Pharmacol Sci 1981;1:75–77.
114. Donaldson J, LaBella FS, and Gesser D. Enhanced autoxidation of dopamine as a possible basis of manganese neurotoxicity. Neurotoxicology 1981;2:53–64.
115. Archibald FS and Fridovich I. Manganese, superoxide dismutase, and oxygen tolerance in some lactic acid bacteria. J Bacteriol 1981;146:928–936.
116. Kono Y, Takahashi MA, and Asada K. Oxidation of manganous pyrophosphate by superoxide radicals and illuminated spinach chloroplasts. Arch Biochem Biophys 1976;174:454–462.
117. Graham DG. Catecholamine toxicity: A proposal for the molecular pathogenesis of manganese neurotoxicity and Parkinson's disease. Neurotoxicology 1984;5: 83–95.
118. Maynard LS and Cotzias GC. The partition of manganese among organs and intracellular organelles of the rat. J Biol Chem 1955;214:489–495.
119. Gavin CE, Gunter KK, and Gunter TE. Manganese and calcium efflux kinetics in brain mitochondria. Relevance to manganese toxicity. Biochem J 1990;266:329–334.
120. Brouillet EP, Shinobu L, McGarvey U, et al. Manganese injection into the rat striatum produces excitotoxic lesions by impairing energy metabolism. Exp Neurol 1993;120:89–94.
121. Cook DG, Fahn S, and Brait KA. Chronic manganese intoxication. Arch Neurol 1974;30:59–64.
122. Rosenstock HA, Simons DG, and Meyer JS. Chronic manganism. Neurologic and laboratory studies during treatment with levodopa. JAMA 1971;217:1354–1358.
123. Greenhouse AH. Manganese intoxication in the United States. Trans Am Neurol Assoc 1971;96:248–249.
124. Lu CS, Huang CC, Chu NS, et al. Levodopa failure in chronic manganism. Neurology 1994;44:1600–1602.
125. Shillito JH, Drinker CK, and Sahgnessy TJ. The problem of nervous and mental sequelae in carbon monoxide poisoning. JAMA 1936;106:669–674.
126. Bour H, Tutin M, and Pasquier P. The central nervous system and carbon monoxide poisoning. I. Clinical data with reference to 20 fatal cases. Prog Brain Res 1967;24:1–30.
127. Meigs JW and Hughes JP. Acute carbon monoxide poisoning; an analysis of one hundred five cases. A M A Arch Ind Hyg Occup Med 1952;6:344–356.
128. Richardson JC and Chambers RA, Heywood PM. Encephalopathies of anoxia and hypoglycemia. Arch Neurol 1959;1:178–182.
129. Smith J and Brandon S. Morbidity from acute carbon monoxide poisoning at three year follow up. Br Med J 1970;1:318–320.
130. Choi IS. Delayed neurologic sequelae in carbon monoxide intoxication. Arch Neurol 1983;40:433–435.
131. Mathieu D, Nolf M, Durocher A, et al. Acute carbon monoxide poisoning. Risk of late sequelae and treatment by hyperbaric oxygen. J Toxicol Clin Toxicol 1985;23:315–324.
132. Norkool DM and Kirkpatrick JN. Treatment of acute carbon monoxide poisoning with hyperbaric oxygen: A review of 115 cases. Ann Emerg Med 1985;14:1168–1171.
133. Lee MS and Marsden CD. Neurological sequelae following carbon monoxide poisoning clinical course and outcome according to the clinical types and brain computed tomography scan findings. Mov Disord 1994;9:550–558.
134. Siesjo BK. Carbon monoxide poisoning: Mechanism of damage, late sequelae and therapy. Clin Toxicol 1985;23:247–248.
135. Min SK. A brain syndrome associated with delayed neuropsychiatric sequelae following acute carbon monoxide intoxication. Acta Psychiatr Scand 1986;73:80–86.
136. Lacey DJ. Neurologic sequelae of acute carbon monoxide intoxication. Am J Dis Child 1981;135:145–147.
137. Ginsberg MD. Delayed neurological deterioration following hypoxia. Adv Neurol 1979;26:21–44.
138. Raskin N and Mullaney OC. The mental and neurological sequelae of carbon monoxide poisoning: Serial investigation 33 years after poisoning. Seishin Shinkeigaku Zasshi 1940;101:592–618.

139. Davous P, Rondot P, Marion MH, et al. Severe chorea after acute carbon monoxide poisoning. J Neurol Neurosurg Psychiatry 1986;49:206–208.
140. Schwartz A, Hennerici M, and Wegener OH. Delayed choreoathetosis following acute carbon monoxide poisoning. Neurology 1985;35:98–99.
141. Kim JS and Lee SA. Myoclonus, delayed sequelae of carbon monoxide poisoning, piracetam trial. Yonsei Med J 1987;28:231–233.
142. Pulst SM, Walshe TM, and Romero JA. Carbon monoxide poisoning with features of Gilles de la Tourette's syndrome. Arch Neurol 1983;40:443–444.
143. Choi IS and Cheon HY. Delayed movement disorders after carbon monoxide poisoning. Eur Neurol 1999;42: 141–144.
144. Hayashi R, Hayashi K, Inoue K, et al. A serial computerized tomographic study of the interval form of CO poisoning. Eur Neurol 1993;33:27–29.
145. Miura T, Mitomo M, Kawai R, et al. CT of the brain in acute carbon monoxide intoxication: Characteristic features and prognosis. AJNR Am J Neuroradiol 1985;6: 739–742.
146. Sawada Y, Takahashi M, Ohashi N, et al. Computerised tomography as an indication of long-term outcome after acute carbon monoxide poisoning. Lancet 1980;1: 783–784.
147. Mimura K, Harada M, Sumiyoshi S, et al. [Long-term follow-up study on sequelae of carbon monoxide poisoning; serial investigation 33 years after poisoning]. Seishin Shinkeigaku Zasshi 1999;101:592–618.
148. Destee A, Courteville V, Devos PH, et al. Computed tomography and acute carbon monoxide poisoning. J Neurol Neurosurg Psychiatry 1985;48:281–282.
149. Jaeckle RS and Nasrallah HA. Major depression and carbon monoxide-induced parkinsonism: Diagnosis, computerized axial tomography, and response to L-dopa. J Nerv Ment Dis 1985;173:503–508.
150. Vieregge P, Klostermann W, Blumm RG, et al. Carbon monoxide poisoning: Clinical, neurophysiological, and brain imaging observations in acute disease and follow-up. J Neurol 1989;236:478–481.
151. Garland H and Pearce J. Neurological complications of carbon monoxide poisoning. Q J Med 1967;36:445–455.
152. Gordon EB. Carbon-Monoxide Encephalopathy. Br Med J 1965;1:1232.
153. Lapresle J and Fardeau M. The central nervous system and carbon monoxide poisoning. II. Anatomical study of brain lesion following intoxication with carbon monoxide. In Bour H and Ledingham IM (eds). Progress in Brain Research. Amsterdam: Elsevier, 1967: 31–74.
154. Jellinger K. Exogenous lesions of the pallidum. In Vinken PJ and Bruyn GW (eds). Handbook of Clinical Neurology. New York: Elsevier, 1986: 465–491.
155. Kobayashi K, Isaki K, Fukutani Y, et al. CT findings of the interval form of carbon monoxide poisoning compared with neuropathological findings. Eur Neurol 1984;23: 34–43.
156. Jefferson JW. Subtle neuropsychiatric sequelae of carbon monoxide intoxication: Two case reports. Am J Psychiatry 1976;133:961–964.
157. Shiraki H. The neuropathology of carbon monoxide poisoning in humans with special reference to the change of globus pallidus. Adv Neurol Sci 1969;133:961–964.
158. Ginsberg MD, Hedley-Whyte ET, and Richardson EP, Jr. Hypoxic-ischemic leukoencephalopathy in man. Arch Neurol 1976;33:5-14.
159. Vogt C and Vogt O. Erkrandungen der Grosshirnrunde im Lichte der Topistik Pathoklise und Pathoarchitektonik. J Psychol Neurol 1922;28:1–171.
160. Friede RL. Chemoarchitecture and neuropathology. In Proceedings of the 4th International Congress on Neuropathology. Stuttgart: G Thieme, 1962: 70–75.
161. Dexter DT, Wells FR, Lees AJ, et al. Increased nigral iron content in post-mortem parkinsonian brain. Lancet 1967;ii:1219–1220.
162. Klawans HL, Stein RW, Tanner CM, et al. A pure parkinsonian syndrome following acute carbon monoxide intoxication. Arch Neurol 1982;39:302–304.
163. Ringel SP, Klawans HL, Jr. Carbon monoxide-induced Parkinsonism. J Neurol Sci 1972;16:245–251.
164. Lewey FH. Neurological, medical and biochemical signs and symptoms indicating chronic industrial carbon disulfide absorption. Ann Intern Med 1941;15:869–883.
165. Frumkin H. Multiple system atrophy following chronic carbon disulfide exposure. Environ Health Perspect 1998;106:611–613.
166. Pentschew A. Intoxications. In Menckler J (ed). Pathology of the Nervous System. New York: McGraw-Hill, 1971: 1618–1650.
167. Peters HA, Levine RL, Matthews CG, et al. Extrapyramidal and other neurologic manifestations associated with carbon disulfide fumigant exposure. Arch Neurol 1988;45:537–540.
168. Peters HA, Levine RL, Matthews CG, et al. Synergistic neurotoxicity of carbon tetrachloride/carbon disulfide (80/20 fumigants) and other pesticides in grain storage workers. Acta Pharmacol Toxicol (Copenh) 1986;59 Suppl 7:535–546.
169. Peters HA, Levine RL, Matthews CG, et al. Carbon disulfide-induced neuropsychiatric changes in grain storage workers. Am J Ind Med 1982;3:373–391.
170. Huang CC, Chu CC, Chen RS, et al. Chronic carbon disulfide encephalopathy. Eur Neurol 1996;36:364–368.
171. Alpers BJ and Lewy FH. Changes in the nervous system following carbon disulfide poisoning in animals and in man. Arch Neurol Psychiatry 1940;44:725–726.
172. Ferraro A, Jervis GA, and Flicker DJ. Neuropathologic changes in experimental carbon disulfide poisoning in cats. Arch Pathol 1941;32:723–738.
173. Bus JS. The relationship of carbon disulfide metabolism to development of toxicity. Neurotoxicology 1985;6: 73–80.
174. Barbeau A and Pourcher E. New data on the genetics of Parkinson's disease. Can J Neurol Sci 1982;9:53–60.
175. Seppalainen AKM and Haltia M. Carbon disulfide. In Spencer RS, Schaumburg HM, eds. Experimental Clinical Neurotoxicology. Baltimore: Williams & Wilkins, 1980: 356–373.
176. Naughton M. Acute cyanide poisoning. Anaesth Intensive Care 1974;2:351–356.

177. Dreisbach RH. Handbook of Poisoning Prevention, Diagnosis and Treatment, 11th ed. Los Altos, CA: Lange Med, 1993.
178. Pentore R, Venneri A, and Nichelli P. Accidental choke-cherry poisoning: Early symptoms and neurological sequelae of an unusual case of cyanide intoxication. Ital J Neurol Sci 1996;17:233–235.
179. Uitti RJ, Rajput AH, Ashenhurst EM, et al. Cyanide-induced parkinsonism: A clinicopathologic report. Neurology 1985;35:921–925.
180. Feldman JM and Feldman MD. Sequelae of attempted suicide by cyanide ingestion: A case report. Int J Psychiatry Med 1990;20:173–179.
181. Rosenberg NL, Myers JA, Martin WR. Cyanide-induced parkinsonism: Clinical, MRI, and 6-fluorodopa PET studies. Neurology 1989;39:142–144.
182. Grandas F, Artieda J, and Obeso JA. Clinical and CT scan findings in a case of cyanide intoxication. Mov Disord 1989;4:188–193.
183. Haymaker W, Ginzler AM, and Ferguson RL. Residual neuropathological effects of cyanide poisoning; a study of the central nervous system of 23 dogs exposed to cyanide compounds. Mil Surg 1952;111:231–246.
184. Von Burg R. Methanol toxicology update. J Appl Toxicol 1994;14:309–313.
185. Bennett IL, Jr., Cary FH, Mitchell GL, Jr., et al. Acute methyl alcohol poisoning: A review based on experiences in an outbreak of 323 cases. Medicine (Baltimore) 1953;32:431–463.
186. Mittal BV, Desai AP, and Khade KR. Methyl alcohol poisoning: An autopsy study of 28 cases. J Postgrad Med 1990;37:9-13.
187. Glazer M and Dross P. Necrosis of the putamen caused by methanol intoxication: MR findings. AJR Am J Roentgenol 1993;160:1105–1106.
188. Gonda A, Gault H, Churchill D, et al. Hemodialysis for methanol intoxication. Am J Med 1978;64:749–758.
189. McLean DR, Jacobs H, and Mielke BW. Methanol poisoning: A clinical and pathological study. Ann Neurol 1980;8:161–167.
190. Guggenheim MA, Couch JR, and Weinberg W. Motor dysfunction as a permanent complication of methanol ingestion. Presentation of a case with a beneficial response to levodopa treatment. Arch Neurol 1971;24:550–554.
191. Davis LE, Adair JC. Parkinsonism from methanol poisoning: Benefit from treatment with anti-Parkinson drugs. Mov Disord 1999;14:520–522.
192. Erlanson P, Fritz H, Hagstam KE, et al. Severe Methanol Intoxication. Acta Med Scand 1965;177:393–408.
193. Potts AM, Praglin J, Farkas I, et al. Studies on the visual toxicity of methanol. VIII. Additional observations on methanol poisoning in the primate test object. Am J Ophthalmol 1955;40:76–83.
194. Ritchie JM. The aliphatic alcohols. In Goodman LS and Gilman A (eds). The Pharmacological Basis of Therapeutics. London: Macmillan, 1970: 135–150.
195. Clay KL, Murphy RC, and Watkins WD. Experimental methanol toxicity in the primate: Analysis of metabolic acidosis. Toxicol Appl Pharmacol 1975;34:49–61.
196. McMartin KE, Makar AB, Martin G, et al. Methanol poisoning. I. The role of formic acid in the development of metabolic acidosis in the monkey and the reversal by 4-methylpyrazole. Biochem Med 1975;13:319–333.
197. Uitti RJ, Snow BJ, Shinotoh H, et al. Parkinsonism induced by solvent abuse. Ann Neurol 1994;35:616–619.
198. Tanner CM. Occupational and environmental causes of parkinsonism. Occup Med 1992;7:503–513.
199. Hageman G, van der Hoek J, van Hout M, et al. Parkinsonism, pyramidal signs, polyneuropathy, and cognitive decline after long-term occupational solvent exposure. J Neurol 1999;246:198–206.
200. Anton-Stephens D. Preliminary observations on the psychiatric uses of chlorpromazine (largactil). J Ment Sci 1954;100:543–557.
201. Lehmann HE and Hanrahan GE. Chlorpromazine; new inhibiting agent for psychomotor excitement and manic states. AMA Arch Neurol Psychiatry 1954;71:227–237.
202. Miller LG and Jankovic J. Neurologic approach to drug-induced movement disorders: A study of 125 patients. South Med J 1990;83:525–532.
203. Ayd FJ, Jr. A survey of drug-induced extrapyramidal reactions. JAMA 1961;175:1054–1060.
204. Koller WC and Hubble JP. Classification of parkinsonism. In Koller WC (ed). Handbook of Parkinson's disease: Marcel Dekker, 1992: 59–104.
205. Hall RA, Jackson RB, and Swain JM. Neurotoxic reactions resulting from chlorpromazine administration. J Am Med Assoc 1956;161:214–218.
206. Chaudhuri KR, Nott J. Drug-Induced Parkinsonism. In Sethi KD (ed). Drug-Induced Movement Disorders. New York: Marcel Dekker, 2004: 61–75.
207. Stephen PJ and Williamson J. Drug-induced parkinsonism in the elderly. Lancet 1984;2:1082–1083.
208. Hoffman WF, Labs SM, and Casey DE. Neuroleptic-induced parkinsonism in older schizophrenics. Biol Psychiatry 1987;22:427–439.
209. Goetz CG. Drug-induced Parkinsonism and idiopathic Parkinson's disease. Arch Neurol 1983;40:325–326.
210. Bateman DN, Rawlins MD, and Simpson JM. Extrapyramidal reactions to prochlorperazine and haloperidol in the United Kingdom. Q J Med 1986;59:549–556.
211. Grimes JD, Hassan MN, and Preston DN. Adverse neurologic effects of metoclopramide. Can Med Assoc J 1982;126:23–25.
212. Miller LG and Jankovic J. Metoclopramide-induced movement disorders. Clinical findings with a review of the literature. Arch Intern Med 1989;149:2486–2492.
213. Sethi KD, Patel B, and Meador KJ. Metoclopramide-induced parkinsonism. South Med J 1989;82:1581–1582.
214. Bateman DN, Darling WM, Boys R, et al. Extrapyramidal reactions to metoclopramide and prochlorperazine. Q J Med 1989;71:307–311.
215. Marsden CD, Tarsy D, and Bladessarini RH. Spontaneous and drug-induced movement disorders. In Benson DF and Blumer D (eds). Psychiatric Aspects of Neurologic Disease. New York: Grune & Stratton, 1975.
216. Hershey LA, Gift T, and Rivera-Calminlin L. Not Parkinson's disease. Lancet 1982;ii:49.
217. Indo T, Ando K. Metoclopramide-induced Parkinsonism. Clinical characteristics of ten cases. Arch Neurol 1982;39:494–496.

218. Akbostanci MC, Atbasoglu EC, and Balaban H. Tardive dyskinesia, mild drug-induced dyskinesia, and drug-induced parkinsonism: Risk factors and topographic distribution. Acta Neurol Belg 1999;99:176–181.
219. Klawans HL, Jr., Bergen D, and Bruyn GW. Prolonged drug-induced Parkinsonism. Confin Neurol 1973;35:368–377.
220. Weiden PJ, Mann JJ, Haas G, et al. Clinical nonrecognition of neuroleptic-induced movement disorders: A cautionary study. Am J Psychiatry 1987;144:1148–1153.
221. Yamamoto M, Ujike H, and Ogawa N. Metoclopramide-induced parkinsonism. Clin Neuropharmacol 1987;10:287–289.
222. Hansen TE, Brown WL, Weigel RM, et al. Underrecognition of tardive dyskinesia and drug-induced parkinsonism by psychiatric residents. Gen Hosp Psychiatry 1992;14:340–344.
223. Crowley TJ, Hoehn MM, Rutledge CO, et al. Dopamine excretion and vulnerability to drug-induced Parkinsonism. Schizophrenic patients. Arch Gen Psychiatry 1978;35:97–104.
224. Korczyn AD and Goldberg GJ. Extrapyramidal effects of neuroleptics. J Neurol Neurosurg Psychiatry 1976;39:866–869.
225. Moleman P, Janzen G, von Bargen BA, et al. Relationship between age and incidence of parkinsonism in psychiatric patients treated with haloperidol. Am J Psychiatry 1986;143:232–234.
226. McClelland HA. Assessment of drugs in schizophrenia. Discussion on assessment of drug-induced extrapyramidal reactions. Br J Clin Pharmacol 1976;3:401–403.
227. Glazer WM, Naftolin F, Moore DC, et al. The relationship of circulating estradiol to tardive dyskinesia in men and postmenopausal women. Psychoneuroendocrinology 1983;8:429–434.
228. Kennedy PF, Hershon HI, and McGuire RJ. Extrapyramidal disorders after prolonged phenothiazine therapy. Br J Psychiatry 1971;118:509–518.
229. Moleman P, Schmitz PJ, and Ladee GA. Extrapyramidal side effects and oral haloperidol: An analysis of explanatory patient and treatment characteristics. J Clin Psychiatry 1982;43:492–496.
230. Crowley TJ, Rutledge CO, Hoehn MM, et al. Low urinary dopamine and prediction of phenothiazine-induced Parkinsonism: A preliminary report. Am J Psychiatry 1976;133:703–706.
231. Metzer WS, Newton JE, Steele RW, et al. HLA antigens in drug-induced parkinsonism. Mov Disord 1989;4:121–128.
232. Parkes JD. Domperidone and Parkinson's disease. Clin Neuropharmacol 1986;9:517–532.
233. Debontridder O. Dystonic reactions after domperidone. Lancet 1980;2:1259.
234. Hornykiewicz O. Parkinsonism induced by dopaminergic antagonists. Adv Neurol 1975;9:155–164.
235. Hausner RS. Amantadine-associated recurrence of psychosis. Am J Psychiatry 1980;137:240–242.
236. Carlsson A, Lindqvist M, and Magnusson T. 3,4-Dihydroxyphenylalanine and 5-hydroxytryptophan as reserpine antagonists. Nature 1957;180:1200.
237. Fahn S. Treatment of tardive dyskinesia: Use of dopamine-depleting agents. Clin Neuropharmacol 1983;6:151–158.
238. Klawans HL, Tanner CM. The reversibility of permanent tardive dyskinesia. Neurology 1983;33 (suppl 2):163.
239. Reches A, Burke RE, Kuhn CM, et al. Tetrabenazine, an amine-depleting drug, also blocks dopamine receptors in rat brain. J Pharmacol Exp Ther 1983;225:515–521.
240. Jankovic J. Tetrabenazine in the treatment of hyperkinetic movement disorders. Adv Neurol 1983;37:277–289.
241. Jankovic J and Orman J. Tetrabenazine therapy of dystonia, chorea, tics, and other dyskinesias. Neurology 1988;38:391–394.
242. Gillman MA and Sandyk R. Parkinsonism induced by methyldopa. S Afr Med J 1984;65:194.
243. Rosenblum AM and Montgomery EB. Exacerbation of parkinsonism by methyldopa. JAMA 1980;244:2727–2728.
244. Fermaglich J and Chase TN. Methyldopa or methyldopahydrazine as levodopa synergists. Lancet 1973;1:1261–1262.
245. Micheli F, Pardal MF, Gatto M, et al. Flunarizine- and cinnarizine-induced extrapyramidal reactions. Neurology 1987;37:881–884.
246. Micheli FE, Pardal MM, Giannaula R, et al. Movement disorders and depression due to flunarizine and cinnarizine. Mov Disord 1989;4:139–146.
247. DeVries DJ and Beart PM. Competitive inhibition by [^{3}H] spiperone binding to D_2 dopamine receptors in striatal homogenates by organic calcium-channel antagonists and plyvalen cations. Eur J Pharmacol 1985;106:133–139.
248. Fadda F, Gessa GL, Mosca E, et al. Different effects of the calcium antagonists nimodipine and flunarizine on dopamine metabolism in the rat brain. J Neural Transm 1989;75:195–200.
249. Marti-Masso JF and Poza JJ. Cinnarizine-induced parkinsonism: Ten years later. Mov Disord 1998;13:453–456.
250. Dick RS and Barold SS. Diltiazem-induced parkinsonism. Am J Med 1989;87:95–96.
251. LeMaire JF, Autret A, Biziere K, al. E. Amiodarone neuropathy: Further arguments for drug-induced neurolipidosis. Eur Neurol 1982;21:65–68.
252. Palakurthy PR, Iyer V, and Meckler RJ. Unusual neurotoxicity associated with amiodarone therapy. Arch Intern Med 1987;147:881–884.
253. Werner EG and Olanow CW. Parkinsonism and amiodarone therapy. Ann Neurol 1989;25:630–632.
254. Kane J, Rifkin A, Quitkin F, et al. Extrapyramidal side effects with lithium treatment. Am J Psychiatry 1978;135:851–853.
255. Tyrer P, Alexander MS, Regan A, et al. An extrapyramidal syndrome after lithium therapy. Br J Psychiatry 1980;136:191–194.
256. Fox JH, Bennett DA, Goetz CG, et al. Induction of parkinsonism by intraventricular bethanechol in a patient with Alzheimer's disease. Neurology 1989;39:1265.
257. Iwasaki Y, Wakata N, and Kinoshita M. Parkinsonism induced by pyridostigmine. Acta Neurol Scand 1988;78:236.
258. Suranyi-Cadotte BE, Nestoros JN, Nair NP, et al. Parkinsonism induced by high doses of diazepam. Biol Psychiatry 1985;20:455–457.
259. Bouchard RH, Pourcher E, and Vincent P. Fluoxetine and extrapyramidal side effects. Am J Psychiatry 1989;146:339–340.

260. Gernaat HB, Van de Woude J, and Touw DJ. Fluoxetine and parkinsonism in patients taking carbamazepine. Am J Psychiatry 1991;148:1604–1605.
261. Tate JL. Extrapyramidal symptoms in a patient taking haloperidol and fluoxetine. Am J Psychiatry 1989;146: 399–400.
262. Teusink JP, Alexopoulos GS, and Shamoian CA. Parkinsonian side effects induced by a monoamine oxidase inhibitor. Am J Psychiatry 1984;141:118–119.
263. Gjerris F. Transitory procaine-induced Parkinsonism. J Neurol Neurosurg Psychiatry 1971;34:20–22.
264. Lieberman AN and Goldstein M. Reversible parkinsonism related to meperidine. N Engl J Med 1985;312:509.
265. Mintz U, Liberman UA, and de Vries A. Parkinsonism syndrome due to cephaloridine. JAMA 1971;216:1200.
266. Bergevin PR, Patwardhan VC, Weissman J, et al. Letter: Neurotoxicity of 5-fluorouracil. Lancet 1975;1:410.
267. Boranic M and Raci F. A Parkinson-like syndrome as side effect of chemotherapy with vincristine and adriamycin in a child with acute leukaemia. Biomedicine 1979;31: 124–125.

CHAPTER 24

Rare Degenerative Syndromes Associated with Parkinsonism

Candan Depboylu, J. Carsten Möller, and Wolfgang H. Oertel

▶ FRONTOTEMPORAL PARKINSONISM LINKED TO CHROMOSOME 17 (FTDP-17)

Frontotemporal dementia (FTD) is one of the most common dementia syndromes and represents a collection of neurodegenerative diseases of frontal and temporal brain regions. About 14% of FTD cases show features of parkinsonism (FTDP).

EPIDEMILIOGY, GENETICS, AND PATHOPHYSIOLOGY

Sporadic or autosomal-dominant familial forms of FTDP have long been associated with mutations in the microtubule-associated protein tau (MAPT).[1] The identification of loss-of-function mutations in progranulin (PGRN) fully resolves a 10-year-old conundrum,[2] namely the genetic basis of FTDP linked to chromosome 17q21, and explains why multiple families linked to this region lack MAPT mutations (60–90%).[3] The facts that PGRN is located 1.7 Mb centromeric of MAPT and that mutations in both genes independently yield indistinguishable clinical phenotypes are presumably an extraordinary coincidence. The main function of MAPT is to stabilize and promote microtubuli assembly by binding to tubulin, which is likely to regulate transport of vesicles and organelles as well as the cell shape and cell motility. Over 100 families with 45 different pathogenic mutations in the gene have been identified worldwide,[4] with the most common mutations accounting for approximately 60% of known cases, being P301L, N279K, and a splice site mutation (exon 10+16). The pathogenetic mechanisms are thought to be related to the altered proportion of tau isoforms (with three amino acid repeats to those with four amino acid repeats) or to the ability of tau to bind microtubules and to promote microtubule assembly.[5] PGRN encodes a widely expressed secreted precursor protein that is cleaved into seven nonidentical cysteine-rich granulin peptides A–G. PGRN and the granulin peptides have mitogenic functions in the regulation of cell growth and cell cycle progression and are involved in multiple physiological processes such as cellular proliferation, survival, and tissue repair and pathological processes including inflammation and tumorogenesis. At least 35 different pathogenic mutations (mostly in exons 2, 10, and 11) have been found, resulting in haploinsufficiency of the PGRN protein by nonsense-mediated transcript decay.[4]

NEUROPATHOLOGY

The brains of FTDP-17 patients are characterized by an atrophy of the frontotemporal cortex and basal ganglia and by a depigmentation of the substantia nigra. Neuronal loss and gliosis are found in affected brain regions. The histopathology of patients with defined mutations is characterized by cytoplasmic neurofibrillary inclusions composed of hyperphosphorylated tau in neurons and glial cells in the cortex, basal ganglia, brain stem nuclei, and white matter (FTDP-17T).[6] In contrast, patients with PGRN mutations have ubiquitin-positive cytoplasmic and intranuclear inclusions in neurons in the frontotemporal cortex, striatum, and hippocampus (FTDP-17U).[7] In both, Pick or Lewy bodies, tangles or plaques are usually not found.

CLINICAL PRESENTATION

It was estimated that there have been reports of about 50–600 FTDP-17T patients, with fewer than 70 individuals still living in 2006.[5] The mean age of disease onset ranges between 25 and 65 years for FTDP-17T and between 45 and 85 years for FTDP-17U, respectively.[8] The disease duration is 3–10 years for FTDP-17T and 1–15 years for FTDP-17U. No sex predilection has been identified. Mutations for FTDP-17T have >95% penetrance, while the penetrance for FTDP-17U is >90% at the age of 70.[8] Despite the differences, FTDP-17T and FTDP-17U share a largely overlapping clinical phenotype. The three major clinical features include motor dysfunctions, cognitive deficits, and behavioral disturbances. Motor symptoms include akinetic-rigid parkinsonism without resting tremor and also dystonia, spasticity, supranuclear gaze palsy, amyotrophy, apraxia, and myoclonus in variable proportions. Cognitive symptoms consist of impaired executive functions and non-fluent aphasia, with a relative preservation of visuospatial orientation and common memory. Behavioral disturbances can be presented as impaired social conduct, hyperorality and hyperphagia, drug abuse, obsessive stereotyped behavior, apathy, as well as psychosis. Neuropathological and clinical manifestations of the disease can be heterogenous, both between and within families carrying the same mutations. A retrospective neuropathologic study reported that clinically, PGRN-positive cases had more frequent language impairment and parkinsonism than PGRN-negative cases.[9] About 30% of PGRN mutation carriers may develop parkinsonism during the course of the disease.[10]

DIAGNOSTICS, DIFFERENTIAL DIAGNOSIS, AND THERAPY

The diagnostic criteria are (a) age at disease onset between the third and sixth decade, (b) rapid disease progression, (c) parkinsonism-plus symptoms, (d) frontotemporal dementia, and (e) behavioral disturbances. FTDP-17 should be considered in the differential diagnosis of patients with a positive family history suggestive of autosomal-dominant inheritance of a neurodegenerative disorder, even if there has been variability in clinical presentations. Genetic counseling should be offered to affected and at-risk individuals. Structural and functional imaging often reveals frontotemporal and basal ganglia atrophies and/or hypoperfusion/hypometabolism. FTDP-17U cases were reported to be associated with more asymmetric frontotemporoparietal atrophy, while FTDP-17T cases show a more symmetric frontotemporal atrophy.[7] Parenchymal signal changes are more seen in FTDP-17U. A history of dream enactment behavior suggesting rapid eye movement (REM) sleep behavior disorder or electrophysiologic features of REM sleep without atonia may exclude the existence of FTDP-17.[11] No biochemical criteria exist for FTDP-17T. FTDP-17U may be predicted by low PGRN levels in plasma.[12] Several diseases are to be considered for differential diagnosis, including sporadic tauopathies, other types of FTD, Parkinson's disease with dementia, dementia with Lewy bodies, Alzheimer's disease, Huntington's disease, and prion disease. The therapy of FTDP-17 is only symptomatic and supportive. The response to levodopa is poor. Psychiatric treatment is usually necessary.

▶ NEURODEGENERATION WITH BRAIN IRON ACCUMULATION (NBIA)

In 1922, a disease in a kindred characterized by gait impairment resulting in rigidity of legs and feet deformity and mental deterioration with juvenile onset was reported.[13] The cause of this rare, heterogenous, and usually autosomal-recessive disease was linked to chromosome 20p13,[14] and has been shown to be a result of mutations in the gene for pantothenate kinase 2 (PANK2).[15] The initial name Hallervorden–Spatz syndrome has been replaced by panthothenate kinase-associated neurodegeneration (PKAN), and more recently this disease has been termed neurodegeneration with brain iron accumulation type one (NBIA-1). NBIA defines a group of progressive extrapyramidal disorders with radiographic evidence of focal iron accumulation in the brain, usually in the basal ganglia. Other NBIA forms (40–50%) include infantile neuroaxonal dystrophy (INAD), neuroferritinopathy, and aceruloplasminemia.

EPIDEMIOLOGY, GENETICS, AND PATHOPHYSIOLOGY

Over 86 mutations in PANK2 have been described, with the G411R and T418M mutations accounting for more than 25% of mutant alleles.[16] Mutations in PANK2 are found in all classical NBIA-1 cases, usually leading to protein truncations, and in one-third of atypical disease, often associated with amino acid changes.[17] PANK2 is ubiquitously expressed, including retina and basal ganglia, and targeted to the mitochondria. It is an essential regulatory enzyme in coenzyme A biosynthesis, catalyzing the cytosolic phosphorylation of pantothenate (vitamin B_5), *N*-pantothenoyl cysteine, and pantotheine. It has been suggested that PANK2 mutations lead to coenzyme A depletion associated with defective membrane biosynthesis.[15] Furthermore, accumulated cysteine, which would normally condense with phosphopantothenate, may form complexes with iron and cause oxidative damage in the brain.[17]

NEUROPATHOLOGY

In the NBIA-1 brain, a rust-brown pigmentation of the globus pallidus, red nucleus, and pars reticulata of substantia nigra occurs. Iron granules are found intracellularly in neurons and glial cells and also extracellularly. A further prominent finding of the disease is a widely distributed distal axonal swelling and dystrophy called spheroids, accompanied by loss of neurons and myelinated fibers as well as gliosis.[18] Lewy body-like alpha-synuclein-positive intraneuronal inclusions, glial inclusions, and rare neurofibrillary tangles can occur.[19]

CLINICAL PRESENTATION

NBIA-1 with early onset and rapid progression reflects the originally reported, classic form of the disease.[13] Mean age of disease onset is 3.4 years. The initial symptom is often gait impairment. The mean disease duration is 11 years.[20] Motor symptoms include extrapyramidal symptoms such as parkinsonism, dystonia, choreoathetosis and tremor, pyramidal signs, and cerebellar ataxia. Ophthalmological symptoms can be present, such as retinitis pigmentosa and optic atrophy. Intellectual impairment is common and is sometimes accompanied by seizures. Atypical patients with PANK2 mutations have a mean age of onset of 13.7 years, frequently present initially with speech problems and feature less severe and more slowly progressive extrapyramidal symptoms. Apart from mental deterioration, personality changes such as impulsivity and violent outbursts, depression, and emotional lability are observed in patients with atypical NBIA-1 and PANK2 mutations.[17] Parkinsonism seems more common in late-onset disease (>20 years), and dystonia is more frequent in cases with younger age of onset (<20 years) with and without PANK2 mutations.[21] A tau-predominant sporadic late-onset form of NBIA-1 has been reported.[22]

DIAGNOSTICS, DIFFERENTIAL DIAGNOSIS, AND THERAPY

The diagnostic criteria are (a) age at disease onset between the first and second decades, (b) progressive course, (c) extrapyramidal syndrome, and supportively (d) pyramidal syndrome, (e) retinopathy, (f) seizures, and (g) cognitive impairment. Magnetic resonance imaging (MRI) shows decreased signal intensity in the globus pallidus and substantia nigra pars reticulata in T_2-weighted images, which is compatible with iron deposits, and a small area of hyperintensity in the internal segment of pallidum, constituting the so-called "eye of the tiger" sign.[23] In all (homozygous and heterozygous) NBIA-1 patients, whether classic or atypical, MRI shows the "eye of the tiger" sign, whereas this pattern has not been observed in atypical patients without PANK2 mutations. Laboratory investigations do not reveal any distinctive abnormalities. Vacuolated circulating lymphocytes containing abnormal cytosomes and sea-blue histiocytes in the bone marrow may be found.[18] HARP syndrome (hypoprebetalipoproteinemia, acanthocytosis, retinitis pigmentosa, pallidal degeneration) presents with similar clinical features of parkinsonism, dystonia, and choreoathetosis and is allelic with PANK2.[24] There is no specific therapy for NBIA-1. Symptomatic management, such as levodopa and dopamine agonists,[18] or pallidal stimulation may be beneficial to patients.[24] Hypothetically, supplementation of panthothenate may ameliorate the symptoms.[17] Single case reports describe a dramatic improvement with pantothenate, but no studies yet have been performed.

INFANTILE NEURAXONAL DYSTROPHY (INAD)

The term NBIA-2 is used for the autosomal-recessive INAD, which is caused to 80% by mutations in the gene of calcium-independent group VIa phospholipase A2 (PLA2G6) on chromosome 22q13.[25] PLA2G6 catalyzes the hydrolysis of glycerophospholipids, generating leukotriene, prostaglandin, and lysophospholipid, and is involved in signal transduction, cell proliferation, and endoplasmic reticulum stress-mediated apoptosis. Defects in PLA2G6 are predicted to disrupt membrane homeostasis. Classical NBIA-2 has an age of disease onset at 1.1 years and an average age of death at 9.4 years. Cases are characterized by mental retardation, early cerebellar ataxia, pyramidal signs, sensory impairment, and visual disturbances. Nerve biopsy may help for diagnosis, as spheroids are found in peripheral nerves like in the brain and spinal cord. Mutation carriers have optic and cerebellar atrophy, and half show brain iron accumulation.[26] Mutations in PLA2G6 have also been described to cause adult-onset levodopa-responsive dystonia–parkinsonism with pyramidal signs, cognitive/psychiatric features, and cerebral and cerebellar atrophy on MRI (but absent iron in the basal ganglia)[27] and also the Karak syndrome (young-onset cerebellar ataxia, chorea, dystonia, and intellectual decline).

NEUROFERRITINOPATHY

Mutations in the ferritin light chain (FTL1) gene on chromosome 19q13 results in an autosomal-dominant disease appropriately termed neuroferritinopathy, which is characterized by late-onset, slowly progressive NBIA.[28] Ferritin has light and heavy chains and stores iron in different cells. Neuroferritinopathy has a typical age at onset between 40 and 55 years and clinically features choreoathetosis, dystonia, spasticity, parkinsonism, and sometimes acute progression. Plasma ferritin is usually reduced. Pathological changes in neuroferritinopathy include reddish-brown discoloration of basal ganglia and ferritin-positive inclusions localized to the globus pallidus, forebrain, and cerebellum. Axonal spheroids are immunoreactive for neurofilaments, ubiquitin, and tau in the globus pallidus, putamen, and white-matter tracts.[29]

ACERULOPLASMINEMIA

Aceruloplasminemia is an autosomal-recessive disorder associated with mutations in the ceruloplasmin gene on chromosome 3q23 resulting in iron overload in the basal ganglia, retina, liver, and pancreas, and decrease in serum iron.[30] Ceruloplasmin has a ferroxidase activity and is involved in iron trafficking in tissues. The clinical triad of aceruloplasminemia includes retinal degeneration, diabetes mellitus, and neurological symptoms in the form of ataxia, blepharospasm, dystonia, tremor, parkinsonism, and chorea in association with cognitive dysfunction and dementia. Typical age at onset is between 30 and 39 years (40% of cases) for diabetes and between 40 and 49 years (71% of cases) for the neurologic manifestations. Pathological accumulation of iron in neurons and glial cells and a loss of neurons in the striatum and in the ganglionic layer of the cerebellum are found. It is suggested that gradient echo and fast-spin echo MRI may distinguish the four subtypes of NBIA.[31] Other differential diagnoses of NBIA include Wilson's disease, Huntington's disease, chorea–acanthocytosis, and neurometabolic disorders.

▶ HEMIPARKINSON–HEMIATROPHY SYNDROME (HPHA)

Hemiatrophy has been reported in association with a variety of neurologic conditions, including parkinsonism. Patients with HPHA have asymmetric parkinsonism with body hemiatrophy on the more affected side.[32] Other characteristics are an early age of onset, ipsilateral dystonia, and a slowly progressive course.[33]

EPIDEMIOLOGY, GENETICS, AND PATHOPHYSIOLOGY

Although no systematic genetic studies have been performed, parkin mutations have been found in one patient with HPHA.[34] Genetic etiology is suggested by the occurrence of HPHA in a pair of twins.[35] A postcentral lesion before 3 years of age most likely causes contralateral body atrophy.[36] Accordingly, it is thought that the occurrence of parkinsonism in HPHA patients is related to an additional subcortical lesion.[32] Neuroradiological evidence of a contralateral brain hemiatrophy in >60% of HPHA patients has been found.[37] Classical pediatric cerebral hemiatrophy, also known as Dyke–Davidoff–Masson syndrome, is a condition characterized by seizures, facial asymmetry, contralateral hemiparesis, and learning difficulties and is due to cerebral injury that may occur in utero or early in life.[38] Since an association between perinatal asphyxia, brain hemiatrophy, and delayed-onset hemidystonia has been shown, HPHA could represent an example of a movement disorder with delayed onset as a consequence of neonatal brain injury[37] or an early childhood brain insult.[33] In support of this point of view, about 50% of HPHA cases reported to have a difficult birth or severe febrile illness in the first few months of life.[35] Dopa-responsive dystonia with hemiatrophy has also been reported.[39] Since dopa-responsive dystonia results from a purely biochemical deficit in the brain, it has been suggested that a deficiency of the nigrostriatal dopamine system may by itself be sufficient to cause body hemiatrophy. However, neonatal ablation of the nigrostriatal pathway does not influence limb development in rats but is markedly attenuated by corticospinal lesions sustained during the neonatal period.[40] Dystonic contractions alone can also not account for body asymmetry, because patients with idiopathic dystonia often have asymmetric symptoms but do not develop body asymmetry.[39] Although over 60 HPHA cases have been described, no postmortem analysis has been published to date.

CLINICAL PRESENTATION

The mean age of onset of parkinsonism ranges between 38 and 49 years. The course of the disease is slowly progressive with a mean duration of disease until initiation of levodopa therapy of 14.2 years. No progression to Hoehn and Yahr stage greater than III has been observed in one study.[33] But a more variable clinical course, for instance with progression from Hoehn and Yahr stage I to stage V during "off" within 2.5 years, has also been reported.[37] Tremor and dystonia are the most initial symptoms in the course of the disease.[35] Apart from the parkinsonian features, pyramidal tract dysfunction ipsilateral to the side of HPHA is present in about 50% of cases.[33] Asymmetric freezing of gait ipsilateral to the side of parkinsonism in HPHA is described.[41] Learning difficulties and mild motor impairment such as walking difficulties can occur during childhood.[35] Psychiatric symptoms are not a major feature of HPHA. The patients can suffer from scoliosis and body hemiatrophy with small and narrow extremities on one side. In some patients the face, arm, and leg are affected, whereas in other patients only the hand is affected. The most likely part of the hand to demonstrate hemiatrophy is the thumb.

DIAGNOSTICS, DIFFERENTIAL DIAGNOSIS, AND THERAPY

The diagnostic criteria are (a) early age of onset between the fourth and fifth decades, (b) slowly progressive course, (d) highly asymmetric parkinsonism with predominant signs on hemiatrophic side, (e) dystonia occurring prior to levodopa therapy, and supportively (f) abnormal birth or early childhood brain history. Brain asymmetry in ventricular, subcortical, or cortical regions may be found by structural imaging, helping to confirm the diagnosis, especially in patients with minimal body asymmetry. Functional imaging may show reduced dopa uptake in the striatum and hypometabolism in the basal ganglia and medial frontal cortex contralateral to the hemiatrophy, suggesting that the clinical manifestations of HPHA arise through a combination of pre- and postsynaptic nigrostriatal dopaminergic dysfunction.[42] Functional imaging might be useful to distinguish HPHA from typical unilateral Parkinson's disease. But this observation is not confirmed by others.[34] Brain hemiatrophy is not correlated to body hemiatrophy.[37] A dominance of the left hemisphere and of the male gender of cerebral hemiatrophy is found.[43] The level of homovanillic acid in the cerebrospinal fluid can be reduced. The majority of HPHA patients have a good-to-moderate response to levodopa therapy[37] and to a combination of amantadine and anticholinergics.[33] A dramatic improvement after subthalamic nucleus stimulation has been reported.[44] In the differential diagnosis a benign, early-onset parkinsonism has to be considered. In the beginning the differential diagnosis may include corticobasal ganglionic degeneration, since HPHA may mimic its early stage.[45]

▶ X-LINKED DYSTONIA–PARKINSONISM SYNDROME (XDP)

This disease is a biphasic movement disorder and occurs endemically in the Philippines.[46] Among the Ilongo-speaking Filipino families, the disease is called "lubag" when intermittent twisting movements are present, "wa'eg" when sustained twisting postures occur, or "sud-sud" (an onomatopoeic term denoting the sound of sandals slapping the pavement) when there is shuffling gait. Hereafter, the disease is referred to as XDP.

EPIDEMIOLOGY, GENETICS, AND PATHOPHYSIOLOGY

As of June 2001, 376 XDP cases have been registered. The prevalence of XDP is 0.34 per 100,000 in the general population, but on the island of Panay the prevalence is 5.24 per 100,000 with highest degrees in the provinces Capiz with 18.88 per 100,000 and Aklan with 7.46 per 100,000.[46] Presumably, the disease originates from a common ancestor on the island, suggesting a single gene mutation. The neuropathological similarity between a patient with XDP and a non-Filipino patient with dystonia suggests that this mutation may not be restricted to the Filipino population.[47] An X-linked recessive mode of inheritance with nearly full penetrance has been suggested. Linkage analyses have assigned the disease locus (DYT3) to chromosome Xq13.1.[48] It should be mentioned that women can also be affected (male-to-female ratio of 93:1), leading to the hypothesis that XDP may be a codominant disorder.[49] Five possible disease-specific sequence changes (DSCs) and a 48-bp deletion have been described in the "multiple transcript system" in the DYT3 critical region.[50] A disease-specific SVA (short interspersed nuclear element, variable number of tandem repeats, and Alu composite) retrotransposon insertion in intron 32 of the TAF1 (TATA-binding protein associated factor 1) gene has been identified at Xq13.1.[51] TAF1 is the largest and the essential component of the TFIID complex in the pathway of RNA polymerase II–mediated gene transcription and regulates transcription of a large number of genes related to cell division and proliferation. XDP brains show significantly decreased expression levels of TAF1 and of the dopamine receptor D_2 gene. Abnormal pattern of DNA methylation in the retrotransposon in the genome from the patient's caudate has been suggested to account for decreased expression of TAF1.[52] It has been postulated that in earlier stages of XDP, severe loss of striosomal GABAergic projection neurons may lead to disinhibition of nigral dopaminergic neurons, resulting in a hyperkinetic dystonia disorder. At the later stage, when parkinsonism predominates, there may be greater involvement of the matrix compartment, leading to reduction of matrix-based projections and resulting in an "extranigral form" of parkinsonism.[53]

NEUROPATHOLOGY

A subtle astrocytosis in a mosaic pattern is found in the atrophic caudate and putamen.[49] The lateral part of the putamen is the most severely gliotic. Gliotic areas also exhibit neuronal loss. Overall, varying degrees of neuronal loss and astrogliosis involving the caudate and putamen are observed.[46]

CLINICAL PRESENTATION

The mean age of onset of XDP for female patients is 52 years, much older than that for men with 39 years. About 50% present with focal dystonia (33% lower extremities; 27% blepharospasm, jaw opening, and closing or tongue protrusion; 25% torticollis, retrocollis, anterocollis, neck stiffness, tremors, or shoulder dystonia; 14% tremors and cramps of the upper extremities). The symptoms usually progress in 98% to involve other body parts, leading to generalized dystonia within 5 years in 84%.[46] Parkinsonism is the initial symptom in 6% of cases.[46] In most patients, dystonia becomes less intense as the 10th year of illness is approached. Then bradykinesia sets in, and a festinating gait, freezing, and masked facies can be observed. Rigidity and cogwheeling, however, are rare. The mean duration of illness until parkinsonism has become predominant is 13.4 years. Other symptoms that have been observed in XDP include chorea, myorhythmia, and myoclonus.[54] A predominant parkinsonism with late-onset or no dystonia has been described.[55] Olfactory dysfunction may occur in XDP patients.[56] Compared with male XDP patients, affected women tend to have a more benign phenotype and milder course. Dystonia, if present, remains mild, nonprogressive, and nondisabling.[57] Primary psychiatric symptoms have not been reported.

DIAGNOSTICS, DIFFERENTIAL DIAGNOSIS, AND THERAPY

The diagnostic criteria are (a) early age of onset between the fourth and fifth decades, (b) progressive course, (c) focal, multifocal, or generalized dystonia, and (d) parkinsonism. Structural imaging may reveal mild cerebral atrophy. At an early disease stage the outer rim of the putamen may feature an increased signal intensity in T_2-weighted MRI images.[46] Later on the atrophy of the caudate and putamen becomes visible. A selective striatal hypometalolism can be determined.[58] Functional imaging may show pre- and postsynaptic nigrostriatal dysfunction.[59] With the exception of an elevated manganese value obtained in the serum of affected Filipino men, laboratory studies showed no abnormalities.[60] Patients are treated with trihexyphenidyl, levodopa, lorazepam, diazepam, or diphenhydramine, either alone or in combination, with no or only moderate improvement of symptoms.[61] Surgical treatment provide partial but no lasting relief.[46] Patients may benefit from the local administration of botulinum toxin. Furthermore, treatment with zolpidem, which selectively binds to the alpha1-subunit of the $GABA_A$ receptor, may improve dystonia.[54] Patients with parkinsonism as only or predominant manifestation may benefit from levodopa therapy.[55] In the differential diagnosis, any of the dystonias associated with parkinsonism should be considered, such as Wilson's disease, NBIA-1, chorea–acanthocytosis, and levodopa-responsive dystonia.

▶ CHOREA-ACANTHOCYTOSIS (CHAC)

Acanthocytes are erythrocytes with changed morphology bearing spicules of variable length and breadth.[62] If they occur in association with neurological symptoms, the term neuroacanthocytosis is used. Four different types of neuroacanthocytosis are known: (a) CHAC, also called Levine–Critchley syndrome,[63,64] (b) autosomal-recessive abetalipoproteinemia, the so-called Bassen–Kornzweig syndrome,[65] (c) familial hypobetalipoproteinemia,[66] and (d) the X-linked McLeod syndrome.[67–69] Sporadic association of acanthocytes has been described, that is, in NBIA-1 and mitochondrial encephalomyopathies, as well as without neurologic association, that is, in uremia, splenectomy, or malnutrition.

EPIDEMIOLOGY, GENETICS, AND PATHOPHYSIOLOGY

The prevalence of CHAC is unknown; in 2005 only approximately 300 cases have been known worldwide.[70] Although considered to be an autosomal-recessive disorder, apparent autosomal-dominant inheritance has been reported. CHAC has been previously linked to chromosome 9q21.[71] The disease-causing gene has been identified as VPS13A (vacuolar protein sorting 13 homolog A), which encodes chorein.[72,73] At least 75 different chorein mutations have been found, indicating a strong allelic heterogeneity with no single mutation causing the majority of cases.[74] Most of them are loss-of-function mutations leading to absence or marked reduction of chorein. The function of chorein remains unclear, but it is thought to be involved in protein trafficking at the trans-Golgi network. Absence of the functional gene product may lead to destabilization of the plasma membrane structure, and hence acanthocytosis.[73] The suggested occurrence of CHAC without acanthocytes may indicate that the gene can be variably expressed in different tissues and may cause neurological abnormalities alone. In a family with features typical of CHAC, an autosomal-dominant transmission, neuronal inclusions immunoreactive to ubiquitin, expanded polyglutamine repeats and torsin A in many areas of the cerebral cortex, and abnormalities of the membrane protein band 3 have been demonstrated.[75] In affected members of this family—characterized by onset in the third and fourth decades with chorea, dystonia, parkinsonism, or progressive cognitive decline with severe cortical and striatal atrophy—trinucleotide repeat expansions in the junctophilin-3 gene on chromosome 16q24.3, confirming a diagnosis of Huntington's disease-like 2, has been identified.[76] Junctophilin-3 appears to play a role in junctional membrane structures and may be involved in calcium regulation.

NEUROPATHOLOGY

CHAC brains show enlargement of the ventricles, particularly of the frontal horns. Caudate and putamen are the most severely affected brain areas showing atrophy, neuronal loss, and gliosis. Depletion of small- and medium-sized striatal neurons is apparent. Involvement of the globus pallidus is also present, and in some cases the thalamus and the anterior horns of spinal cord show neuronal loss and mild gliosis.[77] In CHAC with parkinsonism the neuronal density in the substantia nigra (particularly in the ventrolateral region) is lower than in CHAC without parkinsonian features and controls.[78]

CLINICAL PRESENTATION

The mean age of onset is 32 years (ranging from 8 to 62 years). The course of the disease is progressive, and death usually occurs after 10–20 years. The most striking symptoms are orofacial dyskinesias and limb chorea,[79] spreading then to the whole body. Akinetic-rigid parkinsonism (about 32% of cases) may occur either with chorea or as a subsequent feature when the hyperkinetic movement disorder subsides.[80,81] Orofacial dyskinesias can cause tongue and lip biting and, very often, interferes with speech and swallowing. Accordingly, involuntary vocalizations are frequently observed. In some cases, the predominant manifestation is dystonia rather than chorea, and tics are noticed. Additionally, hypo- or areflexia is repeatedly found. Several ocular motor deficits in patients with CHAC that involve fixation stability, saccades, and pursuit can be found.[70] In many cases muscle wasting occurs, and an axonal neuropathy is observed.[82] Moreover, >30% of patients suffered from seizures, and in >50% of the cases cognitive impairment, psychiatric features, and personality change are seen.[83] The most consistent psychiatric symptoms are personality change with impulsive and distractable behavior, apathy, and loss of insight. Additionally, depression, anxiety, paranoid delusions, and obsessive-compulsive features can occur. There is no obvious association between the degree of acanthocytosis and the severity of the neurologic disability. The clinical manifestation and presentation of the disease can be heterogenous between sisters of different ages carrying the same mutations,[84] as well as in monozygotic twins.[85]

DIAGNOSTICS, DIFFERENTIAL DIAGNOSIS, AND THERAPY

The diagnostic criteria are (a) age of onset between the third and fifth decades, (b) progressive course, (c) appearance of a hypokinetic and/or hyperkinetic extrapyramidal syndrome, (d) psychiatric symptoms, and supportively (e) seizure and (f) peripheral neuropathy. Structural imaging reveals cortical or occasional caudate atrophy[82] as well as parenchymal signal abnormalities in the caudate and lentiform nuclei.[83] Functional imaging shows cerebral hypoperfusion and hypometabolism with altered striatal signal intensity,[86] and loss of caudate and putamen D_2 receptors.[87] Presynaptic dopaminergic impairment is also found.[85] Significant acanthocytosis is defined by the presence of >3% acanthocytes (up to 80%) in peripheral blood smears in >85% of cases. Acanthocytes have to be thoroughly distinguished from echinocytes. Scanning electron microscopy may be helpful in measuring the extent of the erythrocyte morphological abnormalities when in doubt.[83] Apart from acanthocytosis, elevated creatine kinase is observed in 85%,[79] higher than that usually seen in neurogenic muscular atrophy, suggesting the presence of a myopathic process in the muscular atrophy of this disease.[88] Other laboratory parameters, especially serum low- or high-density lipoproteins, show usually no abnormalities, unlike abetalipoproteinemia or familial hypobetalipoproteinemia. The therapy is symptomatic. Parkinsonian symptoms do not respond to high dosages of levodopa,[81] and the response of the involuntary movements to drug treatment is generally poor. Severe trunk spasms may improve by bilateral thalamic stimulation.[89] The most important diseases to be considered for differential diagnosis of CHAC include Huntington's disease, Gilles de la Tourette syndrome, also Friedreich ataxia, and other forms of young-onset extrapyramidal syndromes, including acanthocytosis-like Huntington's disease-like 2, NBIA-1, or HARP syndrome. The existence of parkinsonism in McLeod syndrome is questionable as the three described cases had been treated with dopamine-blocking agents.[68]

▶ PALLIDONIGROLUYSIAN DEGENERATION (PNLD)

A progressive degeneration of the globus pallidus alone or in association with the substantia nigra (PND) and/or the nucleus subthalamicus (of Luys; PLD or PNLD) is observed in a rare familial or sporadically occurring movement disorder clinically defined by a slowly progressive course and a wide variety of extrapyramidal symptoms. The first clinical description of a case with sporadic pallidal degeneration, most often reported in the literature as Hunt's syndrome, was associated with dystonic postures and superimposed involuntary movements.[90] This category of disorders with predominant affection of the pallidonigroluysian system has previously been classified into four distinct groups: (a) pure pallidal atrophy, (b) pure pallidoluysian atrophy, (c) extended forms of pallidal degeneration (involving the striatum and/or the substantia nigra), and (d) combinations of pallidal and pallidoluysian atrophy with other system degenerations.[91] For instance, the separately described pallidopyramidal disease (see below) can be considered a member of this group.[91] Furthermore, the relation of the familial pallidonigral system degeneration with cystic damage to the diseases discussed here is not known.[92] Finally, in a small number of cases there is evidence of a possibly different movement disorder, characterized by the isolated degeneration of the external pallidum or status marmoratus of the basal ganglia in association with the occurrence of intraneuronal polyglucosan bodies.[93]

EPIDEMIOLOGY, GENETICS, AND PATHOPHYSIOLOGY

No epidemiological data are available due to the small number of investigated cases. In most of the reported families the condition appears to be of autosomal-recessive inheritance.[91] The mutation N279K in the MAPT gene has been described in PNLD.[94] This mutation has been also found in a family with pallidopontonigral degeneration and in a family with dementia and supranuclear palsy.[95] The pathogenesis is not exactly known. The discovery of a mutation in the gene and the histopathological demonstration of hyperphosphorylated tau in PNLD suggest that this disorder is a tauopathy.[94,96] It can therefore be speculated that PNLD is related to FTDP-17T (see above). It is not clear whether pallidal degeneration, PLD, and PND degeneration are tauopathies as well.

NEUROPATHOLOGY

A progressive loss of nerve cells and fibers accompanied by proportional gliosis, particularly in the globus pallidus and the subthalamic nucleus, has been found.[91] The changes may vary in their extent. In rare instances they might be associated with further degenerative lesions in other extrapyramidal, motor neuron, or spinocerebellar systems. A pure pallidal degeneration with gliosis and locally differing neuronal loss is reported.[97] In another case of pure pallidal degeneration,[97] morphometric analysis reveals a shrinkage of the globus pallidus externus to 59% of normal and of the globus pallidus internus to 37% of normal, but with no obvious neuronal loss. Bilateral symmetrical loss of neurons and myelin with gliosis mainly in the outer pallidum is observed with pallor of the ansa lenticularis and atrophy of subthalamic nucleus in PLD.[98] In PNLD bilateral marked neuronal loss and gliosis are restrictedly observed in the globus pallidus, substantia nigra, and nucleus subthalamicus with the appearance of tau-positive argyrophilic fibrous structures related to glia.[99] These changes are consistent with the findings observed in the various (extended) forms of this group of neurodegenerative disorders. Other observations include the occurrence of corpora amylacea throughout the brain and brown granular deposits showing a positive reaction to iron in the degenerated nuclei and the striatum in PNLD.[100,101] Hyperphosphorylated tau is found in PNLD.[96]

CLINICAL PRESENTATION

The disorders demonstrate an insidious onset and a slowly progressive course. Age of onset in familial cases is between 5 and 40 years, and in sporadic cases between 30 and 64 years. In pure pallidal degeneration the clinical picture is characterized by the development of progressive choreoathetotic hyperkinesias with axial dystonia, followed by the appearance of progressive rigidity. Finally, the involuntary movements are overcome by permanent rigidity, and the patients become bedridden.[91] In contrast, pallidal degeneration with an extreme slowness of movements without rigidity as the main symptom is also reported.[102] In PLD, additional symptoms are torticollis, head tremor, and distal movements with or without a ballistic component.[91] A presentation with 20 years of progressive generalized dystonia, dysarthria, gait disorder, vertical gaze palsy, and bradykinesia in PLD has been described.[103] Onset in PNLD is mostly with frozen gait and akinesia,[104] and the most apparent symptoms are progressive akinesia and rigidity with little or no tremor.[91] Vertical or upward gaze palsy, nuchal stiffness, dysarthria, and dysphagia appear in the later stage of the disease in most cases, and dementia occurs in 50% of cases.[104] A PNLD case with rapidly progressive hemidystonia has also been reported.[105] Progressive pure akinesia with no other parkinsonian features such as tremor or rigidity might be also associated with PNLD.[99] In conclusion, a wide spectrum of different clinical manifestations exists, depending on the spatial and temporal pattern of affection of the distinct brain areas. Consequently, because of their rarity, the clinical correlates of the distinct forms are still not well described. Familial occurrence of the combination of progressive rigidity and choreoathetosis or torsion dystonia with an early onset may suggest one of the subtypes of progressive pallidal degenerations. The disorders may be accompanied by mental deterioration, but intellectual impairment may be absent, whereas personality change and aggressiveness have been observed in advanced disease stages.[91] A history of psychosis has been described in several cases.[100,101] Recently, pathologically confirmed cases with progressive supranuclear palsy (PSP) with additional features of PNLD have been compared to PSP alone.[106] PSP-PNLD cases are younger, had longer disease duration, and more often are not initially diagnosed with PSP; in the end, they do not differ from PSP with respect to any major clinical feature. The clinical course of PSP-PNLD, however, is different, with earlier gait abnormalities and difficulty with handwriting, but later falls, rigidity, and dysphagia than PSP. Pathologically, the same types of lesions are detected in both PSP and PSP-PNLD, but there are differences in the distribution and density of tau pathology, with less tau pathology in motor cortex, striatum, pontine nuclei, and cerebellum, but more neuronal loss in the nucleus subthalamicus in PSP-PNLD.[106]

DIAGNOSTICS, DIFFERENTIAL DIAGNOSIS, AND THERAPY

The diagnostic criteria are (a) age of onset between the third and sixth decades, (b) progressive course, and (c) extrapyramidal symptoms. The diagnosis of these rare conditions can only be proven by means of postmortem examination. Sequencing of the MAPT gene, if available, should be performed. Structural imaging in younger patients is usually normal,[91] or shows minimal atrophy of the brain stem and dilation of the brain stem and of the sylvian fissure.[102] In a patient with PLD no abnormalities have been found.[103] Increased signal intensity in the pallidum and substantia nigra in a PNLD patient with adult-onset hemidystonia has been described in T_2-MRI.[105] In the same patient contralateral cortical hyperperfusion and hypermetabolism have been observed.[105] Routine laboratory data are unremarkable. Treatment with levodopa has produced only equivocal improvement of the movement disorder.[102,107] However, patients with dystonic symptoms may benefit from baclofen.[103] Possible differential diagnoses include juvenile parkinsonism, idiopathic torsion dystonia, NBIA-1, atypical parkinsonism such as PSP, and corticobasal ganglionic degeneration and others.

▶ PALLIDOPYRAMIDAL DISEASE (PPD)

Pallidopyramidal disease is thought to be an autosomal-recessive disorder with a clinical picture consisting of parkinsonism and pyramidal tract signs.[108–111] Furthermore, a syndrome that is closely related but not identical to PPD is reported. It is called Kufor-Rakeb syndrome and additionally characterized by supranuclear upgaze paresis and dementia.[112] The disease locus for Kufor-Rakeb syndrome has been mapped to chromosome 1p36.[113] Recently, the disease gene has been identified as a lysosomal type 5 P-type ATPase (ATP13A2), and subsequently Kufor-Rakeb syndrome has been classified among the familial Parkinson's diseases (PARK9).[114]

EPIDEMIOLOGY, GENETICS, AND PATHOPHYSIOLOGY

It has been suggested that PPD is recessively inherited.[111] PPD has been associated with the homozygous mutation R378G in the FBXO7 (F-box only protein 7) gene on chromosome 22q12 in one family with autosomal-recessive inheritance.[115] F-box, named after cyclin F, in which it was originally observed, binds SKP1. F-box proteins, such as FBXO7, are components of modular E3 ubiquitin protein ligases called SCFs (SKP1, cullin, F-box proteins), which function in phosphorylation-dependent ubiquitination. The exact pathogenesis of PPD is unknown.

NEUROPATHOLOGY

Until now only one autopsy in a nonfamilial patient 50 years after onset has been performed.[108] A pallor of the pallidal segments, slight shrinkage, and cellular change of the substantia nigra, a thinning of the ansa lenticularis, and early demyelination of the pyramids and crossed pyramidal tracts are observed. The latter extend from the lower parts of the medulla oblongata into the spinal cord.

CLINICAL PRESENTATION

In general, disease onset occurs during the second or the early third decade. The classical parkinsonian features, including rigidity, bradykinesia, hypomimia, and monotone speech, are observed in all cases. Pyramidal tract signs, consisting of Babinski signs, hyperreflexia, spastic muscle tone, and extensor plantar responses, are also found. The occurrence of pyramidal tract signs can precede the appearance of extrapyramidal symptoms by up to 20 years.[115] The progression of the disorder is slow; ambulatory patients after 10–13 years of disease are reported.[109] No diurnal variation is observed. Additional symptoms such as horizontal nystagmus, intention tremor, poor memory, and impaired intelligence can occur.[108] One case with additional features such as blepharospasm, rapid worsening of bradykinesia, stiffness, and postural instability confining to bed is also described. Psychiatric symptoms have not been observed in this syndrome, except one case with impaired intelligence.[108]

DIAGNOSTICS, DIFFERENTIALDIAGNOSIS, AND THERAPY

The diagnostic criteria are (a) age of onset between the second and third decades, (b) parkinsonism, and (c) pyramidal tract signs. The diagnostic possibilities are limited. Evidence of isolated extrapyramidal and pyramidal signs and normal laboratory and neuroradiologic investigations in a young adult are suggestive of PPD. Structural imaging may show no abnormalities[111] or bilateral calcifications in the basal ganglia.[116] Patients suffering from Kufor-Rakeb syndrome show, in contrast, generalized atrophy with pronounced atrophy of the lentiform nuclei and the pyramids.[112] Functional imaging in PPD may show dopaminergic denervation of the striatum,[117] and a decrease in benzodiazepine receptor density in the precentral gyrus and the mesial frontal cortex.[118] Hypoperfusion in frontoparietal and temporal cortical areas and basal ganglia in one hemisphere has been noted.[119] No biochemical criteria for diagnosis are known. Extrapyramidal symptoms improve with levodopa therapy. Typically, the pyramidal symptoms are not influenced by this treatment. However, a worsening of pyramidal tract signs due to the medication regimen is reported.[110] Response to levodopa is somewhat variable; most patients respond rapidly to low doses with improvement persisting for a long period. After many years of treatment, "wearing-off" phenomena occur. The daily dose of levodopa used in the patients is high.[111] Possible differential diagnoses are juvenile parkinsonism and levodopa-responsive dystonia.

▶ RETT SYNDROME (RS)

RS is a progressive neurological developmental disorder, which is reported almost exclusively in females and characterized by a wide spectrum of motor and behavioral abnormalities.[120–123] The most typical symptoms are stereotyped movements and gait disturbance. Furthermore, parkinsonism and hyperkinetic disorders can be associated with RS.

EPIDEMIOLOGY, GENETICS, AND PATHOPHYSIOLOGY

The prevalence of RS in females is estimated to be 1 in 10,000–20,000. It has been proposed that RS is the result of an X-linked-dominant mutation with mortality for hemizygous males with each case representing a new mutation.[124] Rarely, classically affected males with somatic mosaicism or an extra X chromosome have been described.[125] The disease locus has been mapped to chromosome Xq28,[126] and mutations in the gene encoding methyl-CpG-binding protein 2 (MeCP2) have been identified as a cause of RS,[127] in females as well as in males. More than 225 mutations have been identified in MeCP2, although eight common loss-of-function mutations (especially T158M, R168X, and R255X) are found in approximately 70% of those fulfilling the consensus criteria.[128] Mutations in the MeCP2 gene have been found in 75–90% of sporadic (representing 99% of all RS cases) and approximately 50% of the rare familial cases[129] as well as in >90% of typical RS and <60% of atypical RS cases, respectively.[128] However, MeCP2 mutations can also be found in individuals lacking the clinical features of RS.[130] Methylation of CpG dinucleotides in genomic DNA represents an epigenetic mechanism of gene expression control. MeCP2 regulates the expression of a wide range of genes and can function as both an activator and a repressor of transcription. Genotype–phenotype studies suggest that the pattern of X-chromosome inactivation has a more prominent effect on clinical severity than the type of mutation.[129] Several females carrying the same mutation display different phenotypes, suggesting that factors other than the type or position of mutations influence the severity of RS. It is hypothesized that dysregulation of MeCP2 in specific neuronal populations impacts the function of other neurons, leading to network abnormalities and possibly secondary neurobehavioral phenotypes.[131] A mutation on chromosome 1 in the gene for netrin G1 protein, which has an important role in the developing central nervous system, particularly in axonal guidance, signalling, and NMDA receptor function, has been shown to be a rare cause of RS.[132] Early infantile epileptic encephalopathy-2 is an Xp22-linked severe, atypical form of RS with infantile spasms, which is caused by a mutation in the cyclin-dependent kinase-like 5 (CDKL5) gene. The expression of CDKL5 overlaps highly with MeCP2 during neural maturation and synaptogenesis, and both can regulate each other, suggesting that both may belong to the same molecular pathway. The phenotype is characterized by early-onset seizures, delayed psychomotor development, hypotonia, scoliosis, microcephaly, lack of speech development, stereotypic hand movements, and repetitive behaviors.[133] A congenital variant of RS may be caused in some cases by mutation in the forkhead box G1 (FOXG1) gene on chromosome 14q13. FOXG1 acts as a transcriptional repressor and is expressed—overlapping with MeCP2—in differentiating cortical compartments. Cases suffer from infantile onset of microcephaly, mental retardation, and peculiar jerky movements.[134]

NEUROPATHOLOGY

Brains of RS cases show diffuse cerebral atrophy with a decrease in weight of 14–34% compared to that of age-matched controls, with increased amounts of lipofuscin and, occasionally, mild astrocytosis. Moreover, mild but inconsistent spongy changes of white matter can be found. Most apparent is a low level of pigmentation of the substantia nigra, whereas the number of nigral neurons seems not to be highly altered.[135] In addition, selective dendritic alterations with no degeneration of pyramidal neurons in the cortex of patients with RS have been reported.[136]

CLINICAL PRESENTATION

RS leads not only to neurological abnormalities but also to dysfunction of other organs.[137] Gastrointestinal complains include constipation and weight loss. Swallowing difficulties are also common. Furthermore, an unusual breathing pattern with central apnea intermixed with hyperventilation is frequently observed. Scoliosis occurs often. Patients with RS have significantly longer corrected QT intervals and T-wave abnormalities on electrocardiograms, which might explain sudden death in RS.[138] A four-stage model for the description of classical RS has been proposed.[123] Stage 1 is defined by developmental stagnation, hypotonia, and deceleration of head growth (onset 0.5–1.5 years). Stage 2 is characterized by loss of functional hand use, stereotypic hand-wringing, loss of expressive language, rapid developmental regression, and occasional seizures (onset 1–4 years). Stage 3 is termed a pseudostationary period because of some restitution of communication, but increasing ataxia, hyperreflexia, and rigidity as well as breathing dysfunction and bruxism are observed. After several years stage 4 develops with the so-called late motor deterioration and growth retardation. With respect to extrapyramidal dysfunction, bruxism (97%), oculogyric crises (63%), and parkinsonism and dystonia (59%) are common features.[139] Myoclonus and choreoathetosis are seen only infrequently. In younger patients (<4 years) hyperkinetic disorders are more evident, whereas in older patients (>8 years) the bradykinetic syndrome tended to predominate. Drooling (75%), rigidity (44%), and bradykinesia (41%) are the most often observed parkinsonian symptoms. Parkinsonism has so far not been included among the diagnostic criteria of classical or variant RS.[130,140] The cardinal neurological symptoms are developmental stagnation followed by dementia, autism, loss of purposeful hand movements, and jerky truncal ataxia in a stage-dependent manner.[122] It has been suggested that the jerky truncal ataxia represents a combination of cerebellar ataxia and myoclonus.[139] Sleep disturbances, mainly in the early stages, are frequently present in RS. They are characterized by an overall increase in daytime sleep and a delayed onset of sleep at night. The initial criteria for the diagnosis of RS[140] have been revised in the light of the advances in the understanding of the molecular biology of RS.[130]

DIAGNOSTICS, DIFFERENTIAL DIAGNOSIS, AND THERAPY

The diagnostic criteria are (a) apparently normal prenatal and perinatal history, (b) largely normal (or delayed) psychomotor development through the first 6 months, (c) normal head circumference at birth, (d) postnatal deceleration of head growth in the majority, (e) loss of purposeful hand skills, (f) stereotypic hand movements, (g) emerging social withdrawal, communication dysfunction, loss of learned words, and cognitive impairment, and (h) impaired or failing locomotion. Supportive criteria include (a) awake disturbances of breathing, (b) bruxism, (c) impaired sleep pattern from early infancy, (d) abnormal muscle tone, (e) peripheral vasomotor disturbances, (f) scoliosis/kyphosis progressing through childhood, (g) growth retardation, and (h) small hands and feet. Diagnostic criteria for variant RS have also been developed.[141] Structural imaging indicates a global hypoplasia of brain with preferential progressive atrophy of the cerebellum,[142] caudate nucleus, and frontocortical area.[143] An increased density of D_2 receptors in the striatum[144] and a presynaptic deficit of nigrostriatal activity can be found by functional imaging.[145] Several areas of hypometabolism with markedly lower metabolism in the occipital lobes occur.[146] It has been proposed that hyperammonemia could be an essential sign of this condition,[120,121] but further investigations have not reproduced the findings of hyperammonemia in most patients.[122] Significant reductions in the metabolites of norepinephrine, dopamine, and serotonin as well as an elevation of biopterin in the cerebrospinal fluid have been constituted the first detected biochemical alterations.[147] Additionally, there is evidence of elevation of lactate, pyruvate, alpha-ketoglutarate, malate, and glutamate in the cerebrospinal fluid.[148,149] There is no specific treatment. Naltrexone appears to provide clinical benefit in the treatment of breathing dysfunction and cognitive impairment.[150] Furthermore, bromocriptine, carnitine, and lamotrigine can be tried to improve certain disease symptoms.[151–153] The relatively normal development during the first 6–18 months of life may allow for presymptomatic therapeutic intervention, especially if newborn screening programs can identify affected females. For differential diagnoses, infantile autism, Angelman syndrome, and other neurodevelopmental disorders with mental retardation and motor impairment are to be considered.

▶ FRAGILE-X TREMOR/ATAXIA SYNDROME (FXTAS)

FXTAS is a multisystem progressive neurodegenerative disorder characterized by extrapyramidal, cognitive, and psychiatric features,[154–156] It is completely distinct from clinical and molecular pathogenic perspectives from the neurodevelopmental disorder fragile-X syndrome (FXS).

EPIDEMIOLOGY, GENETICS, AND PATHOPHYSIOLOGY

FXS, FXTAS, and premature ovarian failure (POF) are caused by expansions of a trinucleotide (CGG)-repeat element over the normal range of 5–44 in the 5′ untranslated region of the FMR1 (fragile-X mental retardation 1) gene,[157,158] which is located on chromosome Xq27.3.[159] Full mutation alleles (>200 repeats) are associated with gene methylation and transcriptional silencing. Premutation alleles (55–200 repeats) are unstable and may expand to full mutation alleles when transmitted maternally. Premutations of FMR1 are frequent in the general population, with estimated prevalences of 1 per 259 females and 1 per 813 males.[160] Expansions of 45–54 repeats (gray-zone expansions) are only mildly unstable and require at least two generations before evolving into a full mutation. FXS is caused by full mutation with consequent absence of the FMR1 protein (FMRP).[161] It has been shown that deletions in FMR1 without a significant sequence expansion can also cause a loss-of-function mutation leading to FXS.[162] POF and FXTAS cases are characterized by premutation FMR1 alleles and normal or slightly reduced FMRP.[154,163] It is hypothesized that the presence of elevated levels of expanded-repeat FMR1 mRNA in premutation carriers has a toxic gain-of-function effect.[158] The penetrance and severity of the neurological disorder is a function of the number of CGG repeats. Moreover, the penetrance increased with age, exceeding 30% for male carriers over the age of 50 years and 50% for men at the age of 70–90 years. Its penetrance in female carriers is 5–10%.[164] The RNA-binding protein FMRP forms a messenger ribonucleoprotein complex that associates with polyribosomes, suggesting that it is involved in translation,[165] often in neuronal dendritic spines, particularly during development, and is particularly regulated by synaptic activity.[166]

NEUROPATHOLOGY

The principal neuropathological characteristic of FXTAS is eosininophilic, ubiquitin-positive inclusions in the nuclei of neurons and astrocytes throughout the brain and spinal cord.[167] The inclusions are tau- and alpha-synuclein-negative, and contain FMR1 mRNA.[168] There is prominent white-matter involvement with patchy loss of axons, myelin, and associated astroglial cells. Nearly all cases studied show spongiosis of the middle cerebellar peduncles and loss of Purkinje cells.[167,169] A strong correlation between repeat size and frequency of intranuclear inclusions and an inverse correlation between repeat size and age at death have been found.[167]

CLINICAL PRESENTATION

Onset occurs usually at 50–70 years. The prevalence is approximately 1:3000.[160] Clinically, FXTAS consists of cerebellar symptoms with progressive intention tremor (70%) and gait ataxia (80–90%) and parkinsonian features presenting with resting tremor (30%), bradykinesia (60%), and rigidity (30–70%).[156,160] Additional features include autonomic dysfunctions such as impotence (80%) and incontinence (30–50%), peripheral neuropathy (60%) with decreased sensation and vibration sense in the distal lower extremities, and lower limb proximal muscle weakness (30%).[156,160] Cognitive changes range from mild frontal executive and memory deficits to global dementia.[170] Common psychiatric symptoms include anxiety, agitation, disinhibition, and depression.[171,172] Furthermore, among affected males, the age at onset of tremor or ataxia inversely correlates with repeat size featuring an earlier onset in those with a higher CGG repeat number.[173] A presentation of FXTAS with essential tremor[174] or rapidly progressive dementia as major symptoms may occur.[175] CGG repeat size is significantly associated with overall motor impairment in premutation carriers.[176]

DIAGNOSTICS, DIFFERENTIAL DIAGNOSIS, AND THERAPY

The diagnostic criteria are (a) age of onset between the fifth and seventh decades, (b) progressive course, (c) cerebellar symptoms, (d) parkinsonism, (e) cognitive decline, and (f) psychiatric features. Supportively, the familial history can be positive. As broad intrafamilial variability of FXTAS exists,[177] testing for FMR1 premutations in familial FXTAS with affected female patients, even in the absence of a family history of mental retardation, should be taken into account due to the great importance of genetic counseling with regard not only to FXTAS but also to fragile X syndrome in the offspring. Neuroradiological features of FXTAS include prominent white-matter disease in the periventricular, subcortical, and middle cerebellar peduncles on T_2-weighted MRI.[178] Increased signal intensities of the middle cerebellar peduncles are a distinctive and common feature of FXTAS.[156,178] Global brain atrophy is most evident in the frontal and parietal regions as well as in the pons and the cerebellum. The degree of brain atrophy is associated with the presence and severity of tremor, ataxia, and CGG repeat size.[178–180] This observation seems not to be true for female premutation carriers. Milder radiographic findings in affected females compared to affected males may suggest that a buffering effect may be present in females.[181] Functional imaging may show altered nigrostriatal dopaminergic function.[182,183] The neurological disorder with the clinical presentation most closely resembling FXTAS is multiple system atrophy. The therapy of FXTAS is symptomatic, with variable benefit from beta-blockers against intention tremor, levodopa against parkinsonism, acetylcholinesterase inhibitors against cognitive decline, venlafaxine against anxiety, and gabapentin against neuropathy.[184]

REFERENCES

1. Hutton M, Lendon CL, Rizzu P, et al. Association of missense and 5'-splice-site mutations in tau with the inherited dementia FTDP-17. Nature 1998;393:702–705.
2. Baker M, Mackenzie IR, Pickering-Brown SM, et al. Mutations in progranulin cause tau-negative frontotemporal dementia linked to chromosome 17. Nature 2006;442: 916–919.
3. Rademakers R, Cruts M, Dermaut B, et al. Tau negative frontal lobe dementia at 17q21: significant finemapping of the candidate region to a 4.8 cM interval. Mol Psychiatry 2002;7:1064–1074.
4. http://www.molgen.ua.ac.be/FTDmutations
5. Wszolek ZK, Tsuboi Y, Ghetti B, et al. Frontotemporal dementia and parkinsonism linked to chromosome 17 (FTDP-17). Orphanet J Rare Dis 2006;1:30.
6. Foster NL, Wilhelmsen K, Sima AA, et al. Frontotemporal dementia and parkinsonism linked to chromosome 17: A consensus conference. Conference Participants. Ann Neurol 1997;41:706–715.
7. Ghetti B, Spina S, Murrell JR, et al. In vivo and postmortem clinicoanatomical correlations in frontotemporal dementia and parkinsonism linked to chromosome 17. Neurodegener Dis 2008;5:215–217.
8. Boeve BF, Hutton M. Refining frontotemporal dementia with parkinsonism linked to chromosome 17: Introducing FTDP-17 (MAPT) and FTDP-17 (PGRN). Arch Neurol 2008;65:460–464.
9. Josephs KA, Ahmed Z, Katsuse O, et al. Neuropathologic features of frontotemporal lobar degeneration with ubiquitin-positive inclusions with progranulin gene (PGRN) mutations. J Neuropathol Exp Neurol 2007;66:142–151.
10. Le Ber I, van der Zee J, Hannequin D, et al. Progranulin null mutations in both sporadic and familial frontotemporal dementia. Hum Mutat 2007;28:846–855.
11. Boeve BF, Lin SC, Strongosky A, et al. Absence of rapid eye movement sleep behavior disorder in 11 members of the pallidopontonigral degeneration kindred. Arch Neurol 2007;63:268–272.
12. Ghidoni R, Benussi L, Glionna M, et al. Low plasma progranulin levels predict progranulin mutations in frontotemporal lobar degeneration. Neurology 2008;71: 1235–1239.
13. Hallervorden J, Spatz H. Eigenartige Erkrankung im extrapyramidalen System mit besonderer Beteiligung des

Globus pallidus und der Substantia nigra. Z Gesamte Neurol Psychiatr 1922;79:254–302.
14. Taylor TD, Litt M, Kramer P, et al. Homozygosity mapping of Hallervorden-Spatz syndrome to chromosome 20p12.3-p13. Nat Genet 1996;14:479–481.
15. Zhou B, Westaway SK, Levinson B, et al. A novel pantothenate kinase gene (PANK2) is defective in Hallervorden-Spatz syndrome. Nat Genet 2001;28:345–349.
16. http://www.genetests.org
17. Hayflick SJ, Westaway SK, Levinson B, et al. Genetic, clinical, and radiographic delineation of Hallervorden-Spatz syndrome. N Engl J Med 2003;348:33–40.
18. Swaiman KF. Hallervorden-Spatz syndrome and brain iron metabolism. Arch Neurol 1991;48:1285–1293.
19. Galvin JE, Giasson B, Hurtig HI, et al. Neurodegeneration with brain iron accumulation, type 1 is characterized by alpha-, beta-, and gamma-synuclein neuropathology. Am J Pathol 2000;157:361–368.
20. Thomas M, Hayflick SJ, Jankovic J. Clinical heterogeneity of neurodegeneration with brain iron accumulation (Hallervorden-Spatz syndrome) and pantothenate kinase-associated neurodegeneration. Mov Disord 2004;19:36–42.
21. Zarranz JJ, Gómez-Esteban JC, Atarés B, et al. Tau-predominant-associated pathology in a sporadic late-onset Hallervorden-Spatz syndrome. Mov Disord 2006;21: 107–111.
22. Dooling EC, Schoene WC, Richardson EP Jr. Hallervorden-Spatz syndrome. Arch Neurol 1974;30:70–83.
23. Rutledge JN, Hilal SK, Silver AJ, et al. Study of movement disorders and brain iron by MR. AJR Am J Roentgenol 1987;149:365–379.
24. Ching KH, Westaway SK, Gitschier J, et al. HARP syndrome is allelic with pantothenate kinase-associated neurodegeneration. Neurology 2002;58:1673–1674.
25. Castelnau P, Cif L, Valente EM, et al. Pallidal stimulation improves pantothenate kinase-associated neurodegeneration. Ann Neurol 2005;57:738–741.
26. Morgan NV, Westaway SK, Morton JE, et al. PLA2G6, encoding a phospholipase A2, is mutated in neurodegenerative disorders with high brain iron. Nat Genet 2006;38:752–754.
27. Gregory A, Westaway SK, Holm IE, et al. Neurodegeneration associated with genetic defects in phospholipase A(2). Neurology 2008;71:1402–1409.
28. Paisan-Ruiz C, Bhatia KP, Li A, et al. Characterization of PLA2G6 as a locus for dystonia-parkinsonism. Ann Neurol 2008;65:19–23.
29. Curtis AR, Fey C, Morris CM, et al. Mutation in the gene encoding ferritin light polypeptide causes dominant adult-onset basal ganglia disease. Nat Genet 2001;28:350–354.
30. Yoshida K, Furihata K, Takeda S, et al. A mutation in the ceruloplasmin gene is associated with systemic hemosiderosis in humans. Nat Genet 1995;9:267–272.
31. McNeill A, Birchall D, Hayflick SJ, et al. T2* and FSE MRI distinguishes four subtypes of neurodegeneration with brain iron accumulation. Neurology 2008;70:1614–1619.
32. Klawans HL. Hemiparkinsonism as a late complication of hemiatrophy: A new syndrome. Neurology 1981;31: 625–628.
33. Buchman AS, Goetz CG, Klawans HL. Hemiparkinsonism with hemiatrophy. Neurology 1988;38:527–530.
34. Pramstaller PP, Künig G, Leenders K, et al. Parkin mutations in a patient with hemiparkinsonism-hemiatrophy: A clinical-genetic and PET study. Neurology 2002;58: 808–810.
35. Wijemanne S, Jankovic J. Hemiparkinsonism-hemiatrophy syndrome. Neurology 2007;69:1585–1594.
36. Penfield W, Robertson JSM. Growth asymmetry due to lesions of the post central cortex. Arch Neurol Psychiatry 1943;50:405–430.
37. Giladi N, Burke RE, Kostic V, et al. Hemiparkinsonism-hemiatrophy syndrome: Clinical and neuroradiologic features. Neurology 1990;40:1731–1734.
38. Aguiar PH, Liu CW, Leitão H, et al. MR and CT imaging in the Dyke-Davidoff-Masson syndrome. Report of three cases and contribution to pathogenesis and differential diagnosis. Arq Neuropsiquiatr 1998;56:803–807.
39. Greene PE, Bressman SB, Ford B, et al. Parkinsonism, dystonia, and hemiatrophy. Mov Disord 2000;15:537–541.
40. Hebb MO, Lang AE, Fletcher PJ, et al. Neonatal ablation of the nigrostriatal dopamine pathway does not influence limb development in rats. Exp Neurol 2002;177:547–556.
41. Lee PH, Joo US, Yong SW, et al. Asymmetric freezing of gait in hemiparkinsonism-hemiatrophy. Neurology 2004;63:E7.
42. Przedborski S, Giladi N, Takikawa S, et al. Metabolic topography of the hemiparkinsonism-hemiatrophy syndrome. Neurology 1994;44:1622–1628.
43. Unal O, Tombul T, Cirak B, et al. Left hemisphere and male sex dominance of cerebral hemiatrophy (Dyke-Davidoff-Masson Syndrome). Clin Imaging 2004;28: 163–165.
44. Jenkins M, Mendonca D, Parrent A, et al. Hemiparkinsonism-somatic hemiatrophy syndrome. Can J Neurol Sci 2002;29:184–187.
45. Giladi N, Fahn S. Hemiparkinsonism-hemiatrophy syndrome may mimic early-stage cortical-basal ganglionic degeneration. Mov Disord 1992;7:384–385.
46. Lee LV, Pascasio FM, Fuentes FD, et al. Torsion dystonia in Panay, Philippines. Adv Neurol 1976;14:137–151.
47. Lee LV, Maranon E, Demaisip C, et al. The natural history of sex-linked recessive dystonia parkinsonism of Panay, Philippines (XDP). Parkinsonism Relat Disord 2002;9: 29–38.
48. Waters CH, Faust PL, Powers J, et al. Neuropathology of lubag (x-linked dystonia parkinsonism). Mov Disord 1993;8:387–390.
49. Németh AH, Nolte D, Dunne E, et al. Refined linkage disequilibrium and physical mapping of the gene locus for X-linked dystonia-parkinsonism (DYT3). Genomics 1999;60:320–329.
50. Waters CH, Takahashi H, Wilhelmsen KC, et al. Phenotypic expression of X-linked dystonia-parkinsonism (lubag) in two women. Neurology 1993;43:1555–1558.
51. Nolte D, Niemann S, Müller U. Specific sequence changes in multiple transcript system DYT3 are associated with X-linked dystonia parkinsonism. Proc Natl Acad Sci U S A 2003;100:10347–10352.
52. Makino S, Kaji R, Ando S, et al. Reduced neuron-specific expression of the TAF1 gene is associated with X-linked dystonia-parkinsonism. Am J Hum Genet 2007;80: 393–406.

53. Goto S, Lee LV, Munoz EL, et al. Functional anatomy of the basal ganglia in X-linked recessive dystonia-parkinsonism. Ann Neurol 2005;58:7–17.
54. Evidente VG, Advincula J, Esteban R, et al. Phenomenology of "Lubag" or X-linked dystonia-parkinsonism. Mov Disord 2002;17:1271–1277.
55. Evidente VG, Gwinn-Hardy K, Hardy J, et al. X-linked dystonia ("Lubag") presenting predominantly with parkinsonism: A more benign phenotype? Mov Disord 2002;17:200–202.
56. Evidente VG, Esteban RP, Hernandez JL, et al. Smell testing is abnormal in 'lubag' or X-linked dystonia-parkinsonism: A pilot study. Parkinsonism Relat Disord 2004;10:407–410.
57. Evidente VG, Nolte D, Niemann S, et al. Phenotypic and molecular analyses of X-linked dystonia-parkinsonism ("lubag") in women. Arch Neurol 2004;61:1956–1959.
58. Tackenberg B, Metz A, Unger M, et al. Nigrostriatal dysfunction in X-linked dystonia-parkinsonism (DYT3). Mov Disord 2007;22:900–902.
59. Eidelberg D, Takikawa S, Wilhelmsen K, et al. Positron emission tomographic findings in Filipino X-linked dystonia-parkinsonism. Ann Neurol 1993;34:185–191.
60. Lee LV, Kupke KG, Caballar-Gonzaga F, et al. The phenotype of the X-linked dystonia-parkinsonism syndrome. An assessment of 42 cases in the Philippines. Medicine (Baltimore) 1991;70:179–187.
61. Evidente VG. Zolpidem improves dystonia in "Lubag" or X-linked dystonia-parkinsonism syndrome. Neurology 2002;58:662–663.
62. Brecher G, Bessis M. Present status of spiculed red cells and their relationship to the discocyte-echinocyte transformation: A critical review. Blood 1972;40:333–344.
63. Levine IM, Estes JW, Looney JM. Hereditary neurological disease with acanthocytosis. A new syndrome. Arch Neurol 1968;19:403–409.
64. Critchley EM, Clark DB, Wikler A. Acanthocytosis and neurological disorder without betalipoproteinemia. Arch Neurol 1968;18:134–140.
65. Kornzweig AL, Bassen FA. Retinitis pigmentosa, acanthrocytosis, and heredodegenerative neuromuscular disease. AMA Arch Ophthalmol 1957;58:183–187.
66. Young SG, Bertics SJ, Curtiss LK, et al. Genetic analysis of a kindred with familial hypobetalipoproteinemia. Evidence for two separate gene defects: One associated with an abnormal apolipoprotein B species, apolipoprotein B-37; and a second associated with low plasma concentrations of apolipoprotein B-100. J Clin Invest 1987;79:1842–1851.
67. Allen FH, Krabbe FMR, Corcoran PA. A new phenotype (McLeod) in the Kell blood group system. Vox Sang 1961;6:555–560.
68. Danek A, Rubio JP, Rampoldi L, et al. McLeod neuroacanthocytosis: Genotype and phenotype. Ann Neurol 2001;50:755–764.
69. Swash M, Schwartz MS, Carter ND, et al. Benign X-linked myopathy with acanthocytes (McLeod syndrome). Its relationship to X-linked muscular dystrophy. Brain 1983;106:717–733.
70. Gradstein L, Danek A, Grafman J, et al. Eye movements in chorea-acanthocytosis. Invest Ophthalmol Vis Sci 2005;46:1979–1987.
71. Rubio JP, Danek A, Stone C, et al. Chorea-acanthocytosis: Genetic linkage to chromosome 9q21. Am J Hum Genet 1997;61:899–908.
72. Ueno S, Maruki Y, Nakamura M, et al. The gene encoding a newly discovered protein, chorein, is mutated in chorea-acanthocytosis. Nat Genet 2001;28:121–122.
73. Rampoldi L, Dobson-Stone C, Rubio JP, et al. A conserved sorting-associated protein is mutant in chorea-acanthocytosis. Nat Genet 2001;28:119–120.
74. Dobson-Stone C, Velayos-Baeza A, Jansen A, et al. Identification of a VPS13A founder mutation in French Canadian families with chorea-acanthocytosis. Neurogenetics 2005;6:151–158.
75. Walker RH, Morgello S, Davidoff-Feldman B, et al. Autosomal dominant chorea-acanthocytosis with polyglutamine-containing euronal inclusions. Neurology 2002;58:1031–1037.
76. Walker RH, Rasmussen A, Rudnicki D, et al. Huntington's disease-like 2 can present as chorea-acanthocytosis. Neurology 2003;61:1002–1004.
77. Rinne JO, Daniel SE, Scaravilli F, et al. The neuropathological features of neuroacanthocytosis. Mov Disord 1994;9:297–304.
78. Rinne JO, Daniel SE, Scaravilli F, et al. Nigral degeneration in neuroacanthocytosis. Neurology 1994;44:1629–1632.
79. Sakai T, Mawatari S, Iwashita H, et al. Choreoacanthocytosis. Clues to clinical diagnosis. Arch Neurol 1981;38:335–338.
80. Yamamoto T, Hirose G, Shimazaki K, et al. Movement disorders of familial neuroacanthocytosis syndrome. Arch Neurol 1982;39:298–301.
81. Spitz MC, Jankovic J, Killian JM. Familial tic disorder, parkinsonism, motor neuron disease, and acanthocytosis: A new syndrome. Neurology 1985;35:366–370.
82. Serra S, Xerra A, Scribano E, et al. Computerized tomography in amyotrophic choreo-acanthocytosis. Neuroradiology 1987;29:480–482.
83. Hardie RJ, Pullon HW, Harding AE, et al. Neuroacanthocytosis. A clinical, haematological and pathological study of 19 cases. Brain 1991;114:13–49.
84. Ruiz-Sandoval JL, Garcia-Navarro V, Chiquete E, et al. Choreoacanthocytosis in a Mexican family. Arch Neurol 2007;64:1661–1664.
85. Müller-Vahl KR, Berding G, Emrich HM, et al. Chorea-acanthocytosis in monozygotic twins: Clinical findings and neuropathological changes as detected by diffusion tensor imaging, FDG-PET and (123)I-beta-CIT-SPECT. J Neurol 2007;254:1081–1088.
86. Tanaka M, Hirai S, Kondo S, et al. Cerebral hypoperfusion and hypometabolism with altered striatal signal intensity in chorea-acanthocytosis: A combined PET and MRI study. Mov Disord 1998;13:100–107.
87. Brooks DJ, Ibanez V, Playford ED, et al. Presynaptic and postsynaptic striatal dopaminergic function in neuroacanthocytosis: A positron emission tomographic study. Ann Neurol 1991;30:166–171.
88. Ohnishi A, Sato Y, Nagara H, et al. Neurogenic muscular atrophy and low density of large myelinated fibres of sural nerve in chorea-acanthocytosis. J Neurol Neurosurg Psychiatry 1981;44:645–648.
89. Burbaud P, Rougier A, Ferrer X, et al. Improvement of severe trunk spasms by bilateral high-frequency stimulation

of the motor thalamus in a patient with chorea-acanthocytosis. Mov Disord 2002;17:204–207.
90. Hunt JR. Progressive atrophy of the globus pallidus (primary atrophy of the pallidal system): A system disease of the paralysis agitans type, characterized by atrophy of the motor cells of the corpus striatum. A contribution to the functions of the corpus striatum. Brain 1917;40:58–148.
91. Jellinger K. Pallidal, pallidonigral, and pallidoluysionigral degenerations including association with thalamic and dendate degenerations. In Vinken PJ, Bruyn GW (eds). Handbook of Clinical Neurology. Amsterdam: Elsevier, pp. 445–463, 1986.
92. McCormick WF, Lemmi H. Familial degeneration of the pallidonigral system. Neurology 1965;15:141–153.
93. Yagishita S, Itoh Y, Nakano T, et al. Pleomorphic intraneuronal polyglucosan bodies mainly restricted to the pallidium. A case report. Acta Neuropathol 1983;62: 159–163.
94. Yasuda M, Kawamata T, Komure O, et al. A mutation in the microtubule-associated protein tau in pallido-nigroluysian degeneration. Neurology 1999;53:864–868.
95. Wszolek ZK, Uitti RJ, Hutton M. A mutation in the microtubule-associated protein tau in pallido-nigroluysian degeneration. Neurology 2000;54:2028–2030.
96. Mori H, Motoi Y, Kobayashi T, et al. Tau accumulation in a patient with pallidonigroluysian atrophy. Neurosci Lett 2001;309(2):89–92.
97. Lange E, Poppe W, Scholtze P. Familial progressive pallidum atrophy. Eur Neurol 1970;3:265–267.
98. van Bogaert L: Aspects cliniques et pathologiques des atrophies pallidales et pallido-luysiennes progressives. J Belge Neurol Psychiatr 1947;47:268–286.
99. Konishi Y, Shirabe T, Katayama S, et al. Autopsy case of pure akinesia showing pallidonigro-luysian atrophy. Neuropathology 2005;25:220–227.
100. Kosaka K, Matsushita M, Oyanagi S, et al. Pallido-nigroluysial atrophy with massive appearance of corpora amylacea in the CNS. Acta Neuropathol 1981;53:169–172.
101. Kawai J, Sasahara M, Hazama F, et al. Pallidonigroluysian degeneration with iron deposition: A study of three autopsy cases. Acta Neuropathol 1993;86:609–616.
102. Aizawa H, Kwak S, Shimizu T, et al. A case of adult onset pure pallidal degeneration. I. Clinical manifestations and neuropathological observations. J Neurol Sci 1991;102:76–82.
103. Wooten GF, Lopes MB, Harris WO, et al. Pallidoluysian atrophy: Dystonia and basal ganglia functional anatomy. Neurology 1993;43:1764–1768.
104. Shimoda M, Hosoda Y, Kato S, et al. Pallidonigroluysian atrophy: Clinicopathological and immunohistochemical studies. Neuropathology 1996;16:21–28.
105. Vercueil L, Hammouti A, Andriantseheno ML, et al. Pallido-Luysio-Nigral atrophy revealed by rapidly progressive hemidystonia: A clinical, radiologic, functional, and neuropathologic study. Mov Disord 2000;15:947–953.
106. Ahmed Z, Josephs KA, Gonzalez J, et al. Clinical and neuropathologic features of progressive supranuclear palsy with severe pallido-nigro-luysial degeneration and axonal dystrophy. Brain 2008;131:460–472.
107. Yamamoto T, Kawamura J, Hashimoto S, et al. Pallido-nigro-luysian atrophy, progressive supranuclear palsy and adult onset Hallervorden-Spatz disease: A case of akinesia as a predominant feature of parkinsonism. J Neurol Sci 1991;101:98–106.
108. Davison C. Pallido-pyramidal disease. J Neuropathol Exp Neurol 1954;13:50–59.
109. Horowitz G, Greenberg J. Pallido-pyramidal syndrome treated with levodopa. J Neurol Neurosurg Psychiatry 1975;38:238–240.
110. Tranchant C, Boulay C, Warter JM. [Pallido-pyramidal syndrome: An unrecognized entity] Rev Neurol (Paris) 1991;147:308–310.
111. Nisipeanu P, Kuritzky A, Korczyn AD. Familial levodopa-responsive parkinsonian-pyramidal syndrome. Mov Disord 1994;9:673–675.
112. Najim al-Din AS, Wriekat A, Mubaidin A, et al. Pallido-pyramidal degeneration, supranuclear upgaze paresis and dementia: Kufor-Rakeb syndrome. Acta Neurol Scand 1994;89:347–352.
113. Hampshire DJ, Roberts E, Crow Y, et al. Kufor-Rakeb syndrome, pallido-pyramidal degeneration with supranuclear upgaze paresis and dementia, maps to 1p36. J Med Genet 2001;38:680–682.
114. Ramirez A, Helmbach A, Gründemann J, et al. Hereditary parkinsonism with dementia is caused by mutations in ATP13A2, encoding a lysosomal type 5 P-type ATPase. Nat Genet 2006;38:1184–1191.
115. Shojaee S, Sina F, Banihosseini SS, et al. Genome-wide linkage analysis of a parkinsonian-pyramidal syndrome pedigree by 500 K SNP arrays. Am J Hum Genet 2008;82:1375–1384.
116. Srivastava T, Goyal V, Singh S, et al. Pallido-pyramidal syndrome with blepharospasm and good response to levodopa. J Neurol 2005;252:1537–1538.
117. Remy P, Hosseini H, Degos JD, et al. Striatal dopaminergic denervation in pallidopyramidal disease demonstrated by positron emission tomography. Ann Neurol 1995;38:954–956.
118. Pradat PF, Dupel-Pottier C, Lacomblez L, et al. Case report of pallido-pyramidal disease with supplementary motor area involvement. Mov Disord 2001;16:762–764.
119. Panagariya A, Sharma B, Dev A. Pallido-pyramidal syndrome: A rare entity. (Letter) Indian J Med Sci 2007;61: 156–157.
120. Rett A. [On an until now unknown disease of a congenital metabolic disorder] Krankenschwester 196619:121–122.
121. Rett A. Cerebral atrophy with hyperammonaemia. In Vinken PJ, Bruyn GW (eds). Handbook of Clinical Neurology. Amsterdam: Elsevier, pp. 305–329, 1977.
122. Hagberg B, Aicardi J, Dias K. A progressive syndrome of autism, dementia, ataxia, and loss of purposeful hand use in girls: Rett's syndrome: Report of 35 cases. Ann Neurol 1983;14:471–479.
123. Hagberg B, Witt-Engerström I. Rett syndrome: A suggested staging system for describing impairment profile with increasing age towards adolescence. Am J Med Genet Suppl 1986;1:47–59.
124. Comings DE. The genetics of Rett syndrome: The consequences of a disorder where every case is a new mutation. Am J Med Genet Suppl 1986;1:383–388.
125. Moog U, Smeets EE, van Roozendaal KE, et al. Neurodevelopmental disorders in males related to the gene causing Rett syndrome in females (MECP2). Eur J Paediatr Neurol 2003;7:5–12.

126. Sirianni N, Naidu S, Pereira J, et al. Rett syndrome: Confirmation of X-linked dominant inheritance, and localization of the gene to Xq28. Am J Hum Genet 1998;63:1552–1558.
127. Amir RE, Van den Veyver IB, Wan M, et al. Rett syndrome is caused by mutations in X-linked MECP2, encoding methyl-CpG-binding protein 2. Nat Genet 1999;23: 185–188.
128. Percy AK, Lane JB, Childers J, et al. Rett syndrome: North American database. J Child Neurol 2007;22:1338–1341.
129. Shahbazian MD, Zoghbi HY. Molecular genetics of Rett syndrome and clinical spectrum of MECP2 mutations. Curr Opin Neurol 2001;14:171–176.
130. Hagberg B, Hanefeld F, Percy A, et al. An update on clinically applicable diagnostic criteria in Rett syndrome. Comments to Rett Syndrome Clinical Criteria Consensus Panel Satellite to European Paediatric Neurology Society Meeting, Baden Baden, Germany, September 2001. Eur J Paediatr Neurol 2002;6:293–297.
131. Chahrour M, Zoghbi HY. The story of Rett syndrome: From clinic to neurobiology. Neuron 2007;56:422–437.
132. Borg I, Freude K, Kübart S, et al. Disruption of Netrin G1 by a balanced chromosome translocation in a girl with Rett syndrome. Eur J Hum Genet 2005;13:921–927.
133. Scala E, Ariani F, Mari F, et al. CDKL5/STK9 is mutated in Rett syndrome variant with infantile spasms. J Med Genet 2005;42:103–107.
134. Ariani F, Hayek G, Rondinella D, et al. FOXG1 is responsible for the congenital variant of Rett syndrome. Am J Hum Genet 2008;83:89–93.
135. Jellinger K, Seitelberger F. Neuropathology of Rett syndrome. Am J Med Genet Suppl 1986;1:259–288.
136. Armstrong D, Dunn JK, Antalffy B, et al. Selective dendritic alterations in the cortex of Rett syndrome. J Neuropathol Exp Neurol 1995;54:195–201.
137. Braddock SR, Braddock BA, Graham JM Jr. Rett syndrome. An update and review for the primary pediatrician. Clin Pediatr (Phila) 1993;32:613–626.
138. Sekul EA, Moak JP, Schultz RJ, et al. Electrocardiographic findings in Rett syndrome: An explanation for sudden death? J Pediatr 1994;125:80–82.
139. FitzGerald PM, Jankovic J, Percy AK. Rett syndrome and associated movement disorders. Mov Disord 1990;5: 195–202.
140. The Rett Syndrome Diagnostic Criteria Work Group. Criteria for Rett syndrome. Ann Neurol 1988,23:425–428.
141. Hagberg BA, Skjeldal OH. Rett variants: A suggested model for inclusion criteria. Pediatr Neurol 1994;11:5–11.
142. Murakami JW, Courchesne E, Haas RH, et al. Cerebellar and cerebral abnormalities in Rett syndrome: A quantitative MR analysis. AJR Am J Roentgenol 1992;159: 177–183.
143. Subramaniam B, Naidu S, Reiss AL. Neuroanatomy in Rett syndrome: Cerebral cortex and posterior fossa. Neurology 1997;48:399–407.
144. Chiron C, Bulteau C, Loc'h C, et al. Dopaminergic D2 receptor SPECT imaging in Rett syndrome: Increase of specific binding in striatum. J Nucl Med 1993;34:1717–1721.
145. Dunn HG, Stoessl AJ, Ho HH, et al. Rett syndrome: Investigation of nine patients, including PET scan. Can J Neurol Sci 2002;29:345–357.
146. Naidu S, Wong DF, Kitt C, et al. Positron emission tomography in the Rett syndrome: Clinical, biochemical and pathological correlates. Brain Dev 1992;14:75–79.
147. Zoghbi HY, Milstien S, Butler IJ, et al. Cerebrospinal fluid biogenic amines and biopterin in Rett syndrome. Ann Neurol 1989;25:56–60.
148. Hamberger A, Gillberg C, Palm A, et al. Elevated CSF glutamate in Rett syndrome. Neuropediatrics 1992;23: 212–313.
149. Matsuishi T, Urabe F, Percy AK, et al. Abnormal carbohydrate metabolism in cerebrospinal fluid in Rett syndrome. J Child Neurol 1994;9:26–30.
150. Percy AK, Glaze DG, Schultz RJ, et al. Rett syndrome: Controlled study of an oral opiate antagonist, naltrexone. Ann Neurol 1994;35:464–470.
151. Kumandas S, Caksen H, Ciftçi A, et al. Lamotrigine in two cases of Rett syndrome. Brain Dev 2001;23:240–242.
152. Plioplys AV, Kasnicka I. L-carnitine as a treatment for Rett syndrome. South Med J 1993;86:1411–1412.
153. Zappella M, Genazzani A, Facchinetti F, et al. Bromocriptine in the Rett syndrome. Brain Dev 1990;12:221–225.
154. Hagerman RJ, Leehey M, Heinrichs W, et al. Intention tremor, parkinsonism, and generalized brain atrophy in male carriers of fragile X. Neurology 2001;57:127–130.
155. Berry-Kravis E, Lewin F, Wuu J, et al. Tremor and ataxia in fragile X premutation carriers: Blinded videotape study. Ann Neurol 2003;53:616–623.
156. Jacquemont S, Hagerman RJ, Leehey M, et al. Fragile X premutation tremor/ataxia syndrome: Molecular, clinical, and neuroimaging correlates. Am J Hum Genet 2003;72:869–878.
157. Verkerk AJ, Pieretti M, Sutcliffe JS, et al. Identification of a gene (FMR-1) containing a CGG repeat coincident with a breakpoint cluster region exhibiting length variation in fragile X syndrome. Cell 1991;65:905–914.
158. Hagerman PJ, Hagerman RJ. The fragile-X premutation: A maturing perspective. Am J Hum Genet 2004;74: 805–816.
159. Krawczun MS, Jenkins EC, Brown WT. Analysis of the fragile-X chromosome: Localization and detection of the fragile site in high resolution preparations. Hum Genet 1985;69:209–211.
160. Jacquemont S, Hagerman RJ, Leehey MA, et al. Penetrance of the fragile X-associated tremor/ataxia syndrome in a premutation carrier population. JAMA 2004;291: 460–469.
161. Kremer EJ, Pritchard M, Lynch M, et al. Mapping of DNA instability at the fragile X to a trinucleotide repeat sequence p(CCG)n. Science 1991;252:1711–1714.
162. Gedeon AK, Baker E, Robinson H, et al. Fragile X syndrome without CCG amplification has an FMR1 deletion. Nat Genet 1992;1:341–314.
163. Allingham-Hawkins DJ, Babul-Hirji R, Chitayat D, et al. Fragile X premutation is a significant risk factor for premature ovarian failure: The International Collaborative POF in Fragile X study - preliminary data. Am J Med Genet 1999;83:322–325.
164. Greco CM, Tassone F, Garcia-Arocena D, et al. Clinical and neuropathologic findings in a woman with the FMR1 premutation and multiple sclerosis. Arch Neurol 2008;65:1114–1116.

165. Jin P, Zarnescu DC, Ceman S, et al. Biochemical and genetic interaction between the fragile X mental retardation protein and the microRNA pathway. Nat Neurosci 2004;7:113–117.
166. Greenough WT, Klintsova AY, Irwin SA, et al. Synaptic regulation of protein synthesis and the fragile X protein. Proc Natl Acad Sci U S A 2001;98:7101–7106.
167. Greco CM, Berman RF, Martin RM, et al. Neuropathology of fragile X-associated tremor/ataxia syndrome (FXTAS). Brain 2006;129:243–255.
168. Tassone F, Iwahashi C, Hagerman PJ. FMR1 RNA within the intranuclear inclusions of fragile X-associated tremor/ataxia syndrome (FXTAS). RNA Biol 2004;1:103–105.
169. Greco CM, Hagerman RJ, Tassone F, et al. Neuronal intranuclear inclusions in a new cerebellar tremor/ataxia syndrome among fragile X carriers. Brain 2002;125:1760–1771.
170. Grigsby J, Brega AG, Jacquemont S, et al. Impairment in the cognitive functioning of men with fragile X-associated tremor/ataxia syndrome (FXTAS). J Neurol Sci 2006;248:227–233.
171. Bacalman S, Farzin F, Bourgeois JA, et al. Psychiatric phenotype of the fragile X-associated tremor/ataxia syndrome (FXTAS) in males: Newly described fronto-subcortical dementia. J Clin Psychiatry 2006;67:87–94.
172. Hessl D, Tassone F, Loesch DZ, et al. Abnormal elevation of FMR1 mRNA is associated with psychological symptoms in individuals with the fragile X premutation. Am J Med Genet B Neuropsychiatr Genet 2005;139:115–121.
173. Tassone F, Adams J, Berry-Kravis EM, et al. CGG repeat length correlates with age of onset of motor signs of the fragile X-associated tremor/ataxia syndrome (FXTAS). Am J Med Genet B Neuropsychiatr Genet 2007;144:566–569.
174. Leehey MA, Munhoz RP, Lang AE, et al. The fragile X premutation presenting as essential tremor. Arch Neurol 2003;60:117–121.
175. Gonçalves MR, Capelli LP, Nitrini R, et al. Atypical clinical course of FXTAS: Rapidly progressive dementia as the major symptom. Neurology 2007;68:1864–1866.
176. Leehey MA, Berry-Kravis E, Goetz CG, et al. FMR1 CGG repeat length predicts motor dysfunction in premutation carriers. Neurology 2008;70:1397–1402.
177. Peters N, Kamm C, Asmus F, et al. Intrafamilial variability in fragile X-associated tremor/ataxia syndrome. Mov Disord 2006;21:98–102.
178. Brunberg JA, Jacquemont S, Hagerman RJ, et al. Fragile X premutation carriers: Characteristic MR imaging findings of adult male patients with progressive cerebellar and cognitive dysfunction. AJNR Am J Neuroradiol 2002;23:1757–1766.
179. Loesch DZ, Churchyard A, Brotchie P, et al. Evidence for, and a spectrum of, neurological involvement in carriers of the fragile X pre-mutation: FXTAS and beyond. Clin Genet 2005;67:412–417.
180. Cohen S, Masyn K, Adams J, et al. Molecular and imaging correlates of the fragile X-associated tremor/ataxia syndrome. Neurology 2006;67:1426–1431.
181. Adams JS, Adams PE, Nguyen D, et al. Volumetric brain changes in females with fragile X-associated tremor/ataxia syndrome (FXTAS). Neurology 2007;69:851–859.
182. Zühlke Ch, Budnik A, Gehlken U, et al. FMR1 premutation as a rare cause of late onset ataxia-evidence for FXTAS in female carriers. J Neurol 2004;251:1418–1419.
183. Ceravolo R, Antonini A, Volterrani D, et al. Dopamine transporter imaging study in parkinsonism occurring in fragile X premutation carriers. Neurology 2005;65:1971–1973.
184. Hall DA, Berry-Kravis E, Hagerman RJ, et al. Symptomatic treatment in the fragile X-associated tremor/ataxia syndrome. Mov Disord 2006;21:1741–1744.

III. TREMOR DISORDERS

CHAPTER 25

Essential Tremor

Kelly E. Lyons

▶ INTRODUCTION

Essential tremor (ET) is the most common cause of tremor and one of the most prevalent movement disorders affecting an estimated 10 million persons in the United States.[1] The first descriptions of tremor date back to ancient times; however, it was not until the 1800s that ET was recognized as a distinct disorder. At that time, it was defined as a disorder that is often hereditary with persistent action tremor without other neurological signs. The term "essential tremor" was first used in the 1800s, but several other terms have been used to describe this disorder throughout the years such as senile tremor, benign tremor, familial tremor, and benign familial tremor. It was not until the later 1900s that the term "essential tremor" was consistently used in the medical literature.[1] In medical terminology, the word "essential" is often used to describe a disorder in which the cause is unknown. Therefore, "essential tremor" refers to a disorder characterized primarily by tremor for which the cause is unknown.

▶ CLINICAL CHARACTERISTICS

PRIMARY CHARACTERISTICS

ET is a neurological disorder characterized primarily by an action tremor including a kinetic tremor occurring during voluntary movement, and/or a postural tremor occurring when the affected body part is held against gravity.[2] Intention tremor, a type of tremor in which the tremor is increased as the limb approaches a target, is also commonly seen in ET.[2] Rest tremor is rarely seen in ET but has been reported in older patients with more advanced disease.[3] During examination, it is important to make certain that the tremulous body part is relaxed and completely supported to assure the observed tremor is truly a resting and not a postural tremor. Tremor frequency usually ranges between 4 and 12 Hz. Older patients tend to have lower frequency tremor between 4 and 8 Hz, while younger patients generally have a higher frequency tremor ranging between 8 and 12 Hz.[4]

DISTRIBUTION

ET affects the upper extremities in approximately 95% of patients, and is generally a bilateral tremor.[5] Hand tremor can cause significant disability in completing activities of daily living such as eating, dressing, drinking, and writing. Handwriting tends to be large and tremulous as opposed to the micrographia seen in PD.[6] ET also affects the head in approximately 34% of patients.[5] Head tremor generally occurs in combination with hand tremor. Less often, head tremor can occur in isolation in ET; however, in these cases, it is important to rule out cervical dystonia as the cause of the tremor. Other body parts that can be affected by ET include the lower extremities (20%), voice (12%), face (5%), and trunk (5%).[5] It is not uncommon to see both the severity of the tremor and the range of body parts affected by the tremor increase as the disease progresses.

AGE OF ONSET AND DISEASE PROGRESSION

ET can affect persons of all ages; however, it is commonly seen in older adults with an estimated 5% of persons 65 years of age and older being affected.[5,7] Some studies have reported a bimodal distribution of the age of onset of ET with a peak around 30–40 years of age and another peak in older adulthood.[8] It has been suggested that age of onset may be earlier in those with a family history of ET compared to sporadic ET[9]; however, age of onset has not been related to clinical or therapeutic outcomes.[6,10] ET is generally considered to be a slowly progressive disorder, but individual variability occurs.[6] The progression of ET can range from a mild tremor present throughout most of life that does not seem to worsen to a mild tremor that slowly becomes more severe, affects additional body parts, and eventually leads to significant disability. Despite its potentially progressive course, ET is generally not associated with increased mortality.[11]

OTHER SYMPTOMS

ET is typically described as a monosymptomatic disorder without other neurological signs or symptoms.[12] It is accepted that mild abnormalities of tone with slight cogwheeling and impairment in tandem gait can be observed in persons with ET.[9,10] In one study, tandem gait abnormalities were seen in 50% of ET patients compared with 28% of age-matched controls.[13] Similarly, in a quantitative assessment of gait in ET patients, abnormalities in tandem gait with increased missteps were reported.[14] Cognitive deficits have generally been considered to be mild. Deficits in verbal fluency, mental set shifting, verbal memory, working memory, visuoperceptual dysfunction, and encoding as well as increased depression have been reported.[15,16] The effects on cognitive function in ET are not clear, and further research is necessary to determine the extent of any potential neuropsychiatric deficits.

INFLUENCING FACTORS

Multiple factors can affect ET. ET is more common and tends to progress with age.[6,11] Other factors such as anxiety, embarrassment, fatigue, temperature extremes, emotional upset or excitement, sexual arousal, and central nervous system stimulants can increase tremor.[6,10] In contrast, alcohol has a significant suppressive effect on ET in the majority of patients. In fact, a response to alcohol has often been used to help confirm the diagnosis of ET.[6] In addition, tremor is generally suppressed during sleep.[6]

▶ EPIDEMIOLOGY

PREVALENCE

Studies examining the prevalence of ET have been conducted throughout the world and have reported quite variable prevalence rates ranging from 0.008 to 22%; however, it is generally reported to be less than 5%.[17] A fairly consistent finding is that those studies examining persons over the age of 40 or, more specifically, those over the age of 65, reported the highest prevalence rates compared to studies examining the entire population (Table 25–1).[9,11,18–34] There are multiple possibilities as to why the range of reported prevalence rates is so large including variable criteria for the diagnosis of ET, method of ascertainment such as door-to-door surveys versus medical record review, different screening criteria used, use of formal neurological examination for all participants versus self-report or screening questionnaires, and the reporting of specific age groups versus the whole population. The variability in these results stresses the importance of conducting well-designed studies

▶ TABLE 25–1. SELECTED PREVALENCE STUDIES OF ESSENTIAL TREMOR

References	Country	Age of Cohort	Prevalence (%)
Snow and colleagues[18]	Canada	All	0.008
Chouza and colleagues[19]	Uruguay	All	0.22
Rajput and colleagues[11]	United States	All	0.31
Hornabrook and Nagurney[20]	New Guinea	All	0.35
Das and colleagues[21]	India	All	0.40
Salemi and colleagues[23]	Italy	All	0.41
Haerer and colleagues[24]	United States	≥40	0.42
Salemi and colleagues[23]	Italy	≥40	1.08
Das and colleagues[22]	India	≥60	1.38
Bharucha and colleagues[25]	India	All	1.59
Hornabrook and Nagurney[20]	New Guinea	≥40	1.64
Larsson and Sjogren[9]	Sweden	All	1.70
Broe and colleagues[26]	Scotland	≥65	1.70
Larsson and Sjogren[9]	Sweden	≥40	3.73
Louis and colleagues[27]	United States	≥65	3.92
Dogu and colleagues[28]	Turkey	≥40	4.00
Bergareche and colleagues[29]	Spain	≥65	4.80
Benito-Leon and colleagues[30]	Spain	≥65	4.80
Rautakorpi and colleagues[31]	Finland	≥40	5.55
Marti-Masso and Poza[32]	Spain	≥39	5.59
Mateo and Gimenez-Roldan[33]	Spain	≥65	9.80
Moghal and colleagues[34]	Canada	≥65	14.0

throughout the world to determine the true prevalence rate of ET.

INCIDENCE

Few studies have examined the incidence rate of ET. A 45-year study based on medical records of all residents in Olmstead County, Minnesota, USA reported an age- and sex-adjusted incidence rate for ET of approximately 24 per 100,000 persons.[11] There were no differences in age-adjusted incidence rates between men (18.3 per 100,000) and women (17.1 per 100,000). In a population-based survey of persons at least 65 years of age in Central Spain, the incidence rate was 616 per 100,000.[35] It was noted that 77% of the incident cases were not diagnosed, which suggests that the actual incidence of ET may be higher as not all persons with ET seek medical care.

▶ ETIOLOGY

GENETICS

Although the tendency for multiple members of the same family to be affected by ET was recognized in the earliest descriptions of ET [1] and has been confirmed in multiple reports thereafter,[6,9,10] a specific gene accounting for the majority of ET cases has not been identified. The percentage of patients that report a family history of ET varies greatly from 17 to 100% with an average of approximately 50%.[36] There are multiple factors that may account for this variability. The first is the manner in which family history information was obtained including self-report of the proband versus a detailed genetic analysis of the family, patient self-report versus interview with each family member, interview of both affected and unaffected individuals, and clinic-based versus community-based populations. In addition, the size of the families investigated, age structure of the family, and the presence of comorbid conditions within the family are important factors in getting accurate reports of family history.

The majority of the research to date suggests an autosomal dominant inheritance pattern for ET. A study of 26 patients with familial ET, 93 first-degree relatives and 38 more distant relatives comprising three generations reported an autosomal dominant inheritance pattern with nearly complete penetrance by 65 years of age and no instances in which ET skipped a generation.[37] Similarly, in a study of 210 ET patients in Sweden including six generations and nine families,[9] an autosomal dominant pattern of inheritance was observed with nearly complete penetrance by the age of 70 and no instances in which ET skipped a generation.

To date, there have been three genetic loci linked to autosomal dominant ET (Table 25–2). Gulcher and colleagues[38] reported 16 Icelandic families with 75 affected family members with linkage to the genetic loci ETM1 at

▶ TABLE 25–2. GENETIC LINKAGE STUDIES IN ESSENTIAL TREMOR

Study	Population	Locus	LOD Scores
Gulcher and colleagues[38]	16 Icelandic families	3q13 (ETM1)	3.71
Higgins and colleagues[39,40]	4 American families	2p22–25 (ETM2)	5.92
Shatunov and colleagues[44]	7 North American families	6p23	2.98

LOD, logarithm of the odds.

chromosome 3q13. However, when this loci was studied in four American families, the linkage was not present.[39] Higgins and colleagues[40] evaluated a large American family of Czechoslovakian descent with 15 affected individuals over four generations and reported linkage to loci ETM2 at chromosome 2p22–25. This linkage was later confirmed by the same researchers in three additional American families[39] and an ET population in Singapore.[41] However, other studies have not confirmed these linkages with the loci on chromosomes 2p or 3q.[42,43] In another report of seven multigenerational North American families with 325 family members and 65 affected with ET, linkage was found on 6p23[44]; however, other studies have failed to demonstrate this association.[45] The results of these studies highlight the heterogeneity of the ET population, the potential complexity of the genetic underpinnings of ET, and the potential for other causative factors.

In order to examine the genetic and environmental influences in ET, Tanner and colleagues [46] examined 16 pairs of ET twins. They reported a concordance ratio in monozygotic twins that was twice that found in dizygotic twins. Although this appears to provide support for a genetic basis of ET, the concordance rate for the monozygotic twins was not 100%, suggesting that other factors may also be involved in the development of ET.

Recently, a genome-wide association study of 452 ET patients and 14,394 controls identified a marker on the LINGO1 gene on chromosome 15q24.3.[47] This is the first association that suggests a relationship between ET and impairments in axonal function. Defects in LINGO1 have the potential to alter neurite outgrowth, mylination, and neuronal survival. Further studies are needed to confirm these results and determine how they may affect the future research and treatment of ET.

ENVIRONMENTAL FACTORS

Although ET is often thought of as a hereditary disorder, on average, only about 50% of patients report a family history of ET[48] and a differentiation between hereditary and sporadic ET has been reported.[37] In an attempt to identify an additional or alternate cause of ET, several studies have examined potential environmental risk factors. β-carboline alkaloids, primarily harmine, and harmane, which are naturally occurring chemicals with the largest concentrations found in well-cooked meats,[49] have been shown in animal studies to cause a tremor similar to ET and, in acute doses, have been shown to cause tremor in humans.[50] In addition, blood harmane levels have been shown to increase in ET patients compared with controls.[51] Exposure to lead has also been examined as a possible risk factor for the development of ET, and preliminary results suggest higher blood lead concentrations in persons with ET compared with controls[52]; however, these findings need further confirmation. Other potential environmental risk factors have been examined, including exposure to pesticides, manganese, and organic solvents, but no associations were found with the development of ET.[53]

▶ PATHOPHYSIOLOGY

ET is postulated to be related to central nervous system dysfunction, but the location and type of dysfunction are not clear. Clinical characteristics, neuroimaging studies, and neuropathology studies suggest that ET involves a dysfunction of the cerebellum and connected structures.[54] Resolution of ET following stroke affecting the cerebellum[55] or thalamus [56] as well as the significant improvement in ET following thalamotomy and deep brain stimulation of the thalamus,[57] all involving the cerebellocortical loop, provides evidence for the involvement of the cerebellum. In addition, the presence of intention tremor and tandem gait abnormalities in many ET patients also suggests involvement of the cerebellum.[58] A positron emission tomography (PET) study demonstrated hypermetabolism of the medulla and thalamus during tremor activation.[59] In another PET study, increased blood flow in the cerebellum was noted with postural tremor.[60] These investigators concluded that ET is the result of oscillations within the olivocerebellar pathway with connections to the thalamus and motor cortex.

Initial neuropathological studies of ET reported no significant pathological changes.[61] More recent studies, using more sophisticated neuropathological techniques, have reported pathological changes most commonly in the cerebellum. In one study, the majority of 33 ET brains demonstrated an increase in cerebellar torpedoes, a decrease in Purkinje cells, Purkinje cell heterotopias, and dendrite swellings compared with control brains. In a minority of ET patients, an increase in brainstem Lewy bodies, particularly in the locus ceruleus, was reported.[62] In another study of 24 ET brains, seven subjects had cerebellar changes including reduced Purkinje cells, cerebellar cortical sclerosis, and an increase in cerebellar gliosis.[63] In addition, eight brains demonstrated neuron loss in the locus ceruleus and five had neuron loss in the substantia nigra. However, when compared with controls, the only significant differences were gliosis in the cerebellum and locus ceruleus depletion. In contrast to the previously discussed report, there was no increase in Lewy bodies between ET brains and controls. These pathological findings support the heterogeneity of ET and highlight the need for further pathological examinations of potential ET brain changes.

▶ DIAGNOSTIC CRITERIA

CLASSIC ESSENTIAL TREMOR

There are currently no definitive tests to confirm the diagnosis of ET. Therefore, the diagnosis of ET is based on the type, presentation, location, and history of the tremor. In addition, family history of tremor and response to alcohol assist in the diagnostic process.[6] The most widely accepted clinical criteria for the diagnosis of classic ET are based on the criteria developed by the Tremor Research Investigation Group and later modified by the Consensus Statement of the Movement Disorder Society on Tremor.[2,64,65] These criteria include core criteria that are required for the diagnosis of ET and secondary criteria that are not mandatory but can be helpful in confirming the diagnosis (Table 25–3).

VARIANTS OF CLASSIC ESSENTIAL TREMOR

Primary Writing Tremor

Primary writing tremor is a form of tremor that occurs only during writing or when the wrist is in the position used for writing.[66] This form of tremor is generally classified as a variant of ET; however, it should be distinguished from writer's cramp, which involves muscle

▶ TABLE 25–3. CLINICAL CRITERIA OF THE DIAGNOSIS OF CLASSIC ESSENTIAL TREMOR[64]

Core criteria
Bilateral action tremor of the hands and forearms without rest tremor
Absence of other neurological signs with the exception of cogwheeling
May have isolated head tremor if no signs of dystonia
Supporting criteria
Tremor duration of greater than 3 years
Positive family history of tremor
Positive response to alcohol

spasms and is generally considered a form of focal dystonia.[67] Electromyographic (EMG) studies usually differentiate these conditions.

Orthostatic Tremor

There is controversy as to whether orthostatic tremor is a variant of ET or a unique tremor disorder.[68] Orthostatic tremor is generally described as an unsteady feeling during standing that resolves while walking. The primary clinical feature is a 13–18 Hz tremor of the quadriceps and gastrocnemius muscles while standing but not while sitting or lying down. The diagnosis can generally be confirmed by EMG.[5]

▶ DIFFERENTIAL DIAGNOSIS

There are multiple tremor disorders that can be confused with ET.[5] Table 25–4 lists the most common differential diagnosis and key clinical features to assist with diagnosis. The most common differential diagnosis are discussed here including Parkinson's disease (PD), drug-induced tremor, cerebellar tremor, and Holmes tremor. Other differential diagnosis include cortical tremor, dystonic tremor, enhanced physiologic tremor, Fragile X syndrome, neuropathic tremor, and psychogenic tremor.

▶ **TABLE 25–4. COMMON DIFFERENTIAL DIAGNOSES OF ESSENTIAL TREMOR**

Tremor Type	Key Diagnostic Characteristics
Cerebellar tremor	Ataxia, intention tremor
Cortical tremor	Action myoclonus, irregular high-frequency postural and kinetic tremor
Drug-induced tremor	Sudden onset, initiation of a new medication
Dystonic tremor	Action tremor, dystonic posturing, focal tremor
Enhanced physiologic tremor	No evidence of neurologic disease, short duration, high-frequency postural tremor
Fragile X	Ataxia, parkinsonism, peripheral neuropathy, cognitive decline, imaging abnormalities
Holmes (midbrain, rubral) tremor	Stroke or trauma, unilateral tremor
Neuropathic tremor	Other signs of peripheral neuropathy
Parkinson's disease	Unilateral tremor, rest tremor, leg tremor, bradykinesia, rigidity, gait and balance disturbance
Psychogenic tremor	Sudden onset, emotional distress, distraction, irregular tremor

PARKINSON'S DISEASE

The most challenging differentiation is between ET and PD, primarily early in the disease process. It has been estimated that the misdiagnosis of ET and PD is approximately 20–30%.[69] There are several clinical features that can assist in making the correct diagnosis.[70] In PD rest tremor is the primary tremor type along with postural tremor and less commonly kinetic tremor, whereas ET is characterized primarily by postural and kinetic tremor with rare rest tremor. Family history is important as ET often has a strong family history affecting persons of multiple generations, whereas a smaller percentage of PD patients report a strong family history. PD generally presents with a unilateral tremor in contrast to ET, which generally presents with a bilateral tremor. Although both types of tremor most commonly affect the upper extremities, in contrast to ET, parkinsonian tremor generally does not occur in the head or voice. Handwriting samples can also be useful in distinguishing between the two disorders.[6] PD is often characterized by micrographia, whereas the writing of persons with ET is often large and tremulous. Additional parkinsonian features include bradykinesia, rigidity, postural instability, shuffling gait, speech, and swallowing problems, which are generally not observed in ET. While alcohol often has a suppressive effect on ET, it generally does not provide benefit for persons with PD.[6] In addition, parkinsonian medications such as carbidopa/levodopa significantly reduce tremor and other features of PD but generally do not benefit those with ET.

Neuroimaging can be used to differentiate ET and PD. DaTSCAN, [123I]-FP-CIT single photon emission computerized tomography (SPECT), has been evaluated as a method to accurately classify parkinsonism, ET, and controls.[71] DaTSCAN uses a radioactive chemical to measure dopamine transporter, which regulates the release of dopamine. It is assumed that if dopamine cells are depleting as in parkinsonian disorders, there would be reduced dopamine transporter in the putamen and caudate when compared with persons with ET or controls in which there is no known decrease in dopamine. In a study of 158 parkinsonian patients, 27 with ET and 35 controls, DaTSCAN results were visually analyzed by a blinded investigator at the testing site and 154 of 158 parkinsonian patients were rated as abnormal whereas 27 of 27 ET patients and 34 of 35 controls were rated as normal. This represents a sensitivity of 97% for the recognition of parkinsonism and a specificity of 100% for ET. In order to test the reliability of these results, additional visual analyses were performed by five independent raters in which 150 of 158 parkinsonian patients were rated as abnormal and 25 of 27 ET and 33 of 35 controls were rated as normal. This represented a sensitively for PD of 95% and specificity for ET of 93%.[71] The DaTSCAN results provide evidence that neuroimaging may be a valuable technique in differentiating between ET and PD; however, it is not currently available in the United States.

DRUG-INDUCED TREMOR

Multiple drugs can cause tremor.[72] It is important to recognize drugs with tremorgenic effects and obtain a complete medication history from the patient. Generally, after discontinuation of the offending agent, the tremor resolves. The diagnosis of drug-induced tremor requires the elimination of other causes of tremor such as neurologic disorders, hyperthyroidism, etc. In addition, a relationship to the initiation of the offending agent and the onset of the tremor should be established. In drug-induced tremor, the symptoms are generally bilateral, have sudden onset, and do not progress unless the dose of the drug is increased. Table 25–5 provides a list of the primary drugs reported to cause tremor.

CEREBELLAR TREMOR

Cerebellar tremor is primarily an intention tremor of the upper or lower extremities with rare postural tremor and no rest tremor.[2,5] It can be unilateral or bilateral and has a frequency of less than 5 Hz. The tremor may also be associated with dysmetria, hypotonia, and ataxia. The most common causes of cerebellar tremor are multiple sclerosis and trauma, and it can also be seen in Wilson's disease.

HOLMES TREMOR

Holmes tremor has also been referred to as rubral or midbrain tremor. It is primarily a rest and intention tremor, although postural tremor may also be present.[2] The tremor is often less rhythmic than other tremors and has a slow frequency of less than 4.5 Hz. Holmes tremor is most often the result of stroke or trauma to the central nervous system.

▶ ASSESSMENT TOOLS

A variety of assessments can be used to aid in the diagnosis and treatment of ET (Table 25–6).[73,74] An accurate measurement of ET can be difficult as tremor severity tends to fluctuate related to both the inherent nature of the tremor and external influences such as the testing environment as well as the mental and emotional state of the patient at the time of testing.[37] The most common means of assessing tremor is the use of subjective rating scales during a routine clinic visit. Assessments can include direct measures of tremor, patient report of impact of tremor, measures of emotional impact of tremor including anxiety and depression, and measures of quality of life.

▶ TABLE 25–5. PRIMARY CAUSES OF DRUG-INDUCED TREMOR

Offending Agent
Adrenaline
Adrenocorticosteroids
Amiodarone
Amitriptyline
Amphotericin B
Caffeine
Calcitonin
Cyclosporin
Cimetidine
Cinnarizine
Cocaine
Co-trimoxazole
Cytarabine
Ecstasy
Epinephrine
Ethanol
Haloperidol
Ifosfamide
Interferon-α
Lithium
Medroxyprogesterone
Metoclopramide
Mexiletine
Nicotine
Procainamide
Reserpine
Salbutamol
Salmeterol
Selective serotonin reuptake inhibitors
Tacrolimus
Tamoxifen
Tetrabenazine
Thalidomide
Theophylline
Thioridazine
Thyroxine
Valproic acid
Vidarabine

The most widely used assessment of tremor is the Fahn-Tolosa-Marin Tremor Rating Scale.[74] This scale has three primary sections. All questions have five possible responses ranging from 0 to 4, with 0 being normal and 4 being the most severe tremor. The first section is a direct assessment of tremor in the face, tongue, voice,

▶ TABLE 25-6. COMMON ASSESSMENT TOOLS FOR ESSENTIAL TREMOR

Clinical rating scales
Scales completed by medical personnel
Fahn-Tolosa-Marin Tremor Rating Scale[74]
Bain Analog Scale of Tremor Severity[75]
Rating of spirals and handwriting[75]
TRG Essential Tremor Rating Assessment Scale (TETRAS)[76,77]
Scales completed by patient/caregiver
Activities of Daily Living Questionnaire[73,75]
Tremor Disability Questionnaire[82]
Assessment of Tremor Related Handicap[73,75]
Quality of Life in Essential Tremor Questionnaire (QUEST)[83]
General assessments of quality of life, mood, depression, anxiety, etc.
Functional performance tests
Water spilled while holding a cup[79]
Water spilled while pouring from one cup to another[74]
Pegboard[73]
Gibson Maze[81]
Physiological assessments
Accelerometry
Digital writing tablets
Electromyography
Gyroscopes

head, trunk, and upper and lower extremities, and in most body parts, it has separate assessments for resting, postural, and kinetic tremor. The second section measures functional ability such as line drawing, spiral drawing, handwriting, and pouring water with both the left and right hands. The final section measures the impact of tremor on activities of daily living including speaking, feeding, drinking, hygiene, dressing, writing, and working. Bain and colleagues[75] developed an analog scale in which the severity of each tremor type (i.e., postural, kinetic, intention, resting) can be rated on a scale from 0 to 10 for each body part affected. In addition, inter- and intrarater reliability, as well as correlations with other measures of tremor, has been shown to be good for rating spirals and handwriting on a scale of 0–10.[75]

More recently, the Tremor Research Group developed the TRG Essential Tremor Rating Assessment Scale (TETRAS) as an assessment tool specific for ET.[76,77] This scale has two sections. The first section is composed of 12 questions based on historical information from the patient. Each question is scored on a 5-point scale from 0 to 4 reflecting the effects of tremor on various activities of daily living and social situations. The second section is a direct measure of tremor completed by a medical professional. Tremor of the head, face, voice, lower extremities and standing (trunk and legs), as well as handwriting and spirals are measured on a 5-point scale ranging from 0 to 4. The ratings for upper extremity tremor are expanded to an 8-point scale ranging from 0 to 4 with assessments of postural tremor in the outstretched and wing-beating positions and kinetic tremor during the finger-to-nose test. In addition, patients perform the "dot" test in which they hold a pencil as close as possible without touching above a dot on a piece of paper for 10 seconds. This question is also scored on an 8-point scale. Reliability and validity testing is currently ongoing for this scale.

Functional performance tests can also be used to evaluate ET. One assessment of postural tremor involves holding 100 ml of water with the elbow supported and flexed at approximately a 20-degree angle for one minute and measuring the amount of water spilled.[78,79] Generally three trials with each hand are performed and a mean is obtained for each hand. Another assessment that measures kinetic tremor is pouring water between two glasses and measuring the amount of water spilled.[74] Louis and colleagues developed a more elaborate assessment of functional ability that includes the performance of 15 daily tasks.[80] These tasks are scored on a scale of 0—4, with 0 being normal and 4 being unable to perform. Other tests such as the 9-hole pegboard test, which measures the time to place pegs into a hole,[73] and the Gibson maze test, which is a more objective measure of drawing spirals,[81] have been used in the assessment of ET.

In addition to directly measuring tremor, it is important to measure the impact of the tremor on the patient's daily life. The Fahn-Tolosa-Marin Tremor Rating Scale[74] and the TETRAS [76] both have assessments of activities of daily living. In addition, the Activities of Daily Living Questionnaire [73,75] is a 25-item patient-completed questionnaire in which the level of disability for various daily tasks is rated on a scale of 0–3. The Tremor Disability Questionnaire[82] is a 36-item patient-completed questionnaire in which 31 daily tasks are listed and the patient is to answer three questions for each task including whether the patient has difficulty with the task, if no difficulty the patient indicates whether they have modified the task, or whether they are less efficient at the task. The final five questions relate to voice tremor, head tremor, leg tremor, and trunk tremor. The Assessment of Tremor Related Handicap[73,75] measures the impact of tremor on nine social activities, taking into account the impact of both embarrassment and physical disability. Finally, the Quality of Life in Essential Tremor (QUEST) questionnaire[83] is a valid and reliable, ET-specific assessment of quality of life examining five domains including communication, work/finances, hobbies/leisure, physical/activities of daily living, and psychosocial issues. In addition to the above-mentioned assessments, general clinical measures of quality of life, depression, anxiety, etc., can be helpful in determining the impact of ET.[84]

There are several physiologic measures of tremor; however, these are less practical for the routine clinical setting and most often used in research.[73] Linear accelerometers are commonly used to measure ET. In addition, short-term and long-term EMG recordings, gyroscopes, computerized tracking systems, and digitized writing tablets have been used to evaluate ET.

▶ TREATMENT

The decision to initiate treatment for ET is based on functional and psychosocial disability, as there is currently no cure and no treatment that slows disease progression. When planning a treatment strategy it is important to assess the presence of not only motor symptoms but also anxiety and embarrassment related to tremor. One study reported that over 50% of ET patients were embarrassed by their tremor and in many cases, embarrassment, regardless of tremor severity, led to the desire for treatment.[85] If tremor is mild and does not cause functional or psychosocial disability, treatment may not be necessary. If tremor is situational and largely isolated to stressful events, treatment may be required on an as-needed basis. On the other hand, if tremor is functionally or psychosocially disabling, daily treatment should be initiated.[86] The most common pharmacological (Table 25–7) and surgical treatments for ET are discussed below, and a proposed treatment strategy is outlined in Figure 25–1.

BETA-ADRENERGIC ANTAGONISTS

Propranolol

Propranolol is the only pharmacologic treatment approved by the United States Food and Drug Administration for ET and is considered a first-line treatment option. Its mechanism of action in ET is unknown, and both central and peripheral sites of action have been proposed.[87, 88] It was first shown to provide benefit for ET in 1968, and since that time, multiple studies using both objective and subjective methods have confirmed its antitremor effects in about 50% of patients.[89] The American Academy of Neurology (AAN) evidence-based review of treatment for ET[90] identified 12 controlled studies of propranolol for upper extremity tremor. As measured by clinical rating scales and accelerometry, a mean improvement of 50% was observed with an average daily dose of 185 mg, ranging from 60 to 320 mg/day. In a dose–response study examining daily dosages from 80 to 800 mg,[91] maximum benefit was achieved with doses from 160 to 320 mg/day and higher doses provided no additional benefit. Reports are less consistent for head and voice tremor, ranging from no effect to some benefit, although the benefit is generally less dramatic than for the upper extremities.[92–95]

▶ TABLE 25–7. POTENTIAL PHARMACOLOGICAL TREATMENT OPTIONS FOR ESSENTIAL TREMOR AND AMERICAN ACADEMY OF NEUROLOGY (AAN) EVIDENCE-BASED TREATMENT CONCLUSIONS[90]

AAN Evidence-Based Conclusions	Treatments
Effective	Propranolol, propranolol long-acting, primidone
Probably effective	Atenolol, sotalol, gabapentin, topiramate
Possibly effective	Nadolol, clonazepam, clozapine, nimodipine, botulinum toxin type A
Evidence for ineffectiveness	Trazodone, acetazolamide, isoniazid, pindolol, methazolamide, mirtazapine, nifedipine, verapamil
Insufficient evidence	Amantadine, glutethimide,olanzapine, clonidine, L-tryptophan/ pyridoxine, phenobarbital, metoprolol, quetiapine, nicardipine, theophylline
Not included in review	Arotinolol, timolol, levetiracetam, zonisamide, pregabalin

Propranolol is available in 10, 20, 40, 60, and 80 mg tablets. It can be used on an as-needed basis for patients with bothersome tremor primarily during stressful situations. In these cases, 20–80 mg of propranolol is generally given about an hour before the stressful event. For daily use, propranolol is initiated at 10 to 60 mg/day in divided doses, and slowly increased as needed. The majority of patients will have benefit at doses up to 120 mg/day; however, if tremor persists without adverse effects, propranolol can be increased up to 320 mg/day as needed. Propranolol is generally well tolerated, with the most common adverse effects including bradycardia, nausea, vomiting, diarrhea, hypotension, drowsiness, paresthesia, lightheadedness, weakness, fatigue, and lethargy. Propranolol is contraindicated in patients taking calcium channel blockers and in those with severe bronchial asthma, sinus bradycardia, cardiogenic block, and high-grade or complete atrioventricular block.

Propranolol is also available as a once-daily, long-acting capsule in strengths of 60, 80, 120, and 160 mg. In a study comparing the immediate- and long-acting

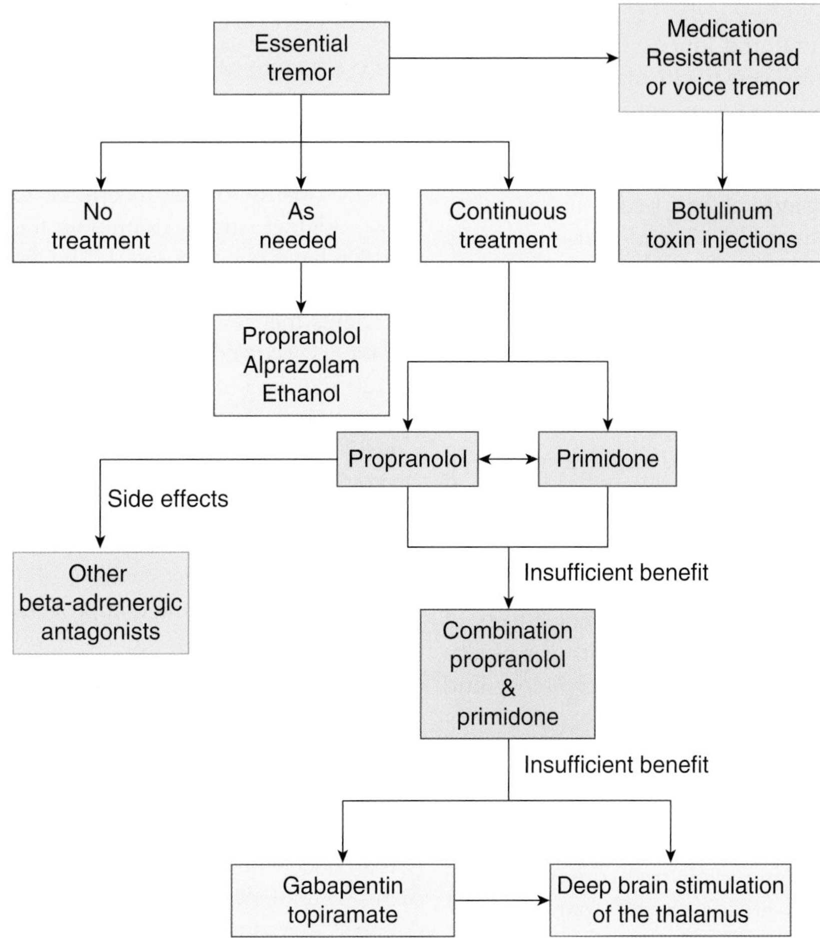

Figure 25–1. Proposed treatment strategy for essential tremor.

formulations, all patients had similar or greater benefit with long-acting propranolol.[96] In addition, in this study, the long-acting formulation was preferred by 67% of patients for tremor control and by 87% for ease of administration. The long-acting formulation is initiated at 60 mg/day and slowly increased as needed.

OTHER BETA-ADRENERGIC ANTAGONISTS

Several other β-adrenergic antagonists have been studied for the treatment of ET; however, none has been shown to be superior to propranolol.[89] In a study comparing metoprolol and propranolol, both treatments provided tremor reduction in approximately 50% of patients; however, when these patients were examined after prolonged use only propranolol resulted in prolonged benefit.[97] Other studies have shown no difference between metoprolol and placebo in controlling tremor.[98,99] Metoprolol is generally initiated at 50 mg/day and the dose can be increased to 200 mg/day in divided doses. Adverse effects are similar to those seen with propranolol.

In a double-blind, crossover study of atenolol (100 mg/day), propranolol (240 mg/day), and placebo, both treatments reduced tremor compared to placebo; however, the majority of patients preferred propranolol to atenolol.[100] In contrast, another study found no differences in tremor reduction between atenolol and placebo.[98] Atenolol is generally initiated at 25 mg once daily and the doses can be gradually increased to 50–150 mg/day. Common adverse effects include lightheadedness, nausea, dry mouth, and sleepiness.

Nadolol is a once-daily β-adrenergic antagonist that was shown in a double-blind, placebo-controlled study to significantly reduce tremor at doses of 120–240 mg/day in patients who also responded to propranolol.[101] Similarly, in a double-blind, placebo-controlled study, sotalol significantly reduced tremor compared with placebo,[98] and in another study, sotalol and propranolol were more effective than atenolol in reducing tremor.[88] The usual dose of sotalol is 80 mg twice a day. In a single-blind, placebo-controlled, crossover study of timolol (10 mg/day) and atenolol (100 mg/day), tremor was reduced with timolol but not atenolol.[102] Similarly, in one study, arotinolol (30 mg/day) was shown to significantly reduce postural and kinetic tremor,[103] and in another study, arotinolol (up to 30 mg/day) and propranolol (up to 160 mg/day) were found to be equally effective in reducing tremor.[104] Arotinolol is generally initiated at 10 mg/day and increased to 30 mg/day as needed. In contrast, pindolol has been shown to be ineffective in the treatment of ET and may potentially increase tremor.[105]

ANTICONVULSANTS

Primidone

Although primidone is not approved for the treatment of ET, it is considered a first-line therapy and multiple studies have demonstrated its benefit in reducing tremor.[90] It is an anticonvulsant metabolized to phenylethylmalonamide and phenobarbital. The mechanism of action of primidone in ET is unknown. The antitremor effects of primidone were first reported in 1981 when it was observed to reduce tremor in a patient with epilepsy and ET.[106] In a study examining low and high dosages of primidone, daily dosages of 250 and 750 mg were compared.[107] Tremor reduction occurred to the same degree with both doses. However, the 750 mg/day dose resulted in significantly more adverse effects. In a study comparing primidone to propranolol, both drugs reduced tremor to a significantly greater degree than placebo, and there was no significant difference between the two drugs.[108] Another study compared propranolol long-acting (80–160 mg/day) and primidone (50–250 mg/day) for one year.[109] Approximately 70% of both groups had tremor reduction of approximately 50%, which was maintained throughout the study. In another study, the effect of primidone (50–1000 mg/day) was examined in untreated and propranolol-treated (mean 260 mg/day) ET patients.[110] All primidone doses of at least 250 mg/day significantly reduced tremor, with no differences between dosages ranging from 250 to 1000 mg/day. In the propranolol-treated patients, a 35% reduction in upper extremity tremor with propranolol was increased to 60–70% when primidone was added, suggesting that combination therapy may provide benefit superior to either drug alone. Although multiple studies have indicated that primidone is effective for upper extremity tremor, there are no consistent reports of improvement in head tremor.[111]

Primidone is generally initiated at 12.5 to 25 mg once a day for 1 week, usually at bedtime. The dose is gradually increased to 50 mg three times a day over 4–6 weeks. Further increases up to 750 mg/day are made as needed, if tolerated. Common side effects of primidone include nausea, dizziness, ataxia, and vertigo. Less common side effects include vomiting, fatigue, impotence, diplopia, polyuria, and skin rash.

Gabapentin

The structure of gabapentin is similar to γ-aminobutyric acid (GABA). Although its mechanism of action in ET is unclear, it has been postulated that it may affect the metabolism or reuptake of GABA as it does not act directly on the GABA receptors. One monotherapy and two adjunct studies examining the effects of gabapentin in ET have been reported. The monotherapy trial was a double-blind, placebo-controlled, crossover study in ET patients that discontinued all previous treatments for ET. Patients received gabapentin (1200 mg/day), propranolol (120 mg/day), or placebo. Based on both tremor rating scales and accelerometry, gabapentin and propranolol resulted in a similar reduction in tremor, both of which provided significantly greater tremor reduction than placebo.[112] In a double-blind, placebo-controlled, crossover, adjunctive study, mean tremor reduction with gabapentin (1800 mg/day) was comparable to placebo. However, one patient did have marked improvement with gabapentin.[113] In a double-blind, placebo-controlled, multiple-dose adjunct study, gabapentin at doses of 1800 and 3600 mg/day similarly and significantly reduced tremor compared with placebo as measured by tremor rating scales but not according to accelerometry.[114] Gabapentin is generally initiated with 100–300 mg at bedtime and gradually increased to 600 mg three times a day. It is generally well tolerated, with the most common adverse effects including somnolence, lethargy, fatigue, decreased libido, dizziness, nervousness, shortness of breath, and nausea.

Topiramate

Topiramate blocks sodium and calcium channels and increases GABA activity; however, the mechanism of action in ET is unclear. Two double-blind, placebo-controlled trials reported significant tremor reduction with topiramate for a portion of ET patients. In the first study,[115] there was a significant reduction in tremor in about 80% of patients at a mean dose of 333 mg/day compared with placebo. However, 38% of the topiramate group withdrew from the study due primarily to dizziness and disorientation. In the first large, multicenter ET clinical drug trial, 223 ET subjects received either topiramate (mean 292 mg/day) or placebo for 6 months.[116] Topiramate significantly reduced tremor by approximately 30% compared to 16% with placebo. However, 32% of the topiramate group compared to 10% of the placebo withdrew from the study due to adverse effects. Topiramate is generally initiated at 25 mg once daily and increased by 25 mg after one week and slowly increased to a maximum of 200 mg twice daily. The majority of patients will have benefit with less than 100 mg/day. Common adverse effects include paresthesias, weight loss, taste perversion, memory difficulty, fatigue, nausea, decreased appetite, and somnolence.

Levetiracetam

Levetiracetam has binding sites exclusively in the central nervous system synaptic plasma membranes. It inhibits synchronous neuronal burst firing but does not affect normal neuronal excitability, suggesting that it may have benefit for ET. Three double-blind, placebo-controlled trials examined levetiracetam for ET and provided inconsistent results. A single-dose study of 1000 mg of levetiracetam reported a significant improvement in hand tremor for up to 2 hours with no significant adverse effects.[117] In contrast, in a 6-week crossover study of levetiracetam up to 3000 mg/day and placebo, there were no significant differences in tremor reduction.[118] However, 43% of patients withdrew while taking levetiracetam and 40% withdrew while taking placebo due to adverse effects. In a second crossover study, levetiracetam at doses up to 3000 mg/day was not significantly different from placebo and tended to result in worsening of tremor.[119] The most common adverse effects in these studies were fatigue, drowsiness, balance difficulties, dizziness, depression, poor concentration, memory problems, nausea, and worsening of tremor. The available data suggest that levetiracetam is not an effective treatment for ET.

Zonisamide

Zonisamide has been recently examined as a potential treatment for ET. It has multiple mechanisms of action, which include blocking sodium and calcium channels and inhibiting carbonic anhydrase. In a double-blind trial subjects received 100 mg/day of zonisamide for 2 weeks followed by an increase to 200 mg/day or placebo.[120] There were no significant differences between zonisamide and placebo according to tremor rating scales, but according to accelerometry, there was a significant reduction in tremor with zonisamide. However, 60% of patients reported no change and 40% reported only minimal improvement with zonisamide. In addition, 30% of the zonisamide group withdrew from the study due to adverse effects, which included fatigue, headache, nausea, diarrhea, and paresthesia. A randomized, crossover study of propranolol (up to 160 mg/day) and zonisamide (up to 200 mg/day) reported a significantly greater reduction in head tremor with zonisamide.[121] The most common adverse effects were sedation, diarrhea, and abdominal pain. There are not enough data at this time to recommend zonisamide as an effective treatment option for ET.

Pregabalin

Pregabalin is an isomer of GABA, and there are minimal data regarding its effect on ET. In a double-blind, placebo-controlled study, pregabalin (up to 600 mg/day) significantly reduced tremor according to accelerometry compared with placebo, and 67% of the pregabalin group compared with 20% of the placebo group reported some improvement in tremor.[122] However, there were no significant differences between pregabalin and placebo on measures of drawing, pouring, or activities of daily living. Approximately one third of the pregabalin group withdrew due to adverse effects, which included dizziness, flu symptoms, and malaise. Further studies are necessary to determine whether pregabalin is an effective treatment for ET.

Benzodiazepines

Benzodiazepines are commonly used in the treatment of ET, particularly in patients with associated anxiety. They bind to GABA receptors and increase GABAergic inhibition at all levels of the central nervous system. Their mechanism of action in ET is unknown. Benzodiazepines can be used on an as-needed basis during stressful situations or they can be used daily; however, long-term use can lead to addiction.[89] There are limited data on the effectiveness of these medications in reducing tremor. In a double-blind, placebo-controlled study, alprazolam (mean 0.75 mg/day) significantly improved tremor compared with placebo and tremor reduction was comparable to that of primidone.[123] The only reported adverse effect of alprazolam was mild sedation. In another double-blind, placebo-controlled study, alprazolam reduced tremor to a significantly greater degree than placebo.[124] The most common adverse effects were transient sedation and fatigue. Alprazolam is generally initiated at 0.125 to 0.25 mg three times a day, and gradually increased as tolerated to 1.5 mg three times a day.

Clonazepam has also been examined for ET in two small studies. In one study, clonazepam (up to 6 mg/day) significantly reduced kinetic tremor in 100% of 14 ET patients.[125] However, in a double-blind, placebo-controlled study, clonazepam (up to 4mg/day) was comparable to placebo and the majority of patients withdrew from the study due to sedation.[126] Clonazepam is generally initiated at 0.25 mg at bedtime and gradually increased as tolerated up to 1.5 mg three times a day.

Alcohols

The ability of ethanol to dramatically and temporarily reduce tremor in the majority of ET patients was described in the late 1940s.[6] This finding was confirmed by a study in which ET patients received intravenous ethanol, which significantly decreased tremor in 100% of those studied, whereas propranolol decreased tremor in 73%.[127] It is not uncommon for ET patients to use ethanol on an as-needed basis prior to a stressful event, before a meal, etc. In fact, reduction in tremor with ethanol has often been used to confirm the diagnosis of ET.[128] However, ethanol use is not recommended as a regular or chronic treatment for ET due to the potential for intoxication, rebound tremor, and addiction.[129] The exact mechanism by which ethanol reduces tremor is unknown. It has been suggested that ethanol may interact with GABA receptors in the cerebellum and reduce the synchronized oscillations in the inferior olive.[130]

In an attempt to provide the reduction of tremor observed with ethanol while avoiding its intoxicating and potentially addictive effects, methylpentynol, a 6-carbon alcohol, was examined for ET but was no more effective than placebo.[131] 1-Octanol, an 8-carbon alcohol that occurs naturally in citrus oils and is approved by the FDA as a food additive, is currently being examined as a treatment of ET.[132,133] In a double-blind, placebo-controlled study of 12 ET patients, a single dose of 1-octanol (1 mg/kg) significantly reduced tremor compared with placebo and antitremor effects were maintained for up to 120 minutes.[132] In an open-label, dose escalation study, ET subjects received a single dose of 1-octanol ranging between 1 and 64 mg/kg.[133] Maximum improvement in drawing spirals, handwriting, and accelerometry occurred after 2 hours. There was also a trend toward a dose effect, with higher doses having a more lasting effect. In the 64 mg/kg group, tremor was reduced by 39% after 4 hours, 55% after 5 hours, and 74% after 6 hours. There were no signs of intoxication in either study. Adverse effects were mild and transient and included asthenia, headache, lethargy, unpleasant taste, nausea, dry mouth, and urinary tract infection. Further research is necessary to confirm the efficacy of 1-octanol in ET, determine the appropriate dose, and expand the duration of action.

MISCELLANEOUS PHARMACOLOGICAL TREATMENTS

Clozapine

Clozapine, an atypical antipsychotic, has been reported to be effective for ET. In a single-dose (12.5 mg/ day), double-blind, crossover study, clozapine reduced tremor by at least 50% in 87% of patients.[134] A significant reduction in tremor was maintained for an average of 16 months. The only adverse effect reported was sedation. The use of clozapine is limited by the potential for agranulocytosis, which can occur in approximately 1% of patients, and mandatory weekly blood monitoring. Common adverse effects with clozapine can include increased salivation, tachycardia, dizziness, constipation, and hypotension. Clozapine is generally initiated at 6.25 mg at bedtime and gradually increased to 75 mg/day as needed

Nimodipine

Nimodipine is a calcium channel blocker shown in one study to be beneficial for ET. A double-blind, placebo-controlled study demonstrated a significant tremor reduction with nimodipine (30 mg four times daily) compared with placebo.[135] Nimodipine is usually given in 30 mg doses four times a day. The most common adverse effects are headache, low blood pressure, and heartburn.

Others

Multiple other pharmacologic agents have been examined in small, often open-label studies for their effects on ET. The majority of these studies were reviewed in the AAN evidence-based guidelines and were found to either have insufficient evidence to determine whether they are beneficial for ET or be ineffective for ET based on currently available studies, and will therefore not be discussed in detail in this review.[90] Treatments found to have insufficient evidence to make a recommendation for effectiveness in ET include amantadine, glutethimide, olanzapine, clonidine, L-tryptophan/pyridoxine, phenobarbital, quetiapine, nicardipine, and theophylline. Trazodone was found to have strong evidence suggesting it is ineffective; acetazolamide, isoniazid, and pindolol were found to have good evidence suggesting their ineffectiveness in ET; and methazolamide, mirtazapine, nifedipine, and verapamil were found to have weak evidence suggesting they are ineffective for ET.

Botulinum Toxin

Botulinum toxin type A blocks the release of acetylcholine from nerve to muscle, and has been examined as a treatment for upper extremity, head, and voice tremor in ET. There are no studies regarding the use of botulinum toxin type B for tremor. In a large, double-blind, multicenter trial, ET patients received injections of botulinum toxin type A (50 or 100 units) or placebo into the wrist flexors and extensors for upper extremity tremor.[136] Postural tremor was significantly reduced with both doses of botulinum toxin; however, there was no effect on kinetic tremor and functional ability was minimally improved. Hand weakness was reported in 30% of patients receiving 50 units and 70% of patients receiving 100 units. Other adverse effects included pain at the injection site, stiffness, cramping, paresthesias, and hematoma.

In a double-blind, placebo-controlled, crossover study of botulinum toxin type A for head tremor, 40 units of botulinum toxin were injected into each sternocleidomastoid muscle and 60 units into each splenius capitis muscle. Moderate to marked improvement was observed in 50% of the patients with botulinum toxin compared with 10% with placebo; however, this improvement was not significantly different than placebo as measured by clinical rating scales.[137] Side effects included neck weakness and injection site pain in most patients.

There are two open-label studies of botulinum toxin type A for essential voice tremor. In one study with injections into the thyroarytenoid, cricothyroid, or thyrohyoid muscles, 67% of patients reported subjective improvement and objective improvements were observed in 50%.[138] In the other study, 30% of ET patients had an objective reduction in voice tremor with bilateral injections compared with 20% with unilateral injections.[139] However, 80% of patients chose to continue receiving injections after the study due to an improvement in vocal effort. The most common adverse effects include a breathy voice quality, hoarseness, and swallowing difficulties, which are often transient.

SURGICAL TREATMENT

Thalamotomy

Thalamotomy is an ablative stereotactic surgical procedure for ET in which a lesion is placed in the ventral intermediate (Vim) nucleus of the thalamus.[140] Multiple open-label studies have demonstrated that thalamotomy significantly reduces upper extremity tremor in up to 90% of ET patients,[89,141] an effect that has been reported to be maintained long term in the majority of patients.[142] The primary disadvantages of thalamotomy are that it is not adjustable or reversible and bilateral procedures can result in significant speech and balance problems. In the 1960s, it was observed that during thalamotomy, the electrical stimulation used for targeting also resulted in tremor reduction.[143,144] This finding led to the implantation of stimulating electrodes into the Vim nucleus of the thalamus as a treatment for ET.[145] Thalamic stimulation has been shown to have comparable efficacy to thalamotomy with fewer adverse effects.[146,147] Therefore, thalamic deep brain stimulation (DBS) has become the surgical treatment of choice for ET.

Gamma Knife Thalamotomy

Gamma knife thalamotomy is a noninvasive radiosurgical procedure that does not require general anesthesia. Several studies have reported significant reduction in tremor in the majority of patients after gamma knife thalamotomy[148,149]; however, serious neurological complications have also been reported.[150] Gamma knife thalamotomy is rarely used in the treatment of ET due to variability in lesion size and location and delay of weeks to months for benefits or potentially severe complications; however, it may be a treatment option in patients who cannot undergo traditional thalamotomy or thalamic stimulation procedures.[90]

Thalamic Deep Brain Stimulation

Deep brain stimulation (DBS) of the ventral intermediate (Vim) nucleus of the thalamus is the surgical treatment of choice for ET. Candidates for Vim DBS are ET patients with medication-resistant disabling tremor without comorbidities precluding surgery. The DBS system provides electrical stimulation to the brain to control tremor. It has three primary components: the lead containing four electrode contacts, which is stereotactically implanted into the brain; the implantable pulse generator (IPG) or system battery, which is generally placed in the chest cavity below the clavicle; and an extension wire, which is tunneled down the neck to connect the lead and IPG. The DBS system is generally programmed 2–4 weeks after surgery and periodically over time to adjust the amplitude, frequency, and pulse width of the stimulation as well as the active contacts to be used, to control tremor and reduce adverse effects.[151]

Multiple studies have demonstrated that Vim DBS results in improvements in hand tremor ranging from 60 to 90%,[152,153] which have been shown to be maintained up to 7 years.[154–156] The improvement in tremor translates into improvements in functional ability and activities of daily living, which range from 35 to 86%. There are no large studies specifically examining head and voice tremor; however, several studies performed to reduce hand tremor have also examined subsequent effects on head and voice tremor.[156–158] In these studies, Vim DBS resulted in improvements in head and voice tremor in some patients, particularly those with bilateral procedures. The improvements in hand, head, and voice tremor as well as functional ability and activities of daily living from several Vim DBS studies are shown in Table 25–8.

Surgical complications generally occur in less than 5% of patients. However, severe complications leading to sustain disability like intraoperative hemorrhage have an incidence of about 0.5–1%. Infection and other problems related with the device are present in about 10% of patients and most commonly include malfunction of device components and extension wire erosion. In addition, the IPG is generally replaced every 3–5 years depending upon stimulation parameters and usage. A rechargeable IPG that has a lifespan of approximately 8 years was approved in 2009. Stimulation adverse effects most commonly include paresthesia, headache, disequilibrium, and dysarthria (more common with bilateral procedures), and are generally mild and resolve with adjustments of stimulation parameters.[159,160]

In conclusion, there are several treatment options for ET. The majority of the pharmacologic treatments are effective in approximately 50% of patients but generally do not completely resolve tremor. Surgical treatment with DBS can significantly reduce tremor in the

▶ **TABLE 25-8. SELECTED STUDIES OF THALAMIC DEEP BRAIN STIMULATION FOR THE TREATMENT OF ESSENTIAL TREMOR (% IMPROVEMENT COMPARED TO BASELINE)**

References	*n* (u/b)	Age (years)	Follow-up (months)	Hand Tremor	Functional Ability/ADLs	Head Tremor	Voice Tremor
Koller et al.[152]	29/0	67	12	~60%	48–63%	—	—
Pahwa et al.[155]	15/7	71	60	75% (u) 65-86% (b)	44-57% (u) 35-57% (b)	—	—
Limousin et al.[153]	28/9	63	12	> 75%	44-80%	15% (u); 85% (b)	33% (u); 40% (b)
Sydow et al.[156]	12/7	62	80	50-70%	37-39%	45% (u); 85% (b)	25% (u); 60% (b)
Koller et al.[157]	20/0	72	12	—	—	50%	—
Koller et al.[157a]	25/0	72	22-69	78%	—	—	—
Putzke et al.[154]	29/23	72	3-36	>83%	>63%	15-51% (u); 39-79% (b)	15-51% (u); 39-79% (b)
Putzke et al.[158]	0/22	70	29	80-91%	69-86%	90-100%	65-100%

u, unilateral; b, bilateral; ADLs, activities of daily living.

majority of patients; however, it is not an option for all patients. In addition to medical and surgical treatments, occupational therapy can be helpful for persons with ET to identify assistive aids to assist with activities of daily living, computer tasks, voice issues, etc. For patients with anxiety or depression, behavioral therapies may be useful. There is still a great need for additional treatment options that can significantly reduce tremor in the majority of ET patients.

▶ SUMMARY

ET is a common movement disorder that can affect persons of all ages, although it is more common with age. Tremor is generally a postural or kinetic tremor of the upper extremities, although it can also affect the head, voice, trunk, and legs. The cause of ET is unknown, although it has been postulated to involve the cerebellum and related brain structures. Multiple members of the same family are often affected by ET, although a specific genetic mutation accounting for the majority of cases has not been identified. There are multiple pharmacological treatments for ET, but even the most effective treatments reduce tremor by approximately 50% in about 50–60% of patients. Surgical treatment with DBS can be extremely effective in reducing tremor in patients with medication-resistant disabling tremor. There is currently a great need to continue research to identify the cause of ET and medications to more effectively reduce tremor.

REFERENCES

1. Louis ED, Broussolle E, Goetz CG, et al. Historical underpinnings of the term essential tremor in the late 19th century. Neurology 2008;71:856–859.
2. Deuschl G, Bain P, Brin M. Consensus statement of the Movement Disorder Society on tremor. Ad Hoc Scientific Committee. Mov Disord 1998;13(Suppl 3):2–23.
3. Rajput AH, Rozdilsky B, Ang L, et al. Significance of parkinsonian manifestations in essential tremor. Can J Neurol Sci 1993;20:114–117.
4. Elble RJ. Essential tremor frequency decreases with time. Neurology 2000;55:1547–1551.
5. Elble RJ. Diagnostic criteria for essential tremor and differential diagnosis. Neurology 2000;54:S2–S6.
6. Critchley M. Observations on essential (heredofamilial) tremor. Brain 1949;72:113–139.
7. Louis ED, Wendt KJ, Ford B. Senile tremor. What is the prevalence and severity of tremor in older adults? Gerontology 2000;46:12–16.
8. Louis ED, Dogu O. Does age of onset in essential tremor have a bimodal distribution? Data from a tertiary referral setting and a population-based study. Neuroepidemiology 2007;29:208–212.
9. Larsson T, Sjogren T. Essential tremor: A clinical and genetic population study. Acta Psychiatr Scand Suppl 1960; 36:1–176.
10. Larsen TA, Calne DB. Essential tremor. Clin Neuropharmacol 1983;6:185–206.
11. Rajput AH, Offord KP, Beard CM, et al.. Essential tremor in Rochester, Minnesota: A 45-year study. J Neurol Neurosurg Psychiatry 1984;47:466–470.
12. Elble RJ. Essential tremor is a monosymptomatic disorder. Mov Disord 2002;17:633–637.
13. Singer C, Sanchez-Ramos J, Weiner WJ. Gait abnormality in essential tremor. Mov Disord 1994;9:193–196.
14. Stolze H, Petersen G, Raethjen J, et al. The gait disorder of advanced essential tremor. Brain 2001;124: 2278–2286.
15. Lombardi WJ, Woolston DJ, Roberts JW, et al. Cognitive deficits in patients with essential tremor. Neurology 2001;57:785–790.
16. Troster AI, Woods SP, Fields JA, et al. Neuropsychological deficits in essential tremor: An expression of cerebello-

thalamo-cortical pathophysiology? Eur J Neurol 2002; 9:143–151.
17. Louis ED, Ottman R, Hauser WA. How common is the most common adult movement disorder? Estimates of the prevalence of essential tremor throughout the world. Mov Disord 1998;13:5–10.
18. Snow B, Wiens M, Hertzman C, Calne D. A community survey of Parkinson's disease. CMAJ 1989;141:418–422.
19. Chouza C, Ketzoian C, Caamano JL, et al. Prevalence of Parkinson's disease in a population of Uruguay. Preliminary results. Adv Neurol 1996;69:13–17.
20. Hornabrook RW, Nagurney JT. Essential tremor in Papua, New Guinea. Brain 1976;99:659–672.
21. Das SK, Banerjee TK, Roy T, Raut DK, Chaudhuri A, Hazra A. Prevalence of essential tremor in the city of Kolkata, India: A house-to-house survey. Eur J Neurol 2009.
22. Das SK, Biswas A, Roy J, et al. Prevalence of major neurological disorders among geriatric population in the metropolitan city of Kolkata. J Assoc Physicians India 2008; 56:175–181.
23. Salemi G, Savettieri G, Rocca WA, et al. Prevalence of essential tremor: A door-to-door survey in Terrasini, Sicily. Sicilian Neuro-Epidemiologic Study Group. Neurology 1994;44:61–64.
24. Haerer AF, Anderson DW, Schoenberg BS. Prevalence of essential tremor. Results from the Copiah County study. Arch Neurol 1982;39:750–751.
25. Bharucha NE, Bharucha EP, Bharucha AE, et al. Prevalence of essential tremor in the Parsi community of Bombay, India. Arch Neurol 1988;45:907–908.
26. Broe GA, Akhtar AJ, Andrews GR, et al. Neurological disorders in the elderly at home. J Neurol Neurosurg Psychiatry 1976;39:362–366.
27. Louis ED, Marder K, Cote L, et al. Differences in the prevalence of essential tremor among elderly African Americans, whites, and Hispanics in northern Manhattan, NY. Arch Neurol 1995;52:1201–1205.
28. Dogu O, Sevim S, Camdeviren H, et al. Prevalence of essential tremor: Door-to-door neurologic exams in Mersin Province, Turkey. Neurology 2003;61:1804–1806.
29. Bergareche A, De La Puente E, Lopez De Munain A, et al. Prevalence of essential tremor: A door-to-door survey in bidasoa, spain. Neuroepidemiology 2001;20: 125–128.
30. Benito-Leon J, Bermejo-Pareja F, Morales JM, et al. Prevalence of essential tremor in three elderly populations of central Spain. Mov Disord 2003;18:389–394.
31. Rautakorpi I, Takala J, Marttila RJ, et al. Essential tremor in a Finnish population. Acta Neurol Scand 1982;66:58–67.
32. Marti-Masso JF, Poza JJ. A new type of epidemiological study: Questionnaire administered by medical personnel. Neuroepidemiology 1992;11:296–298.
33. Mateo D, Gimenez-Roldan S. Essential tremor in the elderly: Incidence in hospital admissions for non-neurologic reasons. Neurologia 1989;4:323–327.
34. Moghal S, Rajput AH, D'Arcy C, et al. Prevalence of movement disorders in elderly community residents. Neuroepidemiology 1994;13:175–178.
35. Benito-Leon J, Bermejo-Pareja F, Louis ED. Incidence of essential tremor in three elderly populations of central Spain. Neurology 2005;64:1721–1725.
36. Findley LJ. Epidemiology and genetics of essential tremor. Neurology 2000;54:S8–S13.
37. Bain PG, Findley LJ, Thompson PD, et al. A study of hereditary essential tremor. Brain 1994;117(Pt 4): 805–824.
38. Gulcher JR, Jonsson P, Kong A, et al. Mapping of a familial essential tremor gene, FET1, to chromosome 3q13. Nat Genet 1997;17:84–87.
39. Higgins JJ, Loveless JM, Jankovic J, et al. Evidence that a gene for essential tremor maps to chromosome 2p in four families. Mov Disord 1998;13:972–977.
40. Higgins JJ, Pho LT, Nee LE. A gene (ETM) for essential tremor maps to chromosome 2p22-p25. Mov Disord 1997;12:859–864.
41. Higgins JJ, Lombardi RQ, Pucilowska J, et al. A variant in the HS1-BP3 gene is associated with familial essential tremor. Neurology 2005;64:417–421.
42. Abbruzzese G, Pigullo S, Di Maria E, et al. Clinical and genetic study of essential tremor in the Italian population. Neurol Sci 2001;22:39–40.
43. Kovach MJ, Ruiz J, Kimonis K, et al. Genetic heterogeneity in autosomal dominant essential tremor. Genet Med 2001; 3:197–199.
44. Shatunov A, Sambuughin N, Jankovic J, et al. Genomewide scans in North American families reveal genetic linkage of essential tremor to a region on chromosome 6p23. Brain 2006;129:2318–2331.
45. Aridon P, Ragonese P, De Fusco M, et al. Further evidence of genetic heterogeneity in familial essential tremor. Parkinsonism Relat Disord 2007.
46. Tanner CM, Goldman SM, Lyons KE, et al. Essential tremor in twins: An assessment of genetic vs environmental determinants of etiology. Neurology 2001;57:1389–1391.
47. Stefansson H, Steinberg S, Petursson H, et al. Variant in the sequence of the LINGO1 gene confers risk of essential tremor. Nat Genet 2009;41:277–279.
48. Louis ED. Etiology of essential tremor: Should we be searching for environmental causes? Mov Disord 2001; 16:822–829.
49. Louis ED, Keating GA, Bogen KT, et al. Dietary epidemiology of essential tremor: Meat consumption and meat cooking practices. Neuroepidemiology 2008;30:161–166.
50. Louis ED, Zheng W, Jurewicz EC, et al. Elevation of blood beta-carboline alkaloids in essential tremor. Neurology 2002;59:1940–1944.
51. Louis ED, Jiang W, Pellegrino KM, et al. Elevated blood harmane (1-methyl-9H-pyrido[3,4-b]indole) concentrations in essential tremor. Neurotoxicology 2008;29: 294–300.
52. Louis ED, Jurewicz EC, Applegate L, et al. Association between essential tremor and blood lead concentration. Environ Health Perspect 2003;111:1707–1711.
53. Louis ED. Environmental epidemiology of essential tremor. Neuroepidemiology 2008;31:139–149.
54. Deuschl G, Raethjen J, Lindemann M, et al. The pathophysiology of tremor. Muscle Nerve 2001;24:716–735.
55. Dupuis MJ, Delwaide PJ, Boucquey D, et al. Homolateral disappearance of essential tremor after cerebellar stroke. Mov Disord 1989;4:183–187.
56. Duncan R, Bone I, Melville ID. Essential tremor cured by infarction adjacent to the thalamus. J Neurol Neurosurg Psychiatry 1988;51:591–592.

57. Lyons KE, Pahwa R. Deep brain stimulation and tremor. Neurotherapeutics 2008;5:331–338.
58. Deuschl G, Wenzelburger R, Loffler K, et al. Essential tremor and cerebellar dysfunction clinical and kinematic analysis of intention tremor. Brain 2000;123 (Pt 8): 1568–1580.
59. Hallett M, Dubinsky RM. Glucose metabolism in the brain of patients with essential tremor. J Neurol Sci 1993; 114:45–48.
60. Colebatch JG, Findley LJ, Frackowiak RS, et al. Preliminary report: Activation of the cerebellum in essential tremor. Lancet 1990;336:1028–1030.
61. Rajput AH, Rozdilsky B, Ang L, et al. Clinicopathologic observations in essential tremor: Report of six cases. Neurology 1991;41:1422–1424.
62. Louis ED, Faust PL, Vonsattel JP, et al. Neuropathological changes in essential tremor: 33 cases compared with 21 controls. Brain 2007;130:3297–3307.
63. Shill HA, Adler CH, Sabbagh MN, et al. Pathologic findings in prospectively ascertained essential tremor subjects. Neurology 2008;70:1452–1455.
64. Bain P, Brin M, Deuschl G, et al. Criteria for the diagnosis of essential tremor. Neurology 2000;54:S7.
65. Findley LJ. Classification of tremors. J Clin Neurophysiol 1996;13:122–132.
66. Bain PG, Findley LJ, Britton TC, et al. Primary writing tremor. Brain 1995;118(Pt 6):1461–1472.
67. Elble RJ, Moody C, Higgins C. Primary writing tremor. A form of focal dystonia? Mov Disord 1990;5:118–126.
68. Bhattacharyya KB, Basu S, Roy AD, et al. Orthostatic tremor: Report of a case and review of the literature. Neurol India 2003;51:91–93.
69. Hughes AJ, Daniel SE, Kilford L, et al. Accuracy of clinical diagnosis of idiopathic Parkinson's disease: A clinicopathological study of 100 cases. J Neurol Neurosurg Psychiatry 1992;55:181–184.
70. Morgan J, Sethi K. Differential Diagnosis. In Pahwa R, Lyons KE (eds). Handbook of Parkinson's Disease, 4th ed. New York: Informa Healthcare, 2007, pp. 29–47.
71. Benamer TS, Patterson J, Grosset DG, et al. Accurate differentiation of parkinsonism and essential tremor using visual assessment of [123I]-FP-CIT SPECT imaging: The [123I]-FP-CIT study group. Mov Disord 2000;15:503–510.
72. Morgan JC, Sethi KD. Drug-induced tremors. Lancet Neurol 2005;4:866–876.
73. Bain PG. Tremor assessment and quality of life measurements. Neurology 2000;54:S26–S29.
74. Fahn S, Tolosa E, Marin C. Clinical rating scale for tremor. In Jankovic J, Tolosa E (eds). Parkinson's Disease and Movement Disorders. Baltimore-Munich: Urban & Schwarzenberg, 1988, pp. 225–234.
75. Bain PG, Findley LJ, Atchison P, et al. Assessing tremor severity. J Neurol Neurosurg Psychiatry 1993;56: 868–873.
76. Elble RJ. Report from a U.S. conference on essential tremor. Mov Disord 2006;21:2052–2061.
77. Elble RJ, Pullman SL, Matsumoto JY, et al. Tremor amplitude is logarithmically related to 4- and 5-point tremor rating scales. Brain 2006;129:2660–2666.
78. Mally J. Aminophylline and essential tremor. Lancet 1989;2:278–279.
79. Bain PG, Mally J, Gresty M, et al. Assessing the impact of essential tremor on upper limb function. J Neurol 1993; 241:54–61.
80. Louis ED, Wendt KJ, Albert SM, et al. Validity of a performance-based test of function in essential tremor. Arch Neurol 1999;56:841–846.
81. Gibson HB. The spiral maze. A psychomotor test with implications for the study of delinquency. Br J Psychol 1964; 55:219–225.
82. Louis ED, Barnes LF, Wendt KJ, et al. Validity and test-retest reliability of a disability questionnaire for essential tremor. Mov Disord 2000;15:516–523.
83. Troster AI, Pahwa R, Fields JA, et al. Quality of life in Essential Tremor Questionnaire (QUEST): Development and initial validation. Parkinsonism Relat Disord 2005; 11:367–373.
84. Louis ED, Barnes L, Albert SM, et al. Correlates of functional disability in essential tremor. Mov Disord 2001; 16:914–920.
85. Louis ED, Rios E. Embarrassment in essential tremor: Prevalence, clinical correlates and therapeutic implications. Parkinsonism Relat Disord 2008.
86. Pahwa R, Lyons KE. Essential tremor: Differential diagnosis and current therapy. Am J Med 2003;115:134–142.
87. Young RR, Growdon JH, Shahani BT. Beta-adrenergic mechanisms in action tremor. N Engl J Med 1975;293:950–953.
88. Jefferson D, Jenner P, Marsden CD. beta-Adrenoreceptor antagonists in essential tremor. J Neurol Neurosurg Psychiatry 1979;42:904–909.
89. Lyons KE, Pahwa R, Comella CL, et al. Benefits and risks of pharmacological treatments for essential tremor. Drug Saf 2003;26:461–481.
90. Zesiewicz TA, Elble R, Louis ED, et al. Practice parameter: Therapies for essential tremor: report of the Quality Standards Subcommittee of the American Academy of Neurology. Neurology 2005;64:2008–2020.
91. Koller WC. Dose-response relationship of propranolol in the treatment of essential tremor. Arch Neurol 1986;43: 42–43.
92. Koller W, Graner D, Mlcoch A. Essential voice tremor: Treatment with propranolol. Neurology 1985;35:106–108.
93. Koller WC. Propranolol therapy for essential tremor of the head. Neurology 1984;34:1077–1079.
94. Calzetti S, Sasso E, Negrotti A, et al. Effect of propranolol in head tremor: Quantitative study following single-dose and sustained drug administration. Clin Neuropharmacol 1992;15:470–476.
95. Massey EW, Paulson GW. Essential vocal tremor: Clinical characteristics and response to therapy. South Med J 1985; 78:316–317.
96. Koller WC. Long-acting propranolol in essential tremor. Neurology 1985;35:108–110.
97. Calzetti S, Findley LJ, Perucca E, et al. Controlled study of metoprolol and propranolol during prolonged administration in patients with essential tremor. J Neurol Neurosurg Psychiatry 1982;45:893–897.
98. Leigh PN, Jefferson D, Twomey A, et al. Beta-adrenoreceptor mechanisms in essential tremor; a double-blind placebo controlled trial of metoprolol, sotalol and atenolol. J Neurol Neurosurg Psychiatry 1983;46: 710–715.

99. Leigh PN, Marsden CD, Twomey A, et al. beta-Adrenoceptor antagonists and essential tremor. Lancet 1981;1:1106.
100. Larsen TA, Teravainen H, Calne DB. Atenolol vs. propranolol in essential tremor. A controlled, quantitative study. Acta Neurol Scand 1982;66:547–554.
101. Koller WC. Nadolol in essential tremor. Neurology 1983;33:1076–1077.
102. Dietrichson P, Espen E. Effects of timolol and atenolol on benign essential tremor: Placebo-controlled studies based on quantitative tremor recording. J Neurol Neurosurg Psychiatry 1981;44:677–683.
103. Kuroda Y, Kakigi R, Shibasaki H. Treatment of essential tremor with arotinolol. Neurology 1988;38:650–652.
104. Lee KS, Kim JS, Kim JW, et al. A multicenter randomized crossover multiple-dose comparison study of arotinolol and propranolol in essential tremor. Parkinsonism Relat Disord 2003;9:341–347.
105. Teravainen H, Larsen A, Fogelholm R. Comparison between the effects of pindolol and propranolol on essential tremor. Neurology 1977;27:439–442.
106. O'Brien MD, Upton AR, Toseland PA. Benign familial tremor treated with primidone. Br Med J (Clin Res Ed) 1981;282:178–180.
107. Serrano-Duenas M. Use of primidone in low doses (250 mg/day) versus high doses (750 mg/day) in the management of essential tremor. Double-blind comparative study with one-year follow-up. Parkinsonism Relat Disord 2003;10:29–33.
108. Gorman WP, Cooper R, Pocock P, et al. A comparison of primidone, propranolol, and placebo in essential tremor, using quantitative analysis. J Neurol Neurosurg Psychiatry 1986;49:64–68.
109. Koller WC, Vetere-Overfield B. Acute and chronic effects of propranolol and primidone in essential tremor. Neurology 1989;39:1587–1588.
110. Koller WC, Royse VL. Efficacy of primidone in essential tremor. Neurology 1986;36:121–124.
111. Findley LJ, Cleeves L, Calzetti S. Primidone in essential tremor of the hands and head: A double blind controlled clinical study. J Neurol Neurosurg Psychiatry 1985;48:911–915.
112. Gironell A, Kulisevsky J, Barbanoj M, et al. A randomized placebo-controlled comparative trial of gabapentin and propranolol in essential tremor. Arch Neurol 1999;56: 475–480.
113. Pahwa R, Lyons K, Hubble JP, et al. Double-blind controlled trial of gabapentin in essential tremor. Mov Disord 1998;13:465–467.
114. Ondo W, Hunter C, Vuong KD, et al. Gabapentin for essential tremor: A multiple-dose, double-blind, placebo-controlled trial. Mov Disord 2000;15:678–682.
115. Connor GS. A double-blind placebo-controlled trial of topiramate treatment for essential tremor. Neurology 2002; 59:132–134.
116. Ondo WG, Jankovic J, Connor GS, et al. Topiramate in essential tremor: A double-blind, placebo-controlled trial. Neurology 2006;66:672–677.
117. Bushara KO, Malik T, Exconde RE. The effect of levetiracetam on essential tremor. Neurology 2005;64:1078–1080.
118. Handforth A, Martin FC. Pilot efficacy and tolerability: A randomized, placebo-controlled trial of levetiracetam for essential tremor. Mov Disord 2004;19:1215–1221.
119. Elble RJ, Lyons KE, Pahwa R. Levetiracetam is not effective for essential tremor. Clin Neuropharmacol 2007;30: 350–356.
120. Zesiewicz TA, Ward CL, Hauser RA, et al. A double-blind placebo-controlled trial of zonisamide (zonegran) in the treatment of essential tremor. Mov Disord 2007;22:279–282.
121. Song IU, Kim JS, Lee SB, et al. Effects of zonisamide on isolated head tremor. Eur J Neurol 2008;15:1212–1215.
122. Zesiewicz TA, Ward CL, Hauser RA, et al. A pilot, double-blind, placebo-controlled trial of pregabalin (Lyrica) in the treatment of essential tremor. Mov Disord 2007; 22:1660–1663.
123. Gunal DI, Afsar N, Bekiroglu N, et al. New alternative agents in essential tremor therapy: Double-blind placebo-controlled study of alprazolam and acetazolamide. Neurol Sci 2000;21:315–317.
124. Huber SJ, Paulson GW. Efficacy of alprazolam for essential tremor. Neurology 1988;38:241–243.
125. Biary N, Koller W. Kinetic predominant essential tremor: Successful treatment with clonazepam. Neurology 1987;37:471–474.
126. Thompson C, Lang A, Parkes JD, et al. A double-blind trial of clonazepam in benign essential tremor. Clin Neuropharmacol 1984;7:83–88.
127. Koller WC, Biary N. Effect of alcohol on tremors: Comparison with propranolol. Neurology 1984;34:221–222.
128. Critchley EM. Essential tremor. Lancet 2007;369:2157.
129. Schroeder D, Nasrallah HA. High alcoholism rate in patients with essential tremor. Am J Psychiatry 1982; 139:1471–1473.
130. Boecker H, Wills AJ, Ceballos-Baumann A, et al. The effect of ethanol on alcohol-responsive essential tremor: A positron emission tomography study. Ann Neurol 1996; 39:650–658.
131. Teravainen H, Huttunen J, Lewitt P. Ineffective treatment of essential tremor with an alcohol, methylpentynol. J Neurol Neurosurg Psychiatry 1986;49:198–199.
132. Bushara KO, Goldstein SR, Grimes GJ Jr,et al. Pilot trial of 1-octanol in essential tremor. Neurology 2004;62:122–124.
133. Shill HA, Bushara KO, Mari Z, et al. Open-label dose-escalation study of oral 1-octanol in patients with essential tremor. Neurology 2004;62:2320–2322.
134. Ceravolo R, Salvetti S, Piccini P, et al. Acute and chronic effects of clozapine in essential tremor. Mov Disord 1999;14:468–472.
135. Biary N, Bahou Y, Sofi MA, et al. The effect of nimodipine on essential tremor. Neurology 1995;45:1523–1525.
136. Brin MF, Lyons KE, Doucette J, et al. A randomized, double masked, controlled trial of botulinum toxin type A in essential hand tremor. Neurology 2001;56:1523–1528.
137. Pahwa R, Busenbark K, Swanson-Hyland EF, et al. Botulinum toxin treatment of essential head tremor. Neurology 1995;45:822–824.
138. Hertegard S, Granqvist S, Lindestad PA. Botulinum toxin injections for essential voice tremor. Ann Otol Rhinol Laryngol 2000;109:204–209.
139. Warrick P, Dromey C, Irish JC, et al. Botulinum toxin for essential tremor of the voice with multiple anatomical sites of tremor: A crossover design study of unilateral versus bilateral injection. Laryngoscope 2000;110: 1366–1374.

140. Ohye C. Thalamotomy for Parkinson's disease. Part 1. Historical background and technique. In Gildenberg P, Tasker R (eds). Textbook of Stereotactic and Functional Neurosurgery. New York: McGraw-Hill, 1998, pp. 1167–1178.
141. Speelman J, Schuurman R, de Bie R, et al. Stereotactic neurosurgery for tremor. Mov Disord 2002;17(Suppl 3): S84–S88.
142. Mohadjer M, Goerke H, Milios E, et al. Long-term results of stereotaxy in the treatment of essential tremor. Stereotact Funct Neurosurg 1990;54–55:125–129.
143. Hassler R, Riechert T, Mundinger F, et al. Physiological observations in stereotaxic operations in extrapyramidal motor disturbances. Brain 1960;83:337–350.
144. Ohye C, Kubota K, Hongo T, et al. Ventrolateral and subventrolateral thalamic stimulation. Motor effects. Arch Neurol 1964;11:427–434.
145. Benabid AL, Pollak P, Gervason C, et al. Long-term suppression of tremor by chronic stimulation of the ventral intermediate thalamic nucleus. Lancet 1991;337:403–406.
146. Schuurman PR, Bosch DA, Bossuyt PM, et al. A comparison of continuous thalamic stimulation and thalamotomy for suppression of severe tremor. N Engl J Med 2000;342:461–468.
147. Pahwa R, Lyons KE, Wilkinson SB, et al. Comparison of thalamotomy to deep brain stimulation of the thalamus in essential tremor. Mov Disord 2001;16:140–143.
148. Young RF, Jacques S, Mark R, et al. Gamma knife thalamotomy for treatment of tremor: Long-term results. J Neurosurg 2000;93(Suppl 3):128–135.
149. Kondziolka D, Ong JG, Lee JY, et al. Gamma Knife thalamotomy for essential tremor. J Neurosurg 2008;108: 111–117.
150. Siderowf A, Gollump SM, Stern MB, et al. Emergence of complex, involuntary movements after gamma knife radiosurgery for essential tremor. Mov Disord 2001;16: 965–967.
151. Lyons KE, Pahwa R. Deep brain stimulation and essential tremor. J Clin Neurophysiol 2004;21:2–5.
152. Koller W, Pahwa R, Busenbark K, et al. High-frequency unilateral thalamic stimulation in the treatment of essential and parkinsonian tremor. Ann Neurol 1997;42: 292–299.
153. Limousin P, Speelman JD, Gielen F, et al. Multicentre European study of thalamic stimulation in parkinsonian and essential tremor. J Neurol Neurosurg Psychiatry 1999;66: 289–296.
154. Putzke JD, Wharen RE Jr, Obwegeser AA, et al. Thalamic deep brain stimulation for essential tremor: Recommendations for long-term outcome analysis. Can J Neurol Sci 2004;31:333–342.
155. Pahwa R, Lyons KE, Wilkinson SB, et al. Long-term evaluation of deep brain stimulation of the thalamus. J Neurosurg 2006;104:506–512.
156. Sydow O, Thobois S, Alesch F, et al. Multicentre European study of thalamic stimulation in essential tremor: A six year follow up. J Neurol Neurosurg Psychiatry 2003;74: 1387–1391.
157. Koller WC, Lyons KE, Wilkinson SB, et al. Efficacy of unilateral deep brain stimulation of the VIM nucleus of the thalamus for essential head tremor. Mov Disord 1999; 14:847–850.
157a. Koller WC, Lyons KE, Wilkinson SB, Troster AI, Pahwa R. Long-term safety and efficacy of unilateral deep brain stimulation of the thalamus in essential tremor. Mov Disord. 2001 May;16(3):464–468
158. Putzke JD, Uitti RJ, Obwegeser AA, et al. Bilateral thalamic deep brain stimulation: Midline tremor control. J Neurol Neurosurg Psychiatry 2005;76:684–690.
159. Lyons KE, Wilkinson SB, Overman J, et al. Surgical and hardware complications of subthalamic stimulation: A series of 160 procedures. Neurology 2004;63:612–616.
160. Videnovic A, Metman LV. Deep brain stimulation for Parkinson's disease: Prevalence of adverse events and need for standardized reporting. Mov Disord 2008;23: 343–349.

CHAPTER 26

Uncommon Forms of Tremor

Shyamal H. Mehta, Kapil D. Sethi, and Bala V. Manyam

Tremor is generally defined as "rhythmic involuntary oscillatory movement of a body part."[1] The amplitude of tremor is not critical to the definition. Tremor is most commonly seen in the upper extremities, but tremor of the lower extremities, head, trunk, lips, chin, tongue, and vocal cords can also occur. Functionally, rest tremor is present when the affected part of the body is in repose and fully supported against gravity, requiring no active muscle contraction.[2] Tremor seen in parkinsonism is typically rest tremor and often assumes a "pill-rolling quality." This tremor typically disappears with onset of movement but, once partial stability is attained in the new position, the tremor returns (re-emergent tremor). When tremor occurs with maintained posture such as holding arms perpendicular to the body, it is called postural tremor. Postural tremor is possibly the most common form of tremor and can be seen in physiological tremor, essential tremor, cerebellar postural tremor, and others. When tremor occurs with movement from one point to another, it is referred to as kinetic tremor. Kinetic tremor that appears near termination of movement is known as terminal kinetic tremor (intention tremor). Kinetic tremor present during specific tasks but absent with other activities involving the same limb is referred to as task-specific tremor (TST). Examples include primary writing tremor, vocal tremor, and orthostatic tremor. Tremor may arise from several anatomic locations within the central nervous system (CNS) or peripheral nervous system, including the cerebral cortex, white matter, basal ganglia, thalamus, midbrain, cerebellum, and peripheral nerves. In physiological tremor, no known lesion is present. Intention tremor is usually caused by damage to the deep cerebellar nuclei (dentate and globose-emboliform) or their efferent pathway to the contralateral ventrolateral thalamus. Alterations in neurotransmitters such as dopamine deficiency (as seen in Parkinson's disease [PD]), excess epinephrine as seen in anxiety, decreased level of substrate such as glucose (hypoglycemia), reduced level of electrolyte (hyponatremia), and excess level of a hormone such as thyroxin (thyrotoxicosis) can induce tremor attesting to the presence of biochemical nonspecificity.

We will begin the discussion with physiological tremor that represents a normal variant as a lead in to uncommon forms of tremor.

▶ PHYSIOLOGICAL TREMOR

Physiological tremor is present in normal people and is usually invisible to the naked eye. It is thought to reflect a mechanical vibration of body parts. It is symptomatic only during activities that require extreme precision. Physiological tremor has two distinct oscillations. The 8–12-Hz level[3] is very resistant to frequency change. Internal loads,[4,5] elastic loads,[5] limb cooling,[6] and torque loads[7] produce less than a 1–2-Hz frequency change. This frequency variability and the intense synchronous motor unit modulation suggest that the neuronal oscillator is responsible for the 8–12-Hz tremor.[6] It occurs during the maintenance of study limb postures and has a low amplitude. The functional significance of this tremor is not known. The mechanical reflex component is the larger of the two distinct oscillations of physiological tremor and is a result of the internal viscous and elastic properties of the limb or some other body part. The two oscillations are superimposed upon a background of irregular fluctuations in muscle force and limb displacement. The frequency of this mechanical reflex oscillation is determined largely by inertia and stiffness of the body part. Consequently, normal elbow tremors have a frequency of 3–5 Hz, wrist tremors 8–12 Hz, and metacarpophalangeal joint tremors 17–30 Hz. Mechanical reflex tremor is a passive oscillation that occurs in response to broad frequency, irregular forces that are produced by asynchronous subtetanic motor unit firing. It has been considered that the component of lower frequency originated from the CNS as a long loop, and that of higher frequency originated from the muscle-spindle loop system as a short loop.[8] Although both oscillations should be considered together, from a practical standpoint the 8–12-Hz due to the neural oscillator seem to have more practical implications. It has been considered that physiological tremor may be a protective measure against unusual limb posture.[9]

Because the physiological tremor has 8–12 Hz, and alpha rhythm in electroencephalogram (EEG) has a similar frequency (7–13 Hz), a common central origin was considered. However, no evidence for this hypothesis was found.[10] Renshaw cells in the spinal cord receive excitatory input from motoneurons, and feed back inhibition to the same motoneuron pool. This recurrent inhibition has been variously suggested as a mechanism for tremor reduction by preventing excessive motoneuron synchronization or alternatively as the generator of ~10 Hz physiological tremor. Using a biophysically based computational model, the authors showed that Renshaw cell recurrent inhibition improved physiological tremor by reducing corticomuscular coupling at 10 Hz.[11] Renshaw cells receive excitatory input from motoneurons, and feed back inhibition to the same motoneuron pool. This recurrent inhibition has been variously suggested as a mechanism for tremor reduction by preventing excessive motoneuron synchronization, or alternatively as the generator of ~10 Hz physiological tremor. The frequency of physiological tremor is not influenced by age. Enhanced physiological tremor can occur under various conditions, including emotional stress, fatigue, exercise, hypoglycemia, thyrotoxicosis, pheochromocytoma, hypothermia, alcohol withdrawal, and by means of drugs such as valproic acid, lithium, neuroleptics, and tricyclic antidepressants. Ethanol can also cause a decrease in the amplitude of physiological tremor.[12] In enhanced physiological tremor, there is no evidence of an underlying neurological disease. It has been considered that the stretch–reflex response to oscillation increases during fatigue and in anxiety and response to the several medications named above and to hormones that produce a modulation of motor unit activity. This is what results in an increase in amplitude, being referred to as "enhanced physiological tremor."[13,14] Physiological tremor was not altered by caffeine in controlled studies.[15] Studies with tremorolytic action of beta-adrenoceptor blockers in physiological and isoprenaline-induced tremor suggested that the tremor activity is exerted via the same $beta_2$-adrenoceptors located in a deep peripheral compartment that is thought to be in the muscle spindles.[16] Intravenous propranolol produces a 34–60% decrease in the amplitude of physiological tremor. There was a delay of about 10 minutes, suggesting that this was the result of formation of a highly specific, centrally acting metabolite of propranolol.[17]

Postanesthetic tremor may manifest as shivering. Electromyography (EMG) studies revealed postanesthetic tremor to be consistent with exacerbated physiological tremor and is considered to be secondary to high levels of circulating catecholamines[18] seldom requiring any treatment.

Physiological tremor can interfere with fine coordinative movements, such as those required for performing microsurgery, watch repair, or diamond cutting. Although knowledge of factors that aggravate physiological tremor should be addressed (e.g., lack of sleep, fatigue, anxiety, etc.), use of a single 40-mg dose of propranolol has been found to be effective. Surgeons who perform microsurgery are known to take such a drug before the start of a procedure.

Next we will discuss uncommon forms of tremor and then talk about the unusual etiologies that may result in tremor.

▶ UNCOMMON FORMS OF TREMOR

CORTICAL TREMOR

Cortical tremor is a rare disorder with the electrophysiological characteristics of cortical myoclonus. It may be inherited and presents with high-frequency, irregular tremor-like postural and action myoclonus. Others are idiopathic and acquired or secondary to diffuse brain pathology and the lesion localization is generally difficult. The term "cortical tremor" was coined by Ikeda and colleagues[19] who described two patients with action and postural 9-Hz tremor with electrophysiological evidence of cortical myoclonus. These patients were refractory to beta-blocker therapy but responded to a combination of valproic acid and clonazepam. The authors concluded that this tremor disorder represented a variant of action-induced myoclonus in the setting of cortical myoclonus. Subsequently, Toro and colleagues[20] described 10 additional cases. The presenting symptom was often tremor or action myoclonus. The etiology was idiopathic in five, Baltic myoclonus in three, and one each of Lafora body disease, postanoxic myoclonus, progressive myoclonic epilepsy of unknown etiology, and opsoclonus myoclonus syndrome. The features common to all patients were abnormal rhythmic bursts on the EMG during voluntary isometric contraction with synchronous activation of agonist and antagonist muscles, alternating periods of near silence, a peak burst frequency of 9–18 Hz with low levels of isometric activation, and an associated cortical potential on EEG back-averaging. Cortical tremor/myoclonus has also been described in association with corticobasal degeneration and celiac disease.[21,22]

DYSTONIC TREMOR

A clear definition of dystonic tremor is still under debate. The Consensus Statement of the Movement Disorder Society on Tremor[1] proposed the following definition: "Tremor in an extremity or body part that is affected by dystonia. Focal tremors, usually have irregular amplitude and variable frequency (mainly less than 7 Hz). Tremor is mainly postural/ kinetic and usually not seen during complete rest." A typical example of dystonic tremor is tremulous spasmodic torticollis or dystonic head tremor. On the contrary, tremor can be associated with dystonia, in which case the tremor occurs in a body part not affected by dystonia. An example is the presence of upper limb postural tremor in a patient with cervical dystonia. In this section, both will be discussed together. Oppenheim[23] described presence of tremor associated with dystonic movements. In a review of 42 patients with idiopathic torsion dystonia, tremor was found in 14%,[24] but occurrence of tremor before manifestation of dystonia is not uncommon.[25,26] In a series of 271 patients with cervical dystonia, 71% had associated tremor.[27] In another series of 308 patients, 10% of the patients with varieties of dystonia had tremor.[28] In an accidental toxic exposure to 2,3,7,8-tetrachlorodibenzo-*p*-dioxin, focal hand dystonia and intention tremor were present in 22 of the 45 patients.[29] Dystonic tremor is also described as postural, localized, and irregular in amplitude, with periodicity absent during muscle relaxation, exacerbated by smooth muscle contraction, and associated frequently with myoclonus. It is considered a distinct entity from essential tremor, as it is irregular, has a broad range of frequencies, and remains localized.[30] Thus, there is considerable confusion on the very nomenclature. Occurrence of dystonia associated with postural tremor of upper extremity secondary to contralateral anterior thalamic infarct is reported.[31] Head tremor is common in cervical dystonia and is more commonly associated with hand tremor and family history of tremor or other movement disorders.[32]

Recently, Schneider and colleagues[33] have drawn attention to a subgroup of patients who have an interesting upper extremity tremor that may be misdiagnosed as PD. This may present as asymmetric resting arm tremor, with impaired arm swing and sometimes facial hypomimia or a jaw tremor. However, these patients do not have a true akinesia with progressive fatigue and reduction of movement amplitude on rapid alternating movements that is characteristic of PD. Moreover, the functional neuroimaging is normal that is inconsistent with PD. These patients may belong to the group of Scans Without Evidence of Dopaminergic Deficits (SWEDDS). The authors felt that these patients represent a form of adult-onset dystonia with predominant dystonic tremor.[33]

Treatment of dystonia with botulinum often results in significant improvement of tremor as seen in cases of cervical dystonia. Deep brain stimulation (DBS) of subthalamic area was beneficial in a patient with tremor and dystonia.[34]

TASK-SPECIFIC TREMOR

TSTs are a rare form of tremor that involves skilled, highly learned motor acts. The tremor occurs only when performing a specific repetitive task unique to each individual. Examples include hair cutting, shaving, putting on makeup, combing hair, use of tools, sewing, use of scissors, putting or rarely golf club swinging, playing a musical instrument, and other activities. Generally, no other associated neurological signs and symptoms are present with the exception of focal dystonia. The frequency of tremor is 5–7 Hz.[35] EMG has shown both an alternating and a roughly synchronous pattern in the antagonistic muscles, but the alternating pattern appears to be more common.[35]

Primary Writing Tremor

Primary writing tremor is the most common form of TST that occurs predominantly during writing but not during other hand tasks. Primary writing tremor was first described by Rothwell and colleagues[36] in a 20-year-old man who presented with tremor while writing. Active pronation of his hand produced several beats of pronation–supination tremor. A burst of tremor could also be elicited by tendon taps to the volar surface of the wrist, to the finger extensors, to pectoralis major, and by means of forcible supination of the wrist delivered by torte motor. The subject's writing difficulty and tremor were temporarily abolished by partial motor point anesthesia of pronator teres. The frequency of this tremor was 4 Hz, and EMG revealed tremor in the muscles of the forearm and arm. Primary writing tremor is considered a form of focal dystonia.[35,37,38] The clinical characteristics of primary writing tremor and focal dystonia of hand (writer's cramp and other occupational cramps) are similar in several respects, as both conditions are more or less task-specific and are not inherited. Patients with primary writing tremor often do not exhibit dystonia. On the contrary, tremor is known to occur in focal dystonia.[39] Photon emission tomography (PET) studies of regional cerebral blood flow on voluntary wrist oscillations of control subjects produced ipsilateral cerebellar activation. Patients with primary writing tremor displayed bilateral cerebellar activation only, whereas those with essential tremor displayed activation in the red nucleus cerebellum and thalamus.[40] Two forms of primary writing tremor have been described. Task-induced tremor is characterized by tremor appearing during writing only (type A, TST). If it occurs when the hand adopts a writing position, the terms position-specific or position-sensitive tremor (type B) have been used.[41]

Several authors have argued that TST is a variant of essential tremor.[37,42,43] However, although essential tremor is generally inherited in an autosomal-dominant fashion, TST is most often sporadic. Clinical and neurophysiological characteristics of TST are too varied. Essential tremor often responds to ethanol, propranolol, and others but not to anticholinergics, whereas the TST is often resistant to pharmacotherapy.

The management of TST is difficult. As already stated the oral pharmacological treatment for TST is disappointing. Botulinum toxin injections have been used with success.[44] Interestingly, in one reported case the cortical mapping using Transcranial magnetic stimulation revealed posterior displacement of hand region that normalized after botulinum toxin injections.[45] Stereotactic thalamotomy centered mainly on the nucleus ventralis intermedius has also been successfully used in treatment of this condition.[46] Also, thalamic stimulation with the electrode lead implanted in the nucleus ventralis intermedius resulted in nearly complete control of primary writing tremor.[47]

Isolated Jaw Tremor

Jaw tremor can be a component of various neurological disorders such as PD, essential tremor, dystonia, branchial myoclonus, hereditary geniospasm, TST, and Whipple's disease, as well as in normal situations such as shivering and subclinical physiological jaw tremor.[48] Rarely, isolated jaw tremor in the absence of any of the above-mentioned causative etiologies has been reported. Tarsy and Ro reported a woman with a focal position-sensitive jaw tremor present when the jaw is held slightly open or while drinking from a cup. EMG recording showed rhythmic 5 Hz alternating tremor involving masseter and digastric muscles with normal reciprocal inhibition. This patient and others respond well to injections of botulinum toxin into specific muscles.[49]

Tremor on Smiling

Recently, Schwingenschuh and colleagues have reported two patients with a bilateral facial tremor that occurs on smiling related to the activation of therisorii muscles. EMG showed a high frequency of 9 Hz. One of the patients had young-onset PD, whereas the other patient did not have any other neurological symptoms or signs except for the tremor.[50]

HOLMES' (MIDBRAIN) TREMOR

In 1904, Gordon Holmes described nine patients with different etiologies (vascular and tumors) all having a characteristic tremor.[51] Because his was one of the first descriptions, the tremor has been eponymously named after him as "Holmes tremor" (HT). (Synonyms: midbrain tremor, rubral tremor, thalamic tremor, myorhythmia, and Benedikt's syndrome.) Although the literature is abundant with various terms such as midbrain tremor, rubral tremor, and myorhythmia, which have been used interchangeably, the term HT is preferred to describe this specific tremor syndrome. This tremor can also be a part of a larger syndrome associated with additional signs and symptoms such as ataxia, nystagmus and ophthalmoplegia, bradykinesia, and apathy. Some characteristics of HT include:[51,52]

1. a tremor of a low frequency usually less than 4.5 Hz, mostly unilateral.
2. tremor is usually of large amplitude and has a certain irregularity to it. It is more prominently seen with action, although may be present at rest and with posture as well.
3. there is considerable delay in the onset of the tremor when compared with the timing of the original insult (from weeks to months).
4. tremor cannot be controlled by volition and only increases in severity with the attempt. It also abates during sleep.

It is widely accepted that HT is a symptomatic tremor, that is, secondary to a lesion. In HT, the lesions usually involve the brainstem/cerebellar and thalamic regions mostly affecting the cerebello-thalamo-cortical and dentato-rubro-olivary pathways, and the dysfunction of the nigrostriatal system may account for the rest component.[53] A PET study of six patients with HT secondary to a contralateral peduncular lesion showed significantly decreased [^{18}F]-fluorodopa uptake in the striatum suggestive of nigrostriatal dysfunction.[54] Also, magnetic resonance imaging (MRI) and dopamine transporter single photon emission computed tomography scan in a patient with the classic HT secondary to midbrain cavernous angioma showed damage to the cerebellorubrothalamic and nigrostriatal pathways.[55] This also suggests a possible pathophysiological interplay between the two pathways in the production of this distinct tremor.

Any lesion that disrupts the above mentioned pathways can produce a HT. Some of the different lesions reported to cause a HT include tumors, vascular insults (i.e., stroke, arteriovenous malformations), hemorrhages, infections including abscesses, multiple sclerosis, and iatrogenic causes (i.e., surgery/gamma-knife procedures or radiation injury) damaging the midbrain, among others. Hence, the diagnostic workup in a patient with HT is directed at detecting the lesion that caused the tremor.

Because HT is usually secondary to an underlying lesion, treating a reversible cause is the most prudent approach. Symptomatic medical treatment involves the use of various drugs such as levodopa, anticholinergics, and clonazepam.[56] Some have also tried propranolol, dopamine agonists, levetiracetam, and valproate with mixed results.[57] A small study by Hallett and colleagues suggested that isoniazid may play a favorable role in treatment of cerebellar outflow tremor such as HT.[58] However, the dosage required is quite high and carries a risk of heptotoxicity. Surgical treatment for medically refractory HT has gained popularity in the recent years. Improvement of tremor in many patients has been noted following stimulation or lesioning of the nucleus ventrointermedius (Vim) of the thalamus as well as with pallidotomy or stimulation.[59–62] Some groups have observed synergistic improvement of the tremor with combining targets such as Vim DBS with subthalamic nucleus DBS, globus pallidus interna pallidotomy, or ventralis oralis anterior (Voa)/posterior (Vop) pallidal receiving area stimulation.[63–65] Also, newer targets are being identified for better tremor control in these patients.

PRIMARY ORTHOSTATIC TREMOR

In orthostatic tremor, also referred to as "shaky leg syndrome," first described by Heilman,[66] there is a subjective feeling of unsteadiness during standing, usually for over 10 seconds. In severe cases falls may occur during walking. Standing may induce visible or palpable fine-amplitude ripping in the leg muscles (gastrocnemius or quadriceps). The diagnosis can be confirmed by a surface EMG recording of the above muscles with the patient standing with a typical 13–18-Hz pattern. Similar tremor can be recorded in all leg and trunk muscles, with the tremor disappearing when patient sits or lies down. Walking, sitting, and lying were unaffected. Standing involved a wide base, but gait was normal. There are no other abnormal neurological signs or symptoms. Patients find it harder to stand still and are forced to take a step to regain balance. Falls and injuries are uncommon, as patients start moving as soon as the sense of imbalance occurs. Within any individual patient the frequency of tremor remains unchanged in all of the muscles examined. Salient features of orthostatic tremor are outlined in Table 26–1.[67] The etiology of this condition is unknown, and it is thought to arise from a central generator in the cerebellum or the brainstem. Gerschlager and colleagues reviewed 41 patients with orthostatic tremor to further elucidate the natural history and symptoms associated with this disorder. They found that ~25% patients had other features such as parkinsonism. Although, OT typically does not progress, Gerschlager and colleagues found that in 15% patients the condition gradually worsened and the tremor moved proximally to involve the trunk and arms.[68] Symptomatic orthostatic tremor in pontine lesions is reported.[69] In some cases slower frequency OT may be a component of parkinsonian tremor and may respond to levodopa.[70] The term pseudo-OT has been employed in this setting.

Case reports of successful response to clonazepam, phenobarbital, primidone, L-dopa, pramipexole, and valproic acid have been reported, whereas response to propranolol and ethanol remains unsatisfactory.[71] In a placebo-controlled, double-blind, crossover trial, three of four patients had complete resolution, and one had significant reduction, of orthostatic tremor on gabapentin (dose range 300–2400 mg/day).[72] Similar results of efficacy of gabapentin in treating orthostatic tremor were reported by Rodrigues and colleagues in a recent study with six patients.[73]

▶ TABLE 26–1. FEATURES OF ORTHOSTATIC TREMOR

	Orthostatic Tremor
Age of onset	Late
Family history of tremor	Rare
Occurrence	Standing
Legs affected	Always
Tremor frequency	14–16 Hz
Paraspinal muscle effected	Always
Response to	
Alcohol	0
Propranolol	0
Clonazepam	++
Phenobarbital	++
Primidone	++
L-Dopa	++
Pramipexole	++
Gabapentin	+++

0, absent; +, fair response; ++, good response; +++, excellent response.

In medically refractory cases DBS of VIM thalamus may be considered.[74,75]

PALATAL TREMOR

The entity formerly termed palatal myoclonus (synonyms: rhythmic palatal myoclonus, oculopalatal myoclonus, palatal nystagmus, brainstem myorhythmia, and palatal myorhythmia) has been renamed palatal tremor.[76] This reclassification more accurately describes the condition.[77] Palatal tremor is divided into two distinct clinical entities: symptomatic palatal tremor, in which rhythmic movements of the soft palate (levator veli palatini) and often other brainstem-innervated or extremity muscles. Symptoms are preceded by brainstem/cerebellar lesion with subsequent hypertrophic degeneration of inferior olive. In essential palatal tremor, patients often complain of a rhythmic ear click. The rhythmic movements of the soft palate mainly involve the tensor veli palatini. No involvement of extremity or eye muscles occurs. No lesions of brainstem, cerebellum, and olive are known.[76]. Table 26–2 gives the criteria for symptomatic and essential forms of palatal tremor. Here, only the symptomatic form will be discussed.

Symptomatic palatal tremor may be often a result of an underlying neurological abnormality, such as a previous brainstem stroke, multiple sclerosis, trauma, or degenerative disease. Thus, it is not surprising that the most consistent clinical finding in these patients is a unilateral or bilateral cerebellar syndrome. On MRI scan,

▶ **TABLE 26–2. CRITERIA FOR SYMPTOMATIC AND ESSENTIAL FORMS OF PALATAL TREMOR**

Criteria	Symptomatic Palatal Tremor	Essential Palatal Tremor
Cause	Cerebrovascular disease, degenerative disease, encephalitis, multiple sclerosis, trauma	Unknown
Anamnestic or clinical evidence of brainstem or cerebellar disease	Present	Absent
Presenting symptoms	Oscillopsia and others related to brainstem or cerebellar disease	Ear clicks
Involvement of muscle groups other than soft palate	Frequently	Rarely
Involvement of eyes	Frequently	Never
Involvement of extremities	Rarely	Never
Involvement of soft palatal muscles	Levator veli palatini	Tensor veli palatini
Activation of brainstem motor nuclei	Ambiguous nucleus or facial nucleus	Trigeminal nucleus
Cessation of symptoms during sleep	No	Yes
Remote effects of palatal tremor on tonic EMG activity	Unilateral or bilateral	None
Brainstem reflexes	Often abnormal, indicating focal brainstem disease	Normal or nonspecific abnormalities
MRI	Inferior olive abnormality	Normal

From ref 76, with permission.

unilateral or bilateral hyperintense signals in the upper medulla are seen, consistent with the gliosis representing olivary pseudohypertrophy.[76] This is considered to be the hallmark for symptomatic palatal tremor. When unilateral olivary abnormality is seen, palatal tremor and cerebellar signs are present contralateral to the side of olivary hypertrophy. Sleep does not abolish symptomatic palatal tremor. Symptomatic palatal tremor results from activation of levator veli palatini muscle, which is innervated by the seventh or ninth cranial nerves. Frequency of palatal tremor is 2 Hz, which is the range of normal firing frequency of inferior olive cells.[78] The tremor rhythm in symptomatic palatal tremor is highly resistant to both external and internal inferences.[79,80] Improvement of palatal tremor following administration of a calcium entry blocking agent, flunarizine, is reported.[81] Botulinum toxin A injected into each tensor veli palatini is reported to be of benefit.[82]

A subgroup of symptomatic palatal tremor comprises of the progressive ataxia and palatal tremor syndrome (PAPT). PAPT syndrome can be subdivided into the sporadic and familial forms. In the sporadic form, progressive cerebellar degeneration is the most common feature along with the typical olivary hyperintensity on T_2-weighted MRI. The familial form is associated with marked brainstem and cervical cord atrophy with corticospinal tract findings, but the typical olivary MRI abnormalities are not seen. A substitution in the glial fibrillary acidic protein (*GFAP*) gene has been reported in the familial from, raising the possibility of Alexander's disease.[83]

VOCAL TREMOR

Vocal tremor (synonyms: voice, tremulous voice, wavy voice, or tremulous, quivering speech) is defined as involuntary, rhythmic, oscillatory movements that affect the vocal musculature in patients with tremor disorders. Vocal tremor is characterized by rhythmic alterations of pitch and loudness of vowels and in some cases with voice arrests, especially during vowel prolongation. The muscles of the sound production mechanism may also be affected, and rhythm alterations in pitch and loudness may be generated.[84]

The "prime generator" of vocal tremor is CNS; the phonatory reflection is typically multifactorial, involving a combination of the extrinsic and intrinsic laryngeal muscles, pharyngeal muscles (including that of the supraglottic structure), and auxiliary respiratory muscles, including the intercostal abdominal muscles and the diaphragm.[84] The frequency of vocal tremor may range from 4 to 8 Hz, with amplitudes of oscillation ranging widely.[85–89] Acoustic analysis has been the primary noninvasive method for quantification of vocal tremor, with most acoustic data obtained by visual inspection of oscillographic displays of the waveform data or graphic record displays of amplitude contours of sustained oral phonation. As a result, the bulk of acoustic data on vocal tremor includes visual quantifiable amplitude oscillations without frequency modulation components.[84,85,87,89]

In isolated vocal tremor, vocalization is tremulous, but no other parts of the body show tremor. It occurs in two variants. The first form is often considered as a form of focal dystonia of the vocal cords, and the second form a variant of essential tremor. In the differential diagnoses of vocal tremor, idiopathic spasmodic dysphonia should be considered. In abductor spasmodic dysphonia caused by intermittent abduction of the vocal folds, patients exhibit a breathy effortful voice quality with abrupt termination of voicing, resulting in aphonic, whispered segments of speech. In adductor spasmodic dysphonia caused by irregular hyperabduction of the vocal folds, patients exhibit a choked, strained-strangled vocal quality, with abrupt initiation and termination of voicing, resulting in short breaks in phonation. Some patients can have a combination of the two. Because many patients with spasmodic dysphonia present with a tremulous voice, differential diagnosis between isolated vocal tremor and spasmodic dysphonia may be difficult. Both respond to botulinum treatment.

Mild vocal tremor may be masked during contextual speech[90] and is referred to as essential vocal tremor. Eleven percent of patients with essential tremor are known to suffer from vocal tremor.[91] In a double-blind study, clonazepam, propranolol, and diazepam treatments were effective for vocal and hand tremor, based on clinical and electrophysiological examinations, although hand tremor was more responsive to these drugs.[92] Koller and colleagues did not find propranolol beneficial in seven patients, compared to placebo in vocal tremor.[93] Koda and Ludlow[94] found that the thyroarytenoid muscle was affected in vocal tremor and suggested that botulinum toxin injections may be beneficial in treating this disorder. One patient with vocal tremor improved following bilateral DBS of the thalamus.[95]

Vocal tremor may occur in PD.[96,97] Despite the recognition of vocal tremor in PD, hypophonia is often the major problem.

In cerebellar diseases, dysarthria and vocal tremor occur simultaneously.[98] Vocal tremor frequency in cerebellar diseases is reported to be 3 Hz, which is similar to that reported for cerebellar and kinetic postural tremor.[99]

MISCELLANEOUS UNUSUAL TREMORS

The rabbit syndrome is a distinctive perioral/mouth tremor most often seen as a complication of neuroleptic treatment but sometimes occurs spontaneously or in association with PD. The tremor may respond well to anticholinergic drugs.[100]

Hereditary chin quivering (geniospasm) is an autosomal-dominant onset disorder (linkage to chromosome 9q) with a high penetrance among families. The tremor is episodic, usually stress-induced and associated with trembling of the chin at a frequency of 8–10 Hz. It should be distinguished from facial myokymia, palatal tremor, and essential tremor affecting the facial muscles. Geniospasm responds well to localized injections of botulinum toxin in the mentalis muscle.[100]

▶ UNUSUAL ETIOLOGIES OF TREMOR

PERIPHERAL NEUROPATHY-ASSOCIATED TREMOR

A variety of tremors has been described in patients with peripheral neuropathy. These include rest tremors, postural tremors, and intention tremors.[101–103] When peripheral neuropathy and essential tremor coexist, it may be difficult to establish the etiology unless essential tremor was clearly present prior to development of symptoms and signs of peripheral neuropathy. The tremor seen in peripheral neuropathy has been described as irregular, rhythmic, proximal, or distal, with a frequency ranging from 3 to 10 Hz. Peripheral neuropathies cause slowing of the nerve conduction. No relationship between the degree of conduction velocity and sensory loss has been found.[102,104] Slowing of nerve conduction would increase the delay in stretch reflex, and this may lead to enhancement of tremor.[105] It was suggested that tremor associated with peripheral neuropathy may be an enhancement of physiological tremor secondary to weakness.[104] This hypothesis has been disputed.[106] It was hypothesized that generation of tremor in peripheral neuropathy may be the result of an abnormality in the CNS. However, most patients with peripheral neuropathy show normal computed tomography (CT)/MRI scans and routine cerebrospinal fluid examination. In dogs (Scottish terriers) with whole-body tremor and ataxia, widespread axonal changes, vacuolation, and gliosis in the white matter of CNS were seen at autopsy.[107] However, the applicability of these findings to humans is limited as no such changes have been reported in humans.

Presence of tremor in Charcot-Marie-Tooth disease was named Roussy-Lévy syndrome. Currently, it is classified as hereditary motor sensory neuropathy (HMSN) type I. Marie observed presence of tremor in HMSN.[108] A detailed evaluation in HMSN type I revealed that tremor was present in 40% of patients. The time from appearance of tremor until onset of disease was 16 years, and the tremor involved mostly hand, followed by arms, legs, and head. Tremor was mostly postural, with rest components but no parkinsonian features. Some patients reported improvement of tremor with alcohol,

TABLE 26–3. TREMOR IN PERIPHERAL NEUROPATHY

Hereditary motor and sensory neuropathy type I (HMSN type I)
Chronic inflammatory demyelinating polyneuropathy (CIDP)
Immunoglobulin M (IgM) chronic paraproteinemic demyelinating polyneuropathy
Guillain-Barré syndrome (recovery stage)
Dystonic tremor secondary to peripheral nerve injury
Diabetic neuropathy
Uremic neuropathy
Neuropathy associated with porphyria
Amiodarone can cause both tremor and peripheral neuropathy
Neuropathy associated with alcoholism

Data modified from ref 105.

and some indicated improvement with propranolol. The authors considered that the pattern of tremor seen in HMSN type I resembles essential tremor. Perhaps HMSN type I and essential tremor are related by linkage of a common gene.[109]

In chronic demyelinating polyneuropathy with IgM paraproteinemia, the incidence of tremor is considered to be 47%.[105] Tremor is often mild, postural, and seen in the hands. When the amplitude is prominent, tremor may be more disabling than weakness. Treatment with gabapentin was reported to be effective in one report.[110] The prevalence of tremor in chronic sensorimotor neuropathy (CIDP) has been reported to vary between 3 and 84%. Tremor may appear during relapse and disappear during remission. Tremor subsides with treatment of CIDP with corticosteroid therapy, either alone or in combination with cytotoxic drug, or plasma exchange.[105] In other conditions of peripheral neuropathy associated with tremor, symptomatic treatment with beta-blockers and other drugs used in essential tremor can be tried. Tremor can also be seen in peripheral neuropathy associated with diabetes mellitus, uremia, and during the recovery phase of Guillain-Barré syndrome and treatment with amiodarone. Symptomatic treatment with drugs used in the treatment of essential tremor may be attempted in tremor associated with peripheral neuropathy.

Table 26–3 lists tremor occurring in various peripheral neuropathies.

FRAGILE X-ASSOCIATED TREMOR/ATAXIA SYNDROME

Fragile-X-associated tremor/ataxia syndrome (FXTAS) is a complex neurological disorder among carriers of expanded alleles (55–200 CGG repeats; premutation range) of the fragile X mental retardation 1 (*FMR1*) gene (OMIM #309550). Clinical features include gait ataxia and intention tremor, associated features include parkinsonism, dysautonomia, peripheral neuropathy, and cognitive decline.[111] In the original report, all five patients with FXTAS had nerve conduction studies consistent with peripheral neuropathy and peripheral neuropathies have been reported in subsequent FXTAS patients at a higher frequency as compared to their age matched controls.[111,112] Approximately 50% of male carriers with the premutation over age 70 are affected by tremor and/or ataxia. Because approximately 1 in 800 males (1 in 250 females) is a carrier in the general population, FXTAS represents a common but underdiagnosed cause of tremor and peripheral neuropathy among older adults.[113] Tremor in FXTAS is multidimensional, involving rest, postural, and kinetic elements. Postural and kinetic tremors are typically more obvious initially and rest tremor sometimes comes on as the condition progresses.[114] For further discussion of the clinical features, pathophysiology and treatment of FXTAS readers are encouraged to read the review by Leehay.[115]

PSYCHOGENIC TREMOR

Occurrence of tremor as a manifestation of hysteria has been known for over a century.[116] Koller and colleagues[117] reported a more detailed study and established diagnostic criteria (Table 26–4). Psychogenic tremor is the most common form (~55%) of all psychogenic movement disorders. Psychogenic tremor has higher incidence in females than males, and, while any age is susceptible, it is less frequently reported in children. The onset is often abrupt. It shows variable amplitude and more importantly a variable frequency. In some cases, the tremor is stimulus sensitive, becoming enhanced with passive movement, light touch, or noise. It typically disappears with distraction. The importance of this finding was emphasized by Campbell, in 1979, when he wrote: "functional or psychogenic tremor disappears when attention is withdrawn from the limb or area involved. I will give $25.00 to the first MD who can prove me wrong."[118] Two other common features are entrainment of the tremor to the frequency of repetitive movement of the opposite limb and their tendency to fatigue during the examination. However, a recent series showed that entrainment is not as common as distractibility and variability.[119] Deuschl and colleagues have emphasized the co-contraction sign of psychogenic tremor. The physician moves a distal joint (usually the wrist) while the tremor is present. The resistance is felt in both directions while the tremor is present. However, the enhanced resistance ceases when the tremor is absent.[120] Electrophysiological studies may aid in identifying and confirming the clinical characteristics mentioned above.[120]

TABLE 26-4. CLINICAL FEATURES OF PSYCHOGENIC TREMOR

Abrupt onset
Static course
Spontaneous remissions
Unclassifiable tremors (complex tremors)
Clinical inconsistencies (selective disabilities)
Changing tremor characteristics
Unresponsiveness to antitremor drugs
Tremor increases with attention
Tremor lessens with distractibility
Responsiveness to placebo
Absence of other neurological signs
Remission with psychotherapy
Multiple somatizations
Multiple undiagnosed conditions
Spontaneous remissions or cures of symptoms
Presence of unphysiological weakness or sensory complaints
No evidence of disease by laboratory or radiographic procedures
Presence of unwitnessed paroxysmal disorders
Employed in allied health professions
Litigation or compensation pending
Presence of secondary gain
Presence of psychiatric disease
Documented functional disturbances in the past

From Ref. 117, with permission.

Tremor is often complex and may occur at rest, with posture or action and combinations thereof. Activities of daily living may not be impaired; patients will appear well-groomed, but when asked to demonstrate, significant changes in handwriting and other tasks can be seen. Symptoms present usually when attention is given to the patient, either during clinical examination or by family members, and disappear when attention is drawn to some other task or when the patient is alone. The direction of tremor may change from supination–pronation orientation to one of flexion–extension.[117] On the contrary, the amplitude may be strikingly consistent in all positions, a pattern rarely encountered in tremor of organic origin. Often, there is a history of symptoms for a year or longer before the patient seeks medical attention. Details in the history are vague and the patient may become hostile when details are inquired into. Location of the tremor and the pattern may vary from one visit to another. Additional nonphysiological neurological findings may or may not be present, such as split tuning fork test, clearly detectable physiological weakness, or other sensory changes.

Psychogenic tremor is not a diagnosis of exclusion. The presence of characteristic features on history and especially clinical examination can permit an accurate diagnosis and avoid unnecessary investigations. Tests are of limited utility in making a diagnosis of psychogenic movement disorders are typically done to rule out organic causes. It is equally important to realize that all tremors can be exaggerated by anxiety.

Electrophysiologic studies for objective assessments of frequency, amplitude, distractibility, and entrainment can be done using EMG studies. Other more sophisticated techniques such as hypnosis and sodium amytal interview have been employed by some.[121] However, the diagnosis remains primarily a clinical one to be made by the movement disorder specialist. In a small number of patients, psychogenic tremor may be superimposed on other organic conditions with a preexisting disorder in which tremor is part of the disease, such as PD, and a clear distinction between the psychogenic and organic component may not always be easy to make.

There are limited data as to the long-term outcome of psychogenic tremor. One large study looked at long-term follow-up of 127 patients with a diagnosis of psychogenic tremor. It was encouraging that 56.6% of patients reported improvement in their tremor. Factors predictable of a favorable outcome were elimination of stressors and patient's perception of effective treatment by the physician.[119]

STROKE-ASSOCIATED TREMOR

The development of tremor subsequent to a thalamic stroke has been known since the time of Dejerine and Roussy.[122] Isolated tremor as a result of stroke is rare. In a review of 62 cases of movement disorders associated with focal lesion in the thalamus and subthalamus, no case of isolated tremor was found.[123] In lesions confined to thalamus, six cases of tremor with a postural and kinetic component have been described.[124–127] Moroo and colleagues[128] described three patients with postural and kinetic tremor with a frequency of 3–4 Hz whose brain MRI scans showed an ischemic lesion in the midthalamus. Ferbert and Gerwig[129] described four patients with tremor, among whom three had associated dystonia, and one hemiparesis. Dethy and colleagues[130] reported a patient with pure motor stroke associated with hemibody tremor involving right upper and lower extremities. Tremor frequency was 5–6 Hz. MRI scan showed ischemic lesion in the left centrum semiovale and the left caudate nucleus. PET scan showed glucose hypermetabolism in the ipsilateral sensory motor cortex. Thalamic ataxia syndrome, in which there are significant cerebellar signs, may be associated with intention tremor. Kim,[131] in a prospective study of 35 patients with delayed onset of movement disorder following thalamic infarct, found that action tremor was not an isolated phenomenon but was often accompanied by dystonia-athetosis-chorea. A case of spontaneous tremor following thalamic/subthalamic infarct that subsided in 24 hours is reported.[132] Defer and colleagues reported a 25-year-old man who had midbrain hemorrhage followed by the development of left rest tremor associated with mild bilateral extrapyramidal symptoms responsive to levodopa. A PET ^{18}F-dopa study showed a large decrease of the Ki value in the right striatum. One year after the stroke a persistent postural component developed.[133] Holmes (midbrain) tremor with its classical appearance secondary to stroke was discussed earlier.

Because tremor is not usually an isolated phenomenon and there are associated neurological deficits, treatment needs to address all segments of a patient's disability. A case of "yes–yes" head tremor following right occipital and bilateral cerebellar infarction that responded to botulinum toxin A is reported.[134] However, in general when there is an associated cerebellar component with the tremor, pharmacotherapy is disappointing. In the absence of a cerebellar component, attempts at treatment may be made by using drugs that are used in the treatment of essential tremor. No controlled studies have been done, so the only approach is to use one drug at a time, reaching the maximum dose and trying another when the previous one is proven to be ineffective.

POSTTRAUMATIC TREMOR

In this section, trauma will refer to physical trauma, such as injury to a structure that was previously intact. An artificial separation of central versus peripheral injury will also be made, even as we remain fully aware of the intimate relationship between the central and peripheral nervous systems. When tremor is noted with a history of injury, there is always an interval of days to years before onset of the tremor. Additionally, there are often associated neurological findings, such as rigidity, hemiparesis, reflex sympathetic dystrophy, and the like, so tremor generally does not occur in isolation. CT or MRI scan may not show lesions that are tiny and at a cellular or subcellular level. In light of these factors and limitations, one can still find evidence in the literature of tremor being precipitated or caused by various injuries. For an excellent review the reader is referred to Curren and Lang.[135]

Most cases of tremor resulting from severe head injury are believed to result from damage to the midbrain. However, in addition to the typical midbrain tremor discussed above, other forms of tremor are well recognized. The association of head trauma with parkinsonism was made in 1929.[136] A year earlier, parkinsonian symptoms, including rest tremor associated with "punch drunk" syndrome caused by multiple head injuries in boxers, were studied.[137] Subsequently, more clear cases of parkinsonism with known head injury were studied.[138–140] Tremor occurring after sudden twisting of the neck that resulted in an intimal tear of the carotid artery, leading to an embolic infarct has been reported.[141] An 18-year-old girl, in a diving accident at a swimming pool, developed ipsilateral tremor in the right upper and lower extremities. The tremor had a kinetic component. The MRI scan showed a lesion in the left ventral lateral thalamus.[142]

Tremor resulting from peripheral nerve injury is rare. There are often other associated neurological abnormalities, such as dystonia or reflex sympathetic dystrophy. In one study of 43 patients with movement disorders associated with reflex sympathetic dystrophy described by Schwartzman and Kerrigan,[143] only 38 demonstrated a history of injury. Deuschl and colleagues[144] found that 12 of their 21 patients showed a distal tremor with a mean frequency of 7.2 Hz, and those researchers considered it as enhanced physiological tremor. On treatment of reflex sympathetic dystrophy, the tremor completely disappeared. Entrapment of the ulnar nerve in Guyon's canal resulted in development of a tremor in the fourth and fifth fingers with disappearance of tremor after surgery in a secretary/typist subjected to repeated hand movement.[145] This illustrates the possibility that peripheral trauma could induce tremor. Pathophysiological mechanisms underlying these phenomena are not entirely known, but functional changes in afferent neuronal input to the spinal cord and secondary affection of higher brainstem and subcortical centers are probably involved.[146]

The issue of posttraumatic movement disorders is often complicated by the presence of litigation. Minor trauma may precipitate psychogenic dystonia and tremor. In fact, we feel that many cases that have been reported in the literature as organic may have a psychogenic basis.[147]

Treatment of the underlying cause such as compression neuropathy or reflex sympathetic dystrophy may be beneficial. However, where a cause cannot be found or where other associated conditions are present, such as lesion of the midbrain, conventional (pharmacological) therapies have been less than satisfactory. Stereotactic thalamotomy has been tried with success.[141] However, because the tremor may be self-limited the surgery be restricted to select cases of disabling tremor. Numerous medications have been studied in the treatment of posttraumatic tremor with variable results. Posttraumatic tremor may respond to clonazepam,[148] propranolol,[149] alone, or in combination with valproic acid.[150]

▶ TREMOR IN SYSTEMIC DISORDERS AND DISEASES

AIDS

Unilateral postural and action tremor resulting from thalamic toxoplasmosis in a patient with AIDS is reported.[151] There appears to be a high incidence of tremor when patients with AIDS are treated with trimethoprim sulfamethoxazole.[151]

HEREDITARY HEMOCHROMATOSIS

Neurological manifestations are rarely described in hereditary hemochromatosis. Whether this is an association by chance or a cause and effect remains to be ascertained. Arm and head tremor are reported to occur rarely. Phlebotomies and symptomatic treatments may not change the course of the disease.[153]

HYPOXIA/HYPOTENSION

The amplitude of tremor may be higher in hypocapnic hypoxia than during eucapnic hypoxia.[154] In one case, prolonged hypotension induced localized delayed anoxic lesions in basal ganglia, resulting in postural tremor along with bradykinesia and gait disturbance. MRI showed low signal intensities in the bilateral caudate nuclei and putamen on the T_1-weighted image and high signal intensities on the T_2-weighted images. PET scan with ^{18}F-FDG revealed a severe decrease in glucose metabolism in bilateral basal ganglia.[155]

PORPHYRIA

Presence of tremor is reported in variegate porphyria.[156] Plasma exchange or erythrocytapheresis may not show any beneficial effects on the clinical or laboratory abnormalities.

THYROID DISORDERS

Tremor is a well-known symptom of thyrotoxicosis. Tremor in thyrotoxicosis is an enhanced physiological tremor that cannot be separated clinically or by an EMG examination. Both types of tremor have similar mechanisms and can be distinguished only by the circumstances responsible for their occurrence and presence of other signs and symptoms related to that particular disorder. Only a moderate correlation between tremor intensity and thyroid hormone level is known.[157] Successful treatment of thyrotoxicosis results in dramatic improvement of tremor. Rarely, tremor resembling orthostatic tremor has been reported in thyrotoxicosis.[158]

WILSON'S DISEASE

Tremor as an initial manifestation of Wilson's disease occurred in 13–32% of patients.[159,160] Because of its relative rarity, the initial manifestation may be hepatic or neurological and the diagnosis may be easily missed. With chelation therapy, dramatic improvement of tremor is reported.[161] The tremor may be proximal resulting in "wing beating tremor" when the arms are held up. One patient presented with dystonic tremor.[162]

▶ TABLE 26-5. MAJOR CATEGORIES OF DRUGS THAT INDUCE OR EXACERBATE TREMOR

Category	Major Drugs Associated With Tremor
Antiarrhythmics	Amiodarone
Antibiotics/antivirals	Trimethoprim/sulfa, vidarabine
Antidepressants/mood stabilizers	Amitriptyline, lithium, selective serotonin reuptake inhibitors (SSRIs)
Antiepileptics	Tiagabine, valproate
Bronchodilators	Albuterol (salbutamol), salmeterol
Chemotherapeutics	α-Interferon, tamoxifen, thalidomide
Drugs of abuse	Alcohol, cocaine, MPTP, MDMA ("Ecstasy"), nicotine
Gastrointestinal drugs	Cimetidine, metoclopramide
Hormones	Epinephrine, thyroxine
Immunosuppressants	Cyclosporine, tacrolimus (FK-506)
Methylxanthines	Caffeine, aminophylline
Neuroleptics	Cinnarizine, haloperidol
Sympathomimetics	Ephedrine, phenylpropanolamine, pseudoephedrine

MPTP, 1-methyl-4-phenyl-1,2,5,6-tetrahydropyridine; MDMA, 3,4-methylenedioxymethamphetamine.

DRUG-OR TOXININDUCED TREMOR

A variety of drugs can result in tremor or an exacerbation of existing tremor. A tremor is considered to be drug-induced if it occurs in a reasonable time frame following drug ingestion. It can have the whole range of clinical presentation of tremor and there could be presence of additional signs depending on the nature of the drug and individual disposition of the patient. Tremor secondary to drugs and toxins can take many forms, including enhanced physiological tremor, precipitated essential tremor, rest tremor secondary to parkinsonism, and tremor of cerebellar syndrome. Tables 26–5 and 26–6 summarize this vast topic.[163]

Toxin-Associated Causes of Tremor

Heavy Metals

Neurotoxic effects from ingestion of metals such as mercury, lead, copper, arsenic, and aluminum are well-known but only a few of these cause tremor.

▶ **TABLE 26-6. MAJOR DRUGS KNOWN TO CAUSE POSTURAL, INTENTION, AND RESTING TREMORS**

Major Category	Typical Examples
Action/Postural	
Antiarrhythmics	Amiodarone, mexiletine, procainamide
Antidepressants/mood stabilizers	Amitriptyline, lithium, SSRIs
Antiepileptics	Valproate
Bronchodilators	Albuterol, salmeterol
Chemotherapeutics	Tamoxifen, Ara-C, ifosfamide
Drugs of abuse	Cocaine, ethanol, MDMA, nicotine
Gastrointestinal drugs	Metoclopramide, cimetidine
Hormones	Thyroxine, calcitonin, medroxyprogesterone
Immunosuppressants	Tacrolimus, cyclosporine, α-interferon
Methylxanthines	Theophylline, caffeine
Neuroleptics/dopamine depleters	Haloperidol, thioridazine, cinnarizine, reserpine tetrabenazine
Intention/Terminal Kinetic	
Major Category	**Typical Examples**
Antibiotics/antivirals/antimycotics	Ara-A
Antidepressants/mood stablilizers	Lithium
Bronchodilators	Albuterol, salmeterol
Chemotherapeutics	Ara-C, ifosfamide
Drugs of abuse	Ethanol
Hormones	Epinephrine
Immunosuppressants	Tacrolimus, cyclosporine
Resting	
Major Category	**Typical Examples**
Antibiotics/antivirals/antimycotics	Trimethoprim/sulfa, amphotericin B
Antidepressants/mood stabilizers	SSRIs, lithium
Antiepileptics	Valproate
Chemotherapeutics	Thalidomide
Drugs of abuse	Cocaine, ethanol, MDMA, MPTP
Gastrointestinal drugs	Metoclopramide
Hormones	Medroxyprogesterone
Neuroleptics/dopamine depleters	Haloperidol, thioridazine, cinnarizine, reserpine, tetrabenazine

MDMA, 3,4-methylenedioxymethamphetamine or "Ecstasy"; SSRIs, selective serotonin reuptake inhibitors; Ara-A, vidarabine; Ara-C, cytarabine.

Mercury can cause toxic effects in three forms: inorganic mercury salts, organic mercury compounds, and metallic mercury. Inorganic mercury salts are water-soluble, irritate the gut, and cause severe kidney damage. Organic mercury compounds are fat-soluble, can cross the blood–brain barrier, and cause neurological damage. Mercury metal poses two dangers. It can be vaporized: the vapor pressure at room temperature is about 100 times the safe amount, so poisoning can occur if mercury metal is spilled into crevices or cracks in the floorboards. Dentists are occasionally poisoned this way. Mercury easily crosses into the brain, and causes tremor, depression, and behavioral disturbances. A second danger from metallic mercury is that it is biotransformed into organic mercury, by bacteria at the bottom of lakes. This can be passed along through seafood and eventually to humans. Mercury was found useful in the treatment of syphilis in the 16th century, leading to increased demands for the mineral and, therefore, to heightened mining activities. Miners were said to remain at work rarely for more than a few years because they developed tremor and vertigo. This was considered possibly a result of the toxicity of mercury.[164] Epidemics of inorganic mercury poisoning have occurred, usually manifested by the appearance of tremor. Chronic inorganic exposure to mercury may lead to fine rapid tremor that affects extremities, head, tongue, eyelids, and voice. The incidence of tremor in felt hat makers was found to be 20% when exposed for more than 20 years. However, in industrial accidents, the incidence has been 50–90%.[164] Organic mercury poisoning was rare before 1953 when industrial pollution in Minamata Bay, Japan, caused an epidemic of mercury poisoning. Ataxic tremor was one of the components. At autopsy, cerebellar atrophy, along with cerebral edema, was seen.[165] A similar syndrome in a single family from Alamagordo, New Mexico, who consumed meat from hogs that were accidentally fed with grain treated with methyl mercury fungicide, has been reported.[166] Onset of intention tremor along with cerebellar signs has been reported in an agricultural worker after the worker consumed cereal seeds treated with mercury derivative.[167] Accidental acute mercury vapor poisoning with high mercury levels in blood and urine in three patients, resulting in tremor, severe pulmonary edema, and coma leading to death, has been reported.[168] Chelating agent British anti-Lewisite (BAL) and *N*-acetyl-DL-penicillamine have been used to treat mercury intoxication.[169]

Chronic exposure to manganese, usually among manganese miners or in smelter accidents leads to a neurological picture of parkinsonism and dystonia with a peculiar gait called cock-walk gait.[171] Rest tremor is rare but an action tremor may be seen. Total parenteral nutritional feeding in a child resulted in tremors and seizures with elevated serum manganese levels. Withdrawal of manganese in the nutritional supplement may result in full recovery.

Tremor is considered a clinical sign of chronic lead exposure. However, the type of tremor and its pathophysiological mechanisms are controversial. Lead neurotoxicity manifests mainly as encephalopathy with irritability, insomnia, memory loss, restlessness, confusion, and hallucinations. Leaded gasoline sniffing leading to lead toxicity in Navajo adolescents resulted in 31% having tremor and ataxia. In addition, their blood lead levels were elevated.[172] Twenty-three men with history of chronic lead exposure showed postural and kinetic tremor. EMG examination showed the frequency to be 12 Hz with characteristics of enhanced physiological tremor.[173] Another single case of postural tremor is reported in a 15-year-old boy who inhaled gasoline for its euphoric effects.[174] Forty-eight of 50 (96%) children and adolescents who chronically sniffed leaded gasoline showed exaggerated deep reflexes, postural tremor, and evidence of cerebellar dysfunction. Forty-nine (98%) had blood lead levels greater than or equal to 40 μg/dL. The mean blood lead levels were significantly higher in those with abnormally brisk deep reflexes and with evidence of cerebellar dysfunction. Thirty-nine patients received chelation therapy. The neurological abnormalities resolved within 8 weeks in all but one patient.[175] The treatment of choice in lead poisoning is chelation with calcium ethylenediaminetetraacetic acid (EDTA).

Insecticides and Herbicides

Chlordecone (kepone), an organochlorine pesticide, is used as an ant and roach pesticide. Exposure to this pesticide in industrial workers resulted in occurrence of tremor. In the severely affected workers, tremor was present, even at rest, whereas, in those patients moderately affected, tremor was described as irregular with a frequency of 12 Hz.[176] In addition, workers exhibited ataxia, weight loss, opsoclonus, pleuritic and joint pains, and abnormalities on liver function tests.[177] The tremors were reproducible in mice,[178,179] and rats. Treatment consists of use of cholestyramine, an anion-exchange resin that would facilitate fecal excretion.[180]

Dichlorodiphenyltrichloroethane (DDT), a residual insecticide, was used worldwide to control mosquitoes, especially in endemic areas where malaria is prevalent, and banned in most places because of its carcinogenicity. DDT is known to produce tremor in experimental animals.[181,182] Inhaling the toxic fumigant, phosphine, 31 crew members aboard a grain freighter exhibited intention tremor, ataxia, diplopia, and other neurological manifestations.[183]

Methylbromide is widely used as a fumigant and is known to produce tremor, ataxia, and myoclonus.[184] Dioxin (referred to as Agent Orange) exposure resulted in postural and intention tremor in 35 of 47 railroad workers during a chemical spillage after damage to a tank car filled with this herbicide. Carbon disulfide, along with carbon tetrachloride, is used as a fumigant. Exposure in 21 grain workers resulted in about half of them developing parkinsonian features, along with resting tremor; the other half developed cerebellar syndrome associated with intention tremor.[185]

Poisoning from herbicides containing glufosinate ammonium used in Japan caused generalized tremor, and dysarthria.[186]

Solvents

Exposure to solvents that contained toluene and methyl ethyl ketone during spray painting in a closed garage resulted in development of intention tremor and other cerebellar signs.[187] Toluene abuse in the form of lacquer sniffing in a 24-year-old man for 5 years resulted in development of tremor with cerebellar signs, with evidence of severe atrophy of cerebellar hemispheres, vermis, and brainstem, as well as mild atrophy of cerebral hemispheres on CT scan.[188] Irreversible cholinesterase inhibitor soman, used as a nerve gas, is known to produce tremor.[189] In ship painters who were chronically exposed to high concentrations of solvents showed a syndrome of acquired blue–yellow color vision deficits, coarse tremor, impaired vibration sensation in the legs, and cognitive impairment.[190] A 30-year-old man with chronic toluene exposure developed visual impairment, horizontal nystagmus, pyramidal tract signs, postural tremor, and sensory disturbance below the level of T_2 dermatome. T_2-weighted images on MRI of the brain had a marked high-intensity appearance in the posterior limbs of the internal capsule, and in the posterior columns and lateral tracts from the cervical through the upper thoracic cord. The lesions probably reflect demyelination and axonal degeneration produced by chronic toluene abuse.[191]

Food-Induced Tremor

A tremor is considered to be food- or beverage-induced if it occurs in a reasonable time frame following ingestion of that particular food or beverage. Tremor secondary to food or beverages can take many forms, including enhanced physiological tremor, precipitated essential tremor, tremor of cerebellar syndrome, or can be associated with peripheral neuropathy. On the contrary, alcohol can suppress essential and certain other forms of tremor.[192]

Coffee, tea, cocoa, and caffeinated soda are sources of caffeine, a stimulant. It is believed that caffeine can induce new onset of tremor or may exacerbate previously existing tremor.[193,194] In a survey of 4558 healthy individuals, 16% reported tremor that was sometimes associated with coffee intake.[195] Individual sensitivity to caffeine may vary. Under experimental conditions, caffeine at 3 mg/kg, but not at 1 mg/kg body weight, significantly increased whole-arm physiological tremor in young adult males with no effect by time of the day.[196]

Alcohol, known to suppress essential tremor and a few other forms of tremor,[192] and withdrawal following chronic ingestion may produce tremor. Alcohol-induced liver disease may result in asterixis and may be coupled with alcohol withdrawal tremor in some patients.[197] Alcohol withdrawal tremor might be a variant of enhanced physiological tremor, most often caused by anxiety or emotional stress. In 40 patients who had alcohol withdrawal tremor, EMG examination performed 1–10 days following alcohol withdrawal to evaluate the pattern, frequency, and amplitude of tremor revealed 8–12 Hz low-amplitude postural tremor with synchronous activity in antagonist muscles. Patients with alcohol withdrawal tremor had significantly higher amplitude tremor compared to patients with anxiety and emotional stress.[198] Alcohol withdrawal tremor is a postural tremor of the upper extremity which, when severe, may spread to other parts of the body (face, tongue, larynx, muscles, and head).[199] Chronic alcoholism results in cerebellar degeneration, in which case a 3-Hz leg tremor and upper extremity tremor have been demonstrated.[200] A variety of movement disorders associated with cirrhosis of the liver occurs in chronic alcoholics and is complicated by portosystemic shunts, resulting in acquired hepatocerebral degeneration. The symptoms include various forms of tremor.[201]

The Chamorro population of the western Pacific islands of Guam and Rota consume palm (*Cycas circinalis*) flour as a staple diet and are known to develop parkinsonism dementia-amyotrophic lateral sclerosis complex that includes rest tremor. The active compound, beta-*N*-methylamino-L-alanine, is considered the underlying cause,[202] but the exact cause is not fully established.

Tobacco is consumed by chewing, smoking, or sniffing. Nicotine affects both the peripheral and CNSs. Nicotine causes tremor in animals[203,204] and is reported to produce tremor in normal individuals.[205,206] However, a controlled study failed to elicit any significant influence of nicotine on either physiological or pathological tremor.[207]

REFERENCES

1. Deuschl G, Bain P, Brin M; Consensus Statement of the Movement Disorder Society on Tremor. Ad hoc scientific committee. Mov Disord 1998;13(Suppl 3):2.
2. Fahn S. Cerebellar tremor: Clinical aspects. In Findley LJ, Capildeo R (eds). Movement Disorders: Tremor. London: Macmillan, 1984, pp. 355–363.
3. Matthews PBC, Muir RB. Comparison of electromyogram spectra with force spectra during human elbow tremor. J Physiol (Lond) 1980;302:427.
4. Fox JR, Randall JE. Relationship between forearm tremor and the biceps electromyogram. J Appl Physiol 1970;29:103.
5. Elble RJ, Randall JE. Mechanistic components of normal hand tremor. Electroencephalogr Clin Neurophysiol 1978;44:72.
6. Elble RJ, Randall JE. Motor-unit activity responsible for 8- to 12-Hz component of human physiological finger tremor. J Neurophysiol 1976;39:370.
7. Sutton GG, Sykes K. The variation of hand tremor with force in healthy subjects. J Physiol (Lond) 1967;191:699.
8. Sakamoto K, Nishida K, Zhou L, et al. Characteristics of physiological tremor in five fingers and evaluations of fatigue of fingers in typing. Ann Physiol Anthropol 1992;11:61.
9. Elke-Okoro ST. Explanation of physiological muscle tremor. Electromyogr Clin Neurophysiol 1994;34:341.
10. Pizzuti GP, Byford GH, Cifaldi S, et al. Finger tremor and the central nervous system. J Biomed Eng 1992;14:356.

11. Williams ER, Baker SN. Renshaw cell recurrent inhibition improves physiological tremor by reducing corticomuscular coupling at 10 Hz. J Neurosci 2009;29:6616.
12. Lakie M, Frymann K, Villagra F, et al. The effect of alcohol on physiological tremor. Exp Physiol 1994;79:273.
13. Hagbarth K-E, Young RR. Participation of the stretch reflex in human physiological tremor. Brain 1979; 102:509.
14. Young RR, Hagbarth K-E. Physiological tremor enhanced by maneuvers affecting the segmental stretch reflex. J Neurol Neurosurg Psychiatry 1980;43:248.
15. Koller W, Cone S, Herbster G. Caffeine and tremor. Neurology 1987;37:169.
16. Abila B, Wilson JF, Marshall RW, et al. The tremorolytic action of beta-adrenoceptor blockers in essential, physiological and isoprenaline-induced tremor is mediated by beta-adrenoceptors located in a deep peripheral compartment. Br J Clin Pharmacol 1985;20:369.
17. Zilm DH. The effect of propranolol on normal physiologic tremor. Electroencephalogr Clin Neurophysiol 1976;41:310.
18. Monso A, Barbal F, Riudeubas J, et al. Electromyographic characteristics of postanesthetic tremor. Esp Anestesiol Reanim 1997;44:324.
19. Ikeda A, Kakigi A, Funai N, et al. Cortical tremor: A variant of cortical reflex myoclonus. Neurology 1990;40:1561.
20. Toro C, Pascual-Leone A, Deuschl G, et al. Cortical tremor: A common manifestation of cortical myoclonus. Neurology 1993;43:2346.
21. Thompson PD, Day BL, Rothwell JC, et al. The myoclonus in corticobasal degeneration. Evidence for two forms of cortical reflex myoclonus. Brain 1994:117(Pt 5):1197.
22. Fung VS, Duggins A, Morris JG, et al. Progressive myoclonic ataxia associated with celiac disease presenting as unilateral cortical tremor and dystonia. Mov Disord 2000;15:732.
23. Oppenheim H. Uber eine eigenartige Kramfkrankheit des kindlichen und jungedichen Alters (Dybasia lordotica progressiva, dystonia musculorum deformans). Neurol Centralbl 1911;30:1090.
24. Marsden CE, Harrison MJG. Idiopathic torsion dystonia (dystonia musculorum deformans): A review of forty-two patients. Brain 1974;97:793.
25. Rivest J, Marsden CD. Trunk and head tremor as isolated manifestations of dystonia. Mov Disord 1990;5:60.
26. Hughes AJ, Lees AJ, Marsden CE. Paroxysmal dystonia head tremor. Mov Disord 1991;6:85.
27. Jankovic J, Leder S, Warner D, et al. Cervical dystonia: Clinical findings and associated movement disorders. Neurology 1991;41:1088.
28. Dubinsky RM. Tremor and dystonia. In Findley LJ, Koller WC (eds). Handbook of Tremor Disorders. New York: Marcel Dekker, 1995, pp. 405–410.
29. Klawans HL. Dystonia and tremor following exposure to 2,3,7,8-tetrachlorodibenzo-*p*-dioxin. Mov Disord 1987;2:255–261.
30. Jedynak CP, Bonnet AM, Agid Y. Tremor and idiopathic dystonia. Mov Disord 1991;6:230.
31. Cho C, Samkoff LM. A lesion of the anterior thalamus producing dystonic tremor of the head. Arch Neurol 2000;57:1353–1355.
32. Pal PK, Samii A, Schulzer M, et al. Head tremor in cervical dystonia. Can J Neurol Sci 2000;27:137.
33. Schneider SA, Edwards MJ, Mir P, et al. Patients with adult-onset dystonic tremor resembling parkinsonian tremor have Scans Without Evidence of Dopaminergic Deficit (SWEDDs). Mov Disord 2007;22:2210.
34. Kitagawa M, Murata J, Kikuchi S, et al. Deep brain stimulation of subthalamic area for severe proximal tremor. Neurology 2000;55:114–116.
35. Elble RJ, Moody C, Higgins C. Primary writing tremor. Mov Disord 5:118, 1990.
36. Rothwell JC, Traub MM, Marsden CD. Primary writing tremor. J Neurol Neurosurg Psychiatry 1979;42:1106.
37. Rosenbaum F, Jankovic J. Focal task-specific tremor and dystonia: Categorization of occupational movement disorders. Neurology 1988;38:522.
38. Lang AE. Writing tremor and writing dystonia. Mov Disord 1990;5:354.
39. Sheehy MP, Marsden CD. Writer's cramp: A focal dystonia. Brain 1982;105:461.
40. Wills AJ, Jenkins IH, Thompson PD, et al. A positron emission tomography study of cerebral activation associated with essential and writing tremor. Arch Neurol 1995;52:299.
41. Bain PG, Findley LJ, Britton TC, et al. Primary writing tremor. Brain 1995;118:1461.
42. Kachi T, Rothwell JC, Cowan JMA, et al. Writing tremor: Its relationship to benign essential tremor. J Neurol Neurosurg Psychiatry 1985;48:545.
43. Koller WC, Martyn B. Writing tremor: Its relationship to essential tremor. J Neurol Neurosurg Psychiatry 1986;49:220.
44. Bain P. Task specific tremor. ITF Newslett 1993;5:3.
45. Byrnes ML, Mastaglia FL, Walters SE, et al. Primary writing tremor: Motor cortex reorganisation and disinhibition. J Clin Neurosci 2005;12:102.
46. Ohye C, Miyazaki M, Hirai T, et al. Primary writing tremor treated by stereotactic selective thalamotomy. J Neurol Neurosurg Psychiatry 1982;45:988.
47. Racette BA, Dowling J, Randle J, et al. Thalamic stimulation for primary writing tremor. J Neurol 2001;248:380.
48. Gonzalez-Alegre P, Kelkar P, Rodnitzky RL. Isolated high-frequency jaw tremor relieved by botulinum toxin injections. Mov Disord 2006;21:1049.
49. Tarsy D, Ro SI. Unusual position-sensitive jaw tremor responsive to botulinum toxin. Mov Disord 2006;21:277.
50. Schwingenschuh P, Cordivari C, Czerny J, et al. Tremor on smiling. Mov Disord 2009;24:1542.
51. Holmes G. On certain tremors in organic cerebral lesions. Brain 1904;27:327.
52. Deuschl G, Bergman H. Pathophysiology of nonparkinsonian tremors. Mov Disord 2002;17(Suppl 3):S41–S48.
53. Vidailhet M, Jedynak CP, Pollak P, et al. Pathology of symptomatic tremors. Mov Disord 1998;13(Suppl 3): 49–54.
54. Remy P, de Recondo A, Defer G, et al. Peduncular 'rubral' tremor and dopaminergic denervation: A PET study. Neurology 1995;45:472.
55. Paviour DC, Jäger HR, Wilkinson L, et al. Holmes tremor: Application of modern neuroimaging techniques. Mov Disord 2006;21:2260.

56. Deuschl G, Volkmann J and Raethjen J. Tremors: Differential diagnosis, pathophysiology and therapy. In: Jankovic J, Tolosa E, editors. Parkinson's Disease and Movement Disorders. 5th ed.Philadelphia, PA: Lippincott, Williams, & Wilkins, 2007, pp. 298–320.
57. Ferlazzo E, Morgante F, Rizzo V, et al. Successful treatment of Holmes tremor by levetiracetam. Mov Disord 2008;23:2101.
58. Hallett M, Lindsey JW, Adelstein BD, et al. Controlled trial of isoniazid therapy for severe postural cerebellar tremor in multiple sclerosis. Neurology 1985;35:1374.
59. Krauss JK, Mohadjer M, Nobbe F, et al. The treatment of posttraumatic tremor by stereotactic surgery. Symptomatic and functional outcome in a series of 35 patients. J Neurosurg 1994;80:810.
60. Alusi SH, Aziz TZ, Glickman S, et al. Stereotactic lesional surgery for the treatment of tremor in multiple sclerosis: A prospective case-controlled study. Brain 2001; 124:1576.
61. Kim MC, Son BC, Miyagi Y, et al. Vim thalamotomy for Holmes tremor secondary to midbrain tumor. J Neurol Neurosurg Psychiatry 2002;73:453.
62. Miyagi Y, Shima F, Ishido K, et al. Postereoventral pallidotomy for midbrain tremor after a pontine hemorrhage. J Neurosurg 1999;91:885.
63. Romanelli P, Bronte-Stewart H, Courtney T, et al. Possible necessity for deep brain stimulation of both the ventralis intermedius and subthalamic nuclei to resolve Holmes tremor. Case report. J Neurosurg 2003;99:566.
64. Goto S, Yamada K. Combination of thalamic Vim stimulation and GPi pallidotomy synergistically abolishes Holmes' tremor. J Neurol Neurosurg Psychiatry 2004;75:1203.
65. Foote KD, Okun MS. Ventralis intermedius plus ventralis oralis anterior and posterior deep brain stimulation for posttraumatic Holmes tremor: Two leads may be better than one: technical note. Neurosurgery 2005;56(2 Suppl):E445.
66. Heilman KM. Orthostatic tremor. Arch Neurol 1984;41:880.
67. Thompson PD. Primary orthostatic tremor. In Findley LJ, Koller WC (eds). Handbook of Tremor Disorders. New York: Marcel Dekker, 1995, pp. 387–399.
68. Gerschlager W, Münchau A, Katzenschlager R, et al. Natural history and syndromic associations of orthostatic tremor: A review of 41 patients. Mov Disord 2004;19:788.
69. Benito-Leon J, Rodriguez J, Orti-Pareja M, et al. Symptomatic orthostatic tremor in pontine lesions. Neurology 1997;49:1439.
70. Thomas A, Bonanni L, Antonini A, et al. Dopa-responsive pseudo-orthostatic tremor in parkinsonism. Mov Disord 2007;22:1652.
71. Cabrera-Valdiva F, Jimenez-Jimenez FJ, Albea EG, et al. Orthostatic tremor: Successful treatment with phenobarbital. Clin Neuropharmacol 1991;14:438.
72. Onofrj M, Thomas A, Paci C, et al. Gabapentin in orthostatic tremor: Results of a double-blind crossover with placebo in four patients. Neurology 1998;51:880.
73. Rodrigues JP, Edwards DJ, Walters SE, et al. Blinded placebo crossover study of gabapentin in primary orthostatic tremor. Mov Disord 2006;21:900.
74. Espay AJ, Duker AP, Chen R, et al. Deep brain stimulation of the ventral intermediate nucleus of the thalamus in medically refractory orthostatic tremor: Preliminary observations. Mov Disord 2008;23:2357.
75. Guridi J, Rodriguez-Oroz MC, Arbizu J, et al. Successful thalamic deep brain stimulation for orthostatic tremor. Mov Disord 2008;23:1808.
76. Deuschl G, Toro C, Valls-Sole J, et al. Symptomatic and essential palatal tremor. Brain 1994;117:775.
77. Hallett M, Shibasaki H, Obeso J. Criteria for the visual identification of myoclonus. Mov Disord 1994;9.
78. Thack WT. Discharge of cerebellar neurons related to two maintained postures and two prompt movements. I. Nuclear cell output. J Neurophysiol 1970;33:527.
79. Schenck E. Die Hirnnervenmyorhythmie, ihre Pathogenese und ihre Stellung im myoklonischen Syndrom. Berlin: Springer Verlag, 1965.
80. Laprsle J. Palatal myoclonus. Adv Neurol 1986;43:265.
81. Cakmur R, Idiman E, Idiman F, et al. Essential palatal tremor successfully treated with flunarizine. Eur Neurol 1997;38:133.
82. Cho JW, Chu K, Jeon BS. Case of essential palatal tremor: Atypical features and remarkable benefit from botulinum toxin injection. Mov Disord 2001;16:779.
83. Samuel M, Torun N, Tuite PJ, et al., Progressive ataxia and palatal tremor (PAPT): Clinical and MRI assessment with review of palatal tremors. Brain 2004;127:1252.
84. Brin MF, Bilitzer A. Vocal tremor. In Findley LJ, Koller WC (eds). Handbook of Tremor Disorders. New York: Marcel Dekker, 1995, pp. 495–520.
85. Brown JR, Simonson J. Organic voice tremor: A tremor of phonation. Neurology 1963;13:520.
86. Lebrun Y, Devreux F, Rousseau JJ, et al. Tremulous speech. Folia Phoniatr 1982;34:134.
87. Ludlow C, Bassich C, Connor N, et al. Phonatory characteristics of vocal fold tremor. J Phonet 1986;14:509.
88. Hachinski VC, Thomsen IV, Buch NH. The nature of primary vocal tremor. Can J Neurol Sci 1975;2:195.
89. Ramig LA, Shipp T. Comparative measures of vocal tremor and vocal vibrato. J Voice 1987;2:162.
90. Aronson AE. Organic (essential) voice tremor. In Aronson AE (ed). Clinical Voice Disorders. New York: Thieme-Stratton, 1980, pp. 108–111.
91. Findley LJ, Gresty MA. Head, facial, and voice tremor. Adv Neurol 1988;239.
92. Massey EW, Paulson G. Essential vocal tremor: Response to therapy. Neurology 1982;32:A113.
93. Koda J, Ludlow CL. An evaluation of laryngeal muscle activation in patients with voice tremor. Otolaryngol Head Neck Surg 1992;107:684.
94. Koller W, Graner D, Mlcoch A. Essential voice tremor: Treatment with propranolol. Neurology 1985;35:106.
95. Yoon MS, Munz M, Sataloff RT, et al. Vocal tremor reduction with deep brain stimulation. Stereotact Funct Neurosurg 1999;72:241.
96. Seguier N, Spira A, Dordain M, et al. Relationship between speech disorders and other clinical manifestations of Parkinson's disease (translated title). Folia Phoniatr 1974;16:108.
97. Logemann J, Fisher H, Boshes B, et al. Frequency and cooccurrence of vocal tract dysfunctions in the speech

of a large sample of Parkinson patients. J Speech Hear Disord 1978;43:47.
98. Ackerman H, Ziegler W. Cerebellar voice tremor: An acoustic analysis. J Neurol Neurosurg Psychiatry 1991;54:74.
99. Silfverskiold BP. A 3 c/sec leg tremor in a "cerebellar" syndrome. Acta Neurol Scand 1977;55:385.
100. Lees AJ. Odd and unusual movement disorders. J Neurol Neurosurg Psychiatry. 2002;72(Suppl 1):I17.
101. Matthews WB, Howell DA, Hughes RC. Relapsing corticosteroid-dependent polyneuritis. J Neurol Neurosurg Psychiatry 1970;33:330.
102. Smith IS, Furness P, Thomas PK. Tremor in peripheral neuropathy. In Findley LF, Capildeo R (eds). Movement Disorders: Tremor. London: Macmillan, 1984, pp. 399–406.
103. Thomas PK. Clinical features and differential diagnosis. In Dyck PJ, Thomas PK, Lambert EH, Bunge R (eds). Peripheral Neuropathy. 2nd ed. Philadelphia: WB Saunders, 1984.
104. Said G, Bathien N, Cesaro P. Peripheral neuropathies and tremor. Neurology 1982;32:480.
105. Smith IS. Tremor in peripheral neuropathy. In Findley LJ, Koller WC (eds). Handbook of Tremor Disorders. New York: Marcel Dekker, 1995, pp. 443–454.
106. Elble RJ. Peripheral neuropathies and tremor. Neurology 1983;33:1389.
107. Van Ham L, Vandevelde M, Desmidt M, et al. A tremor syndrome with a central axonopathy in Scottish terriers. J Vet Intern Med 1994;8:290.
108. Marie MP. Forme speciale de nevrite interstitielle hypergrophique progressive de l'enfance. Rev Neurol (Paris) 1906;14:557.
109. Cardoso, FEC, Jankovic J. Hereditary motor-sensory neuropathy and movement disorders. Muscle Nerve 1993;16:904.
110. Saverino A, Solaro C, Capello E, et al. Tremor associated with benign IgM paraproteinaemic neuropathy successfully treated with gabapentin. Mov Disord 2001;16:967.
111. Hagerman RJ, Leehey M, Heinrichs W, et al. Intention tremor, parkinsonism, and generalized brain atrophy in male carriers of fragile X. Neurology. 2001;57:127.
112. Berry-Kravis E, Goetz CG, Leehey MA, et al. Neuropathic features in fragile X premutation carriers. Am J Med Genet. 2007;143A:19.
113. Dombrowski C, Levesque ML, Morel ML, et al. Premutation and intermediate-size FMR1 alleles in 10,572 males from the general population: Loss of an AGG interruption is a late event in the generation of fragile X syndrome alleles. Hum Mol Genet. 2002;11:371.
114. Berry-Kravis E, Abrams L, Coffey SM, et al. Fragile X-associated tremor/ataxia syndrome: Clinical features, genetics, and testing guidelines. Mov Disord. 2007; 22:2018.
115. Leehay MA. Fragile X-associated tremor/ataxia syndrome: Clinical phenotype, diagnosis, and treatment. J Investig Med. 2009;57:830-833.
116. Gowers WR. Disease of the Nervous System. Philadelphia: Blakiston, 1888.
117. Koller W, Lang A, Vetere-Overfield B, et al. Psychogenic tremors. Neurology 1989;39:1094.
118. Campbell J. The shortest paper. Neurology 1979;29: 1633.
119. Jankovic J, Vuong KD, Thomas M. Psychogenic tremor: Long-term outcome. CNS Spectr 2006;11:501.
120. Deuschl G, Raethjen J, Lucking CH, et al. The diagnosis and physiology of psychogenic tremor. In Hallett M, Fahn S, Jankovic J, Lang AE, Cloninger CR, Yodofsky SC (eds). Psychogenic Movement Disorders. Philadelphia: Lippincott, Williams, & Wilkins, 2005, pp. 265–273.
121. Lang AE. General overview of psychogenic movement disorders: Epidemiology, diagnosis and prognosis. In Hallett M, Fahn S, Jankovic J, Lang AE, Cloninger CR, Yodofsky SC (eds). Psychogenic Movement Disorders. Lippincott Williams, & Wilkins, 2006, pp. 35–41.
122. Dejerine J, Roussy G. Le syndrome thalamique. Rev Neurol 1906;12:521.
123. Lee MS, Marsden CD. Movement disorders following lesions of the thalamus or subthalamic region. Mov Disord 1994;9:493.
124. Marsden CD, Obeso JA, Zarranz JJ, et al. The anatomical basis of symptomatic dystonia. Brain 1985;108:463.
125. Pettigrew LC, Jankovic J. Hemidystonia: A report of 22 patients and a review of the literature. J Neurol Neurosurg Psychiatry 1985;48:650.
126. Schlitt M, Brown JW, Zeiger HE, et al. Appendicular tremor as a late complication of intracerebral hemorrhage. Surg Neurol 1986;25:181.
127. Kim JS. Delayed onset of hand tremor caused by cerebral infarction. Stroke 1992;23:292.
128. Moroo I, Hirayama K, Kohima S. Involuntary movements caused by thalamic lesion. Rinsho Shinkeigaku 1994;34:805.
129. Ferbert, Gerwig M. Tremor due to stroke. Mov Disord 1993;8:179.
130. Dethy S, Luxen A, Bidaut LM, et al. Hemibody tremor related to stroke. Stroke 1993;24:2094.
131. Kim JS. Delayed onset mixed involuntary movements after thalamic stroke: Clinical, radiological and pathophysiological findings. Brain 2001;124:299.
132. Kao YF, Shih PY, Chen WH. An unusual concomitant tremor and myoclonus after a contralateral infarct at thalamus and subthalamic nucleus. Kaohsiung J Med Sci 1999;15:562.
133. Defer GL, Remy P, Malapert D, et al. Rest tremor and extrapyramidal symptoms after midbrain haemorrhage: Clinical and ^{18}F-dopa PET evaluation. J Neurol Neurosurg Psychiatry 1994;57:987.
134. Finsterer J, Muellbacher W, Mamoli B. Yes/yes head tremor without appendicular tremor after bilateral cerebellar infarction. J Neurol Sci 1996;139:242.
135. Curren TG, Lang AE. Trauma and tremor. In Findley LJ, Koller WC (eds). Handbook of Tremor Disorders. New York: Marcel Dekker, 1995.
136. Crouzon O, Justin-Besancon L. Le parkinsonisme traumatique. Presse Med 1929 ;37:1325.
137. Martland HS. Punch drunk. J Am Med Assoc 1928;91:1103.
138. Lindenberg R. Die Schadigungmechanismen der Substantia Nigra bei Hirntraumen und das Problem des posttraumatischen Parkinsonismus. Dtsch Z Nervenheilkd 1964;185:637.
139. Nayermouri T. Postraumatic parkinsonism. Surg Neurol 1985;24:263.

140. Bruetsch WL, DeArmond M. The parkinsonian syndrome due to trauma. A clinico-anatomical study of a case. J Nerv Ment Dis 1935;81:531.
141. Andrew J, Fowler CJ, Harrison MJG, et al. Post-traumatic tremor due to vascular injury and its treatment by stereotactic thalamotomy. J Neurol Neurosurg Psychiatry 1982;45:560.
142. Qureshi F, Morales A, Elble RJ. Tremor due to infarction in the ventrolateral thalamus. Mov Disord 1996;11:440.
143. Schwartzman RJ, Kerrigan J. The movement disorder of reflex sympathetic dystrophy. Neurology 1990; 40:57.
144. Deuschl G, Blumberg H, Lucking CH. Tremor in reflex sympathetic dystrophy. Arch Neurol 1991;48:1247.
145. Streib EW. Distal ulnar neuropathy as a cause of finger tremor: A case report. Neurology 1990;40:153.
146. Nobrega JC, Campos CR, Limongi JC, et al. Movement disorders induced by peripheral trauma. Arq Neuropsiquiatr 2002;60:17.
147. Morgan JC, Sethi KD, Lang AE. Fixed dystonia and tremor in complex regional pain syndrome. Neurology 2005;64:2162.
148. Biary N, Koller WC. Kinetic predominant essential tremor: Successful treatment with clonazepam. Neurology 1988;37:471.
149. Ellison PH. Propranolol for severe post-head injury action tremor. Neurology 1978;28:197.
150. Obeso JA, Narbona J. Post-traumatic tremor and myoclonic jerking. J Neurol Neurosurg Psychiatry 1983;46:788.
151. Micheli F, Granana N, Scorticati MC, et al. Unilateral postural and action tremor resulting from thalamic toxoplasmosis in a patient with acquired immunodeficiency syndrome. Mov Disord 1997;12:1096.
152. Aboulafia DM. Tremors associated with trimethoprimsulfamethoxazole therapy in a patient with AIDS: Case report and review. Clin Infect Dis 1996;22:598.
153. Demarquay G, Setiey A, Morel Y, et al. Clinical report of three patients with hereditary hemochromatosis and movement disorders. Mov Disord 2000;15:1204.
154. Krause WL, Leiter JC, Marsh Tenney S, et al. Acute hypoxia activates human 8–12 Hz physiological tremor. Respir Physiol 2000;123:131.
155. Takahashi W, Ohnuki Y, Takizawa S, et al. Neuroimaging on delayed postanoxic encephalopathy with lesions localized in basal ganglia. Clin Imaging 1998;22:188
156. Aizawa T, Hiramatsu K, Ohtsuka H, et al. Defective hepatic anion transport in variegate porphyria. Am J Gastroenterol 1987;82:1180.
157. Milanov I, Sheinkova G. Clinical and electromyographic examination of tremor in patients with thyrotoxicosis. Int J Clin Pract 2000;54:364.
158. Tan EK, Lo YL, Chan LL. Graves disease and isolated orthostatic tremor. Neurology 2008;70:1497.
159. Saito T. Presenting symptoms and natural history of Wilson disease. Eur J Pediatr 1987;146:261.
160. Brewer GJ, Yuzbasiyan-Gurkan V. Wilson's disease. Medicine 1992;71:139.
161. Frucht S, Sun D, Schiff N, et al. Arm tremor secondary to Wilson's disease. Mov Disord 1998;13:351.
162. Nicholl DJ, Ferenci P, Polli C, et al. Wilson's disease presenting in a family with an apparent dominant history of tremor. J Neurol Neurosurg Psychiatry 2001;70:514.
163. Morgan JC, Sethi KD. Drug-induced tremors. Lancet Neurology 2005;4:866.
164. Greenhouse AH. Heavy metals and the nervous system. Clin Neuropharmacol 1982;5:45.
165. Kurland L, Faro S, Siedler H. Minamata disease: The outbreak of a neurologic disorder in Minamata, Japan and its relationship to the ingestion of seafood contaminated by mercuric compounds. World Neurol 1960;1:370.
166. Nelson N, Byerly TC, Kolbye AC, et al. Hazards of mercury: Special report to the secretary's pesticide advisory committee, Department of Health, Education and Welfare. Environ Res 1971;4:1.
167. Lefevre JP, Gil R. Encephalopathy due to organomercuric compounds (translated title). Sem Hop 1977;53:165.
168. Jaeger A, Tempe JD, Haegy JM, et al. Accidental acute mercury vapor poisoning. Vet Hum Toxicol 1979;21(Suppl):62.
169. Kark RA, Poskanzer D, Bullock J, et al. Mercury poisoning and its treatment with *N*-acetyl-D,L-penicillamine. N Engl J Med 1971;185:10.
170. Komaki H, Maisawa S, Sugai K, et al. Tremor and seizures associated with chronic manganese intoxication. Brain Dev 1999;21:122.
171. Lee JW. Manganese intoxication. Arch Neurol 2000; 57:597.
172. Coulehan JL, Hirsch W, Brillman J, et al. Gasoline sniffing and lead toxicity in Navajo adolescents. Pediatrics 1983;71:113.
173. Milanov I, Kolev P. Clinical and electromyographic examinations of patients with tremor after chronic occupational lead exposure. Occup Med 2001;51:157.
174. Goldings AS, Stewart RM. Organic lead encephalopathy: Behavioral change and movement disorder following gasoline inhalation. J Clin Psychol 1982;43:70.
175. Seshia SS, Rjani KR, Boeckx RL, et al. The neurological manifestations of chronic inhalation of leaded gasoline. Dev Med Child Neurol 1978;20:323.
176. Gerhart JM, Hong JS, Uphouse LL, et al. Chlordecone-induced tremor: Quantification and pharmacological analysis. Toxicol Appl Pharmacol 1982;66:234.
177. Taylor JR, Selhorst JB, Houff SA, et al. Chlordecone intoxication of man. I: Clinical observations. Neurology 1978;28:626.
178. Huang TP, Ho IK, Mehendale HM. Assessment of neurotoxicity induced by oral administration of chlordecone (Kepone) in the mouse. Neurotoxicology 1981;2:113.
179. Reiter LW, Kidd K, Ledbetter G, et al. Comparative behavioral toxicology of mirex and kepone in the rat. Toxicol Appl Pharmacol 1977;41:143.
180. Cohn WJ, Boylan JJ, Blanke RV, et al. Treatment of chlordecone (Kepone) toxicity with cholestyramine. N Engl J Med 1978;198:243.
181. Hietanen E, Vainio H. Effect of administration route on DDT on acute toxicity and on drug biotransformation in various rodents. Arch Environ Contam Toxicol 1976;4:201.
182. Kashyap SK, Nigam SK, Karnik AB, et al. Carcinogenicity of DDT (dichlorodiphenyltrichloroethane) in pure inbred Swiss mice. Int J Cancer 1977;19:725.
183. Wilson R, Lovejoy FH, Jaeger RJ, et al. Acute phosphine poisoning aboard a grain freighter: Epidemiologic,

clinical, and pathological findings. J Am Med Assoc 1980;244:148.

184. Zatuchni J, Hong K. Methyl bromide poisoning seen initially as psychosis. Arch Neurol 1981;38:529.
185. Peters HA, Levine RL, Matthews CG, et al. Extrapyramidal and other neurologic manifestations associated with carbon disulfide fumigant exposure. Arch Neurol 1988;45:537.
186. Hirose Y, Kobayashi M, Koyama K, et al. A toxicokinetic analysis in a patient with acute glufosinate poisoning. Hum Exp Toxicol 1999;18:305.
187. Welch L, Kirschner H, Heath A, et al. Chronic neuropsychological and neurological impairment following acute exposure to a solvent mixture of toluene and methyl ethyl ketone (MEK). J Toxicol Clin Toxicol 1991;29:435.
188. Poungvarin N. Multifocal brain damage due to lacquer sniffing: The first case report of Thailand. J Med Assoc Thailand 1991;74:296.
189. Buccafusco JJ, Heithold DL, Chon SH. Long-term behavioral and learning abnormalities produced by the irreversible cholinesterase inhibitor soman: Effect of a standard pretreatment regimen and clonidine. Toxicol Lett 1990;52:319.
190. Dick F, Semple S, Chen R, et al. Neurological deficits in solvent-exposed painters: A syndrome including impaired colour vision, cognitive defects, tremor and loss of vibration sensation. Q J Med 2000;93:655.
191. Sakai T, Honda S, Kuzuhara S. Encephalomyelopathy demonstrated on MRI in a case of chronic toluene intoxication. Rinsho Shinkeigaku 2000;40:571.
192. Rajput AH, Jamison H, Hirsh S, Quraishi A. Relative efficacy of alcohol and propranolol in action tremor. Can J Neurol Sci 1975;2:31.
193. Jankovic J, Fahn S. Physiologic and pathologic tremors. Ann Intern Med 1980;73:460.
194. Larsen TA, Calne DB. Essential tremor. Clin Neuropharmacol 1983;6:185.
195. Shirlow MJ, Matheers CS. A study of caffeine consumption and symptoms: Indigestion, palpitations, tremor, headache, and insomnia. Int J Epidemiol 1985; 14:239.
196. Miller LS, Lombardo TW, Fowler SC. Caffeine, but not time of day, increases whole-arm physiological tremor in non-smoking moderate users. Clin Exp Pharmacol Physiol 1998;25:131.
197. Leavitt S, Tyler HR. Studies in asterixis. Arch Neurol 1964;10:360.
198. Milanov I, Toteva S, Georgiev D. Alcohol withdrawal tremor. Electromyogr Clin Neurophysiol 1996;36:15.
199. Koller W, O'Hara R, Durus W, et al. Tremor in chronic alcoholism. Neurology 1985;35:1660.
200. Silverskoid BP. Romberg's test in the cerebellar syndrome occurring in chronic alcoholism. Acta Neurol Scand 1969;45:292.
201. Victor M, Adams RD, Cole IM. The acquired (non-Wilsonian) type of chronic hepatocerebral degeneration. Medicine (Baltimore) 1965;44:345.
202. Spencer PS, Nunn PB, Hu J, et al. Guam amyotrophic lateral sclerosis-parkinsonism-dementia linked to a plant excitant. Science 1987;237:517.
203. Bovet D, Longo VG. The action of nicotine-induced tremors of substances effective in parkinsonism. J Pharmacol Exp Ther 1951;102:22.
204. Cahen RL, Thomas JM, Tvede KM. Nicotinolytic drugs. II: Action of adrenergic blocking agents on nicotine-induced tremors. J Pharmacol Exp Ther 1953;107:424.
205. Stiffmaln SM, Fritz ER, Maltese J, et al. Effects of cigarette smoking and oral nicotine on hand tremor. Clin Pharmacol Ther 1983;33:800.
206. Lippold OC, Williams EJ, Wilson CG. Finger tremor and cigarette smoking. Br J Clin Pharmacol 1980;10:83.
207. Zdonczyk D, Royse V, Koller WC. Nicotine and tremor. Clin Neuropharmacol 1988;11:282.

CHAPTER 27

Pathophysiology of Tremor

Rodger J. Elble

Tremor is an approximately rhythmic, roughly sinusoidal involuntary movement. Despite more than a century of clinical and laboratory investigations, no tremor is understood completely. Common and uncommon forms of tremor are reviewed in this chapter, and two basic questions are addressed for each form: what is the source of oscillation and why does the oscillation occur.

▶ PHYSIOLOGICAL TREMOR

Physiological tremor is barely visible to the unaided eye and is symptomatic only during activities that require extreme precision. Physiological tremor consists of two distinct oscillations: mechanical reflex (MR) and 8–12 Hz, which are superimposed upon a background of irregular fluctuations in muscle force and limb displacement.[1,2] These background irregularities have a frequency of 0–15 Hz and are produced by motor units that fire near their threshold.[3] The low-pass filtering property of skeletal muscle attenuates the amplitude of these irregularities at frequencies above 3–5 Hz.[4]

The MR component of physiological tremor is much larger than the 8–12-Hz component and is exhibited by everyone. The MR component is a passive mechanical oscillation that is produced by the underdamped inertial, viscous, and elastic properties of the limbs and other body parts. Participation of the stretch reflex is evident only when physiological tremor is enhanced by fatigue, anxiety, or drugs.[5,6] The mechanical attributes of most body parts are such that damped oscillations occur in response to pulsatile perturbations. The frequency of these MR oscillations ω is determined largely by the inertia I and stiffness K of the body part, according to the formula $\omega \approx \sqrt{K/I}$. Consequently, normal elbow tremor has a frequency, 3–5 Hz, which is lower than the 8–12-Hz frequency of wrist tremor because the forearm has much greater inertia than the hand.[7] Similarly, the finger has even less inertia, so the frequency of metacarpophalangeal joint tremor is 17–30 Hz.[8] Voluntary co-contraction of muscles about a joint produces a slight increase in tremor frequency due to the increased joint stiffness. Conversely, relaxation of the joint causes the frequency of MR tremor to fall.

The mechanical properties of the body are not sufficient to cause tremor. One or more sources of mechanical energy are required to force or perturb a limb into oscillation at a frequency determined by limb inertia and stiffness. Voluntary muscle contraction contains irregularities in subtetanic motor-unit firing that perturb the limb continuously and randomly. The ejection of blood at cardiac systole provides additional perturbations of the limbs. Such cardioballistics account for nearly all of physiological tremor at rest but only a fraction of physiological postural and kinetic tremor.[2,9]

Under normal circumstances, somatosensory receptors (e.g., muscle spindles) respond to the mechanical oscillations of physiological tremor, but the response is usually too weak to entrain motoneurons at the frequency of tremor. Consequently, the power spectrum of rectified-filtered electromyography (EMG) is essentially flat during normal steady muscle contraction (Fig. 27–1). The stretch-reflex response to oscillation increases during fatigue and anxiety and in response to some medications, producing a modulation of motor-unit activity and so-called enhanced physiological tremor (Fig. 27–1).[5,6,10] This involvement of the stretch-reflex can increase tremor or suppress it, depending on the dynamics of the reflex loop and limb mechanics.[11] Thus, MR oscillation is minimized when the natural frequency of the mechanical system is far removed from the natural frequencies of associated stretch-reflex pathways.

In contrast to the MR oscillation, the 8–12-Hz component of physiological tremor is always associated with modulation of motor-unit activity, even when the 8–12-Hz tremor is much smaller than the MR oscillation (Fig. 27–1). Participating motor units are entrained at 8–12 Hz, regardless of their mean frequency of discharge.[1,12] The 8–12-Hz and MR oscillations are easily distinguished by their response to inertial and elastic loads. The frequency of 8–12 Hz tremor changes less than 1 Hz when inertial or elastic loads are attached to the limb. By contrast, the frequency of MR oscillation is proportional to $\sqrt{K/I}$.[8,13] Furthermore, the frequency of 8–12 Hz tremor is independent of stretch-reflex loop time and muscle twitch properties.[12,14,15] For these reasons, the 8–12-Hz tremor is believed to originate in an oscillating neuronal network within the central nervous system and,

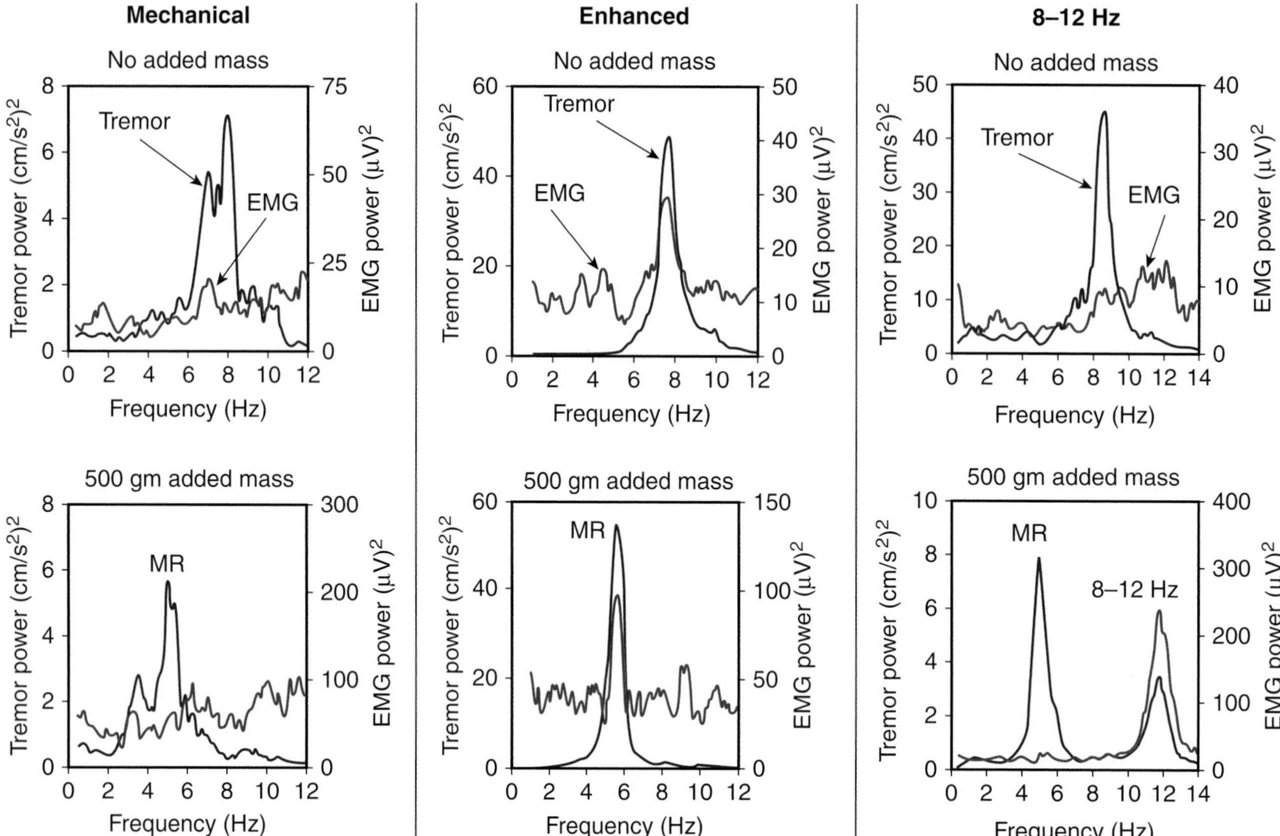

Figure 27–1. Fourier power spectra of normal MR tremor (mechanical), enhanced physiological tremor due to thyrotoxicosis (enhanced) and physiological tremor with a prominent 8–12-Hz component (8–12 Hz). Postural hand tremor was recorded a miniature accelerometer (blue lines), and rectified-filtered EMG of the extensor carpi radialis brevis was recorded with skin electrodes (red lines). Note how a 500-g load on the hand reduced normal and enhanced MR tremor. By contrast, the 8–12-Hz tremor increased in amplitude, but its frequency did not change.

therefore, referred to as the central neurogenic component of physiological tremor. There is now convincing evidence that this 8–12-Hz tremor emerges from oscillation in the cerebello-thalamo-cortical loop.[16,17]

▶ GENERAL PROPERTIES OF PATHOLOGICAL TREMORS

The segmental stretch-reflex and limb mechanics comprise the final common pathway for all forms of tremor (Fig. 27–2) and, therefore, can influence the frequency or amplitude of a tremor, depending on its origin. The frequency of normal MR tremor is largely a function of limb inertia and stiffness and is easily changed by added inertia or stiffness because there is little involvement of segmental and long-loop reflexes. However, tremors with greater involvement of segmental and long-loop (e.g., transcortical) sensorimotor pathways have frequencies that are relatively less dependent on limb mechanics and more on reflex loop dynamics (e.g., loop time).[18,19] Consequently, the frequencies of enhanced physiological tremor and cerebellar tremor are altered less by mechanical loads than the frequency of normal MR tremor.[10,20] Tremors originating from central oscillators have frequencies that are independent of limb mechanics and reflex arc length, except in the hypothetical and pathological situation when the stretch reflex is so strong relative to the central oscillator that the central oscillator becomes entrained by stretch-reflex oscillation.[19] An example of this situation would be the entrainment of tremor by pathological clonus. Nevertheless, if tremor frequency is independent of limb inertia *and* reflex-arc length, the source of tremor is a central oscillator. Parkinson tremor, essential tremor (ET), primary writing tremor, palatal tremor, Holmes tremor, dystonic tremor, and orthostatic tremor are examples of central oscillation.[21]

Motor pathways are sufficiently integrated that no source of tremor can be isolated completely from the effects of sensory feedback. Consequently, peripheral stretch-reflex manipulations can reset the phase and entrain the frequency of tremors even when they emerge from central sources of oscillation.[22–26] Similarly,

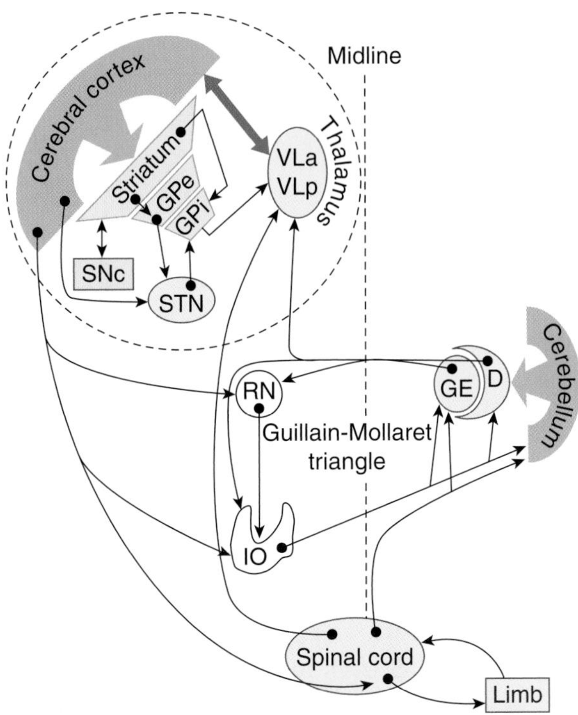

Figure 27–2. This schematic diagram illustrates the pathways that have been implicated in the various tremors discussed in this chapter. D = dentate nucleus; GE = globose and emboliform nuclei; GPe and GPi = globus pallidus externa and interna; RN = red nucleus; RetN = reticular nuclei; SNc = substantia nigra pars compacta; STN = subthalamic nucleus; IO = inferior olive; VLa and VLp = anterior and posterior ventrolateral thalamic nuclei; and VLp is also called Vim.

a central oscillator can resonate with the MR system, if their natural frequencies are similar.[24] For example, Parkinson and essential hand tremors have frequencies that are similar to the MR frequency of the wrist, so there is less mechanical limitation of the tremor than would occur if these tremors had much higher frequencies. The 14–18-Hz frequency of orthostatic tremor is much higher than the natural MR frequency of the lower limbs, so this tremor is difficult to see unless it undergoes subharmonic reduction to 7–9 Hz. Similar dynamical interactions undoubtedly occur between the central oscillators of pathological tremors and the central neural pathways to which the oscillators are connected. Resonance between a tremor oscillator and other parts of the central nervous system probably plays an important role in determining the amplitude and distribution of pathological tremors.[27]

Magnetic stimulation of the contralateral motor cortex can reset the phase of ET, Parkinson tremor, and normal rapid alternating wrist movements.[28,29] These observations prove that the motor cortex can influence a tremor but do not reveal the anatomical origin of tremor.

Positron emission tomography (PET) has revealed increased cerebellar blood flow in patients with many forms of tremor, including Parkinson tremor, writing tremor, orthostatic tremor, and ET.[30] The cerebellum receives abundant somatosensory feedback and projects directly or indirectly to all parts of the motor system except the basal ganglia. Thus, cerebellar hyperactivity is a nonspecific abnormality and could be a consequence of tremor rather than its cause.

Nucleus ventralis intermedius (Vim) of the ventrolateral thalamus has been the preferred stereotactic surgical site for treating essential, Parkinson, cerebellar, rubral, task specific, and orthostatic tremors,[31–35] even though Vim receives inputs from cerebellum and ascending spinal sensory tracts and only sparse input from the internal pallidum (Fig. 27–2).[36–39] It is unclear whether Vim is the primary source of oscillation for any of these tremor disorders. Nevertheless, the oscillatory properties and anatomical connections of Vim could facilitate the development of pathological oscillation originating from virtually any location in the motor system. This may explain why Vim is a nonspecific Achilles heel for most forms of pathological tremor.

ESSENTIAL TREMOR

ET is the most common form of pathological tremor. ET begins at any age but is most common in older people, having a prevalence of approximately 5% in people over the age of 65.[40] Many patients have a family history that is compatible with mendelian-dominant inheritance. However, genetic linkage studies have failed to identify a gene, even though several promising loci have been found.[41] Consequently, many or perhaps most patients with ET may have polygenic inheritance, analogous to the genetics of restless leg syndrome.

ET affects the hands in nearly all cases and frequently affects the head (at least 34%), face/jaw (approximately 7%), voice (approximately 12%), tongue (approximately 30%), trunk (approximately 5%), and lower limbs (approximately 30%).[42,43] ET is a postural tremor with a variable kinetic component. Patients with advanced ET exhibit intention tremor and impaired tandem walking, consistent with impaired cerebellar function.[21] Tremor in repose is uncommon and observed only in the most advanced patients, who are typically older. The complex pill-rolling hand movements of Parkinson tremor are not seen in ET.[42]

The fundamental electrophysiological abnormality of ET is an abnormal entrainment of motor-unit firing at the frequency of tremor, which is typically 4–8 Hz. Many observations suggest that motor-unit entrainment emerges from oscillation in thalamocortical and olivocerebellar pathways.[21] Lesions of the cerebellum, basis pontis, and thalamus have abolished or reduced ET. These observations are consistent with the notion that

ET depends critically on the corticospinal tract and on cerebellar pathways projecting via the ventrolateral thalamus (Vim) to motor cortex.

Louis and coworkers have found abnormally high numbers of axonal torpedoes in the deep cerebellar white matter and reduced numbers of Purkinje cells in the cerebellar cortex of patients with ET.[44,45] PET studies of patients with ET revealed increased olivary glucose utilization and increased blood flow in the cerebellum, red nucleus, and thalamus.[30] The electroencephalogram (EEG) contains cortical rhythmicity that is correlated with ET,[46] and functional magnetic resonance imaging (MRI) studies have disclosed increased blood flow bilaterally in the cerebellar hemispheres, dentate nucleus, and red nucleus and contralaterally in the globus pallidus, thalamus, and primary sensorimotor cortex.[30] Harmaline and related beta-carboline alkaloids enhance the inhibition-rebound properties of olivary neurons and other neurons, causing increased rhythmicity and neuronal entrainment, and the tremor produced by harmaline resembles ET.

The neurophysiological properties of ET are consistent with a central source of oscillation that is influenced by somatosensory reflex pathways. Mechanical loads have little effect on the frequency of ET (Fig. 27–3), thereby distinguishing this tremor from enhanced physiological tremor.[47] Cooling the upper extremity reduces tremor amplitude but does not change tremor frequency.[48] Patients with ET exhibit normal MR properties, and MR oscillation and ET can exhibit mutual frequency entrainment and resonance if their frequencies are similar.[49] When a mechanical load separates the MR and ETs, resonance and entrainment are abolished, resulting in reduced tremor amplitude and a more clear demonstration of the frequency of ET (best measured in the rectified-filtered EMG spectrum; Fig. 27–3).

Tremor amplitude bears a logarithmic relationship with the intensity and frequency of motor-unit entrainment, according to the equation: $\log(\textit{amplitude}) = -2.3\log(\textit{frequency}) + 2.3\log(\textit{intensity}) + 10$.[50] The frequency–amplitude relationship (slope approximately –2) of ET is predicted by the second-order low-pass filtering properties of skeletal muscle.[4] This relationship also predicts that tremor amplitude could be significantly reduced by increasing tremor frequency.

Mild high-frequency ET is similar to the 8–12 Hz component of physiological tremor, so these tremors could emerge from the same central oscillator.[51] However, oscillators in the frequency range of ET are found throughout the nervous system, and the similarities between ET and the 8–12 Hz physiological tremor could be fortuitous.[52] Nevertheless, patients within the same family commonly exhibit tremors with different frequencies, ranging from 4 to 12 Hz, and tremor frequency is strongly correlated with the patient's age (in years), according to the equation: $\textit{frequency} \approx 0.07\,\textit{age} + 10$.[53] The tremor frequency decreases at a rate of approximately 0.07 Hz per year, in the average patient.[53] This drop in tremor frequency presumably is related to age-related changes in the nervous system or to progression of the underlying pathophysiology.[53,54]

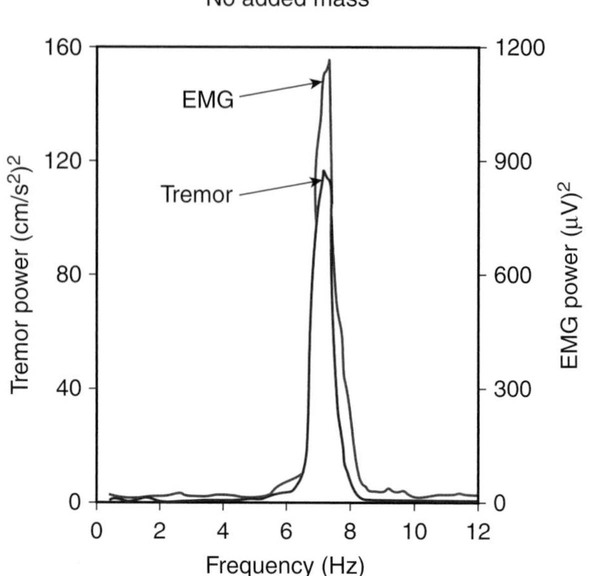

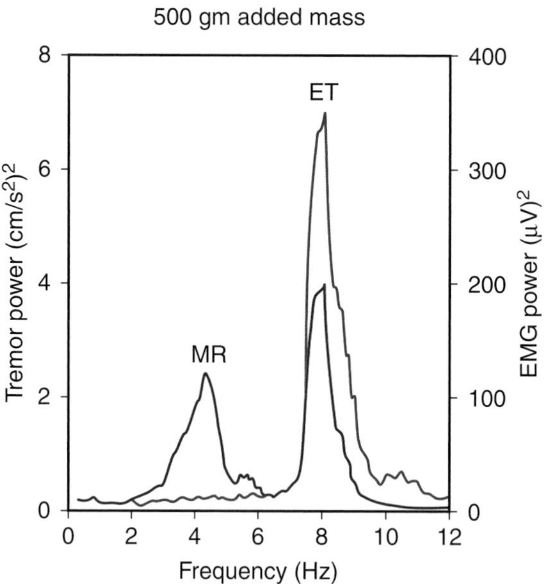

Figure 27–3. Fourier power spectra of postural hand tremor recorded from a 57-year-old woman with mild familial tremor. Hand tremor was recorded with a miniature accelerometer (blue lines), and extensor digitorum brevis EMG was recorded with skin electrodes (red lines). Note the single large spectral peak in tremor and EMG (no added mass). Mass loading reduced the frequency of the MR oscillation to 4 Hz, leaving the ET at 8 Hz (500 g added mass). This precluded any resonance between the two oscillations, so the overall amplitude of tremor was reduced.

Ethanol, primidone, and beta-adrenergic blockers suppress ET by mechanisms that are poorly understood.[55] Based on the harmaline model, ethanol and primidone could have direct actions on the neuronal oscillator or could uncouple the oscillation from segmental spinal pathways. Beta-blockers act peripherally, possibly by reducing the sensitivity of sensory receptors (e.g., muscle spindles) and by increasing the low-pass filtering properties of skeletal muscle. A central mode of action is also possible. None of these treatments is specific for ET.

Stereotactic thalamotomy and deep brain stimulation (DBS) in Vim are the most effective treatments for ET (Chapter 25), but their mechanisms of action are unclear. One possibility is that tremor is reduced by interrupting resonant oscillation in the thalamocortical loop. This might occur regardless of the primary site of tremorogenic oscillation. An alternative possibility is that the tremorogenic oscillation emerges from the Vim, motor cortex or thalamocortical loop, but this possibility is at odds with the recent observation that stimulation of neighboring subthalamic structures is more effective than stimulation of Vim.[56]

Several investigators have found that subthalamic DBS is effective in ET.[57,58] The critical target in this anatomically compact area is unclear and could be the subthalamic nucleus, zona incerta, or prelemniscal radiation, which carries cerebellar and somatosensory afferents to the ventrolateral thalamus.[58] Parkinson tremor and ET both respond to subthalamic DBS when these diseases occur in the same patient.[59] These observations raise the possibility that tremorogenic oscillation in the basal ganglia could participate in the pathogenesis of ET.

PARKINSONIAN TREMOR

Rest tremor in the upper or lower extremities is the most specific feature of Parkinson disease. Action tremor (i.e., postural tremor or kinetic tremor) is also common and may result from a re-emergent rest tremor or may exist independently of rest tremor.[60] There is no compelling reason to hypothesize different sources of oscillation for Parkinson action tremor and rest tremor. Both forms of tremor occur in monkeys after destruction of the substantia nigra pars compacta with intracarotid injections of MTPT (1-methyl-4-phenyl-1,2,3,6-tetrahydropyridine).[61]

The principal pathology of Parkinson disease is a loss of dopaminergic cells in the substantia nigra pars compacta, and this deficit is probably sufficient to produce Parkinson tremor.[62] Neurons in the motor cortex,[63] ventrolateral thalamus,[64,65] globus pallidus,[66] and subthalamic nucleus[67–70] oscillate intermittently in correlation with tremor, and a stereotactic lesion or high-frequency stimulation in any of these locations suppresses tremor (Fig. 27–2). The cerebellum is active in patients with Parkinson tremor, but the cerebellum is not necessary for the production of rest tremor.[71] Thus, many parts of the motor system are clearly involved, and the principal source of oscillation is unclear. Their collective oscillation, rather than individual oscillation, may be necessary for Parkinson rest tremor.[72,73]

Vim is the most effective stereotactic surgical site in the thalamus for treating Parkinson tremor even though Vim receives inputs from cerebellum and ascending spinal sensory tracts and only sparse input from the internal pallidum.[37–39] Stereotactic destruction and DBS of the posteroventrolateral internal pallidum and the subthalamus are effective treatments for tremor,[74] but the thalamic receiving nucleus of the internal pallidum, ventralis oralis posterior (Vop; also known as ventralis lateralis anterior: VLa; Fig. 30–2), is not an effective target.[75] How can these paradoxical surgical and anatomical data be reconciled? Of note is recent evidence that the inputs to Vop and Vim (both part of VL) are not completely segregated, and both nuclei project to and receive considerable input from supplementary and primary motor cortices.[39,76] Therefore, these overlapping corticothalamocortical projections could mediate entrainment of the pallidothalamic and cerebellothalamic pathways through resonance within the thalamocortical loops.[69] Furthermore, the subthalamic area, neighboring the ventrolateral thalamus, contains the subthalamus, zona incerta, pallidothalamic fibers, and cerebellothalamic fibers, which are all potential players in tremorogenesis.[77,78] Consequently, the interpretation of surgical data, in the context of tremorogenesis, is still controversial.

CEREBELLAR INTENTION TREMOR

Gordon Holmes used the terms static tremor and intention tremor to describe the tremors that he observed in patients with cerebellar lesions.[79] This discussion is devoted to intention tremor, which is most common.

The rhythm and amplitude of cerebellar intention tremor are often irregular, and proximal limb muscles are usually involved more than distal ones. The frequency of cerebellar intention tremor is commonly cited as 3–5 Hz, but animal and human studies have shown that tremor frequency is influenced by reflex arc length and by the inertia and stiffness of the body part.[20,80] These observations are consistent with the mechanistic involvement of somatosensory feedback loops. However, instability in these loops is probably not the sole source of tremor because upper extremity deafferentation in decerebellate monkeys does not eliminate the 2–4-Hz intention tremor that occurs with cerebellar ablation alone.[81] The preservation of tremor following somatosensory deafferentation is probably due to the participation of visual feedback[82] and thalamocortical oscillation[83] in tremorogenesis.

Classic intention tremor occurs in humans with lesions in the cerebellum or in the brachium conjunctivum pathway from the deep cerebellar nuclei to the contral-

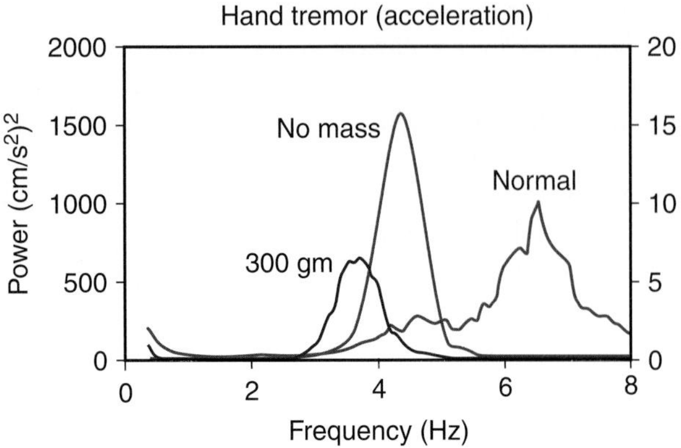

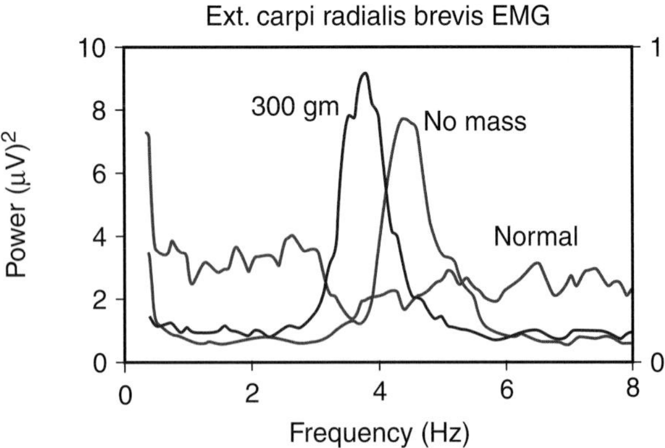

Figure 27–4. Fourier power spectra of hand tremor and rectified-filtered forearm EMG that were recorded from an 8-year-old girl who suffered from a small infarct in the contralateral ventrolateral thalamus. With horizontal posture, she exhibited normal physiologic tremor (normal; right vertical axis) with no entrainment of motor units in the extensor carpi radialis brevis (statistically flat spectrum). However, her tremor increased substantially when she pointed at a fixed target without moving her hand, and prominent tremor-related bursts of EMG occurred in the forearm muscles, producing an EMG spectral peak at the frequency of tremor. This abnormal tremor occurred at a lower frequency (no mass), and the frequency of this abnormal tremor decreased further with mass loading (300 g). However, the change in frequency with mass loading was not as great as seen in normal people (Fig. 27–1). Similar abnormal tremor was evident when writing, drawing and performing finger-to-nose testing.

ateral ventrolateral thalamus (Fig. 27–2).[84,85] Small lesions in the vicinity of the ventrolateral thalamus may produce intention tremor with no other signs of ataxia.[84,85] An 8-year-old girl with a ventrolateral infarct and contralateral intention tremor was reported by Qureshi and coworkers, and this tremor exhibited the properties of a MR oscillation (Fig. 27–4).

A 3–5-Hz intention tremor occurs in the ipsilateral extremities of laboratory primates with lesions in the deep cerebellar nuclei (dentate, globose, and emboliform) or in the outflow tracts of these nuclei (superior cerebellar peduncle; brachium conjunctivum). The critical nuclear lesion appears to be the globose-emboliform (interpositus).[86] Tremulous modulation of neuronal activity occurs in the motor cortex, somatosensory cortex, interpositus nucleus, and somatosensory afferents of monkeys but does not occur in the dentate nucleus, which receives no somatosensory feedback.[20,87] These observations are consistent with the hypothesis that cerebellar tremor is produced by abnormal oscillation in transcortical and transcerebellar sensorimotor feedback loops. Changes in stiffness and inertia influence the frequency of cerebellar tremor less than the frequency of physiological tremor (MR component) because transcortical and transcerebellar sensorimotor loops are heavily involved in cerebellar tremor but not in physiological tremor.

Normal rapid limb movements toward a target are decelerated with a burst of antagonist muscle contraction. Target overshoot and limb oscillation occur when this antagonist activity is delayed or inappropriately sized. Patients with cerebellar damage exhibit delayed antagonist muscle activation and terminal oscillation.[87,88] Cerebellar damage impairs the feedforward control of movement, so that available sensory information and prior experience are not used effectively in the formulation of antagonist muscle activity before the target is reached. Instead, limb movement is guided more by sensory feedback control.[87] Sensory feedback control is too slow and imprecise to prevent ataxia and tremor. Feedforward control (i.e., anticipatory deceleration) of movement is necessary, and the cerebellum plays a critical role in this aspect of motor control.

Elble and coworkers found that tremor-related interpositus bursts in a rhesus monkey occurred an average 12.5 ms after the agonist EMG bursts.[20] Murphy and coworkers found that motor cortex and interpositus were activated nearly simultaneously by agonist muscle stretch.[89] Therefore, the interpositus bursts occurred too late to drive the agonist muscle. Instead, interpositus could be involved in limiting agonist activity through an inhibitory pathway, or it could drive the subsequent burst of antagonist EMG. Li Volsi and colleagues found that agonist pyramidal tract neurons in the cat were inhibited by the interpositus-thalamocortical pathway, but the antagonist pyramidal tract neurons were either excited or excited and then inhibited.[90] These observations support the notion that the cerebellum plays a critical role in the feedforward control of antagonist activation, which decelerates the limb in a smooth and accurate approach to the intended destination. The participation of these transcortical pathways explains why repetitive transcranial magnetic stimulation of motor cortex produces a cerebellar-like tremor in normal people.[91]

Classic cerebellar intention tremor exhibits a crescendo increase in amplitude as the limb approaches

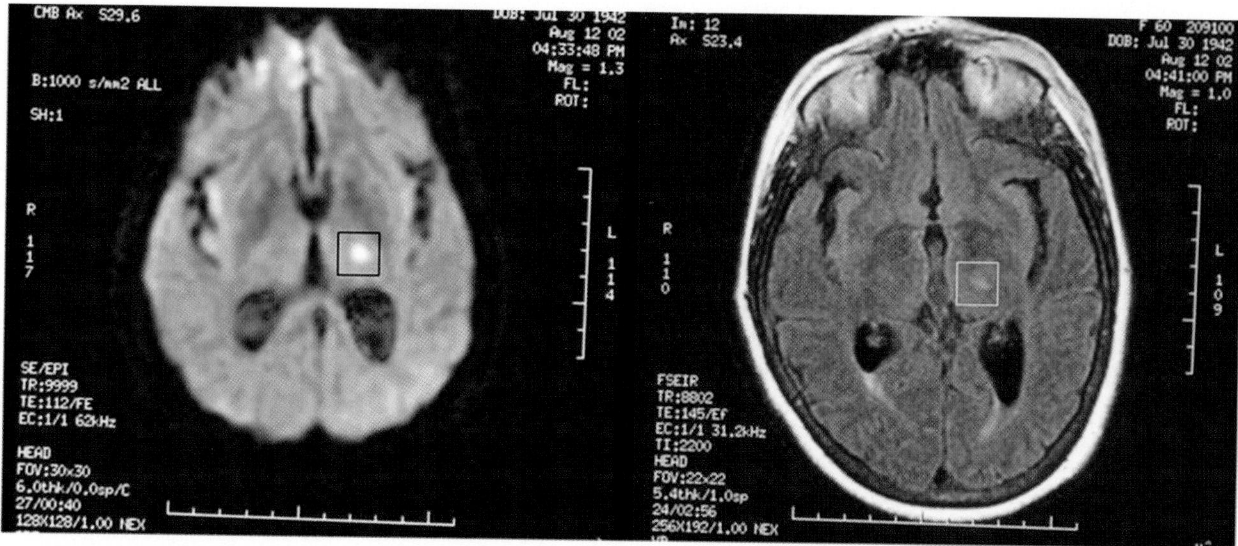

Figure 27–5. A 60-year-old woman developed a severe Holmes tremor in her right upper limb one month after this small thalamic infarct. A follow-up MRI scan was normal. Left image is diffusion weighted MRI, and the right image is FLAIR.

its target. The mechanism of this dramatic terminal accentuation of tremor is unclear. A contribution from a central source of oscillation is likely (e.g., the inferior olive, thalamus, or brainstem reticular formation). The Guillain-Mollaret triangle and other excitatory brainstem-cerebellar loops could contribute to the crescendo, nearly paroxysmal features of cerebellar intention tremor.[92,93] Resonance in the ventrolateral thalamocortical loop could also contribute in this manner, and this would explain why Vim and the neighboring cerebellothalamic fibers are effective stereotactic targets for intention tremor.[56]

HOLMES (RUBRAL) TREMOR

Holmes tremor is a striking combination of 2–5-Hz rest, postural, and kinetic tremor of an extremity. Frequencies as high as 7 Hz have been reported, and the frequency may vary with posture and movement.[94,95] This unusual tremor has been called rubral tremor because it is often caused by lesions in the vicinity of the red nucleus (Fig. 27–2). However, lesions in the vicinity of the ventrolateral thalamus also cause this tremor (Fig. 27–5), and isolated lesions in the red nucleus are not tremorogenic. Combined impairment of the neighboring cerebellothalamic and nigrostriatal or pallidothalamic fiber tracts is probably required and explains the peculiar rest, postural, and kinetic features.[83,96,97] Consequently, participants of the 1997 Tremor Symposium in Kiel, Germany proposed to abolish the term rubral tremor and adopt the term Holmes tremor, which has gained widespread use.[98]

In some patients, Holmes tremor may be little more than a combination of parkinsonian rest and cerebellar intention tremors because some patients have reduced striatal ^{18}F-fluorodopa uptake, and virtually all patients have damage to the cerebellothalamic pathway.[95] Reduced striatal ^{18}F-fluorodopa uptake explains why levodopa and dopaminergic agonists occasionally are beneficial. However, Holmes tremor, like cerebellar intention tremor, is usually refractory to pharmacotherapy.

Holmes tremor usually begins weeks to months after thalamic or midbrain trauma or stroke. Therefore, secondary or compensatory changes in nervous system function probably participate in tremorogenesis. The nature of these deleterious secondary changes is unclear,

Holmes tremor responds to stereotactic thalamotomy and DBS in Vim, but for reasons already discussed, this response contributes little to our understanding of this tremor.[31,99]

PALATAL TREMOR

Palatal tremor (also known as palatal myoclonus) consists of vertical oscillations of the soft palate at 1–3 Hz. Higher frequencies are rarely encountered. There are two forms of palatal tremor, symptomatic and essential, which differ clinically and pathophysiologically. *Symptomatic palatal tremor* occurs in patients with damage to in the dentato-olivary pathway (Fig. 27–2), which causes secondary hypertrophic olivary degeneration (hence the name symptomatic palatal tremor).[100] This anatomical abnormality is visible with MRI (Fig. 27–6).[101,102] The palatal movements of symptomatic palatal tremor are usually asymptomatic but occasionally cause an ear click by moving the eustachian tube. Symptomatic palatal tremor

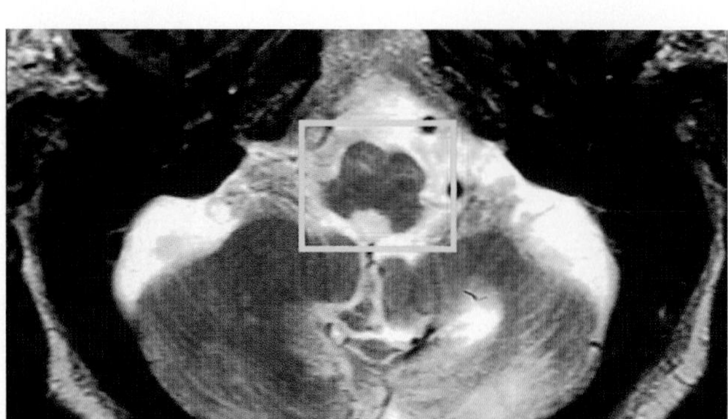

Figure 27-6. This T_2-weighted MRI reveals right olivary hypertrophy secondary to an old left cerebellar infarct.

is nearly always associated with other brainstem and cerebellar signs, depending on the nature and extent of underlying pathology.[100] Synchronous movements of the tongue, floor of the mouth, larynx, face, diaphragm, intercostal muscles, eyes, extremities, and trunk may also occur.

Essential palatal tremor causes an annoying ear click but no other neurological signs or symptoms, and the pathophysiology of essential palatal tremor is a complete mystery.[100] The ear click of essential palatal tremor is produced by movements of the eustachian tube that are caused by contraction of the tensor veli palatini, which can be suppressed with botulinum toxin injection. By contrast, the levator veli palatini muscle is rhythmically active in symptomatic palatal myoclonus, and its contraction usually does not cause an ear click.[103,104]

Clinicopathological studies have repeatedly found dentato-olivary pathway damage in stroke patients with symptomatic palatal myoclonus. This leads to secondary hypertrophic olivary degeneration and palatal myoclonus weeks to months after the initial ictus.[101,102,105] Many investigators believe that the hypertrophied olives oscillate at 1–3 Hz, producing abnormal movements at the same frequency. However, the data supporting this hypothesis are largely inferential and inconclusive. Electrophysiological studies of olivary hypertrophy in a laboratory animal with palatal myoclonus have not been done.[93]

Hong and coworkers recently proposed a novel hypothesis explaining the delayed development of symptomatic palatal tremor following damage to the cerebello-olivary pathway.[106] They reasoned that damage to this pathway produces olivary hypertrophy and loss of GABAergic inhibition of the gap junctions among olivary neurons. The net result is 1–2-Hz oscillation and greater synchrony among olivary neurons. This oscillation initially produces no symptoms, but the persistent synchronous 1–2-Hz climbing fiber input to the cerebellar cortex eventually alters the interaction between interneurons and Purkinje cells in the cerebellar cortex, resulting in enhanced Purkinje cell excitability. The enhanced excitability eventually amplifies the olivary oscillation to a level that produces palatal tremor. In effect, the cerebellar cortex learns to oscillate.

Symptomatic palatal myoclonus is associated with at least three forms of extremity tremor. An asymptomatic tremor is produced by periodic inhibition of limb muscles at 1–3 Hz, time-locked to the palatal movements.[107] These brief periods of inhibition cause irregularities in muscle force that perturb the limb, producing an enhanced MR tremor. The other two forms of tremor are associated with palatal myoclonus, but it is not clear that these tremors emerge from the same source of oscillation. Masucci and Kurtzke described five patients with symptomatic palatal myoclonus and a 2–4-Hz rest tremor of the limbs that persisted during posture and movement.[108] All of their patients had signs of extensive brainstem damage, and only one of the five patients had tremor that was synchronous with the palatal movements. Masucci and coworkers also described a 1–3-Hz mixed rest and action tremor, which they called *myorhythmia*.[109] This tremor involved various combinations of one or more extremities, the trunk, head, face, pharynx, jaw, tongue, and eyes, and the affected body parts seemed to oscillate synchronously in some patients and asynchronously in others.

Miyagi and colleagues described a 49-year-old man who developed disabling right upper extremity action tremor and palatal myoclonus 4 months after a hemorrhage in the left pontine tegmentum.[110] The distal postural tremor responded to Vim stimulation, but the proximal intention tremor did not. A subsequent left posteroventral pallidotomy greatly suppressed this tremor. This observation suggests that the effect of pallidotomy is not specific for Parkinson tremor and that lesions in the dentato-olivary pathway can lead to tremorogenic participation of the basal ganglia.

STROKE-INDUCED TREMOR

Tremor frequently follows strokes in the midbrain, superior cerebellar peduncle, and cerebellum, but tremor is a surprisingly uncommon complication of strokes elsewhere in the nervous system. Tremor in the absence of other neurological signs is a very rare. Holmes tremor and palatal tremor are the best known examples of tremor following stroke. These tremors and others following stroke typically begin weeks to months after the ictus, so secondary neuronal changes are probably involved.[85,111,112] An exception to this rule is intention tremor that often develops immediately following damage to the cerebellothalamic pathway.

A review of 240 published cases of focal lesions in the basal ganglia revealed only three cases of tremor, one of which resembled Parkinson rest tremor.[111,113] Strokes in the ventrolateral thalamus have produced contralateral action tremor,[112] parkinsonian rest tremor,[111] and intention tremor,[84,85] but in most cases, the tremor following ventrolateral thalamic strokes is associated with dystonia.[114]

TREMOR DUE TO PERIPHERAL NERVE PATHOLOGY

Patients with acquired and hereditary peripheral neuropathies frequently exhibit symptomatic 3–10-Hz action tremors. These tremors are usually less rhythmic than ET although some patients with hereditary neuropathy have tremor that is indistinguishable from ET.[115] The action tremor in many patients behaves like an abnormal MR oscillation, resembling enhanced physiological tremor or cerebellar tremor.[116]

The frequency and amplitude of most neuropathic tremors bear no relationship to the degree of sensory loss or velocity of nerve conduction, and the underlying illnesses in most patients do not cause damage to the central nervous system.[116–118] Deleterious compensatory changes in central nervous system function probably cause abnormal oscillation to emerge from otherwise normal sensorimotor pathways, resulting in symptomatic tremor. The cerebellum has been implicated, but the details are far from clear.[119] Central reorganization in response to altered peripheral sensorimotor function is also hypothesized to cause the rare heterogeneous tremors that occur weeks to months after peripheral nerve trauma.[120]

TASK-SPECIFIC, FOCAL, AND DYSTONIC TREMORS

Patients with *primary writing tremor* exhibit severe tremor during the act of writing but experience little or no tremor during other activities. The frequency of primary writing tremor is not altered by mechanical loads, suggesting a central source of oscillation.[121] As in many other tremor disorders, patients with primary writing tremor exhibit bilaterally increased cerebellar activity, as measured with $H_2^{15}O$ PET.[122]

It is unclear whether primary writing tremor is a variant of focal dystonia, a variant of ET, or a separate disease entity.[121,123-125] Dystonic muscle contractions are commonly tremulous, and writer's cramp is no exception.[126–128] The dystonia in patients with tremulous writer's cramp can be very subtle and difficult or impossible to distinguish from compensatory posturing aimed at stabilizing the hand. It seems likely that some or possibly all cases of isolated writing tremor are a focal task-specific dystonia (i.e., tremor-predominant writer's cramp). ET can be relatively task specific during writing but is probably never completely task specific. Nevertheless, the relationships between primary writing tremor, ET and dystonia will not be resolved until specific biomarkers for these conditions are found.

Isolated *tremors of the voice, chin, tongue, and smile* have been described, but these conditions are sufficiently rare that their nosology is unclear.[98] Like primary writing tremor, these less common task-specific and focal tremors may be variants of dystonia, variants of ET or separate entities.[42] Isolated tremor of the head is commonly due to cervical dystonia, but it may also be a manifestation of ET.[98,128,129]

ORTHOSTATIC TREMOR

Orthostatic tremor is an unusual 14–18-Hz postural tremor that develops in the lower extremities and torso within seconds of assuming quiet erect stance.[130–134] This tremor was initially believed to be restricted to the lower limbs and torso, but it is now clear that the tremor is generalized and nearly synchronous throughout the body.[134] The widespread synchrony and 14–18-Hz rhythmicity are easily demonstrated with EMG (Fig. 27–7). This high-frequency tremor is usually symptomatic to the patient but barely visible to the examiner. Within seconds to minutes of continued standing, the frequency of body tremor may change to a 7–9-Hz subharmonic oscillation that is more symptomatic and visible.

Patients with orthostatic tremor complain of unsteadiness while standing and are often unaware of a tremor, per se. There is increasing evidence that the strong high-frequency oscillation entrains proprioceptive feedback to a degree that precludes or reduces normal feedback. Hence, patients feel unsteady, particularly when standing with eyes closed.[135]

Although ET affects the lower extremities in 30–45% of patients,[136] the unusually high frequency of orthostatic tremor (14–18 Hz) and the marked synchrony among ipsilateral and contralateral muscles are never seen in ET. Orthostatic tremor is a distinct entity, not a variant of ET.[47,98]

The pathophysiology of orthostatic tremor has been studied extensively, but our understanding of this tremor is still incomplete. Orthostatic tremor must emerge from a central source of oscillation because the 14–18-Hz frequency of orthostatic tremor is too high to originate in a lower extremity reflex loop, and a central source of oscillation is needed to produce the dramatic rhythmicity and synchrony of this tremor in muscles of the limbs, torso and cranium. Involvement of cranial muscles suggests an oscillator above the spinal cord.[134] Like many other tremors, orthostatic tremor is associated with increased cerebellar blood flow, as measured with $H_2^{15}O$ PET.[137] Oscillation in the posterior fossa, with involvement of the motor cortex, is supported by transcranial magnetic and electrical stimulation studies.[138,139]

Guridi and coworkers recently treated a patient with Vim DBS and produced complete suppression of

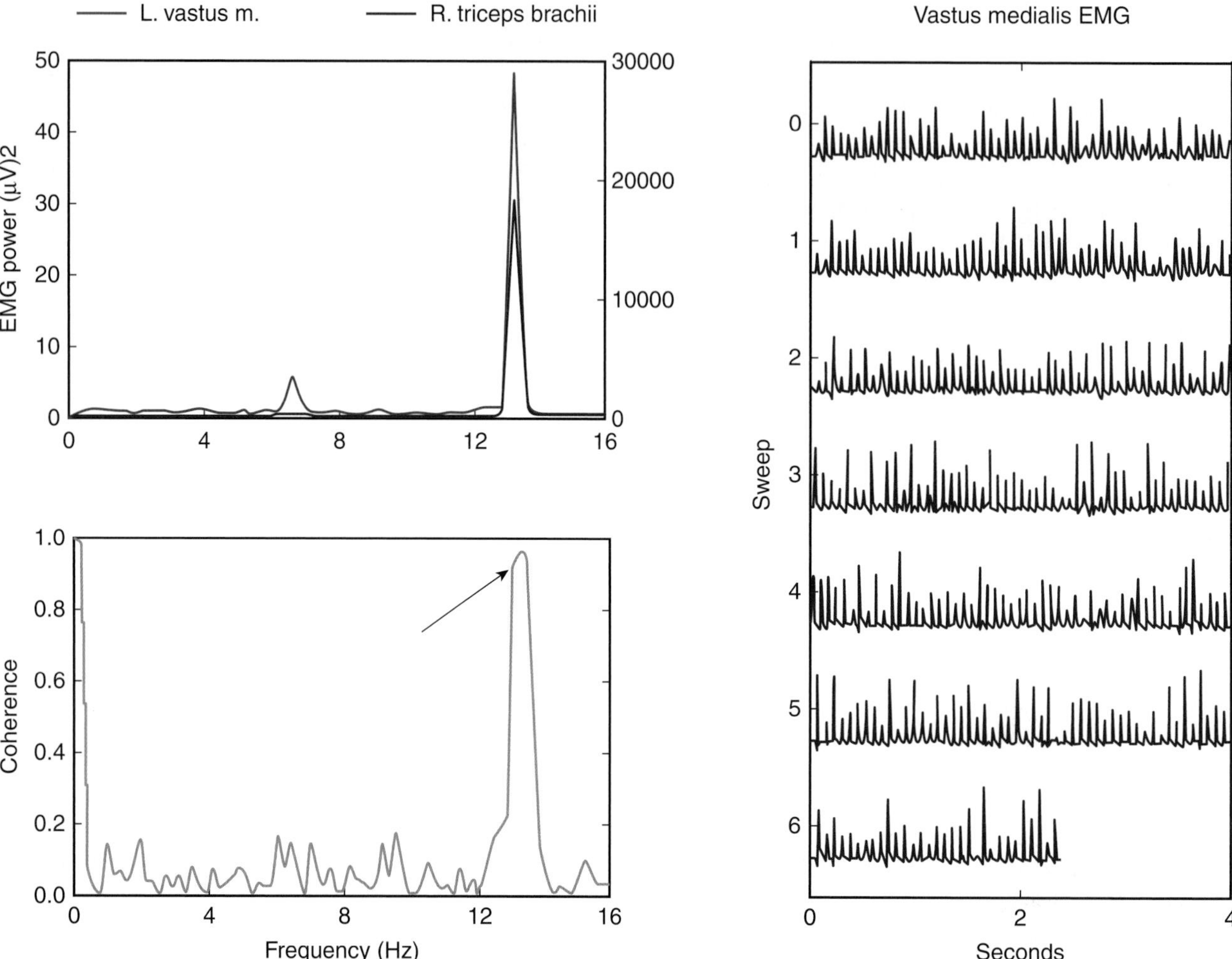

Figure 27–7. EMG was recorded with skin electrodes from the left vastus medialis and right triceps brachii of a patient with orthostatic tremor while he stood and leaned on a table with his hands. Consecutive 4-second recordings (sweeps) of vastus medialis rectified-filtered EMG are shown on the right, illustrating the very rhythmic motor unit discharge at 13.5 Hz. This rhythmicity produced a prominent 13.5-Hz peak in Fourier power spectra **(left upper graph)**, and the coherence (linear correlation squared) between the two muscles is nearly 1.0 **(arrow; left lower graph)**.

the tremor.[35] Rhythmic cortical EEG activity was phase-locked with the tremor, and FDG-PET revealed bilateral motor cortex and cerebellar vermis hypermetabolism. These data clearly demonstrate involvement of the thalamocortical loop, as well as cerebellar pathways, in the pathogenesis of orthostatic tremor.

▶ CORTICAL TREMOR

An irregular 7–14-Hz action tremor, resembling ET, occurs in patients with cortical myoclonus and is called cortical tremor (Fig. 27–8).[140–142] Many investigators prefer the term rhythmic cortical myoclonus, which acknowledges the underlying pathophysiology.[143] Cortical tremor can be acquired or hereditary and occurs most commonly in patients with asterixis. The enhanced C-reflex and giant sensory-evoked potentials in many patients are consistent with the presence of enhanced cortical irritability and transcortical reflexes. An EEG transient preceding the EMG bursts of cortical tremor has been demonstrated with EEG back-averaging.[141,144,145] Thus, the 7–14-Hz oscillation of cortical tremor probably emerges from abnormal cortical oscillation. Cortical tremor generally responds to the same drugs used for cortical myoclonus, such as clonazepam and levetiracetam.[146]

▶ DRUG-INDUCED TREMOR

Many drugs produce parkinsonian rest tremor (neuroleptics), postural tremor (beta-adrenergic agonists, valproic acid, thyroxin, tricyclic antidepressants, and methylxanthines), kinetic tremor (lithium), and combinations

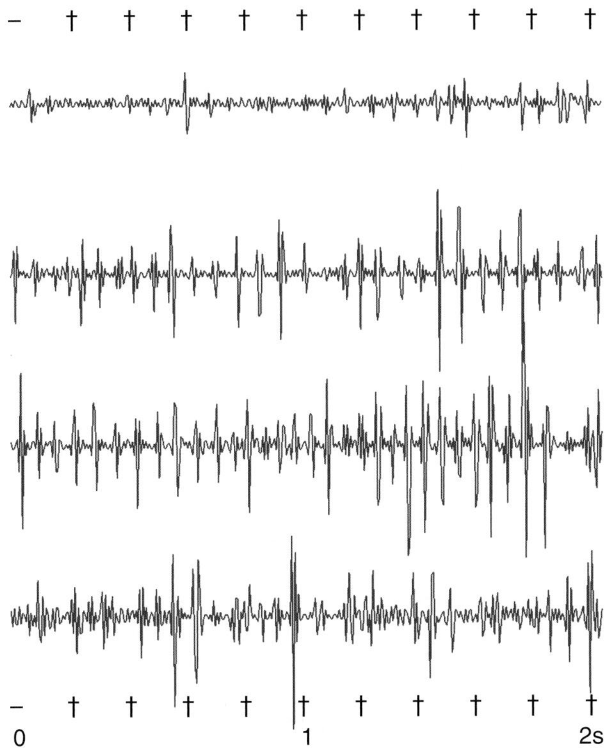

Figure 27–8. Four consecutive 2-second sweeps of EMG were recorded from the extensor carpi radialis brevis of a woman with cortical tremor due to corticobasal degeneration. Note the wide variation in the amplitude of the EMG bursts and the less dramatic variability in tremor frequency. Clinically, the tremor appeared very irregular.

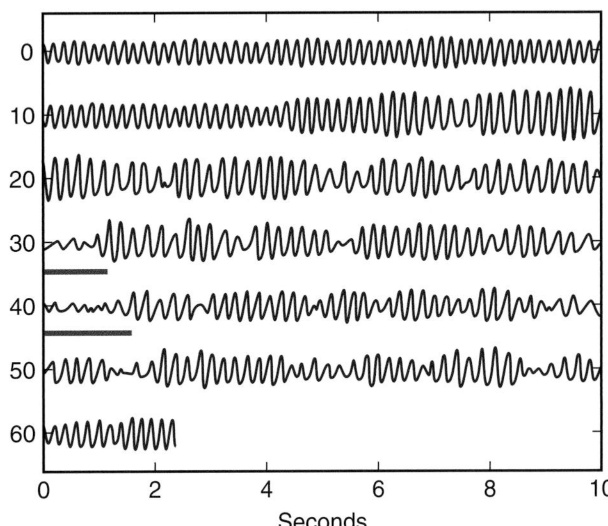

Figure 27–9. Consecutive 10-second sweeps (top to bottom) of right hand movement were recorded with an accelerometer from a man with psychogenic tremor in the right hand. He had no other neurologic signs or symptoms. After 20 seconds (during the third sweep), the man was asked to rhythmically tap his left index finger to his thumb. He performed this task very intermittently and with inexplicable difficulty, except when his right hand was not shaking or when he tapped at the frequency of his tremor. The performance of left finger tapping at other frequencies caused his tremor to stop (horizontal red bars) or change to the frequency of finger tapping (not shown).

thereof (lithium, amiodarone, and valproic acid).[147] Little is known about the mechanisms of these tremors. Amiodarone- and lithium-induced tremors are particularly noteworthy because they are occasionally irreversible.[148–152] Persistent lithium-induced tremor and ataxia are caused by neuronal loss and gliosis of the cerebellar cortex and dentate nuclei.[153] It has long been suspected but never proven that people with subclinical ET and subclinical Parkinson disease are more susceptible to tremorogenic drugs.[154]

▶ PSYCHOGENIC TREMOR

There are two basic types of psychogenic tremor: coherent type and co-contraction type. These two forms of psychogenic tremor are equally common, and electrophysiology is useful in their diagnosis.[155]

The coherent type is produced by a conscious or subconscious rhythmic movement of the affected joint. The tremor frequency is usually about 6 Hz or less because voluntary rhythmic movement at higher frequencies is very difficult and exhausting. People with the coherent form of psychogenic tremor cannot rhythmically move the same or contralateral extremity at a different frequency, except at subharmonics of the psychogenic tremor frequency. The performance of a voluntary rapid rhythmic movement either suppresses psychogenic tremor or causes its frequency to shift to that of the voluntary movement. Poly-EMG and accelerometry are useful in capturing the frequency shifts and interruptions that occur in psychogenic tremor during voluntary movements (Fig. 27–9).[156]

In the co-contraction type of psychogenic tremor, patients consciously or subconsciously coactivate the muscles of the affected body part, which produces an enhanced physiological tremor or physiological clonus.[157] In the hands, one typically sees a 7–10-Hz tremor that is independent (not synchronous) with tremor in the contralateral limb. This tremor occurs only when there is abnormally increased joint stiffness, produced by coactivation of the forearm muscles. This dependence of tremor on coactivation is demonstrated during passive manipulation of the wrist; the amplitude of tremor is proportional to the degree of coactivation ("coactivation sign"), and the tremor stops during interruptions in coactivation.

▶ CONCLUSION

The motor system contains a vast array of central and peripheral feedback loops, oscillating neuronal networks, and underdamped body mechanics. The complex integration of these sources of oscillation has made the elucidation of all tremors exceedingly difficult. Some tremors may emerge from the interaction of two or more anatomical structures, such that the identification of a single anatomical source of tremor is not possible. Nevertheless, considerable progress has been made, and many patients with disabling tremors are now the beneficiaries of a large and rapidly growing research effort.

▶ ACKNOWLEDGMENTS

Supported by NS20973 from the National Institute of Neurological Disorders and Stroke and by the Spastic Paralysis Research Foundation of Kiwanis International, Illinois-Eastern Iowa District.

REFERENCES

1. Elble RJ, Randall JE. Motor-unit activity responsible for 8- to 12-Hz component of human physiological finger tremor. J Neurophysiol 1976;39:370–383.
2. Elble RJ, Randall JE. Mechanistic components of normal hand tremor. Electroencephalogr Clin Neurophysiol 1978;44:72–82.
3. Freund HJ. Motor unit and muscle activity in voluntary motor control. Physiol Rev 1983;63:387–436.
4. Milner-Brown HS, Stein RB, Yemm R. The contractile properties of human motor units during voluntary isometric contractions. J Physiol (Lond) 1973;228:285–306.
5. Hagbarth K-E, Young RR. Participation of the stretch reflex in human physiological tremor. Brain 1979;102:509–526.
6. Young RR, Hagbarth K-E. Physiological tremor enhanced by maneuvers affecting the segmental stretch reflex. J Neurol Neurosurg Psychiatry 1980;43:248–256.
7. Fox JR, Randall JE. Relationship between forearm tremor and the biceps electromyogram. J Appl Physiol 1970;29:103–108.
8. Stiles RN, Randall JE. Mechanical factors in human tremor frequency. J Appl Physiol 1967;23:324–330.
9. Brumlik J, Yap C-B. *Normal Tremor: A Comparative Study*. Springfield, IL: Charles C. Thomas, 1970.
10. Stiles RN. Mechanical and neural feedback factors in postural hand tremor of normal subjects. J Neurophysiol 1980;44:40–59.
11. Rack PMH. Limitations of somatosensory feedback in control of posture and movement. In Brooks V B (ed). Handbook of Physiology: The Nervous System, Motor Control. Baltimore, MD: Williams & Wilkins, 1981, pp. 229–256.
12. Kakuda N, Nagaoka M, Wessberg J. Common modulation of motor unit pairs during slow wrist movement in man. J Physiol (Lond) 1999;520:929–940.
13. Lakie M, Walsh EG, Wright GW. Passive mechanical properties of the wrist and physiological tremor. J Neurol Neurosurg Psychiatry 1986;49:669–676.
14. Brown TI, Rack PM, Ross HF. Different types of tremor in the human thumb. J Physiol 1982;332:113–123.
15. Wessberg J, Vallbo ÅB. Pulsatile motor output in human finger movements is not dependent on the stretch reflex. J Physiol (Lond) 1996;493:895–908.
16. Raethjen J, Lindemann M, Dumpelmann M, et al. Corticomuscular coherence in the 6-15 Hz band: Is the cortex involved in the generation of physiologic tremor? Exp Brain Res 2002;142:32–40.
17. Schnitzler A, Timmermann L, Gross J. Physiological and pathological oscillatory networks in the human motor system. J Physiol (Paris) 2006;99:3–7.
18. Stein RB, Oguztöreli MN. Tremor and other oscillations in neuromuscular systems. Biol Cybern 1976;22:147–157.
19. Wenderoth N, Bock O. Load dependence of simulated central tremor. Biol Cybern 1999;80:285–290.
20. Elble RJ, Schieber MH, Thach WT, Jr. Activity of muscle spindles, motor cortex and cerebellar nuclei during action tremor. Brain Res 323:330–334,.
21. Deuschl G, Bergman H. Pathophysiology of nonparkinsonian tremors. Mov Disord 2002;17(Suppl 3):S41–S48.
22. Rack PMH, Ross HF. The role of reflexes in the resting tremor of Parkinson's disease. Brain 1986;109:115–141.
23. Britton TC, Thompson PD, Day BL, et al. 'Resetting' of postural tremors at the wrist with mechanical stretches in Parkinson's disease, essential tremor, and normal subjects mimicking tremor. Ann Neurol 1992;31: 507–514.
24. Elble RJ, Higgins C, Hughes L. Phase resetting and frequency entrainment of essential tremor. Exp Neurol 1992;116:355–361.
25. Britton TC, Thompson PD, Day BL, et al. Modulation of postural tremors at the wrist by supramaximal electrical median nerve shocks in essential tremor, Parkinson's disease and normal subjects mimicking tremor. J Neurol Neurosurg Psychiatry 1993;56:1085–1089.
26. Bock O, Wenderoth N. Dependence of peripheral tremor on mechanical perturbations: Modeling study. Biol Cybern 1999;80:103–108.
27. Elble RJ. Central mechanisms of tremor. J Clin Neurophysiol 1996;13:133–144.
28. Britton TC, Thompson PD, Day BL, et al. Modulation of postural wrist tremors by magnetic stimulation of the motor cortex in patients with PD and essential tremor and in normal subjects mimicking tremor. Ann Neurol 1993;33:473–479.
29. Pascual-Leone A, Valls-Solé J, Toro C, et al. Resetting of essential tremor and postural tremor in Parkinson's disease with transcranial magnetic stimulation. Muscle Nerve 1994;17:800–807.
30. Boecker H, Brooks DJ. Functional imaging of tremor. Mov Disord 1998;13:64–72.
31. Andrew J, Fowler CJ, Harrison MJ. Tremor after head injury and its treatment by stereotaxic surgery. J Neurol Neurosurg Psychiatry 1982;45:815–819.
32. Ohye C, Miyazaki M, Hirai T, et al. Primary writing tremor treated by stereotactic selective thalamotomy. J Neurol Neurosurg Psychiatry 1982;45:988–997.
33. Schuurman PR, Bosch DA, Bossuyt PM, et al. A comparison of continuous thalamic stimulation and thalamotomy for suppression of severe tremor [see comments]. N Engl J Med 2000;342:461–468.

34. Krauss JK, Simpson RK, Jr., Ondo WG, et al. Concepts and methods in chronic thalamic stimulation for treatment of tremor: technique and application. Neurosurgery 2001;48:535–541; discussion 541–533.
35. Guridi J, Rodriguez-Oroz MC, Arbizu J, et al. Successful thalamic deep brain stimulation for orthostatic tremor. Mov Disord 2008;23:1808–1811.
36. Hirai T, Jones EG. A new parcellation of the human thalamus on the basis of histochemical staining. Brain Res Brain Res Rev 1989;14:1–34.
37. Ohye C, Shibazaki T, Hirai T, et al. Further physiological observations on the ventralis intermedius neurons in the human thalamus. J Neurophysiol 1989;61:488–500.
38. Inase M, Tanji J. Thalamic distribution of projection neurons to the primary motor cortex relative to afferent terminal fields from the globus pallidus in the macaque monkey. J Comp Neurol 1995;353:415–426.
39. Sakai ST, Inase M, Tanji J. Comparison of cerebellothalamic and pallidothalamic projections in the monkey (Macaca fuscata): a double anterograde labeling study. J Comp Neurol 1996;368:215–228.
40. Louis ED: Essential tremor. Lancet Neurol 2005;4: 100–110.
41. Deng H, Le W, Jankovic J. Genetics of essential tremor. Brain 2007;130(Pt 6):1456–1464.
42. Elble RJ. Diagnostic criteria for essential tremor and differential diagnosis. Neurology 2000;54:S2–S6.
43. Whaley NR, Putzke JD, Baba Y, et al. Essential tremor: Phenotypic expression in a clinical cohort. Parkinsonism Relat Disord. 2007;13:333–339.
44. Louis ED, Faust PL, Vonsattel JP, et al. Neuropathological changes in essential tremor: 33 cases compared with 21 controls. Brain 2007;130:3297–3307.
45. Axelrad JE, Louis ED, Honig LS, et al. Reduced Purkinje cell number in essential tremor: A postmortem study. Arch Neurol 2008;65:101–107.
46. Hellwig B, Häussler S, Schelter B, et al. Tremor-correlated cortical activity in essential tremor. Lancet 2001;357: 519–523.
47. Deuschl G, Elble RJ. The pathophysiology of essential tremor. Neurology 2000;54:S14-S20.
48. Lakie M, Walsh EG, Arblaster LA, et al. Limb temperature and human tremors. J Neurol Neurosurg Psychiatry 1994;57:35–42.
49. Elble RJ, Higgins C, Moody CJ. Stretch reflex oscillations and essential tremor. J Neurol Neurosurg Psychiatry 1987;50:691–698.
50. Elble RJ, Higgins C, Leffler K, et al. Factors influencing the amplitude and frequency of essential tremor [published erratum appears in Mov Disord 1995 May;10(3):411]. Mov Disord 1994;9:589–596.
51. Elble RJ. Physiologic and essential tremor. Neurology 1986;36:225–231.
52. Elble RJ, Higgins C, Elble S. Electrophysiologic transition from physiologic tremor to essential tremor. Mov Disord 2005;20:1038–1042.
53. Elble RJ. Essential tremor frequency decreases with time. Neurology 2000;55:1547–1551.
54. Elble RJ. The role of aging in the clinical expression of essential tremor. Exp Gerontol 1995;30:337–347.
55. Zesiewicz TA, Elble R, Louis ED, et al. Practice parameter: therapies for essential tremor: report of the Quality Standards Subcommittee of the American Academy of Neurology. Neurology 2005;64:2008–2020.
56. Herzog J, Hamel W, Wenzelburger R, et al. Kinematic analysis of thalamic versus subthalamic neurostimulation in postural and intention tremor. Brain 2007;130:1608–1625.
57. Murata J, Kitagawa M, Uesugi H, et al. Electrical stimulation of the posterior subthalamic area for the treatment of intractable proximal tremor. J Neurosurg 2003;99:708–715.
58. Plaha P, Patel NK, Gill SS. Stimulation of the subthalamic region for essential tremor. J Neurosurg 2004;101:48–54.
59. Stover NP, Okun MS, Evatt ML, et al. Stimulation of the subthalamic nucleus in a patient with Parkinson disease and essential tremor. Arch Neurol 2005;62:141–143.
60. Jankovic J, Schwartz KS, Ondo W. Re-emergent tremor of Parkinson's disease. J Neurol Neurosurg Psychiatry 1999;67:646–650.
61. Bergman H, Raz A, Feingold A, et al. Physiology of MPTP tremor. Mov Disord 1998;13:29–34.
62. Tetrud JW, Langston JW. MPTP-induced parkinsonism and tremor. In Findley LJ, Koller WC (eds). Handbook of Tremor Disorders. New York: Marcel Dekker, 1995, pp. 319–350.
63. Volkmann J, Joliot M, Mogilner A, et al. Central motor loop oscillations in parkinsonian resting tremor revealed by magnetoencephalography. Neurology 1996;46:1359–1370.
64. Lenz FA, Kwan HC, Martin RL, et al. Single unit analysis of the human ventral thalamic nuclear group. Tremor-related activity in functionally identified cells. Brain 1994;117:531–543.
65. Hua S, Reich SG, Zirh AT, et al. The role of the thalamus and basal ganglia in parkinsonian tremor. Mov Disord 1998;13:40–42.
66. Hurtado JM, Gray CM, Tamas LB, et al. Dynamics of tremor-related oscillations in the human globus pallidus: a single case study. Proc Natl Acad Sci U S A 1999;96: 1674–1679.
67. Hutchison WD, Allan RJ, Opitz H, et al. Neurophysiological identification of the subthalamic nucleus in surgery for Parkinson's disease. Ann Neurol 1998;44:622–628.
68. Levy R, Hutchison WD, Lozano AM, et al. High-frequency synchronization of neuronal activity in the subthalamic nucleus of parkinsonian patients with limb tremor. J Neurosci 2000;20:7766–7775.
69. Magnin M, Morel A, Jeanmonod D. Single-unit analysis of the pallidum, thalamus and subthalamic nucleus in parkinsonian patients. Neuroscience 2000;96:549–564.
70. Magarinos-Ascone CM, Figueiras-Mendez R, Riva-Meana C, et al. Subthalamic neuron activity related to tremor and movement in Parkinson's disease. Eur J Neurosci 2000;12:2597–2607.
71. Deuschl G, Wilms H, Krack P, et al. Function of the cerebellum in Parkinsonian rest tremor and Holmes' tremor. Ann Neurol 1999;46:126–128.
72. Wichmann T, Bergman H, DeLong MR. The primate subthalamic nucleus. III. Changes in motor behavior and neuronal activity in the internal pallidum induced by subthalamic inactivation in the MPTP model of parkinsonism. J Neurophysiol 1994;72:521–530.
73. Elble RJ. Origins of tremor. Lancet 2000;355:1113–1114.
74. Krack P, Poepping M, Weinert D, et al. Thalamic, pallidal, or subthalamic surgery for Parkinson's disease? J Neurol 2000;247(Suppl 2):II122–134.

75. Bakay RAE, Vitek JL, DeLong MR. Thalamotomy for tremor. Neurosurgical Operative Atlas 1992;2:299–312.
76. Stepniewska I, Preuss TM, Kaas JH. Thalamic connections of the primary motor cortex (M1) of owl monkeys. J Comp Neurol 1994;349:558–582.
77. Herzog J, Fietzek U, Hamel W, et al. Most effective stimulation site in subthalamic deep brain stimulation for Parkinson's disease. Mov Disord 2004;19:1050–1054.
78. Plaha P, Ben-Shlomo Y, Patel NK, et al. Stimulation of the caudal zona incerta is superior to stimulation of the subthalamic nucleus in improving contralateral parkinsonism. Brain 2006;129:1732–1747.
79. Holmes G. The symptoms of acute cerebellar injuries due to gunshot injuries. Brain 1917;40:461–535.
80. Vilis T, Hore J. Effects of changes in mechanical state of limb on cerebellar intention tremor. J Neurophysiol 1977;40:1214–1224.
81. Gilman S, Carr D, Hollenberg J. Kinematic effects of deafferentation and cerebellar ablation. Brain 1976;99: 311–330.
82. Sanes JN, LeWitt PA, Mauritz K-H. Visual and mechanical control of postural and kinetic tremor in cerebellar system disorders. J Neurol Neurosurg Psychiatry 1988;51: 934–943.
83. Elble RJ. Animal models of action tremor. Mov Disord 1998;13:35–39.
84. Bastian AJ, Thach WT. Cerebellar outflow lesions: A comparison of movement deficits resulting from lesions at the levels of the cerebellum and thalamus. Ann Neurol 1995;38:881–892.
85. Qureshi F, Morales A, Elble RJ. Tremor due to infarction in the ventrolateral thalamus. Mov Disord 1996;11: 440–444.
86. Thach WT, Goodkin HP, Keating JG. The cerebellum and the adaptive coordination of movement. Ann Rev Neurosci 1992;15:403–442.
87. Hore J, Vilis T. A cerebellar-dependent efference copy mechanism for generating appropriate muscle responses to limb perturbations. In Bloedel JR, Dichgans J, Precht W (eds). Cerebellar Functions. Berlin: Springer-Verlag, 1984, pp. 24–35.
88. Diener H-C, Dichgans J. Pathophysiology of cerebellar ataxia. Mov Disord 1992;7:95–109.
89. Murphy JT, Kwan HC, MacKay WA, et al. Physiological basis of cerebellar dysmetria. Can J Neurol Sci 1975;2: 279–284.
90. Li Volsi G, Pacitti C, Perciavalle V, et al. Interpositus nucleus influences on pyramidal tract neurons in the cat. Neuroscience. 1982;7:1929–1936.
91. Topka H, Mescheriakov S, Boose A, et al. A cerebellar-like terminal and postural tremor induced in normal man by transcranial magnetic stimulation. Brain 1999;122: 1551–1562.
92. Houk JC, Keifer J, Barto AG. Distributed motor commands in the limb premotor network. Trends Neurosci 1993;16:27–33.
93. De Zeeuw CI, Simpson JI, Hoogenraad CC, et al. Microcircuitry and function of the inferior olive. Trends Neurosci 1998;21:391–400.
94. Nakamura R, Kamakura K, Tadano Y, et al. MR imaging findings of tremors associated with lesions in cerebellar outflow tracts: Report of two cases. Mov Disord 1993;8:209–212.
95. Remy P, de Recondo A, Defer G, et al. Peduncular "rubral" tremor and dopaminergic denervation: A PET study. Neurology 1995;45:472–477.
96. Holmes G. On certain tremors in organic cerebral lesions. Brain 1904;27:327–375.
97. Ohye C, Shibazaki T, Hirai T, et al. A special role of the parvocellular red nucleus in lesion-induced spontaneous tremor in monkeys. Behav Brain Res 1988;28:241–243.
98. Deuschl G, Bain P, Brin M. Consensus statement of the Movement Disorder Society on Tremor. Ad Hoc Scientific Committee. Mov Disord 1998;13:2–23.
99. Goldman MS, Kelly PJ. The surgical treatment of tremor. In Findley LJ, Koller WC (eds). Handbook of Tremor Disorders. New York: Marcel Dekker, 1995, pp. 521–562.
100. Deuschl G, Mischke G, Schenck E, et al. Symptomatic and essential rhythmic palatal myoclonus. Brain 1990;113:1645–1672.
101. Birbamer G, Buchberger W, Kampfl A, et al. Early detection of post-traumatic olivary hypertrophy by MRI. J Neurol 1993;240:407–409.
102. Uchino A, Hasuo K, Uchida K, et al. Olivary degeneration after cerebellar or brain stem haemorrhage: MRI. Neuroradiology. 1993;35:335–338.
103. Deuschl G, Toro C, Hallett M. Symptomatic and essential palatal tremor. 2. Differences of palatal movements. Mov Disord 1994;9:676–678.
104. Deuschl G, Toro C, Valls-Sole J, et al. Symptomatic and essential palatal tremor. 1. Clinical, physiological and MRI analysis. Brain 1994;117:775–788.
105. Birbamer G, Gerstenbrand F, Kofler M, et al. Post-traumatic segmental myoclonus associated with bilateral olivary hypertrophy. Acta Neurol Scand 1993;87:505–509.
106. Hong S, Leigh RJ, Zee DS, et al. Inferior olive hypertrophy and cerebellar learning are both needed to explain ocular oscillations in oculopalatal tremor. Prog Brain Res 2008;171:219–226.
107. Elble RJ. Inhibition of forearm EMG by palatal myoclonus. Mov Disord 1991;6:324–329.
108. Masucci E, Kurtzke J. Palatal myoclonus associated with extremity tremor. J Neurol 1989;236:474–477.
109. Masucci EF, Kurtzke JF, Saini N. Myorhythmia: a widespread movement disorder. Clinicopathological correlations. Brain 1984;107:53–79.
110. Miyagi Y, Shima F, Ishido K, et al. Posteroventral pallidotomy for midbrain tremor after a pontine hemorrhage. J Neurosurg 1999;91:885–888.
111. Kim JS. Delayed onset hand tremor caused by cerebral infarction. Stroke 1992;23:292–294.
112. Ferbert A, Gerwig M. Tremor due to stroke. Mov Disord 1993;8:179–182.
113. Bhatia KP, Marsden CD. The behavioural and motor consequences of focal lesions of the basal ganglia in man. Brain 1994;117:859–876.
114. Lee MS, Marsden CD. Movement disorders following lesions of the thalamus or subthalamic region. Mov Disord 1994;9:493–507.
115. Shahani BT: Tremor associated with peripheral neuropathy. In Findley LJ, Capildeo R (eds). Movement Disorders: Tremor. London: Macmillan, 1984, pp. 389–398.

116. Smith IS, Kahn SN, Lacey BW, et al. Chronic demyelinating neuropathy associated with benign IgM paraproteinaemia. Brain 1983;106:169–195.
117. Said G, Bathien N, Cesaro P. Peripheral neuropathies and tremor. Neurology 1982;32:480–485.
118. Dalakas MC, Teravainen H, Engel WK. Tremor as a feature of chronic relapsing and dysgammaglobulinemic polyneuropathies. Incidence and management. Arch Neurol 1984;41:711–714.
119. Bain PG, Britton TC, Jenkins IH, et al. Tremor associated with benign IgM paraproteinaemic neuropathy. Brain 1996;119:789–799.
120. Cardoso F, Jankovic J. Peripherally induced tremor and parkinsonism. Arch Neurol 1995;52:263–270.
121. Elble RJ, Moody C, Higgins C. Primary writing tremor. A form of focal dystonia? Mov Disord 1990;5:118–126.
122. Wills AJ, Jenkins IH, Thompson PD, et al. A positron emission tomography study of cerebral activation associated with essential and writing tremor. Arch Neurol 1995;52:299–305.
123. Rothwell JC, Traub MM, Marsden CD. Primary writing tremor. J Neurol Neurosurg Psychiatry. 1979;42: 1106–1114.
124. Ravits J, Hallett M, Baker M, et al. Primary writing tremor and myoclonic writer's cramp. Neurology 1985;35: 1387–1391.
125. Rosenbaum F, Jankovic J. Focal task-specific tremor and dystonia: Categorization of occupational movement disorders. Neurology 1988;38:522–527.
126. Yanagisawa N, Goto A, Narabayashi H. Familial dystonia musculorum deformans and tremor. J Neurol Sci 1972;16:125–136.
127. Sheehy MP, Marsden CD. Writers' cramp-a focal dystonia. Brain 1982;105:461–480.
128. Deuschl G, Heinen F, Kleedorfer B, et al. Clinical and polymyographic investigation of spasmodic torticollis. J Neurol 1992;239:9–15.
129. Rivest J, Marsden CD. Trunk and head tremor as isolated manifestations of dystonia. Mov Disord 1990;5:60–65.
130. Heilman KM. Orthostatic tremor. Arch Neurol 1984;41: 880–881.
131. Thompson PD, Rothwell JC, Day BL, et al. The physiology of orthostatic tremor. Arch Neurol 1986;43:584–587.
132. Kelly JJ, Sharbrough FW. EMG in orthostatic tremor. Neurology. 1987;37:1434.
133. McManis PG, Sharbrough FW. Orthostatic tremor: Clinical and electrophysiologic characteristics. Muscle Nerve 1993;16:1254–1260.
134. Köster B, Lauk M, Timmer J, et al. Involvement of cranial muscles and high intermuscular coherence in orthostatic tremor. Ann Neurol 1999;45:384–388.
135. Fung VS, Sauner D, Day BL. A dissociation between subjective and objective unsteadiness in primary orthostatic tremor. Brain 2001;124:322–330.
136. Bain PG, Findley LJ, Thompson PD, et al. A study of hereditary essential tremor. Brain 1994;117:805–824.
137. Wills AJ, Thompson PD, Findley LJ, et al. A positron emission tomography study of primary orthostatic tremor. Neurology 1996;46:747–752.
138. Tsai CH, Semmler JG, Kimber TE, et al. Modulation of primary orthostatic tremor by magnetic stimulation over the motor cortex. J Neurol Neurosurg Psychiatry 1998;64:33–36.
139. Wu YR, Ashby P, Lang AE. Orthostatic tremor arises from an oscillator in the posterior fossa. Mov Disord 2001;16:272–279.
140. Ikeda A, Kakigi R, Funai N, et al. Cortical tremor: A variant of cortical reflex myoclonus. *Neurology*. 40:1561–1565,1990.
141. Toro C, Pascual-Leone A, Deuschl G, et al. Cortical tremor. A common manifestation of cortical myoclonus. Neurology 1993;43:2346–2353.
142. Oguni E, Hayashi A, Ishii A, et al. A case of cortical tremor as a variant of cortical reflex myoclonus. Eur Neurol 1995;35:63–64.
143. Young RR. What is a tremor? Neurology 2002;58: 165–166.
144. Terada K, Ikeda A, Mima T, et al. Familial cortical myoclonic tremor as a unique form of cortical reflex myoclonus. Mov Disord 1997;12:370–377.
145. Okuma Y, Shimo Y, Shimura H, et al. Familial cortical tremor with epilepsy: An under-recognized familial tremor. Clin Neurol Neurosurg 1998;100:75–78.
146. Bourdain F, Apartis E, Trocello JM, et al. Clinical analysis in familial cortical myoclonic tremor allows differential diagnosis with essential tremor. Mov Disord 2006;21: 599–608.
147. Morgan JC, Sethi KD. Drug-induced tremors. Lancet Neurol 2005;4:866–876.
148. Prien RF, Caffey EM, Jr., Klett CJ. Lithium carbonate. A survey of the history and current status of lithium in treating mood disorders. Dis Nerv Syst 1971;32:521–531.
149. Donaldson IM, Cuningham J. Persisting neurologic sequelae of lithium carbonate therapy. Arch Neurol 1983;40:747–751.
150. Charness ME, Morady F, Scheinman MM. Frequent neurologic toxicity associated with amiodarone therapy. Neurology 1984;34:669–671.
151. Palakurthy PR, Iyer V, Meckler RJ. Unusual neurotoxicity associated with amiodarone therapy. Arch Intern Med 1987;147:881–884.
152. Werner EG, Olanow CW. Parkinsonism and amiodarone therapy. Ann Neurol 1989;25:630–632.
153. Schneider JA, Mirra SS. Neuropathologic correlates of persistent neurologic deficit in lithium intoxication. Ann Neurol 1994;36:928–931.
154. Burn DJ, Brooks DJ. Nigral dysfunction in drug-induced parkinsonism: An ^{18}F-dopa PET study. Neurology 1993;43:552–556.
155. Raethjen J, Kopper F, Govindan RB, et al. Two different pathogenetic mechanisms in psychogenic tremor. Neurology 2004;63:812–815.
156. McAuley J, Rothwell J. Identification of psychogenic, dystonic, and other organic tremors by a coherence entrainment test. Mov Disord 2004;19:253–267.
157. Deuschl G, Köster B, Lücking CH, et al. Diagnostic and pathophysiological aspects of psychogenic tremors. Mov Disord 1998;13:294–302.

CHAPTER 28

Genetic Forms of Dystonia

Susan B. Bressman

Genetic causes have long been suspected in many subtypes of dystonia. The earliest descriptions of early-onset primary dystonia in the first decades of the 20th century contained important clues to its genetic etiology. In recent decades, advances in molecular biology have led to the identification of an increasing number of genes for both primary and secondary dystonia subtypes. The identification of dystonia genes has, in turn, led to a clearer understanding of dystonia and to important changes in both clinical and basic science approaches to dystonia. With the advent of gene discovery, further investigations into the basic pathogenic mechanisms of dystonia using cellular and animal models have become possible, our understanding of the phenotypic spectrum of gene expression has been broadened, and the way that neurologists diagnose and counsel patients with dystonia has been altered. Ultimately, a more complete understanding of the genetic causes of dystonia and their mechanisms holds the promise of rational, targeted therapies.

▶ CLASSIFICATION OF DYSTONIA

Dystonia is a clinically defined movement disorder characterized by involuntary sustained postures and repetitive movements that result from co-contraction of agonist and antagonist muscles.[1] Dystonia is a clinically and etiologically heterogeneous condition. The clinical spectrum of dystonia is very broad, ranging from generalized, disabling contractions, which are much more common in those with early-onset disease, to localized or focal involvement, most commonly seen in those with adult-onset symptoms; focal adult-onset dystonia typically affects the cervical muscles (e.g., torticollis), cranial muscles (e.g., blepharospasm, hemifacial spasm, spasmodic dysphonia), or the arm (e.g., writer's cramp).

Dystonia can be classified according to age of onset (early-onset versus late-onset), distribution (focal, segmental, multifocal, or generalized), and etiology (primary or secondary). When classified by etiology, dystonia is divided into the two broad categories: primary torsion dystonia (PTD, previously named idiopathic torsion dystonia), and secondary (nonprimary) dystonia. PTD is defined as a syndrome in which dystonia is the only neurological clinical sign (except for tremor), and in which there is no evidence of a neurodegenerative process or an acquired cause. The primary dystonias include both early-onset and adult-onset forms. Early-onset dystonia typically first affects a limb and then spreads, whereas late-onset dystonia typically starts in the cervical, cranial, or brachial muscles and usually remains focal or segmental. Adult-onset dystonia (which most commonly affects the cervical muscles) constitutes the great majority of primary dystonia. The PTDs were previously termed "idiopathic torsion dystonia" because of the lack of etiology or consistent pathological or neurochemical abnormality. However, with the determination of genetic etiologies of "idiopathic" dystonia, beginning with the identification of the *DYT1* gene in 1997, the term "primary" has since replaced "idiopathic."

Secondary dystonias include all nonprimary dystonia subtypes; many have neurological signs other than dystonia and anatomic or biochemical changes involving the basal ganglia. The secondary dystonias can be subdivided into those with acquired etiologies, due to inherited neurodegenerative diseases, and the dystonia plus syndromes, due to hereditary nondegenerative neurological disorders that differ from primary dystonia because there are characteristic clinical features other than dystonia, such as parkinsonism or myoclonus (see DYSTONIA PLUS SYNDROMES). Finally, dystonia may be a feature of other movement disorders, including the degenerative parkinsonian disorders and other dyskinetic movement disorders, including tic disorders (dystonic tics) and the paroxysmal dyskinesias (PKD, paroxysmal nonkinesigenic dyskinesia [PNKD], paroxysmal exertion-induced dyskinesia [PED]) (see Table 28–1).

This chapter focuses on genetic forms of early-onset primary dystonia and the dystonia plus syndromes. Genetic etiologies have also been identified in many inherited neurodegenerative diseases associated with secondary dystonia, as well as in a family with adult-onset primary dystonia (DYT7). The secondary dystonias and adult-onset primary dystonias are discussed in detail in later chapters.

▶ TABLE 28-1. **CLASSIFICATION OF DYSTONIA BY ETIOLOGY**

I. Primary Dystonia (formerly idiopathic): Dystonia is the only movement disorder, and there is no secondary etiology.
1. Early onset: Onset in childhood or adolescence (up to 26 years), usually limb onset with spread to other regions.
   - DYT1
   - Other genes not yet identified (e.g., autosomal-recessive DYT2).
2. Mixed phenotype: Primarily early usually with onset in neck, cranial muscles, or arm, with spread to other regions
   - DYT6 (THAP1), identified in Mennonite kindreds and also other families of European ancestry, dysarthria a common feature
   - DYT13 (gene not identified): One Italian family with segmental cervical and cranial muscle involvement
   - DYT17 (gene not identified): One Lebanese family
3. Adult onset (>26 years), usually onset in neck, cranial muscles, or arm; remains focal or segmental
   - DYT7 (gene not identified): in a German family with torticollis
   - Other genes and causes not yet identified

II. Secondary Dystonia

A. Dystonia associated with hereditary neurological syndromes

1. **Dystonia plus syndromes:** inherited neurological syndromes with no evidence of neurodegeneration; features other than dystonia are present.
   DRD
   - Most due to GTP cyclohydrolase I (*GCH1*) mutations (*DYT5*)
   - TH mutations
   - Other biopterin-deficient states

   MD
   - Many familial cases are due to SGCE mutations (*DYT11*)
   - Due to *DYT15* on Chr18 in one family; gene not identified

   RDP
   - Due to ATP1A3 mutations (*DYT*12)

   Dystonia-parkinsonism
   - Due to PRKRA (DYT16)
2. **Heredodegenerative disorders:** inherited neurological disorders associated with neurodegeneration.
   Autosomal dominant
      HD
      Machado-Joseph's disease/SCA3 disease
      Other SCA subtypes (e.g., SCA 2, 6, 17)
      Familial basal ganglia calcifications (Fahr's)
      DRPLA
      Neuroferritinopathy, etc.
   Autosomal recessive
      Juvenile parkinsonism (Parkin)
      Wilson's
      Glutaric acidemia
      NBIA/PKAN/Hallervorden-Spatz disease
      Gangliosidoses (GM1, GM2)
      Metachromatic leukodystrophy
      Homocystinuria
      Propionic acidemia
      Methylmalonic aciduria
      Dystonic lipidosis/Neimann Pick type C (NPC1)
      Ceroid-lipofuscinosis
      AT
      Ataxia with vitamin E deficiency
      Recessive ataxia with ocular apraxia
      Neuroacanthocytosis
      Neuronal intranuclear inclusion disease (NIID), etc.
   X-linked recessive
      Lubag (X-linked dystonia-parkinsonism, *DYT*3)
      Lesch–Nylan syndrome
      Deafness/dystonia
      Pelizaeus-Merzbacher disease

(continued)

▶ TABLE 28-1. CONTINUED

Mitochondrial
- MERRF/MELAS
- Leber's disease

B. Dystonia due to acquired/exogenous causes
- Perinatal cerebral injury
- Encephalitis, infectious, and postinfectious
- Paraneoplastic
- Head trauma
- Pontine myelinolysis
- Primary antiphospholipid syndrome
- Stroke
- Tumor
- Multiple sclerosis
- Cervical cord injury or lesion
- Peripheral injury
- Complex regional pain syndrome
- Drugs
  - Especially dopamine receptor blockers: acute and tardive dystonic syndromes
- Toxins

C. Dystonia due to degenerative parkinsonian disorders
- PD
- PSP
- MSA
- CBGD

D. Dystonia as a feature of other dyskinetic disorders
- Tics (dystonic tics)
- Paroxysmal dyskinesia disorders
  - PKD (*DYT 10*/EKD1, EKD2)
  - PNKD (*DYT*8)
  - CSE (*DYT* 9)

DRD, dopa-responsive dystonia; TH, tyrosine hydroxylase; MD, myoclonus-dystonia; SGCE, ε-sarcoglycan; RDP, rapid-onset dystonia-parkinsonism; HD, Huntington's disease; DRPLA, dentato-rubral pallido-luisian atrophy; AT, ataxia-telangiectasia; NIID, neuronal intranuclear inclusion disease; MERRF/MELAS, mitochondrial encephalopathy with ragged red fibers/mitochondrial encephalopathy with lactic acidosis; PD, Parkinson disease; PSP, progressive supranuclear palsy; MSA, multisystem atrophy; CBGD, cortico-basal-ganglionic degeneration.

▶ MOLECULAR CLASSIFICATION OF DYSTONIA

There is no unified genetic classification that systematically catalogues both primary and secondary dystonia; there is, however, a genetic classification based on HUGO/Genome Database nomenclature (http://www.genenames.org) that designates DYT/dystonia loci. It includes all the loci for PTD, a subset of loci for secondary dystonia, and also includes loci for the paroxysmal dyskinesias (see Table 28–2). This classification system designates *DYT* genes in chronological order of either clinical description or gene mapping of specific dystonia syndromes. It currently lists DYT1-18. (The locus initially designated DYT14 was later found to be identical to DYT5, so that there is now no DYT14; see DOPA-RESPONSIVE DYSTONIA.) The HUGO DYT designations are not as clinically useful as the classification schema by etiology or clinical features, as the molecular designations are organized solely by chronological order of discovery, and therefore include dystonias of various clinical and etiological subtypes without distinction: primary dystonias (*DYT1*, *DYT6*, *DYT7*, *DYT13*), some forms of secondary dystonia (*DYT3*), and the dystonia plus syndromes (*DYT5*, *DYT11*, *DYT12*, *DYT15*). They also include the paroxysmal dyskinesia syndromes (*DYT8*, *DYT9*, *DYT10*), which are usually clinically classified as paroxysmal dyskinetic disorders rather than as dystonias.

Two of the primary dystonia genes have been identified: *DYT1* (*TOR1A*)[2] and *DYT6*,[3] and five other nonprimary *DYT* genes have been identified: *DYT3* (X-linked dystonia-parkinsonism, or "Lubag")[4]; *DYT5* (now relabeled *GCH1*)[5]; *DYT11* (*SGCE*)[6]; *DYT12* (*ATP1A3*)[7]; and *DYT16* (*PRKRA*).[8] A gene (*MR-1*) has also been identified for *DYT8*, a paroxysmal dyskinesia disorder,[9] and *DYT18* refers to PED occurring in association with a mutation in the *GLUT1* transporter gene, *SLC2A1*.[9,10] Loci for most of the other HUGO DYT subtypes have been identified. The exceptions are DYT2, autosomal-recessive dystonia in the Spanish Roma population,[11] and *DYT4*, whispering dysphonia,[12] which have been clinically described but for which no locus has been established.

▶ **TABLE 28-2. MOLECULAR CLASSIFICATION OF DYSTONIA**

Designation	Dystonia type	Inheritance	Gene locus	Gene/Product	OMIM number
DYT1	Early-onset PTD	Autosomal dominant	9q	GAG deletion in DYT1 coding for torsinA	128100
DYT2	Autosomal-recessive early-onset TD	Autosomal recessive	Unknown	Unknown	224500
DYT3	X-linked dystonia-parkinsonism; "lubag"	X-chromo-somal recessive	Xq	TAF1/DYT3	314250
DYT4	"Non-DYT1" whispering dysphonia, in 1 family	Autosomal dominant	Unknown	Unknown	128101
DYT5/DYT14	Dopa-responsive dystonia (Segawa disease)	Autosomal dominant	14q	GTP-cyclohydrolase1	128230
		Autosomal recessive			
			11p	Tyrosine hydroxylase	
DYT6	Adolescent/early adult -onset TD of mixed type	Autosomal dominant	8p	Unknown	602629
DYT7	Adult-onset focal TD (cervical, cranial, brachial)	Autosomal dominant	18p	Unknown	602124
DYT8	PNKD	Autosomal dominant	2q	Myofibrillo-genesis regulator 1 (MR-1)	118800
DYT9	Paroxysmal choreoathetosis with episodic ataxia and spasticity	Autosomal dominant	1p	Unknown	601042
DYT10	Paroxysmal kinesigenic choreoathetosis	Autosomal dominant	16p-q	Unknown	128200
DYT11	Myoclonus-dystonia	Autosomal dominant	7q	ε-Sarcoglycan (SGCE)	159900
DYT12	Rapid-onset dystonia parkinsonism	Autosomal dominant	19q	Na/K ATPase α-3 (ATP1A3)	128235
DYT13	Early- and late-onset cervical/cranial dystonia (in one Italian family)	Autosomal dominant	1p	Unknown	607671
DYT15	Myoclonus-dystonia	Autosomal dominant	18p	Unknown	607488
DYT16	Dystonia-parkinsonism	Autosomal recessive	2q	PRKRA	612067
DYT17	Adolescent-onset focal/ segmental dystonia (in 1 Lebanese family)	Autosomal recessive	20p-q	Unknown	612406
DYT18	PED; (with hemolytic anemia)	Autosomal dominant	1p	SLC2A1	612126

PED, Paroxysmal exertion-induced dyskinesia; PNKD, paroxysmal nonkinesigenic dyskinesia; PTD, primary torsion dystonia.

▶ EARLY-ONSET PRIMARY TORSION DYSTONIAS

DYT1

Early-onset PTD

Early-onset PTD usually begins in childhood or adolescence with a cutoff variously defined as before 22 or 26 years. Typically, dystonia starts in a limb with leg dystonia having an earlier age-onset than arm. Regardless of which limb is first affected, the dystonia often spreads to other regions, and the likelihood of spread is closely associated with the age at onset (the earlier the onset the more likely the dystonia will spread).[13] Two major genes have been identified that cause early-onset PTD; *DYT1* and *DYT6*. There are phenotypic differences but also overlap between these genetic subtypes. *DYT1* predominantly involves the legs, arms, and axial muscles, and gait and writing are often significantly affected; *DYT6* more frequently affects the arms, cervical and cranial muscles, and speech rather than gait is a significant source of disability (see below). These early-onset subtypes contrast to adult-onset primary dystonia, which typically presents in cervical and cranial muscles rather than in the limbs and usually remains focal or segmental, that is, the dystonia does not spread widely to other body sites.

DYT1

History

The first description of early-onset dystonia was in 1908 by Schwalbe, who described an Eastern European family of Ashkenazi Jewish descent in which three siblings were affected with what we now know to be childhood-onset dystonia.[14] The term dystonia was not yet coined, and Schwalbe used the term "chronic cramps." He also described the movements as hysterical in origin. In 1911, Oppenheim reported the same disorder,[15] but argued for an organic basis and invented the term dystonia, naming the condition "dystonia musculorum deformans." In recognition of his contribution, this form of dystonia, later discovered to be DYT1 dystonia, also carries the name Oppenheim's dystonia. In his report, Oppenheim did not recognize that the disorder was inherited. This was pointed out in another report later that same year.[16] Thus, the earliest descriptions of early-onset primary dystonia contained important clues to its genetic etiology. But progress toward further understanding of the inherited nature of the disorder was stymied for over the next half a century, in part, due to nosologic confusion by authors who lumped together what we now categorize as primary and secondary dystonias. In a landmark article in 1967, Zeman and Dyken[17] analyzed pedigrees of 253 primary dystonia cases and reached two important conclusions about the genetics of the disorder that have since been definitively confirmed: that the disorder is inherited as an autosomal-dominant trait with reduced penetrance, and they estimated a five-fold increased gene frequency in Ashkenazi Jews compared to non-Jews. In subsequent decades, further astute clinical observation and disease classification, led by David Marsden[18,19] and Stanley Fahn,[20] together with the application of new molecular advances and genetic epidemiological tools,[21–23] laid the foundation for the current era of gene discovery in dystonia, which began with the identification of the gene for DYT1 dystonia in 1997, now called *TOR1A* in the HUGO classification.[2]

DYT1 Epidemiology

DYT1 is an important cause of early-onset PTD; most clinic-based studies of generalized childhood and adolescent onset dystonia find that about 50% of non-Jewish and 90% of Ashkenazi Jewish cases are due to mutations in the *TORA* gene.[24,25] The disease frequency of DYT1 dystonia is estimated to be 1:3000 to 1:9000 (with a gene frequency of 1:2000–1:6000) in Ashkenazi Jews, and 1:9000 to 1:36,000 in the non-Jewish population. The increased disease frequency in Ashkenazi Jews is likely the result of a founder mutation in the gene postulated to have occurred in the 1600s in Lithuania or Byelorussia.[26] Although patients with early-onset PTD who are Ashkenazi Jewish are more likely to have a *DYT1* mutation, DYT1 dystonia is also present in non-Jewish populations throughout the world,[27] including Eastern and Western Europe, South America, and Asia. The rate of de novo DYT1 mutations is not known, but these have been reported in Mennonite, non-Jewish Russian, and Danish individuals.[28] DYT1 dystonia should therefore be considered in the differential diagnosis of all early-onset PTD, regardless of ethnic background.

DYT1 Clinical features

The great majority of people with DYT1 dystonia develop symptoms within a window of early onset, after age 3 and before age 26, with the mean age of onset at 13 years. A small proportion begins later in life; many of the reported late-onset cases (as late as 64 years) were identified through family studies, and most of these individuals had brachial dystonia that was not medically diagnosed previously.

DYT1 dystonia first affects a limb in over 90% of cases (arm or leg equally), and one or more limbs are almost always affected.[25] The dystonia rarely starts in the neck (3.3%) or larynx (2.2%). Approximately 67% of patients progress over 5–10 years to a generalized (spread of dystonia to both legs or to one leg and the trunk) or multifocal distribution, with the rest having either segmental (12%) or focal (21%) involvement. Spread to cervical or cranial muscles is less common (about 25–35% and 10–20%, respectively). In fact, in one study of early-onset primary dystonia, cranial involvement was the best clinical predictor of *non*-DYT1 status.[29]

In those whose disease remains focal, the arm is the body site most commonly affected. Cervical or cranial muscles have been reported as isolated affected sites,[25,30,31] but this is rare. Accordingly, one study of patients with early-onset cervical dystonia failed to find any patients with the *DYT1* mutation,[24] and *DYT1* has very rarely been found to cause adult-onset focal dystonia.

Dystonic tremor may be a feature of DYT1 dystonia and may be occasionally misdiagnosed as essential tremor (ET), although the presence of dystonia at other body sites and the directionality and irregularity of the tremor often helps to clarify the diagnosis.

DYT1 Genetics

TOR1A, the gene responsible for DYT1 dystonia , is located on chromosome 9q34 and encodes the protein torsinA, a 332 amino acid (37 kDa) protein. To date, despite extensive screening, only one clearly pathogenic mutation of TOR1A has been identified, that is, all DYT1 dystonia is due to a single recurring mutation: an in-frame GAG deletion in exon 5 of TOR1A. This deletion results in the loss of a pair of glutamic acid residues in the C-terminal region of the protein[2]. Three other variations in the TOR1A gene have been found that change the amino acid sequence, but none have been definitively associated with disease.[32–34] A fourth variation, a polymorphism in the coding sequence for residue 216 that encodes aspartic acid in 88% and histidine in 12% of alleles in control populations, has recently been identified as a genetic modifier of clinical disease expression in DYT1 mutation carriers, as discussed below.

Reduced Penetrance and Variable Expressivity of the DYT1 Mutation

The DYT1 mutation is inherited in an autosomal-dominant pattern with reduced penetrance of 30% in both Ashkenazi and non-Jewish families,[27] that is, 70% of individuals who carry the DYT1 mutation have no definite signs of dystonia. Among the 30% of gene carriers who do manifest dystonia, clinical symptoms are variable. Although young age of onset and onset in a limb are relatively homogeneous features in all cases of DYT1 dystonia, there is remarkable heterogeneity in the degree of severity and spread of dystonia, even within affected members of the same family. Opal and colleagues[35] reported a DYT1 family in which dystonia ranged in severity from a child with dystonic storm leading to death in the second decade to a family member with onset of dystonia at age 64, with other family members with dystonia of all distributions, including focal, segmental, multifocal, and generalized. The reason for reduced penetrance is not known, and the identification of genetic and environmental modifying factors is a current field of active investigation.

A recent study by Risch and colleagues[36] identified the first evidence of an intragenic modifier of DYT1 dystonia penetrance. They assessed the DYT1 D216H variant in 119 GAG deletion carriers with dystonia ("manifesting carriers"), 113 deletion carriers without dystonia ("nonmanifesting carriers"), and 197 controls. They found a significantly increased frequency of the D216H allele (encoding histidine rather than aspartate) in nonmanifesting carriers and a decreased frequency of this allele in manifesting carriers compared to controls. Analysis of haplotypes demonstrated a highly protective effect of the D216H allele in *trans* with the GAG deletion, and there was suggestive evidence that the D216 allele in *cis* is required for disease to be penetrant. Although these findings established, for the first time, a clinically relevant gene modifier of DYT1 dystonia, this genetic variant has a relatively small role in explaining the overall reduced penetrance of DYT1 dystonia, as the protective H allele is not common (occurring at most in 20% of the population) and can therefore explain the reduced penetrance in only a small proportion of cases (approximately 5%). There must be other, yet-to-be identified disease modifying factors, genetic or environmental, to explain the overall reduced penetrance of DYT1.

DYT1 Endophenotypes

With the identification of the gene for DYT1 dystonia, it has also become possible to explore DYT1 endophenotypes or biomarkers using imaging, electrophysiological, and other techniques to measure subclinical traits. Nonmanifesting mutation carriers (i.e., those without overt dystonia), a group constituting 70% of those with the mutation, can be studied in comparison to both their non-mutation carrier family members and to those who do manifest dystonia. The psychiatric expression of the DYT1 mutation was investigated using this approach, with the finding that both manifesting and nonmanifesting gene carriers had the same increased risk for early-onset major depression when compared with their noncarrier family members.[37] Other subtle clinical changes noted in nonmanifesting carriers include deficiencies in sequence learning[38] and "probable" dystonia on clinical examination. Functional imaging (FDG-PET) studies have demonstrated a characteristic pattern of glucose utilization, with increased metabolism in the basal ganglia, cerebellum, and supplementary motor cortex in both manifesting and nonmanifesting gene carriers.[39–41] Other imaging studies have found decreased striatal D2 receptor binding[42] and microstructural changes in the subgyral white matter of the sensorimotor cortex[41] in both manifesting and nonmanifesting carriers. Electrophysiological studies have also identified genotype-associated abnormalities, such as reduced intracortical inhibition and a shortened cortical silent period as well as higher tactile and visuotactile temporal discrimination thresholds and temporal order judgments.[43,44] These types of studies strongly support the presence of a wider clinical expression, with abnormal brain processing and associated structural brain changes in DYT1 mutation carriers regardless of overt motor signs of dystonia, thereby expanding the notion of penetrance and phenotype.

TorsinA and Dystonia Pathogenesis

TorsinA, the protein encoded by the *DYT1* gene, is a member of the AAA+ superfamily (ATPases Associated with a variety of cellular Activities), a family of chaperone proteins that mediate conformational changes in target proteins and perform a variety of functions including degradation of proteins, membrane trafficking, vesicle fusion and organelle movement, cytoskeletal dynamics, and correct folding of nascent proteins.[45,46] Although the precise role of torsinA remains unknown, in vivo and in vitro studies suggest that torsinA may perform several of these roles.

TorsinA is widely distributed in the brain, with intense expression in the substantia nigra dopamine neurons, cerebellar Purkinje cells, thalamus, globus pallidus, hippocampal formation, and cerebral cortex.[47–50] It is restricted to neurons, and in the normal state it localizes to the lumen of the endoplasmic reticulum. It is also found in most cells in the body,[2] although its role in extracerebral cells is unknown and has of yet not been explored.

Most pathological studies of DYT1 brains have not detected specific changes in torsinA labeling or evidence of degeneration. One study, however, of four DYT1 brains found ubiquitin-positive perinuclear inclusion bodies in the midbrain reticular formation and periaqueductal gray.[51] Although this finding remains to be confirmed, animal models show similar brainstem inclusions (see below).

In cellular models of GAG-deleted torsinA, there is aberrant localization of the mutant protein, with redistribution from the ER to the nuclear envelope[52,53]; and mutant torsinA is associated with abnormal morphology and apparent thickening of the nuclear envelope. Its aberrant localization and interactions may result in stress-induced abnormalities, including dopamine release.[54,55] Mutant torsinA has also been shown to interfere with cytoskeletal events, which may affect development of neuronal pathways.[56] Additionally, recent studies demonstrate differences in the degradation pathways of normal and mutant torsinA.[57,58]

The role of dopamine in the pathogenesis of DYT1 dystonia remains uncertain. Parkinsonism is not a feature of the DYT1 phenotype, and no clear or consistent response to dopaminergic therapy occurs in patients with DYT1 dystonia. Biochemically, dopamine concentration is normal in DYT1 except for a 50% reduction in dopamine and homovanilic acid in the rostral portions of the putamen and caudate in one case[59] and a possible increase in striatal dopamine turnover in three cases.[60] Two studies have found co-localization of torsinA and α-synuclein immunoreactivity in Lewy bodies, suggestive of a role for torsinA in dopamine transmission.[61,62]

DYT1 Animal Models

Mouse models of DYT1 include both engineered lines in which the endogenous mouse locus is modified, and transgenic models in which the human mutant torsinA gene is randomly inserted into the mouse genome and overexpressed via genetic promoters.

In one transgenic model about 40% of the mice show hyperactivity, circling, and abnormal movement, and also have abnormal levels of dopamine metabolites and aggregates in the brainstem similar to those reported in DYT1 human brains.[63] Another transgenic model does not show an overt movement disorder, but these animals do exhibit impaired motor sequence learning.[64]

In the mice in which the endogenous locus is modified, the knockin (KI) mice bearing the 3base pair (bp) deletion in the heterozygous state, analogous to human DYT1 dystonia, manifest hyperactivity, difficulty in beam walking, and have abnormal levels of dopamine metabolites, though they do not have overt dystonic posturing. They also have brainstem neuronal aggregates, consistent with the findings in human pathologic studies.[51] In contrast, mice that are either homozygous KI or knockout for the deletion die at birth, suggesting that the pathogenic deletion in DYT1 dystonia causes a loss of function of the torsinA protein. A knockdown mouse model, in which expression of torsinA is reduced, displays a phenotype similar to the heterozygous KI mice, further supporting a loss of function model, as deletion of torsinA is not necessary to produce the pathogenic phenotype. It is possible that the loss of function is the result of a "dominant negative effect" whereby the mutant protein interferes with the wild-type protein, implying that RNA interference may be used therapeutically to block aggregate formation and restore cellular function of torsinA.[65]

▶ NON-DYT1 EARLY-ONSET PRIMARY DYSTONIA

There remains a large group of early-onset primary dystonia, especially among non-Jewish populations, which is not due to the DYT1 GAG deletion. To date, two genetic loci, *DYT6*[66] and *DYT13*,[67] have been mapped in families with autosomal-dominant transmission and reduced penetrance of non-DYT1 primary dystonia. The *DYT6* locus was mapped in a large Amish Mennonite kindred, and DYT13 was mapped in a single Italian family, and most recently, the DYT6 gene, *THAP1*, was identified.[3]

Overall clinical features in these two families differ from DYT1 (although features in any single family member may overlap with DYT1). In both, average age of onset is in adolescence, although a higher proportion appears to have onset after age 21. More importantly, in contrast to DYT1, the phenotypes in both the DYT6 and DYT13 families are marked by prominent cranial and cervical muscle involvement with variable spread. The term "mixed" dystonia has been applied to these phenotypes to distinguish them from both the typical early-onset phenotype associated with DYT1 and from typical late-onset focal dystonia.

DYT6

The DYT6 gene, *THAP1*, is the most recently identified dystonia gene.[3] A founder mutation was detected in the Amish-Mennonite families in which the DYT6 locus was first mapped, but a second mutation was identified in a German family without Amish-Mennonite ancestry, providing the first evidence that this gene has a broader role in dystonia outside of the Amish-Mennonite population. The Amish-Mennonite founder mutation is a heterozygous 5-bp (GGGTT) insertion followed by a

3-bp deletion (AAC) in exon 2 of the THAP1 gene. The mutation causes a frameshift at position 44 of the protein, resulting in a premature stop codon at position 73. The mutation found in the non-Mennonite family was also in exon 2, and consists of a 241 T-to-C substitution, resulting in the replacement of a phenylalanine with a leucine in a highly conserved and functionally significant region of the THAP1 protein. THAP1 is a member of a family of cellular factors sharing a highly conserved THAP domain, which is an atypical zinc finger. Associated with its DNA-binding domain, THAP1 regulates endothelial cell proliferation. In addition to the THAP domain at the N-terminus, THAP1 possesses a nuclear localization signal at its C-terminus. One proposed disease mechanism is that DYT6 mutations disrupt DNA binding and produce transcriptional dysregulation.

DYT6 dystonia is characterized by a relatively early but broad age of onset (median 13 years, range 2–49 years). The body regions first affected include brachial, cranial, and cervical muscles. In contrast to DYT1, onset at the leg occurs in only 10%. The dystonia usually progresses, but the degree of progression is variable. Although the legs are ultimately affected in approximately 50%, significant gait disturbance is uncommon. Unlike DYT1, most patients with DYT6 dystonia have disabling cranial dustonia involving facial, jaw, lingual and laryngeal muscles, and speech is affected in about two-thirds. DYT6 is inherited in an autosomal-dominant pattern with reduced penetrance of about 60%.

Although *THAP1* was initially thought to have a limited role, different *THAP1* mutations in families with diverse ancestries have now been identified.[68,69] In a study that screened for *THAP1* mutations in families with early-onset, non-DYT1, nonfocal primary dystonia, 9 of 36 families (25%) had *THAP1* mutations.[68] Most were of German, Irish, or Italian ancestry. One family had the Amish-Mennonite founder mutation, and the other eight families each had novel, potentially truncating or missense mutations. This screening study suggests that mutations in *THAP1* underlie a substantial proportion of early-onset primary dystonia in non-DYT1 families. It also confirmed the clinical features characteristic of affected individuals with *THAP1* mutations, including limb and cranial involvement, with speech frequently affected. Determining the pathogenic mechanisms of this gene mutation, and its ultimate import in other dystonia populations, including adult-onset focal populations, will be important next research steps.

DYT13

The *DYT13* locus on chromosome 18p was mapped in an Italian family; thus far other families definitively linked to this region have not been reported and gene is not yet identified. The average age of onset of dystonia is in adolescence (mean = 15.6 years, range 5–43).[70] Body regions first affected include neck, neck with cranial muscles, and arm. Only 2 of the 11 individuals developed leg dystonia, and similar to DYT6, disability due to leg dystonia was mild. There was less laryngeal involvement in DYT13 than in DYT6.

Late-onset PTD

The majority of primary dystonia is adult-onset and is about 9 to 10 times more prevalent than early-onset dystonia. Late-onset dystonia typically starts in cervical, brachial, or cranial muscles and either remains focal or spreads only to a segmental distribution, with very rare generalization. Focal cervical dystonia constitutes approximately half of all adult-onset cases, with blepharospasm and writer's cramp making up the two other largest groups.

Most cases of PTD are sporadic, and lack a clear pattern of inheritance. When a family history is present, late-onset PTD often appears to have autosomal-dominant inheritance[71,72] with reduced penetrance. However, most studies show that penetrance is even more reduced than in early-onset dystonia (about 12–15% compared to 30–40%). An alternative explanation for these observations is that penetrance may be higher in a subset of the late-onset PTD population, with the remainder of late-onset cases being sporadic. Consistent with the notion of increased penetrance in a subset of late-onset PTD are descriptions of large families with more highly penetrant autosomal-dominant disease.[73,74] A study of one such family with adult-onset torticollis resulted in the mapping of DYT7.[75] However, DYT7 has been excluded in other clinically similar families,[76] suggesting the existence of still other loci for adult-onset focal PTD.

Because the majority of adult-onset dystonia patients do not have many affected relatives, association studies using cases and controls have been employed to find genetic risk factors. Several studies found that a polymorphism in the D5 dopamine receptor gene is associated with adult-onset torticollis and blepharospasm,[77,78] but the role of this gene as a susceptibility factor remains to be elucidated. Other recent studies have found an association of adult-onset primary dystonia with a *DYT1* haplotype in the Icelandic and Italian populations[79,80] but not in Germany and the United States.[79,81] Thus, for the great majority of adult-onset PTD, genetic causation remains to be clarified.

▶ DYSTONIA PLUS SYNDROMES

Dystonia Plus Syndromes are a subcategory of the inherited forms of secondary dystonia. This category includes three clinically defined syndromes: dopa-responsive dystonia (DRD), myoclonus-dystonia (MD), and rapid-onset dystonia-parkinsonism (RDP).

These disorders are placed in their own category, distinct from primary dystonia and other inherited secondary dystonias because these disorders share features of each of those groups. As in the primary dystonias, there is no evidence of neurodegeneration or frank neuroimaging abnormalities, but as in secondary dystonia, these disorders do have characteristic neurological features other than dystonia, specifically parkinsonism in DRD and RDP, and myoclonus in MD. All three of these disorders have known genetic etiologies, and they have been designated in the HUGO nomenclature as DYT5 (DRD), DYT11 and 15 (MD), and DYT12 (RDP). Although pathological studies in these disorders are limited, current evidence supports the principle of pathogenic genetic defects that result in functional brain changes that are not associated with progressive neuronal death.

DOPA-RESPONSIVE DYSTONIA (DRD, DYT5, SEGAWA DISEASE)

The classic form of DRD was first described in 1976 by Segawa and colleagues,[82] who called the disorder "hereditary progressive dystonia with diurnal variation," and mentioned that it responded to levodopa. Classic DRD is consequently also known as Segawa disease. Independently in the same year, Allen and Knopp[83] described a form of hereditary childhood dystonia with features of parkinsonism, which showed sustained response to levodopa and anticholinergic medication. Since these initial descriptions, the clinical spectrum of the disorder has broadened, but the defining feature for all clinical subtypes of DRD is a dramatic and sustained response to low-dosage levodopa, making the preferred label for all forms of this disorder DRD, thereby emphasizing the appropriate treatment. It is critical to recognize this disorder, as it is so easily and effectively treated. If left untreated, patients can be left with severe motor disability, whereas with treatment they are typically fully symptom-free indefinitely.[20]

DRD Clinical Features

DRD is an early-onset dystonia, typically presenting in mid-childhood (5–6 years) with dystonia affecting gait, usually due to dystonia of the foot or leg. A frequent presenting symptom is therefore a peculiar gait, especially walking on the toes, or a stiff-legged gait with plantar flexion and eversion. Consequently, this disorder can be misdiagnosed as spastic diplegic cerebral palsy. Arm dystonia, hyperreflexia, extensor plantar reflexes, and parkinsonism (bradykinesia, postural instability) are also common features. Symptoms are often diurnal, worsening as the day progresses and improving after sleep, though not all patients with DRD have this diurnal fluctuation pattern.

Over time, the clinical spectrum of this disorder has broadened and has been found to include a wide variety of phenotypes, not all of them characterized by limb dystonia, including adult-onset parkinsonism,[84] adult-onset oromandibular dystonia,[85] developmental delay and spasticity mimicking cerebral palsy,[86] scoliosis,[87] generalized hypotonia with proximal weakness,[88] and neonatal onset of rigidity, tremor, and dystonia.[89]

As stated, the hallmark feature for all clinical subtypes is a dramatic and sustained response to low-dose levodopa therapy (50–200 mg/day). Rarely (especially in those cases with compound heterozygous mutations or adult-onset symptoms) the dose required may be more substantial. Some DRD patients may also have an excellent response to anticholinergics (e.g., trihexyphenidyl).[90] Patients will still respond dramatically to low doses of levodopa even if levodopa therapy is delayed for many years.[91]

Adverse motor effects of long-term levodopa therapy, such as wearing-off or motor fluctuations do not occur in DRD.[84,91] Dyskinesias may appear at the beginning of levodopa therapy, but subside after a dose reduction and do not reappear when the dose is gradually increased.

DRD Genetics

DRD is genetically heterogeneous, that is, it has been found to be associated with mutations of more than one gene, and within single genes, numerous pathogenic mutations have been identified. The genetic basis for many cases of DRD is a number of heterozygous mutations in the GTP cyclohydrolase 1 (*GCH1*) gene located on chromosome 14.[5,92,93] DRD related to *GCH1* (DYT5) is transmitted in an autosomal-dominant pattern with incomplete and sex-related penetrance. For unclear reasons, female carriers of *GCH1* mutations appear to manifest dystonia two to four times as frequently as males with a mutation.[94] Many *GCH1* mutations are unique and new mutations appear to occur commonly. (A registry of mutations is available at http://www.bh4.org/biomdb1.html.)

Although *GCH1* mutations have been found to account for many cases of DRD, up to 40% of patients with DRD have no identifiable mutations in the coding exons of *GCH1*. Other mutations in the gene, that is, those in noncoding regions, including mutations in promoter or regulatory sequences, as well as deletions, may account for some of the mutation negative cases. And, in fact, in one study in which rigorous screening was done using sequence analysis of coding exons in combination with quantitative duplex PCR, mutations were identified in 87% of cases.[95] No additional loci for autosomal-dominant DRD are known to date. A DRD family originally designated as DYT14 was initially reported to not be linked to the *GCH1* locus, but upon clinical recategorization, a family member was later found to be linked and to have a deletion of *GCH1*.[96] The *DYT14* locus is therefore no longer listed in the current HUGO nomenclature, as it is identical to DYT5.

Compound heterozygous mutations of *GCH1* have been identified in two patients, one of whom had a more severe form of the disease with developmental motor delay, truncal hypotonia, intermittent dystonic extension of the legs, progressing by 1 year to generalized dystonia with oculogyric crises; the other compound heterozygote had a clinical course similar to typical dominantly inherited GTPCH deficiency.[97] Different genetic defects have been identified in autosomal-recessive forms of DRD, as described below.

GCH1 DRD Pathogenesis

GTP cyclohydrolase 1 is the first and rate-limiting enzyme in the synthesis of tetrahydrobiopterin (BH4), which is an essential cofactor for tyrosine hydroxylase (TH) and thus is essential for dopamine synthesis. TH is also essential for epinephrine and norepinephrine production, and BH4 is also an essential cofactor for tryptophan hydroxylase, which is essential for serotonin synthesis, and phenylalanine hydroxylase, which converts phenylalanine into tyrosine, but it is not currently understood why the disorder manifests with symptoms related primarily to dopamine deficiency (Fig. 28–1).

Autosomal-recessive Forms of DRD

It has become evident that some cases of DRD are due to autosomal-recessive mutations in genes encoding enzymes other than *GCH1* that are involved in dopamine synthesis, including TH,[98] 6-pyruvoyltetrahydropterin synthase,[99] and sepiapterin reductase.[100] Classically, the clinical picture in these recessively inherited conditions is much more severe than in GCH1 DRD, as the typical forms of these disorders (unlike autosomal-dominant GCH1) manifest symptoms reflective of deficiencies of serotonin or norepinephrin in addition to dopamine deficiency. Symptoms can include hypotonia, severe bradykinesia, drooling, ptosis, miosis, oculogyria, cognitive impairment, and seizures. These more severe phenotypes may have some response to levodopa, but symptoms do not resolve to the dramatic extent that they typically do in GCH1 DRD. However, mild phenotypes of these enzyme defects have been reported that may be completely responsive to levodopa, with phenotypes including typical DRD signs, mild spastic paraplegia, and exercise-induced stiffness.[101]

An important disease that mimics DRD and therefore needs to be considered in the differential diagnosis

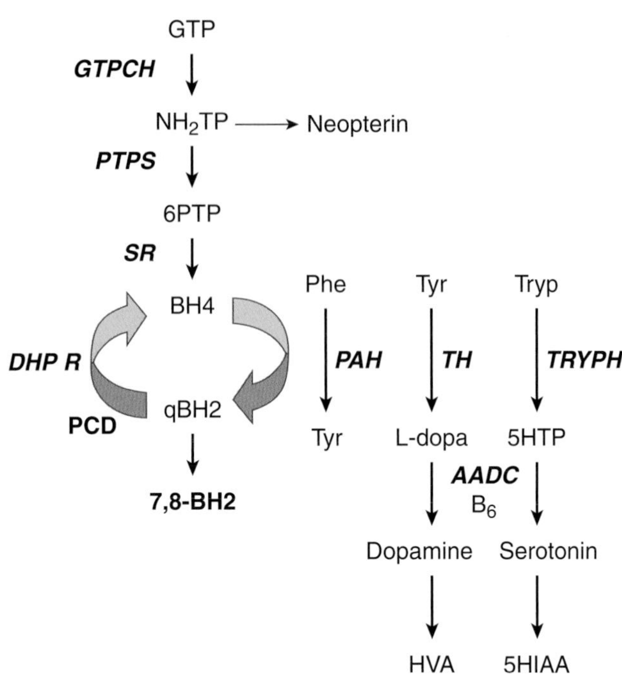

Figure 28–1. Synthesis and catabolism of dopamine and serotonin. Dopamine and serotonin are formed from the amino acids tyrosine and tryptophan, respectively. Their synthesis also requires two cofactors. BH4 (tetrahydrobiopterin) is formed in a three-step pathway from GTP and is the cofactor for tyrosine hydroxylase and tryptophan hydroxylase. It is also required for the activity of PAH. The second cofactor is pyridoxal 5′-phosphate (B_6), which is required for AADC activity. Following release of dopamine and serotonin, they are rapidly metabolized to form HVA and 5HIAA, respectively; these metabolites are measured in spinal fluid and provide an indication of the overall turnover of these neurotransmitters. GTPCH, GTP cyclohydrolase; 6PTPS, 6-pyruvoyltetrahydropterin synthase; SR, sepiapterin reductase; PCD, pterin a-carbinolamine dehydratase; DHPR, dihydropteridine reductase, NH2TP: dihydroneopterin triphosphate; 6PTP, 6-pyruvoyltetrahydropterin; qBH2, quinonoid dihydrobiopterin; 7,8-BH2, 7,8-dihydrobiopterin; Phe, phenylalanine; Tyr, tyrosine; Tryp, tryptophan; PAH, phenylalanine hydroxylase; TH, tyrosine hydroxylase; TRYPH, tryptophan hydroxylase; 5HTP, 5-hydroxytryptophan; B6, pyridoxal 5′-phosphate. (Reproduced with permission from Hyland K. Inherited disorders affecting dopamine and serotonin: Critical neurotransmitters derived from aromatic amino acids. J Nutr 2007;137:1568S-1572S.)

is dystonia due to homozygous mutations in the juvenile parkinsonism *parkin* gene,[102,103] which causes early-onset autosomal-recessive parkinsonism and dystonia. The presence of early, prominent parkinsonism and severe dyskinesias with levodopa therapy generally favors *parkin* mutations rather than DRD (see Table 28–3).

▶ **TABLE 28-3. FEATURES DIFFERENTIATING DRD (GCH1), PTD (DYT1), AND JUVENILE PARKINSONISM**

	Dopa-responsive Dystonia (GCH1)	Early-onset PTD (DYT1)	Juvenile Parkinsonism PARK2 (Parkin)
Age of onset	Childhood, 5–6 years (infancy to sixth decade)	Childhood–adolescence (mean onset 13 years; range 4 years to seventh decade; uncommon <6 and >26 years)	Adolescence (7 years to sixth decade)
Gender	Predominantly female	Equal	Predominantly male
Initial sign	Foot/leg dystonia, gait disorder	Arm or leg dystonia	Foot/leg > hand/arm dystonia, rest tremor, akinsia/rigidity
Dystonia	Throughout	Throughout	At onset
Diurnal pattern	Sometimes	No	May occur but usually not dramatic
Sleep benefit	Sometimes	No	Yes
Bradykinesia	Sometimes (may be mild)	No	Yes
Postural instability	Sometimes	No	Yes
Gait	Abnormal	Abnormal if leg or trunk is affected	Abnormal
Anticholinergic response	Yes	Yes	Yes
Levodopa responsive	Yes	No or mild-moderate	Yes
Levodopa dosage	Very low	High	Moderate to high
Dyskinesias	With high-dose levodopa	Unknown	Prominent
Fluoro-DOPA PET	Normal or borderline	Normal	Decreased
β-CIT SPECT	Normal	Normal	Decreased
CSF			
HVA	Decreased	Normal	Decreased
Neopterin	Markedly decreased	Normal	Moderately decreased
Biopterin	Decreased	Normal	Decreased
Prognosis	Sustained excellent response to levodopa with near-complete resolution of symptoms in most	Progression then usually plateaus	Slow-to-moderate progression
Gene	Heterozygous mutations in GCH1	Heterozygous GAG deletion in DYT1	Homozygous or compound heterozygous PARKIN mutations
Testing	Screening for GCH1 mutations in select laboratories	Gene test commercially available	Screening for some PARKIN mutations in select laboratories

PTD, primary torsion dystonia; SPECT, single photon emission computed tomography; CSF, cerebral spinal fluid; HVA, homovanillic acid.

Functional imaging techniques can be helpful in distinguishing *parkin*-associated juvenile parkinsonism from DRD, as discussed below.

DRD Diagnosis

The heterogeneity and multitude of DRD mutations makes genetic diagnosis complex and therefore cumbersome in the clinical setting. In approximately 15% of cases, mutations or deletions in *GCH1* may not be detected even by rigorous screening methods,[95] so that a negative genetic test does not conclusively rule out a diagnosis of DRD. Diagnosis of DRD is therefore currently made by clinical features, most important of which is the excellent and sustained response of symptoms to levodopa. A levodopa trial is therefore critical in all cases with any degree of suspicion of DRD.

Lumbar puncture with analysis of cerebral spinal fluid (CSF) neurotransmitters may be useful to distinguish juvenile parkinsonism from classic DRD and TH deficiency, which can sometimes be difficult to distinguish on clinical grounds, as they are all levodopa responsive. In classic DRD, both neopterin and tetrahydrobiopterin (BH4) are reduced, in TH deficiency neopterin and BH4 are normal, and in juvenile parkinsonism (*parkin*) BH4 may be decreased but neopterin is normal. Phenylalanine loading to assess activity of phenylalanine hydroxylase may be a good marker, but appears to have limited sensitivity.

Functional imaging with either fluorodopa PET scan or ^{123}I-β-CIT single photon emission computed tomography can also discriminate DRD from juvenile Parkinson disease. Fluorodopa PET is normal in DRD and shows reduced F-dopa uptake in *parkin*-associated disease. ^{123}I-β-CIT, a sensitive marker of dopamine uptake sites, is also normal in DRD and abnormal in Parkinson disease.[104,105] Biochemically, GCH1 activity as well as low biopterin and neopterin can be measured in cytokine-stimulated fibroblasts.[106] When more readily available, this test may also have clinical utility in distinguishing DRD from early-onset parkinsonism and other forms of early-onset PTD.

MYOCLONUS-DYSTONIA (DYT11, DYT15)

Myoclonus is characterized by fast, lightning-like jerks. It may be isolated or occur in association with other movement disorders, particularly dystonia. Patients with DYT1 and other primary dystonias may have quick dystonic movements[107] and can have occasional superimposed myoclonic jerks. In contrast, MD is a distinct genetic disorder in which early-onset, prominent myoclonus is the primary inherited feature, which may occur with or without dystonia. The dystonia in MD is usually mild. There are no other associated neurological features such as ataxia or dementia. The presence of seizures was initially considered to be an exclusionary criterion, but epilepsy has since been found to be associated with genetically proven MD. Rarely, dystonia can be the only feature of MD.[108]

Symptom onset is usually in the first or second decade. Males and females are equally affected in most, though not all, families. The neck and arms are the most commonly involved sites, typically causing difficulties with activities such as eating and writing. Bulbar or trunk muscles can also be affected, and truncal myoclonus can cause falls. Leg involvement can occur but is less common, except for in the very young, in whom leg involvement may be the initial feature.[6] The myoclonus may occur as isolated jerks at rest and also as more complex, oscillatory or pseudorhythmic bursts. The overflow phenomenon, in which myoclonus or dystonia increases in one affected body part with activity of a different body part, is a characteristic feature. Neurophysiological studies support a subcortical origin of the myoclonus.[109] The disorder tends to plateau in adulthood, and the myoclonus may improve dramatically with alcohol. Psychiatric symptoms, particularly obsessive–compulsive disorder and major depressive disorder are prominent in family members, and the former has been reported even in individuals without motor symptoms.[110]

MD Genetics

The pattern of inheritance of familial MD appears to be autosomal dominant with reduced penetrance and variable expressivity. It also appears to be consistent with a maternal imprinting mechanism, that is, the maternal allele of the affected gene is selectively silenced, so that most individuals who inherit the gene from their father manifest symptoms while those who inherit the gene from their mother are usually not symptomatic.

An MD locus on chromosome 7q21 (DYT11) was mapped in a North American family with 10 affected individuals with clinical features typical for the disorder.[111] This locus was then confirmed and narrowed in other MD families,[112] and in 2001, based on the findings of different loss of function mutations in six families, the gene was identified as ε-sarcoglycan (SGCE).[113] The sarcoglycans are a family of genes that encode components of the dystrophin–glycoprotein complex. Mutations in α-, β-, γ-, and δ-sarcoglycan produce recessive muscular limb-girdle dystrophy. SGCE, however, is expressed widely in the brain in neurons of the cerebral cortex, basal ganglia, hippocampus, cerebellum, and the olfactory bulb, and it is located at the plasma membrane. Although the exact protein function and mechanism by which the mutated protein produces MD remains unknown, studies in a cellular model have demonstrated that mutations in SGCE can impair trafficking of the protein to the plasma membrane. TorsinA and the ubiquitin proteasome system may also play a role in the recognition and processing of misfolded SGCE.[114]

The proportion of MD and clinically related phenotypes that is due to SGCE mutations is still under study. SGCE mutations have been confirmed in many other families with MD, including the original large kindred showing linkage to the 7q region. However, SGCE mutations do not account for all familial MD and probably are not responsible for most sporadic, nonfamilial MD cases. However, it is likely that with the addition of gene dosaging methods for deletions, the rate of detectable mutations would be increased. To date, one other gene locus for MD has been mapped in one family to chromosome 18p (DYT15).[115]

RAPID-ONSET DYSTONIA-PARKINSONISM (RDP, DYT12)

RDP is a rare disorder described in several unrelated families in the United States and Europe.[7] It is characterized by both dystonia and parkinsonism that is usually sudden and rapid in onset, beginning over hours to days, often after a major stressor. Symptom onset may, however, be more insidious, with a subsequent period of rapid worsening. After the initial rapid onset or period of worsening, symptoms may plateau or rarely improve.[7,116] Onset is usually in adolescence or early adulthood. Motor features may include dystonia–parkinsonism–hyperreflexia or dystonia alone.

The dystonia is characterized by prominent bulbar features of dysarthria and facial grimacing, which may mimic the cranial dystonia (including risus sardonicus) seen in Wilson's disease. The dystonia is usually tonic, with relatively sustained dystonic limb posturing. The parkinsonian features of bradykinesia, with waxy, effortful rapid successive movements, and postural instability are prominent. Seizures, depression, and social phobia have been reported. CSF homovanillic acid (HVA), a dopamine metabolite, is reduced in some patients, but neuroimaging and pathology do not suggest nigral degeneration, and RDP is generally refractory to treatment, including levodopa.

Inheritance is autosomal dominant with reduced penetrance, and de novo mutations have been observed. The gene has been mapped to chromosome 19q13 (DYT12) and identified as the *ATP1A3* gene, which codes for the sodium potassium transporting ATPase α-3 chain, a catalytic subunit of the sodium-potassium pump.[117] However, only 21% of newly described families with the clinical syndrome had a mutation in the *ATP1A3* gene.[7]

▶ CLINICAL APPROACH TO GENETIC TESTING IN DYSTONIA

Despite the likely genetic etiology of primary dystonia, a negative family history is not uncommon. This is predominantly due to the markedly reduced penetrance (about 15% for adult-onset forms and 30% for early-onset) of dystonia genes, and to their variable expression, with mild cases frequently going unrecognized. Additionally, new mutations also account for a proportion of DYT1 and other autosomal-dominant genetic forms of dystonia in which there is no family history; nonpaternity can also be a factor. In recessive forms of dystonia, family history is often negative, and other clues such as consanguinity need to be pursued in taking a family history.

Based on current findings it is therefore reasonable to assume a genetic etiology for most early-onset PTD, regardless of family history. Many early-onset patients (especially those starting in childhood or adolescence with dystonia in an arm or leg, or of Ashkenazi descent) will have the DYT1 mutation. Because all DYT1 dystonia appears to be due to the same GAG deletion, screening is relatively easy. The test is commercially available and as stated, should be considered the first diagnostic test to apply to all primary dystonia patients (whether Ashkenazi, non-Ashkenazi Jewish, or non-Jewish, with (a) onset by age 26 or (b) when age of onset is uncertain (especially in patients with writer's cramp/arm involvement, as it may be very difficult to accurately determine when writing problems first begin). DYT1 testing should also be done for those with later onset PTD who have a relative with early onset.[25]

Clinical screening of the DYT6 gene, *THAP1*, is not yet available at the time of this writing, but is expected to become available in the near future. Although the proportion of early-onset PTD due to DYT6 remains to be determined, initial study suggests a significant proportion of early-onset non-DYT1 patients will have mutations, especially if there is prominent speech involvement (see above section on DYT6).

Commercial genetic testing is also available for many genetic causes of primary plus dystonia.

Additionally, some genetic causes of dystonia have been mapped, but the genes remain to be identified (e.g., DYT7, 13, 15); this limits evaluation of these genetic causes to linkage analysis in suitably large families, which is only performed on a research basis. To obtain up-to-date information regarding genetic testing sites (and also clinically relevant reviews) a highly recommended online resource is http://www.geneclinics.org.

Before diagnostic gene testing is done, genetic counseling is highly recommended to provide a format for discussion of the implications of either a positive or a negative test result. For instance, if a test is negative, a genetic etiology is not necessarily excluded, and this needs to be explained clearly to the patient and their family. For example, mutations in *GCH1* and in SGCE do not explain all inherited cases of DRD and MD, respectively. It is also important to keep in mind that a positive genetic test impacts other at-risk family members. These family members, even if asymptomatic, may wish to undergo carrier testing, and genetic counseling for all asymptomatic family members must be done before testing.

For autosomal-dominant disorders with markedly reduced penetrance and very variable expression, as is the case in many forms of primary dystonia, the psychological and social implications of genetic testing are complex, and therefore require considerable time for patient and family education and counseling.

REFERENCES

1. Fahn S, Bressman SB, Marsden CD. Classification of dystonia. Adv Neurol 1998;78:1–10.
2. Ozelius LJ, Hewett JW, Page CE, et al. The early-onset torsion dystonia gene (DYT1) encodes an ATP-binding protein. Nat Genet 1997;17(1):40–48.
3. Fuchs T, Gavarini S, Saunders-Pullman R, et al. Mutations in the THAP1 gene are responsible for DYT6 primary torsion dystonia. Nat Genet 2009;41(3):286–288.
4. Nolte D, Niemann S, Muller U. Specific sequence changes in multiple transcript system DYT3 are associated with X-linked dystonia parkinsonism. Proc Natl Acad Sci U S A 2003;100(18):10347–10352.
5. Ichinose H, Ohye T, Takahashi E, et al. Hereditary progressive dystonia with marked diurnal fluctuation caused by mutations in the GTP cyclohydrolase I gene. Nat Genet. 1994 Nov;8(3):236–42.
6. Asmus F, Zimprich A, Tezenas Du Montcel S, et al. Myoclonus-dystonia syndrome: Epsilon-sarcoglycan mutations and phenotype. Ann Neurol 2002;52(4):489–492.

7. Brashear A, Dobyns WB, de Carvalho Aguiar P, et al. The phenotypic spectrum of rapid-onset dystonia-parkinsonism (RDP) and mutations in the ATP1A3 gene. Brain 2007;130(Pt 3):828–835.
8. Camargos S, Scholz S, Simon-Sanchez J, et al. DYT16, a novel young-onset dystonia-parkinsonism disorder: Identification of a segregating mutation in the stress-response protein PRKRA. Lancet Neurol 2008;7(3):207–215.
9. Rainier S, Thomas D, Tokarz D, et al. Myofibrillogenesis regulator 1 gene mutations cause paroxysmal dystonic choreoathetosis. Arch Neurol 2004;61(7):1025–1029.
10. Weber YG, Storch A, Wuttke TV, et al. GLUT1 mutations are a cause of paroxysmal exertion-induced dyskinesias and induce hemolytic anemia by a cation leak. J Clin Invest 2008;118(6):2157–2168.
11. Gimenez-Roldan S, Delgado G, Marin M, et al. Hereditary torsion dystonia in gypsies. Adv Neurol 1988;50:73–81.
12. Parker N. Hereditary whispering dysphonia. J Neurol Neurosurg Psychiatry 1985;48(3):218–224.
13. Greene P, Kang UJ, Fahn S. Spread of symptoms in idiopathic torsion dystonia. Mov Disord 1995;10(2):143–152.
14. Schwalbe W. Eine eigentumliche tonische Krampform mit hysteriscehn Symptomen. Medicin and chirurgie. 1908.
15. Oppenheim H. Uber eine eigenartige Krampfkrankheit des kindlichen und jegendlichen. Alters (dysbasia lordotica progressiva, dystonia musculorum deformans). Neurol Centralbr. 1911;75:323–345.
16. Flateau E, Sterlinge W. Profressiver Torsionspasms bie Kindern. Z Gesamte Neurol Psychiatr. 1911;7:586–612.
17. Zeman W, Dyken P. Dystonia musculorum deformans. clinical, genetic and pathoanatomical studies. Psychiatr Neurol Neurochir 1967;70(2):77–121.
18. Marsden CD, Harrison MJ. Idiopathic torsion dystonia (dystonia musculorum deformans). A review of forty-two patients. Brain 1974;97(4):793–810.
19. Marsden CD, Harrison MJ, Bundey S. Natural history of idiopathic torsion dystonia. Adv Neurol 1976;14:177–87.
20. Fahn S. Concept and classification of dystonia. Adv Neurol 1988;50:1–8.
21. Bressman SB, de Leon D, Brin MF, et al. Idiopathic dystonia among Ashkenazi Jews: Evidence for autosomal dominant inheritance. Ann Neurol 1989;26(5):612–620.
22. Risch NJ, Bressman SB, deLeon D, et al. Segregation analysis of idiopathic torsion dystonia in Ashkenazi Jews suggests autosomal dominant inheritance. Am J Hum Genet 1990;46(3):533–538.
23. Pauls DL, Korczyn AD. Complex segregation analysis of dystonia pedigrees suggests autosomal dominant inheritance. Neurology 1990;40(7):1107–1110.
24. Valente EM, Warner TT, Jarman PR, et al. The role of DYT1 in primary torsion dystonia in europe. Brain 1998;121(Pt 12):2335–2339.
25. Bressman SB, Sabatti C, Raymond D, et al. The DYT1 phenotype and guidelines for diagnostic testing. Neurology 2000;54(9):1746–1752.
26. Risch N, de Leon D, Ozelius L, et al. Genetic analysis of idiopathic torsion dystonia in Ashkenazi Jews and their recent descent from a small founder population. Nat Genet 1995;9(2):152–159.
27. Waxman SG. Molecular Neurology. Burlington, MA: Elsevier Academic Press; 2007.
28. Klein C, Brin MF, de Leon D, et al. De novo mutations (GAG deletion) in the DYT1 gene in two non-Jewish patients with early-onset dystonia. Hum Mol Genet 1998;7(7):1133–1136.
29. Fasano A, Nardocci N, Elia AE, et al. Non-DYT1 early-onset primary torsion dystonia: Comparison with DYT1 phenotype and review of the literature. Mov Disord 2006;21(9):1411–1418.
30. Tuffery-Giraud S, Cavalier L, Roubertie A, et al. No evidence of allelic heterogeneity in the DYT1 gene of European patients with early onset torsion dystonia. J Med Genet 2001;38(10):E35.
31. Leube B, Kessler KR, Ferbert A, et al. Phenotypic variability of the DYT1 mutation in German dystonia patients. Acta Neurol Scand 1999;99(4):248–251.
32. Leung JC, Klein C, Friedman J, et al. Novel mutation in the TOR1A (DYT1) gene in atypical early onset dystonia and polymorphisms in dystonia and early onset parkinsonism. Neurogenetics 2001;3(3):133–143.
33. Kabakci K, Hedrich K, Leung JC, et al. Mutations in DYT1: Extension of the phenotypic and mutational spectrum. Neurology 2004;62(3):395–400.
34. Zirn B, Grundmann K, Huppke P, et al. Novel TOR1A mutation p.Arg288Gln in early-onset dystonia (DYT1). J Neurol Neurosurg Psychiatry 2008;79(12):1327–1330.
35. Opal P, Tintner R, Jankovic J, et al. Intrafamilial phenotypic variability of the DYT1 dystonia: From asymptomatic TOR1A gene carrier status to dystonic storm. Mov Disord 2002;17(2):339–345.
36. Risch NJ, Bressman SB, Senthil G, et al. Intragenic cis and trans modification of genetic susceptibility in DYT1 torsion dystonia. Am J Hum Genet 2007;80(6):1188–1193.
37. Heiman GA, Ottman R, Saunders-Pullman RJ. Increased risk for recurrent major depression in DYT1 dystonia mutation carriers. Neurology 2004;63(4):631–637.
38. Ghilardi MF, Carbon M, Silvestri G, et al. Impaired sequence learning in carriers of the DYT1 dystonia mutation. Ann Neurol 2003;54(1):102–109.
39. Eidelberg D, Moeller JR, Antonini A, et al. Functional brain networks in DYT1 dystonia. Ann Neurol 1998;44(3):303–312.
40. Carbon M, Kingsley PB, Tang C, et al. Microstructural white matter changes in primary torsion dystonia. Mov Disord 2008;23(2):234–239.
41. Carbon M, Kingsley PB, Su S, et al. Microstructural white matter changes in carriers of the DYT1 gene mutation. Ann Neurol 2004;56(2):283–286.
42. Asanuma K, Ma Y, Okulski J, et al. Decreased striatal D2 receptor binding in non-manifesting carriers of the DYT1 dystonia mutation. Neurology 2005;64(2):347–349.
43. Edwards MJ, Huang YZ, Wood NW, et al. Different patterns of electrophysiological deficits in manifesting and non-manifesting carriers of the DYT1 gene mutation. Brain 2003;126(Pt 9):2074–2080.
44. Fiorio M, Gambarin M, Valente EM, et al. Defective temporal processing of sensory stimuli in DYT1 mutation carriers: A new endophenotype of dystonia? Brain 2007;130(Pt 1):134–142.
45. Vale RD. AAA proteins. lords of the ring. J Cell Biol 2000;150(1):F13–F19.
46. Hanson PI, Whiteheart SW. AAA+ proteins: Have engine, will work. Nat Rev Mol Cell Biol 2005;6(7):519–529.

47. Augood SJ, Penney Jr JB, Friberg IK, et al. Expression of the early-onset torsion dystonia gene (DYT1) in human brain. Ann Neurol 1998;43(5):669–673.
48. Augood SJ, Martin DM, Ozelius LJ, et al. Distribution of the mRNAs encoding torsinA and torsinB in the normal adult human brain. Ann Neurol 1999;46(5):761–769.
49. Shashidharan P, Kramer BC, Walker RH, et al. Immunohistochemical localization and distribution of torsinA in normal human and rat brain. Brain Res 2000;853(2):197–206.
50. Konakova M, Huynh DP, Yong W, et al. Cellular distribution of torsin A and torsin B in normal human brain. Arch Neurol 2001;58(6):921–927.
51. McNaught KS, Kapustin A, Jackson T, et al. Brainstem pathology in DYT1 primary torsion dystonia. Ann Neurol 2004;56(4):540–547.
52. Naismith TV, Heuser JE, Breakefield XO, et al. TorsinA in the nuclear envelope. Proc Natl Acad Sci U S A 2004;101(20):7612–7617.
53. Goodchild RE, Dauer WT. Mislocalization to the nuclear envelope: An effect of the dystonia-causing torsinA mutation. Proc Natl Acad Sci U S A 2004;101(3):847–852.
54. Torres GE, Sweeney AL, Beaulieu JM, et al. Effect of torsinA on membrane proteins reveals a loss of function and a dominant-negative phenotype of the dystonia-associated DeltaE-torsinA mutant. Proc Natl Acad Sci U S A 2004;101(44):15650–15655.
55. Misbahuddin A, Placzek MR, Taanman JW, et al. Mutant torsinA, which causes early-onset primary torsion dystonia, is redistributed to membranous structures enriched in vesicular monoamine transporter in cultured human SH-SY5Y cells. Mov Disord 2005;20(4):432–440.
56. Hewett JW, Zeng J, Niland BP, et al. Dystonia-causing mutant torsinA inhibits cell adhesion and neurite extension through interference with cytoskeletal dynamics. Neurobiol Dis 2006;22(1):98–111.
57. Giles LM, Chen J, Li L, et al. Dystonia-associated mutations cause premature degradation of torsinA protein and cell-type-specific mislocalization to the nuclear envelope. Hum Mol Genet 2008;17(17):2712–2722.
58. Gordon KL, Gonzalez-Alegre P. Consequences of the DYT1 mutation on torsinA oligomerization and degradation. Neuroscience 2008;157(3):588–595.
59. Furukawa Y, Hornykiewicz O, Fahn S, et al. Striatal dopamine in early-onset primary torsion dystonia with the DYT1 mutation. Neurology 2000;54(5):1193–1195.
60. Augood SJ, Hollingsworth Z, Albers DS, et al. Dopamine transmission in DYT1 dystonia: A biochemical and autoradiographical study. Neurology 2002;59(3):445–448.
61. Shashidharan P, Good PF, Hsu A, et al. TorsinA accumulation in lewy bodies in sporadic parkinson's disease. Brain Res 2000;877(2):379–381.
62. Sharma N, Hewett J, Ozelius LJ, et al. A close association of torsinA and alpha-synuclein in lewy bodies: A fluorescence resonance energy transfer study. Am J Pathol 2001;159(1):339–344.
63. Shashidharan P, Sandu D, Potla U, et al. Transgenic mouse model of early-onset DYT1 dystonia. Hum Mol Genet 2005;14(1):125–133.
64. Sharma N, Baxter MG, Petravicz J, et al. Impaired motor learning in mice expressing torsinA with the DYT1 dystonia mutation. J Neurosci 2005;25(22):5351–5355.
65. Gonzalez-Alegre P. The inherited dystonias. Semin Neurol 2007;27(2):151–158.
66. Almasy L, Bressman SB, Raymond D, et al. Idiopathic torsion dystonia linked to chromosome 8 in two mennonite families. Ann Neurol 1997;42(4):670–673.
67. Valente EM, Bentivoglio AR, Cassetta E, et al. Identification of a novel primary torsion dystonia locus (DYT13) on chromosome 1p36 in an italian family with cranial-cervical or upper limb onset. Neurol Sci 2001;22(1):95–96.
68. Bressman SB, Raymond D, Fuchs T, et al. Mutations in THAP1 (DYT6) in early-onset dystonia: A genetic screening study. Lancet Neurol 2009;8(5):441–446.
69. Djarmati A, Schneider SA, Lohmann K, et al. Mutations in THAP1 (DYT6) and generalised dystonia with prominent spasmodic dysphonia: A genetic screening study. Lancet Neurol 2009;8(5):447–452.
70. Bentivoglio AR, Ialongo T, Contarino MF et al. Phenotypic characterization of DYT13 primary torsion dystonia. Mov Disord 2004;19(2):200–206.
71. Waddy HM, Fletcher NA, Harding AE, et al. A genetic study of idiopathic focal dystonias. Ann Neurol 1991; 29(3):320–324.
72. Defazio G, Livrea P, Guanti G, et al. Genetic contribution to idiopathic adult-onset blepharospasm and cranial-cervical dystonia. Eur Neurol 1993;33(5):345–350.
73. Bressman SB, Warner TT, Almasy L, et al. Exclusion of the DYT1 locus in familial torticollis. Ann Neurol 1996;40(4):681–684.
74. Munchau A, Valente EM, Davis MB, et al. A Yorkshire family with adult-onset cranio-cervical primary torsion dystonia. Mov Disord 2000;15(5):954–959.
75. Leube B, Rudnicki D, Ratzlaff T, et al. Idiopathic torsion dystonia: Assignment of a gene to chromosome 18p in a German family with adult onset, autosomal dominant inheritance and purely focal distribution. Hum Mol Genet 1996;5(10):1673–1677.
76. Jarman PR, del Grosso N, Valente EM, et al. Primary torsion dystonia: The search for genes is not over. J Neurol Neurosurg Psychiatry 1999;67(3):395–397.
77. Placzek MR, Misbahuddin A, Chaudhuri KR, et al. Cervical dystonia is associated with a polymorphism in the dopamine (D5) receptor gene. J Neurol Neurosurg Psychiatry 2001;71(2):262–264.
78. Misbahuddin A, Placzek MR, Chaudhuri KR, et al. A polymorphism in the dopamine receptor DRD5 is associated with blepharospasm. Neurology 2002;58(1):124–126.
79. Clarimon J, Brancati F, Peckham E, et al. Assessing the role of DRD5 and DYT1 in two different case-control series with primary blepharospasm. Mov Disord 2007;22(2):162–166.
80. Clarimon J, Asgeirsson H, Singleton A, et al. Torsin A haplotype predisposes to idiopathic dystonia. Ann Neurol 2005;57(5):765–767.
81. Hague S, Klaffke S, Clarimon J, et al. Lack of association with TorsinA haplotype in German patients with sporadic dystonia. Neurology 2006;66(6):951–952.
82. Segawa M, Hosaka A, Miyagawa F, et al. Hereditary progressive dystonia with marked diurnal fluctuation. Adv Neurol 1976;14:215–233.
83. Allen N, Knopp W. Hereditary parkinsonism-dystonia with sustained control by L-DOPA and anticholinergic medication. Adv Neurol 1976;14:201–213.

84. Nygaard TG, Takahashi H, Heiman GA, et al. Long-term treatment response and fluorodopa positron emission tomographic scanning of parkinsonism in a family with dopa-responsive dystonia. Ann Neurol 1992;32(5):603–608.
85. Steinberger D, Topka H, Fischer D, et al. GCH1 mutation in a patient with adult-onset oromandibular dystonia. Neurology 1999;52(4):877–879.
86. Nygaard TG, Waran SP, Levine RA, et al. Dopa-responsive dystonia simulating cerebral palsy. Pediatr Neurol 1994; 11(3):236–240.
87. Furukawa Y, Kish SJ, Lang AE. Scoliosis in a dopa-responsive dystonia family with a mutation of the GTP cyclohydrolase I gene. Neurology 2000;54(11):2187.
88. Kong CK, Ko CH, Tong SF, et al. Atypical presentation of dopa-responsive dystonia: Generalized hypotonia and proximal weakness. Neurology 2001;57(6):1121–1124.
89. Nardocci N, Zorzi G, Blau N, et al. Neonatal dopa-responsive extrapyramidal syndrome in twins with recessive GTPCH deficiency. Neurology 2003;60(2):335–337.
90. Jarman PR, Bandmann O, Marsden CD, et al. GTP cyclohydrolase I mutations in patients with dystonia responsive to anticholinergic drugs. J Neurol Neurosurg Psychiatry 1997;63(3):304–308.
91. Harwood G, Hierons R, Fletcher NA, et al. Lessons from a remarkable family with dopa-responsive dystonia. J Neurol Neurosurg Psychiatry 1994;57(4):460–463.
92. Hagenah J, Saunders-Pullman R, Hedrich K, et al. High mutation rate in dopa-responsive dystonia: Detection with comprehensive GCHI screening. Neurology 2005;64(5):908–911.
93. Ichinose H, Suzuki T, Inagaki H, et al. Molecular genetics of dopa-responsive dystonia. Biol Chem 1999;380(12):1355–1364.
94. Furukawa Y, Lang AE, Trugman JM, et al. Gender-related penetrance and de novo GTP-cyclohydrolase I gene mutations in dopa-responsive dystonia. Neurology 1998;50(4):1015–1020.
95. Hagenah J, Saunders-Pullman R, Hedrich K, et al. High mutation rate in dopa-responsive dystonia: Detection with comprehensive GCHI screening. Neurology 2005;-64(5):908–911.
96. Wider C, Melquist S, Hauf M, et al. Study of a swiss dopa-responsive dystonia family with a deletion in GCH1: Redefining DYT14 as DYT5. Neurology 2008;70(16 Pt 2):-1377–1383.
97. Furukawa Y. Update on dopa-responsive dystonia: Locus heterogeneity and biochemical features. Adv Neurol 2004;94:127–138.
98. van den Heuvel LP, Luiten B, Smeitink JA, et al. A common point mutation in the tyrosine hydroxylase gene in autosomal recessive L-DOPA-responsive dystonia in the dutch population. Hum Genet 1998;102(6):644–646.
99. Hanihara T, Inoue K, Kawanishi C, et al. 6-Pyruvoyl-tetrahydropterin synthase deficiency with generalized dystonia and diurnal fluctuation of symptoms: A clinical and molecular study. Mov Disord 1997;12(3):408–411.
100. steinberger D, Blau N, Goriuonov D, et al. Heterozygous mutation in 5'-untranslated region of sepiapterin reductase gene (SPR) in a patient with dopa-responsive dystonia. Neurogenetics 2004;5(3):187–190.
101. Furukawa Y, Graf WD, Wong H, et al. Dopa-responsive dystonia simulating spastic paraplegia due to tyrosine hydroxylase (TH) gene mutations. Neurology 2001;-56(2):260–263.
102. Tassin J, Durr A, Bonnet AM, et al. Levodopa-responsive dystonia. GTP cyclohydrolase I or parkin mutations? Brain 2000;123(Pt 6):1112–1121.
103. Khan NL, Graham E, Critchley P, et al. Parkin disease: A phenotypic study of a large case series. Brain 2003;126(Pt 6):1279–1292.
104. Snow BJ, Nygaard TG, Takahashi H, et al. Positron emission tomographic studies of dopa-responsive dystonia and early-onset idiopathic parkinsonism. Ann Neurol 1993;34(5):733–738.
105. Naumann M, Pirker W, Reiners K, et al. 123I]beta-CIT single-photon emission tomography in DOPA-responsive dystonia. Mov Disord 1997;12(3):448–451.
106. Bonafe L, Thony B, Leimbacher W, et al. Diagnosis of dopa-responsive dystonia and other tetrahydrobiopterin disorders by the study of biopterin metabolism in fibroblasts. Clin Chem 2001;47(3):477–485.
107. Obeso JA, Rothwell JC, Lang AE, et al. Myoclonic dystonia. Neurology 1983;33(7):825–830.
108. Kyllerman M, Forsgren L, Sanner G, et al. Alcohol-responsive myoclonic dystonia in a large family: Dominant inheritance and phenotypic variation. Mov Disord 1990;5(4):270–279.
109. Marelli C, Canafoglia L, Zibordi F, et al. A neurophysiological study of myoclonus in patients with DYT11 myoclonus-dystonia syndrome. Mov Disord 2008;23(14):-2041–2048.
110. Hess CW, Raymond D, Aguiar Pde C, et al. Myoclonus-dystonia, obsessive-compulsive disorder, and alcohol dependence in SGCE mutation carriers. Neurology. 2007;68(7):522–524.
111. Nygaard TG, Raymond D, Chen C, et al. Localization of a gene for myoclonus-dystonia to chromosome 7q21-q31. Ann Neurol 1999;46(5):794–798.
112. Vidailhet M, Tassin J, Durif F, et al. A major locus for several phenotypes of myoclonus--Dystonia on chromosome 7q. Neurology 2001;56(9):1213–1216.
113. Zimprich A, Grabowski M, Asmus F, et al. Mutations in the gene encoding epsilon-sarcoglycan cause myoclonus-dystonia syndrome. Nat Genet 2001;29(1):66–69.
114. Esapa CT, Waite A, Locke M, et al. SGCE missense mutations that cause myoclonus-dystonia syndrome impair epsilon-sarcoglycan trafficking to the plasma membrane: Modulation by ubiquitination and torsinA. Hum Mol Genet 2007;16(3):327–342.
115. Han F, Racacho L, Lang AE, et al. Refinement of the DYT15 locus in myoclonus dystonia. Mov Disord 2007;22(6):888–892.
116. McKeon A, Ozelius LJ, Hardiman O, et al. Heterogeneity of presentation and outcome in the Irish rapid-onset dystonia-parkinsonism kindred. Mov Disord 2007;22(9): 1325–1327.
117. de Carvalho Aguiar P, Sweadner KJ, Penniston JT, et al. Mutations in the Na^+/K^+-ATPase alpha3 gene ATP1A3 are associated with rapid-onset dystonia parkinsonism. Neuron 2004;43(2):169–175.

CHAPTER 29

Adult-Onset Idiopathic Focal Dystonias

Maria. J. Martí and Eduardo S. Tolosa

Dystonia is characterized by involuntary muscular contractions causing twisting movements and abnormal postures. As described in the previous chapter, dystonia can be classified into primary (dystonic movements and postures in the absence of other motor neurological abnormalities, with the exception of tremor) and secondary forms (environmental causes or symptomatic; dystonia plus syndromes and heredodegenerative diseases).[1] In other chapters in this book, childhood-onset PTD (Chapter 31) and the symptomatic dystonias (Chapter 34) are covered in detail.

The clinical spectrum of PTD in adults is considerably different from that observed in childhood (Table 29–1). It generally involves the upper body—the cranial musculature, neck, or arm—and the spasms tend to remain focal or spread only to the adjacent musculature. In this chapter we cover PTD of adult onset, discussing the clinical manifestations of the various focal dystonias and current thoughts on the underlying pathophysiology.

Most adult-onset focal dystonias (AOFDs) are sporadic, although, on occasion, more than one member in a family may have a focal dystonia. Table 29–2 lists the terminology used to describe the various forms of AOFD. The AOFDs are much more common than previously recognized. Their prevalence has been estimated by Nutt and colleagues,[13] in the population living in Rochester, Minnesota, at 30 per 100,000, compared to generalized PTD at 3.4 per 100,000. A study in the western area of Tottori Prefecture in Japan encountered a lower prevalence (6.2 per 100,000) for focal dystonias than in western countries.[14] A study of primary dystonia in several European countries showed a prevalence rate of 152 per million, with the majority being focal dystonia (117 per million).[15] The reasons for these geographical differences in prevalence are unclear and may reflect the difficulty in identifying cases: patients with focal dystonias may go undiagnosed, and others do not seek medical help. Although the prevalence of generalized PTD is higher among the Ashkenazi Jewish population, this is not the case for AOFD.[16]

▶ TABLE 29–1. EARLY-ONSET VERSUS LATE-ONSET DYSTONTA

Early-Onset
Onset <age 26
Frequently starts in one leg
Commonly becomes generalized with involvement of the trunk
Usually hereditary
Adult-Onset
Onset >26
Focal onset
Tends to remain focal
Spreads to neighboring regions (segmental dystonia) in 20% of cases
Usually sporadic

▶ TABLE 29–2. AOFD SYNDROMES

Muscle Groups Involved	Terminology
A. Orbicularis oculi and neighboring facial muscles	Essential BSP, dystonic BSP
B. Peribuccal muscles and platysma	Lower facial dystonia
C. Lower facial, masticatory, pharyngeal, and lingual muscles	OMD syndrome
D. A plus B or A plus C	Meige's syndrome, BSP-OMD syndrome
E. Laryngeal muscles	Laryngeal dystonia, spasmodic dysphonia
F. Cervical muscles	Cervical dystonia, ST
G. Hand, forearm, arm and leg muscles	LD, WC, TSD, musician's dystonia, athlete's TSD

AOFD, adult-onset focal dystonia; BSP, blepharospasm; OMD, oromandibular dystonia; ST, spasmodic torticollis; LD, limb dystonia; WC, writer's cramp; TSD, task-specific dystonia.

▶ CLINICAL FEATURES OF THE ADULT-ONSET FOCAL DYSTONIAS

FEATURES COMMON TO THE VARIOUS AOFD

Prolonged muscle contractions producing sustained abnormal movements or postures are the clinical hallmark of dystonia. In the AOFD, such spasms are limited to a single body region, with clinical symptoms depending primarily on the group of muscles involved.[17–19]

Characteristics common to the various focal dystonias of adulthood are shown in Table 29–3. AOFD typically have their onset in the fourth or fifth decades but can also begin much earlier, and they typically affect women more than men (3:1). The onset is generally insidious, with symptoms varying depending on the body region involved and degree of spasm intensity. Dystonias occurring in adult life usually progress during the first few years after the initial manifestations. Symptoms at onset can be intermittent, appearing only during times of emotional stress or without any apparent reason, but eventually they become steadily present. The time from onset to maximal disability, though, can vary considerably from patient to patient; in some patients, intense disabling spasms develop in just a few days or weeks, whereas in others the disorder continues to spread slowly 10–15 years after onset. Some studies have suggested that different type of focal dystonia onset confers different risks of spread. So, patients presenting with blepharospasm (BSP) have a higher risk of spread during the 5 first years of illness than those with onset in the neck or upper extremities.[20]

Remissions, either partial or complete, can occur in all of the AOFD, almost always during the first 2–3 years from onset, and are always transient, lasting for days to months. At times, symptoms can recur in a different area of the body than was affected originally. Remissions are more common in patients with spasmodic torticollis (ST) than with other types of AOFD, and they occur more often in those patients with an earlier age of onset.[17–19,21]

Similar to generalized PTD of childhood, in AOFD symptoms at onset usually appear during movement (action dystonia) and disappear when the affected body part is at rest. With the passage of time, dystonic movements may involve muscles not normally used in a task or movement. In writer's cramp (WC), for example, this phenomenon, which is called "overflow," produces the characteristic posture of elevation of the elbow and abduction of the shoulder. In some patients, dystonia is triggered by actions in other parts of the body, as excessive unwanted movements to attempts at voluntary movements (e.g., dystonic movements appearing in the affected arm in a patient with WC when the patient is attempting to write with the healthy hand).

Primary dystonia often starts as a task-specific dystonia (TSD). With progression, however, the dystonic movements may appear with other activities. As an example, in patients with limb dystonia (LD), dystonic cramps may occur initially only when writing but later also when using the hands for other tasks such as eating or sawing. In some patients with spasmodic dysphonia, laryngeal spasms occur initially only when the patient is speaking but not when singing or whispering; however, eventually they may be triggered by these actions as well. As the disease progresses, dystonia also may appear even at rest and, if left untreated, may evolve into fixed postures that eventually cause permanent contractures, as can be seen in long-standing untreated cervical dystonia.

Although dystonic spasms are usually continuous, the timing and intensity of the movements can be influenced by various factors. Emotional stress and fatigue typically worsen dystonia, whereas rest and relaxation improve the spasms and they disappear during sleep. Some patients notice that certain "sensory tricks" can transiently reduce their dystonia. This reduction in dystonia by tactile or proprioceptive stimuli is a feature almost unique to dystonic movements.[22] Touching the back of the head or chin with one or more fingers, for example, allows some patients with torticollis to straighten their head, and gently leaning on the wall when standing may eliminate truncal dystonia transiently.

In addition to prolonged dystonic spasms, patients with AOFD, like those with generalized dystonias, can exhibit other types of involuntary movements. In some patients, rapid movements resembling myoclonus occur. Obeso and colleagues[23] have described myoclonus occurring in patients with idiopathic dystonia that occurs irregularly, is seen mostly on voluntary muscle activation, and is superimposed on dystonic muscle spasms. These rapid movements can cause diagnostic confusion in some cases. Rhythmic, tremor-like movements are not uncommon in patients with dystonia, especially when

▶ TABLE 29–3. CLINICAL FEATURES COMMON TO THE VARIOUS ADULT-ONSET FOCAL DYSTONIAS

Onset generally in fourth to sixth decades
Female predominance
Insidious onset, gradual progression during the first few years
Spread to neighboring regions not uncommon but almost never generalizes
Remissions infrequent but can occur in the early years
Worsened by emotional stress and fatigue
Improved by relaxation and rest
Sensory "tricks" transiently improve dystonic spasms
Tremor is common: focal "dystonic" tremor or essential-like tremor

the patient attempts to actively resist the involuntary movements. This focal, action-type tremor is generally irregular and slow, and is called dystonic tremor.[24] Occasionally, it may precede the onset of dystonia, as described by Rivest and Marsden,[25] or it may be the only manifestation of the dystonic disorder.

Another type of tremor encountered in the primary dystonias, in up to 20% of patients in some series, is one that resembles essential tremor and is frequently observed in both hands, even though they may not be affected by dystonic spasms, or in the head. It is a regular tremor, generally of modest amplitude, and has been reported in torticollis, WC, Meige's syndrome, and other focal dystonias.[24,26,27] True essential tremor has been said to occur commonly in patients with primary dystonias, but it is not clear whether this type of postural tremor is a form of essential tremor, or whether it is an expression of some dystonia-related physiological abnormality. The finding that families with essential tremor do not have the DYT1 mutation, as determined by means of linkage analysis, indicates that the two disorders are not genetically identical.[28] Mild parkinsonism has been described in some of the AOFD, such as Meige's syndrome and WC.[27]

BLEPHAROSPASM

Patients with BSP have intermittent or sustained bilateral eyelid closure as a result of involuntary contractions of the orbicularis oculi muscles. Mild spasms of the frontalis and the middle and lower facial muscles also occur frequently. When the spasms are limited to the orbital or periorbital muscles, it is frequently called essential or dystonic BSP. The association of BSP with oromandibular dystonia (OMD) is called cranial dystonia, or Meige's syndrome, because it was the French neurologist Henri Meige who, in 1910, first described in detail this syndrome, calling it "spasm facial median."[29,30] BSP affects women more than men and has its onset in about the sixth decade of life.

Patients with BSP, which may begin in one eye only, complain of eye discomfort, involuntary eye closure, eye narrowing, or inability to open the eyes. Common complaints at onset are excessive blinking, eye irritation, burning, and photophobia, similar to symptoms of ocular surface, lid margin, and tear film disorders. Both light intensity[31] and the wavelength of light [32] have been reported to be the basis of the photophobia in these patients. BSP patients have variable degrees of difficulty with tasks such as reading, watching television, or driving, and they are frequently disabled, both occupationally and socially, by the spasms and the resulting functional blindness.[29–30,33–35]

Spasms of eye closure are generally aggravated by stress and disappear during sleep. BSP also is worsened by exposure to bright light, and for this reason most patients with BSP wear dark glasses. Other actions that frequently worsen the spasms are looking upward, walking, and reading and, less commonly driving, watching television, or looking downward. Maneuvers or tricks that alleviate some patients include talking, lying down, humming or singing, yawning, laughing, pressure on the eyebrows or the temple, chewing, and opening the mouth.

▶ TABLE 29–4. EYELID DYSFUNCTION IN 17 PATIENTS WITH DYSTONIC BSP

Eyelid Dysfunction	No. of Patients*
Clonic spasms	17 (3)
Dystonic spasms	9 (6)
"Apraxia" of lid opening	11 (3)
Tonic orbicularis contractions	8 (3)
Reflex BSP	6 (2)

BSP, blepharospasm.
*In parentheses is the number of patients in whom the specific type of eyelid dysfunction is the only or the predominant one.
Source: Data modified from Tolosa and Marti.[36]

There are several clinical presentations of BSP[36] (Table 29–4). In the dystonic variety, the more common type, the spasms are prolonged, lasting for several seconds or even minutes, and the eyebrows are displaced downward, below the superior orbital rim (Charcot's sign). In the clonic form, the repetitive spasms of eye closure (blepharoclonus) are fast and resemble normal blinking. In some patients, as a result of contractions of the pretarsal part of the orbicularis oculi, BSP mimics apraxia of lid opening.[36–39] In these patients, the eyes are closed in the absence of overt spasm, and the patient cannot initiate or sustain eye opening. Elevation of the eyebrows, as a result of contraction of the frontalis muscles in an effort by the patient to open the eyelids, is common in this form of BSP (Fig. 29–1). Patients with this type of spasm frequently try to open the eyes with their fingers, pulling the lids apart. At times, reflex BSP is also present, and such attempts to open the eyes manually are met with increasing resistance by stronger spasms of the orbicularis oculi.[40] Yet, in other patients, a persistent narrowing of the palpebral fissure without complete eye closure is observed. The different types of spasms described here can be seen in a given BSP patient but sometimes can occur in isolation.

In most patients, dystonia spreads during the initial 5 years of onset of BSP. Previous head or face trauma with loss of consciousness, age at the onset of BSP, and female sex have been independently associated with an increased risk of spread.[41]

OROMANDIBULAR DYSTONIA

OMD affects women more than men, and the mean age of symptoms onset is between 50 and 60 years of age.[42]

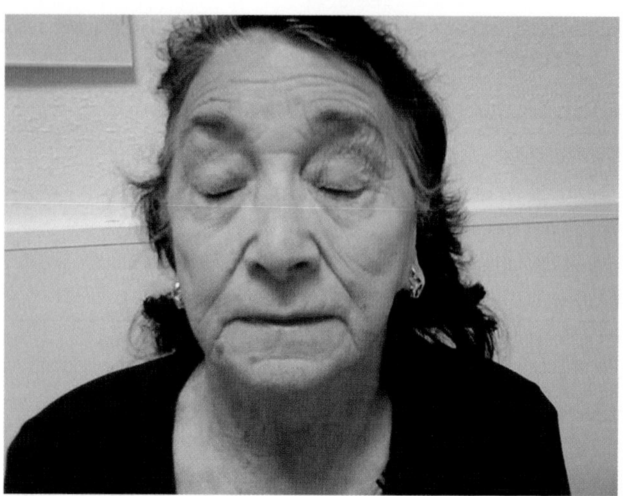

Figure 29–1. "Apraxia" of lid opening in patient with blepharospasm. Oribuclaris oculi spasms are not clearly evident. The patient tries to open the eyes with vigorous frontalis contraction.

In patients with OMD, spasms occur in the region of the jaw, lower face, and mouth.[43–45] Involvement of the masticatory muscles frequently produces spasms of jaw closure or opening, jaw protrusion, lateral deviation, or a combination of these movements. Spasms of jaw closure associated with involuntary contractions of the temporalis muscle and the masseters can produce trismus and bruxism. Involuntary contractions of the lower facial muscles result in spasms of lip tightening, involuntary retraction of the corners of the mouth, and lip pursing. Platysmal contractions are also common. Lingual dystonia is manifested by lateral or upper deviation of the tongue, as well as by tongue protrusion. OMD in isolation is a relatively uncommon form of dystonia, but it is usually very disabling, causing jaw pain, dysarthria, and difficulty chewing and eating. Sensory tricks in OMD include touching the chin, chewing gum, biting on a toothpick, talking, and applying pressure in the submental area. In some patients, OMD is triggered by actions such as biting, chewing, or speaking.

In patients with OMD, spasms frequently occur in adjacent regions, and anterocollis, dysphonia, contraction of the nasalis muscles, and BSP are commonly present. In a study of 162 patients with OMD, 57.4% had associated cervical dystonia, 50% blepharospasms, 21% LD, 16% hand tremor, and 9.9% laringeal dystonia.[42]

SPASMODIC DYSPHONIA (LARYNGEAL DYSTONIA)

Spasmodic dysphonia (SD) occurs between 30 and 50 years of age and, like other AOFD, affects women more than men. It was originally described, by Traube in 1871,[46] as "a spastic form of nervous hoarseness" and was wrongly considered to be a psychogenic disorder until recently. Even today, many patients are referred to psychiatrists because the correct diagnosis is not made when the patient presents for treatment. Dystonic spasms in SD occur during speech (action-specific dystonia, and TSD), whereas the muscles and anatomic structures of the larynx are normal during rest. There are two types of SD:[47–51] adductor SD, which is caused by irregular hyperadduction of the vocal cords, and abductor SD, which is characterized by contraction of the posterior cricoarytenoid muscles during the action of speaking, resulting in inappropriate abduction of the vocal cords. Patients with adductor SD exhibit a choked, strained, staccato, strangled voice quality with abrupt initiation, and termination of vocalization, resulting in short breaks in phonation. There is decreased smoothness of speech, which becomes less intelligible. Usually, singing is less affected than speaking, except in severe cases.

Abductor SD is much less frequent. Patients exhibit a breathy, effortful voice, resulting in aphonic whispered segments of speech.[52] The voice is reduced in loudness, and speech is difficult to understand.

Onset of symptoms in SD is usually gradual, at times following an upper respiratory infection and during either occupational or emotional stress.[53] The initial complaints are increased effort and loss of voice and pitch control, at times only during stress. After 1–2 years of progression, the disease tends to stabilize and become chronic. Maneuvers or tricks that ameliorate SD are usually not as obvious as in other focal dystonias, but some patients report improving transiently when they press their hand on the back of their head,[54] or press their hand on their abdomen. Also, speech can improve briefly after a yawn or a sneeze. Laughing, coughing, or crying does not become affected, but, in 20–30% percent of patients, dystonia occurs elsewhere, usually in the cranial or cervical region. About 20% of patients have an irregular, audible dystonic voice tremor that can, at times, precede the appearance of the dystonic laryngeal spasms.

A more uncommon type of laryngeal dystonia is adductor breathing laryngeal dystonia. Patients with this type of dystonia have inspiratory stridor, which may range from mild to severe but without voice abnormalities. The stridor disappears during sleep and resumes after awakening. Patients can experience breathing difficulties, mainly during eating or speaking, and sometimes they also have respiratory dysrhythmia with diaphragmatic contractions. On laringoscopy, the vocal folds have paradoxical movements that result in a narrow glotic space during inspiration.[55]

SPASMODIC TORTICOLLIS (CERVICAL DYSTONIA)

Dystonia of the neck muscles results in a condition characterized by abnormal head and neck posture commonly referred to as ST. Patients with ST experience jerky movements of the head and intermittent or constant head deviation at rest. Deviation of the head can take any combination of directions: lateral rotation of the head (torticollis), frequently associated with a head tilt, is the most common,[56–58] but there can be head tilt alone (laterocollis), anterocollis, retrocollis as well as lateral or sagittal shift. Frequently, the shoulder is elevated on the side toward which the chin is pointing, and a mild degree of dystonia can be detected commonly in the proximal muscles of the limbs on the same side. According to one study, scoliosis is present in nearly 40% of patients with ST.[57] Unlike other focal dystonias, the incidence of pain in ST is remarkably high (over two thirds of the patients) and contributes to disability.[56–58] Pain is most frequent in patients with constant head deviation, and, although it is usually localized in the neck, patients can develop secondary cervical radiculopathy (over 30% of patients in some series) and experience pain radiating into the arm. Head tremor, considered of a dystonic tremor, and/or hand tremor (essential tremor), occur in about one third of ST patients.[56,59,60]

Sensory tricks used by torticollis patients to reduce the intensity of spasms include touching of the chin, face, or occiput. One such trick, called "geste antagonistique," consists of correction of head position when a very light touch or pressure is applied to the chin, cheek, or elsewhere in the head contralateral to the direction of the head turn. This trick was used in the past as evidence for a psychogenic basis for ST, although it is now recognized as a component of the physiology of ST. Symptoms frequently lessen when the patient lies down in bed, and they worsen when the patient walks and/or is under stress. In addition to cervical dystonia, about 20% of ST patients exhibit cranial (e.g., BSP) or arm-hand dystonia, which is usually mild.

Reported female-to-male ratios for idiopathic ST are approximately 2:1. Mean age at onset is between 38 and 42 years, with most cases clustering in the fourth through the sixth decades.[61] Severity of dystonia tends to progress during the first months or years of the illness, and the dystonic spasms can later spread to the oromandibular region or arm and, exceptionally, the leg. Even though ST is mild in some patients, it is usually disabling, interfering with the patient's daily activities and causing frequent pain. In patients with long-standing cervical dystonia, contractures may develop and fixed deformities may occur.

Although most cases of cervical dystonia are of unknown cause, ST has been described after neck trauma. Some of these posttraumatic cases differ clinically from the more typical cases of idiopathic cervical dystonia because of the presence of marked limitation of range of motion, absence of geste antagonistique, and lack of improvement after sleep.[62,63]

About 10% of patients experience brief spontaneous remission of symptoms, and another 10%, mostly with an earlier age at onset, experience a longer period of remission (2–3 years) that occurs usually during the first 5 years of the illness.[64–66]Remission may be more common in some familial forms of ST. Recently a series of 76 patients with young-onset cervical dystonia has been reported.[67] The mean age at onset was 21 and a familial history of dystonia or tremor was found in 26% of cases. The incidence of dystonia affecting other contiguous areas and spread to involve the legs was similar to that observed in late-onset cervical dystonia. A distinctive feature was a high incidence of sustained spontaneous remissions (30%), but in all cases dystonia relapsed after a variable period.

LIMB DYSTONIA

LD is characterized by involuntary contractions of limb musculature that result in twisting and repetitive movements or abnormal postures in the extremities. LD can affect the leg or the arm and can be focal, as in WC, or segmental, as when involving the arm and the neck (brachial) or leg and trunk (crural). It is always present in patients with generalized dystonia and in hemidystonia, when the upper and the lower extremities on one side are affected.[68,69]

Idiopathic LDs are frequently action dystonias, superimposed on voluntary movements such as writing, using eating utensils, or walking. As the disease progresses, the dystonic postures become more sustained and fixed, even more so when they occur in the legs. When occurring in the arm, distal involvement is more common in the form of wrist flexion, ulnar deviation, and supination. However, elevation, internal rotation, and abduction of the arm can occur also. In some patients the arm pulls behind the patient's back spontaneously.[18]

Many upper extremity LDs are task-specific, that is, they occur exclusively or primarily when the patient performs a specific task. The most frequent task-specific dystonia of the arm is WC, but, in addition to writing, a large number of dystonia-inducing tasks have been reported in musicians[70,71] (e.g., guitarists, trumpet players) or sportsmen (e.g., golfers, snooker players, dart throwers).[68,72]

Symptoms of WC appear as soon as the pen is picked up or after a few words of writing. It usually presents as a forceful exaggeration of the usual grip of the pen, but in other instances hyperextension of the fingers may prevent the pen from being held in the hand. The wrist can show hyperextension or flexion, or forced supination or pronation. Arm and shoulder involvement can also occur. Writing is jerky, shaky, and laborious, and it may be accompanied by a sensation of tension and discomfort in the forearm. At times, frank pain is associated with writing. Frequently, writing becomes impossible after a few words. Classically, patients with WC can manage to write on a wallboard. Some patients find relief by stabilizing the writing hand by holding it with the contralateral one or by using thicker writing devices.[73–76]

WC is classified as "simple" when dystonia occurs only when writing, and as "dystonic" when the spasms appear with other hand tasks, such as using a screwdriver or shaving. WC may evolve from simple to dystonic in about one third of cases but, generally, the severity of the condition remains relatively unchanged. Extension of dystonia to other adjacent or more distant body regions can occur over months to years after onset of symptoms. In about 25% of patients who try to write with the noninvolved hand, bilateral WC develops.[66] As with other dystonias, tremor occurs in about one third of the cases. It can be a postural symmetrical hand tremor or a tremor triggered by writing. In such cases the differentiation with primary writing tremor, a form of task-specific tremor, can be quite difficult.[77,78]

It is not clear whether extensive writing can cause WC. It is likely that patients who write frequently will recognize their symptoms earlier and will seek early medical attention.[65] WC can be the earliest manifestation of generalized torsion dystonia, but it can also represent the presenting complaint of neurological disorders, such as Parkinson's disease or progressive supranuclear palsy.[79–82]

In patients with WC, several electrophysiological abnormalities have been found, and these are shared with other task-specific dystonias (see Ref. 83 for review). Co-contraction of antagonist muscles occurs, such that movement can be undertaken only with the greatest of effort. There is lack of selectivity in attempts to perform independent finger movements, and neural activation may spread ("overflow") to involve muscles not normally used in the task of writing (e.g., abduction of the shoulder). Failure to activate the appropriate muscles may also occur. These findings highlight the fact that patients have more problems with voluntary actions than with involuntary muscle spasm.

Dystonia occurring in the lower extremities usually affects distal joints, principally the ankle, with plantar flexion and inversion of the foot. The sole of the foot can also cup and the toes can flex. Initially, foot dystonia occurs only when one is walking, being absent with the limb at rest. Frequently, running, walking in tandem, or walking backward fails to trigger the abnormal posture. The initial equinovarus posture that occurs when the patient is walking may evolve into a fixed dystonic posture, commonly causing plantar flexion, extension of the knee, and extension, internal rotation, and abduction of the hip.

When lower extremity LD occurs in childhood, it usually heralds the onset of early-generalized dystonia.[84] When lower extremity LD occurs after the age of 20, it suggests the possibility of focal central nervous system structural disease. Also, when dystonia affects the foot in an adult, the possibility of Parkinson's disease or another parkinsonian syndrome should be considered because kinesigenic foot dystonia is an early sign of young-onset Parkinson's disease.[80]

Primary dystonia affecting exclusively one foot or leg has been rarely reported. Recently, Schneider and colleagues.[85] reported a series of 17 patients with lower LD in whom a specific cause was excluded after an average of symptoms duration of 5 years. Age at onset ranged from 30 to 72 years. The more frequent patterns of dystonia were plantar flexion of the toes and foot inversion, which were activated by standing or walking. In contrast to what happen in children, in these cases dystonia almost never extended to other body regions. Singer and Papapetropoulus[86] have also described four patients with onset of focal food dystonia at age ranging between 44 and 74 years. Again, after a mean follow-up of 6 years dystonia remained focal. Foot dystonia appeared mainly during walking and subsided at rest, causing moderate physical impairment.

The lower limb is the more frequent body part involved in cases presenting with fixed dystonia. In this syndrome features of either complex regional pain syndrome or psychogenic dystonia overlap. Usually fixed dystonia occurs after a peripheral injury and pain is present in the majority of cases. Investigations are typically normal and some patients fulfilled criteria for somatization disorder. However, transcranial magnetic stimulation studies show abnormal cortical excitability, similar to those reported in typical mobile dystonia.[87]

OTHER TASK-SPECIFIC DYSTONIAS

In addition to WC, other TSD have been described in milkers, seamstresses, cobblers, shoemakers, musicians, and others whose work involves frequent repetitive movements.[68,88] This population of individuals who repeatedly overuse their limbs is also more predisposed to nerve entrapments and muscle and joint disorders. This may lead to some clinical confusion. Tasks capable of inducing action dystonia almost always require either highly repetitive movements or extreme motor precision. The majority of TSD involve the upper limb and, rarely, the leg, probably because the use of the lower limb for precise repetitive tasks is unusual. They have been described in knife sharpeners, dancers, tradesmen, cyclists, sewing machine workers, and cello players.

Telegraphist cramp, found in one study to affect 14% of 516 telegraphists,[89] has been progressively disappearing since the introduction of the modern telephone. It is likely that typist's cramp will become more prevalent with the expansion of keyboard-dependent telecommunication. Musicians, with the years of practice and repetition of precise and complicated movements required to achieve professional status, are prone to overuse syndromes, and as many as 15% of professional musicians may be suffering from overuse syndromes.[70] These focal dystonias are particularly devastating. They can occur in musicians using almost any kind of instrument, but are more common in piano players. Newmark and Hochberg,[71] evaluated the focal motor syndromes in 57 instrumental musicians and noted three stereotyped afflictions: (1) flexion of fourth and fifth fingers in pianists, (2) flexion of the third finger in guitarists, and (3) extension of the third finger in clarinetists. The disabilities in these patients were not progressive. In brass instrumentalists, as well as in double-reed players, musician's dystonia may involve the peribuccal and cervical muscles. Frucht and colleagues reported the clinical observations in 26 brass and woodwind players affected with embouchure dystonia (the pattern of lip, jaw, and tongue muscles used to control the flow of air into a mouthpiece). Initial symptoms were limited to one range of notes or style of playing, eventually progressing without remission, although a percentage of patients reported fluctuations in their symptoms.[90]

Musician's cramps are usually refractory to medical treatment, rest, or physical therapy. Alteration of playing technique may help some patients. The response to botulinum toxin injections is generally insufficient because, for professional musicians, even a marked response to treatment is of no benefit when the abilities needed to play professionally are not maintained.

Athlete's TSD can occur in golfers and other sportsmen, such as tennis players, snooker players, or dart throwers. Golfer's TSD (the "yips") may affect as many as 28% of golfers, more commonly afflicting those who have more cumulative years of golfing.[72] Involuntary movements emerge particularly during putting, but are much less evident during chipping or driving.[91] As in patients with other TSD, golfers with the yips use complementary strategies, such as changing hand preference. About one fourth of them report that other activities can be similarly affected.

OTHER FOCAL DYSTONIAS

Rarely, isolated dystonia of the pharyngeal muscles occurs causing dysphagia (dystonic dysphagia). Disability in these patients may be severe, and surgical section of the crycopharyngeus muscle may be needed to improve swallowing.[92–94] Patients with dystonic dysphagia frequently have OMD or neck dystonia as well. Isolated lingual dystonia is very rare,[95] but lingual dystonia can certainly be the most prominent manifestation of OMD. Another AOFD occasionally encountered is truncal dystonia. In these patients, continuous or repetitive spasms cause flexion, extension, scoliosis, or torsion of the trunk.[92] As with other focal dystonias, spasms at onset may occur only when walking or standing but, eventually, they can be present even when the patient is lying down. In some patients, spasms are rapid enough to resemble myoclonus, and this has been referred to as "woodpecker dystonia." Extension to adjacent regions can occur, such as retrocollis, involvement of proximal limb muscles, or pelvic involvement (so-called copulatory dystonia). Sensory tricks that improve truncal dystonia include gently leaning against the wall when standing, pressing in the back of the neck, or pressing on the hips.

Abdominal wall dystonia (belly dancer's dyskinesia) has been described,[96] and Caviness and colleagues[97] have reported a group of patients with focal or segmental dyskinesias affecting the ears, back, shoulder girdle, abdomen, and pelvic girdle that closely resemble focal dystonias. In these patients the movements were slow, sinuous, semirhythmic, and associated with long-duration bursts of electromyogram (EMG) activity in neurophysiological studies. Peripheral trauma may have played a role in the pathogenesis of the movements in some patients.

▶ ETIOLOGY

The cause of AOFD remains unknown in the majority of cases. As discussed in the preceding chapter, several genetic mutations that may cause familial forms of AOFD have been identified, including DYT6, DYT7, and DYT13, but these are collectively rare and account for only a small proportion of AOFD. There is evidence that suggests that there are additional genetic triggers for AOFD that remain to be discovered. A role for heredity in AOFD is suggested by the observed familial cases of orofacial dystonia, WC, and ST,[105,106] and the reports of Meige's syndrome and cervical dystonia in apparently identical twins.[107] Furthermore, several large studies of focal dystonias have reported positive family histories, ranging from 2 to 15% of patients.[108] Affected relatives displayed focal and segmental signs but not generalized dystonia. Waddy and colleagues[109] found that 25% of 40 non-Jewish patients with focal dystonia had relatives in whom dystonia could be identified. Defazio and colleagues made similar observations in a family study of 29 patients with BSP and craniocervical dystonia.[110]

Autoimmune disorders, such as thyroid disease, systemic lupus erythematosus, rheumatoid arthritis, or myasthenia gravis, have been associated with primary dystonia.[35,121] Nilaver and colleagues,[122] however, could not find anticentral nervous system antibodies in the serum of 11 patients with cranial dystonia, using the direct immunoperoxidase technique. More recently, a study directed to detect basal ganglia-specific antibodies in serum of seven patients with primary BSP also failed to find them.[123] Use of sympathicomimetic drugs, eye color, and focal brainstem and diencephalic lesions have been associated with the focal dystonias only in occasional patients. Therefore, they are not widely accepted as risk factors.

Several studies have indicated that dystonia may be precipitated by peripheral factors such as overuse, misuse, or trauma.[124] Fletcher and colleagues[125] showed that peripheral trauma may trigger dystonia in carriers of the ITD gene. A similar phenomenon in isolated BSP is suggested by the finding that up to 12% of patients report the occurrence of ocular trauma or lesion before the onset of the movement disorder.[126] Peripheral trauma has also been reported in 5–12% of patients with cervical dystonia,[127,128] occurring 3–6 months before the onset of symptoms. Similarly, cases of OMD have occurred soon after facial lacerations and dental work.[129] Laryngitis can precede spasmodic dysphonia.[130] Occasionally, focal LD may be associated with extremity injury, such as electrical injury,[131] or with reflex sympathetic dystrophy. Tremor and dystonia are the movement disorders most often associated with reflex sympathetic dystrophy ("causalgia-dystonia syndrome"),[132,133] and it almost always develops after peripheral trauma. In these cases the development of pain may be of importance.

Peripheral factors are also generally accepted to play a role in a variety of occupational or TSD, such as WC, typist's cramp, or the focal dystonias occurring in musicians or sportsmen. A recently described case of OMD occurring in an auctioneer is another example of a focal dystonia that was possibly related to muscle overuse.[134] Inzelberg and colleagues[135] found a highly significant relationship between motor dominance and the laterality of limb onset in ITD patients, which suggests that the preferred use of a limb may trigger the onset of dystonia.

The exact role of muscle overuse or trauma in the genesis of dystonia remains to be clarified. A study by Fletcher and colleagues[136] did not support the notion that trauma is important in idiopathic dystonia. In their study of 71 patients with ITD and 71 matched controls investigating the role of environmental factors in the development of the disorder, trauma was no more frequent among patients than among control subjects, either in the year preceding the onset of dystonia in the index patients or at any other time. It is unlikely that trauma alone is sufficient for dystonia to develop because, if this were the case, dystonia would be much more common. It has been postulated that trauma may trigger the expression of a previously subclinical or very mild dystonia or trigger dystonia only in patients with preexisting susceptibility, perhaps on a genetic basis.[17,124,137] A recently developed rat model has supported these concepts. A combination of partial dopaminergic cell destruction in the substantia nigra and a lesion on the zygomatic branch of the facial nerve lead the animal to present spontaneous spasms of eyelid closure. Individually, both of these lesions produced a hyperexcitability of the blink reflex, but BSP was only observed when they were performed on the same animal. This model suggested that a subclinical loss of striatal dopamine confers a susceptibility to developing dystonia, which can be apparent when an external insult occurs.[138]

It has been suggested that complex movement disorders such as dystonia, occurring after a peripheral nerve or spinal nerve root lesion, are generated by reorganization of spinal motor circuitry or by changes in supraspinal somatosensory integration that result in altered basal ganglia function.[138] Some authors believe that there may be a psychogenic basis for many cases of posttraumatic dystonia.[139]

▶ ANATOMIC SUBSTRATE AND PATHOPHYSIOLOGY OF THE FOCAL DYSTONIAS

Autopsy studies have been performed in 16 patients with presumed idiopathic cranial dystonia. No significant abnormalities were found in four; one had an "incidental" small angioma of the pons, and the other patients had relatively nonspecific abnormalities.[140,141] Mosaic neuronal cell loss and gliosis have been seen in two patients,[142] and three patients have been reported as having cell loss and gliosis of the substantia nigra pars compacta and other brainstem nuclei.[143,144] In two of these patients, abundant Lewy bodies were present. Lesions in the basal ganglia, thalamus, cerebral cortex, diencephalon, and brainstem have been reported to be associated with some of the focal dystonias.[145,146]

Recently Holton and colleagues have described six patients with focal and segmental adult-onset dystonia.[147] Unlike what has been described in patients with DYT1 dystonia,[148] these investigators were unable to detect brainstem perinuclear inclusion bodies, except for some ubiquitine-immunereactive inclusions in subependymal regions in both patients and controls. There was also no loss of the striatal striosome compartment. One case had Alzheimer pathology and brainstem predominant Lewy bodies inclusions.

Mostly based on the correlations that exist between the secondary dystonias and lesions of the putamen and thalamus, it is currently believed that the focal dystonias result from an abnormality in the basal ganglia. Dynamic imaging studies, using positron emission tomography (PET), showed hypometabolism in the caudate and lentiform nucleus, and in the frontal projection fields of the mediodorsal thalamic nucleus.[149] Hence, functional disturbance in the basal ganglia and their frontal connections is thought to be the underlying cause of the dystonias. In Meige's syndrome, relative glucose hypermetabolism of the putamen was detected.[150] In addition, bilateral relative increments in glucose utilization for the thalamus and primary sensorimotor cortices has been observed. When the subjects are studied during sleep, the same pattern of hypermetabolism is present, even though no dystonic spasms are occurring.[151] Recently, some PET studies using ^{18}F-fluorodeoxyglucose (FDG) or regional cerebral blood flow (rCBF) measuring methods have shown abnormalities in the activation pattern of cortical structures. In a recent study, CBF was measured using $H^{15}{}_2O$ and PET, at rest and during movement, in a group of six patients with ITD, one of whom had isolated WC. Results demonstrated overactivity of the striatum and its frontal association projection areas. Reduced activity in motor executive areas was also detected.[152] Using rCBF PET, Ibañez and colleagues[153] studied seven patients with WC during rest and performing different tasks with the right hand. Patients showed a deficient activation of the sensorimotor and premotor cortex and decreased correlation between premotor cortical regions and putamen, suggesting a dysfunction of the premotor cortical network. Similar results, with decreased activation of the primary sensory motor area, were observed in patients with BSP in response to vibration.[154] Hutchinson and colleagues[155] used FDG PET to investigate the metabolic topography of BSP in six patients. During wakefulness, patients showed hypermetabolism of the cerebellum and pons compared with controls. While asleep, the BSP group exhibited superomediofrontal hypometabolism, in a region associated with cortical control of eyelid movements.

Measures of the index binding in putamen of the dopaminergic radioligand ^{18}F-spiperone in patients with facial dystonia and WC were 29% lower in patients than in controls, suggesting abnormality of dopaminergic receptors in primary dystonia.[156]

Studies with proton magnetic resonance spectroscopy in patients with BSP[157] and torticollis[158] showed a reduction in *N*-acetylaspartate (NAA)/choline and NAA/creatine ratios in the lentiform nucleus, indicating neuronal dysfunction in this region. By contrast, no differences in metabolite levels were seen in another study comparing normal subjects and patients with primary focal hand dystonia.[159]

Studies using voxel-based morphometry in patients with blepharospasm, cervical and focal hand dystonia showed changes in grey matter density in several brain areas.[160–163] A common finding was a bilateral increase in grey matter density in primary somatosensory and motor cortex with abnormalities in subcortical structures like the basal ganglia.

Functional magnetic resonance imaging studies have shown that patients with BSP and focal hand dystonia display overactivity of the primary sensorimotor cortex and the caudal part of SMA.[164–166] Under specific dystonia inducing tasks, overactivation in cerebellum and premotor areas have also been seen.[167] Taken together these studies suggest abnormalities in cortex and brainstem in addition to basal ganglia dysfunction.

Recently, using diffusion tensor imaging Fabbrini and colleagues found abnormalities in the right prefrontal cortex associated to duration of botulinum toxin treatment in 18 patients with cervical dystonia, suggesting the presence of brain white matter ultrastructural changes.[168]

How dysfunction of the basal ganglia results in dystonia is unclear. In dystonia, basal ganglia dysfunction may result in an inability to target inhibition to opposite sets of neurons in the cortex, thus producing excessive motor output, particularly during movement.[16] Ridding and colleagues[169] have reported that ipsilateral cortico-cortical inhibition is abnormal in patients with WC, which could represent a disturbance in the excitability of local intracortical inhibitory interneurons. Decreased intracortical inhibition related to hand muscles has also been reported in patients who have BSP without hand dystonia.[170] This suggests increased exitability of the cortical hand motor areas. In a patient with unilateral focal dystonia resulting from a lesion of the contralateral putamen, Hanajima and colleagues[171] detected, using double cortical stimulation techniques, hyperexcitability of the motor cortex ipsilateral to the putaminal lesion, with normal excitability of the sensory cortex. In a study investigating cortical excitability using high-intensity transcortical magnetic stimulation, Curra and colleagues[172] elicited an abnormally short cortical silent period in facial muscles in patients with cranial dystonia, suggesting a reduced excitability of cortical inhibitory interneurons in the motor cortex. A consequence of decreased inhibition is a loss of surround inhibition that may explain the overflow phenomenon seen in patients.[173]

In addition to these alterations in the cortex, many reflex abnormalities have been described in dystonic patients, and these are greatest in muscles affected by dystonia. In cranial, laryngeal, and cervical dystonia, blink reflex and masseter inhibitory reflex abnormalities have been clearly documented, suggesting that both excitatory and inhibitory interneuronal pathways in the brainstem are perturbed.[174–176] In many of the focal dystonias, such as ST or spasmodic dysphonia, subclinical abnormalities of the blink reflexes generally occur, suggesting that the clinical abnormalities are not a consequence of the abnormalities observed in these tests. Also, treatment with botulinum toxin markedly improves BSP and ST, but clinical improvement is not accompanied by a concomitant normalization of the blink reflex excitability curve in these patients.[177,178]

Another example of abnormal brain stem interneuronal excitability is the finding of reduced exteroceptive inhibition of the sternocleidomastoid muscle after a supra- or infraorbital nerve stimulus.[179,180] Vestibular abnormalities have also been reported in ST, but they could be secondary to the abnormal head position.[181,182] Reciprocal inhibition has been extensively studied in dystonia. It refers to the active inhibition of activity in antagonist muscles during voluntary contraction of the agonist. In LD, reciprocal inhibition studied in the flexor and extensor muscles of the forearm is reduced.[183,184]

A similar abnormality has been detected in patients with ST and with BSP, even though there was no clinical involvement of forearm muscles.

Although there is no deficit of sensation in dystonia, there are some phenomena relating to the sensory system, such as overuse or trauma preceding dystonia, which could indicate that there are sensory disturbances in dystonia that can contribute to generate, maintain or suppress the dystonic movements. In a study investigating how sensory tricks diminish the dystonic symptoms, we examined the effects on blink reflex and its recovery curve by touching the face with the finger in eight patients with BSP.[185] This maneuver increased the amplitude of R_1 and reduced the area of R_2. This reduction of R_2 could be caused by sensory gating of trigeminal afferents, thereby lowering the gain of trigeminofacial reflexes and contributing to transit benefit induced by sensory tricks. Stimulation of spindle afferents obtained by tonic vibration of the tendon or the belly muscle can induce dystonia in patients with WC, which can be improved with partial lidocaine block of the muscle.[186] Recently, using neurophysiological techniques tactile temporal discrimination deficits have been described in patients with AOFD.[187,188] The abnormalities were not thought to be of clinically significant. Sensory dysfunction can also been demonstrated with somatosensory evoked potential testing[189] and can be present in both hand of patients with focal hand dystonia.[190]

The picture that emerges from all of these physiological studies is that the brainstem and spinal interneuron circuitry are functioning abnormally in patients with focal dystonias, resulting in a change in the tonic control of reflex excitability. An abnormal input from the basal ganglia via cortical or subcortical connections on brainstem and spinal interneurons could result in these static abnormalities. Such changes might produce particular problems during movement, when activity in specific reflex pathways is normally well regulated according to the task being performed.[83]

▶ DIFFERENTIAL DIAGNOSIS AND INVESTIGATIONS IN PATIENTS WITH FOCAL DYSTONIAS

Most focal dystonias prove to be idiopathic, regardless of the location. Occasionally, a known cause can be identified. Although the list of such secondary or symptomatic dystonias is quite extensive,[69,191] symptomatic focal dystonias clinically similar to idiopathic ones are not common. Nevertheless, the distinction between idiopathic and symptomatic forms is important to give patients an appropriate prognosis and genetic counseling. Most importantly, adequate treatment of some of the symptomatic dystonias, when appropriately diagnosed, can result in a cure or avoid progression to a more generalized disorder, as could be the case in dystonia associated with Wilson's disease.

The most common cause of symptomatic AOFD is tardive dystonia induced by chronic neuroleptic administration.[192,193] Cases of tardive dystonia can be identical to those of BSP, OMD, cervical dystonia, spasmodic dysphonia, or idiopathic truncal dystonia, and can sometimes only be differentiated from the idiopathic dystonias by the history of neuroleptic use.[36] Tardive dystonia does not usually lead to WC. Also relatively common in movement disorder clinics are focal dystonias induced by L-dopa in Parkinson's disease,[194] and those occurring in the setting of the various degenerative parkinsonian syndromes. Kinesigenic foot dystonia can be the presenting manifestation of untreated young-onset Parkinson's disease,[195,196] and WC, torticollis, OMD, and BSP have been described as preceding the onset of otherwise typical Parkinson's disease by variable periods, from months up to several years (see Ref. 105 for review). LD and BSP can also be the presenting manifestations of progressive supranuclear palsy,[197] and focal dystonia was described as a prominent presenting feature in a group of patients with hereditary or sporadic cerebellar ataxia.[198] When a focal dystonia is the presenting feature of one of these syndromes, when other neurological findings are not yet present, it is usually impossible to differentiate it from one of the "idiopathic" dystonias on clinical grounds.

Focal dystonic spasms similar to the primary ones have been described secondary to focal hemispheric brain pathology and to brainstem/diencephalic lesions in patients with stroke, multiple sclerosis, or hydrocephalus. We have also seen prominent focal dystonia, either as the initial manifestation or during the course of disorders such as head trauma, kernicterus, delayed-onset dystonia, Hallervorden-Spatz disease, Tourette's syndrome, Huntington's disease, Wilson's disease, and acquired nonwilsonian hepatocerebral degeneration and the degenerative cerebellar ataxias.[124,199] Focal LD has also been encountered in patients with cerebellar lesions.[200,201]

A large part of the clinical investigations in a patient with AOFD is directed to uncover a possible cause for the disorder. Historical features can be quite useful in ruling out certain etiological factors. A history of exposure to drugs or toxins must be sought diligently. Antidopaminergic drugs, such as the neuroleptics, antiemetics, or some antivertiginous agents can cause tardive focal dystonias that can be otherwise indistinguishable from idiopathic ones. Toxins such as manganese and methanol can cause similar symptoms, usually after an initial neurological insult. In a number of instances, symptomatic dystonia appears months to years after the initial cerebral insult.[202,203] Delayed-onset dystonias can occur in adolescence that are related to birth asphyxia,[204] but this phenomenon can be observed also with central pontine myelinolysis[205] and cyanide intoxication.[206] A history of recent trauma, in the same body region as the focal dystonia, or head trauma, suggests a posttraumatic dystonia.[127,137] Details of the onset, distribution, and clinical characteristics of the dystonic spasms is sometimes helpful in diagnosing a symptomatic dystonia. A focal dystonia of abrupt onset suggests a structural nervous system lesion or a psychogenic etiology. Idiopathic dystonias are typically action-induced at onset, followed by overflow dystonia and, eventually, are present at rest. Dystonia at rest, even from the beginning, strongly suggests a secondary dystonia.

In primary dystonia, the only neurological abnormality is the presence of dystonic postures and movements. Such movements are tremoric at times and exceptionally myoclonic. There is no associated oculomotor abnormality, ataxia, dementia, seizures, weakness, atrophy, or spasticity. However, many of the symptomatic dystonias are associated with some of these neurological findings and, therefore, their presence strongly suggests that one is dealing with such a case. The presence of stereotypes—repetitive, patterned, seemingly purposeful but purposeless movements, such as repetitive tongue protrusion ("fly-catching" tongue movements) or the "bon-bon" sign (roving movements of the tongue inside the mouth)—in patients with otherwise typical BSP, for example, strongly suggests the diagnosis of tardive dystonia. The absence of such neurological abnormalities, however, does not exclude the possibility of symptomatic dystonia, which may present as pure dystonia. Equally important in the evaluation of a patient with focal dystonia are the findings on general physical examination, which can even be diagnostic of a specific disorder; for example, the presence of a Kayser-Fleischer ring indicates Wilson's disease.

Careful clinical evaluation of the dystonic spasm is always necessary, particularly if the patient is a candidate for botulinum toxin treatment. In some patients, diagnosis may not be possible on simple inspection because dystonia may not be present at all times. In these cases, certain clinical maneuvers may bring out the dystonic spasms and allow for a precise diagnosis. Shining a bright light in front of the patient's eyes or asking the patient to open and close the eyes repeatedly[35] may, for example, trigger BSP. Dystonic tremor, which may be treated successfully with botulinum toxin, may have to be brought out by asking the patient to adopt a certain position (e.g., trying to oppose the dystonic spasms). In general, an attempt has to be made to find the position with the most severe dystonia, instructing the patient to position the affected body region so as to show maximal abnormality. The patient should always be examined while standing, walking, sitting, and lying down. In patients with LD or cervical dystonia, passive movements of the affected region may help in localizing the contracting muscles and in determining the full range of motion or the presence of contractures.

Palpation of the contracting muscles is also useful in localizing involved muscles and in estimating muscle mass, and it helps in detecting points of tenderness.

Psychogenic dystonia can be most difficult to diagnose in an adult, but it can occur particularly in certain subsets of dystonia, such as adult-onset lower LD, paroxysmal dystonia, and adductor laryngeal dystonia. Certain historical or examination features, such as a large number of somatic complaints, abrupt onset, presence of false weakness, or incongruous movements not fitting with typical organic dystonia, provide clues that suggest a psychogenic etiology[207] (see Chapter 55).

In addition to psychogenic causes, a number of other disorders in which abnormal postures occur but are not associated with underlying inappropriate muscle contraction should be differentiated from dystonia. Conditions simulating focal dystonia[55] can be orthopedic (an atlantoaxial subluxation, for example, can lead to an abnormal head posture that mimics torticollis) or neurological (such as posterior fossa tumors, syringomyelia, or extraocular muscle palsies), producing abnormal head or spine postures. Muscle contractures occurring in neurological patients or after orthopedic injuries may also pose difficult diagnostic problems, and infectious, inflammatory, and neoplastic involvement of the soft-tissue structures of the head and neck may simulate cervical dystonia.[208]

In the investigation of patients with AOFD presumed to be idiopathic, there is little need for laboratory or neuroimaging tests because a symptomatic cause is almost never found. When the patient is under 40 years of age, investigations for Wilson's disease should be conducted (see Chapter 48), but older patients with typical focal dystonias require no further workup unless new or atypical features appear on follow-up, particularly when the disorder has been present for several months or longer.

REFERENCES

1. Fahn S, Bressman SB, Marsden CD. Classification of dystonia. In Fahn S, Marsden CD, DeLOng MR (eds). Dsytonia 3: Advances in Neurology, Vol 78. Philadelphia, PA: Lippincott-Raven, 1998, pp: 1–10.
2. Bugalho P, Correa B, Guimaraes J, Xavier M. Set-shifting and behavioral dysfunction in primary focal dystonia. Mov Disord 2008;23:200–206.
3. Kramer PL, DeLeon D, Ozelius L, et al. Dystonia gene in Ashkenazi Jewish population is located on chromosome 9q32–34. Ann Neurol 1990;27:114–120.
4. Opal P, Tintner R, Jankovic J, et al. Intrafamilial phenotypic variability of the DYT1 dystonia: From asymptomatic TORIA gene carrier status to dystonic storm. Mov Disord 2002;17:339–345.
5. Chinnery PF, Reading PJ, McCarthy EL, et al. Late-onset axial jerky dystonia due to DYT1 deletion. Mov Disord 2002;17:196–198.

6. Almasy L, Bressman SB, Raymond D, et al. Idiopathic torsion dystonia linked to chromosoma 8 in two Mennonite families. Ann Neurol 1997;42:670–673.
7. Leube B, Rudnicki D, Ratzlaff T, et al. Idiopathic torsion dystonia: Assignment of a gene to chromosoma 18p in a german family with adult onset, autosomal dominant inheritance and purely focal distribution. Hum Mol Genet 1996;5:1673–1677.
8. Bressman SB, Warner TT, Almasy L, et al. Exclusion of the DYT1 locus in familial torticollis. Ann Neurol 1996; 40(4):681–684.
9. Cassetta E, Del Grosso N, Bentivoglio AR, et al. Italian family with cranial cervical dystonia: Clinical and genetic study. Mov Disord 1999;14:820–825.
10. Bentivoglio AR, Ialongo T, Contarino MF, et al. Phenotipic characteritzation of DYT13 primary torsion dystonia. Mov Disord 2004;19:200–206.
11. Valente EM, Bentivoglio AR, Cassetta E, et al. DYT13, a novel primary torsión dystonia locus, maps to cromosoma 1p36.13-36.32 in a Italian family with crnial-cervical or upper-limb onset. Ann Neurol 2001;49:362–366.
12. Holmgren G, Ozelius L, Forsgren L, et al. Adult onset idiopathic torsion dystonia is excluded from the DYT1 region (9q34) in a Swedish family. J Neurol Neurosurg Psychiatry 1995;59:178–181.
13. Nutt JG, Muenter MD, Aronson A, et al. Epidemiology of focal and generalized dystonia in Rochester, Minnesota. Mov Disord 1988;3:188–194.
14. Nakashima K, Kusumi M, Inoue Y, et al. Prevalence of focal dystonias in the Western area of Tottori prefecture in Japan. Mov Disord 1995;10:440–443.
15. The Epidemiological Study of Dystonia in Europe (ESDE) Collaborative Group. A prevalence study of primary dystonia in eight European countries. J Neurol 2000;247: 787–792.
16. Fahn S. Generalized dystonia. In Tsui JK, Calne DB (eds). Handbook of Dystonia. New York, NY: Marcel Dekker, 1995, pp. 193–211.
17. Jankovic J, Fahn S. Dystonic disorders. In Jankovic J, Tolosa E (eds). Parkinson's Disease and Movement Disorders, 2nd ed. Baltimore, MD: Williams & Wilkins, 1993, pp. 337–374.
18. Fahn S. Dystonia, in Jankovic J, Hallett M (eds). Therapy with Botulinum Toxin. New York, NY: Marcel Dekker, 1994, pp. 173–189.
19. Marsden CD. The focal dystonias. Clin Neuropharmacol 1986;9(suppl 2):49–60.
20. Abbruzzese G, Berardelli A, Girlanda P, et al. Long-term assessment of the risk of spread in primary late-onset focal dystonia. J Neurol Neurosurg Psychiatry 2008; 79:392–396.
21. Friedman A, Fahn S. Spontaneous remissions in spasmodic torticollis. Neurology 1986;36:398–400.
22. Rothwell JC, Obeso JA, Day BL, et al. Pathophysiology of dystonias. In Desmedt JE (ed). Motor Control Mechanisms in Health and Disease. New York, NY: Raven Press, 1983, pp. 851–863.
23. Obeso JA, Rothwell JC, Lang AE, et al. Myoclonic dystonia. Neurology 1983;33:825–830.
24. Cleeves L, Findley J, Marsden D. Odd tremors. In Marsden D, Fahn S (eds). Movement Disorders 3. Oxford: Butterworth-Heinemann, 1994, pp. 434–453.
25. Rivest J, Marsden D. Trunk and head tremor as isolated manifestation of dystonia. Mov Disord 1990;5:60–65.
26. Patterson RM, Little SC. Spasmodic torticollis. J Nerv Ment Dis 1943;98:571–599.
27. Sheehy MP, Marsden CD. Writer's cramp: A focal dystonia. Brain 1982;105:461–480.
28. Conway D, Bain PG, Warner TT, et al. Linkage analysis with chromosome-9 markers in hereditary essential tremor. Mov Disord 1993;8:374–376.
29. Tolosa ES. Clinical features of Meige's disease (idiopathic orofacial dystonia): A report of 17 cases. Arch Neurol 1981;38:147–151.
30. Tolosa ES, Klawans HL. Meige's disease: A clinical form of facial convulsion bilateral and medial. Arch Neurol 1979;36:635–637.
31. Adams WH, Digre KB, Patel BC, et al. Evaluation of light sensitivity in benign essential blepharospasm. Am J Ophtalmol 2006;142:82–87.
32. Herz NL, Yen MT. Modulation of sensory photophobia in essential blepharospasm with chromatic lenses. Ophtalmology 2005;112:2208–2211.
33. Grandas F, Elston JS, Quinn N, et al. Blepharospasm: A review of 264 patients. J Neurol Neurosurg Psychiatry 1988;51:767–772.
34. Marsden CD. The problem of adult-onset idiopathic torsion dystonia and other isolated dyskinesias in adult life (including blepharospasm, oromandibular dystonia, dystonic writer's cramp and torticollis, or axial dystonia). Adv Neurol 1976;14:259–276.
35. Jankovic J, Ford J. Blepharospasm and orofacial-cervical dystonia: Clinical and pharmacological findings in 100 patients. Ann Neurol 1983;13:402–411.
36. Tolosa E, Martí MJ. Blepharospasm-oromandibular dystonia syndrome (Meige's syndrome): Clinical aspects. Adv Neurol 1988;49:73–84.
37. Tolosa E, Kulisevsky J, Martí MJ. Apraxia of lid opening in dystonic blepharospasm. IV International Meeting of the Benign Essential Blepharospasm Research Foundation, Barcelona, Spain, 1986.
38. Tolosa E, Kulisevsky J, Martí MJ. "Apraxia" of lid opening in essential blepharospasm. XXXVIIII Reunión de la American Academy of Neurology, New York, 1987.
39. Elston JS. A new variant of blepharospasm. J Neurol Neurosurg Psychiatry 1992;55:369–371.
40. Obeso JA, Artieda J, Marsden CD. Stretch reflex blepharospasm. Neurology 1985;35:1378–1380.
41. Defazio G, Berardelli A, Abbruzzese G, et al. Risk factors for spread of primary adult onset blepharospasm: A multicentre investigation of the Italian movement disorders study group. J Neurol Neurosurg Psychiatry 1999;67: 613–619.
42. Tan EK, Jancovic J. Botulinum toxin A in patients with oromandibular dystonia: long-term follow-up. Neurology 1999;53:2102–2107.
43. Marsden CD. Blepharospasm-oromandibular dystonia syndrome (Breughel's syndrome): A variant of adult-onset torsion dystonia? J Neurol Neurosurg Psychiatry 1976; 39:1204–1209.
44. Cardoso F, Jankovic J. Oromandibular dystonia. In Ching Tsiu JK, Calne DB (eds) . Handbook of Dystonia. New York, NY: Marcel Dekker, 1995, pp. 181–192.

45. Brin MF, Blitzer A, Herman S, et al. Oromandibular dystonia: Treatment of 96 patients with botulinum toxin type A. In Jankovic J, Hallett M (eds). Therapy with Botulinum Toxin. New York, NY: Marcel Dekker, 1994, pp. 429–436.
46. Traube L. Zur Lehre von den Larynxaffectionen beim Ileotyphus. Berlin: Verlag Von August Hirschwald, 1871.
47. Ludlow CL. The spasmodic dysphonias: Speech, movement, and physiological characteristics. In Ching Tsui JK, Calne DB (eds). Handbook of Dystonia. New York, NY: Marcel Dekker, 1995, pp. 159–180.
48. Aronson AE. Clinical Voice Disorders. New York, NY: Thieme, 1985.
49. Blitzer A, Brin MF, Fahn S, et al. Clinical and laboratory characteristics of focal laryngeal dystonia: Study of 110 cases. Laryngoscope 1988;98:636–640.
50. Rosenfield DB. Spasmodic dysphonia. Adv Neurol 1988;49: 317–328.
51. Ludlow CL, Naunton RF, Terada S, et al. Successful treatment of selected cases of abductor spasmodic dysphonia using botulinum toxin injection. Otolaryngol Head Neck Surg 1991;104:849–855.
52. Hartman DE, Aronson AE. Clinical investigations of intermittent breathy dysphonia. J Speech Hear Disord 1991;46: 428–432.
53. Izdebski K, Dedo HH, Boles L. Spastic dysphonia: A patient profile of 200 cases. Am J Otolaryngol 1984;5: 7–14.
54. Aronson AB, Petersen HW, Litin EM. Voice symptomatology in functional dysphonia and aphonia. J Speech Hear Disord 1964;29:367–380.
55. Grillone GA, Blitzer A, Brin MF, et al. Treatment of adductor laryngeal dystonia with botulinum toxin type A. Laryngoscope 1994;104:30–32.
56. Tsui JKC. Cervical dystonia. In Tsui JKC, Calne DB (eds). Handbook of Dystonia. New York, NY: Marcel Dekker, 1995, pp. 115–127.
57. Jankovic J, Leder S, Warner D, et al. Cervical dystonia: Clinical findings and associated movement disorders. Neurology 1991;41:1088–1091.
58. Chan J, Brin MF, Fahn S. Idiopathic cervical dystonia: Clinical characteristics. Mov Disord 1991; 6:119–126.
59. Couch JR. Dystonia and tremor in spasmodic torticollis. Adv Neurol 1976;14:245–258.
60. Duane DD. Spasmodic torticollis: Clinical and biologic features and their implications for focal dystonia. Adv Neurol 1988;50:473–492.
61. Duane DD. Spasmodic torticollis. Adv Neurol 1988;49: 135–150.
62. Truong DD, Dubinsky R, Hermanowicz N, et al. Posttraumatic torticollis. Arch Neurol 1991;48:221–223.
63. Schott GD. The relationship of peripheral trauma and pain to dystonia. J Neurol Neurosurg Psychiatry 1985;48: 698–701.
64. Lowenstein DH, Aminoff MJ. The clinical course of spasmodic torticollis. Neurology 1988;38:530–532.
65. Jahanshahi M, Marion MH, Marsden CD. Natural history of adult-onset idiopathic torticollis. Arch Neurol 1990;47:548.
66. Friedman A, Fahn S. Spontaneous remission in spasmodic torticollis. Neurology 1986;36:398–400.
67. Koukouni V, Martino D, Arabia G, et al. The entity of young onset primary cervical dystonia. Mov Disord 2007;22:843–847.
68. Uitti RJ, Vingerhoets FJG, Tsui JKC. Limb dystonia., In Tsui JKC, Calne DB (eds). Handbook of Dystonia. New York, NY: Marcel Dekker, 1995, pp. 143–158.
69. Fahn S, Marsden CD, Calne DB. Classification and investigation of dystonia. In Marsden CD, Fahn S (eds). Movement Disorders 2. London: Butterworth, 1987, pp. 332–358.
70. Lockwood AH. Medical problems in musicians. N Engl J Med 1989;320:221–227.
71. Newmark J, Hochberg FH. Isolated painless manual incoordination in 57 musicians. J Neurol Neurosurg Psychiatry 1987;50:291–295.
72. McDaniel KD, Cummings JL, Shain S. The "yips": A focal dystonia in golfers. Neurology 1989;39:192–195.
73. Sheehy MP, Marden CD. Writer's cramp: A focal dystonia. Brain 1982;105:462–480.
74. Marsden CD, Sheehy MP. Writer's cramp. Trends Neurosci 1990;13:148–153.
75. Sheehy MP, Rothwell JC, Marsden CD. Writer's cramp. Adv Neurol 1988;50:457–472.
76. Ludolph AC, Windgassen K. Klinische Untersuchungen zum Schreibkrampf bei 30 Patienten. Nervenarzt 1992; 8:462–466.
77. Rothwell JC, Traub MM, Marsden CD. Primary writing tremor. J Neurol Neurosurg Psychiatry 1979;42:1106–1114.
78. Rosenbaum F, Jankovic J. Focal task-specific tremor and dystonia: Categorization of occupational movement disorders. Neurology 1988;38:522–527.
79. Quinn N, Critchley P, Marsden CD. Young onset Parkinson's disease. Mov Disord 1987;2:73–91.
80. Poewe WH, Lees AJ, Stern GM. Dystonia in Parkinson's disease: Clinical and pharmacological features. Ann Neurol 1988;23:73–78.
81. Rivest J, Quinn N, Marsden CD. Dystonia in Parkinson's disease, multiple system atrophy, and progressive supranuclear palsy. Neurology 1990;40:1571–1578.
82. Rafal RD, Friedman JH. Limb dystonia in progressive supranu-clear palsy. Neurology 1987;37:1546–1549.
83. Rothwell JC. The physiology of dystonia. In Tsui JKC, Calne DB (eds). Handbook of Dystonia. New York, NY: Marcel Dekker, 1995, pp. 59–76.
84. Marsden CD, Harrison MJG, Bundey S. Natural history of idiopathic torsion dystonia. In Eldridge R, Fahn S (eds). Dystonia. New York, NY: Raven Press, 1976, pp. 177–187.
85. Schneider SA, Edwards MJ, Grill SE, et al. Adult-onset lower limb dystonia. Mov Disord 2006;21:767–771.
86. Singer C, Papapetropoulus S. Adult-onset focal foot dystonia. Parkinsonism Relat Disord 2006;12:57–60.
87. Avanzino L, Martino D, van de Warrenburg B, et al. Cortical exitability is abnormal in the patients with "fixed dystonia" syndrome. Mov Disord 2008;25:646–652.
88. Gowers WR. A Manual of Diseases of the Nervous System. London: Churchill, 1888, p. 656.
89. Ferguson D. An Australian study of telegraphist's cramp. Br J Int Med 1971;28:280–285.
90. Frucht SJ, Fahn S, Greene PE, et al. The natural history of embouchure dystonia. Mov Disord 2001;16:899–906.

91. Cohen A. Putting on the agony. Nurs Mirror Midwives J 1976;143:72.
92. Marsden CD. The focal dystonias. Clin Neuropharmacol 1986;9(suppl 2):S49–S60.
93. Marsden CD. Dystonia: The spectrum of the disease. In Yahr M (ed). The Basal Ganglia. New York: Raven Press, 1976, pp. 351–367.
94. Marsden CD. Blepharospasm-oromandibular dystonia syndrome (Breughel's syndrome). J Neurol Neurosurg Psychiatry 1976;39:1204–1209.
95. Robertson-Hoffman DE, Mark MH, Sage JL. Isolated lingualpalatal dystonia. Mov Disord 1991;6:177–179.
96. Iliceto G, Thompson PD, Day BL, et al. Diaphragmatic flutter, the moving umbilicus syndrome, and "belly dancer's" dyskinesia. Mov Disord 1990;5:1522.
97. Caviness JN, Gabellini A, Kneebone CS, et al. Unusual focal dyskinesias: The ears, the shoulders, the back, and the abdomen. Mov Disord 1994;9:531–538.
98. Ozelius L, Kramer PL, Moskowitz CB, et al. Human gene for torsion dystonia on chromosome 9q32–34. Neuron 1989;2:1427–1434.
99. Fletcher NA, Harding AE, Marsden CD. A genetic study of idiopathic torsion dystonia in the UK. Brain 1990;113: 379–395.
100. Bressman SB, De Leon D, Brin MF, et al. Idiopathic torsion dystonia among Ashkenazi Jews: Evidence for autosomal dominant inheritance. Ann Neurol 1989;26:612–620.
101. Risch NJ, Bressman SB, De Leon D, et al. Segregation analysis of idiopathic torsion dystonia in Ashkenazi Jews suggests autosomal dominant inheritance. Am J Hum Genet 1990;46:533–538.
102. Gasser T, Windgassen K, Bereznai B, et al. Phenotypic expression of the DYT1 mutation: A family with writer's cramp of juvenile onset. Ann Neurol 1998;44:126–128.
103. Kamm C, Asmus F, Mueller J, et al. Strong genetic evidence for association of TOR1A/TOR1B with idiophatic dystonia. Neurology 2006; 67:1857–1859.
104. Hage S, Klaffkle S, Clarimon J, et al. Lack of association with Torsin A haplotypes in German patient with sporadic dystonia. Neurology 2006;67:951–952.
105. Chan J, Brin MF, Fahn S. Idiopathic cervical dystonia: Clinical characteristics. Mov Disord 1991;6:119–126.
106. De Leon D, Heiman G, Brin MF, et al. Genetic factors in spastic dysphonia. Neurology 1990;40(suppl 1):142.
107. Comella CL, Klawans HL. Meige's syndrome in twins. Neurology 1988;38(suppl 1):315.
108. Kramer PL, Bressman SB, Fahn S, et al. The genetics of dystonia. In Tsui JKC, Calne DB (eds). Handbook of Dystonia. New York, NY: Marcel Dekker, 1995, pp. 43–58.
109. Waddy HM, Fletcher NA, Harding AE, et al. A genetic study of idiopathic focal dystonias. Ann Neurol 1991; 29:320–324.
110. Defazio G, Livrea P, Leon A, et al. Antineuronal antibodies in cranial dystonia. Mov Disord 1991;6:183–184.
111. Brancati F, Defazio G, Caputo V, et al. Novel Italian family supports clinical and genetic heterogeneity of primary adult-onset torsion dystonia. Mov Disord 2002;17: 392–397.
112. Münchau A, Valente EM, Davis MB, et al. A Yorkshire family with adult-onset cranio-cervical primary torsion dystonia. Mov Disord. 2000;15:954–959.
113. Leube B, Rudnicki D, Ratzlaff T, et al. Idiopathic torsion dystonia: Assignment of a gene to chromosome 18p in a German family with adult onset, autosomal dominant inheritance and purely focal distribution. Hum Mol Genet 1996;5:1673–1677.
114. Almasy L, Bressman SB, Raymond D, et al. Idiopathic torsion dystonia linked to chromosome 8 in two mennonite families. Ann Neurol 1997;42:670–673.
115. Bentivoglio AR, Del Grosso N, Valente EM. Non-DTY1 dystonia in a large Italian family. J Neurol Neurosurg Psychiatry 1997;62:357–360.
116. Valente EM, Bentivoglio AR, Cassetta E, et al. Identification of a novel primary torsion dystonia locus (DYT13) on chromosome 1p36 in an Italian family with cranial-cervical or upper limb onset. Neurol Sci 2001;22:95–96.
117. Plazcek MR, Misbauddin A, Chaudhuri KR, et al. Cervical dystonia is associated with a polymorphism in the dopamine (D5) receptor gene. J Neurol Neurosurg Psychiatry 2001;71:262–264.
118. Bathia KP, Warner TT. A polymorphism in the dopamine receptor DRD5 is associated with blepharospasm. Neurology 2002;58:124–126.
119. Brancati F, Valente EM, Castori M, et al. Role of the dopamine D5 receptor (DRD5) as a susceptibility gene for cervical dystonia. J Neurol Neurosurg Psychiatry 2003;74:665–666.
120. Clarimon J, Brancati F, Peckham E, et al. Assessing the role of DRD5 and DYT1 in two different case-control series with primary blepharospasm. Mov Disord 2007;22: 162–166.
121. Jankovic J, Patten BM. Blepharospasm and autoimmune diseases. Mov Disord 1987;2:159–163.
122. Nilaver G, Whitling S, Nutt JG. Autoimmune etiology for cranial dystonia. Mov Disord 1990;5:179–180.
123. Ramachandran V, Church A, Giovannoni G, et al. Anti-basal ganglia antibodies are absent in patients with primary blepharospasm. Neurology 2002;58:150.
124. Tolosa E, Kulisevski J. The pathophysiology of dystonia. In Quinn NP, Jenner PG (eds). Disorders of Movement. Clinical, Pharmacological and Physiological Aspects. London: Academic Press, 1989, pp. 251–262.
125. Fletcher NA, Harding AE, Marsden CD. The relationship between trauma and idiopathic torsion dystonia. J Neurol Neurosurg Psychiatry 1991;54:713–717.
126. Grandas F, Elston J, Quinn N, et al. Blepharospasm: A review of 264 patients. J Neurol Neurosurg Psychiatry 1988;51:767–772.
127. Jankovic J, Van Der Linden C. Dystonia and tremor induced by peripheral trauma: Predisposing factors. J Neurol Neurosurg Psychiatry 1988;51:1512–1519.
128. Truong DD, Dubinsky R, Hermanowicz N, et al. Posttraumatic torticollis. Arch Neurol 1991;48:221–223.
129. Brin MF, Fahn S, Bressman SB, et al. Dystonia precipitated by peripheral trauma. Neurology 1986; 36(suppl 1):119.
130. Ludlow CL. The spasmodic dysphonias: Speech, movement, and physiological characteristics. In Tsui JKC, Calne DB (eds). Handbook of Dystonia. New York, NY: Marcel Dekker, 1995, pp. 159–180.
131. Tarsy D, Sudarsky L, Charness ME. Limb dystonia following electrical injury. Mov Disord 1994;9:230–232.

132. Schott GD. Induction of involuntary movements by peripheral trauma: An analogy with causalgia. Lancet 1986; 2:712–715.
133. Bhatia KP, Bhatt MH, Marsden CD. The causalgia-dystonia syndrome. Brain 1993;116:834–851.
134. Scolding NJ, Smith SM, Sturman S, et al. Auctioneer's jaw: A case of occupational oromandibular dystonia. Mov Disord 1995;10:508–509.
135. Inzelberg R, Zilber N, Kahana E, Korczyn AD. Laterality of onset in idiopathic torsion dystonia. Mov Disord 1993; 8:327–330.
136. Fletcher NA, Harding AE, Marsden CD. A case-control study of idiopathic torsion dystonia. Mov Disord 1993; 6:304–309.
137. Marsden CD. Peripheral movement disorders. In Marsden CD, Fahn S (eds). Movement Disorders 3. Oxford: Butterworth-Heinemann, 1994, pp. 406–417.
138. Schicatano EJ, Basso MA, Evinger C. Animal model explains the origins of the cranial dystonia benign essential blepharospasm. J Neurophysiol 1997;77:2842–2846.
139. Lang AE, Fahn S. Movement disorders of RSD. Neurology 1990;40:1476–1477.
140. Garcia-Albea E, Franch O, Muñoz D. Breughel's syndrome: Report of a case with postmortem studies. J Neurol Neurosurg Psychiatry 1981;44:437–440.
141. Jankovic J. Pharmacologic approach to blepharospasm and cranial-cervical dystonia. Adv Ophthalmol Plast Reconstr Surg 1985;4:211–217.
142. Altrocchi PH, Forno LS. Spontaneous oral-facial dyskinesia: Neuropathology of a case. Neurology 1983; 33: 802–805.
143. Kulisevsky J, Marti MJ, Ferrer I, et al. Meige syndrome: Neuropathology of a case. Mov Disord 1988;3:170–175.
144. Zweig RM, Hedreen JC, Jankel WR. Pathology in brainstem regions of individuals with primary dystonia. Neurology 1988;38:702–706.
145. Rothwell JC, Obeso JA. The anatomical and physiological basis of torsion dystonia. In Marsden CD, Fahn S (eds). Movement Disorders 2. London: Butterworths, 1987, pp. 313–331.
146. Jankovic J. Blepharospasm with basal ganglia lesions. Arch Neurol 1986;43:866–868.
147. Holton JL, Schneider SA, Ganesharajah T, et al. Neuropathology of primary adult-onset dystonia. Neurology 2008; 70:695–699.
148. McNaught KS, Kapustin A, Jackson T, et al. Brainstem pathology in primary torsion dystonia. Ann Neurol 2004; 56:540–547.
149. Karbe H, Holthoff VA, Rudolf J. Positron emission tomography demonstrates frontal cortex and basal ganglia hypometabolism in dystonia. Neurology 1992; 42:1540–1544.
150. Fife TD, Hutchinson M, Woods RP, et al. Motor system hypermetabolism in Meige's syndrome. Neurology 1993; 43(suppl 4):A409-A410.
151. Hutchinson M, Fife TD, Woods RP, et al. Glucose metabolism in Meige's syndrome in wakefulness and sleep. J Cereb Blood Flow Metab 1993;13(suppl 1):S370.
152. Ceballos-Baumann O, Passingham RE, Warner T, et al. Over-active prefrontal and underactive motor cortical areas in idiopathic dystonia. Ann Neurol 1995;37:363–372.
153. Ibañez V, Sadato N, Karp B, et al. Deficient activation of the motor cortical network in patients with writer's cramp. Neurology 1999;53:96–105.
154. Feiwell RJ, Black KJ, McGee-Minnich LA, et al. Diminished regional cerebral blood flow response to vibration in patients with blepharospasm. Neurology 1999;52: 291–297.
155. Hutchinson M, Nakamura T, Moeller JR, et al. The metabolic topography of essential blepharospasm. A focal dystonia with general implications. Neurology 2000; 55:673–677.
156. Perlmutter JS, Stambuk MK, Markham J, et al. Decreased [^{18}F] spiperone binding in putamen in idiopathic focal dystonia. J Neurosci 1997;17:843–850.
157. Federico F, Simone IL, Lucivero V, et al. Proton magnetic resonance spectroscopy in primary blepharospasm. Neurology 1998;51:892–895.
158. Federico F, Lucivero V, Simone IL, et al. Proton MR spectroscopy in idiophatic spasmodic torticollis. Neuroradiology 2001; 43:532–536.
159. Naumann M, Warmuth-Metz M, Hillerer C, et al. Magnetic resonance spectroscopy of lentiform nucleus in the primary focal hand dystonia. Mov Disord 1998; 13: 929–933.
160. Draganski B, Thun-Hohenstein C, Bogdahn U, et al. "Motor circuit" gray matter changes in idiopathic cervical dystonia. Neurology 2003;11:1228–1231.
161. Garraux G, Bauer A, Hanakawa T, et al. Changes in brain anatomy in focal hand dystonia. Ann Neurol 2004; 55:736–739.
162. Etgen T, Muhlau M, Gaser C, et al. Bilateral grey matter increase in the putamen in the primary blepharospasm. J Neurol Neurosurg Psychiatry 2006;77:1017–1020.
163. Egger K, Mueller J, Schocke M, et al. Voxel based morphometry reveals specific grey matter changes in primary dystonia. Mov Disord 2007;22:1538- 1542.
164. Oga T, Honda M, Toma K, et al. Abnormal cortical mechanisms of voluntary muscle relaxation in patients with writer's cramp: An fMRI study. Brain 2002; 125:895–903.
165. Baker RS, Andersen AH, Morecraft RJ, et al. A functional magnetic resonance imaging study in patients with bening essential blepharospasm. J Neurophtalmol 2003; 23:11–15.
166. Dresel C, Haslinger B, Castrop F, et al. Silent event-related fMRI reveals deficient motor and enhanced somatosensory activation in orofacial dystonia. Brain 2006; 129:36–46.
167. Berg D, Prreibisch C, Hofmann E, et al. Cerebral activation pattern in primary writing tremor. J Neurol Neurosurg Psychiatry 2000;69:780–786.
168. Fabbrini G, Pantano P, Totaro P, et al. Diffusor tensor imaging in patients with primary cervical dystonia and in patients with blepharospasm. Eur J Neurol 2008; 15: 185–189.
169. Ridding MC, Sheean G, Rothwell JC, et al. Changes in the balance between motor cortical excitation and inhibition in focal, task specific dystonia. J Neurol Neurosurg Psychiatry 1995;59:493–498.
170. Sommer M, Ruge D, Tergau F, et al. Intracortical excitability in the hand motor representation in hand dystonia and blepharospasm. Mov Disord 2002;17:1017–1025.

171. Hanajima R, Ugawa Y, Masuda N, et al. Changes of motor cortical excitability in a patient with unilateral focal dystonia due a lesion of the contralateral putamen. Mov Disord 1994;9(suppl 1):43.
172. Curra A, Romaniello A, Berardelli A, et al. Shortened cortical silent period in facial muscles of patients with cranial dystonia. Neurology 2000;54:130–135.
173. Sohn Y, Hallet M. Disturbed surround inhibition in focal hand dystonia. Ann Neurol 2004;56:595–599.
174. Tolosa ES, Montserrat L. Depressed blink reflex habituation in dystonia blepharospasm. Neurology 1985;35:271.
175. Berardelli A, Rothwell JC, Day BL, et al. Pathophysiology of blepharospasm and oromandibular dystonia. Brain 1985;108:593–608.
176. Tolosa E, Montserrat L, Bayes A. Blink reflex studies in focal dystonias: Enhanced excitability of brainstem interneurones in cranial dystonia and spasmodic torticollis. Mov Disord 1988;3:61–69.
177. Valls J, Tolosa E, Ribera G. Neurophysiological observation on the effects of botulinum toxin treatment in patients with dystonic blepharospasm. J Neurol Neurosurg Psychiatry 1991;54:310–313.
178. Valls J, Tolosa E, Martí MJ, et al. Treatment with botulinum toxin injection does not change brainstem interneuronal excitability in patients with cervical dystonia. Clin Neuropharmacol 1994;17:229–235.
179. Carella F, Ciano C, Musicco M, et al. Exteroceptive reflexes in dystonia: A study of the recovery cycle of the R2 component of the blink reflex and of the exteroceptive suppression of the contracting sternocleidomastoid muscle in blepharospasm and torticollis. Mov Disord 1994; 9:183–187.
180. Quartarone A, Girlanda P, Di Lazzaro V, et al. Short latency trigemino-sternocleidomastoid response in muscles in patients with spasmodic torticollis and blepharospasm. Clin Neurophysiol 2000;111:1672–1677.
181. Münchau A, Bronstein AM. Role of the vestibular system in the pathophysiology of spasmodic torticollis. J Neurol Neurosurg Psychiatry 2001;71:285–288.
182. Colebatch JG, Di Lazzaro V, Quartarone A, et al. Click-evoked vestibulocollic reflexes in torticollis. Mov Disord 1995;10:455–459.
183. Nakashima K, Rothwell JC, Day BL, et al. Reciprocal inhibition in writer's and other occupational cramps and hemiparesis due to stroke. Brain 1989;112:681–697.
184. Panizza ME, Hallett M, Nilson J. Reciprocal inhibition in patients with hand cramps. Neurology 1991;41:553–556.
185. Gomez-Wong E, Marti MJ, Cossu G, et al. The "geste antagonistique" induces transient modulation of the blink reflex in human patients with blepharospasm. Neurosci Lett 1998;252:125–128.
186. Kaji R, Rothwell JC, Katayama M, et al. Tonic vibration reflex and muscle afferent block in writer's cramp. Ann Neurol 1995;38:155–162.
187. Fiorio M, Tinazzi M, Scontrini A, et al. Tactile temporal discrimination in patients with blepharospasm. J Neurol Neurosurg Psychiatry 2008;79:796–798.
188. Bara-Jimenez W, Shelton P, Sanger TD, et al. Sensori discrimination capabilities in patients with focal hand dystonia. Ann Neurol 2000;47:377–380.
189. Bara-Jimenez W, Catalan MJ, Hallet M, et al. Abnormal somatosensory homunculus in dystonia of the hand. Ann Neurol 1998;44:828–831.
190. Meunier S, Garnero L, Ducorps A, et al. Human brain mapping in dystonia reveals both endophenotypic traits and adaptative reorganization. Ann Neurol 2001;50: 521–527.
191. Calne DB, Lang AE. Secondary dystonia. Adv Neurol 1988;50:9–34.
192. Weiner WJ, Nausieda PA, Glanz RH. Meige syndrome (blepharospasm-oromandibular dystonia) after long term neuroleptic therapy. Neurology 1981;31:1555–1556.
193. Burke RE, Fahn S, Jankovic J, et al. Tardive dystonia: Late onset and persistent dystonia caused by antipsychotic drugs. Neurology 1982;32:1335–1346.
194. Weiner W, Nausieda P. Meige's syndrome during long-term dopaminergic therapy in Parkinson's disease. Arch Neurol 1982;39:451–452.
195. Gershanik OS, Leist A. Juvenile onset Parkinson's disease. Adv Neurol 1986;45:213–216.
196. Poewe WH, Lees AJ, Stern GM. Dystonia in Parkinson's disease: Clinical and pharmacological features. Ann Neurol 1988;23:73–79.
197. Leger JM, Girault JA, Bolgert F. Deux cas de dystonie isolee d'un membre superieur inagurant une maladie de Steele-Richardson-Olszweski. Rev Neurol (Paris) 1987; 143:140–142.
198. Fletcher NA, Stell R, Harding A, et al. Degenerative cerebellar ataxia and focal dystonia. Mov Disord 1988;3: 336–342.
199. Tolosa E, Kulisevsky J, Fahn S. Meige syndrome: Primary and secondary forms. Adv Neurol 1988;50:509–516.
200. Muñoz E, Tolosa E. Upper-limb dystonia secondary to a mid-brain hemorrhage. Mov Disord 1996;11:96–99.
201. Alarcon F, Muñoz E, Tolosa E. Focal limb dystonia in a patient with a cerebellar mass. Arch Neurol 2001; 58:1125–1227.
202. Chu N-S, Huang C-C, Lu C-S, Calne DB. Dystonia caused by toxins. In Ching Tsui JK, Calne BC (eds). Handbook of Dystonia. New York, NY: Marcel Dekker, 1995, pp. 241–265.
203. LeWitt PA, Martin SD. Dystonia and hypokinesia with putaminal necrosis after methanol intoxication. Clin Neuropharmacol 1988;11:61.
204. Burke RE, Fahn S, Gold AP. Delayed-onset dystonia in patients with "static" encephalopathy. J Neurol Neurosurg Psychiatry 1980; 43:789.
205. Maraganore DM, Folger WN, Swanson JW, et al. Movement disorders as sequelae of central pontine myelinolysis: Report of three cases. Mov Disord 1992;7: 142–148.
206. Grandas F, Artieda J, Obeso JA. Clinical and CT scan findings in a case of cyanide intoxication. Mov Disord 1989; 4:188.
207. Fahn S, Williams DT. Psychogenic dystonia. Adv Neurol 1988;50:431–455.
208. Lang AE, Weiner WJ. Symptomatic dystonia. In Lang E, Weiner WJ (eds). Movement Disorders: A Comprehensive Survey. Mount Kisko, NY: Futura, 1989.

CHAPTER 30

Treatment of Dystonia

Octavian R. Adam and Joseph Jankovic

▶ INTRODUCTION

CLASSIFICATION AND ETIOLOGY OF DYSTONIA

The term "dystonia" was coined by Oppenheim in 1911[1] in his description of "dystonia musculorum deformans," even though he was not the first to recognize this hyperkinetic movement disorder. The word *dystonia*, originally from modern Latin and then adapted from German *dystonie*, derived from *dys*- and the Greek term *–tonos*, which has a musical connotation, meaning stretching, tension raising of voice, pitch.[2] The term "dystonia" is used to describe a hyperkinetic movement disorder manifested by repetitive muscle contractions causing abnormal, but patterned, movements, or postures.

Dystonias are classified by various criteria. Their distribution may be generalized, segmental, hemibody, multifocal, and focal. Dystonias may be primary (without any other neurological deficit), or secondary, in which case it may be accompanied by other neurological features such myoclonus or parkinsonism; the latter "dystonia plus" disorders are often caused by structural lesions involving the basal ganglia or may be associated with heredodegenerative disorders.[3] The genetics and pathophysiology of dystonia are described in the preceding chapters in this volume, and in recent reviews.[4]

CLINICAL ASSESSMENT OF DYSTONIA

Several clinical scales have been developed to aid in the objective assessment of dystonia and its response to therapeutic interventions. The Burke–Fahn–Marsden Dystonia Rating Scale (BFMDRS)[5] is used most frequently. Other scales used chiefly for assessment of generalized dystonias include the Unified Dystonia Rating Scale (UDRS) designed by the Dystonia Study Group and the Global Dystonia Scale (GDS).[6] These three scales showed excellent internal consistency and good to excellent correlation among raters.[6] Toronto Western Spasmodic Torticolis Rating Scale (TWSTRS) was developed for assessment of cervical dystonia (CD). [7] The Jankovic Rating Scale (JRS), which assesses the severity and frequency of involuntary eyelid contractions in patients with blepharospasm and the self-rating response scale Blepharospasm Disability Index (BSDI) have been found to correlate well with each other.[8]

MEDICAL TREATMENT OF DYSTONIA

The treatment of dystonia is largely geared toward symptomatic relief as there is no cure or even neuroprotective strategies for dystonia to date. Strategies for treatment may be divided into pharmacological, botulinum neurotoxin (BoNT) chemodenervation, and surgery, either peripheral or central (stereotactic). Many patients are treated, at least initially, with pharmacological therapy, but it is important to note that the use of these medications are based largely on clinical experience and custom and that none of the pharmacological approaches are supported by strong clinical trial-based evidence for efficacy. There is, however, strong (Class I and Class II) evidence from randomized controlled trials for the efficacy of BoNT in forms of focal dystonia (Simpson, 2008).[9]

ADJUNCTS TO MEDICAL TREATMENT

In addition to medical treatment, physical and occupational therapy play an important role in the overall quality of life and disability of patients with dystonia. A range of motion exercises are important in preventing or minimizing contractures. Custom-fitted braces are often used not only to improve postures but also to serve as a sensory trick, providing sensory input that mimics the *geste antagoniste*. On the basis of the notion that overuse results in cortical changes causing occupational dystonia, several studies investigated the use of splints to immobilize the upper limb.[10,11] However, we caution against immobilization techniques as such treatment can result in worsening dystonia or may even trigger peripherally induced dystonia.[12] Other types of therapy advocate the avoidance of specific movement patterns with the dystonic limb, similar to the main affected task, reducing the amount of task-associated movement behavior.[13] Also, sensory training through 30–60 minutes daily of Braille reading in patients with focal hand dystonia has been reported to provide sustained improvement at one year follow up.[14] Transcranial magnetic stimulation (TMS) has also been shown to improve temporarily focal hand dystonia,[15–17] generalized secondary dystonia[18] and CD.[19] Transcutaneous electrical stimulation (TENS) was found effective and the improvement was apparently maintained at 3 weeks of treatment in a double blind study of 10 patients with writer's cramp.[20] External shock wave therapy shown to reduce hypertonicity in patients with upper motor neuron syndrome may also have some benefit in treating dystonia.[21] Evidence, based on well-designed controlled trials, that alternative treatments such as acupuncture, relaxation techniques, homeopathy, or massage are effective, is lacking.

▶ PHARMACOLOGICAL TREATMENT OF DYSTONIA

DOPAMINERGIC THERAPY

Although dysfunction of the dopaminergic system has been implicated in the etiology of several forms of dystonia (see Chapter 28), studies of the effect of levodopa and other dopaminergic drugs in the treatment of generalized dystonia have yielded contradictory results, most likely with some of the positive outcomes being attributable to placebo response.[22] In a review of dopaminergic treatment in generalized and focal dystonia, 35% of patients with generalized dystonia had some improvement with levodopa (open trials), while 19% of patients worsened.[23]

The exception to this overall modest response to dopaminergic therapy in dystonia is the distinct syndrome of dopa-responsive dystonia (DRD). DRD was first described by Segawa[24] in young girls who presented with dystonia with diurnal variation that responded dramatically to levodopa. As is described in detail in Chapter 28, DRD is a genetic form of dystonia-plus syndrome, which may be caused by one of several different mutations. The most common mutation involves the GCH1 gene that encodes GTP-cyclohydrolase 1, the rate-limiting enzyme in tetrahydrobiopterin synthesis, which is the essential cofactor for tyrosine hydrolase.[25] The symptoms of DRD usually start in childhood (on average 6 years old) with lower extremity action-induced dystonia that invariably generalizes.[26] Typical features include gait impairment, diurnal fluctuation, with a restorative effect of sleep, bradykinesia, rigidity, and postural instability.[27] Levodopa is a very effective treatment for DRD, its conversion to dopamine not being dependent on tetrahydrobiopterin. Patients with DRD usually respond to small dosages of levodopa in combination with a decarboxylase inhibitor, and, in contrast to young-onset Parkinson's disease, rarely develop dyskinesias.[28] Other treatments for DRD, generally less effective than levodopa, include anticholinergics, dopamine receptor agonists, tricyclic agents, and carbamazepine.[24] Because of the heterogeneity of the clinical presentation of DRD and its response to levodopa, a therapeutic trial with levodopa is advised in all childhood-onset dystonias.

ANTIDOPAMINERGIC THERAPIES

Treatments that block dopaminergic transmission have also been used in dystonia. Antidopaminergic drugs include dopamine receptor blocking drugs (neuroleptics) and dopamine depleting agents. The typical neuroleptic drugs, such as haloperidol, are generally viewed as carrying a high risk of parkinsonism and tardive phenomena due to their high affinity for the D_2 receptors and are not commonly used in the treatment of dystonia. Risperidone, marketed as an "atypical" neuroleptic (despite a fairly high affinity for D_2 receptors and a propensity to cause tardive dyskinesia), was reported to decrease both the duration and the amplitude of abnormal movements in segmental and generalized dystonia.[29,30] Clozapine, an atypical neuroleptic with a very favorable D_4:D_2 receptor affinity ratio and high affinity for serotonergic 5-HT2A receptors, has been used with some benefit in small numbers of patients who have failed other therapies. In an open-label study of clozapine, five patients with either generalized or severe focal dystonia completely or partially refractory to other medications were treated.[31] The initial dosage of 12.5 mg/day was increased by 25 mg/day, as tolerated, up to maximum 900 mg/day. Patients remained on the maximally tolerated dose for 2 weeks and demonstrated an improvement of 25–35%. However, frequent limiting side effects included orthostatic hypotension and tachycardia, sedation, hallucinations, vivid dreams, and epileptiform activity on EEG (managed by lowering the dose). None of the patients developed leucopenia. However, in an open label study of six patients with cervical dystonia (CD), clozapine was found to be ineffective.[32] While clozapine can potentially offer some improvement in resistant cases of dystonia, with functional benefits, the mandatory weekly white cell count and the frequent occurrence of side effects make this treatment a challenge for both the patient and the physician and should be reserved for refractory cases of severe dystonia.

Dopamine-depleting drugs, which include reserpine and tetrabenazine, do not carry the risk of tardive side effects, but may nevertheless cause acute dystonic reactions. Reserpine is seldom used because of its dual peripheral and central actions and long duration of effect, leading to orthostatic hypotension and a variety of other side effects. Tetrabenazine was recently approved by the Food and Drug Administration (FDA) for the treatment of chorea associated with Huntington disease. It has been shown in both small double-blind studies[33] and large open-label studies[34,35] to be an effective treatment for dystonia. The most common side effects in the chronic treatment with tetrabenazine are drowsiness (25.9%), parkinsonism (16.1%), and akathisia (7.7%).[36] Tetrabenazine may worsen depression in patients with a preexisting history of depression.[37]

ANTICHOLINERGIC THERAPY

Anticholinergics block the action of acetylcholine on the muscarinic receptors in the central nervous system. Trihexyphenidyl, originally used in the treatment of Parkinson's disease, was introduced as an antidystonia drug in 1983.[38] It was shown in both double-blind, placebo-controlled[39] and open-label[40,41] trials to be effective in segmental and generalized dystonias in children and young adults. There are no controlled trials of trihexyphenidyl in adults with generalized dystonia. The best clinical benefit is achieved if the treatment is started within 5 years of symptom onset.[42] Children tolerate higher dosages better than adults do, and therefore respond better to the treatment. Another commonly used anticholinergic agent is benztropine. Common side effects to all anticholinergics are dry mouth, blurry vision, and urinary retention. Some of these side effects can be lessened by the coadministration of peripherally acting anticholinesterase (pyridostygmine), as well as synthetic saliva and eye drops with pilocarpine. Dose-limiting side effects that usually result in the discontinuation of the drug include cognitive decline, confusion, and visual hallucinations.[43]

GABAERGIC THERAPIES: BACLOFEN

Oral Baclofen

Baclofen is a presynaptic GABA agonist, and, as such, it reduces spinal neuron excitability. There are no control studies of baclofen in dystonia. However, several retrospective studies support the effectiveness of baclofen in dystonia in children and adolescents[44–46] and in dystonia associated with Parkinson's disease.[47] The treatment with oral baclofen resulted in a remarkable improvement in symptoms, especially gait, in 30% of 31 children and adolescents.[46] The response to baclofen in adults with dystonia was less impressive.[42]

Intrathecal Baclofen

Baclofen can also be administered by direct infusion into the spinal subarachnoid space, using implantable mechanical pumps. There are several uncontrolled studies demonstrating the effect of intrathecal baclofen in dystonia.[48–52] The response of patients to intrathecal baclofen is initially tested by a bolus infusion. If an acceptable therapeutic response is obtained, surgical implantation of a pump and catheter can be considered. After the implantation, the effects are usually observed after a latency of 2–3 days. In dystonia, higher dosages of intrathecal baclofen are needed than are used in the treatment of spasticity, the other major indication for baclofen pump implantation. The need for higher doses may reflect the need to deliver the drug to the brain, rather than just to the spinal cord. For this reason, intraventricular baclofen pumps have been developed and used with good preliminary results, achieving higher cortical concentrations with lower dosages, but further studies are needed.[53]

BENZODIAZEPINES AND OTHER DRUGS

Even though there are no controlled trials assessing the efficacy of benzodiazepines in dystonia, they are frequently used as ancillary, nonspecific muscle relaxants. Particularly clonazepam, among other benzodiazepines, has been used effectively in the treatment of blepharospasm, dystonic choreoathetosis, CD, secondary dystonia, myoclonic dystonia.[42,54–56]

Mexiletine, an antiarrhythmic drug related to lidocaine was found to be effective in the treatment of CD in two small open-label studies[57,58] Two-thirds of patients experienced tolerable and manageable adverse effects such as heartburn, dizziness, ataxia, dysarthria, and tremor.[57] Strong correlation between the serum and CSF levels of mexiletine suggest an effective CNS penetration. Mexiletine was also shown to improve blepharospasm.[59]

Carbamazepine was reported to be of some benefit in treating torsion dystonia.[60,61] Levetiracetam is another antiepileptic that has shown mixed results in the treatment of segmental and generalized dystonia,[62,63] craniovervical dystonia,[64,65] and CD.[66]

Alcohol has been used traditionally as a test for myoclonus dystonia,[67] and has shown improvement as an intravenous infusion in CD, but not in generalized dystonia, cranial-cervical dystonia, or tardive dystonia.[68] Both lithium[69] and nabilone[70] were found ineffective in double-blind, placebo-controlled studies despite earlier encouraging reports.

Clonidine[71] and riluzole[72] were also considered in the treatment of dystonia, but without solid evidence for efficacy.

▶ CHEMODENERVATION TREATMENT WITH BOTULINUM TOXIN

BOTULINUM NEUROTOXINS

Botulinum neurotoxins (BoNTs), produced by *Clostridium botulinum*, consists of a family of immunologically distinct neurotoxic proteins sharing similar structure and function, chiefly inhibiting the release of acetylcholine from the presynaptic terminal into the neuromuscular junction.[73] There are seven BoNT serotypes (A, B, C, D, E, F, and G). They are synthesized as relatively inactive single-chain polypeptides with a molecular mass of approximately 150 kDa. Activation of the neurotoxins occurs upon proteolytic cleavage into 100 kDa heavy and 50 kDa light chains, which remain linked by a single disulfide bond. The heavy chain facilitates the binding to the presynaptic membrane of motor nerve terminals, while the light chains each cleave specific members of the SNARE (soluble *N*-ethyl-maleimide-sensitive fusion protein attachment receptor) protein family (Table 30–1). The SNARE proteins are found in association with the synaptic vesicles or presynaptic membrane of cholinergic nerve terminals, and are essential for the fusion of vesicles to the synaptic membrane and release of acetylcholine. Thus, the enzymatic activity of the BoNT light chains is a very effective means of inhibiting cholinergic neurotransmission.[74]

FORMS OF BOTULINUM TOXIN

There are currently four commercial preparations of BoNT serotype A (BoNT/A) available: Botox (Allergan, Inc., Irvine, CA), Dysport (Ipsen Limited, Slough, Berkshire, UK), Xeomin (Merz Pharmaceutical, Germany), and Hengli (Lanzhou Institute of Biological Products, China). BoNT/A (Botox) was approved by the FDA for the treatment of blepharospasm, strabismus, and other facial nerve disorders (1989) and CD (2000). There is one commercial preparation of BoNT/B (Myobloc, Neurobloc in some countries). It was approved by the FDA for the treatment of CD in 2000.

CLINICAL EFFECTS OF BoNT

In the early 1990s, several open-label and placebo-controlled studies demonstrated the effectiveness of BoNT/A in the treatment of CD with mild and transient side effects reported, such as dysphagia, neck weakness, and local pain.[75–79] In a double-blind, placebo-controlled study of 55 BoNT naïve patients treated with Botox, 61% improved after treatment.[76] Open-label studies show a more robust response (approximately 90%) not only because of the added placebo effect, but also because of larger dosages and fewer restrictions in muscle selection.

In clinical use, the typical latency to onset of improvement after BoNT injection is 1 week, and the duration of maximum effect averages 3–4 months. In most cases, repeated injections are required every 4–6 months. Longitudinal studies have shown that treatment with BoNT in CD not only corrects the abnormal posture and movement, but also reduces pain (84% with first injection),[78] prevents contractures and possibly

▶ TABLE 30–1. DIFFERENCES IN THE BoNT SEROTYPES

Type of Toxin	Presynaptic Membrane Receptor	Substrate		Reference
A	SV2C	SNAP-25	Presynaptic plasma membrane	(184) (185) (186)
B	Synaptotagmin I, II	Synaptobrevin (VAMP)	Vesicle-associated membrane protein	(184) (187) (188)
C	Not identified	SNAP-25 Syntaxin	Presynaptic plasma membrane	(189)
D	Not identified	VAMP	Vesicle-associated membrane protein	(190)
E	Not identified	SNAP-25	Presynaptic plasma membrane	(190)
F	Not identified	VAMP	Vesicle-associated membrane protein	(188)
G	Synaptotagmin I, II	VAMP		(191) (73)

SNAP, synaptosome-associated protein; VAMP, vesicle-associated membrane protein.

degenerative changes of the cervical spine,[80] and reduces depression and disability.[81] Most patients note marked improvements within 2–3 weeks after injection, but the therapeutic effect may not stabilize and the impact on quality of life may not be fully appreciated until after several treatment visits.[82] BoNT treatment appears to be equally effective in "simple" rotational torticollis and in more complex forms of CD.[82] BoNT/A was found to be more effective than trihexyphenidyl in the treatment of CD in a comparison trial.[83]

The side effects of BoNT/A in the treatment of CD are generally mild, transitory, and fully reversible, and include neck weakness (8.4%) and local pain (6.5%).[84] According to a prospective study analyzing the frequency, severity, and radiologic features of swallowing abnormalities following treatment with Botox in CD, 50% of patients developed new radiologic abnormalities following Botox, but only 33% had clinical symptoms of dysphagia.[85] The latency was 5.3 days (range 1–10 days), and duration of 15.8 days (range 4–42 days). The most severe cases required a change to liquid diet for 2–3 weeks. The severity of the new dysphagia symptoms correlated highly with the severity of new radiologic pharyngeal abnormalities. Therefore, videofluoroscopic swallowing studies may be used for patients with severe clinical symptoms as an objective measure to assess the possibility of aspiration.

COMPARATIVE EFFECTIVENESS OF BoNT FORMULATIONS

Clinical trials of BoNT naïve patients established that both Botox[76] and Dysport[83,86] are effective in the treatment of CD. In the first US multicenter, double-blind, randomized, controlled trial assessing the safety and efficacy of Dysport in CD, 80 patients were randomly assigned to receive one treatment with Dysport (500 units) or placebo.[87] Dysport was significantly more efficacious than placebo at weeks 4, 8, and 12 as assessed by the TWSTRS (10-point vs. 3.8-point reduction in total score, respectively, at week 4; $P \leq 0.013$). Of participants in the Dysport group, 38% showed positive treatment response, compared with 16% in the placebo group (95% CI, 0.02–0.41). The median duration of response to Dysport was 18.5 weeks. Side effects were generally similar in the two treatment groups; only blurred vision and weakness occurred significantly more often with Dysport. Dysport was also studied in patients previously exposed to Botox.[88] The adverse event profiles of the two preparations did not differ significantly, except dysphagia, which seemed to be slightly more prevalent in the Dysport group. The dose equivalence between the two preparations remains a matter of debate, since the methods used in the manufacturing process differ, but generally one unit of Botox is equivalent to 2–4 units of Dysport.[89,90]

Following positive safety data from the first study of BoNT/B on humans[91] the efficacy of Myobloc in CD was confirmed in controlled clinical trials of patients previously treated with BoNT/A (Botox), either responders[92,93] or secondarily nonresponders.[94] The two serotypes, A (Botox) and B (Myobloc) were compared in a double-blind randomized study, concluding that both treatment groups had the same maximum efficacy (as evaluated by TWSTRS at 4 weeks) and comparable effect duration (slightly longer with A, extending the clinical benefit by 2 weeks).[95] The incidence and severity of dry mouth and dysphagia were higher in the B group; however, the higher frequency of dysphagia was found to correlate with the dry mouth, suggesting a reporting bias. The study used a 1 (Botox):40 (Myobloc) dose ratio. The suspected higher incidence of autonomic side effects of Myobloc was confirmed in a double-blind, randomized study, comparing the effect of BoNT on salivary production.[96] This finding may be potentially explained by a higher affinity of BoNT/B to the cholinergic terminals.

IMMUNORESISTANCE TO BoNT

The development of blocking antibodies directed to the heavy chain of BoNT (immunogenicity) is one of the major reasons of secondary nonresponsiveness to BoNT therapy. There are several methods of assessing immunoresistance to BoNT. Standard tests, such as the mouse lethality assay (MLA) and mouse protection assay (MPA),[97] are expensive and not readily available. Simple tests, such as the unilateral eyebrow (UBI) or frontalis injections (FTAT), are very informative in clinical practice.[98] Other similar clinical tests include the ninhydrin sweat test.[99] The UBI test consists of injecting 20 U of Botox (1000 U of Myobloc), by convention into the right eyebrow. After 1 to 2 weeks, the patient is instructed to look in the mirror and frown. Symmetrical medial eyebrow contractions indicate that the right medial eyebrow muscles (procerus and corrugator) are not paralyzed, thus suggesting immunoresistance. In a prospective, open-label, multicenter study, immunoresistance was assessed by BoNT/A neutralizing antibodies using the MPA and clinical resistance was assessed with a test injection of 20 U of BoNT/A placed unilaterally into either the frontalis (FTAT) or corrugator muscle (UBI).[100] Of 326 subjects enrolled 251 (77%) completed the study. Subjects received a median of 9 BoNT/A treatments, with mean doses per session ranging from 148.4 to 213.0 units over a mean of 2.5 years (range: 3.2 months–4.2 years). Only 4/326 (1.2%) subjects tested positive for antibodies in the MPA. Three of these subjects stopped responding clinically to BoNT/A (of whom one also showed clinical resistance in the FTAT), and one continued to respond.

The frequency of immunogenicity was once reported to be as high as 18% of patients treated with the "original" preparation of Botox[82,101] but the immunogenicity has been largely reduced by the development of the "current" Botox. Its lower protein content (5 ng protein/100 units), compared with the "original" formulation (25 ng protein/100 units) has been associated with a reduction in the risk of antibody formation by a factor of six, while maintaining the same efficacy (latency, peak effect, response duration) and comparable side effect rate.[102] In a study of 110 patients treated with the "current" Botox formulation for poststroke spasticity, only 0.6% developed antibodies.[103] The anamnestic immunologic response to BoNT/A can wane (after average 30 months), but can be reactivated by repeat BoNT/A treatments.[104]

Another type of BoNT/A (Xeomin) was developed by Merz Pharmaceutical, Germany, as a highly purified and free of any accessorial complexing proteins, presumably to minimize immunogenicity. Several trials have been conducted in Europe and Israel, concluding noninferior efficacy, comparable safety profiles, similar onset of action, duration and waning of effect in the treatment of CD and blepharospasm compared with Botox, at a conversion ratio of 1:1. It has not been associated with any biological relevant immunogenicity in animal models.[105]

BoNT/B (Myobloc) was found to have a higher antigenicity than BoNT/A. The higher immunogenicity of BoNT/B (Myobloc) is probably related to its significant lower specific biological activity (5.0 MU/ng BNT) (low antigenicity is described by a high specific biological activity) than the BoNT/A preparations (Botox: 60MU/ngBNT, Dysport: 100MU/ng BTN, Xeomin: 167 MU/ng BTN).[106] This is supported by the findings from a multicenter observational study of patients treated with BoNT/B.[107] A third of the patients who were negative for BoNT/B antibodies at baseline became positive for BoNT/B antibodies at last visit. Thus, the high antigenicity of BoNT/B limits its long-term efficacy. In an effort to minimize the development of immunogenicity, "booster" administrations need to be avoided, and patients should receive the minimum dose needed for optimal benefit, thus limiting protein loading. Besides immunogenicity, other reasons for reduced responsiveness include change in the pattern of dystonia or downregulation of the substrate protein assuming that the dosage used is optimal.[108]

USE OF BoNT IN FOCAL DYSTONIA

Blepharospasm

Blepharospasm was one of the first indications for the treatment with BoNT approved by the FDA in 1989. The main scale used for reliable assessment of blepharospasm in clinical trials is the Jankovic Rating Scale (JRS). The efficacy of BoNT/A was confirmed by two double-blind studies[109,110] utilizing Botox, and one multicenter double-blind trial of Dysport[111] with an improvement rate of 72%, latency of 3.7 days, and an effect duration of 12.5 weeks.[109] Side effects included blurry vision, ecchymosis, lacrimation, ptosis, and diplopia. The different preparations of BoNT/A are equally effective in blepharospasm at conversion rates of 1 (Botox): 4 (Dysport),[112,113] 1 (Botox): 1 (Xeomin),[114] 1 (Botox): 1 (Prosigne),[115] with similar effect duration, latency, and side effects. Several studies addressed specific techniques to minimize the occurrence of side effects. The injection of the pretarsal portion is more effective, lasts longer, and is associated with a lower risk for ptosis compared with the technique of injecting the preseptal portion.[116] Also, avoiding the middle two-thirds of the lower eyelid minimizes the risk of diplopia, which may be the result of inferior oblique weakness.[117] In addition to antibody formation, other reasons for failure of blepharospasm patients to respond appropriately to BoNT include underdosing, improper injection technique, and presence of eyelid opening apraxia.[118]

Oromandibular Dystonia

Oromandibular dystonia encompasses a group of dystonias involving the masticatory, lingual, and pharyngeal muscles. The abnormal muscle activity results in jaw opening, closing, and deviation movements that are difficult to treat. As with most focal dystonias, there is no effective medical treatment with the exception of BoNT. The muscles injected are usually the masseters and temporalis in jaw closure dystonia, submental complex (geniohyoid, mylohyoid, digastric), and lateral pterygoid in jaw opening dystonia.[119] In a large study evaluating the efficacy of BoNT in oromandibular dystonia, 162 patients were treated with BoNT/A.[120] Using a severity scale (0–4), definite functional improvement, in particular in chewing and speaking, was reported in 67.9% of patients, with a mean total duration of clinical improvements of 16.4 ± 7.1 weeks, 31.5% of patients reported some form of complication, the most common being dysphagia (10.2% of visits) and dysarthria (0.9% of visits). In a different study[121] of 96 patients with oromandibular dystonia treated with BoNT/A, there were fewer reported side effects (15% of patients) utilizing smaller dosages by EMG guided technique. However, the rate of functional improvement was not as robust (37–45%). Bruxism, which can accompany or occur independently of oromandibular dystonia, is also amenable to the treatment with BoNT, with a response rate of 88.9% in an open-label study of 18 patients.[122] However, double blind, placebo-controlled trials are lacking.

Limb Dystonia

BoNT has also been found to be effective in the treatment of focal limb dystonias, although this is more difficult to establish in clinical trials. Most of the studies of the treatment of BoNT in focal limb dystonia involve the upper extremity. They include primary limb dystonias, such as writer's cramp, and occupational dystonias, such as those plaguing many musicians.[123] The results are mixed, mostly because of lack of standardized and reliable outcome measures, and variability in the injection technique. Several blinded, placebo-controlled studies, using different outcome measures (subjective, handwriting analysis, visual analog scale, video scoring, etc.) confirmed the efficacy of BoNT/A,[124] for both preparations of Dysport[125] and Botox.[125,126] In one double-blind, placebo-controlled study of 10 patients with hand dystonia (6 with writer's cramp, 2 with stenographer's cramp, and 2 with musician's cramp), 6 had an improvement after treatment with Botox. The most common side effect is hand weakness,[127] the risk being higher when the forearm extensors are injected. Although injection techniques have been studied in several trials, there is not enough evidence to support the superiority of EMG guidance,[128] or the advantage of EMG versus stimulation for muscle localization.[129]

Laryngeal Dystonia

Laryngeal dystonia caused by abnormal contractions of the thyroarytenoid muscles (adductor type) is more common than the abnormal contraction of the cricoarytenoid muscles (abductor type). The former is characterized by a "strained" voice, while the latter by a "breathy" voice. A double-blinded randomized study found significant benefit in seven patients injected percutaneously with Botox compared with saline, with mild side effects consisting of excessive breathiness, mild bleeding, and vocal cord edema.[130] Several injection techniques have been proven effective in the adductor type: percutaneously, EMG-guided, either unilaterally[119] or bilaterally,[131] and via indirect laryngoscopy.[132] The unilateral EMG-guided percutaneously administered Botox into the thyroarytenoid muscles was as effective and with fewer side effects than smaller amounts injected bilaterally, using the same technique.[133] Additional voice therapy[134] or 30-minute voice rest[135] following the BoNT injections may prolong the benefit. As opposed to the adductor type, where the benefit averages 90%, the less common abductor laryngeal dystonia poses more technical difficulties, the BoNT treatment being less effective (66.7%).[136] There is no other effective therapeutic alternative to the treatment with BoNT, the successful treatment of laryngeal dystonia depending on the careful direct examination of the vocal cords by direct laryngoscopy to exclude other abnormalities of the vocal cords, and on the skills of the treating physician.

LONG-TERM EFFECTS OF BoNT IN DYSTONIA

In conclusion, chemodenervation with BoNT in focal dystonias represents the treatment of choice for many patients, being effective and safe. According to one of the longest follow-up studies that followed patients treated with BoNT for 12 years, the latency and effect duration of BoNT with chronic treatment did not change over time; however, the efficacy (peak duration and global effect) and the BoNT dose per visit increased since the initial visit.[101] A meta-analysis of 36 randomized controlled trial of BoNT/A (Botox) involving a total of 2309 patients found a 25% (353/1425) rate of mild and moderate adverse effects in the BoNT/A treated group compared with 15% (133/884) in the controlled group.[137] None of the studies reported any severe adverse events. Focal weakness was the only adverse event that occurred significantly more often with the BoNT/A treatment than control demonstrating that the formulation of BoNT/A has a favorable safety profile across a broad spectrum of therapeutic uses, mild to moderate adverse events were reported in about 25% in the BoNT/A-treated group.

▶ SURGICAL APPROACHES TO DYSTONIA

PERIPHERAL NERVE AND MUSCLE SURGERY

Even though the treatment with BoNT is effective and has a high rate of success, a minority of patients with CD remains refractory and require alternative therapy. Several surgical procedures have been used in the treatment of refractory CD. The intradural anterior rhizotomy consists of intradural sectioning of the upper cervical anterior nerve roots and the spinal accessory nerve roots. In a retrospective study of 58 patients with refractory spasmodic torticolis, 49 (85%) had a marked improvement in their condition and 30 (64%) had become free of pain.[138]

The extradural ramisectomy involves sectioning of the posterior primary divisions of the cervical nerve roots and the branches of the spinal accessory nerve to the sternocleidomastoidian muscle.[139] This procedure may provide moderate to complete return to normal function in about a third of patients, as reported in a retrospective, open-label study of 16 patients with disabling torticolis, followed at 5 years after undergoing ramisectomy; however, six patients required a second intervention, and one required a third.[140]

Selective peripheral denervation may provide benefit in as high as 87% of cases of CD,[140] with minimal risks of atrophy of the denervated muscle and local skin anesthesia. Patients with imaging evidence of moderate to severe cervical degenerative changes seem to respond poorly to selective peripheral denervation.[141] Myectomy/myotomy of trapezius muscle in patients with severe cervical dystonia, unresponsive to conservative management has been reported to improve posture and pain postoperatively and can be used as adjunct in other peripheral surgical procedures in patients with marked laterocollis and dystonic elevation and anterior rotation of the shoulder.[142] In general, peripheral surgical procedures seem to be safe and effective in refractory cases of CD. In a retrospective study of 46 patients with CD who underwent 70 procedures (33 intradural rhizotomies, 21 extradural ramisectomies, 22 myectomy/myotomy single or combined) the global outcome (0: none–4: excellent) was excellent in 9 patients (21%), marked in 12 (27%), moderate in 9 (21%), mild in 9 (21%), and no improvement in 5(11%). Patients with excellent outcome generally underwent on average a higher number of surgeries than those patients who achieved no benefit.[139] Many of the studies of the different surgical procedures in CD were retrospective, using different outcome scales, often criticized, and comparing the different techniques remains problematic. Therefore, it is difficult to estimate the importance of different peripheral surgical procedures in the treatment of CD.

Peripheral surgical interventions for other focal dystonias are very seldom used today, because of the effective treatment with BoNT. Before myectomy became available, peripheral facial neurectomy was the surgical treatment of choice for blepharospasm. However, because of the high recurrence rate (75.9%) and associated complications (lower face paralysis, lagophthalmos, persistent Bell's phenomenon, eyelid drop, ectropion, corneal exposure, accumulation of parotid secretions),[143] this procedure is reserved for the very few cases refractory to BoNT and myectomy. Myectomy refers to the surgical resection of the eyelid protractor muscles (orbicularis oculi, procerus, corrugator, and depressor supercilii), being better tolerated, with fewer side effects and lower recurrence rates than peripheral facial neurectomy.[144] Frontalis sling surgery[145] is another option for patients with blepharospasm. Other peripheral surgical procedures such as recurrent laryngeal nerve section[146] as treatment for spasmodic dysphonia, and spinal cord stimulation for cervical dystonia[147] are rarely used.

Deep Brain Stimulation (DBS) Surgical Treatment

Functional surgery has been used in the treatment of both generalized and focal dystonias, as a rationale for the abnormally active direct and indirect basal ganglia pathways. Abnormal dystonic movements respond to the ablation of the internal segment of the globus pallidus (GPi)[148–150] and ventral intermediate thalamic nucleus (Vim).[151] DBS of the GPi has become the preferred technique for dystonia because of the lower rates of complications, adjustable stimulation parameters, and reversibility of the procedure.

DBS FOR GENERALIZED DYSTONIA

Since the medical management of generalized dystonias is largely unsatisfactory (with few exceptions) and BoNT treatment is unreasonable due to the high dosage required, deep brain stimulation is often considered early in the course of treatment. The most common target remains the GPi. In one study, 53 patients with generalized dystonia of various etiologies that were treated with bilateral GPi DBS were followed for 1 year and evaluated with the BFMDRS.[151] Patients with primary generalized dystonia had a good response, with 71% improvement in BFMDRS in patients with a DYT-1 genetically confirmed diagnosis, and 74% in primary generalized dystonia of unknown origin. Patients with secondary dystonia had a more modest response of only 31%. The same cohort was followed at 2 years, with a sustained response of the primary generalized dystonia patients, irrespective of their DYT-1 status.[152] Children had a greater improvement than adults on the clinical scores, but not on the functional BFMDRS. Similar positive results of bilateral GPi DBS were obtained in a multicenter study of 22 patients with an improvement in the BFMDRS from a mean of 46.3 ± 21.3 before surgery to 21.0 ± 14.1 at 12 months ($P < 0.001$).[153] In addition, the improvement in disability was also sustained. Except for an increase in mean pulse width from 77 ± 30 μsec at 3 months to 139±130 μsec at 12 months, there were minor changes in the frequency (majority at 130 Hz) and mean voltage (3.8 ± 0.9 V at 3 months and 3.7 ± 1.0 V at 12 months). In a 3-year follow-up, motor improvement observed at 1 year (51%) was maintained at 3 years (58%) and the authors concluded that "bilateral pallidal stimulation provides sustained motor benefit after 3 years."[154] In a study involving French centers, bilateral DBS of ventral GPi was associated with a 42% reduction in the BFMDRS score; whereas, DBS of dorsal GPi resulted in less predictable effects.[155] Most studies use a combination of high frequency (>100 Hz) and broad pulse width (>120 μsec),[151–153,156] but lower stimulation frequencies (60 Hz) with similar success rate may have the advantage of prolonging the battery life.[157]

In addition to the location of the active electrode,[158,159] other factors may influence the response of patients with generalized dystonia to GPi DBS, such as age of onset (children have a better response), overall BFMDRS scale (patients with higher scores had less robust postoperative responses), and GPi volume (the greater the GPi volume, particularly the right, the greater degree of improvement).[160] GPi DBS remains a relatively safe procedure. In a study of 40 patients with generalized and segmental dystonia implanted with DBS in the GPi bilaterally and assessed with either neurostimulation or sham stimulation at 3 months, the change from baseline in the mean BFMDRS scale was significantly greater in the neurostimulation group (–15.8 ± 14.1 points) than in the sham-stimulation group (–1.4 ± 3.8 points, $P < 0.001$), with a total of 22 adverse events in 19 patients.[161] In addition to having a favorable risk-benefit ratio, DBS has a favorable impact on the quality of life.[162]

DBS IN FOCAL DYSTONIA

In contrast to generalized dystonia, where BoNT treatment is limited by technical aspects (high dose, selection of muscles etc.), focal dystonias have a high response rate to the treatment with BoNT. However, in a minority of refractory cases, GPi DBS may represent an alternative. Small sample studies assessed the efficacy of GPi DBS in CD. In one study, 8 patients with complex CD (3 with CD in the context of a generalized movement disorder) resistant to other forms of treatment, including BoNT, underwent bilateral GPi DBS.[163] Three patients also had spinal surgery for secondary cervical myelopathy. The adjustment of DBS was time consuming in some cases, with a mean number of visits of 8.8 at 12 months postoperatively. The full benefit was delayed for several months of chronic stimulation, with an improvement of 63% on the severity score, 60% on the disability score, and 50% on the pain score of a modified TWSTRS at 20 months. In a longer follow up study of 10 patients with refractory CD treated with bilateral GPi DBS, the TWSTRS total scores improved by 56.8% at 6-months, with no additional improvement at the last available follow-up at 31.9 ± 20.9 months (163). However, the study was open-label, the rater not being blinded. Patients with phasic contractions improved more rapidly than patients with tonic contractions. As with generalized dystonia, higher stimulation settings are preferred as more effective in the pallidal stimulation in CD (164).

The response of medically refractory craniocervical dystonia to GPi DBS was also assessed in a pilot study of 6 patients.[166] At six months, the BFMDRS total score showed a 72% mean trend toward improvement ($P < 0.06$), with a total TWSTRS amelioration of 54% ($P < 0.043$). However, worsening of motor function was noticed in nondystonic preoperatively normal extremities, not associated with aberrant lead placement near the internal capsule.[167] These adverse events were responsive to turning the stimulator off.

DBS IN SECONDARY DYSTONIA

GPi DBS was also used in segmental,[168] tardive,[169,170] and secondary dystonias.[171] Pantothenate kinase-associated neurodegeneration[172–174] and X-linked dystonia-parkinsonism[175] have also been reported to respond to GPi DBS. Ventral intermediate thalamic nucleus (Vim) DBS has been reported effective in the treatment of myoclonus-dystonia,[176] and writer's cramp.[177]

LONG-TERM OUTCOMES OF DBS FOR DYSTONIA

Longer retrospective analyses confirm the efficacy and safety of GPi DBS in the treatment of dystonia.[178,179] According to a long-term follow up of dystonia patients (2 with generalized dystonia, 4 with cervical dystonia, one with paroxysmal dystonia, one with hemidystonia, one with craniocervical dystonia) pallidal (thalamic in paroxysmal dystonia) stimulation resulted in a positive change within days of surgery, but the full benefit was achieved at 6 months, remained stable at 3 years, and was maintained at the last follow up visit, which was between 5 and 10 years postoperatively.[176] Only one patient (paroxysmal dystonia) with thalamic DBS lost effectiveness, which was regained with replacement of the DBS in the GPi. There is emerging evidence that the subthalamic nucleus may also be a suitable target for medically refractory dystonia.[180–182]

▶ TREATMENT OF DYSTONIC STORM

The dystonic storm, or status dystonicus, is a neurological emergency consisting of severe episodes of generalized dystonia and rigidity. First reported in an 8-year-old boy with autosomal dominant dystonia,[183] this potentially fatal complication can occur in primary or secondary dystonias. Severe complications include bulbar and ventilatory complications, rhabdomyolysis, acute renal failure, and hyperpyrexia. The urgent treatment is imperative, and it is usually conducted in an intensive care unit with aggressive respiratory and hemodynamic support, muscle paralysis and sedation. Some cases may require the triple "Marsden cocktail" of a dopamine blocker (pimozide), dopamine depleting drug (tetrabenazine) and anticholinergic (benzhexol)[42] or variations. Other treatment options for this emergency include intrathecal baclofen and pallidal deep brain stimulation.[184]

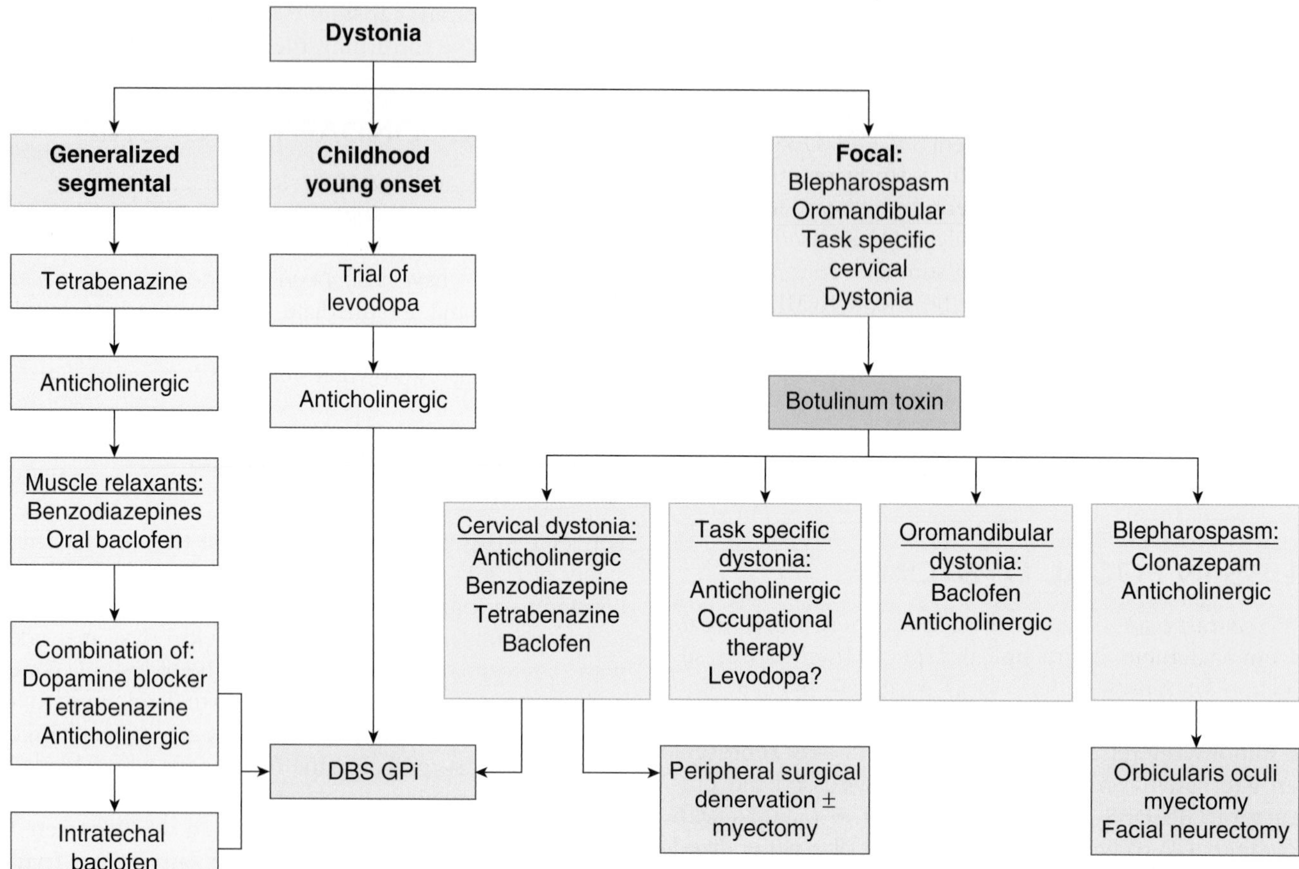

Figure 30–1. Dystonia treatment algorithm.

▶ CONCLUSIONS

The treatment for dystonia remains focused on symptomatic relief. There is no generally accepted algorithm for the treatment of dystonia; however, there are several useful clinical guidelines (Fig. 30–1): dystonia with onset in childhood merits a levodopa trial; the treatment of choice for focal dystonias is BoNT; GPi DBS is generally considered effective and safe, but should be considered only for patients with disabling dystonia that fails to respond to optimal medical therapy.

REFERENCES

1. Oppenheim H. Über eine eigenartige Krampfkrankheit des kindlichen und jungendlichen Alters (Dysbasia lordotica progressive, Dystonia musculorum defromans). Neurologisches Zentralblatt 1911;30:1090.
2. Pearce JM. Dystonia. Eur Neurol 2005;53:151.
3. Jankovic J. Dystonia. Phenomenology, Classification, Etiology, Pathology, Biochemistry, and Genetics. In Fahn S and Jankovic J (eds), Principles and Practice of Movement Disorders. New York: Churchill Livingston Elsevier, 2007, p. 307.
4. Breakfield XO, Blood A, Li Y, Hallett M, et al. The pathophysiological basis of dystonias. Nat Rev Neuroscience 2008;9:222.
5. Burke RE, Fahn S, Marsden CD, et al. Validity and reliability of a rating scale for the primary torsion dystonia. Neurology 1985;35:73.
6. Comella C, Leurgans S, Wuu J, et al. Rating scales for dystonia: A multicenter assessment. Mov Disord 2003;18:303.
7. Consky E, Lang A. Clinical assessment of patients with cervical dystonia. In Jankovic J, Hallett M (eds), Therapy with Botulinum Toxin, New York: Marcel Dekker, 1994, p. 211.
8. Jankovic J, Kenney C, Grafe S, et al. Relationship between various clinical outcome assessments in patients with blepharospasm. Mov Disord 2009;24:407.
9. Simpson DM, Blitzer A, Brashear A, et al. Therapeutics and Technology Assessment Subcommittee of the American Academy of Neurology. Department of Neurology, Mount Sinai Medical Center, New York, NY, USA. Neurology. 2008 May 6;70(19):1699–1706.
10. Candia V, Elbert T, Altenmüller E, et al. Constraint-induced movement therapy for focal hand dystonia in musicians. Lancet 1999;353:42.
11. Priori A, Pesenti A, Cappellari A, et al. Limb immobilization for the treatment of focal occupational dystonia. Neurology 2001;57:405.

12. Jankovic J. Can peripheral trauma induce dystonia and other movement disorders? Yes!. Mov Disord 2001;16:7.
13. Candia V, Rosset-Llobet J, Elbert T, et al. Changing the brain through therapy for musicians' hand dystonia. Ann N Y Acad Sci 2005;1060:335.
14. Zeuner KE, Hallett M. Sensory training as treatment for focal hand dystonia: A 1-year follow-up. Mov Disord 2003;18:1044.
15. Siebner HR, Tormos JM, Ceballos-Baumann AO, et al. Low-frequency repetitive transcranial magnetic stimulation of the motor cortex in writer's cramp. Neurology 1999;52:529.
16. Murase N, Rothwell JC, Kaji R, et al. Subthreshold low-frequency repetitive transcranial magnetic stimulation over the premotor cortex modulates writer's cramp. Brain 2005;128:104.
17. Borich M, Arora S, Kimberley TJ. Lasting effects of repeated rTMS application in focal hand dystonia. Restor Neurol Neurosci 2009;27:55.
18. Lefaucheur JP, Fénelon G, Ménard-Lefaucheur I, et al. Low-frequency repetitive TMS of premotor cortex can reduce painful axial spasms in generalized secondary dystonia: A pilot study of three patients. Neurophysiol Clin 2004;34:141.
19. Allam N, Brasil-Neto JP, Brandão P, et al. Relief of primary cervical dystonia symptoms by low frequency transcranial magnetic stimulation of the premotor cortex: Case report. Arq Neuropsiquiatr 2007;65:697.
20. Tinazzi M, Farina S, Bhatia K, et al. TENS for the treatment of writer's cramp dystonia: A randomized, placebo-controlled study. Neurology 2005;64:1946.
21. Trompetto C, Avanzino L, Bove M, et al. External shock waves therapy in dystonia: Preliminary results. Eur J Neurol. 2009 Jan 27. [Epub ahead of print].
22. Balash Y, Giladi N. Efficacy of pharmacological treatment of dystonia: Evidence-based review including meta-analysis of the effect of botulinum toxin and other cure options. Eur J Neurol 2004;11:361.
23. Lang A. Dopamine agonists in the treatment of dystonia. Clin Neuropharmacol 1985;8:38.
24. Segawa M, Ohmi K, Itoh S, et al. Childhood basal ganglia disease with remarkable response to l-DOPA. Shinryo 1971;24:667.
25. Furukawa Y. Update on dopa-responsive dystonia: Locus heterogeneity and biochemical features. Adv Neurol 2004;94:127.
26. Nygaard TG, Marsden CD, Fahn S. Dopa-responsive dystonia: Long-term treatment response and prognosis. Neurology 1991;41:174.
27. Nygaard TG. Dopa-responsive dystonia. Delineation of the clinical syndrome and clues to pathogenesis. Adv Neurol 1993;60:577.
28. Hwang WJ, Calne DB, Tsui JK, et al. The long-term response to levodopa in dopa-responsive dystonia. Parkinsonism Relat Disord 2001;8:1.
29. Zuddas A, Cianchetti C. Efficacy of risperidone in idiopathic segmental dystonia. Lancet 1996;347:127.
30. Grassi E, Latorraca S, Piacentini S, et al. Risperidone in idiopathic and symptomatic dystonia: Preliminary experience. Neurol Sci 2000;21:121.
31. Karp BI, Goldstein SR, Chen R, et al. An open trial of clozapine for dystonia. Mov Disord 1999;14: 652.
32. Thiel A, Dressler D, Kistel C, et al. Clozapine treatment of spasmodic torticolis, Neurology 1994;44:957.
33. Jankovic J. Treatment of hyperkinetic movement disorders with tetrabenazine: A double-blind crossover study. Ann Neurol 1982;11:41.
34. Jankovic J, Orman J. Tetrabenazine therapy of dystonia, chorea, tics, and other dyskinesias. Neurology 1988;38:391.
35. Jankovic J, Beach J. Long-term effects of tetrabenazine in hyperkinetic movement disorders. Neurology 1997;48:358.
36. Kenney C, Hunter C, Jankovic J. Long-term tolerability of tetrabenazine in the treatment of hyperkinetic movement disorders. Mov Disord 2007;22:193.
37. Kenney C, Hunter C, Mejia N, et al. Is history of depression a contraindication to treatment with tetrabenazine? Clin Neuropharmacol 2006;29:259.
38. Fahn S. High dosage anticholinergic therapy in dystonia. Neurology 1983;33:1255.
39. Burke RE, Fahn S, Marsden CD. Torsion dystonia: A double-blind, prospective trial of high-dosage trihexyphenidyl. Neurology 1986;36:160.
40. Sanger TD, Bastian A, Brunstrom J, et al. Prospective open-label clinical trial of trihexyphenidyl in children with secondary dystonia due to cerebral palsy. J Child Neurol 2007;22:530.
41. Marsden CD, Marion MH, Quinn N. The treatment of severe dystonia in children and adults. J Neurol Neurosurg Psychiatry 1984;47:1166.
42. Greene P, Shale H, Fahn S. Analysis of open-label trials in torsion dystonia using high dosages of anticholinergics and other drugs. Mov Disord 1988;3:46.
43. Taylor AE, Lang AE, Saint-Cyr JA, et al. Cognitive processes in idiopathic dystonia treated with high-dose anticholinergic therapy: Implications for treatment strategies Clin Neuropharmacol 1991;14:62.
44. Anca MH, Falic Zaccai T, Badarna S, et al. Natural history of Oppenheim's Dystonia (DYT1) in Israel. J Child Neurol 2003;18:325.
45. Greene PE, Fahn S. Baclofen in the treatment of idiopathic dystonia in children. Mov Disord 1992;7:48.
46. Greene P. Baclofen in the treatment of dystonia. Clin Neuropharmacol 1992;15:276.
47. Jankovic J, Tintner R. Dystonia and parkinsonism. Parkinsonism Relat Disord 2001;8:109.
48. Hou JG, Ondo W, Jankovic J. Intrathecal baclofen for dystonia. Mov Disord 2001;16:1201.
49. Albright AL, Barry MJ, Shafton DH, et al. Intrathecal baclofen for generalized dystonia. Dev Med Child Neurol 2001;43:652.
50. Paret G, Tirosh R, Ben Zeev B, et al. Intrathecal baclofen for severe torsion dystonia in a child. Acta Paediatr 1996;85:635.
51. Penn RD, Gianino, York MM. Intrathecal baclofen for motor disorders. Mov Disord 1995;10:657.
52. Narayan RK, Loubser PG, Jankovic J, et al. Intrathecal baclofen for intractable axial dystonia. Neurology.1991;41:1141.
53. Albright AL, Ferson SS. Intraventricular baclofen for dystonia: Techniques and outcomes. J Neurosurg Pediatr 2009;3:11.

54. Jankovic J, Ford J. Blepharospasm and orofacial-cervical dystonia: Clinical and pharmacological findings in 100 patients. Ann Neurol 1983;13:402.
55. Hughes AJ, Lees AJ, Marsden CD. Paroxysmal dystonic head tremor. Mov Disord 1991;6:85.
56. Obeso JA, Rothwell JC, Lang AE, et al. Myoclonic dystonia. Neurology 1983;33:825.
57. Ohara S, Hayashi R, Momoi H, et al. Mexiletine in the treatment of Spasmodic Torticolis, Mov Disord 1998;13:934.
58. Lucetti C, Nutti A, Gambaccini G, et al. Mexiletine in the treatment of torticolis and generalized dystonia. Clinical Neuropharmacology 2000;23:186.
59. Ohara S, Tsuyuzaki J, Hayashi R. Mexiletine in the treatment of blepharospasm: Experience with the first three patients. Mov Disord 1999;14:173.
60. Isgreen WP, Fahn S, Barrett RE, et al. Carbamazepine in torsion in dystonia. Adv Neurol 1976;14:411.
61. Garg BP. Dystonia musculorum deformans: Implications of therapeutic response to levodopa and carbamazepine. Arch Neurol 1982;39:376.
62. Hering S, Wenning GK, Seppi K, et al. An open trial of levetiracetam for segmental and generalized dystonia. Mov Disord 2007;22:1649.
63. Sullivan KL, Hauser RA, Louis ED, et al. dystonia. Parkinsonism Relat Disord 2005;11:469.
64. Yardimci N, Karatas M, Kilinc M, et al. Levetiracetam in Meige's syndrome. Acta Neurol Scand 2006;114:63.
65. Zesiewicz TA, Louis ED, Sullivan KL, et al. Substantial improvement in a Meige's syndrome patient with levetiracetam treatment. Mov Disord 2004;19:1518.
66. Tarsy D, Ryan RK, Ro SI. An open-label trial of levetiracetam for treatment of cervical dystonia. Mov Disord 2006;21:734.
67. Quinn NP, Rothwell JC, Thompson PD, et al. Hereditary myoclonic dystonia, hereditary torsion dystonia and hereditary essential myoclonus: An area of confusion. Adv Neurol 1988;50:391.
68. Biary N, Koller W. Effect of alcohol on dystonia. Neurology 1985;35:239.
69. Koller WC, Biary N. Lithium ineffective in dystonia. Ann Neurol 1983;13:579.
70. Fox SH, Kellett M, Moore AP, et al. Randomised, double blind, placebo-controlled trial to assess the potential of cannabinoid receptor stimulation in the treatment of dystonia. Mov Disord 2002;17:145.
71. Riker DK, Hurtig H, Lake CR, et al. Open trial of clonidine in dystoniamusculorum defromans. Abstr Soc Neurosci 1982;8:563.
72. Muller J, Wenning GK, Wissel J et al. Riluzole therapy in cervical dystonia. Mov Disord 2002;17:198.
73. Jankovic J. Treatment of dystonia. In Fahn S, Jankovic J, Hallett M, Jenner P. (eds). Principles and Practice of Movement Disorders, New York: Churchill Livingston Elsevier, 2007 p. 345.
74. Foster K. Engineered toxin: New therapeutics. Toxicon 2009 Mar 2 [Epub ahead of print].
75. Blackie JD, Lees AJ. Botulinum toxin treatment in spasmodic torticollis. J Neurol Neurosurg Psychiatry 1990;53:640.
76. Greene P, Kang U, Fahn S, et al. Double-blind, placebo controlled trial of botulinum toxin injection for the treatment of spasmodic torticollis. Neurology 1990;40:1213.
77. Lorentz IT, Subramanian SS, Yiannikas C. Treatment of idiopathic spasmodic torticollis with botulinum toxin A: A double-blind study on twenty-three patients. Mov Disord 1991;6:145.
78. Poewe W, Schelosky L, Kleedorfer B, et al. Treatment of spasmodic torticollis with local injections of botulinum toxin. J Neurol 1992;239:21.
79. Jankovic J, Schwartz KS. Botulinum toxin injections for cervical dystonia. Neurology 1990;41:277.
80. Jankovic J. Botulinum toxin therapy for cervical dystonia. Neurotox Res 2006;9:145.
81. Jahanhashi M, Marsden CD . Psychological functioning before and after treatment of torticollis with botulinum toxin. J Neurol Neurosurg Psychiatry 1992;55:229.
82. Kessler KR, Skutta M, Benecke R. Long-term treatment of cervical dystonia with botulinum toxin A: Efficacy, safety, and antibody frequency. J Neurol 1999;246:265.
83. Brans JW, Lindeboom R, Snoek JW, et al. Botulinum toxin versus trihexyphenidyl in cervical dystonia: A prospective, randomized, double-blind controlled trial. Neurology 1996;46:1066.
84. Comella CL, Jankovic J, Daggett S, et al. Interim results of an observational study of neutralizing antibody formation with the current preparation of botulinum toxin type A in the treatment for cervical dystonia. Neurology 2004;62(suppl 5):A511.
85. Comella CL, Tanner CM, DeFoor-Hill L, et al. Dysphagia after botulinum toxin injections for spasmodic torticolis: Clinical and radiologic findings. Neurology 1992;42:1307.
86. Poewe W, Deuschl G, Nebe A, et al. What is the optimal dose of botulinum toxin A in the treatment of cervical dystonia? Results of a double blind, placebo controlled, dose ranging study using Dysport. German Dystonia Study Group. J Neurol Neurosurg Psychiatry 1998;64:13.
87. Truong D, Duane DD, Jankovic J, et al. Efficacy and safety of botulinum type A toxin (Dysport) in cervical dystonia: Results of the first US randomized, double-blind, placebo-controlled study. Mov Disord 2005;20:783.
88. Odergren T, Hjaltason H, Kaakkola S, et al. A double blind, randomized, parallel group study to investigate the dose equivalence of Dysport® and Botox® in the treatment of cervical dystonia. J Neurol Neurosurg Psychiatry 1998;64:6.
89. Kranz G, Haubenberger D, Voller B, (et al). Respective potencies of Botox and Dysport in a human skin model: A randomized, double-blind study. Mov Disord 2009;30:231.
90. Marchetti A, Magar R, Findley L, et al. Retrospective evaluation of the dose of Dysport® and BOTOX® in the management of cervical dystonia and blepharospasm: The REAL DOSE study. Mov Disord 2005;20:937.
91. Tsui JKC, Hayward M, Mak EKM, et al. Botulinum toxin type B in the treatment of cervical dystonia: A pilot study. Neurology 1995;45:2109.
92. Brashear A, Lew MF, Dykstra DD, et al. Safety and efficacy of NeuroBloc (botulinum toxin type B) in type A-responsive cervical dystonia. Neurology 1999;53:1439.
93. Lew MF, Adornato BT, Duane DD, et al. Botulinum toxin type B: A double-blind, placebo-controlled, safety and efficacy study in cervical dystonia. Neurology 1997;49:701.

94. Brin MF, Lew MF, Adler CH, et al. Safety and efficacy of NeuroBloc (botulinum toxin type B) in type A-resistant cervical dystonia. Neurology 1999;53:1431.
95. Comella CL, Jankovic J, Shannon KM, et al. Comparison of botulinum toxin serotypes A and B for the treatment of cervical dystonia. Neurology 2005;65:1423.
96. Tintner R, Gross R, Winzer UF, et al. Autonomic function after botulinum toxin type A or B: A double-blind, randomized trial. Neurology 2005;65:765.
97. Dressler D, Dirnberger G, Bhatia K, et al. Botulinum toxin antibody testing: Comparison between the mouse protection assay and the mouse lethality assay. Mov Disord 2000;15:973.
98. Jankovic J. Botulinum toxin in clinical practice. J Neurol Neurosurg Psychiatry 2004;75:951.
99. Voller B, Moraru E, Auff E, et al. Ninhydrin sweat test: A simple method for detecting antibodies neutralizing botulinum toxin type A. Mov Disord 2004;19:943.
100. Brin MF, Comella CL, Jankovic J, et al. CD-017 BoNTA Study Group. Long-term treatment with botulinum toxin type A in cervical dystonia has low immunogenicity by mouse protection assay. Mov Disord 2008; 23:1353.
101. Mejia NI, Vuong KD, Jankovic J. Long-term botulinum toxin efficacy, safety and immunogenicity. Mov Disord 2005;20:592.
102. Jankovic J, Vuong KD, Ahsan J. Comparison of efficacy and immunogenicity of original versus current botulinum toxin in cervical dystonia. Neurology 2003;60:1186.
103. Turkel CC, Dru RM, Daggett S, et al. Neutralizing antibody formation is rare following repeated injections of a low-protein formulation of botulinum toxin type A (BTX-A) in patients with post-stroke spasticity. Neurology 2002;58(suppl 7):A316.
104. Sankhla C, Jankovic J, Duane D. Variability in the immunologic and clinical response in dystonic patients immunoresistant to botulinum toxin injections. Movement Disorders 1998;13:150.
105. Jost WH, Blumel J, Graft S. Botulinum Neurotoxin Type A Free of Complexing Proteins (Xeomin) in Focal Dystonia. Drugs 2007;67:669.
106. Dressler D, Hallett M. Immunological aspects of Botox, Dysport and Myobloc/Neurobloc. Eur J Neurol 2006; 13(suppl. 1):11.
107. Jankovic J, Hunter C, Dolimbek BZ, (et al). Clinico-immunologic aspects of botulinum toxin type B treatment of cervical dystonia. Neurology 2006;67:2233.
108. Jankovic J. Schwartz KS. Clinical correlates of response to botulinum toxin injections. Arch Neurol 1991;48:1253.
109. Jankovic J, Orman J. Botulinum toxin A for cranial-cervical dystonia: A double-blind, placebo-controlled study. Neurology 1987;37:616.
110. Girlanda P, Quartarone A, Sinicropi S, et al. Unilateral injection of botulinum toxin in blepharospasm: Single fiber electromyography and blink reflex study. Mov Disord 1996;11:27.
111. Truong D, Comella C, Fernandez HH, et al. Efficacy and safety of purified botulinum toxin type A (Dysport) for the treatment of benign essential blepharospasm: A randomized, placebo-controlled, phase II trial. Parkinsonism Relat Disord 2008;14:407.
112. Nussgens Z, Roggenkamper P. Comparison of two botulinum-toxin preparations in the treatment of essential blepharospasm. Graefes Arch Clin Exp Ophthalmol 1997;235:197.
113. Sampaio C, Ferreira JJ, Simões F, et al. DYSBOT: A single-blind, randomized parallel study to determine whether any differences can be detected in the efficacy and tolerability of two formulations of botulinum toxin type A—Dysport and Botox—assuming a ratio of 4:1. Mov Disord 1997;12:1013.
114. Roggenkamper P, Jost WH, Bihari K, et al. Efficacy and safety of a new Botulinum Toxin Type A free of complexing proteins in the treatment of blepharospasm. J Neural Transm 2006;113:303.
115. Rieder CR, Schestatsky P, Socal MP, et al. A double-blind, randomized, crossover study of Prosigne versus Botox in patients with blepharospasm and hemifacial spasm. Clin Neuropharmacol 2007;30:39.
116. Cakmur R, Ozturk V, Uzunel F, et al. Comparison of preseptal and pretarsal injections of botulinum toxin in the treatment of blepharospasm and hemifacial spasm. J Neurol 2002;249:64.
117. Frueh BR, Nelson CC, Kapustiak JF, et al. The effect of omitting botulinum toxin from the lower eyelid in blepharospasm treatment. Am J Ophthalmol 1988; 106:45.
118. Kenney C, Jankovic J. Botulinum toxin in the treatment of blepharospasm and hemifacial spasm. J Neural Transm 2008;115:585.
119. Jankovic J, Schwartz K, Donovan D. Botulinum toxin treatment of cranial-cervical dystonia, spasmodic dysphonia, other focal dystonias and hemifacial spasm. J Neurol Neurosurg Psychiatry 1990;53:633.
120. Tan EK, Jankovic J. Botulinum toxin A in patients with oromandibular dystonia. Neurology 1999;53:2102.
121. Brin MF, Blitzer A, Herman S, et al. Oromandibular dystonia: Treatment of 96 patients with botulinum toxin A, in Jankovic J, Hallett M (eds.), Therapy with Botulinum Toxin. New York: Marcel Dekker, 1994, p. 429.
122. Jankovic J, Ashoori A. Movement disorders in musicians. Mov Disord 2008;14:1957.
123. Yoshimura DM, Aminoff MJ, Olney RK. Botulinum toxin therapy for limb dystonias. Neurology 1992;42:627.
124. Kruisdijk JJ, Koelman JH, Ongerboer de Visser BW, et al. Botulinum toxin for writer's cramp: A randomised, placebo-controlled trial and 1-year follow-up. J Neurol Neurosurg Psychiatry 2007;78:264.
125. Tsui JK, Bhatt M, Calne S, et al. Botulinum toxin in the treatment of writer's cramp: A double-blind study. Neurology 1993;43:183.
126. Cole R, Hallett M, Cohen LG. Double-blind trial of botulinum toxin for treatment of focal hand dystonia. Mov Disord 1995;10:466.
127. Jankovic J, Schwartz K. Use of botulinum toxin in the treatment of hand dystonia. J Hand Surg [Am] 1993;18:883.
128. Molloy FM, Shill HA, Kaelin-Lang A, et al. Accuracy of muscle localization without EMG: Implications for treatment of limb dystonia. Neurology 2002;58:805..
129. Geenen C, Consky E, Ashby P. Localizing muscles for botulinum toxin treatment of focal hand dystonia. Can J Neurol Sci 1996;23:194.

130. Truong DD, Rontal M, Rolnick M, et al. Double-blind controlled study of botulinum toxin in adductor spasmodic dysphonia. Laryngoscope 1991;101:630.
131. Brin M, Blitzer A, Stewart C, et al. Treatment of spasmodic dysphonia (laryngeal dystonia) with local injections of botulinum toxin: Review and technical aspects, in Neurological Disorders of the Larynx, edited by Blitzer A, Brin M, Sasaki C, et al. New York, Thieme Medical Publishers, 1992 p. 214.
132. Ford C, Bless D, Lowery J. Indirect laryngoscopy approach for injection of botulinum toxin in spasmodic dysphonia. Otolaryngol Head Neck Surg 1990;103:752.
133. Adams SG, Hunt EJ, Irish JC, et al. Comparison of botulinum toxin injection procedures in adductor spasmodic dysphonia. J Otolaryngol 1995;24:345.
134. Murry T, Woodson GE. Combined-modality treatment of adductor spasmodic dysphonia with botulinum toxin and voice therapy. J Voice 1995;9:460.
135. Wong DL, Adams SG, Irish JC, et al. Effect of neuromuscular activity on the response to botulinum toxin injections in spasmodic dysphonia. J Otolaryngol 1995;24:209.
136. Blitzer A, Brin MF, Stewart CF. Botulinum toxin management of spasmodic dysphonia (laryngeal dystonia): A 12-year experience in more than 900 patients. Laryngoscope 1998;108:1435.
137. Naumann M, Jankovic J. Safety of botulinum toxin type A: A systematic review and meta-analysis. Current Medical Research and Opinion 2004;20:981.
138. Friedman AH, Nashold BS Jr, Sharp R, et al. Treatment of spasmodic torticollis with intradural selective rhizotomies. J Neurosurg 1993;78:46.
139. Krauss JK, Toups EG, Jankovic J, et al. Functional and symptomatic outcome of surgical treatment of cervical dystonia. J Neurol Neurosurg Psychiatry 1997;63:642.
140. Bertrand CM. Selective peripheral denervation for spasmodic torticollis: Surgical technique, results, and observations in 260 cases. Surg Neurol 1993;40:96.
141. Chawda SJ, Munchau A, Johnson D, et al. Pattern of premature degenerative changes of the cervical spine in patients with spasmodic torticollis and the impact on the outcome of selective peripheral denervation. J Neurol Neurosurg Psychiatry 2000;68:465.
142. Krauss JK, Koller R, Burgunder JM. Partial myotomy/myectomy of the trapezius muscle with an asleep-awake-asleep anesthetic technique for treatment of cervical dystonia. J Neurosurg 1999;91:889.
143. Grandas F, Elston J, Quinn N, et al. Blepharsospasm: A review of 264 patients. J Neurol Neurosurg Psychiatry 1988;51:767.
144. McCord CD Jr, Coles WH, Shore JW, et al. Treatment of essential blepharospasm. I. Comparision of facial nerve avulsion and eyebrow-eyelid muscle stripping procedure. Arch Ophthalmol 1984;102:266.
145. Wabbels B, Roggenkamper P. Long-term follow up of patients with frontalis sling operation in the treatment of essential blepharospasm unresponsive to botulinum toxin therapy. Graefes Arch Clin Exp Ophthalmol 2007;245:45.
146. Dedo HH, Behlau MS. Resurrent laryngeal nerve section for spasmodic dysphonia: 5- to 14-year preliminary results in the first 300 patients. Ann Otol Rhinol Laryngol 1991;100:274.
147. Goetz CG, Penn RD, Tanner CM. Efficacy of cervical cord stimulation in dystonia. Adv Neurol 1988;50:645.
148. Vitek JL, Chockkan V, Zhang JY, et al. Neuronal activity in the basal ganglia in patients with generalized dystonia and hemiballismus. Ann Neurol 1999;46:22.
149. Ondo WG, Desaloms JM, Jankovic J, et al. Pallidotomy for generalized dystonia. Mov Disord 1998;13:693.
150. Lozano AM, Kumar R, Gross RE, et al. Globus pallidus internus pallidotomy for generalized dystonia. Mov Disord 1997;12:865.
151. Cif L, El Fertit H, Vayssiere N, et al. Treatment of dystonic syndromes by chronic electrical stimulation of the internal globus pallidus. J Neurosurg Sci 2003;47:52.
152. Coubes P, Cif L, El Fertit H, et al. Electrical stimulation of the globus pallidus internus in patients with primary generalized dystonia: Long-term results. J Neurosurg 2004;101:189.
153. Vidailhet M, Vercueil L, Houeto JL, et al. Bilateral deep-brain stimulation of the globus pallidus in primary generalized dystonia. N Engl J Med 2005;352:459.
154. Vidailhet M, Vercueil L, Houeto JL, et al. Bilateral, pallidal, deep-brain stimulation in primary generalised dystonia: A prospective 3 year follow-up study. Lancet Neurol 2007;6:223.
155. Houeto JL, Yelnik J, Bardinet E, et al. Acute deep-brain stimulation of the internal and external globus pallidus in primary dystonia: Functional mapping of the pallidum. Arch Neurol 2007;64:1281.
156. Diamond A, Shahed J, Azher S, et al. Globus pallidus deep brain stimulation in dystonia. Mov Disord 2006;21:692.
157. Alterman RL, Miravite J, Weisz D, et al. Sixty hertz pallidal deep brain stimulation for primary torsion dystonia. Neurology 2007;69:681.
158. Starr PA, Turner RS, Rau G, et al. Microelectrode-guided implantation of deep brain stimulators into the globus pallidus internus for dystonia: Techniques, electrode locations, and outcomes. J Neurosurg 2006;104:488.
159. Tisch S, Zrinzo L, Limousin P, et al. The effect of electrode contact location on clinical efficacy of pallidal deep brain stimulation in primary generalised dystonia. J Neurol Neurosurg Psychiatry 2007;78: 1314.
160. Vasques X, Cif L, Gonzales V, et al. Factors predicting improvement in primary generalized dystonia treated by pallidal deep brain stimulation. Mov Disord 6 Feb 2009. [Epub ahead of print].
161. Kupsch A, Benecke R, Muller J, et al. Pallidal deep-brain stimulation in primary generalized or segmental dystonia. N Engl J Med 2006;355:1978.
162. Mueller J, Skogseid IM, Benecke R, et al. Pallidal deep brain stimulation improves quality of life in segmental and generalized dystonia: Results from a prospective, randomized sham-controlled trial. Mov Disord 2008;23:131.
163. Krauss JK, Loher TJ, Pohle T, et al. Pallidal deep brain stimulation in patients with cervical dystonia and severe cervical dyskinesias with cervical myelopathy. J Neurol Neurosurg Psychiatry 2002;72: 249.
164. Hung SW, Hamani C, Lozano AM, et al. Long-term outcome of bilateral pallidal deep brain stimulation for primary cervical dystonia. Neurology 2007;68:457.
165. Moro E, Piboolnurak P, Arenovich T, et al. Pallidal stimulation in cervical dystonia: Clinical implications of acute

changes in stimulation parameters. Eur J Neurol 2009 Jan 15 [Epub ahead of print].
166. Ostrem J, Marks, W, Voltz M, et al. Pallidal deep brain stimulation in patients with cranial-cervical dystonia (Meige syndrome). Mov Disord 2007;13:1885.
167. Berman B, Starr P, Marks W, et al. Induction of bradykinesia with pallidal deep brain stimulation in patients with cranial-cervical dystonia. Stereotact Funct Neurosurg 2009;87:37.
168. Wohrle JC, Weigel R, Grips E, et al. Risperidone-responsive segmental dystonia and pallidal deep brain stimulation. Neurology 2003;61:546.
169. Trottenberg T, Paul G, Meissner W, et al. Pallidal and thalamic neurostimulation in severe tardive dystonia. J Neurol Neurosurg Psychiatry 2001;70:557.
170. Sako W, Goto S, Shimazu H, et al. Bilateral deep brain stimulation of the globus pallidus internus in tardive dystonia. Mov Disord 2008;23:1929.
171. Pretto TE, Dalvi A, Kang UJ, et al. A prospective blinded evaluation of deep brain stimulation for the treatment of secondary dystonia and primary torticollis syndromes. J Neurosurg 2009;109:405.
172. Mikati MA, Yehya A, Darwish H, et al. Deep brain stimulation as a mode of treatment of early onset pantothenate kinase-associated neurodegeneration. Eur J Paediatr Neurol 2009;13:61.
173. Krause M, Fogel W, Tronnier V, et al. Long-term benefit to pallidal deep brain stimulation in a case of dystonia secondary to pantothenate kinase-associated neurodegeneration.Mov Disord 2006;21:2255.
174. Castelnau P, Cif L, Valente EM, et al. Pallidal stimulation improves pantothenate kinase-associated neurodegeneration. Ann Neurol 2005;57:738.
175. Evidente VG, Lyons MK, Wheeler M, et al. First case of X-linked dystonia-parkinsonism ("Lubag") to demonstrate a response to bilateral pallidal stimulation. Mov Disord 2007;22:1790.
176. Trottenberg T, Meissner W, Arnold G, et al. Neurostimulation of the ventral intermediate thalamic nucleus in inherited myoclonus-dystonia syndrome. Mov Disord 2001;16:769.
177. Fukaya C, Katayama Y, Kano T, et al. Thalamic deep brain stimulation for writer's cramp. J Neurosurg 2007;107:977.
178. Mehrkens JH, Bötzel K, Steude U, et al. Long-term efficacy and safety of chronic pallidus internnus stimulation in different types of primary dystonia. Stereotact Funct Neurosurg 2009;87:8.
179. Loher TJ, Capelle HH, Laelin-Lang A, et al. Deep brain stimulation for dystonia: Outcome at a long-term follow up. J Neurol 2008;255:881.
180. Novak KE, Nenonene EK, Bernstein LP, et al. Successful bilateral subthalamic nucleus stimulation for segmental dystonia after unilateral pallidotomy. Stereotact Funct Neurosurg 2008;86:80.
181. Kleiner-Fisman G, Liang GS, Moberg PJ, et al. Subthalamic nucleus deep brain stimulation for severe idiopathic dystonia: Impact on severity, neuropsychological status, and quality of life. J Neurosurg 2007;107:29.
182. Sun B, Chen S, Zhan S, et al. Subthalamic nucleus stimulation for primary dystonia and tardive dystonia. Acta Neurochir Suppl 2007;97:207.
183. Jankovic J, Penn AS. Severe dystonia and myoglobinuria. Neurology 1982;32:1195.
184. Manji H, Howard RS, Miller DH, et al. Status dystonicus: The syndrome and its management. Brain 1998;121:243.
185. Blasi J, Chapman E, Link E, et al. Botulinum neurotoxin A selectively cleaves the synaptic protein SNAP-25. Nature 1993;365:104.
186. Dong M, Yeh F, Tepp W, et al. SV2 is the protein receptor for botulinum neurotoxin A. Science 2006;312:592.
187. Mahrhold S, Rummel A, Bigalke H, et al. The synaptic vesicle protein 2C mediates the uptake of botulinum neurotoxin A into phrenic nerves. FEBS Lett 2006; 580:2011.
188. Dong M, Richards D, Goodnough M, et al. Synaptogamin I and II meciate entry of botulinum neurotoxin B into cells. J Cell Biol 2003;162:1293.
189. Rummel A, Eichner T, Weil T, et al. Identification of the protein receptor binding site of botulinum neurotoxins B and G proves the double-receptor concept. Proc Natl Acad Sci U S A 2007;104:359.
190. Blasi J. Chapman E, Yamasaki S, et al. Botulinum neurotoxin C1 blocks neurotransmitter release by means of cleaving HPC-A/syntaxin. EMBO J 1993;12:4821.
191. Schiavo G, Rossetto O, Catsicas S, et al. Identification of the nerve terminal targets of botulinum neurotoxin serotypes A,D, and E. J Biol Chem 1993;268:23784.
192. Rummel A, Karnath T, Henke T, et al.. Synaptogamins I and II act as nerve cell receptors for botulinum neurotoxin G. J Biol Chem 2004;279:30865.

CHAPTER 31

Symptomatic Dystonias

J.L. Lopez-Sendon, S. Cantarero, C. Tabernero, A.V. Vázquez, and J.G. de Yébenes

▶ DEFINITION OF SECONDARY OR SYMPTOMATIC DYSTONIA

The concept of symptomatic or secondary dystonia, as opposed to primary or idiopathic dystonia, emerged in the medical literature as a class of dystonias of known etiology. Perinatal brain injury was the most representative cause of symptomatic dystonia. More recently, different focal brain lesions, neurodegenerations, metabolic disorders of the nervous system, and drugs and chemicals have been recognized as causes of dystonia.

As opposed to primary dystonia, secondary dystonia is considered to be "often accompanied by other neurological deficits,"[1,2] to "begin suddenly at rest and occur at rest from the onset,"[3] and to be associated with different known hereditary and environmental causes.[4] (Table 31–1) These differential criteria are relative since there is a great clinical diversity of secondary dystonias. This chapter discusses the dystonic syndromes secondary to focal, degenerative, metabolic, or chemical insult to the nervous system as well as the pseudodystonias of organic and psychogenic origin. The main clinical characteristics of secondary dystonia, as well as clues for the differential diagnosis, are summarized in Tables 31–2 and 31–3.

▶ SYMPTOMATIC DYSTONIA RELATED TO FOCAL BRAIN LESIONS

In spite of recent improvements in prenatal care and delivery throughout the world, the most frequent cause of dystonia secondary to focal brain lesions is cerebral palsy (Fig. 31–1).[5,6] With modern neuroimaging techniques it is not uncommon to find focal brain lesions, frequently perinatal vascular injury, in patients with dystonia, occasionally unaware of perinatal brain damage. Focal brain lesions are responsible for the great majority of cases of hemidystonia.[7-16]

▶ TABLE 31–1. ETIOLOGIC CLASSIFICATION OF SECONDARY DYSTONIA

Secondary Dystonias
A. Caused by focal brain lesions
B. Associated with degeneration of the central nervous system
C. Resulting from metabolic disorders of the central nervous system
D. Produced by drugs and chemicals

▶ RELEVANT BRAIN STRUCTURES INVOLVED IN DYSTONIA

Identification of the brain structures involved in dystonia is based on neuroimaging and pathology.[7] Magnetic resonance imaging (MRI) and positron emission tomography (PET) are more sensitive than computed tomography (CT). Three regions are most often involved: the basal ganglia, thalamus, and brain stem.[7] Focal dystonia has been also rarely described in patients with lesions of the parietal cortex,[8,9] and the cerebellum.[10]

The role of basal ganglia damage in dystonia is firmly established. Putaminal lesions are the most frequent cause of hemidystonia (Fig. 31–2).[7,11–13] Even some patients with idiopathic dystonia have a T_2 signal alteration in the putamen in high-field MRI.[14] The caudate nucleus is occasionally involved in limb dystonia. Pallidal lesions with gliosis due to kernicterus cause symptomatic dystonia in childhood. Thalamic lesions are also a cause of secondary dystonia. Limb dystonia may appear after stereotaxic thalamotomy for the treatment of tremor,[15] and dystonia.[16] In summary, symptomatic dystonia due to focal brain lesions suggests that the structural basis of dystonia lies in the basal ganglia-thalamocortical motor circuit; this has led to the current concept of dystonia as a dysfunction of this loop.

Evidence of brain stem lesions inducing dystonia (i.e., cranial dystonia) is supported by neuroimaging, neurophysiological studies, and clinical physiopathological associations.[17–24] Neuropathological results are not consistent.[25–31] Although it has not yet been possible to localize accurately a responsible nucleus or neuronal circuit, brain stem projections to and from the basal ganglia are most probably involved.

▶ **TABLE 31–2. DIFFERENTIAL DIAGNOSIS OF SYMPTOMATIC DYSTONIAS**

Disease	Inheritance	Type of Dystonia	Age at Onset	Clinical Findings	Neuroimaging	Diagnosis
Focal brain lesions	Sporadic	Hemidystonia, focal	Children, young adults	Corticospinal and brain stem signs	Focal lesion	Clinical/MRI
PD	Mostly sporadic	Focal	Adults	Tremor, ARS	Normal (nigral T_2 shortening)	Clinical
PSP	Mostly sporadic	Axial	Mature senile	Gaze palsy, ARS	Midbrain tectal atrophy	Clinicopathological
CBD	Sporadic	Limb	Mature senile	Apraxia, myoclonus, alien limb	Asymmetric cerebral atrophy	Clinicopathological
MSA	Sporadic	Axial	Mature senile	ARS, autonomic, cerebellar	OPCA, T_2 putaminal hypointensity in SDS and SND	Pathology
Huntington's disease	AD	Generalized	Young adults	Chorea, dementia	Caudate and cortical atrophy	Genetic, IT_{15} CAG expansion
Neuroacanthocytosis	AR sporadic	Orolingual, generalized	Young adults	Chorea, amyotrophy, epilepsy	Caudate atrophy	Acanthocytes
Wilson's disease	AR	Generalized	Children, young adults	Tremor, psychiatric, dysarthria	Putaminal, thalamic dentate, brain stem, T_2 high signal	K-F rings, Cu^{2+} levels, ceruloplasmin gene defects of chromosome 13
Neurodegeneration with brain iron accumulation	AR	Multifocal, generalized	Children, young adults	Corticospinal, dementia	Pallidal T_2 hypointensity ("eye of the tiger" sign)	Pathology
Fahr's syndrome	AD/AR/ sporadic	Generalized hemidystonia	Adults	ARS, corticospinal, ataxia, dementia	Basal ganglia striking calcifications	Imaging (exclusion diagnosis)
Ataxia telangiectasia	AR	Generalized	Children	Ataxia, neuropathy	Cerebellar atrophy	Clinical, low levels IgA
Machado-Joseph	AD	Multifocal, generalized	Children, young adults	Ataxia, ophthalmoplegia, amyotrophy	Cerebellar atrophy	Genetic, CAG expansion 14q
Dentatorubro-pallidoluysian atrophy	AD	Generalized	Adults	Ataxia, dementia, myoclonus	Brain stem, cerebellum Alt signal	Genetic, CAG expansion 21p
Intraneuronal inclusion	Sporadic	Focal, generalized	Children, young adults	Corticospinal, ataxia, dementia		Pathology (rectal biopsy)
Rett syndrome	Sporadic (females)	Focal	Children	Autism, stereotypy, epilepsy	Brain atrophy	Clinical
GM1 gangliosidosis, type 3	AR	Generalized	Children, young adults	Ataxia, corticospinal (no dementing)	Basal ganglia lesions	β-D-galactosidase

GM2 gangliosidosis	AR	Generalized	Children, young adults	Corticospinal, epilepsy, blindness	T_2 high signal in the basal ganglia, severe atrophy	Hexosaminidase
Niemann-Pick type C	AR	Generalized	Children	Dementia, gaze palsy, epilepsy		Defective cholesterol esterification/ sphingomyelinase
Metachromatic leukodystrophy	AR	Generalized	Children	Dementia, psychiatric symptoms	White matter, diffuse confluent T_2 high signal	Aryl sulfatase A
Ceroid lipofuscinosis/ Kufs disease	AR	Focal (cranial) hemidystonia	Children, young adults	Dementia, ataxia, epilepsy	T_2 low signal in thalami and striata	Pathology (rectal biopsy)
Leigh's syndrome	AR	Generalized	Children	Hypotonia, ataxia, optic atrophy	Striatal lucencies (T_2 basal ganglia hyperintensities)	Pyruvic acid and alanine levels, mtDNA mutations, cytochrome *c* oxidase activity
Glutaric aciduria I	AR	Generalized	Children	Encephalopathic crisis, mental retardation	Frontotemporal atrophy, enlarged Sylvian fissures	Glutaric acid in urine, glutaryl-CoA dehydrogenase
Methylmalonic aciduria	AR	Generalized	Children	Acute encephalopathy	Pallidal T_2 hyperintensity	Chromatography of organic acids, methylmalonyl-CoA mutase
Homocystinuria	AR	Generalized	Children	Focal deficits, mental retardation	Focal ischemic lesions, sinus thrombosis	AA chromatography
Hartnup's disease	AR	Generalized, paroxysmal	Children	Mental retardation, recurrent ataxia, and behavioral alterations	White matter T_2 hyperintensity	AA chromatography
Lesch-Nyhan syndrome	X-linked	Generalized	Children	Mental retardation, self-mutilation		Hypoxanthine-guanine phosphoribosyl transferase

Abbreviations: AA, amino acid; AD, autosomal-dominant inheritance; AR, autosomal-recessive inheritance; ARS, akinetic-rigid syndrome; CBD, corticobasal degeneration; K-F rings, Kayser–Fleisher rings; MRI, magnetic resonance imaging; mtDNA, mitochondrial DNA OPCA, olivopontocerebellar atrophy; SDS, Shy-Drager syndrome; SND, Striatonigral degeneration.

▶ TABLE 31–3. DIAGNOSTIC CLUES TO SECONDARY DYSTONIA

Clinical Clues in the Most Common Symptomatic Dystonias	Most Likely Clinical Diagnosis
I. Dystonia in Children	
A. Dystonia associated with focal neurological signs and perinatal brain injury, ectopia lentis, skeletal deformities, mental retardation	Dystonic cerebral palsy, homocystinuria
B. Dystonia after acute encephalopathy associated with macrocephaly, tetraparesis, dysphagia, dysarthria, optic atrophy, hypotonia, tetraparesis, ataxia, dysphagia, dysarthria	Glutaric aciduria, methylmalonic aciduria, Leigh's syndrome
C. Acute dystonia, without any other neurological symptoms	Intake of neuroleptics, antiemetics, catecholamine releasers, antiepileptics, and other drugs and chemicals
D. Fixed congenital focal dystonia	Musculoskeletal deformities
E. Dystonia associated with other neurological deficits, spinocerebellar deficits, tetraparesis, blindness, and seizures	GM1 gangliosidosis
F. Dystonia associated with spasticity, exaggerated startle reaction and seizures, skeletal deformities, mental retardation associated with automutilation, urinary stones, and hyperuricemia	GM2 gangliosidosis, Niemann–Pick disease, Lesch–Nyhan syndrome
II. Dystonia in Adolescents and Adults	
A. Dystonia associated with akinetic-rigid syndromes, foot dystonia, axial dystonia mostly in extension, gaze palsy, dysphagia, dysarthria, gait disturbance, anterocollis, poor response to L-dopa, autonomic disturbances, asymmetric hand dystonia with myoclonus, generalized dystonia with akinetic-rigid syndrome in children and young adults	PD, PSP MSA, CBD, mitochondrial, encephalopathy
B. Dystonia associated with chorea and oromandibular dystonia	Neuroacanthocytosis
C. Dystonia associated with ataxia, Autosomal-dominant disease with ataxia, dementia, dysarthria, ophthalmoplegia, dystonia and akinetic-rigid syndromes, rhythmic dystonia, and hemidystonia	Machado–Joseph disease, MSA, drug-induced, focal putaminal lesions
Clues from MRI Findings	**Most likely Clinical Diagnosis**
A. Pattern of atrophy	
Frontotemporal atrophy with Sylvian enlargement, cerebellar atrophy, caudate atrophy, midbrain atrophy, asymmetric frontoparietal atrophy	Glutaric aciduria, MSA, Machado–Joseph, ataxia telangiectasia, HD, neuroacanthocytosis, PSP, CBD
B. T_2 high-intensity signal	
1. Putaminal	Focal vascular lesion, WD, Leigh's disease, GM2 gangliosidosis, cyanide
2. Pallidal	Methylmalonic aciduria, carbon monoxide, methyl alcohol
3. White matter	Metachromatic leukodystrophy, homocystinuria, Hartnup's disease
C. Low-intensity signal	
1. Putaminal	MSA, Kufs' disease, calcification of the basal ganglia
2. Pallidal	Neurodegeneration with brain iron accumulation

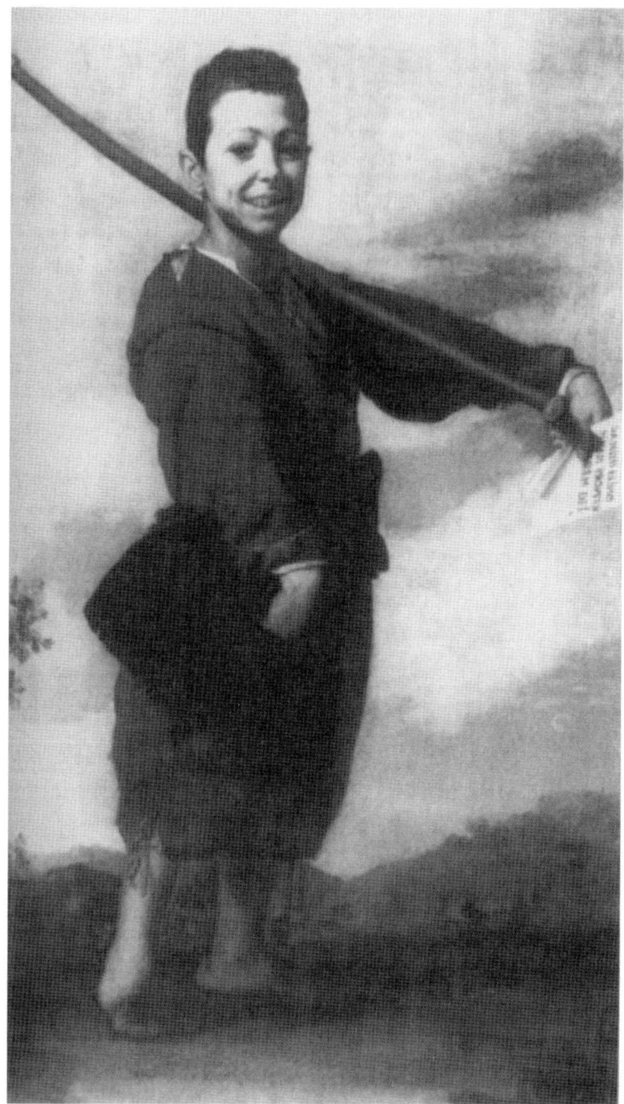

Figure 31–1. The limp child. Hemidystonia in cerebral palsy, documented by J. Ribera (1591–1652) in 1642. (The Louvre, Paris)

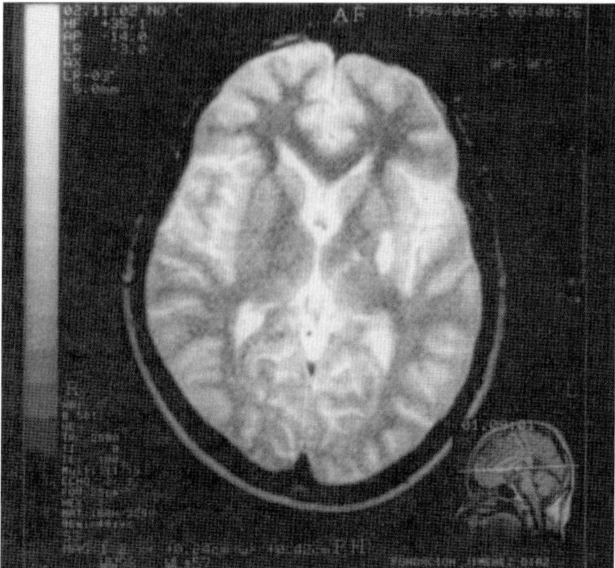

Figure 31–2. MRI scan showing left perinatal putaminal hemorrhage in a patient with right hemiparesis and right hemidystonia.

Recent neurophysiological and neuropharmacological studies have suggested that, without downplaying the protagonistic role of the basal ganglia, other brain regions such as the cerebellum and the cerebral cortex play a role in dystonia.[32–34] In focal hand dystonia, it has been observed a reduced cortical inhibition.[41] In animal models of dystonia activation of the cerebellum or lesion of the striatum has been found to aggravate dystonia.[42,43]

TYPE OF BRAIN LESION

Dystonia may appear after almost any properly placed focal lesion (i.e., in the basal ganglia, thalamus, or brain stem) (Table 31–4), although the most common cause of dystonia of focal origin is vascular injury. Diffuse brain injuries (anoxia, kernicterus, hydrocephalus, etc.) may produce a selective involvement of the structures mentioned earlier (Fig. 31–3) Focal lesions (vascular malformation, tumor) located away from these regions (basal ganglia, thalami, brain stem) may produce dystonia by indirect mechanisms, most probably related to compression or steal phenomena.[8,9] Demyelinating lesions inducing dystonia are most often located at the brain stem level. Individual features, including age and genetic susceptibility, are distinctly relevant for the different phenotypic expression of similar lesions.[8,12] Secondary dystonia due to basal ganglia and thalamic injuries is much more frequent when the insult takes place in the perinatal period and earlier years of life than in adulthood (Fig. 31–4).[2,35–39] Brain injury in young children is associated with longer latency to onset of subsequent movement disorder, a greater tendency to development of generalized dystonia, and a greater probability of altered handedness.[40] An increased vulnerability of the striatum during development, related to different arrangement of matrix/striosomes or to a high level of excitatory neurotransmission at this stage, could be a possible explanation. Age-related differences reflect different grades of neuronal plasticity and different compensatory potential of particular neuronal circuits. The role of genetic susceptibility is well documented in drug-induced dystonia, but unknown in dystonia induced by focal lesions.

▶ TABLE 31–4. SYMPTOMATIC DYSTONIA RESULTING FROM FOCAL LESIONS OF THE NERVOUS SYSTEM

A. Focal lesion of the basal ganglia, thalamus, and brain stem
   1. Vascular
      a. Infarction
      b. Hemorrhage
      c. Vascular malformation
      d. Vasculitis (systemic lupus erythematosus, primary antiphospholipid syndrome, Behçet's syndrome, Sjögren syndrome, isolated angiitis of the central nervous system)
      e. Migraine
   2. Head trauma
   3. Tumor and cysts: astrocytoma, lymphoma, glioma, porencephalic cyst, subarachnoid cyst, metastasis
   4. Infection: HIV and related infections, tuberculosis, viral
   5. Multiple sclerosis
   6. Syringomyelia, cerebellar ectopia

B. Diffuse lesions with prominent damage of the basal ganglia, thalamus, or brain stem
   1. Anoxia and energy failure: perinatal asphyxia, cardiac arrest, toxins
   2. Kernicterus
   3. Hydrocephalus
   4. Metabolic disorders: hyponatremia, hypernatremia, dehydration, hypoparathyroidism, hypoglycemia
   5. Hepatocerebral degeneration
   6. Paraneoplastic syndrome
   7. Hemiparkinsonism–hemiatrophy syndrome

C. Superficial lesions, with unclear effects on the basal ganglia, thalamus or brain stem
   1. Subdural hematoma
   2. Pachygyria

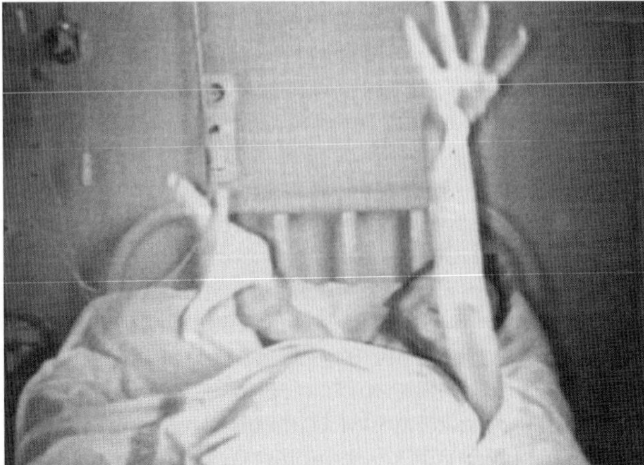

Figure 32–3. Generalized dystonia in a patient with AIDS and cerebral toxoplasmosis.

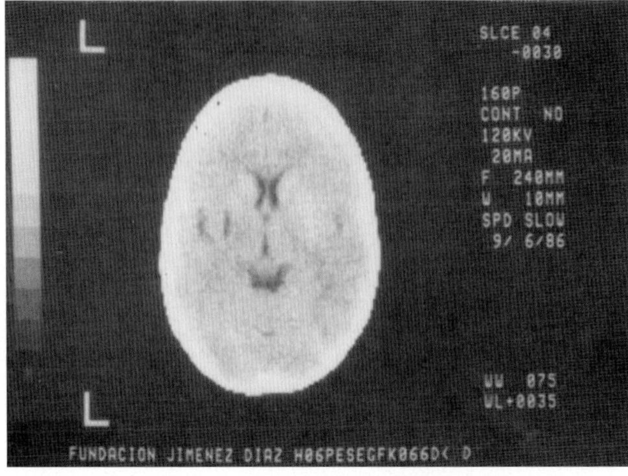

Figure 31–4. CT scan showing right putaminal infarction in an 8-year-old girl with acute lymphocytic leukemia and left hemidystonia.

▶ ANATOMOCLINICAL CORRELATION

There is a certain correlation between the topographic localization of the lesion and the pattern of dystonia:

- Putaminal lesion: hemidystonia or limb dystonia
- Thalamic lesion: hand dystonia
- Brain stem lesion: blepharospasm, Meige's syndrome

However, in some cases, it is difficult to establish which the most relevant lesion is.[41] Cranial dystonia with putaminal lesions,[28,42,43] cranial dystonia and hemidystonia with thalamic lesions,[21,44] and oromandibular dystonia with lesion in head of caudate nucleus are some of the exceptions to this oversimplified scheme. Unilateral diencephalic or brain stem lesions produce bilateral symmetric blepharospasm,[21] although a case of a left rostral diencephalic-brain stem lesion with ipsilateral blepharospasm and contralateral hemidystonia has been reported.[24]

▶ DELAYED ONSET AND INDEPENDENT PROGRESSION

Some of the most characteristic and intriguing features of dystonia secondary to focal brain lesions are the time delay from injury to the appearance of the movement disorder and its posterior independent progression.

It is unlikely that delayed onset is related to the recovery of an associated corticospinal tract lesion[45] since in many cases dystonia appears without previous hemiparesis. Three alternative physiopathological mechanisms—denervation hypersensitivity,[17] aberrant sprouting of the damaged neurons,[42,46] and secondary retrograde degeneration[47]—have been proposed.

DYSTONIA RELATED TO PERIPHERAL INJURY

The relationship between peripheral trauma and dystonia is quite controversial.[48,49] In genetically predisposed individuals (i.e., asymptomatic carriers of the gene for idiopathic torsion dystonia), peripheral trauma may trigger the onset of the dystonia.[50–52] However, it is not proved that peripheral injury induces dystonia through alteration of the sensory input to the central nervous system (CNS) or changes of the central processing. Some peculiarities of peripherally induced dystonia[53–58] set it apart from other symptomatic dystonias:

- Short latency of onset (days)
- Present at rest from the start and persists during sleep
- No "geste antagonistique"
- No overflow
- Fixed postures with limitation of range of motion
- Little response to anticholinergics or botulinum toxin
- Associated causalgia and reflex sympathetic dystrophy
- Associated hypertrophy of individual muscles[58]

Direct nerve injury or surgery, entrapment neuropathies, and electrical injury have been related to the onset of dystonia. Usually, the same region that receives the injury develops the dystonia;[67] hence, local ocular disease is associated to blepharospasm, dental procedures to oromandibular dystonia,[60] whiplash and other neck injuries to cervical dystonia, limb injury to limb dystonia, and posttraumatic abnormal postures and muscle hypertrophy in shoulder after local minor injury.[59] In some cases, occupational cramps may be related to repetitive microtraumatisms; hence, they could be considered as a kind of peripherally induced dystonia. The role of peripheral trauma in dystonia may be underlined by the frequency of occupational dystonia in certain professionals (laryngeal dystonia in teachers, hand dystonia in string or piano players, oromandibular dystonia in wind players). In most cases, these professionals do not record important trauma but only excessive use of the muscles involved in the dystonic phenomenon. It has been recently reported that in some cases of occupational dystonia there is an abnormal lack of physiological inhibition of somatotosensory-evoked potentials in the parietal cortex.[60] It has also been shown that prolonged immobilization of the dystonic extremity produces persistent improvement in occupational dystonia.[61] These data may support the hypothesis of excessive facilitation of muscle contraction in dystonia triggered by lack of inhibition or plasticity of neuronal circuits in response to trauma or overuse of certain muscles but there is still controversy on this topic.[62]

DYSTONIA IN NEURODEGENERATIVE DISORDERS

Dystonia is a common symptom of neurodegenerative disorders, especially those involving the basal ganglia. In most of these diseases, dystonia is associated with other manifestations of the clinical picture. However, in some instances, dystonia may be the unique, most relevant, or first clinical symptom of the neurodegenerative disorder and, therefore, it may be misdiagnosed as idiopathic torsion dystonia.

▶ DYSTONIA IN AKINETIC-RIGID SYNDROMES

PARKINSON'S DISEASE (PD)

Three points deserve discussion regarding dystonia and PD: (1) the presence of dystonia in untreated PD, (2) the evidence of dystonia and parkinsonism as different phenotypic expressions of the same disorders, and (3) the appearance of dystonia as a complication of therapy in PD.

Dystonia is not uncommon in untreated PD, especially in patients with early onset of clinical symptoms. Adult-onset foot dystonia should raise the possibility of PD.[63,64] The foot is often deviated in equinovarus, with 2nd to 5th toes flexed and the great toe dorsiflexed (the so-called striatal toe); this is a typical action dystonia or kinesogenic dystonia, and the deviation worsens with walking (see Chapter 13). Less frequently, dystonia occurs in the upper extremity in untreated patients with PD, and it is most frequently characterized by cubital deviation, metacarpophalangeal flexion, proximal interphalangeal extension, and distal interphalangeal extension. There are some isolated clinical reports of untreated patients suffering blepharospasm, oromandibular dystonia, hemidystonia, writer's cramp, and cervical dystonia,[65,66] and there is a neuropathologically confirmed case of PD with Meige's syndrome.[67] If we consider isolated scoliosis as a symptom of dystonia, then this disorder would be even more frequent in patients with PD.[68] Some authors consider anismus, which is a result of abnormal puborectalis muscle contraction, as a form of dystonia[69] common in PD.

Dystonia and parkinsonism coexist as different clinical manifestations of the same disease in a number of hereditary conditions, including autosomal-dominant familial parkinsonism related to synuclein mutations,[70] L-dopa-responsive dystonia,[71,72] juvenile parkinsonism,[73,74] early-onset parkinsonism with gliosis of the substantia nigra,[75] and other conditions.

In addition, dystonia occurs in patients under treatment for PD as a complication of the treatment. Off-period dystonia occurs more frequently in the morning (early-morning dystonia), after the nocturnal period of L-dopa deprivation, or at moments when the patient is akinetic in the interval between two doses of medication (off-period dystonia). Dystonia also occurs as a side effect of L-dopa treatment at times when the antiparkinsonian effect is present. Peak-effect dyskinesia and, more frequently, biphasic dyskinesia are occasionally characterized by repetitive dystonia of the extremities (see Chapter 14). Dystonia has also been reported in patients with PD treated with deep brain stimulation (DBS).[76]

PROGRESSIVE SUPRANUCLEAR PALSY (PSP)

Oculofaciocervical dystonia[77] is frequent in PSP, which is characterized by akinetic-rigid syndrome, supranuclear gaze palsy, early gait problems, dysphagia, dysarthria, and a variable disturbance of cognitive function, most frequently consistent with apathy and frontal lobe dysfunction. Familial PSP has been described,[78,79] but the gene that causes it is unknown since the PSP-like families already described and related to mutations of tau gene in chromosome 17[80] are better classified as familial frontotemporal dementia with parkinsonism. Axial dystonia is characterized by hyperextended neck and trunk. Facial expression[81] is related to tonic dystonic contraction of frontal and oromandibular muscles, which, together with the fixed eyes, make the patients exhibit "stare gaze." Facial dystonia is often induced by speech. Blepharospasm, often associated with eyelid apraxia, has been described in PSP.[82] Upper limb dystonia, although less typical in PSP, was present in some autopsy-proven cases,[77,80,83–87] as well as in another pathologically confirmed patient from our group[78] (see Chapter 19).

CORTICOBASAL DEGENERATION (CBD)

Since the original report by Rebeiz and colleagues,[88] increasing numbers of patients are being described. The disorder characteristically combines an asymmetric akinetic-rigid syndrome, dystonia, and myoclonus with focal cortical dysfunction. The pathological examination discloses frontoparietal and basal ganglia asymmetrical atrophy, and swollen achromatic neurons (see Chapter 45).

Dystonia was present in 83 % of 36 patients suspected of having CBD, after a mean evolution of 5.2 years[89] and in 59 % of 66 patients in another larger series with a shorter follow up.[90] In CBD, contrary to PSP, dystonia is fairly asymmetric and involves mainly the most affected arm, leading to an adducted and flexed posture with clawed fingers.

MULTIPLE-SYSTEM ATROPHY (MSA)

MSA is characterized by a varied combination of clinical symptoms related to the degeneration of several neuronal systems, including the nigrostriatal pathway, striatum, cerebellum, autonomic nervous system. It can be divided in two categories depending on the predominant clinical feature: MSA with predominant parkinsonism (MSA-P) and MSA with predominant cerebellar ataxia (MSA-C). Autonomic dysfunction should be present to meet the diagnostic criteria of MSA[91]

The frequency of dystonia in MSA is variable. Quinn suggests that around 50% of his patients with MSA, as confirmed by pathology, had anterocollis.[69] Berciano[92] reported the presence of "involuntary movements" in 40% of patients with familial MSA-C (formerly OPCA) and 18% with sporadic MSA-C. Description of these involuntary movements lacks precise details for most of these patients. Some of them had chorea, probably related to lesions of the subthalamic nucleus; others, including the initial patient described by Menzel,[93] had torticollis. In 1 case, this torticollis was attributed to atrophy of the vestibuloreticular system.[94] A large clinicopathological study of more than 200 cases of pathology proven MSA has confirmed the presence of dystonia in at least 12 % of patients with MSA. The most common localization was anterocollis.[95]

▶ DYSTONIA IN CHOREIC SYNDROMES

HUNTINGTON'S DISEASE (HD)

Dystonia is a frequent clinical symptom in (HD). In patients with late-onset and rapid chorea, dystonia occurs most often as a complication of treatment with neuroleptics. In juvenile patients, hypokinesia, rigidity, hypomimia, bradykinesia, and dystonia are the motor signs.[96] In many patients with classical forms, initial rapid chorea disappears with the progression of the illness and is substituted for or accompanied by dystonia. In an epidemiological study, dystonia occurred in 95% of patients and was directly related to the disease progression and antidopaminergic drugs. In 12% of 127 adult-onset HD patients, dystonia was the main finding, and it appeared mainly in those with younger age of onset (see Chapter 36).

▶ OTHER HUNTINGTON-LIKE DISORDERS

Several diseases resemble HD but have no alteration of the Huntingtin gene and are collectively named as HD-like I to IV.[97] In so-called Huntington disease-like 3 (HDL-3), an autosomal-recessive early-onset disease develops in the first decade, with dystonia as a feature.[98,99]

A dominantly inherited disease due to mutations of the gene encoding the ferritin light polypeptide produces choreoathetosis, dystonia, spasticity, and rigidity, with onset between ages of 40 and 55. Cavitation of basal ganglia is found on MRI.[100]

Benign hereditary chorea is an autosomal-dominant disorder with chorea and dystonia in some cases not associated with intellectual deterioration.[101] It has been mapped to chromosome 14q.[102] The responsible gene has been identified as the thyroid transcription factor 1.[103]

▶ NEUROACANTHOCYTOSIS

Three neurological disorders associate with acanthocytosis: hypobetalipoproteinemia or Basen–Kornzweig disease, McLeod syndrome, and choreoacanthocytosis.

Hypobetalipoproteinemia is mainly a spinocerebellar syndrome associated with peripheral neuropathy and retinitis pigmentosa.

McLeod syndrome is usually considered a red blood cell disorder in which X chromosome mutations cause a dysfunction of an erythrocyte membrane protein Kx. It associates to a benign myopathy. However, the phenotype can be similar to choreoacanthocytosis, including dystonia. Caudate atrophy can be found in late disease, but early presymptomatic hypometabolism in caudate nucleus has been found.[104] The clinical manifestations of neuroacanthocytosis usually start in the third decade as orobuccolinguofacial hyperkinesia, lip-smacking, vocalizations, and even orolingual action dystonia, leading to lip and tongue automutilation. Thereafter, a generalized chorea develops, often a mixture of chorea and dystonia. In 30% of patients, there is no cognitive deterioration. About one-half of patients suffer epileptic seizures. Most of them present a motor polyneuropathy with distal amyotrophy and pes cavus. The clinical diagnosis is confirmed by the finding of acanthocytes, usually more than 20% of red blood cells, in fresh or saline-incubated blood smears. The neuropathology shows atrophy of the basal ganglia, maximal in caudate nucleus and preferentially affecting small neurons.[105] Neuronal loss also involves the anterior horn of the spinal cord in some cases. The muscle shows denervation, and peripheral nerve shows axonal degeneration with demyelination.

Kito and colleagues[106] described increased norepinephrine in the cerebrospinal fluid and low urinary excretion of dihydroxyphenylacetic acid. De Yebenes and colleagues[107,108] found moderately decreased striatal levels of dopamine, as well as a great elevation of norepinephrine levels, suggesting that dystonia may be related to disequilibrium of dopamine/norepinephrine neurotransmission in the basal ganglia. Choreoacanthocytosis is inherited in most cases as an autosomal-recessive complex movement disorder. Linkage has been found to chromosome 9q21.[109] The gene responsible for this disease has been recently identified, independently, by two groups;[110,111] the protein, called chorein, is considered to play a key role in protein sorting.

▶ DENTATORUBROPALLIDOLUYSIAN ATROPHY

In this disease, there is degeneration of cerebellar efferent (dentatorubral) and pallidoluysian systems. It is an unusual disease, initially described in Europe by Titica and Van Bogaert in 1946,[112] but most of the actual cases are from Japan. The genetic defect has been located on chromosome 12p as an expansion of the trinucleotide CAG.[113] Iizuka[114] described three clinical types: an ataxo-choreoathetoid, a pseudo-Huntington, and a third type combining myoclonic epilepsy with ataxia. Now that genetic diagnosis is possible, two main clinical groups have been described: adult-onset (at 20 years or older) with ataxia, choreoathetosis, and dementia; and juvenile-onset (before 20 years), with a progressive myoclonic epilepsy added to the previous symptoms.[115] As in HD, paternal transmission correlates with larger expansions of the repeat and earlier presentation.[116] Dystonia has been described, but not as an isolated or prominent manifestation.

▶ DYSTONIA IN BASAL GANGLIA DISORDERS

WILSON'S DISEASE (WD)

This is an autosomal-recessive systemic disease related to abnormal metabolism of copper with mutations of an ATPase, located on chromosome 13q; ATPase plays a very important role in the metabolism of copper, transferring copper ions from apoceruloplasmin to ceruloplasmin. Tissue damage is a result of copper accumulation. In 217 patients reviewed by Walshe,[117] 43% started with hepatic disease and 42% with CNS involvement, including 2 patients with initial psychiatric symptoms. In the patients with neurological onset, tremor in the upper extremities, dysarthria, dystonia, and athetosis were, in that order, the most frequent presenting manifestations. Dystonia also appears during the evolution of the disease, producing bizarre posturing that may affect the four limbs and the trunk (Fig. 31–5). In a clinicoradiological correlation study of 16 symptomatic patients with WD, 11 of them, presenting with dystonia, had putaminal lesions in MRI.[118] When considering the differential diagnosis of a patient with dystonia, it is of prime importance to consider and screen for WD, because it is a treatable condition in which the reversibility of the clinical symptoms

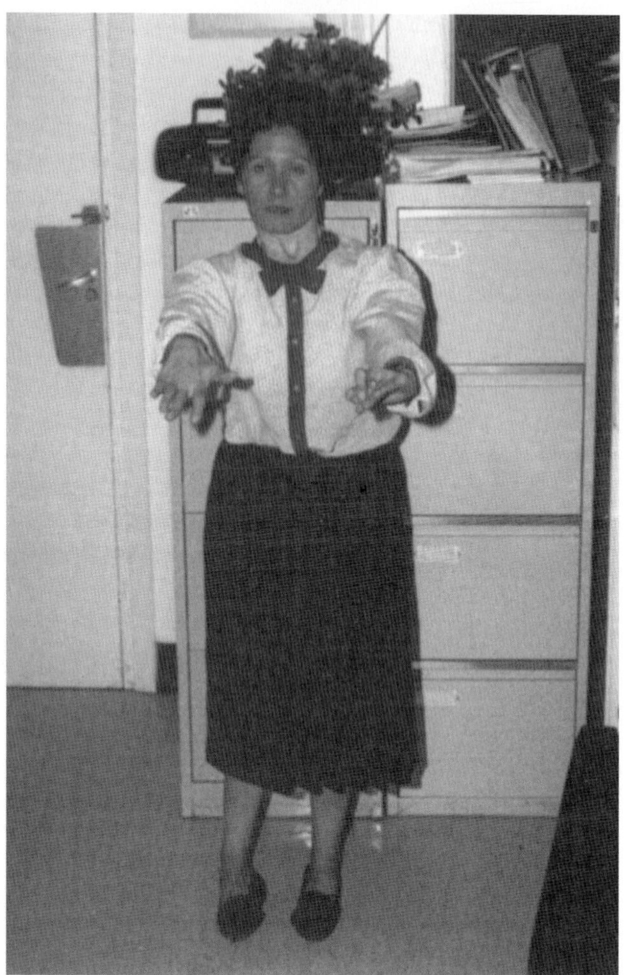

Figure 31–5. Generalized dystonia in Wilson's disease.

may depend on when definitive therapy is initiated (see also Chapter 46).

▶ DISORDERS OF IRON METABOLISM IN BRAIN: NEURODEGENERATION WITH BRAIN IRON ACCUMULATION (NBIA) AND NEUROFERRITINOPATHY

Seitelberger classified the primary neuroaxonal dystrophies, including NBIA (formerly called Hallevorden–Spatz disease), infantile neuroaxonal dystrophy (INAD), late infantile and juvenile neuroaxonal dystrophy, and neuroaxonal leukodystrophy. The pathological marker in this group of related disorders is neuroaxonal dystrophy or axonal spheroid. In INAD, the clinical symptoms develop at the end of the first year or during the second year of life and are characterized by psychomotor retardation, spasticity and rigidity, loss of vision and hearing, autonomic signs, and death between 3 and 6 years of age. Dystonia may occur with the progression of the disease, especially in cases with long evolution.[119] Pathological involvement is widespread but is most prominent in the posterior spinal horns and the dorsal bulbomedullary nuclei, the pallidum, substantia nigra and other brain stem nuclei, and cerebellar cortex. There is an excess of ferric pigment. Gliosis and long-tract degeneration take place.

NBIA is an autosomal-recessive disorder related to a mutation in the pantothenate kinase 2 gene (PANK-2).[120] Neuropathology is characterized by iron deposition in the pallidum and substantia nigra, pars reticularis, and widespread axonal spheroid formation neuroaxonal dystrophy. Of 64 pathologically confirmed cases, 8 presented with dystonia, and 41 more suffered dystonia during evolution of the disease.[121] Generalized dystonia was the most frequent presentation, but it could appear as focal or segmental cranial and upper limb dystonia (Fig. 31–6). Dystonia may be associated with tics and other movement disorders in NBIA.[122,123] An isolated case of treatment of dystonia in NBIA with stereotactic pallidotomy has been described.[124]

Neuroferritinopathy is another form of neurodegeneration associated with brain iron accumulation, sometimes termed NBIA2. It is an autosomal dominant disorder related to mutation of the ferritin light chain. Its most important clinical features are characterized by

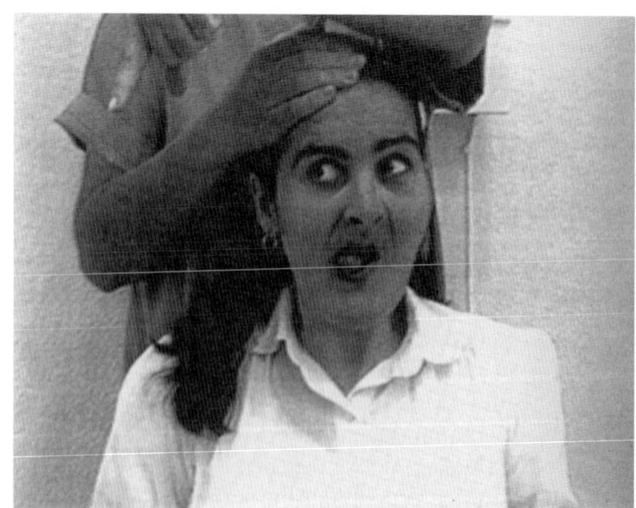

Figure 31–6. Orolinguomandibular dystonia in a patient with Hallervorden-Spatz disease and generalized dystonia related to two mutations, in combined heterozygosis, in exons 5 and 6 of the PANK2 gene, which produce the amino acid changes I391T and G411R, respectively, of the PANK2 protein.

adult onset generalized dystonia and choreoathetosis and, more rarely, parkinsonism.[125–130]

▶ CALCIFICATION OF THE BASAL GANGLIA (CBG)

CBG occurs in up to 30 sporadic and hereditary diseases, and is often associated with different movement disorders, including parkinsonism, chorea, and dystonia. Abnormal parathyroid function is frequently associated with CBG, but there are cases without any evidence of biochemical or humoral abnormalities of calcium and phosphorus metbolism. These idiopathic cases are often called Fahr's disease; this can be hereditary or sporadic and diagnosis is by exclusion. A long series of familial and sporadic cases found movement disorders the most frequent neurological manifestation of CBG: parkinsonism accounted for 57%, chorea 19%, tremor 8%, dystonia 8%, athetosis 5%, and orofacial dyskinesia 3%. This study found a relationship between volume of calcification and clinical status.[131] There are reports of familial dystonia as the main manifestation of this disease. The patients reported by Caraceni and colleagues[132] were two brothers with cranial dystonia or limb dystonia. Larsen and colleagues[133] reported a family with idiopathic CBG and autosomal-dominant segmental dystonia.

Two sporadic cases with isolated calcification of the globus pallidus have been described.[134] Both patients had cognitive dysfunction, amnesia state, perceptual distortions, complex visual hallucinations, and myoclonus. Patient 1 manifested depression, auditory hallucinations, anxiety, paranoia, and postural tremor; patient 2 manifested multifocal dystonia with dystonic tremor. These cases suggest specific involvement of the pallidal pathways in hallucinations, myoclonus, and dystonia.

In a family with CBG, a linkage to chromosome 14q and genetic anticipation have been found. Interestingly the proband started with writing tremor and hand dystonia.[135]

No specific therapy (aside from symptomatic) exists for Fahr's disease, but there is a single case reported that benefited from etidronate.[136]

▶ PROGRESSIVE PALLIDAL DEGENERATIONS

These rare diseases have been subdivided into four groups according to the pathological findings:[137] (1) "pure" pallidal atrophy, (2) "pure" pallidoluysian atrophy, (3) "extended" forms with nigral, striatal, or dentate nucleus involvement, including pallidoluysionigral atrophy, (4) combinations of (1) and (2), with thalamic, pyramidal, or spinal motor lesion.

Given the small number of cases, precise clinicopathological correlation has not been possible, but prominent generalized or focal dystonia, together with akinetic-rigid syndromes, is the most common clinical manifestation. Dystonia was described in patients with pure pallidal and pallidoluysian atrophies by Van Bogaert.[138] A patient reported by Wooten and colleagues[139] had progressive generalized dystonia, dysarthria, and supranuclear gaze palsy. Pathological examination disclosed a pure pallidoluysian atrophy; hence, the authors attributed the symptoms to damage of the indirect pathway and increased inhibition of internal pallidum.

▶ INTRANUCLEAR NEURONAL INCLUSION DISEASE

This is a rare disorder characterized by developmental delay and movement disorders, including dystonia and parkinsonism, with onset from 3 to 30 years of age, most frequently in childhood,[140] but also in adults.[141] The pathological marker is a round autofluorescent eosinophilic inclusion body found in neurons of different regions, more abundant in the basal ganglia but also involving other structures such as the motor neurons, autonomic system, and myenteric plexus. Ante-mortem diagnosis is possible by means of rectal biopsy.[142]

▶ RETT SYNDROME

Rett Syndrome is devastating progressive disorder observed in mostly in young girls. This disease characteristically combines psychomotor regression, loss of purposeful use of the hands and stereotypia, ataxia and apraxia of gait, and acquired microcephaly. Mutations in the X chromosome gene encoding methyl-CpG-binding protein 2 are the cause of Rett syndrome.[143] Phenotypical variability in females is explained by skewed X chromosome inactivation and by the type of mutations. It was previously considered that only females were affected, but there are a few affected males whose phenotype is more severe as in neonatal encephalopathy.[144]

Abnormal levels of 5-hydroxyindoleacetic acid and catecholamine metabolites are found in the cerebrospinal fluid. Dystonia is included among the diagnostic criteria.[145] Fitzgerald and colleagues[146] found that the presence of movement disorders in 32 patients with Rett syndrome was common, and increased with age. The disease usually evolves with age from hyperkinetic to hypokinetic patterns. Dystonia, most frequently crural, was present in 59% of patients. Bruxism was the most common movement disorder after gait abnormality and stereotyped movements of the hands. Oculogyric crises occurred in 63% of cases (see Chapter 25).

The presence of dystonia in Machado–Joseph disease is much more common than in other familial spinocerebellar degenerations.[158] This is attributed to the much more frequent involvement of subthalamopallidal pathways in Machado-Joseph disease, in comparison to other degenerative ataxias.

▶ DYSTONIA IN HEREDITARY ATAXIAS

Dystonia can be found in some hereditary ataxias and can aid specific diagnosis.[147] In autosomal-dominant ataxias, dystonia is very suggestive of spinocerebellar atrophy type 3 (SCA-3) and DRPLA, but it could occur in other SCA sub-types. Two young patients of the only SCA-12 family reported suffered lower extremity dystonia.[148] In recessive ataxia, dystonia is common in ataxia telangiectasia but not found in the more frequent Friedreich ataxia, although there is one report of head dystonic tremor.[149] Dystonia is also common in non-Friedreich recessive ataxia with ocular apraxia.[150]

▶ MACHADO–JOSEPH DISEASE (SCA-3)

This is an autosomal-dominant spinocerebellar degeneration, mainly affecting families descending from ancestors in the Portuguese islands of the Azores. The clinical manifestations have been classified into different phenotypes. Coutinho and Andrade[151] suggested three clinical subtypes according to the clinical symptoms present, in addition to a common ataxic disorder: type I with earliest onset and predominant pyramidal-extrapyramidal signs; type II, the most common, with middle-aged onset and cerebellar plus pyramidal manifestations; and type III of later onset, with cerebellar features and distal amyotrophy. Barbeau and colleagues[152] reviewed 138 patients with this disease and concluded, based on the continuity of the clinical symptoms in the three subtypes, that this disease was a single clinical entity. The pathological examination usually discloses spinal degeneration affecting anterior horn cells and Clarke's column, and neuronal loss in the dentate nucleus and substantia nigra pars compacta (hence, the name nigrospinodentatal degeneration).[153] A GAG expansion has been found on chromosome 14q in Japanese cases[154,155] Dystonia was present in 20% of the 82 patients reported by Freire Gonzalves and colleagues,[156] and involved the hands, feet, face, or neck most commonly, but it was rarely generalized and severe. Dystonia appeared mostly in the younger group. The patient of Lang and colleagues[157] with a double genetic load, also had an early onset with generalized dystonia.

▶ ATAXIA TELANGIECTASIA

This is an autosomal-recessive hereditary disorder associated with abnormalities of DNA repair. It is clinically characterized by progressive ataxia in childhood, ocular and auricular telangiectasia, increased frequency of respiratory infections resulting from absent or low IgA levels, and increased frequency of malignancies. In most of these patients, dystonia is severe, although often not recognized because of the severity of the cerebellar symptoms.[159] After a few years of normal development, affected children develop progressive ataxia of gait, which progressively involves the trunk and upper extremities. Independent gait is progressively more difficult and requires special walkers. Dystonia appears early in the course of the disease,[160–163] but usually after the ataxia; most frequently, it is generalized and further disturbs ambulation (Fig. 31–7). Ocular apraxia, slow saccades, and polyneuropathy may complicate the clinical picture. Severe intellectual deterioration is not typical of this disorder. Telangiectatic lesions appear at about 3–5 years of age, and may disappear after several years of progression of the disease. Therefore, there may be patients with ataxia telangiectasia with severe dystonia and no prominent telangiectasia in late stages of the disease. Death occurs as a complication of bronchopulmonary infection or neoplasm, usually a lymphoma.

The pathology of ataxia telangiectasia involves mainly the cerebellar cortex, in which there is a loss of neurons, and the pigmented brain stem nuclei, including the substantia nigra and locus ceruleus, which occasionally show Lewy bodies.[164] There is demyelinating neuropathy as also loss of fibers in the posterior columns and spinocerebellar tracts.

▶ DYSTONIA IN OTHER NEURODEGENERATIONS

XERODERMA PIGMENTOSUM

The main manifestations of this entity are dermatological, with photosensitivity and skin malignancies, but in some patients, neurological manifestations appear with combinations of mental retardation, seizures, spasticity, deafness, ataxia, chorea, dystonia, and axonal sensory neuropathy.[165] There is a defect in DNA repair, as

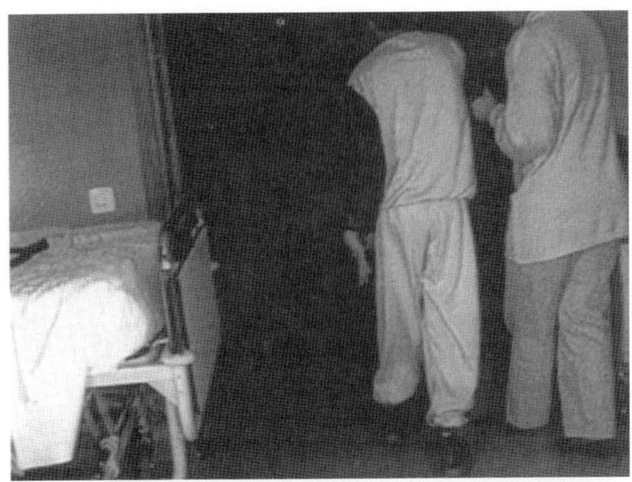

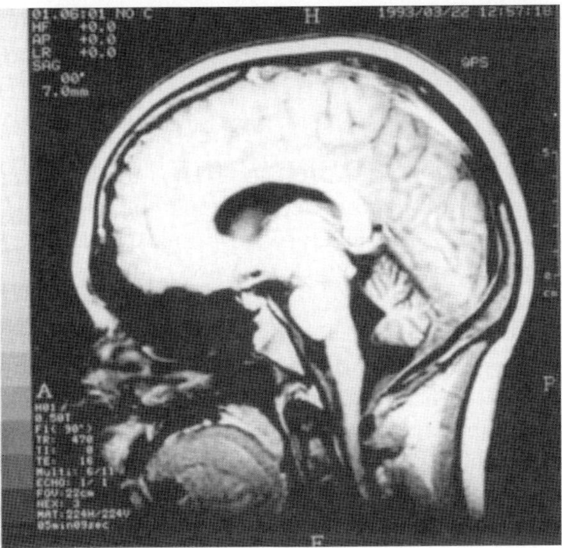

Figure 31–7. *Top*: Generalized dystonia in ataxia telangiectasia. *Bottom:* MRI scan showing cerebellar atrophy in ataxia telangiectasia.

in ataxia telangiectasia. The inheritance is autosomal-recessive. The gene locus has been mapped to 9q in the xeroderma pigmentosum gene.

WOLFRAM'S SYNDROME

Although mainly described as an association of diabetes mellitus, diabetes insipidus, optic atrophy, and deafness, with autosomal-recessive transmission, Wolfram's syndrome can also be associated with several neurological manifestations. These occur usually late in the course, and consist of ataxia, dizziness, mental and conduct alterations, seizures, tremor and dystonia, areflexia, tonic pupils, and neurogenic bladder.[166] A specific gene in chromosome 4p16.1 has been found with different mutations.[167]

▶ DYSTONIA IN METABOLIC DISORDERS

DISORDERS OF LIPID METABOLISM

GM1 Gangliosidosis

Dystonia can appear in disorders of lipid metabolism in children and adults. GM1 gangliosidosis is an autosomal-recessive disorder related to a deficiency in β-galactosidase, leading to intraneuronal storage of GM1 and visceral deposit of compounds with a β-galactose terminal. GM1 gangliosidosis is clinically characterized by visceromegaly, intellectual impairment, dysmorphism, and a cherry-red spot in the macular region in children. The infantile form, or GM1 type 1, begins at birth or in the first months of life. Affected infants display coarse facial features, and skeletal deformities similar to those seen in Hurler's disease. They develop blindness, quadriplegia, and seizures, and they usually die before 2 years of age. Type 2 GM1 begins between 6 and 18 months of age. The course is slower, with gait disturbance, mental deterioration, seizures, optic atrophy with a macular cherry-red spot, and late acoustic startle. No marked skeletal deformities are present. Type 3 GM1 gangliosidosis presents between 2 and 27 years of age, with variable manifestations, including a spinocerebellar deficit, dystonia, and myopathy.[168–170]

In adults, GM1 gangliosidosis is characterized by dystonia and early-onset parkinsonism, lack of mental deterioration, and prolonged survival.[171] Atrophy of the head of the caudate nucleus was found in CT scans of two patients,[169,170] and bilateral putaminal lesions on MRI were seen in other patients.[170] Pathological examination of 1 patient revealed depletion of neurons and intracytoplasmic accumulation of storage material in the basal ganglia, amygdala, and cerebellum.[169] Adult GM1, or type 3, gangliosidosis occurs with partial deficiencies of β-galactosidase activity (total lack of activity is associated with the infantile phenotype; partial, 5–15%, enzyme activity is associated with adult forms; activity high than 15% does not produce neurological symptoms). In these patients dystonia and parkinsonism could be the most relevant clinical findings.[172]

GM2 Gangliosidosis

This disease is due to intraneuronal accumulation of GM2 to 100–300 times the normal levels. The cause of the disease is a deficiency in lysosomal hexosaminidase inherited as an autosomal-recessive trait. It is more frequent among Ashkenazis from East Europe.

The symptoms start in infancy. The first symptoms are jerks in response to loud and sudden noises. Quick deterioration of developmental acquisitions takes place and few infants reach sitting position. Blindness, spasticity, and convulsions appear, and about 90% of these children have a cherry-red spot uni- or bilaterally. Some children develop macrocephaly related to neuronal storage. Survival after the second year of life is rare.

Diagnosis is made by measuring blood and leukocyte hexosaminidase activity. This test shows the heterogeneity of the disease. There are three isoenzymes (A, B, and S), differing in their quaternary structure: hexosaminidiase A is a trimer (a1 b2), hexosaminidase B a tetramer (b2 b2), and hexosaminidase S a dimer (a2). There are different mutations of the locus. In classic Tay–Sachs, or B variant, A and S isoenzymes are not functional, and normal hexosaminidase B is unable to hydrolyze gangliosides. In Sandhoff's disease (O variant), a mutation of the gene coding for B chain on chromosome 5 (5q13) reduces both A and B isoenzymes. In the AB variant, hexosaminidase A and B levels are normal but the disease is related to a deficit in an activator protein. Individuals with the same enzymatic variants present with similar phenotypes.[171] The parents are heterozygous and it is possible to do a prenatal diagnosis through chorionic biopsy. There is another variant, B1, which is a rare form characterized by the presence of a mutation in the hexosaminidase A gene, leading to a defect in the catalytic region of the alpha-subunit of hexosaminidase A (heterodimer). The mutated hexosaminidase A has almost normal activity against the natural synthetic substrates but is unable to hydrolyse GM2 ganglioside and sulfated synthetic substrates. There is a report that describes two cases of this variant; both cases presented regression of mental skills, leading to dementia, epilepsy, quadriplegia, and dystonic involuntary movements.[173] There is no effective treatment available, although transplantation of bone marrow and genetic engineering have been attempted.

Most children with classic infantile GM2 gangliosidosis develop an aggressive disease, with spastic tetraparesis, seizures and, blindness. Dystonia may appear late in the course of the disease. In juvenile GM2 and in chronic GM2, or adult form, dystonia may appear as the presenting clinical feature,[174–177] and, if so, dystonia involves primary the legs (Fig. 31–8). Some of the juvenile and chronic forms present clinical pictures resembling spinocerebellar degeneration and motor neuron disease.[178]

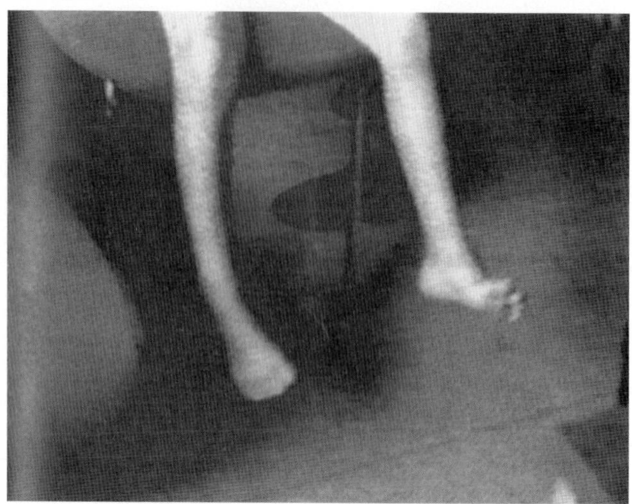

Figure 31–8. Foot dystonia in an 8-year-old patient with generalized dystonia resulting from GM2 gangliosidosis.

▶ NIEMANN–PICK DISEASE AND RELATED DISORDERS

This is a heterogeneous group of conditions linked by an accumulation of sphingomyelin in the reticuloendothelial system. Spence and Callahan[179] divided it into group I, including former types A and B, with sphingomyelinase deficiency, and group II, including types C, D, and E without precise enzymatic deficit

The main neurological manifestations in Niemann–Pick type A are myoclonic seizures, spasticity, and blindness. Type B disease is also termed visceral or not neuronopathic because only occasionally do neurological signs develop. No primary metabolic defect has been identified for types C and D. Sphingomyelinase activity is normal in most tissues and only in three-quarters of patients is it decreased in cultured fibroblasts. However, there is a constant defective cholesterol esterification[180] and excessive lysosomal filipin staining in cultured skin fibroblasts.[181,182] The initial manifestation is transient neonatal cholestatic icterus, which relapses in 20% of patients, returns in the first months of life, and leads to death. Surviving patients develop neurological symptoms. Severe cases with onset before 3 years suffer a devastating neurological deterioration and may not develop ophthalmoplegia. Patients with later onset present with a very characteristic supranuclear or vertical gaze palsy, mental deterioration, gait disorder, cerebellar ataxia, and dystonia. So-called juvenile dystonic lipidosis may be included in type C Niemann–Pick.[183]

▶ METACHROMATIC LEUKODYSTROPHY

Deficiency of cerebroside sulfatase leads to sulfatide accumulation. Different mutations underlie the late infantile and adult forms; the juvenile form seems to be related to compound heterozygosity.[184] Rare cases due to mutation in an activator protein[185] have also been reported. Juvenile forms present between 4 and 10 years of age, with schizophrenia-like psychosis, deterioration of the cognitive functions, personality changes, depression, and dementia.[186] Nerve conduction velocity may be normal and a dystonic phenotype has been described.[187]

▶ CEROID LIPOFUSCINOSIS

This group of diseases is marked by the storage of lipopigments in nervous and other tissues.[177] So far, eight subtypes have been described with different clinical features, age at onset, and gene defects, identified so far in five of these sub-types. Accumulation takes place in lysosomal-like structures, and the finding of a high concentration of dolichols is supportive of the lysosomal nature of these cytosomes. The infantile form (Santavuori–Haltia disease), rare outside Finland, has been mapped to chromosome 1p32, and the gene defect is related to palmitoyl thiol esterase. Other clinical forms include a late infantile form, a juvenile form (Vogt–Spielmeyer or Batten disease), and an adult form (Kufs' disease), without visual failure and presenting with myoclonic epilepsy, dementia and behavioral disturbances, and extrapyramidal signs, mainly facial dyskinesias.[188]

▶ PELIZAEUS–MERZBACHER DISEASE

This disorder has been related to a severe deficiency in myelin-specific lipids caused by a lack of two types of lipoproteins: proteolipid protein, and DM20 transcripts from the proteolipid protein gene. The mutations of these genes are very varied: deletions, loss of function, and missense mutations to additional copies of the gene.[189] Two clinical forms of the disorder have been described: type I is X-linked and starts in infancy; type II is X-linked or autosomal-recessive. The pathology shows a partial to total absence of myelination. In type I, myelin is preserved in internal capsule and subcortical U fibers. Clinical manifestations include ataxia, nystagmus, and hypotonia, and later dystonia progressing slowly. In type II, there is a severe psychomotor retardation.[190]

▶ DISORDERS OF ENERGY PRODUCTION

MITOCHONDRIAL ENCEPHALOMYOPATHIES

Movement disorders, including dystonia, are present in patients with mitochondrial encephalopathies.[191,192] Truong and colleagues[193] reviewed 85 patients with mitochondrial myopathies and found that 9 had movement disorders, most frequently myoclonus,[192] but there was generalized dystonia preceded by mild parkinsonism in 1 case, and associated with strokes in another patient.

Generalized dystonia was reported in a patient with suspected mitochondrial myopathy and putaminal hypodensities,[194] in some individuals of a family with patients affected by Leber's hereditary optic neuropathy, and others with childhood-onset dystonia.[195] There is a report of 1 patient with writer's cramp who progressed over 5 years to dystonia in facial muscles and lower limbs with a 3,243 mitochondrial DNA mutation.[196]

SUBACUTE NECROTIZING ENCEPHALOMYELOPATHY, OR LEIGH'S SYNDROME

Leigh's disease is characterized by intermittent or progressive neurological deterioration after normal development during the first year of life. Children lose their motor acquisitions and develop hypotonia, ataxia, corticospinal tract signs, optic atrophy, dystonia, dysphagia, and dysarthria with relative intellectual preservation. Dystonia is the most common movement disorder in Leigh's disease.[197,198] It may be the principal clinical manifestation in infants,[199] and it is occasionally associated with other movement disorders, including rigidity, tremor, chorea, hypokinesia, myoclonus, and tics. Some patients resemble the primary torsion dystonia phenotype. Neuroradiologic studies show basal ganglia lesions[198] in putamen, caudate, substantia nigra, and globus pallidus, in the majority of the patients. MRI is very helpful since it shows in nearly all cases the symmetric lesions of basal ganglia and brain stem. This pattern of striatal lucencies is consistent with the pathologic findings. The pathology of Leigh's disease is characterized by extensive damage of the brain stem and basal ganglia. There is spongiosis of the neuropil and capillary proliferation, but extensive leukoencephalopathy or gray cortical damage are uncommon. Leigh's disease is an autosomal-recessive disorder related to abnormalities of the pyruvate kinase complex. The activity of this enzyme in fibroblasts is low, and the blood levels of pyruvate and alanine are usually high. The most common enzymatic defect found in these patients is a reduction of the activity of cytochrome *c* oxidase. The juvenile forms present dystonia and movement disorders as protagonistic clinical elements.[200]

Two other disorders related to energy production, Leber's disease and bilateral striatal necrosis, occasionally overlap with Leigh's disease. Therefore, it has been suggested that a variety of energy production disorders, including subacute necrotizing encephalomyelopathy, bilateral striatal necrosis, and Leber's disease, may be grouped under the title of Leigh's syndrome.[201,202] Leber's hereditary optic neuropathy is an X-linked inherited disorder related to different mutations of the mitochondrial genome. Striatal lucencies are present in dystonic patients with Leigh's disease, Leber's hereditary optic neuropathy, and other conditions. In some cases, no biochemical abnormality is found, although some of these may be variants of Leigh's disease. Mutations at point 14459 of the NADH dehydrogenase subunit 6 gene are associated with maternally inherited Leber's hereditary optic neuropathy and dystonia,[203] but there is a report that describes 3 complex I-deficient patients from two separate pedigrees who presented with Leigh's disease, with no evidence of family history of Leber's hereditary optic neuropathy or dystonia.[204]

There is a wide variety of clinical presentations, ranging from adult-onset blindness to pediatric dystonia and basal ganglial degeneration in patients with this mutation. Severe nucleotide substitutions are generally new mutations that cause pediatric diseases such as Leigh's syndrome and dystonia. Mitochondrial DNA rearrangements also cause a variety of phenotypes.[205,206]

▶ MOHR–TRANEBJAERG SYNDROME

This is an X-linked recessive disorder with childhood-onset deafness and adult-onset progressive dystonia, spasticity, and optic atrophy.[207] It has been related to mutations in a protein (DDP) related to protein import to mitochondria.[208,209]

▶ DISORDERS OF ORGANIC AND AMINO ACID METABOLISM

GLUTARIC ACIDURIA TYPE I

Glutaric aciduria type I is a rare autosomal-recessive disease due to a deficiency in glutaryl-CoA dehydrogenase. Homozygous patients have an abnormal degradation of tryptophan, lysine, and hydroxylysine; some of these homozygotes may be clinically asymptomatic. Patients develop their symptoms in infancy. Many of these individuals present generalized dystonia, which occasionally may appear after recovery from an acute episode of diffuse encephalopathy. Other patients follow a progressive course leading to similar manifestations. Generalized dystonia is the main manifestation, being present in 77% of 57 cases.[210] Imaging studies show a characteristic frontotemporal atrophy with enlargement of the Sylvian fissures.[211] MRI shows involvement of the putamina. PET shows lesions in the head of the caudate nuclei and decreased uptake in the cerebral cortex and thalamus.[212] The pathology reveals a severe loss of cells in the basal ganglia, especially in the putamen.[213] Diagnosis is made by measurement of glutaric acid in urine or cerebrospinal fluid. Dietetic treatment with restriction of tryptophan and lysine reduces the levels of glutaric acid; if recognized in the presymptomatic stage, early institution of treatment may prevent the onset of neurological symptoms.[214,215]

METHYLMALONIC ACIDURIA

This is an autosomal-recessive aciduria due to abnormal catabolism of methylmalonic acid. Acute neurological symptoms develop during the first years of life, including generalized dystonia, dysphagia, dysarthria, and different degrees of tetraparesis. These symptoms are considered to be a metabolic stroke involving the globus pallidus and the internal capsule.[216–220] Recent reports on the neurological deficits present in children with different mutations of the enzyme methylmalonyl-CoA mutase suggest that there is a phenotypic pleomorphism without a consistent pattern of neurological injury, and that acidosis and metabolic imbalance are not necessary preconditions for significant neurological morbidity in methylmalonic aciduria. Analysis of urinary organic acids reveals a massive amount of methylmalonic acid. Some patients obtain relief from dystonic symptoms with L-dopa.[219]

FUMARASE DEFICIENCY

This is an inborn error of the tricarboxylic acid cycle characterized by progressive encephalopathy, dysmorphic facial features,[221] dystonia, leukopenia, and neutropenia. MRI shows multiple abnormalities, including diffuse polymicrogyria, decreased cerebral white matter, large ventricles, and open opercula. Elevation of lactate in the cerebrospinal fluid and high fumarate excretion in the urine provide clues for the investigation of the cytosolic and mitochondrial fumarase isoenzymes. In two recently reported cases,[222] the analysis of fumarase cDNA demonstrated that both patients were homozygous for a missense mutation, a G955-C transversion, predicting a Glu319-Gln substitution. This substitution occurred in a highly conserved region of the fumarase cDNA. Both parents exhibited half the expected fumarase activity in their lymphocytes and were found to be heterozygous for this substitution.

HOMOCYSTINURIA

Homozygous patients for cystathionine β-synthase deficiency present ectopia lentis, ocular and skeletal deformities, mental retardation, and vascular occlusions sometimes affecting the brain vessels. Occasionally dystonia has been described in homocystinuria,[223–227] sometimes in adulthood,[228] and could be due to vascular damage to the basal ganglia. It is also possible that dystonia develops as a metabolic complication[216] through enhanced excitotoxic neurotransmission via stimulation of the glutamate receptors by homocysteinic acid or by alteration of the levels of taurine in the basal ganglia. It has also been reported that the fluctuating dystonia that takes place during metabolic decompensation in patients with homocystinuria is related to the levels of sulfur containing amino acids in brain.[229]

HARTNUP'S DISEASE

This disease is characterized by a recurrent personality disorder and cerebellar ataxia, together with a failure to thrive and an intermittent cutaneous rash resembling pellagra. Onset occurs in late infancy and early childhood. Darras and colleagues[230] described a patient with intermittent focal dystonia. Tamoush and colleagues reported two patients with dystonic features.[231] The biochemical deficit is characterized by a defect in the transport of large neutral amino acids.

▶ ABNORMALITIES OF PURINE METABOLISM

LESCH–NYHAN SYNDROME

This is an X-linked disorder of purine metabolism related to reduced activity of the enzyme hypoxanthine-guanine phosphoribosyl transferase (HGPRT). The clinical features are characterized by normal development up to the age of 6–12 months, followed by developmental delay, mental retardation, spasticity, a variety of movement disorders, most prominently dystonia, and automutilation. The patients have high blood levels of uric acid and enhanced urinary elimination of uric acid, which often produces "sandy urine" and urinary stones. Frequent complications of hyperuricemia include gout and tophus. The diagnosis is performed by measurement of HGPRT activity in fibroblasts or red blood cells.

HGPRT deficiency may be complete (Lesch–Nyhan syndrome) or partial (Kelley–Seegmiller syndrome). In a recent series[232] of four patients with complete HGPRT deficiency and four with incomplete enzymatic defect, it was found that the eight patients with Lesch–Nyhan syndrome presented choreoathetosis, corticospinal motor system dysfunction, mental retardation, and signs of self-mutilation. The patients with Kelley–Seegmiller syndrome were heterogeneous: two patients had psychomotor retardation with spasticity, one was mentally retarded with generalized dystonia, and one patient had only gout with no neurologic manifestations. There is a report that describes a Lesch–Nyhan variant that presented with dystonia, ataxia, near-normal intelligence, and no self-mutilation.[233] A mutation was identified in exon 3 of the gene coding for HGPRT (substitution of guanine with thymine), conditioning the substitution of the normal glycine by valine (HGPRT Madrid).[234] Affected patients have abnormally few dopaminergic nerve terminals and cell bodies; this includes all dopaminergic pathways and is not restricted to the basal ganglia. These dopaminergic deficits contribute to the characteristic neuropsychiatric manifestations of the disease.[235]

▶ DYSTONIA DUE TO PHYSICAL AND CHEMICAL AGENTS

Head trauma, which can produce dystonia secondary to focal lesions of the nervous system, and peripheral trauma, which can trigger the development of focal dystonias in individuals at risk, are physical injuries that can produce dystonia. In addition, other physical agents have been reported to induce dystonia. Electrical injuries may produce dystonia, often located in limbs but also in other locations.[236–239] Dystonia induced by physical agents has also been described as an occupational disease in users of lasers and in survivors of the Chernobyl radiation leakage.[240,241] The pathogenesis of dystonia in these cases has been attributed to radiation-induced lesions of small blood vessels in the brain; the clinical description of these cases is far from clear. Most of these reports are in the Russian literature and the word "dystonia" is used with different meanings, including disturbances compatible with dystonia, others with autonomic symptoms, as well as psychogenic disorders.

Dystonia induced by chemicals is common.[242–245] Therapeutic agents, with a variety of pharmacological actions, produce dystonia as an acute side effect of the pharmacological treatment, or as a persistent, and often permanent, complication. Many of these compounds modify the metabolism of the brain monoamines dopamine, norepinephrine, serotonin, and acetylcholine. Most frequently, dopamine-stimulating agents, such as L-dopa and dopamine agonists, induce acute dystonia, particularly in patients with akinetic-rigid syndromes, but there are reports of persistent, and occasionally paroxysmal, dystonia after intake of cocaine, amphetamine, and related compounds.[246,247] Dopamine receptor blockers produce acute and persistent dystonia. Acute dystonic reactions occur frequently with typical neuroleptics, less frequently with atypical neuroleptics, and with frequently used benzamide derivatives, and antihistaminics. These acute dystonic reactions, which are occasionally life-threatening and always alarming, respond very well to treatment with anticholinergics, which sometimes should be administered intravenously. Persistent dystonia was described in the French literature of the 1950s as a late (hence the name "tardive") complication of the treatment of schizophrenic patients with chlorpromazine, and is a frequent complication of long-term neuroleptic treatment (Fig. 31–9). However, the adjective "tardive" meaning "late" is misleading since the condition

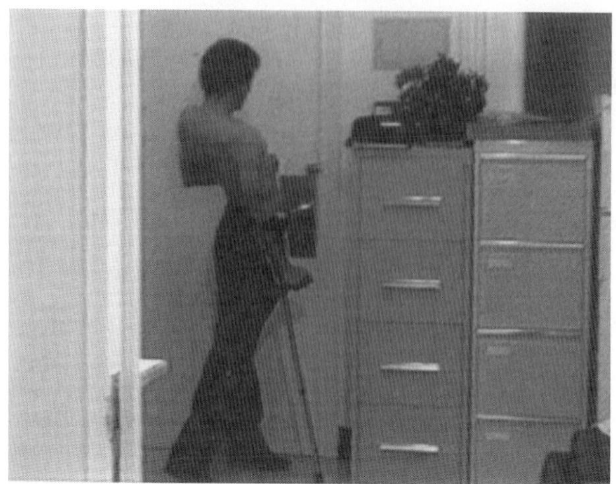

Figure 31–9. Generalized persistent dystonia induced by neuroleptics.

occasionally occurs very early. The mechanism usually proposed is dopamine receptor blockage, especially D2 receptors, but other neurotransmitters and neuropeptides have also been implicated.[248–250] Atypical neuroleptics were initially considered free of risk of tardive symptoms but, with the exception of clozapine, these drugs may not be completely innocents.[251]

Persistent dystonia is very difficult to treat.[252–256] Not infrequently, it is produced by drugs of doubtful indication. Therefore, prevention, early recognition of symptoms, and discontinuation of the offending medication, whenever possible, are the first steps in the treatment of drug-induced dystonia. Other drugs implicated in producing dystonia are some antiepileptic drugs, anxiolytics, and others (usually sporadic or isolated reports). A list of drugs that produce dystonia is given in Table 31–5.

▶ TABLE 31–5. DRUGS AND CHEMICALS IMPLICATED IN DRUG-INDUCED DYSTONIA

	Acute Dystonia	Persistent Dystonia
I. THERAPEUTIC AGENTS		
A. Dopamine receptor blockers		
Classic neuroleptics	•••	••
Atypical neuroleptics[276–301]	•	•
Substituted benzamides[302–314]	•••	•
Catecholamine depletors[315,316]	•	
B. Antihistaminics (with dopamine receptor blocking properties)		
Thiethylperazine[317]	•	
Prochlorperazine[318]	•	
Diphenhydramine[319,320]	•	
C. Catecholamine stimulating agents		
L-Dopa[321–327]	•	•
Dopamine agonists[328–330]	•	
Cocaine[331–334]	•	
Catecholamine releasers[335–338]	•	•
Tricyclic antidepressants[339–341]	•	•
Monoamine oxidase inhibitors[342]	•	
Ergotamine[343,344]	•	•
D. 5-HT stimulating agents		
Selective serotonin reuptake inhibitors[345–355]	•	•
m-chlorophenyl-piperazine[356]	•	
E. Acetylcholine stimulators		
Acetylcholinesterase inhibitors[357,358]	•	
F. Anxiolytics		
Buspirone[359,360]	•	
Fluspirene[361–364]	•	
Bromazepam[365]	•	
Midazolam[366]	•	
Diazepam[367]	•	
G. Antiepileptic drugs		
Carbamazepine[368,369]	•	•
Phenytoin[370,371]	•	•
Phenobarbital[372]	•	

(continued)

TABLE 31-5. (CONTINUED)

	Acute Dystonia	Persistent Dystonia
Gabapentine[373,374]	•	
Tiagabine[375]	•	
H. Other		
Anesthetics[376–379]	•	
Disulfiram[380–382]	•	•
Erythromycin[383]	•	
Chloroquine[384]	•	
Flecainide[385]	•	•
Ranitidine[386,387]	•	
Cimetidine[388]	•	
Sumatriptan[389,390]	•	
Meperidine[391]	•	
Flunarizine and cinnarizine[392]	•	•
Bromvalerylurea[393]	•	•
5-Fluorouracil and doxorubicin[394]		•
Lithium[395]	•	•
Betahistine[396]	•	
II. NEUROTOXIC CHEMICALS		
A. Minerals		
Manganese[257,258]	•	
Copper[259]	•	
Mercury[260]	•	
B. Organic compounds		
Methyl alcohol[261]	•	
Cyanide[262–264]	•	
Carbon monoxide[265,266]	•	
Carbon disulfide[397]	•	
C. Plant derivatives and pesticides		
Ergotmycotoxin[267,268]	•	
Poisoning from mildew-infected sugar cane[269,270]	•	
Fenthion	•	

Dystonia is produced by toxic environmental agents. Manganese produces dystonia and parkinsonism, related to degeneration of the striatum and pallidum, in miners as well as in patients with chronic liver disease.[257,258] Dystonia has also been attributed to high copper levels in 1 patient with cholestatic liver disease.[259] Organic mercury poisoning produces choreoathetosis, parkinsonism, and occasionally dystonic reactions.[260] Organic compounds, including methanol,[261] cyanide,[262–264] and carbon monoxide,[265,266] also produce dystonia. The mechanism usually implicated is cellular hypoxia from mitochondrial damage, or generation of free radicals.

Dystonia may be caused by plant derivatives. The best known of these diseases is epidemic ergotism, which associates to focal and generalized dystonia, epilepsy, stroke, and peripheral ischemia of the limbs (Fig. 31–10).[267,268] Mycotoxin poisoning (3-nitropropionic acid) from mildew-infected sugar cane produces encephalopathy and dystonia[269,270] in the developing world.

PSYCHOGENIC DYSTONIAS

Although about 40% of patients with dystonia are misdiagnosed with psychogenic disorders at a certain stage, less than 3% of our patients have dystonia of psychogenic etiology. This distinction is especially difficult in psychotic patients.[271] These patients do not belong to a single group, but can be subdivided into different subtypes, which occasionally overlap.

Munchausen's syndrome simulating dystonia[272] is characterized by a chronic factitious disorder consistent with clinical symptoms that are under the patient's voluntary control and depend on the medical knowledge of the subject. This behavior is intended to ensure that the affected individual is permanently dependent

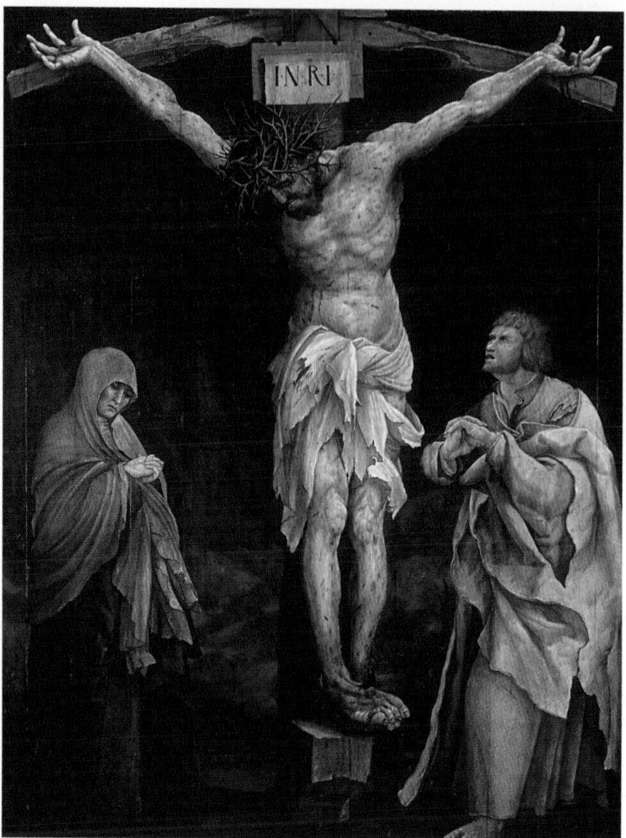

Figure 31–10. Foot dystonia in a patient with epidemic ergotism. The painting was done by M. Grunewald (c 1455–1528), about 1523. The model was probably a patient with epidemic ergotism contacted by Grunewald during his work for the Antonin friars at the Monastery of Issenheim. *(Tauberbischofstein Museum, Karlsruhe, Germany.)*

on medical care, and may cause unjustified, aggressive, and occasionally risky, medical treatments. Malingering is characterized by consciously simulated illness in order to obtain social or economic compensation. Hysteria or conversion disorders are characterized by no conscious production of symptoms.

In general, psychogenic dystonia can be differentiated from genuine dystonia by several clinical characteristics, including the presence of associated atypical weakness or sensory complaints, fixed postures, and lack of modification of the movement disorder by action or sensory tricks. The pattern of movement changes inconsistently in different situations and in the presence or absence of medical and nursing staff or, at times, when the patient believes they are not being observed. There is worsening by stress, improvement by relaxation and psychotherapy, and disappearance by revelation of the nature of the disorder.[273–275] Such disorders can persist for a long time (Table 31–6).

▶ PSEUDODYSTONIAS OF ORGANIC ORIGIN

These disorders are characterized by abnormal postures or movements related to musculoskeletal deformities, or are performed to compensate for pain or abnormal function of different elements of the central or peripheral nervous system. These disorders may be confounded with focal or segmental dystonias since they are restricted to a part of the body. The correct diagnosis can be made by taking into consideration the fixed nature of the abnormality, the lack of improvement with sensory tricks, and the absence of aggravation by action. A list of organic disorders simulating dystonias is given in Table 31–7.

▶ **TABLE 31–6. CLINICAL CHARACTERISTICS OF GENUINE DYSTONIA, PSYCHOGENIC DYSTONIA, AND PSEUDODYSTONIA**

	Dystonia	Psychogenic Dystonia	Pseudodystonia
Socioeconomic benefit	+/–	+++	+/–
Atypical symptoms (weakness, sensory complaints)	+/–	+++	+/–
Triggered/worsened by action	+++	–	–
Triggered/worsened by stress	++	+++	+/–
Fixed dystonia	+	+++	+++
Improved by sensory tricks or geste antagonistic	+++	–	–
Improved by relaxation	++	+++	–
Abnormal imaging findings	+/–	–	++

–, negative; +/–, questionable; +, positive; ++, very positive; +++, very characteristic.

▶ TABLE 31-7. **PSEUDODYSTONIA OF ORGANIC ORIGIN**

A. Disorders simulating blepharospasm Eyelid apraxia Palpebral ptosis B. Disorders simulating oromandibular dystonia Trismus C. Disorders simulating cervical dystonia 1. Osteoarticular Subluxation of the atlantoaxial articulation Klippel-Feil abnormality Platybasia and basilar imprecision Cervical hemivertebra Damage, absence or laxity of the cervical ligaments 2. Muscular Congenital or acquired muscle weakness Muscle fibrosis following local radiation therapy 3. Soft tissue Neck mass 4. Neurological Posterior fossa tumor or cyst Diplopia, mainly cranial nerve IV palsy Vestibular lesions Syringomyelia, syringobulbia Tonsillar herniation of any cause, including Arnold-Chiari syndrome	D. Disorders simulating brachial dystonia Carpal tunnel syndrome and other painful neuropathies Hyperventilation E. Disorders simulating trunk dystonia 1. Osteoarticular Bony abnormalities causing kyphosis, lordosis or scoliosis 2. Neuromuscular Myopathies or neuropathies Opisthotonos Muscle cramps Stiff-person syndrome Isaac's syndrome Compensatory postures due to visceral or anorectal pain F. Disorders simulating leg dystonia 1. Osteoarticular Asymmetry, bony abnormalities 2. Neuromuscular Spasticity, muscle cramps Restless legs Focal tetanus

REFERENCES

1. Calne DB and Lang AE. Secondary dystonia. Adv Neurol 1988;50:9–33.
2. Hartmann A, Pogarell O, andOertel WH. Secondary dystonias. J Neurol 245:511-518, 1998.
3. Jankovic J and Fahn S. Dystonic disorders. In Jankovic J and Tolosa E (eds), Parkinson's Disease and Movement Disorders. Baltimore: Williams & Wilkins, 1993, pp 337–374.
4. Fahn S. Dystonia: Where next? In Quinn NP, Jenner PG (eds), Disorders of Movement. New York: Academic Press, 1989, pp 349–357.
5. Dooling EC, Adams RD. The pathologic anatomy of posthemiplegic athetosis. Brain 1975;98:29–48.
6. Gracia Cruz A, Ortega Perez M, and Hernandez Lara J. Cerebral palsy with dystonic components. A presentation of nine cases. Rev Neurol 1999;29:591.
7. Marsden CD, Obeso JA, and Zarranz JJ. The anatomical basis of symptomatic dystonia. Brain 108:463–483, 1985.
8. Krauss JK, Mohakjer M, Nobbe F, et al. Hemidystonia due to a contralateral parietooccipital metastasis: Disappearance after removal of the mass lesion. Neurology 1991;41:1519–1520.
9. Coria F, Blanco Martin AI, and Rivas Vilas MD. Pseudodystonic hand posturing contralateral to a metastasis of the parietal association cortex. Neurologia 2000;15:362–365.
10. Alarcon F, Tolosa E, and Muñoz E: Focal limb dystonia in a patient with a cerebellar mass. Arch Neurol 2001;58:1125–1127.
11. Menkes JH and Curren J. Clinical and MR correlates in children with extrapyramidal cerebral palsy. Am J Neuroradiol 1994;15:451–457.
12. Krystkowiak P, Martinat P, Defebvre L, et al. Dystonia after striatopallidal and thalamic stroke: Clinicoradiological correlations and pathophysiological mechanisms. J Neurol Neurosurg Psychiatry 1998;65: 703–708.
13. Kelley RE and Jain PK. Hyperkinetic movement disorders caused by corpus striatum infarcts: brain MRI/CT findings in three cases. J Neuroimaging 2000;10:22–26.
14. Schneider S, Feifel E, Ott D, et al. Prolonged MRI T2 times of the lentiform nucleus in idiopathic spasmodic torticollis. Neurology 1994;44:846–850.
15. Krauss JK, Mohadjer M, Nobbe F, Mundinger F. The treatment of post traumatic tremor by stereotactic surgery. Symptomatic and functional outcome in a series of 35 patients. J Neurosurg 1994;80:810–819.
16. Yamashiro K and Tasker RR. Stereotactic thalamotomy for dystonic patients. Stereotact Funct Neurosurg 1993;60: 81–85.
17. Jankovic J and Patel SC. Blepharospasm associated with brainstem lesions. Neurology 1983;33:1237–1240.
18. Lang AE and Sharpe JA. Blepharospasm associated with palatal myoclonus [letter]. Neurology 1984;34:1522.
19. Sandyk R, Gillman MA. Blepharospasm associated with communicating hydrocephalus [letter]. Neurology 1984;34:1522–1523.
20. Jankovic J. Blepharospasm associated with palatal myoclonus and communicating hydrocephalus [letter]. Neurology 1984;34:1523–1525.
21. Powers JM. Blepharospasm due to unilateral diencephalon infarction. Neurology 1985;35:283–284.
22. Jankovic J. Blepharospasm with basal ganglia lesions [letter]. Arch Neurol 1986;43:866–868.

23. Day TJ, Lefroy RB, Mastaglia FL. Meige's syndrome and palatal myoclonus associated to brainstem stroke. A common mechanism? J Neurol Neurosurg Psychiatry 1986;48:1324–1325.
24. Leenders KL, Frackowiack RSJ, Quinn N, et al. Ipsilateral blepharospasm and contralateral hemidystonia and parkinsonism in a patient with a unilateral rostral brainstem-thalamic lesion: Structural and functional abnormalities studied with CT, MRI and PET scanning. Mov Disord 1986;1:151–158.
25. Salerno SM, Kurlan R, Joy SE, et al. Dystonia in central pontine myelinolysis without evidence of extrapontine myelinolysis. J Neurol Neurosurg Psychiatry 1993;56: 1221–1223.
26. García-Albea E, Franch O, Muñoz D, et al. Brueghel's syndrome, report of a case with post-mortem study. J Neurol Neurosurg Psychiatry 1981;44:437–440.
27. Gibb WRG, Lees AJ, and Marsden CD. Pathological report of four patients presenting with cranial dystonias. Mov Disord 1988;3:211–221.
28. Altrocchi PH and Forno LS. Spontaneous oral-facial dyskinesia: Neuropathology of a case. Neurology 1983;33:802–805.
29. Zweigg RM, Jankel WR, Whitehouse MF, et al. Brainstem pathology in dystonia. Neurology 1986;36(suppl 1):74–75.
30. Kulisevsky J, Marti MJ, Ferrer I, Tolosa E. Meige syndrome: Neuropathology of a case. Mov Disord 1988;3:170–175.
31. Mark MH, Sage JI, Dickson DW, et al. Meige syndrome in the spectrum of Lewy body disease. Neurology 1994;44:1432–1436.
32. Hanajima R, Okabe S, Terao Y, et al. Difference in intracortical inhibition of the motor cortex between cortical myoclonus and focal hand dystonia. Clin Neurophysiol 2008;119(6):1400–1407.
33. Neychev VK, Fan X, Mitev VI, et al. The basal ganglia and cerebellum interact in the expression of dystonic movement. Brain 2008;131(Pt 9):2499–2509.
34. Quartarone A, Rizzo V, and Morgante F. Clinical features of dystonia: A pathophysiological revisitation. Curr Opin Neurol 2008;21(4):484–490.
35. Grimes JD, Hassan MN, Quarrington AM, et al. Delayedonset post-hemiplegic dystonia: CT demonstration of basal ganglia pathology. Neurology 1982;32:1033–1035.
36. Russo LS. Focal dystonia and lacunar infarction of the basal ganglia. Arch Neurol 1983;40:61–62.
37. Keane JR and Young JA. Blepharospasm with bilateral basal ganglia infarction. Arch Neurol 1985;42:1206–1208.
38. Giroud M and Dumas R. Dystonie secondaire, un infarctus putamino-capsulo-caud chez l'enfant. Rev Neurol (Paris) 1988;144:375–377.
39. Picard A, Elghozi D, Schuman-Clacy E, et al. Troubles du langage de type sous-cortical et hemidystonie sequelles d'un infarctus putamino-caude datant de la premiere enfance. Rev Neurol (Paris) 1989;145:73–75.
40. Burton L, Scott PhD, and Jankovic J. Delayed-onset progressive movement disorders after static brain lesions. Neurology 1996;46:68–74.
41. Bhatt MH, Obeso JA, and Marsden CD: Time course of post anoxic dystonic syndromes. Neurology 1993;43:314–317.
42. Saint Hilaire MH, Burke RE, Bressman SB, et al. Delayed-onset dystonia due to perinatal or early childhood asphyxia. Neurology 1991;41:216–222.
43. Larumbe R, Vaamonde J, Artieda J, et al. Blepharospasm associated with anoxic damage of the basal ganglia during cardiac surgery. Mov Disord 1993;8:198–200.
44. Chiang CY and Lu CS. Delayed-onset posthemiplegic dystonia and imitation synkinesia [letter]. J Neurol Neurosurg Psychiatry 1990;53:623.
45. Factor SA, Sanchez-Ramos J, and Weiner WJ. Delayed-onset dystonia associated with corticospinal tract dysfunction. Mov Disord 1988;3:201–210.
46. Burke RE, Fahn S, and Gold AP. Delayed-onset dystonia in patients with "static" encephalopathy. J Neurol Neurosurg Psychiatry 1982;43:789–797.
47. Münchau A, Mathen D, Cox T, et al. Unilateral lesions of the globus pallidus: Report of four patients presenting with focal or segmental dystonia. J Neurol Neurosurg Psychiatry 2000;69:494–498
48. Jankovic J. Can peripheral trauma induce dystonia and other movement disorders? Yes! Mov Disord 2001;16:7–12.
49. Weiner WJ. Can peripheral trauma induce dystonia? No! Mov Disord 2001;16:13–22.
50. Fletcher NA, Harding AE, and Marsden CD. The relationship between trauma and idiopathic torsion dystonia. J Neurol Neurosurg Psychiatry 1991;54:713–717.
51. Sankhla C, Lai EC, and Jankovic J. Peripherally induced oromandibular dystonia. J Neurol Neurosurg Psychiatry 1998;65:722–728.
52. Frucht S, Fahn S, and Ford B. Focal task-specific dystonia induced by peripheral trauma. Mov Disord 2000;15: 348–350.
53. Schott GD. The relationship of peripheral trauma and pain to dystonia. J Neurol Neurosurg Psychiatry 1985;48: 698–701.
54. Jankovic J and Van der Linden C. Dystonia and tremor induced by peripheral trauma: Predisposing factors. J Neurol Neurosurg Psychiatry 1988;51:1512–1519.
55. Truong DD, Dubinsky R, Hermanowicz N, et al. Posttraumatic torticollis. Arch Neurol 1991;48:221–223.
56. Goldman S and Ahlskog JE. Posttraumatic cervical dystonia. Mayo Clin Proc 1993;68:443–448.
57. Foley-Nolan D, Kinirons M, Coughlan RJ, O'Connor P: Post-whiplash dystonia well controlled by transcutaneous electrical nervous stimulation (TENS): Case report. J Trauma 1990;30: 909–910.
58. Jankovic J. Post-traumatic movement disorders: Central and peripheral mechanisms. Neurology 1994;44:2006–2014.
59. Thyagarajan D, Kompoliti K, and Ford B. Post-traumatic shoulder dystonia: persistent abnormal postures of the shoulder after minor trauma. Neurology 1998;51: 1205–1207.
60. Murase N, Kaji R, Shimazu H, et al. Abnormal premovement gating of somatosensory input in writer's cramp. Brain 2000;123:1813–1829.
61. Jankovic J. Post-traumatic movement disorders: Central and peripheral mechanisms. Neurology 1994;44: 2006–2014.
62. Reich SG, Weiner WJ, and Morgan JC. Progression of dystonia in complex regional pain syndrome. Neurology 2005;64: 2162–2163.
63. Lees AJ, Hardie RJ, and Stern GM. Kinesigenic foot dystonia as a presenting feature of Parkinson's disease. J Neurol Neurosurg Psychiatry 1984;47:885.

64. Poewe W, Lees AJ, Steiger D, et al. Foot dystonia in Parkinson's disease: Clinical phenomenology and neuropharmacology. Adv Neurol 1986;45:357–360.
65. LeWitt PA, Burns RS, and Newman RP. Dystonia in untreated Parkinsonism. Clin Neuropharmacol 1986;9: 293–297.
66. Katchen M and Duvoisin RC. Parkinsonism following dystonia in three patients. Mov Disord 1986;1:151–157.
67. Mark MH, Sage JI, Dickson DW, Heikkila RE, Manzino L, Schwarz KO, Duvoisin RC. Neurology 1994 Aug;44(8) 1432–6
68. Grimes JD, Hassan MN, Halle D, et al. Clinical and radiographic features of scoliosis in Parkinson's disease. Adv Neurol 1986;45:353–355.
69. Mathers SE, Kempster PA, Swash M, et al. Constipation and paradoxical puborectalis contraction in anismus and Parkinson's disease: A dystonic phenomenon? J Neurol Neurosurg Psychiatry 1988;51:1503–1507.
70. Golbe LI, Di Iorio G, Bonavita V, et al. A large kindred with autosomal dominant Parkinson's disease. Ann Neurol 1990;27:276–282.
71. De Yebenes JG, Moskowitz C, Fahn S, et al. Long-term treatment with levodopa in a family with autosomal dominant torsion dystonia. Adv Neurol 1988;50:101–111.
72. Nygaard TG, Trugman JM, de Yebenes JG, et al. DOPA responsive dystonia: The spectrum of clinical manifestations in a large North American family. Neurology 1990;40:253–257.
73. Yokochi M. Nosological concept of juvenile parkinsonism with reference to the DOPA-responsive syndrome. Adv Neurol 1993;60:548–552.
74. Bastos Lima A, Levy A, Castro Galdas A, et al. Parkinson's disease before age 30. Adv Neurol 1993;60:553–561.
75. Dwork AJ, Balmaceda C, Fazzini EA, et al. Dominantly inherited, early-onset parkinsonism: Neuropathology of a new form. Neurology 1993;43:69–74.
76. Tolosa E and Compta Y. Dystonia in Parkinsons disease. J Neurol 2006;253 (suppl 7): VII/7–VII/1.
77. Probst A and Dufresne JJ. Paralysie supranuclaire progressive ou dystonie oculo facio cervicale. Schweiz Arch Neurol Neurochir Psychiatr 1975;116:107–134.
78. Constantino A and Bolton CF. The face in progressive supranuclear palsy. Neurology 1985;35(suppl 1):161.
79. Jackson JA, Jankovic J, Ford J. Progressive supranuclear palsy: Clinical features and response to treatment in 16 patients. Ann Neurol 1983;13:237–278.
80. Steele JC, Richardson JC, and Olszewsky J. Progressive supranuclear palsy. Arch Neurol 1964;10:333–359.
81. Weimann RL. Heterogeneous degeneration of the central nervous system associated with peripheral neuropathy. Neurology 1967;17:507–603.
82. Steele JC. Progressive supranuclear palsy. Brain 1972;95:693–704.
83. Ratal RD and Fredman JH. Limb dystonia in progressive supra-nuclear palsy. Neurology 1987;37:1546–1548.
84. Kurihara T, Landau WM, and Torack RM. Progressive supranuclear palsy with action myoclonus, seizures. Neurology 1974;24:219–223.
85. Leger JM, Girault JA, and Bolgert F. Deux cas de dystonie isole d'un membre superieur inagurant una maladie de Steele Richardson Olszewsky. Rev Neurol (Paris) 1987;143:140–142.
86. Fenelon G, Guillard A, Romanet S, et al. Les signes parkinsoniens du syndrome de Steele-Richardson-Olszewsky. Rev Neurol (Paris) 1993;149:69–64.
87. De Yebenes JG, Sarasa JL, Daniel SE, et al. Familial progressive supranuclear palsy. Brain 1995 ;118:1095–1103.
88. Rebeiz JJ, Kolondy EH, and Richardson EP. Corticodentatonigral degeneration with neuronal achromasia. Arch Neurol 1968;18:20–33.
89. Lee MS, Thompson PD, and Marsden CD. Corticobasal degeneration: A clinical study of 36 cases. Brain 1994;117:1183–1196.
90. Vanek Z and Jankovic J. Dystonia in corticobasal degeneration. Mov Disord 2001;16(2):252–257.
91. Gilman S, Wenning GK, Brooks DJ, et al. Second consensus statement on the diagnosis of multiple system atrophy. *Neurology* 2008;71:670–676.
92. Berciano J. Olivopontocerebellar atrophy. In Jankovic J and Tolosa E (eds), Parkinson's Disease and Movement Disorders. Baltimore: Williams & Wilkins, 1993, pp. 163–189.
93. Menzel P. Beitrage zur Kenntnigs der hereditarien Ataxie und Kleinhinrnatrophie. Arch Psychiatr Nervenkr 1891;22:160–190.
94. Neumann MA. Pontocerebellar atrophy combined with vestibular reticular degeneration. J Neuropathol Exp Neurol 1977;36:321–337.
95. Wenning GB, Tison F, Ben Shlomo Y, et al. Multiple System Atrophy: A Review of 203 Pathologically Proven Cases. Mov Disord 1997;12(2):133–147.
96. Bruyn GW and Went LN. Huntington's chorea. In Vinken PJ, Bruyn GW, Klawans HL (eds), Handbook of Clinical Neurology: Extrapyramidal Disorders, Vol 5. Amsterdam: Elsevier, 1986, pp. 255–266.
97. Wild EJ and Tabrizi SJ. Huntington's disease phenocopy syndromes. Curr Opin Neurol 2007;20:681–687.
98. Al-Tahan AY, Divarkaran MP, Kambouris M, et al. A novel autosomal recessive "Huntington's disease-like" neurodegenerative disorder in a Saudi family. Saudi Med J 1999;20:85–89.
99. Kambouris M, Bohlega S, Al T, et al. Localization of the gene for a novel autosomal recessive neurodegenerative Huntington-like disorder to 4p15.3. Am J Hum Genet 2000;66:445–452.
100. Curtis ARJ, Fey C, Morris C, et al. Mutation in the gene encoding ferritin light polypeptide causes dominant adult-onset basal ganglia disease. Nat Genet 2001;28: 350–354.
101. Schady W and Meara RJ. Hereditary progressive chorea without dementia. J Neurol Neurosurg Psychiatry 1988;51:295–297.
102. de Vries BBA, Arts WFM, Breedveld G, et al. Benign hereditary chorea of early onset maps to chromosome 14q. Am J Hum Genet 2000;66:136–142.
103. Mahajnah M, Inbar D, Steinmetz A, et al. Benign hereditary chorea: Clinical, neuroimaging, and genetic findings. J Child Neurol 2007;22:1231–1234.
104. Oechsner M, Buchert R, Beyer W, et al. Reduction of striatal glucose metabolism in McLeod choreoacanthocytosis. J Neurol Neurosurg Psychiatry 2001;70:517–520.
105. Rinne JO, Daniels E, Scaravilli F, et al. Neuropathological features of neuroacanthocytosis. Mov Disord 1994;9: 297–304.

106. Kito S, Itoga E, Hiroshige Y, et al. A pedigree of amyotrophic chorea with acanthocytosis. Arch Neurol 1980;37:514–517.
107. De Yebenes JG, Vazquez A, Martinez A, et al. Biochemical findings in symptomatic dystonias. Adv Neurol 1988;50:167–175.
108. De Yebenes JG, Brin MF, Mena MA, et al. Neurochemical findings in neuroacanthocytosis. Mov Disord 1988;3:300–312.
109. Rubio JP, Danek A, Stone C, et al. Chorea-acanthocytosis: Genetic linkage to chromosome 9q21. Am J Hum Genet 1997;61:899–908.
110. Rampoldi L, Dobson-Stone C, Rubio JP, et al. A conserved sorting-associated protein is mutant in chorea-acanthocytosis. Nat Genet 2001;28:119–120.
111. Ueno S, Maruki Y, Nakamura M, et al. The gene encoding a newly discovered protein, chorein, is mutated in chorea-acanthocytosis. Nat Genet 2001;28:121–122.
112. Titica J and Van Bogaert L. Heredodegenerative hemiballismus: A contribution to the question of primary atrophy of the corpus Luysii. Brain 1946;69:251–263.
113. Nagafuchi S, Yanagisawa H, and Sato K. Dentatorubral and pallidoluysian atrophy expansion of an unstable CAG trinucleotide on chromosome 12p. Nat Genet 1994;6:14–18.
114. Iizuka R, Hirayama K, and Maehara K. Dentato-rubropallidoluysian atrophy: A clinico-pathological study. J Neurol Neurosurg Psychiatry 1984;47:1288–1298.
115. Komure O, Sano A, and Nishino N. DNA analysis in hereditary dentatorubral-pallidoluysian atrophy: Correlation between CAG repeat length and phenotypic variation and the molecular basis of anticipation. Neurology 1995;45:143–149.
116. Sano A, Yamamuchi N, Kakimoto Y. Anticipation in hereditary dentatorubral-pallidoluysian atrophy. Hum Genet 1994;93:699–702.
117. Walshe JM: Wilson's disease. In Vinken PJ, et al. (eds), Handbook of Clinical Neurology. Amsterdam: Elsevier, 1986, pp. 223–238.
118. Magalhaes AC, Caramelli P, Menezes JR, et al. Wilson's disease: MRI with clinical correlation. Neuroradiology 1994;36:97–100.
119. Simonati A, Trevisan C, Salviati A, et al. Neuroaxonal dystrophy with dystonia and pallidal involvement. Neuropediatrics 1999;30:151–154.
120. Zhou B, Westaway SK, Levinson B, et al. A novel pantothenate kinase gene (PANK2) is defective in Hallervorden-Spatz syndrome. Nat Genet 2001;28:345–349.
121. Dooling EC, Schoene WC, and Richardson EP. Hallervorden-Spatz syndrome. Arch Neurol 1974;30:70–83.
122. Nardocci N, Rumi V, Combi ML, et al. Complex tics, stereotypies, and compulsive behavior as clinical presentation of a juvenile progressive dystonia suggestive of Hallervorden-Spatz disease. Mov Disord 1994;9:369–371.
123. Hayflick SJ, Westaway SK, Levinson B, et al. Genetic, clinical, and radiographic delineation of Hallervorden–Spatz syndrome. N Engl J Med 2003;348:33–40.
124. Justesen CR, Penn RD, Kroin JS, et al. Stereotactic pallidotomy in a child with Hallervorden-Spatz disease. Case report. J Neurosurg 1999;90:551–554.
125. Crompton DE, Chinnery PF, Fey C, et al. Neuroferritinopathy: a window on the role of iron in neurodegeneration. Blood Cells Mol Dis 2002;29(3):522–531.
126. Chinnery PF, Curtis AR, Fey C, et al. Neuroferritinopathy in a French family with late onset dominant dystonia. J Med Genet 2003;40(5.
127. Crompton DE, Chinnery PF, Bates D, et al. Spectrum of movement disorders in neuroferritinopathy. Mov Disord 2005;20(1):9599.
128. Mir P, Edwards MJ, Curtis AR, et a;. Adult-onset generalized dystonia due to a mutation in the neuroferritinopathy gene. Mov Disord 2005;20(2):243–235.
129. Burn J and Chinnery PF. Neuroferritinopathy. Semin Pediatr Neurol 2006;13(3):176–181.
130. Chinnery PF, Crompton DE, Birchall D, et al. Clinical features and natural history of neuroferritinopathy caused by the FTL1 460InsA mutation. Brain 2007:110–119.
131. Manyam BV, Walters AS, and Narla KR. Bilateral striopallidodentate calcinosis: Clinical characteristics of patients seen in a registry. Mov Disord 2001;16:258–264.
132. Caraceni T, Broggi G, and Avanzini G. Familial idiopathic basal ganglia calcifications exhibiting "dystonia musculorum deformans". Eur Neurol 1974;12:351–359.
133. Larsen TA, Dunn HG, Jan JE, et al. Dystonia and calcification of the basal ganglia. Neurology 1985;35:533–537.
134. Lauterbach EC, Spears TE, Prewett MJ, et al. Neuropsychiatric disorders, myoclonus, and dystonia in calcification of basal ganglia pathways. Biol Psychiatry 1994;35:345–351.
135. Geschwind DH, Loginov M, and Stern JM. Identification of a locus on chromosome 14q for idiopathic basal ganglia calcification (Fahr disease). Am J Hum Genet 1999;65:764–772.
136. Loeb JA. Functional improvement in a patient with cerebral calcinosis using a bisphosphonate. Mov Disord 1998;13:345–349.
137. Jellinger K. Pallidal, pallidonigral and pallidoluysonigral degeneration including association with thalamic and dentate degeneration. In Vinken PJ, Bruyn GW, and Klawans HL (eds), Handbook of Clinical Neurology: Extrapyramidal Disorders. Vol 5. Amsterdam: Elsevier, 1986, pp. 445–464.
138. Van Bogaert L. Aspects cliniques et pathologiques des atrophies pallidales et pallido-luysiennes progressives. J Neurol Neurosurg Psychiatry 1946;9:125–157.
139. Wooten GF, Lopes MB, Harris WO, et al. Pallidoluysian atrophy: Dystonia and basal ganglia functional anatomy. Neurology 1993;43:1764–1768.
140. Haltia M, Somer H, and Palo J. Neuronal intranuclear inclusion disease in identical twins. Ann Neurol 1984;15:316–321.
141. Muñoz-García D and Ludwin SK. Adult onset neuronal intranuclear hyaline inclusion disease. Neurology 1986;36:785–790.
142. Goutieres F, Mikol F, and Aicardi J. Neuronal intranuclear inclusion disease in a child: Diagnoses by rectal biopsy. Ann Neurol 1990;27:103–106.
143. Amir RE, Wan M, van den Veyver IB, et al. Rett syndrome is caused by mutations in X-linked MECP2, encoding methyl-CpG-binding protein 2. Nat Genet 1999;23:185–188.

144. Shahbazian MD and Zoghbi HY. Molecular genetics of Rett syndrome and clinical spectrum of MECP2 mutations. Curr Opin Neurol 2001;14:171–176.
145. The Rett syndrome Diagnostic Criteria Study Group. Diagnostic criteria for Rett syndrome. Ann Neurol 1988;23:425–428.
146. Fitzgerald PM, Jankovic J, and Percy AK. Rett syndrome and associated movement disorders. Mov Disord 1990;5:195–202.
147. Subramony SH and Filla A. Autosomal dominant spinocerebellar ataxias ad infinitum? Neurology 2001;56:287–289.
148. Hearn E, Holmes SE, Calvert PC, et al. SCA-12: Tremor with cerebellar and cortical atrophy is associated with a CAG repeat expansion. Neurology 2001;56:299–303.
149. Wali GM. Friedreich ataxia associated with dystonic head tremor provoked by prolonged exercise. Mov Disord 2000;15:1298–1299.
150. Barbot C, Coutinho P, Chorao R, et al. Recessive ataxia with ocular apraxia: Review of 22 Portuguese patients. Arch Neurol 2001;58:201–205.
151. Coutinho P and Andrade C. Autosomal dominant system degeneration in Portuguese families of the Azores islands. Neurology 1978;28:703–709.
152. Barbeau A, Roy M, and Cunha L. The natural history of Machado-Joseph disease. Can J Neurol Sci 1984;11: 510–525.
153. Woods B and Schaumburg H. Nigro-spino-dentatal degeneration with nuclear ophthalmoplegia: A unique and partially treatable clinicopathological entity. J Neurol Sci 1972;17:149–166.
154. Takiyama Y, Oyanagi S, Kawashima S, et al. A clinical and pathologic study of a large Japanese family with Machado-Joseph disease tightly linked to the DNA markers on chromosome 14q. Neurology 1994;44:1302–1308.
155. Kawaguchi Y, Okamoto T, and Taniwaki M. CAG expansions in a novel gene for Machado-Joseph disease at chromosome 14q32.1. Nat Genet 1994;8:221–227.
156. Freire Gonzalves A, Dinis M, and Ferro MA.Machado-Joseph disease. In Berciano J (ed), Ataxias y Paraplegias Hereditarias: Aspectos Clínicos y Genéticos. Madrid: Ergon, 1993, pp. 189–202.
157. Lang AE, Rogaeva EA, Tsuda T, et al. Homozygous inheritance of the Machado-Joseph disease gene. Ann Neurol 1994;36:443–447.
158. Schols L, Peters S, Szymanski S, et al. Extrapyramidal motor signs in degenerative ataxias. Arch Neurol 2000;57:1495–1500.
159. Bodesteiner JB, Goldblum RM, and Goldman AS. Progressive dystonia masking ataxia telangiectasia. Arch Neurol 1980;37:464–465.
160. Aguilera T and Negrete O. Un caso de ataxia telangiectasia. Rev Clin Esp 1967;107:51–54.
161. Castroviejo P, Rodriguez-Costa T, and Ojeda Casas A. Ataxia telangiectasia, presentacion de dos casos con agammaglobulinemia. Rev Clin Esp 1968;109:439–444.
162. Garcia-Urra D, Campos J, Varela de Seijas E, et al. Movement disorders in ataxia telangiectasia. Neurology 1989;39:321.
163. Garcia-Ruiz P, Garcia-Urra D, and Jimenez-Jimenez FJ. Movimientos anormales en ataxia telangiectasia. Arch Neurobiol 1993;56:30–33.
164. Agamanolis DP and Greenstein JI. Ataxia telangiectasia. J Neuropathol Exp Neurol 1979;38:475.
165. Robbins JH, Kraemer KH, and Lutzer MA. Xeroderma pigmentosum: An inherited disease with sun sensitivity, multiple cutaneous neoplasm and abnormal DNA repair. Ann Intern Med 1974;80:221–248.
166. Rando TA, Horton JL, and Layder BB. Wolfram syndrome: Evidence of a neurodegenerative disease by magnetic resonance imaging. Neurology 1986;36:438–440.
167. Hardy EL, Khanim F, Torres R, et al. Clinical and molecular genetic analysis of 19 Wolfram syndrome kindreds demonstrating a wide spectrum of mutations in WFS1. Am J Hum Genet 1999;65:1279–1290.
168. Goldman JE, Katz D, and Rapin I. Chronic GM1 gangliosidosis presenting as dystonia: I. Clinical and pathological features. Ann Neurol 1981;9:465–475.
169. Guazzi GC, D'Amore I, Van Hoff F, et al. Type 3 (chronic) GM1 gangliosidosis presenting as infanto choreo athetotic dementia, without epilepsy in three sisters. Neurology 1988;38:1124–1127.
170. Uyama E, Terasaki T, Watanabe S, et al. Type 3 GM1 gangliosidosis: Characteristic MRI findings correlated with dystonia. Acta Neurol Scand 1992;86:609–615.
171. Federico A, Palmeri S, Malandrini A, et al. The clinical aspects of adult hexosaminidase deficiencies. Dev Neurosci 1991;13:280–287.
172. Roze E, Paschke E, and Lopez N. Dystonia and Parkinsonism in GM1 Type 3 Gangliosidosis. Mov Disord, 2005;20:1366–1369.
173. Eirís J, ChabÁs A, Coll MJ, et al. Fenotipo infantil tardío y juvenil de la variante B1 de gangliosidosis GM2. Rev Neurol 1999;29:435–438.
174. Meek D, Wolfe LS, Andermann E, et al. Juvenile progressive dystonia: A new phenotype of GM2 gangliosiodsis. Ann Neurol 1984;15:348–352.
175. Hardie RJ, Young EP, and Morgan-Hughes JA. Hexosaminidase A deficiency presenting as juvenile progressive dystonia. J Neurol Neurosurg Psychiatry 1988;51:446–447.
176. Hardie RJ and Morgan-Hughes JA. Dystonia in GM2 gangliosidosis. Mov Disord 1992;7:390–391.
177. Nardocci N, Bertagnolio B, Rumi V, et al. Progressive dystonia symptomatic of juvenile GM2 gangliosidosis. 1992;Mov Disord 7:64–67.
178. Johnson WG. The clinical spectrum of hexosaminidase deficiency diseases. Neurology 1981;31:1453–1456.
179. Spence MW an dCallahan JW. Sphingomyelin cholesterol lipidoses: The Niemann Pick group of diseases. In Scriver CR, Beaudet Al, Sly WS, Valle D (eds), The Metabolic Basis of Inherited Disease, 6th ed. New York: McGraw-Hill, 1989, pp. 1655–1676.
180. Varier MT, Wenger DA, Comly ME, et al. Niemann Pick disease group C: Clinical variability and diagnosis based on defective cholesterol sterification: A collaborative study of 70 patients. Clin Genet 1988;33: 311–348.
181. Uc EY, Wenger DA, and Jankovic J. Niemann-Pick disease type C: Two cases and an update. Mov Disord 2000;15:1199–1203.
182. Watanabe Y, Akoboshi S, Ishida G, et al. Increased levels of GM2 ganglioside in fibroblasts from a patient

with juvenile Niemann-Pick disease type C. Brain Dev 1998;20:95–97.
183. Martin JJ, Loventhal A, Luteric C, Varier MT: Juvenile dystonic lipidosis (variant of Niemann Pick disease type C). J Neurol Sci 1984;66:33–45.
184. Pollen A, Fluharty AL, Fluharty EB, et al. Molecular basis of different forms of metachromatic leucodystrophy. N Engl J Med 1991;324:18–22.
185. Inui K, Emmett M and Wenger DA. Immunological evidence for deficiency in an activator protein for sulfatide sulfatase in a variant form of metachromatic leukodystrophy. Proc Natl Acad Sci U S A 1983;80:3074–3076.
186. Mihaljevic-Peles A, Jakkovljevis M, Milicevic Z, et al. Low arylsulphatase A activity in the development of psychiatric disorders. Neuropsychobiology 2001;43:75–78.
187. Berkovic SF, Carpenter S, Andermann F, et al. "Kufs" disease: A critical reappraisal. Brain 1988;111:27–62.
188. Simonati A, Santorum E, Tessa A, et al. A CLN2 gene nonsense mutation is associated with severe caudade atrophy and dystonia in LINCL. Neuropediatrics 2000;31: 199–201.
189. Yool DA, Edgar JM, Montague P, et al. The proteolipid protein gene and myelin disorders in man and animal models. Hum Mol Genet 2000;9:987–992.
190. Boulloche J and Aicardi A. Pelizaeus-Merzbacher disease: Clinical and nosological study. J Child Neurol 1986;1: 233–239.
191. Harding AE and Shapira A. Mitochondrial disease and movement disorders. In Jankovic J, Tolosa E (eds), Parkinson's Disease and Movement Disorders. Baltimore: Williams & Wilkins, 1993, pp. 569–583.
192. Hanna MG and Bhatia KP. Movement disorders and mitochondrial dysfunction. Curr Opin Neurol 1997;10:351–356.
193. Truong DD, Harding AE, and Scaravilli F. Movement disorders in mitochondrial myopathies: A report of nine cases with two autopsy studies. Mov Disord 1990;5: 109–117.
194. Bercovic SF, Karpati G, Carpenter S, et al. Progressive dystonia with bilateral putaminal hypodensities. Arch Neurol 1987;44:1184–1187.
195. Novotny EJ, Singh G, Wallace DC, et al. Leber's disease and dystonia: A mitochondrial disease. Neurology 1986;36:1053–1060.
196. Sudarski L, Plotkin GM, Logigian EL, et al. Dystonia as a presenting feature of the 3243 mitochondrial DNA mutation. Mov Disord 1999;14:488–491.
197. Macaya A, Munell F, Burke RE, et al. Disorders of movement in Leigh syndrome. Neuropediatrics 1993;24:60–67.
198. Lera G, Bhatia K, and Marsden CD. Dystonia as the major manifestation of Leigh's syndrome. Mov Disord 1994;9:642–649.
199. Munoz-Hiraldo ME, Martinez-Bermejo A, Gutierrez-Molina M, et al. Distonia como manifestacion principal en el sindrome de Leigh del lactante. An Esp Pediatr 1993;38:348–350.
200. Whetsell WO and Plaitakis A. Leigh's disease in an adult: Evidence of an "inhibitory factor" in family members. Ann Neurol 1978;3:529–534.
201. Leuzzi V, Bertini E, De Negri AM, et al. Bilateral striatal necrosis, dystonia and optic atrophy in two siblings. J Neurol Neurosurg Psychiatry 1992;55:16–19.
202. Bruyn GW, Bots GTAM, Went LN, et al. Hereditary optic neuropathy: Neuropathological findings. J Neurol Sci 1992;113:55–61.
203. Jun AS, Brown MD, and Walance DC. A mitochondrial DNA mutation at nucleotide pair 14459 of the NADH dehydrogenase subunit 6 gene associated with maternally inherited Leber hereditary optic neuropathy and dystonia. Proc Natl Acad Sci U S A 1994;91:6206–6210.
204. Kirby DM, Hons BS, Kahler SG, et al. Leigh disease caused by the mitochondrial DNA G14459A mutation in unrelated families. Ann Neurol 2000;48:102–104.
205. Walance DC. Mitochondrial DNA mutations in diseases of energy metabolism. J Bioeneg Biomembr 1994;26: 241–250.
206. Walance DC. Mitochondrial DNA sequence variation in human evolution and disease. Proc Natl Acad Sci U S A 1994;91:8739–8746.
207. Tranebjaerg L, Schwartz C, Eriksen H, et al. A new X linked recessive deafness syndrome with blindness, dystonia, fractures, and mental deficiency is linked to Xq22. J Med Genet 1995;32: 257–263.
208. Jin H, Kendall E, Freeman TC, et al. The human family of deafness dystonia peptide (DDP) related mitochondrial import proteins. Genomics 1999;61:259–267.
209. Koehler CM, Leuenberger D, Merchant S, et al. Human deafness dystonia syndrome is a mitochondrial disease. Proc Natl Acad Sci U S A 1999;96:2141–2146.
210. Kyllerman M, Skjeldal OH, Lundberg M, et al. Dystonia and dyskinesia in glutaric aciduria type I: Clinical heterogeneity and therapeutic considerations. Mov Disord 1994;9:22–30.
211. Voll R, Hoffmann GF, Lipinski CG, et al. Die Glutarazidamie/Glutarazidurie I as differential Diagnose der Chorea Minor. Klin Peadiatr 1993;205:124–126.
212. Al-Essa M, Bakheet S, Patay Z, et al. Fluoro-2-deoxyglucose (18FDG) PET scan of the brain in glutaric aciduria type 1: Clinical and MRI correlations. Brain Dev 1998;20:295–301.
213. Chow CW, Haan EA, Goodman SI, et al. Neuropathology of glutaric acidemia type I. Acta Neuropathol (Berl) 1988;75:590–594.
214. Lawrence Wolf B, Herberg KP, Hoffmann GF, et al. Entwicklung der Hirnatrophie. Therapie und Therapieuberwachung bei Glutarazidurie Typ 1 (Glutaryl-CoA Dehydrogenase-Mangel). Klin Paediatr 1993;205: 23–29.
215. Hauser SE and Peters H. Glutaric aciduria type I: An under-diagnosed cause of encephalopathy and dystonia-dyskinesia syndrome in children. J Paediatr Child Health 1998;34:302–304.
216. Heindenreich R, Natowicz M, Hainline BE, et al. Acute extrapyamidal syndrome in methylmalonic acidemia: "Metabolic stroke" involving the globus pallidus. J Pediatr 1988;113:1022–1027.
217. Roodhooft AM, Baumgartner ER, Martin JJ, et al. Symmetrical necrosis of the basal ganglia in methylmalonic acidemia. Eur J Pediatr 1990;149:582–584.
218. de Sousa C, Piesowicz AT, Brett EM, et al. Focal changes in the globi pallidi associated with neurological dysfunction in methylmalonic acidemia. Neuropediatrics 1989;20:119–201.

219. Shimoizumi H, Okabe I, Kodama H, et al. [Methylmalonic acidemia with bilateral MRI high intensities of the globus pallidus]. No To Hattatsu 1993;25:554–557.
220. Andreula CF, Blasi RD, and Carella A. CT and MR studies of methylmalonic acidemia. Am J Neuroradiol 1991;12:410–412.
221. Kerrigan JF, Aleck KA, Tarby TJ, et al. Fumaric aciduria: Clinical and imaging features. Ann Neurol 2000;47:583–588.
222. Bourgeron T, Chretien D, Poggi Bach J, et al. Mutation of the fumarase gene in two siblings with progressive encephalopathy and fumarase deficiency. J Clin Invest 1994;93:2514–2518.
223. Hagberg B, Hambraeus L, and Bensch K. A case of homocystinuria with a dystonia neurological syndrome. Neuropadiatrie 1970;1:337–343.
224. Davous P, Rondot P: Homocystinuria and dystonia. J Neurol Neurosurg Psychiatry 1983;46:283–286.
225. Arbour L, Rosenblatt B, Clow C, et al. Postoperative dystonia in a female patient with homocystinuria. J Pediatr 1988;113:863–864.
226. Kempster PA, Brenton DP, Gale AN, Stern GM: Dystonia in homocystinuria. J Neurol Neurosurg Psychiatry 1988;51:859–862.
227. Bernardelli A, Thompson PD, Zacagnini M, et al. Two sisters with generalized dystonia associated with homocystinuria. Mov Disord 1991;6:163–165.
228. Wada Y, Kita Y, Yamamoto T, et al. Homocystinuria with generalized chorea and other movement disorders: A case report. No To Shinkei 2000;52:629–631.
229. Sinclair AJ, Barling L, and Nightingale S. Recurrent Dystonia in homocystinuria: A metabolic pathogenesis. Mov Disord 2006;21:1780–1782.
230. Darras BT, Ampola MG, Dietz WH, Gilmore HE: Intermittent dystonia in Hartnup disease. Pediatr Neurol 1989;5:118–120.
231. Tamoush A, Alpers PH, Feigin RD, et al. Hartnup disease: Clinical, pathological and biochemical observations. Arch Neurol 1976;33:797–807.
232. Jankovic J, Caskey TC, Stout JT, et al. Lesch Nyhan syndrome: A study of motor behavior and CSF monoamine turnover. Ann Neurol 1988;23:466–469.
233. Adler CH and Wrabetz L. Lesch-Nyhan variant: Dystonia, ataxia, near-normal intelligence, and no self mutilation. Mov Disord 1996;11:583–584.
234. Garcia Puig J, Mateos FA, Jimenez ML, et al: Espectro clinico de la deficiencia de hipoxantina-guanina fosforribosiltransferasa: Estudio de 12 pacientes. Med Clin (Barc) 1994;14(102):681–687.
235. Ernst M, Zametkin AJ, Matochik JA, et al. Presynaptic dopaminergic deficits in Lesch-Nyhan disease. N Engl J Med 1996;334:1568–1572.
236. Adler CH and Caviness JN. Dystonia secondary to electrical injury: Surface electromyographic evaluation and implications for the organicity of the condition. J Neurol Sci 1997;148:187–192.
237. Ondo W. Lingual dystonia following electrical injury. Mov Disord 1997;12:253.
238. Boonkongchuen P an dLees A. Case of torticollis following electrical injury. Mov Disord 1996;11:109, .
239. Tarsy D, Sudarsky L, and Charness ME. Limb dystonia following electric injury. Mov Disord 1994;9:230–232.
240. Panchenko EN, Kazakova SE, Safonova EF: Nervnye narusheniia u likvidatorov avarii na Chernobyl'skoi AES, podvergavshikhsia vozdeistviiu ioniziruiushchego izlucheniia v malykh dozakh. Vrach Delo 1993;8: 13–16.
241. Ushkova IN and Koshelev NF. Kliniko-gigienicheskie i eksperimental'nye obosnovaniia nozologii lazernoi bolezni. Vrach Delo 1994;2:63–68.
242. Friedman J and Standaert DG. Dystonia and its disorders. Neurol Clin 2001;19:681–705.
243. Van Harten P, Hoek HW, and Kahn RS. Acute dystonia induced by drug treatment. BMJ 1999;319:623–626.
244. Llau ME, Senard JM, Rascol O, et al. Therapie 1995;50: 425–427.
245. Jankovic J. Tardive syndromes and other drug-induced movement disorders. Clin Neuropharmacol 1995;18: 197–214.
246. Gay CT and Ryan SG. Paroxysmal kinesigenic dystonia after methylphenidate administration. J Child Neurol 1994;9:45–46.
247. Humphreys A and Tanner AR. Acute dystonic drug reaction or tetanus? An unusual consequence of a 'Whizz' overdose. Hum Exp Toxicol 1994;13:311–312.
248. Saltz B, Woerner MG, Robinson DG, et al. Side effects of antipsychotic drugs. Postgrad Med 2000;107:169–178.
249. Kiriakakis V, Bhatia KP, Quinn NP, et al. The natural history of tardive dystonia. A long -term follow up study of 107 cases. Brain 1998;121:2053–2066.
250. Van Harten PN, Hoek HW, Matroos GE, et al: Intermittent neuroleptic treatment and risk for tardive dyskinesia: Curaçao Extrapyramidal Syndromes Study III. Am J Psychiatry 1998;155:565–567.
251. Tarsy D and Baldessarini RJ. Epidemiology of Tardive Dyskinesia: Is Risk Declining With Modern Antipsychotics? Mov Disord 2006;21: 589–598.
252. Soares KVS, McGrath JJ: Anticholinergic medication for neuroleptic-induced tardive dyskinesia. Cochrane Library 2001:Issue 1.
253. Caligiuri MR, Jeste DV, and Lacro JP. Antipsychotic-induced movement disorders in the elderly: epidemiology and treatment recommendations. Drugs Aging 2000;17:363–384.
254. Simpson GM. The treatment of tardive dyskinesia and tardive dystonia. J Clin Psychiatry 2000;61(suppl 4): 39–44.
255. Burke RE, Fahn S, Jankovic J, et al. Tardive dystonia: Late onset and persistent dystonia caused by antipsychotic drugs. Neurology 1982;32:1335–1346.
256. Giménez Roldán S, Mateo D, and Bartolome P. Tardive dystonia and severe tardive dyskinesia. Acta Psychiat Scand 1985;71:488–494.
257. Barbeau A, Inoue N, and Cloutier T. Role of manganese in dystonia. Adv Neurol 1976;14:339–352.
258. Pal PK, Samii A, and Calne DB. Manganese neurotoxicity: A review of clinical features, imaging and pathology. Neurotoxicology 1999;20:227–238.
259. Danks DM. Copper-induced dystonia secondary to cholestatic liver disease. Lancet 1990;335:410.
260. Janavs JL and Aminoff MJ. Dystonia and chorea in acquired systemic disorders. J Neurol Neurosurg Psychiatry 1998;65:436–444.

261. Ross DR. Methanol induced dystonia. Can J Neurol Sci 1990;97:155–162.
262. Borgohain R, Singh AK, Radhakrishna H, et al. Delayed onset generalised dystonia after cyanide poisoning. Clin Neurol Neurosurg 1995;97:213–215.
263. Valenzuela R, Court J, and Godoy J. Delayed cyanide induced dystonia. J Neurol Neurosurg Psychiatry 1992;55:198–199.
264. Carella F, Grassi MP, Savoiardo M, et al. Dystonic-parkinsonian syndrome after cyanide poisoning: Clinical and MRI findings. J Neurol Neurosurg Psychiatry 1988;51:1345–1348.
265. Choi IS and Cheon HY. Delayed movement disorders after carbon monoxide poisoning. Eur Neurol 1999;42:141–144.
266. Choi IS. Delayed neurologic sequelae in carbon monoxide intoxication. Arch Neurol 1983;40:433–435.
267. De Yebenes JG and de Yebenes PG. La distonia en la pintura de Matias Grunewald. El ergotismo epidemico en la baja Edad Media. Arch Neurobiol 1991;54:37–40.
268. Quinn NP. Dystonia in epidemic ergotism. Neurology 1983;33:1267.
269. He F, Zhang S, Quian F, and Zhang C. Delayed dystonia with striatal CT lucencies induced by a mycotoxin (3-nitropropionic acid). Neurology 1995;45:2178–2183.
270. Spencer PS, Ludolph AC, and Kisby GE. Neurologic diseases associated with use of plant components with toxic potential. Environ Res 1993;62:106–113.
271. Thornton A, McKenna PJ. Acute dystonic reaction complicated by psychotic phenomena. Br J Psychiatry 1994;164:115–118.
272. Batshaw ML, Wachtel RC, Deckel AW, et al. Munchausen's syndrome simulating torsion dystonia. N Engl J Med 1985;312:1437–1439.
273. Marsden D. Psychogenic problems associated with dystonia. Adv Neurol 1995;65:319–326.
274. Factor SA, Podskalny GD, and Molho ES. Psychogenic movement disorders: Frequency, clinical profile, and characteristics. J Neurol Neurosurg Psychiatry 1995;59: 406–412.
275. Feinstein A, Stergiopoulos V, Fine J, et al. Psychiatric outcome in patients with a psychogenic movement disorder: A prospective study. Neuropsychiatry Neuropsychol Behav Neurol 2001;14:169–176.
276. Owens DG: Extrapyramidal side effects and tolerability of risperidone: A review. J Clin Psychiatry 1994;55(suppl):29–35.
277. Casey DE. Motor and mental aspects of acute extrapyramidal syndromes. Acta Psychiatr Scand Suppl 1994;380: 14–20.
278. Khanna R, Damodaran SS, and Chakraborty SP. Overflow movements may predict neuroleptic-induced dystonia. Biol Psychiatry 1994;35:491–492.
279. Malhotra AK, Litman RE, and Pickar D. Adverse effects of antipsychotic drugs. Drug Saf 1993;9:429–436.
280. Sachdev P. Risk factors for tardive dystonia: A case control comparison with tardive dyskinesia. Acta Psychiatr Scand 1993;88:98–103.
281. Sachdev P. Clinical characteristics of 15 patients with tardive dystonia. Am J Psychiatry 1993;150:498–500.
282. Meltzer LT, Christoffersen CL, Serpa KA, et al. Lack of involvement of haloperidol-sensitive sigma binding sites in modulation of dopamine neuronal activity and induction of dystonias by antipsychotic drugs. Neuropharmacology 1992;31:961–967.
283. Yassa R, Nastase C, Dupont D, et al. Tardive dyskinesia in elderly psychiatric patients: A 5-year study. Am J Psychiatry 1992;149:1206–1211.
284. Chiu H, Shum P, Lau J, et al: Prevalence of tardive dyskinesia, tardive dystonia, and respiratory dyskinesia among Chinese psychiatric patients in Hong Kong. Am J Psychiatry 1992;149: 1081–1085.
285. Khanna R, Das A, and Damodaran SS. Prospective study of neuroleptic-induced dystonia in mania and schizophrenia. Am J Psychiatry 1992;149:511–513.
286. Wojcik JD, Falk WE, Fink JS, et al: A review of 32 cases of tardive dystonia. Am J Psychiatry 1991;148:1055–1059.
287. Matsumoto RR, Hemstreet MK, and Lai NL. Drug specificity of pharmacological dystonia. Pharmacol Biochem Behav 1990;36:151–155.
288. Shorten GD, Srithran S, and Hendron M. Pseudo-tetanus following trifluoperazine. Ulster Med J 1990;59:221–222.
289. Ernst M, Gonzalez NM, and Campbell M. Acute dystonic reaction with low-dose pimozide. J Am Acad Child Adolesc Psychiatry 1993;32:640–642.
290. Vaamonde J, GonzÁlez JM, HernÁndez A, et al. Writer's cramp induced by olanzapine. J Neurol 2001;248:422.
291. Jonnalagada JR and Norton JW. Acute dystonia with quetiapine. Clin Neuropharmacol 2000;23:229–230.
292. Dunayevich E and Strakowski S. Olanzapine-induced tardive dystonia. Am J Psychiatry 1999;156:1662.
293. Vercueil L and Foucher J. Risperidone-induced tardive dystonia and psychosis. Lancet 1999;353:981.
294. Krebs MO and Olie JP. Tardive dystonia induced by risperidone. Can J Psychiatry 1999;44:507–508.
295. Simpson GM and Lindemayer JP. Extrapyramidal symptoms in patients treated with risperidone. J Clin Psychopharmacol 1997;17:194–201.
296. Tollefson GD, Beasley CM, Tamura RN, et al. Blind, controlled, long-term study of the comparative incidence of treatment-emergent tardive dyskinesia with olanzapine or haloperidol. Am J Psychiatry 1997;154: 1248–1253.
297. Faulk R, Gilmore JH, Jensen EW, et al. Risperidone-induced dystonic reaction. Am J Psychiatry 1996;153:577.
298. Miller LG and Jankovic J. Neurologic approach to drug-induced movement disorders: A study of 125 patients. South Med J 1990;83:525–532.
299. Dickson R, Williams R, and Dalby JT. Dystonic reaction and relapse with clozapine discontinuation and risperidone initiation. Can J Psychiatry 1994;39:184.
300. Thomas P, Lalaux N, Vaiva G, et al. Dose-dependent stuttering and dystonia in a patient taking clozapine. Am J Psychiatry 1994;151:1096.
301. Kastrup O, Gastpar M, and Schwarz M. Acute dystonia due to clozapine. J Neurol Neurosurg Psychiatry 1994; 57:119.
302. Ganzini L, Casey DE, Hoffman F, et al. The prevalence of metoclopramide-induced tardive dyskinesia and acute extrapyramidal movement disorders. Arch Intern Med 1993;153:1469–1475.
303. Sempere AP, Mola S, Flores J. Distonia tardia tras la administración de clebopride. Rev Neurol 1997;25:2060.

304. Angelini L, Zorzi G, Rumi V, et al. Transient paroxysmal dystonia in an infant possibly induced by cisapride. Ital J Neurol Sci 1996;17:157–159.
305. Cory DA. Adverse reaction to metoclopramide during enteroclysis. AJR Am J Roentgenol 1994;163:480.
306. Guala A, Mittino D, Ghini T, et al. Le distonie da metoclopramide sono familiari? Pediatr Med Chir 1992;14: 617–618.
307. Guala A, Mittino D, Fabbrocini P, Ghini T. Familial metoclopramide-induced dystonic reactions. Mov Disord 1992;7:385–386.
308. Lauterbach EC. Haloperidol-induced dystonia and parkinsonism on discontinuing metoclopramide: Implications for differential thalamocortical activity. J Clin Psychopharmacol 1992;12:442–443.
309. Gabellini AS, Pezzoli A, De Massis P, et al. Veralipride-induced tardive dystonia in a patient with bipolar psychosis. Ital J Neurol Sci 1992;13:621–623.
310. Linazasoro G, Marti Masso JF, Olasagasti B: Acute dystonia induced by sulpiride. Clin Neuropharmacol 1991;14: 463–464.
311. Factor SA and Matthews MK. Persistent extrapyramidal syndrome with dystonia and rigidity caused by combined metoclopramide and prochlorperazine therapy. South Med J 1991;84:626–628.
312. Bonuccelli U, Nocchiero A, Napolitano A, et al. Domperidone-induced acute dystonia and polycystic ovary syndrome. Mov Disord 1991;6:79–81.
313. Miller LG and Jankovic J. Sulpiride-induced tardive dystonia. Mov Disord 1990;5:83–84.
314. Tait P, Balzer R, and Buchanan N. Metoclopramide side effects in children. Med J Aust 1990;152:387.
315. McCann UD, Penetar DM, and Belenky G. Acute dystonic reaction in normal humans caused by catecholamine depletion. Clin Neuropharmacol 1990;13:565–568.
316. Burke RE, Reches A, Traub MM, et al: Tetrabenazine induces acute dystonic reactions. Ann Neurol 1985;17: 200–202.
317. Jimenez Jimenez FJ, Vazquez A, Garcia Ruiz P, et al. Chronic hemidystonia following acute dystonic reaction to thiethylperazine. J Neurol Neurosurg Psychiatry 1991;54:562.
318. Olsen JC, Keng JA, Clark JA: Frequency of adverse reactions to prochlorperazine in the ED. Am J Emerg Med S 2000;18:609–611.
319. Joseph MM and King WD. Dystonic reaction following recommended use of cold syrup. Ann Emerg Med 1995;26:749–751.
320. Etzel JV. Diphenhydramine-induced acute dystonia. Pharmacotherapy 1994;14:492–496.
321. Fahn S. The spectrum of levodopa-induced dyskinesias. Ann Neurol 2000;47(suppl 1):S1–S11.
322. Bejjani BB, Arnulf I, Damier P, et al. Levodopa-induced dyskinesias in Parkinson's disease: Is sensitization reversible? Ann Neurol 2000;47:655–658.
323. Zimmerman TR Jr, Sage JI, Lang AE, et al. Severe evening dyskinesias in advanced Parkinson's disease: Clinical description, relation to plasma levodopa, and treatment. Mov Disord 1994;9:173–177.
324. Marconi R, Lefebvre Caparros D, Bonnet AM, et al. Levodopainduced dyskinesias in Parkinson's disease: Phenomenology and pathophysiology. Mov Disord 1994;9:2–12 .
325. Bravi D, Mouradian MM, Roberts JW, et al: End-of-dose dystonia in Parkinson's disease. Neurology 1993;43: 2130–2131.
326. Rupniak NM, Boyce S, Steventon MJ, et al. Dystonia induced by combined treatment with L-DOPA and MK-801 in parkinsonian monkeys. Ann Neurol 1992;32:103–105.
327. Mark MH, Sage JI: Levodopa-associated hemifacial dystonia. Mov Disord 6:383, 1991.
328. Leiguarda R, Merello M, Sabe L, et al. Bromocriptine-induced dystonia in patients with aphasia and hemiparesis. Neurology 1993;43:2319–2322.
329. Peacock L, Lublin H, and Gerlach J. The effects of dopamine D1 and D2 receptor agonists and antagonists in monkeys withdrawn from long-term neuroleptic treatment. Eur J Pharmacol 1990;186:49–59.
330. Mitchell IJ, Luquin R, Boyce S, et al: Neural mechanisms of dystonia: Evidence from a 2-deoxyglucose uptake study in a primate model of dopamine agonist-induced dystonia. Mov Disord 1990;5:49–54.
331. Van Harten N, Van Trier J, Horwitz EH, et al. Cocaine as a risk factor of neuroleptic-induced acute dystonia. J Clin Psychiatry 1998;59:128–130.
332. Cardoso FE and Jankovic J. Cocaine-related movement disorders. Mov Disord 1993;8:175–178.
333. Hegarty AM, Lipton RB, Merriam AE, et al. Cocaine as a risk factor for acute dystonic reactions. Neurology 1991;41:1670–1672.
334. Farrell PE, Diehl AK: Acute dystonic reaction to crack cocaine. Ann Emerg Med 20:322, 1991.
335. Heath HW, Allen JK: Acute dystonia following standard doses of cold medicine containing phenylpropanolamine. Clin Pediatr 1997;36:57–58.
336. Prior A, Bertolasi L, Berardelli A, Manfredi M: Acute dystonic reactions to ecstasy. Mov Disord 1995;10:353.
337. Thiel A and Dressler D. Dyskinesias possibly induced by norpseudoephedrine. J Neurol 1994;241:167–169.
338. Capstick C, Checkley S, Gray J, et al. Dystonia induced by amphetamine and haloperidol. Br J Psychiatry 1994;165:276.
339. Vandel P, Bonin B, Leveque E, et al: Tricyclic antidepressant-induced extrapyramidal side effects. Eur Neuropsychopharmacol 1997;7:207–212.
340. Ornadel D, Barnes EA,and Dick DJ: Acute dystonia due to amitryptiline. J Neurol Neurosurg Psychiatry 1992;55:414.
341. Matot JP, Ziegler M, Olie JP, et al. Amoxapine. An antidepressant responsible for extrapyramidal side effects? Therapie 1985;40:187–190.
342. Jarecke CR and Reid PJ. Acute dystonic reaction induced by a monoamine oxidase inhibitor. J Clin Psychopharmacol 1990;10:144–145.
343. Olson WL. Dystonia and reflex sympathetic dystrophy induced by ergotamine. Mov Disord 1992;7:188–189.
344. Merello MJ, Nogues MA, Leiguarda RC, et al. Dystonia and reflex sympathetic dystrophy induced by ergo-tamine. Mov Disord 1992;7:188–189.
345. Gerber PE and Lynd LD. Selective serotonin-reuptake inhibitor-induced movement disorders. Ann Pharmacother 1998;32:692–698.

346. Lauterbach EC, Meyer JM, and Simpson GM: Clinical manifestations of dystonia and dyskinesia after SSRI administration. J Clin Psychiatry 1997;58:403–404.
347. Poyurovsky M, Schneidman M, and Weizman A. Successful treatment of fluoxetin-induced dystonia with low dose mianserin. Mov Disord 1997;12:1102–1104.
348. Pies RW.Must we now consider SRIs as neuroleptics? J Clin Psychopharmacol 1997;17:443–445.
349. Leo RJ.Movement disorders associated with the serotonin selective reuptake inhibitors. J Clin Psychiatry 1996;57:449–454.
350. Shihabuddin L and Rapport D. Sertraline and extrapyramidal side effects. Am J Psychiatry 1994;151:288.
351. Dave M. Fluoxetine-associated dystonia. Am J Psychiatry 1994;151:149.
352. George MS and Trimble MR. Dystonic reaction associated with fluvoxamine. J Clin Psychopharmacol 1993;13: 220–221.
353. Rio J, Molins A, Viguera ML, et al. Distonia aguda por fluoxetina. Med Clin (Barc) 1992;99:436–437.
354. Lock JD, Gwirtsman HE, and Targ EF: Possible adverse drug interactions between fluoxetine and other psychotropics. J Clin Psychopharmacol 1990;10: 383–384.
355. Reccoppa L, Welch WA, and Ware MR. Acute dystonia and fluoxetine. J Clin Psychiatry 1990;51:487.
356. Adityanjee and Lindenmeyer JP. Precipitation of dystonia by m-CPP in a schizophrenic patient treated with haloperidol. Am J Psychiatry 1993;150:837–838.
357. Miyaoka T, Seno H, Yamamori C, et al. Pisa syndrome due to a cholinesterase inhibitor (donepezil): A case report. J Clin Psychiatry 2001;62:573–574.
358. Kwak YT, Han IW, and Baik J. Relation between cholinesterase inhibitor and Pisa syndrome. Lancet 2000;355:2222.
359. LeWitt PA, Walters A, Hening W, et al. Persistent movement disorders induced by buspirone. Mov Disord 1993;8:331–334.
360. Boylan K. Persistent dystonia associated with buspirone. Neurology 1990;40:1904.
361. Kappler J, Menges C, Ferbert A, et al. Schwere "Spat" Dystonie nach "Neuroleptanxiolyse" mit Fluspirilen. Nervenarzt 1994;65:668.
362. Stones M, Kennie DC, and Fulton JD. Dystonic dysphagia associated with fluspirilene. BMJ 1990;301:668–669.
363. Rittmann M and Steegmanns Schwarz I: Schwere Spatdystonie unter Fluspirilen. Dtsch Med Wochenschr 1991;116:1613.
364. Laux G and Gunreben G. Schwere Spatdystonie unter Fluspirilen. Dtsch Med Wochenschr 1991;116:977–980.
365. Perez Trullen JM, Modrego Pardo PJ, Vazquez Andre M, et al. Bromazepam-induced dystonia. Biomed Pharmacother 1992;46:375–376.
366. Tolarek IH and Ford MJ. Acute dystonia induced by midazolam and abolished by flumazenil. BMJ 1990;300:614.
367. Lee JW. Persistent dystonia associated with carbamazepine therapy: A case report. N Z Med J 1994;107: 360–361.
368. Lee JW. Persistent dystonia associated with carbamazepine therapy: A case report. N Z Med J 1994;107:360–361.
369. Soman P, Jain S, Rajsekhar V, et al. Dystonia: A rare manifestation of carbamazepine toxicity. Postgrad Med J 1994;70:54–55.
370. Reynolds EH and Trimble MR. Adverse neuropsychiatric effects of anticonvulsant drugs. Drugs 1985;29:570–581.
371. Moss W, Ojukwu C, and Chiriboga CA. Phenytoin-induced movement disorder. Unilateral presentation in a child and response to diphenhydramine. Clin Pediatr (Phila) 1994;33:634–638.
372. Lacayo A and Mitra N. Report of a case of phenobarbital-induced dystonia. Clin Pediatr (Phila) 1992;31:252.
373. Palomeras E, Sanz P, Cano A, et al. Dystonia in a patient treated with propranolol and gabapentin. Arch Neurol 2000;57:570–571.
374. Reeves AL, So EL, Sharbrough FW, et al. Movement disorder associated with the use of gabapentin. Epilepsia 1996;37:988–990.
375. Wolanczyk T and Grabowska A. Transient dystonia in three patients treated with tiagabine. Epilepsia 2001;42:944–946.
376. Bernard JM, Le Roux D, Pereon Y: Acute dystonia during sevofluorane induction. Anesthesiology 1999;90: 1215–1216.
377. Hussein G, Olejniczak P, Carey M, et al. Propofol-induced dystonia: A case report and a review of the literature. Clin Res Regul Affairs 1999;16:175–181.
378. Reddy RV, Moorthy SS, Dierdorf SF, et al. Excitatory effects and electroencephalographic correlation of etomidate, thiopental, methohexital, and propofol. Anesth Analg 1993;77:1008–1011.
379. Mets B. Acute dystonia after alfentanil in untreated Parkinson's disease. Anesth Analg 1991;72:557–558.
380. Riley D. Disulfiram induced dystonia. Mov Disord 1992;7:188–192.
381. Riley D. Pallidal and putaminal lesions resulting from disulfiram intoxication. Mov Disord 1991;6:166–170.
382. Krauss JK, Mohadjer M, Wakhlo AK, et al. Dystonia and akinesia due to pallidoputaminal lesions after disulfiram intoxication. Mov Disord 1991;6:166–170.
383. Brady W and Hall K. Erythromycin-related dystonic reaction. Am J Emerg Med 1992;10:616.
384. Achumba JI, Ette E, Thomas WO, et al. Chloroquine-induced acute dystonic reactions in the presence of metronidazole. Drug Intell Clin Pharm 1988;22:308–310.
385. Miller LG and Jankovic J. Persistent dystonia possibly induced by flecainide. Mov Disord 1992;7:62–63.
386. Kapur V, Barber KR, and Peddireddy R. Ranitidine-induced acute dystonia. Am J Emerg Med 1999;17:258–260.
387. Davis BJ, Aull EA, Granner MA, et al. Ranitidine-induced cranial dystonia. Clin Neuropharmacol 1994;17:489–491.
388. Peiris RS and Peckler BF. Cimetidine-induced dystonic reaction. J Emerg Med 2001;21:27–29.
389. Oterino A and Pascual J. Sumatriptan-induced axial dystonia in a patient with cluster headache. Cephalalgia 1998;18:360–361.
390. Lopez M, Ferrer C, and Bernacer B. Akathisia and acute dystonia induced by sumatriptan. J Neurol 1997;244: 131–133.
391. Saneto RP, Fitch JA, and Cohen BH. Acute neurotoxicity of meperidine in an infant. Pediatr Neurol 1996;14: 339–341.

392. Micheli FE, Fernandez MM, and Giannaula R. Movement disorders and depression due to flunarizine and cinnarizine. Mov Disord 1989;4:139–146.
393. Kawakami T, Takiyama Y, Yanaka I, et al: Chronic bromvalerylurea intoxication: Dystonic posture and cerebellar ataxia due to nonsteroidal anti-inflammatory drug abuse. Intern Med 1998;37:788–791.
394. Brashear A and Siemers E. Focal dystonia after chemotherapy: A case series. J Neurooncol 1997;34:163–167.
395. Ghadirian A, Annable L, Belanger MC, et al. A cross-sectional study of parkinsonism and tardive dyskinesia in lithium-treated affective disordered patients. J Clin Psychiatry 1996;57:22–28.
396. Mascias J, Perez OS, Chaverri D, et al. Distonia aguda secundaria a tratamiento ccon betahistina. Neurologia 2000;15:417.
397. Frumkin H. Multiple system atrophy following chronic carbon disulfide exposure. Environ Health Perspect 1998;106:611–613.

IV. CHOREATIC DISORDERS: HUNTINGTON'S DISEASE

CHAPTER 32

Genetics and Molecular Biology of Huntington's Disease

James F. Gusella, Marcy E. Macdonald, and Vanessa C. Wheeler

▶ HISTORY AND EPIDEMIOLOGY

In 1872, George Huntington described a unique ailment involving characteristic involuntary movements that begin insidiously, usually in middle age, and progress gradually until the victim is consumed by full-blown chorea.[1] His description was based on his observations of families with the disorder in his clinical practice as a family physician in East Hampton, on Long Island, New York. As members of the same families had been cared for by his father and grandfather, who were also physicians, Huntington was attuned to the inherited nature of the peculiar disorder. He described frequent transmission of the defect from either an affected mother or an affected father to offspring, with no skipping of generations. Huntington also noted that "if by any chance these children go through life without it, the thread is broken and the children and great grandchildren of the original shakers may rest assured that they are free from the disease." This pattern of transmission was recognized as the result of a mendelian autosomal-dominant defect by Osler in 1908.[2] Indeed, Vessie[3] later traced many of the Long Island families to immigrants from Bures, England, who landed in New England in 1649, confirming Huntington's description of this hereditary chorea as "an heirloom from generations away back in the dim past." George Huntington's accurate, lucid, and succinct description of this nightmarish affliction led to its appellation of Huntington's chorea, subsequently changed to Huntington's disease (HD), as its manifestations are not limited to loss of motor control.

Although Huntington believed that the disorder existed only in eastern Long Island, it is now known to be widespread throughout the world. The prevalence is highest in populations of western European ancestry, in which 4–7 persons/100,000 are affected.[4] However, the actual disease gene frequency is 2.5–3 times higher, as HD typically has its onset only in midlife, and, at any given time, two thirds of gene carriers have yet to become symptomatic. The prevalence is relatively consistent across Europe and in other regions of the world that have populations of western European descent, with the exception of Finland, where a significantly lower rate reflects this population's restricted genetic origin. HD is also seen in Africans and Asians, although with a much lower prevalence.

Many of the early studies of HD concentrated on its familial nature, documenting large kindreds in which the defect was passed from generation to generation. HD, as an autosomal-dominant disorder, is transmitted equally from males and females, and both sexes have a 50:50 chance of inheriting the defect. The disease gene is highly penetrant, but onset is variable, ranging from early childhood to late in life. As most cases manifest in middle age, the *HD* gene is often passed on to children before the parent is aware of the disorder. The rare cases of juvenile onset (<15 years of age) are usually inherited from an affected father.[5,6]

HD is currently untreatable, except for palliative care, and its victims are condemned to slow, inexorable progression of their disease that ends in death 10–20 years after onset. The progression of the motor symptoms of HD is accompanied by intellectual decline and psychiatric alterations, all of which are ultimately due to a selective loss of neurons in the brain. The most prominent region affected is the striatum, where medium-sized spiny neurons are lost along the posteroanterior, dorsoventral, and mediolateral axes, leading to destruction of the architecture of the caudate nucleus.[7]

▶ GENETIC LINKAGE APPROACH

The high penetrance, late onset, and characteristic clinical manifestations, which combine to produce large identifiable disease families (Fig. 32–1), made this disorder the ideal candidate for pioneering a novel strategy that emerged in the early 1980s for establishing the chromosomal location of a genetic defect.[8] This approach relied on merging the tenets of mendelian inheritance with the power of recombinant DNA technology, using naturally occurring variations in DNA

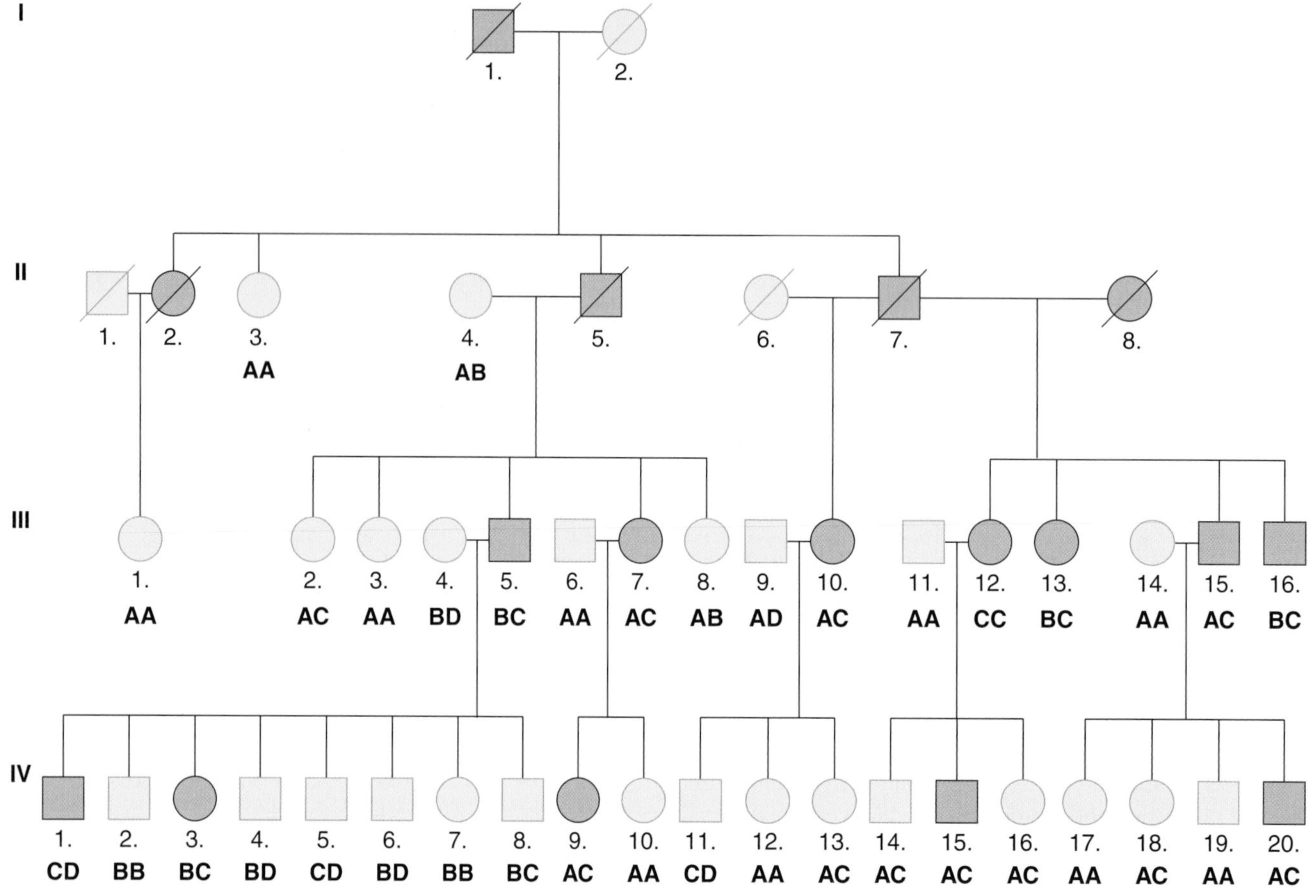

Figure 32–1. An idealized HD pedigree showing cosegregation of *D4S10* with the disorder. An imaginary four generation (I–IV) HD pedigree is shown with genotypes for the *D4S10* marker (four alleles: A, B, C, D) shown under the symbol for each living family member. In each generation, the family members are numbered sequentially. Circles and squares denote females and males, respectively. Slashed symbols indicate deceased individuals. Filled symbols represent those individuals clinically diagnosed with HD. Individuals II–5 and II–7 are monozygotic twins. The disorder is segregating in this pedigree with the C allele of *D4S10*. As this marker displays 4% recombination with *HD*, all individuals who inherit the C allele from their affected parent have a 96% chance of also having inherited the *HD* defect. Individual II–8 is an HD-affected individual who married into the pedigree and, with II–7, produced progeny at risk of having two copies of the *HD* defect.

sequence as highly informative genetic markers to search for genetic linkage with the disease gene. The goal was to discover a polymorphic DNA marker that co-segregates with the disorder in families and thereby infers the presence of the disease gene in the same chromosomal vicinity. It would then be possible to identify the genetic defect on the basis of its chromosomal location, without any additional knowledge of its biochemical nature.

Previous genetic linkage studies of *HD* (the Huntington's disease gene) had used a limited panel of expressed polymorphic systems, blood group antigens, and serum enzymes that permitted only 15% of the autosomal genome to be searched.[9] The concept of DNA markers offered a potential route to making the remaining 85% of the genome accessible to examination, but only a handful of DNA markers had been described. These were restriction fragment-length polymorphisms (RFLPs), detected by using single-copy human DNA clones to probe genomic DNA blots for variations in restriction fragment size that reflected differences in the primary DNA sequence. As RFLP markers were generated, they were tested for genetic linkage to *HD* in two large pedigrees, one of American and one of Venezuelan origin. In 1983, success came quickly, as one of the initial 13 RFLP markers tested revealed strong genetic linkage to the disorder[10] (see Fig. 32–1). This marker, *D4S10*, consisting of two *Hind*III polymorphisms detected by an anonymous DNA probe (G8), placed *HD* on the short arm of chromosome 4 (Fig. 32–2). There were no crossovers between the marker and *HD*, either in a large section of the Venezuela pedigree or in the

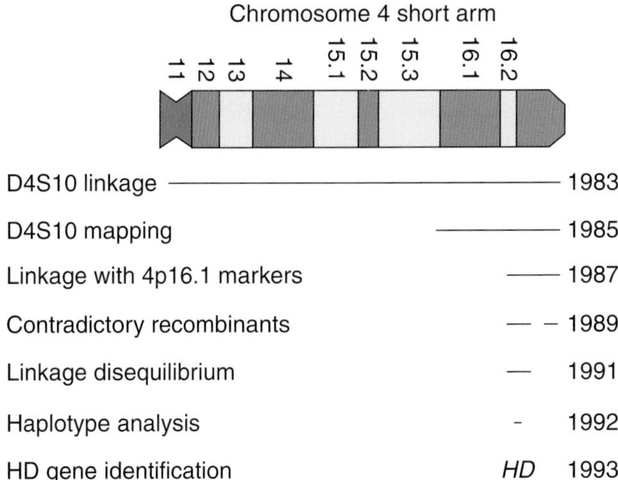

Figure 32–2. Progressive narrowing of the *HD* gene search. In 1983, genetic linkage with *D4S10* assigned the *HD* gene to chromosome 4. The horizontal lines below the schematic diagram of the chromosome 4 short arm depict the chronology of the *HD* search (1983–1993), as the candidate region was progressively narrowed using the techniques listed and described in the text.

independent American HD family with 14 affected members, producing odds of greater than 100 million to 1 in favor of genetic linkage. This was the first example of mapping a genetic defect to a human chromosome using only genetic linkage to a DNA polymorphism, without any prior clue to the disease gene's nature or location. This approach was replicated subsequently in a host of different disorders and has become increasingly sophisticated as newer and more informative markers were elaborated, the human genetic map became increasingly detailed and the human genome was eventually sequenced. Indeed, the success of the linkage strategy, and the opportunities that it created for isolating disease genes via their chromosomal location, provided a major impetus for undertaking the Human Genome Initiative to map and sequence the human genome.

▶ GENETIC AND PHYSICAL MAPPING OF THE *HD* REGION

The anonymous DNA marker, *D4S10*, genetically linked to *HD*, was initially assigned to chromosome 4 by hybridization of the G8 probe to a panel of human × mouse somatic cell hybrid lines that had segregated various human chromosomes.[10] The marker was then regionally assigned to the terminal cytogenetic band of the chromosome 4 short arm, because it was hemizygous (present in a single copy) in patients with Wolf–Hirschhorn syndrome, a congenital anomaly caused by heterozygous deletion on 4p.[11] Several groups later confirmed this assignment by in situ hybridization to metaphase chromosomes.[12–14] Genotyping of HD families revealed that the *HD* gene is located on chromosome 4 in all of the families tested, yielding no evidence of other genes that can cause both the clinical symptoms and neuropathological correlates of HD (nonallelic heterogeneity).[15] These same investigations made HD the first genetic disorder in man established to be completely dominant. Several individuals who were homozygous for the *HD* defect, having inherited a disease allele from both parents, were found to be clinically indistinguishable from typical heterozygous *HD* gene carriers.[16,17] This surprising result indicated that, in *HD* heterozygotes, the remaining normal allele does not act to delay the disease process or alter its manifestation, and two doses of the defective gene are not significantly more damaging than a single dose.

The position of the *HD* defect relative to the cytogenetic map could be determined only indirectly, by linkage analysis with *D4S10* and other surrounding DNA markers. *HD* and *D4S10* displayed 4% recombination, placing the disease gene within about 4×10^6 base pairs (bp) of DNA either centromeric or telomeric to the DNA marker (Fig. 32–2). DNA markers were identified centromeric to *D4S10* in 4p16, using Wolf–Hirschhorn patients with different extents of 4p16 deletion. When the highly polymorphic 4p16.1 marker *RAF1P1* (then known as *RAF2*) was typed in the same HD kindreds as *D4S10*, it revealed additional crossovers, indicating that the disease gene must be located telomeric to both DNA markers.[18] This assigned the *HD* gene to the 4p16.3 subband, between *D4S10* and the short-arm telomere, a segment corresponding to about 0.2% of the genome, or 6 million bp of DNA (Fig. 32–2).

The chromosomal localization of the *HD* gene, and, subsequently, many other genetic defects, created the need to improve standard mapping methods and develop new techniques to clone genes based on their map location, without a knowledge of the protein defect involved. As with the DNA marker linkage approach, the search for the *HD* gene also acted as the proving ground for several of these technologies. The initial stages of more detailed mapping in 4p16.3 were aided by the construction of regional somatic cell hybrid panels that permitted rapid assignment and ordering of new DNA probes to several regions of 4p16.[19,20] These hybrid panels acted as a backbone upon which more sophisticated approaches, such as radiation hybrid mapping[21,22] and pulsed-field gel electrophoresis,[23] could be appended. Numerous novel sources of DNA probes, including phage libraries of flow-sorted chromosome 4 DNA, chromosome 4-enriched somatic cell hybrid genomic libraries, chromosome "jumping" libraries, *Not* I "linking" clones, P1 clones, yeast artificial chromosome clones, combined with pulsed-field gel electrophoresis, and somatic cell hybrid mapping eventually produced a physical map that spanned 5×10^6 bp in 4p16.3 (Fig. 32–2).[24–26]

Because the *HD* gene had been assigned to 4p16.3, using only genetic linkage techniques, and because there was no physical rearrangement of the region associated with the disorder, the only means of locating the defect on the physical map was to construct a parallel genetic map by tracking the inheritance of informative DNA markers through normal and HD pedigrees. Although RFLP markers, like *D4S10*, were used initially, successive generations of newer, more informative markers were added to the map as they emerged. First, variable numbers of tandem repeat (VNTR) markers, detected like RFLPs by DNA blotting but displaying many different potential restriction fragment sizes as a result of variation in the copy number and, therefore, length, of a repeated DNA motif located between two restriction sites, were found to be particularly frequent in telomeric regions like 4p16.[27,28] Later, the advent of the polymerase chain reaction (PCR) permitted the easy use of simple-sequence repeats (SSR), di-, tri-, and tetranucleotide repeat, varying in repeat unit number, as highly informative multiallele polymorphisms.[29,30] The genetic map of 4p16.3 was anchored to the physical map by DNA sites common to both, revealing that the 5×10^6 bp of DNA between *D4S10* and *D4S90* in 4p16.3 spanned 6% recombination.[31–33] However, there was a striking difference between the apparent distance between markers suggested by the genetic map and their actual separation on the physical map. Markers located within a 300–400-kb genetic "hot spot" immediately telomeric to *D4S10* revealed far more recombination than expected, such that this small physical interval accounted for more than one-half of the genetic distance of the entire 4p16.3 genetic map.[31] The remaining segment between *D4S125* and the telomere spans at least 4 Mb of physical distance but shows only 2.6% recombination.

In the absence of a physical benchmark, such as a deletion or translocation, to precisely position the disease gene within the linked segment, genetic crossovers between 4p16.3 DNA markers and the disease gene in HD families remained the only potential route to defining the DNA segment containing the defect. The success of this strategy depends on unequivocal diagnosis of the disorder in affected individuals, on accurate DNA typing, and on the frequency of double, as opposed to single, crossovers on HD chromosomes. *HD* was readily mapped beyond the "hot spot" of increased recombination telomeric to *D4S10*, as most crossovers with the defect occurred within this interval. However, the position of the disease gene in the remaining 3.5×10^6 of the physical map was not so easily discerned, as several genetic events in well-defined HD pedigrees yielded contradictory implications concerning its location.[32,34] Initially, a few diagnosed individuals in well-defined HD pedigrees were found to possess only marker alleles characteristic of the affected parent's normal chromosome. These events, in which no evidence of marker–marker crossover was seen, suggested that *HD* must be located in the telomeric 100-kb segment of the chromosome, beyond all informative DNA markers then available. However, several other HD cases were subsequently discovered that predicted a location closer to *D4S10*, as markers in the terminal 1.5×10^6 bp of the chromosome showed crossover with *HD*, whereas markers in the 2.5×10^6 bp telomeric to *D4S10* did not. Thus, the two classes of apparent recombination events implied mutually exclusive locations for the defect (Fig. 32–2).

One explanation for this genetic conundrum was the possibility of double recombination in the latter cases, with the chromosome switching back to the HD version telomeric to the final marker (*D4S142*) in the terminal 100 kb predicted by former events. This scenario led to the isolation of the entire segment between *D4S142* and the telomere of an HD chromosome as a yeast artificial chromosome (YAC).[35] Analysis of this DNA was complicated by the presence of subtelomeric repeat sequences and by sequence similarities to acrocentric chromosomes.[36] No evidence was found for a double crossover or for the presence of genes that could cause HD. Mounting evidence (see below) gradually favored the internal region of 4p16.3 as the site of the *HD* gene, but an explanation for the apparent crossovers that predicted this telomeric location had to await the identification of the genetic defect. Pulsed-field gel mapping initially produced a long-range physical map spanning the 2.5×10^6 bp of this internal region, which was subsequently isolated as overlapping clone sets, first of YACs and later of cosmids.[23–26]

▶ MINIMIZING THE CANDIDATE REGION WITH HISTORICAL RECOMBINATIONS

With genetic recombination having failed to provide a single, unequivocal site for the HD gene, innovative genetic strategies were required to progress with the search. The observation that some markers in the internal 4p16.3 segment displayed allele association with HD implicated this region as the site of the defect and provided the opportunity for a more powerful approach to localizing it.[37,38] Certain alleles for *D4S95* and *D4S98* RFLPs were more frequently represented on HD chromosomes than expected from their frequency on normal chromosomes. This was presumed to be a result of the presence of these alleles on the original chromosome 4 that underwent an *HD* mutation, with an insufficient number of subsequent generations to return the markers to their equilibrium frequencies. A comprehensive analysis of 4p16.3 DNA markers revealed the patterns of allele association to be quite complex.[39] Markers with evident allele association were interspersed on the physical map with sites that showed no association with HD. This supported the view that the current pool of HD chromosomes reflects more than one independent *HD* mutation or primordial chromosome. It also suggested that if HD chromosomes could be grouped

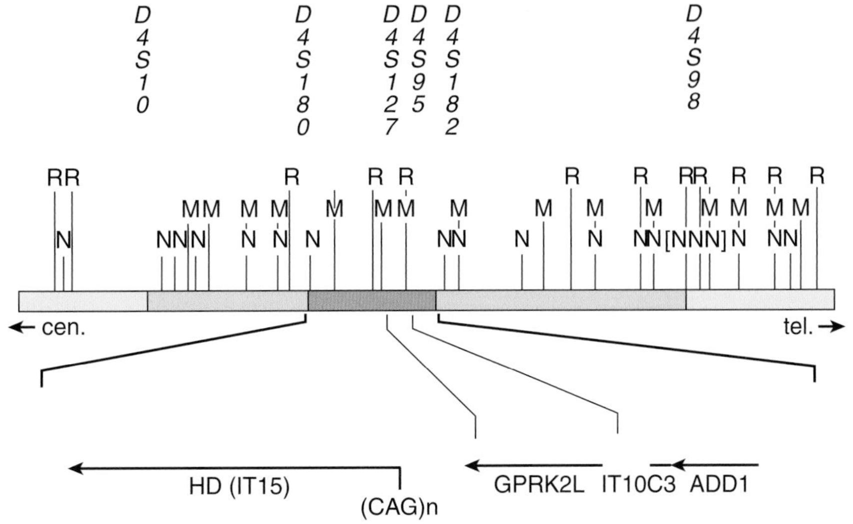

Figure 32–3. Isolation of *HD* candidate gene from the region of haplotype sharing. The long-range restriction enzyme map of 3 × 10^6 bp of the central portion of 4p16.3 is shown, with the progressively narrowing candidate region denoted by increasing intensity of shading. The unshaded region was eliminated by recombination events in HD families, placing the defect within the region between the DNA markers *D4S10* and D4S98. Initial haplotype analysis placed the defect in the 500-kb segment between DNA markers D4S180 and D4S182. Candidate genes from this region are depicted below the map. Detailed haplotype analysis eventually narrowed the search to the interval of darkest shading, targeting the search to the 5′ end of the *IT15* gene. This proved to contain the *HD* defect as an unstable, expanded CAG trinucleotide repeat (CAG)n. R, *NruI* site; M, *MluI* site; N, *NotI* site; cen., centromeric direction; tel., telomeric direction.

based on their mutational ancestry, the identification of a minimum cluster of shared marker alleles of 4p16.3 might pinpoint the location of the genetic defect.

The implementation of this novel approach was feasible because of the emergence of VNTR and SSR markers with a sufficiently large array of alleles to discriminate many potential primordial haplotypes.[40] Haplotype analysis unearthed evidence for a multitude of independent *HD* mutations, with 78 HD chromosomes exhibiting 26 different haplotypes within the region of maximal linkage disequilibrium, around *D4S127* and *D4S95*. The most frequent *HD* haplotype accounted for about one third of HD chromosomes, and the initial assessment of decay in strength of linkage disequilibrium within this class of chromosomes predicted a most likely location for *HD* in the 500-kb region between *D4S180* and *D4S182* (Figs. 32–2 and 32–3).

▶ IDENTIFICATION OF THE HD DEFECT

A set of overlapping cosmid clones between *D4S180* and *D4S182* acted as the source of genomic DNA for exon amplification, a novel approach for identifying candidate genes that took advantage of the splicing signals bordering exons to permit rapid and efficient isolation of the small proportion of genomic DNA that codes for proteins. This strategy identified a number of candidate genes[41–43]: *ADD1*, encoding α-adducin, a protein that participates in organizing the actin–spectrin cytoskeletal lattice; *IT10C3*, a probable small-molecule transporter with similarity to the tetracycline efflux proteins of *Escherichia coli*; *GPRK2L*, a G protein-coupled receptor kinase; and several anonymous genes with no similarity to previously described sequences (Fig. 32–3). Scanning of the full coding sequence of the first three candidates revealed no evidence of abnormalities or sequence differences specific to HD. Similarly, examination of the genomic segment spanned by each of these genes failed to disclose any alteration on disease chromosomes, with the exception of one report that mistakenly interpreted a rare Alu repeat sequence insertion within an intron of *ADD1* in two individuals as causative of HD.[44] This change was relegated to the status of a rare polymorphism by the discovery of the actual *HD* defect that had emerged from investigation of IT15, one of the anonymous candidate transcripts.[45]

Continued haplotype analysis with markers in the *D4S180–D4S182* interval, particularly a codon deletion polymorphism in the very long IT15 transcript, refined the size of the candidate region as additional HD chromosomes, previously thought to be unrelated, were exposed to belong to the most common haplotype class, based on sharing of a small segment of 150 kb immediately centromeric to *D4S95* (Fig. 32–3). This finding, which represented the ultimate distillation of the genetic approach, targeted the search for the defect to the extreme 5′ end of IT15. The culmination of the location cloning strategy came in 1993 with the discovery of an

Normal HD cDNA sequence Normal huntingtin in sequence	1	ATGGCGACCCTGGAAAAGCTGATGAAGGCCTTCGAGTCCCTCAAGTCCTTCCAGCAGCAGCAG Met Ala Thr Leu Glu Lys Leu Met Lys Ala Phe Glu Ser Leu Lys Ser Phe Gln Gln Gln Gln
Expanded disease CAG segment **Insert in disease huntingtin**		**CAGCAGCAGCAGCAGCAGCAGCAGCAGCAGCAGCAGCAGCAGCAGCAGCAGCAGCAGCAGCAG** **GlnGlnGlnGlnGlnGlnGlnGlnGlnGlnGlnGlnGlnGlnGlnGlnGlnGlnGlnGlnGln**
Normal HD cDNA sequence Normal huntingtin sequence	22	CAGCAGCAGCAGCAGCAGCAGCAGCAGCAGCAGCAGCAGCAGCAGCAGCAGCAACAGCCGCCACCG GlnGlnGlnGlnGlnGlnGlnGlnGlnGlnGlnGlnGlnGlnGlnGlnGlnGlnProProPro
Normal HD cDNA sequence Normal huntingtin sequence	43	CCGCCGCCGCCGCCGCCGCCTCCTCAGCTTCCTCAGCCGCCGCCGCAGGCACAGCCGCTGCTG ProProProProProProProProGlnLeuProGlnProProProGlnAlaGlnProLeuLeu
Normal HD cDNA sequence Normal huntingtin sequence	64	CCTCAGCCGCAGCCGCCCCCGCCGCCGCCCCCGCCGCCACCCGGCCCGGCTGTGGCTGAGGAG ProGlnProGlnProProProProProProProProProProGlyProAlaValAlaGluGlu
Normal HD cDNA sequence Normal huntingtin sequence	85	CCGCTGCACCGACCAAAGAAAGAACTTTCAGCTACC -->+ 9,141 bases ProLeuHisArgProLysGluLeuSerAlaThr -->+ 3,047 amino acids

Figure 32–4. The N-terminal sequence of huntingtin encoded by the 5′ end of the *HD* gene. The huntingtin cDNA 5′ coding sequence for a normal allele is shown above the amino acids (1–96) specified by each codon. This normal allele produces a huntingtin protein with 22 consecutive glutamine (Gln) residues. The effect of the *HD* mutation is shown as an inserted sequence of an additional 21 CAG repeats, encoding 21 Gln residues.

expanded, unstable trinucleotide repeat with the sequence CAG as the cause of HD (Fig. 32–4).[46]

▶ CHARACTERISTICS OF THE CAG REPEAT

The *HD* CAG repeat on normal chromosomes is polymorphic, ranging from 6 to 34 units (Fig. 32–5), and is inherited in a mendelian fashion.[47,48] Adjacent to the CAG trinucleotide stretch is a segment of consecutive CCG codons that is also polymorphic, varying from 6 to 12 repeat units.[49] The CCG alleles are also inherited in a mendelian fashion but show strong linkage disequilibrium in HD, as more than 90% of disease chromosomes have seven CCG units.[50] The CAG repeat of disease chromosomes is expanded, ranging from 36 to more than 100 units (Fig. 32–5). By contrast with the normal CAG alleles and with the CCG repeat, the *HD* CAG alleles do not show mendelian inheritance. Rather, they change in length, becoming either shorter or longer, when passed to progeny from either a male or a female parent (Fig. 32–6). In most cases, the magnitude of the changes is small (<6 repeat units), with a bias toward repeat length increases, but fathers sometimes transmit alleles with larger expansions, up to a doubling or more in the number of CAG units[48] and extremely rare, dramatic *HD* CAG expansions have been transmitted from mothers.[51,52]

The different allele sizes among progeny of male *HD* mutation carriers are reflected in similar variation in DNA prepared from sperm, although the normal alleles in these individuals remain identical in blood and sperm DNA.[53] Paternal *HD* CAG repeat expansions are found at many stages during spermatogenesis with a substantial fraction of changes already present in premeiotic spermatogonia.[54] *HD* CAG repeat variation is

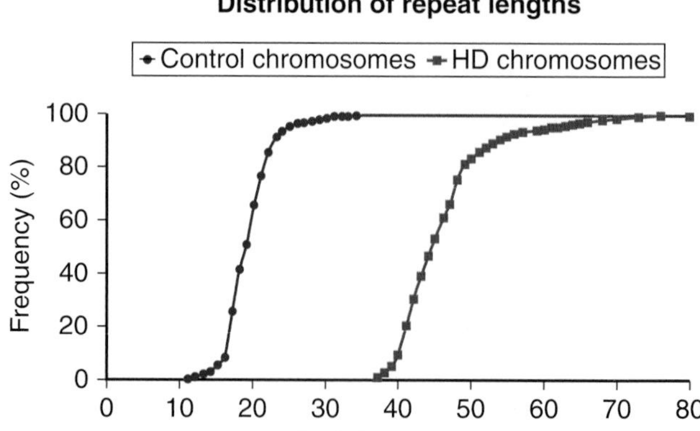

Figure 32–5. The cumulative distribution of CAG repeat lengths on HD and normal chromosomes. The frequency of CAG allele sizes on normal (circles) and disease (squares) chromosomes determined in Ref. 154 is depicted as a cumulative distribution for each.

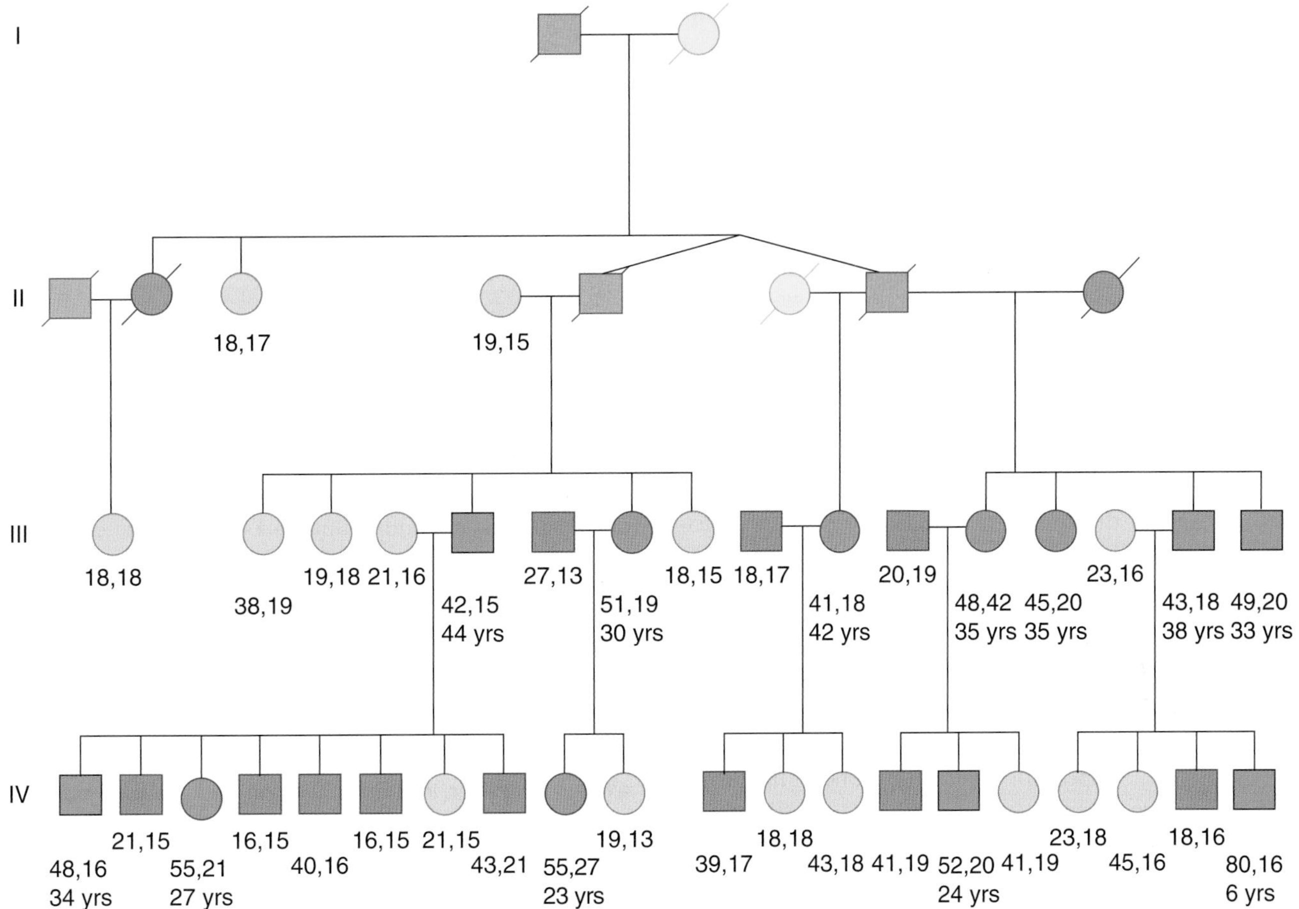

Figure 32–6. CAG repeat lengths and age of onset in the idealized HD pedigree. The same pedigree shown in Fig. 33–1 is displayed with CAG repeat length for both alleles (larger allele shown first by convention) under each symbol. For those individuals who are symptomatic, age of onset (in years) is also shown. Of the 4 progeny who were potential HD homozygotes, only the eldest possesses two *HD* alleles with CAG repeat lengths of 48 and 42, respectively. Juvenile onset has occurred in the youngest member of the pedigree in generation IV, because of an *HD* allele with 80 CAG units, whereas the eldest member of generation III remains asymptomatic with an *HD* allele of 38 CAG repeats.

also expected to occur in HD oogenesis, but this has not yet been demonstrated directly. In both male and female transmissions intergenerational instability is determined largely by the initial *HD* CAG repeat length, but is not significantly influenced by either parental age or disease status.[55] However, not all *HD* alleles of a given CAG length are equally unstable, implying that genetic factors other than *HD* CAG repeat length influence instability, consistent with the significant sibling-to-sibling correlation in repeat instability.[55] Moreover, certain haplotypes associated with HD chromosomes are also overrepresented among chromosomes bearing high-normal (27–35 CAGs) alleles, from which expansion to disease-causing CAG lengths occurs, suggesting that there may be DNA sequences that act *in cis* to the CAG repeat that influence repeat instability.[56]

In comparison with sperm DNA, *HD* CAG length variation in the DNA of somatic tissues, such as blood, is relatively circumscribed.[53,57–59] For example, several pairs of identical twins have been shown to possess repeats of identical length in blood-derived lymphoblastoid cells,[53] as well as blood DNA, including the lengths of mosaic alleles.[60] However, sensitive small pool-PCR methods have revealed extensive *HD* CAG expansion in postmortem brain that correlates with cell type-specific vulnerability.[61–64] These methods also reveal some instability in buccal cells,[65] suggesting that *HD* CAG length variation in somatic tissues may be more widespread.

The constitutive *HD* CAG repeat length is a major determinant of somatic instability, though instability can differ between individuals with identical repeat lengths, implicating modifiers. Longer somatic expansions in the brain are associated with earlier neurological onset,[64] suggesting that somatic expansion in target tissues may hasten the disease process. Interestingly, in some juvenile-onset HD individuals decreases in the number of CAG units have been observed in the cerebellum,[57] a brain region that is relatively insensitive to the pathological effects of the mutation.

▶ CLINICAL CORRELATES OF CAG REPEAT LENGTH

After the cloning of the *HD* gene, a plethora of reports analyzed the CAG repeat in cohorts of individuals with a clinical diagnosis of HD.[47] In all studies, the vast majority of patients possessed a CAG repeat in the expanded size range, attesting to the universality of this mutational mechanism of HD in many races, nationalities, and ethnic groups. In some studies, a number of HD-diagnosed individuals did not possess an expanded CAG allele, but careful analysis of one such data set showed that the majority of these can be explained as sample mix-ups, laboratory errors, or erroneous diagnoses based on atypical features.[66] The latter category is well-established to exist, based on the absence of HD-like neuropathology in a small percentage of postmortem brains from individuals with a clinical diagnosis of HD.

As almost all cases of HD are familial, the disorder has traditionally been viewed as having a very low rate of new mutation. Support for this notion came in the failure of the few sporadic cases to meet stringent criteria for new mutation status, including absence of disease in elderly parents, proof of paternity, and disease transmission. The linkage disequilibrium approach used in the search for the *HD* gene provided the first evidence that new mutations to HD do occur, as the many different 4p16.3 haplotypes on HD chromosomes indicated independent origins for some chromosomes.[40] Identification of the *HD* CAG repeat has provided a direct genetic test of whether sporadic cases of HD-like symptoms are a result of new mutations. Indeed, sporadic cases with classic HD symptoms display an expanded CAG repeat in the HD size range.[46,67,68] Interestingly, their unaffected relatives who have the same chromosome possess a CAG repeat that is intermediate between the size ranges associated with normal and HD chromosomes. Several cases of HD new mutation have occurred on a chromosome bearing the major *HD* haplotype, that shared by one third of HD chromosomes. This indicates that many of the HD families with this major haplotype may share a common ancestor who was not in fact affected with the disorder. Chromosomes with intermediate alleles on this and other haplotype backgrounds thus represent a reservoir from which new sporadic HD cases may arise. The complement of the clinical HD studies is the analysis of postmortem brain tissue, in which HD neuropathology has been documented. In a study of 310 brains assessed for HD neuropathology, using the grading system of Vonsattel and colleagues,[7] only three were found not to have an expanded CAG repeat.[47] Examination of the clinical records in these three cases revealed numerous features atypical of HD, suggesting a distinct

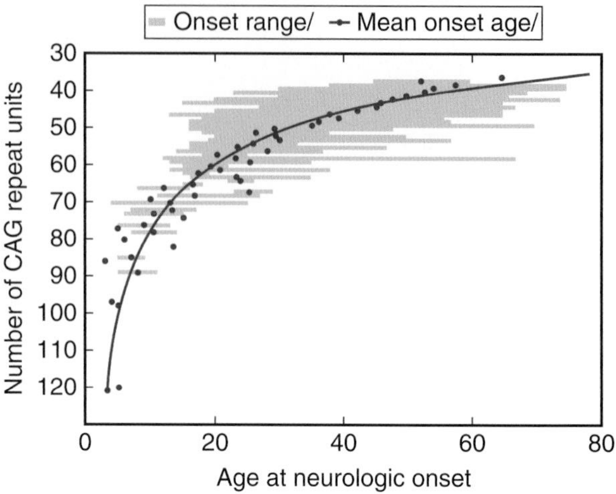

Figure 32–7. Inverse correlation between onset age and CAG repeat length. Published age at onset data for 1070 HD patients were used to calculate the average age at onset associated with any given repeat length. This mean age at onset (filled circles) and the associated range of onset ages (shaded bars) are plotted against CAG repeat length with curve fitting by power regression. A highly significant inverse correlation (r = −0.87, P < 0.00001) between age at onset of neurological symptoms and CAG repeat length occurs across all *HD* alleles. However, in the adult-onset age group, there is a very wide range of possible ages of onset associated with any given repeat length, precluding its use in predicting the timing of the disorder in individual cases.

disorder. Consequently, use of a combination of clinical and neuropathological criteria to assign a diagnosis of HD yields a collection of cases that all display an expanded CAG allele. If another type of mutation, either at the *HD* locus or elsewhere in the genome, can cause the same constellation of clinical and neuropathological features typically associated with HD, then it is quite rare.

Before the identification of the *HD* defect, family studies had established that inheritance of the *HD* defect invariably produced the disorder but with significant variation in clinical presentation. The most dramatic example is the manifestation of HD in juveniles in some cases of paternal (and rarely maternal) transmission of the defect. The nature of the *HD* mutation has explained much of this variation, including the effect of paternal inheritance, as there is a strong inverse correlation between CAG repeat length and age at onset of neurological symptoms (Fig. 32–7) in all populations examined.[69] The increased magnitude of size changes in spermatogenesis dictates that paternal transmissions are the major source of the long CAG repeats that underlie juvenile onset.

The assessment of neurological onset and, to an even greater degree, psychiatric onset, has been viewed as prone to considerable subjective error. However, inverse correlations of CAG repeat length with age at onset of both neurological and psychiatric symptoms and with the objective parameter, age at death, are evident even when clinical data are contributed by many independent reporting physicians from different areas.[69] About one-half of the variation in age at onset and death is explained by CAG repeat length, as there can be significant differences between individual patients with identical *HD* alleles, presumably because of modifying factors, such as interacting genes, environmental influences, or stochastic events. The question as to whether rate of progression also varies with repeat length is more complicated, as studies comparing CAG repeat with functional decline have been in conflict.[70–74] The result may depend on the particular measures of progression that are used as neuropathological severity clearly increases with CAG repeat length.[75,76] However, if duration from onset of motor symptoms to patient death is used as a measure, CAG length has little or no effect, indicating the predominance of factors other than the *HD* gene in determining this duration.[77]

A number of studies have demonstrated measurable motor signs, cognitive impairment, psychiatric disturbances, striatal and cortical volume loss, as well as functional brain changes that are detectable before the characteristic neurological symptoms that support accepted clinical diagnosis of HD.[78–93] Notably, the ongoing, longitudinal Neurobiological Predictors of Huntington's Disease (PREDICT-HD) study, engaged in prospectively characterizing clinical and biological markers in HD has found detectable changes in cognitive, motor, psychiatric, and imaging measures in individuals 10–20 years before their predicted time of clinical diagnosis. Further refined clinical phenotyping in the future may well reveal changes that occur even earlier.

▶ STRUCTURE AND EXPRESSION OF THE HD GENE

The *HD* CAG repeat is located in exon 1 of a 67-exon gene, 17 codons downstream from the initiator ATG.[45] The gene is transcribed in a telomere-to-centromere orientation and encodes a protein of more than 3140 amino acids named huntingtin.[46] The CAG repeat produces a polymorphic segment of consecutive glutamine residues, adjacent to a set of proline residues encoded by the CCG repeat. Huntington's molecular function is not known. Its sequence is not closely related to other proteins but shows a high degree of structurally driven evolutionary conservation that is detectable throughout vertebrates and in a wide variety of lower organisms.[94–104] No huntingtin homologues have been discovered in yeast or plants. Interestingly, the most evolutionarily divergent segment is the polyglutamine–polyproline stretch, encoded by the adjacent CAG and CCG repeats. The normal human gene encodes 12–36 glutamines, whereas the pig, rat, mouse, zebrafish, and pufferfish genes, respectively, encode 18, 8, 7, 4, and 4 glutamines at the equivalent location in the protein. The human glutamine segment is followed by a region of 42 amino acids that includes 29 prolines. The corresponding regions of pig, rat, and mouse huntingtins have 27, 28, and 27 prolines of 35, 36, and 35 residues, respectively, whereas zebrafish and pufferfish huntingtins have only 1 or 2 prolines, respectively, out of 4 residues. These comparisons suggest that the long polyglutamine and polyproline segments are not essential for huntingtin's most fundamental normal functions but may have evolved a modulatory role as vertebrate evolution progressed.

The sequence of huntingtin protein contributed to the definition of a new protein domain, termed HEAT for its presence in huntingtin, elongation factor 3, protein phosphatase 2A, and yeast TOR1.[105] HEAT motifs do not show strong sequence conservation, but appear structurally to represent two α-helices separated by a nonhelical linker. They are typically found in tandem arrays, such as in the PP2A PR65/A subunit and β-importin, which are entirely composed of 15 and 19 HEAT repeats, respectively. The crystal structures of these proteins reveal that tandem HEATs can form a flexible solenoid structure that provides a binding surface to act as a scaffold in bringing together interacting proteins.[106] Huntingtin was originally reported to have 10 HEAT repeats in three different locations in the protein, with the three near its N-terminus being the most evolutionarily conserved.[105] However, further analysis has revealed that all huntingtins, across a diverse array of organisms through evolution, are largely made up of HEAT-like sequences, perhaps explaining the absence of other notable functional domains, and suggesting that Huntington's normal function is as a scaffold or carrier of multiple protein partners.[103] Recently, it has been demonstrated that huntingtin is composed of two large α-helical domains linked by a hinge region, a structure that supports structural flexibility leading to multiple protein conformations.[107]

Huntingtin is expressed widely in both neural and nonneural (e.g., kidney, liver, lymphoblast, lung, heart, etc.) tissues based on studies of both mRNA and protein, suggesting that its normal function is not confined to cells in the areas of HD neuropathology. Antisera against the N-terminal peptide encoded 5′ to the CAG stretch have provided direct evidence that the CAG repeat is translated, as they react with the same large ~350-kDa Western blot band detected by antisera raised against C-terminal regions.[108–111] The size change caused by the expanded CAG of the disease allele permits normal and HD isoforms of huntingtin to be distinguished by sodium dodecyl sulfate-polyacrylamide gel electrophoresis. Cell fractionation experiments have indicated that huntingtin is a protein principally found in the cytoplasm, although it is capable of shuttling to and from the nucleus.[109,112]

Different anti-huntingtin antibodies reveal different patterns of localization, suggesting that either the corresponding epitopes may be accessible or hidden, depending on the protein complex containing huntingtin, and/or the protein can undergo conformational changes, consistent with a flexible solenoid structure, depending on its modifications or binding partners.[112,113] Immunocytochemical localization of huntingtin in rat, monkey, and human brain tissues has shown that the pattern of huntingtin expression does not parallel the regions of HD neuropathology.[110,111,114] Thus, the neuronal target cells that succumb to the effects of the *HD* defect represent only a small subset of the neural and nonneural cell populations that actually express the mutant protein.

▶ OTHER POLYGLUTAMINE NEURODEGENERATIVE DISORDERS

Several other neurodegenerative disorders (Fig. 32–8) are also caused by expanded trinucleotide repeats and show striking genetic similarities with HD.[115] In each case, a normally polymorphic CAG repeat is expanded and unstable on disease chromosomes, with the onset of the neurological symptoms beginning only above a threshold CAG repeat length, which can be lower or higher than the ~35 CAGs required in HD. The CAG repeat is located within the coding sequence of the respective gene, predicting an altered protein with an extended stretch of consecutive glutamine residues. Hence, these disorders have been grouped with HD under the term "polyglutamine neurodegenerative disorders." In each, a different pattern of neuronal cell loss results from the CAG expansion mutation. Most strikingly, in every disorder there is a strong negative correlation between CAG repeat length and age at onset of neurological symptoms, supporting a common fundamental mechanism. The similarity in the mutational mechanism but with quite different early patterns of neuronal cell loss in each polyglutamine disorder suggests that the specificity of neuronal vulnerability and the precise trigger of pathogenesis are dependent on the nature of the protein containing the polyglutamine, likely because in each disorder the polyglutamine tract modulates activity of the host protein, perhaps enhancing it as in HD.

▶ MECHANISM OF ACTION OF THE HD DEFECT

Although the precise mechanism of action of the *HD* defect is not certain, much has been learned since the cloning of the disease gene and some significant pos-

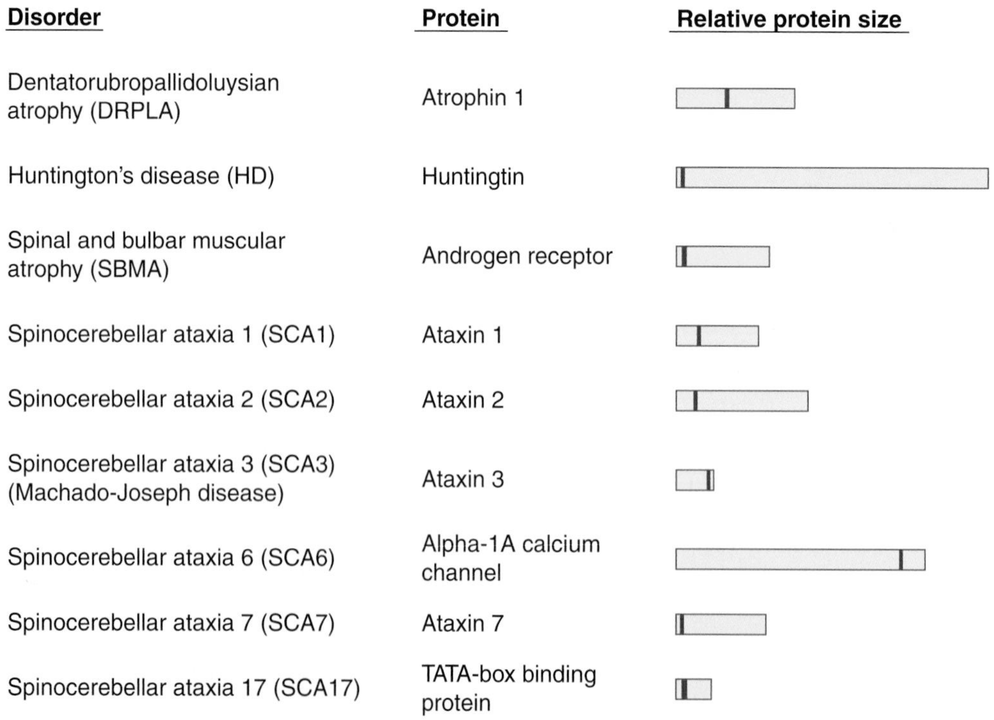

Disorder	Protein	Relative protein size
Dentatorubropallidoluysian atrophy (DRPLA)	Atrophin 1	
Huntington's disease (HD)	Huntingtin	
Spinal and bulbar muscular atrophy (SBMA)	Androgen receptor	
Spinocerebellar ataxia 1 (SCA1)	Ataxin 1	
Spinocerebellar ataxia 2 (SCA2)	Ataxin 2	
Spinocerebellar ataxia 3 (SCA3) (Machado-Joseph disease)	Ataxin 3	
Spinocerebellar ataxia 6 (SCA6)	Alpha-1A calcium channel	
Spinocerebellar ataxia 7 (SCA7)	Ataxin 7	
Spinocerebellar ataxia 17 (SCA17)	TATA-box binding protein	

Figure 32–8. Neurodegenerative disorders caused by translated expanded CAG trinucleotide repeats. Nine polyglutamine neurodegenerative disorders are listed with the name of the corresponding protein. The relative size of each protein is shown as a box to the right, with the location of the polyglutamine tract denoted by a vertical black line.

sibilities have been ruled out. The expanded CAG repeat does not drastically alter transcription of the *HD* gene, as huntingtin mRNA is expressed at comparable levels from the disease and normal alleles.[45,116] Similarly, the ability to distinguish mutant and normal huntingtin based on electrophoretic mobility has revealed that the defect does not prevent translation of the mRNA. Thus, the lack of transcriptional and translational effects suggests that the *HD* defect acts through the altered structure of huntingtin and its extended polyglutamine segment.

The lengthened polyglutamine stretch does not cause HD by simply eliminating huntingtin's activity, as there is direct genetic evidence in both man and mouse that disruption of this gene does not produce disease symptoms. In humans, individuals with an *HD* gene translocation that eliminates 50% of huntingtin production do not develop HD.[45] Similarly, mice with one copy of the *HD* gene homologue (*Hdh*) inactivated by targeted mutagenesis show no abnormality.[117,118] However, homozygosity for complete inactivation of the mouse gene leads to death early in embryonic life, before development of the nervous system, which is in sharp contrast with the adult-onset neuropathology in humans.[117,118] The mouse experiments establish that huntingtin activity is essential for normal development. Thus, the existence of adult individuals homozygous for an expanded CAG allele indicates that the *HD* mutation does not simply remove huntingtin's normal activity.

Instead, HD pathogenesis appears to involve a "gain of function," in which the lengthened polyglutamine segment confers a new property on the protein, which could include a novel activity, an increase in an existing activity, or deregulation of an existing activity. Genotype–phenotype studies relating CAG repeat length with age at neurological onset in HD patients dictate a number of criteria for this "gain of function" and the fundamental mechanism that triggers the disorder.[115] Investigations of heterozygous HD patients indicate that the disease-initiating mechanism requires a threshold glutamine tract length (if it is to cause disease in a typical human lifespan), is progressively more severe above that length, and is dominant over normal huntingtin. As individuals who possess two mutant *HD* alleles (HD homozygotes), and consequently no normal *HD* allele, do not show earlier onset than equivalent HD heterozygotes, the "gain of function" mechanism is insensitive to the presence or absence of normal huntingtin and is much more sensitive to increasing polyglutamine length than huntingtin concentration. Finally, the comparison of HD with the other polyglutamine neurodegenerative disorders indicates that the deleterious effect of the polyglutamine tract achieves its neuronal specificity due to its being presented in the context of the huntingtin protein, because of the protein's structure, localization/interactions, or inherent activity.

Huntingtin's precise normal functions remain to be solved at the molecular level. However, knowledge of these functions is likely to be critical for understanding the disease, as the genetic data are consistent with their modulation by the length of the polyglutamine repeat. Indeed, expansion of the polyglutamine tract to cause HD may simply represent the extreme of a normal modulatory role for the polyglutamine tract that could act in both the normal and expanded size ranges. Molecular biological and biochemical analyses have indicated that huntingtin, especially at its N-terminus, can interact with more than three dozen different proteins, including transcription factors, cytoskeletal components, proteins involved in intracellular trafficking, and others.[119] Similarly, cell biological studies have suggested huntingtin involvement in a wide range of processes, though few of these have assessed the full-length protein or the effect of the polyglutamine tract length. However, where the latter have been examined, a modulatory role for the polyglutamine region is supported. For example, in human lymphoblasts, the ratio of ATP/ADP is correlated with the length of the *HD* CAG repeat, implicating huntingtin in regulation of some aspect of energy metabolism.[120] This possibility is consistent with findings from genetically modified mice that produce huntingtin with no polyglutamine tract. These mice are fully viable with only minor motor and behavioral differences, but fibroblasts derived from them have increased ATP levels and senesce prematurely.[121] Recently, the first direct measurement of a biochemical activity of huntingtin has been achieved in vitro.[107] Huntingtin enhances the activity of polycomb repressive complex 2, a protein complex that regulates transcription by methylation of histones. As predicted, this activity of huntingtin was increased by expanding the length of the polyglutamine tract, suggesting that subtly altered transcriptional repression could play a role in triggering the disorder. As a potential scaffold for diverse protein complexes, it is likely that huntingtin also serves other functions as a facilitator, some of which may also be enhanced by the expansion of the polyglutamine tract and be candidates for causing the lifelong pathway of pathogenic changes that is HD.

▶ MODIFIERS OF *HD* PATHOGENESIS

Although the presence of an expanded CAG tract in the *HD* gene is required to trigger HD pathogenesis, it is not the only genetic factor that determines disease manifestations. For example, the age at motor onset is primarily determined by the length of the CAG tract, but the variance remaining after accounting for this factor remains highly heritable. As onset of characteristic neurological symptoms underlies the clinical diagnosis of HD, it is evident that variation in other genes can alter the course of the disorder and likely that genetic factors may also contribute to the degree and nature of psychiatric and cognitive involvement. The search for genetic modifiers has focused on candidate pathways/processes potentially involved in HD pathogenesis but not yet produced definitive results that can be exploited for therapeutic purposes, though it has provided strong evidence against particular players. For example, many investigators have used neurobiological and molecular approaches to explore the potential participation of brain-derived neurotrophic factor (BDNF) in HD. However, genetic studies of a functional protein polymorphism that alters the activity of BDNF have showed that this activity is not a significant factor in determining the rate of HD pathogenesis before diagnosis as it has no effect on altering age at neurological onset.[122–124]

Many other genes have been similarly analyzed with a number of reported positive results that appear to implicate such processes as glutamatergic transmission (*GRIK2, GRIN2A, GRIN2B*), protein degradation (*UCHL1*), gene transcription (*TCERG1, TP53*), stress response/apoptosis (*DFFB, MAP3K5, MAP2K6*), lipoprotein metabolism (*APOE*), axonal trafficking (*HAP1*), folate metabolism (*MTHFR*), and energy metabolism (*PPARGC1A*) as having small effects on age-at-motor onset.[125] However, negative studies have also been reported for many of these genes and definitive confirmation has remained elusive in most cases. Similarly, the precise mechanism by which the genetic variation might act is unknown for these potential modifiers. For example, *GRIK2*, the earliest reported genetic modifier that was shown in multiple studies to harbor a particular allele of TAA trinucleotide repeat polymorphisms in the 3′ untranslated region that is associated with earlier onset of HD[126,127] has been investigated using genetic strategies.[128] The findings have revealed that the potential modifier effect is not due to functional changes in the coding sequence, promoter, or introns of the *GRIK2* gene, but rather to the TAA repeat itself, but the mechanistic consequence of this polymorphism on *GRIK2* expression remains enigmatic. In most other cases, the modifier effect has been attributed to individual single nucleotide polymorphisms (SNPs) without any delineation of the specific functional SNP responsible or its effect on gene expression.

Advances in genetic technologies that permit the scanning of SNPs across the entire genome for association with variation in disease phenotypes offer tremendous promise for identifying genetic modifiers in HD. Most importantly, like the original search for the *HD* gene itself, these techniques offer an unbiased approach to the search for modifiers so that investigators need not be limited to prior knowledge and are able to discover the unexpected, as was the case with the discovery of huntingtin itself. Genomewide association and linkage scans can be expected to reveal genetic modifiers that act at various stages of the pathogenic process, from the initial trigger and long preclinical phase through the appearance and progression of individual disease symptoms. Importantly, identifying these genetic factors capable of altering the HD disease process should provide the basis for therapeutic intervention by targeting pathways/processes already validated in humans.

▶ MODELING THE GENETICS OF *HD* IN THE MOUSE

The well-defined genetic lesion in HD has permitted the construction by a number of laboratories of precise genetic models of HD, in which the expanded CAG tract has been inserted by "knock-in" technology into the homologous mouse gene (*Hdh*).[129–133] Longer CAG alleles in the endogenous mouse gene display gametic instability, although the distribution of size changes is somewhat different from that seen in human gametogenesis.[129,132,134] The precise genetic models express full-length mutant huntingtin at normal physiological levels in a tissue pattern comparable to wild-type huntingtin. The mutant huntingtin is functional in development, as it fully rescues the embryonic lethality of *Hdh* null "knock-out" alleles.[133] Moreover, other engineered mice displaying either globally reduced huntingtin expression or elimination of huntingtin expression in selected populations of adult neurons have revealed a postembryonic role for huntingtin in neurogenesis,[133,135] and in the maintenance of adult neurons.[136] Defects in neither of these are seen in mice either heterozygous, hemizygous or homozygous for mutant *Hdh* alleles expressing full-length mutant huntingtin with glutamine tract lengths that are associated with adult onset or juvenile onset in man.

While the mutant huntingtin in these mice effectively replaces the function of wild-type huntingtin, it also appears to possess a "gain of function" property that fulfills all of the genetic criteria for participation in the initiation of HD pathogenesis, including striatal specificity.[137–140] The knock-in mice display a series of subtle, progressive phenotypes staged across the entire lifespan. At a few weeks of life, a subset of the huntingtin protein in striatal neurons becomes more apparent in the nucleus and begins to disappear from the cytoplasm. This redistribution of huntingtin staining progresses, with apparent accumulation of full-length huntingtin in the nucleus and is followed over the ensuing 2 years by a series of histological and biochemical changes that include alterations in gene expression, energy metabolism, cellular signaling, eventual appearance of N-terminal huntingtin fragment and nuclear inclusions, and, late in life, evidence for dysfunctional degenerating neurons. *Hdh* knock-in mice also display early motor and cognitive abnormalities.[141–146] Similar findings have been derived with transgenic mice expressing full-length human mutant huntingtin from a modified human YAC clone.[147,148]

Notably, different rates of some of the progressive phenotypes in knock-in mice on different inbred genetic backgrounds[149] provide the opportunity to search in an unbiased manner across the genome for genetic modifiers that act very early in the HD pathogenic process.

These precise genetic knock-in models of HD argue that the process of pathogenesis is a long one that is time-dependent, rather than developmental-stage dependent, and that the lifespan of the mouse is insufficient to reproduce the full 1–2 decade course of the disorder in humans. Rather, these mice appear to model presymptomatic HD, with deleterious consequences first resulting from expression of full-length mutant huntingtin. Interestingly, the progressive phenotypes that the mice display raise the likelihood that other features of huntingtin may participate downstream in the pathogenic pathway to accelerate the demise of the vulnerable neuronal cells. For example, in vulnerable neurons CAG repeat instability is eventually detected that would be expected to produce mutant huntingtin with even longer polyglutamine tracts than those in the inherited allele.[132,139] This potential for increasing the severity of the triggering mechanism has received some support from CAG instability measured in post-mortem HD brain,[61–64,150] the association of longer CAG repeat lengths in brain with earlier disease onset[64] and from the demonstration that, in the mice, DNA repair enzymes Msh2 and Msh3, which are required for repeat instability, are genetic modifiers of the progressive phenotypes.[151,152] Similarly, the eventual appearance of nuclear inclusions suggests that cleavage of huntingtin later in the disease process may reduce the beneficial effects of its normal activities,[153–156] which have been suggested to be antiapoptotic, and introduce the deleterious effects of N-terminal mutant fragment. The former is consistent with one suggestion that symptomatic progression may be accelerated in HD homozygotes.[157]

▶ CLINICAL CONSEQUENCES: DIAGNOSIS

The major impact of molecular biology on clinical care of HD has so far been the capacity to perform predictive testing, determining whether asymptomatic individuals born "at risk" because of a parent with HD have, in fact, inherited the defect. The discovery of DNA markers for HD in 1983 made it possible to perform presymptomatic or prenatal diagnostic testing for some interested individuals. However, the test was cumbersome and prone to various forms of inaccuracy, as it required tracing genetically linked markers through several related family members, at least one of whom was clinically affected. Thus, it was only applicable to at-risk individuals for whom several family members were able and willing to donate their DNA. This newfound ability to predict the future presence of a devastating, untreatable neurological disorder in a currently unaffected individual raised numerous ethical dilemmas that were debated at length. Pilot testing programs began cautiously, with a heavy emphasis on counseling both before and after delivery of the test result.[158–160] A high level of psychological and emotional support was built in because of the potentially calamitous consequences of a positive test result in a disorder with psychiatric disturbances and the lack of a precedent for determining ability to cope with such information. This experience led to the establishment of formal guidelines sanctioned by the International Huntington Association (IHA) and by the World Federation of Neurology (WFN) to ensure ethical administration of predictive testing.[161] This precedent has become an increasingly important guide, as genetic defects have been found in numerous other late-onset human disorders, including the other CAG repeat diseases referred to above.

The discovery of the nature of the genetic defect in HD has revolutionized the technical aspects of predictive testing, providing an inexpensive method that can be applied to any at-risk individual, without the critical need for DNA from relatives. CAG repeat measurement can also be applied to prenatal testing for confirmation of a clinical diagnosis of HD and for differential diagnosis in difficult cases (Fig. 32–9). Similarly, assaying for the CAG expansion or for linked markers can be used for perimplantation genetic diagnosis of HD, permitting individuals to bear children free of the defect, even in cases where the at risk parent chooses not to receive their own molecular diagnosis.[162–172] Although direct assay of CAG length is more accurate and more widely applicable than the former linkage test, the essential nature of the information being obtained remains the same. Thus, the IHA-WFN guidelines remain in force, revised to take into account the nature of direct testing.[173]

Despite the improvement in the testing procedure, there remain complicating factors that must be considered in applying CAG repeat measurement to disease prediction. Alleles low in the HD range (36–39 units) are sometimes nonpenetrant within a typical lifespan.[174] Moreover, chromosomes from unaffected members of the rare "new mutation" families can possess high "normal" alleles (29–35 units) whose potential for giving rise to abnormalities in extremely long-lived individuals or to longer alleles in children where they may cause HD symptoms is difficult to accurately assess.[46,55,66,68,175,176] Indeed, there may be no precise border between chromosomes that cause HD and those that do not, as modifying factors become paramount in determining onset for alleles low in the HD range. Moreover, potential gametic instability of alleles high in the "normal" range must be taken into account in counseling potential parents with such alleles. Thus, alleles in the high "normal" and low HD ranges represent dilemmas for predictive testing of at-risk individuals and for assessing the potential risk of transmitting HD. Recent

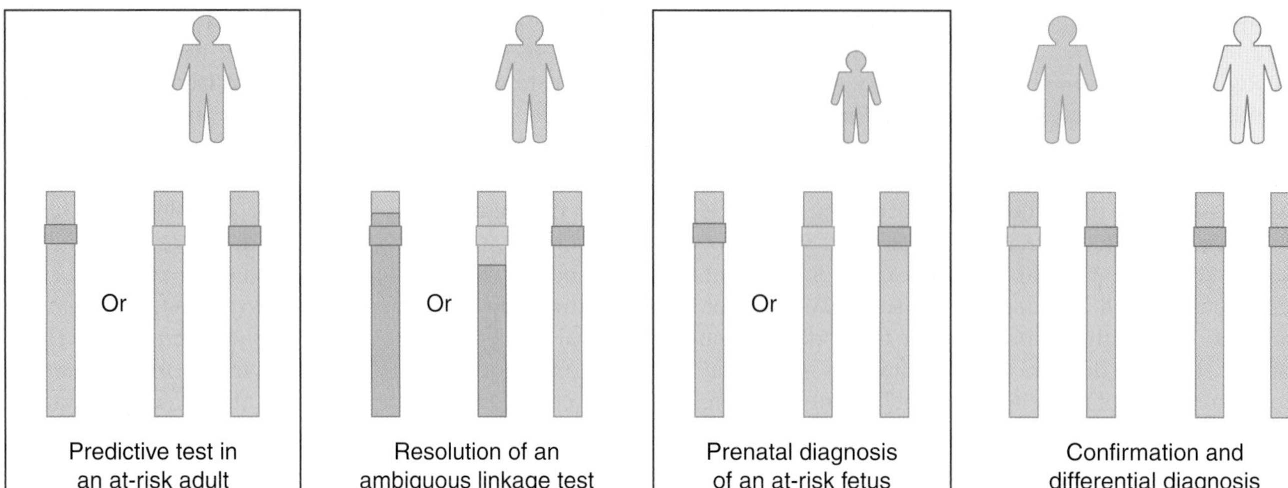

Figure 32–9. Applications of molecular diagnosis. A schematic diagram is shown to illustrate the clinical uses of direct measurement of CAG repeats. An expanded CAG repeat is depicted by a black box on one chromosome. The normal allele is denoted by an unfilled box. CAG repeat measurement distinguishes between normal and HD chromosomes in predictive testing of "at-risk" individuals, including those who have received an ambiguous result from the *HD* linkage test because of recombination between the markers and the disease gene. CAG repeat length can also provide prenatal diagnosis in at-risk pregnancies and is of value in confirming or refuting the clinical diagnosis of HD in atypical or difficult cases.

widely varying assessments of the risk of expansion of high normal alleles (sometimes referred to erroneously as "intermediate" alleles) into the disease-associated range[175–177] suggest that a more thorough understanding of the instability of high normal alleles is critically needed to reliably guide clinical counseling.

A second consideration in using the CAG assay for predictive testing derives from the linkage studies aimed at delineating the *HD* candidate region. As noted above, several clinically diagnosed individuals in different HD pedigrees yielded marker genotypes characteristic of the normal chromosome from the corresponding affected parent, confusing the localization of the defect by predicting a second candidate region.[32,34] Discovery of the *HD* CAG mutation permitted resolution of this genetic conundrum. Despite the presence of expanded trinucleotide repeats in all other affected members of these HD families, the exceptional individuals had only normal alleles. Thus, these individuals appear to have another movement disorder mistakenly diagnosed as HD because of an extensive family history. Such cases can be expected to occur at a low frequency in families undergoing presymptomatic testing. The fact that a negative HD test does not exclude the future occurrence of another movement disorder should be conveyed to at-risk individuals.

Finally, the strong inverse correlation between age at onset and CAG repeat length raises special problems in delivering the results of the *HD* CAG test.[178] Every HD test that yields an allele in the established disease range can be considered diagnostic of the future onset of the disorder. However, despite the precision with which the number of CAG units can be measured, the CAG length cannot be considered an accurate predictor of age at onset in any individual case, because the range of ages at onset observed for any particular repeat length is far too extensive to make such predictions meaningful. Though mathematical modeling has permitted a quantification of the age and CAG-length dependent risk of initial motor symptoms,[179] these estimates are more appropriate for planning clinical trials than for predictive clinical testing. Effective communication of the dubious prognostic value of CAG length for each at-risk individual represents another significant challenge for genetic counselors dealing with this disorder.

Although delivery of the HD predictive test has become more practical and experience with its associated genetic counseling has grown, many at-risk individuals choose not to undergo testing. Despite its reduced cost, increased accuracy, and wider applicability, the CAG repeat test shares the major drawback of the linkage test: nothing can yet be done to prevent the disease in those found to carry the defective gene. Without an effective treatment, the predictive test is a mixed blessing.

▶ CLINICAL CONSEQUENCES: PROSPECTS FOR THERAPY

Over the past 20 years, molecular biology has brought us to identification of HD's primary defect, and, while it has yet to define precisely its biochemical mechanism, it has revealed numerous targets for development of potential therapies. Overall, the findings are consistent with a disease course in which the first biochemical abnormality, which remains to be identified, is triggered by expression of full-length mutant protein and leads over a long period of time to progressive debilitation of individual neurons which eventually begin to cleave retained nuclear huntingtin and accumulate nuclear inclusions before neuronal death. Consequently, potential rational treatments can be considered at various levels. If possible, eliminating the expression of mutant huntingtin, which is being explored via RNA interference and antisense oligonucleotide approaches, would clearly be effective, but would require continued expression of wild-type huntingtin for neuronal maintenance. Specific *HD* locus SNPs overrepresented on HD chromosomes may offer the potential for specific targeting of the mutant allele.[56,180,181] Understanding the mechanisms underlying *HD* CAG repeat instability may provide an alternative therapeutic strategy directed at the mutant allele itself by reducing CAG length. Interfering directly with the gain of function conferred by the expanded polyglutamine segment might also prevent triggering of the pathogenic pathway. Once triggered, treatments aimed at correcting the biochemical alterations that occur require precisely defining these targets. Perhaps the most hopeful strategy in this regard is to use genetics to unlock the information inherent in HD patients themselves, by identifying genetic modifiers that can lead the search for small molecule therapeutic interventions aimed at the most effective targets. However, general processes implicated in cellular and animal systems as likely to participate in the disease, especially at later stages, suggest that boosting energy metabolism, general neuroprotectants, modulating protein degradation via the ubiquitin-proteasome-mediated or autophagy-mediated pathway, modulating gene transcription, and inhibiting the enzymes that lead to huntingtin cleavage and apoptosis might provide treatments. Finally, once neuronal cells have been lost, treatment options would appear to be limited to preventing further damage and possibly replacing function via neuronal implants. The latter strategy as a longer term hope has received a boost in recent years by developments that permit the generation of pluripotent stem cells from somatic cells and the subsequent redifferentiation into neuronal and other populations.[182]

Currently, the testing of potential therapies is limited to individuals close to or after clinical diagnosis in which measures of dysfunction are relatively well established and accepted. However, the ideal intervention for HD would be targeted early in the pathogenic process before clinical diagnosis. To test such interventions will require biomarkers that reflect the ongoing pathogenic process in individuals before diagnosis. Fortunately, unlike most other disorders, genetic analysis provides an extremely reliable method to identify those who will eventually be clinically diagnosed with HD, permitting their detailed scrutiny decades before formal clinical diagnosis. Moreover, the length of the *HD* CAG repeat in mutation-positive individuals also provides a predictor of the severity of the pathogenic process that increases the power and precision of the search for modifiers. As a result, observational studies, such as the large PREDICT-HD and TRACK-HD studies, are beginning to define alterations decades before the neurological abnormalities required for diagnosis, and confirming that HD pathogenesis is a lifelong process, initiated by the presence of the expanded CAG tract.[88,183] Hopefully, the singular mutational mechanism in HD will sow the seeds of its own destruction in the power that it holds for generating insights into the disorder, clues to effective treatment targets and biomarkers of disease to enable prediagnosis testing of potential therapies in preventative therapeutic trials.

REFERENCES

1. Huntington G. On chorea. Med Surg Rep 1872;26:317.
2. Osler, W. Historical note on hereditary chorea. In Browning W (ed). Neurographs. Vol. 1. Brooklyn, NY: Albert C. Huntington, 1908, pp. 113–116.
3. Vessie, PR. On the transmission of Huntington's chorea for 300 years: The Bures family group. J Nerv Ment Dis 1932;76:553.
4. Harper PS. The epidemiology of Huntington's disease. Hum Genet 1992;89:365.
5. Bird ED, Caro AJ, Pilling JB. A sex related factor in the inheritance of Huntington's chorea. Ann Hum Genet 1974;37:255.
6. Merritt AD, Conneally PM, Rahman NF, et al. Juvenile Huntington's chorea. In Barbeau A, TR Brunette (ed). Progress in Neurogenetics. Amsterdam: Excerpta Medica Foundation, 1969, pp. 645–650.
7. Vonsattel JP, Myers RH, Stevens TJ, et al. Neuropathological classification of Huntington's disease. J Neuropathol Exp Neurol 1985;44:559.
8. Gusella JF. DNA polymorphism and human disease. Annu Rev Biochem 1986;55:831.
9. Pericak-Vance MA, Conneally PM, Merritt AD, et al. Genetic linkage studies in Huntington disease. Cytogenet Cell Genet 1978;22:640.
10. Gusella JF, Wexler NS, Conneally PM, et al. A polymorphic DNA marker genetically linked to Huntington's disease. Nature 1983;306:234.
11. Gusella JF, Tanzi RE, Bader PI, et al. Deletion of Huntington's disease-linked G8 (*D4S10*) locus in Wolf-Hirschhorn syndrome. Nature 1985;318:75.
12. Landegent JE, Jansen in de Wal N, Fisser-Groen YM, et al. Fine mapping of the Huntington disease linked *D4S10* locus by non-radioactive in situ hybridization. Hum Genet 1986;73:354.
13. Wang HS, Greenberg CR, Hewitt J, et al. Subregional assignment of the linked marker G8 (*D4S10*) for Huntington disease to chromosome 4p16.1-16.3. Am J Hum Genet 1986;39:392.

14. Zabel BU, Naylor SL, Sakaguchi AY, et al. Mapping of the DNA locus *D4S10* and the linked Huntington's disease gene to 4p16--p15. Cytogenet Cell Genet 1986;42:187.
15. Conneally PM, Haines JL, Tanzi RE, et al. Huntington disease: No evidence for locus heterogeneity. Genomics 1989;5:304.
16. Myers RH, Leavitt J, Farrer LA, et al. Homozygote for Huntington disease. Am J Hum Genet 1989;45:615.
17. Wexler NS, Young AB, Tanzi RE, et al.: Homozygotes for Huntington's disease. Nature 1987;326:194.
18. Gilliam TC, Tanzi RE, Haines JL, et al. Localization of the Huntington's disease gene to a small segment of chromosome 4 flanked by *D4S10* and the telomere. Cell 1987;50:565.
19. MacDonald ME, Anderson MA, Gilliam TC, et al. A somatic cell hybrid panel for localizing DNA segments near the Huntington's disease gene. Genomics 1987;1:29.
20. Smith B, Skarecky D, Bengtsson U, et al. Isolation of DNA markers in the direction of the Huntington disease gene from the G8 locus. Am J Hum Genet 1988;42:335.
21. Altherr MR, Plummer S, Bates G, et al. Radiation hybrid map spanning the Huntington disease gene region of chromosome 4. Genomics 1992;13:1040.
22. Doucette-Stamm LA, Riba L, Handelin B, et al. Generation and characterization of irradiation hybrids of human chromosome 4. Somat Cell Mol Genet 1991;17:471.
23. Bucan M, Zimmer M, Whaley WL, et al. Physical maps of 4p16.3, the area expected to contain the Huntington disease mutation. Genomics 1990;6:1.
24. Bates GP, MacDonald ME, Baxendale S, et al. Defined physical limits of the Huntington disease gene candidate region. Am J Hum Genet 1991;49:7.
25. Bates GP, Valdes J, Hummerich H, et al. Characterization of a yeast artificial chromosome contig spanning the Huntington's disease gene candidate region. Nat Genet 1992;1:180.
26. Baxendale S, MacDonald ME, Mott R, et al. A cosmid contig and high resolution restriction map of the 2 megabase region containing the Huntington's disease gene. Nat Genet 1993;4:181.
27. MacDonald ME, Cheng SV, Zimmer M, et al. Clustering of multiallele DNA markers near the Huntington's disease gene. J Clin Invest 1989;84:1013.
28. Wasmuth JJ, Hewitt J, Smith B, et al. A highly polymorphic locus very tightly linked to the Huntington's disease gene. Nature 1988;332:734.
29. Tagle DA, Blanchard-McQuate KL, Valdes J, et al. Dinucleotide repeat polymorphism in the Huntington's disease region at the D4S182 locus. Hum Mol Genet 1993;2:489.
30. Taylor SA, Barnes GT, MacDonald ME, et al. A dinucleotide repeat polymorphism at the D4S127 locus. Hum Mol Genet 1992;1:142.
31. Allitto BA, MacDonald ME, Bucan M, et al. Increased recombination adjacent to the Huntington disease-linked *D4S10* marker. Genomics 1991;9:104.
32. MacDonald ME, Haines JL, Zimmer M, et al. Recombination events suggest potential sites for the Huntington's disease gene. Neuron 1989;3:183.
33. Youngman S, Sarfarazi M, Bucan M, et al. A new DNA marker (D4S90) is located terminally on the short arm of chromosome 4, close to the Huntington disease gene. Genomics 1989;5:802.
34. Robbins C, Theilmann J, Youngman S, et al. Evidence from family studies that the gene causing Huntington disease is telomeric to D4S95 and D4S90. Am J Hum Genet 1989;44:422.
35. Bates GP, MacDonald ME, Baxendale S, et al. A yeast artificial chromosome telomere clone spanning a possible location of the Huntington disease gene. Am J Hum Genet 1990;46:762.
36. Youngman S, Bates GP, Williams S, et al. The telomeric 60 kb of chromosome arm 4p is homologous to telomeric regions on 13p, 15p, 21p, and 22p. Genomics 1992;14:350.
37. Snell RG, Lazarou LP, Youngman S, et al. Linkage disequilibrium in Huntington's disease: An improved localisation for the gene. J Med Genet 1989;26:673.
38. Theilmann J, Kanani S, Shiang R, et al. Non-random association between alleles detected at D4S95 and D4S98 and the Huntington's disease gene. J Med Genet 1989;26:676.
39. MacDonald ME, Lin C, Srinidhi L, et al. Complex patterns of linkage disequilibrium in the Huntington disease region. Am J Hum Genet 1991;49:723.
40. MacDonald ME, Novelletto A, Lin C, et al. The Huntington's disease candidate region exhibits many different haplotypes. Nat Genet 1992;1:99.
41. Ambrose C, James M, Barnes G, et al. A novel G protein-coupled receptor kinase gene cloned from 4p16.3. Hum Mol Genet 1992;1:697.
42. Duyao MP, Taylor SA, Buckler AJ, et al. A gene from chromosome 4p16.3 with similarity to a superfamily of transporter proteins. Hum Mol Genet 1993;2:673.
43. Taylor SA, Snell RG, Buckler A, et al. Cloning of the alpha-adducin gene from the Huntington's disease candidate region of chromosome 4 by exon amplification. Nat Genet 1992;2:223.
44. Goldberg YP, Rommens JM, Andrew SE, et al. Identification of an Alu retrotransposition event in close proximity to a strong candidate gene for Huntington's disease. Nature 1993;362:370.
45. Ambrose CM, Duyao MP, Barnes G, et al. Structure and expression of the Huntington's disease gene: evidence against simple inactivation due to an expanded CAG repeat. Somat Cell Mol Genet 1994;20:27.
46. Huntington's Disease Collaborative Research Group. A novel gene containing a trinucleotide repeat that is expanded and unstable on Huntington's disease chromosomes. The Huntington's Disease Collaborative Research Group. Cell 1993;72:971.
47. Gusella JF, MacDonald ME. Huntington's disease: CAG genetics expands neurobiology. Curr Opin Neurobiol 1995;5:656.
48. Gusella JF, MacDonald ME. Huntington's disease. Semin Cell Biol 1995;6:21.
49. Rubinsztein DC, Barton DE, Davison BC, et al. Analysis of the huntingtin gene reveals a trinucleotide-length polymorphism in the region of the gene that contains two CCG-rich stretches and a correlation between decreased age of onset of Huntington's disease and CAG repeat number. Hum Mol Genet 1993;2:1713.

50. Andrew SE, Goldberg YP, Theilmann J, et al. A CCG repeat polymorphism adjacent to the CAG repeat in the Huntington disease gene: Implications for diagnostic accuracy and predictive testing. Hum Mol Genet 1994;3:65.
51. Nahhas FA, Garbern J, Krajewski KM, et al. Juvenile onset Huntington disease resulting from a very large maternal expansion. Am J Med Genet A 2005;137A:328.
52. Papapetropoulos S, Lopez-Alberola R, Baumbach L, et al. Case of maternally transmitted juvenile Huntington's disease with a very large trinucleotide repeat. Mov Disord 2005;20:1380.
53. MacDonald ME, Barnes G, Srinidhi J, et al. Gametic but not somatic instability of CAG repeat length in Huntington's disease. J Med Genet 1993;30:982.
54. Yoon SR, Dubeau L, de Young M, et al. Huntington disease expansion mutations in humans can occur before meiosis is completed. Proc Natl Acad Sci U S A 2003;100:8834.
55. Wheeler VC, Persichetti F, McNeil SM, et al. Factors associated with HD CAG repeat instability in Huntington disease. J Med Genet 2007;44:695.
56. Warby SC, Montpetit A, Hayden AR, et al. CAG expansion in the Huntington disease gene is associated with a specific and targetable predisposing haplogroup. Am J Hum Genet 2009;84:351.
57. Telenius H, Kremer B, Goldberg YP, et al. Somatic and gonadal mosaicism of the Huntington disease gene CAG repeat in brain and sperm. Nat Genet 1994;6:409.
58. De Rooij KE, De Koning Gans PA, Roos RA, et al. Somatic expansion of the (CAG)n repeat in Huntington disease brains. Hum Genet 1995;95:270.
59. Zuhlke C, Riess O, Bockel B, et al. Mitotic stability and meiotic variability of the (CAG)n repeat in the Huntington disease gene. Hum Mol Genet 1993;2:2063.
60. Norremolle A, Hasholt L, Petersen CB, et al. Mosaicism of the CAG repeat sequence in the Huntington disease gene in a pair of monozygotic twins. Am J Med Genet A 2004;130A:154.
61. Shelbourne PF, Keller-McGandy C, Bi WL, et al. Triplet repeat mutation length gains correlate with cell-type specific vulnerability in Huntington disease brain. Hum Mol Genet 2007;16:1133.
62. Kennedy L, Evans E, Chen CM, et al. Dramatic tissue-specific mutation length increases are an early molecular event in Huntington disease pathogenesis. Hum Mol Genet 2003;12:3359.
63. Gonitel R, Moffitt H, Sathasivam K, et al. DNA instability in postmitotic neurons. Proc Natl Acad Sci U S A 2008;105:3467.
64. Swami M, Hendricks AE, Gillis T, et al. Somatic expansion of the Huntington's disease CAG repeat in the brain is associated with an earlier age of disease onset. Hum Mol Genet 2009;18:3039.
65. Veitch NJ, Ennis M, McAbney JP, et al. Inherited CAG. CTG allele length is a major modifier of somatic mutation length variability in Huntington disease. DNA Repair (Amst) 2007;6:789.
66. Andrew SE, Goldberg YP, Kremer B, et al. Huntington disease without CAG expansion: Phenocopies or errors in assignment? Am J Hum Genet 1994;54:852.
67. Goldberg YP, Kremer B, Andrew SE, et al. Molecular analysis of new mutations for Huntington's disease: Intermediate alleles and sex of origin effects. Nat Genet 1993;5:174.
68. Myers RH, MacDonald ME, Koroshetz WJ, et al. De novo expansion of a (CAG)n repeat in sporadic Huntington's disease. Nat Genet 1993;5:168.
69. Persichetti F, Srinidhi J, Kanaley L, et al. Huntington's disease CAG trinucleotide repeats in pathologically confirmed post-mortem brains. Neurobiol Dis 1994;1:159.
70. Brandt J, Bylsma FW, Gross R, et al. Trinucleotide repeat length and clinical progression in Huntington's disease. Neurology 1996;46:527.
71. Illarioshkin SN, Igarashi S, Onodera O, et al. Trinucleotide repeat length and rate of progression of Huntington's disease. Ann Neurol 1994;36:630.
72. Kieburtz K, MacDonald M, Shih C, et al. Trinucleotide repeat length and progression of illness in Huntington's disease. J Med Genet 1994;31:872.
73. Marder K, Sandler S, Lechich A, et al. Relationship between CAG repeat length and late-stage outcomes in Huntington's disease. Neurology 2002;59:1622.
74. Squitieri F, Cannella M, Simonelli, M. CAG mutation effect on rate of progression in Huntington's disease. Neurol Sci 2002;23(Suppl 2):S107.
75. Furtado S, Suchowersky O, Rewcastle B, et al. Relationship between trinucleotide repeats and neuropathological changes in Huntington's disease. Ann Neurol 1996;39:132.
76. Penney JB Jr, Vonsattel JP, MacDonald ME, et al. CAG repeat number governs the development rate of pathology in Huntington's disease. Ann Neurol 1997;41:689.
77. Gusella JF, McNeil S, Persichetti F, et al. Huntington's disease. Cold Spring Harb Symp Quant Biol 1996, 61:615.
78. Aylward EH, Sparks BF, Field KM, et al. Onset and rate of striatal atrophy in preclinical Huntington disease. Neurology 2004;63:66.
79. Beglinger LJ, Paulsen JS, Watson DB, et al. Obsessive and compulsive symptoms in prediagnosed Huntington's disease. J Clin Psychiatry 2008;69:1758.
80. Biglan KM, Ross CA, Langbehn DR, et al. Motor abnormalities in premanifest persons with Huntington's disease: The PREDICT-HD study. Mov Disord 2009;24:1763.
81. Diamond R, White RF, Myers RH, et al. Evidence of presymptomatic cognitive decline in Huntington's disease. J Clin Exp Neuropsychol 1992;14:961.
82. Duff K, Paulsen JS, Beglinger LJ, et al. Psychiatric symptoms in Huntington's disease before diagnosis: The predict-HD study. Biol Psychiatry 2007;62:1341.
83. Johnson SA, Stout JC, Solomon AC, et al. Beyond disgust: Impaired recognition of negative emotions prior to diagnosis in Huntington's disease. Brain 2007;130:1732.
84. Julien CL, Thompson JC, Wild S, et al. Psychiatric disorders in preclinical Huntington's disease. J Neurol Neurosurg Psychiatry 2007;78:939.
85. Kirkwood SC, Siemers E, Stout JC, et al. Longitudinal cognitive and motor changes among presymptomatic Huntington disease gene carriers. Arch Neurol 1999; 56:563.
86. Kloppel S, Chu C, Tan GC, et al. Automatic detection of preclinical neurodegeneration: Presymptomatic Huntington disease. Neurology 2009;72:426.

87. Kloppel S, Draganski B, Siebner HR, et al. Functional compensation of motor function in pre-symptomatic Huntington's disease. Brain 2009;132:1624.
88. Paulsen JS, Langbehn DR, Stout JC, et al. Detection of Huntington's disease decades before diagnosis: The Predict-HD study. J Neurol Neurosurg Psychiatry 2008;79:874.
89. Paulsen JS, Zimbelman JL, Hinton SC, et al. fMRI biomarker of early neuronal dysfunction in presymptomatic Huntington's Disease. AJNR Am J Neuroradiol 2004;25:1715.
90. Reading SA, Dziorny AC, Peroutka LA, et al. Functional brain changes in presymptomatic Huntington's disease. Ann Neurol 2004;55:879.
91. Rosas HD, Hevelone ND, Zaleta AK, et al. Regional cortical thinning in preclinical Huntington disease and its relationship to cognition. Neurology 2005;65:745.
92. Siemers E, Foroud T, Bill DJ, et al. Motor changes in presymptomatic Huntington disease gene carriers. Arch Neurol 1996;53:487.
93. Solomon AC, Stout JC, Johnson SA, et al. Verbal episodic memory declines prior to diagnosis in Huntington's disease. Neuropsychologia 2007;45:1767.
94. Barnes GT, Duyao MP, Ambrose CM, et al. Mouse Huntington's disease gene homolog (Hdh). Somat Cell Mol Genet 1994;20:87.
95. Baxendale S, Abdulla S, Elgar G, et al. Comparative sequence analysis of the human and pufferfish Huntington's disease genes. Nat Genet 1995;10:67.
96. Candiani S, Pestarino M, Cattaneo E, et al. Characterization, developmental expression and evolutionary features of the huntingtin gene in the amphioxus Branchiostoma floridae. BMC Dev Biol 2007;7:127.
97. Gissi C, Pesole G, Cattaneo E, et al. Huntingtin gene evolution in Chordata and its peculiar features in the ascidian Ciona genus. BMC Genomics 2006;7:288.
98. Karlovich CA, John RM, Ramirez L, et al. Characterization of the Huntington's disease (HD) gene homologue in the zebrafish Danio rerio. Gene 1998;217:117.
99. Li Z, Karlovich CA, Fish MP, et al. A putative Drosophila homolog of the Huntington's disease gene. Hum Mol Genet 1999;8:1807.
100. Lin B, Nasir J, MacDonald H, et al. Sequence of the murine Huntington disease gene: Evidence for conservation, alternate splicing and polymorphism in a triplet (CCG) repeat [corrected]. Hum Mol Genet 1994;3:85.
101. Matsuyama N, Hadano S, Onoe K, et al. Identification and characterization of the miniature pig Huntington's disease gene homolog: Evidence for conservation and polymorphism in the CAG triplet repeat. Genomics 2000;69:72.
102. Schmitt I, Bachner D, Megow D, et al. Expression of the Huntington disease gene in rodents: Cloning the rat homologue and evidence for downregulation in non-neuronal tissues during development. Hum Mol Genet 1995;4:1173.
103. Takano H, Gusella JF. The predominantly HEAT-like motif structure of huntingtin and its association and coincident nuclear entry with dorsal, an NF-kB/Rel/dorsal family transcription factor. BMC Neurosci 2002;3:15.
104. Tartari M, Gissi C, Lo Sardo V, et al. Phylogenetic comparison of huntingtin homologues reveals the appearance of a primitive polyQ in sea urchin. Mol Biol Evol 2008;25:330.
105. Andrade MA, Bork P. HEAT repeats in the Huntington's disease protein. Nat Genet 1995;11:115.
106. Kobe B, Gleichmann T, Horne J, et al. Turn up the HEAT. Structure 1999;7:R91.
107. Seong IS, Woda JM, Song JJ, et al. Huntingtin facilitates polycomb repressive complex 2. Hum Mol Genet 2009.
108. Jou YS, Myers, RM. Evidence from antibody studies that the CAG repeat in the Huntington disease gene is expressed in the protein. Hum Mol Genet 1995;4:465.
109. Persichetti F, Ambrose CM, Ge P, et al. Normal and expanded Huntington's disease gene alleles produce distinguishable proteins due to translation across the CAG repeat. Mol Med 1995;1:374.
110. Sharp AH, Loev SJ, Schilling G, et al. Widespread expression of Huntington's disease gene (IT15) protein product. Neuron 1995;14:1065.
111. Trottier Y, Devys D, Imbert G, et al. Cellular localization of the Huntington's disease protein and discrimination of the normal and mutated form. Nat Genet 1995;10:104.
112. Trettel F, Rigamonti D, Hilditch-Maguire P, et al. Dominant phenotypes produced by the HD mutation in STHdh(Q111) striatal cells. Hum Mol Genet 2000; 9:2799.
113. Persichetti F, Trettel F, Huang CC, et al. Mutant huntingtin forms in vivo complexes with distinct context-dependent conformations of the polyglutamine segment. Neurobiol Dis 1999;6:364.
114. DiFiglia M, Sapp E, Chase K, et al. Huntingtin is a cytoplasmic protein associated with vesicles in human and rat brain neurons. Neuron 1995;14:1075.
115. Gusella JF, MacDonald, ME. Molecular genetics: Unmasking polyglutamine triggers in neurodegenerative disease. Nat Rev Neurosci 2000;1:109.
116. Stine OC, Li SH, Pleasant N, et al. Expression of the mutant allele of IT-15 (the HD gene) in striatum and cortex of Huntington's disease patients. Hum Mol Genet 1995;4:15.
117. Duyao MP, Auerbach AB, Ryan A, et al. Inactivation of the mouse Huntington's disease gene homolog Hdh. Science 1995;269:407.
118. Zeitlin S, Liu JP, Chapman DL, et al. Increased apoptosis and early embryonic lethality in mice nullizygous for the Huntington's disease gene homologue. Nat Genet 1995;11:155.
119. Gusella JF, MacDonald ME. Huntingtin: a single bait hooks many species. Curr Opin Neurobiol 1998;8:425.
120. Seong IS, Ivanova E, Lee JM, et al. HD CAG repeat implicates a dominant property of huntingtin in mitochondrial energy metabolism. Hum Mol Genet 2005;14:2871.
121. Clabough EB, Zeitlin, SO. Deletion of the triplet repeat encoding polyglutamine within the mouse Huntington's disease gene results in subtle behavioral/motor phenotypes in vivo and elevated levels of ATP with cellular senescence in vitro. Hum Mol Genet 2006; 15:607.
122. Di Maria E, Marasco A, Tartari M, et al. No evidence of association between BDNF gene variants and age-at-onset of Huntington's disease. Neurobiol Dis 2006;24:274.
123. Kishikawa S, Li JL, Gillis T, et al. Brain-derived neurotrophic factor does not influence age at neurologic onset of Huntington's disease. Neurobiol Dis 2006;24:280.

124. Metzger S, Bauer P, Tomiuk J, et al. Genetic analysis of candidate genes modifying the age-at-onset in Huntington's disease. Hum Genet 2006;120:285.
125. Gusella JF, Macdonald ME. Huntington's disease: the case for genetic modifiers. Genome Med 2009;1:80.
126. MacDonald ME, Vonsattel JP, Shrinidhi J, et al. Evidence for the GluR6 gene associated with younger onset age of Huntington's disease. Neurology 1999;53:1330.
127. Rubinsztein DC, Leggo J, Chiano M, et al. Genotypes at the GluR6 kainate receptor locus are associated with variation in the age of onset of Huntington disease. Proc Natl Acad Sci U S A 1997;94:3872.
128. Zeng W, Gillis T, Hakky M, et al. Genetic analysis of the GRIK2 modifier effect in Huntington's disease. BMC Neurosci 2006;7:62.
129. Ishiguro H, Yamada K, Sawada H, et al. Age-dependent and tissue-specific CAG repeat instability occurs in mouse knock-in for a mutant Huntington's disease gene. J Neurosci Res 2001;65:289.
130. Lin CH, Tallaksen-Greene S, Chien WM, et al. Neurological abnormalities in a knock-in mouse model of Huntington's disease. Hum Mol Genet 2001;10:137.
131. Menalled LB, Sison JD, Wu Y, et al. Early motor dysfunction and striosomal distribution of huntingtin microaggregates in Huntington's disease knock-in mice. J Neurosci 2002;22:8266.
132. Shelbourne PF, Killeen N, Hevner RF, et al. A Huntington's disease CAG expansion at the murine Hdh locus is unstable and associated with behavioural abnormalities in mice. Hum Mol Genet 1999;8:763.
133. White JK, Auerbach W, Duyao MP, et al. Huntingtin is required for neurogenesis and is not impaired by the Huntington's disease CAG expansion. Nat Genet 1997;17:404.
134. Wheeler VC, Auerbach W, White JK, et al. Length-dependent gametic CAG repeat instability in the Huntington's disease knock-in mouse. Hum Mol Genet 1999;8:115.
135. Auerbach W, Hurlbert MS, Hilditch-Maguire P, et al. The HD mutation causes progressive lethal neurological disease in mice expressing reduced levels of huntingtin. Hum Mol Genet 2001;10:2515.
136. Dragatsis I, Levine MS, Zeitlin S. Inactivation of Hdh in the brain and testis results in progressive neurodegeneration and sterility in mice. Nat Genet 2000;26:300.
137. Fossale E, Wheeler VC, Vrbanac V, et al. Identification of a presymptomatic molecular phenotype in Hdh CAG knock-in mice. Hum Mol Genet 2002;11:2233.
138. Gines S, Seong IS, Fossale E, et al. Specific progressive cAMP reduction implicates energy deficit in presymptomatic Huntington's disease knock-in mice. Hum Mol Genet 2003;12:497.
139. Wheeler VC, Gutekunst CA, Vrbanac V, et al. Early phenotypes that presage late-onset neurodegenerative disease allow testing of modifiers in Hdh CAG knock-in mice. Hum Mol Genet 2002;11:633.
140. Wheeler VC, White JK, Gutekunst CA, et al. Long glutamine tracts cause nuclear localization of a novel form of huntingtin in medium spiny striatal neurons in HdhQ92 and HdhQ111 knock-in mice. Hum Mol Genet 2000;9:503.
141. Brooks SP, Betteridge H, Trueman RC, et al. Selective extra-dimensional set shifting deficit in a knock-in mouse model of Huntington's disease. Brain Res Bull 2006;69:452.
142. Hickey MA, Kosmalska A, Enayati J, et al. Extensive early motor and non-motor behavioral deficits are followed by striatal neuronal loss in knock-in Huntington's disease mice. Neuroscience 2008;157:280.
143. Menalled L, El-Khodor BF, Patry M, et al. Systematic behavioral evaluation of Huntington's disease transgenic and knock-in mouse models. Neurobiol Dis 2009;35:319.
144. Trueman RC, Brooks SP, Jones L, et al. The operant serial implicit learning task reveals early onset motor learning deficits in the Hdh knock-in mouse model of Huntington's disease. Eur J Neurosci 2007;25:551.
145. Trueman RC, Brooks SP, Jones L, et al. Time course of choice reaction time deficits in the Hdh(Q92) knock-in mouse model of Huntington's disease in the operant serial implicit learning task (SILT). Behav Brain Res 2008;189:317.
146. Trueman RC, Brooks SP, Jones L, et al. Rule learning, visuospatial function and motor performance in the Hdh(Q92) knock-in mouse model of Huntington's disease. Behav Brain Res 2009;203:215.
147. Hodgson JG, Agopyan N, Gutekunst CA, et al. A YAC mouse model for Huntington's disease with full-length mutant huntingtin, cytoplasmic toxicity, and selective striatal neurodegeneration. Neuron 1999;23:181.
148. Hodgson JG, Smith DJ, McCutcheon K, et al. Human huntingtin derived from YAC transgenes compensates for loss of murine huntingtin by rescue of the embryonic lethal phenotype. Hum Mol Genet 1996;5:1875.
149. Lloret A, Dragileva E, Teed A, et al. Genetic background modifies nuclear mutant huntingtin accumulation and HD CAG repeat instability in Huntington's disease knock-in mice. Hum Mol Genet 2006;15:2015.
150. Kono Y, Agawa Y, Watanabe Y, et al. Analysis of the CAG repeat number in a patient with Huntington's disease. Intern Med 1999;38:407.
151. Wheeler VC, Lebel LA, Vrbanac V, et al. Mismatch repair gene Msh2 modifies the timing of early disease in Hdh(Q111) striatum. Hum Mol Genet 2003;12:273.
152. Dragileva E, Hendricks A, Teed A, et al. Intergenerational and striatal CAG repeat instability in Huntington's disease knock-in mice involve different DNA repair genes. Neurobiol Dis 2009;33:37.
153. Hilditch-Maguire P, Trettel F, Passani LA, et al. Huntingtin: An iron-regulated protein essential for normal nuclear and perinuclear organelles. Hum Mol Genet 2000;9:2789.
154. Rigamonti D, Bauer JH, De-Fraja C, et al. Wild-type huntingtin protects from apoptosis upstream of caspase-3. J Neurosci 2000;20:3705.
155. Rigamonti D, Sipione S, Goffredo D, et al. Huntingtin's neuroprotective activity occurs via inhibition of procaspase-9 processing. J Biol Chem 2001;276:14545.
156. Zuccato C, Ciammola A, Rigamonti D, et al. Loss of huntingtin-mediated BDNF gene transcription in Huntington's disease. Science 2001;293:493.
157. Squitieri F, Gellera C, Cannella M, et al. Homozygosity for CAG mutation in Huntington disease is associated with a more severe clinical course. Brain 2003;126:946.

158. Brandt J, Quaid KA, Folstein SE, et al. Presymptomatic diagnosis of delayed-onset disease with linked DNA markers. The experience in Huntington's disease. JAMA 1989;261:3108.
159. Meissen GJ, Myers RH, Mastromauro CA, et al. Predictive testing for Huntington's disease with use of a linked DNA marker. N Engl J Med 1988;318:535.
160. Wiggins S, Whyte P, Huggins M, et al. The psychological consequences of predictive testing for Huntington's disease. Canadian Collaborative Study of Predictive Testing. N Engl J Med 1992;327:1401.
161. Went L. Ethical issues policy statement on Huntington's disease molecular genetics predictive test. International Huntington Association. World Federation of Neurology. J Med Genet 1990;27:34.
162. Alberola TM, Bautista-Llacer R, Fernandez E, et al. Preimplantation genetic diagnosis of P450 oxidoreductase deficiency and Huntington Disease using three different molecular approaches simultaneously. J Assist Reprod Genet 2009;26:263.
163. Chow JF, Yeung WS, Lau EY, et al. Singleton birth after preimplantation genetic diagnosis for Huntington disease using whole genome amplification. Fertil Steril 2009;92:828 e7.
164. Evers-Kiebooms G, Nys K, Harper P, et al. Predictive DNA-testing for Huntington's disease and reproductive decision making: a European collaborative study. Eur J Hum Genet 2002;10:167.
165. Jasper MJ, Hu DG, Liebelt J, et al. Singleton births after routine preimplantation genetic diagnosis using exclusion testing (D4S43 and D4S126) for Huntington's disease. Fertil Steril 2006;85:597.
166. Lashwood A, Flinter F. Clinical and counselling implications of preimplantation genetic diagnosis for Huntington's disease in the UK. Hum Fertil (Camb) 2001;4:235.
167. Moutou C, Gardes N, Viville S. New tools for preimplantation genetic diagnosis of Huntington's disease and their clinical applications. Eur J Hum Genet 2004;12:1007.
168. Pecina A, Lozano Arana MD, Garcia-Lozano JC, et al. One-step multiplex polymerase chain reaction for preimplantation genetic diagnosis of Huntington disease. Fertil Steril, 2009.
169. Sermon K, De Rijcke M, Lissens W, et al. Preimplantation genetic diagnosis for Huntington's disease with exclusion testing. Eur J Hum Genet 2002;10:591.
170. Sermon K, Goossens V, Seneca S, et al. Preimplantation diagnosis for Huntington's disease (HD): Clinical application and analysis of the HD expansion in affected embryos. Prenat Diagn 1998;18:1427.
171. Sermon K, Seneca S, De Rycke M, et al. PGD in the lab for triplet repeat diseases—Myotonic dystrophy, Huntington's disease and Fragile-X syndrome. Mol Cell Endocrinol 2001;183(Suppl 1):S77.
172. Stern HJ, Harton GL, Sisson ME, et al. Non-disclosing preimplantation genetic diagnosis for Huntington disease. Prenat Diagn 2002;22:503.
173. International Huntington Association (IHA) and the World Federation of Neurology (WFN) Research Group on Huntington's Chorea: Guidelines for the molecular genetics predictive test in Huntington's disease. Neurology 1994;44:1533.
174. McNeil SM, Novelletto A, Srinidhi J, et al. Reduced penetrance of the Huntington's disease mutation. Hum Mol Genet 1977;6:775.
175. Hendricks AE, Latourelle JC, Lunetta KL, et al. Estimating the probability of de novo HD cases from transmissions of expanded penetrant CAG alleles in the Huntington disease gene from male carriers of high normal alleles (27-35 CAG). Am J Med Genet A 2009;149A:1375.
176. Semaka A, Collins JA, Hayden MR. Unstable familial transmissions of Huntington disease alleles with 27–35 CAG repeats (intermediate alleles). Am J Med Genet B Neuropsychiatr Genet 2009.
177. Brocklebank D, Gayan J, Andresen JM, et al. Repeat instability in the 27–39 CAG range of the HD gene in the Venezuelan kindreds: Counseling implications. Am J Med Genet B Neuropsychiatr Genet 2009;150B:425.
178. Duyao M, Ambrose C, Myers R, et al. Trinucleotide repeat length instability and age of onset in Huntington's disease. Nat Genet 1993;4:387.
179. Langbehn DR, Brinkman RR, Falush D, et al. A new model for prediction of the age of onset and penetrance for Huntington's disease based on CAG length. Clin Genet 2004;65:267.
180. Lombardi MS, Jaspers L, Spronkmans C, et al. A majority of Huntington's disease patients may be treatable by individualized allele-specific RNA interference. Exp Neurol 2009;217:312.
181. Pfister EL, Kennington L, Straubhaar J, et al. Five siRNAs targeting three SNPs may provide therapy for three-quarters of Huntington's disease patients. Curr Biol 2009;19:774.
182. Park IH, Arora N, Huo H, et al. Disease-specific induced pluripotent stem cells. Cell 2008;134:877.
183. Tabrizi SJ, Langbehn DR, Leavitt BR, et al. Biological and clinical manifestations of Huntington's disease in the longitudinal TRACK-HD study: Cross-sectional analysis of baseline data. Lancet Neurol 2009;8:791.

CHAPTER 33

Clinical Features and Treatment of Huntington's Disease

Sarah Wahlster and Jang-Ho J. Cha

Chorea is essentially a disease of the nervous system. The name "chorea" is given to the disease on account of the dancing propensities of those who are affected by it, and it is a very appropriate designation... The hereditary chorea, as I shall call it, is confined to certain and fortunately a few families, and has been transmitted to them, an heirloom from generations away back in the dim past. It is spoken of by those in whose veins the seeds of the disease are known to exist, with a kind of horror, and not at all alluded to except, through dire necessity, when it is mentioned as "that disorder." It is attended generally by all the symptoms of common chorea, only in an aggravated degree, hardly ever manifesting itself until adult or middle life, and then coming on gradually but surely, increasing by degrees, and often occupying years in its development, until the hapless sufferer is but a quivering wreck of his former self...I have never known a recovery or even an amelioration of symptoms in this form of chorea; when once it begins it clings to the bitter end.—George Huntington, 1872[1]

▶ INTRODUCTION

In 1872, George Huntington provided one of the first descriptions of the disease that was subsequently named after him. His essay was based on his own clinical experience combined with his grandfather's and father's observations of several afflicted families in East Hampton, Long Island.[1] As a physician he followed these patients with great interest. He published his famous essay only at age 21; this manuscript remained his sole significant publication.[2]

It was not until over a century later that the genetic mutation causing HD was localized to chromosome 4p16.3 in 1983.[3] The defective gene and the nature of its mutation were identified in 1993 in a unique collaborative effort.[4] The discovery of the gene was rendered possible by the analysis of a large HD population in Venezuela. This kindred, thought to be the largest HD population in the world, live in the state of Zulia in the region of Lake Maracaibo, and comprise more than 18,149 individuals spanning 10 generations. Besides the enormous significance in identifying the HD mutation and for genetic research in general, the analysis of the Venezuelan population allowed a detailed description of the clinical picture and natural history of the disease.[5,6]

In the United States, HD affects approximately 30,000 people (5–10 per 100,000) with another estimated 150,000 at risk for developing the disease. There is a similar and rather uniform prevalence of HD throughout Europe, ranging between 4 and 7 per 100,000 with no clear distribution patterns over the continent. Particularly low rates of HD are encountered in Finland and Japan. Very high frequencies in Latin American countries neighboring Venezuela are probable. Obvious gender disparities among different countries and racial preponderances have not been observed.[7]

▶ DISEASE-CAUSING MUTATION

The genetic defect causing HD was assigned to chromosome 4 in 1983 in one of the first successful linkage analyses using polymorphic DNA markers.[3] The mutation accounting for the disease lies in the *IT15* (interesting transcript 15) gene, subsequently renamed Huntingtin (HTT). Huntingtin is a large protein with a molecular weight of approximately 350 kDa, encompassing 3144 amino acids. Its structure does not share any homology with other known proteins.[4] The gene for huntingtin comprises 67 exons, and the mutation is an expansion of the cytosine–adenine–guanosine (CAG) repeat in exon 1 coding for an abnormally large polyglutamine tract. The normal range of CAG repeats is between 7 and 34 triplets. Repeat lengths greater than 40 repeats invariably cause the disease. Intermediate CAG lengths between 35 and 39 may cause HD in some instances.[8–13] HD is part of a growing family of disorders caused by exonic CAG expansions that share multiple genetic and clinical features (Table 33–1). Each of the diseases displays a progressive neurodegenerative course and wide phenotypic variations between affected individuals. The

▶ TABLE 33–1. **CAG TRIPLET REPEAT EXPANSION DISEASES**

Disease	Affected Gene	Chr. Locus	Inh.	Repeat ranges		Clinical Features
				Normal	Disease	
Spinobulbar muscular atrophy (SBMA)/ Kennedy's disease	Androgen receptor (AR)	Xq11-12	XLR	13-30	38-62	Neurological: Limb-girdle muscle weakness (CK ↑), prominent muscle cramps, fasciculations (esp. facial and perioral), bulbar dysfunction (jaw drop), dysarthria, dysphagia, sensory neuronopathy (abnormal nerve conduction studies) with mild sensory impairment. Systemic/endocrine: Gynecomastia, testicular atrophy, feminization, infertility, diabetes mellitus. *Female heterozygous carriers can present with mild late-onset neuromuscular symptoms.*
Huntington's disease (HD)	Huntingtin (HTT)	4p16.3	AD	6-34	40-121	As reviewed within this chapter.
Dentatorubro-pallido-luysian atrophy (DRP-LA)/Haw River Syndrome (HRS)	Atrophin 1 (ATN1)	12p13.31	AD	7-23	49-88	Chorea, ataxia, myoclonic epilepsy, dystonia, parkinsionism, psychosis, dementia. Mostly observed within people of Japanese descent. Also described in African American family as Haw River Syndrome with extensive subcortical white matter demyelination and basal ganglia (BG) calcifications.
Spinocerebellar ataxia-1 (SCA 1)	Ataxin 1 (ATXN1)	6p23	AD	25-36	39-81	Spinocerebellar (SC) symptoms with prominent oculomotor abnormalities, UMN signs, behavioral disorders, dysphagia, peripheral neuropathy, autonomic impairment. Extrapyramidal symptoms and dementia are rare and occur late.
Spinocerebellar ataxia-2 (SCA 2)	Ataxin 2 (ATXN2)	12q24.12	AD	15-24	35-64, 200	SC symptoms, severe saccadic slowing, early and prominent gaze palsies, areflexia, hypotonus, impaired proprioception, muscle cramps, tremor, early dementia. With >200 repeats: infancy onset, retinitis pigmentosa.
Spinocerebellar ataxia-3 (SCA 3)/ Machado-Joseph Disease (MJD)	Ataxin 3 (ATXN3)	14q24.3-q31	AD	12-41	61-84	Most common AD cerebellar ataxia, high clinical variability (several subtypes). SC symptoms with oculomotor abnormalities, visual disturbances, dysphagia, UMN/ LMN signs and extrapyramidal features. Prominent facial/lingual fasciculations. Characteristic: Lid retraction → bulging eyes, persistent stare. Restless leg syndrome and sleep disturbances are frequent, dementia is rather atypical.

(continued)

▶ **TABLE 33–1. (CONTINUED)**

Disease	Affected Gene	Chr. Locus	Inh.	Repeat ranges		Clinical Features
				Normal	Disease	
Spinocerebellar ataxia-6 (SCA 6)	∝-1a Ca channel (CACNA1A) P/Q type Ca channel	19p13	AD	4-20	21-30	Almost pure cerebellar syndrome. Slow progression with episodic fluctuations. Horizontal (and some vertical) nystagmus. Same gene is also linked to Episodic Ataxia type 2 and Familial Hemiplegic Migraine (different mutations), overlap of symptoms between the diseases.
Spinocerebellar ataxia-7* (SCA 7)	Ataxin 7 (ATXN7)	3p12-13	AD	7-19	37-220	SC symptoms, irreversible bilateral visual loss (pigmentary macular degeneration), UMN signs. Childhood onset form: rapid and severe course, seizures, myoclonus, cardiac involvement, early visual loss, extremely large repeats. Adult onset: Ataxia predominant, later visual loss.
Spinocerebellar ataxia-8 (SCA 8) *Bidirectional transcription*	Ataxin 8 (ATXN8)-CTG/ Ataxin 8 Opposite Strand (ATXN8OS)-CAG	13q21	AD	15-34	89-240	Almost pure cerebellar syndrome. Dramatic repeat instability, expansions mostly observed with maternal transmission, possible contractions with paternal transmission). Extremely large repeats (800 bp) may be associated with an absence of clinical symptoms
Spinocerebellar ataxia-17 (SCA 17)	TATA-box binding protein (TBP)	6q27	AD	25-42	49-63	SC symptoms + prominent dementia, psychiatric symptoms, extrapyramidal features

Chr, chromosome; Inh, inheritance; AD, autosomal-dominant; XLR, X-linked recessive.

initial manifestation is typically in adult midlife with a wide variability. A negative correlation exists between the repeat length and the age of onset. Anticipation can occur as the gene is passed on to successive generations. Except for spinobulbar muscular atrophy (SBMA), which is inherited in an X-linked recessive manner, they are all inherited in an autosomal dominant fashion.

The function of normal huntingtin is unknown although it appears to be essential for development given that knockout mice die at embryonic stages.[14–16] Huntingtin is ubiquitously expressed with particularly high levels in the brain as well as the lung, ovaries, testis, skeletal muscle, and pancreas;[17] however, the disease primarily presents with neurological deficits.

▶ CLINICAL FEATURES

Huntington's disease is a neurodegenerative disease. It is inherited in an autosomal dominant fashion with complete penetrance. The major symptoms consist of the classic triad of a movement disorder, behavioral disturbance, and cognitive decline. There is a large heterogeneity in the manifestations of the disease in regard to the range of severity, predominant features, age of onset, and rate of clinical progression.

The peak age of adult-onset HD is in the fourth and fifth decade of life. The major determinant of age on onset is the length of the causative triplet CAG repeats with longer repeat lengths leading to a younger age at onset[8,9,12,18–20] (Fig. 33–1). The CAG repeat length is accountable for about 70% of the variability in age of onset,[19] suggesting additional genetic or environmental modifiers.

Homozygotes were initially thought to be similarly affected as heterozygotes,[21,22] supporting the hypothesis that expanded repeat-length huntingtin incurs a toxic gain-of-function. However, recent studies suggest that homozygotes may have slightly faster progression of motor, cognitive and behavioral features, and more

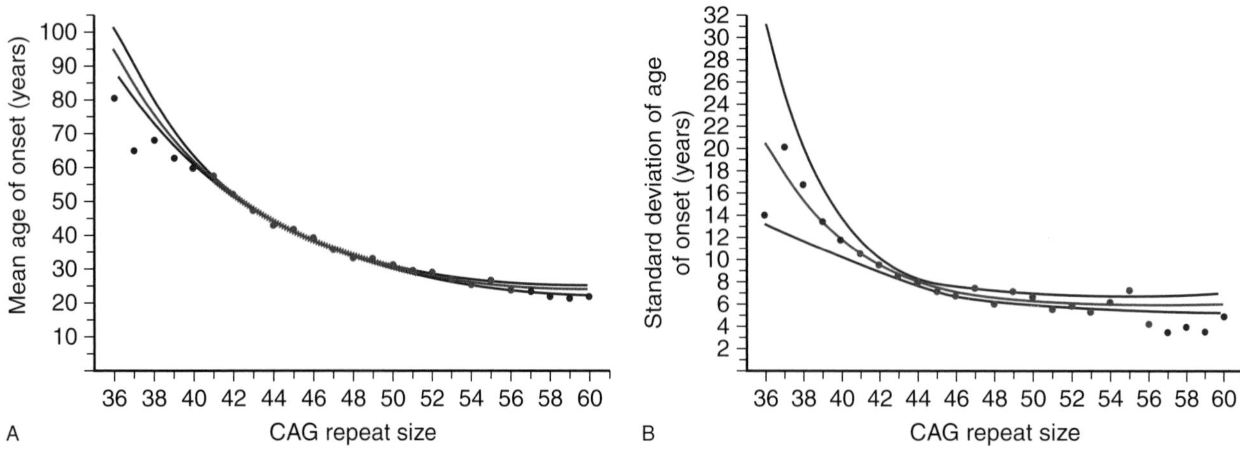

Figure 33–1. Relationship between CAG repeat length and age of onset in HD.[19] Population estimates of the mean age of onset (A) and standard deviation of the age of onset (B) for CAG repeat lengths 36–60. The symbols and solid line indicate the range of data that was used to fit the exponential curves. The O symbols and long dashed lines indicate CAG lengths for which the model's predictions were extrapolated. Small dashed lines indicate 95% confidence intervals, larger spaces between dashes indicate the region where the model's predictions were extrapolated.

pronounced neuropathological involvement, challenging the notion that HD is a purely dominant disease.[23]

The initial manifestation of disease varies among individuals. Subtle cognitive and behavioral changes that are often thought to precede the motor symptoms may be hard to capture. Given the progressive and insidious nature of the disease, it might be more appropriate to think of a "zone of onset" rather than a distinct age. The average duration of the disease is 15–20 years with wide variability. Main causes of mortality include pneumonia and cardiovascular disease. Pneumonia is often a direct consequence of the disease as a result of immobility and declining cognitive status in conjunction with swallowing difficulties.[24]

▶ NEUROPATHOLOGY

The most dramatic changes in HD are encountered in the neostriatum that consists of the caudate nucleus and putamen (Fig. 33–2). Severe striatal neuronal loss and reactive fibrillary astrocytosis are the pathological hallmark of the disease. Striatal medium spiny projection neurons degenerate selectively, whereas interneurons are relatively spared until the later stages of disease. The changes in the striatum exhibit a distinct pattern as the disease progresses. Degeneration is initially most pronounced in the tail of the caudate and the caudal portion of the putamen and progresses in a caudorostral and a mediolateral direction. Vonsattel and colleagues[25] distinguished five grades (0–4) of neuropathological involvement based on gross and microscopic findings in the striatum (Table 33–2). The classification is derived from findings at two different coronal levels: CAP (level caudate–accumbens–putamen) and GP (level globus pallidus). The Vonsattel grades correlate closely with CAG length,[26,27] clinical severity and the involvement of other brain regions. Grades 3 and 4 were found to be accompanied by pronounced atrophy of nonstriatal structures including the GP, cortex, thalamus, the subthalamic nucleus (STN), the substantia nigra and in some instances the cerebellum.[28]

The cortex in HD sustains a preferential loss of large pyramidal projection neurons in the deep cortical layers with a relative sparing of local circuits.[29–31] Recent neu-

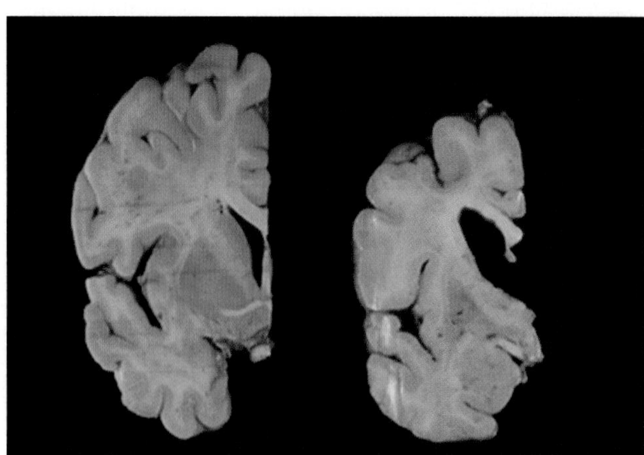

Figure 33–2. Neuropathology of HD: macroscopic features. Macroscopically visible changes in the HD brain (B) in comparison to a normal brain (A)—the HD brain displays global cerebral atrophy. The caudate nucleus is displaced, discolorated, and shrunken in size; the lateral ventricles are correspondingly enlarged.

▶ TABLE 33–2. **VONSATTEL CLASSIFICATION**

Grade	Pathological Correlate	
0	Substantial clinical evidence for HD, ideally along with a positive family history; however, no macroscopic or microscopic abnormalities related to HD	
1	Macroscopic: No distinguishable alterations in the striatum	Microscopic: CN: Evidence of mild to moderate FA and ND (medial > lateral) PUT: Evidence of mild FA (dorsal > rostral)
2	Macroscopic: Mild atrophy of the CN and PUT. The convex medial contour of the CN's head and the IC are still retained. The lateral ventricle is slightly enlarged.	Microscopic: CN: Evidence of moderate-to-severe FA and ND (medial > lateral) PUT: Evidence of mild-to-moderate FA and ND (dorsal > rostral) GP: Mild FA
3	Macroscopic: Moderate-to-severe atrophy of the CN and PUT. The CN head shows some yellow-brown discoloration and its medial outline is now forming a straight line. The anterior horn of the lateral ventricle is correspondingly enlarged. The GP is mildly decreased in size. The IC is about half of its normal thickness and its medial part is also in a straight-line configuration.	Microscopic: CN: Evidence of severe FA and ND (medial > lateral), difference between involvement of medial and lateral division less pronounced compared to Grades 1 and 2 PUT: Evidence of severe FA and ND (dorsal > rostral) GP: Evidence of mild-to-moderate FA and ND in the GPe, GPi mostly unremarkable NA: Evidence of slight FA and ND in a few instances.
4	Macroscopic: Very severe atrophy of the CN. The CN head is extremely shrunken, yellow-brown in discoloration and it's medial outline appears concave. The anterior horn of the lateral ventricle is correspondingly enlarged. The PUT is severely affected, also displaying a concave medial outline. The GP displays moderate atrophy with an indistinct external medullary lamina. The NA is mildly involved. The IC is also medially concave and its thickness is decreased to approximately one third.	Microscopic: CN: Evidence of extremely severe and diffuse FA and ND PUT: Evidence of extremely severe and diffuse FA and ND GP: Evidence of mild-to-moderate FA and ND in both the GPe and GPi NA: Evidence of mild-to-moderate FA (esp. dorsally) and slight ND L

CN, caudate nucleus; FA, fibrillary astrocytosis; GP, globus pallidus; GPe, globus pallidus external segment (lateral segment); GPi, globus pallidus internal segment (medial segment); IC, internal capsule; NA, nucleus accumbens; ND, neuronal depletion; PUT, putamen.

roimaging studies have described a progressive thinning of the cortex that occurs in topographically selective patterns.[32] In general, HD brains are found to demonstrate a prominent atrophy on autopsy with a particular involvement of the frontal lobes. The mean brain weight declines from 1350 to less than 1100 g. In addition to corticostriatal atrophy, a distinctive amount of volumetric white matter loss is observed.[28]

▶ MOVEMENT DISORDER

The movement disorder in Huntington's disease comprises both involuntary movements as well as an abnormality of normal movements. The coexisting hyperkinetic and hypokinetic components of the movement disorder are thought to be caused by the degeneration of striatal neurons and reflect the involvement of both the direct and indirect pathways in accordance with the current basal ganglia model (Fig. 33–3).

Patients are mostly hyperreflexic early on; plantar response signs and Babinski signs occur in late stages. Spasticity may occur and additionally interfere with motor function. HD patients frequently exhibit a tremor with postural, action, and resting components.[5]

HYPERKINESIAS

Chorea

The term "chorea" is derived from the greek word *χορεία*, an ancient Greek circle dance. Chorea is an ex-

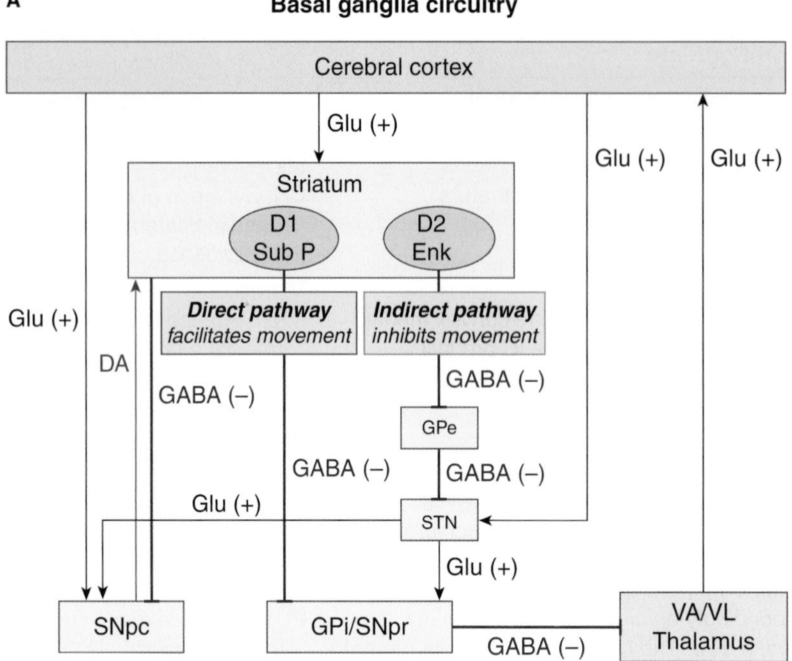

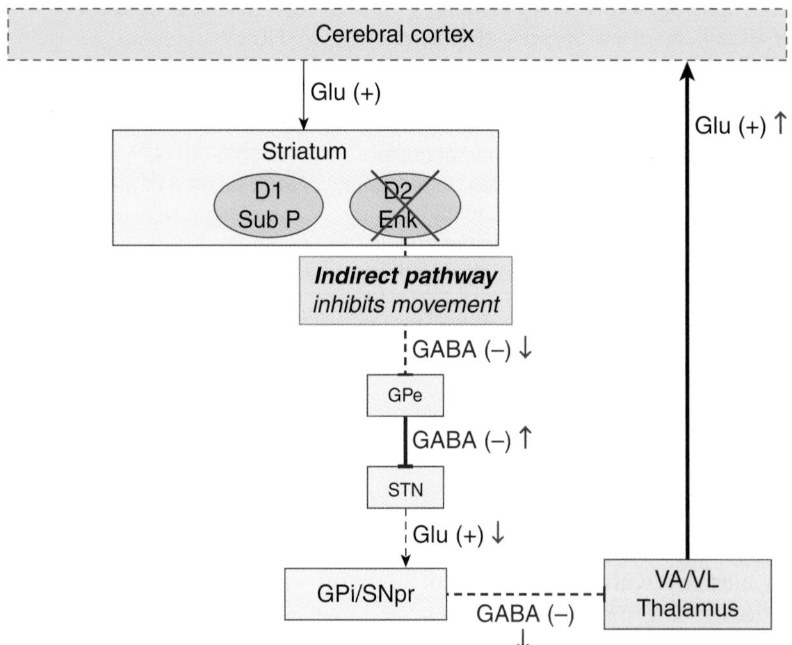

Figure 33–3. Basal ganglia model in HD pathogenesis. (A) Overview of the basal ganglia circuitry. (B) Early HD: Disruption of the indirect pathway → disinhibition of the thalamus → excessive cortical stimulation → increased movements. (C) Late HD: Additional disruption of the direct pathway → inhibition of the thalamus → lack of cortical stimulation → decreased movements.
Arrows: black = glutamatergic (excitatory) pathways; blue = GABAergic (inhibitory) pathways; purple = dopaminergic (both excitatory/inhibitory) pathways.

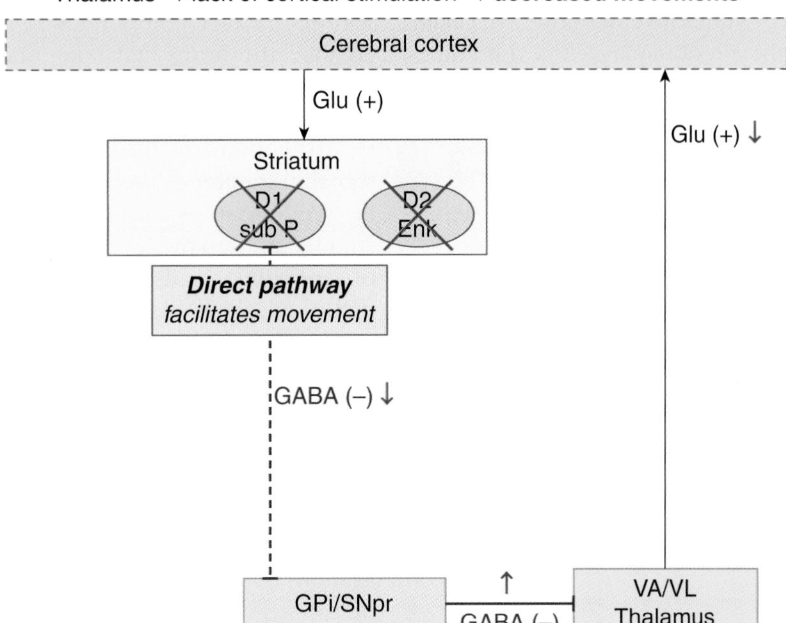

Figure 33–3. (Continued)

cessive, rapid, irregular, uncontrolled movement. It occurs spontaneously and randomly throughout the whole body, seeming to move from one part of the body to another. All skeletal muscles may be involved, including the respiratory, pharyngeal, and laryngeal musculature. Chorea is not typically repetitive or rhythmic, and in its initial manifestation usually not disabling.[33] However as the visually most striking symptom, chorea can frequently expose the patient to social stigmatization. Some patients report that they can feel the movements building up and initially they may be able to suppress them. Patients occasionally superimpose voluntarily semipurposeful movements to the choreiform movements to mask them, a phenomenon referred to as *parakinesia*. At a later stage, patients often develop a certain habituation toward their movements and may not even be consciously aware of them.

Patients with chorea exhibit motor impersistence, failing to maintain a sustained posture. When asked to protrude the tongue, patients are often unable to keep it outside as it snaps back ("harlequin's tongue"). Upon attempting to grip an object, they alternately squeeze and release ("milkmaid's grip") and often tend to drop the object. Chorea appears less frequently in the deep stages of sleep.[34] As the amplitude and frequency of the movements increases chorea can interfere with the patients' ability to ambulate independently. Chorea tends to diminish in the later stages of the disease.

The neuropathological correlate of chorea is characterized by a selective loss of striatal neurons projecting to the external segment of the GP and an interruption of the "indirect pathway" of the basal ganglia circuit. Loss of these neurons decreases tonic inhibitory input on the motor cortex resulting in increased movement.[35–39]

Athetosis and Ballismus

Chorea often occurs concomitantly with athetosis and is then referred to as choreoathetosis. Athetosis (*Greek—not fixed*) is considered to be a slower form of chorea that has an additional writhing component, resembling the twisting movements of a snake. The writhing appearance may be caused by superimposed dystonia. Ballism/ballismus (*Greek—jumping about, dancing*) is a severe manifestation of chorea in which the movements have a violent, flinging quality. Ballism mostly involves the axial and proximal appendicular musculature and typically appears as rotatory, wild flailing movements of the extremities. It is frequently confined to one side of the body and then referred to as hemiballismus. Hemiballismus is thought to emanate from the STN either by direct impairment of the STN or as a result of disrupted circuits, for example through lost inhibition by the external globus pallidus (GPe).

Tics and Myoclonus

Patients can present with other hyperkinesias such as motor and vocal tics, often resembling Tourette's syndrome.[40–42] Excessive bruxism, which involves grinding of the teeth and jaw-clenching, may occur.[42,43] Myoclonus is mostly observed in bradykinetic forms of the disease, typically associated with a juvenile onset, but has also been reported as the predominant clinical feature in adults.[44–46]

EYE MOVEMENT ABNORMALITIES

Oculomotor deficits are among the earliest motor manifestations of HD[5] and can also be observed in gene-positive individuals several years before clinical diagnosis,[6, 47–50] whereas deficits in executing voluntary saccades[48] and perturbed optokinetic nystagmus (OKN) are characteristic early changes.[51] Attempts at initiating voluntary saccades are frequently accompanied by compensatory head thrusts and eye blinks ("oculomotor apraxia").[52] Saccadic reaction time increases as the disease progresses.[53] The range of voluntary eye movements decreases with the vertical component being more strongly affected than the horizontal component. In advanced cases with a marked restriction of voluntary gaze saccades often fall short of the target (hypometria).[52]

In contrast to the striking deficits in voluntary internally triggered saccades, externally triggered "reflexive" saccades to suddenly appearing novel visual stimuli are relatively spared.[49, 50, 52, 54] This consistent observation stands in accordance with the neuropathological profile of HD, suggesting a stronger involvement of frontobasal pathways in the face of less affected parieto-occipital circuits (Fig. 33–4). Patients with HD frequently experience difficulties in maintaining fixation.[52] Steady gaze is commonly disrupted by

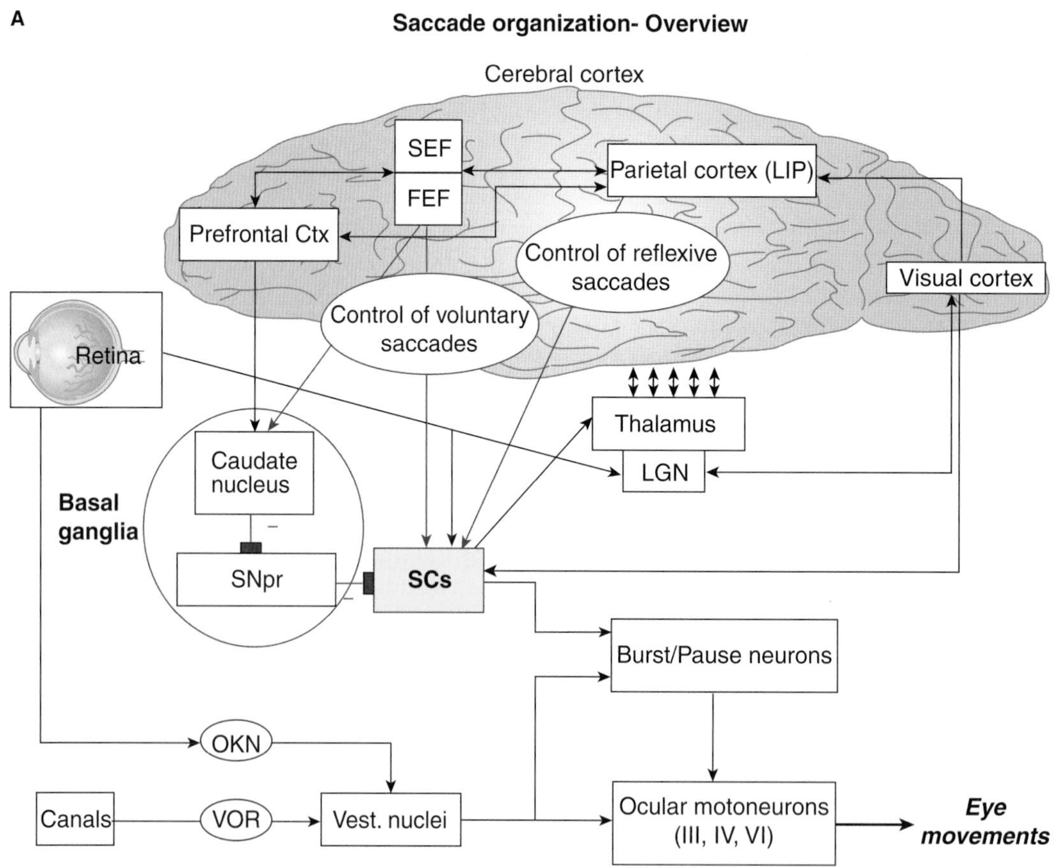

Figure 33–4. Pathways saccadic control in HD. (A) Organization of saccades. The superior colliculi (SC) are thought to control the release of saccades. The SC receive convergent input from different cerebral cortical areas and the basal ganglia. Voluntary saccades are thought to be regulated by pathways from the frontal eye field (FEF) to the SC. Also, the FEFs send projections to the caudate nucleus (CN), which inhibits the substantia nigra pars reticulata (SNpr). Reflexive saccades are thought to be mediated by connections between the lateral interparietal (LIP) area and the SC. (B) Disruption of saccadic organization secondary to frontostriatal atrophy in HD. The SNpr exerts a tonic inhibition on the SC. The degeneration of caudate neurons leads to a loss of the disinhibition that is needed for the saccades to be allowed. Also, the direct FEF-SC connections may be lost because of frontal cortical atrophy in HD.
Arrows: red = main pathways involved in voluntary/internally triggered saccade initiation; blue = main pathways involved in reflexive/externally triggered saccade initiation.

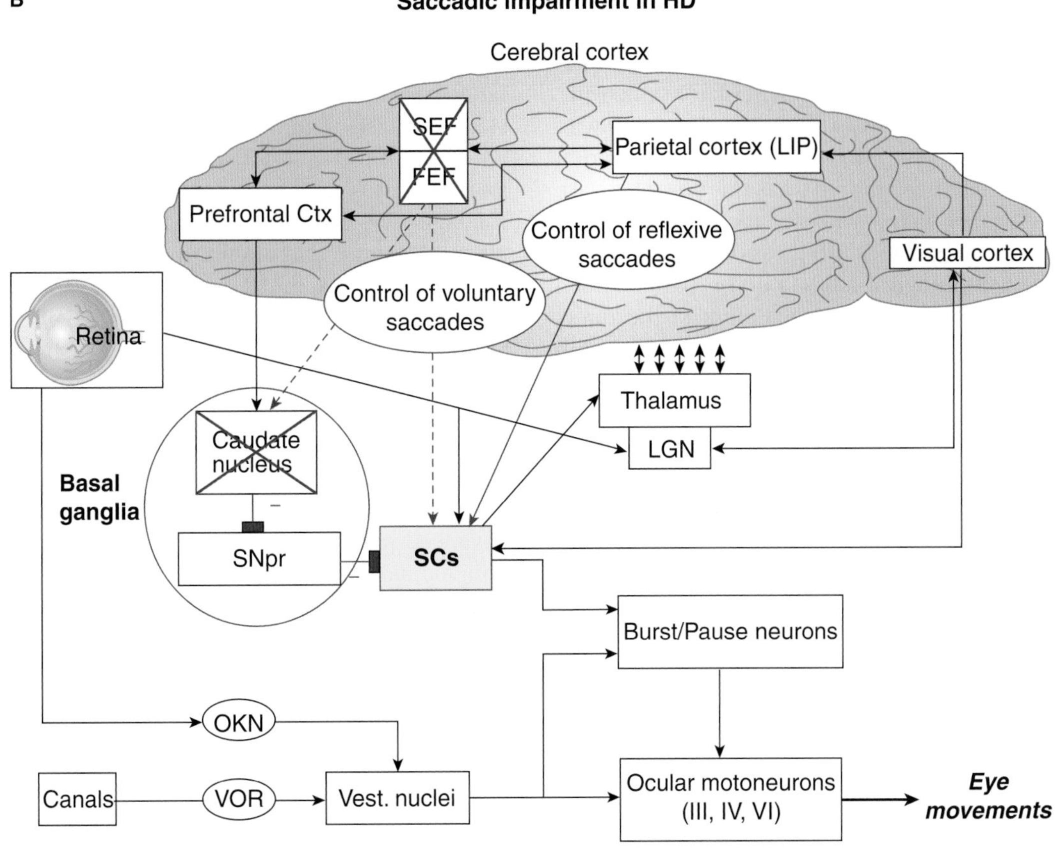

Figure 33–4. (Continued)

small extraneous saccades (<3 degrees in amplitude). These "square wave jerks" are very sensitive changes in HD; they persist in total darkness and can occur up to 10 times/minute. Fixation is also disrupted by large extraneous saccades (>10 degrees) that take the eye off the target and become more pronounced as the disease progresses.[55] OKN is impaired in all directions with the vertical component being affected earlier,[56] the vestibulo-ocular reflex (VOR) is relatively spared. Smooth pursuit of eye movements becomes disrupted in more advanced cases of HD.

FINE MOTOR COORDINATION

Concomitant with eye movement abnormalities, loss of fine motor control is one of the early motor manifestations ("soft signs") of HD.[5] Impairment of finger tapping and the slowing of rapid alternating movements (dysdiadochokinesia) can be observed in prediagnostic gene carriers.[6] Lack of coordination is present, frequently leading to over- or undershooting when the patient is trying to reach a certain goal (dysmetria). Ataxia is a rather atypical feature but may occur rarely in conjunction with pronounced cerebellar atrophy,[57,58] and is mostly seen in juveniles and younger patients.[28]

DYSARTHRIA AND DYSPHAGIA

Dysarthria is a common and prominent feature of HD that is thought to result from interplay of impaired coordination between laryngeal, pharyngeal and respiratory muscles, speech motor deficits attributable to slowed movement execution, and superimposed chorea. Speech difficulties are present early on and worsen during the course of the disease. Patients are frequently hypophonic. Other speech deficits include syllable repetition, displaced articulation and an increased variability of utterance duration and voice-onset-time.[59] In advanced stages, the speech becomes truncated and hardly intelligible; some patients are anarthric. Dysphagia emerges as the disease progresses and becomes severe in the final stages of the illness. The impairment in swallowing contributes to weight loss. Frequent choking makes the patients prone to aspiration and resulting pneumonia, which is the most frequent cause of death in HD.

DYSTONIA AND PARKINSONISM

Dystonia and parkinsonism may be present in early stages and surface increasingly in the course of the disease. In the later stages choreic movements generally tend to diminish as dystonia and parkinsonism predominate.[60,61] Patients with the juvenile form of HD frequently present with rigidity and bradykinesia as the predominant motor symptoms. In rare instances pronounced parkinsonism at onset with paucity of chorea can also been seen in the adult form of HD. This manifestation is referred to as the Westphal variant and is associated with a younger age of onset, larger repeat sizes, and faster clinical progression.[33,58,62]

The neuropathological correlate for parkinsonian features can be explained by involvement of the direct pathway in the basal ganglia circuit. In patients with the akinetic-rigid form of HD, there is additional loss of the striatal neurons projecting to the medial segment of the pallidum (GPi) in the absence of neuronal degeneration in the substantia nigra.[37] Functional imaging studies have shown more pronounced reductions of dopamine D1 and D2 receptors in patients with predominantly rigid manifestations of HD.[63]

GAIT DIFFICULTIES

Gait instability is a major concern in patients with HD because it predisposes for falls and subsequent injuries. Abnormalities of gait and posture are evident in HD patients early on and become increasingly pronounced, eventually limiting the patients' independence and frequently resulting in nursing home placement.[64] Subtle gait difficulties that can already be seen in gene-positive at-risk individuals include decreased velocity and stride length. The impairments worsen with time and correlate to the predicted age of onset.[65]

Observers such as family members and friends frequently remark that the patients have a "drunk appearance" when walking. Decreased speed of walking, wide-based station, imbalance, and increased trunk sway is seen, with patients often exhibiting large lateral deviations. The gait disorder in HD is in some aspects similar to a parkinsonian gait with small shuffling steps, difficulty in initiation of locomotion, reduced associated movements of the arms and difficulties in turning. Tandem gait becomes impaired in advanced disease stages.[66,67] Worsening gait correlates with disease severity and significantly impacts the individuals' functional capacity.[68,69]

▶ COGNITIVE AND PSYCHIATRIC ABNORMALITIES

The cognitive profile in HD exhibits a subcortical pattern. The most prominent deficits involve executive dysfunction and impairments in attention and concentration,[70–72] corresponding with the strong involvement of frontostriatal circuits in HD pathology. These deficits are tightly interlaced with the affective symptoms in HD.[73] Cognitive impairment in HD is thought to occur before the onset of motor symptoms,[74,75] and poses an important feature of functional decline,[76,77] Patients with HD experience difficulties in performing simultaneous or sequential movements, and the development of adequate movement strategies is perturbed.[78] These impairments of complex psychomotor skills and tasks requiring integrative cognitive processing are thought to be sensitive measures of disease progression in early stages accompanied by changes upon neuroimaging.[70,71] Tests that are aimed at measuring executive tasks, planning, and attention and thus best capture the cognitive deficits in HD include the Tower of Hanoi/London task, the modified Wisconsin Card Sorting Test, Stroop Color Word Interference Task, Verbal Fluency, and Symbol Digit Modalities Test. The latter three tests are part of the cognitive subscale of the Unified Huntington's Disease Rating Scale (UHDRS) In contrast to patients with Alzheimer's disease, semantic memory appears to be relatively spared in HD patients with some decline at very advanced stages.[70,71,79,80] Global cognition--as measured by Mini Mental State Examination--is also well preserved until the later stages of the disease.[70,71]

EMOTION RECOGNITION

It has been reported that individuals with HD display marked deficits in recognizing facial emotions, in particular those reflecting negative nuances. This feature appears to be an early correlate of the disease and has also been found in preclinical carriers of the HD gene.[81–84] Impairments in accurate recognition of facial expressions have been observed for disgust, anger, fear, sadness but also surprise.[85–89] Most studies have observed a disproportionately severe deficit for disgust recognition in premanifest[81,82,84] and manifest HD carriers.[81,86,88,89] Functional neuroimaging studies have implicated the anterior insular cortex and the basal ganglia in the ability to recognize disgust.[90–92] Impairments in recognizing facial expressions of disgust are also seen in other disorders with basal ganglia pathology, including Wilson's disease[89] and obsessive–compulsive disorder (OCD).[93] These defects in processing emotions may play a role in the disrupted demeanor encountered in many HD patients and explain social deviations such as inadequate social interactions, poor temper control, and neglect of personal hygiene.

ANOSOGNOSIA

Patients often exhibit a distorted self-perception and an extreme lack of insight regarding their own disease. They are frequently in denial of the extent of their condition: in particular they tend to persistently underestimate the degree of their dysexecutive behavior.[94] Self-assessments of their functioning state and their mood are often contradictory to the impression of caregivers. These discrepancies between caregivers and patients especially occur in conjunction with poor cognition.[95] Patients with HD have been observed to have poor judgment.[96] However, patients' judgment seems more impaired in respect to themselves while they are still being able to accurately reflect upon others.[94]

BEHAVIORAL DISTURBANCES

Alteration in behavior and psychiatric manifestations are highly common in HD and they are thought to precede the motor symptoms by an estimated 10 years.[97] In the absence of a clear family history patients with HD may be often misdiagnosed and first come to attention in the context of psychiatric disease. It may be particularly difficult to determine the onset of behavioral disturbance as a manifestation of the HD pathology, mainly because of a rather insidious development of personality changes. Also it is often hard to separate whether certain behavioral deviations are part of the disease or may rather be attributed to a disrupted social background and a consequence of experiencing the familial impact of HD. However, subtle subclinical psychiatric symptoms occur at a significantly higher rate in gene carriers than in individuals who do not show the repeat expansion.[97]

PERSONALITY CHANGES

A wide variety of behavioral disturbances is known to occur in HD patients, the most prevalent symptoms being dysphoria, irritability, apathy, anxiety as well as loss of energy and initiative. Neglect of self-care and personal hygiene, emotional blunting, self-centered demanding behavior, poor temper control, and verbal outbursts are also frequently encountered.[18,98]

DEPRESSION

HD patients are particularly vulnerable to depression with prevalence estimates ranging between 40 and 60%.[98–100] Depression is the most frequent psychiatric onset symptom[100] and thought to be one of the major factors that influence the quality of life in HD patients.[101] Many aspects are thought to contribute to the development of depression including the burden of carrying a fatal disease, the implications upon carrier or symptomatic disease detection in other members of the family, and the psychological burden of caring for a family member with HD. When compared with gene-negative individuals, *HD* gene carriers were reported to have a significantly higher rate of depressive symptoms.[102] Moreover, distinct neuropathological changes that accompany HD correlate with the development of behavioral and mood changes. These observations altogether implicate depression as a primary disease manifestation.[103]

PSYCHOSIS

In the absence of a family history of HD, patients with prominent psychotic symptoms as their initial manifestation are often misdiagnosed as having schizophrenia. The psychotic manifestations of the disease are a major concern in the lives of HD patients and their families, posing a potential threat to both the patients themselves and their surroundings. Dangerous and violent actions deriving from delusional thoughts and hallucinations markedly impair the ability to live a normal life and destabilize social structures of an HD family resulting in involuntary hospitalizations and the need for a placement in a skilled care facility.

Prevalence estimates of schizophrenia-like psychosis in Huntington's disease patients range from 5 to 25%,[99,104] which is markedly higher than the prevalence of 1% for schizophrenia in the general population. Delusions, hallucinations, and disruption of formal thought processes have been observed. Several studies of cases with psychotic features have revealed a familial aggregation of schizophrenia-like syndromes in HD patients.[105–108]

OBSESSIVE–COMPULSIVE SYMPTOMS

Recent studies in large patient samples have revealed a frequent incidence of obsessions and compulsions in HD patients.[76,109] HD patients with obsessive–compulsive symptoms show more pronounced deficits in neuropsychological tests, in particular a greater impairment of executive function.[110] Obsessive and compulsive symptoms have been described in the context of auto- and heteroaggressive behavior, excessive hand-washing and cleanliness, drinking, smoking, skin scraping, knitting, lip and finger biting, head banging, singing, dancing, chasing cars, pathological gambling, cleanliness, and even homicidal ideation[96,111,112] and as such additionally compromise the patient's ability to interact in a socially appropriate manner.

Frontostriatal pathology has been implicated in idiopathic OCD by numerous neuropsychological and imaging studies.[113,114] Moreover, OCD has been reported to evolve in association with lesions of both the caudate and the pallidus as well as with frontal lobe impairment.[96] These findings altogether suggest that the frontal-caudate-pallidal circuit plays a crucial role in impulse and behavioral control by regulating excitatory subcortical output to the cortex and provide an explanation for the association between HD and obsessive–compulsive syndromes.

SEXUAL BEHAVIOR

Up to 85% of men and up to 75% of women with HD experience sexual problems and deviations of sexual behavior are frequently encountered.[115] Both hypo- and hypersexual disorders occur with hypoactive sexual disorder being the most common manifestation. Hyposexual problems comprise reduced or absent libido, inhibited orgasm--especially in male patients--and domestic sexual hypoactivity. Hypersexuality and disinhibited sexual behavior have been reported in a range between 5 and 30% of patients with HD.[99,115,116]

George Huntington observed an increased sexual interest in two of his patients that he documented in his description as follows: *"I know of two married men, whose wives are living, and who are constantly making love to some young lady, not seeming to be aware that there is any impropriety in it. They are suffering from chorea to such an extent that they can hardly walk, and would be thought, by a stranger, to be intoxicated. They are men of about 50 years of age, but never let an opportunity to flirt with a girl go past unimproved. The effect is ridiculous in the extreme."*[1]

Paraphilias that have been reported in patients with HD include morbid sexual jealousy, homosexual assault, promiscuity, child perversity, obscene phone calls, exhibitionism, sodomy as well as incestuous thoughts and behavior.[115]

SUICIDALITY

The increased predisposition to suicidal behavior was recognized and captured by George Huntington in his original description: *"The tendency to insanity, and sometimes that form of insanity which leads to suicide, is marked. I know of several instances of suicide of people suffering from this form of chorea, or who belonged to families in which the disease existed."*[1]

Suicide rates in HD have been estimated to range between 5 and 8.5% in various studies with suicide attempt rates ranging up to 30%. These rates have consistently been several times larger than in the normal corresponding population. Suicide rates are also increased among relatives of HD patients with an unknown carrier status and healthy family members.[24,117–119] This fact not only reflects the burden of being at risk for the disease, but also relates to instabilities that result from growing up in an HD family. Suicide has been observed to occur most frequently in the early and middle stages of manifest HD.[118] When investigating the rate of suicidal ideation in a large sample (>4000) of individuals diagnosed with HD, the critical period for suicidal thoughts were immediately before receiving the formal diagnosis of HD (23.5%) and in stage II of the disease (16.3%), as independence diminishes.[120] Risk factors for suicidal behavior comprise depression, the lack of offspring, being single or divorced. There tends to be an accumulation of suicides within families.[121]

▶ OTHER FEATURES

METABOLIC DEFECTS

A cumulative body of evidence suggests a central role for mitochondrial dysfunction in the primary pathology of HD.[122–128] Findings in toxin mouse models and measurements of mitochondrial enzyme activity imply that impairments in energy metabolism may cause the HD phenotype as a result of enhanced susceptibility to oxidative damage with subsequent excitotoxicity-mediated neuronal degeneration.

Patients with HD often appear cachectic. They typically tend to lose weight despite increased food intake.[129–131] Weight loss can partially be attributed to higher energy expenditure due to the increased movements[132,133] as weight loss has been shown to correlate with pronounced chorea.[33,134] Persons with the HD mutation are also noted to have lower body mass indices (BMIs) at very early and even premanifest stages, when chorea is not present or yet minimal in comparison to control subjects, supporting the hypothesis of primary metabolic derangement.[129] The rate of weight loss increases with higher CAG number that indicates a hypermetabolic state in conjunction with the HD mutation.[135,136] The weight loss seems to reflect the progression of the pathology in HD, as a high BMI has been shown to be a good prognostic factor, associated with longer durations of the disease.[137] In the late stages of HD, swallowing problems additionally impair the ability to maintain an adequate caloric intake. Multiple factors seem to synergistically predispose patients to the increased wasting in HD, including mitochondrial dysfunction and endocrine deregulations with superimposed contributing factors such as depression, excessive movements, and feeding difficulty.

ENDOCRINE ABNORMALITIES

In addition to striatal and cortical atrophy, cell death also occurs in the hypothalamus at early stages of the disease with pronounced cell loss and astrocytosis in the lateral tuberal nucleus and loss of orexin- and somatostatin-containing cell populations.[138–141] Increases in urine cortisol correlating with disease progression have been observed in HD patients; these changes may contribute to symptoms such as muscle wasting, diabetes, and mood changes.[142] Further endocrine changes that have been reported in HD patients include elevated vasopressin levels in conjunction with increased thirst and drinking,[143] high ghrelin and low leptin levels,[144,145] as well as reduced testosterone and luteinizing hormone levels in male patients.

DIABETES

An increased prevalence of diabetes has been observed in HD patients.[146] Normoglycemic HD patients exhibit an increased insulin resistance, resembling the profile of diabetes mellitus type II in the absence of lipid abnormalities or a high BMI.[147] The pathophysiology of diabetes in HD is not completely understood, with both pancreatic and hypothalamic etiologies being possible underlying mechanisms. However, pancreatic biopsies from a small number of HD patients found pancreatic islet cells to be unaffected with normal levels of insulin transcripts.[148]

SLEEP

A high rate of sleep problems has been reported in HD patients with prevalence rates ranging around 90%, often negatively affecting the caregivers' sleep and the relationship with caregivers.[149] Patients report frequent insomnia, nocturnal awakenings and excessive daytime sleepiness.[150,151] Patients generally have an earlier sleep onset[150] and early awakening.[149] The reduction of sleep efficiency is accompanied by underlying electroencephalographic abnormalities revealing perturbed sleep architecture. An increased proportion of stage I sleep and a high spindle density have been observed, whereas REM sleep duration and the amount of slow wave sleep are found to be reduced.[150,152–154] These findings altogether suggest a more superficial and shallow sleep in HD patients. Reduced REM sleep duration has been seen in gene carriers that were yet free from motor symptoms.[150] Sources of sleep dysregulation include hypothalamic pathology, excessive movements and restlessness, as well as mood changes such as depression and anxiety.

IMMUNOLOGICAL FEATURES

There is a growing body of evidence suggests that a widespread abnormal activation of the immune system in HD patients, occurring both in the central nervous system (CNS) as well as in the periphery. Upregulated immune responses were observed in the CNS in the form of microglial activation corresponding with disease severity.[155–158] In addition, alterations in the peripheral immune profile were reported in the form of hyperactive monocytes and macrophages. Cytokine levels (IL-6, -8, -4, -5, -10, and TNF-α) are increased both centrally and peripherally, whereas immunoglobulin levels are normal. These findings suggest selective changes in the innate (IL-6 and -8) and adaptive (IL-4 and -10) immune response in the face of spared humoral immune pathways. Microglial cells as well as monocytes express mutant huntingtin.[159,160] PET studies demonstrate evidence of activated microglia correlating with disease severity in HD patients[155] as well as presymptomatic individuals.[157]

AUTONOMIC DYSFUNCTION

Imbalances of the autonomic nervous system (ANS) are present in the early stages of HD. Both the sympathetic and the parasympathetic components of the ANS display deficits. Patients have impairments of skin sweat regulation, consistent with sympathetic dysregulation.[161] They also may experience orthostatic disturbances and had decreased variability of the heart rate during exertion and postural changes.[161–164] Reduced vagal modulation of neurocardiogenic responses reflects parasympathetic dysfunction and makes patients prone to orthostatic impairment and syncope. With the parasympathetic branch being more affected, there is a relative sympathetic predominance in HD.[161–163] The overall raised sympathetic activity may increase the susceptibility to cardiovascular arrhythmias that could contribute to the cardiovascular mortality in HD. Primary or secondary sites of ANS functions that have shown histopathological involvement in patients with HD include the hypothalamus, brainstem (dorsal vagal nuclei), cerebral cortex, thalamus, and intermediolateral column cells in the spinal cord.

OLFACTION

Similar to other neurodegenerative diseases, disturbance in olfactory function is a consistently encountered early symptom in HD. Deficits comprise both absolute odor detection as well as odor discrimination and are morphologically correlated with the entorhinal cortex, thalamus, parahippocampal gyrus, and caudate nucleus.[165–167]

CANCER RISK

An interesting observation was made when investigating the major causes of mortality captured in the Danish registry. Individuals with HD had a decreased overall incidence of cancer for all different subtypes of cancer except for cancer of the buccal mucosa/pharynx. The incidence was also lower when compared to unaffected relatives, minimizing the impact of environmental influences.[24,168] One of the hypotheses for this phenomenon is that growth and proliferation of cancer cells are arrested in individuals carrying an expanded CAG sequence because the expanded polyglutamine tract in huntingtin predisposes to cell death. Interestingly, a similar relationship between CAG numbers and cancer risk has been reported in connection with the androgen receptor (AR), the gene that is mutated in SBMA (Kennedy's disease). Several studies found a decrease of the relative risk for prostate cancer, recurrence and a higher age of onset associated with a higher number of CAG repeats in the polyglutamine tract of AR.[169,170]

▶ JUVENILE-ONSET HD

When HD was first described by George Huntington, it was thought to "manifest itself as a grave disease only in adult life".[1] However, it is now known that HD can occur in individuals as young as 2 years of age.[171] Per definition, "juvenile HD" has onset of symptoms before 20 years of age. The juvenile form is estimated to account for 5–10% of all HD cases with less than 1% of

HD patients presenting with symptoms before 10 years of age.[172] The number of CAG repeats length is usually greater than 60[173] and can range up to over 200.[13,174] In the majority of cases (80–90%), juvenile-onset HD is inherited from the affected fathers. This tendency for paternal transmission can be attributed to a propensity for large CAG repeat expansions during male gametogenesis as a result of increased meiotic instability,[9,175–178] a phenomenon referred to as anticipation. Sons and daughters are equally affected. In contrast to the adult-onset form, there is often a predominance of hypokinetic features such as parkinsonism and dystonia. The dystonia can be very severe and resistant to therapy. Some patients develop a fine postural tremor of the trunk and limbs. Ataxia and other cerebellar signs are more frequently seen than in adult patients and can significantly impair the ability to ambulate.[179] In 25–30% of cases there is a tendency for epileptic seizures that are usually of the generalized or myoclonic type. The severity and frequency of seizures varies widely. Epileptiform abnormalities are considerably more common than in the adult forms with polyspikes and waves being the most remarkable finding on EEG.[180]

Chorea is uncommon in juvenile-onset HD, especially in children who develop symptoms in the first decade of life. Patients with a more adolescent onset are more likely to exhibit clinical characteristics similar to the adult form. Severe behavioral disturbances, often requiring medical or legal intervention, may be the first symptom in a teenager.[171] The cognitive status is slightly better preserved in patients with juvenile-onset HD. Speech and language delays are early manifestations of juvenile-onset HD.[181] Although similar brain regions are affected in juvenile and adult-onset HD, the degree of atrophy is more pronounced in juvenile-onset cases, suggesting a more aggressive course.[182] Although some longitudinal clinical studies suggest that juvenile-onset HD patients progress more rapidly than adult-onset patients[5,137] Roos and colleagues[183] did not find a difference in disease duration when describing a large patient population.

▶ DIAGNOSIS

The genetic test for Huntington's disease has been shown to be highly sensitive (98.8%) and specific (100%).[184] In the presence of a positive gene test and clinical symptoms, the diagnosis of HD is indisputable. However, testing rates among individuals at risk for the mutation remain low and are estimated between 5 and 10%. The major reasons for these low numbers are the reluctance to live with the knowledge of developing a dreadful and incurable disease and preferment to live with the uncertainty, but also fear of stigmatization and isolation. Especially in the United States, health insurance problems are a great concern.[185] The implementation of the Genetic Information Nondiscrimination Act in 2008 should help in this regard.

It should be noted that a positive genetic test is quite different than a clinical diagnosis of manifest HD. Indeed, patients carrying the gene mutation may be neurologically normal for decades. Although initial clinical presentations of HD could be cognitive or psychiatric, the presence of an extrapyramidal movement disorder is much more specific in making the diagnosis of clinical manifestation of HD. In the setting of a secure family history of HD, obtaining a genetic test may not be obligatory in making the diagnosis.

Other hereditary neurodegenerative diseases should be considered in the setting of a negative gene test in conjunction with clinical symptoms and a positive family history. An overview of genetic conditions that may resemble HD closely is provided in Table 33–3. Other causes of abnormal movements in combination with neuropsychiatric abnormalities include structural brain lesions as well as metabolic, autoimmune, and infectious/parainfectious conditions. Toxic exposures, substance abuse, and medication effects should also be considered. Psychiatric illnesses with psychotic features and elements of pseudodementia have strong overlaps with the behavioral phenotype encountered in HD. Tardive dyskinesia, a consequence of antipsychotic treatment, may closely resemble the chorea of HD.

▶ TREATMENT

HD remains an incurable disease to date. There are no treatments that can prevent the disease onset or slow the progression. The main focus of clinical care in HD currently rests on symptomatic therapy and supportive measures to enhance the quality of life for patients and their families.

To manage the complex clinical picture and the grave psychosocial implications of the disease patients should receive support from a multidisciplinary team including neurologists, psychiatrists, psychologists, geneticists, physical therapists, speech therapists, nutritionists, and social workers. Patients and caregivers require careful assistance in long-term planning decisions and questions regarding skilled care facility placement, disability evaluations, terminal care measures, and legal issues. If possible, the patients' families should be tightly integrated in the process of care and also have access to psychological and genetic counseling as well as support groups. Patients should be encouraged to maintain a high level of physical and mental activity as far as they are able to. Environmental enrichment has been shown to slow the disease progression in mouse models[186,187] and is widely presumed to have a beneficial impact in humans as well.

▶ **TABLE 33–3. HEREDITARY DISEASES RESEMBLING HUNTINGTON'S DISEASE**

Mode of Inheritance	Disease	Mutation/Affected Gene	Characteristic Features
Autosomal dominant	Huntington's disease-like illnesses (HDL) types –1, –2, and –4 *~ 1% of suspected HD cases are gene negative → 'HD phenocopies'*	HDL-1: 8-octapeptide repeat insertion in the prion protein gene (PRNP), Chr. 20p12 HDL-2: CTG/CAG repeat expansion in the Junctophilin 3 (*JPH3*) gene, Chr. 16q24 HDL-4: equals SCA 17 (Table 33–1)	HDL-1 inherited prion disease with relatively early onset, long course and prominent cognitive decline HDL-2: Mostly observed in people with African heritage, in some cases acanthocytes on blood smear HDL-4: Equals SCA 17 (Table 33–1)
	Dentatorubropallido-luysian atrophy (DRPLA)/ Haw-river syndrome (HRS)	CAG triplet expansion in the Atrophin 1 (ATN1) gene, Chr. 12p13.31 (Table 33–1)	Onset, course and symptoms similar as in HD. Can also present with seizures and myoclonus. Most common in people of Japanese descent. HRS: African American family with same mutation, in addition extensive subcortical white matter demyelination and BG calcifications.
	Spinocerebellar ataxias (SCA) *currently 28 subtypes identified*	Genetically heterogenous, SCA-1,-2,-3,-6,-7,-8 and -17 are CAG repeat expansion diseases (Table 33–1)	Midlife onset. Spinocerebellar degeneration with gait ataxia, dysarthria, oculomotor abnormalities. High clinical variability, depending on subtype additional symptoms (also see Table 33–1). SCA-2, -3 and -17 resemble HD most closely.
	Neuroferritinopathy (Adult-onset basal ganglia disease)	Ferritin light chain (FTL) gene*, Chr. 9q13.3 –q13.4 → abnormal iron accumulation in the BG	Midlife onset. Chorea, parkinsionism, spasticity. Cognitive decline may occur. Classic: speech-related orofacial dystonia → prominent dysarthria (dysarthrophonia). Serum ferritin levels ↓, MRI/CT: BG cavitation and iron accumulation.
	Benign hereditary chorea (BHC)	Thyroid transcription factor-1 (TITF1) gene*, Chr. 14q13, possibly additional mutations	Childhood onset. Chorea, delayed motor milestones, dyarthria, dystonia. Mostly normal cognition. Usually not or only slowly progressive, can improve during adulthood. Thyroid/lung abnormalities may be present.
	Idiopathic basal ganglia calcification (IBGC)-1	Genetically heterogeneous, mostly linked to Chr. 14q	Midlife onset. Often associated with low Ca or PTH metabolic disorders. Incomplete penetrance and autosomal recessive/sporadic forms have been reported. Diagnosis is difficult since BG calcifications are nonspecific.
	Acute intermittent porphyria (AIP)	Porphobilinogen-deaminase (*PBGD*) gene* (Chr. 11q23.3) → impaired heme biosynthesis → accumulation of toxic precursors	Onset: 18–40 years. Episodic attacks (can be triggered by medications), abdominal cramps, constipation, wide range of psychiatric disorders, peripheral and autonomic neuropathies, may manifest with tremor and other movement disorders, seizures. ↑ urinary excretion of the PBGD precursors δ-aminolevulinic acid (ALA) and porphobilinogen (PBG)

(continued)

▶ **TABLE 33–3. (CONTINUED)**

Mode of Inheritance	Disease	Mutation/Affected Gene	Characteristic Features
Autosomal recessive	Wilson's disease/ hepatolenticular degeneration	*ATP7B* gene* (Chr. 13q14.3-q21.1) → impaired Cu transport → accumulation of Cu in various tissues (liver, cornea, BG)	Onset: typically late adolescence-early adulthood, clinically highly heterogeneous. Symptoms comprise: Hepatic failure, wide variety of movement disorders (esp. prominent dysarthria, flapping tremor, incoordination) and psychiatric disturbances, Kayser–Fleischer ring, sunflower cataracts, arthropathies, renal tubular acidosis, chondrocalcinosis, rarely cardiomyopathy. Serum ceruloplasmin ↓, 24-h Cu excretion ↑. 'Panda' sign on MRI/CT.
	HDL-3	Presumably localized to 4p15.3	Extremely rare, so far only observed in a few families.
	Chorea-acanthocytosis	VPS13A gene* (Chr. 9q21) encoding for Chorein	Midlife onset. Mimics HD closely, characteristic: Orofacial dystonia and tics with tongue protrusion/lip-biting. Seizures in up to 50% of cases. Distal amyotrophy, CK ↑, peripheral neuropathy. Acanthocytes on blood smear.
	Pantothenate kinase associated neuro-degeneration (PKAN)	*PANK 2* (pantothenate kinase 2) gene*, Chr 20p13 →Accumulation of iron in the BG	Onset: usually childhood/ adolescence, also adult-onset forms. Progressive dementia, extrapyramidal signs, significant dysarthria, typically early and prominent dystonia, often visual disturbances because of pigmentary retinopathy/optic atrophy, seizures. "Eye of the tiger" sign on MRI. Acanthocytes may be seen on blood smear.
X-linked recessive	McLeod syndrome	Kell blood group precursor gene*, Chr.Xp21.2-p21.1	Onset: sixth decade, slowly progressive course. Chorea, tics, seizures, late dementia/behavioral changes can occur, mypopathy, peripheral neuropathy, CK ↑, cardiomyopathy, hepatosplenomegaly, hemolytic anemia. Acanthocytes on blood smear.
	Lesch–Nyhan disease	HPRT (hypo-xanthine-guanine-phosphoribo-syltransferase) gene*, Chr. Xq26-q27.2 → impaired purine metabolism, overproduction of uric acid.	Early childhood onset. Cognitive impairment, behavioral disturbances (self-mutilation), motor dysfunction (predominantly dystonia, variety of extrapyramidal features and UMN signs), hyperuricemia (→ nephrolithiasis, renal failure, gouty arthritis), growth retardation, megaloblastic anemia

*Genetically heterogenous mutations. BG, basal ganglia.

SYMPTOMATIC INTERVENTION

The efficacy of symptomatic treatments is limited by the impermanence of beneficial impacts and a wide range of side effects. In the European HD REGISTRY network, a database comprising 2128 HD patients, 84% were reported to receive pharmacological treatment. The main indications were depression (50%), and chorea (28%), as well as irritability and aggression (13%), sleep disturbances (9%), and psychosis (7%).[188] Table 33–4 provides an overview of commonly prescribed drugs in HD. The use of most of these medications has not been supported by randomized clinical trials. HD patients display a prominent variability regarding the response to drugs and the manifestation of side effects, and, as such, therapy needs to be individualized. Fluctuations may occur in a patient over time and paradoxical reactions are not uncommon, making careful titration of doses and strict monitoring of adverse effects a necessity.

TREATING THE MOVEMENT DISORDER

Chorea is typically not the main source of functional impairment in HD. The indication to treat chorea is given when the movements are perceived as stigmatizing or disabling. Antidopaminergic drugs are the current mainstay of therapy; both dopamine receptor antagonists (typical and atypical neuroleptics) and dopamine-depleting agents (tetrabenazine, reserpine) are thought to be effective in diminishing chorea. Dopamine receptor antagonists have a long history of clinical use in HD for both chorea and psychotic symptoms, and they are especially useful for patients who exhibit both features. The conventional neuroleptic haloperidol is well-established as an antichorea treatment in the hands of experienced physicians. Surprisingly, the effect of haloperidol on movements has never been investigated in a larger controlled clinical trial, and smaller studies have been inconclusive.[189–192] The same statement holds true for other conventional antipsychotics. The newer atypical neuroleptics (e.g., clozapine, olanzapine, quetiapine, risperidone) have shown some significant improvements of UHDRS motor scores in small open-label trials.[193–197] Patients on neuroleptics must be carefully monitored for adverse reactions such as extrapyramidal and anticholinergic side effects, metabolic syndrome, as well as agranulocytosis with clozapine treatment.

The dopamine depleting drugs are thought to exert their effect by inhibiting vesicular monoamine transporters (VMATs) and blocking the uptake and storage of dopamine and norepinephrine into synaptic vesicles. Although tetrabenazine (TBZ) reversibly binds to the central VMAT2 receptor, the alkaloid reserpine irreversibly inhibits both VMAT1/2 receptors. Peripheral side effects caused by the VMAT1 binding as well as the considerably longer half-life make reserpine less favorable compared

▶ TABLE 33–4. SYMPTOMATIC TREATMENTS COMMONLY USED IN HD

Symptom	Medication
Chorea	**Dopamine receptor antagonists**
	Typical Antipsychotics
	Haloperidol (Haldol)
	Fluphenazine (Prolixin)
	Thioridazine (Mellaril)
	Atypical Antipsychotics
	Clozapine (Clozaril)
	Olanzapine (Zyprexa)
	Quetiapine (Seroquel)
	Risperidone (Risperdal)
	Zisprasidone (Geodon)
	Dopamine-depleting drugs
	Tetrabenazine (Xenazine)
	Glutamate antagonists
	Amantadine (Symmetrel)
	Riluzole (Rilutek)
	GABA agonists
	Baclofen (Lioresal)
	Valproic acid (Depakote)
	Benzodiazepines
	Clonazepam (Klonopin)
	Alprazolam (Xanax)
Depression	**Selective Serotonin Reuptake Inhibitors (SSRIs)**
	Fluoxetine (Prozac)
	Citalopram (Celexa)
	Sertraline (Zoloft)
	Paroxetine (Paxil)
	Fluvoxamine (Luvox)
	Selective Serotonin Noradrenaline
	Reuptake Inhibitors (SNARIs)
	Venlafaxine (Effexor)
	Tricyclic Antidepressants (TCAs)
	Nortryptiline (Pamelor)
	Amitryptiline (Elavil)
	Monoamine Oxidase Inhibitors
	Phenelezine (Nardil)
	Isocarboxazid (Marplan)
	Aminoketones
	Bupropion (Wellbutrin)
Psychosis	**Typical/Atypical Antipsychotics (as reviewed above)**
Dementia	**Choline Esterase Inhibitors**
	Donezepil (Aricept)
	Rivastigmine (Exelon)
	Galantamine (Razadyne)
	Glutamate antagonists
	Memantine (Namenda)

to TBZ. The efficacy of TBZ has been documented in a series of studies[198–201] and was recently confirmed in a randomized controlled trial.[202]

On the basis of the "excitotoxin theory," which attributes neurodegeneration in HD to a relative excess of excitatory neurotransmitters, several antiglutamatergic agents have tested for neuroprotective and symptomatic effects. Amantadine, riluzole, and remacemide have demonstrated some transient antichoreic effects.[203–209] Although the benefits of these drugs remain to be confirmed in larger trials, they may be prescribed when antidopaminergics are ineffective or contraindicated.

An alternative approach to suppressing chorea has been sought in enhancing GABAergic neurotransmission. The clinical use of baclofen and benzodiazepines in HD is not well documented and has only shown limited success.[210–212] In some patients, benzodiazepines such as diazepam and clonazepam, have both antichoreic and anxiolytic effects.

The doses for antichorea drugs should be titrated slowly to the minimal effective dose and individualized for each patient. The necessity of medication should be reassessed as chorea tends to diminish over the disease course.

HD patients with predominant parkinsonian features may benefit from dopaminergic agents. Both L-DOPA and dopamine agonists have been shown to elicit improvements as documented in several case reports.[213–217] However, they should be used with caution as they may exacerbate chorea and dystonia, as well as provoke hallucinations and psychosis. The treatment of dystonia in HD is difficult and has been poorly investigated. Although dystonic features are a source of functional impairment, there are no trials assessing potential interventions for dystonia.

TREATING THE COGNITIVE DYSFUNCTION

There are only sparse data regarding beneficial interventions with respect to the cognitive decline in HD. In several open-label studies cholinesterase inhibitors proved ineffective.[218–221] Nonpharmacological treatments, such as simplifying preexisting regimens, are useful. Reducing distractions and focusing on one task at a time are helpful in counteracting distractibility.

TREATING THE BEHAVIORAL SYMPTOMS

Personality changes and behavioral deviations exert a big impact on patients' and families' lives, often evoking the desire for treatment. Depression represents the most frequently treated feature in HD.[188] Despite this prevalent demand and use there are no large controlled trials that document the efficacy of any antidepressant medication in HD. There are also no data on how different antidepressants compare regarding their benefits and risks in HD. Electroconvulsive therapy may be considered in patients with severe depression that is resistant to pharmacotherapy.[222]

Most behavioral symptoms in HD such as psychosis, irritability, bipolar illness, and OCD are treated as they would be in non-HD patients. There are no studies investigating these drugs specifically for HD patients.

SURGICAL INTERVENTIONS

There are only sparse case reports on deep brain stimulation (DBS) treatment in HD and no reports on the long-term efficacy. Bilateral GPi (globus pallidus, internal segment) stimulation has been shown to cause an improvement in choreoathetosis, dystonia, and oculomotor symptoms at frequencies 40 and 130 Hz, which could be sustained over 1 year. Stimulation at 130 Hz provoked worsening of bradykinetic features.[223–225] Because DBS carries no benefit regarding the neuropsychiatric features and may even worsen cognition,[223] the risk-to-benefit ratio for undergoing such an invasive surgical procedure is overall suboptimal for HD patients.

Fetal striatal transplantation has been performed in a small number of patients in an attempt to replace the degenerated neurons. Improvement or stabilization of motor and cognitive symptoms was noted in some of the patients in correlation with increased brain activity on neuroimaging.[226–228] However, these effects could not be sustained over a longer period.[193] Further advances in cell replacement therapy may be reached with induced pluripotent stem (iPS) cells. The discovery that human somatic cells can be reprogrammed into a pluripotent state[229] holds promise to ameliorate regenerative techniques by circumventing immunological barriers associated with fetal tissue.

▶ PERSPECTIVES

There has been significant progress since George Huntington's description of the malady that now bears his name. Mutant forms of the huntingtin protein cause neurodegeneration, predominantly in the caudate–putamen, resulting in symptoms that affect movement, cognition, and psychiatric functioning. Although current treatments are limited to targeting symptoms, future therapies, guided by better understanding of disease pathogenesis, will aim to slow disease progression and eventually cure this devastating disorder.

REFERENCES

1. Huntington G. On chorea. George Huntington, M.D. J Neuropsychiatry Clin Neurosci 2003;15(1):109–112.

2. Durbach N, Hayden MR. George Huntington: the man behind the eponym. J Med Genet 1993;30(5):406–409.
3. Gusella JF, Wexler NS, Conneally PM, et al. A polymorphic DNA marker genetically linked to Huntington's disease. Nature 1983;306(5940):234–238.
4. The Huntington's Disease Collaborative Research Group. A novel gene containing a trinucleotide repeat that is expanded and unstable on Huntington's disease chromosomes. Cell 1993;72(6):971–983.
5. Young AB, Shoulson I, Penney JB, et al. Huntington's disease in Venezuela: Neurologic features and functional decline. Neurology 1986;36(2):244–249.
6. Penney JB Jr, Young AB, Shoulson I, et al. Huntington's disease in Venezuela: 7 years of follow-up on symptomatic and asymptomatic individuals. Mov Disord 1990;5(2):93–99.
7. Harper PS. The epidemiology of Huntington's disease. Hum Genet 1992;89(4):365–376.
8. Andrew SE, Goldberg YP, Kremer B, et al. The relationship between trinucleotide (CAG) repeat length and clinical features of Huntington's disease. Nat Genet 1993;4(4):398–403.
9. Duyao M, Ambrose C, Myers R, et al. Trinucleotide repeat length instability and age of onset in Huntington's disease. Nat Genet 1993;4(4):387–392.
10. Persichetti F, Srinidhi J, Kanaley L, et al. Huntington's disease CAG trinucleotide repeats in pathologically confirmed post-mortem brains. Neurobiol Dis 1994;1(3): 159–166.
11. Rubinsztein DC, Leggo J, Goodburn S, et al. Study of the Huntington's disease (HD) gene CAG repeats in schizophrenic patients shows overlap of the normal and HD affected ranges but absence of correlation with schizophrenia. J Med Genet 1994;31(9):690–693.
12. Snell RG, MacMillan JC, Cheadle JP, et al. Relationship between trinucleotide repeat expansion and phenotypic variation in Huntington's disease. Nat Genet 1993;4(4):393–397.
13. Zuhlke C, Riess O, Schroder K, et al. Expansion of the (CAG)n repeat causing Huntington's disease in 352 patients of German origin. Hum Mol Genet 1993;2(9): 1467–1469.
14. Zeitlin S, Liu JP, Chapman DL, et al. Increased apoptosis and early embryonic lethality in mice nullizygous for the Huntington's disease gene homologue. Nat Genet 1995;11(2):155–163.
15. Nasir J, Floresco SB, O'Kusky JR, et al. Targeted disruption of the Huntington's disease gene results in embryonic lethality and behavioral and morphological changes in heterozygotes. 1995;Cell 81(5):811–823.
16. Duyao MP, Auerbach AB, Ryan A, et al. Inactivation of the mouse Huntington's disease gene homolog Hdh. Science 1995;269(5222):407–410.
17. Li SH, Schilling G, Young WS 3rd, et al. Huntington's disease gene (IT15) is widely expressed in human and rat tissues. Neuron 1993;11(5):985–993.
18. Craufurd D, Dodge A. Mutation size and age at onset in Huntington's disease. J Med Genet 1993;30(12): 1008–1011.
19. Langbehn DR, Brinkman RR, Falush D, et al. A new model for prediction of the age of onset and penetrance for Huntington's disease based on CAG length. Clin Genet 2004;65(4):267–277.
20. Stine OC, Pleasant N, Franz ML, et al. Correlation between the onset age of Huntington's disease and length of the trinucleotide repeat in IT-15. Hum Mol Genet 1993;2(10):1547–1549.
21. Wexler NS, Young AB, Tanzi RE, et al. Homozygotes for Huntington's disease. Nature 1987;326(6109):194–197.
22. Myers RH, Leavitt J, Farrer LA, et al. Homozygote for Huntington disease. Am J Hum Genet 1989;45(4):615–618.
23. Squitieri F, Gellera C, Cannella M, et al. Homozygosity for CAG mutation in Huntington disease is associated with a more severe clinical course. Brain 2003;126(Pt 4):946–955.
24. Sorensen SA, Fenger K. Causes of death in patients with Huntington's disease and in unaffected first degree relatives. J Med Genet 1992;29(12):911–914.
25. Vonsattel JP, Myers RH, Stevens TJ, et al. Neuropathological classification of Huntington's disease. J Neuropathol Exp Neurol 1985;44(6):559–577.
26. Furtado S, Suchowersky O, Rewcastle B, et al. Relationship between trinucleotide repeats and neuropathological changes in Huntington's disease. Ann Neurol 1996;39(1):132–136.
27. Penney JB Jr, Vonsattel JP, MacDonald ME, et al. CAG repeat number governs the development rate of pathology in Huntington's disease. Ann Neurol 1997;41(5):689–692.
28. Vonsattel JP, DiFiglia M. Huntington disease. J Neuropathol Exp Neurol 1998;57(5):369–384.
29. Cudkowicz M, Kowall NW. Degeneration of pyramidal projection neurons in Huntington's disease cortex. Ann Neurol 1990;27(2):200–204.
30. Sotrel A, Paskevich PA, Kiely DK, et al. Morphometric analysis of the prefrontal cortex in Huntington's disease. Neurology 1991;41(7):1117–1123.
31. Sotrel A, Williams RS, Kaufmann WE, et al. Evidence for neuronal degeneration and dendritic plasticity in cortical pyramidal neurons of Huntington's disease: A quantitative Golgi study. Neurology 1993;43(10):2088–2096.
32. Rosas HD, Salat DH, Lee SY, et al. Cerebral cortex and the clinical expression of Huntington's disease: complexity and heterogeneity. Brain 2008;131(Pt 4):1057–1068.
33. Mahant N, McCusker EA, Byth K, et al. Huntington's disease: clinical correlates of disability and progression. Neurology 2003;61(8):1085–1092.
34. Fish DR, Sawyers D, Allen PJ, et al. The effect of sleep on the dyskinetic movements of Parkinson's disease, Gilles de la Tourette syndrome, Huntington's disease, and torsion dystonia. Arch Neurol 1991;48(2):210–214.
35. Albin RL. Selective neurodegeneration in Huntington's disease. Ann Neurol 1995;38(6):835–836.
36. Albin RL, Reiner A, Anderson KD, et al. Preferential loss of striato-external pallidal projection neurons in presymptomatic Huntington's disease. Ann Neurol 1992;31(4): 425–430.
37. Albin RL, Reiner A, Anderson KD, et al. Striatal and nigral neuron subpopulations in rigid Huntington's disease: Implications for the functional anatomy of chorea and rigidity-akinesia. Ann Neurol 1990;27(4):357–365.
38. Reiner A, Albin RL, Anderson KD, et al. Differential loss of striatal projection neurons in Huntington disease. Proc Natl Acad Sci U S A 1988;85(15):5733–5737.

39. Storey E, Beal MF. Neurochemical substrates of rigidity and chorea in Huntington's disease. Brain 1993;116 (Pt 5):1201–1222.
40. Jankovic J, Ashizawa T. Tourettism associated with Huntington's disease. 1995;Mov Disord 10(1):103–105.
41. Angelini L, Sgro V, Erba A, et al. Tourettism as clinical presentation of Huntington's disease with onset in childhood. Ital J Neurol Sci 1998;19(6):383–385.
42. Alonso H, Cubo-Delgado E, Mateos-Beato MP, et al. Huntington's disease mimicking Tourette syndrome. Rev Neurol 2004;39(10):927–929.
43. Tan EK, Jankovic J, Ondo W. Bruxism in Huntington's disease. Mov Disord 2000;15(1):171–173.
44. Carella F, Scaioli V, Ciano C, et al. Adult onset myoclonic Huntington's disease. Mov Disord 1993;8(2):201–205.
45. Thompson PD, Bhatia KP, Brown P, et al. Cortical myoclonus in Huntington's disease. Mov Disord 1994;9(6): 633–641.
46. Vogel CM, Drury I, Terry LC, et al. Myoclonus in adult Huntington's disease. Ann Neurol 1991;29(2):213–215.
47. Blekher T, Johnson SA, Marshall J, et al. Saccades in presymptomatic and early stages of Huntington disease. Neurology 2006;67(3):394–399.
48. Golding CV, Danchaivijitr C, Hodgson TL, et al. Identification of an oculomotor biomarker of preclinical Huntington disease. Neurology 2006;67(3):485–487.
49. Hicks SL, Robert MP, Golding CV, et al. Oculomotor deficits indicate the progression of Huntington's disease. Prog Brain Res 2008;171:555–558.
50. Blekher TM, Yee RD, Kirkwood SC, et al. Oculomotor control in asymptomatic and recently diagnosed individuals with the genetic marker for Huntington's disease. Vision Res 2004;44(23):2729–2736.
51. Kirkwood SC, Siemers E, Bond C, et al. Confirmation of subtle motor changes among presymptomatic carriers of the Huntington disease gene. Arch Neurol 2000;57(7):1040–1044.
52. Leigh RJ, Newman SA, Folstein SE, et al. Abnormal ocular motor control in Huntington's disease. Neurology 1983;33(10):1268–1275.
53. Peltsch A, Hoffman A, Armstrong I, et al. Saccadic impairments in Huntington's disease. Exp Brain Res 2008;186(3):457–469.
54. Tian JR, Zee DS, Lasker AG, et al. Saccades in Huntington's disease: Predictive tracking and interaction between release of fixation and initiation of saccades. Neurology 1991;41(6):875–881.
55. Lasker AG, Zee DS, Hain TC, et al. Saccades in Huntington's disease: initiation defects and distractibility. Neurology 1987;37(3):364–370.
56. Rubin AJ, King WM, Reinbold KA, et al. Quantitative longitudinal assessment of saccades in Huntington's disease. J Clin Neuroophthalmol 1993;13(1):59–66.
57. Rodda RA. Cerebellar atrophy in Huntington's disease. J Neurol Sci 1981;50(1):147–157.
58. Squitieri F, Berardelli A, Nargi E, et al. Atypical movement disorders in the early stages of Huntington's disease: Clinical and genetic analysis. Clin Genet 2000;58(1):50–56.
59. Hertrich I, Ackermann H. Acoustic analysis of speech timing in Huntington's disease. Brain Lang 1994;47(2): 182–196.
60. Feigin A, Kieburtz K, Bordwell K, et al. Functional decline in Huntington's disease. Mov Disord 1995;10(2): 211–214.
61. Young AB, Penney JB, Starosta-Rubinstein S, et al. PET scan investigations of Huntington's disease: cerebral metabolic correlates of neurological features and functional decline. Ann Neurol 1986;20(3):296–303.
62. Louis ED, Anderson KE, Moskowitz C, et al. Dystonia-predominant adult-onset Huntington disease: association between motor phenotype and age of onset in adults. Arch Neurol 2000;57(9):1326–1330.
63. Sanchez-Pernaute R, Kunig G, del Barrio Alba A, et al. Bradykinesia in early Huntington's disease. Neurology 2000;54(1):119–125.
64. Wheelock VL, Tempkin T, Marder K, et al. Predictors of nursing home placement in Huntington disease. Neurology 2003;60(6):998–1001.
65. Rao AK, Quinn L, Marder KS. Reliability of spatiotemporal gait outcome measures in Huntington's disease. Mov Disord 2005;20(8):1033–1037.
66. Grimbergen YA, Knol MJ, Bloem BR, et al. Falls and gait disturbances in Huntington's disease. Mov Disord 2008;23(7):970–976.
67. Koller WC, Trimble J. The gait abnormality of Huntington's disease. Neurology 1985;35(10):1450–1454.
68. Hausdorff JM, Cudkowicz ME, Firtion R, et al. Gait variability and basal ganglia disorders: stride-to-stride variations of gait cycle timing in Parkinson's disease and Huntington's disease. Mov Disord 1998;13(3):428–437.
69. Hausdorff JM, Mitchell SL, Firtion R, et al. Altered fractal dynamics of gait: Reduced stride-interval correlations with aging and Huntington's disease. J Appl Physiol 1997;82(1):262–269.
70. Bamford KA, Caine ED, Kido DK, et al. A prospective evaluation of cognitive decline in early Huntington's disease: Functional and radiographic correlates. Neurology 1995;45(10):1867–1873.
71. Ho AK, Sahakian BJ, Brown RG, et al. Profile of cognitive progression in early Huntington's disease. Neurology 2003;61(12):1702–1706.
72. Lange KW, Sahakian BJ, Quinn NP, et al. Comparison of executive and visuospatial memory function in Huntington's disease and dementia of Alzheimer type matched for degree of dementia. J Neurol Neurosurg Psychiatry 1995;58(5):598–606.
73. Hamilton JM, Salmon DP, Corey-Bloom J, et al. Behavioural abnormalities contribute to functional decline in Huntington's disease. J Neurol Neurosurg Psychiatry 2003;74(1):120–122.
74. Lawrence AD, Hodges JR, Rosser AE, et al. Evidence for specific cognitive deficits in preclinical Huntington's disease. Brain 1998;121(Pt 7):1329–1341.
75. Paulsen JS, Zhao H, Stout JC, et al. Clinical markers of early disease in persons near onset of Huntington's disease. Neurology 2001;57(4):658–662.
76. Marder K, Zhao H, Myers RH, et al. Rate of functional decline in Huntington's disease. Huntington Study Group. Neurology 2000;54(2):452–458.
77. Nehl C, Paulsen JS. Cognitive and psychiatric aspects of Huntington disease contribute to functional capacity. J Nerv Ment Dis 2004;192(1):72–74.

78. Quinn L, Reilmann R, Marder K, et al. Altered movement trajectories and force control during object transport in Huntington's disease. Mov Disord 2001;16(3):469–480.
79. Hodges JR, Salmon DP, Butters N. Differential impairment of semantic and episodic memory in Alzheimer's and Huntington's diseases: A controlled prospective study. J Neurol Neurosurg Psychiatry 1990;53(12):1089–1095.
80. Rohrer D, Salmon DP, Wixted JT, et al. The disparate effects of Alzheimer's disease and Huntington's disease on semantic memory. Neuropsychology 1999;13(3): 381–388.
81. Gray JM, Young AW, Barker WA, et al. Impaired recognition of disgust in Huntington's disease gene carriers. Brain 1997;120(Pt 11):2029–2038.
82. Hennenlotter A, Schroeder U, Erhard P, et al. Neural correlates associated with impaired disgust processing in pre-symptomatic Huntington's disease. Brain 2004;127(Pt 6):1446–1453.
83. Johnson SA, Stout JC, Solomon AC, et al. Beyond disgust: impaired recognition of negative emotions prior to diagnosis in Huntington's disease. Brain 2007;130(Pt 7):1732–1744.
84. Sprengelmeyer R, Schroeder U, Young AW, et al. Disgust in pre-clinical Huntington's disease: A longitudinal study. Neuropsychologia 2006;44(4):518–533.
85. Milders M, Crawford JR, Lamb A, et al. Differential deficits in expression recognition in gene-carriers and patients with Huntington's disease. Neuropsychologia 2003;41(11):1484–1492.
86. Montagne B, Schutters S, Westenberg HG, et al. Reduced sensitivity in the recognition of anger and disgust in social anxiety disorder. Cogn Neuropsychiatry 2006;11(4): 389–401.
87. Snowden JS, Austin NA, Sembi S, et al. Emotion recognition in Huntington's disease and frontotemporal dementia. Neuropsychologia 2008;46(11):2638–2649.
88. Sprengelmeyer R, Young AW, Calder AJ, et al. Loss of disgust. Perception of faces and emotions in Huntington's disease. Brain 1996;119(Pt 5):1647–1665.
89. Wang K, Hoosain R, Yang RM, et al. Impairment of recognition of disgust in Chinese with Huntington's or Wilson's disease. Neuropsychologia 2003;41(5):527–537.
90. Phillips ML, Young AW, Scott SK, et al. Neural responses to facial and vocal expressions of fear and disgust. Proc Biol Sci 1998;265(1408):1809–1817.
91. Phillips ML, Young AW, Senior C, et al. A specific neural substrate for perceiving facial expressions of disgust. Nature 1997;389(6650):495–498.
92. Sprengelmeyer R, Rausch M, Eysel UT, et al. Neural structures associated with recognition of facial expressions of basic emotions. Proc Biol Sci 1998;265(1409):1927–1931.
93. Sprengelmeyer R, Young AW, Pundt I, et al. Disgust implicated in obsessive-compulsive disorder. Proc Biol Sci 1997;264(1389):1767–1773.
94. Ho AK, Robbins AO, Barker RA. Huntington's disease patients have selective problems with insight. Mov Disord 2006;21(3):385–389.
95. Chatterjee A, Anderson KE, Moskowitz CB, et al. A comparison of self-report and caregiver assessment of depression, apathy, and irritability in Huntington's disease. J Neuropsychiatry Clin Neurosci 2005;17(3):378–383.
96. Cummings JL, Cunningham K. Obsessive-compulsive disorder in Huntington's disease. Biol Psychiatry 1992;31(3):263–270.
97. Duff K, Paulsen JS, Beglinger LJ, et al. Psychiatric symptoms in Huntington's disease before diagnosis: The predict-HD study. Biol Psychiatry 2007;62(12): 1341–1346.
98. Paulsen JS, Ready RE, Hamilton JM, et al. Neuropsychiatric aspects of Huntington's disease. J Neurol Neurosurg Psychiatry 2001;71(3):310–314.
99. Craufurd D, Thompson JC, Snowden JS. Behavioral changes in Huntington Disease. Neuropsychiatry Neuropsychol Behav Neurol 2001;14(4):219–226.
100. Di Maio L, Squitieri F, Napolitano G, et al. Onset symptoms in 510 patients with Huntington's disease. J Med Genet 1993;30(4):289–292.
101. Ho AK, Gilbert AS, Mason SL, et al. Health-related quality of life in Huntington's disease: Which factors matter most? Mov Disord. 2009 Mar 15;24(4):574–578.
102. Julien CL, Thompson JC, Wild S, et al. Psychiatric disorders in preclinical Huntington's disease. J Neurol Neurosurg Psychiatry 2007;78(9):939–943.
103. Mayberg HS, Starkstein SE, Peyser CE, et al. Paralimbic frontal lobe hypometabolism in depression associated with Huntington's disease. Neurology 1992;42(9): 1791–1797.
104. De Marchi N, Mennella R. Huntington's disease and its association with psychopathology. Harv Rev Psychiatry 2000;7(5):278–289.
105. Correa BB, Xavier M, Guimaraes J. Association of Huntington's disease and schizophrenia-like psychosis in a Huntington's disease pedigree. Clin Pract Epidemol Ment Health 2006;2:1.
106. Jardri R, Medjkane F, Cuisset JM, et al. Huntington's disease presenting as a depressive disorder with psychotic features. J Am Acad Child Adolesc Psychiatry 2007;46(3):307–308.
107. Tsuang D, Almqvist EW, Lipe H, et al. Familial aggregation of psychotic symptoms in Huntington's disease. Am J Psychiatry 2000;157(12):1955–1959.
108. Tsuang D, DiGiacomo L, Lipe H, et al. Familial aggregation of schizophrenia-like symptoms in Huntington's disease. Am J Med Genet 1998;81(4):323–327.
109. Beglinger LJ, Langbehn DR, Duff K, et al. Probability of obsessive and compulsive symptoms in Huntington's disease. Biol Psychiatry 2007;61(3):415–418.
110. Anderson KE, Louis ED, Stern Y, et al. Cognitive correlates of obsessive and compulsive symptoms in Huntington's disease. Am J Psychiatry 2001;158(5):799–801.
111. De Marchi N, Morris M, Mennella R, et al. Association of obsessive-compulsive disorder and pathological gambling with Huntington's disease in an Italian pedigree: Possible association with Huntington's disease mutation. Acta Psychiatr Scand 1998;97(1):62–65.
112. Patzold T, Brune M. Obsessive compulsive disorder in Huntington disease: a case of isolated obsessions successfully treated with sertraline. Neuropsychiatry Neuropsychol Behav Neurol 2002;15(3):216–219.
113. Robinson D, Wu H, Munne RA, et al. Reduced caudate nucleus volume in obsessive-compulsive disorder. Arch Gen Psychiatry 1995;52(5):393–398.

114. Saxena S, Rauch SL. Functional neuroimaging and the neuroanatomy of obsessive-compulsive disorder. Psychiatr Clin North Am 2000;23(3):563–586.
115. Schmidt EZ, Bonelli RM. Sexuality in Huntington's disease. Wien Med Wochenschr 2008;158(3–4):78–83.
116. Fedoroff JP, Peyser C, Franz ML, et al. Sexual disorders in Huntington's disease. J Neuropsychiatry Clin Neurosci 1994;6(2):147–153.
117. Di Maio L, Squitieri F, Napolitano G, et al. Suicide risk in Huntington's disease. J Med Genet 1993;30(4): 293–295.
118. Farrer LA. Suicide and attempted suicide in Huntington disease: implications for preclinical testing of persons at risk. Am J Med Genet 1986;24(2):305–311.
119. Schoenfeld M, Myers RH, Cupples LA, et al. Increased rate of suicide among patients with Huntington's disease. J Neurol Neurosurg Psychiatry 1984;47(12):1283–1287.
120. Paulsen JS, Hoth KF, Nehl C, et al. Critical periods of suicide risk in Huntington's disease. Am J Psychiatry 2005;162(4):725–731.
121. Lipe H, Schultz A, Bird TD. Risk factors for suicide in Huntingtons disease: A retrospective case controlled study. Am J Med Genet 1993;48(4):231–233.
122. Beal MF, Brouillet E, Jenkins B, et al. Age-dependent striatal excitotoxic lesions produced by the endogenous mitochondrial inhibitor malonate. J Neurochem 1993;61(3):1147–1150.
123. Beal MF, Brouillet E, Jenkins BG, et al. Neurochemical and histologic characterization of striatal excitotoxic lesions produced by the mitochondrial toxin 3-nitropropionic acid. J Neurosci 1993;13(10):4181–4192.
124. Brouillet E, Jenkins BG, Hyman BT, et al. Age-dependent vulnerability of the striatum to the mitochondrial toxin 3-nitropropionic acid. J Neurochem 1993;60(1):356–359.
125. Browne SE, Bowling AC, MacGarvey U, et al. Oxidative damage and metabolic dysfunction in Huntington's disease: Selective vulnerability of the basal ganglia. Ann Neurol 1997;41(5):646–653.
126. Gu M, Gash MT, Mann VM, et al. Mitochondrial defect in Huntington's disease caudate nucleus. Ann Neurol 1996;39(3):385–389.
127. Jenkins BG, Koroshetz WJ, Beal MF, et al. Evidence for impairment of energy metabolism in vivo in Huntington's disease using localized 1H NMR spectroscopy. Neurology 1993;43(12):2689–2695.
128. Koroshetz WJ, Jenkins BG, Rosen BR, et al. Energy metabolism defects in Huntington's disease and effects of coenzyme Q10. Ann Neurol 1997;41(2):160–165.
129. Djousse L, Knowlton B, Cupples LA, et al. Weight loss in early stage of Huntington's disease. Neurology 2002;59(9):1325–1330.
130. Sanberg PR, Fibiger HC, Mark RF. Body weight and dietary factors in Huntington's disease patients compared with matched controls. Med J Aust 1981;1(8):407–409.
131. Trejo A, Tarrats RM, Alonso ME, et al. Assessment of the nutrition status of patients with Huntington's disease. Nutrition 2004;20(2):192–196.
132. Gaba AM, Zhang K, Marder K, et al. Energy balance in early-stage Huntington disease. Am J Clin Nutr 2005;81(6):1335–1341.
133. Pratley RE, Salbe AD, Ravussin E, et al. Higher sedentary energy expenditure in patients with Huntington's disease. Ann Neurol 2000;47(1):64–70.
134. Hamilton JM, Wolfson T, Peavy GM, et al. Rate and correlates of weight change in Huntington's disease. J Neurol Neurosurg Psychiatry 2004;75(2):209–212.
135. Aziz NA, van der Burg JM, Landwehrmeyer GB, et al. Weight loss in Huntington disease increases with higher CAG repeat number. Neurology 2008;71(19): 1506–1513.
136. Marder K, Zhao H, Eberly S, et al. Dietary intake in adults at risk for Huntington disease: Analysis of PHAROS research participants. Neurology 2009;73(5):385–392.
137. Myers RH, Sax DS, Koroshetz WJ, et al. Factors associated with slow progression in Huntington's disease. Arch Neurol 1991;48(8):800–804.
138. Kassubek J, Juengling FD, Kioschies T, et al. Topography of cerebral atrophy in early Huntington's disease: A voxel based morphometric MRI study. J Neurol Neurosurg Psychiatry 2004;75(2):213–220.
139. Kremer HP, Roos RA, Dingjan G, et al. Atrophy of the hypothalamic lateral tuberal nucleus in Huntington's disease. J Neuropathol Exp Neurol 1990;49(4): 371–382.
140. Kremer HP, Roos RA, Dingjan GM, et al. The hypothalamic lateral tuberal nucleus and the characteristics of neuronal loss in Huntington's disease. Neurosci Lett 1991;132(1):101–104.
141. Petersen A, Gil J, Maat-Schieman ML, et al. Orexin loss in Huntington's disease. Hum Mol Genet 2005;14(1): 39–47.
142. Bjorkqvist M, Petersen A, Bacos K, et al. Progressive alterations in the hypothalamic-pituitary-adrenal axis in the R6/2 transgenic mouse model of Huntington's disease. Hum Mol Genet 2006;15(10):1713–1721.
143. Wood NI, Goodman AO, van der Burg JM, et al. Increased thirst and drinking in Huntington's disease and the R6/2 mouse. Brain Res Bull 2008;76(1–2):70–79.
144. Politis M, Pavese N, Tai YF, et al. Hypothalamic involvement in Huntington's disease: an in vivo PET study. Brain 131(Pt 11):2860–2869, 2008.
145. Popovic V, Svetel M, Djurovic M, et al. Circulating and cerebrospinal fluid ghrelin and leptin: potential role in altered body weight in Huntington's disease. Eur J Endocrinol 2004;151(4):451–455.
146. Farrer LA. Diabetes mellitus in Huntington disease. Clin Genet 27(1):62–67, 1985.
147. Lalic NM, Maric J, Svetel M, et al. Glucose homeostasis in Huntington disease: Abnormalities in insulin sensitivity and early-phase insulin secretion. Arch Neurol 2008;65(4):476–480.
148. Bacos K, Bjorkqvist M, Petersen A, et al. Islet beta-cell area and hormone expression are unaltered in Huntington's disease. Histochem Cell Biol 2008;129(5): 623–629.
149. Taylor N, Bramble D. Sleep disturbance and Huntingdon's disease. Br J Psychiatry 1997;171:393.
150. Arnulf I, Nielsen J, Lohmann E, et al. Rapid eye movement sleep disturbances in Huntington disease. Arch Neurol 2008;65(4):482–488.

151. Videnovic A, Leurgans S, Fan W, Jaglin J, Shannon KM. Daytime somnolence and nocturnal sleep disturbances in Huntington disease. Parkinsonism Relat Disord, 2009 Jul;15(6):471–474. Epub 2008 Nov 28.
152. Emser W, Brenner M, Stober T, et al. Changes in nocturnal sleep in Huntington's and Parkinson's disease. J Neurol 1988;235(3):177–179.
153. Wiegand M, Moller AA, Lauer CJ, et al. Nocturnal sleep in Huntington's disease. J Neurol 1991;238(4): 203–208.
154. Silvestri R, Raffaele M, De Domenico P, et al. Sleep features in Tourette's syndrome, neuroacanthocytosis and Huntington's chorea. Neurophysiol Clin 1995,25(2): 66–77.
155. Pavese N, Gerhard A, Tai YF, et al. Microglial activation correlates with severity in Huntington disease: A clinical and PET study. Neurology 2006;66(11):1638–1643.
156. Sapp E, Kegel KB, Aronin N, et al. Early and progressive accumulation of reactive microglia in the Huntington disease brain. J Neuropathol Exp Neurol 2001;60(2): 161–172.
157. Tai YF, Pavese N, Gerhard A, et al. Microglial activation in presymptomatic Huntington's disease gene carriers. Brain 2007;130(Pt 7):1759–1766.
158. Tai YF, Pavese N, Gerhard A, et al. Imaging microglial activation in Huntington's disease. Brain Res Bull 2007;72(2–3):148–151.
159. Shin JY, Fang ZH, Yu ZX, et al. Expression of mutant huntingtin in glial cells contributes to neuronal excitotoxicity. 2005;J Cell Biol 171(6):1001–1012.
160. Bjorkqvist M, Wild EJ, Thiele J, et al. A novel pathogenic pathway of immune activation detectable before clinical onset in Huntington's disease. J Exp Med 2008;205(8):1869–1877.
161. Sharma KR, Romano JG, Ayyar DR, et al. Sympathetic skin response and heart rate variability in patients with Huntington disease. Arch Neurol 1999;56(10):1248–1252.
162. Andrich J, Schmitz T, Saft C, et al. Autonomic nervous system function in Huntington's disease. J Neurol Neurosurg Psychiatry 2002;72(6):726–731.
163. Bar KJ, Boettger MK, Andrich J, et al. Cardiovagal modulation upon postural change is altered in Huntington's disease. Eur J Neurol 2008;15(8):869–871.
164. Kobal J, Meglic B, Mesec A, et al. Early sympathetic hyperactivity in Huntington's disease. Eur J Neurol 2004;11(12):842–848.
165. Barrios FA, Gonzalez L, Favila R, et al. Olfaction and neurodegeneration in HD. Neuroreport 2007;18(1):73–76.
166. Hamilton JM, Murphy C, Paulsen JS. Odor detection, learning, and memory in Huntington's disease. J Int Neuropsychol Soc 1999;5(7):609–615.
167. Lazic SE, Goodman AO, Grote HE, et al. Olfactory abnormalities in Huntington's disease: Decreased plasticity in the primary olfactory cortex of R6/1 transgenic mice and reduced olfactory discrimination in patients. Brain Res 2007;1151:219–226.
168. Sorensen SA, Fenger K, Olsen JH. Significantly lower incidence of cancer among patients with Huntington disease: An apoptotic effect of an expanded polyglutamine tract? Cancer 1999;86(7):1342–1346.
169. Giovannucci E, Stampfer MJ, Krithivas K, et al. The CAG repeat within the androgen receptor gene and its relationship to prostate cancer. Proc Natl Acad Sci U S A 1997;94(7):3320–3323.
170. Stanford JL, Just JJ, Gibbs M, et al. Polymorphic repeats in the androgen receptor gene: molecular markers of prostate cancer risk. Cancer Res 1997;57(6):1194–1198.
171. Nance MA, Myers RH. Juvenile onset Huntington's disease--Clinical and research perspectives. Ment Retard Dev Disabil Res Rev 2001;7(3):153–157.
172. Rasmussen A, Macias R, Yescas P, et al. Huntington disease in children: Genotype-phenotype correlation. Neuropediatrics 2000;31(4):190–194.
173. Gusella JF, MacDonald ME. Huntington's disease and repeating trinucleotides. N Engl J Med 1994;330(20): 1450–1451.
174. Nance MA, Mathias-Hagen V, Breningstall G, et al. Analysis of a very large trinucleotide repeat in a patient with juvenile Huntington's disease. Neurology 1999;52(2): 392–394.
175. Leeflang EP, Zhang L, Tavare S, et al. Single sperm analysis of the trinucleotide repeats in the Huntington's disease gene: Quantification of the mutation frequency spectrum. Hum Mol Genet 1995;4(9):1519–1526.
176. MacDonald ME, Barnes G, Srinidhi J, et al. Gametic but not somatic instability of CAG repeat length in Huntington's disease. J Med Genet 1993;30(12):982–986.
177. Telenius H, Almqvist E, Kremer B, et al. Somatic mosaicism in sperm is associated with intergenerational (CAG)n changes in Huntington disease. Hum Mol Genet 1995;4(2):189–195.
178. Telenius H, Kremer HP, Theilmann J, et al. Molecular analysis of juvenile Huntington disease: the major influence on (CAG)n repeat length is the sex of the affected parent. Hum Mol Genet 1993;2(10): 1535–1540.
179. Squitieri F, Pustorino G, Cannella M, et al. Highly disabling cerebellar presentation in Huntington disease. Eur J Neurol 2003;10(4):443–444.
180. Landau ME, Cannard KR. EEG characteristics in juvenile Huntington's disease: a case report and review of the literature. Epileptic Disord 2003;5(3):145–148.
181. Yoon G, Kramer J, Zanko A, et al. Speech and language delay are early manifestations of juvenile-onset Huntington disease. Neurology 2006;67(7):1265–1267.
182. Myers RH, Vonsattel JP, Stevens TJ, et al. Clinical and neuropathologic assessment of severity in Huntington's disease. Neurology 1988;38(3):341–347.
183. Roos RA, Hermans J, Vegter-van der Vlis M, et al. Duration of illness in Huntington's disease is not related to age at onset. J Neurol Neurosurg Psychiatry 1993;56(1): 98–100.
184. Kremer B, Goldberg P, Andrew SE, et al. A worldwide study of the Huntington's disease mutation. The sensitivity and specificity of measuring CAG repeats. N Engl J Med 1994;330(20):1401–1406.
185. Oster E, Dorsey ER, Bausch J, et al. Fear of health insurance loss among individuals at risk for Huntington disease. Am J Med Genet A 2008;146A(16): 2070–2077.

186. Hockly E, Cordery PM, Woodman B, et al. Environmental enrichment slows disease progression in R6/2 Huntington's disease mice. Ann Neurol 2002;51(2):235–242.
187. van Dellen A, Blakemore C, Deacon R, et al. Delaying the onset of Huntington's in mice. Nature 2000;404(6779): 721–722.
188. Priller J, Ecker D, Landwehrmeyer B, et al. A Europe-wide assessment of current medication choices in Huntington's disease. Mov Disord 2008;23(12):1788.
189. Barr AN, Fischer JH, Koller WC, et al. Serum haloperidol concentration and choreiform movements in Huntington's disease. Neurology 1988;38(1):84–88.
190. Girotti F, Carella F, Scigliano G, et al. Effect of neuroleptic treatment on involuntary movements and motor performances in Huntington's disease. J Neurol Neurosurg Psychiatry 1984;47(8):848–852.
191. Leonard DP, Kidson MA, Brown JG, et al. A double blind trial of lithium carbonate and haloperidol in Huntington's chorea. Aust N Z J Psychiatry 1975;9(2):115–118.
192. Leonard DP, Kidson MA, Shannon PJ, et al. Letter: Double-blind trial of lithium carbonate and haloperidol in Huntington's chorea. Lancet 1974;2(7890): 1208–1209.
193. Bachoud-Levi AC, Gaura V, Brugieres P, et al. Effect of fetal neural transplants in patients with Huntington's disease 6 years after surgery: A long-term follow-up study. Lancet Neurol 2006;5(4):303–309.
194. Bonelli RM, Mahnert FA, Niederwieser G. Olanzapine for Huntington's disease: An open label study. Clin Neuropharmacol 2002;25(5):263–265.
195. Bonelli RM, Niederwieser G, Diez J, et al. Riluzole and olanzapine in Huntington's disease. Eur J Neurol 2002;9(2):183–184.
196. Bonuccelli U, Ceravolo R, Maremmani C, et al. Clozapine in Huntington's chorea. Neurology 1994;44(5):821–823.
197. Duff K, Beglinger LJ, O'Rourke ME, et al. Risperidone and the treatment of psychiatric, motor, and cognitive symptoms in Huntington's disease. Ann Clin Psychiatry 2008;20(1):1–3.
198. Jankovic J, Beach J. Long-term effects of tetrabenazine in hyperkinetic movement disorders. Neurology 1997;48(2):358–362.
199. Kenney C, Hunter C, Davidson A, et al. Short-term effects of tetrabenazine on chorea associated with Huntington's disease. Mov Disord 2007;22(1):10–13.
200. Ondo WG, Tintner R, Thomas M, et al. Tetrabenazine treatment for Huntington's disease-associated chorea. Clin Neuropharmacol 2002;25(6):300–302.
201. Paleacu D, Giladi N, Moore O, et al. Tetrabenazine treatment in movement disorders. Clin Neuropharmacol 2004;27(5):230–233.
202. Huntington Study Group. Tetrabenazine as antichorea therapy in Huntington disease: A randomized controlled trial. Neurology 2006;66(3):366–372.
203. Huntington Study Group. A randomized, placebo-controlled trial of coenzyme Q10 and remacemide in Huntington's disease. Neurology 2001;57(3):397–404.
204. Heckmann JM, Legg P, Sklar D, et al. IV amantadine improves chorea in Huntington's disease: An acute randomized, controlled study. Neurology 2004;63(3):597–598; author reply 597–598.
205. Lucetti C, Del Dotto P, Gambaccini G, et al. IV amantadine improves chorea in Huntington's disease: An acute randomized, controlled study. Neurology 2003;60(12):1995–1997.
206. Lucetti C, Gambaccini G, Bernardini S, et al. Amantadine in Huntington's disease: Open-label video-blinded study. Neurol Sci 2002;23(Suppl 2):S83-S84.
207. Rosas HD, Koroshetz WJ, Jenkins BG, et al. Riluzole therapy in Huntington's disease (HD). Mov Disord 1999;14(2):326–330.
208. Seppi K, Mueller J, Bodner T, et al. Riluzole in Huntington's disease (HD): An open label study with one year follow up. J Neurol 2001;248(10):866–869.
209. Verhagen Metman L, Morris MJ, Farmer C, et al. Huntington's disease: A randomized, controlled trial using the NMDA-antagonist amantadine. Neurology 2002;59(5): 694–699.
210. Anden NE, Dalen P, Johansson B. Baclofen and lithium in Huntington's chorea. Lancet 1973;2(7820):93.
211. Shoulson I, Odoroff C, Oakes D, et al. A controlled clinical trial of baclofen as protective therapy in early Huntington's disease. Ann Neurol 1989;25(3):252–259.
212. Stewart JT. Treatment of Huntington's disease with clonazepam. South Med J 81(1):102, 1988.
213. Bird MT, Paulson GW. The rigid form of Huntington's chorea. Neurology 1971;21(3):271–276.
214. Bonelli RM, Niederwieser G, Diez J, et al. Pramipexole ameliorates neurologic and psychiatric symptoms in a Westphal variant of Huntington's disease. Clin Neuropharmacol 2002;25(1):58–60.
215. Jongen PJ, Renier WO, Gabreels FJ. Seven cases of Huntington's disease in childhood and levodopa induced improvement in the hypokinetic--Rigid form. Clin Neurol Neurosurg 1980;82(4):251–261.
216. Racette BA, Perlmutter JS. Levodopa responsive parkinsonism in an adult with Huntington's disease. J Neurol Neurosurg Psychiatry 1998;65(4):577–579.
217. Reuter I, Hu MT, Andrews TC, et al. Late onset levodopa responsive Huntington's disease with minimal chorea masquerading as Parkinson plus syndrome. J Neurol Neurosurg Psychiatry 2000;68(2):238–241.
218. de Tommaso M, Specchio N, Sciruicchio V, et al. Effects of rivastigmine on motor and cognitive impairment in Huntington's disease. Mov Disord 2004;19(12):1516–1518.
219. de Tommaso M, Difruscolo O, Sciruicchio V, et al. Two years' follow-up of rivastigmine treatment in Huntington disease. Clin Neuropharmacol 2007;30(1):43–46.
220. Fernandez HH, Friedman JH, Grace J, et al. Donepezil for Huntington's disease. Mov Disord 2000;15(1):173–176.
221. Rot U, Kobal J, Sever A, et al. Rivastigmine in the treatment of Huntington's disease. Eur J Neurol 2002;9(6):689–690.
222. Ranen NG, Peyser CE, Folstein SE. ECT as a treatment for depression in Huntington's disease. J Neuropsychiatry Clin Neurosci 1994;6(2):154–159.
223. Fasano A, Mazzone P, Piano C, et al. GPi-DBS in Huntington's disease: Results on motor function and cognition in a 72-year-old case. Mov Disord 2008;23(9):1289–1292.
224. Fawcett AP, Moro E, Lang AE, et al. Pallidal deep brain stimulation influences both reflexive and voluntary saccades in Huntington's disease. Mov Disord 2005;20(3): 371–377.

225. Moro E, Lang AE, Strafella AP, et al. Bilateral globus pallidus stimulation for Huntington's disease. Ann Neurol 2004;56(2):290–294.
226. Bachoud-Levi AC, Remy P, Nguyen JP, et al. Motor and cognitive improvements in patients with Huntington's disease after neural transplantation. Lancet 2000;356(9246):1975–1979.
227. Hauser RA, Furtado S, Cimino CR, et al. Bilateral human fetal striatal transplantation in Huntington's disease. Neurology 2002;58(5):687–695.
228. Philpott LM, Kopyov OV, Lee AJ, et al. Neuropsychological functioning following fetal striatal transplantation in Huntington's chorea: Three case presentations. Cell Transplant 1997;6(3):203–212.
229. Takahashi K, Tanabe K, Ohnuki M, et al. Induction of pluripotent stem cells from adult human fibroblasts by defined factors. Cell 2007;131(5):861–872.

CHAPTER 34

Neuropathology and Pathophysiology of Huntington's Disease

Steven M. Hersch, H. Diana Rosas, and Robert J. Ferrante

Huntington's disease (HD) is a neurodegenerative disorder related to a mutation occurring in the coding region of the IT15 gene on chromosome 4. The average age of onset is about 40 years; however, the range is extremely broad, with pediatric and late-life onsets not infrequent. The genetic mutation consists of expansion of a polymorphic trinucleotide (CAG) repeat, near the 5′ end of the gene, that normally ranges from about 17 to 30 copies. Individuals with more than 37 repeats develop HD, with the largest numbers (greater than 60) correlating with juvenile onset of HD. Genetic anticipation occurs such that the affected offspring of males have an increased probability of developing the disease at an earlier age than their fathers. The IT15 gene codes for a protein named huntingtin, which is highly interactive with many other proteins and may have many functions, including new ones conferred by the repeat expansion. In individuals heterozygous for HD, both normal huntingtin and huntingtin containing an expanded polyglutamine tract, transcribed by the CAG expansion, are expressed. The relationship between this abnormal protein and neuropathology and pathogenesis has been studied extensively since the gene was discovered and evidence points to complex contributions from the mutant protein, its proteolytic fragments, and dysfunction of the normal protein in neuronal degeneration and death. The mutation is thus considered to lead to both gain of function and loss of function alterations in cellular biochemistry, which lead progressively to neurodegeneration and cell death. A hallmark of HD is the presence of insoluble aggregates of huntingtin,[1] which can occur in neuronal nuclei, cytoplasm, and processes[2] and which consists of heterogeneous mixtures of mutant and normal huntingtin and a variety of other proteins. Most evidence suggests that the toxicity of mutant huntingtin resides in its soluble interactions as a holoprotein, as fragments, or as soluble oligomers. While much has been learned, many questions remain, particularly which interactions of mutant huntingtin and which of its forms are most important for pathogenesis. The clinical expression of HD is characteristic, though variable, and consists of progressively disordered movement, behavior, and cognition. The specific symptoms and progression of HD can be related directly to its neuropathology (Fig. 34–1), which is characterized by relatively selective loss of specific neuronal populations in a variety of brain regions. Basal ganglia pathology has been the most thoroughly characterized and has been central to the development of animal models and hypotheses about the circuitry involved in chorea and about potential mechanisms of neuronal death in HD. Pathology in other brain regions has not been studied as extensively but is very widespread and more significant than the customary focus on basal ganglia might suggest and contributes importantly to the clinical phenotype of HD. Outside the brain, molecular and biochemical alterations have been identified; however, their clinical significance is unknown. This review focuses on research occurring in the last 25 years,

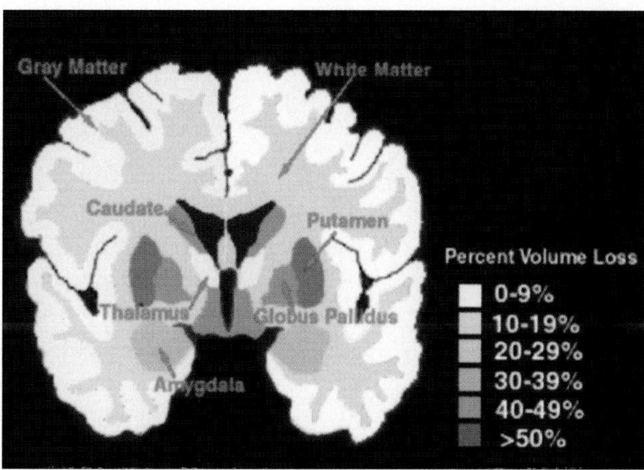

Figure 34–1. MRI brain segmentation. Composite representation of volume loss occurring in the brains of 18 individuals in the early stages of HD. In addition to the expected marked atrophy of the striatum, significant volume loss is also evident in the globus pallidus, amygdala, hypothalamus, and cortical white and gray matters.

during which the identification of the causative genetic mutation, the development of many genetic cellular and animal models, and new methods in quantitative anatomy, neuroimaging, immunocytochemistry, biochemistry, and molecular biology have converged to produce an explosion of new knowledge and ideas about HD.

▶ NEUROPATHOLOGY

STRIATUM

Gross and Histologic Pathology

The most severe neuropathology in HD occurs within the neostriatum, in which there is gross atrophy of the caudate nucleus and putamen, accompanied by marked neuronal loss, astrogliosis (Fig. 34–2), and reactive microgliosis.[3–6] The striatal astrogliosis appears to reflect relative astrocyte survival in a shrinking striatum,[7] rather than a primary or reactive astrocytosis. However, progressive microgliosis has been detected recently using a positron emission tomography ligand[8,9] that suggests some level of active inflammation in the striatum. Oligodendrogliosis also accompanies neuronal loss,[10] most likely an artifact of their relative preservation. The extent of gross striatal pathology, neuronal loss, and gliosis provides a basis for grading the severity of HD pathology (grades 0–4),[11] which also correlates with the extent of clinical disability (Fig. 34–3). Grade 0 cases have a strong clinical and familial history or genetic test indicating HD but no detectable histological neuropathology at autopsy.

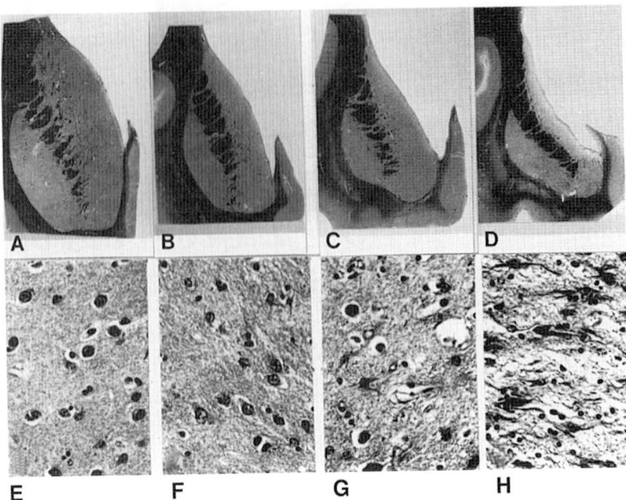

Figure 34–3. Coronal sections through the level of the caudate nucleus and putamen, demonstrating the grades of severity of striatal involvement. A normal specimen is represented in (**A**). No gross striatal atrophy is observed in grades 0 and 1. In grade 2 (**B**), there is striatal atrophy, but the caudate nucleus remains convex. In grade 3 (**C**), striatal atrophy is more severe, with the caudate nucleus flat. In grade 4 (**D**), striatal atrophy is most severe, with the medial surface concave. Concomitant with the severity of gross atrophy observed in grades 2, 3, and 4, progressive neuronal loss and astrogliosis occur within the caudate nucleus and putamen in (**F**, **G**, and **H**), respectively. There is a dorsoventral gradient of cell death, with the dorsal striatum most severely involved.

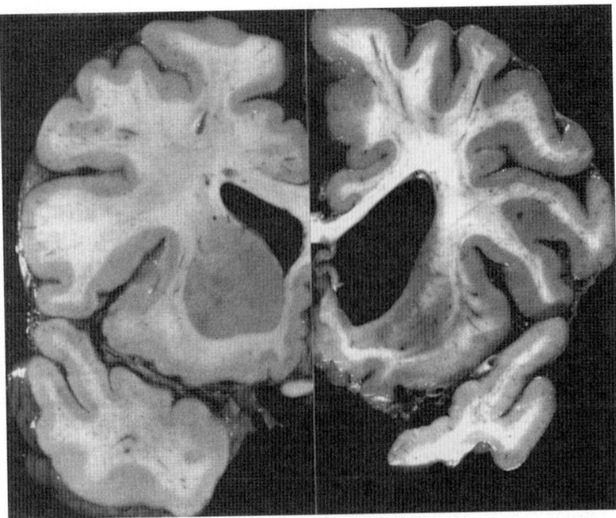

Figure 34–2. Photomicrographs of fixed cerebral hemispheres from a 58-year-old female with HD (*right*) and an age-matched normal specimen (*left*) at a coronal level through the rostral striatum. Note the marked atrophy of the caudate nucleus and putamen, along with cortical atrophy and white matter loss in HD.

In grade 1 cases, neuropathological changes can be detected microscopically with as much as 50% depletion of striatal neurons but without gross atrophy. In more severe grades (2–4), gross atrophy, neuronal depletion, and gliosis are progressively more pronounced, and pallidal pathology becomes evident. In the most severe grade (4), more than 90% of striatal neurons are lost, and microscopy predominantly reveals astrocytes. There is a dorsal-to-ventral, anterior-to-posterior, and medial-to-lateral progression of neuronal death, with the dorsomedial striatum affected earliest and relative sparing of the ventral striatum and nucleus accumbens.[11,12] Neuropathology predates symptoms by many years. Postmortem evaluations of individuals at risk for HD who died prior to the onset of symptoms have revealed striatal atrophy, widespread huntingtin aggregation, and oligodendrogliosis in the presence of neuronal loss.[2,13] Similarly, quantitative magnetic resonance imaging (MRI) analysis has revealed striatal volume atrophy in presymptomatic individuals at known genetic risk for developing HD. [14–16] In fact, by the time the earliest clinical symptoms are detectable, the striatum has diminished in volume by about 50%. The magnitude of the CAG repeat expansion correlates with the magnitude of striatal volume loss, suggesting that the rate of progression of striatal pathology is faster in individuals with higher numbers of repeats.[17–19]

Selective Neuronal Loss and Preservation

Quantitative microscopic studies demonstrating relative preservation of large striatal neurons and severe loss of medium-sized striatal neurons provided early evidence for selective neuronal degeneration in the neostriatum.[7,20] Since then, extensive biochemical, tissue-binding, immunocytochemical, and genomic studies of HD brain tissue have demonstrated marked disparities, with loss versus preservation of a variety of neurochemical substances within the basal ganglia, suggesting that the destructive process is not equally expressed in all striatal neurons and that there is a selective pattern of neuronal vulnerability. Neuropathology is accompanied by selective but profound alterations in gene transcription that reflect degenerative and compensatory processes, some of which likely worsen pathology.[21]

Medium spiny neurons are inhibitory projection neurons that use γ-aminobutyric acid (GABA) as their primary neurotransmitter, and they comprise more than 80% of all striatal neurons. Reductions in GABA, its synthetic enzyme glutamic acid decarboxylase, and its degradative enzyme GABA transaminase in the neostriatum were among the earliest neurochemical changes detected in HD and could be correlated with loss of medium spiny neurons.[22–26] Medium spiny neurons have further been shown to be depleted in HD based on the loss of substance P,[27] enkephalin, calcineurin,[28] calbindin,[29–31] histamine H_2 receptors,[32] dopamine receptors,[33,34] cannabinoid receptors,[35] and adenosine A_{2A} receptors[36] (Fig. 34–4). Medium spiny neurons can be divided into two populations based upon both connectional and neurochemical differences. One subpopulation expresses D_1 dopamine receptors and the cotransmitter substance P, and projects primarily to the internal segment of the globus pallidus (GPi) and the substantia nigra pars reticulata (SNr). The other population expresses the D_2 dopamine receptor and enkephalin and projects primarily to the external segment of the globus pallidus (GPe).[37] All of these markers of striatal projection neurons and their axonal projections are progressively lost in HD, correlating with the degeneration and loss of medium spiny neurons.[38–43] Among the early changes are losses in cannabinoid CB1, D_2, and adenosine A_{2A} receptors in the striatum and GPe, followed later by a loss of D_1, with all of these receptors being profoundly lost as HD progresses.[44] Recent evidence, especially in transgenic mouse models of HD, suggests that there are many selective neurochemical alterations due to transcriptional dysfunction that predates neuronal loss and provides neurochemical bases for neuronal dysfunction prior to neuronal loss.[45]

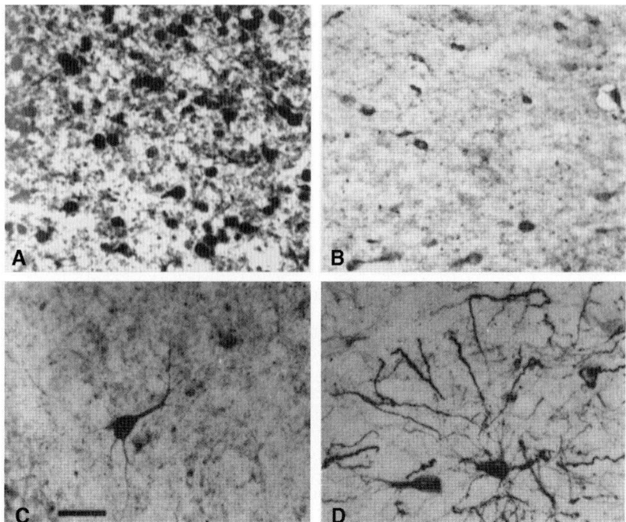

Figure 34–4. Calbindin-positive spiny striatal neurons in normal (**A** and **C**) and HD (**B** and **D**) caudate nucleus. The number of immunoreactive neurons is significantly reduced in HD. Degenerative alterations of this neuronal population, as demonstrated in Golgi preparations (see Fig. 34–6), are observed in (**D**). There is a distal shift in dendritic staining in HD.

Although both populations of medium spiny neurons are lost, there is evidence that, particularly in the early stages of HD, striatal neurons projecting to the GPe are preferentially lost in comparison to striatal neurons projecting to the GPi.[46–48] It has been suggested that this differential loss of striatal projections leads to imbalanced activity in the so-called direct and indirect pathways, causing chorea.[49–51] More specifically, the release of the GPe from inhibitory striatal input is hypothesized to result in excessive inhibition of the subthalamic nucleus, which, in turn, causes decreased activation of the GPi and reduced inhibition of the thalamus, leading to increased cortical excitation and chorea. Consistent with this hypothesis, bicuculline blockade of the GABAergic input to the GPe causes chorea in primates.[52] Furthermore, more equal loss of neurons projecting to both GPi and GPe may be associated with the occurrence of the rigid-akinetic variant of HD,[47] which usually occurs in juveniles. This model has been very useful but is probably oversimplified, because it does not account for the heterogeneity of the disease or such findings as increased thalamic levels of GABA,[48] for simultaneous pathology in other parts of the circuit, or for the finding that the D_1 dopamine receptor is reduced more than D_2 in the striatum and in the termination zones of striatal afferents.[33,34] This latter finding is contrary to what would be predicted, based on the changes in substance P and enkephalin.

In addition to medium spiny neurons, there are a variety of interneurons in the striatum, expressing other

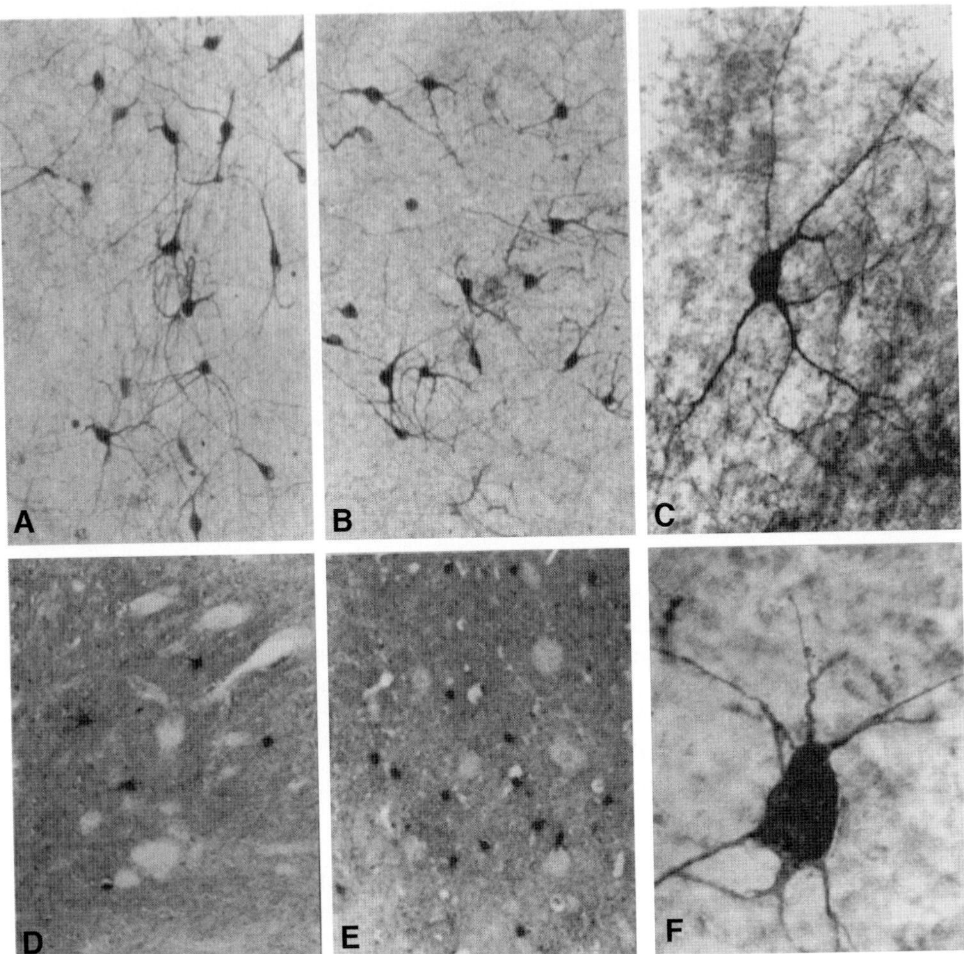

Figure 34–5. Photomicrographs of aspiny striatal neuron populations, which are relatively spared in HD. Medium-sized NADPH-diaphorase striatal neurons are represented in (**A–C**), with normal staining found in (**A**) and preservation in an HD case demonstrated in (**B**). Large acetylcholinesterase striatal neurons are demonstrated in (**D–F**). (**D**) demonstrates the normal density of these neurons, while (**E**) demonstrates that their numbers increase in HD as a result of survival in a shrinking striatum. The density of both neuronal types is significantly increased in HD.

neuroactive substances. Those interneurons that have been studied appear resistant to the neurodegeneration that occurs in HD (Fig. 34–5). These include several types of large- and medium-sized aspiny or sparsely spiny neurons, including one type that expresses somatostatin and neuropeptide Y and can be visualized by NADPH-diaphorase histochemistry,[53] a type of substance P-expressing neuron,[54] large cholinergic interneurons,[55] and calretinin-expressing interneurons.[56] There is a striking persistence of somatostatin and neuropeptide Y,[57,58] and of the somatostatin/neuropeptide Y/NADPH-diaphorase neurons that express them in both caudate nucleus and putamen in HD.[59,60,61,62] The density of these neurons is actually increased four- to fivefold, reflecting the combined effects of both neuronal sparing and tissue shrinkage. The preservation of large cholinergic interneurons likely accounts for the increased ratio of large to small neurons seen in morphometric studies[7,20] of the striatum in HD and also for the preservation of acetylcholinesterase activity.[63] Levels of choline acetyltransferase, the synthetic enzyme for acetylcholine, by contrast, are progressively reduced.[24,55] This may be a result of loss of local postsynaptic targets for cholinergic neurons, most of which are spiny dendrites,[64] and of subsequent reduction in their axons and in acetylcholine synthesis. The preservation of classes of neurons has been invaluable experimentally, providing a means for determining whether animal models of HD reproduce the selective vulnerability that occurs in human HD.

Neuronal Remodeling and Degeneration

Alterations in the dendritic structure of several types of neurons vulnerable in HD have suggested that both proliferative and degenerative alterations occur in a prolonged process before cell death finally ensues. Whether these alterations reflect a primary abnormality in the

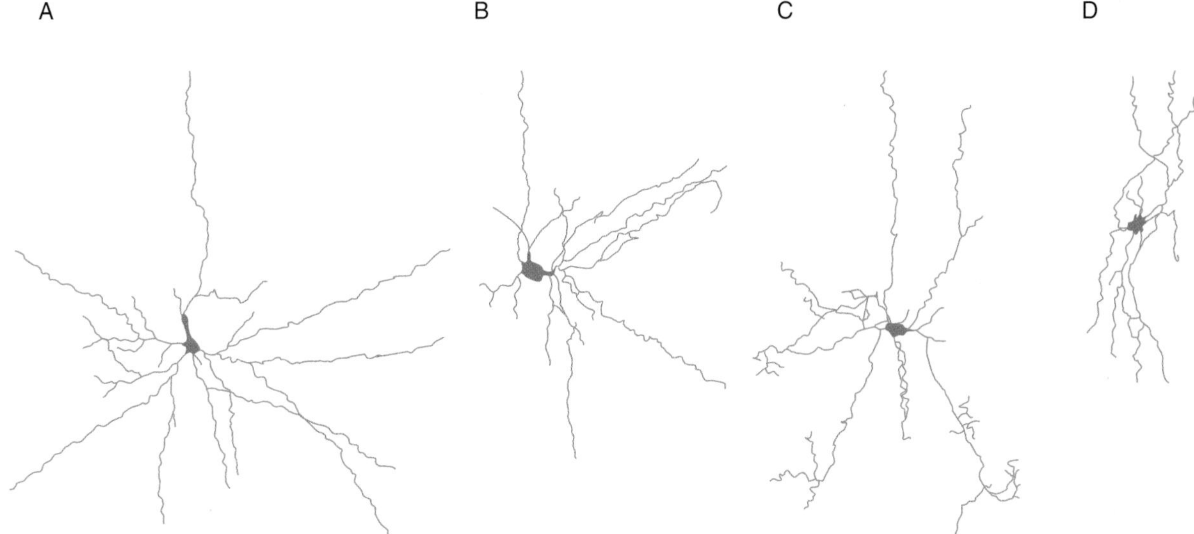

Figure 34–6. Camera lucida drawings of representative spiny striatal neurons in normal (**A**), moderate grades of HD (**B** and **C**), and severe grades of HD (**D**). Normal spiny neurons have 3–7 primary dendrites, which centrifugally radiate from the soma. In moderate grades of HD, the dysmorphic alterations are proliferative. There is an increase in spine density with short-segment branching and terminal dendritic curving. In severe grades of HD, the changes are degenerative, consisting of truncated dendritic arbors, focal swellings, and marked spine loss.

regulation of dendritic architecture or a secondary compensation and decompensation is unknown; however, they likely represent significant functional changes in the neurophysiology of striatal neurons. Early morphological alterations of spiny striatal neurons have been described using Golgi and calbindin immunocytochemical methods (Fig. 34–6).[65,66] Proliferative changes, found primarily in moderate grades of HD, include prominent recurving of distal dendritic segments, short-segment branching along the length of dendrites, and increased numbers and size of dendritic spines. Degenerative alterations, found primarily in more severe cases, consist of truncated dendritic arbors, focal dendritic swelling, and marked spine loss. The relative extent to which enkephalin and substance P subsets develop proliferative changes is not known. It is also not known whether such alterations also occur in striatal interneurons that are spared in HD. These newly formed dendritic arbors and increased numbers of dendritic spines may form functional connections and represent a plastic increase in postsynaptic surfaces in compensation for lost neurons. It has been suggested that the resulting increase in synapses could facilitate neuronal excitability and exacerbate excitotoxic cell death.[66] Plastic degenerative alterations in dendritic structure have also been reported in transgenic mouse models of HD.[67,68,69] Once neurons become unable to compensate for the stresses they undergo, they degenerate in a process with some similarities to apoptosis and to autophagic cell death.[70,71,72] The morphology of the cell death, which has been best examined in HD transgenic mouse models (Fig. 34–7), includes cellular and nuclear shrinkage, irregular cell and nuclear envelopes, chromatin clumping, accumulations of degradation organelles and deposits (lysosomes, autophagasomes, lipofuscin), mild endoplasmic reticulum swelling, and mitochondrial degeneration. Unlike neuronal apoptosis or excitotoxic cell death, the nuclear membrane does not break down until very late, smooth dense spherical chromatin balls are not formed, and apoptotic bodies are not seen.[73] Perhaps transcriptional dysfunction (see later) prevents the complete expression of more typical genetic cell death programs. Progressive oxidative damage to cellular molecules and organelles starts early and may accelerate pathology.[74] Although the features of degeneration have been best studied in the striatum, degeneration in other brain regions seems indistinguishable.

Striosome and Matrix Pathology

The striatum is also composed of chemically and connectionally heterogeneous compartments termed patches or striosomes and matrix.[37,75] Striosomes consist of discrete areas distributed throughout the striatum in which opiate receptors, substance P, met-enkephalin, and cholecystokinin are concentrated. The intervening matrix is enriched in somatostatin, neuropeptide Y, NADPH-diaphorase, calbindin, choline acetyltransferase, acetylcholinesterase, and cytochrome oxidase. Although the striosome-matrix compartments, as determined by acetylcholinesterase[76,77] or by calbindin immunocytochemistry,[30,78] persist in the striatum in HD, the total area of the matrix is reduced, whereas the total area of striosomes is unchanged (Fig. 34–8). These findings are consistent with the preferential loss of striatal D_1 receptors[33,34] but would be unexpected when

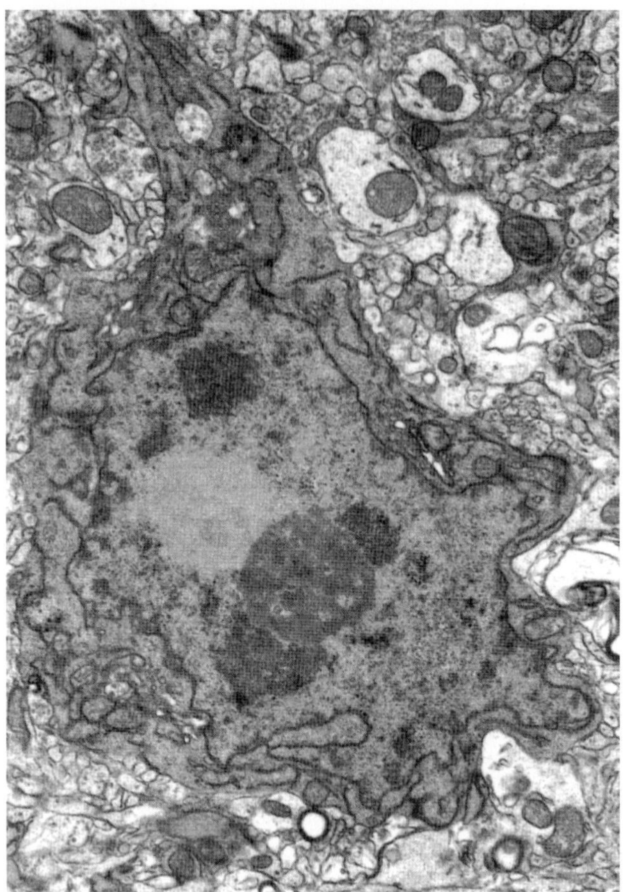

Figure 34–7. Electron micrograph of a degenerating striatal neuron from the R6/2 transgenic mouse, demonstrating typical features of cell death in HD models with shrinkage, loss of round cellular and nuclear contours, nuclear invaginations, chromatin clumping, and mild swelling of organelles. The pale nuclear mass is a nuclear aggregate.

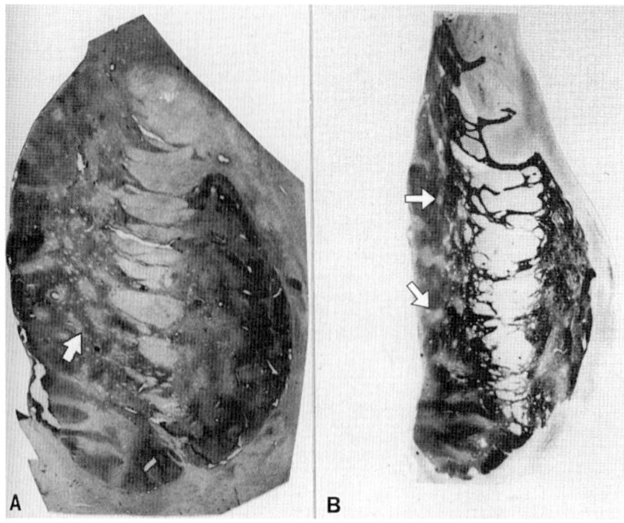

Figure 34–8. Acetylcholinesterase staining in the striatum in normal (**A**) and severe (**B**) HD. The intensity of staining is heterogeneous, with lighter-stained areas (*arrows*) referred to as patches, and the intervening more intensely stained area referred to as the matrix. There is a significant reduction in the matrix compartment, in comparison to that of the total area of patch compartments in HD.

striatal neurons projecting to the GPe are preferentially lost. Because both types of projection neurons are actually admixed in the striatum,[79] patterns of connectivity may not relate quite exactly to striosome/matrix organization. Recent findings suggest that heterogeneity in striosome and matrix pathology occurs between individuals and that striosome involvement (as measured by GABA(A) receptor expression) is associated with mood disorders occurring in HD patients.[80]

GLOBUS PALLIDUS

Pallidal atrophy and gliosis have long been recognized to occur in HD;[11,81] however, its extent is probably underappreciated. In a standard-setting quantitative study,[7] Lange and colleagues determined that both the GPe and GPi can lose more than 50% of volume and more than 40% of neurons, while glia increase both in concentration and in absolute number (Fig. 34–9). These authors felt that pallidal degeneration is more likely a result of primary degeneration of pallidal neurons than of a transneuronal consequence of striatal atrophy. As they also pointed out, pallidal degeneration and loss of pallidal projections have not been sufficiently considered in models attempting to explain chorea. Most studies concerned with pallidal pathology in HD have focused more on

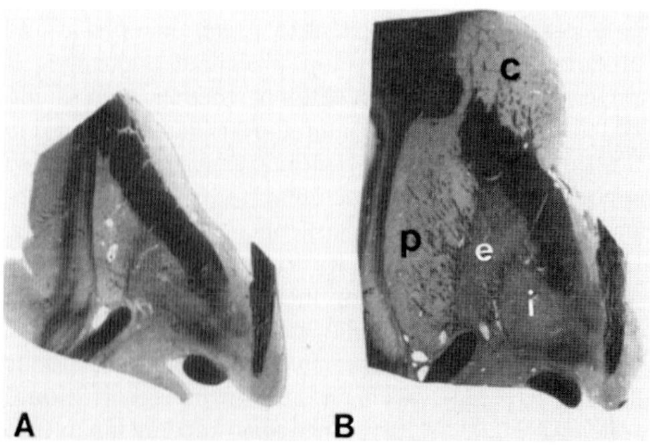

Figure 34–9. Coronal sections through the globus pallidus in HD (**A**) and a normal age-matched specimen (**B**) stained for myelin. The caudate nucleus (*c*) is reduced to a thin ribbon, whereas the putamen (*p*), GPi (*i*) and GPe (*e*) are severely atrophic in HD.

striatopallidal afferents than on pallidal neurons or their projections. Inhibitory striatal afferents project differentially to the GPi and GPe and coat pallidal dendrites with terminals. Striatopallidal neurons expressing substance P project primarily to the GPi, whereas those expressing enkephalin project primarily to the GPe.[37] As discussed earlier, there has been some evidence of preferential loss of GPe afferents in choreatic HD, based primarily on the differential loss of substance P and enkephalin immunoreactivity.[46–48,82] Whether these results were in any way affected by pallidal neuron loss is unknown.

SUBSTANTIA NIGRA

Loss of striatonigral fibers, as well as nigral neurons, has previously been reported to occur in HD.[6,83,84] There have been two quantitative studies of nigral pathology in HD, using distinct methods that may explain the differences in their results.[85,86] Both studies found substantial atrophy and gliosis of both the pars compacta (SNc) and pars reticulata (SNr), with a loss in cross-sectional area of as much as 40% (Fig. 34–10). Ferrante and colleagues observed that the SNr, however, had a greater area loss than the SNc. Both studies also reported that nonpigmented neurons were reduced in both nigral zones and by as much as 45%. Oyanagi and colleagues found that pigmented neurons were reduced by about 50% medially and laterally but were preserved centrally, whereas Ferrante and colleagues found pigmented neurons to be relatively spared with an increase in number resulting from their preservation in a shrinking SNc. The loss of nonpigmented cells may be quite relevant to the development of motor symptoms, because these neurons are the source of nigral afferents to the thalamus, superior colliculus, and brain stem. The relative preservation of pigmented neurons is consistent with some preservation of dopaminergic nigrostriatal projections,[57] although there is evidence of significant loss of nigrostriatal terminals, especially in HD patients with a rigid-akinetic syndrome.[87] The topography of nigral atrophy did not correlate with the dorsomedial-to-ventrolateral pattern of striatal atrophy,[85] suggesting that nigral cell loss cannot be fully explained by loss of striatonigral afferents. However, the possibility of transneuronal degeneration remains because striatal excitotoxic lesions in rodents can cause subsequent neuronal degeneration in the SNr.[88] Interestingly, because the neuronal loss can be prevented by administration of a specific GABA agonist, neuronal death may be related to the loss of inhibitory GABAergic input with subsequent excessive excitation of SNr neurons.

THALAMUS

Until recently, there has been limited study of thalamic pathology in HD, although its presence has been acknowledged. Dom and colleagues,[89] who examined the

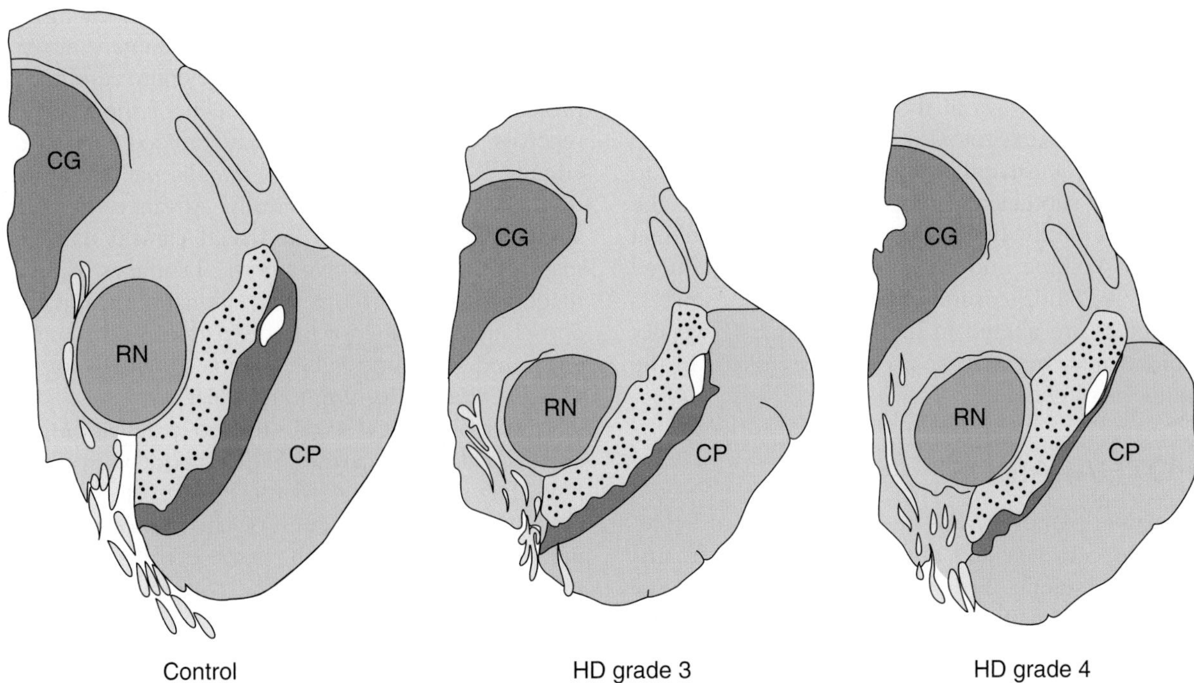

Figure 34–10. Sections through the substantia nigra at the level of the red nucleus (RN) and third nerve in normal control and grades 3 and 4 HD. The total area of the SNc (stippled area) and SNr (solid black area) is significantly reduced in HD, with the SNr most severely involved and the SNc relatively spared.

ventrolateral thalamus in seven cases of HD, performed the first specific study. Because the basal ganglia outflow directed to the frontal cortex is relayed by the ventrolateral thalamus, pathology in this nucleus may be quite relevant to the movement disorders occurring in HD. These investigators found that 50% of small neurons disappeared, whereas large neurons were not altered. If these small thalamic neurons are inhibitory interneurons, their loss could be related to thalamic disinhibition. Increased levels of thalamic GABA in HD,[48] however, are not consistent with this hypothesis, unless it can somehow be viewed as a compensatory upregulation of GABA. The centromedian–parafascicular complex, which is the major source of thalamostriatal afferents, was found to undergo a loss of 55% of neurons along with marked astrogliosis.[90] In contrast, the mediodorsal nucleus, which is not directly connected to the striatum but projects to the frontal cortex, was found to undergo a loss of 23.8% of neurons and a modest gliosis.[91] Perhaps these differences reflect the relative severity of neuropathology affecting striatal and frontal cortex circuitry. Clearly, further study of thalamic neuropathology would help clarify its contribution to HD symptoms.

SUBTHALAMUS

The subthalamus is an extremely interesting nucleus with respect to HD. Subthalamic strokes have long been known to cause ballistic involuntary movements that are very similar to those of chorea. The subthalamus is also postulated to be excessively inhibited in HD, leading to alterations in pallidothalamic excitation, as previously outlined, which may be the basis for chorea. Furthermore, the subthalamus gives rise to one of the few excitatory pathways in the basal ganglia and thus may be relevant in excitotoxic cell death (see section on pathophysiology). Nevertheless, little has been added to knowledge of subthalamic pathology in HD since the morphometric study by Lange et al., who found that subthalamic volume and neuron number are reduced by about 25%.[7] Studies examining how neurotransmitters and receptors are altered in the subthalamus have not been performed, but may help elucidate its role in the pathogenesis of chorea.

HYPOTHALAMUS

Hypothalamic pathology has been postulated to be related to the cachexia and autonomic disturbance that occurs in HD patients. Bruyn noted significant neuronal loss and gliosis in the supraoptic nucleus and lateral hypothalamic nucleus.[81] In the only quantitative studies of hypothalamic pathology, Kremer and colleagues[92,93] found up to 90% neuronal loss in the lateral tuberal nucleus, which was worse in patients developing motor symptoms at an early age. The percentage of astrocytes did not change, whereas oligodendrocytes were reduced by 40%. It was further postulated that the high levels of glutamate receptors normally present in the lateral tuberal nucleus render these neurons selectively susceptible to excitotoxic cell death.[92] Although little is known about the normal function of the lateral tuberal nucleus, the possibility that its degeneration underlies the catabolic state that frequently occurs in HD patients is intriguing. Furthermore, because cell loss is so severe, this nucleus may have value in experimental investigations of cell death and neuroprotection in HD. In the lateral hypothalamus, losses of orexin containing neurons in human HD and transgenic mice have also been described.[94]

CEREBRAL CORTEX

Cerebral cortical atrophy and degeneration has long been recognized as occurring in HD.[95,96] Its extent, clinical significance, and relationship to striatal degeneration have emerged as important issues in understanding and treating HD. For example, the cortex is the most important source of glutamatergic projections to the striatum, which have been implicated in excitotoxic contributions to degeneration, and it is also the source of trophic factors, particularly brain-derived neurotrophic factor (BDNF), critical for maintaining striatal neurons and which huntingtin may play a direct role in regulating.[97] Although the relative roles of the cerebral cortex and basal ganglia in psychiatric, behavioral, and cognitive symptoms of HD are difficult to separate, there should be little doubt that cortical degeneration is at least involved in personality change, cognitive symptoms, voluntary motor dyscontrol, and spasticity. Because the entire cerebral cortex projects to the striatum and much of the frontal lobe receives the outflow of striatopallido–thalamocortical circuits,[98,99] cortical and basal ganglia pathology may be difficult to distinguish clinically. Advances in neuroimaging analytic methods in which clinical data can be mapped onto the involved cortical surfaces has recently made it possible to correlate regional cortical pathology and clinical features of the disease and substantiate the early and profound relationships between cortical involvement and the symptoms of HD.

Most preclinical studies related to developing potential medical or surgical therapies aimed at neuroprotection have focused on the striatum; however, should treatments preserve the striatum but not the cortex, many of the worst symptoms of the disease will still occur. The interrelationships between the cortex and striatum are complicated and may change depending upon the progression of HD. It is unclear whether preserving the striatum selectively can benefit the cortex; however, the cortex has both trophic and toxic influences on the striatum. At one extreme, experimental removal of the cortex is significantly protective of the underlying striatum in

HD mouse models.[100] Thus striatal degeneration likely occurs because of a mixture of the endogenous toxicity of the mutant huntingtin protein within striatal neurons as well as the exogenous stressors delivered by the cortex through the massive corticostriatal innervation. This two-hit model could help explain the particular vulnerability of the striatum.

Gross and Regional Neuropathology

Generalized cortical atrophy is readily apparent at autopsy (Fig. 34–2) and is a major component of the 15–30% loss in brain weight that occurs in HD.[101,102] Gross and regional cortical atrophy was first studied planimetrically by several investigators. Lange[101] reported an overall cortical shrinkage of 15% in 5 cases of HD, and noted that atrophy occurred the least in frontal regions and the most in occipital association areas (30%). De la Monte and colleagues[102] studied 30 HD brains and demonstrated a 20–30% overall reduction in the cross-sectional area of cerebral cortex, accompanied by a 29–34% reduction in subcortical white matter. Thinning of the cortical gray matter ranged from 9% to 16%, perhaps explaining why obvious cortical pathology is easily missed when individual sections are examined. The severity of atrophy occurring in the cortex, as well as in the striatum and thalamus, correlates with the clinical progression of the disease.[11,102] With increasing pathological grades of HD, brain weight declines, ventricular volume increases, cerebral atrophy increases, and the cortical ribbon thins. Depression and dementia correspond to the extent of both cortical and basal ganglia atrophy.

While cortical atrophy is widespread in advanced disease, it is becoming clear that some cortical areas undergo earlier and more pronounced atrophy than others. A recent post-mortem study demonstrated especially pronounced degenerative changes in medial postcentral cortex and occipital isocortex (areas 18 and 19); another volumetric study of seven late-stage cases found shrinkage of all cortical lobes, averaging 19%, with sparing of the medial temporal lobe.[103] Gray matter volume loss averaged 23% and white matter 13%. Interestingly, the CAG repeat number in these cases correlated with cortical atrophy divided by age of death but not with striatal atrophy, suggesting that cortical atrophy may be a better marker for disease progression than striatal atrophy, which likely loses linearity because it is so severe early in the disease.[104] Although neuroimaging research has also focused on the striatum,[19,105,106] new MRI analytical methods capable of detecting more subtle cortical changes suggest a mixture of areas predictably affected and areas more variably affected as well as a temporal pattern in which some areas are affected earlier and others later.[107] Thinning of the cortex has been found in pre-manifest carriers more than a decade prior to expected onset,[108] with progression occurring in a selective manner as disease advances (Fig. 34–11). Early changes occur in sensori-motor regions,[109] occipital isocortex (areas 18 and 19), the precuneus, prepyriform cortex, cingulate cortex,[101] superior temporal regions, dorsolateral prefrontal cortex (areas 8, 9, 10, and 46)[110–112] and perihippocampal cortex, including entorhinal and transentorhinal regions.[113,114] In pre-manifest HD, cortical thinning ranges between 5% and 15%; in early symptomatic HD several cortical regions thin by more than 20%. Cortical thinning appears to be both regionally and individually variable, suggesting not only that the cortex is affected early in the disease, but that regional selectivity may explain some of the variability in the clinical symptoms of HD.[115]

Significant changes in cortical white matter have also been reported. In postmortem studies of advanced HD, more than 30% of the volume of the white matter has been reported lost,[101] although microscopic abnormalities have not been reported using conventional methods.[116] Several imaging studies (Fig. 34–12) have now reported significant loss of white matter volume early, becoming more extensive with disease progression. Newer methods, including diffusion imaging, have suggested region-specific involvement of white matter, including specific disruptions of corticocortical[117] and corticostriatal,[118–120] connections that appear to echo the spatial distribution of cortical atrophy and that suggest that altered cortical connectivity may also play an important role in clinical symptoms.

Functional MRI and PET studies (Fig. 34–13) have demonstrated altered patterns of cerebral activation in gene carriers.[121,122] With PET, radioactive tracers are used to measure glucose metabolism or receptor density. Reductions of ^{18}F-fluorodeoxyglucose and in postsynaptic D_1 and D_2 receptor densities, as measured by radiolabeled ^{11}C-raclopride or ^{11}C-beta-CIT, respectively, have been reported in the striatum and in areas of cortex, and were found to correlate with duration of symptoms or with cognitive performance.[123] Similar alterations have been reported in individuals who were known genetic mutation carriers but who did not have motor symptoms and in whom there was no measurable change in striatal volumes,[124–126] suggesting that neuronal dysfunction occurs prior to measurable morphometric changes and may be used to identify transition to clinical symptoms. This is illustrated in Fig. 34–14, which utilizes a statistical modeling approach, the scaled subprofile model, and principal components analysis, to identify significant patterns of regional metabolic covariation in regional cerebral metabolic rates for glucose in presymptomatic as compared with healthy control groups.

Laminar and Cellular Neuropathology

The laminar pattern of cerebral cortical degeneration in HD has been studied qualitatively, with varying

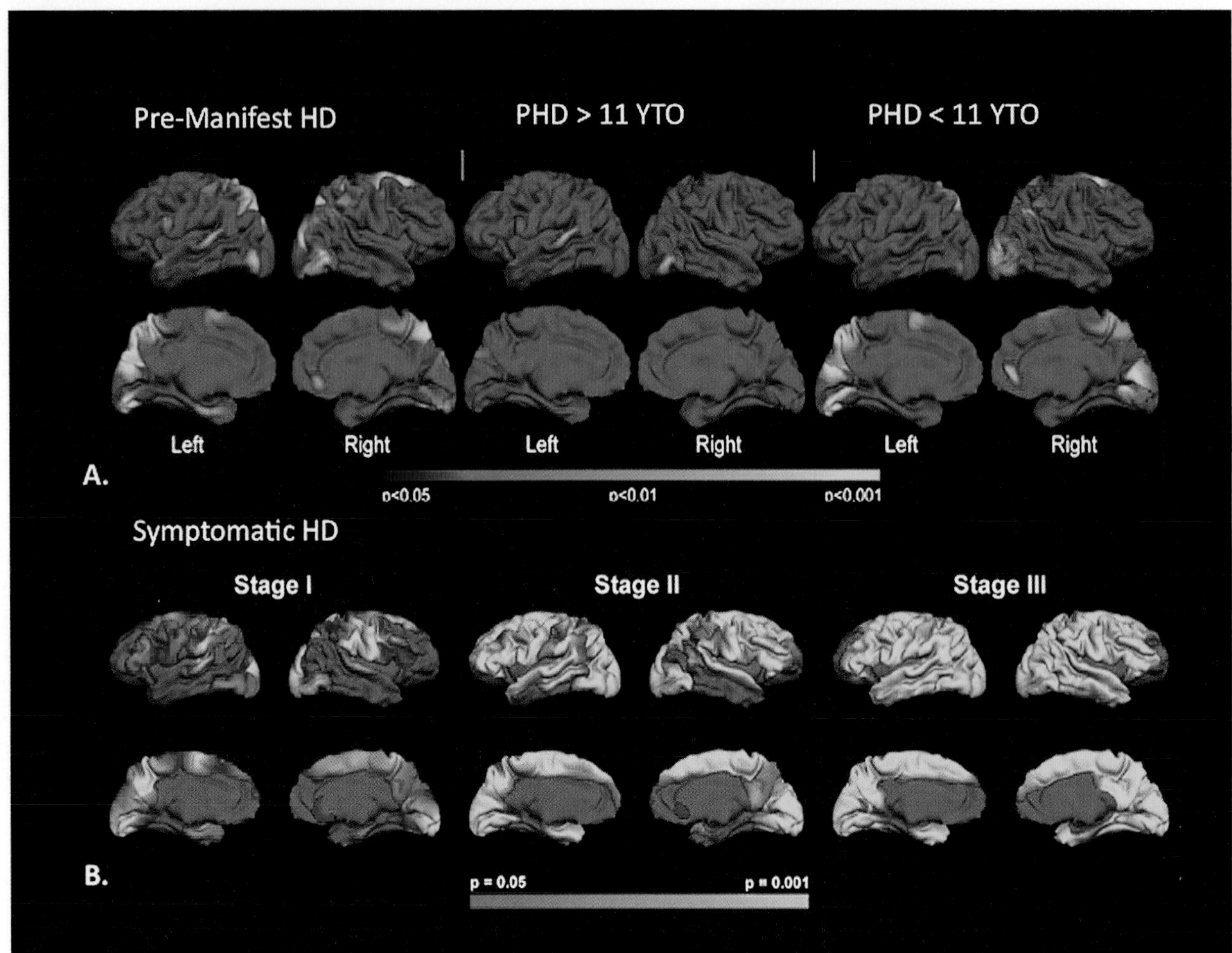

Figure 34–11. Cortical thinning in vivo determined by MRI in pre-manifest HD (PHD, *top panel*) and in symptomatic HD (*bottom panel*). Early cortical changes are present more than a decade prior to expected onset in gene carriers, involving primarily primary cortical areas. Cortical involvement progressively involves unimodal and higher association cortical regions, but remains regionally selective until later stages where diffuse cortical thinning is present.

results. McCaughey[127] described diffuse degeneration through layers III, V, and VI, with some patchy involvement of IV. In four pediatric cases,[128] cortical degeneration appeared pan-laminar. Forno and Jose[83] observed layer III to be the most severely affected in a series of adults. Roizin and colleagues[129] found that the middle layers of cortex were most affected in some cases, whereas the deeper layers were most affected in others. Bruyn and colleagues[6] later reported that layers III and V, and sometimes IV, had the most neuronal loss.

Quantitative studies have been performed more recently in a variety of brain regions, mostly in the frontal lobes.[108–111,130,131,133] The most consistent findings have been loss of volume and neurons in layers III, V, and VI. The concentration of neurons in these layers may not change,[109–111] however, indicating that cortical neuronal loss is proportional to cortical volume loss. Only one study has used unbiased counting methods, which permit estimating total numbers of neurons and glia.[131] The mean neuronal loss in the entire left cortical hemisphere was 33%, and was most pronounced in the supragranular layers. Interestingly, regional atrophy varied, with the primary sensory areas seemingly most affected, followed by prefrontal and premoter areas, while temporal association areas were only subtly affected. Astrocyte and oligodendrocyte concentrations, though not necessarily absolute numbers,[132] increase dramatically, especially in layers III–VI (Fig. 34–15). These increases likely indicate glial survival in a shrinking cortex and not reactive gliosis, because cortical glial fibrillary acidic protein staining does not increase.[132] The size of cortical neurons also declines in HD, suggesting selective loss or shrinkage of larger pyramidal cells (Fig. 34–10). Although there have been differing interpretations of these data, cortical cell loss is clearly not confined to neurons projecting to the striatum, which consist of a limited population of medium-sized

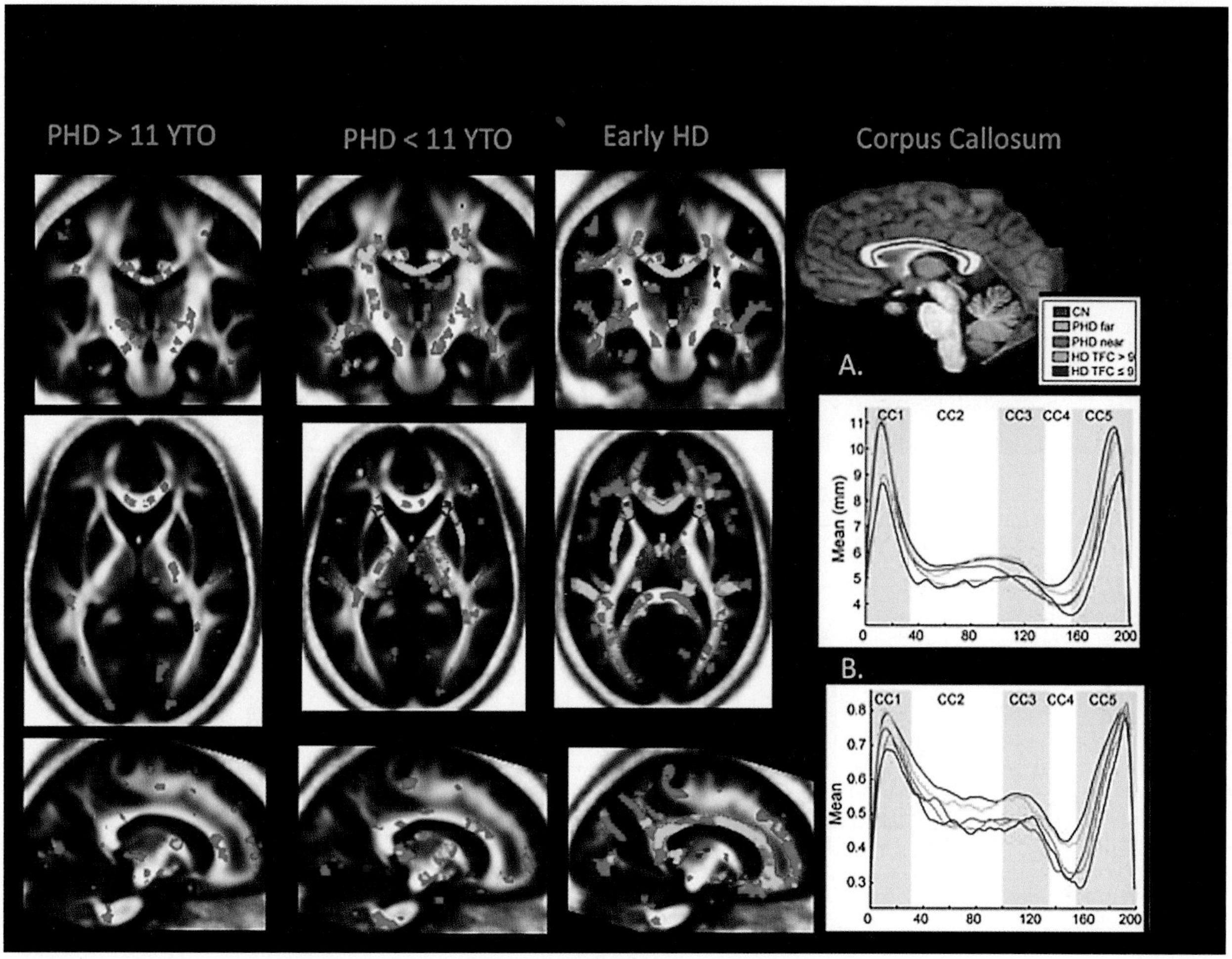

Figure 34–12. Diffusion weighted imaging (DWI) demonstrating early and progressive white matter and corpus callosum (CC) pathology in HD. *Left*: DWI reveals early white matter changes in presymptomatic gene carriers (PHD) more than 10 years prior to expected onset (YTO) which progresses as subjects become closer to onset and develop symptoms. White matter disease is regionally selective, with significant changes in the corpus callosum, posterior limb of the internal capsule, external capsule, and splenium. Right: The thickness of the CC is progressively reduced in presymptomatic and early symptomatic patients, especially inmore posterior regions (CC3–CC5).

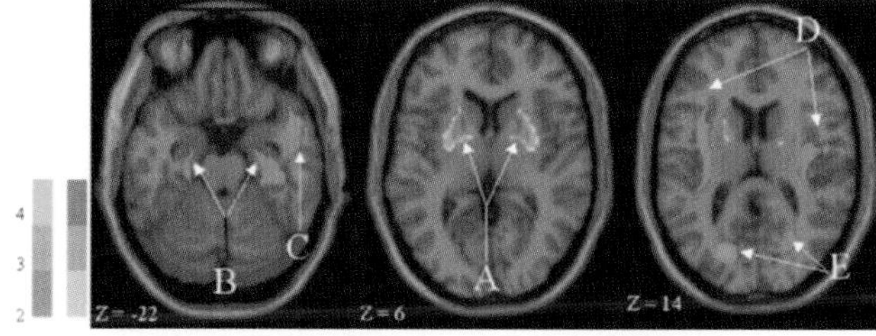

Figure 34–13. Voxel-based network analysis utilizing a principal component analysis applied to flourodeoxyglucose/PET scans from a group of 12 presymptomatic HD gene carriers and 11 age-matched controls. The first principal component discriminated the HD gene carriers from controls *($P < 0.005$)*, and was characterized by hypometabolism in bilateral striatum (**A**), covarying with hypermetabolism in bilateral hippocampi (**B**), right superior temporal gyrus (**C**), bilateral insula (**D**), and cuneus (**E**). (*Courtesy of Andy Feigin.*)

pyramidal cells located deep in layer III and superficially in layer V. Thus, retrograde degeneration of corticostriatal neurons cannot readily account for cortical atrophy. These studies also suggest that there is relative sparing of cortical interneurons, which typically are small neurons. Further evidence for this includes data indicating that substance P-expressing interneurons are spared,[133] and that cortical concentrations of GABA, somatostatin, neuropeptide Y, cholecystokinin, and vasoactive intestinal polypeptide, which are expressed by interneurons, are all elevated in HD.[134–136] Cerebral cortical pyramidal cells have also been shown, by means of Golgi staining, to develop increased numbers of dendrites and dendritic spines whereas others appear to have degenerative changes,[137] suggesting that proliferative and degenerative changes occur in these neurons before cell death.

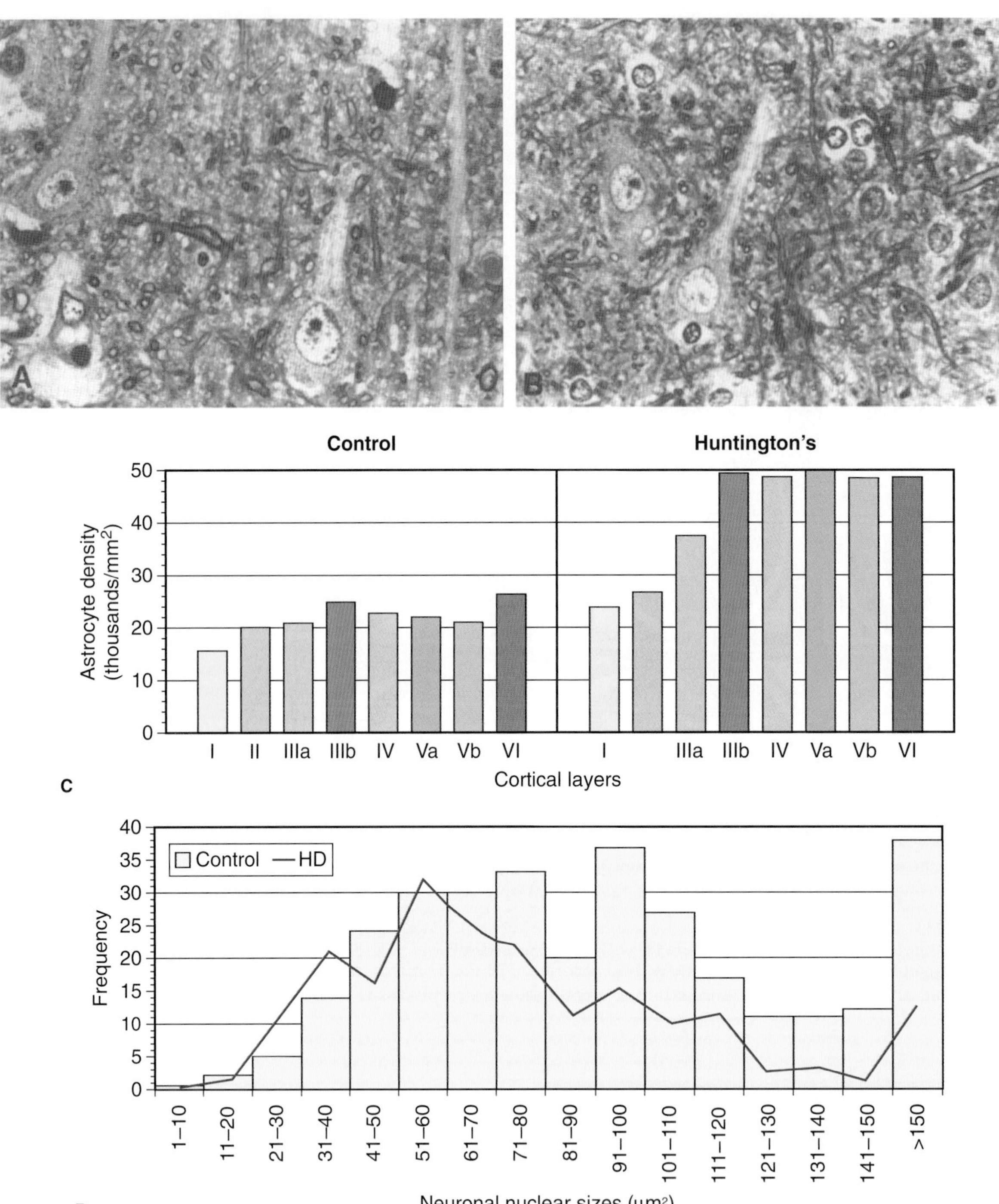

Figure 34–14. Toluidine blue-stained 2-μm sections from control (**A**) and HD (**B**) primary motor cortex. Normal-appearing pyramidal cells are visible in each. The HD case, however, contains many more astrocytes, as well as nuclear ghosts from degenerated neurons. Quantitative data (**C**) demonstrate that the density of astrocytes is more than doubled in layers III–VI. Measurement of nuclear diameters demonstrates that surviving neurons are smaller than control neurons and that the largest neurons seem to have disappeared.

Neurochemistry

Many neurochemical alterations in the cerebral cortex in HD have been identified. Two laboratories[26,138] found that glutamate, the putative neurotransmitter of pyramidal cells, and GABA, a marker for inhibitory cortical interneurons, are reduced in the cerebral cortex. In contrast, Storey and colleagues showed glutamate and aspartate to increase in most areas of cortex that they examined.[137] Unlike the striatum, *N*-methyl-D-aspartate (NMDA) receptor binding

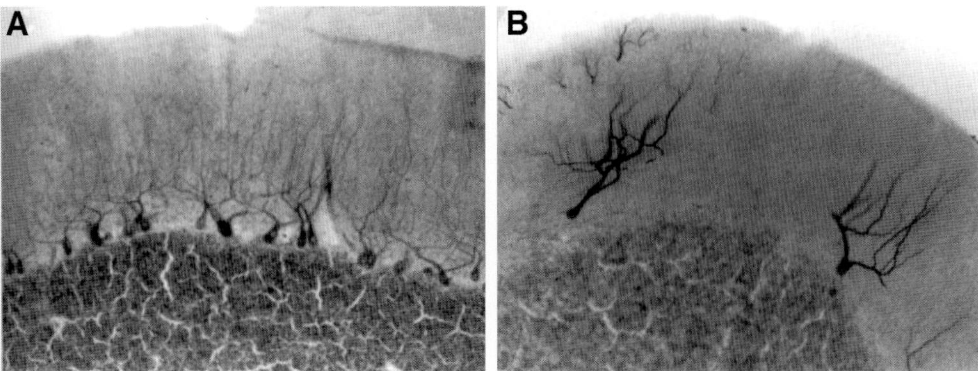

Figure 34–15. Immunocytochemistry in control (**A**) and HD cerebellum (**B**), using antihuntingtin antibodies. Purkinje cell drop-out is evident in the HD case (**B**), as is remodeling of the dendritic trees of those that survive.

is unchanged in cortex, whereas oc-amino-3-hydroxy-5-methyl-4-isoxazole propionic acid (AMPA) and kainate receptor binding is reduced in layer VI.[139] Hassel has shown that glutamate uptake may also be reduced in cortex, which can also affect glutamate levels, receptor levels, and excitotoxicity.[140] Such studies may offer evidence of selective vulnerability of distinct neuronal types; however, biochemical changes can be difficult to interpret without a detailed understanding of the underlying anatomic changes. For example, glutamate could be reduced from loss of neurons, loss of glutamatergic afferents, or alteration of glutamate transport, or metabolism in the absence of degenerative change. Understanding how the expression of glutamate receptors is altered in the cortex in HD may help explain altered cortical levels of glutamate. Whether cortical alterations in glutamate levels or glutamate receptors play a role in excitotoxic cell death in the cerebral cortex or in the striatum, via corticostriatal projections, is an unresolved question. Neurochemical markers of cortical interneurons have also been studied, including cholecystokinin, vasoactive intestinal peptide, neuropeptide Y, and somatostatin, which remain stable or increase, suggesting relative preservation of the interneurons expressing them.[141]

While there has long been an interest in alterations in neurotransmitter systems, there has also been a growing interest in other types of molecules that might reflect many other normal and pathologic cellular processes. BDNF mRNA and protein levels are reduced in HD cortex.[142] Proteins involved in synaptic vesicle release and recycling, SNAP 25 and rabphilin, are reduced selectively.[143] A range of mRNAs have been identified as selectively increased or decreased in the cortex in HD,[144] with severity corresponding regionally to cortical thinning maps.

CEREBELLUM AND BRAIN STEM

Reports of cerebellar involvement in HD have been variable, with cerebellar atrophy being reported in some pediatric and adult cases.[106,145–147] At a cellular level, Purkinje cell loss has been the primary consistent finding;[6] however, thinning of the granule cell layer has also been observed and has been taken to indicate loss of this cell type as well.[129] One quantitative study[148] examined Purkinje cell loss in 17 HD cases of unknown grade. More than one-half had a reduction in Purkinje cell density greater than 50%. With huntingtin immunocytochemistry, we have also noted severe loss of Purkinje cells in advanced grades of HD (Fig. 34–14). In addition, proliferative and degenerative changes are visible in Purkinje cells. Dentate cell loss and gliosis and involvement of cerebellar efferent and afferent pathways have also been noted.[6,148] The clinical significance of cerebellar atrophy is difficult to gauge, as involuntary movements and dystonia may obscure the cardinal signs of cerebellar dysfunction. Nevertheless, contributions to gait ataxia, postural instability, dysrhythmic voluntary movements, altered speech cadence, and disordered eye movements are all possible. Since cerebellar pathology does seem late, cerebellar tissue is often used as a less-affected brain tissue in studies using HD brain.

Brain stem alterations in HD have received almost no attention in the last two decades, so there is little to add to the review of Bruyn and colleagues[6] from 1979, in which severe degeneration of the superior and inferior olivary, lateral vestibular, dorsal vagal, and hypoglossal nuclei was noted. Additional significant regions of neuropathology from the earlier literature include the red nucleus, the basis pontis, and the spinal cord.[5,6,83,149]

▶ MOLECULAR PATHOLOGY AND PATHOPHYSIOLOGY

EXCITOTOXIC STRESS

The initial observations suggesting that excitotoxicity may play a role in HD were made by McGeers[63] and Coyle and Schwarcz.[150] Both sets of investigators showed that injections of the glutamate agonist kainic acid produced axon-sparing lesions of the striatum resembling HD. This model was refined by the use of selective NMDA agonists, such as quinolinic acid,[57,151,152] which cause medium spiny neurons to degenerate (astrogliosis) but are sparing of NADPH-diaphorase and cholinergic interneurons. Chronic lesions result in significantly increased striatal atrophy, more closely replicating the neuropathology of HD.[153,154] Furthermore, in monkeys, quinolinic acid excitotoxic lesions lead to hyperkinesis and dopamine agonist-induced chorea.[114,137] The close match of these models with HD neuropathology strongly suggested an excitotoxic mechanism of cell death. Selective depletion of NMDA receptors in the putamen in HD suggested that neurons expressing this glutamate receptor are selectively vulnerable.[155] However, alterations in other types of glutamate receptors also occur.[156,157] Because increased glutamate levels, abnormal functioning of glutamate receptors, or the significant presence of endogenous excitotoxins have not been demonstrated in the striatum in HD, a basis for why excitotoxicity should occur has been elusive. Studies using transgenic mouse models of HD have identified increased NMDA receptor sensitivity,[158,159] possible alterations in glutamate transporter function,[160] and altered corticostriatal physiology as possible mechanisms.[161] Neurons weakened by the toxic effects of mutant huntingtin may simply be unable to tolerate the stress of normal synaptic activity.

It is well established that striatal excitotoxic lesions depend on corticostriatal glutamatergic inputs. There is also a substantial evidence indicating that striatal excitotoxic lesions are dependent on dopaminergic inputs from the substantia nigra.[162–165] Nigrostriatal dopaminergic neurotransmission is altered in HD, based on early and dramatic changes in related receptors, and may contribute to striatal vulnerability in HD. More directly, released dopamine can be a stressor to striatal neurons through oxidative mechanisms, as well as by presynaptic modulation of glutamate release.[166] It is very plausible that both cortical and nigral afferents contribute to the enhanced vulnerability of the striatum that is observed in HD. Importantly, glutamate antagonists have been neuroprotective in transgenic mouse models of HD, providing preclinical validation for excitotoxicity as a therapeutic target.[167–169] The evidence for excitotoxicity contributing to the pathogenesis of HD remains compelling enough to justify medication trials in human HD,[170] despite the recent failure of the NMDA receptor antagonist remacemide to be neuroprotective in one such trial.[171]

ENERGY DEPLETION AND OXIDATIVE STRESS

An hypothesis explaining the pattern of degeneration in HD has evolved that suggests that impaired energy metabolism may be involved in the degenerative process.[172–175] Several studies have suggested that altered energy metabolism occurs in HD. Cytochrome oxidase (complex IV) activity is reduced in striatum;[176] complex I activity is reduced in platelets[177] and muscle;[178] and complex II/III activity is reduced in the caudate nucleus and putamen.[156,179] Levels of oxidative damage to DNA, proteins, and lipids are also increased in the HD striatum.[156,180] Increased lactate, a marker for metabolic stress, has been demonstrated in HD cortex and striatum in vivo by means of MRS.[181] These studies in HD suggest that metabolic dysfunction does occur, but it has been difficult to discern whether it is a secondary marker of degeneration or related to the pathophysiology of neuronal death. New studies in lymphoblasts from HD patients suggest that early mitochondrial dysfunction due to the presence of mutant huntingtin precedes degeneration.[182,183] Experimentally, energy (adenosine triphosphatase) depletion, which has recently been demonstrated to occur in a presymptomatic knock-in mouse model of HD,[184] can produce partial membrane depolarization and removal of the voltage-dependent magnesium block of the NMDA-linked calcium channel.[185] The open calcium channel could then permit normal amounts of glutamate to produce a heightened NMDA receptor response, which, in turn, could cause excitotoxic cell death. Animal studies show that striatal injection of mitochondrial toxins, such as the succinic dehydrogenase inhibitors 3-nitropropionic acid (3-NP) and malonic acid, produces selective neuronal loss identical to that produced by NMDA agonists and identical to the neuropathological pattern in HD, as well as analogous motor symptoms (Fig. 34–16)[186–188] Importantly, mitochondrial toxin-induced striatal pathology is dramatically reduced by NMDA receptor blockade, as well as by antioxidants and free radical scavengers.[189,190] This further strengthens the hypothesis of a metabolic defect underlying selective excitotoxicity,[191] and provides a rationale for treating HD with protectants against oxygen free-radical activity, such as OPC-14117 and coenzyme Q_{10},[192] as well as energy buffers such as creatine.[193,194]

The generation of reactive oxygen species is a normal by-product of cellular respiration, mediated by mitochondria. Accumulation of reactive oxygen species in neurons and subsequent oxidative stress are normally blocked by endogenous free radical scavengers, such as glutathione and superoxide dismutase, preventing molecular damage. In HD, the generation of reactive oxygen species and the resulting oxidative stress may play a central role in neurodegeneration. Multiple lines of evidence implicate oxidative stress in the etiology of neuronal death in HD.[195] Studies of the postmortem human HD brain show increased levels of oxidative damage. These include increased cytoplasmic lipofuscin, DNA strand breaks, and the accumulation of oxidative markers in DNA bases, along with other cellular macromolecules

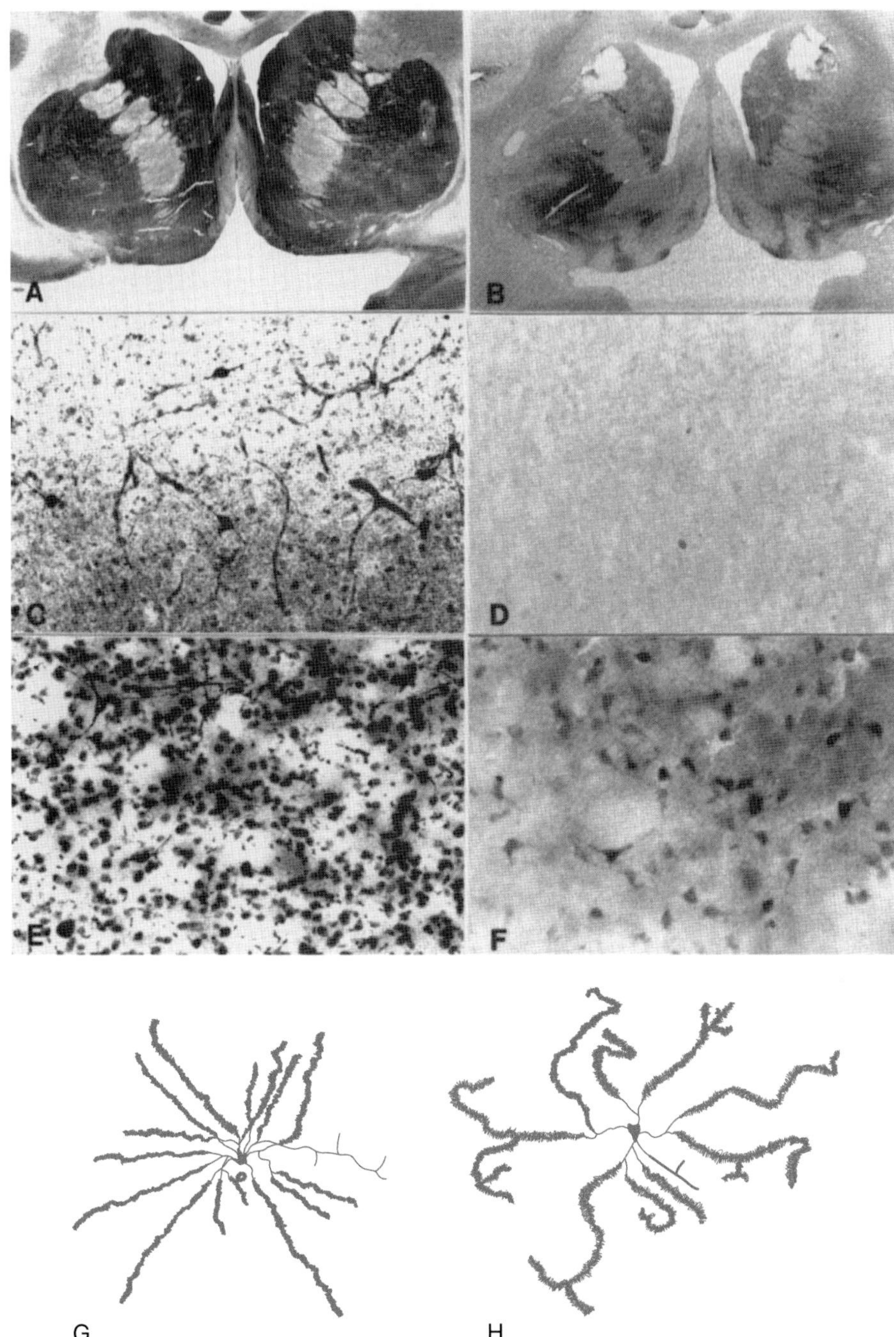

Figure 34–16. Histopathological alterations observed in a 3-NP-treated primate. Gross lesions are found in the dorsal aspect of the caudate nucleus and putamen in Nissl- and calbindin-stained sections through the striatum (**A** and **B**, respectively). There is a dorsoventral gradient of neuronal loss, with the dorsal striatum more severely involved. Only aspiny NADPH-diaphorase neurons persist in the dorsal striatum (**C**), with few spiny calbindin neurons (**D**). All neuronal populations are better preserved in the ventral striatum (**E** and **F**). Similar dysmorphic alterations, as observed in HD, are found in treated animals (**H**) in comparison to controls (**G**) (From Brouillet et al.,[188] used with permission.)

associated with protein nitration and lipid oxidative damage.[181] Lipofuscin is an intracellular deposit associated with cellular aging and is the product of unsaturated fatty acid peroxidation. Lipofuscin increases at a greater rate under oxidative stress. The abnormal accumulation of lipofuscin has long been reported in HD brain. A marked increase in lipofuscin within both cortical and striatal neurons occurs in patients with HD, with little or no presence of lipofuscin in spared NADPH diaphorase neurons in the caudate nucleus.[196]

DNA damage results from excess free radicals in HD leading to epigenetic responses, induction of DNA repair pathways, mutagenesis, and DNA fragmentation as neurons die. DNA fragmentation is increased in HD patients and correlates with CAG repeat length. There are significant increases in DNA fragmentation in human HD striatal and cortical neurons compared with levels of DNA fragmentation in age-matched control brains.[197,198] Mitochondrial DNA may be even more susceptible than nuclear DNA to fragmentation. The oxidation of either nuclear or mitochondrial DNA results in the formation of a variety of nucleotide adducts that induce DNA repair, which may not always successful. Base excision repair releases oxidized nucleotides, such as the stable metabolite 8-hydroxy-2-deoxyguanosine (8OH2dG). Striking increases in 8OH2dG levels in nuclear DNA occur in the caudate nucleus in postmortem tissue from HD patients as well as in mitochondrial DNA from the parietal cortex.[199] In addition, 8OH2dG levels are markedly elevated in CSF, plasma, and urine (its route of elimination) providing a peripheral biomarker of CNS oxidative damage and neurodegeneration.[200] The DNA repair that occurs following guanine oxidation has also been associated with the somatic expansion of the CAG repeat that occurs in HD brain and may play a role in accelerating pathogenesis.[201]

Many additional markers of oxidative damage, including heme oxygenase (an inducible isoform that occurs in response to oxidative stress), 3-nitrotyrosine (a marker for peroxynitrite-mediated protein nitration), and malondialdehyde (a marker for oxidative damage to lipids), are elevated in human HD striatum and cortex compared with age-matched control brain specimens. The extent and intensity of these markers mirror the dorsoventral pattern of progressive neuronal loss in the neostriatum, with increased immunoreactive expression in the dorsal striatum compared with the less severely affected ventral striatum.[181,200] Similarly, colorimetric assays demonstrate significant increases in malondialdehyde and 4-hydroxynonenal brain levels, almost eightfold greater than in control subjects.[202]

^{1}H-MRS has been a tool for the measurement of brain metabolites and has been particularly useful in the determination of key substrates in oxidative and intermediary metabolism. Increased concentrations of lactate (Fig. 34–17), a marker of energetic defects, and choline, a glial marker, which may represent neuronal membrane breakdown and liberation of glycerylphosphocholine, have been reported in the striatum, and occipital and frontal regions.[203] Decreased levels of *N*-acetyl aspartate (NAA, a neuronal marker) have been reported in the striatum, most likely reflecting neuronal loss, or which may reflect impaired mitochondrial energy production as inhibitors of the mitochondrial respiratory chain have been shown to result in lower NAA concentrations.

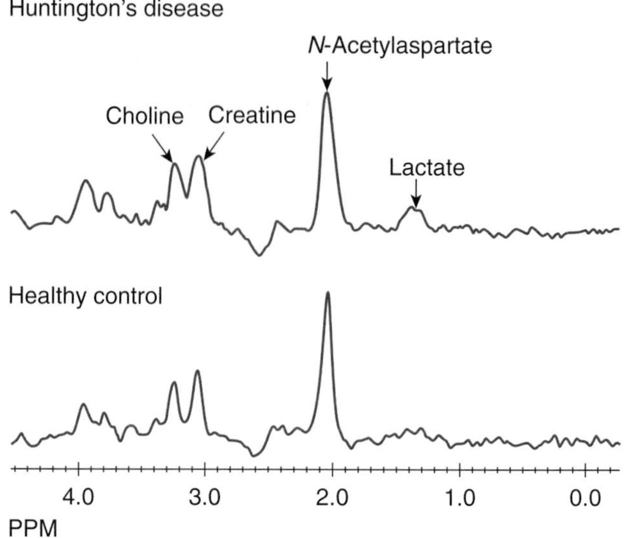

Figure 34–17. ^{1}H-MRS spectra of supplementary motor cortex, comparing an individual with HD (*top*) and a control subject (*bottom*). Lactate is elevated in the HD subject compared with the healthy control, suggesting an energetic defect.

Increases in glutamine have been postulated in humans and reported in transgenic mouse models of HD; however, it is impossible to separate glutamate from glutamine using 1.5-T field strengths, but this could likely be done using higher field strengths. ^{31}P studies of skeletal muscle have shown reduced phosphocreatine/inorganic phosphate ratios in symptomatic HD, suggesting a role for a more global mitochondrial dysfunction in HD.[204] ^{13}C studies have been performed in transgenic mouse models, with potential to provide important information on the specific nature of the metabolic defect in humans with HD.

Proapoptotic signaling cascades initiated by mHtt and linked to mitochondrial stresses may play a role in mHtt-induced striatal neurodegeneration. In apoptotic-induced cell death, signaling cascades activate multiple proteases that destroy proteins essential for neuronal survival, along with a concurrent activation of genes involved in cell suicide.[205] The primary constituents of the apoptotic cascade are the cysteine proteases known as caspases. There are at least four initiator caspases, and at least three effector caspases, including caspases -3, -6, and -7. Expanded polyglutamine stretches have been shown to sequentially activate the initiator caspases. There is increasing evidence implicating apoptosis-mediated cell death in the pathogenesis of neurodegenerative diseases.[206] One important event in the apoptotic cascade is the release of cytochrome *c* by mitochondria into the cytoplasm, activating caspase-9 and leading to the subsequent activation of downstream executioner caspases.

NORMAL AND MUTANT HUNTINGTIN PROTEINS AND PATHOGENESIS

Huntingtin and RNA

Huntingtin mRNA is normally distributed in diverse tissues in humans and rats and is expressed predominantly in neurons within the brain.[207–209] All neurons appear to express huntingtin mRNA, and there is no apparent correlation within particular types of neurons between levels of mRNA and their vulnerability to cell death. Because mRNA for both the normal and mutant alleles is produced by individuals with HD, and because known "knockout" mutations affecting one HD allele do not cause the HD phenotype,[210–212] simple gene inactivation is unlikely to underlie disease pathogenesis. Because mRNA for the mutant allele is expressed in HD brain in amounts similar to that of the normal allele,[213] an alteration in transcription is also unlikely to be pathogenic. The remaining possibilities are that the genetic mutation affects ribosomal translation, or that it acts at the protein level to alter the normal function of huntingtin. RNA-binding proteins, which are tissue-specific and have been demonstrated to interact with the huntingtin CAG repeat,[214] could affect translation and also the intracellular localization of huntingtin mRNA. Nevertheless, inactivation of one allele does not cause HD, and so it would be difficult for a translational block to account in large part for disease pathogenesis. MicroRNAs, however, can be affected by mutant huntingtin or its downstream effects and selectively affect post-transcription processes.[215,216]

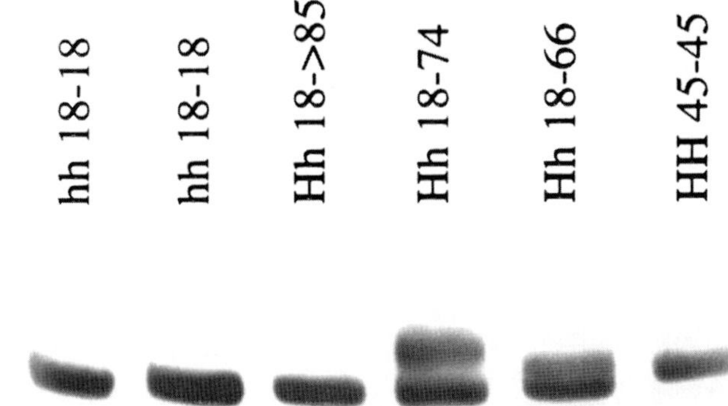

Figure 34–18. Western blot, using monoclonal antihuntingtin antibodies of lymphoblast lysates from control (hh) patients, heterozygote HD patients (Hh), and a homozygote HD patient (HH). The numbers correspond to the number of CAG repeats contained in each huntingtin allele. A single band is detected in control and homozygote cases because the alleles have identical numbers of repeats; however, the homozygote is at a higher molecular weight. Two bands are visible in each of the heterozygote cases, corresponding to the differing molecular weights of normal and mutant huntingtin. This immunoblot demonstrates that both normal and mutant forms of huntingtin are expressed in tissue from HD patients. (From Gutekunst et al.[218] Used with permission.)

Huntingtin Protein

The normal functions of huntingtin remain uncertain. Current hypotheses have been based on its subcellular localization and on its interactions with large numbers of known proteins. Subcellular fractionation reveals that huntingtin is found primarily in soluble fractions, and its relative levels in various tissues and brain areas correspond to the levels of its mRNA.[217] Both normal and mutant proteins are expressed in cell lines and tissues from HD patients (Fig. 34–18). Immunocytochemistry[218–221] (Fig. 34–19) indicates that huntingtin is located in neurons throughout the brain, with high levels evident in cortical pyramidal cells, cerebellar Purkinje cells, and large striatal interneurons, among others. Striatal medium spiny neurons are also well labeled, whereas medium-sized neurons in other brain regions may be quite variable. There are significant levels of huntingtin in the striatum, with heterogeneous expression evident both in medium spiny neurons and in interneurons such that more vulnerable neuronal populations appear to have relatively higher levels of huntingtin protein.[222] Subcellular localization of huntingtin is consistent with a primarily cytosolic protein found most abundantly in somatodendritic regions, but with some presence in axons as well as in the nucleus (Fig. 34–20). Huntingtin appears to associate particularly with dendritic microtubules and membrane-bound organelles, including mitochondria, transport vesicles, synaptic vesicles, and components of the endocytic system.[222–224] These localization studies have suggested a possible role for huntingtin in the transport, homeostasis, or function of organelles, with mitochondrial, synaptic, and endosomal–lysosomal systems all being of particular importance. Dysfunction in these pathways could conceivably impair their cytoskeletal anchoring, transport, function, or turnover. Interactions at the protein level between huntingtin and many proteins associated with these organelles and with intracellular transport have suggested a scaffolding function in which huntingtin plays a role in complex protein–protein/organelle interactions. The availability of mutant huntingtin at these functional sites, however, is not well understood, and it is possible that mutant huntingtin is significantly redistributed, for example to insoluble aggregates and to the nucleus. Although normal huntingtin is not abundant in the nucleus, normal and mutant huntingtin so avidly interact with so many proteins involved in transcription that it could play a normal role in transcriptional regulation.

Like most proteins, huntingtin undergoes a number of post-translational modifications that modulate its interactions, intracellular locations, and metabolism, including ubiquitination,[225] palmitoylation,[226] acetylation,[227]

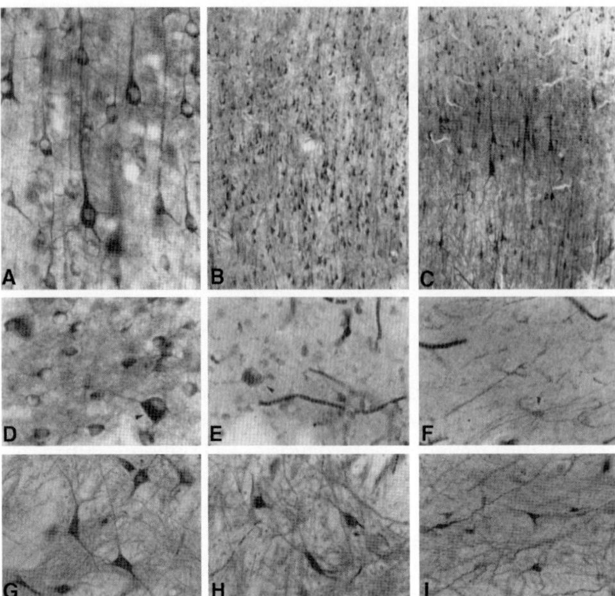

Figure 34–19 FCImmunocytochemistry using monoclonal antihuntingtin antibodies in sections from monkeys (first column), from human controls (middle column), and from human HD cases (last column). The first row is from frontal cortex (**A–C**), the second row is from caudate nucleus (**D–F**), and the third row is from globus pallidus (**G–I**). As a result of optimal fixation, the monkey tissue is better stained and permits better resolution of cellular detail. In each region, neurons are well stained, glia are unstained, nuclei are not labeled, and most label is somatodendritic, with some additional staining of axons and more diffuse staining of the neuropil. In cerebral cortex (**A–C**), pyramidal cells are most prominently stained. In normal monkey (**D**) and human (**E**) caudate nucleus, medium-sized neurons and large interneurons (*arrows*) are visible. In HD (**F**), only one neuron (*arrow*) is visible, which appears to be an aspiny interneuron. GPe and GPi neurons are also well stained in monkey (**G**) and human (**H**), although they appear shrunken in HD (**I**). (Several of these micrographs were from Gutekunst et al.,[218] used with permission.)

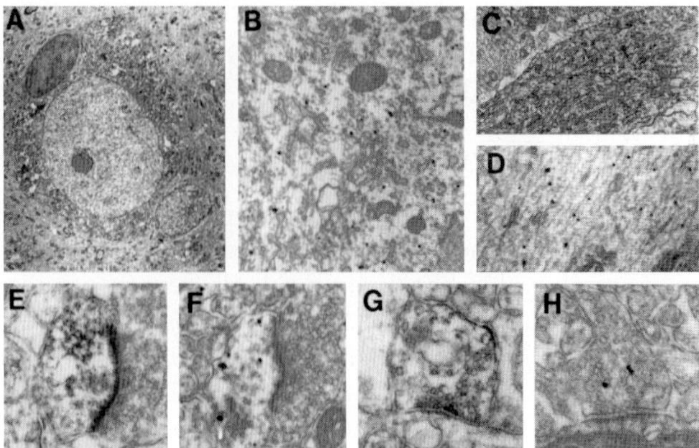

Figure 34–20 Electron microscopic immunocytochemistry of huntingtin in monkeys, using the diffusible reaction product diaminobenzidine (DAB) (**A**,**C**,**E**,**G**) and immunogold (**B**,**D**,**F**,**H**), which permits much higher spatial resolution. DAB reaction product is visible in the perikaryon of a cortical pyramidal cell (*center*), but not in an adjacent astrocyte (*bottom right*) or oligodendrocyte (*top left*). All nuclei are unlabeled. At a higher magnification, immunogold particles are primarily free in the cytoplasm and are not associated with endoplasmic reticulum or Golgi apparatus, suggesting that the protein is synthesized by free ribosomes. A Purkinje cell dendrite (**C**), in longitudinal section, is filled with reaction product, which coats all its organelles but appears to associate particularly with its microtubules. Immunogold labeling of another Purkinje cell dendrite (**D**) shows many immunogold particles contacting microtubules. A DAB-labeled dendritic spine (**E**) from the putamen is diffusely filled with reaction product, which also appears to label the postsynaptic density; however, with immunogold labeling (**F**), neither plasma membrane nor postsynaptic density labeling is seen. Axon terminals from the cerebellum (**G**) and cerebral cortex (**H**) are also shown. DAB coats the membrane, synaptic vesicles, and presynaptic density. In contrast, immunogold particles appear to associate primarily with synaptic vesicles but not with the presynaptic density or membrane. (Several of these micrographs were reproduced from Gutekunst et al.[218] and were used with permission.)

sumoylation,[228] and phosphorylation.[229–232] These modifications can promote or diminish huntingtin's toxicity by regulating its location to pathologic locations or by modulating its turnover. These modifications may also be promising upstream therapeutic targets.

While a toxic gain of function due to mutant huntingtin has been considered to be a means through which the HD genetic mutation causes neurotoxicity, there is also increasing evidence that a loss of the normal functions of huntingtin may also play roles in the pathogenesis of HD. Wild-type huntingtin is itself protective,[233–235] and its reduction might reduce levels of needed neurotrophic factors, such as brain-derived neurotrophic factor (BDNF),[91] or compromise some of its normal functions. There is substantial evidence that the loss of BDNF might contribute to degeneration and that this may be a consequence of transcriptional suppression. There is a reported loss of huntingtin-mediated BDNF gene transcription in HD. In addition, the reduction in cortical BDNF messenger correlates with the progression of the disease in R6/2 mice, whereas the function BDNF may play in disease onset in human HD is less clear.

Mutant Huntingtin Aggregation and HD Pathogenesis

The mutation that causes HD is a polyglutamine expansion that changes the amino acid sequence of huntingtin and causes a conformational change, as shown by the ability of antibodies to completely discriminate the normal and mutated forms.[236,237] It had been hypothesized that long polyglutamine stretches self-associate, either internally by forming hairpin loops or with other polyglutamine-containing molecules,[238] and thereby engage in aberrant molecular interactions. Mutant huntingtin also undergoes proteolytic processing, releasing persistent *N*-terminal fragments containing the polyglutamine tract, which may be more toxic than the holoprotein. These fragments form macromolecular aggregates with themselves and with other proteins, which become ubiquitinated (targeting them for proteasomal degradation), insoluble, and large enough to be visible in the processes, cytoplasm, and nuclei of neurons.[1] Huntingtin aggregates are readily detected in histologic sections by antibodies against polyglutamines, *N*-terminal huntingtin epitopes, or ubiquitin. They have not been observed to persist in the extracellular space after the degeneration of the neurons containing them. They can be found all over the brain and are especially frequent in cortical regions and relatively infrequent in the striatum (Fig. 34–21).[226,239] This has alternately been interpreted as a reflection of neurons having different capacities to metabolize huntingtin, different vulnerabilities such that more vulnerable neurons die before aggregates are more appreciable, or aggregation being neuroprotective. In human HD brain, the great majority of huntingtin aggregates are in dendrites, dendritic spines, and axons with a small proportion in neuronal somata and nuclei (Fig. 34–22).[226] Few are identifiable in glia. Many of the proteins that interact with huntingtin can also be found sequestered in the aggregates, and this sequestration is a potential means of diminishing functional levels of needed proteins.

Aggregation of the *N*-terminus fragments of huntingtin is CAG length-dependent, occurring once the polyglutamine tract is about 39 amino acids long and increasing with greater lengths.[239–241] Thus, it has been hypothesized that aggregation may be the trigger for a toxic gain of function leading to neurodegeneration. Since similar inclusions have been seen in other triple repeat disorders, including dentatorubropallidoluysian atrophy,[242] spinocerebellar ataxia (SCA) types SCA1,[243] SCA3,[244] and SCA7,[245] and spinal and bulbar muscular atrophy,[246] protein aggregates have been proposed to be the common cause of neurodegeneration.[247,248] Many studies, however, have cast doubt on whether insoluble aggregates directly cause neurodegeneration. Huntingtin aggregates are relatively infrequent in the striatum in cases of HD compared with other brain regions.[2] Striatal interneurons resistant to neurodegeneration are far more likely to have huntingtin aggregates than the vulnerable medium spiny neurons.[249] It has been relatively difficult to show neuronal death in the R6/2 transgenic mouse model of HD in which huntingtin aggregates appear early and are extraordinarily large and frequent.[250] In a transgenic model utilizing a polyglutamine expansion to

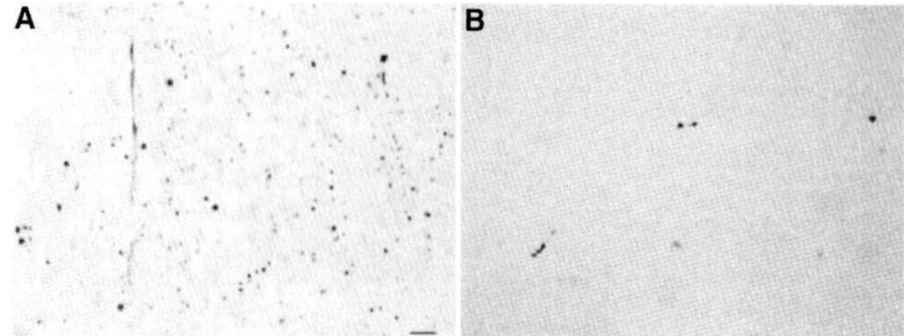

Figure 34–21 Huntingtin immunocytochemistry in the cerebral cortex and striatum of a presymptomatic individual using an antibody selective for aggregated mutant protein (EM48). There are many more huntingtin aggregates in the cortex (**A**) than in the striatum (**B**). Most aggregates are in neuronal processes, which they appear to loosely fill before condensing into more punctate forms.

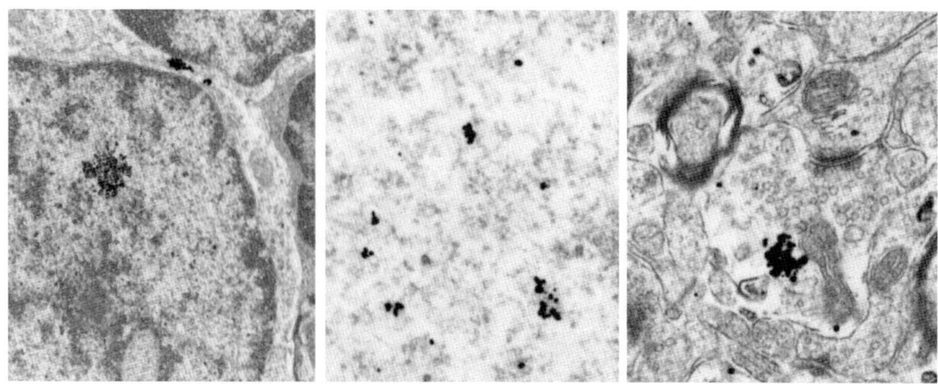

Figure 34–22 Electron micrographs of huntingtin aggregates in HD transgenic mice labeled with EM48 immunogold. *Left:* nuclear and cytoplasmic aggregates in a cerebellar granule cell. *Center:* microaggregates in the nucleus of striatal neuron that might still represent soluble intermediates. *Right:* a neuropil aggregate in an axon terminal.

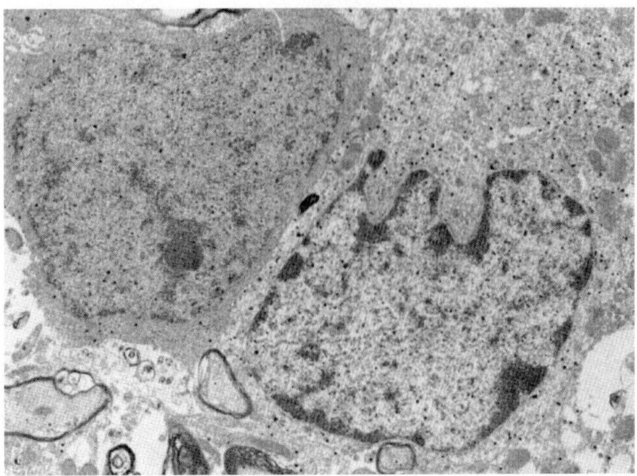

Figure 34–23 Electron micrograph of degenerating striatal neurons from a transgenic mouse model of HD containing nuclear and cytoplasmic microaggregates labeled by EM48 immunogold.

cause an unrelated cytoplasmic protein to translocate to the nucleus and aggregate, there was no evidence for neuronal death.[251] A variety of in vitro studies have dissociated the presence of huntingtin aggregates from cell death.[252–254] In transgenic models of SCA1, nuclear but not aggregated ataxin-1 is responsible for the neurodegenerative phenotype.[255] Thus, it is likely that macroscopic huntingtin aggregates represent a relatively benign cellular sequestration of a protein fragment that cannot be readily broken down and might even be protective.[256–258] Aggregation of huntingtin *N*-terminal fragments, however, has not yet been ruled out as a contributor to cell death.[259] One possibility is that there are soluble aggregated intermediates (microaggregates) (Fig. 34–23) that are toxic but which do not correlate with the presence of macroscopic insoluble aggregates.[260,261] However, it is far more likely that aggregation is not the only new property of huntingtin triggered at the CAG length transition.

Protein–Protein Interactions of Mutant Huntingtin and Pathogenesis

It is widely assumed that the toxic effects of mutant huntingtin are exerted through abnormal interactions that it has with proteins that it normally relates to or with proteins that unexpectedly relate to it as a result of its altered conformation or mislocation. A large number of proteins that huntingtin normally interacts with have been identified.[262] A number of these can be related to intracellular transport of organelles, including huntingtin-associated protein 1,[263–266] a protein analogous to the yeast cytoskeleton-associated protein Sla2p (huntingtin-interacting protein 1, or HIP1),[267–269] and HIP14, a protein related to endocytosis and endosome transport.[270] Other interacting proteins, such as glyceraldehyde phosphate dehydrogenase,[271] an unidentified calmodulin-associated protein,[272] and CIP4,[273] play roles in signal transduction and metabolism.

An extensive and important group of huntingtin interactions are with proteins related to gene transcription.[274–280] There is growing evidence of early transcriptional dysfunction in cellular and animal models of HD,[281] and reversing this has become a major therapeutic focus. Associated with the transcription dysregulation in HD are epigenetic changes that could contribute further to transcriptional dysfunction and pathogenesis. Histone modifications, leading to chromatin remodeling, impact transcription through altered nucleosome dynamics.[282] Changes in histone methylation, acetylation, and ubiquitylation favoring transcriptional repression have all been identified in HD models or HD brain or blood, which regulate transcription factor access to promoter regions in DNA[283,284] Huntingtin itself has also been found to bind to DNA, directly,[285] perhaps providing another direct means of complicating transcription.

Additional interactions are with processive or proteolytic enzymes, such as an ubiquitin-conjugating enzyme,[286] transglutaminases that can crosslink glutamine residues,[287] caspases,[288–290] and calpains,[291,292] which have been implicated in the production of toxic fragments of mutant huntingtin,[293] all of which are also being considered as therapeutic targets. Additionally, polyglutamines may impair proteasome function and their own proteolysis,[294,295] further perturbing cellular homeostasis. Some of the huntingtin protein–protein interactions vary with the length of the huntingtin polyglutamine tract and are thus stronger candidates for being affected by the HD genetic mutation. Huntingtin therefore has many possible molecular interactions, the disruption of which might be relevant to neurodegeneration.

REFERENCES

1. DiFiglia M, Sapp E, Chase KO, et al. Aggregation of huntingtin in neuronal intranuclear inclusions and dystrophic neurites in brain. Science 1997;277:1990–1993.
2. Gutekunst CA, Li SH, Yi H, et al. Nuclear and neuropil aggregates in Huntington's disease: Relationship to neuropathology. J Neurosci 1999;19:2522–2534.
3. Sapp E, Kegel KB, Aronin N, et al. Early and progressive accumulation of reactive microglia in the Huntington disease brain. J Neuropathol Exp Neurol 2001;60:161–172.
4. Singhrao SK, Neal JW, Morgan BP, et al. Increased complement biosynthesis by microglia and complement activation on neurons in Huntington's disease. Exp Neurol 1999;159:362–376.
5. Bruyn GW. Huntington's chorea. Historical, clinical and laboratory synopsis. In Vinken PJ and Bruyn GW (eds). Handbook of Clinical Neurology, Vol. 6. Amsterdam: Elsevier, 1968, pp. 298–378.

6. Bruyn G, Bots G, and Dom R. Huntington's chorea: Current neuropathological status. Adv Neurol 1979;23: 83–93.
7. Lange H, Thorner G, Hopf A, et al. Morphometric studies of the neuropathological changes in choreatic diseases. J Neurol Sci 1976;28:401–425.
8. Tai YF, Pavese N, Gerhard A, et al. Microglial activation in presymptomatic Huntington's disease gene carriers. Brain 2007;130(pt 7):1759–1766.
9. Pavese N, Gerhard A, Tai YF, et al. Microglial activation correlates with severity in Huntington disease: A clinical and PET study. Neurology 2006;66(11):1638–1643.
10. Myers RH, Vonsattel JP, Paskevich PA, et al. Decreased neuronal and increased oligodendroglial densities in Huntington's disease caudate nucleus. J Neuropathol Exp Neurol 1991;50:729–742.
11. Vonsattel JP, Myers RH, Stevens TJ, et al. Neuropathological classification of Huntington's disease. J Neuropathol Exp Neurol 1985;44:559–577.
12. Roos RA, Pruyt JF, de Vries J, et al. Neuronal distribution in the putamen in Huntington's disease. J Neurol Neurosurg Psychiatry 1985;48:422–425.
13. Gomez-Tortosa E, MacDonald ME, Friend JC, et al. Quantitative neuropathological changes in presymptomatic Huntington's disease. Ann Neurol 2001;49:29–34.
14. Aylward EH, Codori AM, Rosenblatt A, et al. Rate of caudate atrophy in presymptomatic and symptomatic stages of Huntington's disease. Mov Disord 2000;15:552–560.
15. Aylward EH, Codori AM, Barta PE, et al. Basal ganglia volume and proximity to onset in presymptomatic Huntington disease. Arch Neurol 1996;53:1293–1296.
16. Thieben MJ, Duggins AJ, Good CD, et al. The distribution of structural neuropathology in pre-clinical Huntington's disease. Brain 2002;125(pt 8):1815–1828.
17. Furtado S, Suchowersky O, Rewcastle B, et al. Relationship between trinucleotide repeats and neuropathological changes in Huntington's disease. Ann Neurol 1996;39:132–136.
18. Penney JB Jr, Vonsattel JP, MacDonald ME, et al. CAG repeat number governs the development rate of pathology in Huntington's disease. Ann Neurol 1997;41:689–692.
19. Rosas HD, Goodman J, Chen YI, et al. Striatal volume loss in HD as measured by MRI and the influence of CAG repeat. Neurology 2001;57:1025–1028.
20. Dom R, Baro F, and Brucher JM. A cytometric study of the putamen in different types of Huntington's chorea. Adv Neurol 1973;1:369–385.
21. Kuhn A, Goldstein DR, Hodges A, et al. Mutant huntingtin's effects on striatal gene expression in mice recapitulate changes observed in human Huntington's disease brain and do not differ with mutant huntingtin length or wild-type huntingtin dosage. Hum Mol Genet 2007; 16(15):1845–1861.
22. Perry TL, Hansen S, and Kloster M. Huntington's chorea. Deficiency of gamma-aminobutyric acid in brain. N Engl J Med 1973;288:337–342.
23. Bird ED and Iversen LL. Huntington's chorea. Postmortem measurement of glutamic acid decarboxylase, choline acetyltransferase and dopamine in basal ganglia. Brain 1974;97:457–472.
24. Spokes EGS. Neurochemical alterations in Huntington's chorea. A study of post-mortem brain tissue. Brain 1980;103:179–210.
25. Carter CJ. Reduced GABA transaminase activity in the Huntington's disease putamen. Neurosci Lett 1984;48: 339–342.
26. Reynolds GP and Pearson SJ. Decreased glutamic acid and increased 5-hydroxytryptamine in Huntington's disease brain. Neurosci Lett 1987;78:233–238.
27. Marshall P, Landis D, Zalneraitis E. Immunocytochemical studies of substance P and leucine-enkephalin in Huntington's disease. Brain Res 1983;289:11–26.
28. Goto S, Hirano A, and Rojas-Corona RR. An immunohistochemical investigation of the human neostriatum in Huntington's disease. Ann Neurol 1989;25:298–304.
29. Ferrante R, Kowall N, and Richardson E Jr. Immunocytochemical localization of calcium binding protein in normal and Huntington's disease striatum. J Neuropathol Exp Neurol 1988;47:352.
30. Seto-Ohshima A, Emson PC, Lawson E, et al. Loss of matrix calcium-binding protein-containing neurons in Huntington's disease. Lancet 1988;i:1252–1255.
31. Augood SJ, Faull RL, and Emson PC. Dopamine D1 and D2 receptor gene expression in the striatum in Huntington's disease. Ann Neurol 1997;42:215–221.
32. Martinez-Mir MI, Pollard H, Moreau J, et al. Loss of striatal histamine H2 receptors in Huntington's chorea but not in Parkinson's disease: comparison with animal models. Synapse 1993;15:209–220.
33. Joyce JN, Lexow N, Bird E, et al. Organization of dopamine D1 and D2 receptors in human striatum: Receptor autoradiographic studies in Huntington's disease and schizophrenia. Synapse 1988;2:546–557.
34. Richfield EK, O'Brien CF, Eskin T, et al. Heterogeneous dopamine receptor changes in early and late Huntington's disease. Neurosci Lett 1991;132:121–126.
35. Richfield EK and Herkenham M. Selective vulnerability in Huntington's disease: Preferential loss of cannabinoid receptors in lateral globus pallidus. Ann Neurol 1994;36:577–584.
36. Martinez-Mir MI, Probst A, and Palacios JM. Adenosine A2 receptors: Selective localization in the human basal ganglia and alterations with disease. Neuroscience 1991;42:697–706.
37. Gerfen C. The neostriatal mosaic: Multiple levels of compartmental organization in the basal ganglia. Annu Rev Neurosci 1992;15:285–320.
38. Kanazawa I, Bird E, O'Connell R, et al. Evidence for the decrease in substance P content of substantia nigra in Huntington's chorea. Brain Res 1977;120:387–392.
39. Gale J, Bird E, Spokes E, et al. Human brain substance P: Distribution in controls and Huntington's chorea. J Neurochem 1978;30:633–634.
40. Emson P, Arregui A, Clement-Jones V, et al. Regional distribution of met-enkephalin and substance P immunoreactivity in normal human brain and in Huntington's disease. Brain Res 1980;199:147–160.
41. Grafe MR, Forno LS, and Eng LF. Immunocytochemical studies of substance P and Met-enkephalin in the basal ganglia and substantia nigra in Huntington's, Parkinson's and Alzheimer's diseases. J Neuropathol Exp Neurol 1985;44:47–59.
42. Waters CM, Peck R, Rossor M, et al. Immunocytochemical studies on the basal ganglia and substantia nigra in

Parkinson's disease and Huntington's chorea. Neuroscience 1988;25:419–438.
43. Beal MF, Ellison DW, Mazurek MF, et al. A detailed examination of substance P in pathologically graded cases of Huntington's disease. J Neurol Sci 1988;84:51–61.
44. Glass M, Dragunow M, and Faull RL. The pattern of neurodegeneration in Huntington's disease: A comparative study of cannabinoid, dopamine, adenosine and GABA(A) receptor alterations in the human basal ganglia in Huntington's disease. Neuroscience 2000;97:505–519.
45. Cha JH, Frey AS, Alsdorf SA, et al. Altered neurotransmitter receptor expression in transgenic mouse models of Huntington's disease. Philos Trans R Soc Lond B Biol Sci 1999;354:981–989.
46. Reiner A, Albin RL, Anderson KD, et al. Differential loss of striatal projection neurons in Huntington disease. Proc Natl Acad Sci U S A 1988;85:5733–5737.
47. Albin RL, Young AB, Penney JB, et al. Abnormalities of striatal projection neurons and N-methyl-D-aspartate receptors in presymptomatic Huntington's disease. N Engl J Med 1990;322:1293–1298.
48. Storey E and Beal MF. Neurochemical substrates of rigidity and chorea in Huntington's disease. Brain 1993;116(pt 5): 1201–1222.
49. Crossman AR. Primate models of dyskinesia: The experimental approach to the study of basal ganglia-related involuntary movement disorders. Neuroscience 1987;21:1–40.
50. Albin R, Young A, and Penney J. The functional anatomy of basal ganglia disorders. Trends Neurosci 1989;12:366–375.
51. DeLong M. Primate models of movement disorders of basal ganglia origin. Trends Neurosci 1990;13:281–285.
52. Crossman A, Mitchell I, Sambrook M, et al. Chorea and myoclonus in the monkey induced by gamma-aminobutyric acid antagonism in the lentiform complex. Brain 1988;111: 1211–1233.
53. Kowall N, Ferrante R, and Martin J. Patterns of cell loss in Huntington's disease. Trends Neurosci 1987;10:24–29.
54. Ferrante R, Kowall N, Martin J, et al. Substance P-containing striatal neurons in Huntington's disease. Exp Neurol 1987;46:375.
55. Ferrante RJ, Beal MF, Kowall NW, et al. Sparing of acetylcholinesterase-containing striatal neurons in Huntington's disease. Brain Res 1987;411:162–166.
56. Cicchetti F, Gould PV, and Parent A. Sparing of striatal neurons coexpressing calretinin and substance P (NK1) receptor in Huntington's disease. Brain Res 1996;730:232–237.
57. Beal M, Kowall N, Ellison D, et al. Replication of the neurochemical characteristics of Huntington's disease by quinolinic acid. Nature 1986;321:168–171.
58. Aronin N, Cooper PE, Lorenz LJ, et al. Somatostatin is increased in the basal ganglia in Huntington's disease. Ann of Neurol 1983;13:519–526.
59. Albin RL, Reiner A, Anderson KD, et al. Striatal and nigral neuron subpopulations in rigid Huntington's disease: Implications for the functional anatomy of chorea and rigidity akinesia. Ann Neurol 1990;27:357–365.
60. Ferrante RJ, Kowall NW, Beal MF, et al. Morphologic and histo-chemical characteristics of a spared subset of striatal neurons in Huntington's disease. J Neuropathol Exp Neurol 1987;46:12–27.
61. Ferrante RJ, Kowall NW, Beal MF, et al. Selective sparing of a class of striatal neurons in Huntington's disease. Science 1985;230:561–563.
62. Dawbarn D, De Quidt ME, and Emson PC. Survival of basal ganglia neuropeptide Y-somatostatin neurones in Huntington's disease. Brain Res 1985;340:251–260.
63. McGeer E and McGeer P. Duplication of biochemical changes of Huntington's chorea by intrastriatal injections of glutamic and kainic acids. Nature 1976;263:517–519.
64. Hersch S, Gutekunst C-A, Rees H, et al. Distribution of m1–4 muscarinic receptor proteins in the rat striatum. Light and electron microscopic immunocytochemistry using subtype specific antibodies. J Neurosci 1994;14:3351–3363.
65. Graveland GA, Williams RS, and DiFiglia M. Evidence for degenerative and regenerative changes in neostriatal spiny neurons in Huntington's disease. Science 1985;227: 770–773.
66. Ferrante RJ, Kowall NW, and Richardson EP Jr. Proliferative and degenerative changes in striatal spiny neurons in Huntington's disease: A combined study using the section-Golgi method and calbindin D28k immunocytochemistry. J Neurosci 1991;11:3877–3887.
67. Guidetti P, Charles V, Chen EY, et al. Early degenerative changes in transgenic mice expressing mutant huntingtin involve dendritic abnormalities but no impairment of mitochondrial energy production. Exp Neurol 2001;169: 340–350.
68. Laforet GA, Sapp E, Chase K, et al. Changes in cortical and striatal neurons predict behavioral and electrophysiological abnormalities in a transgenic murine model of Huntington's disease. J Neurosci 2001;21:9112–9123.
69. Klapstein GJ, Fisher RS, Zanjani H, et al. Electrophysiological and morphological changes in striatal spiny neurons in R6/2 Huntington's disease transgenic mice. J Neurophysiol 2001;86:2667–2677.
70. Butterworth NJ, Williams L, Bullock JY, et al. Trinucleotide (CAG) repeat length is positively correlated with the degree of DNA fragmentation in Huntington's disease striatum. Neuroscience 1998;87:49–53.
71. Portera-Cailliau C, Hedreen JC, Price DL, et al. Evidence for apoptotic cell death in Huntington disease and excitotoxic animal models.J Neurosci 1995;15(5 pt 2): 3775–3787.
72. Kiechle T, Dedeoglu A, Kubilus J, et al. Cytochrome C and caspase-9 expression in Huntington's disease. Neuromol Med 2002;1:183–195.
73. Dikranian K, Ishimaru MJ, Tenkova T, et al. Apoptosis in the in vivo mammalian forebrain. Neurobiol Dis 2001;8: 359–379.
74. Browne SE, Ferrante RJ, and Beal MF. Oxidative stress in Huntington's disease. Brain Pathol 1999;9(1):147–163.
75. Graybiel A. Neurotransmitters and neuromodulators in the basal ganglia. Trends Neurosci 1990;13:244–254.
76. Ferrante RJ, Kowall NW, Richardson EP Jr, et al. Topography of enkephalin, substance P and acetylcholinesterase staining in Huntington's disease striatum. Neurosci Lett 1986;71:283–288.
77. Ferrante RJ and Kowall NW. Tyrosine hydroxylase-like immunoreactivity is distributed in the matrix compartment of normal human and Huntington's disease striatum. Brain Res 1987;416:141–146.

78. Kiyama H, Seto-Ohshima A, and Emson PC. Calbindin D28K as a marker for the degeneration of the striatonigral pathway in Huntington's disease. Brain Res 1990;525: 209–214.
79. Hersch S, Ciliax B, Gutekunst C-A, et al. Electron microscopic analysis of D1 and D2 dopamine receptor proteins in the dorsal striatum and their synaptic relationships with motor corticostriatal afferents. J Neurosci 1995;15:5222–5237.
80. Tippett LJ, Waldvogel HJ, Thomas SJ, et al. Striosomes and mood dysfunction in Huntington's disease. Brain 2007;130(pt 1):206–221.
81. Bruyn G. Neuropathological changes in Huntington's chorea. Adv Neurol 1973;1:399–403.
82. Sapp E, Ge P, Aizawa H, et al. Evidence for a preferential loss of enkephalin immunoreactivity in the external globus pallidus in low grade Huntington's disease using high resolution image analysis. Neurosci 1995;64:397–404.
83. Forno LS and Jose C. Huntington's chorea: A pathological study. Adv Neurol 1973;1:453–470.
84. Bugiani O, Tabaton M, and Cammarata S. Huntington's disease: Survival of large striatal neurons in the rigid variant. Ann Neurol 1984;15:154–156.
85. Oyanagi K, Takeda S, Takahashi H, et al. A quantitative investigation of the substantia nigra in Huntington's disease. Ann Neurol 1989;26:13–19.
86. Ferrante R, Kowall N, Richardson EJ. Neuronal and neuropil loss in the substantia nigra in Huntington's disease. J Neuropathol Exp Neurol 1989;48:380.
87. Bohnen NI, Koeppe RA, Meyer P, et al. Decreased striatal monoaminergic terminals in Huntington disease. Neurology 2000;54:1753–1759.
88. Saji M and Reis D. Delayed transneuronal death of substantia nigra neurons prevented by gamma-aminobutyric acid. Science 1987;235:66–69.
89. Dom R, Malfroid M, and Baro F. Neuropathology of Huntington's chorea. Studies of the ventrobasal complex of the thalamus. Neurology 1976;26:64–68.
90. Heinsen H, Rub U, Gangnus D, et al. Nerve cell loss in the thalamic centromedian-parafascicular complex in patients with Huntington's disease. Acta Neuropathol (Berl) 1996;91:161–168.
91. Heinsen H, Rub U, Bauer M, et al. Nerve cell loss in the thalamic mediodorsal nucleus in Huntington's disease. Acta Neuropathol (Berl) 97:613–622, 1999.
92. Kremer HP, Roos RA, Dingjan GM, et al. The hypothalamic lateral tuberal nucleus and the characteristics of neuronal loss in Huntington's disease. Neurosci Lett 1991;132: 101–104.
93. Kremer HP, Roos RA, Dingjan G, et al. Atrophy of the hypothalamic lateral tuberal nucleus in Huntington's disease. J Neuropathol Exp Neurol 1990;49:371–382.
94. Petersen A, Gil J, Maat-Schieman ML, et al. Orexin loss in Huntington's disease. Hum Mol Genet 2005;14(1):39–47.
95. Alzheimer A. Über die anatomische Grunglage der Huntingtonschen Chorea und der choreatischen bewegungen Überhaupt. Neurol Zentral 1911;30:891–892.
96. Hallervorden J. Huntingtonsche chorea (chorea chronica progressiva herditaria). In Lubarsch O, et al. (eds). Handbuch der speziellen pathologischen Anatomie und Histologie. Springer: Berlin, 1957, pp. 793–822.
97. Zuccato C, Ciammola A, Rigamonti D, et al. Loss of huntingtin-mediated BDNF gene transcription in Huntington's disease. Science 2001;293:493–498.
98. Alexander GE, Delong MR, Strick PL. Parallel organization of functionally segregated circuits linking basal ganglia and cortex. Annu Rev Neurosci 1986;9:357–381.
99. Alexander GE, Crutcher MD, and DeLong MR. Basal gangliathalamocortical circuits: Parallel substrates for motor, oculo-motor, "prefrontal" and "limbic" functions. Prog Brain Res 1990;85:119–146.
100. Stack EC, Dedeoglu A, Smith KM, et al. Neuroprotective effects of synaptic modulation in Huntington's disease R6/2 mice. J Neurosci 2007;27(47):12908–12915.
101. Lange HW. Quantitative changes of telencephalon, diencephalon, and mesencephalon in Huntington's chorea, postencephalic, and idiopathic Parkinson's disease. Verh Anat Ges 1981;75:923–925.
102. De la Monte SM, Vonsattel JP, and Richardson EP Jr. Morphometric demonstration of atrophic changes in the cerebral cortex, white matter, and neostriatum in Huntington's disease. J Neuropathol Exp Neurol 1988;47:516–525.
103. Halliday GM, McRitchie DA, Macdonald V, et al. Regional specificity of brain atrophy in Huntington's disease. Exp Neurol 1998;154:663–672.
104. Sieradzan K, Mann DM, Dodge A. Clinical presentation and patterns of regional cerebral atrophy related to the length of trinucleotide repeat expansion in patients with adult onset Huntington's disease. Neurosci Lett 1997;225:45–48.
105. Aylward EH, Brandt J, Codori AM, et al. Reduced basal ganglia volume associated with the gene for Huntington's disease in asymptomatic at-risk persons. Neurology 1994;44:823–828.
106. Aylward EH, Li Q, Stine OC, et al. Longitudinal change in basal ganglia volume in patients with Huntington's disease. Neurology 1997;48:394–399.
107. Rosas HD, Liu AK, Hersch S, et al. Regional and progressive thinning of the cortical ribbon in Huntington's disease. Neurology 2002;58:695–701.
108. Rosas HD, Salat DH, Lee SY, et al.Complexity and heterogeneity: What drives the ever-changing brain in Huntington's disease? Ann N Y Acad Sci 2008;1147:196–205.
109. Hersch S, Gutekunst C-A, Rosenfeld V, et al. A Quantitative morphometric study of the cerebral cortex in Huntington's disease. World Fed Neurol (Abs), 1991.
110. Sotrel A, Paskevich PA, Kiely DK, et al. Morphometric analysis of the prefrontal cortex in Huntington's disease. Neurology 1991;41:1117–1123.
111. Hedreen JC, Peyser CE, Folstein SE, et al. Neuronal loss in layers V and VI of cerebral cortex in Huntington's disease. Neurosci Lett 1991;133:257–261.
112. Rajkowska G, Selemon L, and Goldman-Rakic P. Morphometric evidence for prefrontal cellular atrophy in advanced Huntington's disease. Soc Neurosci Abstr 1993;19:838.
113. Braak H and Braak E. Allocortical involvement in Huntington's disease. Neuropathol Appl Neurobiol 1992;18: 539–547.
114. Braak H, Del Tredici K, Bohl J, et al. Pathological changes in the parahippocampal region in select non-Alzheimer's dementias. Ann N Y Acad Sci 2000;911:221–239.

115. Rosas HD, Salat DH, Lee SY, et al. Cerebral cortex and the clinical expression of Huntington's disease: Complexity and heterogeneity. Brain 2008;131(pt 4):1057–1068.
116. Vonsattel JP, Keller C, and Pilar Amaya MD. Neuropathology of Huntington's disease. Handb Clin Neurol 2008;89:599–618.
117. Rosas HD, Tuch DS, Hevelone ND, et al. Diffusion tensor imaging in presymptomatic and early Huntington's disease: Selective white matter pathology and its relationship to clinical measures. Mov Disord 2006;21(9): 1317–1325.
118. Kloppel S, Draganski B, Golding CV, et l. White matter connections reflect changes in voluntary-guided saccades in pre-symptomatic Huntington's disease. Brain 2008; 131(pt 1):196–204.
119. Reading SA, Yassa MA, Bakker A, et al. Regional white matter change in pre-symptomatic Huntington's disease: A diffusion tensor imaging study. Psychiatry Res 2005;140(1):55–62.
120. Weaver KE, Richards TL, Liang O, et al. Longitudinal diffusion tensor imaging in Huntington's Disease. Exp Neurol 2009;216(2):525–529.
121. Clark VP, Lai S, Deckel AW. Altered functional MRI responses in Huntington's disease. Neuroreport 2002;13:703–706.
122. Aron AR, Schlaghecken F, Fletcher PC, et al. Inhibition of subliminally primed responses is mediated by the caudate and thalamus: Evidence from functional MRI and Huntington's disease. Brain 2003;126(pt 3):713–723.
123. Backman L, Robins-Wahlin TB, Lundin A, et al. Cognitive deficits in Huntington's disease are predicted by dopaminergic PET markers and brain volumes. Brain 1997;120(pt 12):2207–2217.
124. Feigin A, Leenders KL, Moeller JR, et al. Metabolic network abnormalities in early Huntington's disease: An [(18)F]FDG PET study. J Nucl Med 2001;42:1591–1595.
125. Antonini A, Leenders KL, Spiegel R, et al. Striatal glucose metabolism and dopamine D2 receptor binding in asymptomatic gene carriers and patients with Huntington's disease. Brain 1996;119(pt 6):2085–2095.
126. Ginovart N, Lundin A, Farde L, et al. PET study of the pre and post-synaptic dopaminergic markers for the neurodegenerative process in Huntington's disease. Brain 1997;120(pt 3):503–514.
127. McCaughey W. The pathologic spectrum of Huntington's chorea. J Nerv Ment Dis 1961;133:91–103.
128. Byers RK, Gilles FH, Fung C. Huntington's disease in children. Neuropathologic study of four cases. Neurology 1973;23:561–569.
129. Roizin L, Kaufman M, Wilson N, et al. Neuropathologic observations in Huntington's chorea. In Zimmerman H (ed). Progress in Neuropathology. New York: Grune & Stratton, 1976, pp. 447–488.
130. Heinsen H, Strik M, Bauer M, et al. Cortical and striatal neurone number in Huntington's disease. Acta Neuropathol 1994;88:320–333.
131. Selemon LD, Rajkowska G, and Goldman-Rakic PS. Elevated neuronal density in prefrontal area 46 in brains from schizophrenic patients: Application of a three-dimensional, stereologic counting method. J Comp Neurol 1998;392: 402–412.
132. Zalneraitis EL, Landis DMA, Richardson EPJ, et al. A comparison of astrocytic structure in cerebral cortex and striatum in Huntington's disease. Neurology 1981 ;31:151 (abstract).
133. Cudkowicz M, Kowall NW. Degeneration of pyramidal projection neurons in Huntington's disease cortex. Ann Neurol 1990;27:200–204.
134. Beal MF, Swartz KJ, Finn SF, et al. Amino acid and neuropeptide neurotransmitters in Huntington's disease cerebellum. Brain Res 1988;454: 393–396.
135. Mazurek MF, Beal MF, Knowlton SF, et al. Elevated concentrations of cholecystokinin and vasoactive intestinal peptide in Huntington's disease postmortem cerebral cortex. Neurology 1989;39(suppl 1):203.
136. Storey E, Kowall NW, Finn SF, et al. The cortical lesion of Huntington's disease: Further neurochemical characterization, and reproduction of some of the histological and neurochemical features by N-methyl-D-aspartate lesions of rat cortex. Ann Neurol 1992;32:526–534.
137. Sotrel A, Paskevich P, Kiely D, et al. Morphometric analysis of the prefrontal cortex in Huntington's disease. Neurology 1991;41:1117–1123.
138. Ellison DW, Beal MF, Mazurek MF, et al. Amino acid neuro-transmitter abnormalities in Huntington's disease and in the quinolinic acid animal model of Huntington's disease. Brain 1987;110:1657–1673.
139. Wagster MV, Hedreen JC, Peyser CE, et al. Selective loss of [3H]kainic acid and [3H]AMPA binding in layer VI of frontal cortex in Huntington's disease. Exp Neurol 1994;127:70–75.
140. Hassel B, Tessler S, Faull RL, et al. Glutamate uptake is reduced in prefrontal cortex in Huntington's disease. Neurochem Res 2008;33(2):232–237.
141. Mazurek MF, Garside S, Beal MF. Cortical peptide changes in Huntington's disease may be independent of striatal degeneration. Ann Neurol 1997;41:540–547.
142. Zuccato C, Marullo M, Conforti P, et al. Systematic assessment of BDNF and its receptor levels in human cortices affected by Huntington's disease. Brain Pathol 2008;18(2): 225–238.
143. Smith R, Klein P, Koc-Schmitz Y, . Loss of SNAP-25 and rabphilin 3a in sensory-motor cortex in Huntington's disease. J Neurochem 2007;103(1):115–123.
144. Hodges A, Strand AD, Aragaki AK, et al. Regional and cellular gene expression changes in human Huntington's disease brain. Hum Mol Genet 2006;15(6):965–977.
145. Markham C, Knox J. Observations on Huntington's chorea in childhood. J Pediatr 1965;67:46–57.
146. Jervis G. Huntington's chorea in childhood. Arch Neurol 1963;9:50–63.
147. Rodda R. Cerebellar atrophy in Huntington's disease. J Neurol Sci 1981;50:147–157.
148. Jeste DV, Barban L, Parisi J. Reduced Purkinje cell density in Huntington's disease. Exp Neurol 1984;85:78–86.
149. McCaughey WTE. The pathologic spectrum of Huntington's chorea. J Nerv Ment Dis 1961;133:91–103.
150. Coyle J, Schwarcz R. Lesions of striatal neurons with kainic acid provides a model for Huntington's chorea. Nature 1976;263:244–246.
151. Ferrante RJ, Kowall NW, Cipolloni PB, et al. Excitotoxin lesions in primates as a model for Huntington's disease.

Histopathologic and neurochemical characterization. Exp Neurol 1993;119:46–71.
152. Beal MF, Kowall NW, Ferrante RJ, et al. Quinolinic acid striatal lesions in primates as a model of Huntington's disease. Ann Neurol 1989;26:137.
153. Beal MF, Ferrante RJ, Swartz KJ, et al. Chronic quinolinic acid lesions in rats closely resemble Huntington's disease. J Neurosci 1991;11:1649–1659.
154. Bazzett TJ, Becker JB, Kaatz KW, et al. Chronic intrastriatal dialytic administration of quinolinic acid produces selective neural degeneration. Exp Neurol 1993;120: 177–185.
155. Young AB, Greenamyre JT, Hollingsworth Z, et al. NMDA receptor losses in putamen from patients with Huntington's disease. Science 1988;241: 981–983.
156. Dure LS, Young AB, Penney JB. Excitatory amino acid binding sites in the caudate nucleus and frontal cortex of Huntington's disease. Ann Neurol 1991;30:785–793.
157. Gutekunst C-A, Hersch S, Wimpey T, et al. Western blot analysis of glutamate receptor subunits in huntington's disease. Soc Neurosci, 1993.
158. Levine MS, Klapstein GJ, Koppel A, et al. Enhanced sensitivity to N-methyl-D-aspartate receptor activation in transgenic and knockin mouse models of Huntington's disease. J Neurosci Res 1999;58:515–532.
159. Zeron MM, Hansson O, Chen N, et al. Increased sensitivity to N-methyl-D-aspartate receptor-mediated excitotoxicity in a mouse model of Huntington's disease. Neuron 2002;33:849–860.
160. Behrens PF, Franz P, Woodman B, et al. Impaired glutamate transport and glutamate-glutamine cycling: Downstream effects of the Huntington mutation. Brain 2002;125(pt 8): 1908–1922.
161. Cepeda C, Hurst RS, Calvert CR, et al. Transient and progressive electrophysiological alterations in the corticostriatal pathway in a mouse model of Huntington's disease. J Neurosci 2003;23:961–969.
162. McGeer EG, McGeer PL, and Singh K. Kainate-induced degeneration of neostriatal neurons: Dependency upon corticostriatal tract. Brain Res 1978;139:381–383.
163. Biziere K and Coyle JT. Effects of cortical ablation on the neurotoxicity and receptor binding of kainic acid in striatum. J Neurosci Res 1979;4:383–398.
164. Meldrum A, Dunnett SB, and Everitt BJ. Role of corticostriatal and nigrostriatal inputs in malonate-induced striatal toxicity. NeuroReport 2001;12:89–89.
165. Stack EC, Dedeoglu A, Smith KM, et al. Neuroprotective effects of synaptic modulation in Huntington's disease R6/2 mice. J Neurosci 2007;27(47):12908–12915.
166. Reynolds DS, Carter RJ, and Morton AJ. Dopamine modulates the susceptibility of striatal neurons to 3-nitropropionic acid in the rat model of Huntington's disease. J Neurosci 1998;18(23):10116–10127.
167. Ferrante RJ, Andreassen OA, Dedeoglu A, et al. Therapeutic effects of coenzyme Q10 and remacemide in transgenic mouse models of Huntington's disease. J Neurosci 2002;22:1592–1599.
168. Schiefer J, Landwehrmeyer GB, Luesse HG, et al. Riluzole prolongs survival time and alters nuclear inclusion formation in a transgenic mouse model of Huntington's disease. Mov Disord 2002;17:748–757.
169. Schilling G, Coonfield ML, Ross CA, et al. Coenzyme Q10 and remacemide hydrochloride ameliorate motor deficits in a Huntington's disease transgenic mouse model. Neurosci Lett 2001;315:149–153.
170. Kieburtz K. Antiglutamate therapies in Huntington's disease. J Neural Transm 1999; Suppl 55:97–102.
171. Group HS. A randomized, placebo-controlled trial of coenzyme Q10 and remacemide in Huntington's disease. Neurology 2001;57:397–404.
172. Beal M. Does impairment of energy metabolism result in excitotoxic neuronal death in neurodegenerative illnesses? Ann Neurol 1992;31:119–130.
173. Beal MF, Hyman BT, Koroshetz W. Do defects in mitochondrial energy metabolism underlie the pathology of neurodegenerative diseases? Trends Neurosci 1993;16:125–131.
174. Albin R, Greenamyre J. Alternative excitotoxic hypotheses. Neurology 1992;42:733–738.
175. Beal MF. Aging, energy, and oxidative stress in neurodegenerative diseases. Ann Neurol 1995;38:357–366.
176. Browne SE, Bowling AC, MacGarvey U, et al. Oxidative damage and metabolic dysfunction in Huntington's disease: Selective vulnerability of the basal ganglia. Ann Neurol 1997;41:646–653.
177. Parker WJ, Boyson SJ, Luder AS, et al. Evidence for a defect in NADH: Ubiquinone oxidoreductase (complex I) in Huntington's disease. Neurology 1990;40:1231–1234.
178. Arenas J, Campos Y, Ribacoba R, et al. Complex I defect in muscle from patients with Huntington's disease. Ann Neurol 1998;43:397–400.
179. Brennan WA Jr, Bird ED, Aprille JR. Regional mitochondrial respiratory activity in Huntington's disease brain. J Neurochem 1985;44:1948–1950.
180. Browne SE, Ferrante RJ, Beal MF. Oxidative stress in Huntington's disease. Brain Pathol 1999;9:147–163.
181. Jenkins B, Koroshetz W, Beal M, et al. Localized proton-NMR spectroscopy in patients with Huntington's disease (HD) demonstrates abnormal lactate levels in occipital cortex: Evidence for compromised metabolism in HD. Neurology 1992;42:223–229.
182. Panov AV, Burke JR, Strittmatter WJ, et al. In vitro effects of polyglutamine tracts on Ca2+-dependent depolarization of rat and human mitochondria: Relevance to Huntington's disease. Arch Biochem Biophys 2003;410:1–6.
183. Panov AV, Gutekunst CA, Leavitt BR, et al. Early mitochondrial calcium defects in Huntington's disease are a direct effect of polyglutamines. Nat Neurosci 2002;5:731–736.
184. Gines S, Seong IS, Fossale E, et al. Specific progressive cAMP reduction implicates energy deficit in presymptomatic Hunting-ton's disease knock-in mice. Hum Mol Genet 2003;12:497–508.
185. Novelli A, Reilly J, Lysko P, et al. Glutamate becomes neurotoxic via the N-methyl-D-aspartate receptor when intracellular energy levels are reduced. Brain Res 1988;451: 205–212.
186. Greene J, Porter R, Eller R, et al. Inhibition of succinate dehydrogenase by malonic acid produces an "excitotoxic" lesion in rat striatum. J Neurochem 1993;61:1151–1154.
187. Beal MF, Brouillet E, Jenkins B, et al. Neurochemical and histologic characterization of striatal excitotoxic lesions produced by the mitochondrial toxin 3-nitropropionic acid. J Neurosci 1993;13:4181–4192.

188. Brouillet E, Hantraye P, Ferrante RJ, et al. Chronic mitochondrial energy impairment produces selective striatal degeneration and abnormal choreiform movements in primates. Proc Natl Acad Sci U S A 1995;92: 7105–7109.
189. Greene J, Greenamyre J: Characterization of the excitotoxic potential of the reversible succinate dehydrogenase inhibitor malonate. J Neurochem 64:430–436, 1995.
190. Beal M, Henshaw D, Jenkins B, et al. Coenzyme Q10 and nicotinamide block striatal lesions produced by the mitochondrial toxin malonate. Ann Neurol 36:882–888.
191. Henshaw R, Jenkins B, Schulz J, et al. Malonate produces striatal lesions by indirect NMDA receptor activation. Brain Res 1994;647:161–166.
192. Huntington Study Group. Safety and tolerability of the free-radical scavenger OPC-14117 in Huntington's disease. Neurology 1998;50:1366–1373.
193. Ferrante RJ, Andreassen OA, Jenkins BG, et al. Neuroprotective effects of creatine in a transgenic mouse model of Huntington's disease. J Neurosci 2000;20:4389–4397.
194. Hersch SM, Gevorkian S, Marder K, et al. . Creatine in Huntington disease is safe, tolerable, bioavailable in brain and reduces serum 8OH2'dG. Neurology 2006;66: 250–252.
195. Stack EC, Matson WR, and Ferrante RJ. Evidence of oxidant damage in Huntington's disease: Translational strategies using antioxidants. Ann N Y Acad Sci 2008;1147: 79–92.
196. Tellez-Nagel I, Johnson AB, and Terry RD. Studies on brain biopsies of patients with Huntington's chorea. J Neuropathol Exp Neurol 1974;33(2):308–332.
197. Browne SE, Ferrante RJ, and Beal MF. Oxidative stress in Huntington's disease. Brain Pathol 1999;9(1):147–163.
198. Butterworth NJ, Williams L, Bullock JY, et al. Trinucleotide (CAG) repeat length is positively correlated with the degree of DNA fragmentation in Huntington's disease striatum. Neuroscience 1998;87(1):49–53.
199. Polidori MC, Mecocci P, Browne SE, et al. Oxidative damage to mitochondrial DNA in Huntington's disease parietal cortex. Neurosci Lett 1999; 272(1):53–56.
200. Kovtun IV, Liu Y, Bjoras M, et al. OGG1 initiates age-dependent CAG trinucleotide expansion in somatic cells. Nature 2007;447(7143):447–452.
201. Stoy N, Mackay GM, Forrest CM, et al. Tryptophan metabolism and oxidative stress in patients with Huntington's disease. J Neurochem 2005;93(3):611–623.
202. Jenkins BG, Koroshetz WJ, Beal MF, et al. Evidence for impairment of energy metabolism in vivo in Huntington's disease using localized 1H NMR spectroscopy. Neurology 1993;43:2689–2695.
203. Lodi R, Schapira AH, Manners D, et al. Abnormal in vivo skeletal muscle energy metabolism in Huntington's disease and dentatorubropallidoluysian atrophy. Ann Neurol 2000;48:72–76.
204. Hengartner MO. The biochemistry of apoptosis. Nature 2000;407:770–776.
205. Friedlander RM. Apoptosis and caspases in neurodegenerative diseases. N Engl J Med 2003; 348:1365–1375.
206. Huntington's Disease Collaborative Research Group. A novel gene containing a trinucleotide repeat that is expanded and unstable on Huntington's disease chromosomes. Cell 1993;72:971–983.
207. Li SH, Schilling G, Young WS, et al. Huntington's disease gene (IT15) is widely expressed in human and rat tissues. Neuron 1993;11:985–993.
208. Strong TV, Tagle DA, Valdes JM, et al. Widespread expression of the human and rat Huntington's disease gene in brain and nonneural tissues. Nat Genet 1993;5: 259–265.
209. Ambrose CM, Duyao MP, Barnes G, et al. Structure and expression of the Huntington's disease gene: Evidence against simple inactivation due to an expanded CAG repeat. Somat Cell Mol Genet 1994;20:27–38.
210. Duyao MP, Auerbach AB, Ryan A, et al. Inactivation of the mouse Huntington's disease gene homolog Hdh. Science 1995;269:407–410.
211. Nasir J, Floresco SB, O'Kusky JR, et al. Targeted disruption of the Huntington's disease gene results in embryonic lethality and behavioral and morphological changes in heterozygotes. Cell 81:811–823.
212. Landwehrmeyer GB, McNeil SM, Dure LS, et al. Huntington's disease gene: Regional and cellular expression in brain of normal and affected individuals. Ann Neurol 1995;37:218–230.
213. Eberwine J, McLaughlin B. Striatal RNA-binding proteins interact with huntingtin mRNA. In Ariano M, Surmeier D (eds). Molecular and Cellular Mechanisms of Neostriatal Function. Austin: RG Landes, 1995, pp. 143–149.
214. Johnson R, Zuccato C, Belyaev D, et al. A microRNA-based gene dysregulation pathway in Huntington's disease. Neurobiol Dis 2008;29(3):438–445.
215. Savas JN, Makusky A, Ottosen S, et al. Huntington's disease protein contributes to RNA-mediated gene silencing through association with Argonaute and P bodies. Proc Natl Acad Sci U S A 2008;105(31):10820–10825.
216. DiFiglia M, Sapp E, Chase K, et al. Huntingtin is a cytoplasmic protein associated with vesicles in human and rat brain neurons. Neuron 1995;14:1075–1081.
217. Hoogeveen AT, Willemsen R, Meyer N, et al. Characterization and localization of the Huntington disease gene product. Hum Mol Genet 1993;2:2069–2073.
218. Gutekunst CA, Levey AI, Heilman CJ, et al. Identification and localization of huntingtin in brain and human lymphoblastoid cell lines with anti-fusion protein antibodies. Proc Natl Acad Sci U S A 1995;92:8710–8714.
219. Sharp AH, Loev SJ, Schilling G, et al. Widespread expression of Huntington's disease gene (IT15) protein product. Neuron 1995;14:1065–1074.
220. Trottier Y, Devys D, Imbert G, et al. Cellular localization of the Huntington's disease protein and discrimination of the normal and mutated form. Nat Genet 1995;10: 104–110.
221. Ferrante R, Gutekunst C-A, Persichetti F, et al. Heterogeneous topographic and cellular distribution of huntingtin expression in the normal human neostriatum. J Neurosci 1997;17:3052–3063.
222. Gutekunst CA, Li SH, Yi H, et al. The cellular and subcellular localization of huntingtin-associated protein 1 (HAP1): Comparison with huntingtin in rat and human. J Neurosci 1998;18:7674–7686.

223. Kegel KB, Kim M, Sapp E, et al. Huntingtin expression stimulates endosomal-lysosomal activity, endosome tubulation, and autophagy. J Neurosci 2000;20:7268–7278.
224. Sieradzan KA, Mechan AO, Jones L, et al. Huntington's disease intranuclear inclusions contain truncated, ubiquitinated huntingtin protein. Exp Neurol 1999; 156(1):92–99.
225. Yanai A, Huang K, Kang R, et al. Palmitoylation of huntingtin by HIP14 is essential for its trafficking and function. Nat Neurosci 2006;9(6):824–831.
226. Jeong HF, Then TJ, Melia JR Jr, et al. Acetylation targets mutant huntingtin to autophagosomes for degradation. Cell 2009;137(1):60–72.
227. Steffan JS, Agrawal N, Pallos J, et al. SUMO modification of Huntingtin and Huntington's disease pathology. Science 2004;304(5667):100–104.
228. Humbert S, Bryson EA, Cordelieres FA, et al. The IGF-1/Akt pathway is neuroprotective in Huntington's disease and involves Huntingtin phosphorylation by Akt. Dev Cell 2002;2(6):831–837.
229. Zala DE, Colin H, Rangone G, et al. Phosphorylation of mutant huntingtin at S421 restores anterograde and retrograde transport in neurons. Hum Mol Genet 2008;17(24):3837–3846.
230. Thompson LM, Aiken CL, Kaltenbach LS, et al. IKK phosphorylates Huntingtin and targets it for degradation by the proteasome and lysosome. J Cell Biol 2009.
231. Aiken CT, Steffan JS, Guerrero CM, et al. Phosphorylation of threonine 3: Implications for Huntingtin aggregation and neurotoxicity. J Biol Chem 2009;284(43):29427–29436.
232. Rigamonti D, Bauer JH, De-Fraja C, et al. Wild-type huntingtin protects from apoptosis upstream of caspase-3. J Neurosci 2000;20:3705–3713.
233. Leavitt BR, Guttman JA, Hodgson JG, et al. Wild-type huntingtin reduces the cellular toxicity of mutant huntingtin in vivo. Am J Hum Genet 2001;68:313–324.
234. Ho LW, Brown R, Maxwell M, et al. Wild type huntingtin reduces the cellular toxicity of mutant huntingtin in mammalian cell models of Huntington's disease. J Med Genet 2001;38:450–452.
235. Li SH and Li XJ. Aggregation of N-terminal huntingtin is dependent on the length of its glutamine repeats. Hum Mol Genet 1998;7:777–782.
236. Trottier Y, Lutz Y, Stevanin G, et al. Polyglutamine expansion as a pathological epitope in Huntington's disease and four dominant cerebellar ataxias. Nature 1995;378: 403–406.
237. Perutz MF, Johnson T, Suzuki M, et al. Glutamine repeats as polar zippers: Their possible role in inherited neurodegenerative diseases. Proc Natl Acad Sci U S A 1994;91: 5355–5358.
238. Maat-Schieman ML, Dorsman JC, Smoor MA, et al. Distribution of inclusions in neuronal nuclei and dystrophic neurites in Huntington disease brain. J Neuropathol Exp Neurol 1999;58:129–137.
239. Scherzinger E, Lurz R, Turmaine M, et al. Huntingtin-encoded polyglutamine expansions form amyloid-like protein aggregates in vitro and in vivo. Cell 1997;90: 549–558.
240. Martindale D, Hackam A, Wieczorek A, et al. Length of huntingtin and its polyglutamine tract influences localization and frequency of intracellular aggregates. Nat Genet 1998;18:150–154.
241. Becher MW, Kotzuk JA, Sharp AH, et al. Intranuclear neuronal inclusions in Huntington's disease and dentatorubral and pallidoluysian atrophy: Correlation between the density of inclusions and IT15 CAG triplet repeat length. Neurobiol Dis 1998;4:387–397.
242. Skinner P, Koshy B, Cummings C, et al. Ataxin-1 with an expanded glutamine tract alters nuclear matrix-associated structures. Nature 1997;389:971–974.
243. Paulson H, Perez M, Trottier Y, et al. Intranuclear inclusions of expanded polyglutamine protein in spinocerebellar ataxia type 3. Neuron 1997;19:333–344.
244. Holmberg M, Duyckaerts C, Durr A, et al. Spinocerebellar ataxia type 7 (SCA7): A neurodegenerative disorder with neuronal intranuclear inclusions. Hum Mol Genet 1998;7:913–918.
245. Li M, Miwa S, Kobayashi Y, et al. Nuclear inclusions of the androgen receptor protein in spinal and bulbar muscular atrophy. Ann Neurol 1998;44:249–254.
246. Ross CA. Intranuclear neuronal inclusions: A common pathogenic mechanism for glutamine-repeat neurodegenerative diseases? Neuron 1997;19:1147–1150.
247. Davies SW, Beardsall, K, Turmaine M, et al. Are neuronal intranuclear inclusions the common neuropathology of triplet-repeat disorders with polyglutamine-repeat expansions? Lancet 1998;351:131–133.
248. Kuemmerle S, Gutekunst CA, Klein AM, et al. Huntington aggregates may not predict neuronal death in Huntington's disease. Ann Neurol 1999;46:842–849.
249. Davies SW, Turmaine M, Cozens BA, et al. Formation of neuronal intranuclear inclusions underlies the neurological dys-function in mice transgenic for the HD mutation. Cell 1997;90:537–548.
250. Ordway J, Tallaksen-Greene S, Gutekunst C-A, et al. Ectopically expressed CAG repeats cause intranuclear inclusions and a progressive late onset neurological phenotype in the mouse. Cell 1997;91:753–763.
251. Saudou F, Finkbeiner S, Devys D, et al. Huntingtin acts in the nucleus to induce apoptosis but death does not correlate with the formation of intranuclear inclusions. Cell 1998;95:55–66.
252. Chun W, Lesort M, Lee M, et al. Mutant huntingtin aggregates do not sensitize cells to apoptotic stressors. FEBS Lett 2002;515:61–65.
253. Kim M, Lee HS, LaForet G, et al. Mutant huntingtin expression in clonal striatal cells: Dissociation of inclusion formation and neuronal survival by caspase inhibition. J Neurosci 1999;19:964–973.
254. Klement I, Skinner P, Kaytor M, et al. Ataxin-1 nuclear localization and aggregation: Role in polyglutamine-induced disease in SCA1 transgenic mice. Cell 1998;95:41–53.
255. Kuemmerle S, Gutekunst CA, Klein AM, et al. Huntington aggregates may not predict neuronal death in Huntington's disease. Ann Neurol 1999;46(6):842–849.
256. Arrasate M, Mitra S, Schweitzer ES, et al. Inclusion body formation reduces levels of mutant huntingtin and the risk of neuronal death. Nature 2004;431(7010):805–810.
257. Taylor JP, Tanaka F, Robitschek J et al. Aggresomes protect cells by enhancing the degradation of toxic

polyglutamine-containing protein. Hum. Mol. Genet 2003;12:749–757)
258. Chen S, Berthelier V, Yang W, et al. Polyglutamine aggregation behavior in vitro supports a recruitment mechanism of cytotoxicity. J Mol Biol 2001;311:173–182.
259. Poirier MA, Li H, Macosko J, et al. Huntingtin spheroids and protofibrils as precursors in polyglutamine fibrilization. J Biol Chem 2002;277:41032–41037.
260. Hodgson J, Agopyan N, Gutekunst C-A, et al. A YAC mouse model for Huntington's disease with full-length mutant huntingtin, cytoplasmic toxicity, and selective striatal neurodegeneration. Neuron 1999;23:181–192.
261. Kaltenbach LS, Romero E, Becklin R, et al. Huntingtin interacting proteins are genetic modifiers of neurodegeneration. PLoS Genet 2007;3(5):e82.
262. Li XJ, Li SH, Sharp AH, et al. A huntingtin-associated protein enriched in brain with implications for pathology. Nature 1995;378:398–402.
263. Li Y, Chin LS, Levey AI, et al. Huntingtin-associated protein 1 interacts with hepatocyte growth factor-regulated tyrosine kinase substrate and functions in endosomal trafficking. J Biol Chem 2002;277:28212–28221.
264. Li SH, Gutekunst CA, Hersch SM, et al. Interaction of huntingtin-associated protein with dynactin P150Glued. J Neurosci 1998;18:1261–1269.
265. Sittler A, Walter S, Wedemeyer N, et al. SH3GL3 associates with the Huntingtin exon 1 protein and promotes the formation of polygln-containing protein aggregates. Mol Cell 1998;2:427–436.
266. Kalchman M, Koide H, McCutcheon K, et al. HIP1, a human homolog of S. cerevisiae Sla2p, interacts with membrane associated huntingtin in the brain. Nat Genet 1997;16: 44–53.
267. Wanker EE, Rovira C, Scherzinger E, et al. HIP-I: A huntingtin interacting protein isolated by the yeast two-hybrid system. Hum Mol Genet 1997;6:487–495.
268. Metzler M, Legendre-Guillemin V, Gan L, et al. HIP1 functions in clathrin-mediated endocytosis through binding to clathrin and adaptor protein 2. J Biol Chem 2001;276: 39271–39276.
269. Singaraja RR, Hadano S, Metzler M, et al. HIP14, a novel ankyrin domain-containing protein, links huntingtin to intracellular trafficking and endocytosis. Hum Mol Genet 2002;11:2815–2828.
270. Burke, JR, Enghild JJ, Martin ME, et al. Huntingtin and DRPLA proteins selectively interact with the enzyme GAPDH. Nat Med 1996;2:347–350.
271. Bao J, Sharp AH, Wagster MV, et al. Expansion of polyglutamine repeat in huntingtin leads to abnormal protein interactions involving calmodulin. Proc Natl Acad Sci U S A 1996;93:5037–5042.
272. Holbert S, Dedeoglu A, Humbert S, et al. Cdc42-interacting protein 4 binds to huntingtin: Neuropathologic and biological evidence for a role in Huntington's disease. Proc Natl Acad Sci U S A 2003;100:2712–2717.
273. Gerber H-P, Seipel K, Georgiev O, et al. Transcriptional activation modulated by homopolymeric glutamine and proline stretches. Science 1994;263:808–811.
274. Passani LA, Bedford MT, Faber PW, et al. Huntingtin's WW domain partners in Huntington's disease post-mortem brain fulfill genetic criteria for direct involvement in Huntington's disease pathogenesis. Hum Mol Genet 2000;9:2175–2182.
275. Boutell JM, Thomas P, Neal JW, et al. Aberrant interactions of transcriptional repressor proteins with the Huntington's disease gene product, huntingtin. Hum Mol Genet 1999;8:1647–1655.
276. Steffan JS, Kazantsev A, Spasic-Boskovic O, et al. The Huntington's disease protein interacts with p53 and CREB-binding protein and represses transcription. Proc Natl Acad Sci U S A 2000;97:6763–6768.
277. Li SH, Cheng AL, Zhou H, et al. Interaction of Huntington disease protein with transcriptional activator Sp1. Mol Cell Biol 2002;22:1277–1287.
278. Holbert S, Denghien I, Kiechle T, et al. The Gln-Ala repeat transcriptional activator CA150 interacts with huntingtin: Neuropathologic and genetic evidence for a role in Huntington's disease pathogenesis. Proc Natl Acad Sci U S A 2001;98:1811–1816.
279. Dunah AW, Jeong H, Griffin A, et al. Sp1 and TAFII130 transcriptional activity disrupted in early Huntington's disease. Science 2002;296:2238–2243.
280. Cha JH. Transcriptional dysregulation in Huntington's disease. Trends Neurosci 2000;23:387–392.
281. Stack EC, Del Signore SJ, Luthi-Carter R, et al. Modulation of nucleosome dynamics in Huntington's disease. Hum Mol Genet 2007;16(10):1164–1175.
282. Sadri-Vakili G and J.H. Cha, Mechanisms of disease: Histone modifications in Huntington's disease. Nat Clin Pract Neurol 2006;2(6):330–338.
283. Sadri-Vakili G, Bouzou B, Benn CL, et al. Yohrling, and J.H. Cha. Histones associated with downregulated genes are hypo-acetylated in Huntington's disease models. Hum Mol Genet 2007;16(11):1293–1306.
284. Benn CL, Sun T, Sadri-Vakili G, et al. Huntingtin modulates transcription, occupies gene promoters in vivo, and binds directly to DNA in a polyglutamine-dependent manner. J Neurosci 2008;28(42):10720–12733.
285. Kalchman MA, Graham RK, Xia G, et al. Huntingtin is ubiquitinated and interacts with a specific ubiquitin-conjugating enzyme. J Biol Chem 1996;271:19385–19394.
286. Cooper AJ, Jeitner TM, Gentile V, et al. Cross linking of polyglutamine domains catalyzed by tissue transglutaminase is greatly favored with pathological-length repeats: Does transglutaminase activity play a role in (CAG)(n)/Q(n)-expansion diseases? Neurochem Int 2002;40:53–67.
287. Goldberg YP, Nicholson DW, Rasper DM, et al. Cleavage of huntingtin by apopain, a proapoptotic cysteine protease, is modulated by the polyglutamine tract. Nat Genet 1996;13:442–449.
288. Wellington CL, Singaraja R, Ellerby L, et al. Inhibiting caspase cleavage of huntingtin reduces toxicity and aggregate formation in neuronal and nonneuronal cells. J Biol Chem 2000;275:19831–19838.
289. Wellington CL, Ellerby LM, Gutekunst CA, et al. Caspase cleavage of mutant huntingtin precedes neurodegeneration in Huntington's disease. J Neurosci 2002;22:7862–7872.
290. Kim YJ, Yi Y, Sapp E, et al. Caspase 3-cleaved N-terminal fragments of wild-type and mutant huntingtin are present in normal and Huntington's disease brains, associate with membranes, and undergo calpain-dependent proteolysis. Proc Natl Acad Sci U S A 2001;98:12784–12789.

291. Gafni J and Ellerby LM. Calpain activation in Huntington's disease. J Neurosci 2002;22:4842–4849.
292. Lunkes A, Lindenberg KS, Ben-Haiem L, et al. Proteases acting on mutant huntingtin generate cleaved products that differentially build up cytoplasmic and nuclear inclusions. Mol Cell 2002;10:259–269.
293. Jana NR, Zemskov EA, Wang G, et al. Altered proteasomal function due to the expression of polyglutamine-expanded truncated N-terminal huntingtin induces apoptosis by caspase activation through mitochondrial cytochrome c release. Hum Mol Genet 2001;10:1049–1059.
294. Waelter S, Boeddrich A, Lurz R, et al. Accumulation of mutant huntingtin fragments in aggresome-like inclusion bodies as a result of insufficient protein degradation. Mol Biol Cell 2001;12:1393–1407.

CHAPTER 35

Tardive Dyskinesia

Stacy Horn and Christopher G. Goetz

The term "tardive dyskinesia" (TD) applies only to abnormal involuntary movements resulting from chronic treatment with agents that block central dopamine receptors. In most instances, these drugs are antipsychotic neuroleptic agents. Nonetheless, other dopaminergic receptor blockers such as metoclopramide are associated with the same disorder.[1] Schoenecker associated oral–facial dyskinesia with chlorpromazine treatment in 1957, yet three decades later a cause-and-effect relationship between neuroleptic therapy and involuntary movements was still questioned.[2,3] The controversy persisted in part because neuroleptics are most commonly used to treat psychosis and agitated senile depression; mannerisms resembling the movements of TD can occur spontaneously in some persons with psychosis and in normal elderly patients.[4]

Nonetheless, the unequivocal occurrence of involuntary movements after chronic neuroleptic therapy in nonpsychotic young adults without other cause for movement disorders[5] leaves no doubt that TD does occur. The 1980 American Psychiatric Association Task Force provided a useful definition of TD as "an abnormal involuntary movement, not including tremor, resulting from treatment with a neuroleptic drug for 3 months in persons with no other identifiable cause for movement disorder."[6] New descriptions add the possibility that tremor might need to be included as a form of TD. This discussion focuses on four topics: phenomenology, epidemiology and natural history, pathophysiology, and treatment of TD.

▶ PHENOMENOLOGY

A variety of movements occur in TD. Most common are rapid unsustained movements variously described as choreic or stereotypic.[7,8] The former term refers to movements that are unpredictable and flow from one body region to another, whereas stereotypic movements are reproducible and regular, remaining generally restricted in their anatomic distribution. Controversy exists currently as to which term is best for most rapid TD movements and the authors have personally seen instances of both, sometimes in the same patient. Any body area may be affected, but the mouth is commonly involved, producing lip-smacking, tongue protrusion, or grimacing. In addition to facial movements, rapid movements of the fingers, hands or more proximal arm, nodding or head-bobbing, pelvic rocking motions, fine movements of the toes, or a nonrhythmic motion of both legs may develop. TD may involve the trunk and diaphragm, sometimes leading to speech disorders[9,10] or even respiratory distress,[11,12] which may rarely be life-threatening.[13,14]

Dystonic movements also occur in TD, either alone or in combination with choreic or stereotypic movements. Dystonic movements are sustained abnormal postures of a body part or parts, induced or increased with use of the affected part, often with superimposed spasm. Although axial dystonia was first reported as a sequel of chronic neuroleptic treatment in 1962,[15] the term "tardive dystonia" was only recently applied to a series of neuroleptic-treated patients,[16] most suffering primarily from axial dystonias.

"Tardive akathisia" is an unpleasant sensation of internal restlessness that is partially relieved by volitional movements occurring in a patient who has received chronic neuroleptics. These movements typically involve the lower extremities.[17] Tardive akathisia is phenomenologically indistinguishable from acute or subacute akathisia, but these latter entities occur when a patient's normal dose is increased, and akathisia occurs within days or weeks. Tardive akathisia occurs after chronic exposure to neuroleptics and a steady or decreasing drug dosage.

Tics and myoclonic movements are also within the potential repertoire of TD, as well as "tardive tremor."[8,18,19] This latter movement disorder is a parkinsonian tremor that develops in the context of a constant or decreasing dose of neuroleptic. Importantly, it does not refer to parkinsonism or mouth tremor (rabbit syndrome) seen with starting neuroleptic medication or with a recent increase in neuroleptic dose. As a group, tardive movements often represent combinations of various movement disorders, so that dystonia and chorea, myoclonus and stereotypy, or dystonia and myoclonus occur together, rather than as isolated phenomena. When a physician encounters a patient with such mixed disorders, drug-induced, and specifically TD, should be carefully considered.

▶ EPIDEMIOLOGY AND NATURAL HISTORY

Despite methodological differences, recent reviews have shown a striking consistency in prevalence estimates of TD.[20] Jeste and Wyatt[21] reviewed 37 studies and, using a weighted mean methodology, found a prevalence of 17.6%. Kane and Smith[22] reviewed 56 studies and found a prevalence of 20%. Although more recent estimates (1981–1986) have been higher, with an average prevalence of 30%, overall, the average prevalence of TD is 15–20%.[23]

Another condition termed spontaneous dyskinesia resembles TD, but occurs independently of neuroleptic treatment. To estimate the true prevalence of TD, the frequency of this movement disorder should be subtracted from those for TD. The prevalence of spontaneous dyskinesia ranges from 0 to 53%.[24] Based on a series of 18 studies carried out between 1966 and 1983, Casey and Gerlach[25] calculated the prevalence rate of TD to be 19.8% and spontaneous dyskinesia as 5.9%. The net difference of 13.9 may, therefore, be a better estimate of the prevalence of TD. A small prospective study of schizophrenic patients attempted to answer the question of prevalence of spontaneous dyskinesia. In this small sample, 27 neuroleptic naïve patients were compared with 36 age-matched controls with neuroleptic exposure. Using the Abnormal Involuntary Movements Scale (AIMS), these investigators found an incidence of spontaneous dyskinesia in 4–11% of patients depending upon the stringency of diagnostic criteria.[26]

Gardos and Cole estimate that the risk for a schizophrenic inpatient developing TD during 1 year of continuous neuroleptic exposure is 4–5%.[27] Cumulative incidence of TD is approximately 10% after 2 years, 15% after 3 years, and 19% after 4 years. This linear increase over the first years of neuroleptic exposure argues against the idea of a period of maximal risk. Incidence estimates in other prospective studies range from 3 to 7%, with an average of approximately 5%.[28]

The above figures do not take into account several putative risk factors related to either the patient or the neuroleptic treatment. The most consistently observed risk factors are age and sex. Several studies have shown that the prevalence of TD is higher in women,[29,30] particularly when they are elderly.[31] Patients with affective disorders appear to be more susceptible to TD than patients with schizophrenia.[32,33] Crane first suggested that TD was more likely to develop in patients with neuroleptic-induced parkinsonism,[34] but this issue has been debated. Likewise, early studies suggested an association between TD and prior brain injury, electroconvulsive therapy (ECT), and lobotomy, but more recent studies have been less certain.[35]

Treatment-related variables such as type of neuroleptic, dose, duration of treatment, and concurrent drug treatment have additionally been studied as putative risk factors for TD. Early reports suggested that piperazine phenothiazines were most likely to result in TD,[36] but subsequent studies[37] have not confirmed this observation. Several studies[38] found that depot fluphenazine increased the prevalence of TD. Dose and duration of neuroleptic exposure have not been established as definite risk factors, but recent studies suggest that high dose[39] and high cumulative dose[40] are risk factors for eventual TD. Other drug exposure, including antiparkinson agents such as anticholinergics, have not been consistently related to an increased risk of TD.[20]

Although most of the risk factors appear to relate to TD regardless of phenomenological form, for tardive dystonia, special risk factor analyses have been performed with case–control methodology. In one study, tardive dystonia was more likely in patients with a prior history of acute neuroleptic-induced dystonia.[41]

If neuroleptics can be discontinued, the signs of TD resolve spontaneously in some patients,[6] transiently worsen in others, and persist in some. Predicting which symptomatic patients have "reversible" rather than "persistent" dyskinesias is at present impossible.[7] Approximately one third of patients with TD on neuroleptics remit within 3 months of discontinuation.[42] Resolution of movements can occur as long as 5 years after neuroleptic withdrawal.[29,43] Some studies suggested that discontinuation shortly after the onset of dyskinesias makes remission more likely, and that remissions are less likely in persons over the age of 60.[44]

In patients who remain on neuroleptics, there is little difference in overall prevalence over a 10-year period. In 63 patients examined at baseline, 5 and 10 years, most TD patients continued to have involuntary movements at all time points. Some patients (15%), however, remitted completely in spite of continued therapy.[45]

▶ PATHOPHYSIOLOGY

The pathophysiology of TD remains unknown, but interaction between dopamine, acetylcholine, γ-aminobutyric acid (GABA) and glutamate systems may be important. In 1973, Klawans[46] proposed that the hyperkinetic movements of TD reflected a relative overactivity of striatal dopaminergic systems and that a reciprocal antagonism existed between striatal cholinergic and dopaminergic systems. He suggested that TD related to denervation hypersensitivity of striatal dopamine receptors, resulting from the "chemical denervation" by the neuroleptic. This behavior was suggested to lead to increased numbers and affinity of D_2 receptors.

In spite of its usefulness, this hypothesis met several problems. For example, in laboratory studies, neuroleptic-induced receptor changes occur within days,[47] whereas movements in TD typically develop after months or years. Second, only about 15–20% of neuroleptic-exposed individuals develop TD,[20] whereas the neuroleptic-related increases in receptor density and sensitivity observed in animals was essentially a universal phenomenon.[48] In animals, neuroleptic-induced changes in motor behavior rarely persisted after drug withdrawal.[48] Finally, attempts to identify receptor changes specifically associated with TD in humans were uniformly inconclusive.

Gunne and Haggstrom[49] proposed that an abnormality of GABA-related striatal neurons caused TD. They observed changes in the GABA-synthesizing enzyme glutamic acid decarboxylase in animals treated with neuroleptics and noted similar changes in humans with TD.[50,51] Although they suggested that neuroleptics specifically injured GABAergic neurons, others have not replicated these findings.[52] Even if GABA changes occur, these changes could reflect increased dopaminergic activity, and thereby be only secondary phenomena.

New interest focuses on the glutamate system and theories of excitotoxins. Basal ganglia function is mediated in part by cortical glutaminergic afferents, which innervate two putaminal GABAergic neuronal populations.[53] Anatomical, physiological, and pharmacological studies suggest that these neuronal populations form specific, parallel efferent pathways that function with peptide cotransmitters.[54] These peptide-specific pathways have been termed "direct" and "indirect" by DeLong, and the "indirect" system[55] has been shown to be dysfunctional in some hyperkinetic disorders. In the "indirect" basal ganglia-thalamocortical circuit, somatotopically organized input from specific cortical areas facilitates striatal GABA/enkephalin (and possibly neurotensin) neurons. These putaminal neurons contain D_2 receptors and are inhibited by nigral dopamine input. They inhibit a second population of GABAergic neurons in the external portion of the globus pallidus. The pallidal GABAergic neurons in turn inhibit excitatory glutaminergic outflow from the subthalamic nucleus to GABA/substance P (and possibly dynorphin) neurons in the internal portion of the globus pallidus. These GABA/substance P/dynorphin cells inhibit thalamic outflow. A parallel "direct" system involves putaminal GABA/substance P neurons and does not include subthalamic nucleus. Studies using 2-deoxyglucose autoradiography in primates suggest that chronic neuroleptics lead to underactivity of the pathway from the subthalamic nucleus to the medial pallidal segment and substantia nigra (pars reticulata), leading ultimately to facilitation of thalamic outflow.[56]

Dysfunction of "indirect" striatal outflow may be consistent with the dopaminergic hypothesis of TD and other forms of chorea.[57] A drug-induced overactivity of dopaminergic function, perhaps via neuroleptic-induced changes in D_2 receptors, could cause excessive inhibition of subthalamic nucleus neurons and functional disinhibition of pallidothalamic outflow. Indirectly, blockade of dopamine receptors and resultant striatal changes could thereby alter expression of peptide co-transmitters. Haloperidol is known to cause alterations of concentrations of several peptide neurotransmitters, including enkephalins and neurotensin, although the clinical sign of such changes is unknown. The unusual temporal course of TD, becoming evident after prolonged exposure and persisting long after drug withdrawal, could in part reflect alterations of these peptide systems. A neurotransmitter system under greater current scrutiny is the cholinergic interneuron pathway in the striatum. Miller and Chouinard[58] reviewed clinical and laboratory evidence to suggest that primary attention to this cell population should not be overshadowed by studies of the dopaminergic system.

Psychiatric researchers have been studying the effects of polymorphisms of the D_2 receptor in schizophrenic patients with regard to therapeutic response.[58] Investigators have studied polymorphisms of dopamine receptors, serotonergic receptors, and cytochrome P450 genes in various ethnic populations with schizophrenia and TD.[59] Zai and colleagues investigated 12 polymorphisms in the *DRD2* gene in 232 whites and African Americans with TD.[60] Two genetypes (C957T and C939T) were found to significantly correlate with the presence of TD. Multiple studies have reported an association between the Ser9Gly *DRD3* gene and TD,[61–69] although these results have not been reproducible across all ethnic populations studied. A case–control trial of 335 Indian patients with schizophrenia and TD evaluated 24 makers from six genes (*DRD1*, *DRD2*, *DRD3*, *DRD4*, *DAT*, and *COMT*).[70] They found a higher incidence of TD in individuals with *DRD4* and *COMT*. The *5-HT2A* gene has been reported by several investigators to be associated with an increased risk of TD.[71–73] These findings, however, were not duplicated in a prospective trial.[74] The -607G/C promotor SNP of 5-HT2C has also been reported to be associated with TD in schizophrenic patients.[75] Finally, cytochrome P450 genes have been studied in schizophrenia and TD. The cytochrome P450 genes are involved in the metabolism of many antipsychotic medications. Polymorphisms that result in poor metabolism of the drugs were associated with a higher development of TD.[76–78] As understanding of the role of genetic polymorphism in the metabolism of medications and their effect upon receptors increases, these tools will likely help determine which medications may be the most effective for treatment with the least amount of side effects. Such studies must cross ethnic and racial groups because different polymorphisms occur across populations.

▶ NEUROIMAGING AND NEUROPATHOLOGY

Magnetic resonance (MR) studies have not revealed differences in size or configuration of basal ganglia or other structures in TD subjects.[79] Kuznetsov and colleagues used proton MR spectroscopy to study 40 patients with TD, spontaneous dyskinesia, antidepressant-treated patients without TD, and normal controls.[80] Subjects with TD or spontaneous dyskinesia had statistically significant reduction in the choline/creatine ratio over normal controls. This reduction suggests decreased membrane phosphatidylcholine turnover and damage to cholinergic neurons. Another study by the same group looked at diffusion-weighted imaging and magnetization transfer imaging in four groups (drug treated with TD, edentulous orodyskinesia, drug treated without TD, and control).[81] Globally different diffusion coefficient values were seen between drug-treated patients with TD and the control group, but the magnetization transfer ratios showed no significant difference. In one study of eight patients with TD using positron emission tomography (PET), D_2 receptor density was not greater than that in age-matched controls.[82] Nine subjects with chronically treated schizophrenia were compared with nine age-matched never-treated controls with schizophrenia for a PET study. The neuroleptic-treated patients were given a 2-week washout period. Each group underwent PET imaging to examine D_2 receptor binding potentials. This small study found a difference in the binding potential in that patients treated with neuroleptic medications had higher D_2 binding.[83] Although most subjects receiving neuroleptic medications have significant psychiatric illness and those not requiring neuroleptic medications are either less severely impaired or have shorter disease duration, additional control groups are needed for full interpretation of these findings. A nonpsychotic group, for instance patients with TD due to other dopamine-blocking agents such as metoclopramide or prochlorperazine used for gastrointestinal tract illness, may serve as a useful comparison group. TD is not associated with a characteristic pathological finding. In some reports, the brains are normal,[83] whereas other reports show inferior olive damage, substantia nigra or nigrostriatal degeneration, or swelling of large neurons of the caudate.[84] In two studies comparing the brains of TD patients to those of controls with similar psychiatric and treatment histories, nonspecific abnormalities were more common in TD.[85,86] Postmortem neurochemical studies found alterations in dopamine concentrations and receptor binding in the brains of persons with schizophrenia, but no specific change correlated with TD.[86]

▶ PREVENTION AND TREATMENT: GENERAL CONSIDERATIONS

CONSERVATIVE USE OF NEUROLEPTICS

TD has no universally effective therapy, and therefore prevention of its development must be the cornerstone of therapy. The first tenet of prevention is to use neuroleptics only when necessary (Table 35–1). The American Psychiatric Association[6] has published useful guidelines. Indications for the short-term use of neuroleptics (6 months or less) included the management of acute psychosis, preoperative medication, control of nausea, and treatment of primary neurological disorders such as Huntington's disease and Tourette's syndrome. Treatment for longer than 6 months was recommended for psychotic patients with objective evidence of continuing psychosis, recurrent psychosis with neuroleptic withdrawal, disabling neurological illnesses requiring chronic treatment, and demonstrated responsiveness to therapy. The continued need for chronic neuroleptic treatment should be regularly reassessed. Neuroleptics should be discontinued when their efficacy is uncertain, and should not be used if other agents can be substituted.

▶ **TABLE 35–1. TREATMENT OF TD REGARDLESS OF PHENOMENOLOGY**

Use neuroleptics only when needed
Withdraw neuroleptics as soon as medically possible
Use lowest possible doses

Although never evaluated in a clinical trial, simple precautions, such as using the lowest effective neuroleptic dose and regularly reevaluating the need for treatment, make intuitive sense.

CHOICE OF NEUROLEPTICS

For decades pharmacologists have searched for a specific antipsychotic drug that acts only at receptors mediating psychosis, without any dopamine-blocking effects elsewhere. This goal has not been achieved, but several "atypical" neuroleptics, most notably, clozapine, have relatively greater effects on limbic than striatal dopamine neurons, and appear to be less associated with TD.[87] Sokoloff and colleagues,[88] using molecular genetic techniques, proposed that a third dopamine receptor (D_3) distributed primarily in anterior, limbic, striatal regions may be important. "Typical" neuroleptics have much stronger affinities for D_2 than for D_3 receptors, whereas "atypical" neuroleptics have only a slightly greater preference for D_2 than for D_3 receptors.[89] If D_3 receptors primarily mediate behavior, rather than motoric function, specific D_3 antagonists should have minimal motoric adverse effects. Although a specific D_3 antagonist is not yet available, use of agents with high D_3 affinity, such as clozapine, sulpiride, thioridazine, olanzapine, and quetiapine may lower the relative risk of TD compared to other neuroleptics. With clozapine, frequent blood counts are necessary to monitor for the possibility of aplastic anemia. It is important to recognize that atypical neu-

▶ **TABLE 35–2. DRUGS ASSOCIATED WITH TD**

Antipsychotic agents (e.g., neuroleptic drugs)
Antidepressants with dopamine-receptor blockade (e.g., amoxapine)
Antinausea medications with dopamine receptor blockade (e.g., metoclopramide)

▶ **TABLE 35–3. TREATMENT OF TD BASED ON PHENOMENOLOGY**

Stereotypies, chorea, tics: reserpine, tetrabenazine, baclofen, benzodiazepines
Dystonia: reserpine, tetrabenazine, anticholinergics, botulinum toxin
Akathisia: reserpine, tetrabenazine, propranolol, opioids

roleptics have also been associated with TD and no neuroleptic is entirely safe.

If a patient is on a neuroleptic and develops early signs of TD, ideally the drug should be stopped immediately. Unfortunately, withdrawal of neuroleptic agents is impossible in the case of many psychotic patients or in disorders like severe Tourette's syndrome in which neuroleptics play a specific therapeutic role. In these cases, the behavioral benefit of continuing neuroleptics must be weighed against the relative neurological risk of TD. Specific data on this question are unclear. In many patients, the movement disorder may not progressively worsen, despite continued therapy.[6] It is well established that TD symptoms will diminish if the neuroleptic dose is increased, as higher medication doses increase blockade of striatal dopamine receptors. The use of the pathogenic agent, however, for the treatment of TD is advised only in life-threatening situations in which all other treatments have failed.

TREATMENT WITH OTHER DRUGS

Because many patients do not have spontaneous remissions of TD, and severe psychosis precludes neuroleptic discontinuation in others, a variety of therapeutic agents have been studied in TD (Table 35–2). Evaluations of all therapeutic regimens are confounded by the inability to distinguish spontaneous remission from treatment-related resolution, the wide variation in age, sex, duration and severity of movements, the lack of universal diagnostic techniques, and the absence of a single standardized rating scale. Also, some studies have treated only patients receiving concurrent neuroleptics, others have treated those no longer taking neuroleptics, and others have mixed the two groups. In the future, pharmacogenetics may play an increasing role in determining the therapeutic medication that best estimates high efficacy for treating psychosis and low risk for TD.

▶ TREATMENT OF SPECIFIC FORMS OF TARDIVE DYSKINESIA

The movements of TD are generally choreic–stereotypic or dystonic, and drug treatment protocols have primarily focused attention on one or the other (Table 35–3). Because many TD patients have a combination of movement types, the treating physician may need to weigh the relative impact of medications on each component of the movement disorder in a patient. Some treatments ameliorate one type of movement disorder while aggravating another.

CHOREIC-STEREOTYPIC MOVEMENTS

Treatments Involving the Dopamine System

The dopamine-depleting agents, reserpine and tetrabenazine, are the treatment of choice for the choreic or stereotypic movements of typical TD.[90] Reserpine depletes presynaptic stores of biogenic amines and is not believed to cause TD. Tetrabenazine, an agent with orphan drug status for Huntington's disease in the United States, also depletes presynaptic stores of biogenic amines but in addition blocks postsynaptic dopamine receptors. Because of this latter action, it could theoretically cause TD. A recent study attempted to answer the question of the efficacy and tolerability of tetrabenazine in the treatment of patients with refractory TD. Twenty patients were studied in this protocol. Each patient was videotaped before and after treatment with tetrabenazine. One patient could not tolerate tetrabenazine due to sedation and was withdrawn from the study. The remaining patients were treated for a mean of 20.3 weeks. The videotapes were then randomized and studied by a blinded rater using AIMS. Videotapes performed after treatment had a significant improvement over pretreatment videotapes. The mean dosage used in this study was 57.9 mg/day. All patients elected to continue treatment with tetrabenazine at the conclusion of the study.[91] Reserpine and tetrabenazine control the movements of TD in the majority of patients and, in some cases, treatment is followed by complete remission of TD.[92] The major side effects of these agents are orthostatic hypotension, depression, and drug-induced parkinsonism. Orthostatic hypotension occurs most commonly in older patients and may be avoided or minimized through the gradual introduction of the drug. Reserpine can be instituted at 0.125–0.25 mg daily and increased by 0.124–0.25 mg weekly, whereas tetrabenazine can be instituted at 25 mg daily and increased by 25 mg weekly or biweekly while monitoring blood pressure. Depression occurs commonly after prolonged (months to years) continuous therapy and generally requires drug discontinuation. Concurrent or latent depression can be severely exacerbated by reserpine and tetrabenazine. The full therapeutic response to a given dose of these agents is not apparent for several weeks and doses as high as 6 mg/day of reserpine may be necessary. Sometimes a neuroleptic will be needed for short-term control of TD during the few weeks when reserpine is being introduced.[93] Long-term experience of tetrabenazine treatment in hyperkinetic movement disorders was recently published.[94] This retrospective chart review examined and documented adverse events of 448 patients. Patients were treated for an average of 2.3 years. Common side effects included drowsiness (25%), parkinsonism (15.4%), depression (7.6%), and akathisia (7.6%). Age was the most reliable predictor of parkinsonism. TD was not described.

Low doses of dopamine agonists designed to activate presynaptic autoreceptors and thereby decrease dopamine release have not been consistently successful.[95] "Desensitizing" dopamine receptors by using increasing doses of L-dopa has not proved regularly beneficial.[96] The monoamine oxidase B inhibitor, selegiline, with putative antioxidant properties along with its dopaminergic facilitation, was tried in a placebo-controlled sample of TD patients, but drug-treated patients fared worse than those receiving placebo.[97] Calcium channel-blocking agents, usually used in cardiac patients, have been suggested to have dopamine-blocking properties, but, in one placebo-controlled study, diltiazem had no efficacy in treating TD.[98] Other studies have suggested that nifedipine and verapamil may be more effective,[99] but better placebo-controlled, and blinded protocols are needed to evaluate this drug class.

In severely disabled patients, particularly those with respiratory or oropharyngeal dyskinesias, withdrawal of the neuroleptic agent may be potentially life-threatening. In such severe cases, a return to neuroleptic medication may be the only feasible therapy. On the other hand, reserpine may be added to a stable dose of the neuroleptic and increased until the movements abate. When movements decrease, the neuroleptic may be slowly withdrawn to keep the dose of the causative agent at its very lowest level. Novel or atypical neuroleptics such as clozapine have been tried at high doses in treating TD, but side effects in the elderly (primarily sedation) preclude its general use.[100] In low doses (50–250 mg/day), clozapine has no significant effect on TD.

Treatments Involving the GABA System

Based on observations that prograbide co-administration with chronic haloperidol can reduce vacuous chewing movements in experimental animals, agents with effects on the GABA system have been tried in TD. The magnitude of benefit achieved with agents that are designed to augment GABA function is generally less than with drugs affecting dopamine systems. However, the therapeutic index is generally greater, so that a short trial with a GABAergic agent is often indicated in mild or moderate TD, before attempting treatment with dopamine-depleting agents. Respiratory depression may accompany overdose with this class of drugs, and the respiratory depressant effect may be additive with other central nervous system depressants, including ethanol. The physician must carefully consider suicide risk and concurrent medications when prescribing these agents.

Small studies have suggested that baclofen,[101] sodium valproate,[102] and γ-vinyl-GABA[103] produce mild improvement in TD, but the effects were inconsistent, short-lasting, or limited by side effects. Of these, baclofen, starting at 5 or 10 mg daily and increasing in 5–10 mg/day increments up to a maximum daily dose of 60–80 mg/day in three or four doses is most likely to be beneficial. In patients receiving concurrent neuroleptics, baclofen may aggravate drug-induced parkinsonism. Sedation is a common adverse effect, and ataxia, confusion, and auditory or visual hallucinations may rarely occur. Abrupt discontinuation should be avoided, because anxiety or hallucinations may occur. Coma, respiratory depression, and seizures may follow severe overdosage.

Benzodiazepines may potentiate central GABA transmission and are mildly beneficial in TD, especially clonazepam and diazepam.[104] Sedation, a common dose-limiting side effect of clonazepam, can be minimized by gradual drug introduction, beginning with 0.5 mg daily and increasing in 0.5–1 mg/week increments. Tolerance for the antidyskinetic effect is common after months of therapy, but Thaker and colleagues[104] found gradual withdrawal followed by a 2-week drug-free period to be associated with renewed efficacy when the drug was reintroduced.

Antioxidant and Other Pharmacological Strategies

A recent focus for studying the pathophysiology of several movement disorders is membrane damage due to free radical formation.[105,106] The antioxidant vitamin, tocopherol, a free radical scavenger, was found to be useful in several short trials of TD,[107,108] but not in all.[109] The dosages used are 400–1200 IU/day. Tocopherol could become an important therapeutic agent if further trials replicate these results. A recent study of 20 patients looked at higher dosages of tocopherol over a 7-month period. In this protocol, 9 patients were treated with tocopherol and 11 patients served as controls using improvement of AIMS scoring as an endpoint. The treatment group was started at 600 mg/day of tocopherol and increased to 1600 mg/day over 7 months. No significant difference in AIMS scores were found until treated patients reached 1600 mg/day.[110] High doses of tocopherol can be associated with increased cardiac risk and coagulation alterations. Careful consideration of patient compliance must be balanced with anticipated clinical benefit in prescribing a high dose of tocopherol. At present, a 2- or 3-week trial of tocopherol in mildly to moderately affected patients could be attempted before other therapeutic regimens, because no risk of treatment-related adverse effects is associated. Higher doses have also been studied with positive effects, but coagulation status and cholesterol levels need to be monitored.[110,111] The effect is not due to changes in neuroleptic drug levels.[111] Although most studies are short term, one has shown maintained improvement for as long as 36 weeks.[112]

Another vitamin therapy under study in tardive dyskinesia is pyridoxine (B_6). Five patients with TD underwent a 4-week open-label trial of pyridoxine at 100 mg/day. Severity of movements was rated using AIMS, Barnes Akathisia Rating Scale (BARS), and the Simpson-Angus Scale (SAS). Four patients had clinically significant improvement using the AIMS scale. No patients had significant side effects from the pyridoxine.[113] A second study was performed testing the efficacy of vitamin B_6 for the treatment of tardive dyskinesia. Fifteen patients with schizophrenia and TD were randomly assigned to treatment or placebo groups and treated for 4 weeks with either placebo or vitamin B_6 in escalating dosages to 400 mg/day. A washout period of 1 week was then instituted with a crossover to treatment or placebo. Patients were evaluated by a blinded rater using the Extrapyramidal Symptom Rating Scale. The treatment group had significant improvement in dyskinesia scores with vitamin B_6 at dosages of 300–400 mg/day.[114] A large double-blind placebo-controlled trial will be needed to determine whether pyridoxine is effective therapy for TD.

Levitaracetam has been studied in small, open-label trials for tardive dyskinesia.[115,116] Both trials showed an improvement in AIMS scores over baseline with one of the trials utilizing blinded videotape ratings. Levitaracetam was well tolerated without any change in psychiatric problems. The most common side effects included drowsiness, confusion, and vertigo. Because levitaracetam is excreted by the kidneys, it does not interfere with the metabolism of hepatically metabolized medications. A large double-blind placebo-controlled trial will be necessary to determine the clinical benefit of levitaracetam in TD.

Van harten reported the improvement in two patients with tongue protrusion from TD with botulinum toxin injections into the genioglossus muscles.[117] Both patients chose to continue treatment with botulinum toxin injections due to improvement in the severity of tongue protrusion movements.

In uncontrolled studies of small numbers of patients, several other agents have been reported to have minimal benefit in TD, including propranolol,[118] clonidine,[119] tryptophan,[120] cyproheptadine,[121] opiates,[122] manganese and niacin,[123] gabapentin,[124] donepezil,[125] and GM1 ganglioside.[126] Lithium was beneficial in some studies,[120] but not in others.[127] Agents affecting the cholinergic system have not had consistent benefit.[7] Buspirone has been used in an open-label trial with statistically significant improvement.[128] With the new interest in neuropeptides, ceruletide has been examined with clinical improvement. The putative advantage to such therapy is its once-weekly administration.[129]

Finally, ECT was reported to both ameliorate TD and increase its occurrence.[130] Because others have noted mood fluctuations to alter the expression of TD,[130,131] these observations may relate to ECT effects on mood more than movement disorders.

SURGICAL THERAPY

Deep brain stimulation has been used to treat a variety of movement disorders. It has been best studied in medication refractory Parkinson's disease, but has been used to treat other refractory movement disorders such as dystonia. Deep brain stimulation involves implantation of electrodes into the basal ganglia. The electrodes are connected to a battery pack. After implantation, adjustments are made to the stimulating electrodes to help control neurological symptoms. Case reports document the effectiveness of deep brain stimulation in medically refractory severe TD, including choreic TD and tardive dystonia.[132] A prospective phase two multicenter study studied the effects of deep brain stimulation in the globus pallidus interna (GPi) in severe TD.[133] Patients were blindly evaluated at 6 months with the Extrapyramidal Symptoms Rate Scale. In 10 patients treated with deep brain stimulation, a mean reduction of 50% in the Extrapyramidal Symptoms Rate Scale at 6 months was seen without any worsening of psychiatric symptoms. These are promising results, but a longer term blinded trial with an increased number of patients will be necessary to determine the long-term success of this treatment.

DYSTONIC MOVEMENTS

Some drugs are useful for dystonic, as well as choreic-stereotypic TD.[16] Like patients with unusual TD, those with tardive dystonia are helped by dopamine-depleting agents such as reserpine and tetrabenazine.[134] Clonazepam[104] and ECT[131] have been reported to be beneficial in a few patients.

In contrast, however, centrally active anticholinergic drugs (muscarinic receptor blockers) are a major therapeutic tool in tardive dystonia,[16] whereas in typical choreic-stereotypic TD, movements worsen when an anticholinergic is given.[46] In patients with both dystonia and typical TD, use of anticholinergics may improve dystonia but worsen other signs. In such cases, the physician should analyze which movements are causing the most pronounced disability. In most instances, other than cosmetic, dystonic movements are more disabling than choreic-stereotypic.

A treatment primarily designed for idiopathic dystonia, but recently applied to other dystonic syndromes, is botulinum toxin (BTX) injection. This biological toxin, when injected directly into overactive muscles, weakens them by decreasing acetylcholine release at the neuromuscular junction. For patients whose tardive dystonia affects primarily one body region, this treatment could be considered.[135] Two serotypes of BTX are currently available for widespread use: BTX-A and BTX-B. BTX-A has been available since the late 1980s and the majority of our clinical experience is with this agent. BTX-B has only been approved since 2000, so our clinical experience with this agent is limited. In patients with combined tardive dystonia and choreic TD movements, BTX can abate the dystonia, whereas other medications focus on the dyskinesias.[136]

In setting an order for medication trials in tardive dystonia, clonazepam or baclofen may be selected first if the dystonia is painful. A trial of anticholinergic agents may be useful in those without prominent choreic or stereotypic movements. Dopamine-depleting agents may be tried as more aggressive treatment in patients without depression. In persons with extreme disability, as is often the case in those with predominantly axial dystonias, neuroleptic agents may be necessary. In this case, careful explanation of the potential for the treatment to aggravate the tardive disorder is recommended. BTX is usually an adjunct medication, supplementing other drugs, and used to focus specific attention to one or two prominently involved body areas.

TARDIVE AKATHISIA

Tardive akathisia is phenomenologically indistinguishable from subacute akathisia accompanying neuroleptic treatment; hence, in patients requiring continued use of neuroleptic agents, a distinction between the two is particularly problematic. Dopamine-depleting agents are useful in tardive akathisia, in doses similar to those used in typical TD.[17] In a few persons, agents useful in treating subacute akathisia may be helpful, such as propranolol (60 mg daily)[137] and opiates (propoxyphene up to 100 mg daily or codeine up to 60 mg daily).[138] In contrast to subacute akathisia, anticholinergic agents are not helpful in tardive akathisia.

▶ FUTURE PERSPECTIVES

Newer imaging techniques have lead to greater understanding of the possible cellular changes that occur in tardive dyskinesia. In the future with increasing numbers of patients undergoing these scans, it may lead to novel treatments focused on neurotransmitter systems other than dopamine. One of the greatest advances is the discovery of pharmacogenomics and receptor variability. The differences in receptors have already helped to determine medical treatments for individuals with psychiatric illness. These same changes have been shown to be associated with increasing incidences of tardive dyskinesia in certain ethnic groups. These receptor changes may explain the variability of tardive dyskinesia and may lead to improved treatments and prevention with further understanding.

REFERENCES

1. Sewell DD, Jeste DV. Metoclopramide-associated tardive dyskinesia: An analysis of 67 cases. Arch Fam Med 1992;1:271–278.
2. Schoenecker VM. Ein eigentümliches Syndrom in oralen Bereich bei megphen Application. Nervenarzt 1957;28: 35–43.
3. Waddington JL. Tardive dyskinesia: A critical re-evaluation of the causal role of neuroleptics and of the dopamine receptor supersensitivity hypothesis. In Callaghan N, Galvin R (eds). Recent Researches in Neurology. London: Pitman, 1984, pp. 34–48.
4. Marsden CD, Tarsy D, Baldessarini RJ. Spontaneous and drug-induced movement disorders in psychotic patients. In Benson DF, Blumer D (eds). Psychiatric Aspects of Neurologic Disease. New York: Grune & Stratton, 1975, pp. 219–265.
5. Klawans HL, Bergen D, Bruyn GW, Paulson GW. Neuroleptic-induced tardive dyskinesia in nonpsychotic patients. Arch Neurol 1974;30:338–339.
6. Baldessarini RJ, Cole JO, Davis JM, et al. Tardive dyskinesia: Summary of a Task Force Report of the American Psychiatric Association. Am J Psychiatry 1980;137:1163–1172.
7. Tanner CM. Drug-induced movement disorders (tardive dyskinesia and dopa-induced dyskinesia). In Vinken PJ, Bruyn GW, Klawans HL (eds). Handbook of Clinical Neurology. Amsterdam: Elsevier, 1986, pp. 185–212.
8. Stacy M, Jankovic J. Tardive dyskinesia. Curr Opin Neurol Neurosurg 1991;4:343–349.
9. Feve A, Angelard B, Benelon G, et al. Postneuroleptic laryngeal dyskinesias: A cause of upper airway obstructive syndrome improved by local injections of botulinum toxin. Mov Disord 1993;7:217–219.
10. Gerratt BR, Goetz CG, Fisher HB. Speech abnormalities in tardive dyskinesia. Arch Neurol 1984;41:273–276.
11. Weiner WJ, Goetz CG, Nausieda PA, Klawans HL. Respiratory dyskinesias: Extrapyramidal dysfunction and dyspnea. Am J Intern Med 1978;88:327–331.
12. Wilcos PG, Bassett A, Jones B, Fleetham JA. Respiratory arrhythmias in patients with tardive dyskinesia. Chest 1994;105:203–207.
13. Casey DE, Rabins P. Tardive dyskinesias as a life-threatening illness. Am J Psychiatry 1978;135:486–488.
14. Feve A, Angelard B, Fenelon G, et al. Postneuroleptic laryngeal dyskinesias: A cause of upper airway obstructive

syndrome improved by local injections of botulinum toxin. Mov Disord 1993;8:217–219.

15. Druckman R, Seelinger D, Thulin B. Chronic involuntary movements induced by phenothiazines. J Nerv Ment Dis 1962;135:69–76.
16. Burke RE, Fahn S, Jankovic J, et al. Tardive dystonia: Late-onset and persistent dystonia caused by anti-psychotic drugs. Neurology 1982;32:1335–1346.
17. Christiansen E, Moller JE, Faurbye A. Neurological investigation of 28 brains from patients with dyskinesia. Acta Psychiatr Scand 1970;46:14–23.
18. Stacy M, Jankovic J. Tardive tremor. Mov Disord 1992;7:75–77.
19. Adler LA, Peselow E, Duncan E, et al. Vitamin E in tardive dyskinesia: Time course of effect after placebo substitution. Psychopharmacol Bull 1993;39:371–374.
20. Khot V, Egan MF, Hyde TM, Wyatt J. Neuroleptics and classic tardive dyskinesia. In Lang AE, Weiner WJ (eds). Drug-Induced Movement Disorders. Kisco: Futura, 1982, pp. 121–166.
21. Jeste DV, Wyatt RJ. Understanding and Treating Tardive Dyskinesia. New York: Guilford Press, 1982.
22. Kane JM, Smith JM. Tardive dyskinesia. Arch Gen Psychiatry 1982;39:473–481.
23. Baldessarini RJ, Cole JO, Davis JM, et al. Tardive Dyskinesia: A Task Force Report. Washington, DC: American Psychiatric Association, 1980.
24. Casey DE, Hansen TE. Spontaneous dyskinesia. In Jeste DV, Wyatt RJ (eds). Neuropsychiatric Movement Disorders. Washington, DC: American Psychiatric Press, 1984, pp. 68–95.
25. Casey DE, Gerlach J. Tardive dyskinesia. Acta Psychiatr Scand 1988;77:369–378.
26. Puri BK, Barnes TR, Chapman JM, et al. Spontaneous dyskinesia in first episode schizophrenia. J Neurol Neurosurg Psychiatry 1999;66:76–78.
27. Gardos G, Cole JO. Overview: Public health issues in tardive dyskinesia. Am J Psychiatry 1980;137:776–781.
28. Chouinard G, Annable L, Ross-Chouinard A, Mercier P. A 5-year prospective longitudinal study of tardive dyskinesia: Factors predicting appearance of new cases. J Clin Psychopharmacol 1988;8(suppl):21–26.
29. Jeste DV, Wyatt RJ. Understanding and Treating Tardive Dyskinesia. New York: Guilford Press, 1982.
30. Byne W, White L, Parella. Tardive dyskinesias in a chronically instutionalized population of elderly schizophrenic patients. Int J Geriatr Psychiatry 1998;13:473–479.
31. Smith JM, Oswald WT, Kucharski LT, Waterman LJ. Tardive dyskinesia: Age and sex differences in hospitalized schizophrenics. Psychopharmacology 1978; 58:207–211.
32. Gardos G, Casey D (eds). Tardive Dyskinesia and Affective Disorders. Washington, DC: American Psychiatric Press, 1983.
33. Yassa R, Nastase C, Dupont D, Thibeau M. Tardive dyskinesia in elderly psychiatric patients: A 5-year study. Am J Psychiatry 1992;149:1206–1211.
34. Crane GE. Persistent dyskinesia. Br J Psychiatry 1973;122:395–405.
35. Gupta S, Egan MF, Hyde TM. An unusual presentation of tardive dyskinesia with prominent involvement of the pectoral musculature. Biol Psychiatry 1993;33:291–292.
36. Gershanik OS. Drug-induced movement disorders. Curr Opin Neurol Neurosurg 1993;6:369–376.
37. Klawans HL, Goetz CG, Perlik S. Tardive dyskinesia: Review and update. Am J Psychiatry 1980;137:900–908.
38. Gardos G, Cole JO, LaBrie RA. Drug variables in the etiology of tardive dyskinesia: Application of discriminant function analysis. In Fahn WE, Smith RC, Davis JM, Domino EF (eds). Tardive Dyskinesia: Research and Treatment. New York: SP Medical and Scientific Books, 1980, pp. 291–296.
39. Morgernstern H, Glazer WM. Identify risk factors for tardive dyskinesia among long-term outpatients maintained with neuroleptic medications. Results of the Yale Tardive Dyskinesia Study. Arch Gen Psychiatry 1993;50: 723–733.
40. Cavallaro R, Regazzetti MG, Mundo E, et al. Tardive dyskinesia outcomes: Clinical and pharmacologic correlates of remission and persistence. Neuropsychopharmacology 1993;8:233–239.
41. Sachdev P. Risk factors for tardive dystonia: A case-control comparison with tardive dyskinesia. Acta Psychiatr Scand 1993;88:98–103.
42. Jeste DV, Jeste SD, Wyatt RJ. Reversible tardive dyskinesia: Implications for therapeutic strategy and prevention of tardive dyskinesia. Mod Probl Pharmacopsychiatry 1983;21:34–48.
43. Klawans HL, Tanner CM. The reversibility of permanent tardive dyskinesia. Neurology 1983;33(Suppl 2):163.
44. Quitkin F, Rifkin A, Gochfeld L, Klein DF. Tardive dyskinesia: Are first signs reversible. Am J Psychiatry 1977;134:84–87.
45. Gardos G, Casey DE, Cole HO, et al. Ten-year outcome of tardive dyskinesia. Am J Psychiatry 1994;151:836–841.
46. Klawans HL. The Pharmacology of Extrapyramidal Movement Disorders. Basel: Karger, 1973.
47. Klawans HL, Rubovits R. The effect of cholinergic and anti-cholinergic agents on tardive dyskinesias. J Neurol Neurosurg Psychiatry 1974;37:941–947.
48. Goetz CG, Klawans HL. Controversies in animal models of tardive dyskinesia. In Marsden CD, Fahn S (eds). Movement Disorders. Boston: Butterworth, 1982, pp. 263–276.
49. Gunne LM, Haggstrom JE. Pathophysiology of tardive dyskinesia. Psychopharmacology 1985;2(Suppl 2): 191–193.
50. Gunne LM, Haggstrom JE, Sjoquist B. Association with persistent neuroleptic-induced dyskinesia of regional changes in brain: GABA synthesis. Nature 1984;309: 347–349.
51. Andersson U, Haggstrom JE, Levin ED, et al. Reduced glutamate decarboxylase activity in the subthalamic nucleus in patients with tardive dyskinesia. Mov Disord 1989;4:37–46.
52. Mithani S, Atmada S, Baimbridge KG, Fubuger HC. Neuroleptic-induced oral dyskinesias: Effects of progabide and lack of correlation with regional changes in glutamic acid decarboxylase and choline acetyl transferase activities. Psychopharmacology 1987;93:94–100.
53. Alexander GE, Crutcher MD. Functional architecture of basal ganglia circuits: Neural substrates of parallel processing. Trends Neurosci 1990;13:266–271.

54. Graybiel AM. Neurotransmitters and neuromodulators in the basal ganglia. Trends Neurosci 1990;13:244–254.
55. DeLong MR. Primate model of movement disorders of basal ganglia origin. Trends Neurosci 1990;13:281–285.
56. Feve A, Angelard B, Fenelon G, et al. Neuroleptic-induced tardive dyskinesia in the Cebus monkey. Mov Disord 1992;7:32–37.
57. Reiner A, Albin RL, Anderson KD, et al. Differential loss of striatal projection neurons in Huntington disease. Proc Natl Acad Sci U S A 1988;85:5733–5737.
58. Miller R, Chouinard G. Loss of striatal cholinergic neurons as a basis for tardive and L-dopa-induced dyskinesias, neuroleptic-induced supersensitivity psychosis and refractory schizophrenia. Biol Psychiatry 1993;34:713–738.
59. Foster A, Miller DD, and Buckley PF. Pharmacogenetics and Schizophrenia. Psychiatr Clin N Am 2007;30:417–435.
60. Zai CC, Hwang RW, De Luca, et al. Association study of tardive dyskinesia and twelve DRD2 polymorphisms in schizophrenia patients. Int J Neuropsychopharmacol 2007 Oct;10(5):639–651.
61. Badri F, Masellis M, Petronis A, et al. Dopamine and serotonin system genes may predict clinical response to clozapine. Am J Hum Genet 1996;59:A247.
62. Steen VM, Lovlie R, MacEwan T, et al. DopamineD3-receptor gene variant and susceptibility to tardive dyskinesia in schizophrenic patients. Mol Psychiatry 1997;2:139–145.
63. Basile VS, Masellis M, Badri F, et al. Association of the Mscl polymorphism of the dopamine D3 receptor gene with tardive dyskinesia in schizophrenia. Neuropsychopharmacology 1999;21:17–27.
64. Segman R, Neeman T, Heresco-Levy U, et al. Genotypic association between the dopamine D3 receptor and tardive dyskinesia in chronic schizophrenia. Mol Psychiatry 1999;4:247–253.
65. Lio Dl, Yeh YC, Chen HM, et al. Association between the Ser9Gly polymorphism of the dopamine D3 receptor gene and tardive dyskinesia in Chinese schizophrenic patients. Neuropsychobiology 2001;44:95–98.
66. Lovlie R, Daly AK, Blennerhassett R, et al. Homozygosity for the Gly-9 variant of the dopamine D3 receptor and risk for tardive dyskinesia in schizophrenic patients. Int J Neuropsychopharmacol 2000;3:61–65.
67. Woo SI, Kim JW, Rha E, et al. Association of the Ser9Gly polymorphism in the dopamine D3 receptor gene with tardive dyskinesia in Korean schizophrenics. Psychiatry Clin Neurosci 2002;56:469–474.
68. Lerer B, Segman RH, Fangerau H, et al. Pharmacogenetics of tardive dyskinesia. Combined analysis of 780 patients supports association with dopamine D3 receptor gene Ser9Gly polymorphism. Neuropsychopharmacology 2002;27:105–119.
69. de Leon J, Susce MT, Pan RM, et al. Polymorphic variations in GSTM1, GSTT1, PgP, CYP2D6, CYP3A5, and dopamine D2 and D3 receptors and their association with tardive dyskinesia in severe mental illness. J Clin Psychopharmacol 2005;25:448–456.
70. Srivastana V, Varma PG, Prasad S, et al. Genetic susceptibility to tardive dyskinesia among schizophrenia: IV role of dopaminergic pathway polymorphisms. Pharmacogenetic Genomics 2006;16:111–117.
71. Segman Rh, Heresco-Levy U, Finkel B, et al. Association between the serotonin 2A receptor gene and tardive dyskinesia in chronic schizophrenia. Mol Psychiatry 2001;6:225–229.
72. Tan EC, Chang SA, Mahendran R, et al. Susceptibility to neuroleptic-induced tardive dyskinesia and the T102C polymorphism in the serotonin type 2A receptor. Biol Psychiatry 2001;50:144–147.
73. Lerer B, Segman Rh, Tan EC, et al. Combined analysis of 635 patients confirms an age related association of serotonin 2A receptor gene with tardive dyskinesia and specificity for non-orofacial subtype. Int J Neuropsychopharmacol 2005;8:411–425.
74. Basile VS, Ozdemir V, Masellis M, et al. Lack of association between serotonin-2A receptor gene (HTR2A) polymorphisms and tardive dyskinesia in schizophrenia. Mol Psychiatry 2001;6:230–234.
75. Zhang ZJ, Zhang XB, Sha WW, et al. Association of polymorphisms in the promoter region of the serotonin 5-HT2C receptor gene with tardive dyskinesia in patients with schizophrenia. Mol Psychiatry 2002;7:670–671.
76. Kapitany T, Meszaros K, Lenzinger E, et al. Geentic polymorphism for drug metabolism (CYP2D6) and tardive dyskinesia in schizophrenia. Schizophr Res 1998;32:101–106.
77. Ohmori O, Suzuki T, Kojima H, et al. Tardive dyskinesia and debrisoquine 4-hydroxylas (CYP2D6) genotype in Japanese schizophrenics. Schizophr Res 1998;32:107–113.
78. Ellingrod VL, Schulz SK, and Arndt S. Association between cytochrome P4502D6 (CYP2D6) genotype, antipsychotic exposure, and abnormal involuntary movement scale (AIMS) score. Psychiatr Genet 2000;10:9–11.
79. Buckley P, O'Callaghan E, Mulvany E. Basal Ganglia T2 relaxation times in schizophrenia: A quantitative magnetic resonance imaging study in relation to tardive dyskinesia. Psychiatry Res 1995;61:95–102.
80. Kuznetsov Y, Khiat A, Blanchet PJ, et al. Proton magnetic resonance spectroscopy study of dyskinesia patients. Mov Dis 2007;22:957–962.
81. Khiat A, Kuznetsov Y, Blanchet PJ, et al. Diffusion-weighted imaging and magnetization transfer imaging of tardive and edentulous orodyskinesia. Mov Dis 2008;23:1281–1285.
82. Blin J, Baron JC, Cambon H, et al. Dyskinesia: PET study. J Neurol Neurosurg Psychiatry 1989;52:1248–1252.
83. Hunter R, Blackwood W, Smith MC. Neuropathological findings in three cases of persistent dyskinesias following phenothiazines. J Neurol Sci 1968;7:263–273.
83. Silverstri S, Seeman MV, Negrete JC, et al. Increased dopamine D2 receptor binding after long-term treatment with antipsychotics in humans: A clinical PET study. Psychopharmacology 2000;152:174–180.
85. Christiansen E, Moller JE, Faurbye A. Neurological investigation of 28 brains from patients with dyskinesia. Acta Psychiatr Scand 1970;46:14–23.
86. Jellinger K. Neuropathologic findings after neuroleptic long-term therapy. In Roizin L, Shiraki H, Grecevic N (eds). Neurotoxicology. New York: Raven Press, 1977, pp. 25–42.
87. Lieberman J, Johns C, Cooper T, et al. Clozapine pharmacology and tardive dyskinesia. Psychopharmacology 1989;99:S54–S59.

88. Sokoloff P, Giros B, Mrtres MP, et al. Molecular cloning and characterization of a novel dopamine receptor (D3) as a target for neuroleptics. Nature 1990;347:146–151.
89. Strange PG. Interesting times for dopamine receptors. Trends Neurosci 1991;14:43–45.
90. Jankovic J, Orman J. Tetrabenazine therapy of dystonia, chorea, tics and other dyskinesias. Neurology 1988;38:391–394.
91. Ondo WG, Hanna PA, Jankovic J. Tetrabenazine treatment for tardive dyskinesia: Assessment by randomized videotape protocol. Am J Psychiatry 1999;156:1279–1281.
92. Lang AE, Marsden CD. Alphamethylparatyrosine and tetrabenazine in movement disorders. Clin Neuropharmacol 1982;5:375–387.
93. Stacy M, Francisco C, Jankovic J. Tardive stereotypy and other movement disorders in tardive dyskinesia. Neurology 1993;43:937–941.
94. Kenney C, Hunter C, Jankovic J. Long-term tolerability of tetrabenazine in the treatment of hyperkinetic movement disorders. Mov Dis 2007;22:193–197.
95. Tamminga CA, Chase TN. Bromocriptine and CF 25–396 in the treatment of tardive dyskinesia. Arch Neurol 1980;37:204–205.
96. Alpert M, Friedhoff A. Clinical application of receptor modification treatment. In Fann WE, Smith RC, Davis JM, Domino EF (eds). Tardive Dyskinesia: Research and Treatment. New York: Spectrum, 1980, pp. 471–474.
97. Goff DC, Renshaw PF, Sarid-Segal O, et al. A placebo-controlled trial of selegiline (L-deprenyl) in the treatment of tardive dyskinesia. Biol Psychiatry 1993;33:700–706.
98. Loonen AJ, Verwey HA, Roels PR, et al. Is diltiazem effective in treating the symptoms of (tardive) dyskinesia in chronic psychiatric inpatients? A negative, double-blind, placebo-controlled trial. J Clin Psychopharmacology 1992;12:39–42.
99. Cates M, Lusk K, Wells BG. Are calcium-channel blockers effective in the treatment of tardive dyskinesia? Ann Pharmacother 1993;27:191–196.
100. Simpson CM, Lee JH, Shrivastava RK. Clozapine and tardive dyskinesia. Psychopharmacologia 1978;56:75–80.
101. Stewart RM, Rollins J, Beckham B, Roffman M. Baclofen in tardive dyskinesia patients maintained on neuroleptics. Clin Neuropharmacol 1982;5:365–373.
102. Nair NPV, Lal S, Schwartz G, Tharundayil JX. Effects of sodium valproate and baclofen in tardive dyskinesia: Clinical and neuroendocrine studies. Adv Biochem Psychopharmacol 1980;24:437–441.
103. Tell GP, Schecter PJ, Koch-Weser J, et al. Effects of gamma vinyl GABA [letter]. N Engl J Med 1981;305:581–582.
104. Thaker GK, Nguyen JA, Strauss ME, et al. Clonazepam treatment of tardive dyskinesia: A practical GABA mimetic strategy. Am J Psychiatry 1990;147:445–451.
105. Lohr JB, Kuczenski R, Bracha HS, et al. Increased indices of free radical activity in the cerebrospinal fluid of patients with tardive dyskinesia. Biol Psychiatry 1990;28: 535–539.
106. Cadet JL. Movement disorders: Therapeutic role of vitamin E. Toxicol Ind Health 1993;9:337–347.
107. Elkashef AM, Ruskin PE, Bacher N, Barrett D. Vitamin E and the treatment of tardive dyskinesia. Am J Psychiatry 1990;147:505–506.
108. Dabiri LM, Pasta D, Darby JK, Mosbacher D. Effectiveness of vitamin E for treatment of long-term tardive dyskinesia. Am J Psychiatry 1994;151:925–926.
109. Shriqui CL, Bradwejn J, Annable L, Jones BD. Vitamin E in the treatment of tardive dyskinesia: A double-blind placebo-controlled study. Am J Psychiatry 1992;149: 391–393.
110. Adler LA, Peselow E, Rotrosen J, et al. Vitamin E treatment of tardive dyskinesia. Am J Psychiatry 1993;150: 1405–1407.
111. Egan MF, Hyde TM, Albers GW, et al. Treatment of tardive dyskinesia with vitamin E. Am J Psychiatry 1992;149: 773–777.
112. Sajjad SH. Vitamin E in the treatment of tardive dyskinesia: A preliminary study over 7 months at different doses. Int Clin Psychopharmacol 1998;13(4):147–155.
113. Lerner V, Kaptsan A, Miodownik, et al. Vitamin B_6 in treatment of tardive dyskinesia: A preliminary case series study. Clin Neuropharmacol 1999;22:241–243.
114. Lerner V, Miodownik C, Kaptsan A, et al. Vitamin B_6 in the treatment of tardive dyskinesia: A double-blind, placebo-controlled, crossover study. Am J Psychiatry 2001;159:1511–1514.
115. Konitsiotis S, Pappa S, Mantas C, et al. Levetiracetam in tardive dyskinesia: An open label study. Mov Dis 2006;21:1219–1221.
116. Meco G, Fabrizio E, Epifanio A, et al. Levetiracetam in tardive dyskinesia. Clin Neuropharmacol 2006;29:265–268.
117. van Harten PN, Hovestadt A. Botulinum toxin as a treatment for tardive dyskinesia. Mov Dis 2006;21: 1276–1277.
118. Bacher NM, Lewis HA. Low dose propranolol in tardive dyskinesia. Am J Psychiatry 1980;137:495–497.
119. Freedman R, Bell J, Kirch D. Clonidine therapy for coexisting psychosis and tardive dyskinesia. Am J Psychiatry 1980;137:629–630.
120. Prange AJ Jr, Wilson IC, Morris CE. Preliminary experience with tryptophan and lithium in the treatment of tardive dyskinesia. Psychopharmacol Bull 1973;9:36–37.
121. Gardos G, Cole JO. Pilot study of cyproheptadine (Periactin) in tardive dyskinesia. Psychopharmacol Bull 1978;14:18–20.
122. Stoessl AJ, Polanski E, Frydryszak H. The opiate antagonist naloxone suppresses a rodent model of tardive dyskinesia. Mov Disord 1993;8:445–452.
123. Kunin RA. Manganese and niacin in the treatment of drug-induced dyskinesia. J Orthomol Psychiatry 1976;5:4–27.
124. Hardoy MC, Hardoy MJ, Carta MG, et al. Gabapentin as a promising treatment for antispychotic-induced movement disorders in schizoaffective and bipolar patients. J Affect Dis 1999;54:315–317.
125. Bergman J, Dwolatzky T, Brettholz I, et al. Beneficial effect of donepezil in the treatment of elderly patients with tardive movement disorders. J Clin Psychiatry 2005;66:107–110.
126. Peselow ED, Irons S, Rotrosen J, et al. GM1 ganglioside as a potential treatment in tardive dyskinesia. Psychopharmacology 1989;25:277–280.
127. Reda FA, Scanlan JM, Escobar JI, et al. Lithium carbonate in the treatment of tardive dyskinesia. Am J Psychiatry 1975;132:560–562.

128. Simpson GM, Branchez MH, Lee HJ. Lithium in tardive dyskinesia. Pharmakopsychiatr Neuropsychopharmakol 1976;9:76–80.
129. Moss LE, Neppe VM, Drevets WC. Buspiron in the treatment of tardive dyskinesia. J Clin Psychopharmacol 1993;13:204–209.
130. Kojima T, Yamauchi T, Miyasaka M, et al. Treatment of tardive dyskinesia with ceruletide: A double-blind, controlled study. Psychiatry Res 1992;43:129–136.
131. Price TRP, Levin R. Effects of electroconvulsive therapy on tardive dyskinesia. Am J Psychiatry 1978;135:991–993.
132. Trottenberg T, Volkmann J, Deuschl G, et al. Treatment of severe tardive dystonia with pallidal deep brain stimulation. Neurology 2005;64:344–346.
133. Damier P, Thobois S, Witjas T, et al. Bilateral deep brain stimulation of the globus pallidus to treat tardive dyskinesia. Arch Gen Pyschiatry 2007;64:170–176.
134. Unrbrand L, Faurbye A. Reversible and irreversible dyskinesia after treatment with perphenazine, chlorpromazine, reserpine and ECT therapy. Psychopharmacologia 1960;1:408–418.
135. Kang JU, Burke RE, Fahn S. Natural history and treatment of tardive dystonia. Mov Disord 1986;1:193–208.
136. Jankovic J, Brin MF. Therapeutic uses of botulinum toxin. N Engl J Med 1991;324:1186–1194.
137. Stip E, Faughnan M, Desjardin I, Labrecque R. Botulinum toxin in a case of severe tardive dyskinesia mixed with dystonia. Br J Psychiatry 1992;161:867–868.

CHAPTER 36

Other Choreatic Disorders

Margery H. Mark

▶ CHOREA

Chorea (Greek for "dance") consists of irregular, unpredictable, brief movements that flow from one body part to another in a nonstereotyped fashion. They may be incorporated, especially in milder cases, into more purposeful movements. They may consist of small twitches or larger jerks of any body part. Choreiform movements rarely occur in isolation; rather, they may be often seen in a spectrum with slower, distal, writhing, sinuous movements called *athetosis*, and described as *choreoathetosis*. In many disorders in which chorea is a feature, it is not uncommon to see other movement disorders as well, particularly dystonia. The converse of speed and amplitude from athetoid movements are *ballistic* movements (i.e., fast and large amplitude), which are usually seen unilaterally as *hemiballism*, although bilateral (*paraballism* or *biballism*) may be encountered. Ballistic movements, the most extreme type of movement disorder, are large amplitude, usually proximal flinging of a limb or body part. Although some investigators separate these disorders, others (including the present author) consider ballism to be a severe form of chorea, and in fact many cases of resolving ballistic movements taper down to chorea.[1]

The prototypic choreic disorder is *Huntington's disease* (HD), discussed in detail in the preceding chapters (see Chapters. 32–34). The phenomenology of chorea in other disorders, both primary and secondary, is essentially the same as in HD; likewise, theories of the pathophysiology of the choreas, for the most part, are very similar. Similarly, Wilson's disease (see Chapter. 42), tardive dyskinesia (see Chapter. 35), and treated Parkinson's disease (see Chapter. 13, and 15) may also demonstrate chorea; the reader is referred to those chapters for more details. In this chapter, we will focus on several clinical entities in which chorea plays a significant role. Other related movement disorders will also be discussed.

▶ THE IMMUNE SYSTEM, HORMONES, AND CHOREA

It has long been recognized that several seemingly unrelated conditions have been uncommonly associated with chorea: rheumatic fever, systemic lupus erythematosus (SLE), and pregnancy (and its flip side, use of oral contraceptives). The pathophysiology of chorea in these conditions may be similar and will be explored below.

SYDENHAM'S CHOREA

In 1686, Thomas Sydenham described the clinical syndrome that now bears his name.[2] Originally called St Vitus dance, as well as chorea minor, acute chorea, and rheumatic chorea, *Sydenham's chorea* (SC) not uncommonly follows rheumatic fever in children and adolescents. Antecedent infection with group A streptococcus is usual, although many patients do not give a history of streptococcal infection; and, as the chorea may occur 6 months or more after infection, antistreptolysin and antistreptococcal antibodies may not be elevated. Adequate antibiotic therapy has dramatically reduced the occurrence of rheumatic fever in the United States, and thus of SC,[3] although it may still be found. It may be seen more often in children from developing countries who lack routine antibiotic care. In fact, a series from Turkey in the mid-1990s showed that acute rheumatic fever is not only still very prevalent in that country, but remains a significant cause of morbidity, and revealed that 20% of patients (45/228) admitted to hospital with rheumatic fever had chorea.[4] Another series of admissions to one hospital in Chile from 1976 to 1989 demonstrated that 16% of attacks of acute rheumatic fever (70/438 in 402 patients) presented with SC.[5]

The clinical syndrome of SC, in addition to the chorea, is characterized by a semiacute illness involving muscular weakness, hypotonia, dysarthria, and behavioral abnormalities. The most common of the behavioral problems is obsessive–compulsive symptomatology, with 82% of individuals affected in one series; nearly half of these children met criteria for frank obsessive–compulsive disorder.[6,7] They also demonstrate increased emotional lability, motoric hyperactivity, irritability, distractibility, and age-regressed behavior. Behavioral symptoms may begin several days to weeks prior to onset of chorea and wax and wane with motor signs.[6] The chorea is usually bilateral, but may be unilateral in about 20% of patients. It may begin either abruptly or insidiously, worsen over 2 to 4 weeks, and usually resolves spontaneously in 3 to 6 months, although some patients may have residual chorea. Recurrences may occur in about 20% of patients, usually within about 2 years,[3,8] and hypothesized to be more likely related to subclinical or autoimmune basal ganglia damage.[9] The vast majority of patients are between 5 and 15 years old at first occurrence, and girls are affected about twice as frequently as boys, especially in the peripubescent ages, suggesting a role for sex hormones in this disorder.[10]

The EEG is often abnormal, with slowing, particularly irregular occipital slowing.[11,12] Neuroimaging studies may shed some light on the pathophysiology (discussed below). Magnetic resonance imaging (MRI) in two cases revealed increased signal on T_2-weighted images in the striatum and globus pallidus, with resolution of signal intensity upon clinical improvement,[13,14] whereas another showed permanent basal ganglia injury.[15] Yet another case demonstrated multiple areas of abnormal signal on MRI, with resultant angiography revealing vasculitis attributed directly to her SC.[16] One analysis of MRI of 24 subjects with SC demonstrated increased size of caudate, putamen, and globus pallidus,[17] suggesting an inflammatory process. Functional neuroimaging, evaluating regional cerebral glucose metabolism using positron emission tomography (FDG-PET), in SC differs from HD and other hereditary choreas. In HD, there is striatal hypometabolism,[18] but in SC, has been seen increased glucose metabolism in bilateral striatum in two girls with Sydenham's and contralaterally in an elderly woman with hemichorea as a residual to adolescent-onset Sydenham's[19,20]; the abnormality on PET was reversible in the girls following clinical improvement. A report of single photon emission computed tomographic (SPECT) scanning in 10 patients with SC demonstrated basal ganglia hyperperfusion in the six most acute cases; the rest were normal.[21]

The chorea in SC responds to dopaminergic blockers (pimozide may be less sedating than haloperidol)[22] or depleters,[23] but, as it tends to be self-limited, should be restricted to those in whom the chorea is so severe as to interfere with function. More recent studies showed more efficacy obtained from valproate and carbamezepine than with haloperidol.[24,25] Corticosteroids, intravenous immunoglobulin, and plasmapheresis may also have a role in the treatment of SC.[12] Antibiotic therapy with penicillin to prevent cardiac dysfunction is usually indicated as well.

A recently described (and still controversial[26]) clinical entity, pediatric autoimmune neuropsychiatric disorders associated with streptococcal infections (PANDAS), may overlap with SC.[27,28] Clinically, while obsessive–compulsive behaviors predominate in both conditions, the movement disorder in PANDAS is more commonly a tic rather than chorea, although chorea occurs. Differentiation of these two disorders may be critical because of divergent therapeutic options: long-term penicillin in SC to reduce the risk of rheumatic heart disease (unnecessary in PANDAS) while plasma exchange, intravenous immunoglobulin, and tonsillectomy have been shown to reduce neuropsychiatric symptom severity in children with PANDAS.[27]

CHOREA GRAVIDARUM

Pregnancy is another nonneurological condition that may rarely present with chorea as *chorea gravidarum* (CG); it is more frequently seen in women with a prior history of SC, or the chorea may be secondary to other conditions (e.g., SLE[29]). It is far less common than when first reviewed in 1932,[30] and morbidity and maternal and fetal mortality have continued to drop with each subsequent decade.[31,32] In the original reports, approximately 60% of women with CG had an antecedent episode of chorea in childhood, almost certainly SC. CG may also herald HD[33] or SLE.[34] It usually resolves without sequelae following delivery. In a single report of a fatal case,[35] neuronal loss and astrocytosis in the striatum, especially the caudate, was found. Although this pathology was nonspecific for CG, it suggests that the chorea has a structural basis in some cases.

Similarly, chorea may occur with the use of estrogens. Chorea following oral contraceptive use has been reported.[36–39] An interesting report[40] describes recurrent chorea in a 61-year-old woman following the use of a topical vaginal cream that contained conjugated estrogen. She had CG when she was younger. As estrogen may affect dopamine receptor sensitivity by upregulating receptors in experimental animals, these reports suggest a role for hormone-induced chorea, especially in the setting of previously damaged basal ganglia.[10,36,41] As with CG, chorea with oral contraceptive use may be the presenting symptom of SLE.[42]

SYSTEMIC LUPUS ERYTHEMATOSUS AND THE ANTIPHOSPHOLIPID ANTIBODY SYNDROME

Of the other systemic disorders that cause chorea, SLE is the most common, although only about 2% of SLE patients have chorea.[43] As with SLE in general, it tends to occur primarily in girls and women, and it occurs more commonly in those with younger onset of their SLE. Chorea may be the sole neurological manifestation preceding the diagnosis of SLE in nearly one quarter of those afflicted.[44] The chorea may last from days to years; it may be episodic and recurrent. It is often unilateral, although it may be generalized. Other neurological manifestations of SLE include stroke, transient ischemic attacks, seizures, migraine, psychosis, and dementia. Diagnosis of SLE is important because of treatment aimed at the more serious and life-threatening complications of this disease. Treatment of the chorea, as in other disorders, may occasionally require antidopaminergics. Steroids and antithrombotic agents such as aspirin and warfarin have also been found to be effective.[45]

A related disorder, *primary antiphospholipid antibody syndrome* (PAPS), has also been associated with chorea.[46] These patients do not fit criteria for SLE. Clinically, PAPS is also associated with, among other things, stroke, transient cerebral ischemia, migraines, recurrent spontaneous abortions, venous thrombosis, cardiac valvular dysfunction, and thrombocytopenia.[47–51] The hallmark is the presence of antiphospholipid antibodies (aPL), consisting of false-positive VDRL, anticardiolipin antibody, and lupus anticoagulant, all of which are also associated with (and were first described in) SLE. These antibodies, both IgG and IgM, inhibit coagulation by interfering with phospholipid-dependent coagulation tests and prolong activated partial thromboplastin time in vitro but are paradoxically associated with thrombosis rather than with bleeding.[52] As with SLE, chorea is more frequently associated with younger age of onset (under 15 in a pan-European cohort of 1000 patients) and female gender.[51] The recently identified anti-β(2)-glycoprotein I antibody[53,54] was found to be higher in cases with chorea, and in some cases, it was the only aPL found on testing, indicating that current evaluations of suspected PAPS or SLE should include anti-β(2)-glycoprotein I antibody testing.

PATHOPHYSIOLOGY: IMMUNE-MEDIATED MECHANISM?

Most interesting is the occurrence of chorea in SC, CG, SLE, PAPS, or without such associations in the presence of aPL.[55] Although thrombotic vascular occlusion is implicated in some cases,[56–58] the current theory of the pathophysiology of chorea in all these disorders in immunological; this is further supported by an MRI study of eight patients with SLE, seven of whom had scans that were negative for lesions in the basal ganglia in the presence of chorea.[59] Many cases of chorea have now been reported with the presence of aPL in SLE[57,60] and PAPS.[61] Interestingly, there are now also cases of SC (or rheumatic fever)[62] and CG and/or oral contraceptive use[63,64] with evidence of aPL, and others with isolated aPL[65,66] who do not meet criteria for either SLE or PAPS. There are further cases with combination of SC, SLE, and aPL with chorea.[67]

As with SC, increased striatal:cortical FDG metabolism measured with PET was found in SLE patients,[68] and in two patients with alternating hemichorea with PAPS, evidence was found on PET for contralateral striatal hypermetabolism.[69,70] These findings, along with similar results in SC,[19,20] and with oral contraceptive use[71] suggest that hypermetabolism in these disorders reflects an autoimmune process, with antibodies directly affecting basal ganglia neurons.[55,71,72] This hypothesis was first supported by the work of Husby and colleagues,[73] who showed that antibodies from both serum and spinal fluid from SC patients cross-reacted with antigens in the cytoplasm of caudate and subthalamic nucleus neurons, and later confirmed by Church and colleagues[74] who demonstrated the presence of anti-basal ganglia antibodies in acute and persistent SC using Western immunoblotting and immunofluorescence techniques. Streptococcal antigens have also been shown to cross-react to neuronal epitopes[75,76] as well as to cardiolipin,[75] further supporting the hypothesis of cross-reactive antibody-mediated inflammation or hypermetabolic dysfunction in these conditions. Nevertheless, while anti-basal ganglia antibodies are associated with 100% of acute cases of SC, only about two thirds of persistent cases have these antibodies, suggesting that the late occurrence of chorea in these patients may be secondary to dopamine hypersensitivity of chronically damaged basal ganglia neurons, likely following induction of an earlier autoimmune antibody response.[77]

▶ HEREDITARY CHOREAS

NEUROACANTHOCYTOSES: CHOREA-ACANTHOCYTOSIS AND MCLEOD'S SYNDROME

Chorea-acanthocytosis (CA) is an uncommon autosomal-recessive disorder recognized since the mid-1960s that has also been called familial amyotrophic chorea, amyotrophic chorea with acanthocytes, and Levine–Critchley's syndrome.[78–84] The more general nomenclature, neuroacanthocytosis (NA), was employed as well, given the wide variety of neurological abnormalities involved, but now should be used more as an umbrella term encompassing CA and the related McLeod's syndrome.[85] CA is characterized by acanthocytosis, normal β-lipoproteins, and multiple movement disorders. Chorea is the most prominent finding, but dystonia (especially lingual action dystonia), motor and vocal tics, and parkinsonism all occur, and may occur in the same individual. Lingual–labial dyskinesias may be so severe as to cause self-mutilation. An axonal sensorimotor polyneuropathy, mostly affecting the distal portion of nerves,[86] is common, along with attendant amyotrophy and, consequently, elevated CPK. Autonomic nervous system involvement, both sympathetic and parasympathetic, has been reported.[87] Decreased or absent reflexes, dysarthria, and dysphagia also occur. Generalized seizures occur in more than half the cases. Cognitive impairment, on the other hand, has been less commonly reported, but mild frontal lobe dysfunction probably exists in at least half of affected individuals.[88–90] Onset is usually in the 20s to 30s, and death occurs, on average, in about 9 years.[89] Some authors propose that NA is, in fact, a heterogeneous group of neurodegenerative disorders, as unusual families have been described, including an autosomal-dominant family with cortical intranuclear inclusions[91]; further, association of some cases with the McLeod's phenotype (a weak expression of Kell blood group antigens), which is X-linked, raised the issue of whether some patients with apparent CA and McLeod's syndrome had the same disease.[92–94] Phenotypically, in McLeod's syndrome, chorea generally occurs in the fifth decade. Facial grimacing and involuntary vocalizations may be present, but lip-biting and facial tics are uncommon, as opposed to CA. Dysphagia is notably absent.[95] Psychiatric signs and symptoms may occur.[96]

As with other disorders, elucidation of genetics has clarified the diagnostic dilemma. Linkage to chromosome 9q21[97] was found in CA, followed by discovery of autosomal-recessive mutations of the gene (***VPS13A***) coding for a new protein, chorein.[98] Chorein is expressed in all human cells, including those in McLeod's syndrome and HD, but not in CA, suggesting a loss of chorein expression as a pathophysiological mechanism in CA.[99] McLeod's syndrome, long known to be X-linked, has more recently been characterized as a disorder in which there is absence of the Kell-binding erythrocyte membrane protein Kx. Kx is encoded by the *XK* gene; several mutations are responsible for the phenotype.[95,96] Molecular genetic analysis, finally, now allows the two syndromes to be distinguished despite phenotypic heterogeneity.[85]

Treatment is symptomatic; the chorea may respond to reduction of dopaminergic transmission (although concomitant parkinsonism may worsen), and seizures should be treated with appropriate anticonvulsants. Levetiracetam as been reported to be very helpful in treating the tics and other movements in CA[100] (as well as the chorea in other disorders[101,102]). In the last decade, some patients with CA have responded successfully to treatment with deep brain stimulation (DBS) of the thalamus[103] and, more recently, of the globus pallidus internus.[104,105] **In all but the case of Guehl and colleagues was high-frequency stimulation necessary to treat the chorea and truncal spasms.**

Pathologically, the findings in the central nervous system are principally confined to the basal ganglia. The caudate and putamen are primarily affected, with neuronal loss and gliosis. The globus pallidus is almost as severely involved. Cortex, subthalamic nucleus, cerebellum, pons, and medulla are generally spared.[89] In cases with prominent parkinsonism, reduced neuronal density in the substantia nigra, primarily the ventrolateral region, has been reported.[106] The pathology of the peripheral nerves reveals a distal axonal neuropathy.[86,107] In a study of the neurochemical findings in the brains of patients with NA, the main abnormality was depletion of dopamine and its metabolites, particularly in the striatum; there were also increases in norepinephrine in putamen and globus pallidus and marked reduction in substance P in striatum and substantia nigra.[108]

Functional neuroimaging with PET in patients with CA[109,110] and McLeod's syndrome[96,111] has demonstrated striatal hypometabolism with FDG, similar to findings in HD.[18] Brooks and colleagues evaluated the presynaptic and postsynaptic dopaminergic system in CA.[112] They found ^{18}F-fluorodopa (^{18}F-dopa) uptake to be normal in caudate and anterior putamen but significantly reduced (in the range of patients with Parkinson's disease) in the posterior putamen. Using ^{11}C-raclopride to evaluate the integrity of striatal D_2 receptors, they found reduction in both caudate and putamen:cerebellum uptake ratios, reflecting a 65% (caudate) and 53% (putamen) loss of D_2-receptor binding sites. Their findings indicate a loss of nigrostriatal dopaminergic projections and of D_2-receptor neurons, and are consistent with a clinical picture of both chorea and parkinsonism in CA.

The erythrocyte abnormalities in CA have been a subject of scrutiny, and some feel that the red cell membrane dysfunction may hold the key to understanding the pathophysiology of this disorder. Although acanthocytes define the disorder (as well as McLeod's syndrome), they are variably seen in CA, and they may be absent in an occasional patient.[107] They are also frequently seen, or can be induced, in obligate heterozygotes.[113] The red blood cells of patients with CA can be induced to form spiny or rounded projections by dilution in normal saline, in vitro aging, or contact with glass.[114] Interestingly, echinocytic transformation is completely reversible by incubation with chlorpromazine. CA erythrocytes also have abnormal membrane-bound fatty acid structures, with increases in palmitic (C16:0) and docosahexaenoic (C22:6) acids and reduction in stearic acid (C18:0).[115] Bosman and coworkers[116,117] have demonstrated abnormal erythrocyte band 3 structure and sulfate flux measurements, indicating anion transport activity is reduced in the erythrocytes of patients with definite CA and with likely CA but without acanthocytes. Their plasma also showed distinct antibrain immunoreactivity. Moreover, band 3 serves as a membrane substrate for tissue transglutaminase, products of which are increased in erythrocytes and muscle in CA patients.[118]

BENIGN HEREDITARY CHOREA

Benign hereditary chorea (BHC), also called hereditary nonprogressive chorea, is another rare disorder. It is primarily symmetric and distal, with onset in childhood and little if any progression beyond adolescence, which may help differentiate it from HD.[119,120] Few other neurological abnormalities are present, with the occasional exception of ataxia, dysarthria, pyramidal tract signs, and postural/action tremor.[121] Although cognitive processes are generally normal, intellectual impairment has been reported in one family.[122] Occasionally, the chorea has been found to be progressive.[123,124] In another sibship in which the basic disorder was compatible with a diagnosis of BHC, monocular horizontal nystagmus (beginning in infancy and remitting in childhood, along with the chorea) and peripheral cataracts were also found. It is questioned whether this is a form of BHC or another familial illness.[125] Some patients with BHC also have familial hypothyroidism and respiratory dysfunction. Functional neuroimaging has not been helpful in differentiating this form of chorea from others. Striatal FDG metabolism was found to be decreased in one study[126] and normal in another,[127] and SPECT imaging in one family show variable results.[128] Although treatment is usually aimed toward dopamine blockade or depletion, one family responded dramatically to levodopa.[129]

The very existence of BHC as a distinct entity had been questioned, even through the new millennium.[130] It is very likely that some families may, in fact, have HD, as in some of the cases with progressive chorea. One family was reported to have the expanded CAG repeat in the *HD* gene, suggesting that some families with so-called "benign" chorea may, in fact, be a phenotypic variant of HD.[131] But the finding in 2000 by de Vries and colleagues of linkage to chromosome 14q,[132] along with subsequent cloning of the gene, a mutation in the thyroid transcription factor 1 (*TITF-1*) gene, a homeodomain-containing transcription factor essential for the organogenesis of the lung, thyroid, and basal ganglia,[133] have put most doubts to rest. Since then, multiple mutations in *TITF-1* have been found, with varying clinical phenotypes.[134–136] Another locus, on chromosome 8 (8q21.3-q23.3) has also been identified in two Japanese families.[137] **Nevertheless, there still remain sporadic and familial cases of BHC with no known genetic link, and etiology must still be explored.**[138]

DENTATORUBROPALLIDOLUYSIAN ATROPHY

An extremely rare autosomal-dominant disorder, *dentatorubropallidoluysian atrophy* (DRPLA) is characterized by its distinctive pathology with extensive cell loss and gliosis in (as its name implies) the dentate nucleus, the red nucleus, the external globus pallidus, and the subthalamic nucleus.[139] DRPLA has a variable phenotypic picture, including chorea, myoclonus, epilepsy, cerebellar ataxia, and dementia, and comprising both juvenile and adult onset. Three clinical subtypes have been proposed: Type I, ataxo-choreoathetoid type; Type II, the pseudo-Huntington type; Type III, the myoclonic–epileptic type.[140] Warner and colleagues,[139] however, suggest that, as phenotypic variation is the rule rather than the exception in autosomal dominantly inherited diseases (as in the hereditary ataxias and the probably mislabeled olivopontocerebellar atrophies[141]) the clinical subclassification is inappropriate and misleading.

The molecular genetic defect of DPRLA is, like HD, a trinucleotide repeat of CAG, with a locus on chromosome 12p, encoding the gene *CTG-B37*, and producing mutations in the protein named atrophin-1.[142–146] Anticipation is a feature of this disorder, as it is in HD, and accounts for the differences in juvenile and adult onsets.[142] The molecular genetics of this disorder become key information in defining syndromes, as in the case of a kindred with the so-called Haw River syndrome,[147] which underwent molecular reevaluation; expanded DRPLA alleles were discovered in this family.[148] Since then, while initial reports of families were not uncommon in Japan, multiple North American and European families have been confirmed by genetic testing.[149–151] Oxidative stress products and reduced of superoxide dismutase expression have been found in postmortem cases of DRPLA.[152] Molecular genetic studies suggest that cleavage of atrophin-1 into a toxic fragment,[153] possibly by caspases (as has been implicated in HD),[154] may be responsible for the pathogenesis of DPRLA.

SENILE CHOREA

Senile chorea is an insidiously developing generalized choreic disorder, primarily involving the limbs, occurring in individuals over 60 with normal mentation, no family history, and no other apparent etiology. It is another unusual and controversial entity, with opinion divided over whether it is a single disorder or a syndrome with multiple etiologies.[155] Few pathological reports exist; a very early study by Alcock[156] described atrophy and cell loss in both the caudate and putamen to a lesser degree than that seen in HD, whereas a modern case examined by Friedman and Ambler demonstrated primarily putaminal cell loss and gliosis, but with caudate sparing.[155] Treatment may follow that of other types of chorea, including the recent approach with pallidal or thalamic DBS.[157]

Some authors have considered senile chorea to be a variant of late-onset HD, whereas others argue that senile chorea is a separate and distinct nosologic entity. One study by Shinotoh and colleagues[158] in which they measured CAG trinucleotide repeat expansion in the *HD* gene in four patients with senile chorea demonstrated normal repeat lengths, supporting the latter theory. On the other hand, in a prospective study by Warren and colleagues[159] of 12 patients followed over a 3-year period, half were ultimately confirmed to have HD; two were found to have PAPS, and one each with hypocalcemia, tardive dyskinesia, and basal ganglia calcification. Only one patient remained undiagnosed after extensive evaluation, leading these authors to conclude that HD remains the most likely cause of senile chorea even in the absence of a family history. Another recent report[160] describes a "typical case" of senile chorea also associated with PAPS, which, with more precise testing, may prove to be, with HD, the most likely etiology of isolated chorea of the elderly.

VASCULAR CHOREA, HEMICHOREA, AND HEMIBALLISMUS

Both generalized chorea and, more commonly, hemichorea and hemiballismus may occur as a result of vascular disease. Classically, hemiballismus was described as a result of a lesion of the subthalamic nucleus[161–163]; it is now known that a variety of lesions in the basal ganglia (and in corticostriatal pathways as well) that interrupt both afferent and efferent subthalamopallidal pathways, detected both at autopsy and with modern neuroimaging, may cause persistent or paroxysmal choreic or ballistic movements, and vascular insults in many areas, including caudate, putamen, thalamus, corona radiata, have been reported.[54,164–178] Vascular etiologies include ischemia, infarction, hemorrhage, and vascular malformations (arteriovenous malformations,[179,180] venous angiomas,[181] and cavernous angiomas[182,183]). Both *hyperglycemia* and *hypoglycemia* may produce hemichorea/hemiballism, generalized chorea, and paroxysmal chorea, presumably also on a vascular basis.[184–193] We will consider the generation of all these types of movements interchangeable. In fact, early authors, including Martin and Alcock,[162] argued that hemiballism was really just an intense, more violent form of hemichorea, and that the ballistic movements generally were more proximal than the choreiform movements. More recent evidence shows that experimental chorea and ballism from different lesions may result in the same reduction in subthalamopallidal activity[194,195] and may also be produced by the same lesion as well,[196,197] further supporting the notion that they result from a common neural mechanism.

Clinically, in the majority of patients with chorea or ballism of vascular etiology, the onset is abrupt. The face is usually spared. Most patients recover spontaneously within 2 to 4 weeks, although some do continue to have choreic movements of long duration. In the interim, if the movements interfere with function, they may respond very well to neuroleptics (low-dose haloperidol) or DA depleters in the short term. Nevertheless, as many of these patients may be elderly, they may be more susceptible to side effects of these drugs such as parkinsonism and tardive dyskinesia. A safer (from the perspective of extrapyramidal adverse effects) and possibly equally effective therapeutic choice is clozapine[198] or other, newer atypical antipsychotics such as quetiapine, olanzapine,[199] and risperidone;[200] similarly, ondansetron has also been reported to provide favorable results.[201] Unlike SC, the response to valproate in vascular hemichorea–hemiballism is variable.[202–204] More promising is treatment with newer anticonvulsants topiramate[205,206] and levetiracetam.[207]

In children with chorea from vascular lesions, thalamic DBS has been successful in reducing movements and improving upper extremity function.[208]

As mentioned above, neuroimaging (CT and especially MRI) are particularly helpful in localizing an anatomic lesion. PET, however, has not shown specific abnormalities. In one study of hemichorea, the contralateral striatum had decreased glucose metabolism and striatal ^{18}F-dopa uptake was normal.[209] Similarly, a SPECT study of one patient with hemichorea–hemiballism in nonketotic hyperglycemia revealed decreased perfusion.[210]

▶ OTHER NEUROLOGICAL AND SYSTEMIC DISEASES

HYPERTHYROIDISM

Chorea secondary to *hyperthyroidism*, an eminently treatable disorder, is rare but may affect about 2% of individuals with hyperthyroidism,[211] although this may be an overestimation. It may be clinically indistinguishable from the chorea of other etiologies and may be bilateral or unilateral, persistent[212–218] or paroxysmal.[219,220] It is generally reversible with normalization of thyroid hormone levels, but may also respond (while still in the hyperthyroid state) to dopaminergic blocking agents.[221] The pathophysiology of hyperthyroid chorea is not understood, but theories include altered function rather than altered structure of the striatum.[1] In view of the seriousness of the disease and the ease of evaluation and treatment, a thyroid screen should be checked in adults who develop chorea, including paroxysmal choreic movements, of otherwise undetermined cause.

POLYCYTHEMIA VERA

Polycythemia vera, a hematological disorder which is more prevalent in men, can rarely be the cause of chorea; interestingly, when it occurs (in less than 1% of cases), it is more common in women (again, invoking a hormonal influence?) and may be the presenting sign of polycythemia in about two thirds of patients.[222] Patients may also demonstrate facial erythrosis or splenomegaly.[223] Onset is usually after 50 and the chorea is generally bilateral and symmetric. It responds to treatment with both reduction of hyperviscosity and antidopaminergics.[224–226] Pathophysiologically, the hyperviscosity may lead to reduced cerebral blood flow with resultant localized ischemia, and the results may be similar to other vascular choreas. As with hyperthyroidism, presentation of chorea in later adulthood should trigger a hematological work-up.

METABOLIC DISORDERS

Other *metabolic* causes of chorea, besides the aforementioned hyperglycemia,[184–188,191–193] hypoglycemia,[189–191] and hyperthyroidism,[207–217] include hyponatremia,[227] hypernatremia,[228] hypocalcemia,[229] hypomagnesemia,[230] hypoparathyroidism,[231–234] hyperparathyroidism,[235] and hepatic encephalopathy (acquired hepatocerebral degeneration).[236–240] Rapid correction of hyponatremia with resultant central pontine myelinolysis has also been reported to be associated with chorea.[241,242]

MULTIPLE SCLEROSIS

Although it too is rare, movement disorders have been reported as a complication of *multiple sclerosis*. Paroxysmal dyskinesias may be the most common presentation and may include choreic movements.[243] Persistent chorea (bilateral or hemichorea) and hemiballism have also been noted to be infrequent accompaniment to multiple sclerosis.[244–248] Demyelinating plaques in the basal ganglia have occasionally been seen.[244,248]

POSTPUMP CHOREA

A little-known entity outside of pediatric cardiovascular services, *postpump chorea* is a not infrequent accompaniment to cardiopulmonary bypass surgery with deep hypothermia for congenital heart disease in children. It was first recognized in 1960[249] and described fully the following year by Bergouignan and colleagues.[250] There have been a number of other reports since, with the incidence of chorea within 2 weeks of surgery varying from 1.2% to 18%, depending on the center.[251–259] Children are from a few months to 3 years old at the time of surgery. They undergo deep hypothermia and there is an association with circulatory arrest. The chorea may resolve within a few months[254,257] or may persist (the longest follow-up of a child with irreversible chorea is >10 years).[257] Most patients with postpump chorea syndrome develop other neurological abnormalities, including seizures (postoperative; occasionally persistent) and developmental delay and cognitive deficits.[253,255,257] The persistent chorea does not respond well to most treatment modalities.[257] Most reports of CT and MRI scans have been normal or show diffuse cerebral atrophy, but a single study with FDG-PET demonstrated hypometabolism in the left frontal lobe.[257] Interestingly, a SPECT evaluation of another child showed nonspecific hypoperfusion of frontal lobe and cerebellum; this child had an unremarkable CT and MRI as well.[258] One long-term follow-up study (from 1986–1995)[260] demonstrated a sudden, transient increase in postoperative chorea that disappeared as they modified treatment strategies in perioperative care. Fifteen patients were followed up and were found to have pervasive deficits in memory, attention, and language; seven of the 15 had persistent chorea.

The pathophysiology of this intriguing disorder is, not surprisingly, unknown. Hypoxic–ischemic damage and thromboembolic infarction in the basal ganglia circuitry has been proposed, especially as this is not uncommon in the setting cardiac bypass surgery.[257] Medlock and colleagues concluded that the absence of structural lesions in the basal ganglia following prolonged chorea suggested a biochemical or microembolic etiology.[257] Another study by Curless and colleagues[259] of three children with postpump chorea found that none had significant intraoperative hypoxemia or hypotension, but all three had hypocapnia and respiratory alkalosis during the rewarming period; they hypothesize that hypocapnia-induced cerebral vasoconstriction may contribute to ischemic damage in critical focal brain areas. In a recent neuropathological examination of two patients, Kupsky and colleagues[261] demonstrated selective neuronal loss and gliosis of the external globus pallidus; areas of the brain usually susceptible to hypoxic–ischemic necrosis were spared. This finding correlates with the older evidence that the globus pallidus bears the brunt of the damage in children who die after cardiac surgery.[249] One other theory proposed for the mechanism of injury here is autoimmune[257]; as with the situation in rheumatic disease,[73] could there be antibodies directed against the basal ganglia in these children? In a slightly different but related story,[262] a child with congenital heart disease received a heart transplant, with deep hypothermia and circulatory arrest, at age 12. Four weeks later, she developed generalized chorea that responded dramatically to corticosteroids, which makes an autoimmune mechanism a reasonable hypothesis. It is unclear whether there is a connection between this case of cardiac transplantation and the chorea developing following bypass surgery. There are no reports of specific aPL being evaluated in any of these cases, which may shed more light on the situation.

OTHER CAUSES: DRUGS, TOXINS, INFECTIONS, NEOPLASMS, AND DEGENERATIVE DISORDERS

A plethora of case reports exist describing the association of chorea with drugs, degenerative disorders, medical conditions, infections, and a variety of other situations. In some instances, there is only a single report to document the connection. Previous authors have compiled extensive lists.[1,263,264] Table 36–1 to Table 36–8 serve to amend and expand those before it with more

▶ **TABLE 36-1. CONDITIONS ASSOCIATED WITH CHOREA AND BALLISM**

Drugs
Hereditary/degenerative disorders
Autoimmune causes of chorea
Autoimmune causes of chorea
Infectious disease, including prions-related, causes of chorea
Systemic, metabolic, endocrinologic, nutritional, and toxic causes of chorea
Other neurological and miscellaneous disorders that can cause chorea

recent references (previously mentioned in text; and refs 265–367). (Accordingly, only those new references will be noted; all others are to be understood as referred to the lists of Weiner and Lang,[1] Duvoisin,[263] or Shoulson.[264]) As with other conditions, treatment of the underlying disease process should be the primary goal in correcting the cause of the chorea.

▶ PAROXYSMAL DYSKINESIAS

Paroxysmal dyskinesias are movement disorders occurring as "attacks" without loss of consciousness, with recovery between attacks. Many of the etiological factors

▶ **TABLE 36-2. DRUGS THAT CAN CAUSE CHOREA DRUGS**

Neuroleptics, dopamine receptor blockers	Calcium-channel blockers
Phenothiazines (e.g., chlorpromazine)	Cinnarizine
Butyrophenones (e.g., haloperidol)	Flunarizine
Thioxanthenes (e.g., thiothixene)	Verapamil[279]
Benzamides (e.g., metoclopramide)	Serotonin-reuptake inhibitors
Atypical antipsychotics (paliperidone,[265] olanzapine[266])	Fluoxetine[280]
Antiparkinson agents	Paroxetine[281]
Levodopa	Other drugs
Dopamine agonists (bromocriptine, pergolide)	Alcohol (intoxication and withdrawal)
Amantadine	Amoxapine
Anticholinergics (including atropine)[267,268]	Artesunate[282]
Anticonvulsants	Baclofen[283]
Phenytoin[269]	Ciprofloxacin[284]
Carbamazepine	Cyclizine
Phenobarbital	Cyclosporine[285]
Ethosuximide	Cyproheptadine,[286] other antihistamines
Valproate[270]	Diazepam-pentobarbital withdrawal287
Lamotrigine[271]	Diazoxide
Gabapentin[272,273]	Digoxin[288]
Stimulants	Interferon-α[289]
Methamphetamine,[274] other amphetamines[275]	Isoniazid
Methylphenidate	Lithium[279,290,291]
Cocaine, crack cocaine ("crack dancing")[276]	Luteinizing hormone-releasing hormone analogue[292]
Caffeine	Methotrexate, intrathecal[293]
Pemoline	Methyldopa
Aminophylline	Modafanil + tranylcypromine[294]
Theophylline[277]	Ondansetron[295]
Steroids	Pentamidine[296]
Anabolic steroids	Ranitidine, cimetidine[297]
Conjugated topical estrogens[40]	Reserpine
Oral contraceptives	Triazolam
Opiates	Tricyclic antidepressants[298]
Methadone[278]	Trimethoprim-sulfamethoxazole299

TABLE 36–3. HEREDITARY/DEGENERATIVE DISORDERS

Alzheimer's disease[300]
Amino acid disorders (glutaric acidemia/aciduria type I,[301] propionic acidemia,[302] cystinuria, homocystinuria, phenylketonuria, Hartnup's disease, argininosuccinicaciduria, ornithine carbamoyltransferase deficiency[303])
Ataxia-telangiectasia[304]
Benign hereditary chorea[120,124,127]
Carbohydrate metabolism (galactosemia, mucopolysaccharidoses, mucolipidoses, pyruvate dehydrogenase deficiency)
Dentatorubropallidoluysian atrophy[139,142–151]
Familial amyotrophic lateral sclerosis[305]
Familial striatal necrosis
Friedreich's ataxia[306,307]
Gilles de la Tourette's syndrome
GLUT-1 deficiency[308]
Hallervorden Spatz (pantothenate kinase-associated neurodegeneration)[309]
Hereditary spinocerebellar ataxias, including Machado–Joseph's disease and SCA type 1[310]
Huntington's disease
Huntington's disease-like 2[311]
Idiopathic basal ganglia calcinosis (Fahr's disease)[312]
Leigh's disease
Lesch–Nyhan's syndrome
Lipidoses (GM_1 and GM_2 gangliosidosis, sphingolipidosis, Gaucher's disease, globoid cell leukodystrophy, metachromatic leukodystrophy, ceroid lipofuscinosis)
MELAS[313]
Mitochondrial encephalomyopathy[314,315]
Multiple system atrophy[316]
Myoclonus epilepsy
Neuroacanthocytoses (chorea-acanthocytosis, McLeod's syndrome)[80–106]
Paroxysmal dyskinesias (PKD, PNKD, PED)
Pelizaeus–Merzbacher's disease
Pick's disease
Progressive supranuclear palsy[317]
Progressive systemic sclerosis[318]
Rett's syndrome[319]
Sea-blue histiocytosis
Sturge–Weber's syndrome
Sulfite-oxidase deficiency
Thyroid hormone transporter defect[320]
Tuberous sclerosis[321]
Wilson's disease
Xeroderma pigmentosum

TABLE 36–4. AUTOIMMUNE CAUSES OF CHOREA

Autoimmune/collagen vascular
Systemic lupus erythematosus[43–45]
Primary antiphospholipid syndrome[47–51]
Rheumatoid arthritis
Behçet's disease[322]
Henoch–Schonlein's syndrome
Periarteritis nodosa
Churg–Straus's syndrome[323]
Hashimoto's thyroiditis[324]
Autoimmune parainfectious
Sydenham's chorea (poststreptococcal)[6,7,12–17,19–25]
PANDAS[28]
Other infections: pertussis, varicella, diphtheria
Serum sickness reaction to tetanus toxoid

already discussed as the causes of choreic and/or ballistic movements can result in paroxysmal chorea as well as persistent movements. Nonepileptic causes of symptomatic paroxysmal chorea include vascular causes,[214,216] hypoglycemia,[190] hyperglycemia,[193] hyperthyroidism,[219,220]

TABLE 36–5. INFECTIOUS DISEASE, INCLUDING PRIONS-RELATED, CAUSES OF CHOREA

Scarlet fever (streptococcal)
Bacterial endocarditis
Typhoid fever
Legionnaires' disease
Lyme disease
Neurosyphilis,[325] meningovascular syphilis[326]
Mycoplasma pneumoniae encephalitis[327]
Encephalitis lethargica (Von Economo's encephalitis)
Viral meningoencephalitis[328] (mumps, measles, varicella, influenza)
Parvovirus B19[329]
Postvaccinial
Infectious mononucleosis
Herpes simplex encephalitis relapse[330,331]
Creutzfeld–Jakob disease[298]
Subacute sclerosing panencephalitis
Mycosis fungoides metastasis[332]
Cysticercosis[333]
Tuberculoma[334]
HIV-related
HIV-1[335–337]
Cryptococcal granuloma[338]
Toxoplasmosis[336,339–341]
Cytomegalovirus encephalitis[326]
Progressive multifocal leukoencephalopathy[336]

TABLE 36-6. SYSTEMIC, METABOLIC, ENDOCRINOLOGIC, NUTRITIONAL, AND TOXIC CAUSES OF CHOREA

Other systemic
Acute intemittent porphyria
Coeliac (celiac) disease[342]
Polycythemia vera[222–226]
Sarcoidosis
Sickle cell anemia
Transitional myeloproliferative disease
Metabolic
Hypoglycemia[189–191] and hyperglycemia[181,184–188]
Hyponatremia and hypernatremia (and central pontine myelinolysis[227,228,241,242])
Hypocalcemia
Hypomagnesemia
Hepatic failure, acquired hepatocerebral degeneration[238]
Renal failure
Endocrine
Hyperthyroidism[211–221]
Hypoparathyroidism,[233] pseudohypoparathyroidism, and hyperparathyroidism
Chorea gravidarum
Addison's disease
Nutritional
Beriberi (thiamine deficiency)
Wernicke's encephalopathy[343]
Pellagra (niacin deficiency)
B_{12} deficiency[344]
Toxins
Carbon monoxide[345]
Lead[346]
Manganese[347]
Mercury
Organophosphate poisoning[348]
Thallium
Toluene (glue-sniffing)

hypoparathyroidism,[231,232] multiple sclerosis,[364] direct infection with human immunodeficiency virus type 1 (HIV)[335] as well as other infections, central and peripheral trauma, kernicterus, and migraine.[326] Paroxysmal dyskinesias may also be seen in other genetic (CA)[368] and systemic (PAPS)[369] causes of chorea, as well as part of a spectrum of other genetic conditions, such as X-linked thyroid transporter hormone mutations.[320]

The original nomenclature of the two major primary forms of paroxysmal dyskinesias, *paroxysmal kinesigenic choreoathetosis* (PKC) and *paroxysmal*

TABLE 36-7. NEOPLASTIC AND CEREBROVASCULAR CAUSES OF CHOREA

Neoplastic
Primary brain tumor
Metastatic brain tumor
Primary CNS lymphoma[349,350]
Acute lymphoblastic leukemia (with lupus anticoagulant)[351]
Paraneoplastic[352,353]
Cerebrovascular
Basal ganglia, subcortical infarcts[166-169,171,172,176]
Basal ganglia, subcortical ischemia[175] (including secondary to hypotension[354])
Basal ganglia, thalamic hemorrhage[170,174]
Carotid stenosis[355]
Epidural hematoma
Subdural hematoma
Moyamoya disease[356–359]
Vascular malformations (arteriovenous malformations,[179,180] venous angioma,[181] cavernous angioma[182,183])

TABLE 36-8. OTHER NEUROLOGICAL AND MISCELLANEOUS DISORDERS THAT CAN CAUSE CHOREA

Head trauma
Peripheral trauma[326]
Cervical disc prolapse/spinal cord compression[360]
CSF leak[361]
Hydrocephalus[362]
Migraine[326,363]
Multiple sclerosis[243,248,364]
Orobuccolingual dyskinesias of aging
Poststatus epilepticus[365]
Senile chorea[155,156,159]
Cerebral palsy
Infantile chorea in bronchopulmonary dysplasia[366]
Kernicterus[326]
Physiological chorea of infancy
Postpump chorea[249–262]
Ventriculoperitoneal shunt[367]

Adapted from Weiner and Lang,[1] Duvoisin,[263] and Shoulson;[264] new additions or updated references only are noted. More than one category may apply to a single condition (e.g., autoimmune and endocrine for chorea gravidarum, autoimmune and neoplastic for acute lymphoblastic leukemia with antiphospholipid antibodies), and some are just difficult to classify (e.g., postpump chorea), but each item will only be listed once.

dystonic choreoathetosis (PDC), have given way to the newer, preferred terms of *paroxysmal kinesigenic dyskinesia* (PKD) and *paroxysmal nonkinesigenic dyskinesia* (PNKD),[370] as the movements may not necessarily be choreoathetotic; in fact, they may be primarily dystonic syndromes, but will be described briefly here nonetheless. Other types of paroxysmal dyskinesias include an *intermediate form* between PKD and PNKD,[1] the rare *paroxysmal exercise-induced dyskinesia* (PED), and *paroxysmal nocturnal or hypnogenic dyskinesia* (PND/PHD).

PKD is precipitated by sudden movements, particularly after coming from a rest position, and by focal movements, stress, excitement, or hyperventilation. Abnormal involuntary movements may span the spectrum of dystonic to choreic to ballistic, but dystonic movements probably predominate; they may be bilateral or unilateral. They usually begin in youth and diminish with age. Attacks may be frequent (100 per day) or rare (2 per year). Consciousness is spared. The attacks usually do not last longer than 2 minutes, and never more than 5 minutes. There is often a prodromal sensation of tightness or tingling and may warn the individual to allow avoidance of the attacks. Although the EEG is normal, patients respond well to low doses of carbamazepine or other anticonvulsants.[1,371–373]

PNKD has similarities to PKD, but differs in that onset is younger (infancy) and duration of the attacks is longer (up to hours). The movements are mostly dystonic, but may be choreic as well. They also differ in precipitating events: in PNKD, it is alcohol and caffeine, as well as sometimes fatigue, stress, or excitement. Frequency is also less than in PKD. Treatment also differs. Anticonvulsants do not usually help, but there is one report of a child improving with gabapentin[374] and another of a family responding to levetiracetam.[375] In PNKD, benzodiazepines are the treatment of choice. Also reportedly effective are acetazolamide and low-dose haloperidol,[1] as well as anticholinergics for more dystonic features of PNKD. More recently, success has been found with DBS of the globus pallidus internus in several patients.[376]

Although the nature of these disorders is intermittent, there have also been recent reports of interictal movement disorders (particularly myoclonus) occurring in patients with paroxysmal dyskinesias.[377,378] Persistent cerebral abnormalities may occur; in a SPECT study on PKC patients, there was interictal hypoperfusion in the posterior regions of the bilateral caudate nuclei.[379]

Recent genetic studies are helping to define these syndromes. PKD is associated in some families with benign familial infantile convulsions (BFIC) in a syndrome termed "ICCA," and linkage has been found on the centromeric region of chromosome 16 (16p12-q12),[380,381] but to date the gene has not been found. This locus is also responsible for the occurrence of familial PKD without BFIC.[382] Linkage was found for several families with PNKD on chromosome 2 (2q31-36),[383] and later found to be associated with mutations in the myofibrillogenesis regulator 1 (MR-1) gene.[384,385] MR-1 may function in the stress response pathway, which may explain PNKD's trigger by alcohol, caffeine, stress, and fatigue.[384]

PED is characterized as episodes of dystonia, particularly of the feet, induced by continuous exercise (e.g., walking or running). It may occur in isolation, or as a spectrum of disease with epilepsy, migraine, cognitive difficulties, and low cerebrospinal fluid glucose.[386,387] Recent genetic studies have demonstrated that PED is associated with mutations in the glucose transporter gene, GLUT1, on the short arm of chromosome 1 (SLC2A1), which is responsible for glucose transport across the blood–brain barrier.[387,388] The movement disorder of PED is hypothesized to result from an exertion-induced energy deficit that may cause episodic dysfunction of the basal ganglia.[388] Antiepileptic drugs are generally unhelpful,[371] but a ketogenic diet in GLUT-1 deficiency syndromes has been shown to be helpful.[389]

PND (or PHD) is now considered a form of frontal lobe epilepsy and is linked to mutations of the neuronal nicotinic acetylcholine receptor genes on chromosome 20 and 15.[371]

The pathophysiology of PKD and possibly other paroxysmal dyskinesias has been suggested to be a channelopathy, with linkage in the region of ion channel genes.[371] Mouse models for paroxysmal dyskinesias have been described.[390,391] The lethargic mouse mutant, which carries a mutation in the CCHB4 gene, encoding the β4 subunit of voltage-regulated calcium channels, has been shown to have transient attacks of severe dyskinetic behavior, often triggered by environmental or chemical influences. Two more mutants, tottering and rocker, also provide further evidence for channelopathies producing paroxysmal dyskinesias.[390,391]

▶ PAINFUL LEGS AND MOVING TOES

Although not a true choreic disorder, we will include the uncommon entity *painful legs and moving toes* in this chapter. First described in 1971,[392] this condition appears to be a peripherally derived movement disorder. The syndrome consists of pain in the affected limb associated with spontaneous, involuntary, and wriggling movements of the toes. The movements may be bilateral or unilateral, continuous or intermittent, occasionally stopping completely for minutes.[392–397] Rarely, the upper limbs may be involved instead of the legs and toes (*pain-*

ful arms and moving fingers),[398,399] or even in addition to the lower limbs.[400] A recent electromyographic study characterized the movements as suggestive of both chorea and dystonia.[401] The disability here is largely from the pain, and rarely from the digit movements. Unfortunately, until recently, almost all treatment modalities, both for hyperkinetic movements and for pain, have been fruitless, except for the occasional reports of success in treating both the pain and the movements with lumbar epidural block with mepivacaine[402] and epidural spinal cord stimulation.[403] Most recently, gabapentin has been reported to help both the pain and movements.[401,404,405]

Painful legs and moving toes frequently occurs in individuals with a history of lumbosacral disease, including spinal nerve root injury, peripheral trauma, or peripheral neuropathy (including HIV-related axonal neuropathy[406,407]), suggesting a peripheral origin for the disorder, but with postulated central nervous system alterations in segmental motor pathways.[408] The severe and unrelenting pain makes the diagnosis clear, despite the disorder's rarity. There also exists a variant, *painless legs and moving toes*, in which the characteristics of the movements are the same, but pain is absent.[408,409] In these patients, the digit movements may be bothersome, and partial relief may be had with injection of botulinum toxin into the toe extensor and flexor muscles (author's personal observations).

▶ CONCLUSIONS

Chorea is a rare manifestation of some very common diseases (vascular disease, hyperthyroidism) as well as a common finding in very rare disorders (CA, DRPLA, BHC). Choreiform movements should alert the physician that any one of a legion of conditions may be responsible, and a thorough physical examination with appropriate laboratory tests are in order. The pathophysiology of chorea is still not understood; but both animal studies and careful observation of clinical phenomena are bringing us closer to elucidating the elusive puzzle of the choreas.

REFERENCES

1. Weiner WJ, Lang AE. Movement Disorders—A Comprehensive Survey. Mount Kisco, New York: Futura Publishing Company, 1989.
2. Sydenham T. The entire works of Thomas Sydenham. London: Sydenham Society, 1848–1850.
3. Nausieda PA, Grossman BJ, Koller WC, Weiner WJ, Klawans HL. Sydenham's chorea: An update. Neurology 1980;30:331–334.
4. Karademir S, Demirceken F, Atalay S, Demiricin G, Sipahi T, Tezic T. Acute rheumatic fever in children in the Ankara area in 1990-1992 and comparison with a previous study in 1980-1989. Acta Paediatr 1994;83:862–865.
5. Figueroa F, Berríos X, Gutiérrez M, et al. Anticardiolipin antibodies in acute rheumatic fever. J Rheumatol 1992;19:1175–1180.
6. Swedo SE, Leonard HL, Schapiro MB, et al. Sydenham's chorea: Physical and psychological symptoms of St Vitus dance. Pediatrics 1993;91:706–713.
7. Swedo SE, Leonard HL. Childhood movement disorders and obsessive–compulsive disorder. J Clin Psychiatry 1994;55(Suppl):32–37.
8. Bird MT, Palkes H, Prensky AL. A follow up study of Sydenham's chorea. Neurology 1976;26:601–606.
9. Korn-Lubetzki I, Brand A, Steiner I. Recurrence of Sydenham chorea: Implications for pathogenesis. Arch Neurol 2004;61(8):1261–1264.
10. Schipper HM. Sex hormones in stroke, chorea, and anticonvulsant therapy. Semin Neurol 1988;8:181–186.
11. Ch'ien LT, Economides AN, Lemmi H. Sydenham's chorea and seizures: Clinical and electroencephalographic studies. Arch Neurol 1978;35:382–385.
12. Swedo SE. Sydenham's chorea: A model for childhood autoimmune neuropsychiatric disorders. JAMA 1994;272:1788–1791.
13. Kienzle GD, Breger RK, Chun RW, Zupanc ML, Sackett JF. Sydenham chorea: MR manifestations in two cases. Am J Neuroradiol 1991;12:73–76.
14. Traill Z, Pike M, Byrne J. Sydenham's chorea: A case showing reversible striatal abnormalities on CT and MRI. Dev Med Child Neurol 1995;37:270–273.
15. Emery ES, Vieco PT. Sydenham chorea: Magnetic resonance imaging reveals permanent basal ganglia injury. Neurology 1997;48:531–533.
16. Ryan MM, Antony JH. Cerebral vasculitis in a case of Sydenham's chorea. J Child Neurol 1999;14:815–818.
17 Giedd JN, Rapoport JL, Kruesi MJP, et al. Sydenham's chorea: Magnetic resonance imaging of the basal ganglia. Neurology 1995;45:2199–2202.
18. Grafton ST, Mazziotta JC, Pahl JJ, et al. Serial changes of cerebral glucose metabolism and caudate size in persons at risk for Huntington's disease. Arch Neurol 1992;49: 1161–1167.
19. Goldman S, Amrom D, Szliwowski HB, et al. Reversible striatal hypermetabolism in a case of Sydenham's chorea. Mov Disord 1993;8:355–358.
20. Weindl A, Kuwert T, Leenders KL, et al. Increased striatal glucose consumption in Sydenham's chorea. Mov Disord 1993;8:437–444.
21. Barsottini OG, Ferraz HB, Seviliano MM, Barbieri A. Brain SPECT imaging in Sydenham's chorea. Braz J Med Biol Res 2002;35:431–436.
22. Shannon KM, Fenichel GM. Pimozide treatment of Sydenham's chorea. Neurology 1990;40:186.
23. Jankovic J, Orman J. Tetrabenazine therapy of dystonia, chorea, tics, and other dyskinesias. Neurology 1988;38: 391–394.
24. Pena J, Mora E, Cardozo J, Molina O, Montiel C. Comparison of the efficacy of carbamazepine, haloperidol and valproic acid in the treatment of children with Sydenham's chorea: Clinical follow-up of 18 patients. Arquiv Neuro-Psiquiatria 2002;60:374–377.
25. Genel F, Arslanoglu S, Uran N, Saylan B. Sydenham's chorea: Clinical findings and comparison of the efficacies

of sodium valproate and carbamazepine regimens. Brain Dev 2002;24:73–76.

26. Gilbert DL, Kurlan R. PANDAS: Horse or zebra? Neurology 2009;73(16):1252–1253.
27. van Toorn R, Weyers HH, Schoeman JF. Distinguishing PANDAS from Sydenham's chorea: Case report and review of the literature. Eur J Paediatr Neurol 2004;8(4): 211–216.
28. Snider LA, Swedo SE. PANDAS: Current status and directions for research. Mol Psychiatry 2004;9(10):900–907.
29. Wolf RE, McBeath JG. Chorea gravidarum in systemic lupus erythematosus. J Rheumatol 1985;12:992–993.
30. Willson P, Preece AA. Chorea gravidarum: A statistical study of 951 collected cases, 846 from the literature and 105 previously unreported. Arch Intern Med 1932;49: 471–533.
31. Beresford OD, Graham AM. Chorea gravidarum. J Obstet Gynaecol Br Emp 1950;57:616–625.
32. Lewis BV, Parsons M. Chorea gravidarum. Lancet 1966;1:284–288.
33. Bolt JM. Abortion and Huntington's chorea. Br Med J 1968;1:840.
34. Donaldson IM, Espiner EA. Disseminated lupus erythematosus presenting as chorea gravidarum. Arch Neurol 1971;25:240–244.
35. Ishikawa K, Kim RC, Givelber H, Collins GH. Chorea gravidarum. Report of a fatal case with neuropathological observations. Arch Neurol 1980;37:429–432.
36. Nausieda PA, Koller WC, Weiner WJ, Klawans HL. Chorea induced by oral contraceptives. Neurology 1979;29: 1605–1609.
37. Galimberti D. Chorea induced by the use of oral contraceptives. Report of a case and review of the literature. Ital J Neurol Sci 1987;8:383–386.
38. Leys D, Destee A, Petit H, Warot P. Chorea associated with oral contraception. J Neurol 1987;235:46–48.
39. Driesen JJ, Wolters EC. Oral contraceptive induced paraballism. Clin Neurol Neurosurg 1987;89:49–51.
40. Caviness JN, Muenter MD. An unusual cause of recurrent chorea. Mov Disord 1991;6:355–357.
41. Hruska RE, Silbergeld EK. Increase dopamine receptor sensitivity after estrogen treatment using the rat rotation model. Science 1980;208:1466–1468.
42. Iskander MK, Khan M. Chorea as the initial presentation of oral contraceptive related systemic lupus erythematosus. J Rheumatol 1989;16:850–851.
43. Gibson T, Myers AR. Nervous system involvement in systemic lupus erythematosus. Ann Rheum Dis 1976;35: 398–406.
44. Bruyn GW, Padberg G. Chorea and systemic lupus erythematosus. Eur Neurol 1984;23:278–290.
45. Feigin A, Kieburtz K, Shoulson I. Treatment of Huntington's disease and other choreic disorders. In: Kurlan R (ed). Treatment of Movement Disorders. Philadelphia, PA: J.B. Lippincott Co., 1995, pp. 337–364.
46. Hughes GRV. Thrombosis, abortion, cerebral disease and the lupus anticoagulant. Br Med J 1983;287:1088–1089.
47. Asherson RA, Khamashta MA, Gil A, et al. Cerebrovascular disease and antiphospholipid antibodies in systemic lupus erythematosus, lupus-like disease, and the primary antiphospholipid syndrome. Am J Med 1989;86:391–399.
48. Asherson RA, Khamashta MA, Ordi-Ros J, et al. The "primary" antiphospholipid syndrome: Major clinical and serological features. Medicine 1989;68:366–374.
49. Levine SR, Welch KM. The spectrum of neurologic disease associated with antiphospholipid antibodies. Lupus anticoagulants and anticardiolipin antibodies. Arch Neurol 1987;44:876–883.
50. Levine SR, Deegan MJ, Futrell N, Welch KMA. Cerebrovascular and neurologic disease associated with antiphospholipid antibodies: 48 cases. Neurology 1990;40:1181–1189.
51. Cervera R, Piette JC, Font J, et al. Antiphospholipid syndrome: Clinical and immunologic manifestations and patterns of disease expression in a cohort of 1,000 patients. Arthritis Rheum 2002;46:1019–1027.
52. Boey ML, Colaco CB, Gharavi AE, et al. Thrombosis in SLE: Striking association with the presence of circulating "lupus" anticoagulant. Br Med J 1983;287:1021–1023.
53. Kumar S, Papalardo E, Sunkureddi P, Najam S, González EB, Pierangeli SS. Isolated elevation of IgA anti-beta2glycoprotein I antibodies with manifestations of antiphospholipid syndrome: A case series of five patients. Lupus 2009;18(11):1011–1014.
54. Avcin T, Benseler SM, Tyrrell PN, Cucnik S, Silverman ED. A follow up study of antiphospholipid antibodies and associated neuropsychiatric manifestations in 137 children with systemic lupus erythematosus. Arthritis Rheum 2008;59(2):206–213.
55. Bouchez B, Arnott G, Hatron PY, Wattel A, Devulder B. Chorée et lupus erythemateux disséminé avec anticoagulant circulant. Trois cas. Rev Neurol 1985;141:571–577.
56. Kirk A, Harding SR. Cardioembolic caudate infarction as a cause of hemichorea in lupus anticoagulant syndrome. Can J Neurol Sci 1993;20:162–164.
57. Asherson RA, Derksen RH, Harris EN, et al. Chorea in systemic lupus erythematosus and "lupus-like" disease: Association with antiphospholipid antibodies. Semin Arthritis Rheum 1987;16:253–259.
58. Kashihara K, Nakashima S, Kohira I, Shohmori T, Fujiwara Y, Kuroda S. Hyperintense basal ganglia on T1-weighted MR images in a patient with central nervous system lupus and chorea. Am J Neuroradiol 1998;19:284–286.
59. Galanaud D, Dormont D, Marsault C, Wechsler B, Piette J-C. Brain MRI in patients with past lupus-associated chorea. Stroke 2000;31:3080–3081.
60. Khamashta MA, Gil A, Anciones B, et al. Chorea in systemic lupus erythematosus: Association with antiphospholipid antibodies. Ann Rheum Dis 1988;47:681–683.
61. Vlachoyiannopoulos PG, Dimou G, Siamopoulou-Mavridou A. Chorea as a manifestation of the antiphospholipid syndrome in childhood. Clin Exp Rheumatol 1991;9: 303–305.
62. de la Fuente Fernandez R. Rheumatic chorea and lupus anticoagulant. J Neurol Neurosurg Psychiatry 1994;57:1545.
63. Lubbe WF, Walker EB. Chorea gravidarum associated with circulating lupus anticoagulant: Successful outcome of pregnancy with prednisone and aspirin therapy. Case report. Br J Obstet Gynaecol 1983;90:487–490.
64. Omdal R, Roalso S. Chorea gravidarum and chorea associated with oral contraceptives—Diseases due to antiphospholipid antibodies? Acta Neurol Scand 1992;86:219–220.

65. Okseter K, Sirnes K. Chorea and lupus anticoagulant: A case report. Acta Neurol Scand 1988;78:206–209.
66. Shimomura T, Takahashi S, Takahashi S. Chorea associated with antiphospholipid antibodies. Clin Neurol 1992;32: 989–993.
67. Besbas N, Damarguc I, Ozen S, Aysun S, Saatci U. Association of antiphospholipid antibodies with systemic lupus erythematosus in a child presenting with chorea: A case report. Eur J Pediatr 1994;153:891–893.
68. Guttman M, Lang AE, Garnett ES, et al. Regional cerebral glucose metabolism in SLE chorea: Further evidence that striatal hypometabolism is not a correlate of chorea. Mov Disord 1987;2:201–210.
69. Furie R, Ishikawa T, Dhawan V, Eidelberg D. Alternating hemichorea in primary antiphospholipid syndrome: Evidence for contralateral striatal hypermetabolism. Neurology 1994;44:2197–2199.
70. Wu SW, Graham B, Gelfand MJ, Gruppo RE, Dinopolous A, Gilbert DL. Clinical and positron emission tomography findings of chorea associated with primary antiphospholipid antibody syndrome. Mov Disord 2007;22(12): 1813–1815.
71. Vela L, Sfakianakis GN, Heros D, Koller W, Singer C. Chorea and contraceptives: Case report with PET study and review of the literature. Mov Disord 2004;19(3):349–352.
72. Miranda M, Cardoso F, Giovannoni G, Church A. Oral contraceptive induced chorea: Another condition associated with anti-basal ganglia antibodies. J Neurol Neurosurg Psychiatry 2004;75(2):327–328.
73. Husby G, van de Rijn I, Zabriskie JB, et al. Antibodies reacting with cytoplasm of subthalamic and caudate nuclei neurons in chorea and acute rheumatic fever. J Exp Med 1976;144:1094–1110.
74. Church AJ, Cardoso F, Dale RC, Lees AJ, Thompson EJ, Giovannoni G. Anti-basal ganglia antibodies in acute and persistent Sydenham's chorea. Neurology 2002;59:227–231.
75. Cunningham MW, Swerlick RA. Polyspecificity of antistreptococcal murine monoclonalantibodies and their implications in autoimmunity. J Exp Med 1986;164: 998–1012.
76. Bronze MS, Dale JB. Epitopes of streptococcal M proteins that evoke antibodies that cross-react with human brain. J Immunol 1993;151:2820–2828.
77. Harrison NA, Church A, Nisbet A, Rudge P, Giovannoni G. Late recurrences of Sydenham's chorea are not associated with anti-basal ganglia antibodies. J Neurol Neurosurg Psychiatry 2004;75:1478–1479.
78. Levine IM, Estes JW, Looney JM. Hereditary neurological disease with acanthocytosis. Arch Neurol 1968;19:403–409.
79. Critchley EMR, Clark DB, Wikler A. Acanthocytosis and neurolgical disorder without abetalipoproteinemia. Arch Neurol 1968;18:134–140.
80. Kito S, Itoga E, Hiroshige Y, Matsumoto N, Miwa S. A pedigree of amyotrophic chorea with acanthocytosis. Arch Neurol 1980;37:514–517.
81. Sakai T, Mawatari S, Iwashita H, Goto I, Kuroiwa Y. Choreoacanthocytosis. Clues to clinical diagnosis. Arch Neurol 1981;38:335–338.
82. Sotaniemi KA. Chorea-acanthocytosis. Neurological disease with acanthocytosis. Acta Neurol Scand 1983;68: 53–56.
83. Sakai T, Iwashita H, Goto I, Kakugawa M. Neuroacanthocytosis syndrome and choreoacanthocytosis (Levine-Critchley syndrome). Neurology 1985;35:1679.
84. Hardie RJ. Acanthocytosis and neurological impairment—A review. Q J Med 1989;71:291–306.
85. Danek A. Progress in molecular chorea diagnosis. McLeod syndrome and chorea acanthocytosis. Nervenarzt 2002;73:564–569.
86. Vita G, Serra S, Dattola R, et al. Peripheral neuropathy in amyotrophic chorea-acanthocytosis. Ann Neurol 1989;26:583–587.
87. Kihara M, Nakashima H, Taki M, Takahashi M, Kawamura Y. A case of chorea-acanthocytosis with dysautonomia; quantitative autonomic deficits using CASS. Autonom Neurosci-Basic Clin 2002;97:42–44.
88. Delecluse F, Deleval J, Gérard J-M, Michotte A, Zegers de Beyl D. Frontal impairment and hypoperfusion in neuroacanthocytosis. Arch Neurol 1991;48:232–234.
89. Rinne JO, Daniel SE, Scaravilli F, Pires M, Harding AE, Marsden CD. The neuropathological features of neuroacanthocytosis. Mov Disord 1994;9:297–304.
90. Hardie RJ, Pullon HWH, Harding AE, et al. Neuroacanthocytosis—A clinical, haematological and pathological study of 19 cases. Brain 1991;114:13–49.
91. Walker RH, Morgello S, Davidoff-Feldman B, et al. Autosomal dominant chorea-acanthocytosis with polyglutamine-containing neuronal inclusions. Neurology 2002 ;58:1031–1037.
92. Witt TN, Danek A, Reiter M, Heim MJ, Dirschinger J, Olsen EG. McLeod syndrome: A distinct form of neuroacanthocytosis—report of 2 cases and literature review with emphasis on neuromuscular manifestations. J Neurol 1992;239:302–306.
93. Takashima H, Sakai T, Iwashita H, et al. A family of McLeod syndrome, masquerading as chorea-acanthocytosis. J Neurol Sci 1994;124:56–60.
94. Malandrini A, Fabrizi GM, Truschi F, et al. Atypical McLeod syndrome manifested as X-linked chorea-acanthocytosis, neuromyopathy and dilated cardiomyopathy: Report of a family. J Neurol Sci 1994;124:89–94.
95. Danek A, Tison F, Rubio J, Oechsner M, Kalckreuth W, Monaco AP. The chorea of McLeod syndrome. Mov Disord 2001;16:882–889.
96. Jung HH, Hergersberg M, Kneifel S, et al. McLeod syndrome: A novel mutation, predominant psychiatric manifestations, and distinct striatal imaging findings. Ann Neurol 2001;49:384–392.
97. Rubio JP, Danek A, Stone C, et al. Chorea-acanthocytosis: Genetic linkage to chromosome 9q21. Am J Hum Genet 1997;61:899–908.
98. Ueno S, Maruki Y, Nakamura M, et al. The gene encoding a newly discovered protein, chorein, is mutated in chorea-acanthocytosis. Nature Genet 2001; 28:121–122.
99. Dobson-Stone C, Velayos-Baeza A, Filippone LA, et al. Chorein detection for the diagnosis of chorea-acanthocytosis. Ann Neurol. 2004;56(2):299–302.
100. Lin FC, Wei LJ, Shih PY. Effect of levetiracetam on truncal tic in neuroacanthocytosis. Acta Neurol Taiwan 2006;15(1): 38–42.
101. Recio MV, Hauser RA, Louis ED, Radhashakar H, Sullivan KL, Zesiewicz TA. Chorea in a patient with cerebral pal-

sy: Treatment with levetiracetam. Mov Disord 2005;20(6): 762–764.
102. Vles GF, Hendriksen JG, Visschers A, Speth L, Nicolai J, Vles JS. Levetiracetam therapy for treatment of choreoathetosis in dyskinetic cerebral palsy. Dev Med Child Neurol 2009;51(6):487–490.
103. Burbaud P, Vital A, Rougier A, et al. Minimal tissue damage after stimulation of the motor thalamus in a case of chorea-acanthocytosis. Neurology 2002;59:1982–1984.
104. Guehl D, Cuny E, Tison F, et al. Deep brain pallidal stimulation for movement disorders in neuroacanthocytosis. Neurology 2007;68(2):160–161.
105. Ruiz PJ, Ayerbe J, Bader B, et al. Deep brain stimulation in chorea acanthocytosis. Mov Disord. 2009;24(10): 1546–1547.
106. Rinne JO, Daniel SE, Scaravilli F, Harding AE, Marsden CD. Nigral degeneration in neuroacanthocytosis. Neurology 1994;44:1629–1632.
107. Malandrini A, Fabrizi GM, Palmeri S, et al. Choreoacanthocytosis-like phenotype without acanthocytes: Clinicopathological case report. A contribution to the knowledge of the functional pathology of the caudate nucleus. Acta Neuropathol 1993;86:651–658.
108. de Yebenes JG, Brin MF, Mena MA, et al. Neurochemical findings in neuroacanthocytosis. Mov Disord 1988;3: 300–312.
109. Dubinsky RM, Hallett M, Levey R, Di Chiro G. Regional brain glucose metabolism in neuroacanthocytosis. Neurology 1989;39:1253–1255.
110. Hosokawa S, Ichiya Y, Kuwabara Y, et al. Positron emission tomography in cases of chorea with different underlying diseases. J Neurol Neurosurg Psychiatry 1987;50; 1284–1287.
111. Oechsner M, Buchert R, Beyer W, Danek A. Reduction of striatal glucose metabolism in McLeod choreoacanthocytosis. J Neurol Neurosurg Psychiatry 2001;70: 517–520.
112. Brooks DJ, Ibanez V, Playford ED, et al. Presynaptic and postsynaptic striatal dopaminergic function in neuroacanthocytosis: A positron emission tomographic study. Ann Neurol 1991;30:166–171.
113. Brin MF, Bressman SB, Fahn S, Resor SR, Weitz J, Sagman DL. Chorea-acanthocytosis: Clinical and laboratory features in five cases [abstract]. Neurology 1985;35 (Suppl 1):110
114. Feinberg TE, Cianci CD, Morrow JS, et al. Diagnostic tests for choreoacanthocytosis. Neurology 1991;41: 1000–1006.
115. Sakai T, Antoku Y, Iwashita H, Goto I, Nagamatsu K, Shii H. Chorea-acanthocytosis: Abnormal composition of covalently bound fatty acids of erythrocyte membrane proteins. Ann Neurol 1991;29:664–669.
116. Kay MM, Goodman J, Lawrence C, Bosman G. Membrane channel protein abnormalities and autoantibodies in neurological disease. Brain Res Bull 1990;24:105–111.
117. Bosman GJ, Bartholmeus IG, De Grip WJ, Horstink MW. Erythrocyte anion transporter and antibrain immunoreactivity in chorea-acanthocytosis. A contribution to etiology, genetics, and diagnosis. Brain Res Bull 1994;33:523–528.
118. Melone MA, Di Fede G, Peluso G,et al. Abnormal accumulation of tTGase products in muscle and erythrocytes of chorea-acanthocytosis patients. J Neuropathol Exp Neurol 2002;61:841–848.
119. Haerer AF, Currier RD, Jackson JF. Hereditary nonprogressive chorea of early onset. N Engl J Med 1967;276: 1220–1224.
120. Wheeler PG, Weaver DD, Dobyns WB. Benign hereditary chorea. Pediatr Neurol 1993;9:337–340.
121. Pincus JH, Chutorian A. Familial benign chorea with intention tremor: A clinical entity. J Pediatr 1967;70:724–729.
122. Leli DA, Furlow TW, Falgout JC. Benign familial chorea: An association with intellectual impairment. J Neurol Neurosurg Psychiatry 1984;47:471474.
123. Behan PO, Bone I. Hereditary chorea without dementia. J Neurol Neurosurg Psychiatry 1977;40:687–691.
124. Schady W, Meara RJ. Hereditary progressive chorea without dementia. J Neurol Neurosurg Psychiatry 1988;51: 295–297.
125. Wheeler PG, Dobyns WB, Plager DA, Ellis FD. Familial remitting chorea, nystagmus, cataracts. Am J Med Genet 1993;47:1215–1217.
126. Suchowersky O, Hayden MR, Martin WRW, et al. Cerebral metabolism of glucose in benign hereditary chorea. Mov Disord 1986;1:33–45.
127. Kuwert T, Lange HW, Langen KJ, et al. Normal striatal glucose consumption in two patients with benign hereditary chorea as measured by positron emission tomography. J Neurol 1990;237:80–84.
128. Mahajnah M, Inbar D, Steinmetz A, Heutink P, Breedveld GJ, Straussberg R. Benign hereditary chorea: Clinical, neuroimaging, and genetic findings. J Child Neurol 2007;22(10):1231–1234.
129. Asmus F, Horber V, Pohlenz J, et al. A novel TITF-1 mutation causes benign hereditary chorea with response to levodopa. Neurology 2005;64(11):1952–1954.
130. Schrag A, Quinn NP, Bhatia KP, Marsden CD. Benign hereditary chorea—Entity or syndrome? Mov Disord 2000; 15:280–288.
131. MacMillan JC, Morrison PJ, Nevin NC, et al. Identification of an expanded CAG repeat in the Huntington's disease gene (IT15) in a family reported to have benign hereditary chorea. J Med Genet 1993;30:1012–1013.
132. de Vries BB, Arts WF, Breedveld GJ, Hoogeboom JJ, Niermeijer MF, Heutink P. Benign hereditary chorea of early onset maps to chromosome 14q. Am J Hum Genet 2000;66: 136–142.
133. Breedveld GJ, van Dongen JW, Danesino C, et al. Mutations in TITF-1 are associated with benign hereditary chorea. Hum Mol Genet 2002;11:971–979.
134. do Carmo Costa M, Costa C, Silva AP, et al. Nonsense mutation in TITF1 in a Portuguese family with benign hereditary chorea. Neurogenetics 2005;6(4):209–215.
135. Provenzano C, Veneziano L, Appleton R, Frontali M, Civitareale D. Functional characterization of a novel mutation in TITF-1 in a patient with benign hereditary chorea. J Neurol Sci 2008;264(1-2):56–62.
136. Glik A, Vuillaume I, Devos D, Inzelberg R. Psychosis, short stature in benign hereditary chorea: A novel thyroid transcription factor-1 mutation. Mov Disord 2008; 23(12):1744–1747.
137. Shimohata T, Hara K, Sanpei K, et al. Novel locus for benign hereditary chorea with adult onset maps

to chromosome 8q21.3 q23.3. Brain 2007;130(Pt 9): 2302–2309.
138. Bauer P, Kreuz FR, Bürk K, et al. Mutations in TITF1 are not relevant to sporadic and familial chorea of unknown cause. Mov Disord 2006;21(10):1734–1737.
139. Warner TT, Lennox GG, Janota I, Harding AE. Autosomal-dominant dentatorubropallidoluysian atrophy in the United Kingdom. Mov Disord 1994;9:289–296.
140. Iizuka R, Hirayama K, Machara K. Dentato-rubro-pallidoluysian atrophy. A clinico-pathological study. J Neurol Neurosurg Psychiatry 1984;47:1288–1298.
141. Mark MH, Sage JI. Olivopontocerebellar atrophy. In: Stern MB, Koller WC (eds). Parkinsonian Syndromes. New York: Marcel Dekker, 1993:43–67.
142. Potter NT, Meyer MA, Zimmerman AW, Eisenstadt ML, Anderson IJ. Molecular and clinical findings in a family with dentatorubral-pallidoluysian atrophy. Ann Neurol 1995;37:273–277.
143. Koide R, Ikeuchi T, Onodera O, et al. Unstable expansion of CAG repeat in hereditary dentatorubral-pallidoluysian atrophy (DRPLA). Nat Genet 1994;6:9–13.
144. Nagafuchi S, Yanagisawa H, Sato K, et al. Dentatorubral and pallidoluysian atrophy expansion of an unstable CAG trinucleotide on chromosome 12p. Nat Genet 1994;6: 14–18.
145. Nagafuchi S, Yanagisawa H, Ohsaki E, et al. Structure and expression of the gene responsible for the triplet repeat disorder, dentatorubral and pallidoluysian atrophy (DRPLA). Nat Genet 1994;8:177–182.
146. Margolis RL, Li SH, Young WS et al. DRPLA gene (atrophin-1) sequence and mRNA expression in human brain. Mol Brain Res 1996;36:219–226.
147. Farmer TW, Wingfield MS, Lynch SA, et al. Ataxia, chorea, seizures, and dementia. Pathologic features of a newly defined familial disorder. Arch Neurol 1989;46: 774–779.
148. Burke JR, Wingfield MS, Lewis KE, et al. The Haw River syndrome: Dentatorubropallidoluysian atrophy (DRPLA) in an African-American family. Nat Genet 1994;7:521–524.
149. Munoz E, Mila M, Sanchez A, et al. Dentatorubropallidoluysian atrophy in a Spanish family: A clinical, radiological, pathological, and genetic study. J Neurol Neurosurg Psychiatry 1999;67:811–814.
150. Becher MW, Rubinsztein DC, Leggo J, et al. Dentatorubral and pallidoluysian atrophy (DRPLA). Clinical and neuropatholgical findings in genetically confirmed North American and European pedigrees. Mov Disord 1997;12: 519–530.
151. Nielesen JE, Sorensen SA, Hasholt L, Norremolle A. Dentatorubral-pallidoluysian atrophy. Clinical features of a five-generation Danish family. Mov Disord 1996;11:533–541.
152. Miyata R, Hayashi M, Tanuma N, Shioda K, Fukatsu R, Mizutani S. Oxidative stress in neurodegeneration in dentatorubral-pallidoluysian atrophy. J Neurol Sci 2008;264 (1-2):133–139.
153. Schilling G, Wood JD, Duan K, et al. Nuclear accumulation of truncated atrophin-1 fragments in a transgenic mouse model of DRPLA. Neuron 1999;24:275–286.
154. Ellerby LM, Andrusiak RL, Wellington Cl, et al. Cleavage of atrophin-1 at caspase site aspartic acid 109 modulates cytotoxicity. J Biol Chem 1999;274:8730–8736.
155. Friedman JH, Ambler M. A case of senile chorea. Mov Disord 1990;5:251–253.
156. Alcock NS. A note on the pathology of senile chorea (non-hereditary). Brain 1936;59:376–387.
157. Yianni J, Nandi D, Bradley K, et al. Senile chorea treated by deep brain stimulation: A clinical, neurophysiological and functional imaging study. Mov Disord 2004;19(5): 597–602.
158. Shinotoh H, Calne DB, Snow B, et al. Normal CAG repeat length in the Huntington's disease gene in senile chorea. Neurology 1994;44:2183-2184.
159. Warren JD, Firgaira F, Thompson EM, Kneebone C, Blumbergs PC, Thompson PD. The causes of sporadic and 'senile' chorea. Aust N Z J Med 1998;28:429–431.
160. Gelosa G, Tremolizzo L, Galbussera A, et al. Narrowing the window for 'senile chorea': A case with primary antiphospholipid syndrome. J Neurol Sci 2009;284 (1-2):211–213
161. Jakob A. Die extrapyramidalen Enkrankungen. Berlin: Springer, 1923.
162. Martin JP, Alcock NS. Hemichorea associated with a lesion of the Corpus Luysii. Brain 1934:504–516.
163. Melamed E, Korn-Lubetzki I, Reches A, Siew F. Hemiballismus: Detection of focal hemorrhage in subthalamic nucleus by CT scan. Ann Neurol 1978;4:582.
164. Martin JP. Hemichorea (hemiballismus) without lesions in the corpus Luysii. Brain 1957;80:1–10.
165. Kase CS, Maulsby GO, deJuan E, Mohr JP. Hemichorea-hemiballism and lacunar infarction of the basal ganglia. Neurology 1981;31:452–455.
166. Folstein S, Abbott M, Moses R, Parlad I, Clark A, Folstein M. A phenocopy of Huntington's disease: Lacunar infarcts of the corpus striatum. Johns Hopkins Med J 1981;148: 104–113.
167. Saris S. Chorea caused by caudate infarction. Arch Neurol 1983;40:590–591.
168. Tabaton M, Mancardi G, Loeb C. Generalized chorea due to bilateral small, deep cerebral infarcts. Neurology 1985;35:588–589.
169. Sethi KD, Nichols FT, Yaghmai F. Generalized chorea due to basal ganglia lacunar infarcts. Mov Disord 1987;2: 61–66.
170. Altafullah I, Pascual-Leone A, Duvall K, Anderson DC, Taylor S. Putaminal hemorrhage accompanied by hemichorea-hemiballism. Stroke 1990;21:1093–1094.
171. Defebvre L, Destee A, Cassim F, Muller JP, Vermersch E. Transient hemiballism and striatal infarction. Stroke 1990; 21:967–968.
172. Destee A, Muller JP, Vermersch P, Pruvo JP, Warot P. Hemiballismus, hemichorea, striatal infarction. Rev Neurol 1990;146:150–152.
173. Bhatia KP, Lera G, Luthert PJ, Marsden CD. Vascular chorea: Case report with pathology. Mov Disord 1994;9:447–450.
174. Freilich RJ, Chambers BR. Choreoathetosis and thalamic haemorrhage. Clin Exp Neurol 1988;25:115–120.
175. Fukui T, Hasegawa Y, Seriyama S, Takeuchi T, Sugita K, Tsukagoshi H. Hemiballism-hemichorea induced by subcortical ischemia. Can J Neurol Sci 1993;20:324–328.
176. Barinagarrementeria F, Vega F, DelBrutto OH. Acute hemichorea due to infarction in the corona radiata. J Neurol 1989;236:371–372.

177. Vidakovic A, Dragasevic N, Kostic VS. Hemiballism: Report of 25 cases. J Neurol Neurosurg Psychiatry 1994;57: 945–949.
178. Calzetti S, Moretti G, Gemignani F, Formentini E, Lechi A. Transient hemiballismus and subclavian steal syndrome. Acta Neurol Belg 1980;80:329–335.
179. Tamaoka A, Sakuta M, Yamada H. Hemichorea-hemiballism caused by arteriovenous malformations in the putamen. J Neurol 1987;234:124–125.
180. Shintani S, Shiozawa Z, Tsunoda S, Shiigai T. Paroxysmal choreoathetosis precipitated by movement, sound and photic stimulation in a case of artero-venous malformation in the parietal lobe. Clin Neurol Neurosurg 1991;93:237–239.
181. Vincent FM. Hyperglycemia-induced hemichoreoathetosis: The presenting manifestation of a vascular malformation of the lenticular nucleus. Neurosurgery 1986;18:787–790.
182. Carpay HA, Arts WF, Kloet A, Hoogland PH, Van Duinen SG. Hemichorea reversible after operation in a boy with cavernous angioma in the head of the caudate nucleus. J Neurol Neurosurg Psychiatry 1994;57:1547–1548.
183. Carella F, Caraceni T, Girotti F. Hemichorea due to a cavernous angioma of the caudate. Case report of an aged patient. Ital J Neurol Sci 1992;13:783–785.
184. Linazasoro G, Urtasun M, Poza JJ, Suárez JA, Martí Massó JF. Generalized chorea induced by nonketotic hyperglycemia. Mov Disord 1993;8:119–120.
185. Lin JJ, Chang MK. Hemiballism–hemichorea and non-ketotic hyperglycaemia. J Neurol Neurosurg Psychiatry 1994; 57:748–750.
186. Nakagawa T, Mitani K, Nagura H, Bando M, Yamanouchi H. Chorea-ballism associated with nonketotic hyperglycemia and presenting with bilateral hyperintensity of the putamen on MR T1-weighted images—A case report. Clin Neurol 1994;34:52–55.
187. Shimomura T, Nozaki Y, Tamura K. Hemichorea-hemiballism associated with nonketotic hyperglycemia and presenting with unilateral hyperintensity of the putamen on MRI T1-weighted images—A case report. Brain Nerve 1995;47:557–561.
188. Broderick JP, Hagen T, Brott T, Tomsick T. Hyperglycemia and hemorrhagic transformation of cerebral infarcts. Stroke 1995;26:484–487.
189. Hefter H, Mayer P, Benecke R. Persistent chorea after recurrent hypoglycemia. Eur Neurol 1993;33:244–247.
190. Newman RP, Kinkel WR. Paroxysmal choreoathetosis due to hypoglycemia. Arch Neurol 1984;41:341–342.
191. Sethi KD, Allen M, Sethi RK, McCord JW. Chorea in hypoglycemia and hyperglycemia [abstract]. Neurology 1990; 40(Suppl 1):337.
192. Stone LA, Armstrong RM. An unusual presentation of diabetes: Hyperglycemia inducing hemiballismus [abstract]. Ann Neurol 1989;26:164.
193. Haan J, Kremer HPH, Padberg G. Paroxysmal choreoathetosis as presenting symptom of diabetes mellitus. J Neurol Neurosurg Psychiatry 1989;52:133.
194. Crossman AR, Sambrook MA, Jackson A. Experimental hemichorea/hemiballismus: Studies on the intracerebral site of action in a drug-induced dyskinesia. Brain 1984;107:579–596.
195. Mitchell IJ, Jackson A, Sambrook MA, Crossman AR. Common neurological mechanism in experimental chorea and hemiballismus in the monkey. Evidence from 2-deoxyglucose autoradiography. Brain Res 1985;339:346–350.
196. Mitchell IJ, Jackson A, Sambrook MA, Crossman AR. The role of the subthalamic nucleus in experimental chorea. Evidence from 2-deoxyglucose metabolic mapping and horseradish peroxidase tracing studies. Brain 1989;112:1533–1548.
197. Crossman AR, Mitchell IJ, Sambrook MA, Jackson A. Chorea and myoclonus in the monkey induced by gamma-aminobutyric acid antagonism in the lentiform complex. The site of drug action and a hypothesis for the neural mechanisms of chorea. Brain 1988;111:1211–1233.
198. Bashir K, Manyam BV. Clozapine for the control of hemiballismus. Clin Neuropharmacol 1994;17:477–480.
199. Safirstein B, Shulman LM, Weiner WJ. Successful treatment of hemichorea with olanzapine. Mov Disord 1999;14: 532–533.
200. Evidente VG, Gwinn-Hardy K, Caviness JN, Alder CH. Risperidone is effective in severe hemichorea/hemiballismus. Mov Disord 1999;14:377–379.
201. Erdinc OO, Ozdemir G, Uysal S, Gucuyener D, Torun S. Improvement of hemichorea with ondansetron. Postgrad Med J 1997;73:127.
202. Chandra V, Wharton S, Spunt AL. Amelioration of hemiballismus with sodium valproate. Ann Neurol 1982; 12:407.
203. Dewey RB Jr, Jankovic J. Hemiballism-hemichorea. Clinical and pharmacologic findings in 21 patients. Arch Neurol 1989;46:862–867.
204. Sethi KD, Patel BP. Inconsistent response to divalproex sodium in hemichorea-hemiballism. Neurology 1990;40:1630–1631.
205. Gatto EM, Uribe Roca C, Raina G, Gorja M, Folgar S, Micheli FE. Vascular hemichorea/hemiballism and topiramate. Mov Disord 2004;19(7):836–838.
206. Driver-Dunckley E, Evidente VG. Hemichorea-hemiballismus may respond to topiramate. Clin Neuropharmacol 2005;28(3):142–144.
207. D'Amelio M, Callari G, Gammino M, et al. Levetiracetam in the treatment of vascular chorea: A case report. Eur J Clin Pharmacol 2005;60(11):835–836.
208. Thompson TP, Kondziolka D, Albright AL. Thalamic stimulation for choreiform movement disorders in children. Report of two cases. J Neurosurg 2000;92:718–721.
209. Otsuka M, Ichiya Y, Kuwabara Y, et al. Cerebral glucose metabolism and ^{18}F-dopa uptake by PET in cases of chorea with or without dementia. J Neurol Sci 1993;115:153–157.
210. Lee EJ, Choi JY, Lee SH.,Song S, Lee YS. Hemichorea-hemiballism in primary diabetic patients: MR correlation. J Comp Asst Tomogr 2002;26:905–911.
211. Logothetic J. Neurologic and muscular manifestations of hyperthyroidism. Arch Neurol 1961;5:533–544.
212. Fidler SM, O'Rourke RA, Buchsbaum HM. Choreoathetosis as a manifestation of thyrotoxicosis. Neurology 1971;21: 55–57.
213. Delwaide PJ, Schoenen J. Hyperthyroidism as a cause of persistent choreic movements. Acta Neurol Scand 1978;58:309–312.
214. Shahar E, Shapiro MS, Shenkman L. Hyperthyroid-induced chorea. Case report and review of the literature. Israel J Med Sci 1988;24:264–266.

215. Ahronheim JC. Hyperthyroid chorea in an elderly woman associated with sole elevation of T3. J Am Geriatr Soc 1988; 36:242–244.
216. Lucantoni C, Grottoli S, Moretti A. Chorea due to hyperthyroidism in old age. A case report. Acta Neurol 1994;16: 129–133.
217. Baba M, Terada A, Hishida R, Matsunaga M, Kawabe Y, Takebe K. Persistent hemichorea associated with thyrotoxicosis. Intern Med 1992;31:1144–1146.
218. Pozzan GB, Battistella PA, Rigon F, et al. Hyperthyroid-induced chorea in an adolescent girl. Brain Dev 1992;14:126–127.
219. Fischbeck KH, Layzer RB. Paroxysmal choreoathetosis associated with thyrotoxicosis. Ann Neurol 1979;6:453–454.
220. Drake ME Jr. Paroxysmal kinesigenic choreoathetosis in hyperthyroidism. Postgrad Med J 1987;63:1089–1090.
221. Klawans HL, Shenker DM, Weiner WJ. Observations on the dopaminergic nature of hyperthyroid chorea. Adv Neurol 1973;1:543–549.
222. Bruyn GW, Padberg G. Chorea and polycythemia. Eur Neurol 1984;23:26–33.
223. Mas JL, Guergen B, Bouche P, Derouesne C, Varet B, Castaigne P. Chorea and polycythaemia. J Neurol 1985;232: 168–171.
224. Rigon G, Baratti M, Quaini F, Calzetti S. Polycythemia chorea. Description of a clinical case. Minerva Med 1987; 78:1325–1329.
225. Cohen AM, Gelvan A, Yarmolovsky A, Djaldetti M. Chorea in polycythemia vera: A rare presentation of hyperviscosity. Blut 1989;58:47–48.
226. Chamouard JM, Smagghe A, Malalanirina BH, Davous P, Poisson M. Chorea disclosing polycythemia and renal adenocarcinoma. Rev Neurol 1992;148:380–382.
227. Tang WY, Gill DS, Chuan PS. Chorea, a manifestation of hyponatremia? Singapore Med J 1981;22:92–93.
228. Sparacio RR, Anziska B, Schutta HS. Hypernatremia and chorea. Neurology 1976;26:46–50.
229. Howdle PD, Bone I, Losowsky MS. Hypocalcemic chorea secondary to malabsorption. Postgrad Med J 1979;55: 560–563.
230. Greenhouse AH. On chorea, lupus erythematosus, and cerebral vasculitis. Arch Intern Med 1966;117:389–393.
231. Tabee-Zadeh MJ, Frame B, Kapphahn K. Kinesiogenic choreoathetosis and idiopathic hypoparathyroidism. N Engl J Med 1972;286:762–763.
232. Soffer D, Licht A, Yaar I, Abramsky O. Paroxysmal choreoathetosis as a presenting symptom in idiopathic hypoparathyroidism. J Neurol Neurosurg Psychiatry 1977; 40:692–694.
233. Kashihara K, Yabuki S. Unilateral choreic movements in idiopathic hypoparathyroidism. Brain Nerve 1992;44: 477–480.
234. Salti I, Paris A, Tannir N, Khouri K. Rapid correction by 1-alpha-hydroxycholecalciferol of hemichorea in surgical hypoparathyroidism. J Neurol Neurosurg Psychiatry 1982; 45:89–90.
235. Rizzo GN, Olanow CW, Roses AD. Chorea in hyperparathyroidism. Report of a case. AMB Rev Assoc Med Bras 1981;27:155–156.
236. Hurwitz LJ, Montgomery AD. Persistent choreoathetotic movements in liver disease. Arch Neurol 1965;13:421–426.
237. Toghill PJ, Johnston AW, Smith JF. Choreoathetosis in porto-systemic encephalopathy. J Neurol Neurosurg Psychiatry 1967;30:358–363.
238. Gerard JM, Vanderhaeghen JJ, Telerman-Toppet N, Coers C. Choreoathetosis with hepato-cerebral degeneration in a patient with a portocaval shunt. Acta Neurol Belg 1973; 73:100–109.
239. Spitaleri DL, Vitolo S, Fasanaro AM, Valiani R. Choreoathetosis. Uncommon manifestation during chronic liver disease with portocaval shunt. Riv Neurol 1983;53:293–299.
240. Yokota T, Tsuchiya K, Umetani K, Furukawa T, Tsukagoshi H. Choreoathetoid movements associated with a splenorenal shunt. J Neurol 1988;235:487–488.
241. Tison FX, Ferrer X, Julien J. Delayed onset movement disorders as a complication of central pontine myelinolysis. Mov Disord 1991;6:171–173.
242. Tsutada T, Hayashi H, Kitano S, Imai T, Nishimura S. A case report of central pontine and extrapontine myelinolysis which occurred during pregnancy and was accompanied by choreic movement. Clin Neurol 1989;29:1294–1297.
243. Roos RA, Wintzen AR, Vielvoye G, Polder TW. Paroxysmal kinesigenic choreoathetosis as presenting symptom of multiple sclerosis. J Neurol Neurosurg Psychiatry 1991;54:657–658.
244. Mouren P, Tatassian A, Toga M, Poinso Y, Blumen G. Etude critique du syndrome hémiballique. Encéphale 1966;55:212–274.
245. Sarkari NBS. Involuntary movements in multiple sclerosis. Br Med J 1968;2:738–740.
246. Bachman DS, Laó-Vélez C, Estanol B. Dystonia and choreoathetosis in multiple sclerosis. Arch Neurol 1976; 33:590.
247. Taff I, Sabato UC, Lehrer G. Choreoathetosis in multiple sclerosis. Clin Neurol Neurosurg 1985;87:41–43.
248. Mao C–C, Gancher ST, Herndon RM. Movement disorders in multiple sclerosis. Mov Disord 1988;3:109–116.
249. Björk VO, Hultquist G. Brain damage in children after deep hypothermia for open-heart surgery. Thorax 1960; 15:284–291.
250. Bergouignan M, Fontan F, Trarieux M, Julien J. Syndromes choreiformes de l'enfant au décours d'interventions cardio-chirurgicales sous hypothermie profonde. Rev Neurol 1961;105:48–60.
251. Brunberg JA, Doty DB, Reilly EL. Choreoathetosis in infants following cardiac surgery with deep hypothermia and circulatory arrest. J Pediatrics 1974;84:232–235.
252. Robinson RO, Samuels M, Pohl KRE. Choreic syndrome after cardiac surgery. Arch Dis Child 1988;63:1466–1469.
253. DeLeon S, Ilbawi M, Arcilla R, et al. Choreoathetosis after deep hypothermia without circulatory arrest. Ann Thorac Surg 1990;50:714–719.
254. Barratt-Boyes BG. Choreoathetosis as a complication of cardiopulmonary bypass. Ann Thorac Surg 1990;50: 693–694.
255. Wical BS, Tomasi LG. A distinictive neurological syndrome after profound hypothermia. Pediatr Neurol 1990; 6:202–205.
256. Wong PC, Barlow CF, Hickey PR, et al. Factors associated with choreoathetosis after cardiopulmonary bypass in children with congenital heart disease. Circulation 1992;86:118–126.

257. Medlock MD, Cruse RS, Winek SJ, et al. A 10-year experience with postpump chorea. Ann Neurol 1993;34: 820–826.
258. Yoshii S, Mohri N, Suzuki S, Kobashiri H. Hashimoto R, Tada Y. Postoperative choreoathetosis in a case of tetralogy of Fallot. J Jpn Assoc Thorac Surg 1995;43:109–112.
259. Curless RG, Katz DA, Perryman RA, Ferrer PL, Gelblum J, Weiner WJ. Choreoathetosis after surgery for congenital heart disease. J Pediatrics 1994;124:737–739.
260. du Plessis A, Bellinger DC, Gauvreau K, et al. Neurologic outcome of choreoathetoid encephalopathy after cardiac surgery. Pediatr Neurol 2002;27:9–17.
261. Kupsky WJ, Drozd MA, Barlow CF. Selective injury of the globus pallidus in children with post-cardiac surgery choreic syndrome. Dev Med Child Neurol 1995;37:135–144.
262. Blunt SB, Brooks DJ, Kennard C. Steroid-responsive chorea in childhood following cardiac transplantation. Mov Disord 1994;9:112–114.
263. Duvoisin RC. Chorea. Semin Neurol 1982;2:351–358.
264. Shoulson I. On chorea. Clin Neuropharmacol 1986;9 (Suppl 2):S85–S99.
265. Hüther R, Gebhart C, Mirisch S, Bäuml J, Förstl H. Choreatic symptoms during and after treatment with paliperidone and escitalopram. Pharmacopsychiatry 2008; 41(5):203–204.
266. Davis LE, Becher MW, Tlomak W, Benson BE, Lee RR, Fisher EC. Persistent choreoathetosis in a fatal olanzapine overdose: Drug kinetics, neuroimaging, and neuropathology. Am J Psychiatry 2005;162(1):28–33.
267. Nomoto M, Thompson PD, Sheehy MP, Quinn NP, Marsden CD. Anticholinergic-induced chorea in the treatment of focal dystonia. Mov Disord 1987;2:53–56.
268. Matsumoto K, Nogaki H, Morimatsu M. A case of choreoathetoid movements induced by anticholinergic drugs, trihexyphenidyl HCl and dosulepin HCl. Jpn J Geriatr 1992;29:686–689.
269. Harrison MB, Lyons GR, Landow ER. Phenytoin and dyskinesias: A report of two cases and review of the literature. Mov Disord 1993;8:19–27.
270. Lancman ME, Asconape JJ, Penry JK. Choreiform movements associated with the use of valproate. Arch Neurol 1994;51:702–704.
271. Zaatreh M, Tennison M, D'Cruz O, Beach RL. Anticonvulsants-induced chorea: A role for pharmacodynamic drug interaction? Seizure 2001;10:596–599.
272. Attupurath R, Aziz R, Wollman D, Muralee S, Tampi RR. Chorea associated with gabapentin use in an elderly man. Am J Geriatr Pharmacother 2009;7(4):220–224.
273. Chudnow RS, Dewey RB Jr, Lawson CR. Choreoathetosis as a side effect of gabapentin therapy in severely neurologically impaired patients. Arch Neurology 1997;54: 910–912.
274. Sperling LS, Horowitz JL. Methamphetamine-induced choreoathetosis and rhabdomyolysis. Ann Intern Med 1994;121:986.
275. Rhee KJ, Albertson TE, Douglas JC. Choreoathetoid disorder associated with amphetamine-like drugs. Am J Emerg Med 1988;6:131–133.
276. Daras M, Koppel BS, Atos-Radzion E. Cocaine-induced choreoathetoid movements ('crack dancing'). Neurology 1994;44:751–752.
277. Stuart AM, Worley LM, Spillane J. Choreiform movements observed in an 8-year-old child following use of an oral theophylline preparation. Clin Pediatr 1992;31:692–694.
278. Bonnet U, Banger M, Wolstein J, Gastpar M. Choreoathetoid movements associated with rapid adjustment to methadone. Pharmacopsychiatry 1998;31:143–145.
279. Helmuth D, Ljaljevic Z, Ramirez L, Meltzer HY. Choreoathetosis induced by verapamil and lithium treatment. J Clin Psychopharmacol 1989;9:454–455.
280. Nielsen AS, Mors O. Choreiform dyskinesia with acute onset and protracted course following fluoxetine treatment. J Clin Psychiatry 1999;60:868–869.
281. Fox GC, Ebeid S, Vincenti G. Paroxetine-induced chorea. Br J Psychiatry 1997;170:193–194.
282. Busari OA, Oligbu G. Chorea in a 29-year-old Nigerian following antimalarial treatment with artesunate. Int J Infect Dis 2008;12(2):221–322.
283. Crystal HA. Baclofen therapy may be associated with chorea in Alzheimer's disease. Ann Neurol 1990;28:839.
284. Azar S, Ramjiani A, Van Gerpen JA. Ciprofloxacin-induced chorea. Mov Disord 2005;20(4):513–514
285. Combarros O, Fabrega E, Polo JM, Berciano J. Cyclosporine-induced chorea after liver transplantation for Wilson's disease. Ann Neurol 1993;33:108–109.
286. Samie MR, Ashton AK. Choreoathetosis induced by cyproheptadine. Mov Disord 1989;4:81–84.
287. Patrick SJ, Snelling LK, Ment LR. Infantile chorea following abrupt withdrawal of diazepam and pentobarbital therapy. J Toxicol Clin Toxicol 1993;31:127–132.
288. Mulder LJ, van der Mast RC, Meerwaldt JD. Generalised chorea due to digoxin toxicity. Br Med J Clin Res Ed 1988; 296:1262.
289. Moulignier A, Allo S, Singer B, Monge-Strauss MF, Zittoun R, Gout O. Sub-cortico-frontal encephalopathy and choreic movements related to recombinant interferon-alpha 2b. Rev Neurol 2002;158:567–572.
290. Matsis PP, Fisher RA, Tasman-Jones C. Acute lithium toxicity—Chorea, hypercalcemia and hyperamylasemia. Aust N Z J Med 1989;19:718–720.
291. Reed SM, Wise MG, Timmerman I. Choreoathetosis: A sign of lithium toxicity. J Neuropsychiatry Clin Neurosci 1989; 1:57–60.
292. Gironell A, de Molina RM, Sancho G, Kulisevsky J. Chorea induced by a luteinizing hormone-releasing hormone analog. J Neurol 2008;255(8):1264–1265.
293. Necioğlu Orken D, Yldrmak Y, Kenangil G, Kandraloğlu N, Forta H, Celik M. Intrathecal methotrexate-induced acute chorea. J Pediatr Hematol Oncol 2009;31(1): 57–58.
294. Vytopil M, Mani R, Adlakha A, Zhu JJ. Acute chorea and hyperthermia after concurrent use of modafinil and tranylcypromine. Am J Psychiatry 2007;164(4):684.
295. Duncan MA, Nikolov NM, O'Kelly B. Acute chorea due to ondansetron in an obstetric patient. Int J Obstet Anesth 2001;10(4):309–311.
296. Sweeney BJ, Edgecombe J, Churchill DR, Miller RF, Harrison MJ. Choreoathetosis/ballismus associated with pentamidine-induced hypoglycemia in a patient with the acquired immunodeficiency syndrome. Arch Neurol 1994;51:723–725.
297. Lehmann AB. Reversible chorea due to ranitidine and cimetidine. Lancet 1988;8603:158.

298. Clarke CE, Bamford JM, House A. Dyskinesia in Creutzfeld-Jakob disease precipitated by antidepressant therapy. Mov Disord 1992;7:86–87.
299. Bua J, Marchetti F, Barbi E, Sarti A, Ventura A. Tremors and chorea induced by trimethoprim-sulfamethoxazole in a child with pneumocystis pneumonia. Pediatr Infect Dis J 2005;24(10):934–935.
300. Fukutani Y, Nakamura I, Kobayashi K, Yamaguchi N, Matsubara R, Kiyota Y. A case of familial juvenile Alzheimer's disease with apallic state at the relatively early stage and various neurological features—A clinicopathological study. Clin Neurol 1989;29:633–638.
301. Voll R, Hoffmann GF, Lipinski CG, Trefz FK, Weisser J. Glutaric acidemia/glutaric aciduria I as differential chorea minor diagnosis. Klin Padiatrie 1993;205:124–126.
302. Sethi KD, Ray R, Roesel RA, et al. Adult-onset chorea and dementia with propionic acidemia. Neurology 1989;39:1343–1345.
303. Wiltshire EJ, Poplawski NK, Harbord MG, Harrison RJ, Fletcher JM. Ornithine carbamoyltransferase deficiency presenting with chorea in a female. J Inher Metabol Dis 2000;23:843–844.
304. Friedman JH, Weitberg A. Ataxia without telangiectasia. Mov Disord 1993;8:223–226.
305. Gamez J, Corbera-Bellalta M, Mila M, López-Lisbona R, Boluda S, Ferrer I. Chorea-ballism associated with familial amyotrophic lateral sclerosis. A clinical, genetic, and neuropathological study. Mov Disord 2008;23(3):434–438.
306. Hanna MG, Davis MB, Sweeney MG, et al. Generalized chorea in two patients harboring the Friedreich's ataxia gene trinucleotide repeat expansion. Mov Disord 1998;13:339–340.
307. Zhu D, Burke C, Leslie A, Nicholson GA. Friedreich's ataxia with chorea and myoclonus caused by a compound heterozygosity for a novel deletion and the trinucleotide GAA expansion. Mov Disord 2002;17:585–589.
308. Friedman JR, Thiele EA, Wang D, et al. Atypical GLUT1 deficiency with prominent movement disorder responsive to ketogenic diet. Mov Disord 2006;21(2):241–245.
309. Hayflick SJ. Unraveling the Hallervorden-Spatz syndrome: Pantothenate kinase-associated neurodegeneration is the name. Curr Opin Pediatr 2003;15(6):572–577.
310. Namekawa M, Takiyama Y, Ando Y. Choreiform movements in spinocerebellar ataxia type 1. J Neurol Sci 2001;187:103–106.
311. Margolis RL, Rudnicki DD, Holmes SE. Huntington's disease like-2: Review and update. Acta Neurol Taiwan 2005;14(1):1–8.
312. Manyam BV, Walters AS, Narla KR. Bilateral striopallidodentate calcinosis: Clinical characteristics of patients seen in a registry. Mov Disord 2001;16:258–264.
313. Nakagaki H, Furuya J, Santa Y, Nagano S, Araki E, Yamada T. A case of MELAS presenting juvenile-onset hyperglycemic chorea-ballism. Rinsho Shinkeigaku 2005;45(7):502–505.
314. Nelson I, Hanna MG, Alsanjari N, Scaravilli F, Morgan-Hughes JA, Harding AE. A new mitochondrial DNA mutation associated with progressive dementia and chorea: A clinical, pathological, and molecular genetic study. Ann Neurol 1995;37:400–403.
315. Truong DD, Harding AE, Scaravilli F, et al. Movement disorders in mitochondrial myopathies: A study of nine cases with two autopsy studies. Mov Disord 1990;5:109–117.
316. Steiger MJ, Pires M, Scaravilli F, Quinn NP, Marsden CD. Hemiballism and chorea in a patient with parkinsonism due to a multisystem degeneration. Mov Disord 1992;7:71–77.
317. Colosimo C, Rossi P, Elia M, Bentivoglio AR, Altavista MC, Albanese A. Transient alternating hemichorea as presenting sign of progressive supranuclear palsy. Ital J Neurol Sci 1991;12:99–101.
318. Seijo Martinez M, Castro del Rio M, Losada Campa A, Varela Freijanes A, Rodriguez M. Chorea as the presenting form of progressive systemic sclerosis. Neurologia 2000;15:304–306.
319. Temudo T, Ramos E, Dias K, et al. Movement disorders in Rett syndrome: An analysis of 60 patients with detected MECP2 mutation and correlation with mutation type. Mov Disord 2008;23(10):1384–1390.
320. Brockmann K, Dumitrescu AM, Best TT, Hanefeld F, Refetoff S. X-linked paroxysmal dyskinesia and severe global retardation caused by defective MCT8 gene. J Neurol 2005;252(6):663–666.
321. Wright RA, Pollock M, Donaldson IM. Chorea and tuberous sclerosis. Mov Disord 1992;7:87–89.
322. Kimura N, Sugihara R, Kimura A, Kumamoto T, Tsuda T. A case of neuro-Behcet's disease presenting with chorea. Rinsho Shinkeigaku 2001;41:45–49.
323. Kok J, Bosseray A, Brion JP, Micoud M, Besson G. Chorea in a child with Churg-Straus syndrome. Stroke 1993;24:1263–1264.
324. Taurin G, Golfier V, Pinel JF, et al. Choreic syndrome due to Hashimoto's encephalopathy. Mov Disord 2002;17:1091–1092.
325. Jones AL, Bouchier IA. A patient with neurosyphilis presenting as chorea. Scot Med J 1993;38:82–84.
326. Blakeley J, Jankovic J. Secondary paroxysmal dyskinesias. Mov Disord 2002;17:726–734.
327. Beskind DL, Keim SM. Choreoathetotic movement disorder in a boy with Mycoplasma pneumoniae encephalitis. Ann Emerg Med 1994;23:1375–1378.
328. Krauss JK, Mohadjer M, Nobbe F, Mundinger F. Bilateral ballismus in children. Child Nerv Syst 1991;7:342–346.
329. Fong CY, de Sousa C. Childhood chorea-encephalopathy associated with human parvovirus B19 infection. Dev Med Child Neurol 2006;48(6):526–528.
330. Gascon GG, al-Jarallah AA, Okamoto E, al Ahdal M, Kessie G, Frayha H. Chorea as a presentation of herpes simplex encephalitis relapse. Brain Dev 1993;15:178–181.
331. Wang HS, Kuo MF, Huang SC, Chou ML. Choreoathetosis as an initial sign of relapsing of herpes simplex encephalitis. Pediatr Neurol 1994;11:341–345.
332. Hengstman GJ, van Rossum MM, van der Kerkhof PC, Bloem BR . Chorea due to mycosis fungoides metastasis. J Neurooncol 2005;73(1):87–88.
333. Bhigjee AI, Kemp T, Cosnett JE. Cerebral cysticercosis presenting with hemichorea. J Neurol Neurosurg Psychiatry 1987;50:1561–1562.
334. Ozer F, Meral H, Aydemir T, Ozturk O. Hemiballism-hemichorea in presentation of cranial tuberculoma. Mov Disord 2006;21(8):1293–1294.

335. Mirsattari SM, Berry ME, Holden JK, Ni W, Nath A, Power C. Paroxysmal dyskinesias in patients with HIV infection. Neurology 1999;52:109–114.
336. Piccolo I, Causarano R, Sterzi R, et al. Chorea in patients with AIDS. Acta Neurol Scand 1999;100:332–336.
337. Gallo BV, Shulman LM, Weiner WJ, Petito CK, Berger JR. HIV encephalitis presenting with severe generalized chorea. Neurology 1996;46:1163–1165.
338. Teive HA, Troiano AR, Cabral NL, Becker N, Werneck LC. Hemichorea-hemiballism associated to cryptococcal granuloma in a patient with AIDS: Case report. Arquiv Neuro-Psiquiatria 2000;58:965–968.
339. Sanchez-Ramos JR, Factor SA, Weiner WJ, Marquez J. Hemichorea-hemiballismus associated with acquired immune deficiency syndrome and cerebral toxoplasmosis. Mov Disord 1989;4:266–273.
340. Pestre P, Milandre L, Farnarier P, Gallais H. Hemichorea in acquired immunodeficiency syndrome. Toxoplasmosis abscess in the striatum. Rev Neurol 1991;147:833–837.
341. Nath A, Hobson DE, Russell A. Movement disorders with cerebral toxoplasmosis and AIDS. Mov Disord 1993;8: 107–112.
342. Pereira AC, Edwards MJ, Buttery PC, et al. Choreic syndrome and coeliac disease: A hitherto unrecognised association. Mov Disord 2004;19(4):478–482.
343. Moodley R, Seebaran AR, Rajput MC. Dystonia and choreo-athetosis in Wernicke's encephalopathy. A case report. S Afr Med J 1989;75:543–544.
344. Pacchetti C, Cristina S, Nappi G. Reversible chorea and focal dystonia in vitamin B12 deficiency. N Engl J Med 2002;347:295.
345. Meucci G, Rossi G, Mazzoni M. A case of transient choreoathetosis with amnesic syndrome after acute carbon monoxide poisoning. Ital J Neurol Sci 1989;10: 513–517.
346. Spitz M, Lucato LT, Haddad MS, Barbosa ER. Choreoathetosis secondary to lead toxicity. Arq Neuropsiquiatr 2008; 66(3A):575–577.
347. de Krom MC, Boreas AM, Hardy EL. Manganese poisoning due to use of Chien Pu Wan tablets. Ned Tijdschr Geneeskd 1994;138:2010–2012.
348. Joubert J, Joubert PH. Chorea and psychiatric changes in organophsophate poisoning. A report of 2 further cases. S Afr Med J 1988;74:32–34.
349. Poewe WH, Kleedorfer B, Willeit J, Gerstenbrand F. Primary CNS lymphoma presenting as a choreic movement disorder followed by segmental dystonia. Mov Disord 1988;3: 320–325.
350. Sakai M, Hashizume Y, Yamamoto H, Kawakami A. An autopsy case of primary cerebral malignant lymphoma initiated with choreoathetosis. Clin Neurol 1990;30: 849–854.
351. Schiff DE, Ortega JA. Chorea, eosinophilia, and lupus anticoagulant associated with acute lymphoblastic leukemia. Pediatr Neurol 1992;8:466–468.
352. Albin RL, Bromberg MB, Penney JB, Knapp R. Chorea and dystonia: A remote effect of carcinoma. Mov Disord 1988:3:162–169.
353. Vernino S, Tuite P, Adler CH, et al. Paraneoplastic chorea associated with CRMP-5 neuronal antibody and lung carcinoma. Ann Neurol 2002;51:625–630.
354. Itoh H, Shibata K, Nitta E, Takamori M. Hemiballism-hemichorea from marked hypotension during spinal anesthesia. Acta Anaesthesiol Scand 1998;42:133–135.
355. Galea I, Norwood F, Phillips MJ, Shearman C, McMonagle P, Gibb WR. Pearls & Oy-sters: Resolution of hemichorea following endarterectomy for severe carotid stenosis. Neurology 2008;71(24):e80–e82.
356. Watanabe K, Negoro T, Maehara M, Takahashi I, Nomura K, Miura K. Moyamoya disease presenting with chorea. Pediatr Neurol 1990;6:40–42.
357. Pavlakis SG, Schneider S, Black K, Gould RJ. Steroid-responsive chorea in moyamoya disease. Mov Disord 1991;6: 347–349.
358. Schmeisser MJ, Unrath A, Otto M, Tumani H, Abler B. Moyamoya disease precipitating Sydenham's chorea in a 19-year-old Caucasian woman. Mov Disord 2009;24(9): 1401–1403.
359. Takanashi J, Sugita K, Honda A, Niimi H. Moyamoya syndrome in a patient with Down's syndrome presenting with chorea. Pediatr Neurol 1993;9:396–398.
360. Tan EK, Lo YL, Chan LL, See SJ, Hong A, Wong MC. Cervical disc prolapse with cord compression presenting with choreoathetosis and dystonia. Neurology 2002;58: 661–662.
361. Mokri B, Ahlskog JE, Luetmer PH. Chorea as a manifestation of spontaneous CSF leak. Neurology 2006;67(8): 1490–1491.
362. Voermans NC, Schutte PJ, Bloem BR. Hydrocephalus induced chorea. J Neurol Neurosurg Psychiatry 2007;78(11): 1284–1285.
363. Yamada K, Harada M, Inoue N, Yoshida S, Morioka M, Kuratsu J. Concurrent hemichorea and migrainous aura—A perfusion study on the basal ganglia using xenon-computed tomography. Mov Disord 2008;23(3): 425–429.
364. Masjuan J, Buisan J, Gimeno A, Alvarez-Cermeno JC. Paroxysmal dyskinesias as the initial manifestation of multiple sclerosis. Neurologia 1998;13:45–48.
365. Fowler WE, Kriel RL, Krach LE. Movement disorders after status epilepticus and other brain injuries. Pediatr Neurol 1992;8:281–284.
366. Hadders-Algra M, Bos AF, Martijn A, Prechtl HF. Infantile chorea in an infant with severe bronchopulmonary dysplasia: An EMG study. Dev Med Child Neurol 1994;36: 177–182.
367. Alakandy LM, Iyer RV, Golash A. Hemichorea, an unusual complication of ventriculoperitoneal shunt. J Clin Neurosci 2008;15(5):599–601
368. Tschopp L, Raina G, Salazar Z, Micheli F. Neuroacanthocytosis and carbamazepine responsive paroxysmal dyskinesias. Parkinsonism Relat Disord 2008;14(5):440–244.
369. Engelen M, Tijssen MA. Paroxysmal non-kinesigenic dyskinesia in antiphospholipid syndrome. Mov Disord 2005;20(1): 111–113.
370. Bhatia KP. The paroxysmal dyskinesias. J Neurol 1999;246: 149–155.
371. Bhatia KP. Familial (idiopathic) paroxysmal dyskinesias: An update. Semin Neurol 2001;21:69–74.
372. Chatterjee A, Louis ED, Frucht S. Levetiracetam in the treatment of paroxysmal kinesiogenic choreoathetosis. Mov Disord 2002;17:614–615.

373. Huang YG, Chen YC, Du F, et al. Topiramate therapy for paroxysmal kinesigenic choreoathetosis. Mov Disord 2005;20(1):75–77.
374. Chudnow RS, Mimbela RA, Owen DB, Roach ES. Gabapentin for familial paroxysmal dystonic choreoathetosis. Neurology 1997;49:1441–1442.
375. Szczałuba K, Jurek M, Szczepanik E, et al. A family with paroxysmal nonkinesigenic dyskinesia: Genetic and treatment issues. Pediatr Neurol 2009;41(2):135–138.
376. Yamada K, Goto S, Soyama N, et al. Complete suppression of paroxysmal nonkinesigenic dyskinesia by globus pallidus internus pallidal stimulation. Mov Disord 2006; 21(4):576–579.
377. Cochen De Cock V, Bourdain F, Apartis E, Trocello JM, Roze E, Vidailhet M. Interictal myoclonus with paroxysmal kinesigenic dyskinesia. Mov Disord 2006;21(9): 1533–1535.
378. De Grandis E, Mir P, Edwards MJ, Quinn NP, Bhatia KP. Paroxysmal dyskinesia with interictal myoclonus and dystonia: A report of two cases. Parkinsonism Relat Disord 2008;14(3):250–252.
379. Joo EY, Hong SB, Tae WS, et al. Perfusion abnormality of the caudate nucleus in patients with paroxysmal kinesigenic choreoathetosis. Eur J Nucl Med Mol Imaging 2005;32(10):1205–1209.
380. Lee WL, Tay A, Ong HT, Goh LM, Monaco AP, Szepetowski P. Association of infantile convulsions with paroxysmal dyskinesias (ICCA syndrome): Confirmation of linkage to human chromosome 16p12-q12 in a Chinese family. Hum Genet 1998;103:608–612.
381. Tomita H, Nagamitsu S, Wakui K, et al. Paroxysmal kinesigenic choreoathetosis locus maps to chromosome 16p11.2-q12.1. Am J Hum Genet 1999;65:1688–1697.
382. Caraballo R, Pavek S, Lemainque A, et al. Linkage of benign familial infantile convulsions to chromosome 16p12-q12 suggests allelism to the infantile convulsions and choreoathetosis syndrome. Am J Hum Genet 2001;68: 788–794.
383. Fouad GT, Servidei S, Durcan S, Bertini E, Ptacek LJ. A gene for familial paroxysmal dyskinesia (FPD1) maps to chromosome 2q. Am J Hum Genet 1996;59:135–139.
384. Lee HY, Xu Y, Huang Y, Ahn AH, et al. The gene for paroxysmal non-kinesigenic dyskinesia encodes an enzyme in a stress response pathway. Hum Mol Genet 2004;13(24): 3161–3170.
385. Ghezzi D, Viscomi C, Ferlini A, et al. Paroxysmal non-kinesigenic dyskinesia is caused by mutations of the MR-1 mitochondrial targeting sequence. Hum Mol Genet 2009;18(6):1058–1064.
386. Kamm C, Mayer P, Sharma M, Niemann G, Gasser T. New family with paroxysmal exercise-induced dystonia and epilepsy. Mov Disord 2007;22(6):873–877.
387. Suls A, Dedeken P, Goffin K, et al. Paroxysmal exercise-induced dyskinesia and epilepsy is due to mutations in SLC2A1, encoding the glucose transporter GLUT1. Brain 2008;131 (Pt 7):1831–1844.
388. Weber YG, Storch A, Wuttke TV, et al. GLUT1 mutations are a cause of paroxysmal exertion-induced dyskinesias and induce hemolytic anemia by a cation leak. J Clin Invest 2008;118(6):2157–2168.
389. Pérez-Dueñas B, Prior C, Ma Q, et al. Childhood chorea with cerebral hypotrophy: A treatable GLUT1 energy failure syndrome. Arch Neurol 2009;66(11):1410–1414.
390. Shirley TL, Rao LM, Hess EJ, Jinnah HA. Paroxysmal dyskinesias in mice. Mov Disord 2008;23(2):259–264.
391. Khan Z, Jinnah HA. Paroxysmal dyskinesias in the lethargic mouse mutant. J Neurosci 2002;22:8193–8200.
392. Spillane JD, Nathan PW, Kelly RE, Marsden CD. Painful legs and moving toes. Brain 1971;94:541–556.
393. Nathan PW. Painful legs and moving toes; evidence on the site of the lesion. J Neurol Neurosurg Psychiatry 1978;41: 934–939.
394. Schott GD. Painful legs and moving toes: The role of trauma. J Neurol Neurosurg Psychiatry 1981;44:344–346.
395. Barrett RE, Singh N, Fahn S. The syndrome of painful legs and moving toes. Neurology 1981;31(suppl 1):79.
396. Wulff CH. Painful legs and moving toes: A report of 3 cases with neurophysiologic studies. Acta Neurol Scand 1982;66:283–287.
397. Schoenen J, Gonce M, Delwaide PJ. Painful legs and moving toes: A syndrome with different pathophysiologic mechanisms. Neurology 1984;34:1108–1112.
398. Funakawa I, Muno Y, Takayanagi T. Painful hand and moving fingers. J Neurol 1987;234:342–343.
399. Verhagen WIM, Horstink WMIM, Notermans SLH. Painful arm and moving fingers. J Neurol Neurosurg Psychiatry 1985; 48:384–385.
400. Ebersbach G, Schelosky L, Schenkel A, Scholz U, Poewe W. Unilateral painful legs and moving toes syndrome with moving fingers—Evidence for distinct oscillators. Mov Disord 1998;13:965–968.
401. Alvarez MV, Driver-Dunckley EE, Caviness JN, Adler CH, Evidente VG. Case series of painful legs and moving toes: Clinical and electrophysiologic observations. Mov Disord 2008;23(14):2062–2066.
402. Okuda Y, Suzuki K, Kitajima T, Masuda R, Asai T. Lumbar epidural block for 'painful legs and moving toes' syndrome: A report of three cases. Pain 1998;78145–147.
403. Takahashi H, Saitoh C, Iwata O, Nanbu T, Takada S, Morita S. Epidural spinal cord stimulation for the treatment of painful legs and moving toes syndrome. Pain 2002;96: 343–345.
404. Aizawa H. Gabapentin for painful legs and moving toes syndrome. Intern Med 2007;46(23):1937.
405. Villarejo A, Porta-Etessam J, Camacho A, et al. Gabapentin for painful legs and moving toes syndrome. Eur Neurol 2004;51(3):180–181.
406. Pitagoras de Mattos J, Oliveira M, Andre C. Painful legs and moving toes associated with neuropathy in HIV-infected patients. Mov Disord 1999;14:1053–1054.
407. Mattos JP, Rosso AL, Correa RB, Novis SA. Movement disorders in 28 HIV-infected patients. Arquiv Neuro-Psiquiatria 2002;60:525–530.
408. Dressler D, Thompson PD, Gledhill RF, Marsden CD. The syndrome of painful leg and moving toes. Mov Disord 1994;9:13–21.
409. Walters AS, Hening WA, Shah SK, Chokroverty S. Painless legs and moving toes: A syndrome related to painful legs and moving toes? Mov Disord 1993;8:377–379.

V. MYOCLONIC DISORDERS

CHAPTER 37

Classification, Clinical Features, and Treatment of Myoclonus

Rafael González-Redondo, Asier Gómez, and José A. Obeso

Myoclonus is a brief muscle jerk caused by neuronal discharges. A sudden and short-lasting interruption of ongoing voluntary muscle contraction may produce a postural pause clinically very similar to myoclonus, hence the term "negative myoclonus." Both forms often share the same etiology, coincide in the same patients, and can even affect the same muscle group.[1] A myoclonic jerk consists of a single muscle discharge but can be repetitive, giving rise to a salvo of muscle activity (Fig. 37–1). The latter is particularly frequent in action myoclonus and interferes severely with the execution of even the most simple motor tasks. For this reason, action myoclonus (both positive and negative types) may be considered among the movement disorder that produces the greatest interference with voluntary movements.

When including all known etiologies, myoclonus has an average annual incidence of 1.3 cases per 100,000.[2]

Myoclonus can be categorized from various points of view (Table 37–1) with no definitive and universally accepted classification. The major categories are clinical presentation, neurophysiological origin, and etiology. According with clinical presentation, myoclonus may occur spontaneously, may be triggered by external stimulation ("reflex"), or may be induced during voluntary muscle activation ("action"). The distribution may be focal, segmental, generalized, or multifocal. The timing of myoclonus can be rhythmic or irregular.

The origin of the abnormal neuronal discharge giving rise to myoclonus can be ascertained as cortical, subcortical (brainstem), or spinal. The etiological

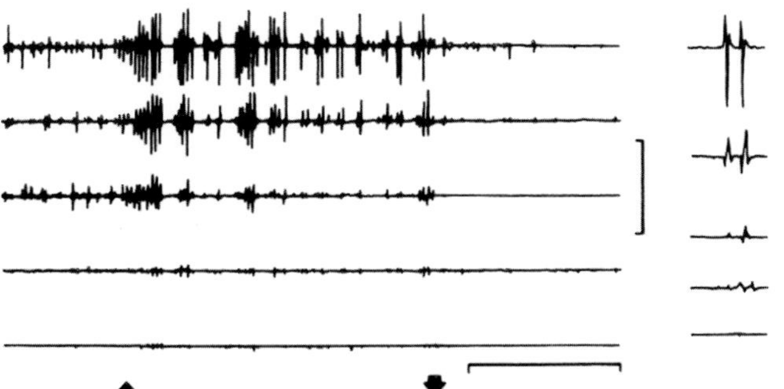

Figure 37–1. EMG recording from several muscles in the right arm of a patient with action myoclonus (Ramsay Hunt syndrome). From top to bottom are deltoid, biceps, triceps, finger extensors, and finger flexors. The horizontal scale bar indicates 2 seconds. The insert on the right shows the EMG discharges in more detail. Scale bar = 100 ms. The salvo of repetitive myoclonic discharges associated with silent periods is clearly seen in the proximal arm muscles. (From Obeso et al.[9] with permission.)

▶ TABLE 37–1. CLASSIFICATION OF MYOCLONUS

Clinical
Presentation
Spontaneous
Action
Reflex
Distribution
Generalized
Multifocal
Segmental
Focal
Neurophysiological origin
Cortical
Subcortical (brainstem)
Spinal
Etiology
Physiological
Essential
Symptomatic
Associated with epilepsy
Associated with other causes

classification of myoclonus has no simple approach and will be discussed in this chapter.

▶ DIFFERENTIATION FROM OTHER MOVEMENT DISORDERS

Myoclonus must be differentiated from other dyskinesias, such as tics, chorea, postural tremor, dystonia, and hemifacial spasm.[3] Tics, as present in Tourette's syndrome, are frequently as brief as myoclonus. The main elements to distinguish between these two categories of muscle jerks include the following. (1) Myoclonus usually interferes notably with voluntary movement and is aggravated by action, whereas tics almost never disrupt motor acts. (2) Tics can be voluntarily suppressed and myoclonus cannot. (3) A high proportion of patients will feel a somesthetic sensation preceding the tic or an internal urgency to produce the movement. Myoclonus is not accompanied by any special sensation. (4) Most forms of myoclonus stop during sleep, whereas tics often persist.

Chorea is a flowing combination of irregular muscle activity. Some of the movements of chorea may look "myoclonic" if taken in isolation, but it is the unpredictable concatenation of different patterns of movement that typifies chorea.

Postural and action tremor, when very severe, may be associated with sudden changes in the amplitude and rhythmicity of the muscle activity, giving rise to a false impression of a myoclonic jerk. This problem may be resolved, when in doubt, by electromyographic (EMG) recording.[4] Slow resting tremor or myorhythmia is difficult to distinguish clinically from rhythmical segmental myoclonus. True myoclonus, even when repetitive and rhythmical, must have a sudden and shocklike onset and end.

Dystonia consists of prolonged muscle spasms, which are longer than those of myoclonus and produce twisting, repetitive movements and abnormal postures.[5] Similarly, the muscle activity of hemifacial spasm lasts longer and provokes sustained, tonic contractions. However, such differentiation might not be so easy in early stages, when only clonic twitching of either the upper or lower facial musculature is present. In such instances, EMG studies are needed to clarify the diagnosis. Typically, EMG recording in dystonia shows long duration (>200 ms) muscle spasms.

It should be kept in mind that myoclonus may coincide with other involuntary movement disorders in the same patients. For instance, some families with essential tremor and myoclonus have been described,[6] myoclonus and dystonia are combined in inherited myoclonic dystonia (Fig. 37–2),[7] and both action and reflex myoclonic jerks may be present in patients with Huntington's chorea.[8] These and other combinations also illustrate the point that the major motor manifestation of a given nosological entity does not imply that other movement disorders cannot be present in such diseases and syndromes. For example, not all the abnormal movements of Tourette's syndrome are tics, nor is chorea the only movement disorder present in Huntington's disease (HD).

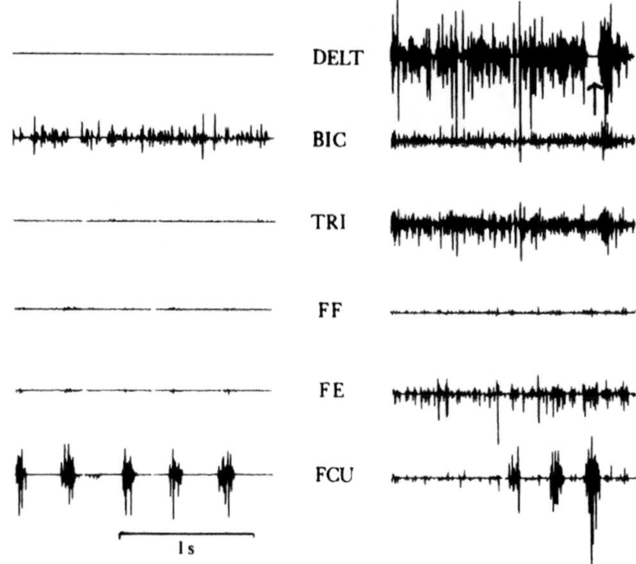

Figure 37–2. EMG recording from the right arm of a patient with myoclonic dystonia. On the left, spontaneous myoclonic activity is present in flexor carpi ulnaris (FCU) at rest. On the right, exaggerated EMG activity is seen in proximal arm muscles (deltoid, biceps, triceps) while the myoclonus persists in FCU. A brief negative myoclonus (asterixis) is indicated by the arrow in deltoid EMG (DELT). BIC, biceps; TRI, triceps; FF, finger flexor muscles; FE, finger extensor muscles. (From Obeso JA, Rothwell JC, Lang AE, Marsden CD: Myoclonic dystonia. Neurology 33:825–830, 1983. Used with permission.)

▶ CLINICAL PRESENTATION

REFLEX MYOCLONUS

Somesthetic, visual, and auditory stimuli, independently and in combination, may trigger myoclonic jerking. Such myoclonus is focal or generalized in distribution. Pinpricking the limbs distally (wrist and palmar surface of the upper limbs and the soles of the feet), as well as flicking the fingers and toes, is probably the most sensitive clinical methods of evoking reflex myoclonus limited to a body area.[9] In some instances, the jerks are so sensitive to somesthetic stimuli that focal myoclonus may become self-perpetuated and simulate spontaneous myoclonus, as in epilepsia partialis continua (EPC), or even look like a tremor. Gaze-evoked myoclonus is a rare form of evoked myoclonus described in relation with brainstem lesions.[10]

Generalized reflex myoclonus to somesthetic stimulation is more commonly obtained by touching or tapping the face, particularly the mentalis zone. Visually triggered reflex myoclonus may be evoked clinically by a threatening stimulus, but more often requires flash stimulation.[11] Auditory stimulation is not a frequent cause of myoclonus, except in children. Both visually and auditorily evoked myoclonus are always generalized. Generalized reflex myoclonus induced by unexpected sounds has to be distinguished from hyperekplexia, which is a pathological exaggeration of the startle response (see below). Neurological conditions in which reflex myoclonus might be a useful clue in the differential diagnosis include corticobasal ganglionic degeneration (CBGD), cerebellar multisystem atrophy (MSA-C), Creutzfeldt–Jakob disease (CJD), and Lafora's body disease.

ACTION MYOCLONUS

This occurs during active muscular contraction and affects both posturally acting muscles and prime movers. Action myoclonus may be focal or segmental, but the most common distribution is multifocal or generalized. This form is undoubtedly the one that produces the greatest disability. This is usually due to the concatenation of several brief and unpredictable muscle discharges (Fig. 37–1), which forces the limbs and trunk to move in unintended directions. The abnormal neuronal activity provoking action myoclonus probably arises from the same areas as those mediating normal motor control mechanisms. Thus, action myoclonus interferes with, prevents, and disrupts very gross voluntary movements to a much greater extent than other movement disorders such as dystonia and tics.

Orthostatic myoclonus has recently been recognized in elderly people.[12] Similar to orthostatic tremor, the pathological EMG activity present during standing improved when sitting or walking. EMG bursts were very brief (<30 ms), irregular, and nonrhythmic with a frequency of 9–15 Hz on standing. Unlike primary orthostatic tremor, coherence analysis demonstrated a lack of synchrony between the right and left legs. The nosology and pathophysiology of this presentation is not well defined and further characterization is needed.

NEGATIVE MYOCLONUS

Negative myoclonus is by definition only present during active muscular contraction and in fact is most frequently combined with positive action myoclonus. There are two major clinical presentations: asterixis and postural lapses.[1] Asterixis is the most common and best-characterized form of negative myoclonus. It consists of a silence of EMG discharges for a short period (50–200 ms), thus producing a brief loss of antigravitational activity and postural control (Fig. 37–2, arrow). Asterixis is usually multifocal in distribution but may affect a muscle group in isolation. Shibasaki and colleagues[13] have described reflex negative myoclonus limited to muscles of one limb. Postural lapses consist of a long-duration EMG silence (200–500 ms), usually occupying axial and proximal muscles of the lower limbs, with a tendency for repetitive appearance over a few seconds.[1] In patients with severe myoclonic encephalopathies, such as postanoxic myoclonus and progressive myoclonic epilepsy (PME), these postural lapses may follow a myoclonic discharge and may actually lead to greater functional disability than the myoclonic discharge.

SPONTANEOUS MYOCLONUS

Spontaneous myoclonus may be focal, multifocal, or generalized, and has several presentations. It may be sporadic and occur unpredictably or coincide with specific moments, such as in normal people with nocturnal myoclonus or in patients with early morning myoclonic epilepsy. In other instances, it may be almost continuously present, as in patients with metabolic encephalopathies or CJD.

RHYTHMIC MYOCLONUS

This is typically spontaneous in presentation, with a focal or segmental distribution. The myoclonic discharge may persist during sleep and is little affected by sensory stimulation. The frequency is variable but usually slow (1–4 Hz). The most common type is spinal myoclonus. Palatal "myoclonus" is nowadays considered a form of tremor, although it continues to be described under the category of myoclonus.[14]

It is important to realize that different myoclonic patterns are often combined in the same subject. For instance, reflex and action myoclonus may coincide and affect the same body region(s); multifocal spontaneous myoclonus, as seen in metabolic encephalopathies, is very commonly aggravated during action; and focal myoclonus may spread to become generalized.

▶ NEUROPHYSIOLOGICAL ORIGIN

This topic is thoroughly covered in Chapter 40, but it will be briefly addressed here because it is important to understand some clinical and therapeutic aspects.

Electrophysiological analysis of myoclonus is mainly aimed at identifying the site of the discharges producing the jerks and the pathophysiological mechanisms involved in their origin. It should be noted that the origin of the discharges producing myoclonus does not necessarily coincide with the topography of the lesion(s) and that, on many occasions, the pathological basis cannot be determined.

The origin of the neuronal discharges giving rise to myoclonus can be divided into three major pathophysiological categories: cortical, subcortical, and spinal myoclonus.

CORTICAL MYOCLONUS

Cortical myoclonus is the most common origin of myoclonus[15] and results from abnormal activity arising in the sensorimotor cortex and spreading down via the corticospinal pathway. The EMG discharge is of short duration (usually 10–50 ms); the somatosensory-evoked potentials (SEPs) are increased in amplitude (20–50 μV) and frequently associated with a reflex muscle response (C-wave) that follows the cortical potential by a short latency of 15–20 ms for the forearm muscles.[9] Back-averaging the electroencephalography (EEG) activity preceding the jerks reveals a biphasic potential over the contralateral sensorimotor cortex preceding the muscle discharge by some 20 ms in the arm and 35 ms in the leg (see Chapter 39).

SUBCORTICAL MYOCLONUS

Subcortical myoclonus indicates that the neuronal discharge originates in structures between the cortex and the spinal cord. The most common type is "reticular reflex myoclonus," (RRM) characterized by generalized jerks, with predominant involvement of proximal limb and axial muscles provoked by sensory stimulation. EMG recording of the spreading of the jerk through different muscles is necessary to determine the brainstem origin (see Chapter 39). The jerks of myoclonic dystonia also constitute an example of subcortical myoclonus.

SPINAL MYOCLONUS

Spinal myoclonus is secondary to abnormal neuronal discharge originating in the spinal cord. It is frequently rhythmical and only exceptionally stimuli-sensitive. Another form is propiospinal myoclonus,[16] in which spontaneous and stimuli-sensitive (tapping) jerks involve mainly the trunk and abdominal muscles. The EMG discharges consist of repetitive bursts with a frequency of 1–7 Hz.

▶ ETIOLOGICAL CLASSIFICATION

Myoclonus may occur in the setting of a wide variety of conditions. Indeed, a list of all causes of myoclonus could be almost as long as the index of a neurology textbook. Accordingly, in many instances, myoclonus is a nonspecific manifestation and is accompanied by many other neurological signs. In such cases, myoclonus is not a key clinical indicator. We shall give detailed attention to those conditions in which myoclonus is a major complaint or the main clinical sign leading to a correct diagnosis.

The etiological classification originally outlined by Marsden and colleagues[17] divided myoclonus into physiological, essential, epileptic, and secondary. It has been widely used and is still valid in some respects. However, the diagnosis of myoclonus from the perspective of neurology and movement disorders specialists has changed, and this classification is no longer useful in clinical practice. Instead, we shall discuss the principal clinical presentations and the most common etiologies of myoclonus. Myoclonus in patients with epilepsy (i.e., myoclonic absences, juvenile myoclonic epilepsy, etc.) as principal clinical problem is not included here.

▶ SEVERE MULTIFOCAL OR GENERALIZED MYOCLONUS

This is the most common clinical presentation in which myoclonus may be overt and the predominant clinical problem. The jerks usually have a multifocal distribution and appear spontaneously, but they may be aggravated by action and be stimulus sensitive.

INHERITED MYOCLONUS (FORMERLY ESSENTIAL MYOCLONUS)

The jerks are usually multifocal, extremely brief (hence the term "lightning"), and aggravated by action. The amplitude and intensity of the jerks are variable. In some patients the jerks are large and almost continuous, provoking severe disability, but in others the amplitude is so small that they interfere only minimally with routine motor acts. The concept about this clinical presentation has changed considerably in the last decade. It is now recognized that what was classically called essential myoclonus is a heterogeneous disorder, which may be sporadic but more often has a genetic basis (hereditary myoclonus). In familial cases, inheritance is autosomal-dominant with variable penetrance and expression, onset occurs in the first two decades of life, severity may be variable within the same family, and all routine laboratory tests and neuroimaging studies are normal.

Although the existence of patients with myoclonus as the only manifestation must be admitted, recent observations indicate that essential myoclonus very often occurs in combination with dystonic postures and movements and shows an extreme sensitivity to alcohol ("alcohol-sensitive myoclonic dystonia").[7] The association of myoclonus and dystonia has been the subject of considerable debate and confusion.[18] The term "myoclonic dystonia" was actually used a long time ago by Davidenkow,[19] and refers to the association of two movement disorders: namely, brief (<100 ms) myoclonic jerking, and long-lasting (>500 ms) dystonic spasms, usually in different muscle groups (Fig. 37–2). This combination also occurs in a low proportion of patients with idiopathic torsion dystonia,[4,18] and also in other clinical settings, such as after trauma and anoxia, or as part of the tardive dyskinesia syndrome. However, the most characteristic, even though infrequent, presentation is that of "inherited myoclonus-dystonia" (IMD) very often exhibiting a very dramatic response to alcohol.[18]

Several families with IMD have been described in recent years.[7] The disease is autosomal-dominant with fairly early onset (<10 years) and mutations in the epsilon-sarcoglycan (SGCE) *DYT11* gene. In such families, phenotypic heterogeneity has been reported within some families with cases demonstrating either dystonia or myoclonus alone.[20] Furthermore, neuropsychiatric features have been reported in several cases such as depression, addiction, attention deficit hyperactivity disorder syndrome, and obsessive–compulsive disorder. Whether alcohol dependency is a result of self-medication or part of the clinical phenotype remains under debate.[21] Spontaneous improvement of myoclonus may occur in 5% or so, and dystonia may improve in adolescence by about 20%.[22,23] SEPs, long-latency reflexes to median and digital nerve stimulation as well as jerk-locked back-averaged EEG have failed to reveal any abnormalities,[2,22,24] in keeping with a subcortical origin. Moreover, transcranial magnetic stimulation studies of motor threshold, intracortical facilitation, and intracortical inhibition have been reported to be normal by the most part.[25,26] These findings contrast with the abnormalities of cortical excitability documented in dystonia, suggesting that indeed the pathophysiology of myoclonic dystonia is distinct and differentiated from idiopathic and inherited torsion dystonia.

PROGRESSIVE MYOCLONIC ENCEPHALOPATHIES

In patients with a progressive myoclonic encephalopathy, the features of myoclonus are not generally distinctive enough to enable the correct identification of the different entities under this title. The key to a correct diagnosis and understanding of the nosology of the progressive myoclonic encephalopathies is the predominant clinical signs associated with myoclonus.

Progressive Myoclonic Encephalopathies With Epilepsy and Dementia

The major clinical features consist of action- and stimuli-sensitive multifocal and generalized myoclonus, tonic–clonic seizures that are difficult to control, and progressive dementia. Age of onset is usually in the first two decades of life, but patients with late onset are occasionally encountered. Other possible signs include ataxia, spasticity, or visual defects. In this setting, the diagnoses to consider are Lafora's disease, myoclonic epilepsy with ragged-red fibers (MERRF), lipofuscinosis (Kufs' disease), and sialidosis. In Japan, dentatorubral-pallidoluysian atrophy (DRPLA) is probably the most common cause of the syndrome.[27] DRPLA is inherited with an autosomal-dominant with incomplete penetrance pattern. The recognition of a gene mutation (CTG-B37) in chromosome 12 producing a CAG triplet expansion has led to the recognition of various clinical presentations for DRPLA worldwide.[28] The phenotype of progressive myoclonus epilepsy is mainly observed in the young-onset (<20 years) presentation.[27]

Electrophysiological analysis of patients with progressive myoclonus encephalopathies frequently indicates a cortical origin for the myoclonus, but this finding is not sufficiently specific to enable a definitive etiological diagnosis to be reached. Equally, neuroimaging studies often show brain atrophy but without any specific sign.

Lafora's disease has a mean age of onset of 14 years (ranging from 5 to 20) and consists of a rapidly progressing dementia, frequent grand mal seizures that are relatively difficult to control, and visual hallucinations. The disease is inherited by autosomal-recessive transmission. There are some 20 mutations reported in a gene coding for a protein known as laforin.[29] Mutations in EPM2A/laforin cause 58% of cases and mutations in EPM2B/malin cause 35% of cases. Accumulating evidence points to Lafora's disease as primarily a disorder of cell death with impaired clearance of misfolded proteins, as shown by ubiquitin-positive aggresomes in HeLa cells transfected with mutated laforin, ubiquitin-positive polyglucosan inclusion bodies, and malin/E3 ubiquitin ligase polyubiquitination of laforin. How polyglucosan inclusion bodies accumulate is still a mystery. A curative therapy for human Lafora's disease with laforin replacement therapy using neutral pegylated immunoliposomes is being investigated.[30]

MERRF is typically suspected in patients with a maternal inheritance pattern, and a clinical picture dominated by myoclonus, epilepsy, and ataxia, associated with other problems such as optic atrophy, deafness, peripheral neuropathy, myocardiopathy, diabetes, hypertension, short stature, and multiple lipomas. Dementia is common, but early development is typically normal. MERRF is a typical example of a respiratory chain/oxidative phosphorylation disease, causing lactic acidosis.[31] Approximately 80–90% of MERRF cases are caused by a heteroplasmic G-to-A point mutation at base pair 8344 in the T_C loop of the *tRNALys* gene (*G8344A* mutations).[32,33]

Neuronal storage diseases are the most frequent cause of progressive myoclonic encephalopathy in children. Tay-Sachs disease (hexosaminidase A deficiency), Sandhoff's disease (hexosaminidase A and B deficiency), infantile neuropathic Gaucher's disease, and the sialidosis are the most common diagnostic entities. Common to all is the generalized, stimuli-sensitive myoclonus and prominent photosensitivity. In the cherry-red-spot myoclonus syndrome (sialidosis type I), SEPs are giant, but the visual-evoked potentials are decreased in amplitude, a rare combination that may have diagnostic value. In adults, Kufs' disease and sialidosis have been described, but are indeed very rare causes of progressive myoclonic encephalopathy.

Slowly Progressive Myoclonic Encephalopathies With Epilepsy

This group is made up of patients with a slowly progressing disease with the combination of action myoclonus, epilepsy, and ataxia, in whom no evidence of mitochondrial or any other abnormality is found.[34] Dementia is not a feature, but mild cognitive impairment may be detected throughout evolution. Proper recognition of these patients has been marred by several factors, the least of which is semantic. Thus, such patients have been labeled as Unverricht–Lundborg's disease, Baltic myoclonus, and Ramsay Hunt syndrome. In fact, various types of neurodegenerations, most of which have cerebellar involvement in common, constitute the underlying pathology of the disease process in most cases. Two major clinical subgroups are now recognized: (1) PME and (2) progressive myoclonic ataxia (PMA).

A genetic basis has been identified for Unverritch-Lundborg's disease resolving most of the previous difficulties in recognizing a given phenotype with a particular disease. The disease has a worldwide spread, but it is more common in Finland where the incidence is 1:20,000 births.[35] Although the condition is frequently dominated by the typical triad (epilepsy, action myoclonus, and ataxia), other clinical features have been reported, such as ocular motor apraxia, dystonia, and rapidly progressive dementia.[2] Likewise, the course of Unverricht–Lundborg's disease is variable between patients[36] with about 50% of patients being able to walk with aids after two to three decades of evolution.[37] Indeed, long-term follow-up has suggested the disease progresses only over a limited period and symptoms may stabilize thereafter.[38]

Cortical SEPs are of large amplitude, photosensitivity is frequent, and the EEG is abnormal. Back-averaging the EEG activity preceding the myoclonus will often show a cortical potential antedating the jerks by a few milliseconds (e.g., 15–20 ms for the upper limb). Magnetic resonance imaging and computed tomography brain scans are normal or show mild atrophy. In a few cases, atrophy of the cerebellum out of proportion with that present supratentorially can be encountered. The diagnosis of Unverricht–Lundborg's disease is confirmed by identifying disease-causing mutations in the cysteine protease inhibitor cystatin B (*CSTB*) gene.[36]

PMA is characterized by action myoclonus with multifocal and occasionally generalized distribution, variable presence of stimuli-induced myoclonus, and ataxia. The latter affects mainly gait in the early stage of evolution but evolves toward a widespread cerebellar syndrome. Clinical assessment of the ataxia is hampered by action myoclonus. It is only after proper drug control of the myoclonus that cerebellar signs may be properly evaluated. Epilepsy is absent or mild and almost always well controlled with the drugs used to treat the myoclonus.[34] Dementia is not a feature of PMA, but changes in mood and depression are relatively common as disability increases due to disease progression. Many cases are sporadic, but familial forms have also been described.[3] Age at onset varies widely from the first to the seventh decade of life. A cortical origin for the myoclonus is demonstrated in about 70% of cases. It remains to be determined whether or not the same genetic defect may give rise to the clinical phenotype of PMA as well as PME.

Mitochondrial disease, MERRF in particular, may have a milder course and show the clinical picture of PMA, including late onset and absent cognitive deficit, but the notion that mitochondrial respiratory chain diseases are the most common etiology of progressive myoclonic syndromes with epilepsy or ataxia is erroneous. In fact, most patients have a neurodegeneration with variable pathological basis. This includes pure spinocerebellar degeneration, spinocerebellar plus dentatorubral degeneration, MSA-C, and DRPLA.[3,34] A deficit of vitamin E (tocopherol) secondary to malabsorption is also a cause of Ramsay Hunt syndrome. Bhatia and colleagues[39] described four patients with sporadic celiac disease coursing without overt malabsorption or malnutritional symptoms with the typical clinical picture of PMA: action and stimuli-sensitive myoclonus, mild ataxia, and infrequent generalized seizures. The myoclonus has all of the electrophysiological characteristics of cortical myoclonus. Stressing a point we made in earlier writings, the pathology of one case revealed Purkinje cell loss in the cerebellum but indemnity of the cortex, thus indicating that cortical myoclonus obeys a disinhibition mechanism.[39]

Slowly Progressive Myoclonic Encephalopathies With Dementia

Alzheimer's disease (AD) may have spontaneous and action-induced generalized myoclonus as a prominent and early sign. This form frequently courses clinically with the triad of myoclonus, dementia, and parkinsonism, and is a frequent cause of diagnostic confusion. In some of these patients, the typical physiological features of cortical myoclonus are present. More often, however, the jerks in AD consist of small amplitude, irregular twitching of the hand muscles, producing a pseudotremulous appearance called "polyminimyoclonus." A slow frontal cortical potential has been recorded preceding these small-amplitude jerks.[39,40]

CBGD (see Chapter 44) is a progressive disorder of asymmetric onset, beginning in the 60s and 70s, and mainly characterized by limb apraxia, alien limb phenomenon, slowness and rigidity, cortical sensory defects, dysarthria and aphasia, hand dystonia, and stimuli-sensitive myoclonus. The evolution of CBGD is slowly progressive. Most patients become bedridden over a period of 5–8 years. Severe cognitive deficit does not occur in the majority of patients, but in about 30% it appears late in the evolution.[41]

The myoclonus of CBGD is a highly characteristic and very frequent (at least 50%),[42] although nonexclusive, feature of this condition. The affected limb, particularly the forearm and hand muscles, shows what appears to be spontaneous, irregular, and practically continuous jerking, aggravated by any attempt to move voluntarily. Careful observation indicates that the apparently spontaneous jerks are actually due to background ongoing muscle activity.[9] Thus, the myoclonic limb will stop moving when complete relaxation is achieved. The most notorious semiological feature of the myoclonus in CBGD is the exquisite sensitivity to sensory stimuli such as light touching, stretching, or even air puffing, the affected hand.[9] These will cause a salvo of muscle jerking that will continue indefinitely unless the explorer can obtain full relaxation of the limb. The extreme tendency for the affected limb to move continuously very often leads to the movement disorder being regarded as tremor,[42] which in addition to the clumsiness and rigidity may lead to an erroneous diagnosis of Parkinson's disease (PD) early in the evolution of the illness. The features of myoclonus in CBGD strongly suggest a cortical origin,[43] but the neurophysiological findings are not totally typical. SEPs are not enlarged, and back-averaging frequently fails to detect a potential preceding the jerks. A distinctive feature of the reflex myoclonus in CBGD is that the latency of the jerks is very short (<40 ms for the forearm and hand muscles).[43]

In HD, action myoclonus is a rare manifestation, but a few patients with genetic and autopsy-proven studies have been described in whom multifocal action myoclonus was the primary manifestation. In one such family,[44] electrophysiological studies showed large SEPs and reflex muscle responses typical of cortical myoclonus, and visual stimulation elicited an EEG pattern consistent with visual reflex myoclonus.[13]

Myoclonus is not a feature of PD, but it may be present in several parkinsonian syndromes, including Lewy body dementia. In this condition, myoclonus has been described in about 15% of patients, but this is in all probability an underestimation because the presence of stimulus-sensitive myoclonus is not generally included as part of the examination.[45] Indeed, focal reflex jerks induced by touching and particularly pin-pricking the wrist and hand ventral area are very frequent in patients with parkinsonism and dementia.[46]

Other causes of severe myoclonus associated with cognitive deficit are viral- or prion-related encephalopathies, particularly CJD, herpes simplex, and subacute sclerosing panencephalitis. The myoclonus in CJD is spontaneous, symmetrical, and generalized. The typical EEG triphasic waves are always present when myoclonus is clinically overt but their relationship is variable. EEG back-averaging shows a widespread negative potential preceding the jerks by some 60 ms. In a few patients, the typical features of cortical reflex myoclonus following somesthetic and photic stimulation have been reported.[43]

In patients with a subacute myoclonic encephalopathy of unknown cause accompanied by cognitive deficit associated or not with other neurological problems (ataxia, seizures, etc.), the diagnostic possibilities include metabolic derangements (renal and liver failure, hyperglycemia, hypokalemia, hyponatremia, etc.), toxic agents (bismuth, methyl bromide, heavy metals), and drugs (antidepressants, antibiotics, phenytoin, cocaine, amphetamine, etc.).

STATIC MYOCLONIC ENCEPHALOPATHIES

Action and spontaneous, multifocal, and/or generalized myoclonus may be extremely disabling in patients who have suffered severe anoxia or head trauma. Posthypoxic myoclonus was described by Lance and Adams[47] and received much attention after the discovery of its dramatic sensitivity to treatment with 5-hydroxytryptophan (5-HTP). However, a high proportion of patients show additional neurological deficits (ataxia, speech difficulties, memory loss, etc.), which reduce the chances of adequate therapeutic control. In their original article, Lance and Adams also described in detail the existence of long EMG silences following the myoclonic jerks. They recognized the importance of these silent periods as being responsible for the postural lapses (negative myoclonus) often seen in posthypoxic myoclonus. The long-term evolution of posthypoxic myoclonus is positive in a majority of patients, in keeping with the nonprogressive nature of the underlying pathology.

▶ FOCAL MYOCLONUS

This section describes conditions characterized by focal or segmental myoclonus that may be spontaneous and rhythmical, may occur in response to sensory stimulation, and/or may occur during action.

FOCAL MYOCLONUS OF THE LIMBS

A "jerking limb" may occur in a wide variety of clinical settings. Lesions located along the neuraxis, including the sensorimotor cerebral cortex, thalamus, mesencephalon, and spinal cord, may be associated with focal myoclonus. However, the major causes to consider here are those affecting the cortex or the spinal cord.

In focal cortical myoclonus, the jerks are restricted to a few muscles with predominant activation of distal and flexor muscles. The most common presentation is during action and provoked by somesthetic stimulation. Stretching the fingers, delicate stimulation such as touching the hand or foot with a feather, and pin-pricking the wrist are all very effective in triggering a salvo of focal myoclonic jerking. In many patients the reflex myoclonus is modality-specific, and only one of the above stimuli is capable of eliciting the myoclonus. Typically, there is neurophysiological evidence of a cortical origin. The condition most likely to be associated with cortical reflex myoclonus of one hand is CBGD.[9,42,43]

Spontaneous and rhythmical presentation is the main characteristic of EPC, which may also be stimuli-sensitive and aggravated by action.[9] The causes of EPC include tumors, arteriovenous malformations, focal encephalitis of Kozhevnikov, abscess, stroke, and disorders of neuronal migration. In a proportion of patients with EPC secondary to ischemia or tumors, the lesion is located subcortically.

Focal stimuli-sensitive myoclonus elicited by stimulation of any of the four limbs is very common in multisystem atrophy with predominant cerebellar impairment (MSA-C).[45–48] However, the presence of reflex myoclonus may well pass unnoticed unless actively investigated. The best type of stimulus consists of pin-pricking the palmar surface of the wrist and the metacarpal region of the index finger while the examiner extends the fingers and wrist. The rate of stimulation must be low (<1/s) to avoid habituation. Small jerks will be seen or felt in the forearm and intrinsic hand muscles. Occasionally, the same stimuli will induce a generalized jerk. SEPs are enhanced in amplitude and usually associated with a reflex muscle discharge, thus having the characteristics of cortical reflex myoclonus. Flash stimulation is also accompanied by reflex jerks in about 50% of patients with MSA-C.[48] In contrast with the common photomyoclonic response more frequently found in patients with epilepsy, visual reflex myoclonus in MSA-C is induced by low-frequency (<10 Hz) flash stimulation, each stimulus being accompanied by a cortical spike that antedates a myoclonic jerk.[13] The origin of the abnormal discharge is in the premotor and motor cortex. The sensitivity to visual stimulus is blocked by L-dopa and dopamine agonists.[13] Because many patients with MSA-C also have parkinsonian features, care must be taken to stop medication for at least 12 hours before conducting the electrophysiological evaluation.

SPINAL MYOCLONUS

Spinal myoclonus is a typical, even though rare, cause of focal and usually rhythmic myoclonus. The most frequent clinical presentation consists of spontaneous, repetitive jerks of one limb, sometimes spreading to adjacent neck and trunk muscles. The frequency of the myoclonus is very variable, from 10 to 50 per minutes. In many reported cases the myoclonus persists during sleep. The most common etiologies are cervical myelopathy (including posttraumatic), tumors, multiple sclerosis, and infections.[49] A rather similar presentation may be observed in patients with evidence of peripheral nerve damage (nerve, plexus, root), with or without accompanying sympathetic changes (Sudeck's atrophy).

FACIAL MYOCLONUS

Twitching of some facial muscles may occur in normal people when tired or after excessive tobacco and alcohol consumption, in hemifacial spasm, and following focal brainstem lesions. In most instances, the EMG pattern is that of myokymia or spasms rather than truly myoclonic. Rhythmic slow movements of the orbicularis oris sometimes spreading to the adjacent musculature leads one to consider Whipple's disease. It may also occur in patients with a lesion of Mollaret triangle even without "palatal myoclonus."[50]

Authentic facial myoclonus without involvement of any other body part is actually rare. The most common condition associated with it is EPC.

AXIAL MYOCLONUS

Segmental and rhythmical myoclonus of the neck and trunk may rarely arise as a consequence of brainstem lesions, Arnold–Chiari malformation, and upper cervical cord damage. Nonrhythmic, repetitive axial flexion, and more rarely extension jerks, occurring spontaneously but aggravated by action and sensitive to stretching, are the major features of "propiospinal myoclonus."[16,51] The EMG shows irregular, brief bursts at a variable frequency of 1–7 Hz. Detailed neurophysiological analysis (see Chapter 39) is necessary to confirm the spinal origin of this uncommon presentation.

▶ GENERALIZED, STIMULI-SENSITIVE MYOCLONUS

In a small proportion of all patients with myoclonus, the main problem consists in whole body jerks triggered by sensory stimuli (sound, touching, stretching, or visual threatening). This clinical presentation may correspond to three different mechanisms: (1) RRM, (2) hyperekplexia, and (3) psychogenic (also see Chapter 39).

RRM is a pathophysiological term describing the origin of myoclonus in the brainstem reticular formation. Anoxia, uremia, liver failure, drugs, and brainstem encephalitis are the major causes of RRM.

Hyperekplexia is the pathological manifestation of startle.[52] Clinical differences from RRM are that the latter may also occur during action, whereas hyperekplexia is always stimuli-induced. Tonic spasms following stimulation may be present in hyperekplexia but are not associated with RRM. Otherwise, precise differentiation of the two conditions requires electrophysiological assessment. Hyperekplexia may be symptomatic or inherited as an autosomal-dominant condition. Hereditary hyperekplexia is a complex genetic disease in which several genes can be implicated, all of them directly or indirectly involved with glycine neurotransmission. Two major proteins involved in hyperekplexia are the strychnine-sensitive glycine receptor (GlyR) and the neuronal glycine transporter GLYT2.[53]

Normal people may, for a variety of reasons, jump and jerk in response to external stimulation mimicking myoclonus and startle.[54] Clinical hints to the diagnosis are the acute onset, variability in the stimuli triggering the jerks, and variable recruitment of the muscles.[55] In such cases, the onset of the EMG discharge is always within the range of normal reaction time.[54]

▶ TREATMENT

Myoclonus is a very disabling movement disorder because it spreads through the same motor pathways that are necessary for normal voluntary movements. The treatment of myoclonus is largely empirical, in so far as there has been little progress in understanding its biochemical basis. Furthermore, only case reports, case series, and a few limited controlled studies support the sparse available evidence regarding efficacy of drug treatments. In this section, the therapeutic possibilities are discussed in accordance with the major clinical presentations, as described above, and the pathophysiological origin of myoclonus regardless of the etiology.

MULTIFOCAL ACTION MYOCLONUS

This is the most incapacitating form and the one requiring the major therapeutic effort. In around 70% of patients with action myoclonus, electrophysiological assessment indicates a cortical origin. This is a very important feature to consider when addressing the pharmacological approach.

1. *Myoclonus secondary to anoxia and trauma.* The initiation of drug treatments in action myoclonus occurred in the 1970s when 5-HTP, the precursor of serotonin, was given to a French patient with postanoxic action myoclonus[56] in whom a large number of drugs had been tried without success and a thalamotomy had also been performed with no benefit. Administration of 5-HTP with carbidopa to prevent peripheral decarboxylation produced a dramatic improvement in the patient. This result led to a number of studies on posthypoxic action myoclonus, which confirmed the therapeutic action of 5-HTP plus carbidopa (100–300/25 mg/day). It was found that the cerebrospinal fluid concentration of the major serotonin metabolite, 5-hydroxyindolacetic acid, was lowered in most of these patients.[57,58] Physiological analysis revealed that patients with postanoxic myoclonus with an excellent response to 5-HTP had RRM, whereas those with a moderate or no response had cortical reflex myoclonus.[57] The failure to control equally well all cases with 5-HTP and the associated side effects (nausea, vomiting, diarrhea, hypotension, and gastrointestinal tract bleeding) led to the examination of other alternative drugs. Clonazepam, sodium valproate, and fluoxetine were found useful.[59] In later years, several patients with action myoclonus have been physiologically and pharmacologically studied, and a general picture of the treatment of severe action myoclonus has emerged.[60]
2. *Treatment of action cortical myoclonus of any etiology.* The major factor recognized as a predictor of the drug responsiveness is the neurophysiological origin. Cortical myoclonus responds exceedingly well to piracetam (8–20 g/day), clonazepam (2–15 mg/day), sodium valproate (1200–3000 mg/day), and primidone (500–1000 mg/day).[61] In the majority of patients with severe, highly disabling action myoclonus, these drugs have to be given in combination to achieve adequate control.[61,62] This is thought to be due to the various mechanisms implicated in the pathophysiology of cortical myoclonus.[9,61] Clonazepam is the most efficient antimyoclonic drug,[60] but piracetam is the first drug to be used because of its excellent tolerance up to 24 g/day.[62,63] All of these drugs are believed to act by increasing g-aminobutyric acid (GABA) activity in the cortex. A reduction of 25–50% of GABA levels has been reported in the cerebrospinal fluid of patients with posthypoxic myoclonus and PME, and GABAergic drugs form the cornerstone of treatment. Of these, sodium valproate (1200–3000 mg/day) is known to increase cortical GABA and potentiate GABA postsynaptic inhibitory activity. Benzodiazepines and barbiturates facilitate GABAergic transmission by effects on the GABA receptor–ionophore com-

plex.[64] In the past few years, the newer antiepileptic agent levetiracetam, an analogue of piracetam, has been tried in a few patients with myoclonus. The response is variable.[65] In our personal experience, not even patients with cortical myoclonus respond as well as to piracetam, but still a few patients may show a dramatic improvement.[65] Treatment with *N*-acetylcysteine (4–6 g/day) in four siblings with Unverricht-Lundborg's disease was associated with dramatic improvement and excellent tolerance.[66] However, a more recent study[67] in three patients failed to support this claim and, in addition, found severe side effects (sensorineural deafness in one patient, and nausea and gastric pain in another).

The degree of symptomatic control achieved in patients with action myoclonus of cortical origin is usually very striking at the beginning of treatment, but the long-term treatment response pattern is variable. Tolerance is a common occurrence. Response to treatment depends on several factors, the most important of which is the underlying disease. Patients with a static encephalopathy (e.g., posthypoxia), in whom myoclonus is the only or major clinical problem, achieve a very long-lasting and adequate control. On the contrary, patients with progressive illness (e.g., MERFF, sialidosis, neurodegenerations, etc.) are very difficult to control for any length of time. An important practical point in the management of such cases is the ease with which generalized seizures may occur when manipulating the drug regimen. Thus, when a given drug treatment is judged inefficient, its withdrawal must be achieved very carefully and slowly. Patients with action myoclonus originating in the brainstem (RRM) or the spinal cord are much less frequent. Clonazepam is the drug of choice in such instances.

The above discussion relates to the treatment of action myoclonus understood as a positive muscle discharge. However, in most patients the jerks are actually a combination of positive and negative (EMG silence) myoclonus.[1] The latter is as incapacitating as the former. However, there has not been any study specifically analyzing the effect of antimyoclonic drugs against negative myoclonus. In many patients, the postural lapses that affect the trunk and proximal leg muscles are the most difficult feature to keep under control.[60,62]

3. *Myoclonic dystonia*. The severity of this condition is variable. It usually carries a relatively benign course, but it can cause significant disability. All classic drugs used for dystonia and myoclonus (clonazepam, anticholinergics, baclofen, litium, carbamazepine, levodopa, valproic acid, piracetam, 5-HTP, etc.) have been unsuccessful, and none comes close to the response induced by alcohol.[68,69] Recently, two patients with myoclonic dystonia due to exonic deletions of ε-sarcoglycan (gene on chromosome 7q21-31,[70]) had significant and sustained improvement with levodopa,[71] suggesting that trials of levodopa should be considered in patients with this condition. In addition, prompted by the alcohol response, a recent open-label study has examined the effects of sodium oxybate in two patients. A 50% clinical improvement was reported, although sedation was a side effect.[65] Finally, deep brain stimulation (DBS) may be a promising option in severe patients. Two cases of sustained benefit have been reported with bilateral DBS of the globus pallidus interna.[72,73] In addition, chronic bilateral thalamic (ventralis intermedius nucleus) stimulation was also reported to be effective in another two patients.[74,75] In general, myoclonus is not a movement disorder sensitive to basal ganglia or thalamic surgery with numerous anecdotic failures.

FOCAL MYOCLONUS OF CORTICAL ORIGIN

Focal myoclonus of cortical origin also responds very well to the drugs discussed above.[9] The only exception is CBGD, but this is a very special pathophysiological type of cortical myoclonus and a rapidly evolving disease.[43,44] In extremely severe cases of cortical myoclonus producing EPC, surgery may be considered after rigorous assessment.

Spinal myoclonus has no specific drug treatment. The best therapeutic approach is to treat the causative condition whenever this is possible. Drugs used with some benefit include clonazepam, carbamazepine, and tetrabenazine. Palatal myoclonus may respond to 5-HTP, trihexyphenidyl (up to 60 mg/day), carbamazepine, and piracetam.

Nocturnal myoclonus, usually involving the legs but occasionally the whole body, may require treatment when very frequent and so severe as to interfere with falling asleep. Clonazepam at a relatively low dose (1–3 mg at bedtime) is very effective for controlling this problem.

▶ CONCLUSIONS

The clinical spectrum of myoclonus is very large and there are numerous different presentations and etiologies. When myoclonus is the major neurological complain, action multifocal or generalized myoclonus is the most frequent type. In such instances, a cortical origin preludes a fairly good response to drugs, which commonly have to be used in combination. Advances in genetic definition of some major myoclonic condidtions, that is, Unverritch-Lundborg's disease or myoclonic dystonia, have occurred and will continue, thus improving the ascertaining and understanding of this movement disorder.

REFERENCES

1. Obeso JA, Artieda J, Burleigh A. Clinical aspects of negative myoclonus. Adv Neurol 1995;67:1–7.
2. Gerschlager W, Brown P. Myoclonus. Curr Opin Neurol 2009;22(4):414–418.
3. Obeso JA, Artieda J, Marsden CD. Different clinical presentations of myoclonus. In Jankovic TE (ed). Parkinson's Disease and Movement Disorders. 2nd ed. Baltimore: Williams & Wilkins; 1993.
4. Obeso JA, Narbona J. Post-traumatic tremor and myoclonic jerking. J Neurol Neurosurg Psychiatry 1983;46(8):788.
5. Rothwell JC, Obeso J. The anatomical and physiological basis of torsion dystonia. In Marsden FS (ed.). Movement Disorders, Vol. 2. London: Butterworth, 1987, pp. 313–331.
6. Mahloudji M, Pikielny RT. Hereditary essential myoclonus. Brain 1967; 90(3):669–674.
7. Quinn NP. Essential myoclonus and myoclonic dystonia. Mov Disord 1996; 11(2):119–124.
8. Vogel CM, Drury I, Terry LC, et al. Myoclonus in adult Huntington's disease. Ann Neurol 1991; 29(2):213–215.
9. Obeso JA, Rothwell JC, Marsden CD. The spectrum of cortical myoclonus. From focal reflex jerks to spontaneous motor epilepsy. Brain 1985; 108 (Pt 1):193–124.
10. Williams DR. Gaze-evoked brainstem myoclonus. Mov Disord 2004; 19(3):346–349.
11. Artieda J, Obeso JA. The pathophysiology and pharmacology of photic cortical reflex myoclonus. Ann Neurol 1993; 34(2):175–184.
12. Glass GA, Ahlskog JE, Matsumoto JY. Orthostatic myoclonus: A contributor to gait decline in selected elderly. Neurology 2007; 68(21):1826–1830.
13. Shibasaki H, Ikeda A, Nagamine T, et al. Cortical reflex negative myoclonus. Brain 1994; 117(Pt 3):477–486.
14. Deuschl G, Toro C, Valls-Solé J, et al. Symptomatic and essential palatal tremor. 1. Clinical, physiological and MRI analysis. Brain 1994; 117(Pt 4):775–788.
15. Caviness JN. Pathophysiology and treatment of myoclonus. Neurol Clin 2009; 27(3):757–777, vii.
16. Brown P, Rothwell JC, Thompson PD, et al. Propriospinal myoclonus: Evidence for spinal "pattern" generators in humans. Mov Disord 1994; 9(5):571–576.
17. Marsden CD, Hallett M, Fahn S. The nosology and pathophysiology of myoclonus. In F.S. Marsden CD (ed.). Movement Disorders, . Vol. 1. 1982, London: Butterworth.
18. Kurlan R, Behr J, Medved L, et al. Myoclonus and dystonia: a family study. Adv Neurol 1988;50:385–389.
19. Davidenkow F. Auf hereditar-abiotrophischer Grundlage akut auf tretende, regressierende und episodische Erkrankungen des Nervensystems und Bemerkungen über die familäre subakute, myoklonische Dystonie. Z Ges Nerol Psychiat 1926;104:596–622.
20. Koukouni V, Valente EM, Cordivari C, et al. Unusual familial presentation of epsilon-sarcoglycan gene mutation with falls and writer's cramp. Mov Disord 2008;23(13):1913–1915.
21. Hess CW, Raymond D, Aguiar PC, et al. Myoclonus-dystonia, obsessive-compulsive disorder, and alcohol dependence in SGCE mutation carriers. Neurology 2007;68(7):522–524.
22. Roze E, Apartis E, Clot F, et al. Myoclonus-dystonia: Clinical and electrophysiologic pattern related to SGCE mutations. Neurology 2008;70(13):1010–1016.
23. Kinugawa K, Vidailhet M, Clot F, et al. Myoclonus-dystonia: an update. Mov Disord 2009;24(4):479–489.
24. Li JY, Cunic DI, Paradiso G, et al. Electrophysiological features of myoclonus-dystonia. Mov Disord 2008;23(14):2055–2061.
25. van der Salm SM, van Rootselaar AF, Foncke EM, et al. Normal cortical excitability in myoclonus-dystonia--A TMS study. Exp Neurol 2009;216(2):300–305.
26. Roze E, Apartis E, Trocello JM. Cortical excitability in DYT-11 positive myoclonus dystonia. Mov Disord 2008;23(5):761–764.
27. Klein C, Liu L, Doheny D, et al. Epsilon-sarcoglycan mutations found in combination with other dystonia gene mutations. Ann Neurol 2002;52(5):675–679.
28. Tsuji S. Dentatorubral-pallidoluysian atrophy: clinical aspects and molecular genetics. Adv Neurol 2002; 89: 231–239.
29. Minassian BA. Progressive myoclonus epilepsy with polyglucosan bodies: Lafora disease. Adv Neurol 2002;89:199–210.
30. Delgado-Escueta AV. Advances in lafora progressive myoclonus epilepsy. Curr Neurol Neurosci Rep 2007;7(5): 428–433.
31. DiMauro S, Hirano M, Kaufmann P, et al. Clinical features and genetics of myoclonic epilepsy with ragged red fibers. Adv Neurol 2002;89:217–229.
32. Melone MA, Tessa A, Petrini S, et al. Revelation of a new mitochondrial DNA mutation (G12147A) in a MELAS/MERFF phenotype. Arch Neurol 2004;61(2):269–272.
33. Shoffner JM, Lott MT, Lezza AM, et al. Myoclonic epilepsy and ragged-red fiber disease (MERRF) is associated with a mitochondrial DNA tRNA(Lys) mutation. Cell 1990;61(6):931–937.
34. Marsden CD, Harding AE, Obeso JA, et al. Progressive myoclonic ataxia (the Ramsay Hunt syndrome). Arch Neurol 1990;47(10):1121–1125.
35. Lehesjoki AE. Clinical features and genetics of Unverricht-Lundborg disease. Adv Neurol 2002;89:193–197.
36. Kalviainen R, Khyuppenen J, Koskenkorva P, et al. Clinical picture of EPM1-Unverricht-Lundborg disease. Epilepsia 2008;49(4):549–556.
37. Chew NK, Mir P, Edwards MJ, et al. The natural history of Unverricht-Lundborg disease: A report of eight genetically proven cases. Mov Disord 2008;23(1):107–113.
38. Magaudda A, Ferlazzo E, Nguyen VH, et al. Unverricht-Lundborg disease, a condition with self-limited progression: Long-term follow-up of 20 patients. Epilepsia 2006;47(5):860–866.
39. Bhatia KP, Brown P, Gregory R, et al. Progressive myoclonic ataxia associated with coeliac disease. The myoclonus

is of cortical origin, but the pathology is in the cerebellum. Brain 1995;118 (Pt 5):1087–1093.
40. Wilkins DE, Hallett M, Berardelli A, et al. Physiologic analysis of the myoclonus of Alzheimer's disease. Neurology 1984;34(7):898–903.
41. Rinne JO, Lee MS, Thompson PD, et al. Corticobasal degeneration. A clinical study of 36 cases. Brain 1994;117 (Pt 5):1183–1196.
42. Thompson PD. Neurodegenerative causes of myoclonus. Adv Neurol 2002;89:31–34.
43. Thompson PD, Day BL, Rothwell JC, et al. The myoclonus in corticobasal degeneration. Evidence for two forms of cortical reflex myoclonus. Brain 1994:117(Pt 5):1197–1207.
44. Thompson PD, Bhatia KP, Brown P, et al. Cortical myoclonus in Huntington's disease. Mov Disord 1994;9(6): 633–641.
45. Shafiq M, Lang AE. Myoclonus in parkinsonian disorders. Adv Neurol 2002:89:77–83.
46. Chen R, Ashby P, Lang AE. Stimulus-sensitive myoclonus in akinetic-rigid syndromes. Brain 1992;115(Pt 6): 1875–1888.
47. Lance JW, Adams RD. The syndrome of intention or action myoclonus as a sequel to hypoxic encephalopathy. Brain 1963:86:111–136.
48. Rodriguez ME, Artieda J, Zubieta JL, et al. Reflex myoclonus in olivopontocerebellar atrophy. J Neurol Neurosurg Psychiatry 1994:57(3):316–319.
49. Jankovic J, Pardo R. Segmental myoclonus. Clinical and pharmacologic study. Arch Neurol 1986;43(10):1025–1031.
50. Lapresle J. Palatal myoclonus. Adv Neurol 1986;43:265–273.
51. Brown P, Thompson PD, Rothwell JC, et al. Axial myoclonus of propriospinal origin. Brain 1991;114(Pt 1A):197–214.
52. Brown P, Rothwell JC, Thompson PD, et al. The hyperekplexias and their relationship to the normal startle reflex. Brain 1991;114(Pt 4):1903–1928.
53. Gimenez C, Zafra F, Lopez-Corcuera B, et al. Molecular bases of hereditary hyperekplexia. Rev Neurol 2008; 47(12):648–652.
54. Thompson PD, Colebatch JG, Brown P, et al. Voluntary stimulus-sensitive jerks and jumps mimicking myoclonus or pathological startle syndromes. Mov Disord 1992;7(3):257–262.
55. Brown P. Neurophysiology of the startle syndrome and hyperekplexia. Adv Neurol 2002;89:153–159.
56. Lhermitte F, Peterfalvi M, Marteau R, et al. Pharmacological analysis of a case of postanoxic intention and action myoclonus. Rev Neurol (Paris) 1971;124(1):21–31.
57. Chadwick D, Hallett M, Harris R, et al. Clinical, biochemical, and physiological features distinguishing myoclonus responsive to 5-hydroxytryptophan, tryptophan with a monoamine oxidase inhibitor, and clonazepam. Brain 1977;100(3):455–487.
58. Van Woert MH, Sethy VH. Therapy of intention myoclonus with L-5-hydroxytryptophan and a peripheral decarboxylase inhibitor, MK 486. Neurology 1975;25(2):135–140.
59. Fahn S. Posthypoxic action myoclonus: Literature review update. Adv Neurol 1986;43:157–169.
60. Frucht SJ. The clinical challenge of posthypoxic myoclonus. Adv Neurol 2002;89:85–88.
61. Obeso JA, Artieda J, Rothwell JC, et al. The treatment of severe action myoclonus. Brain 1989;112(Pt 3):765–777.
62. Obeso JA, Artieda J, Quinn N, et al. Piracetam in the treatment of different types of myoclonus. Clin Neuropharmacol 1988;11(6):529–536.
63. Brown P, Steiger MJ, Thompson PD, et al. Effectiveness of piracetam in cortical myoclonus. Mov Disord 1993;8(1):63–68.
64. Caviness JN, Brown P. Myoclonus: current concepts and recent advances. Lancet Neurol 2004;3(10):598–607.
65. Frucht SJ, Louis ED, Chuang C, et al. A pilot tolerability and efficacy study of levetiracetam in patients with chronic myoclonus. Neurology 2001;57(6):1112–1114.
66. Hurd RW, Wilder BJ, Helveston WR, et al. Treatment of four siblings with progressive myoclonus epilepsy of the Unverricht-Lundborg type with *N*-acetylcysteine. Neurology 1996;47(5):1264–1268.
67. Edwards MJ, Hargreaves IP, Heales SJ, et al. *N*-Acetylcysteine and Unverricht-Lundborg disease: Variable response and possible side effects. Neurology 2002;59(9):1447–1449.
68. Chang VC, Frucht SJ. Myoclonus. Curr Treat Options Neurol 2008;10(3):222–229.
69. Pueschel SM, Friedman JH, Shetty T. Myoclonic dystonia. Childs Nerv Syst 1992;8(2):61–66.
70. Nygaard TG, Raymond D, Chen C, et al. Localization of a gene for myoclonus-dystonia to chromosome 7q21-q31. Ann Neurol 1999;46(5):794–798.
71. Luciano MS, Ozelius L, Sims K, et al. Responsiveness to levodopa in epsilon-sarcoglycan deletions. Mov Disord 2009;24(3):425–428.
72. Cif L, Valente EM, Hemm S, et al. Deep brain stimulation in myoclonus-dystonia syndrome. Mov Disord 2004; 19(6):724–727.
73. Magarinos-Ascone CM, Regidor I, Martinez-Castrillo JC, et al. Pallidal stimulation relieves myoclonus-dystonia syndrome. J Neurol Neurosurg Psychiatry 2005;76(7): 989–991.
74. Kuncel AM, Turner DA, Ozelius LJ, et al. Myoclonus and tremor response to thalamic deep brain stimulation parameters in a patient with inherited myoclonus-dystonia syndrome. Clin Neurol Neurosurg 2009;111(3):303–306.
75. Trottenberg T, Meissner W, Kabus C, et al. Neurostimulation of the ventral intermediate thalamic nucleus in inherited myoclonus-dystonia syndrome. Mov Disord 2001; 16(4):769–771.

CHAPTER 38

Pathophysiology of Myoclonic Disorders

Camilo Toro and Mark Hallett

▶ INTRODUCTION

The electrophysiological study of myoclonic movements touches on the interests of clinical electrophysiologists, epileptologists, movement disorders specialists, and sleep medicine specialists alike. As early as 1935, Gibbs and colleagues[1] had described patients with spike-and-wave discharges in the electroencephalogram (EEG), with muscle jerking at the same rate as the EEG spikes. Grinker and colleagues[2] are credited with the first description of polyspike discharges in the EEG, with close association to myoclonic jerking in patients with progressive myoclonic epilepsy. In 1946, Dawson[3] produced a detailed description of the relationship between EEG spikes and muscle jerks in patients with myoclonus, reporting also, in some of his patients, the possibility of inducing myoclonic jerks by tendon tapping. One year later, Dawson himself demonstrated not only the first recording of somatosensory-evoked potentials (SEPs) from the scalp in humans,[4] but also that the SEPs in patients with myoclonus could be grossly exaggerated in amplitude.[5]

Electrophysiological studies aid in making the diagnosis and provide insight into the pathophysiology of myoclonus.[6–10] The field has grown steadily as technological advances and new experimental techniques have emerged over the last decades. The electrophysiological assessment of myoclonus serves as a prototypical example of the valuable insights to be gained in the understanding of movement disorder pathophysiology by the application of clinical and experimental electrophysiological methods.

▶ ELECTROPHYSIOLOGICAL METHODS IN THE STUDY OF MYOCLONUS

POLYGRAPHIC EMG

Electromyographic (EMG) activity is a direct measure of α motor neuron activity, thus providing information on the nature of the central nervous system events that generate involuntary movements of myoclonus. Multichannel surface EMG is a powerful tool to evaluate the quick involuntary movements of myoclonus and distinguish them from other movement disorders. There is no predefined protocol to conduct a polygraphic EMG study in a patient with myoclonus, but rather, the study design should be guided by the particular patient's clinical presentation and by the questions at hand.[6] When possible, polygraphic EMG should be recorded simultaneously with EEG in the same session. The selection of muscles to record should follow a general logic. Generally, it is recommended to sample agonist/antagonist muscle pairs acting on a given joint. It is also desirable to perform bilateral recordings of homologous muscles. Proximal and distal muscle groups in a given limb give additional information on the axial versus distal character of the involuntary muscle activation. Often, there is a desire to study the order of muscle activation and the velocity of the "wave" of activation in myoclonic movements, thus reflecting on the pathway of spread.[11–13] In those cases, muscles representing multiple levels of the neuroaxis from upper brain stem motor nuclei to lower spinal cord levels myotomes are recorded simultaneously. Polygraphic recordings are often conducted under conditions of rest, posture, actions, and stimuli that elicit the involuntary movements. Nowadays, most studies are collected and stored in digital media for off-line analysis.

Valuable information is contained in polygraphic EMG recordings of myoclonus including whether the observed motor phenomena is the result of positive event (EMG burst) or negative motor phenomena (EMG silence).[14,15] Myoclonus EMG burst duration itself is a useful piece of information differentiating various types of myoclonus and separating myoclonus from fragments of other movement disorders.[6] Synchronous versus alternating agonist/antagonist activation pattern is also helpful in determining the origin and type of myoclonus. Bilateral synchronicity, proximal versus distal predominance, spread pattern and overall frequency, consistency, and reproducibility of findings across the entire recording session are valuable pieces of information.

It is important to keep in mind that some disorders of the peripheral nervous system may also give rise to involuntary movements. These include fasciculations, tetany, myokymia, and neuromyotonic discharges and, generally, best studied with needle EMG examination.[7]

EEG AND MEG METHODS

In the study of myoclonus pathophysiology, there is an interest in determining whether there is a participation of cortical structures, specially the somatosensory cortical regions to myoclonic twitches, and, if so, what is the spatial localization and time relationship of the cortical activation to the myoclonus occurrence.

Electrocortical activity recorded by EEG and MEG methods emerges from the spatial and temporal summation local field potentials from local ionic currents generated by depolarization of cortical apical dendrites. Given the properties of electrical potentials and magnetic fields, the geometry of the cortical ribbon and the skull shape and conductivity, scalp recorded EEG signal is biased to represent local activation of apical dendrites perpendicularly oriented to the surface of the skull, whereas MEG is biased to represent dendritic currents from cortical segments oriented tangential to the skull surface.[16,17] These two techniques can be viewed in many respects as complementary.[18,19] From a practical perspective, EEG is widely available in most clinical settings and the instrumentation is relatively simple. MEG, on the other hand, requires a fairly significant infrastructure making it impractical for routine clinical use. On the other hand, MEG recordings have many technical advantages. MEG signal is "reference-independent," and magnetic fields are free of the troublesome "smearing" effect of the skull and scalp on electrical fields. These factors remove many ambiguities in the process of localizing the neuronal sources that might be implicated in the genesis of myoclonus.[16]

In the evaluation of myoclonus electrophysiology, EEG and MEG signals undergo further processing to enhance the signal-to-noise ratio or to extract signal features not readily appreciable on routine recordings.

1. Back-averaging: Averaging of EEG (or MEG) activity time-locked to the onset of myoclonic EMG bursts is known as back-averaging or "jerk-locked" averaging. This technique is used to establish the presence, location, and characteristics of cortical activity correlated (time-locked) to the onset of the myoclonic bursts.[8,9,20,21] A similar averaging procedure but one that is time-locked to the onset of EMG silent periods can be applied to the study of negative myoclonus (silent period-locked averaging).[14,15,22–24] In conventional myoclonus studies, the sampled EEG or MEG epochs should include at least 100 ms of data before myoclonus EMG onset. The exact number of averaged epochs may vary, depending on the signal-to-noise ratio. Much longer premyoclonus time segments (1–2 seconds) and proper reference and filter parameters should be used when searching for a *Bereitschaftspotential* (BP) in suspected cases of psychogenic myoclonus.[25,26] Most laboratories conducting electrophysiological studies of myoclonus record the EEG (or MEG) and EMG signals onto digital media and conduct the analysis "offline." This offers the advantage of post hoc sorting of different myoclonic events and better control of artifact rejection. Multiple scalp and EMG leads are desirable. For diagnostic purposes, the use of back-averaging may not be necessary in patients who have clear-cut spikes discharges time-locked to myoclonic EMG bursts. But even in this situation, back-averaging may provide more detailed information on the topography and features of the epileptiform paroxysms that best correlate with the myoclonic movements.[7]
2. Evoked responses: The cortical correlates to somatosensory stimulation could be grossly exaggerated and sometimes abnormally configured in some patients with cortical myoclonus.[5,27] This finding is often referred to as a giant SEP. SEPs and their magnetic counterpart, somatosensory-evoked magnetic fields (SEMFs), can be elicited in response to a variety of somatosensory stimuli including peripheral nerve stimulation, cutaneous stimulation, tapping, or joint stretching.[28]
3. Advanced signal analysis methods: The bioelectrical signals (EEG/MEG and EMG) collected in the course of a myoclonus study could be subject to more complex analysis beyond simple averaging. Measures of corticocortical and corticomuscular network connectivity can be explored with various methods such as coherence analysis. These measures are useful in highlighting the degree to which two cortical areas or a cortical area and a pool of α motor neurons (reflected in their EMG output) co-vary with each other.[29] Implicit in this correlation is also a temporal dimension that serves to establish a direction of information flow and time lag between signal pairs.[29] The reactivity of central (Rolandic) rhythms in response to movement preparation, execution, and termination has been studied extensively in normal subjects and subjects with other movement disorders under the term of Event-Related Desynchronization and Synchronization (ERD/ERS).[30–34] Information on these phenomena in myoclonic disorders is emerging.[35]

REFLEX STUDIES

Reflex studies are particularly valuable in evaluating myoclonus and other movement disorders that exhibit a stimulus-dependent or stimulus-reflex component. Somatosensory and photic-reflex myoclonus and hyperekplexia fit into this category.

Long latency reflex (LLR) is the term often used to refer to reflex muscle activity following stimulation of a mixed nerve beyond the direct muscle response

(M response) and the monosynaptic Hoffman reflex (H response). There is a fair degree of complexity in taxonomy and techniques used to elicit these reflexes. For example, when stimulating the median nerve and recording at the thenar eminence, it is possible to record up to three components of the LLR based on their latency (LLR-I, LLR-II, and LLR-III).[36] Of these three, only the LLR-II is consistently recorded in normal subjects. The LLR-II response, however, is of low amplitude and requires rectification and averaging for proper identification. The LLR-I is of particular interest in some forms of myoclonus as, often, it is greatly enhanced and correlates with the clinical phenomena of sensory-reflex myoclonus. Sutton and Mayer, who first characterized this phenomenon in patients with myoclonus, named it the C-reflex inferring a transcortical-mediated long-loop reflex.[37] The latency of the C-reflex (LLR-I) for upper extremity muscles is approximately 36–50 ms after the stimulus given to the hand and 60–70 ms when the reflex is elicited and recorded in lower extremities. When studying this reflex in a clinical setting, care should be exerted not to confuse the C-reflex with other normal reflex EMG responses.

The normal features of the audiogenic startle response have been well characterized and enable proper recognition of this physiological phenomenon and can be contrasted to pathological startle.[38,39] In the normal audiogenic startle, there is a stereotyped bilaterally symmetric pattern with an invariable early blink; other craniocervical muscles almost always are activated, but recruitment of limb muscles is variable. Onset latencies of EMG activity are 20–40 ms in the orbicularis oculi, 35–80 ms in masseter and sternocleidomastoid, 50–100 ms in biceps brachii, 100–125 ms in hamstrings and quadriceps, and 130–140 ms in tibialis anterior. The latency of the response in abductor pollicis brevis is much delayed compared to what would be expected from the latency of the response in the biceps.[39,40] The delay is likely due to the fact that startle is mediated by a reticulospinal pathway that has weak connections to distal muscles. There is synchronous activation of antagonist muscles with EMG burst durations of 50–400 ms, shortening with habituation. Prepulse stimulation with a low-intensity conditioning stimulus has also an effect on startle response and habituation.[41,42] Cranial reflexes have been studied in patients with hyperekplexia disorders and stiff person syndrome.[43,44] The head retraction reflex, for example, is a vestigial withdrawal reflex that might be exaggerated in some patients with stiff person and other acquired and neurodegenerative movement disorders.[45]

TRANSCRANIAL MAGNETIC STIMULATION

Transcranial magnetic stimulation (TMS) is a useful technique to evaluate cortical excitatory and inhibitory mechanisms and their role in the genesis of myoclonus. The induction of an electrical current by a rapidly changing magnetic field is the physical principle behind TMS. In TMS, a coil of fine wire encased in plastic is applied over the scalp. The discharge of a large capacitor generates a rapid change in current along the coil windings creating a brief but large magnetic field. The shape of the field is defined by many factors including the shape and size of the coil. The magnetic field induces an electrical current capable of safely activating neuronal tissue with relatively minor discomfort, thus providing a technique for noninvasive cortical stimulation.[46,47] TMS results in both excitatory and inhibitory influences over the stimulated cortex. When applied over the motor cortex at rest, single pulse TMS can be used to probe motor cortex thresholds by quantifying the stimulation intensity required to generate an excitatory descending volley traveling the pyramidal tract and capable of inducing an motor-evoked potential (MEP). After eliciting an MEP, the stimulated cortical area is rendered temporarily less excitable. In normal subjects, this phenomenon relies on intact intracortical inhibition.[48] TMS applied over the motor cortex during a tonic contraction generates a contralateral silent period that reflects inhibitory intracortical influences[49] as well as an ipsilateral silent period reflective of transcallosal inhibition.[50] Paired-pulse TMS can be used to probe the recovery of cortical excitability or to study the effects of a weak conditioning pulse on a test stimulus.[51] Repetitive TMS (rTMS) delivers trains of stimulation at predefined rates highlighting different aspect of excitatory or inhibitory effects of TMS on cortical function over longer periods and can be used to explore more complex aspects of behavior, learning, cortical plasticity, cortical organization, and even therapeutic roles.[52]

▶ PHYSIOLOGICAL CLASSIFICATION OF MYOCLONUS

From a clinical perspective, myoclonus refers to quick muscle jerks, either irregular or rhythmic, and almost always arising from the central nervous system. This phenomenological definition is relatively nonspecific. On the other hand, understanding the origin and mechanisms of propagation of myoclonic activity using electrophysiological techniques provides valuable information on myoclonus pathophysiology. From a topographical perspective, myoclonus can be classified as focal, involving only a few adjacent muscles, generalized, involving many or most of the muscles in the body, or multifocal, involving many muscles but in different jerks.[8] Myoclonus can be spontaneous, can be activated or accentuated by voluntary movement (action myoclonus), and can be activated or accentuated by sensory stimulation (reflex myoclonus).[9,20,53,54] In the differential diagnosis of myoclonus, the principal features that favor myoclonus are the quickness and fragmentary nature of the resulting movements and the incapacity to voluntary suppress them.[53] Some simple tics may look identical to myoclonus and cannot be visually distinguished. Another disorder that could be confused with myoclonus is tremor, because some forms of myoclonus are rhythmic.[55] Conversely, some tremors, despite a regular frequency, have variable displacement and EMG burst amplitude, thus, exhibiting an irregular appearance not unlike that of myoclonus.[53]

The concept of positive and negative myoclonus is one of pathophysiological relevance. Quick muscle jerks, the clinical hallmark of myoclonus, could arise from either brief EMG activation (positive myoclonus) or brief sudden cessation of tonic EMG output (negative myoclonus). Asterixis is the clinical term used to describe negative myoclonus. It was first described by Adams and Foley[56] in patients with hepatic encephalopathy, but it is known now to represent a nonspecific neurological finding associated with a multitude of disturbances.

There are several useful schemes for classifying myoclonus.[8] For the purposes of therapy, it is valuable to consider both an etiological classification and a physiological classification. The etiological and physiological classifications of myoclonus may not always overlap. An etiological classification of myoclonus provides guidance for treatment of the underlying metabolic, infectious or toxic derangement, and it has clear implications in the prognosis and counseling of patients and relatives of afflicted individuals. The physiological classification of myoclonus, on the other hand, searches for the site and mechanism of origin of the symptoms, the precipitating factors, and the pathways of spread. Myoclonic disorders, with strikingly different etiological, genetic, and prognostic implications, may fall into the same physiological group, sharing relatively homogeneous electrophysiological properties pointing to common physiological derangement and means of expression.[9,10,20,55,57] These findings, in turn, may aid the selection of the most appropriate symptomatic therapy, may serve as a quantitative tool for evaluating efficacy and mechanisms of action of antimyoclonic medications[58–64] and may aid in the early recognition of patients at risk for some myoclonic disorders, even before clinically symptomatic, perhaps allowing for earlier interventions.[65,66]

Halliday[67] can be credited with the first comprehensive attempt to classify the myoclonias, based on their electrophysiological correlates. He divided myoclonus into three main groups: pyramidal, extrapyramidal and segmental. Pyramidal myoclonus encompassed those myoclonic disorders characterized by a brief burst of EMG activity associated with an EEG correlate. Because of the short latency between the EEG event and the EMG burst (15–40 ms), he proposed an origin in the cortex propagated via the pyramidal tract. In extrapyramidal myoclonus, Halliday included those myoclonic movements in which the EEG events were less obvious and the EMG bursts were of longer duration. He considered the movements seen in subacute sclerosing panencephalitis as a prototypical example of this group. The loose association between EEG and EMG and the long and variable length of EMG bursts suggested to Halliday an extrapyramidal site of origin. Segmental myoclonus was used by Halliday to denote myoclonus, often symmetrical and rhythmic, confined to discrete brainstem segments or spinal cord myotomes and arising from brainstem or spinal cord damage as a result of trauma, infection or neoplasm.

From an electrophysiological perspective, myoclonus is classified in two broad groups (Table 38–1). By conceptualizing epileptic myoclonus as a fragment of epilepsy, myoclonus can be divided into epileptic and nonepileptic types.[21,68] The physiological characteristics of epileptic myoclonus are EMG burst length of 10–50 ms, synchronous antagonist activity and an EEG correlate. Nonepileptic myoclonus shows EMG burst lengths of 50–300 ms, synchronous or asynchronous antagonist activity and no EEG correlate. The classification of myoclonus into epileptic and nonepileptic groups has a value beyond simple taxonomic curiosity. Response to anticonvulsant agents and other antimyoclonic medications appears to be closely linked to the physiological features of the myoclonus.[58,59,61] This classification scheme of myoclonus can be equally applied to positive and negative myoclonus. In fact, it can be postulated that epileptic negative and positive myoclonus are parts of the same phenomenon.[15,69–71] During the abnormal cortical discharge, positive and negative influences on motor activity are generated. These influences may differ in their time of maximal expression, threshold for clinical manifestation, their time course, pathways of spread, their sensitivity to medications, and sensitivity to different physiological states such as sleep–wake cycles and fatigue.[15]

▶ TABLE 38–1. PHYSIOLOGICAL CLASSIFICATION OF MYOCLONUS

Epileptic myoclonus
Cortical reflex myoclonus
Reticular reflex myoclonus
Primary generalized epileptic myoclonus
Cortical tremor
Photic cortical reflex myoclonus
Nonepileptic myoclonus
Normal physiological phenomena (e.g., hypnic jerk)
Essential myoclonus, including myoclonus-dystonia
Palatal myoclonus (tremor)
Spinal myoclonus, including propriospinal myoclonus
Peripheral myoclonus
Exaggerated startle
Orthostatic myoclonus
Periodic limb movements in sleep
Psychogenic myoclonus

The terms cortical and subcortical myoclonus are used to classify myoclonus according to the presumed location in the nervous system for the myoclonus generator.[8] The terms cortical and subcortical myoclonus are often used almost interchangeably with epileptic and nonepileptic myoclonus, respectively. However, this is not always true. Reticular reflex myoclonus, classified as epileptic myoclonus, originates from abnormal paroxysmal discharges in the brainstem reticular formation and thus has a subcortical origin.[11,72] The origin of all nonepileptic myoclonias is not known, and it is in fact possible that one or more have cortical origin. For example, a strong argument could be made that psychogenic myoclonus has a cortical origin and a nonepileptic mechanism.

EPILEPTIC MYOCLONUS

Cortical reflex myoclonus is a fragment of focal or partial epilepsy.[21] Each myoclonic jerk involves only a few adjacent muscles, but involvement of larger body segments can occur. The disorder is commonly multifocal and is accentuated by action and sensory stimulation. The EEG reveals a focal positive–negative event over the sensorimotor cortex contralateral to the jerk preceding both spontaneous and reflex-induced myoclonic jerks. With stimulus sensitivity, C-reflexes (the EMG correlate of reflex myoclonus) are easily elicited and are correlated with giant SEPs. The EEG event associated with reflex jerks is a giant P1–N2 component of the SEP (Fig. 38–1).[21,27,60] Often, the P1–N2 has exactly the same topography as the

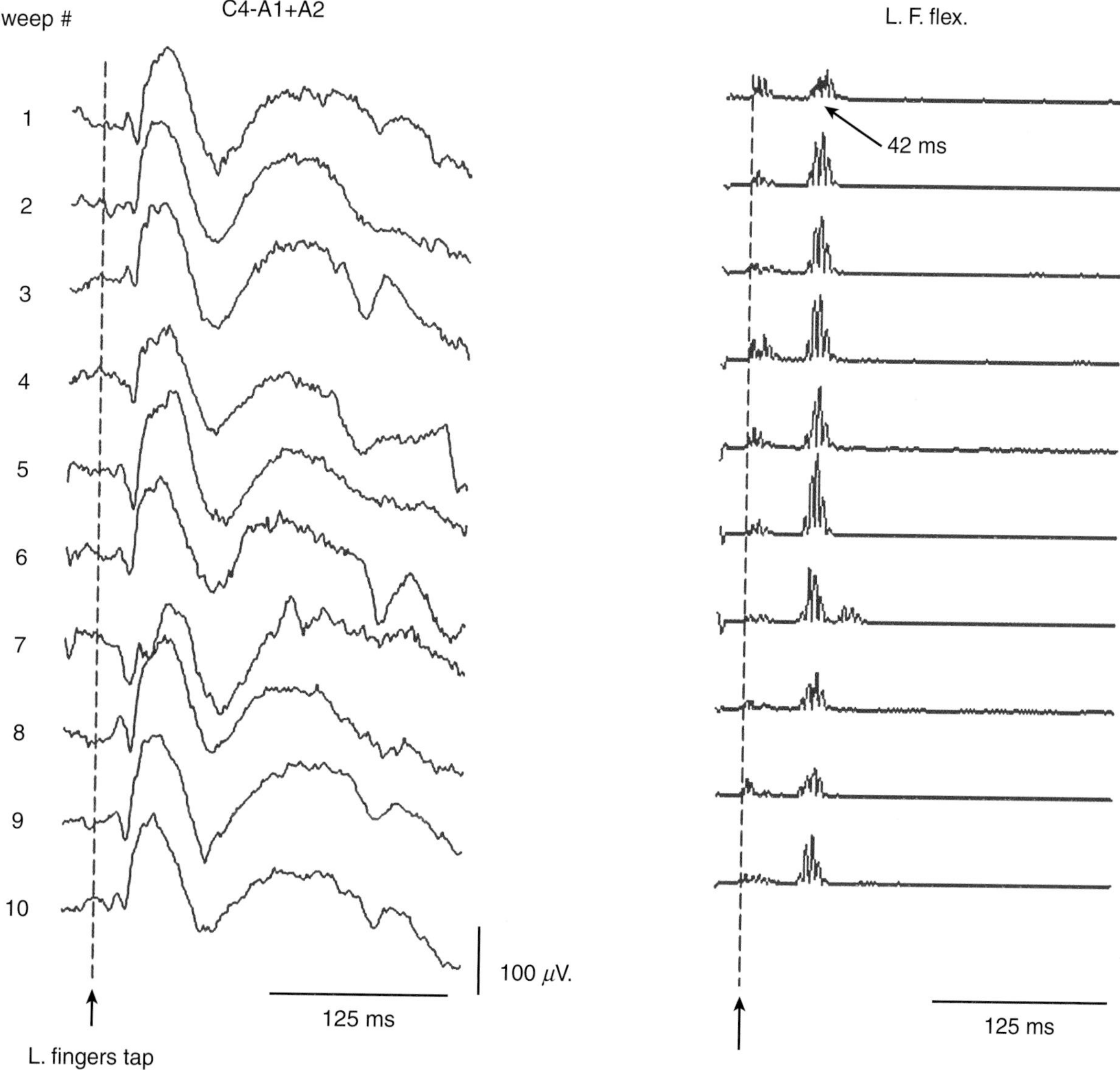

Figure 38–1. Giant SEPs in a patient with cortical sensory-reflex myoclonus. Individual taps to the fingers on the left hand (indicated by the vertical dashed line) give rise to a giant SEP responses discernible in single trials at the C4 electrode. The morphology of the SEPs is akin to epileptiform paroxysms. There is a reflex EMG response (C-reflex) in the left finger flexors at about 42.0 ms in response to each tap.

positive–negative event preceding the spontaneous myoclonus, but at times there are some differences.[9,27,60,73,74] An additional feature of epileptic myoclonus is that, when the cranial nerve muscles are involved, *the timing of onset of activation follows a rostrocaudal sequence consistent with a descending corticospinal volley;* that is, the masseter (fifth cranial nerve) is active before the orbicularis oculi (seventh cranial nerve), which is itself active before the sternocleidomastoid (11th cranial nerve) (Fig. 38–2).[68]

Reticular reflex myoclonus is regarded as a fragment of generalized epilepsy.[11] Myoclonic muscle jerks are usually generalized, with greater activation of proximal than distal and flexor more than extensor muscles. Voluntary action and sensory stimulation increase the jerking. This disorder has the following features: (1) There are brief generalized EMG bursts, lasting 10–30 ms and triggered by sensory stimulation, such as touch or muscle stretch, or by action: (2) The EEG correlates, when present, are not time-locked to the muscle activation: (3) The pattern of EMG activation in cranial nerve muscles indicates that the *sternocleidomastoid muscle is activated first and the other cranial nerve muscles activate in reverse numerical order.* It is as if the front of activation originates in proximity to the motor nucleus of the 11th cranial nerve and travels bidirectionally along the neuroaxis.[11] Reticular reflex myoclonus can be seen in patients with postanoxic myoclonus and in other toxic–metabolic encephalopathies associated with myoclonus, such as uremia.[72] In cats, urea infusions give rise to this form of myoclonus. Depth electrode recordings in this animal model of myoclonus have defined the origin of the abnormal discharge in the nucleus reticularis gigantocellularis.[75]

Both cortical and reticular reflex myoclonus may be seen in the same patient.[68,76] Clinically, there will be both multifocal and generalized jerks and physiological analysis will reveal features of both disorders.

Primary generalized epileptic myoclonus is a fragment of primary generalized epilepsy.[21] The most common clinical manifestation is small, focal jerks, often involving only the fingers; thus, the myoclonus is sometimes called minipolymyoclonus.[77] The term minipolymyoclonus was originally coined to refer to small jerks seen in patients with motor neuron disease. Minipolymyoclonus of central origin and minipolymyoclonus of peripheral origin have a similar clinical appearance, and they are most easily separated by the company they keep. One has associated seizures, whereas the other has progressive muscle weakness and denervation, with marked EMG changes. A second clinical presentation of primary generalized epileptic myoclonus consists of generalized, synchronized whole-body jerks not unlike those seen with reticular reflex myoclonus. The EEG correlate is a slow, bilateral frontocentrally predominant negativity similar to the wave of a primary generalized paroxysm.[77]

Cortical tremor is closely related to cortical myoclonus. As a clinical syndrome, the term cortical tremor

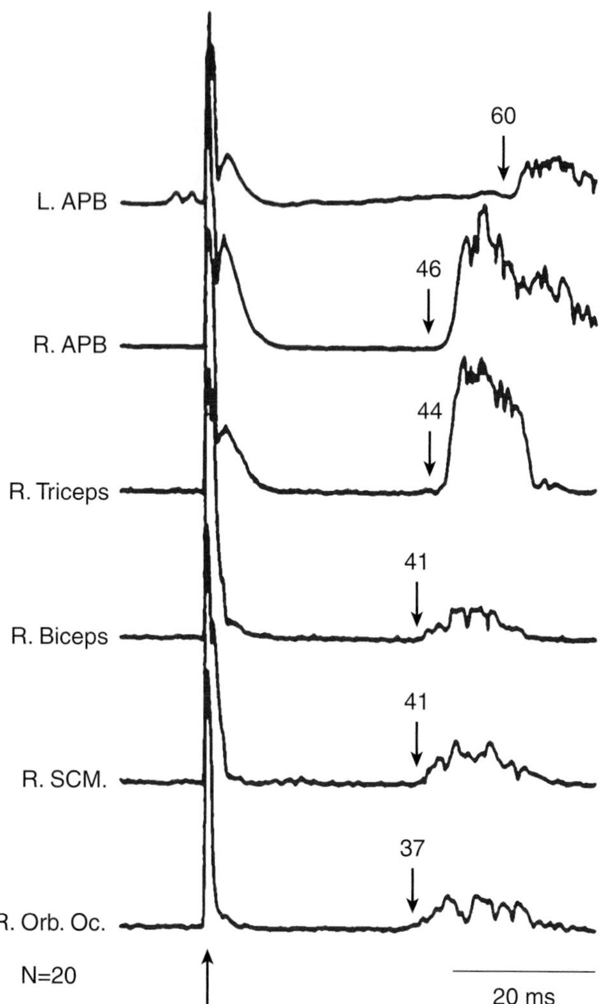

Figure 38–2. Polygraphic average (n = 20) of rectified EMG reflex responses to stimulation of the right median nerve in a patient with cortical reflex myoclonus. In this patient, focal stimulation often resulted in generalized body twitches. The latency of activation of the different muscles is consistent with a rostrocaudal pattern of activation with muscles innervated by the highest cranial nerves activating first. R, right; L, left; APB, abductor pollicis brevis muscle; SCM, sternocleidomastoid muscle; Orb. Oc, orbicularis oculi. Activation of the L. APB follows activation of the R. APB by about 15 ms. This difference probably represents a delay related to transcallosal spread of the activation from the left to the right hemisphere.

is most commonly associated with the condition now known as familial cortical myoclonic tremor with epilepsy (FCMTE).[78] This disorder was first reported less than two decades ago and has been previously reported under many other names (autosomal-dominant cortical myoclonus and epilepsy , benign adult familial myoclonic epilepsy, familial adult myoclonic epilepsy, familial cortical myoclonic tremor, familial cortical tremor with epilepsy, familial essential myoclonus and epilepsy, familial benign myoclonus epilepsy of adult onset, and heredofamilial tremor and epilepsy).[79–88] FCMTE has several characteristics that distinguish it from other forms of tremor disorders. Tremor is usually the first symptom to develop with fast rhythmic jerks of small amplitude involving fingers and hands. The surface EMG studies demonstrate repetitive, 8–13 Hz frequency bursts of 50 ms duration, which can be induced by posture.[80] Polyspike-and-wave patterns are common in patients and unaffected relatives in routine EEG. Giant cortical SEPs produced by median nerve stimulation are present in most patients. Stimulation of median nerve also demonstrates a C-reflex in most cases. Jerk-locked back-averaging of the EEG triggered by tremor-related EMG bursts revealed a cortical potential preceding the myoclonic jerks in over half of the patients. Epilepsy in the form of generalized tonic–clonic type, absence, myoclonic seizures, or complex partial seizures is the second most common symptom.[88] All families with FCMTE show an autosomal-dominant pattern of inheritance, but the genetic analysis of these families shows heterogeneity.[88] Electrodiagnostic criteria are essential in confirming this diagnosis.[80] Patients with otherwise typical cortical myoclonus, regardless of their etiology, may experience tremor of the activated limbs when asked to perform an isometric effort.[55]

Detailed studies of photic cortical reflex myoclonus show that it has an origin in a hyperexcitable motor cortex and is driven by an occipital response of normal appearance.[61,89] There is a remarkable similarity in these findings and those of the myoclonus in the photosensitive baboon *Papio papio*.[90–93] Intermittent light stimulation in the photosensitive baboon gives rise to frontocentral paroxysmal discharges. The surface-positive component of the cortical discharge precedes activation of the orbicularis oculi by 4 ms, the masseter by 7 ms, the biceps by 8 ms, and the paraspinal muscles by 24 ms. These results are consistent with a pyramidal tract route of spread. Unit recordings indicate areas 4 and 6 of the cortex with the highest levels of activity.[93] Recordings from subcortical structures show that their involvement is always secondary to the cortical activation. Failure of intracortical recurrent inhibition seems to be responsible, at least in part, for these findings.[91]

Epileptic myoclonus has been recognized in several disease states not conventionally conceived of as part of the myoclonic or epileptic syndromes. Cortical myoclonus has been reported in corticobasal degeneration (CBD),[60,94,95] Alzheimer's disease,[57,77,96] Parkinson disease,[97–99] Huntington's disease,[100,101] multiple system atrophy-cerebellar type (MSA-C),[102,103] progressive pallido-ponto-nigral degeneration,[104,105] and progressive supranuclear palsy.[106] Epileptic myoclonus is also reported in the late-onset myoclonic epilepsy in Down's syndrome associated with Alzheimer's pathology.[107,108]

NONEPILEPTIC MYOCLONUS

Some myoclonic movements reflect normal physiological phenomena. One such phenomenon is the hypnic jerk experienced by all people at times while drowsy and falling off to sleep.[8]

Essential myoclonus is a term that is used for those patients whose sole neurological abnormality is myoclonus and who specifically do not have seizures, dementia, or ataxia.[8] The EEG and other laboratory investigations should be normal. Familial cases as well as sporadic cases are seen. Ballistic movement overflow myoclonus is one type of essential myoclonus that has been seen as an autosomal-dominant disorder.[8] The myoclonus is generalized, appears to occur seldom at rest, and is clearly induced by action. The EMG is characterized by the ballistic "triphasic" EMG pattern with alternating activity in antagonist muscles (although more tonic EMG patterns might also be seen).[109] There is clinical overlap of essential myoclonus, essential tremor, and myoclonus-dystonia (M-D); all of which are often alcohol-sensitive. In some families, all these different manifestations may be the product of the same genetic abnormality. Inherited M-D is an autosomal-dominant disorder characterized by myoclonus and dystonia that often improves with alcohol. The disorder is caused by mutations in the epsilon-sarcoglycan gene (*DYT11*).[110–112] Jerk-locked back-averaged EEG does not reveal any preceding cortical correlates, the median nerve SEPs are not enlarged and the C-reflex is not exaggerated, all in support of a subcortical nonepileptic origin.[112,113]

Palatal myoclonus, now preferentially called palatal tremor, is the prototypical rhythmic focal myoclonic disorder.[114–117] Palatal tremor is thought to encompass at least two separate disorders: essential palatal tremor (EPT), in which involuntary palatal movements are associated with ear clicks, and symptomatic palatal tremor (SPT), which is when palatal movements develop in the context of cerebellar or brainstem pathology.[117–119] The soft palate involvement differs in the two groups. The palatal movements are consistent with activation of the tensor veli palatini muscle (anterior soft palate) in EPT and of the levator veli palatini muscle (posterior soft palate) in SPT.[116] Palatal movements, unilaterally or bilaterally, occur at 1.5–3 Hz. In SPT, palatal movements may be accompanied by synchronous movements of adjacent muscles, such as the external ocular muscles, tongue, larynx, face, neck, diaphragm, or even limb muscles. During sleep, EPT stops, whereas SPT continues, with only slight variations in the tremor rate. The palatal tremor cycle exerts remote effects on the tonic EMG activity of the upper and lower extremities only in patients with SPT. In SPT, cerebellar dysfunction ipsilateral to the palatal tremor may be a result, in part, of abnormal function of the contralateral inferior olive, which most often appears hypertrophied on magnetic resonance imaging (MRI) images.

In EPT, contractions of the tensor veli palatini muscle collapses and releases the Eustachian tubes openings giving raise to ear click sounds.[120–122] The pathophysiological basis of EPT remains unclear.[115] Bulbar myoclonus or branchial myoclonus is the term often used to describe myoclonic movements of tongue or neck.[114] More recently, some authors have suggested that EPT may be a more heterogeneous group of patients,[123] some of which might have psychogenic palatal tremor.[124–126]

Spinal myoclonus is more commonly rhythmic than arrhythmic.[8,67] Involved regions can be one limb, one limb and adjacent trunk, or both legs. Focal lesions of the spinal cord giving rise to spinal myoclonus include infection, degenerative disease, tumor, cervical myelopathy, and demyelinating disease, and it may follow spinal anesthesia or the introduction of contrast media into the cerebrospinal fluid. Another form of spinal myoclonus is propriospinal myoclonus.[13,127] This is clinically characterized by axial jerks that are nonrhythmic and lead to symmetric flexion of neck, trunk, hips, and knees. Jerks can be spontaneous or stimulus-induced. By polygraphic EMG studies, it can be demonstrated that the myoclonus starts in the midthoracic region and propagates slowly, at about 5 m/s, both rostrally and caudally.[128,129] Propriospinal myoclonus and psychogenic axial myoclonic movements could be difficult to separate clinically and electrophysiologically.[130–132]

Peripheral myoclonus has been reported, but it is not clear that this is always distinct from fasciculation or myokymia. Signs of acute or chronic denervation in the involved muscles characterize peripheral myoclonus. Cases have been reported with lesions of nerve, brachial plexus, and nerve root.[7,8,133] As there can be secondary central nervous system changes following peripheral injury, even if an obvious lesion is peripheral, the myoclonus may still arise centrally.[134]

Exaggerated startle is being increasingly recognized clinically as a form of myoclonus.[39,40] The normal startle consists of a quick muscular response to a surprise stimulus. An exaggerated startle consists of a response that is too large in magnitude, too widespread or too complex, but, most importantly, it is abnormal by virtue of its lack of normal habituation. A normal startle reaction should not take place when the stimulus is not a surprise and should habituate fairly quickly to low-intensity or repeated stimuli. There has been considerable confusion in the literature as to which myoclonic phenomena are truly exaggerated startle reflexes. One source of confusion, for example, is stimulus-sensitive myoclonus, which might be difficult to distinguish purely on clinical grounds from exaggerated startle. Creutzfeldt–Jakob disease is commonly said to be characterized by an exaggerated startle, but the stimulus-induced response is a myoclonic jerk.[8,130] Studies have shown that hyperekplexia or startle disease is characterized by a truly exaggerated startle.[135] A specific mutation affecting the structure of the α subunit of the glycine receptor has been identified in some of these patients.[136] Mutations in other components of the glycine receptor or even components of presynaptic glycine function have been recognized in other patients. Benzodiazepines are fairly effective symptomatic treatment. Startle epilepsy is a disorder consisting of epilepsy after a startle. The interesting syndrome known by many names, including jumping Frenchmen, Myriachit, and Latah,[137,138] appears also to be initiated with a startle-like reaction, but often followed by a variety of more complex behaviors including coprolalia and stereotyped complex movements. The physiology of Latah has never been investigated in detail and some authorities believe it to be a psychogenic disorder.

Nocturnal myoclonic movements might represent several different phenomena, including the hypnic jerk, periodic limb movements in sleep (PLMS), and excessive fragmentary myoclonus in nonrapid eye movement (NREM) sleep. Myoclonus associated with epilepsy, intention myoclonus associated with semivolitional movements, and segmental myoclonus might also occur in sleep but are not primarily nocturnal.[8] PLMS are characterized by a pattern that is unmistakable. EMG bursts lasting 500–2000 ms (really out of the myoclonus range), come every 10–30 s most prominent in the tibialis anterior muscles. The two sides of the body can be activated independently, simultaneously, or even alternately. They occur in NREM sleep but can occur also in drowsiness, when the patient can be fully conscious of their occurrence.[139] PLMS movements may be the result of disinhibition of spinal cord flexor reflexes.[140]

Orthostatic myoclonus is a term recently introduced to describe myoclonus that appears in the lower extremity muscles only upon standing. The majority of patients with this disorder presents with gait difficulties suggestive of parkinsonism or gait apraxia. Unlike orthostatic tremor, the EMG bursts associated with orthostatic myoclonus are slower (7–10 Hz) and lack the monotonic intrinsic rhythmicity typical of orthostatic tremor.[141] A complete characterization of the physiological features of orthostatic myoclonus is lacking. In terms of gait abnormalities in myoclonus, however, it is important to note that many patients with otherwise typical generalized cortical myoclonus exhibit an abnormal rhythmic "bouncing" stance. This phenomenon most likely originates from a mixture of alternating positive and negative myoclonic of lower extremity muscles involved in postural control.[15]

Myoclonus can also be psychogenic. Monday and Jankovic[142] reported on the clinical features of 18 such patients. The myoclonus was present for 1–110 months; it was segmental in 10 patients, generalized in 7 patients, and focal in 1 patient. Stress precipitated or exacerbated the myoclonic movements in 15 patients; 14 had a definite increase in myoclonic activity during periods of anxiety. The following findings helped to establish the psychogenic nature of the myoclonus: (1) clinical features incongruous with "organic" myoclonus, (2) evidence of underlying psychopathology, (3) an improvement with distraction or placebo, and (4) the presence of incongruous sensory loss or false weakness. More than one half of all their patients with adequate follow-up improved after gaining insight into the psychogenic mechanisms of their movement disorder. Physiological investigation in psychogenic myoclonus can be helpful.[130] Reports have demonstrated the presence of a BP or "readiness potential" preceding movement onset in most of these patients.[25,26] A second useful physiological test in a patient suspected of psychogenic reflex myoclonus is to examine the latencies of the reflex EMG response to stimulation. In psychogenic disease, the responses are highly variable and later that than the fastest voluntary reaction time, and certainly, much longer than those of the C-reflex.

▶ ELECTROPHYSIOLOGICAL FINDINGS ACROSS THE SPECTRUM OF MYOCLONUS

POLYGRAPHIC EMG

A unique generalizable feature across the broad spectrum of myoclonus is that myoclonus arises from abnormal muscle activation in the form of short (50–300 ms) EMG bursts (positive myoclonus).[6] Less often, myoclonus is the result of brief interruptions of ongoing tonic EMG (negative myoclonus).[14,15,143] In both instances, abnormal EMG activity leads to a brief displacement of the involved body segment and/or disruption of posture. The polygraphic study of the EMG activity alone provides useful information in classifying and understanding the pathophysiology of myoclonus. EMG bursts of brief duration (50 ms or less) are almost exclusively seen in epileptic myoclonus. Discharges approaching 150 ms are typical of nonepileptic myoclonus. Rapid movements with EMG bursts lasting between 150 and 300 ms are often seen as fragments of other movement disorders, such as dystonia. The temporal relation of activation of different muscles involved in a generalized twitch also provides information on the type of myoclonus. A rostrocaudal "wave" of activation, beginning with the uppermost motor cranial nerves and progressing in a descending fashion along the neuroaxis with a conduction velocity appropriate for the pyramidal tract, is typical of epileptic myoclonus originating in the cortex[68] (Fig. 38–2). A pattern of activation initiating with the sternocleidomastoid muscle and progressing with the activation of both rostrally and caudally innervated muscles is typical for reticular reflex myoclonus.[11,72,144,145] Slow propagation of muscle activation, often beginning in midthoraxic musculature is the hallmark of propriospinal myoclonus. Proximal muscles are most often involved in nonepileptic myoclonus. Synchronous activation of distal agonist/antagonist pairs is the rule in epileptic myoclonus. Inconsistent patterns and timing of muscle activation may hint a psychogenic movement disorder.[130]

The latency differences between homologous muscles in the upper and lower extremities and among muscles innervated by different segments along the neuroaxis may also provide insight into intracortical and transcallosal spread of activation[12,146] (Fig. 38-2).

ROUTINE EEG

For a practitioner, the most common encounter with the electrophysiology of myoclonus occurs usually in the setting of studies involving routine EEG using additional EMG monitoring leads. A similar procedure is routinely used in polygraphic sleep recordings when sleep-related movement disorders are suspected. The presence of well-defined spike, spike-wave, or polyspike discharges in close association with the bursts of EMG activation may indicate an epileptic mechanism. Other encephalopathies not necessarily regarded as epileptic in nature may also show EEG events time-locked to myoclonus, as is the case in Creutzfeldt–Jakob disease.[147] In some patients, despite an obvious epileptic disorder, the routine EEG may not reveal a distinct abnormality associated with myoclonic movements. Many patients with epilepsia partialis continua (EPC) may not have a distinct EEG/EMG correlation.[20,148,149] This may be related, in part, to the specific three-dimensional arrangement of the involved cortical mantle generating tangential dipoles or to involvement of a relatively small area of cortical area lacking the "critical mass" necessary to project an abnormality to the scalp with amplitude discernible from the background EEG signal. Under these circumstances, back-averaging of EEG to the EMG burst may help identify the location and characteristics of EEG abnormalities related to the movements (Fig. 38–3). The EEG itself is also of value in the diagnosis and follow-up of patients with metabolic or degenerative forms of myoclonic disorders.[10] Occipital and Rolandic spikes, as well as paroxysms of generalized spikes and polyspikes, are often seen in the setting of the syndrome of progressive myoclonic epilepsy.[10] Progressive deterioration of background rhythms may parallel disease progression.[10,150]

EEG/MEG BACK-AVERAGING

A cortical participation in the genesis of myoclonus is indicated by the presence of a reproducible EEG potential that precedes the onset of the myoclonic EMG activity. The prototypical finding is the presence of a myoclonus-related cortical spike.[9,68] This is usually in the form of a positive–negative, biphasic sharp EEG potential time-locked to the myoclonus. In most cases, the spike is located over the central region contralateral to the upper extremity muscle used to drive the averaging when the myoclonus is focal or multifocal. The early-positive peak of the spike precedes the EMG onset in upper extremity muscles by about 15–25 ms and for the lower extremity by about 40 ms (Fig. 38–3).

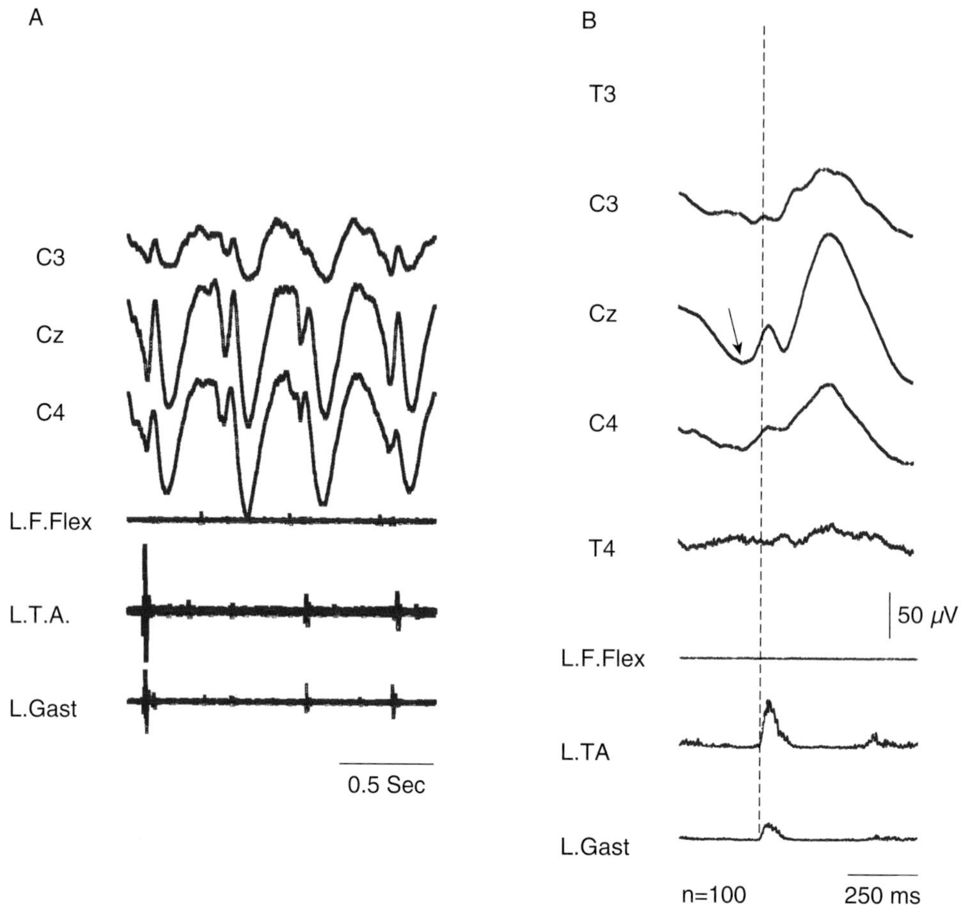

Figure 38–3. (A) Polygraphic EEG and EMG recording in a patient with EPC manifested as irregular twitching of the left foot and nearly continuous spike/wave discharges over the right central and vertex area. (B) Back-averaging of 100 EEG epochs aligned to the onset of myoclonic twitches of the left tibialis anterior muscle (L.TA). Compared to the raw recordings, a much more discrete surface-positive potential emerges over the vertex area (indicated by the arrow) with a latency of 40 ms preceding the EMG twitches. Recording of the left gastrocnemius muscle (L. Gast.) shows a synchronous activation to that of the L.TA muscle. Abnormal myoclonic activity did not spread to the left finger flexors (L.F. Flex).

These latencies are compatible with the corticospinal conduction times for the hand and foot muscles, respectively. Other patterns of myoclonus-related EEG activity have been described. These include monophasic and triphasic EEG potentials, or even more complex sets of wavelets time-locked to the myoclonus[55] (Fig. 38–4).

There is well-defined homuncular representation of EEG correlates of cortical myoclonus. The discharge is maximal over the vertex when myoclonus is recorded from the lower extremities,[151] and more lateral for EEG correlates associated with upper extremity myoclonus (Figs. 39-3 and 39-4). When the myoclonic movements are generalized or bilaterally synchronous, the EEG discharge is widespread with a vertex maximum.[55] In some patients with cortical myoclonus, the initial cortical discharge, spontaneous or reflex, spreads to adjacent motor cortical areas or to homologous areas in the other hemisphere. A high degree of spread characterizes subjects with a tendency to experience generalized myoclonic twitches and frequent seizures.[12]

Ugawa and colleagues [14, 22] described the EEG correlates of asterixis, using the silent period-locked averaging technique in patients with well-defined postural lapses associated with EMG silent periods. The silent periods in these patients were classified in two forms. In type I, silent periods were associated with a complete cessation of background EMG activity, lasting 50–100 ms. The second form, type II, was characterized by a primarily negative event that was associated with a brief and discrete but definite burst of EMG activity that occurred before the silence. Only type II silent periods were preceded by well-defined EEG discharges. The discharges were localized to the contralateral central regions and preceded the event by 20–30 ms. Similar findings have been reported in other patients.[15]

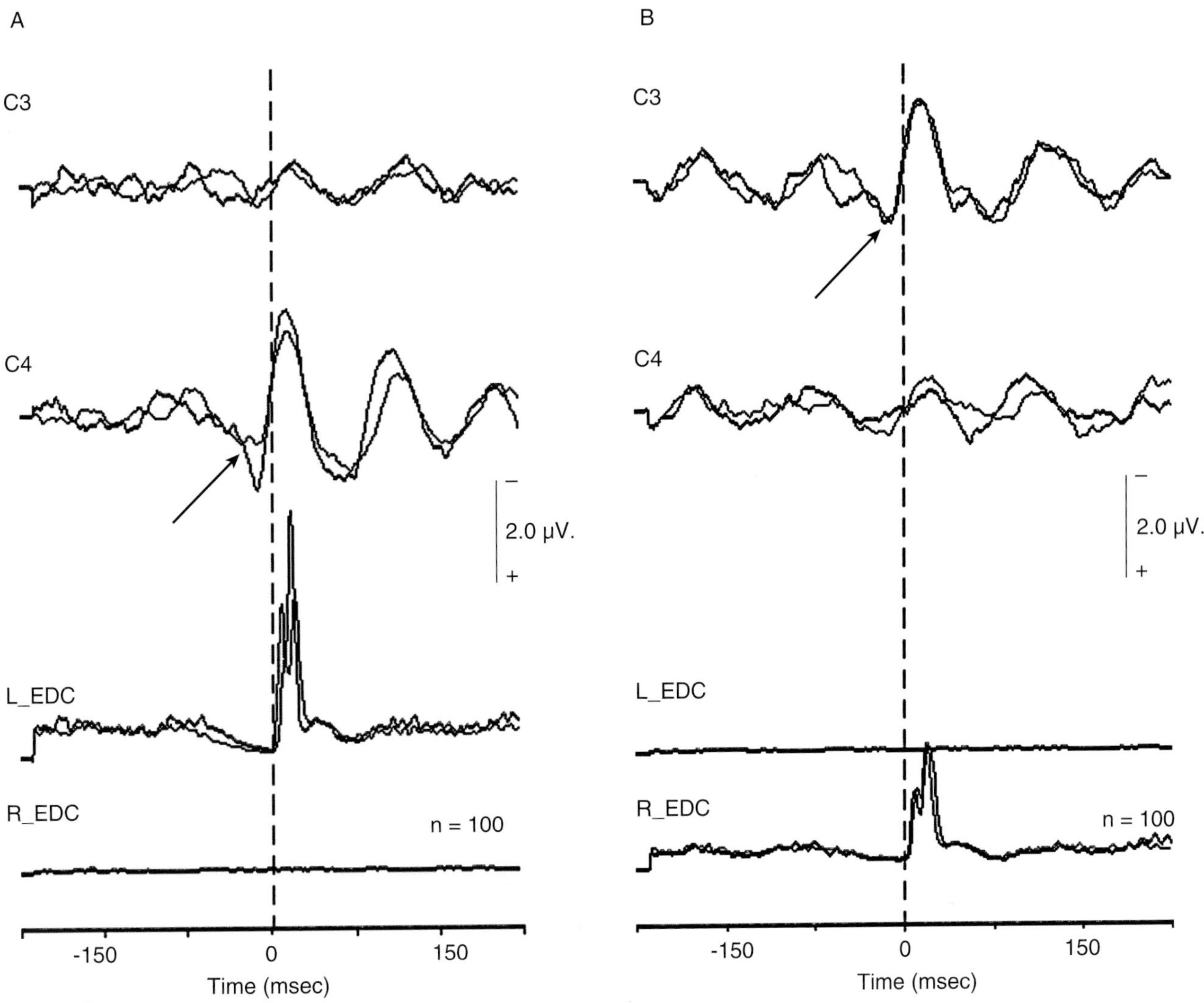

Figure 38–4. Results of back-averaging of EEG activity (reference independent reconstruction) related to myoclonic twitches of the left extensor digitorum communis (L_EDC) (Panel A) and the right extensor digitorum communis (R_EDC) (Panel B) in a patient with cortical myoclonus. A reproducible and somatotopically well-organized series of wavelets beginning shortly before movement onset are evident. These wavelets are preceded by a surface-positive deflection (oblique arrows) before myoclonus EMG onset.

Epileptiform discharges preceding negative myoclonus have been reported in children with epilepsy.[23,24,152] The presenting symptoms in these patients were tremulousness or postural lapses of tonically activated muscles and rare convulsions. The EEG showed focal epileptiform discharges on average 30–50 ms before the onset of the EMG silence. It remains undetermined as to when the EEG discharge of positive and negative myoclonus is consistently different. The C-reflex elicited by electrical stimulation of the median nerve is sometimes present in patients with negative myoclonus. Rare patients may show negative myoclonus in response to sensory stimulation (sensory-reflex asterixis)[15,153] (Fig. 38–5).

Negative myoclonus of subcortical origin may have a completely different pathophysiology. Type I silent periods, without an EEG correlate, may originate primarily from subcortical structures, although this is not known. The high coexistence of type I and type II silent periods in the same patient population may indicate that important cortical–subcortical interactions are operative in the genesis of negative myoclonus.[15,70]

SOMATOSENSORY-EVOKED POTENTIALS AND SOMATOSENSORY-EVOKED MAGNETIC FIELDS

Since Dawson's initial observations in 1947,[5] it has been well known that a subgroup of patients with myoclonus have a grossly enhanced SEP amplitude.[9,27,60]) "Giant

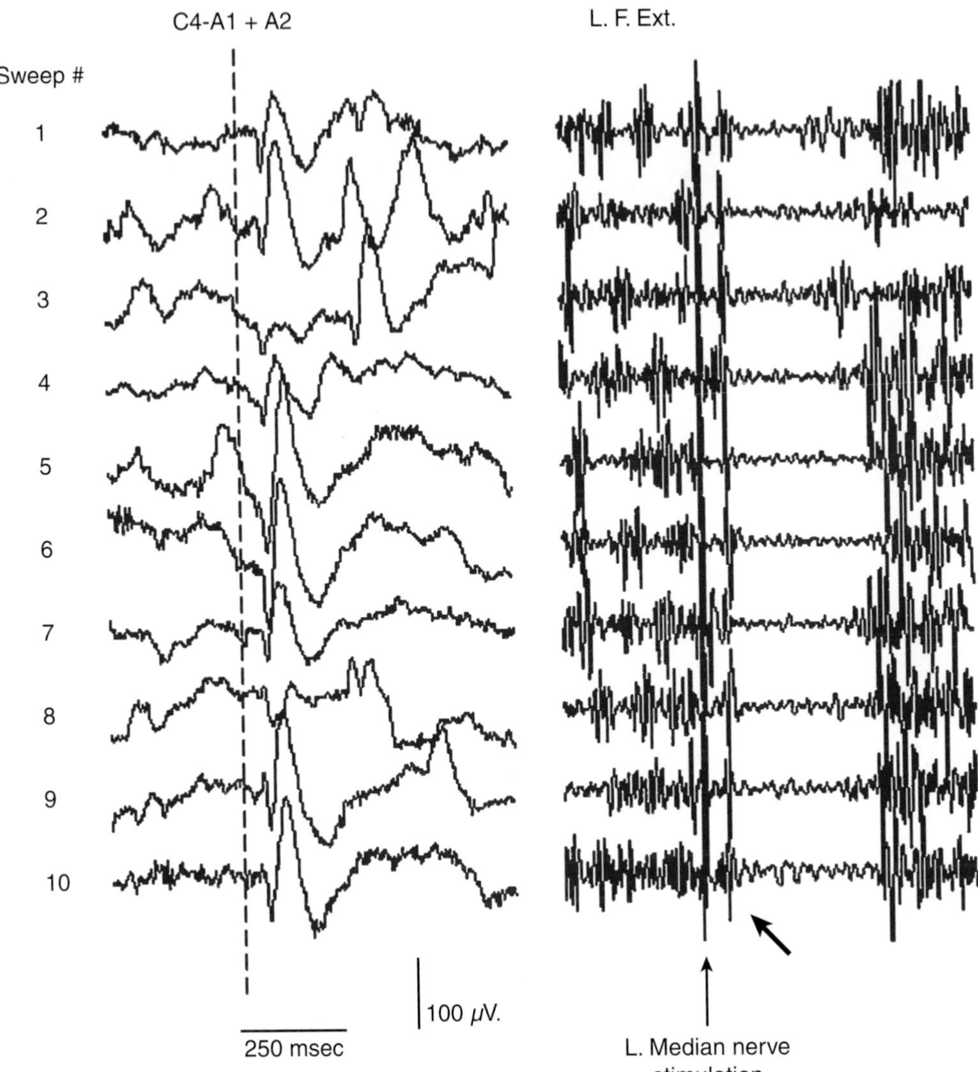

Figure 38–5. Ten epochs of EEG activity recorded from the right central region (C4) and surface EMG activity recorded from the left finger extensor muscles (L.F. Ext.) in a patient with sensory-reflex asterixis. The patient has been asked to hold her hands outstretched in the air against gravity while the left median nerve was electrically stimulated at motor threshold at 0.2 Hz frequency. Epochs were aligned to electrical stimulation. Electrical stimulation produced in most epochs a large-amplitude response (giant SEP), which resembles an epileptic spike. Median nerve stimulation induced a brief myoclonic burst consistent with a C-reflex (oblique arrow) followed by a 250–300-ms period of EMG suppression clinically associated with a postural lapse typical for asterixis.

SEP" is the term generally used to describe this abnormality in patients with cortical myoclonus. Giant SEPs deviate from normal SEPs not only in their amplitude but also in the distortion of the waveform components (Fig. 38–1). The waveform morphology in giant SEPs is usually "simplified" into three large amplitude peaks. Naming the waveforms according to their polarity and sequence (N1, P1, N2, etc.), rather than according to the more conventional terminology (N20, P25/P30, N35, etc.), is favored by some authors.[60] When labeled by its polarity, the N1 component is usually normal in amplitude and has latency comparable to that of the N20 component of regular SEPs. In contrast, the P1 and N2 components are enlarged in magnitude and usually are delayed, when compared to those of normal SEPs.[9,60] A N1/P1 or a P1/N2 amplitude greater than 10 μV and measured at the contralateral central region in ear-referenced recordings is considered a "giant" response.[9] In many patients, giant SEPs resemble typical spike-wave paroxysms (Figs. 39-1 and 39-5). Giant SEPs are often associated with a reflex myoclonic jerk at a latency of approximately 45 ms in hand muscles after median nerve stimulation (C-reflex).[9,60,37,154] The coexistence of these two is the hallmark of sensory-reflex cortical myoclonus. The striking resemblance in latency and morphology of the giant SEP-C-reflex complex to the myoclonus-related cortical spike suggests that both originate from common cortical mechanisms.

The generator of the giant SEP resides in, or in close proximity to, the central sulcus.[27,73,155] Because the subcortical components and the first cortical component (N1) are usually normal in amplitude, it can be suggested that an abnormality in intracortical inhibition after the arrival of the first volley of thalamocortical activity might be responsible for the abnormal activation of surrounding cortex which, in turn, leads to enlargement of both the giant SEP responses and activation of descending motor outputs leading to the C-reflex.[9,60]

The use of paired somatosensory stimuli at variable intervals has been used to trace the excitability cycle of the sensorimotor cortex in cortical myoclonus.[156,157] Patients with cortical myoclonus tend to show a "triphasic" cycle of initial depression of cortical excitability, followed within 20–80 ms by a period of increased excitability, and a subsequent period of depression with recovery of the baseline excitability after 300 ms.[157] There is evidence suggesting that this cycle may be heavily weighted toward inhibition in patients presenting with epileptic negative myoclonus.[153]

Giant SEPs are variably present in patients with negative myoclonus. The recovery curve of SEP amplitude to paired somatosensory stimuli in patients with epileptic negative myoclonus shows a more prominent inhibition, compared to that of patients with positive myoclonus.[153]

MEG has proven valuable in pinpointing the critical role of the motor cortex in the generation of the giant SEP response in cortical myoclonus.[158,159] and to the contribution of other cortical generators to the genesis of myoclonic phenomena.[151,158–161]

ADVANCED SIGNAL ANALYSIS

Increased corticocortical and corticomuscular coherency in patients with epileptic myoclonus indicates an abnormally enhanced and somatotopically organized coupling of motor cortical neurons and spinal motor neurons, most likely as a result of deficient inhibition[29,71,146,162–165] (Fig. 38–6). Corticomuscular coherence does not appear

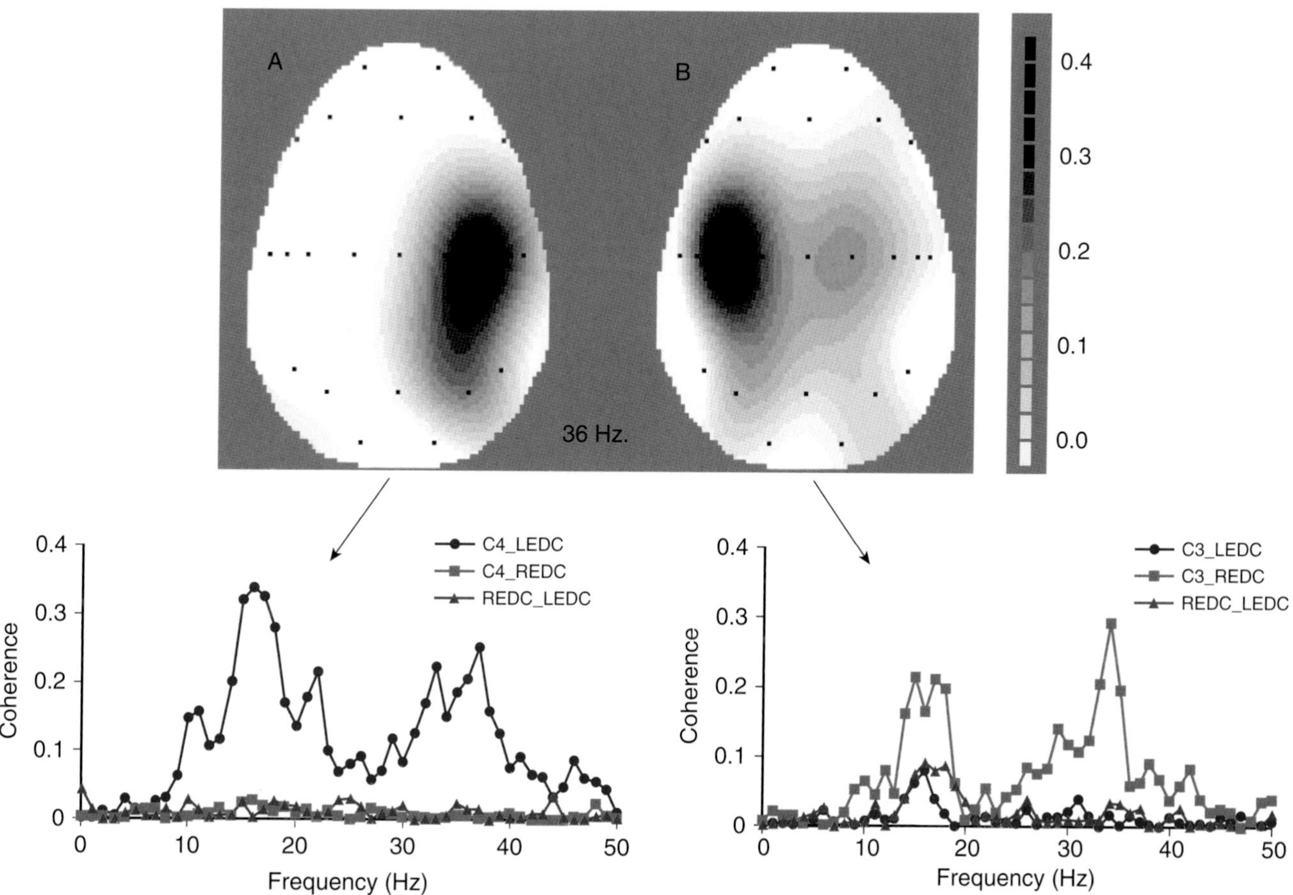

Figure 38–6. Topographical scalp distribution of corticomuscular coherence at 36 Hz calculated during a 2-minute isometric effort between scalp electrodes arranged according to the 10–20 system and the left extensor digitorum communis (L EDC) (Panel A) and the right extensor digitorum communis (R EDC) (Panel B) in a patient with action-induced cortical myoclonus. In the lower panels, corticomuscular and musculomuscular coherence plots are represented for the two conditions.

to be enhanced in patients with nonepileptic myoclonus. For example, in M-D, corticomuscular coherence is not enhanced and musculomuscular coherence was only enhanced at lower frequencies (1–4 Hz), a feature typical for other dystonia syndromes.[166,167]

MEG rhythmic oscillations over the motor cortex in patients with progressive myoclonic epilepsy exhibit distinctly abnormal reactivity to stimulation,[168,169] and confirm the EEG finding of abnormally enhanced level of corticomuscular coherency indicative of impaired inhibition.[29,71,146,162–165,170–172]

α-Range ERD, a measure of cortical activation, was of larger magnitude and more widely spread than controls in patients with Unverricht–Lundborg disease, whereas postmovement ERS, a signal thought to represent cortical deactivation, was absent or reduced in patients.[35] These findings suggest an overall functional abnormality of cortical and perhaps corticothalamic circuitry in this patient group.

REFLEX STUDIES

In many patients with generalized cortical myoclonus, certain types of somatosensory stimulation will readily produce a C-reflex response not present in normal subjects. The latency of the reflex is about twice that of the first cortical component of the SEPs (18–25 ms in upper limb and 30–35 ms in lower limb)[9] (Fig. 38–1). In cases of cortical reflex myoclonus, the C-reflex is the result of abnormal activity in a cortical loop. This loop would involve fast-conducting tracts up to the sensory cortex, using the posterior column, lemniscal, and thalamocortical pathways. The events in the cortex might generate a giant SEPs and activate the motor cortex via corticocortical connections, in turn, leads to a rapid descending discharge to the α motor neurons. In rare patients, the reflex may only occur in response to cutaneous stimuli, whereas in others it occurs in response only to passive stretch.[37,154] A direct relationship between the amplitude of the giant SEP and the presence of a reflex myoclonic jerk has been established.[60] These two events, however, appear to be differentially affected by pharmacological interventions such as lisuride or clonazepam.[60]

As with the LLRs after mixed nerve stimulation, purely cutaneous nerve stimulation also induces a series of excitatory and inhibitory effects on a tonically activated muscle of the same limb. These responses have been explored in parkinsonian syndromes with reflex myoclonus as an associated symptom.[173] In their study, patients with myoclonus in the context of Parkinson disease or multiple-system atrophy revealed facilitation of one of the components of the response (E2 component). Patients with CBD, on the other hand, had a grossly exaggerated and shorter latency response than the E2. This finding, along with the fact that SEPs are not enlarged in CBD, suggests myoclonus in CBD behaves uniquely.[94,173,174] The basis for the underlying difference is not clear, but the data suggest that physiological studies could have a role in establishing a differential diagnosis in neurodegenerative syndromes with parkinsonism and myoclonus.

TRANSCRANIAL MAGNETIC STIMULATION

Resting motor thresholds to TMS could be low in those cortical myoclonic patients with a tendency to experience generalized twitches and seizures, but the motor threshold might be high, even higher than in normal subjects, in those patients with only focal twitches and no seizures.[175] Cortical excitability is enhanced in cortical myoclonus when TMS is presented with a concomitant somatosensory stimulus.[175,176] The recovery of cortical excitability after TMS can be probed with pairs of cortical stimuli, and it has been shown to be abnormally modulated in patients with cortical myoclonus as a result of abnormal intracortical inhibition.[175–178] Patients with cortical myoclonus and the tendency to have generalized and multifocal twitches and frequent seizures exhibit a deficient intra- and transcortical inhibition to paired stimuli[175] and a tendency for spread of their cortical EEG discharges.[12] Restoration of intracortical inhibition by low-frequency rTMS (1.0 Hz rTMS) could serve as strategy to treat cortical myoclonus.[178–180] Intracortical inhibition is normal in patients with inherited M-D,[113] a disorder in the subcortical myoclonus category. TMS studies may also serve as tools to study the mechanism of action of antimyoclonic agents.[181]

▶ SUMMARY AND CONCLUSIONS

Over the last 50 years, the development and application of electrophysiological methods has substantially expanded the knowledge of the functional and anatomical substrate underlying myoclonus. Likewise, myoclonus, as a disease model, has enriched the understanding of motor system function[29,40,182,183] and its relationship to other neurological disorders.[65,152,184] We anticipate the field will continue to evolve toward unifying principles that fully incorporate all aspects of myoclonus from electrophysiological and clinical phenotypes to biochemical and molecular principles. Newer methodologies, such as functional MRI are beginning to open new avenues in the study of myoclonus. It has become possible, for example, to study regional cerebral blood flow changes in relation to myoclonus by using the EMG signals associated with myoclonic activity to model the BOLD signal changes in fMRI.[185,186] These techniques, combined with improved source imaging of EEG and MEG signal, more elaborate TMS paradigms, and advanced models of the network interactions among the structures involved in myoclonus generation, are likely to greatly enhance our understanding of myoclonus pathophysiology.[71,163,171] Beyond its obvious clinical value, the electrophysiological evaluation of myoclonus will continue to be a fertile area on which to explore questions relevant to human motor function in health and disease.

REFERENCES

1. Gibbs FAD, H. Lennox WG. The electro-encephalogram in epilepsy and in conditions of impaired conciousness. Arch Neurol Psychiatry 1935;34:1133.
2. Grinker RR, Serota H, Stein SI. Myoclonic epilepsy. Arch Neurol Psychiatry 1938;40:968.
3. Dawson GD. The relation between the electroencephalogram and muscle action potentials in certain convulsive states. J Neurol Neurosurg Psychiatry 1946;9:5.
4. Dawson GD. Cerebral responses to electrical stimulation of peripheral nerve in man. J Neurol Neurosurg Psychiatry 1947;10:134.
5. Dawson GD. Investigations on a patient subject to myoclonic seizures after sensory stimulation. J Neurol Neurosurg Psychiatry 1947;10:141.
6. Hallett M. Analysis of abnormal voluntary and involuntary movements with surface electromyography. Adv Neurol 1983;39:907.
7. Hallett M. Electrophysiologic evaluation of movement disorders. In Aminoff MJ (ed). Electrodiagnosis in Clinical Neurology. New York: Churchill Livingstone, 1992, p. 403.
8. Marsden CD, Hallett M, Fahn S. The nosology and pathophysiology of myoclonus. In Marsden CD, Fahn F (eds). Neurology 2: Movement Disorders. London: Butterworths, 1982, p. 196.
9. Shibasaki H, Yamashita Y, Kuroiwa Y. Electroencephalographic studies myoclonus. Brain 1978:101:447.
10. So N, Berkovic S, Andermann F, et al. Myoclonus epilepsy and ragged-red fibres (MERRF). 2. Electrophysiological studies and comparison with other progressive myoclonus epilepsies. Brain 1989;112:1261.
11. Hallett M, Chadwick D, Adam J, et al. Reticular reflex myoclonus: A physiological type of human post-hypoxic myoclonus. J Neurol Neurosurg Psychiatry 1977;40:253.
12. Brown P, Day BL, Rothwell JC, et al. Intrahemispheric and interhemispheric spread of cerebral cortical myoclonic activity and its relevance to epilepsy. Brain 1991;114:2333.
13. Brown P, Thompson PD, Rothwell JC, et al. Axial myoclonus of propriospinal origin. Brain 1991;114:197.
14. Ugawa Y, Genba K, Shimpo T, et al. Onset and offset of electromyographic (EMG) silence in asterixis. J Neurol Neurosurg Psychiatry 1990;53:260,.
15. Toro C, Hallett M, Rothwell JC, et al. Physiology of negative myoclonus. Adv Neurol 1995;67:211.
16. Hamalainen MS. Basic principles of magnetoencephalography. Acta Radiol Suppl 1991;377:58.
17. Hamalainen MS. Magnetoencephalography: A tool for functional brain imaging. Brain Topogr 1992;5:95.
18. Molins A, Stufflebeam SM, Brown EN, et al. Quantification of the benefit from integrating MEG and EEG data in minimum l2-norm estimation. Neuroimage 2008;42:1069.
19. Sharon D, Hamalainen MS, Tootell RB, et al. The advantage of combining MEG and EEG: comparison to fMRI in focally stimulated visual cortex. Neuroimage 2007;36:1225.
20. Obeso JA, Rothwell JC, Marsden CD. The spectrum of cortical myoclonus. From focal reflex jerks to spontaneous motor epilepsy. Brain 1985;108:193.
21. Hallett M. Myoclonus: relation to epilepsy. Epilepsia 1985; 26(Suppl 1):S67.
22. Ugawa Y, Shimpo T, Mannen T. Physiological analysis of asterixis: Silent period locked averaging. J Neurol Neurosurg Psychiatry 1989;52:89.
23. Yokota T, Tsukagoshi H. Cortical activity-associated negative myoclonus. J Neurol Sci 1992;111:77.
24. Guerrini R, Dravet C, Genton P, et al. Epileptic negative myoclonus. Neurology 1993;43:1078.
25. Toro C, Torres F. Electrophysiological correlates of a paroxysmal movement disorder. Ann Neurol 1986;20:731.
26. Terada K, Ikeda A, Van Ness PC, et al. Presence of Bereitschaftspotential preceding psychogenic myoclonus: Clinical application of jerk-locked back averaging. J Neurol Neurosurg Psychiatry 1995;58:745.
27. Shibasaki H, Yamashita Y, Neshige R, et al. Pathogenesis of giant somatosensory evoked potentials in progressive myoclonic epilepsy. Brain 1985;108:225.
28. Mima T, Terada K, Ikeda A, et al. Afferent mechanism of cortical myoclonus studied by proprioception-related SEPs. Electroencephalogr Clin Neurophysiol 1997;104:51.
29. Brown P. Cortical drives to human muscle: The Piper and related rhythms. Prog Neurobiol 2000;60:97.
30. Pfurtscheller G, Andrew C. Event-Related changes of band power and coherence: Methodology and interpretation. J Clin Neurophysiol 1999;16:512.
31. Pfurtscheller G, Lopes da Silva FH. Event-related EEG/MEG synchronization and desynchronization: Basic principles. Clin Neurophysiol 1999;110:1842.
32. Toro C, Deuschl G, Thatcher R, et al. Event-related desynchronization and movement-related cortical potentials on the ECoG and EEG. Electroencephalogr Clin Neurophysiol 1994;93:380.
33. Crone NE, Miglioretti DL, Gordon B, et al. Functional mapping of human sensorimotor cortex with electrocorticographic spectral analysis. II. Event-related synchronization in the gamma band. Brain 1998;121:2301.
34. Crone NE, Miglioretti DL, Gordon B, et al. Functional mapping of human sensorimotor cortex with electrocorticographic spectral analysis. I. Alpha and beta event-related desynchronization. Brain 1998;121:2271.
35. Visani E, Agazzi P, Canafoglia L, et al. Movement-related des ynchronization-synchronization (ERD/ERS) in patients with Unverricht-Lundborg disease. Neuroimage 2006;33:161.
36. Deuschl G, Lucking CH. Physiology and clinical applications of hand muscle reflexes. Electroencephalogr Clin Neurophysiol Suppl 1990;41:84.
37. Sutton GGM, RF. Focal reflex myoclonus. J Neurol Neurosurg Psychiatry 1974;37:207.
38. Wilkins DE, Hallett M, Wess MM. Audiogenic startle reflex of man and its relationship to startle syndromes. A review. Brain 1986;109:561.
39. Matsumoto J, Fuhr P, Nigro M, et al. Physiological abnormalities in hereditary hyperekplexia. Ann Neurol 1992; 32:41.

40. Brown P, Rothwell JC, Thompson PD, et al. The hyperekplexias and their relationship to the normal startle reflex. Brain 1991;114:1903.
41. Arnfred SM, Lind NM, Hansen AK, et al. Pre-pulse inhibition of the acoustic startle eye-blink in the Gottingen minipig. Behav Brain Res 2004;151:295.
42. Hall FS, Huang S, Fong G. Effects of isolation-rearing on acoustic startle and pre-pulse inhibition in Wistar and fawn hooded rats. Ann N Y Acad Sci 1997;821:542.
43. Khasani S, Becker K, Meinck HM. Hyperekplexia and stiff-man syndrome: Abnormal brainstem reflexes suggest a physiological relationship. J Neurol Neurosurg Psychiatry 2004;75:1265.
44. Molloy FM, Dalakas MC, Floeter MK. Increased brainstem excitability in stiff-person syndrome. Neurology 2002; 59:449.
45. Berger C, Meinck HM. Head retraction reflex in stiff-man syndrome and related disorders. Mov Disord 2003; 18:906.
46. Rothwell JC. Physiological studies of electric and magnetic stimulation of the human brain. Electroencephalogr Clin Neurophysiol Suppl 1991;43:29.
47. Rothwell JC, Thompson PD, Day BL, et al. Stimulation of the human motor cortex through the scalp. Exp Physiol 1991;76:159.
48. Fuhr P, Agostino R, Hallett M. Spinal motor neuron excitability during the silent period after cortical stimulation. Electroencephalogr Clin Neurophysiol 1991;81:257.
49. Wilson SA, Lockwood RJ, Thickbroom GW, et al. The muscle silent period following transcranial magnetic cortical stimulation. J Neurol Sci 1993;114:216.
50. Wassermann EM, Fuhr P, Cohen LG, et al. Effects of transcranial magnetic stimulation on ipsilateral muscles. Neurology 1991;41:1795.
51. Valls-Sole J, Pascual-Leone A, Wassermann EM, et al. Human motor evoked responses to paired transcranial magnetic stimuli. Electroencephalogr Clin Neurophysiol 1992;85:355.
52. Hallett M. Transcranial magnetic stimulation: A primer. Neuron 2007;55:187.
53. Hallett M, Topka H. In Brandt T, Caplan LR, Dichgans J, et al. (eds). Myoclonus in Neurological Disorders: Course and Treatment. San Diego: Academic Press, 2003, p. 1221.
54. Lance JW, Adams RD. The syndrome of intention or action myoclonus as a sequel to hypoxic encephalopathy. Brain 1963;86:111.
55. Toro C, Pascual-Leone A, Deuschl G, et al. Cortical tremor. A common manifestation of cortical myoclonus. Neurology 1993;43:2346.
56. Adams RDF, JM. The neurological changes in the more common types of severe liver disease. Trans Neurol Assoc 1949;74:217.
57. Thompson PD. Neurodegenerative causes of myoclonus. Adv Neurol 2002;89:31.
58. Brown P, Steiger MJ, Thompson PD, et al. Effectiveness of piracetam in cortical myoclonus. Mov Disord 1993;8:63.
59. Chadwick D, Hallett M, Harris R, et al. Clinical, biochemical, and physiological features distinguishing myoclonus responsive to 5-hydroxytryptophan, tryptophan with a monoamine oxidase inhibitor, and clonazepam. Brain 1977;100:455.
60. Rothwell JC, Obeso JA, Marsden CD. On the significance of giant somatosensory evoked potentials in cortical myoclonus. J Neurol Neurosurg Psychiatry 1984;47:33.
61. Artieda J, Obeso JA. The pathophysiology and pharmacology of photic cortical reflex myoclonus. Ann Neurol 1993;34:175.
62. Ikeda A, Shibasaki H, Tashiro K, et al. Clinical trial of piracetam in patients with myoclonus: Nationwide multiinstitution study in Japan. The Myoclonus/Piracetam Study Group. Mov Disord 1996;11:691.
63. Fedi M, Reutens, D, Dubeau, F, et al. Long-term efficacy and safety of piracetam in the treatment of progressive myoclonus epilepsy. Arch Neurol 2001;58:781.
64. Frucht SJ, Louis ED, Chuang C, et al. A pilot tolerability and efficacy study of levetiracetam in patients with chronic myoclonus. Neurology 2001;57:1112.
65. Garvey MA, Toro C, Goldstein S, et al. Somatosensory evoked potentials as a marker of disease burden in type 3 Gaucher disease. Neurology 2001;56:391.
66. Liepert J, Haueisen J, Hegemann S, et al. Disinhibition of somatosensory and motor cortex in mitochondriopathy without myoclonus. Clin Neurophysiol 2001;112:917.
67. Halliday AM. The electrophysiological study of myoclonus in man. Brain 1967;90:241.
68. Hallett M, Chadwick D, Marsden CD. Cortical reflex myoclonus. Neurology 1979;29:1107.
69. Ikeda A, Ohara S, Matsumoto R, et al. Role of primary sensorimotor cortices in generating inhibitory motor response in humans. Brain 2000;123:1710.
70. Ugawa Y, Hanajima R, Terao Y, et al. Exaggerated 16-20 Hz motor cortical oscillation in patients with positive or negative myoclonus. Clin Neurophysiol 2003;114:1278.
71. Kristeva R, Popa T, Chakarov V, et al. Cortico-muscular coupling in a patient with postural myoclonus. Neurosci Lett 2004;366:259.
72. Chadwick D, French AT. Uraemic myoclonus: An example of reticular reflex myoclonus? J Neurol Neurosurg Psychiatry 1979;42:52.
73. Shibasaki H, Kakigi R, Ikeda A. Scalp topography of giant SEP and pre-myoclonus spike in cortical reflex myoclonus. Electroencephalogr Clin Neurophysiol 1991; 81:31.
74. Deuschl G, Ebner A, Hammers R, et al. Differences of cortical activation in spontaneous and reflex myoclonias. Electroencephalogr Clin Neurophysiol. 1991;80:326.
75. Zuckerman EG, Glasser GH. Urea-induced myoclonic seizures. Arch Neurol 1972;27:14.
76. Thompson PD, Maertens de Noordhout A, Day BL, et al. Clinical and electrophysiological observations in postanoxic myoclonus. In Crossman AR, Sambrook MA (eds). Neuronal Mechanisms in Disorders of Movement. London: John Libbey, 1989, p. 375.
77. Hallett M, Wilkins DE. Myoclonus in Alzheimer's disease and minipolymyoclonus. Adv Neurol 1986;43:399.
78. van Rootselaar AF, van Schaik IN, van den Maagdenberg AM, et al. Familial cortical myoclonic tremor with epilepsy: A single syndromic classification for a group of pedigrees bearing common features. Mov Disord 2005; 20:665.
79. Okuma Y, Shimo Y, Hatori K, et al. Familial cortical tremor with epilepsy. Parkinsonism Relat Disord 1997;3:83.

80. Terada K, Ikeda A, Mima T, et al. Familial cortical myoclonic tremor as a unique form of cortical reflex myoclonus. Mov Disord. 1997;12:370.
81. Elia M, Musumeci SA, Ferri R, et al. Familial cortical tremor, epilepsy, and mental retardation: A distinct clinical entity? Arch Neurol. 1998;55:1569.
82. Okuma Y, Shimo Y, Shimura H, et al. Familial cortical tremor with epilepsy: An under-recognized familial tremor. Clin Neurol Neurosurg. 1998;100:75.
83. van Rootselaar F, Callenbach PM, Hottenga JJ, et al. A Dutch family with 'familial cortical tremor with epilepsy'. Clinical characteristics and exclusion of linkage to chromosome 8q23.3-q24.1. J Neurol. 2002;249:829.
84. van Rootselaar AF, Aronica E, Jansen Steur EN, et al. Familial cortical tremor with epilepsy and cerebellar pathological findings. Mov Disord. 2004;19:213.
85. Striano P, Madia F, Minetti C, et al. Electroclinical and genetic findings in a family with cortical tremor, myoclonus, and epilepsy. Epilepsia 2005;46:1993.
86. Striano P, Zara F, Striano S. Autosomal dominant cortical tremor, myoclonus and epilepsy: Many syndromes, one phenotype. Acta Neurol Scand 2005;111:211.
87. Gardella E, Tinuper P, Marini C, et al. Autosomal dominant early-onset cortical myoclonus, photic-induced myoclonus, and epilepsy in a large pedigree. Epilepsia 2006;47:1643.
88. Regragui W, Gerdelat-Mas A, Simonetta-Moreau M. Cortical tremor (FCMTE: familial cortical myoclonic tremor with epilepsy). Neurophysiol Clin 2006;36:345.
89. Rubboli G, Meletti S, Gardella E, et al. Photic reflex myoclonus: A neurophysiological study in progressive myoclonus epilepsies. Epilepsia 1999;40(Suppl 4):50.
90. Brailowsky S. Myoclonus in Papio papio. Mov Disord 1991;6:98.
91. Naquet R, Meldrum BS. Myoclonus induced by intermittent light stimulation in the baboon: Neurophysiological and neuropharmacological approaches. Adv Neurol 1986;43:611.
92. Rektor I, Bryere P, Silva-Barrat C, et al. Stimulus-sensitive myoclonus of the baboon Papio papio: Pharmacological studies reveal interactions between benzodiazepines and the central cholinergic system. Exp Neurol 1986;91:13.
93. Fischer-Williams M, Poncet M, Riche D, et al. Light-induced epilepsy in the baboon, Papio papio: Cortical and depth recordings. Electroencephalogr Clin Neurophysiol 1968;25:557.
94. Thompson PD, Day BL, Rothwell JC, et al. The myoclonus in corticobasal degeneration. Evidence for two forms of cortical reflex myoclonus. Brain 1994;117:1197.
95. Thompson PD. Myoclonus in corticobasal degeneration. Clin Neurosci 1995;3:203
96. Wilkins DE, Hallett M, Berardelli A, et al. Physiologic analysis of the myoclonus of Alzheimer's disease. Neurology 1984;34:898.
97. Caviness, JN, Adler, CH, Newman, S, et al. Cortical myoclonus in levodopa-responsive parkinsonism. Mov Disord 1998;13:540.
98. Caviness JN, Adler CH, Beach TG, et al. Small-amplitude cortical myoclonus in Parkinson's disease: Physiology and clinical observations. Mov Disord 2002;17:657.
99. Caviness JN, Adler CH, Beach TG, et al. Myoclonus in Lewy body disorders. Adv Neurol 2002;89:23.
100. Caviness JN, Kurth M. Cortical myoclonus in Huntington's disease associated with an enlarged somatosensory evoked potential. Mov Disord 1997;12:1046.
101. Thompson PD, Bhatia KP, Brown P, et al. Cortical myoclonus in Huntington's disease. Mov Disord. 1994;9:633.
102. Rodriguez ME, Artieda J, Zubieta JL, et al. Reflex myoclonus in olivopontocerebellar atrophy. J Neurol Neurosurg Psychiatry 1994;57:316.
103. Lou JS, Valls-Sole J, Toro C, et al. Facial action myoclonus in patients with olivopontocerebellar atrophy. Mov Disord 1994;9:223.
104. Wszolek ZK, Lagerlund TD, Steg RE, et al. Clinical neurophysiologic findings in patients with rapidly progressive familial parkinsonism and dementia with pallido-ponto-nigral degeneration. Electroencephalogr Clin Neurophysiol 1998;107:213.
105. Caviness JN, Wszolek ZK. Myoclonus in pallido-ponto-nigral degeneration. Adv Neurol 2002;89:35.
106. Kofler M, Muller J, Reggiani L, et al. Somatosensory evoked potentials in progressive supranuclear palsy. J Neurol Sci 2000;179:85.
107. Moller JC, Hamer HM, Oertel WH, et al. Late-onset myoclonic epilepsy in Down's syndrome (LOMEDS). Seizure 2002;11(Suppl A):303.
108. Crespel A, Gonzalez V, Coubes P, et al. Senile myoclonic epilepsy of Genton: Two cases in Down syndrome with dementia and late onset epilepsy. Epilepsy Res 2007;77:165.
109. Hallett M, Chadwick D, Marsden CD. Ballistic movement overflow myoclonus a form of essential myoclonus. Brain 1977;100:299.
110. Roze E, Apartis E, Trocello JM. Cortical excitability in DYT-11 positive myoclonus dystonia. Mov Disord 2008; 23:761.
111. Klein C, Ozelius LJ. Dystonia: Clinical features, genetics, and treatment. Curr Opin Neurol 2002;15:491.
112. Li JY, Cunic DI, Paradiso G, et al. Electrophysiological features of myoclonus-dystonia. Mov Disord 2008;23:2055.
113. Roze E, Apartis E, Clot F, et al. Myoclonus-dystonia: Clinical and electrophysiologic pattern related to SGCE mutations. Neurology. 2008;70:1010.
114. Dubinsky RM, Hallett M. Palatal myoclonus and facial involvement in other types of myoclonus. Adv Neurol 1988;49:263.
115. Deuschl G, Mischke G, Schenck E, et al. Symptomatic and essential rhythmic palatal myoclonus. Brain 1990;113:1645.
116. Deuschl G, Toro C, Hallett M. Symptomatic and essential palatal tremor. 2. Differences of palatal movements. Mov Disord 1994;9:676.
117. Deuschl G, Toro C, Valls-Sole J, et al. Symptomatic and essential palatal tremor. 1. Clinical, physiological and MRI analysis. Brain 1994;117:775.
118. Deuschl G, Jost S, Schumacher M. Symptomatic palatal tremor is associated with signs of cerebellar dysfunction. J Neurol 1996;243:553.
119. Deuschl G, Toro C, Valls-Sole J, et al. Symptomatic and essential palatal tremor. 3. Abnormal motor learning. J Neurol Neurosurg Psychiatry 1996;60:520.
120. Deuschl G, Lohle E, Heinen F, et al. Ear click in palatal tremor: Its origin and treatment with botulinum toxin. Neurology 1991;41:1677.

121. Jero J, Salmi T. Palatal myoclonus and clicking tinnitus in a 12-year-old girl--Case report. Acta Otolaryngol Suppl 2000;543:61.
122. Penney SE, Bruce IA, Saeed SR. Botulinum toxin is effective and safe for palatal tremor: A report of five cases and a review of the literature. J Neurol 2006;253:857.
123. Zadikoff C, Lang AE, Klein C. The 'essentials' of essential palatal tremor: A reappraisal of the nosology. Brain 2006;129:832.
124. Leventon G, Man A, Floru S. Isolated psychogenic palatal myoclonus as a cause of objective tinnitus. Acta Otolaryngol 1968;65:391.
125. Williams DR. Psychogenic palatal tremor. Mov Disord 2004;19:333.
126. Pirio Richardson S, Mari Z, Matsuhashi M, et al. Psychogenic palatal tremor. Mov Disord 2006;21:274.
127. Brown P, Thompson PD, Rothwell JC, et al. Paroxysmal axial spasms of spinal origin. Mov Disord 1991;6:43.
128. Chokroverty S, Walters A, Zimmerman T, et al. Propriospinal myoclonus: a neurophysiologic analysis. Neurology 1992;42:1591.
129. Brown P, Rothwell JC, Thompson PD, et al. Propriospinal myoclonus: Evidence for spinal "pattern" generators in humans. Mov Disord 1994;9:571.
130. Thompson PD, Colebatch JG, Brown P, et al. Voluntary stimulus-sensitive jerks and jumps mimicking myoclonus or pathological startle syndromes. Mov Disord 1992;7:257.
131. Williams DR, Cowey M, Tuck K, et al. Psychogenic propriospinal myoclonus. Mov Disord 2008;23:1312.
132. Kang SY, Sohn YH. Electromyography patterns of propriospinal myoclonus can be mimicked voluntarily. Mov Disord 2006;21:1241.
133. Evidente VG, Caviness JN. Myoclonus of peripheral origin. J Neurol Neurosurg Psychiatry 1999;66:123.
134. Tyvaert L, Krystkowiak P, Cassim F, et al. Myoclonus of peripheral origin: Two case reports. Mov Disord 2008; 24:274.
135. Brown P. Neurophysiology of the startle syndrome and hyperekplexia. Adv Neurol 2002;89:153.
136. Becker L, von Wegerer J, Schenkel J, et al. Disease-specific human glycine receptor alpha1 subunit causes hyperekplexia phenotype and impaired glycine- and GABA(A)-receptor transmission in transgenic mice. J Neurosci 2002; 22:2505.
137. Prince R, Tcheng-Laroche F. Culture-bound syndromes and international disease classifications. Cult Med Psychiatry 1987;11:3.
138. Massey EW. Goosey patients: Relationship to jumping Frenchmen, Myriachit, Latah and tic convulsif. N C Med J 1984;45:556.
139. Hening WA, Walters AS, Chokroverty S. Movement disorders and sleep. In Chokroverty SMD (ed). Movement Disorders. Great Neck, NY: PMA Publishing, 1990, p. 127.
140. Bara-Jimenez W, Aksu M, Graham B, et al. Periodic limb movements in sleep: State-dependent excitability of the spinal flexor reflex. Neurology 2000;54:1609.
141. Glass GA, Ahlskog JE, Matsumoto JY. Orthostatic myoclonus: A contributor to gait decline in selected elderly. Neurology 2007;68:1826.
142. Monday K, Jankovic J. Psychogenic myoclonus. Neurology 1993;43:349.
143. Shahani BT, Young RR. Asterixis: A disorder of the neural mechanisms underlying sustained muscle contraction. In Shahani M (ed). The Motor System: Neurophysiological and Muscle Mechanisms. Amsterdam: Elsevier, 1976, p. 301.
144. Brown P, Thompson PD, Rothwell JC, et al. A case of postanoxic encephalopathy with cortical action and brainstem reticular reflex myoclonus. Mov Disord 1991;6:139.
145. Hallett M. Physiology of human posthypoxic myoclonus. Mov Disord 2000;15(Suppl 1):8.
146. Brown P, Farmer SF, Halliday DM, et al. Coherent cortical and muscle discharge in cortical myoclonus. Brain 1999;122(Pt 3):461.
147. Shibasaki H, Motomura S, Yamashita Y, et al. Periodic synchronous discharge and myoclonus in Creutzfeldt-Jakob disease: Diagnostic application of jerk-locked averaging method. Ann Neurol 1981;9:150.
148. Kugelberg E, Widen L. Epilepsia partialis continua. Electroencephalogr Clin Neurophysiol 1954;6:503.
149. Thomas JE, Reagan TJ, Klass DW. Epilepsia partialis continua: A review of 32 cases. Arch Neurol 1977;34:266.
150. Reese K, Toro C, Malow B, et al. Progression of the EEG in Lafora-body disease. Am J EEG Tech 1993;33:229.
151. Oishi A, Tobimatsu S, Ochi H, et al. Paradoxical lateralization of parasagittal spikes revealed by back averaging of EEG and MEG in a case with epilepsia partialis continua. J Neurol Sci 2002;193:151.
152. Cirignotta F, Lugaresi E. Partial motor epilepsy with "negative myoclonus". Epilepsia 1991;32:54.
153. Shibasaki H, Ikeda A, Nagamine T, et al. Cortical reflex negative myoclonus. Brain 1994;117(Pt 3):477.
154. Sutton, GG: Receptors in focal reflex myoclonus. J Neurol Neurosurg Psychiatry 1975;38:505.
155. Cowan JM, Rothwell JC, Wise, RJ, et al. Electrophysiological and positron emission studies in a patient with cortical myoclonus, epilepsia partialis continua and motor epilepsy. J Neurol Neurosurg Psychiatry 1986;49:796.
156. Shibasaki H, Neshige R, Hashiba Y. Cortical excitability after myoclonus: Jerk-locked somatosensory evoked potentials. Neurology 1985;35:36.
157. Ugawa Y, Genba K, Shimpo T, et al. Somatosensory evoked potential recovery (SEP-R) in myoclonic patients. Electroencephalogr Clin Neurophysiol 1991;80:21.
158. Mima T, Nagamine T, Ikeda A, et al. Pathogenesis of cortical myoclonus studied by magnetoencephalography. Ann Neurol 1998;43:598.
159. Mima T, Nagamine T, Nishitani N, et al. Cortical myoclonus: Sensorimotor hyperexcitability. Neurology 1998; 50:933.
160. Ugawa Y, Uesaka Y, Terao Y, et al. Pathophysiology of sensorimotor cortex in cortical myoclonus. Clin Neurosci 1995;3:198.
161. Shigeto H, Tobimatsu S, Morioka T, et al. Jerk-locked back averaging and dipole source localization of magnetoencephalographic transients in a patient with epilepsia partialis continua. Electroencephalogr Clin Neurophysiol 1997;103:440.
162. Marsden JF, Ashby P, Rothwell JC, et al. Phase relationships between cortical and muscle oscillations in cortical myoclonus: Electrocorticographic assessment in a single case. Clin Neurophysiol 2000;111:2170.

163. Grosse P, Guerrini R, Parmeggiani L, et al. Abnormal corticomuscular and intermuscular coupling in high-frequency rhythmic myoclonus. Brain 2003;126:326.
164. Grosse P, Kuhn A, Cordivari C, et al. Coherence analysis in the myoclonus of corticobasal degeneration. Mov Disord 2003;18:1345.
165. Panzica F, Canafoglia L, Franceschetti S, et al. Movement-activated myoclonus in genetically defined progressive myoclonic epilepsies: EEG-EMG relationship estimated using autoregressive models. Clin Neurophysiol 2003;114:1041.
166. Foncke EM, Bour LJ, Speelman JD, et al. Local field potentials and oscillatory activity of the internal globus pallidus in myoclonus-dystonia. Mov Disord 2007;22:369.
167. Foncke EM, Bour LJ, van der Meer JN, et al. Abnormal low frequency drive in myoclonus-dystonia patients correlates with presence of dystonia. Mov Disord 2007;22:1299.
168. Silen T, Forss N, Jensen O, et al. Abnormal reactivity of the approximately 20-Hz motor cortex rhythm in Unverricht Lundborg type progressive myoclonus epilepsy. Neuroimage 2000;12:707.
169. Karhu J, Hari R, Paetau R, et al. Cortical reactivity in progressive myoclonus epilepsy. Electroencephalogr Clin Neurophysiol 1994;90:93.
170. Silen T, Forss N, Salenius S, et al. Oscillatory cortical drive to isometrically contracting muscle in Unverricht-Lundborg type progressive myoclonus epilepsy (ULD). Clin Neurophysiol 2002;113:1973.
171. Silen T, Karjalainen T, Lehesjoki AE, et al. Cortical sensorimotor alterations in Unverricht-Lundborg disease patients without generalized seizures. Neurosci Lett 2002;323:101.
172. Caviness JN, Adler CH, Sabbagh MN, et al. Abnormal corticomuscular coherence is associated with the small amplitude cortical myoclonus in Parkinson's disease. Mov Disord 2003;18:1157.
173. Chen R, Ashby P, Lang AE. Stimulus-sensitive myoclonus in akinetic-rigid syndromes. Brain 1992;115:1875.
174. Lu CS, Ikeda A, Terada K, et al. Electrophysiological studies of early stage corticobasal degeneration. Mov Disord 1998;13:140.
175. Reutens DC, Puce A, Berkovic SF. Cortical hyperexcitability in progressive myoclonus epilepsy: A study with transcranial magnetic stimulation. Neurology 1993;43:186.
176. Manganotti P, Tamburin S, Zanette G, et al. Hyperexcitable cortical responses in progressive myoclonic epilepsy: A TMS study. Neurology 2001;57:1793.
177. Manganotti P, Tamburin S, Bongiovanni LG, et al. Motor responses to afferent stimulation in juvenile myoclonic epilepsy. Epilepsia 2004;45:77.
178. Lefaucheur JP. Myoclonus and transcranial magnetic stimulation. Neurophysiol Clin 2006;36:293.
179. Houdayer E, Devanne H, Tyvaert, L et al. Low frequency repetitive transcranial magnetic stimulation over premotor cortex can improve cortical tremor. Clin Neurophysiol 2007;118:1557.
180. Rossi, S Ulivelli, M Bartalini, S et al. Reduction of cortical myoclonus-related epileptic activity following slow-frequency rTMS. Neuroreport 2004;15:293.
181. Wischer S, Paulus W, Sommer M, et al. Piracetam affects facilitatory I-wave interaction in the human motor cortex. Clin Neurophysiol 2001;112:275.
182. Brown P. Cortical myoclonus: An insight into the organization of normal movement in man. Clin Neurosci 1995; 3:193.
183. Cantello R, Civardi C, Cavalli A, et al. Effects of a photic input on the human cortico-motoneuron connection. Clin Neurophysiol 2000;111:1981.
184. Celesia GG, Parmeggiani L, Brigell M. Dipole source localization in a case of epilepsia partialis continua without premyoclonic EEG spikes. Electroencephalogr Clin Neurophysiol 1994;90:316.
185. Richardson MP, Grosse P, Allen PJ, et al. BOLD correlates of EMG spectral density in cortical myoclonus: Description of method and case report. Neuroimage 2006; 32:558.
186. van Rootselaar AF, Maurits NM, Renken R, et al. Simultaneous EMG-functional MRI recordings can directly relate hyperkinetic movements to brain activity. Hum Brain Mapp 2008;29:1430.

CHAPTER 39

Tourette Syndrome and Related Disorders

Jorge L. Juncos

In his now famous 1885 publication, George Gilles de la Tourette described the illness that now bears his name. He reported nine patients with motor and vocal tics, some of whom had echophenomena and coprolalia (vide infra).[1] Up to the past few decades Tourette syndrome (TS) was viewed as a rare and disabling condition with bizarre symptoms and unknown etiology. Although our understanding of the disorder is still incomplete, it has improved considerably as a result of the body of clinical, neuroscience, imaging, and genetic data that has accumulated since. This new knowledge has led to a paradigm shift in the thinking about TS, and to more informed and effective approaches to the illness. This research and resulting evolution in our clinical approaches to patients with TS are the foci of this chapter.

▶ CLINICAL FEATURES

TICS AND THE DIAGNOSIS OF TS

Tics are the primary motor abnormality and diagnostic signature of TS, and the reason for which the syndrome is sometimes referred to as a "movement disorders." Tics are recurrent, nonrhythmic, stereotyped movements (motor tics) or sounds (phonic tics). Complex phonations involving words or phrases or the use of language are termed vocal tics. In contrast to some other involuntary movements, tics are not constant (except when severe), and occur in a background of otherwise normal motor function. Motor and phonic/vocal tics may take a variety of forms and can be divided conceptually into simple and complex (see Table 39–1). Motor tics can affect any part of the body but they typically begin in the eyelids or face, and may later involve other muscle groups with an apparent rostrocaudal migration during development with constant waxing and wanning.[2]

Simple motor tics are sudden, brief, isolated movements such as an eye blink, a shoulder shrug, or a head jerk. Although most simple motor tics are fast and abrupt, some comprise sustained, tonic movements (e.g., neck twisting, abdominal or buttock tightening) and are termed "dystonic tics". They include painless oculogyric eye movements, blepharospasm, and dystonic neck and back movements (see Table 39–2).[3,4]

Complex motor tics consist of more coordinated and complicated movements that may appear purposeful. Examples include touching, smelling, jumping, copropraxia (obscene gestures), and echopraxia (mimicking movements performed by others). Motor tics usually recur in the same part of the body but multiple body regions can also be involved. Over time, tics often recede from one body part only to emerge elsewhere.[2,5,6]

Vocal tics can range from simple words (e.g., "pain," "get it out"), to complex, inappropriate, or obscene language (coprolalia) present in only a minority of patients

▶ TABLE 39–1. CLINICAL HETEROGENEITY OF TS

- I. The Tic Disorder
  - A. Tic types
    1. Simple motor tics
    2. Simple phonic or vocal tics
    3. Complex motor tics
    4. Complex vocal tics
    5. Tic variants
       - a. Dystonic tics
       - b. Sensory tics
  - B. Tic Disorder Syndromes
    1. Tourette syndrome
    2. Chronic tic disorder (motor or vocal)
    3. Transient tic disorder
  - C. Tic severity
- II. The Behavioral Disorder
  - A. Obsessive compulsive behavior/disorders (OCD)
  - B. Attention deficit hyperactivity disorder (ADHD)
  - C. Anxiety disorders
  - D. Impulse control disorders
  - E. Conduct disorder and rage attacks
  - F. Other behavioral disturbances

▶ **TABLE 39–2. TIC PHENOMENOLOGY**

	Motor	Vocal	Sensory
Simple	Frequent blinking	Sniffing	Burning sensations
	Blepharospasm	Grunting	Tightness
	Grimacing	Throat clearing	Muscle heaviness
	Pouting	Barking	Tingling
	Jaw opening	Growling	Itching
	Head jerking	Coughing	Impulsions
	Shoulder shrugging	Moaning	
	Fist clenching	Humming	
Complex	Head twisting or shaking	Panting	Inner tension
	Spitting	Belching	Pain syndromes:
	Hitting (self, others)	Stuttering	• Premonitory
	Jumping, kicking	Echolalia	• Exertional
	Squatting	Coprolalia	• Secondary to prolonged voluntary tic suppression
	Pelvic/abdominal thrusting	Palilalia	"Phantom tics"

but potentially very disabling (see Table 39–2). Coprolalia has been linked to anxiety and OCD in some cases.

Sensory Experiences Associated With Tics

Tics can be associated with a surprisingly broad array of sensory experiences. First, any external and internal sensory experiences can aggravate tics. External experiences can involve events leading to excitation, distress, or pain. Internal sensory experiences (e.g., tightness, numbness, tingling, pain, or even pleasant sensations) may precede, accompany, or follow the movements or vocalization.[7,8] Sensory experiences preceding tics, so-called premonitory urges, are reported by 41–92% of patients.[5,9]

The term "sensory tic" was introduced by Shapiro et al. in 1988.[10] It refers to recurrent somatic sensations in various parts of the body that evoke a dysphoric feeling. Sensory tics may or may not cause the patient to respond *intentionally* with a movement or vocalization that can partially and temporarily alleviate the abnormal sensation.[10] Sensory tics commonly affect the face, head, and neck areas, with the limbs being less often involved.[8] It is rare for sensory tics to occur in the absence of a motor or vocal tic. In a case followed by the author for more than 12 years, the patient presented at age 12 with "arm claudication" while swimming. This sensation was not associated with a corresponding motor tic in that limb, although she did have motor tics involving the face and neck. Unlike her motor tics, this sensory tic was not controlled with modest doses of dopamine blockers. After an extensive negative vascular workup, the arm claudication finally responded by <30% to higher doses of the same dopamine agents used to control motor tics. After 7 years this symptom gradually disappeared.

DSM-IVR Diagnostic Criteria

The fourth (1994) version of the *Diagnostic and Statistical Manual of Psychiatry (DSM-IV)*[11] lists the following diagnostic criteria for TS:

1. Both multiple motor and one or more vocal tics have been present at some time during the illness, although not necessarily concurrently.
2. The tics occur many times a day (usually in bouts) nearly every day or intermittently throughout a period of more than 1 year, and during this period, there was never a tic-free period of more than 3 consecutive months.
3. The disturbance causes marked distress or significant impairment in social, occupational, or other important areas of functioning.
4. The onset is before age 18 years.
5. The disturbance is not due to the direct physiological effects of a substance (e.g., stimulants) or a general medical condition (e.g., Huntington's disease or post viral encephalitis).

Are Tics Voluntary or Involuntary?

Motor tics have traditionally been interpreted as involuntary because they are not associated with the negative premotor electroencephalographic (EEG) potential (Bereitschaftspotential) normally linked to voluntary movement.[12] More recently, it has been reported that not all voluntary movements are necessarily preceded by these potentials.[13] When asked directly, many patients report that the tics are under "voluntary control".[14] More specifically, motor tics that occur in response to premonitory urges are interpreted by patients as a voluntary act to relieve the urge.[14] The term "unvoluntary" was recently coined in an effort to reconcile the dichotomy that underlies the terms voluntary and involuntary in this setting.[15] *Unvoluntary* refers to an "automatic movement performed without conscious effort," such as scratching in response to an itch.[15] The automaticity of this response may help differentiate these automatic responses from the voluntary response to a sensory tic.

In contrast to motor and vocal tics, sensory tics are involuntary and often unwelcome.[8] More complex sensations or affects associated with tics have been referred to as "complex sensory tics".[16] It is unclear, however, whether these complex phenomena are themselves related to the more involved co-morbid conditions such as obsessions and compulsions. For instance, Karp and Hallett recently described a patient whose tics were associated with out-of-body sensations that were relieved by intentional movements, or tics, directed at the object in question.[17] These "phantom tics" may represent a continuum with obsession and compulsions.

BEHAVIORAL COMORBIDITIES

Tics are often accompanied by a variety of behavioral disturbances. Some of these, like obsessive-compulsive disorder (OCD), are recognized as part of the illness. It is less certain whether behaviors such as attention deficit hyperactivity disorder (ADHD) and the others discussed below are an intrinsic part of the illness, the product of genetic segregation, or the consequence of environmental influences on the disorders. Complex tics involving self-mutilation, for instance, may be a secondary derivate of co-existing OCD or ADHD. Behavioral therapies aim to help the individual unlearn these behaviors or, better yet, prevent their acquisition through early intervention.

Studies have demonstrated that the incidence of OCD in TS patients is about 50%.[18–20] Common examples of OC symptoms include compulsive checking, counting, perfectionism, and obsessive worries or fears. About half of patients with TS will also evidence symptoms of ADHD. These symptoms include inattention, distractibility, impulsivity, and hyperactivity.[21] Other behavioral disturbances sometimes linked to TS include anxiety disorders, conduct disorder, depression, mania, stuttering, obesity, and alcoholism.[22] At present, the extent of this broader spectrum of behaviors and its relationship to TS remains controversial.[23–25]

Their relationship to TS notwithstanding, when present, these behaviors rapidly acquire major importance in the management of the illness. Tics tend to draw attention away from these behaviors, which may be the real reason why the tic control is poor. This confusion leads to the targeting and prioritization of the wrong symptom, typically the tic. Tic severity, however, is often dependent on the stress brought about by the co-morbidities. Examples of such behaviors include personality traits such as argumentativeness, defensiveness, negativism, and impulsiveness, which often accompany ADHD. Self-injurious behavior occurs in 17–22% of patients with TS.[26] These behaviors include head banging, slapping, punching and self-biting. This type of behavior has been linked to high levels of obsessionality and hostility. Other socially inappropriate behaviors occasionally seen in TS are verbally abusive language and obscene/inappropriate gestures.[27]

Aggressive behaviors are also fairly common in TS. It is reported that 25–70% of TS patients have anger control problems, mood liability, and/or recurrent rage attacks.[28–30] Aggression in TS correlates well with co-morbid psychiatric symptoms.[31] The relationship to tic severity is less clear, although coprolalia and copropraxia are closely associated with aggressive behaviors.[32–34] When present, these behaviors are perhaps the most significant impediment to the management of TS. Although these behaviors are almost always multifactorial, the most common conditions associated with aggressive behaviors in TS are co-existing ADHD and OCD.[30,31] When the source of aggression is untreated ADHD, stimulants may play a long-term role in the management but rarely help in the acute setting. The immediate target symptoms in these situations are irritability, anger outburst, and other conduct problems. Behavioral interventions to control the behavior of the patient, as much as the behavior of those around him/her, are imperative. Alpha-adrenergic agonists such as clonidine and guanfacine can reduce aggressive behaviors in children with conduct disorders (CD) and oppositional defiant disorders (ODD), both of which are common in ADHD.[35] When the source of aggression is anxiety and OCD, judiciously titrated use of selective serotonin reuptake inhibitors, anticonvulsants, atypical antipsychotics, and β-blockers has been tried with limited success.[36,37]

Needless to say, differentiating between the multiple factors that play a role in aggression in TS can be a daunting task. Accordingly, a thorough neuropsychiatric evaluation is necessary to begin rational management that establishes clear goals and prioritizes targets to help parents orchestrate an appropriate response to the provocations. Psychosocial triggers, substance abuse, and drug-induced side effects need to be identified and addressed quickly. Management involves a team effort with family psychotherapy individualized use of one or more agents from the above medications groups in the hands of an experienced therapist.

Learning disabilities are another major limiting factor in the ability of these children to adapt to their environment. Comings et al.[22] reported that 13% of 246 children with TS attended classes for emotional or learning disabilities. Kadesjoe et al.[38] reported that 36% of children with TS (21 of 58) had some type of reading disorder. Children with co-morbid ADHD were more likely to receive special education services than those with tics alone. Finally, Spencer et al. showed that youngsters with TS+ADHD had higher rates of special class placements than those with TS alone.[39] These data have the limitation of small sample size and the analysis does not correct for selection bias. However, current consensus is that neuropsychologic and scholastic problems should always be suspected when a child with TS is having behavioral problems in school.

SLEEP DISTURBANCES

Sleep-related complaints are common in TS.[40] These include insomnia, fragmented sleep, periodic leg movements, and daytime somnolence.[41] Polysomnographic contributions to the study of TS are limited.[40] A few have shown a higher percentage of stage III/IV sleep and decreased rapid eye movement sleep compared to controls.[40] Although these findings fail to explain the rate of sleep disruption in TS, they suggest that disordered arousal may be playing a role. Two tantalizing studies suggest that disorders of arousal, such as somnambulism and night terrors, are more common in TS than in controls.[42,43] It can be speculated that disordered arousal may be the sleep cycle equivalent of the "gating" abnormalities postulated that will be covered in the Neurobilogy section below. This hypothesis predicts that, just like tics may not disappear during sleep, TS patients are more likely than controls to "be driven" by urges associated with dreaming (e.g., sleep walking or somnambulism). The mechanisms for these intrusions into normal sleep have yet to be defined, but as they appear related to tic severity,[41] striato-thalamic dysregulation has been proposed as a common mechanism for these sleep phenomena and tics.[44]

▶ EPIDEMIOLOGY

Tourette syndrome has been identified in all races and appears to be uniformly distributed across socioeconomic classes.[10] There is a 3:1 male predominance among patients with TS.[10] However, if one considers OCD to be an alternative clinical expression of the condition (see below), the gender ratio is nearly equal.[45] The clinical features appear to be uniform among different cultural groups, except that coprolalia is particularly uncommon in Japanese patients.[10] Traditionally, TS has been viewed as a rare disorder. However, recent evidence suggests that it is much more common than generally appreciated. An accurate lifetime prevalence rate for TS has not been established. Past estimates, ranging from 0.03 percent to 1.6 percent,[46] have been based largely on case series of patients referred for medical evaluation, or on data obtained from questionnaires without direct clinical examinations. Systematic analysis of large TS kindreds using a family study method in which all available members are directly interviewed and examined indicates that most cases of TS are mild and do not come to medical attention, and that the disorder is often unrecognized and misdiagnosed by physicians.[46,47] Furthermore, studies of the prevalence of TS have been restricted to an analysis of the tic disorder, and mounting evidence (see below) indicates that behavioral disorders, including OCD and ADHD, may be the only clinical manifestations of illness in some individuals.[19,45] This phenotypic extension of TS remains controversial.[23,25]

Looking at it from the other direction, epidemiologic surveys of school-age children have identified tic rates ranging from 4 percent to 50 percent.[48,49] Many of these are probably transient tic disorders, not TS, as the authors did not examine the clinical characteristics of tics (e.g., presence of motor and vocal types, duration of at least 1 year) necessary to satisfy the criteria for TS.

It is reassuring, however, that the above estimates of the prevalence of TS in relatively small samples are congruent with findings in the first national, population-based study of individuals <18 years.[50] Those results suggest an overall prevalence of 3.0 TS cases per 1000 subjects.[50] The diagnosis of TS was approximately three times as likely in boys compared to girls and twice as likely in the age group 12–17 compared with those age 6–11.[50] A limitation of this study lies in the data collection, which relied on telephone questionnaires administered to parents.

Taken together, current evidence suggests that TS and related tic disorders are quite common in the general childhood population. For the most part, they appear to represent mild, nondisabling conditions that do not lead to medical attention or therapy. Tics tend be linked to childhood school problems; thus its more useful role in the general population may be to use the tic as a trigger to raise concern about potential scholastic problems.

▶ DIFFERENTIAL DIAGNOSIS

The clinical features of tics have been extensively studied in primary tic disorders such as TS, but not in other conditions in which tics are a secondary manifestation. For the purposes of this chapter, we will discuss primary and secondary tics together because, phenomenologically, there is no evidence that there are significant differences between them.

Tics can be differentiated from hyperkinesias by their suppressibility, distractibility, suggestibility, their tendency to persist during sleep, and the associated premonitory symptoms mentioned above (see Table 39–3). Unlike tics and perhaps chorea, other movement disorders are seldom suppressible or perceived by patients as "voluntary." Note that voluntary control may be difficult

▶ **TABLE 39–3. RESPONSE OF PATIENTS WITH SELECT MOVEMENT DISORDERS TO QUESTIONS REGARDING SUBJECTIVE PERCEPTION AND OTHER MANEUVERS[a]**

	Subjective Perception	Premonitory Urges	Distraction	Suppression	Effect of Selected Movements
Tics	Vol or Invol	Yes	↓		Usually ↓
Myoclonus	Invol	No	0 or ↑	0	Commonly ↑
Chorea	Invol	No	0 or ↑	±	Variable
Akathitic movements	Vol	Yes	↓	++	↓
Orofacial tardive dyskinesia	Invol	No	↑	++	Commonly ↑
Drug-induced dyskinesia	Invol	No	↑	++	Commonly ↑
Psychogenic movements	Invol	± Yes[b]	↓	±	Usually ↓[b]
Tremors	Invol	No	0 or ↑	In PD: ++; in others: 0	± ↑
Dystonia	Invol	No	0 or ↑	±	Commonly ↑

[a]This important information should be elicited in the course of the history. "Vol" and "Invol" refer to the patients' interpretation of the activity as voluntary or not. The direction of the arrow refers to an increase or a decrease in movement; the thickness of the arrow is an arbitrary representation of the intensity of this change. 0, no change; ±, variable change; +, ++, +++, mild, moderate, or marked suppressibility, respectively.
[b]This is highly variable from patient to patient.
Source: Modified with permission from Lang AE. Clinical phenomenology of tic disorders: selected aspects. Adv Neurol 1992;58:27.

to assess in children. Table 39–3 also illustrates other aspects of the history and physical exam that may help differentiate tics from other movement disorders.

Additional features that help differentiate tics from hyperkinesias are their onset, the rostrocaudal spread noted above, their variability, course, and, to some extent, the company they keep in terms of associated comorbidities. For instance, over the course of primary tic disorders, the severity of tics typically waxes and wanes, with predictable crises during adolescence. Tics may temporarily "disappear" or, more likely, become barely noticeable for extended periods, only to recur unprovoked, or triggered by life stressors. The character of the tics can also change from time to time, more typically over the course of years. For example, excessive blinking or grimacing in childhood may transform into intermittent nose flaring and grunting in adolescence or into neck jerking in adulthood. Compounding this intrinsic variability are the profound effects that stress, stimulants, and other drugs can have on tics. Sensitivity to drugs, unfortunately, does not help differentiate tics from other hyperkinesis.

Dyskinesias (hyperkinesias) that may be difficult to differentiate from tics include myoclonus, chorea, akathisia, tardive dyskinesia, L-dopa-induced dyskinesia, the nonspecific movements (stereotypies) encountered in psychotic patients, and psychogenic movement disorders. Dystonic tics can be differentiated from dystonia by the company they keep; that is, they seldom occur in the absence of clonic or tonic tics. Compared to other tics, dystonic tics are more commonly associated with uncomfortable sensations that are relieved by movements.[3,5] Unlike myoclonus, a patient with tics would not be expected to lose motor control while executing a task such as holding a glass, as is the case with myoclonus.

Chorea and tics are hard to differentiate phenomenologically because both are quick, involuntary movements. However, chorea is less suppressible and is not associated with premonitory urges. Chorea, unlike tics, consists of a dance-like flow of "irregularly irregular" finger, limb, trunk, or facial movements that ebb or cease during sleep. Tics are seldom mistaken for tremors, which are, in contrast to tics, regular and oscillatory in nature. Tardive dyskinesia can be distinguished from tics by drug history and a typical pattern of predominant orobuccolingual involvement. Interestingly, in TS, tardive dyskinesia in response to chronic neuroleptic therapy appears to be exceedingly rare.

Other movements superficially resembling tics include mannerisms, disorders of excessive startle, and hyperplexia. Mannerisms are physiological tics or patterned sequential movements that are commonly outgrown during childhood. Although they appear in normal children, they are commonly associated with mental subnormality.

▶ NATURAL COURSE

Tics typically present in childhood or adolescence and may be transient or last a lifetime. With aging, most tics tend to reach a stable plateau or "disappear," meaning they reach clinically or esthetically insignificant levels.[51–53]

Erenberg found that 73 percent of adult TS subjects reported that over a period of years their tics had either lessened considerably or almost disappeared.[51] Bruun followed 136 TS patients from 5 to 15 years and found that tic severity lessened over time, with 59 percent rated mild-moderate initially and 91 percent rated so at follow-up.[54] Over time, 28 percent came off medications and

52 percent reported spontaneous improvement. Shapiro and Shapiro observed that 5–8 percent of TS patients recover completely and permanently in adolescence; tics become less severe in 35 percent of cases during adolescence, and less severe in "most patients" in adulthood.[55] Thus, many patients with TS experience an improvement or resolution of tics after adolescence.

While the natural course of the tic disorder in TS has received considerable attention, little investigative work has focused on the co-morbidities. Comings and Comings have suggested that, for many children with TS, symptoms of ADHD precede the appearance of tics by an average of 2.5 years.[56] Park et al. found it unusual for ADHD or OCD to be absent at the time of initial diagnosis of TS and then to appear later on, with only 4–6 percent of patients following this course.[57] On the other hand, disruptive behaviors (20%) and school problems (13%) did tend to emerge some time after the diagnosis.

▶ ETIOLOGY AND PATHOGENESIS

GENETICS

Tourette syndrome and chronic motor tic disorder (CMT) have been established as familial entities with a genetic basis subject to environmental and epigenetic factors. The evidence for this is based on multigenerational family studies and more recent linkage and segregation studies that corroborate the original observations.[45,58,59] In addition, twin studies reveal a higher concordance rate for TS among monozygotic compared to dizygotic twins.[60]

Association studies of TS in relation to "candidate genes" like those involved in dopamine or serotonin transmission have thus far proven negative. These genes may ultimate prove to be important modifiers of the trait. Segregation studies ask which model of inheritance best fits the data. Early analysis of this data suggested that TS may have an autosomal dominant mode of transmission and variable penetrance.[45,58,61] Subsequent studies have not borne this out, however.[62–64] To try to solve this dilemma, the current strategy is to find susceptibility genes and variants using genome-wide association studies (GWAS) where few assumptions about inheritance are made a priori. These studies, which require larger data sets than those needed in segregation studies, are underway.

Completed segregation studies in multigenerational families and sib pairs have identified chromosomal regions that may contain genes coding for TS in chromosome 2 and chromosome 17q.[62] These regions are undergoing fine mapping.[65] State et al. identified *SLITRK1* as a candidate gene responsible for TS in one individual with GTS and an inversion in chromosome 13 (q31.1; q33.1).[65] This gene has been associated with abnormal axonal-dendritic development in embryonic mouse cells. Although *SLITRK1* is not a major causal gene for GTS (i.e., no other cases so far), its investigation may shed light on our understanding of the gene-based neural correlates of TS. These advances notwithstanding, the role of these genes or their products in the inheritance and/or pathophysiology of TS remains to be elucidated.

In light of the remaining gaps in our knowledge of the genetics of TS, the information provided here cannot be viewed as genetic counseling. Rather these are proposed questions to consider when consulting a trained genetics counselor. The main question is: What is the risk for a poor quality of life in TS? The question is not: What is my genetic risk of having a child with TS? Are the parents asking about the risk of having tics or of having co-morbid conditions? When a person with TS is identified, the relative risk of having another relative with TS in the family is 15–35%.[59] It is important to recognize, however, that TS has a wide range of outcomes the vast majority of which are good. As noted in the *Natural History* section, the neurobiology of tics makes them peak during adolescence and subside thereafter. This natural history is adulterated when the person has multiple co-morbidities the stress of which can perpetuate the disability associated with tics. Little information is available on the risk of inheriting co-morbid conditions in TS. Nonetheless, the real risk of poor outcomes to individuals with TS may come from poor parenting, poor school and peer relationships, and the untreated adult psychopathology that may surround individual cases. To keep these inheritance factors in perspective, it is important to remember that most children and adults with good coping skills and moderate self-control can manage their illness well.

NEUROBIOLOGY

While genetic factors are now recognized as most important in the development of TS and related tic disorders, investigators continue to search for underlying neuroanatomical and neurochemical disturbances that may be part of the gene expression involved in the pathogenesis of TS symptoms. These would be appropriate targets for therapeutic intervention. Several lines of evidence have supported the notion that striatal dopamine receptor hyperexpression or sensitivity may underlie the tic disorder: (1) dopamine receptor antagonists are the most effective drugs for suppressing tics; (2) tics may be exacerbated by dopaminomimetic medications such as amphetamines; and (3) reduced levels of the dopamine metabolite homovanillic acid have been identified in the cerebrospinal fluid of patients with TS.[66]

Pathological reports are sorely lacking. One report describes absent staining for dynorphin in the globus pallidus of the postmortem brain of a patient with TS.[67] Other reports indicate that drugs affecting the endogenous opioid system may too influence the symptoms of TS.[68–70] Other pathological reports revealed reduced concentrations of adenosine 3′,5′-monophosphate (cyclic AMP) in the cerebral cortex and suggests a possible dysfunction of secondary neurochemical messengers.[71]

Other authors have suggested that sex hormone influences on brain development and function may be important in the pathogenesis of TS.[72,73]

These pathological data notwithstanding, neurobiological substrate of tics remains unknown. From a physiologic perspective, tic and other TS symptoms are thought to involve abnormalities in cortico-striato-thalamic circuits that are modulated by ascending monoaminergic pathways.[74] Evidence for this has been obtained in part from autopsies in neurologic conditions with secondary tic manifestation. For instance, tics have been described as a late sequelae of encephalitis lethargica (i.e., postencephalitic parkinsonism) where there is extensive pathological involvement of the ascending monoaminergic pathways, the midbrain tegmentum, and the periaqueductal gray.[75,76] In these cases the resulting dopaminergic denervation of the basal ganglia leads to "postsynaptic dopamine hypersensitivity," which can lead to tics when combined with the extensive mid-brain pathology of postencephalitic parkinsonism.[75]

Striatal regions forming part of the above circuits, such as the caudate and putamen, are thought to be involved in the generation of motor tics. Vocal tics may involve nonmotor circuits such as those projecting to the prefrontal and limbic cortices.[77,78] Unlike the striatum, which receives dopaminergic innervation from the pars compacta of the substantia nigra, these nonmotor circuits receive dopaminergic projections from the ventral tegmental area of the midbrain.[77] The cortical projections of these circuits include the prefrontal cortex, the cingulate gyrus, the entorhinal cortex, the olfactory tubercle, the amygdala, and selected regions of the midbrain tegmentum. Experiments in primates indicate that manipulations of the cingulate gyrus and other limbic forebrain regions can lead to changes in vocalization.[79,80] The cingulate gyrus is of particular interest in that it connects cortical and limbic structures involved in vocalization and other functions.[24] Other limbic structures have also been associated with obsessions and compulsions, in primary tic disorders and postencephalitic parkinsonism.[75]

Morphometric neuroanatomic studies of these structures, using high-resolution magnetic resonance imaging, support the view that there are basal ganglia abnormalities in TS.[81, 82] The studies indicate that children and adults with TS have reduced volumes in the region of the left lenticular nucleus (globus pallidus and putamen), compared to those of age-matched controls.[81,82] Because the left hemisphere is typically larger than the right, TS subjects seem to exhibit significant attenuation in the normal interhemispheric asymmetry seen in controls. This lack or loss of asymmetry may be more striking in individuals with comorbid TS and ADD.[82,83]

Positron emission tomography studies using ^{18}F-fluorodeoxyglucose suggest that, in TS, there is decreased metabolic activity in subcortical regions, including basal ganglia and limbic cortices. Areas exhibiting decreased metabolic activity include the orbital, frontal, and superior insular cortices, the mesial temporal cortex, and the striatum. Regions exhibiting increased metabolic rate include the premotor regions (lateral premotor and supplementary motor areas), the rolandic cortices, and the postrolandic sensory association areas.[84] These regions are connected by the motor/limbic striato-thalamic circuit mentioned above.[77] More importantly, it seems that the functional metabolic relationship between these regions is altered in TS compared to that of controls.

Much like the morphometric studies discussed above, the alterations in these functional relationships gravitate around the ventral striatum, including the globus pallidus. In TS, striatal metabolic changes are positively coupled to the metabolic rates in overlying cortical regions.[84] In normal subjects, this relationship is negatively correlated; that is, if the metabolic activity in the ventral striatum increases, it is expected to decrease in the corresponding target cortical regions. This has led to speculation that, in TS, there is functional cortical-subcortical "short-circuiting" between these regions, leading to failure of "gating" responsible for the coupling of motor and limbic cortical regions through the ventral striatum.[84] Clinically, this may lead to inability to suppress activity generated anywhere within the motor/limbic striato-thalamic circuitry. Depending on where in the circuitry this activity originates, the patient may present with inability to control motor impulses (tics, compulsions), failure to control sensory overload (ADD), or intrusive thoughts and impulsions (obsessive-compulsive disorder, OCD). Using auditory and visual startle responses as a model of sensorimotor "gating" by striatal outflow, animal experiments have produced evidence that support this hypothesis.[85] Startle responses are profoundly affected by dopaminergic transmission in the basal ganglia, thereby tying this model to what is known about the pharmacology of tics and TS (see below).

Detailed electrophysiological studies provide little insight into the pathogenesis of tics. A number of EEG studies have failed to document consistent abnormalities in subjects with TS.[87, 88] Bergen et al. reported a 34 percent incidence of nonspecific EEG abnormalities in a random selection of 38 TS patients, most of which could be attributed to coexisting so-called "soft neurologic signs".[87] Only 2 patients exhibited epileptiform activity, and none reported seizures.[87] Neufeld et al. examined quantitative EEGs in 48 consecutive patients with TS and concluded that "there was no significant difference between TS patients and matched controls."[88] Krumholz et al. examined the EEG, and the visual, brainstem, and auditory-evoked responses (n = 17) in 40 TS patients and found no "diagnostic or therapeutic value to justify their routine use in this syndrome."[89]

Dysfunction of central dopaminergic pathways is suspected as playing a role in the pathophysiology of TS.[74,90] In experimental animals, dopamine and acetylcholine play complementary and often reciprocal roles.[93] Given this interaction in the striatum, an alternative hypothesis is that tics may result in part from dysfunction in cerebral cholinergic systems.[91,92] According to this hypothesis, evidence for central dopaminergic "hyperfunction" in TS could be mediated by cholinergic "hypofunction." In man, clinical evidence suggests that dopaminergic transmission can be enhanced by cholinergic antagonists.[93] Examples of this include improvement in hypodopaminergic states such as neuroleptic-induced extrapyramidal syndromes and Parkinson's disease, to cholinergic antagonists. Conversely, cholinergic agonists may alleviate hyperdopaminergic states, such as tics and chorea.[16]

Indirect evidence for abnormal cholinergic transmission in TS has been obtained through a series of pharmacological experiments. For instance, oral anticholinergic agents have a definite but variable effect on tics.[94] Most studies support the view that augmentation of central cholinergic transmission relieves tics and possibly other symptoms of TS.[91,92] Accordingly, several purported cholinomimetics have been investigated as possible alternatives to the standard dopamine-blocking strategies in TS.[16] The results have been limited by the agents used which, like choline and lecithin, are poorly tolerated or have poor central nervous system penetration.[91,95]

Serotonin is another potentially important neurotransmitter in the pathogenesis of tic disorders and, in particular, TS. Most of its relevance to TS appears to be in its relationship to anxiety and OCD symptomatology, for serotonergic agents have proven moderately effective.[16] (see OCD therapy below).

Finally, key questions for which there are still only speculative answers are: Where in the supposedly abnormal motor/limbic striato-thalamic circuits does this abnormal activity originate? What sustains, and at the same time, what makes this activity so variable? These questions force us again to examine the key role that the ventral striatum, dopamine, and the overlying cortices play in transforming motivation into action by serving as an interface between the above motor circuits, the limbic system, and the hypothalamus.[86] But if tics are involuntary (or "unvoluntary," as discussed above) as suggested above, then theories regarding motivation, decision-making, and action that underlie the above neurophysiologic assumptions may turn out to be of limited value in the understanding of tics.

▶ THERAPY

The management of patients with TS can be both challenging and rewarding. The initial step is to identify the clinical features that are interfering most with daily activities and direct therapy at those "target" symptoms (Table 39–3). The most important target symptom is not always the tic, and this differentiation is not always obvious. For instance, in cases with co-morbid ADHD or OCD targeting behaviors associated with these conditions, or symptoms of depression, anxiety, may be a more productive approach than addressing the tics first.

TREATMENT OF TICS

General

Most patients with mild tics who have made positive adjustments in their lives to the presence of tics can avoid the use of medications. Educating patients, family members, peers, and school personnel regarding the nature of TS, restructuring the educational environment, and supportive counseling are measures that may be sufficient to avoid drug therapy. Pharmacotherapy should be considered once it is determined that the tics are functionally disabling and not remediable to psychosocial interventions. The goal in treating tics is generally to achieve "satisfactory" suppression or control rather than to attempt to make the patient completely free of tics.

Pharmacotherapy

For the patient with mild or moderate tics, treatment is usually initiated with an alpha-agonist. Clonidine is initiated at 0.05 mg at bedtime, and the dosage is increased by 0.05 mg every few days until satisfactory control of tics is achieved or unacceptable side effects are encountered. Most patients respond to 1 tablet (0.1 mg) 3 times per day (before and after school and at bedtime for children), but the maintenance dose should be the lowest one that gives satisfactory suppression of tics. When necessary, higher doses of clonidine (generally up to 0.6 mg/day) can be used, letting adverse effects (usually sedation) be the dose-limiting factor. Transdermal clonidine is an alternative dosing form, particularly for children who cannot swallow pills, but this formulation often causes skin irritation and may fall off. Guanfacine is a newer alpha-agonist that has the advantages of single daily dosing and causing less sedation than clonidine.[96] This drug has become the first-choice alpha-agonist for many clinicians. It is initiated at 0.5–1 mg at bedtime and gradually titrated as needed to a maximum dosage of 4 mg. A new long-acting formulation of guanfacine, Intuniv®, was recently approved for the treatment of ADHD and may ultimately play a role in TS. Finally, note that the higher doses ranges of these drugs may play a role in the management of aggression in TS (see above).

If an alpha-2 agonist alone is insufficient, antipsychotics can be used to complement or replace this first step. If clonidine or guanfacine is to be discontinued, the drug should be tapered over 7–10 days in order to avoid rebound tachycardia and/or blood pressure elevation.

The newer so-called atypical antipsychotics have generally supplanted the traditional neuroleptic antipsychotics as second-line tic suppressants (after the alpha-agonists)

▶ **TABLE 39–4. PHARMACOLOGIC TREATMENT OF TICS**

Tics
Alpha-agonists: clonidine (oral, transdermal), guanfacine, or Intuniv®
Atypical antipsychotics: risperidal, aripiprazole, ziprasidone, olanzapine
Typical antipsychotics: haloperidol, pimozide, fluphenazine
Tetrabenazine
Calcium channel blockers
Botulinum toxin

due to better side-effect profiles. The atypical agents can generally be given in a single bedtime dose. Those atypical antipsychotics with reported tic-suppressing actions include risperidone (0.25–16 mg/day), aripiprazole (1-15 mg/d), ziprasidone (20–200 mg/day) and olanzapine (2.5–15 mg/day). These drugs, though effective, can be sedating and may be associated with significant weight gain. They may also have an anxiolytic effect and may augment the effect of SSRIs on OCD symptoms.

If the atypical antipsychotic proves ineffective or poorly tolerated, a trial of a typical antipsychotic may be of use. They are generally less sedating and may be associated with less weight gain than some of the atypical antipsychotics. They are, however, more associated with extrapyramidal symptoms (EPS) of which akathisia may be the most insidious becoming a direct contributor to anxiety and a drive to OCD symptoms. The rate of tardive dyskinesia seems to be lower in TS than in other populations. There is no explanation for this observation. Haloperidol remains one of the most commonly used classical antipsychotics for the treatment of tics. The drug is initiated at 0.25 mg at bedtime, increasing as necessary; most patients have a favorable response at ≤2 mg/day usually given at bedtime. Alternatives in this category are pimozide, fluphenazine, or, in cases of high sensitivity to EPS, other lower-potency antipsychotics. In patients with very severe tics, it makes sense to initiate therapy with an antipsychotic rather than an alpha-agonist, at least until the tics and the situation can be controlled. Also helpful are local intramuscular injections of botulinum toxin. These are particular helpful in patients with painful dystonia and other potentially serious tics such as "head snapping" tics.[97] Please see Table 39–4 for other medications that have proven helpful in the management of tics.

Behavioral Therapy of Tics

Our improved understanding of the cognitive processes involved in the generation of tics led to the development of a comprehensive behavioral intervention (CIBIT).[98] The therapy is based on the use of function-based, individualized interventions to address external factors, and habit reversal strategies to address internal factors known to aggravate tics.[99–104] An early dividend of this cognitive work in TS has been the refuting of myths that would have made the development of modern behavioral therapies for the management of tics difficult.[105–107] Some of these disproven assumptions are: (a) suppression of tics leads to a rebound effect; (b) suppression of one tic leads to other tics; and (c) focusing on tics invariably aggravates them.[99] The new knowledge and the results of the study described below support the view that tics are very responsive to the environment, and, as such, can be modified in a positive or negative manner through environmental manipulations. Most effective are the manipulations addressing the reaction of others (e.g., parents, family, teachers, peers) to the tics in a child. These reactions can build or damage the child's self image and cognitive strategies used to cope with the tics and other symptoms of TS. Over time the severity of tics becomes in part the consequence of the learned constructs to internal and external environmental challenges. When the environmental challenge can be changed, CIBIT teaches subjects how to recognize and handle the antecedents (e.g., urges) and address the social consequences of the tic. When indicated, it teaches to escape the consequence by leaving the provoking circumstance without relinquishing responsibility for the task in question. When the environment cannot be easily modified, the patient is taught relaxation strategies, scheduled activity breaks, and cognitive restructuring through the therapy.[98] For more information on these techniques, please see Woods et al. from the series Treatments That Work.[108]

The above study of CIBIT for the treatment of tics was a randomized, controlled trial of 126 children with TS (or CMT) randomized to receive CIBIT or control supportive therapy with education for 10 weeks. CIBIT led to a significantly greater decrease on the Yale Global Tic Severity Scale (change in score from 25 to 17) compared to the control intervention (25 to 21; $P<0.001$), and to more improvement in the Clinical Global Impressions-Improvement scale (52.5% vs 18.5% of subjects improved in each group; $P < 0.001$). Treatment was well received and continued to have benefit participants 6 months after completion of the treatment sessions. [98] For more information on this intervention the reader is referred to the Tourette Syndrome Association (www.tsa-usa.org) and to Woods et al.[108]

Other Behavioral Therapies

Early psychodynamic theories about TS in this century resulted in stigmatization of patients, ineffective therapies, and rejection of psychological therapies among many in the TS community.[109] The advances in the psychology of tics noted above and advances in the understanding of TS behavioral co-morbidities now provide excellent evidence for the use of behavioral therapy in the

▶ TABLE 39–5. PHARMACOLOGIC TREATMENT OF TS COMORBIDITIES

Attention Deficit Hyperactivity Disorder
Alpha-2 agonists: clonidine (oral, transdermal), guanfacine
Stimulants: methylphenidate (methyphenidate, Concerta®, Metadate CR®, Adderall®): Nonstimulant (atomoxetine)
Aggression and rage attacks in ADHD (no controlled data in TS)
Alpha-2 agonists, desipramine, mood stabilizers, antipsychotics
Obsessive-Compulsive Behavior
Serotonin reuptake inhibitors: fluoxetine, fluvoxamine, paroxetine, clomipramine, others. Augmentation strategies with select typical and atypical antipsychotics.

Note: Behavioral therapies are important to consider in many instances but are beyond the scope of this chapter.

treatment of anxiety disorders, OCD, and ADHD.[28,110–112] Comprehensive coverage of the behavioral treatment of OCD and ADHD in TS is beyond the scope of this chapter. Instead the author will summarize some of the general pharmacologic strategies used to treat these disorders in TS without implying that pharmacologic approaches should be the first or only strategy. These therapeutic decisions need to be individualized. In principle, however, behavioral therapy and environmental manipulations should be considered before pharmacotherapy, particularly in children.

TREATMENT OF ATTENTION DEFICIT HYPERACTIVITY DISORDER (ADHD)

When ADHD is the target symptom in TS, the question is how best to manage ADHD-associated symptoms without aggravating the tics. For this, alpha-2 agonists such as clonidine or guanfacine are useful starting medications (see Table 39–5).[96] When alpha-2 agonists are not enough to control the distractibility, impulsivity, hyperactivity, and irritability of ADHD, stimulant have proven more effective. The main ones are methylphenidate and dexedrine and their derivatives available in short-, intermediate-, and long-acting forms. Although treatment with stimulants may exacerbate tics in some patients, the occasional worsening of tics may be tolerable when the medication is started at a low dose and titrated slowly, probably more slowly than usual in ADHD without tics. When effective, the improvement in attention and the control hyperactivity can result in a significant reduction in the symptom-associated stress, and thus a secondary reduction in tics.[113,114] Double-blind placebo-controlled studies of the treatment of ADHD in TS using methylphenidate with or without clonidine, [115] or in a separate study, the non-stimulant atamoxetine, have shown clinically significant improvement in ADHD symptoms with no significant worsening, and often an improvement in tics.[116] In these studies patients were carefully selected such that the results may not generalize to ADHD symptoms in all patients with tics, particularly during acute flare-up of TS-associated symptoms.[117, 118] If tics are worsened by stimulant therapy, an alpha-agonist or an antipsychotic can be added. If the tic exacerbation is tolerable, time should be given for this initial reaction to extinguish using the lowest tolerable dose of the stimulant. Clearly, if the tics continue to escalate, the stimulant will need to be discontinued. The use of the MAO inhibitor selegiline has proven helpful in a few studies. [119] There is no information on the use of the new amphetamine pro-drug, lisdexamfetamine, in the treatment of ADHD in TS.

Finally, there is recent evidence that rage attacks and other aggressive behaviors in ADHD and pervasive developmental delay can be controlled with alpha-2 agonists.[120–123] Whether this applies to similar behaviors in TS, with or without ADHD, remains to be seen.

TREATMENT OF OBSESSIVE COMPULSIVE DISORDER (OCD)

Antidepressant drugs that inhibit serotonin reuptake, including fluoxetine, fluvoxamine, paroxetine, clomipramine among others, may be effective for the treatment of OCD associated with TS.[124, 125] Cognitive behavioral therapy by an experienced therapist has also been proven to be highly effective in the management of OCD. Its effect can be additive to that of pharmacotherapy, and thus the two approaches in conjunction may offer the best benefit to patients. Psychosurgical approaches have been used for rare patients severely disabled by OCD who had inadequate responses to psychotherapy and medications.[126, 127]

DEEP BRAIN STIMULATION

In the last 7 years there has been increasing interest in the use of psychosurgery for the treatment of severe cases of TS not responsive to aggressive behavioral and medical therapy.[128–133] Early use of stereotactic lesions in TS (e.g., stereotactic coagulation of the rostral intralaminar and medial thalamic nuclei, lesions of the cerebellar dentate nucleus, and frontal lobotomies)[134] proved to have dubious benefit and unacceptable risks and was discontinued.[135–137] Based on this, there was skepticism and apprehension when deep brain stimulation (DBS) was introduced in 2007 for use in TS. There were additional doubts regarding the use of a single target site in the brain to control the sometimes complex symptomatology of TS. These doubts were not helped by the fact that even the centers pioneering this surgery could not agree on an ideal target site.[129,135,138–142]

These doubts notwithstanding, results from stimulation of the various proposed target sites began to show fairly consistent and positive results across targets.[131–133,136,139] These generally positive results support the idea that TS is a circuit disorder much like other neuropsychiatric disorders involving cortico-striatal-thalamic circuits (see Neurobiology section).[143]

Since these initial reports, ongoing work using psychosurgery in OCD and the DBS experience in multiple other movement disorders have shown that this technique can be practiced safely. Controversy still exists on the use of DBS in patients with self-mutilation.[142, 144] On the one hand, these may be the patients who need the procedure most; on the other, if the symptoms do not improve rapidly, they may be at high risk of damaging the equipment and in the process sustaining serious injury.[145] This early experience suggests that, in carefully selected cases, these behaviors may also benefit from DBS.[137,146–148] The initial concern that the co-morbidities of TS may worsen following DBS have been partially swayed with the observation that anxiety and OC symptoms may also improve.[130–133,135]

Visser-Vandewalle pioneered DBS of the medial thalamus in TS based on the hypothesis that this region provides physiologic gating to the basal ganglia.[128] The most widely used target to date is the centrum medianum and parafascicular nuclei of the thalamus. In the studies that have used this target, improvement in tics and OCD symptomatology has been in the order of 72–90% for up to 5 years after the surgery. Similar results have been reported in a larger cohorts by Servello and Porta et al. in Italy,[131,133] and Misuounas et al. in a controlled study out of Cleveland, USA.[132]

There is still concern that reports coming out of these large and experienced clinics may not reflect those from smaller sites the results of which may not be published. There are also many stressors that can aggravate tics not all of which may be related to the physiology of cortico-striato-thalamic circuits. Family and financial stressors, issues of codependency, ongoing negative reinforcement by loved ones, and the pernicious effect of chronic disability are all factors that influence the severity of tics and need to be taken in consideration before surgical decisions are made. Are our current screening procedures for surgical candidates adequately screening for these? Undoubtedly, different results may also be the result of differing target sites and coordinates used within each target. DBS programming issues for now appear to be less of a factor in the results. The field as a whole, prematurely or not, appears to be moving in the direction tailoring the surgery to the specific patient needs, with the two leading sites being the medial thalamus and the globus pallidum internus, depending on the degree to which anxiety plays a role in the symptomatology.[101,133,135,144]

The Tourette syndrome association published interim guidelines and expectation in the selection of potential candidates and on the use of DBS for the treatment of TS.[149] These guidelines are currently being revised in light of the experience since 1996. For now the best candidates seem to be adult TS patients with severe motor and/or phonic tics unresponsive to aggressive conventional treatment. OCD and anxiety disorders are not exclusionary criteria but carefully screening for and management of associated psychopathology is essential. Exclusion criteria include the presence of co-morbidities severe enough to overshadow the tic disorder. Some of these include substance abuse, axis II diagnosis, and a history of poor compliance. In sum, the field remains in desperate need of animal models in which to test hypothesis and refine surgical approaches, as was the case with the development of modern stereotactic surgery in Parkinson's disease.[150, 151] The field is also in need of better surgical target definitions, a more comprehensive survey of bad outcomes, and larger controlled studies of DBS in TS.

Finally, and as noted above, a most important aspect of treating TS is education of the patient, family, and significant others in the person's life. This education should include the tic, and where relevant, its co-morbidities. A variety of educational brochures, videotapes, and other materials are available from the Tourette Syndrome Association (www.tsa-usa.org). A local TS support group may be of great benefit to patients and family members. Individual, group, or family counseling may be helpful in facilitating a healthy adaptation to the illness and its symptoms. Specific psychoeducational assessments and therapy are often needed for children with school problems. This therapy may need to involve teachers and other school personnel.

▶ ACKNOWLEDGMENT

The author would like to thank Joash Lazarus, MD, for his valuable help with the preparation of this manuscript.

REFERENCES

1. de la Tourette G. Etude sur une affection nerveuse characterisee par de l'incoordination motrice accompagnee d'echlalie et de coprolalie. In Friedhoff AJ, Chase TN (eds); Goetz CG, Klawans HL (trans). Advances in Neurology, Vol 35. New York: Raven Press, 1982, pp. 1–16.
2. Leckman J, Cohen D. Tourette's Syndrome: Tics, Obsessions, Compulsions: Developmental Psychopatholgy and Clinical Care, Vol 155–176. New York: Wiley, 1999.
3. Jankovic J, Stone L. Dystonic tics in patients with Tourette's syndrome. Mov Disord 1991;6:248–252.
4. Stone LA, Jankovic J. The coexistance of tics and dystonia. Arch Neurol 1991;48:862–865.

5. Kurlan R. Tourette's syndrome: current concepts. Neurology 1989;39(12):1625–1630.
6. Scahill LD, Leckman JF, Marek KL. Sensory phenomena in Tourette's syndrome. Adv Neurol 1995;65:273–280.
7. Cohen AJ, Leckman JF. Sensory phenomena associated with Gilles de la Tourette's syndrome. J Clin Psychiatry 1992;53(9):319–323.
8. Leckman JF, Walker DE, Cohen DJ. Premonitory urges in Tourette's syndrome. Am J Psychiatry 1993;150:98–102.
9. Bliss J. Sensory experiances of Gilles de la Tourette syndrome. Arch Gen Psychiatry 1980;37:1343–1347.
10. Shapiro A, Shapiro E, Young J, Feinberg T. Gilles de la Tourette Syndrome, 2nd ed. New York: Raven Press, 1988.
11. APA. Diagnostic and Statistical Manual of Mental Disorders, 4th Edition (DSM-IV), 4th ed. Washington, DC: American Psychiatric Association, 1994.
12. Obeso JA, Rothwell JC, Marsden CD. Simple tics in Gilles de la Tourete's syndrome are not prefaced by a normal premovement EEG potential. J Neurol Neurosurg Psychiatry 1981;14:735–738.
13. Papa SM, Artieda J, Obeso JA. Cortical activity preceding self-initiated and externally triggered voluntary movement. Mov Disord 1991;6:217–224.
14. Lang A. Patient perception of tics and other movement disorders. Neurology 1991;41:223–238.
15. Fahn S. Motor and vocal tics. In Kurlan R (ed). Handbook of Tourette Syndrome and Related Tic and Behavioral Disorders. New York: Marcell Dekker, 1993, pp. 3–16.
16. Jankovic J. The neurology of tics. In Marsden CD, Fahn S (ed). Movement Disorders. London: Butterworth, 1987. pp. 383–405.
17. Karp BI, Hallet M. Extracorporeal "phantom tics" in Tourette's syndrome. Neurology 1996;46:38–40.
18. Frankel M, Cummings JL, Robertson MM, Trimble MR, Hill MA, Benson DF. Obsessions and compulsions in Gilles de la Tourette's syndrome. Neurology 1986;36(3):378–382.
19. Pauls DL, Hurst CR, Kruger SD, Leckman JF, Kidd KK, Cohen DJ. Gilles de la Tourette's syndrome and attention deficit disorder with hyperactivity. Evidence against a genetic relationship. Arch Gen Psychiatry 1986;43(12):1177–1179.
20. Como P. Neuropsychological testing. In Kurlan R. (ed). Handbook of Tourette's Syndrome and Related Tic and Behavioral Disorders. Marcel Dekker New York, 1993, pp. 221–239.
21. Comings DE, Comings BG. Tourette's syndrome and attention deficit disorder with hyperactivity: are they genetically related? J Am Acad Child Psychiatry 1984;23(2):138–146.
22. Comings DE, Comings BG. A controlled study of Tourette syndrome. Attention deficit disorder, learning disorders,and school problems. Am J Hum Genet 1987;41:701–741.
23. Cohen D. Gilles de la Tourette's syndrome and attention deficit disorder with hyperactivity: Evidence against a genetic relationship? Arch Gen Psychiatry 1986;43: 1177–1179.
24. Pauls DL, Cohen DJ, Kidd KK, Leckman JF. Tourette syndrome and neuropsychiatric disorders: Is there a genetic relationship? Am J Hum Genet 1988;43(2):206–217.
25. Kurlan R. What is the spectrum of Tourette's syndrome? Curr Opin Neurol Neurosurg 1988;1:294–298.
26. Robertson MM, Yakeley JW. Obsessive-compulsive disorder and self-injurious behavior. In Kurlan R (ed). Handbook of Tourette's Syndrome and Related Tic and Behavioral Disorders. Marcel Dekker New York, 1993, pp. 45–87.
27. Kurlan R, Daragjati C, Como PG, et al. Non-obscene complex socially inappropriate behavior in Tourette's syndrome. J Neuropsychiatry Clin Neurosci 1996;8(3):311–317.
28. King R, Scahill L. Emotional and behavioral difficulties associated with Tourette syndrome. In Cohen D, Goetz C, Jankovic J (eds). Tourette Syndrome. Philadelphia, PA: Lippincott Williams & Wilkins, 2001, pp. 79–88.
29. Budman CL, Bruun RD, Park KS, Lesser M, Olson M. Explosive outbursts in children with Tourette's disorder. J Am Acad Child Adolesc Psychiatry. 2000;39:1270–1276.
30. Freeman R, Radt D, Burd L. An international perspective on Tourette syndrome: selected findings from 3500 cases in 22 countries. Dev Med Child 2000;42:436–447.
31. Wand RR, Matazow GS, Shady GA, Furer P, Staley D. Tourette syndrome: associated symptoms and most disabling features. Neurosci Biobehav Rev 1993;17(3): 271–275.
32. DeGroot C, Janus M, Bornstein R. Clinical predictors of psychopathology in children and adolescents with Tourette syndrome. J Psychiatr Res 1995;29:59–70.
33. Nolan E, sverd J, Gadow K. Associated pathology in children with both ADHD and chronic tic disorder. J Am Acad Child Adolesc Psychiatry 1996;35:1622–1630.
34. Robertson M, Trimble M, Lees A. The psychopathology of the Gilles de la Tourette Syndrome. A phenomenological analysis. Br J Psychiatry 1988;152:383–390.
35. Connor D, Glatt S, Lopez I. Psychopharmacology and aggression I. A Meta-analysis of stimulant effects on overt/covert aggression-related behavior in ADHD. J Am Acad Child Adoles Psychiatry 2002;41:253–261.
36. Campbell M, Gonzales N, Silva R. The pharmacological treatment of conduct disorder and rage outbursts. Psychiatr Clin North Am 1992;15:69–85.
37. Pallanti S, Baldini RN, Friedberg J. Psychobiology of impulse-control disorders not otherwise specified (NOS). In D'Haenen H, J dB, Willner P (eds). Biological Psychiatry. New York: John Wiley & Sons, 2000.
38. Kadesjoe B, Gilbert C. Tourette's disorder: Epidemiology and comorbidity in primary school children. J Am Acad Child Adolesc Psychiatry 2000;39:548–555.
39. Spencer T, Biederman J, Wilens TE, Faraone SV. Adults with attention-deficit/hyperactivity disorder: a controversial diagnosis. J Clin Psychiatry 1998;59(Suppl 7):59–68.
40. Glaze DG, Frost JD, Jankovic J. Sleep in Gilles de la Tourette's syndrome. Neurology 1983;33:586–592.
41. Kirov R, Kinkelbur J, Banaschewski T, Rothenberger A. Sleep patterns in children with attention-deficit/hyperactivity disorder, tic disorder, and comorbidity. J Child Psychol Psychiatry 2007;48(6):561–570.
42. Bock RD, Goldberger L. Tonic, phasic and cortical arousal in Gilles de la Tourette's syndrome. J Neurol Neurosurg Psychiatry 1985;48:535–544.
43. Gabor B, Matthewes WS, Ferrari M. Disorders of arousal in Gilles de la Tourette's syndrome. Neurology 1984;33: 586–592.
44. Trajanovic NN, Voloh I, Shapiro CM, Sandor P. REM sleep behaviour disorder in a child with Tourette's syndrome. Can J Neurol Sci 2004;31(4):572–575.

45. Pauls DL, Leckman JF. The inheritance of Gilles de la Tourette's syndrome and associated behaviors. Evidence for autosomal dominant transmission. N Engl J Med 16 1986;315(16):993–997.
46. Kurlan R, Behr J, Medved L, Shoulson I, Pauls D, Kidd KK. Severity of Tourette's syndrome in one large kindred. Implication for determination of disease prevalence rate. Arch Neurol 1987;44(3):268–269.
47. McMahon WM, Leppert M, Filloux F, van de Wetering BJ, Hasstedt S. Tourette symptoms in 161 related family members. Adv Neurol 1992;58:159–165.
48. Lapouse R, Monk MA. Behavior deviations in a representative sample of children: Variation by sex, age, race, social class and family size. Am J Orthopsychiatry 1964;34:436–446.
49. Macfarlane JW, Allen L, Honzik MP. A developmental study of the behavior problems of normal children between twenty-one months and fourteen years. Publ Child Dev Univ Calif 1954;2:1–222.
50. Scahill L, Bitsko R, Visser S, Blumberg S. Prevalence of diagnosed tourette syndrome in persons aged 6-17 years. MMWR 2009;58(21):581–585.
51. Erenberg G, Cruse RP, Rothner AD. The natural history of Tourette syndrome: A follow -up study. Ann Neurol 1987;22:383–385.
52. Goetz CG, Tanner CM, Stebbin GT, Leipzy G, Carr WE. Adult ticks in Gilles de la Tourette's syndrome: Description and risk factors. Neurology 1992;42:784–788.
53. Leckman JF, Towbin KE, Ort SI, Cohen DJ. Clinical assessment of tic disorder severity. In: Cohen DJ, Bruun RD, Leckman JF (eds). Tourette's Syndrome and Tic Disorders New York: Wiley, 1988, pp. 55–78.
54. Bruun R. The natural history of Tourette's syndrome. Tourette's Syndrome and Tic Disorders: Clinical Understanding and Treatment. New York: Wiley, 1988, pp. 21–39.
55. Shapiro E, Shapiro A. Gilles de la Tourette Syndrome and tic disorders. The Harvard Medical School Mental Health Letter. 1989;5.
56. Comings DE, Comings BG. Tourette syndrome: clinical and psychological aspects of 250 cases. Am J Hum Genet 1985;37:435–450.
57. Park S, Como PG, Cui L, Kurlan R. The early course of the Tourette's syndrome clinical spectrum. Neurology 1993;43(9):1712–1715.
58. Pauls DL. An update on the genetics of Gilles de la Tourette syndrome. J Psychosom Res 2003;55(1):7–12.
59. Walkup J, LaBuda M, Singer HS. Family study and segregation analysis of Tourette syndrome: evidence for a mixed model of inheritance. Am J Hum Genet 1996;59: 684–693.
60. Price RA, Kidd KK, Cohen DJ, Pauls DL, Leckman JF. A twin study of Tourette syndrome. Arch Gen Psychiatry 1985;42(8):815–820.
61. Eapen V, Pauls D, Robertson M. Evidence for autosomal dominant transmission in Tourete's Syndrome—United Kingdom Cohort Study. Br J Psychiatry 1993;162: 593–596.
62. Genetics; TSAICf. Genome scan for Tourette disorder in affected-sibling-pair and multigenerational families. Am J Hum Genet 2007;80(2):265–272.
63. Alsobrook JP, 2nd, Pauls DL. The genetics of Tourette syndrome. Neurol Clin 1997;15(2):381–393.
64. O'Rourke JA, Scharf JM, Yu D, Pauls DL. The genetics of Tourette syndrome: A review. J Psychosom Res 2009;67(6):533–545.
65. State MW, Greally JM, Cuker A, et al. Epigenetic abnormalities associated with a chromosome 18(q21-q22) inversion and a Gilles de la Tourette syndrome phenotype. Proc Natl Acad Sci U S A 2003;100(8):4684–4689.
66. Singer HS, Butler IJ, Tune LE, Seifert WJ, Coyle JT. Dopaminergic dsyfunction in Tourette syndrome. Ann Neurol 1982;12(4):361–366.
67. Haber SN, Kowall NW, Vonsattel JP, Bird ED, Richardson EP, Jr. Gilles de la Tourette's syndrome. A postmortem neuropathological and immunohistochemical study. J Neurol Sci 1986;75(2):225–241.
68. Gilman M, Sandyk R. The endogenous opiod system in Gilles de la Tourette's syndrome. Med Hypotheses 1986;19:371–378.
69. Kurlan R, Majumdar L, Deeley C, Mudholkar GS, Plumb S, Como PG. A controlled trial of propoxyphene and naltrexone in patients with Tourette's syndrome. Ann Neurol 1991;30(1):19–23.
70. Lichter D, Majumdar L, Kurlan R. Opiate withdrawal unmasks Tourette's syndrome. Clin Neuropharmacol 1988;11(6):559–564.
71. Singer HS, Hahn IH, Krowiak E, Nelson E, Moran T. Tourette's syndrome: a neurochemical analysis of postmortem cortical brain tissue. Ann Neurol 1990;27(4): 443–446.
72. Kurlan R. The pathogenesis of Tourette's syndrome. A possible role for hormonal and excitatory neurotransmitter influences in brain development. Arch Neurol 1992;49(8):874–876.
73. Peterson BS, Leckman JF, Scahill L, et al. Steroid hormones and CNS sexual dimorphisms modulate symptom expression in Tourette's syndrome. Psychoneuroendocrinology 1992;17(6):553–563.
74. Singer HS. Neurobiological issues in Tourette syndrome. Brain Dev 1994;16:353–364.
75. Devinsky O. Neuroanatomy of Gilles de la Tourette's syndrome: Possible midbrain involvement. Arch Neurol 1983;40:508–514.
76. Sacks OW. Acquired Tourettism in adult life. Adv Neurol 1982;35:89–92.
77. Alexander GE, Crutcher MD, DeLong MR. Basal ganglia-thalamocortical circuits: Parallel substrates for motor, oculomotor, "prefrontal" and "limbic" functions. Prog Brain Res. 1990;85:119–146.
78. Alexander GE, DeLong MR, Strick PL. Parallel organization of functionally segregated circuits linking basal ganglia and cortex. Annu Rev Neurosci 1986;9:357–381.
79. Baleydier C, Mauquierre F. The duality of the cingulate gyrus in monkey. Brain 1980;103:525–554.
80. Muller-Perus P, Jurgens U. Projections from then "cingular" vocalization area in the squirrel monkey. Brain Res 1976;103:29–43.
81. Peterson B, Riddle MA, Cohen DJ, et al. Reduced basal ganglia volumes in Tourette's syndrome usin three dimentional reconstruction techniques from magnetic resonance images. Neurology 1993;43:941–948.

82. Singer HS, Reiss AL, Brown JE, et al. Volumetric MRI changes in basal ganglia of children with Tourette's syndrome. Neurology 1993;43(5):950–956.
83. Witelson SF. Clinical neurology as data for basic neuroscience: Tourette's syndrome and the human motor system. Neurology 1993;43:859–861.
84. Stoetter B, Braun AR, Randolph C, et al. Functional neuroanatomy of Tourette syndrome. Limbic-motor interactions studied with FDG PET. Adv Neurol 1992;58(213): 213–226.
85. Swerdlow NB, Caine SB, Geyer MA. Regionally selective effects of intracerebral dopamine infusion on sensorimotor gating of the startle reflex in rats. Psychopharmacology 1992;108:189–195.
86. Mogenson GJ, Jones DL, Chi YY. From motivation to action:Functional interface between the limbic system and the motor system. Prog Neurobiol 1980;14:69–97.
87. Bergen D, Tanner C, Wilson R. The electroencephalogram in Tourette syndrome. Ann Neurol 1982;11:382–385.
88. Neufeld MY, Berger Y, Chapman J, Korcyzn. Routine and quantitative EEG analysis in Gilles de la Tourette's syndrome. Neurology 1990;40:1837–1839.
89. Krumholz A, Singer HS, Niedermyer E, Burnite R, Harris K. Electrophysiological studies in Tourette's syndrome. Ann Neurol 1983;14:638–641.
90. Messiha FS. Biochemical pharmacology of Gilles de la Tourette's syndrome. Neurosci Biobehav Rev 1988;12: 295–305.
91. Barbeau A. Cholinergic treatment in Tourette syndrome. N Engl J Med 1980;302:1310–1311.
92. Sandyk R. Cholinergic mechanisms in Gilles de la Tourette's syndrome. Int J Neurosci 1995;81:95–100.
93. Guyenet PG, Agid Y, Javoy F, Beaujouan JC, Rossier J, Glowinski J. Effects of dopaminergic receptor agonists and antagonists on the activity of neo-striatal cholinergic system. Brain Res 1975;84:227–244.
94. Tanner CM, Goetz CG, Klawans HL. Cholinergic mechanisms in Tourette's syndrome. Neurology 1982;32: 1315–1317.
95. Polinsky RJ, Ebert MH, Caine ED, Ludlow C, Bassich CJ. Cholinergic treatment in the Tourette's syndrome. N Engl J Med 1980;302:1310–1311.
96. Chappell PB, Riddle MA, Scahill L, et al. Guanfacine treatment of comorbid attention-deficit hyperactivity disorder and Tourette's syndrome: Preliminary clinical experience. J Am Acad Child Adolesc Psychiatry 1995;34(9): 1140–1146.
97. Jankovic J. Tics in other neurological disorders. In Dekker M (ed). Handbook of Tourette's Syndrome and Related Tic and Behavioral Disorders. New York; 1993:167–182.
98. Piacentini J, Woods DW, Scahill L, et al. Behavior therapy for children with Tourette disorder: a randomized controlled trial. JAMA 2010;303(19):1929–1937.
99. Franklin SA, Walther MR, Woods DW. Behavioral interventions for tic disorders. Psychiatr Clin of North Am 2010;33(3):641–655.
100. Himle MB, Woods DW, Piacentini JC, Walkup JT. Brief review of habit reversal training for Tourette syndrome. J Child Neurol 2006;21(8):719–725.
101. Wetterneck CT, Woods DW. An evaluation of the effectiveness of exposure and response prevention on repetitive behaviors associated with Tourette's syndrome. J Appl Behav Anal 2006;39(4):441–444.
102. Woods DW, Twohig MP, Flessner CA, Roloff TJ. Treatment of vocal tics in children with Tourette syndrome: investigating the efficacy of habit reversal. J Appl Behav Anal 2003;36(1):109–112.
103. Wilhelm S, Deckersbach T, Coffey B. Habit reversal versus supportive psychotherapy for Tourette's disorder: A randomized controlled trial. Am J Psychiatry 2003;160:1175–1177.
104. O'Connor KP, Laverdure A, Taillon A, Stip E, Borgeat F, Lavoie M. Cognitive behavioral management of Tourette's syndrome and chronic tic disorder in medicated and unmedicated samples. Behav Res Ther 2009;47(12):1090–1095.
105. Turpin G. The behavioral management of tic disorders: A critical review. Adv Behavior Res Ther 1983;5:203–245.
106. Savicki V, Carlin A. Behavioral treatment of Gilles de la Tourette syndrome. Int J Child Psychother 1972(1): 97–109.
107. Burd L, Kerbeshian J. Treatment-generated problems associated with behavior modification in Tourette disorder. Dev Med Child Neurol 1987;29(6):831–833.
108. Woods DW, Piacentini JC, Chang SW, et al. Managing Tourette Syndrome: A Behavioral Intervention for Children and Adults. Vol Therapist Guide, 1st ed. New York: Oxford University Press, 2008.
109. Peterson A, Azrin N. An evaluation of behavioral treatments for Tourette syndrome. Behav Res Ther 1992;30:167–174.
110. Peterson A, Campise R, Azrin N. Behavioral and pharmacological treatments for tic and habit disorders: A review. J Dev Behav Pediatr 1994;15:430–441.
111. Piacentini J, Chang S. Behavioral treatments for Tourette syndrome and tic disorders: State of the art. Adv Neurol 2001 2001;85:319–331.
112. Ghanizadeh A, Mosallaei S. Psychiatric disorders and behavioral problems in children and adolescents with Tourette syndrome. Brain Dev 2009;31(1):15–19.
113. Robertson MM, Eapen V. Pharmacologic controversy of CNS stimulants in Gilles de la Tourette's syndrome. Clin Neuropharmacol 1992;15:408–425.
114. Kurlan R. Treatment of attention-deficit hyperactivity disorder in children with Tourette's syndrome (TACT Trial). Ann Neurol 2000;48:953.
115. Tourette Syndrome Study Group. Treatment of ADHD in children with tics: a randomized controlled trial. Neurology 2002;58(4):527–536.
116. Spencer TJ, Sallee FR, Gilbert DL, et al. Atomoxetine treatment of ADHD in children with comorbid Tourette syndrome. J Atten Disord 2008;11(4):470–481.
117. Kurlan R. Tourette's syndrome: are stimulants safe? Curr Neurol Neurosci Rep 2003;3(4):285–288.
118. Gadow KD, Sverd J. Stimulants for ADHD in child patients with Tourette's syndrome: The issue of relative risk. J Dev Behav Pediatr 1990;11(5):269–271; discussion 272.
119. Jankovic J. Deprenyl in attention deficit associated with Tourette's syndrome. Arch Neurol 1993;50(3):286–288.
120. Bhatara VS, Carrera J. Medications for aggressiveness. J Am Acad Child Adolesc Psychiatry 1994;33(2):282–283.

121. Connor DF, Barkley RA, Davis HT. A pilot study of methylphenidate, clonidine, or the combination in ADHD comorbid with aggressive oppositional defiant or conduct disorder. Clin Pediatr 2000;39(1):15–25.
122. Rugino TA, Janvier YMCINJCNA, Pmid. Aripiprazole in children and adolescents: Clinical experience. J Child Neurol 2005;20(7):603–610.
123. Wilens TE, Spencer TJ, Swanson JM, Connor DF, Cantwell DCINJAACAPD, Pmid. Combining methylphenidate and clonidine: a clinically sound medication option. J Am Acad Child Adolesc Psychiatry 1999;38(5):614–619; discussion 619–622.
124. Como PG, Kurlan R. An open-label trial of fluoxetine for obsessive-compulsive disorder in Gilles de la Tourette's syndrome. Neurology 1991;41(6):872–874.
125. Kurlan R. Handbook of Tourette's Syndrome and Related Tic and Behavioral Disorders. New York: Marcel Dekker, 1993.
126. Kurlan JF, Kersun J, Ballantine HT Jr., Caine ED. Neurosurgical treatment of severe obsessive-compulsive disorder associated with Tourette's syndrome. Mov Disord 1990;5(2):152–155.
127. Robertson M, Doran M, Trimble M, Lees AJ. The treatment of Gilles de la Tourette syndrome by limbic leucotomy. J Neurol Neurosurg Psychiatry 1990;53(8):691–694.
128. Visser-Vandewalle V, Temel Y, Boon P, et al. Chronic bilateral thalamic stimulation: A new therapeutic approach in intractable Tourette syndrome. Report of three cases. J Neurosurg 2003;99(6):1094–1100.
129. Ackermans L, Temel Y, Cath D, et al. Deep brain stimulation in Tourette's syndrome: two targets? Mov Disord 2006;21(5):709–713.
130. Temel Y, Visser-Vandewalle V. Surgery in Tourette syndrome. Mov Disord 2004;19(1):3–14.
131. Servello D, Porta M, Sassi M, Brambilla A, Robertson MMCINJNNPF, Pmid. Deep brain stimulation in 18 patients with severe Gilles de la Tourette syndrome refractory to treatment: the surgery and stimulation. J Neurol Neurosurg Psychiatry 2008;79(2):136–142.
132. Maciunas RJ, Maddux BN, Riley DE, et al. Prospective randomized double-blind trial of bilateral thalamic deep brain stimulation in adults with Tourette syndrome. J Neurosurg 2007;107(5):1004–1014.
133. Porta M, Sassi M, Ali F, Cavanna AE, Servello D. Neurosurgical treatment for Gilles de la Tourette syndrome: The Italian perspective. J Psychosom Res 2009;67(6): 585–590.
134. Robertson M, Doran M, Trimble M, Less AJ. The treatment of Gilles de la Tourette syndrome by limbic leucotomy. J Neurol Neurosurg Psychiatry 1990;53:691–694.
135. Visser-Vandewalle V. DBS in tourette syndrome: Rationale, current status and future prospects. Acta Neurochir Suppl 2007;97(Pt 2):215–222.
136. Visser-Vandewalle V, Temel Y, van der Linden C, Ackermans L, Beuls E. Deep brain stimulation in movement disorders. The applications reconsidered. Acta Neurol Belg 2004;104(1):33–36.
137. Kuhn J, Gaebel W, Klosterkoetter J, Woopen C. Deep brain stimulation as a new therapeutic approach in therapy-resistant mental disorders: Ethical aspects of investigational treatment. Eur Arch Psychiatr Clin Neurosci 2009;259(Suppl 2):S135-S141.
138. Houeto JL, Karachi C, Mallet L, et al. Tourette's syndrome and deep brain stimulation. J Neurol Neurosurg Psychiatry 2005;76(7):992–995.
139. Welter ML, Mallet L, Houeto JL, et al. Internal pallidal and thalamic stimulation in patients with Tourette syndrome. Arch Neurol 2008;65(7):952–957.
140. Zabek M, Sobstyl M, Koziara H, Dzierzecki S. Deep brain stimulation of the right nucleus accumbens in a patient with Tourette syndrome. Case report. Neurol Neurochir Pol 2008;42(6):554–559.
141. Dueck A, Wolters A, Wunsch K, et al. Deep brain stimulation of globus pallidus internus in a 16-year-old boy with severe tourette syndrome and mental retardation. Neuropediatrics 2009;40(5):239–242.
142. Mink JW. Clinical review of DBS for Tourette Syndrome. Front Biosci 2009;1:72–76.
143. DeLong M, Wichmann T. Changing views of basal ganglia circuits and circuit disorders. Clinical EEG and neuroscience : official journal of the EEG and Clinical Neuroscience Society (ENCS). 2010;41(2):61–67.
144. Neuner I, Podoll K, Janouschek H, Michel TM, Sheldrick AJ, Schneider F. From psychosurgery to neuromodulation: deep brain stimulation for intractable Tourette syndrome. World J Biol Psychiatry 2009;10(4 Pt 2):366–376.
145. Okun MS, Fernandez HH, Foote KD, Murphy TK, Goodman WKCONJNNPF, Pmid. Avoiding deep brain stimulation failures in Tourette syndrome. J Neurol Neurosurg Psychiatry 2008;79(2):111–112.
146. Ackermans L, Temel Y, Visser-Vandewalle V. Deep brain stimulation in Tourette's Syndrome. Neurotherapeutics 2008;5(2):339–344.
147. Idris Z, Ghani AR, Mar W, et al. Intracerebral haematomas after deep brain stimulation surgery in a patient with Tourette syndrome and low factor XIIIA activity. J Clin Neurosci 2010;17(10):1343–1344.
148. Porta M, Servello D, Sassi M, et al. Issues related to deep brain stimulation for treatment-refractory Tourette's syndrome. Eur Neurol 2009;62(5):264–273.
149. Mink JW, Walkup J, Frey KA, et al. Patient selection and assessment recommendations for deep brain stimulation in Tourette syndrome. Mov Disord 2006;21(11): 1831–1838.
150. Bergman HT, Wichmann HT, Karmon B, DeLong MR. The primate subthalamic nucleus. II. Neuronal activity in the MPTP model of parkinsonism. J. Neurophysiol 1994;72:507–520.
151. DeLong MR. Primate models of movement disorders of basal ganglia origin. TINS 1990;13:281–285.

CHAPTER 40

The Molecular Genetics of the Ataxias

George R. Wilmot, S.H. Subramony, and Henry L. Paulson

The inherited ataxias are a group of disorders characterized by incoordination and loss of balance. Many are accompanied by other neurological symptoms depending on the extent to which pathology extends beyond the cerebellar circuitry. With few exceptions, they are progressive, neurodegenerative disorders that often lead to significant debilitation and death.

Recent years have seen dramatic advances in our understanding of the genetic causes of the inherited ataxias, and with that, our ability to diagnose and classify specific genetic conditions has greatly increased.[1–5] But the rapid rate of new discoveries also makes it difficult to keep abreast of the current "state of the art" in diagnosis, much less the myriad scientific advances in the field. In April 2009, a search of Online Mendelian Inheritance in Man (OMIM) at the NCBI website (http://www.ncbi.nlm.nih.gov/) returned 728 entries for the search word "ataxia." Clearly, this massive amount of information must be prioritized to understand it. As with other recent reviews,[2–4,6] here we address the primary ataxic disorders that are most clinically relevant based on their prevalence, ease of diagnosis, or response to treatment. Because this list is not exhaustive, other sources of information should be sought when necessary. Two very good online sources of frequently updated information are OMIM and Genetests (http://www.genetests.org/) a NIH funded Web site that provides information about genetic diseases including commercial and research based genetic testing. Genetests represents the single best site at which to find accurate, updated information on a wide range of hereditary ataxias.

▶ CLINICAL APPROACH

Although there is no set clinical approach to the inherited ataxias, most specialists tend to use similar strategies when evaluating and treating someone who presents with a gait disorder that might fall into this category of disease (see Fig. 40–1). As with most clinical algorithms, the approach outlined in Fig. 40–1 represents a post-hoc conceptualization of these strategies rather than a rigid procedural prescription.

DIAGNOSIS

After ensuring that the patient truly suffers from ataxia, diagnostic considerations turn to separating the inherited ataxias from acquired conditions that are potentially treatable. If there is a clear family history of the disease, an inherited cause should be suspected and then investigated after considering the inheritance pattern. Acquired causes include a number of structural, nutritional, endocrine, toxic, paraneoplastic, and inflammatory conditions, some of which can be easily identified and possibly treated (e.g., vitamin E deficiency). Of particular interest are those that are hard to distinguish from some of the inherited ataxias. Patients in this subgroup of acquired ataxia tend to have slowly developing symptoms, nonspecific magnetic resonance imaging (MRI) changes (e.g., cerebellar atrophy), and normal routine laboratory values. In this subgroup, it is often prudent to consider toxic causes, to look for "gluten ataxia" with antigliadin and antiendomyseal antibodies,[7,8] and to check antiglutamic acid decarboxylase antibodies, which can be associated with cerebellar degeneration even without symptoms of stiff-person syndrome. If there is no family history and the onset of symptoms is subacute, inherited causes are unlikely and consideration should turn towards paraneoplastic and other inflammatory conditions.

Is the patient's disease inherited? The answer to this important question is obvious when a strong family history is present. But what about the patient who has a negative family history? In this case, it is important to keep in mind the potential explanations for genetic etiologies presenting with a negative family history (Table 40–1). In taking a good family history, accurate information should be obtained on all relatives (alive and dead) in three generations; this should include questions about age at symptom onset and age at death, consanguinity, spontaneous abortions, ethnic origin, and of course inquiries into relevant symptoms. Broad-based questioning is best (i.e., asking about walking, balance and coordination rather than "ataxia"). Even within individual families, many inherited ataxias display wide phenotypic variation that can make detection of a positive family history difficult, so careful, detailed questioning is required.

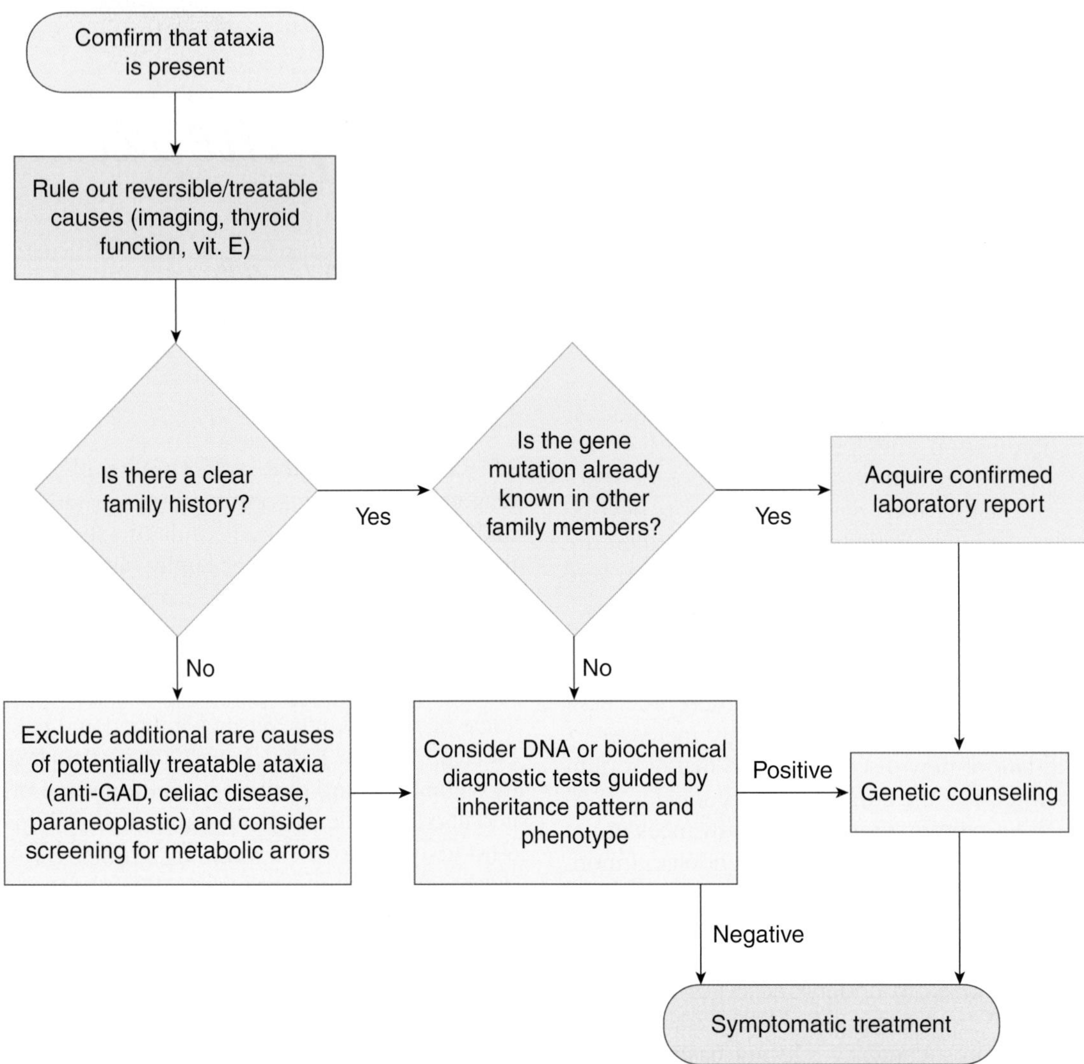

Figure 40–1. General clinical approach to the ataxic patient. GAD, glutamic acid decarboxylase.

One source of phenotypic variation in many inherited ataxias is genetic anticipation, which refers to an unusual feature of inheritance in which successive generations tend to become increasingly affected either through higher penetrance (the likelihood that a person possessing the mutation will have the disease) or higher expressivity (earlier age of onset or more severe disease). The molecular basis of genetic anticipation stems from the dynamic nature of expanded polynucleotide repeats, the type of mutation that underlies the most common hereditary ataxias (see Table 40–2). In most such diseases, the repeat expansion is an enlarged trinucleotide repeat that is prone to expand further upon germline transmission. Therefore, affected persons in successive generations tend to have earlier onset disease, sometimes even manifesting disease before the transmitting parent does. Particularly marked anticipation has been noted in spinocerebellar ataxia type 7 (SCA7), spinocerebellar ataxia type 2 (SCA2) and dentatorubropallidoluysian atrophy (DRPLA).

On average, only 1 out of 4 offspring will inherit an autosomal-recessive disease from their heterozygous

TABLE 40–1. REASONS FOR A NEGATIVE FAMILY HISTORY IN HEREDITARY DISORDERS

Inadequately obtained family history
Autosomal-recessive or X-linked inheritance
Reduced penetrance
Genetic anticipation
Phenotypic variability
New mutation
False paternity
Early death of affected relative

▶ TABLE 40–2. COMMERCIALLY AVAILABLE DNA TESTS FOR ATAXIAS CAUSED BY REPEAT EXPANSION DISEASES

Disease	Repeat Type	Normal Alleles	Disease-Causing Alleles	Comments
SCA1	CAG/polyQ	6–44	39–91	Intermediate alleles (36–44) should be tested for CAA interruptions
SCA2	CAG/polyQ	14–31	32–>400	Intermediate alleles (32–35) have reduced penetrance; 37–39 repeats most common
SCA3	CAG/polyQ	12–43	52–86	Low end of pathogenic range may not be associated with ataxia (45–51 reduced penetrance)
SCA6	CAG/polyQ	4–18	20–33	Expansions smaller than in other poly Q diseases
SCA7	CAG/polyQ	4–19	37–>400	34–36 repeat have reduce penetrance
SCA8	CTG/CAG	15–50	~75–>1300	Variable penetrance; highest penetrance with repeats of 80–250; bidirectional expression of repeat
SCA10	Intronic ATTCT	10–29	~800–4500	
SCA12	CAG	4–32	51–78	Possible bidirectional expression of expanded repeat
SCA17	CAG/polyQ	25–42	45–66	Reduced penetrance for repeats of 43–48
DRPLA	CAG/polyQ	6–35	49–93	
FRDA	Intronic GAA	5–33	66–1700	~95% have expansions on both alleles; remainder are compound heterozygotes (i.e. one expansion, one point mutation).
FXTAS	CGG	5–40	55–200	Premutation size repeat in FMR1 gene

carrier parents, thus the physician frequently does not obtain a positive family history in recessive disorders. By expanding the pedigree over many generations, the likelihood of identifying other family members with the disease increases, but practical limitations come into play and evidence of familial involvement can therefore be hard to find.

For many reasons, accurately diagnosing a progressive ataxia is important and helpful to affected persons. It can lead to specific therapy (if not now, then perhaps in the future), allow for accurate counseling (genetic, psychiatric, and prognostic) and provide greater peace of mind for the patient. Patients suffering from ataxia may have visited many physicians who were not able to establish a diagnosis, and so become frustrated by their mysterious condition, sometimes fearing the unknown (e.g., is this life threatening?) more than the actual disease itself. The value of accurate diagnosis should not be underestimated, even when no specific therapies exist for the potential diseases.

Should all patients with a progressive ataxic syndrome be genetically screened for known ataxia mutations? Opinions differ among ataxia experts, but one reasonable approach is outlined in Fig. 40–2. One factor driving this decision is that several studies of patients with sporadic ataxia found that 5–15% actually have one of the known ataxia-associated mutations, most commonly Friedreich's ataxia (FRDA) or SCA6.[9–12] While these study outcomes may be biased by referral patterns and the skill and knowledge of the examining neurologists, the important point that some patients with apparently sporadic ataxia actually have an inherited disease cannot be denied.

Table 40–2 outlines hereditary ataxias caused by dynamic repeat expansions for which commercial tests are currently available. Many other hereditary ataxias caused by "conventional" mutations also can be tested commercially. We caution that this list changes frequently. Thus, the reader is encouraged to visit Genetests (http://www.genetests.org/) for updates to this list, which inevitably will occur.

SYMPTOMATIC TREATMENT

Unlike extrapyramidal symptoms, ataxia rarely responds to pharmacological intervention. This should not be surprising, since motor coordination depends on the precise integration of multiple neural events and circuits

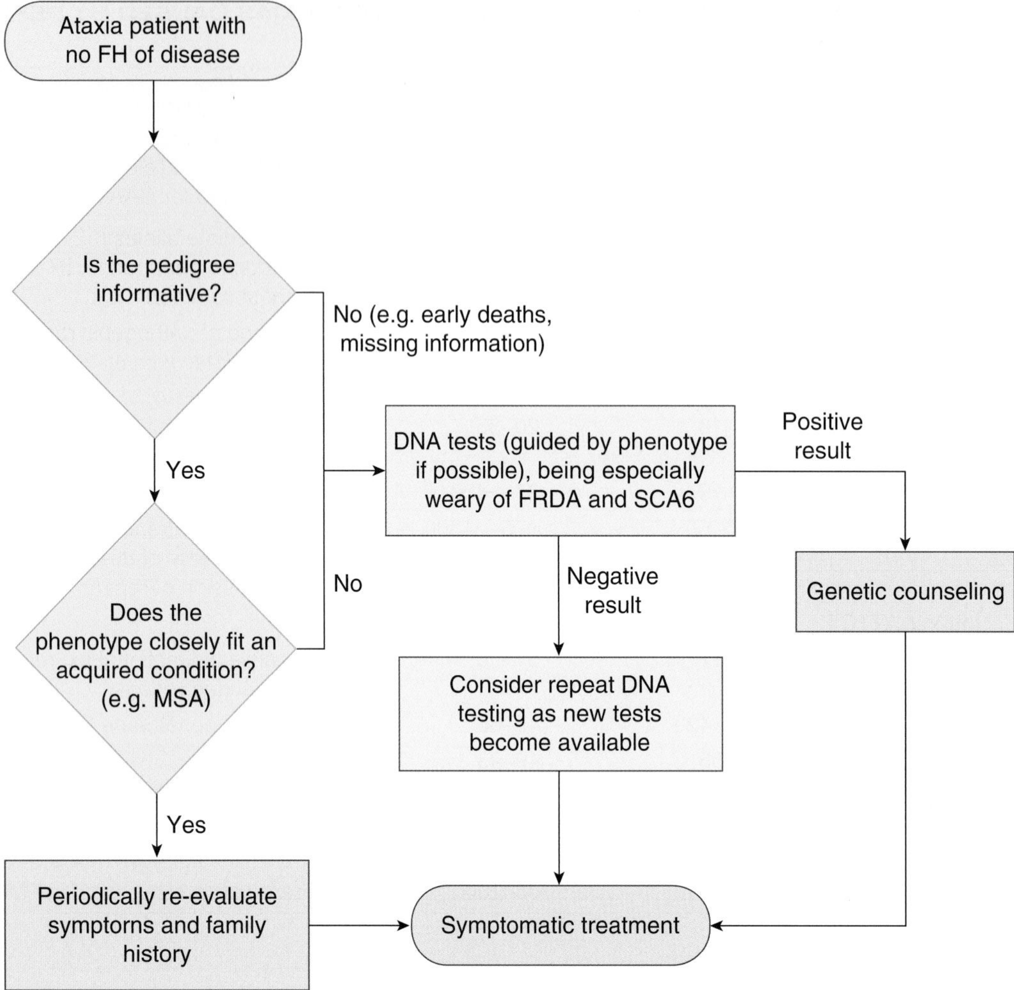

Figure 40–2. Strategy for DNA testing in ataxia patients without a family history of ataxia. MSA, multiple-system atrophy; FRDA, Friedreich's ataxia.

encompassing a variety of neurochemical systems. The limited reports showing the benefit of a particular agent ([13–16] reviewed in[2,17]) should be interpreted cautiously, taking into account the difficulties in accurately quantifying ataxia and the limited reproducibility of their findings.[18–20] An exciting exception is Friedreich ataxia, where insights into disease mechanisms are leading to therapy (reviewed later in this chapter). As more is learned about electrophysiological abnormalities in various hereditary ataxias, specific ion channels or signaling cascades may surface as molecular targets for symptomatic or preventive treatment.

Unlike ataxia, some of the associated neurological symptoms may respond well to currently available medications. Extrapyramidal symptoms accompany ataxia in a variety of ataxic syndromes, and these may respond to standard treatment with dopaminergic agents, anticholinergic medications, or botox injections.[21–23] Neurogenic urinary dysfunction occurs often and typically responds well to treatment with oxybutynin or tolterodine. Sleep disturbances, particularly restless legs syndrome, are common in the SCAs and usually respond to conventional treatment.[24,25]

Psychiatric disturbances should be sought in all ataxic patients and treated appropriately. Depression is common and often contributes significantly to lowered quality of life. Depending on the degree of disability, social difficulties may be significant and contribute markedly to affective dysfunction, so it is often imperative to include psychiatric counseling as part of the treatment. Psychosis and anxiety are less common, but when present should be treated as in any other patient.

SUPPORTIVE CARE AND REHABILITATION

Many different approaches may be required to maximize the daily functioning of an ataxic patient. Mobility is usually the prime issue, but swallowing function is often disturbed and requires careful monitoring and, potentially, intervention with a feeding tube. Evaluation and training for canes, walkers, and/or wheelchairs become necessary in most patients. Orthotics may be required, particularly in patients with superimposed weakness. Balance rehabilitation has been used successfully for vestibular disorders and may benefit ataxia as well.[26] It is unfortunate that so few studies have been published on balance rehabilitation in ataxia, especially in light of the dearth of pharmacological treatment options.

▶ COUNSELING

In addition to the general benefit of psychiatric counseling, genetic counseling can specifically address issues related to inherited ataxias. Many patients do not understand the genetic probabilities of passing on the disease and want to know more for family planning purposes. Should they adopt? Should their spouse be tested? Is prenatal diagnosis available? These are all important questions that can be addressed by a genetic counselor. One of the most confusing topics is whether presymptomatic testing should be sought in at-risk family members. Some issues are nearly identical between Huntington's disease (HD) and many of the most common autosomal dominant ataxias, since they share with HD the molecular pathogenic mechanism of expanded CAG repeats. An extensive literature exists on this topic in HD.[27,28]

▶ AUTOSOMAL-DOMINANT ATAXIAS

Years before the discovery of causative gene mutations, Harding coined the term "autosomal-dominant cerebellar ataxia" (ADCA), and defined ADCA subtypes based on clinical criteria (type 1, cerebellar signs with additional neurological features; type 2, with visual loss; type 3, pure cerebellar dysfunction).[29] Although the ADCA classification of dominant ataxias is still sometimes seen in the literature, the current scheme of SCA classification by genotype is much more informative and should be used in lieu of the ADCA classification.

Within the ataxia field, the term "spinocerebellar ataxia" (SCA) is usually reserved for the nonepisodic autosomal–dominant ataxias. We still do not know how many different gene mutations cause SCA, but at present nearly 30 loci and 18 causative genes have been found. In most populations, known gene mutations account for the majority of cases of SCA,[9,11,30–34] so that any newly discovered genes and loci will represent relatively rare causes of SCA. The relative prevalence of each type of SCA varies in different ethnic populations; for example, among SCA patients, SCA1, and SCA2 are seen much more frequently in the UK[31] than in Japan.[32] Recent evidence suggests that the relative prevalence of some of the repeat expansion SCAs among different populations may be explained by the frequency of large normal alleles, which presumably are more likely to expand into the pathogenic range.[34,35]

The high degree of phenotypic overlap between the SCAs limits the clinician's ability to predict genotype based on phenotype. Some clinical features tend to suggest specific SCAs (Table 40–3) and can be used to guide DNA testing, but the accuracy of this approach is currently limited. Continued systematic acquisition of detailed clinical features may eventually lead to increased accuracy.

Among the nonepisodic dominant ataxias, gene mutations have been identified for SCA1–3, 5–8, 10–17, 20, 27, and DRPLA. The first ataxias to be identified, and still the most common, are repeat expansion diseases. All but one of the dominantly inherited repeat expansion ataxias are caused by trinucleotide repeat expansions (the exception is SCA10 with its pentanucleotide expansion). More recently, "conventional" mutations (missense and frameshift mutations, and gene deletions) have been identified in specific dominant ataxias. The major episodic ataxias identified thus far, EA1 and EA2, are caused by point mutations in ion channel genes and share many characteristics with other channelopathies.[36]

SPINOCEREBELLAR ATAXIA TYPE 1 (SCA1)

Patients with this disorder most often present in the third or fourth decades of life, but a wide variation in age of onset may be seen, including juvenile onset. At the earliest stages, there may be only a mild gait imbalance but, with time, progressive gait and limb ataxia, dysarthria, and bulbar dysfunction ensue. Nystagmus is often present early in the disease, but eventually saccadic slowing and gaze palsies may develop and nystagmus may diminish. Likewise, hyperreflexia is most common early in the course of the disease and then later turn to hyporeflexia due to the development of peripheral neuropathy.[37–39] Mild extrapyramidal features such as chorea may develop in advanced patients, but these findings are usually less common and less severe than with SCA2 or SCA3. Cognitive impairment can also occur late in the disease.[40] Weakness and atrophy of the face and tongue occur along with severe dysphagia, and reflect a progressive bulbar dysfunction that is associated with significant morbidity and mortality, most often by way of respiratory failure. The duration of the disease from onset until death range from ~10–15 years.

In the past 15 years, there have been remarkable strides in our scientific understanding of the SCAs, with Orr, Zoghbi and their colleagues leading the way with their studies of SCA1. In 1993, Orr and colleagues identified an expansion of a normally polymorphic CAG repeat within the *ATXN1* gene as the disease-causing mutation in this disorder.[41] Because the CAG triplet codes for glutamine, the crucial molecular defect appears to be a toxic gain-of-function caused by an enlarged tract of

TABLE 40-3. CLINICAL FEATURES SUGGESTING SPECIFIC SCA GENOTYPES

Genotype	Phenotype
SCA1	Pyramidal signs, hypermetric saccades
SCA2	Slow saccades, hyporeflexia, tremor, occasional dementia
SCA3	High intrafamilial variability, extrapyramidal signs, gaze-evoked nystagmus, hypometric saccades, peripheral neuropathy, parkinsonism
SCA4	Sensory neuropathy, slow course
SCA5	Mild, slow progression, pure cerebellar
SCA6	Relatively pure cerebellar ataxia, downbeat nystagmus, episodic symptoms, slow progression
SCA7	Visual loss, slow saccades, dramatic anticipation
SCA8	Dorsal column sensation loss, pyramidal signs
SCA10	Seizures, dementia
SCA11	Mild ataxia
SCA12	Early tremor, dementia
SCA13	Short stature, mild mental retardation
SCA14	Myoclonus
SCA15/16	Mild, slow progression; tremor
SCA17	Dementia, extrapyramidal signs
DRPLA	Seizures, myoclonus, chorea, dementia, dramatic anticipation
EA1	Episodic ataxia (seconds to minutes), myokymia, no vertigo
EA2	Episodic ataxia and vertigo (minutes to hours), response to acetazolamide

glutamine residues within the encoded protein, ataxin-1. SCA1 and other diseases with glutamine repeat-coding CAG expansions are therefore sometimes referred to as "polyglutamine diseases."[42,43] Seven dominant ataxias represent polyglutamine diseases, all caused by entirely different disease proteins (see Fig. 40–3).

Ataxin-1 is believed to function as a nuclear corepressor that modulates gene expression.[44] Normal individuals have CAG lengths of 6–44 repeats. In normal alleles of 21 or more repeats, the CAG tract is interrupted 1–3 times by CAT triplets that code for histidine rather than glutamine.[45] In contrast, affected individuals have uninterrupted repeat sizes of 39–91 repeats.[41,46,47] As with the other inherited ataxias caused by repeat expansions, the relatively inexpensive DNA test for SCA1 utilizes the polymerase chain reaction (PCR) to amplify the repeat and determine its size. For individuals with intermediate-sized repeats (36–44), a specific restriction digestion of the PCR product can be utilized to test for the presence of CAA interruptions, thereby distinguishing normal from disease-associated alleles in this size range.[45] Uninterrupted repeat lengths of 36–38 have not yet been reported to cause the disease, but on transmission to offspring may expand into the disease-causing range.

While the details of SCA1 pathophysiology are not fully elucidated, polyglutamine expansion alters the conformational state of mutant ataxin-1, leading it to engage in altered protein interactions that ultimately prove deleterious to neurons.[48] Phosphorylation of the disease protein is essential for toxicity, thus one rational approach to therapy may be to inhibit the responsible kinase once it has been identified. Exploiting RNA interference to suppress mutant ataxin-1 expression is another possible route to preventive therapy, provided that RNAi delivery to the brain can be achieved safely and efficiently.[49] A recent trial in SCA1 knock-in mice showed a modest therapeutic benefit from lithium,[50] a drug with multiple potential modes of action; this intriguing finding has led to the current phase 1 tolerability study of lithium in SCA1 subjects.

SPINOCEREBELLAR ATAXIA TYPE 2 (SCA2)

This disease was first identified in the Cuban population,[51] but has subsequently been described in other populations. SCA2 has been found to be the most common autosomal-dominant ataxia in Italy,[52] the UK, and India;[53] in other populations it is less common.[30] Clinical variability is somewhat higher than with SCA1 but the clinical presentations often overlap.[37] Age of onset is centered around the fourth decade but varies widely. Ataxia and dysarthria are always present, but dramatically slowed saccadic velocities, tremor, chorea/dystonia, hyporeflexia, and dementia may also occur, particularly later in the course of the disease.[54]

SCA2 is caused by an expansion of a CAG repeat in the *ATXN2* gene.[55–57] Unlike most other triplet repeat diseases, the size of normal SCA2 alleles is not very polymorphic; approximately 95% of the normal alleles have either 22 or 23.

Intermediate-sized alleles (32–35 repeats) may or may not be pathogenic, and the factors that promote penetrance are poorly understood. One potential modifier of age of onset is polyQ repeat variation in the CACNA1A gene.[58] CAA interruptions of the SCA2 repeat occur, but for SCA2 these interruptions do not clearly distinguish normal and disease-associated alleles from within the intermediate range. The interruptions are CAA triplets, which, like CAG, encode glutamine and therefore will not alter the protein sequence. Uninterrupted

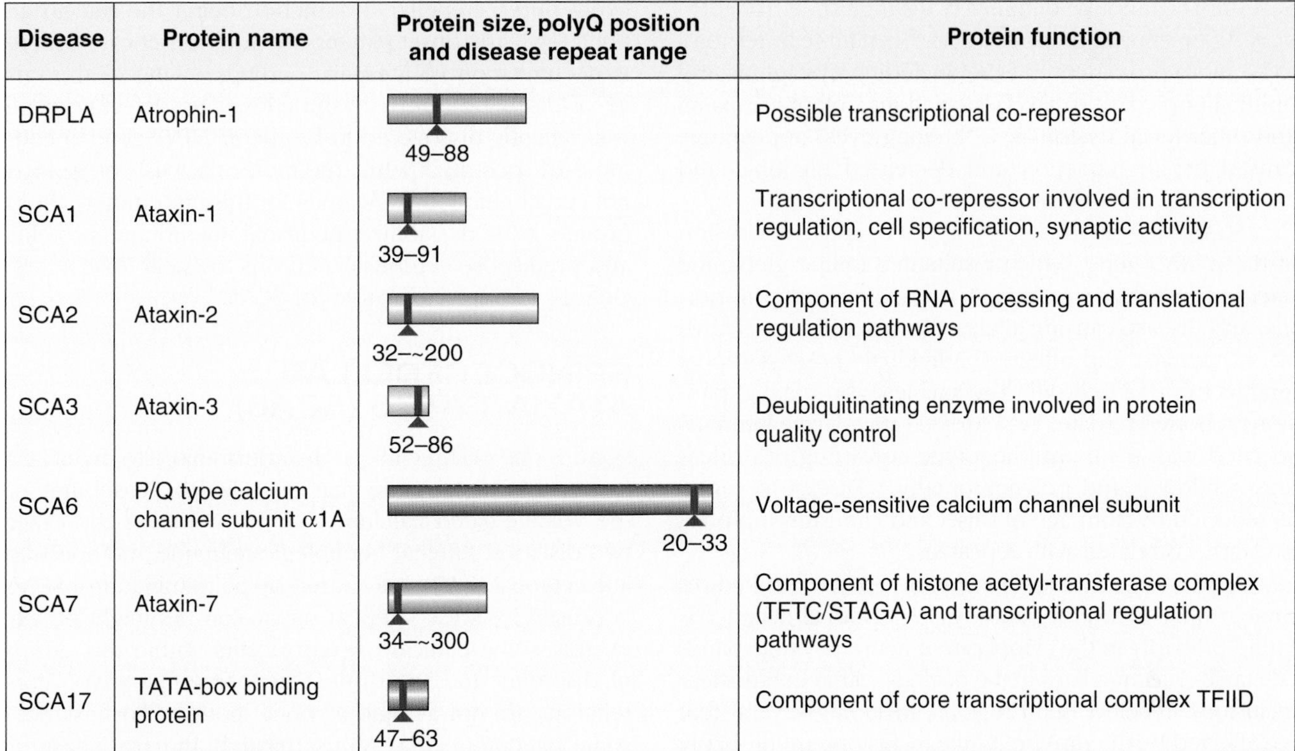

Disease	Protein name	Protein size, polyQ position and disease repeat range	Protein function
DRPLA	Atrophin-1	49–88	Possible transcriptional co-repressor
SCA1	Ataxin-1	39–91	Transcriptional co-repressor involved in transcription regulation, cell specification, synaptic activity
SCA2	Ataxin-2	32–~200	Component of RNA processing and translational regulation pathways
SCA3	Ataxin-3	52–86	Deubiquitinating enzyme involved in protein quality control
SCA6	P/Q type calcium channel subunit α1A	20–33	Voltage-sensitive calcium channel subunit
SCA7	Ataxin-7	34–~300	Component of histone acetyl-transferase complex (TFTC/STAGA) and transcriptional regulation pathways
SCA17	TATA-box binding protein	47–63	Component of core transcriptional complex TFIID

Figure 40–3. Polyglutamine ataxias. Shown are schematic illustrations of the disease proteins that contain expanded polyglutamine in the indicated SCAs. Red bar indicates the point in each protein where the expansion is found, below which the range of pathogenic repeats is indicated for each protein. As suggested by their differing colors, the disease causing proteins are unrelated.

repeats are likely to be more prone to expansion upon transmission to offspring, however.[59]

A largely cytoplasmic protein, the SCA2 disease protein ataxin-2 is associated with ER pathways and recently has been linked to RNA metabolism.[60] How the expansion alters its function is currently unknown. Early studies failed to find evidence of the nuclear inclusions found in most other polyglutamine diseases,[61] but more recent experiments have provided evidence of nuclear accumulation as well as nonubiquitinated microaggregates in the cytoplasm.

Expansions of 36 or more repeats are disease causing, and most often occur as uninterrupted repeats of 36–64 units long. Recently very large expansions (200–500) have been associated with severe early-onset disease. These very large expansions are difficult to detect with the standard SCA2 PCR test, but are identifiable with a southern blot assay.[62]

SPINOCEREBELLAR ATAXIA TYPE 3 (SCA3)/MACHADO-JOSEPH DISEASE (MJD)

MJD was initially described among Portuguese Azorean families as an autosomal-dominant degenerative ataxia with remarkable phenotypic variability.[63] After the identification of the responsible mutation,[64] it became clear that this disorder is in fact the same as SCA3, a separately described dominant ataxia originally thought to have less phenotypic variability.

In the early clinical descriptions of Portuguese MJD patients three phenotypes were identified: type 1 (spastic-rigid syndrome with bradykinesia and dystonia and relatively little ataxia), type 2 (the most common type, with ataxia and upper motor neuron signs), and type 3 (ataxia and peripheral neuropathy). A type 4 (relatively pure parkinsonism) has also been described.[22] In general, type 1 is more typical of early-onset patients and type 3 of later-onset patients. The usefulness of these distinctions is debatable since all types can occur within a single family and individuals may progress from one type to another. Nevertheless, their recognition highlights the significant clinical variability seen in this disease, often much more than in other SCAs.

The age of onset and disease duration in SCA3/MJD are similar to that in SCA1 and SCA2, although usually with more variability. Most SCA3/MJD patients present with early gait ataxia and dysarthria and progressively lose ambulation, eventually dying from respiratory problems related to their severe debilitation. Although

SCA3/MJD cannot be definitively distinguished from other SCAs on clinical grounds alone,[37] certain features tend to be more prominent in SCA3 including nystagmus and ophthalmoplegia, facial fasciculations, blepharospasm and other facial dystonias, a "bulging eyes" appearance caused by lid retraction and decreased blinking, and prominent parkinsonism.

SCA3/MJD is caused by a CAG repeat expansion in the *ATXN3* gene, which results in a longer glutamine tract in the ataxin-3 protein. There is no overlap in normal and disease-causing alleles; normal individuals have 12–43 repeats, and affected individuals possess repeat lengths from 52 to 86.[65,66] The smallest abnormal expansions reported to date, 52–54 repeat units, have been associated with a variant phenotype consisting of restless legs syndrome and polyneuropathy.[67] Disease severity, as reflected by both age of onset and clinical symptoms, is clearly correlated with repeat size.

Ataxin-3 is a deubiquitinating enzyme linked to protein quality control pathways.[1,43,68] Normal ataxin-3 is found primarily in the cytoplasm of neurons, but expanded ataxin-3 accumulates in the nucleus within intranuclear inclusions in select brain regions, including several that are affected by the disease. While inclusions are probably not directly pathogenic structures, they do suggest that a problem in protein accumulation and aggregation underlies toxicity. By virtue of its ubiquitin-linked activities, normal ataxin-3 also localizes to nuclear inclusions seen in other disease states and in the normal aging process.

SPINOCEREBELLAR ATAXIA TYPE 4 (SCA4)

This rare SCA follows a relatively benign course characterized by ataxia and a sensory axonal neuropathy.[69] Pyramidal signs may also be present. As with other inherited neuropathies, patients often have minimal symptoms despite significant EMG/NCS abnormalities and physical examination findings of sensory loss. The responsible gene is unknown but has been localized to 16q22.1.[69] Since the causative gene mutation still has not yet been found, the only way to confirm a diagnosis of SCA4 is through linkage analysis. A Japanese family with a pure cerebellar syndrome localizing to the same region has been reported,[69,70] so sensory neuropathy may not be universal in this disease.

SPINOCEREBELLAR ATAXIA TYPE 5 (SCA5)

This ataxia has been referred to as "Lincoln ataxia" because it was described in a family descended from the grandparents of President Lincoln.[71] Though rare, it has also been described in an additional French family.[72] The onset of SCA5 is usually in the third to fourth decade and the clinical course is typically slow, with relatively pure cerebellar dysfunction being the rule in all but a few early onset patients. In adult-onset cases, there is no limitation of lifespan, perhaps owing to the rarity of disabling bulbar dysfunction. The defective gene was recently discovered to be the *SPTBN2* gene encoding ß-III spectrin.[73] While the molecular basis of SCA5 is not certain, haploinsufficiency for this important scaffold protein may destabilize neuronal membrane proteins and predispose cerebellar neurons to excitotoxic stress. Genetic testing is available for SCA5.

SPINOCEREBELLAR ATAXIA TYPE 6 (SCA6)

SCA6 is one of three allelic disorders linked to mutations in the CACNA1A gene that encodes the α-subunit of the voltage-gated calcium channel. Whereas the other two diseases, familial hemiplegic migraine and episodic ataxia type 2 (EA2), are caused by point mutations, SCA6 is caused by a CAG repeat expansion. As might be expected, some clinical overlap occurs within this group of disorders and the distinct genotype-phenotype correlations are not as rigid as once thought. For instance, some patients with SCA6 go through an early phase of episodic symptoms that can include tinnitus, nausea, vertigo, ataxia, dysarthria, and visual disturbances prior to the development of progressive ataxia.[74,75] Episodic symptoms may persist into the progressive phase. In addition, EA2 patients often have interictal signs of cerebellar dysfunction that can worsen over time.

SCA6 is usually a pure cerebellar syndrome. More widespread dysfunction can occur, however, especially in patients with long-standing disease.[76] Therefore, findings such as ophthalmoplegia, sensory disturbances, reflex changes, and extrapyramidal features do not exclude a diagnosis of SCA6. Although there is some overlap between the SCAs, the eye movement abnormalities of SCA6 include prominent nystagmus (often downbeat) and saccadic pursuits,[77] which may suggest a diagnosis of SCA6. SCA6 is significantly more common than SCA4 or SCA5 and therefore is most likely to be the correct diagnosis in patients with pure cerebellar features.

After FRDA, SCA6 is the most commonly found gene mutation when apparently sporadic ataxia cases are genetically screened (~5% of cases).[76,78–80] This likely reflects the typically mild features, episodic tendencies, and late onset of SCA6, all of which can allow a positive family history to go unnoticed. New mutations are probably not a strong contributor to the prevalence of SCA6 among sporadic cases; indeed, cases of bona fide new SCA6 mutations are so rare as to be reportable.

SCA6 differs from the other common SCAs (e.g., SCAs 1, 2, 3, 8) in certain respects. The age of onset in SCA6 tends to be later and the course more benign. In addition, since the affected gene is an ion channel subunit and polyglutamine expansion may affect channel function, clinical features of a channelopathy (e.g., episodic symptoms) may contribute to the phenotype. The pathologically expanded CAG repeat is shorter than other SCA gene expansions and is much more stably transmitted between generations. With regard to molecular features of SCA6, the disease protein is membrane-bound rather than cytoplasmic or nuclear, as in the other SCAs. The mechanism underlying disease may include alterations in channel properties and abnormal accumulation and/or proteolysis of the mutant protein within Purkinje cells.[81,82]

SPINOCEREBELLAR ATAXIA TYPE 7 (SCA7)

The distinguishing, nonataxic feature of SCA7 is a progressive retinopathy that leads to blindness. The process starts as a macular degeneration with a pigmented central core extending into the periphery with time. When it does begin, visual failure is in the central field and night vision is spared. Dyschromotopsia in the blue-yellow axis can be found years before symptomatic visual failure.

Other than retinopathy, the neurological features of SCA7 overlap with those of other SCAs. In one large series of SCA7 patients, ataxia, dysarthria, decreased visual acuity, upper motor neuron signs, vibratory sensory loss, and eye movement abnormalities (typically slowed saccades, and ophthalmoplegia) were seen in most patients. Axonal neuropathy, auditory impairment, rigidity, and dementia were also present in at least 10% of the patients. Nystagmus and hyporeflexia were seen in less than 5% of cases.

The SCA7 repeat displays greater meiotic instability than does any other polyglutamine disease repeat.[83] Particularly with paternal transmission, an average gain of more than 20 repeats occurs between generations.[101] Very large expansions can occur through paternal transmission, causing severe infantile disease with cardiac involvement and early death.[84] Survival after disease onset can range from a few months in these infantile cases to over 30 years in adult patients with small expansions.[83]

The SCA7 gene encodes the protein ataxin-7,[17,85] which is one component of a transcriptional complex that regulates gene expression. As with many other polyglutamine diseases, nuclear inclusion bodies have been observed in the SCA7 brain but their role in pathogenesis is unclear.

SPINOCEREBELLAR ATAXIA TYPE 8 (SCA8)

Some intrigue and controversy surround SCA8, largely due to its unusual mutational features and its variable penetrance.[86,87] The disorder usually does not limit lifespan, and patients often exhibit upper motor neuron signs and vibration sense loss in addition to ataxia and dysarthria.[88,89]

The mutation associated with SCA8 is an unstable CAG/CTG repeat that occurs at the 3′ end of a fully processed RNA transcript that does not encode a known protein.[90] The repeat is very unstable upon intergenerational transmission and can expand by hundreds of repeats when maternally inherited.[89] In contrast, paternal transmission tends to result in contractions. The repeat may be expressed in both directions hence we report it as a CAG/CTG repeat.

Several studies have now shown that large SCA8 expansions can occur in unaffected controls as well as in unaffected family members of ataxia patients harboring SCA8 expansions.[89,91] This nonabsolute segregation of the expansion with the disease implies either that the SCA8 repeat is not itself pathogenic or that other factors affect its penetrance. Haplotype analysis favors the latter interpretation, although controversy will probably remain until those factors are clearly defined. Importantly, not all SCA8 expansions are associated with progressive ataxia. Thus, one needs to use caution when interpreting a positive SCA8 gene test result. The mechanism of pathogenesis in SCA8 is debated, with recent studies suggesting bidirectional expression across the repeat leading both to an RNA-mediated toxicity and to a protein (polyglutamine) mediated toxicity.[92]

SPINOCEREBELLAR ATAXIA TYPE 10 (SCA10)

SCA9 has not been assigned, so the next dominant ataxia is SCA10. Published reports initially found SCA10 only in the Mexican population,[93] but it has since been recognized in other parts of the world.[94,95] SCA10 may present a pure cerebellar syndrome with seizures, but pyramidal signs, ocular dyskinesia, cognitive impairment, and polyneuropathy have also been described.[96] In addition, affected members of one family had cardiac, hepatic, and hematological manifestations in addition to ataxia. The responsible mutation is an ATTCT pentanucleotide repeat expansion that occurs in the intron of the *ATXN10* gene.[93,95] The mutation can reach phenomenally large lengths (up to 4500 repeats), larger than other known microsatellite expansion. In a study of two SCA10 families manifesting with distinct seizure frequencies,[94] one displayed uninterrupted ATTCT expansions, while in the second family the expansion was interrupted by nonconsensus repeat units differing in length and sequence. This finding challenges the convention that disease-causing microsatellite expansions consist only of uninterrupted pure repeats and suggests that the purity of the expanded repeat element may be a disease modifier in SCA10. The pathophysiology of SCA10 may relate to other disorders in which the repeat expansions reside in nontranslated portions of the transcript.

SPINOCEREBELLAR ATAXIA TYPE 11 (SCA11)

A mild ataxia with hyperreflexia has been described in two British families and localized to chromosome 15q14-21.3.[97] This SCA represents a relatively "pure" cerebellar syndrome with mild pyramidal signs. The genetic basis was recently discovered to be mutations in the tau tubulin kinase gene, TTBK2.[98] Genetic testing is available for SCA11.

SPINOCEREBELLAR ATAXIA TYPE 12 (SCA12)

Patients with SCA12 typically present with limb tremor in their fourth decade and then progress to develop cerebellar dysfunction and ultimately dementia. The responsible mutation has been identified as a CAG repeat expansion in the 5 region of the gene PPP2R2B, which encodes a brain-specific regulatory subunit of the protein phosphatase PP2A.[99,100] Nonaffected control alleles possess 9–31 repeats, and pathogenic alleles range from 55 to 78 repeats. SCA12 has been found to be very rare in most populations,[59,101,102] but it is one of the more common SCAs in India.[103] The mechanism by which the expansion causes disease is unknown, and may involve bidirectional expression across the repeat. PPP2R2B recently was shown to be a proapoptotic factor that mediates stress-induced mitochondrial fission in neurons. Conceivably, then, an imbalance in levels of this protein might contribute to disease pathogenesis.

SPINOCEREBELLAR ATAXIA TYPE 13 (SCA13)

This rare, dominant ataxia has a widely varied age of onset, including in childhood, with delayed motor development and mental retardation being part of the clinical picture in some affected persons.[104] The ataxia is accompanied by dysarthria, nystagmus, and occasionally hyperreflexia. The MRI usually shows cerebellar and pontine atrophy. SCA13 is caused by mutations in the KCNC3 gene encoding a voltage-gated potassium channel subunit.[105] Genetic testing is available for SCA13.

SPINOCEREBELLAR ATAXIA TYPE 14 (SCA14)

Although SCA14 is not caused by an expanded repeat, it still shows wide phenotypic variability.[43,106] Most affected individuals develop slowly progressive ataxia with dysarthria in early adulthood. In late onset cases, SCA14 can manifest as a relatively pure cerebellar ataxia. In earlier onset cases, however, the ataxia can be accompanied by facial myokymia, hyperreflexia, axial myoclonus, dystonia, and vibratory sensory loss. SCA14 is usually compatible with a normal life span, though affected persons can become wheelchair-bound. SCA14 is caused by mutations in the PRKCG gene encoding a serine-threonine protein kinase, PKC-gamma. Genetic testing is available for SCA14, but in contrast to the expanded repeat ataxias, SCA14 gene testing requires sequencing of all exons and flanking sequences in the disease gene.

SPINOCEREBELLAR ATAXIA TYPE 15/16 (SCA15/16)

It recently became clear that these two diseases are allelic (i.e., the mutation is in the same gene so they are the same disease). It is a slowly progressive, pure cerebellar ataxia described in Australian and Japanese families.[107] Dysarthria, horizontal gaze-evoked nystagmus, and impaired smooth movement of the eyes are present in some patients, and roughly one third of the patients have a head tremor. SCA15/16 is caused by mutations in the IPTR gene.[108] IP3 receptors are abundantly expressed in cerebellar Purkinje cells, where they are likely important to electrophysiological properties and calcium homeostasis. Currently, only research based genetic testing is available for SCA15/16.

SPINOCEREBELLAR ATAXIA TYPE 17 (SCA17)

Even in the early days of the polyglutamine disease story it was recognized that certain proteins, including many transcription factors, normally possess polyglutamine tracts. In fact, an antibody raised to one of these proteins, TATA-binding protein (TBP), was found to recognize the expanded polyglutamine tracts in many SCA mutant proteins and has been utilized by researchers for many purposes, including the discovery of new SCA genes. As might be expected, the TBP gene was kept in mind as a candidate gene when new SCAs were sought, and in 1999, a patient was described in which a polyglutamine expansion in TBP appeared to be the causative mutation.[109] Additional families in Japan and many other countries have since been confirmed to have this mutation.[34,110]

Originally described in Japan, SCA17 is rare in the United States. More than any other known SCA, SCA17 manifests with widespread cerebral and cerebellar dysfunction. Affected persons typically present in young to mid-adulthood with progressive gait and limb ataxia that is usually accompanied by dementia, psychiatric symptoms, and varying extrapyramidal features including parkinsonism, tremor, dystonia, and occasional chorea. In some cases, ataxia is not even the most prominent feature. Seizures have been reported in some patients. Consistent with the more global neurological phenotype, the MRI findings in SCA17 include diffuse cerebral and cerebellar atrophy. The ataxia of SCA17 is accompanied by greater intellectual decline and extrapyramidal features (bradykinesia and dystonia) than other SCAs. In some cases, SCA17 can even resemble Huntington disease.

SPINOCEREBELLAR ATAXIA TYPE 18 (SCA18)

An Irish American family was reported with a progressive ataxic disorder with prominent motor and sensory features.[111] Age of onset in this family occurs in the second and third decades, with gait difficulty being the most common initial symptom. Other features included dysmetria, hyporeflexia, muscle weakness and atrophy, and decreased vibratory and proprioceptive sense. The disease gene has not been identified for this disorder,[111] termed by the authors as "sensorimotor neuropathy with ataxia" or SMNA.

SPINOCEREBELLAR ATAXIA TYPE 19 (SCA19)

In the Dutch family in which this SCA was identified, affected individuals displayed a late onset, slowly progressive cerebellar ataxia with hyporeflexia, frontal lobe dysfunction, and occasional postural head tremor and myoclonic movements. The genetic locus, mapped to a broad region of chromosome 1,[112] overlaps with the locus for SCA22, suggesting that these two SCAs may be due to mutations in the same gene.

SPINOCEREBELLAR ATAXIA TYPE 20 (SCA20)

Reported in a single Australian family, SCA20 has a distinctive, slowly progressive phenotype with dysarthria rather than gait ataxia as the initial symptom, accompanied by palatal tremor, hypermetric saccades, and early dentate calcification in the cerebellum. Recently a 260-kb duplication on chromosome 11 was discovered as the apparent genetic defect.[113] This represents the first genomic duplication as a cause of ataxia. Currently, only research-based genetic testing is available for SCA20.

SPINOCEREBELLAR ATAXIA TYPE 21 (SCA21)

SCA21 was reported in a French family in whom affected members showed variable symptoms of cerebellar ataxia, limb ataxia and akinesia, dysarthria, dysgraphia, hyporeflexia, postural tremor, rigidity, resting tremor, cognitive impairment, and cerebellar atrophy. The locus has been mapped to chromosome 7 but the disease gene has not been found.[114]

SPINOCEREBELLAR ATAXIA TYPE 22 (SCA22)

The chromosome 1 locus for SCA22 overlaps with that of SCA19, suggesting that they could be due to mutations in the same gene (neither disease gene has been found). In the reported family,[115] all affected individuals had a slowly progressive, pure cerebellar ataxia with variable dysarthria and hyporeflexia, with age of onset ranging from 10 to 46 years. MRI has shown homogeneous cerebellar atrophy without brainstem involvement.

SPINOCEREBELLAR ATAXIA TYPE 23 (SCA23)

In the single Dutch family in which this ataxia has been reported, disease manifests as a late onset, slowly progressive, isolated ataxia.[116] The disease locus maps to chromosome 20 but the disease gene has not been identified.

SPINOCEREBELLAR ATAXIA TYPE 24 (SCA25)

The cerebellar ataxia in SCA25 is associated with a severe sensory neuropathy and has shown intrafamilial variability, including a Friedreich ataxialike syndrome in some members of the French family in which it has been identified. SCA25 has been mapped to chromosome 2p,[117] but the disease gene has not yet been found.

SPINOCEREBELLAR ATAXIA TYPE 26 (SCA26)

This form of ataxia was identified in kindred of Norwegian ancestry with pure cerebellar ataxia. All affected family members have slowly progressive cerebellar ataxia, with age of onset ranging from 26 to 60 years. Brain MRI has shown atrophy confined to the cerebellum, and neuropathological findings have revealed isolated Purkinje cell degeneration. The locus maps to 19p13.3, near the disease genes for Cayman ataxia and SCA6, but the disease gene has not yet been identified.[118]

SPINOCEREBELLAR ATAXIA TYPE 27 (SCA27)

This early onset ataxia was initially described in a Dutch family. Affected individuals manifest first with hand tremor in childhood followed by progressive ataxia, cognitive difficulties, and psychiatric problems in the second and third decades of life. A heterozygous mutation was found in the *FGF14* gene encoding fibroblast growth factor 14.[119] A second mutation in FGF14 has been reported in a young man with mental retardation and ataxia. In FGF knockout mice, which are ataxic, cerebellar Purkinje neurons have reduced spontaneous firing associated with reduced expression of the sodium channel protein, Nav1.6.[120] Together, these observations suggest that deficiency of FGF14 impairs spontaneous and repetitive firing in Purkinje neurons by altering the expression of sodium channels. Genetic testing is available for SCA27.

SPINOCEREBELLAR ATAXIA TYPE 28 (SCA28)

The SCA28 locus has been mapped to chromosome 18p11.22 in an Italian family. Affected individuals develop juvenile onset, slowly progressive ataxia, dysarthria, hyperreflexia, nystagmus, and ophthalmoparesis. The causative gene may have been found at the time of writing [121], though this requires confirmation.

DENTATORUBROPALLIDOLUYSIAN ATROPHY (DRPLA)

DRPLA is characterized by wide phenotypic variability that encompasses ataxia, myoclonus, choreoathetosis, psychiatric disturbances, epilepsy, and dementia. The age of presentation correlates with the clinical features. Patients with onset before age 20 nearly always have seizures and often display a progressive myoclonic epilepsy phenotype. In contrast, older onset individuals typically develop ataxia with choreoathetosis and dementia. DRPLA is most prevalent in Japan and the second most common dominant ataxia in Portugal, yet quite rare in the United States. One well-characterized African American family in North Carolina has a phenotypic variant known as the Haw River Syndrome, in which seizures and cerebral calcifications accompany the ataxia.

The disease is most commonly seen in Japan, but rare cases are seen in other populations[32,35,122] Like SCA7, DRPLA can show marked anticipation, particularly with paternal transmission.[123] This anticipation is consistent with the mutation, an unstable CAG expansion that results in a polyglutamine expansion in the atrophin-1 protein,[124,125] Atrophin-1 is a nuclear receptor corepressor that regulates gene expression.[126] Ubiquitinated neuronal intranuclear inclusions containing the mutant protein are seen in the disease, as in other polyglutamine diseases, but these represent only part of the story explaining pathogenesis.[127]

EPISODIC ATAXIA TYPE 1 (EA1)

EA1 typically presents during childhood or adolescence and is characterized by brief attacks of ataxia lasting seconds to minutes that are often precipitated by startle or exercise.[36] Vertigo is not present. Interictal myokymia is also a feature of the disease, which is caused by mutations (usually missense) in the voltage-gated potassium channel gene KCNA1.[40] Mutations in this gene can also cause isolated myokymia, myokymia with partial epilepsy, and EA with partial epilepsy. Some patients with EA1 benefit from treatment with acetozolamide, phenytoin, or carbamazepine.

EPISODIC ATAXIA TYPE 2 (EA2)

EA2 is caused by mutations in the CACNA1A gene encoding the α1A voltage-dependent calcium channel subunit.[128] It is distinguished from EA1 by longer episodes of ataxia and dysarthria that also can include vertigo, nausea, oscillopsia, and diplopia. Mild interictal abnormalities in cerebellar function exist and usually progress with time in accord with the progressive midline cerebellar atrophy that occurs in the disease. Although startle does not precipitate attacks, physical and emotional stress may do so, and alcohol and caffeine can increase the likelihood of an attack. Acetazolamide is helpful in reducing the frequency and severity of attacks.[129]

Two other disorders are caused by mutations in the CACNA1A gene: SCA6 and familial hemiplegic migraine (FHM). EA2 mutations appear to cause a loss of P/Q-type calcium channel activity, usually by truncation,[130] whereas FHM mutations are typically missense, and SCA6 is caused by a polyglutamine expansion. The distinction between these disorders is somewhat blurred by clinical overlap. That is to say, FHM patients can have mild cerebellar atrophy, EA2 patients can have migraines, and SCA6 patients can have episodic symptoms.

OTHER AUTOSOMAL-DOMINANT ATAXIAS

Ataxia may be a prominent feature of other dominantly inherited diseases. Specific neurodegenerative causes that should be kept in mind include certain prion diseases[131,132] and certain hereditary spastic paraplegias.[133] Nondegenerative, dominantly inherited diseases (e.g., Von Hippel-Lindau syndrome) may also present with ataxia.

▶ AUTOSOMAL-RECESSIVE ATAXIAS

FRIEDREICH'S ATAXIA (FRDA)

FRDA is the most common known inherited ataxia,[134–136] with a prevalence estimated at approximately 1:30,000–50,000 among Caucasians. Because of a founder effect of the ancestral mutation, the disease is almost exclusively found among people of European, North African, Middle Eastern, and Indian descent.[137] Before the discovery of the FRDA gene mutation the clinical features of the disease were believed to be rather homogeneous: progressive ataxia with onset before age 25, dysarthria within 5 years from onset, areflexia in lower limbs, extensor plantar responses, and neurophysiological evidence of an axonal sensory neuropathy, often with vibration and/or proprioceptive sensation loss.[138] While these features are still found in most FRDA patients, the availability of a specific gene test has extended the phenotype to include unusual features such as late onset (even up to the sixth and seventh decades), hyperreflexia, and spastic ataxia.[134,139] Because of this widened phenotype, genetic testing for FRDA should not be reserved for early-onset classic cases, but rather should be performed in most cases of otherwise unexplained ataxia. Currently, FA is highest on the list of recessively inherited ataxias that a physician needs to consider carefully when evaluating an adult with slowly progressive ataxia of unknown origin without a family history of similar disease.

Extraneuronal manifestations of FRDA include cardiomyopathy, diabetes, and scoliosis. The extent of cardiomyopathy varies greatly from patient to patient, but it is likely that virtually every patient with FRDA has microscopic cardiac pathology. Electrocardiographic (ECG) changes (most often aberrant repolarization) are common but not universal and do not correlate well with cardiac hypertrophy, the most common form of cardiomyopathy.[140] Although symptoms of overt heart failure are seen in only ~10–15% of patients, a higher percentage would likely be seen if it were not for the limited mobility of patients with advanced FRDA. Long-standing disease is clearly associated with more severe cardiac involvement.[141] At the time of diagnosis, all FRDA patients should have an ECG and echocardiogram, and these should be repeated every few months to few years depending on the extent of disease. Mild glucose intolerance has been reported in approximately 50% of FRDA patients and diabetes in 20%, but these percentages are likely to be overestimates because ascertainment of atypically mild or late-onset FRDA was impossible prior to the gene test. Interestingly, carriers of the FRDA gene mutation show increased incidence of glucose intolerance, although they have no neurological or cardiac abnormalities.

The mutation implicated in FRDA is a GAA expansion in intron 1 of the *FXN* gene,[142] which encodes the mitochondrial protein frataxin. The expansion causes much less frataxin to be produced in FRDA patients.[143] Most patients are homozygous for the expansion, but ~3–4% is compound heterozygotes with an expansion on one allele and a point mutation on the other.[144] In an adult ataxic patient with no other identifiable cause of ataxia, the presence of a single FA expansion should lead the physician to consider sequencing of the FXN gene to exclude a rare point mutation in the second allele.

A great deal of research has sought to define the pathophysiology of FRDA.[136,145–147] Frataxin deficiency leads to abnormal intracellular iron metabolism, defects in oxidative phosphorylation, increased oxidant stress, and alterations in the synthesis of iron–sulfur cluster proteins.[148–150] that are essential for electron transport in mitochondria. Accordingly, many treatment efforts have focused on antioxidant therapy. Idebenone, an antioxidant analogue of coenzyme Q_{10}, has shown benefit in numerous trials, particularly for the cardiomyopathy.[151–157] This medication should be offered to all FRDA patients. A combination of coenzyme Q_{10} (400 mg/day) and vitamin E (2100 mg/day) also appeared to reduce the metabolic abnormalities in muscles of FRDA patients, but whether combination treatment with these or other agents will be beneficial in FRDA is not yet known.[152,157]

ATAXIA TELANGIECTASIA (AT)

Ataxia telangiectasia (AT) is probably the second most common cause of early onset progressive ataxia and one of several ataxia disorders caused by mutations that impair DNA repair.[158,159] Usually presenting early in childhood, AT is characterized by telangiectasias, immune deficiencies, and a predisposition to malignancy in addition to the progressive neurological deficits.[159,160] The disease usually results in wheelchair dependence by the 2nd decade and death by early adulthood, most often by recurrent sinopulmonary infections and/or lymphoreticular malignancy.[161] Survival into mid- to late adulthood can occur rarely.

Neurologically, patients usually present with progressive ataxia and dysarthria with facial hypotonia and drooling. Oculomotor abnormalities occur relatively early and are characterized by difficulties in initiating voluntary eye movements (oculomotor apraxia) and fixation instability. Other abnormalities may then develop such as myoclonic jerking, dystonia and/or choreoathetosis, upgoing toes, and dorsal column sensory loss. Later signs may include areflexia and muscle atrophy, indicating peripheral nerve and lower motor neuron involvement. Cognitive function appears to be minimally affected.[162]

The nonneurological features of AT can aid greatly in the diagnosis of this disorder. Oculocutaneous telangiectasias occur in over 95% of patients, typically 2–4 years after the onset of ataxia. α-Fetoprotein (AFP) levels are usually elevated and variable immunodeficiencies occur as a result of incomplete development of the thymus.[162] Recurrent sinopulmonary infections commonly result from the immunodeficiency. Malignancies occur in almost 40% of AT patients, of which 85% are leukemia or lymphoma.[161] Endocrine defects, including gonadal abnormalities and insulin-resistant diabetes, may be seen, and signs of accelerated aging ("progeria") can also be present. Radiation sensitivity occurs and can be assayed in cell culture. These clinical features, supported by laboratory evaluation of AFP levels, immunodeficiency, and sometimes characteristic chromosomal abnormalities,[163] are relied upon to establish the diagnosis. Because of the large size of the affected gene and the large number of known mutations, direct genetic testing is not routinely performed except in certain populations that have high probability of founder mutations.

Disease manifestations in AT are a consequence of the cellular and molecular defects that exist in patients with loss-of-function mutations in the ATM gene. The ATM gene product is a protein kinase that serves as a master regulator of the cellular response to certain kinds of DNA damage.[159] AT cells are defective in recognizing and repairing double-strand breaks and therefore do not adequately initiate repair. As a result, problems with DNA replication, altered cell cycle checkpoints, and abnormalities in apoptosis lead to the malignant transformation and neurodegeneration seen in disease. Heterozygote carriers may be at increased risk for solid tumors even though they display no neurological phenotype.[164]

There is no specific treatment for the primary abnormality of AT, but many secondary clinical features will respond to conventional therapy. Because of the fundamental cellular and molecular defects of the disease, special care needs to be taken in AT patients (e.g., immunization with killed vaccines, limiting radiation exposure, and reducing chemotherapy doses). Treatment by physicians who are very familiar with AT patients is therefore recommended.

ATAXIAS ASSOCIATED WITH VITAMIN E DEFICIENCY

Mutations in the α-tocopherol transfer protein (α-TTP) gene are responsible for ataxia with vitamin E deficiency (AVED), a syndrome with clinical manifestations similar to those of FRDA but with a lower incidence of cardiomyopathy. α-TTP is synthesized in the liver and normally functions to transfer vitamin E to a circulating plasma lipoprotein. AVED mutations lead to a loss of α-TTP activity; this results in reduced plasma vitamin E levels. Plasma levels of vitamin E can be used as a screen for AVED, and replacement of vitamin E by oral administration may lead to clinical stabilization and perhaps mild improvement, at least early in the disease process.

The neurological features of abetalipoproteinemia (ABL, Bassen–Kornzweig syndrome) also resemble those of FRDA. The underlying defect appears to be genetically heterogeneous, but one identified mutation occurs in a subunit of the microsomal triglyceride transfer protein.[165] Physiologically, ABL is characterized by the absence of plasma lipoproteins containing apolipoprotein B, and this results in fat malabsorption and decreased levels of the fat-soluble vitamins. Vitamin E deficiency probably contributes to the progressive neurodegeneration and the development of pigmentary retinal degeneration. Additional diagnostic clues include the presence of acanthocytes in a peripheral blood smear and low serum cholesterol. The diagnosis can be established by a characteristic abnormality on serum protein electrophoresis.

ATAXIA WITH OCULOMOTOR APRAXIA-1 (AOA1)

The phenotype of this disorder resembles AT but without the extraneuronal features.[108,166] The incidence and phenotypic spectrum of this mutation are not yet fully known, but in some populations (e.g., Portugal and Japan), it may be one of the most prevalent autosomal-recessive ataxias.[167–169] Patients present in childhood with slowly progressive ataxia, oculomotor apraxia, and areflexia progressing to severe axonal neuropathy. Chorea may be present but tends to diminish over time.[167] The disease gene codes for aprataxin, a nuclear protein implicated in DNA repair.[168,170,171] Hypoalbuminemia and hypercholesterolemia occur late in the disease; while they are not universally present in these disorders, their presence in a patient with early-onset ataxia suggests AOA1. DNA testing is commercially available.

ATAXIA WITH OCULOMOTOR APRAXIA-2 (AOA2)

AOA2 is characterized by slowly progressive gait and truncal ataxia beginning between ages 3 and 30 years.[171,172] The ataxia is accompanied by tremor, dysarthria, and severe peripheral sensorimotor neuropathy with hyporeflexia. Nystagmus and impaired visual pursuits are common, but only about half of AOA2 patients have oculomotor apraxia. Some patients exhibit dystonic posturing of the hands, choreiform movements, and titubation or postural tremor. Typically, brain MRI shows marked cerebellar atrophy, EMG confirms axonal neuropathy, serum -fetoprotein is usually elevated, and cholesterol may also be elevated. Neuropathological examination has shown marked cerebellar atrophy with loss of Purkinje cells and severe demyelination in the spinal cord. The differential diagnosis includes AOA1, AT, and FA. AOA2 is caused by mutations in the *SETX* gene, which encodes the protein, senataxin. Senataxin is a DNA/RNA helicase involved in the DNA damage response. DNA testing is commercially available.

AUTOSOMAL-RECESSIVE SPASTIC ATAXIA OF CHARLEVOIX-SAGUENAY

This is a relatively rare cause of ataxia first identified in the Charlevoix-Saguenay region of Quebec, where the incidence is quite high.[173,174] Cases from other populations have now been reported.[175,176] Clinically, the disease manifests as an early-onset ataxia with spasticity and later development of distal amyotrophy. Marked saccadic breakdown occurs on horizontal smooth pursuit eye movements. Nerve conduction velocities are low, indicating myelination abnormalities. On fundoscopy, characteristic myelinated fibers usually can be seen in the nerve fiber layer of the retina. The disease gene encodes the protein sacsin, which appears to be a molecular chaperone that may function in protein folding.[177,178]

AUTOSOMAL RECESSIVE CEREBELLAR ATAXIA TYPE 1 (ARCA1, ALSO KNOWN AS RECESSIVE ATAXIA OF BEAUCE)

ARCA1 represents the first genetically identified form of recessively inherited, "pure" cerebellar ataxia.[179] It is a slowly progressive cerebellar ataxia beginning between late teen years and mid life (ages 17–46). Over time, patients may exhibit lower limb hyperreflexia and minor abnormalities in ocular saccades and pursuit, but it remains a pure cerebellar disorder. Disease progresses slowly, resulting in moderate disability and a normal lifespan. Brain MRI shows marked diffuse cerebellar atrophy; nerve conductions studies are normal. Genetic confirmation of mutations in the responsible gene, Syne-1/Nesprin-1, is currently available only on a research basis. Syne-1 is a nuclear envelope scaffolding protein.

SPINOCEREBELLAR ATAXIA WITH AXONAL NEUROPATHY (SCAN)

This rare disease is characterized by early-onset ataxia, axonal neuropathy, mild hypercholesterolemia, borderline hypoalbuminemia, and spared intellectual functioning. Unlike AT and the AOAs, it has not been associated with malignancies or oculomotor apraxia, respectively. The mutation causing this disease occurs in the gene encoding tyrosyl-DNA phosphodiesterase I (TDP1) and appears to cause a loss of function.[180] While details of pathogenesis still need to be elucidated, the association of ataxia with alterations in DNA repair pathways in many ataxias (also seen in AT, AOAs, Cockayne syndrome, xeroderma pigmentosum) is clearly more than an intriguing coincidence.

INBORN ERRORS OF METABOLISM

Table 43–4 lists some of the inborn errors of metabolism that may have ataxia as one of their neurological features. In addition to the disorders listed in that table, cerebrotendinous xanthomatosis should be mentioned because of the readily identifiable association of xanthomatous swelling of tendons (particularly the Achilles) with ataxia and the ease of diagnostic confirmation by documenting elevated cholestanol levels. In general, ataxia is rarely seen in isolation in the inborn metabolic errors, and often there are systemic features that suggest a metabolic workup may be indicated, but these clues cannot always be counted on. Adult-onset metabolic errors are particularly difficult to diagnose because they are often not considered in the differential diagnosis. Broad-based metabolic screening of lysosomal enzymes, organic and amino acids, mucopolysaccharides, and oligosaccharides may pick up many of these disorders.

DiMauro and colleagues reported a series of ataxia patients who have very low levels of coenzyme Q_{10} in muscle biopsy specimens, some of whom responded to coenzyme Q_{10} replacement therapy.[181] Seizures and cognitive impairment can accompany the ataxia. It has since become clear that coenzyme Q_{10} deficiency due to various genetic causes can result in ataxia.[182–185]

OTHER AUTOSOMAL-RECESSIVE ATAXIAS

Clinical descriptions of many other recessive ataxias have appeared in the literature under the description "early-onset inherited ataxias." Many of these disorders are described in only a few patients and have not been linked to specific chromosomal loci, and therefore may represent phenotypes rather than actual diseases. Congenital cerebellar ataxia, which would be classified as an early-onset inherited ataxia, includes several specific syndromes of cerebellar hypoplasia. Early-onset ataxia with retained reflexes is another example of a heterogeneous grouping of multiple disorders (mainly atypical FRDA cases) rather than an individual disease. Finally, progressive myoclonus epilepsies such as EPM1 (also known as Baltic myoclonus or Undverricht-Lundborg disease) and EPM2 (Lafora disease) often present with ataxia late in their course.

▶ X-LINKED ATAXIAS

Sideroblastic anemia with ataxia is caused by mutations in the ABC7 gene, which encodes a putative mitochondrial iron transporter.[186] Patients usually present early in life with ataxia and a microcytic, hypochromic anemia. Usually there is little progression of their ataxia.

▶ THE FRAGILE X PREMUTATION TREMOR/ATAXIA SYNDROME (FXTAS)

Fragile X syndrome, the most common cause of inherited mental retardation, results from a CGG repeat expansion in the five untranslated region of the FMR1 gene located on the X chromosome. Intriguingly, males who carry "premutation"-sized Fragile X repeats can develop a late-life tremor/ataxia syndrome known as FXTAS.[187–189]

The tremor usually resembles essential tremor but the accompanying ataxia is distinctly unusual for benign essential tremor. FXTAS can be accompanied by cognitive disturbances and/or parkinsonism and rarely by features of multiple system atrophy. The brain MRI typically shows characteristic T_2-weighted signal abnormalities in the middle cerebellar peduncles and cerebellar white matter. Note that most elderly men with essential tremor, which is a very common age-related disorder, do *not* have the Fragile X premutation. But in the elderly, tremulous man who also displays ataxia, or who has a grandson with mental retardation, screening for the premutation is recommended. Keep in mind that the identification of a premutation in the grandfather has profound implications for his daughters and their children. Why? FMR1 premutations tend to expand into the full range upon transmission, thus the grandson of a premutation carrier is at high risk for having Fragile X mental retardation.

Pathologically, ubiquitin-positive inclusion bodies are seen in neurons and glia. The molecular mechanism resulting in neurodegeneration remains poorly understood, but almost certainly reflects RNA-mediated toxicity.

▶ MITOCHONDRIAL ATAXIAS

In individuals with ataxia associated with hearing loss, retinopathy, myopathy, neuropathy, and/or diabetes, especially when there is the suggestion of maternal inheritance, the clinician should consider a primary mitochondrial disorder as the cause. Several well-described syndromes are caused by mutations in mitochondrial DNA (mtDNA). The names of these syndromes, all maternally inherited and highly variable in severity and phenotype, provide clues to the major features in each disease: myoclonic epilepsy and ragged red fiber syndrome (MERRF); mitochondrial encephalopathy, lactic acidosis, and stroke syndrome (MELAS); and neuropathy, ataxia, and retinitis pigmentosa (NARP). Of these three, NARP is most commonly associated with ataxia. Straightforward genetic tests exist for these and other mtDNA mutations. Mutations at various points within the small mitochondrial genome can cause widely varying disease that sometimes includes prominent ataxia. For example, mutations in the ATPase 6 gene can cause different diseases, ranging from infantile-onset maternally inherited Leigh syndrome to an adult-onset disorder with mild ataxia and retinitis pigmentosa. This broad phenotypic spectrum reflects the varying degree of heteroplasmy (the relative mix of mutated and normal mitochondria) in different individuals.

Laboratory clues to mitochondrial disorders include elevated serum and CSF lactate, elevated serum creatine kinase, and evidence of enzymatic and histochemical abnormalities on muscle biopsy. Classic mitochondrial disorders display maternal inheritance because the genetic defect resides in the mitochondrial organelle. Many mitochondrial proteins, however, are encoded by the nuclear genome. Thus, mutations in nuclear-encoded genes essential for mitochondrial function can cause similar neurodegenerative disease. In these cases, disease may occur sporadically or in an autosomal dominant or recessive manner. Recent studies suggest that mutations in the nuclear-encoded polymerase gamma (POLG) are a more common cause of progressive ataxia than anticipated, and should be considered even when there are not overt signs and lab findings to suggest a mitochondrial defect.[190–192] While the classic clinical presentation of sensory ataxia with neuropathy, dysarthria, and ophthalmoparesis (SANDO) will suggest POLG defects as a possible cause (or more rarely a mutation in the twinkle-helicase gene), the spectrum of ataxia with POLG mutations is likely broader than this classical presentation.

▶ SUMMARY

Single gene defects that cause ataxia have been clinically characterized and molecularly defined at a remarkably rapid pace over the past 15 years. Each new disease gene description adds to the complexity of the field even as it clarifies previous assumptions and, paradoxically, occasionally generates new uncertainty. For example, when shouldn't we test for FRDA now that we know that it can present in middle age and with spasticity? Diagnostically, the description of new syndromes outpaces our ability to test for them efficiently and economically. Advances in molecular genetics will continue to improve this situation, but only to a point. For example, DNA tests for disorders that are caused by a variety of mutations in very large genes will likely continue to be difficult (and therefore expensive) to perform, and in some cases will remain confined to the research laboratory. Thus, we must continue to rely on our clinical acumen as a vital ally.

The rapid identification of gene mutations that cause Mendelian ataxic disorders is an exciting manifestation of the early "postgenomic" era of genetics. But many diseases are not inherited in a simple Mendelian fashion, but rather through complex and subtle ways by multiple genes. Complex genetic mechanisms may explain features of many of the ataxias: the increased intrafamilial incidence of gluten sensitivity and other autoimmune-mediated ataxias; the variation in disease severity and age of onset in the single gene ataxias; and the incomplete disease penetrance in disorders such as SCA8. One real value of recent advances in molecular genetics may lie in defining complex genetic influences such as these.

Therapeutically, much more progress needs to be made as we pursue treatments for ataxias. Symptomatic improvement (e.g., increasing coordination) is simply not an easily achievable goal for the ataxias as it is for many extrapyramidal disorders. On the other hand, neuroprotection may be achievable for various ataxias, and a concerted effort must be made toward that goal. We can only hope that the very recent, promising therapeutic advances in Friedreich's ataxia, which derived from mechanistic insights made possible by the discovery of the disease gene, are a harbinger of future success in other hereditary ataxias.

REFERENCES

1. Soong BW and Paulson HL. Spinocerebellar ataxias: An update. Curr Opin Neurol 2007;20(4):438–446.
2. Perlman SL. Ataxias. Clin Geriatr Med 2006;22(4): 859–877, vii.
3. Fogel BL and Perlman S. Clinical features and molecular genetics of autosomal recessive cerebellar ataxias. Lancet Neurol 2007;6(3):245–257.
4. Klockgether T. Parkinsonism and related disorders. Ataxias. Parkinsonism Relat Disord 2007;13(suppl 3): S391–S394.
5. Maschke M, et al. Clinical feature profile of spinocerebellar ataxia type 1–8 predicts genetically defined subtypes. Mov Disord 2005;20(11):405–1412.
6. Durr A and Brice A. Clinical and genetic aspects of spinocerebellar degeneration. Curr Opin Neurol 2000;13(4): 407–413.
7. Burk K. et al. Sporadic cerebellar ataxia associated with gluten sensitivity. Brain 2001;124(Pt 5):1013–1019.
8. Hadjivassiliou M, Grunewald RA, and Davies-Jones GA. Gluten sensitivity as a neurological illness. J Neurol Neurosurg Psychiatry 2002;72(5):560–563.
9. Moseley ML, et al. Incidence of dominant spinocerebellar and Friedreich triplet repeats among 361 ataxia families. Neurology 1998;51(6):1666–1671.
10. Futamura N, et al. CAG repeat expansions in patients with sporadic cerebellar ataxia. Acta Neurol Scand 1998; 98(1):55–59.
11. Kim JY, et al. Molecular analysis of Spinocerebellar ataxias in Koreans: Frequencies and reference ranges of SCA1, SCA2, SCA3, SCA6, and SCA7. Mol Cells 2001;12(3): 336–341.
12. Mori M, et al. A genetic epidemiological study of spinocerebellar ataxias in Tottori prefecture Japan. Neuroepidemiology 2001;20(2):144–149.
13. Botez MI, et al. Treatment of Friedreich's ataxia with amantadine. Neurology 1989;39(5):749–750.
14. Trouillas P, et al. Buspirone, a 5-hydroxytryptamine1A agonist, is active in cerebellar ataxia. Results of a double-blind drug placebo study in patients with cerebellar cortical atrophy. Arch Neurol 1997;54(6):749–752.
15. Sorbi S, et al. Double-blind, crossover, placebo-controlled clinical trial with L-acetylcarnitine in patients with degenerative cerebellar ataxia. Clin Neuropharmacol 2000; 23(2):114–118.
16. Takei A, et al. Beneficial effects of tandospirone on ataxia of a patient with Machado-Joseph disease. Psychiatry Clin Neurosci 2002;56(2):181–185.
17. Garden GA and La Spada AR. Molecular pathogenesis and cellular pathology of spinocerebellar ataxia type 7 neurodegeneration. Cerebellum 2008;7(2):138–149.
18. Filla A, et al. A double-blind cross-over trial of amantadine hydrochloride in Friedreich's ataxia. Can J Neurol Sci 1993;20(1):52–55.
19. Schulte T, et al. Double-blind crossover trial of trimethoprim-sulfamethoxazole in spinocerebellar ataxia type 3/Machado-Joseph disease. Arch Neurol 2001;58(9): 1451–1457.
20. Hassin-Baer S, Korczyn AD, and Giladi N. An open trial of amantadine and buspirone for cerebellar ataxia: A disappointment. J Neural Transm 2000;107(10):1187–1189.
21. Gwinn-Hardy K, et al. Spinocerebellar ataxia type 2 with parkinsonism in ethnic Chinese. Neurology 2000;55(6): 800–805.
22. Gwinn-Hardy K. et al. Spinocerebellar ataxia type 3 phenotypically resembling parkinson disease in a black family. Arch Neurol 2001;58(2):296–299.
23. Schols L, et al. Extrapyramidal motor signs in degenerative ataxias. Arch Neurol 2000;57(10):1495–1500.
24. Schols L, et al. Sleep disturbance in spinocerebellar ataxias: Is the SCA3 mutation a cause of restless legs syndrome? Neurology 1998;51(6):1603–1607.
25. Abele M, et al. Restless legs syndrome in spinocerebellar ataxia types 1, 2, and 3. J Neurol 2001;248(4):311–314.
26. Krebs DE, McGibbon CA, and Goldvasser D. Analysis of postural perturbation responses. IEEE Trans Neural Syst Rehabil Eng 2001;9(1):76–80.
27. Visintainer CL, Matthias-Hagen V, and Nance MA. Anonymous predictive testing for Huntington's disease in the United States. Genet Test 2001;5(3):213–218.
28. Evers-Kiebooms G, et al. Predictive DNA-testing for Huntington's disease and reproductive decision making: A European collaborative study. Eur J Hum Genet 2002; 10(3):167–176.
29. Harding AE. The clinical features and classification of the late onset autosomal dominant cerebellar ataxias. A study of 11 families, including descendants of the 'the Drew family of Walworth'. Brain 1982;105(pt 1):1–28.
30. Storey E, et al. Frequency of spinocerebellar ataxia types 1, 2, 3, 6, and 7 in Australian patients with spinocerebellar ataxia. Am J Med Genet 2000;95(4):351–357.
31. Giunti P, et al. The role of the SCA2 trinucleotide repeat expansion in 89 autosomal dominant cerebellar ataxia families. Frequency, clinical and genetic correlates. Brain 1998;121(pt 3):459–467.
32. Watanabe H, et al. Frequency analysis of autosomal dominant cerebellar ataxias in Japanese patients and clinical characterization of spinocerebellar ataxia type 6. Clin Genet 1998;53(1):13–19.
33. Lopes-Cendes I, et al. Frequency of the different mutations causing spinocerebellar ataxia (SCA1, SCA2, MJD/ SCA3 and DRPLA) in a large group of Brazilian patients. Arq Neuropsiquiatr 1997;55(3B):519–529.
34. Silveira I, et al. Trinucleotide repeats in 202 families with ataxia: a small expanded (CAG)n allele at the SCA17 locus. Arch Neurol 2002;59(4):623–629.
35. Takano H, et al. Close associations between prevalences of dominantly inherited spinocerebellar ataxias with CAG-repeat expansions and frequencies of large normal

CAG alleles in Japanese and Caucasian populations. Am J Hum Genet 1998;63(4):1060–1066.
36. Jen JC. Hereditary episodic ataxias. Ann N Y Acad Sci 2008; 1142:250–253.
37. Burk K. et al. Autosomal dominant cerebellar ataxia type I clinical features and MRI in families with SCA1, SCA2 and SCA3. Brain 1996;119(pt 5):1497–1505.
38. Schols L, et al. Spinocerebellar ataxia type 1: Clinical and neurophysiological characteristics in German kindreds. Acta Neurol Scand 1995;92(6):478–485.
39. Schols L, et al. Autosomal dominant cerebellar ataxia: phenotypic differences in genetically defined subtypes? Ann Neurol 1997;42(6):924–932.
40. Burk K, et al. Executive dysfunction in spinocerebellar ataxia type 1. Eur Neurol 2001;46(1):43–48.
41. Orr HT, et al. Expansion of an unstable trinucleotide CAG repeat in spinocerebellar ataxia type 1. Nat Genet 1993; 4(3):221–226.
42. Orr HT and Zoghbi HY. Trinucleotide repeat disorders. Annu Rev Neurosci 2007;30:575–621.
43. Williams AJ and Paulson HL. Polyglutamine neurodegeneration: Protein misfolding revisited. Trends Neurosci 2008;31(10):521–528.
44. Zoghbi HY and Orr HT. Pathogenic mechanisms of a polyglutamine-mediated neurodegenerative disease, spinocerebellar ataxia type 1. J Biol Chem 2009;284(12): 7425–7429.
45. Zuhlke C, et al. Spinocerebellar ataxia type 1 (SCA1): Phenotype-genotype correlation studies in intermediate alleles. Eur J Hum Genet 2002;10(3):204–209.
46. Limprasert P, et al. Comparative studies of the CAG repeats in the spinocerebellar ataxia type 1 (SCA1) gene. Am J Med Genet 1997;74(5):488–493.
47. Ranum LP, et al. Molecular and clinical correlations in spinocerebellar ataxia type I: Evidence for familial effects on the age at onset. Am J Hum Genet 1994;55(2):244–252.
48. Lim J, et al. Opposing effects of polyglutamine expansion on native protein complexes contribute to SCA1. Nature 2008;452(7188):713–718.
49. Gonzalez-Alegre P and Paulson HL. Technology insight: Therapeutic RNA interference: How far from the neurology clinic? Nat Clin Pract Neurol 2007;3(7):394–404.
50. Watase K, et al. Lithium therapy improves neurological function and hippocampal dendritic arborization in a spinocerebellar ataxia type 1 mouse model. PLoS Med 2007;4(5):e182.
51. Orozco G, et al. Dominantly inherited olivopontocerebellar atrophy from eastern Cuba. Clinical, neuropathological, and biochemical findings. J Neurol Sci 1989;93(1):37–50.
52. Filla A, et al. Relative frequencies of CAG expansions in spinocerebellar ataxia and dentatorubropallidoluysian atrophy in 116 Italian families. Eur Neurol 2000;44(1): 31–36.
53. Saleem Q, et al. Molecular analysis of autosomal dominant hereditary ataxias in the Indian population: high frequency of SCA2 and evidence for a common founder mutation. Hum Genet 2000;106(2):179–187.
54. Geschwind DH, et al. The prevalence and wide clinical spectrum of the spinocerebellar ataxia type 2 trinucleotide repeat in patients with autosomal dominant cerebellar ataxia. Am J Hum Genet 1997;60(4):842–850.
55. Imbert G, et al. Cloning of the gene for spinocerebellar ataxia 2 reveals a locus with high sensitivity to expanded CAG/glutamine repeats. Nat Genet 1996;14(3): 285–291.
56. Sanpei K. et al. Identification of the spinocerebellar ataxia type 2 gene using a direct identification of repeat expansion and cloning technique, DIRECT. Nat Genet 1996;14(3):277–284.
57. Pulst SM, et al. Moderate expansion of a normally biallelic trinucleotide repeat in spinocerebellar ataxia type 2. Nat Genet 1996;14(3):269–276.
58. Pulst SM, et al. Spinocerebellar ataxia type 2: PolyQ repeat variation in the CACNA1A calcium channel modifies age of onset. Brain 2005;128(Pt 10):2297–2303.
59. Schols L, et al. Genetic background of apparently idiopathic sporadic cerebellar ataxia. Hum Genet 2000;107(2): 132–137.
60. Nonhoff U, et al. Ataxin-2 interacts with the DEAD/H-box RNA helicase DDX6 and interferes with P-bodies and stress granules. Mol Biol Cell 2007;18(4):1385–1396.
61. Huynh DP, et al. Nuclear localization or inclusion body formation of ataxin-2 are not necessary for SCA2 pathogenesis in mouse or human. Nat Genet 2000;26(1):44–50.
62. Mao R, et al. Childhood-onset ataxia: Testing for large CAG-repeats in SCA2 and SCA7. Am J Med Genet 2002;110(4): 338–345.
63. Nakano KK, Dawson DM, and Spence A. Machado disease. A hereditary ataxia in Portuguese emigrants to Massachusetts. Neurology 1972;22(1):49–55.
64. Kawaguchi Y, et al. CAG expansions in a novel gene for Machado-Joseph disease at chromosome 14q32.1. Nat Genet 1994;8(3):221–228.
65. Cancel G, et al. Marked phenotypic heterogeneity associated with expansion of a CAG repeat sequence at the spinocerebellar ataxia 3/Machado-Joseph disease locus. Am J Hum Genet 1995;57(4):809–816.
66. Silveira I, et al. Analysis of SCA1, DRPLA, MJD, SCA2, and SCA6 CAG repeats in 48 Portuguese ataxia families. Am J Med Genet 1998;81(2):134–138.
67. van Alfen N, et al. Intermediate CAG repeat lengths (53,54) for MJD/SCA3 are associated with an abnormal phenotype. Ann Neurol 2001;49(6):805–807.
68. Todi SV, et al. Ubiquitination directly enhances activity of the deubiquitinating enzyme ataxin-3. Embo J 2009;28(4): 372–382.
69. Flanigan K, et al. Autosomal dominant spinocerebellar ataxia with sensory axonal neuropathy (SCA4): Clinical description and genetic localization to chromosome 16q22.1. Am J Hum Genet 1996;59(2):392–399.
70. Takashima M, et al. A linkage disequilibrium at the candidate gene locus for 16q-linked autosomal dominant cerebellar ataxia type III in Japan. J Hum Genet 2001;46(4):167–171.
71. Ranum LP, et al. Spinocerebellar ataxia type 5 in a family descended from the grandparents of President Lincoln maps to chromosome 11. Nat Genet 1994;8(3): 280–284.
72. Stevanin G, et al. Clinical and MRI findings in spinocerebellar ataxia type 5. Neurology 1999;53(6):1355–1357.
73. Ikeda Y, et al. Spectrin mutations cause spinocerebellar ataxia type 5. Nat Genet 2006;38(2):184–190.

74. Yabe I, et al. [Initial symptoms and mode of neurological progression in spinocerebellar ataxia type 6 (SCA6)]. Rinsho Shinkeigaku 1998;38(6):489–494.
75. Geschwind DH, et al., Spinocerebellar ataxia type 6. Frequency of the mutation and genotype-phenotype correlations. Neurology 1997;49(5):1247–1251.
76. Ikeuchi T, et al. Spinocerebellar ataxia type 6: CAG repeat expansion in alpha1A voltage-dependent calcium channel gene and clinical variations in Japanese population. Ann Neurol 1997;42(6):879–884.
77. Buttner N, et al. Oculomotor phenotypes in autosomal dominant ataxias. Arch Neurol 1998;55(10):1353–1357.
78. Riess O, et al. SCA6 is caused by moderate CAG expansion in the alpha1A-voltage-dependent calcium channel gene. Hum Mol Genet 1997;6(8):1289–1293.
79. Zhuchenko O, et al. Autosomal dominant cerebellar ataxia (SCA6) associated with small polyglutamine expansions in the alpha 1A-voltage-dependent calcium channel. Nat Genet 1997;15(1):62–69.
80. Matsumura R, et al. Spinocerebellar ataxia type 6. Molecular and clinical features of 35 Japanese patients including one homozygous for the CAG repeat expansion. Neurology 1997;49(5):1238–1243.
81. Watase K, et al. Spinocerebellar ataxia type 6 knockin mice develop a progressive neuronal dysfunction with age-dependent accumulation of mutant CaV2.1 channels. Proc Natl Acad Sci U S A 2008;105(33):11987–11992.
82. Kordasiewicz HB and Gomez CM. Molecular pathogenesis of spinocerebellar ataxia type 6. Neurotherapeutics 2007;4(2):285–294.
83. David G, et al. Molecular and clinical correlations in autosomal dominant cerebellar ataxia with progressive macular dystrophy (SCA7). Hum Mol Genet 1998;7(2): 165–170.
84. Hsieh M, et al. Identification of the spinocerebellar ataxia type 7 mutation in Taiwan: Application of PCR-based Southern blot. J Neurol 2000;247(8):623–629.
85. David G, et al. Cloning of the SCA7 gene reveals a highly unstable CAG repeat expansion. Nat Genet 1997;17(1): 65–70.
86. Vincent, J.B., et al. An unstable trinucleotide-repeat region on chromosome 13 implicated in spinocerebellar ataxia: a common expansion locus. Am J Hum Genet, 2000 66(3):819–829.
87. Sobrido MJ, et al. SCA8 repeat expansions in ataxia: a controversial association. Neurology 2001;57(7):1310–1312.
88. Juvonen V, et al. Clinical and genetic findings in Finnish ataxia patients with the spinocerebellar ataxia 8 repeat expansion. Ann Neurol 2000;48(3):354–361.
89. Day JW, et al. Spinocerebellar ataxia type 8: clinical features in a large family. Neurology 2000;55(5):649–657.
90. Koob MD, et al. An untranslated CTG expansion causes a novel form of spinocerebellar ataxia (SCA8). Nat Genet 1999;21(4):379–384.
91. Nemes JP, et al. The SCA8 transcript is an antisense RNA to a brain-specific transcript encoding a novel actin-binding protein (KLHL1). Hum Mol Genet 2000; 9(10):1543–1551.
92. Ikeda Y, Daughters RS and Ranum LP. Bidirectional expression of the SCA8 expansion mutation: One mutation, two genes. Cerebellum 2008;7(2):150–158.
93. Matsuura T, et al. Large expansion of the ATTCT pentanucleotide repeat in spinocerebellar ataxia type 10. Nat Genet 2000;26(2):191–194.
94. Teive HA, et al. Clinical phenotype of Brazilian families with spinocerebellar ataxia 10. Neurology 2004;63(8): 1509–1512.
95. Wakamiya M, et al. The role of ataxin 10 in the pathogenesis of spinocerebellar ataxia type 10. Neurology 2006;67(4):607–613.
96. Rasmussen A, et al. Clinical and genetic analysis of four Mexican families with spinocerebellar ataxia type 10. Ann Neurol 2001;50(2):234–239.
97. Worth PF, et al. Autosomal dominant cerebellar ataxia type III: linkage in a large British family to a 7.6-cM region on chromosome 15q14-21.3. Am J Hum Genet 1999;65(2):420–426.
98. Houlden H, et al. Mutations in TTBK2, encoding a kinase implicated in tau phosphorylation, segregate with spinocerebellar ataxia type 11. Nat Genet 2007;39(12): 1434–1436.
99. Holmes SE, et al. SCA12: an unusual mutation leads to an unusual spinocerebellar ataxia. Brain Res Bull 2001;56 (3–4):397–403.
100. Holmes SE, et al. Expansion of a novel CAG trinucleotide repeat in the 5' region of PPP2R2B is associated with SCA12. Nat Genet 1999;23(4):391–392.
101. Maruyama H, et al. Difference in disease-free survival curve and regional distribution according to subtype of spinocerebellar ataxia: A study of 1,286 Japanese patients. Am J Med Genet 2002;114(5):578–583.
102. Cholfin JA, et al. The SCA12 mutation as a rare cause of spinocerebellar ataxia. Arch Neurol 2001;58(11): 1833–1835.
103. Srivastava AK, et al. Molecular and clinical correlation in five Indian families with spinocerebellar ataxia 12. Ann Neurol 2001;50(6):796–800.
104. Waters MF and Pulst SM. Sca13. Cerebellum 2008;7(2): 165–169.
105. Waters MF, et al. Mutations in voltage-gated potassium channel KCNC3 cause degenerative and developmental central nervous system phenotypes. Nat Genet 2006;38(4):447–451.
106. Klebe S, et al. New mutations in protein kinase Cgamma associated with spinocerebellar ataxia type 14. Ann Neurol 2005;58(5):720–729.
107. Storey E, et al. A new autosomal dominant pure cerebellar ataxia. Neurology 2001;57(10):1913–1915.
108. Hara K, et al. Total deletion and a missense mutation of ITPR1 in Japanese SCA15 families. Neurology 2008; 71(8):547–551.
109. Koide R, et al. A neurological disease caused by an expanded CAG trinucleotide repeat in the TATA-binding protein gene: A new polyglutamine disease? Hum Mol Genet 1999;8(11):2047–2053.
110. Nakamura K, et al. SCA17, a novel autosomal dominant cerebellar ataxia caused by an expanded polyglutamine in TATA-binding protein. Hum Mol Genet 2001;10(14):1441–1448.
111. Brkanac Z, et al. Autosomal dominant sensory/motor neuropathy with Ataxia (SMNA): Linkage to chromosome 7q22-q32. Am J Med Genet 2002;114(4):450–457.

112. Schelhaas HJ and van de Warrenburg BP. Clinical, psychological, and genetic characteristics of spinocerebellar ataxia type 19 (SCA19). Cerebellum 2005;4(1):51–54.
113. Knight MA, et al. A duplication at chromosome 11q12.2-11q12.3 is associated with spinocerebellar ataxia type 20. Hum Mol Genet 2008;17(24):3847–3853.
114. Delplanque J, et al. Slowly progressive spinocerebellar ataxia with extrapyramidal signs and mild cognitive impairment (SCA21). Cerebellum 2008;7(2):179–183.
115. Chung MY, et al. A novel autosomal dominant spinocerebellar ataxia (SCA22) linked to chromosome 1p21-q23. Brain 2003;126(pt 6):1293–1299.
116. Verbeek DS, Spinocerebellar ataxia Type 23: A genetic update. Cerebellum 2008.
117. Stevanin G, et al. Spinocerebellar ataxia with sensory neuropathy (SCA25). Cerebellum 2005;4(1):58–61.
118. Yu GY, et al. Spinocerebellar ataxia type 26 maps to chromosome 19p13.3 adjacent to SCA6. Ann Neurol 2005; 57(3):349–354.
119. Brusse E, et al. Spinocerebellar ataxia associated with a mutation in the fibroblast growth factor 14 gene (SCA27): A new phenotype. Mov Disord 2006;21(3):396–401.
120. Shakkottai VG, et al. FGF14 regulates the intrinsic excitability of cerebellar Purkinje neurons. Neurobiol Dis 2009;33(1):81–88.
121. Mariotti C, et al. Spinocerebellar ataxia type 28: A novel autosomal dominant cerebellar ataxia characterized by slow progression and ophthalmoparesis. Cerebellum, 2008;7(2):184–188.
122. Burke JR, et al. The Haw River syndrome: Dentatorubropallidoluysian atrophy (DRPLA) in an African-American family. Nat Genet 1994;7(4):521–524.
123. Komure O, et al. DNA analysis in hereditary dentatorubral-pallidoluysian atrophy: Correlation between CAG repeat length and phenotypic variation and the molecular basis of anticipation. Neurology 1995;45(1):143–149.
124. Koide R, et al. Unstable expansion of CAG repeat in hereditary dentatorubral-pallidoluysian atrophy (DRPLA). Nat Genet 1994;6(1):9–13.
125. Nagafuchi S, et al. Dentatorubral and pallidoluysian atrophy expansion of an unstable CAG trinucleotide on chromosome 12p. Nat Genet 1994;6(1):14–18.
126. Wang L and Tsai CC. Atrophin proteins: An overview of a new class of nuclear receptor corepressors. Nucl Recept Signal 2008;6:e009.
127. Yamada M, et al. Polyglutamine disease: Recent advances in the neuropathology of dentatorubral-pallidoluysian atrophy. Neuropathology 2006;26(4):346–351.
128. Ophoff RA, et al. Familial hemiplegic migraine and episodic ataxia type-2 are caused by mutations in the Ca2+ channel gene CACNL1A4. Cell 1996;87(3):543–552.
129. Zasorin NL, Baloh RW, and Myers LB. Acetazolamide-responsive episodic ataxia syndrome. Neurology 1983;33(9): 1212–1214.
130. Denier C, et al. High prevalence of CACNA1A truncations and broader clinical spectrum in episodic ataxia type 2. Neurology 1999;52(9):1816–1821.
131. Liou HH, et al. Is ataxic gait the predominant presenting manifestation of Creutzfeldt-Jakob disease? Experience of 14 Chinese cases from Taiwan. J Neurol Sci 1996;140 (1–2):53–60.
132. Berciano J, et al. Ataxic type of Creutzfeldt-Jakob disease with disproportionate enlargement of the fourth ventricle: a serial CT study. J Neurol Neurosurg Psychiatry 1997; 62(3):295–297.
133. Depienne C, et al. Hereditary spastic paraplegias: an update. Curr Opin Neurol, 2007;20(6):674–680.
134. Bhidayasiri R, et al. Late-onset Friedreich ataxia: phenotypic analysis, magnetic resonance imaging findings, and review of the literature. Arch Neurol 2005;62(12): 1865–1869.
135. Schulz JB, et al. Diagnosis and treatment of Friedreich ataxia: A European perspective. Nat Rev Neurol 2009;5(4): 222–234.
136. Pandolfo M. Friedreich ataxia. Arch Neurol 2008;65(10): 1296–1303.
137. Labuda M, et al. Unique origin and specific ethnic distribution of the Friedreich ataxia GAA expansion. Neurology 2000;54(12):2322–2324.
138. Harding AE. Friedreich's ataxia: A clinical and genetic study of 90 families with an analysis of early diagnostic criteria and intrafamilial clustering of clinical features. Brain 1981;104(3):589–620.
139. Schols L, et al. Friedreich's ataxia. Revision of the phenotype according to molecular genetics. Brain 1997;120(pt 12): 2131–2140.
140. Dutka DP, et al. Marked variation in the cardiomyopathy associated with Friedreich's ataxia. Heart 1999;81(2):141–147.
141. Harding AE and Hewer RL. The heart disease of Friedreich's ataxia: A clinical and electrocardiographic study of 115 patients, with an analysis of serial electrocardiographic changes in 30 cases. Q J Med 1983;52(208):489–502.
142. Campuzano V, et al. Friedreich's ataxia: Autosomal recessive disease caused by an intronic GAA triplet repeat expansion. Science 1996;271(5254):1423–1427.
143. Campuzano V, et al. Frataxin is reduced in Friedreich ataxia patients and is associated with mitochondrial membranes. Hum Mol Genet 1997;6(11):1771–1780.
144. Cossee M, et al. Friedreich's ataxia: point mutations and clinical presentation of compound heterozygotes. Ann Neurol 1999;45(2):200–206.
145. Seznec H, et al. Friedreich ataxia: the oxidative stress paradox. Hum Mol Genet 2005;14(4):463–474.
146. Seznec H, et al. Idebenone delays the onset of cardiac functional alteration without correction of Fe-S enzymes deficit in a mouse model for Friedreich ataxia. Hum Mol Genet 2004;13(10):1017–1024.
147. Rai M, et al. HDAC inhibitors correct frataxin deficiency in a Friedreich ataxia mouse model. PLoS ONE, 2008; 3(4):e1958.
148. Rotig A, et al. Aconitase and mitochondrial iron-sulphur protein deficiency in Friedreich ataxia. Nat Genet 1997; 17(2):215–217.
149. Schulz JB, et al. Oxidative stress in patients with Friedreich ataxia. Neurology 2000;55(11):1719–1721.
150. Emond M, et al. Increased levels of plasma malondialdehyde in Friedreich ataxia. Neurology 2000;55(11):1752–1753.
151. Ribai P, et al. Neurological, cardiological, and oculomotor progression in 104 patients with Friedreich ataxia during long-term follow-up. Arch Neurol 2007;64(4):558–564.
152. Tsou AY, et al. Pharmacotherapy for friedreich ataxia. CNS Drugs 2009;23(3):213–223.

153. Pineda M, et al. Idebenone treatment in paediatric and adult patients with Friedreich ataxia: long-term follow-up. Eur J Paediatr Neurol 2008;12(6):470–475.
154. Di Prospero NA, et al. Neurological effects of high-dose idebenone in patients with Friedreich's ataxia: A randomised, placebo-controlled trial. Lancet Neurol 2007; 6(10):878–886.
155. Rustin P, et al. Idebenone treatment in Friedreich patients: one-year-long randomized placebo-controlled trial. Neurology 2004;62(3):524–525; author reply 525; discussion 525.
156. Mariotti C, et al. Idebenone treatment in Friedreich patients: One-year-long randomized placebo-controlled trial. Neurology 2003;60(10):1676–1679.
157. Tonon C and Lodi R. Idebenone in Friedreich's ataxia. Expert Opin Pharmacother 2008;9(13):2327–2337.
158. Caldecott KW. Single-strand break repair and genetic disease. Nat Rev Genet 2008;9(8):619–631.
159. Biton S, Barzilai A, and Shiloh Y. The neurological phenotype of ataxia-telangiectasia: solving a persistent puzzle. DNA Repair (Amst) 2008;7(7):1028–1038.
160. Woods CG and Taylor AM. Ataxia telangiectasia in the British Isles: The clinical and laboratory features of 70 affected individuals. Q J Med 1992;82(298):169–179.
161. Morrell D, Cromartie E, and Swift M. Mortality and cancer incidence in 263 patients with ataxia-telangiectasia. J Natl Cancer Inst 1986;77(1):89–92.
162. Perlman S, et al. Ataxia telangiectasia and its variants, in Manto MU. In M. Pandolfo (ed). The Cerebellum and Its Disorders. Cambridge University Press, 2002, pp. 531–731.
163. Stumm M, et al. High frequency of spontaneous translocations revealed by FISH in cells from patients with the cancer-prone syndromes ataxia telangiectasia and Nijmegen breakage syndrome. Cytogenet Cell Genet 2001;92(3–4): 186–191.
164. Concannon P. ATM heterozygosity and cancer risk. Nat Genet 2002;32(1):89–90.
165. Sharp D, et al. Cloning and gene defects in microsomal triglyceride transfer protein associated with abetalipoproteinaemia. Nature 1993;365(6441):65–69.
166. Nemeth AH, et al. Autosomal recessive cerebellar ataxia with oculomotor apraxia (ataxia-telangiectasia-like syndrome) is linked to chromosome 9q34. Am J Hum Genet 2000;67(5):1320–1326.
167. Shimazaki H, et al. Early-onset ataxia with ocular motor apraxia and hypoalbuminemia: The aprataxin gene mutations. Neurology 2002;59(4):590–595.
168. Moreira MC, et al. The gene mutated in ataxia-ocular apraxia 1 encodes the new HIT/Zn-finger protein aprataxin. Nat Genet 2001;29(2):189–193.
169. Barbot C, et al. Recessive ataxia with ocular apraxia: review of 22 Portuguese patients. Arch Neurol 2001;58(2): 201–205.
170. Date H, et al. Early-onset ataxia with ocular motor apraxia and hypoalbuminemia is caused by mutations in a new HIT superfamily gene. Nat Genet 2001;29(2):184–188.
171. Le Ber I, et al. Frequency and phenotypic spectrum of ataxia with oculomotor apraxia 2: A clinical and genetic study in 18 patients. Brain 2004;127(pt 4):759–767.
172. Tazir M, et al. Ataxia with oculomotor apraxia type 2: A clinical and genetic study of 19 patients. J Neurol Sci 2009;278(1–2):77–81.
173. Bouchard JP, et al. Autosomal recessive spastic ataxia of Charlevoix-Saguenay. Neuromuscul Disord 1998;8(7): 474–479.
174. Scriver CR, Human genetics: lessons from Quebec populations. Annu Rev Genomics Hum Genet 2001;2:69–101.
175. Gucuyener K, et al. Autosomal recessive spastic ataxia of Charlevoix-Saguenay in two unrelated Turkish families. Neuropediatrics 2001 32(3):142–146.
176. Vermeer S, et al. ARSACS in the Dutch population: a frequent cause of early-onset cerebellar ataxia. Neurogenetics 2008;9(3):207–214.
177. Engert JC, et al. ARSACS, a spastic ataxia common in northeastern Quebec, is caused by mutations in a new gene encoding an 11.5-kb ORF. Nat Genet 2000;24(2):120–125.
178. Parfitt D, et al. The ataxia protein sacsin is a functional co-chaperone that protects against polyglutamine-expanded ataxin-1 Human Molecular Genetics 2009;18(9): 1556–1565.
179. Dupre N, et al. Clinical and genetic study of autosomal recessive cerebellar ataxia type 1. Ann Neurol 2007;62(1):93–98.
180. Takashima H, et al. Mutation of TDP1, encoding a topoisomerase I-dependent DNA damage repair enzyme, in spinocerebellar ataxia with axonal neuropathy. Nat Genet 2002;32(2):267–272.
181. Musumeci O, et al. Familial cerebellar ataxia with muscle coenzyme Q10 deficiency. Neurology 2001;56(7): 849–855.
182. Quinzii CM, Hirano M, and DiMauro S. CoQ10 deficiency diseases in adults. Mitochondrion 2007;7(suppl):S122–126.
183. Montero R, et al. Clinical, biochemical and molecular aspects of cerebellar ataxia and Coenzyme Q10 deficiency. Cerebellum 2007;6(2):118–122.
184. Mollet J, et al. CABC1 gene mutations cause ubiquinone deficiency with cerebellar ataxia and seizures. Am J Hum Genet 2008;82(3):623–630.
185. Lagier-Tourenne C, et al. ADCK3, an ancestral kinase, is mutated in a form of recessive ataxia associated with coenzyme Q10 deficiency. Am J Hum Genet 2008;82(3):661–672.
186. Allikmets R, et al. Mutation of a putative mitochondrial iron transporter gene (ABC7) in X-linked sideroblastic anemia and ataxia (XLSA/A). Hum Mol Genet 1999;8(5):743–749.
187. Hagerman RJ, et al. Intention tremor, parkinsonism, and generalized brain atrophy in male carriers of fragile X. Neurology 2001;57(1):127–130.
188. Shan G, Xu S, and Jin P. FXTAS: a bad RNA and a hope for a cure. Expert Opin Biol Ther 2008;8(3):249–253.
189. Berry-Kravis E, et al. Fragile X-associated tremor/ataxia syndrome: clinical features, genetics, and testing guidelines. Mov Disord 2007;22(14):2018–2030, quiz 2140.
190. Wong LJ, et al. Molecular and clinical genetics of mitochondrial diseases due to POLG mutations. Hum Mutat 2008;29(9):E150–E172.
191. Winterthun S, et al. Autosomal recessive mitochondrial ataxic syndrome due to mitochondrial polymerase gamma mutations. Neurology 2005;64(7):1204–1208.
192. Van Goethem G, et al. POLG mutations in neurodegenerative disorders with ataxia but no muscle involvement. Neurology 2004;63(7):1251–1257.

CHAPTER 41

Physiology and Pathophysiology of the Cerebellum, and Rehabilitation Strategies After Cerebellar Injury

W. Thomas Thach

▶ BEHAVIORAL SIGNS OF CEREBELLAR DAMAGE

At the turn of the last century, Flourens and Luciani in animals and Babinski and Holmes in humans described behavioral deficits caused by focal cerebellar lesions, and they speculated about the causal mechanism. Perhaps most influential were the studies of Gordon Holmes, who meticulously documented the movement deficits associated with cerebellar gunshot wounds in World War I.[1,2] He insisted that these deficits may be attributed to cerebellar disease only in patients who have normal strength and somesthesis. Yet even he accepted that weakness/"asthenia" may sometimes occur transiently and acutely.

1. **Ataxia** is a condition that involves lack of coordination between movements of body parts. The term is often used in reference to gait or movement of a specific body part, as in "ataxic arm movements."
2. **Dysmetria** is an inability to make a movement of the appropriate distance. Hypometria is undershooting a target, and hypermetria is overshooting a target. Patients with cerebellar damage tend to make hypermetric movements when they move rapidly and hypo metric movements when they move more slowly and wish to be accurate.
3. **Dysdiadochokinesia** is an inability to make rapidly alternating movements of a limb. It appears to reflect abnormal agonist-antagonist control.
4. **Asynergia** is an inability to combine the movements of individual Limb segments into a coordinated, multisegmental movement.
5. **Hypotonia** is an abnormally decreased muscle tone. It is manifest as a decreased resistance to passive movement, so that a limb swings freely upon external perturbation. Hypotonia often limited to the acute phase of cerebellar disease.
6. **Nystagmus** is an involuntary and rhythmic eye movement that usually consists of a slow and a fast phase. In a unilateral cerebellar lesion, the fast phase of nystagmus is toward the side of the lesion.
7. **Action tremor, or intention tremor**, is an involuntary oscillation that occurs during limb movement and disappears when the limb is at rest. Cerebellar action tremor is generally of high amplitude and low frequency (3–5 Hz). **Titubation** is a tremor of the entire trunk during stance and gait. Lesions of cerebellar target structures (e.g., the red nucleus and the thalamus) often result in cerebellar outflow tremor, or postural tremor. Most prominent when a limb is actively held in a static posture, postural tremor attenuates during limb movement and disappears when the limb is at rest.

As to the mechanism for these deficits, both Luciani and Holmes ascribed to a theory of deficient cerebellar tonic excitatory reinforcement of targets in spinal cord, brain stem, and (via thalamus) cerebral cortex. This thinking was followed by Derek Denny-Brown, and in turn by Sid Gilman.[3] In this view, the signature clinical feature is hypotonia, which is fundamental to all the other deficits.[4] Nonetheless, all of the aforementioned accepted that, given time, even hypotonia may diminish. This in turn was interpreted as an indication that "cerebellar deficits are compensated for, to a considerable extent, by other structures in the brain if sufficient time is given.[5]

By contrast, Flourens[6] and Babinski[7,8] inferred that the deficits were due to an entirely different mechanism,

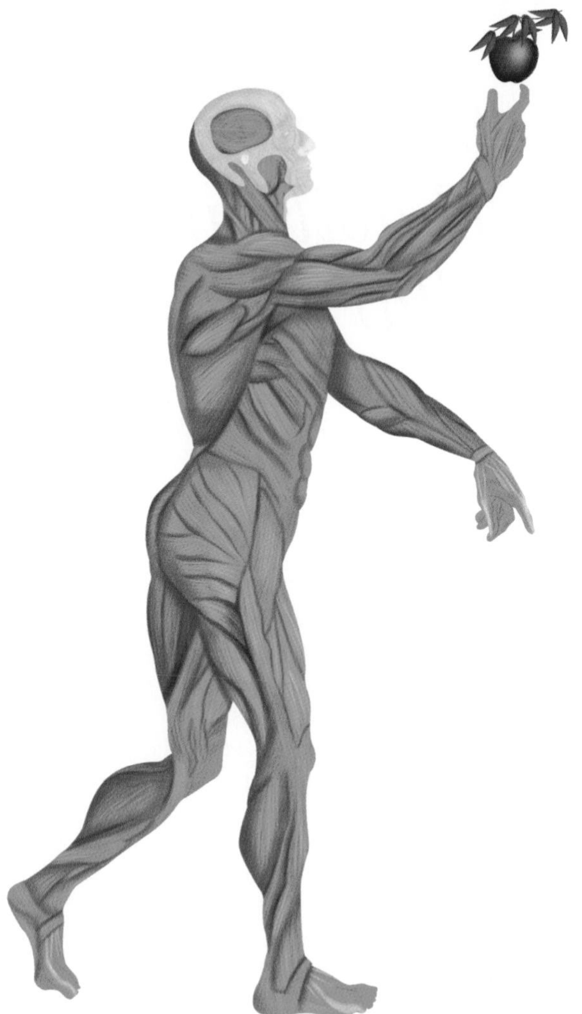

Figure 41–1. Movement coordination = learning of combinations of motor elements. There are 206 bones, many joints, and 650 or so muscles in the adult human. Most movements involve many bones, muscles, and joints. Coordination requires that these elements be combined so that they: (1) start at the correct time, (2) stop at the correct time, (3) contract with the correct amount of force, each element proportionate to do all others. This combining is so complex that it apparently must be done "automatically" without having to think about it. It is therefore something that must be learned through repeated trial and error practice. (From Vesalius A. De Humani corporis fabrica libri septem [On the fabric of the human body in seven books] Muscles 1543; (Pt 2):174. With appreciation to the Bernard Becker Library at Washington University School of Medicine, St. Louis, Missouri.)

one that was quintessential to the cerebellum, which could *not* be compensated by other parts of the nervous system. Their fundamental principle was one of the coordination of the many muscles, joints, and body segments that may be *uniquely combined* in any one of a great variety of movements (Fig. 41–1). Subsequent work has caused this view to gain favor: (1) the anatomy and physiology of the cerebellum appear uniquely capable of linking together simple movement components into compound complex movements; (2) this process appears to be learned and stored within the cerebellum through trial and error repetition of the movement; (3) the same appears to hold for purely mental movements including speech, and possibly other cognitive functions as well. These features are next reviewed in detail.

▶ ASSESSING CEREBELLAR FUNCTION

THE DEEP NUCLEI GENERATE THE EXCITATORY OUTPUT OF THE CEREBELLUM

All of the cerebellum's output is produced by the deep cerebellar nuclei and vestibular nuclei (Fig. 41–2). The deep nuclei exert control over movement of ipsilateral parts of the body. Nearly every motor center of the central nervous system (CNS) receives input from the deep nuclei, including the spinal cord, the vestibular, reticular, and red nuclei, the superior colliculus, and (via the thalamus) the primary motor and premotor cortices, the primary and secondary frontal eye fields, and even the prefrontal cortex. The projections from the deep nuclei to these centers are for the most part glutamatergic and excitatory. An exception is a set of small GABAergic neurons in the deep nuclei which make inhibitory projections to the inferior olivary complex These inhibitory neurons are important in maintaining stability of cerebellar learning functions (see later). All cerebellar target structures receive other excitatory inputs in addition to those from the cerebellum (see above). There are no direct projections from the deep nuclei to the basal ganglia.

In the absence of movement, deep nuclear cells fire at maintained rates of approximately 40–50 Hz.[9–12] During movement, their firing rates increase and decrease above and below their baseline. Through these variations in firing rate, the cerebellum modulates the activity of downstream motor pattern generators (MPGs). In addition, increases in cerebellar nuclear firing rate precede and help increase the discharge frequency in MPGs, thus facilitating the initiation of movement.

PURKINJE CELLS OF THE CEREBELLAR CORTEX INHIBIT THE DEEP NUCLEAR CELLS

Purkinje cells (Pc) are the only output of the cerebellar cortex (Fig. 41–2). Their axons project topographically onto the neurons of the deep nuclei and inhibit

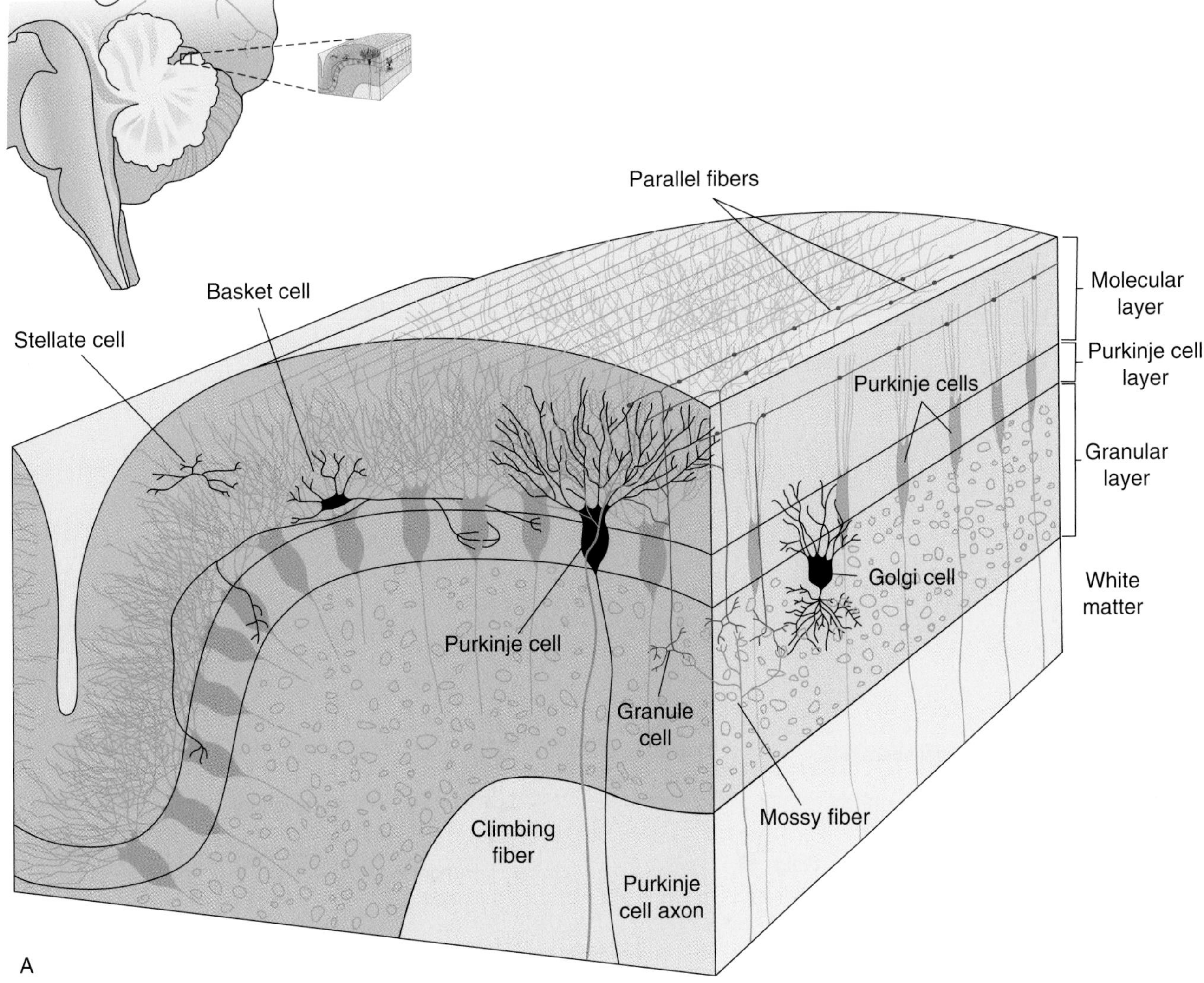

Figure 41–2. (A) The cerebellar cortex is organized into three layers and contains five types of neurons. A vertical section of a single cerebellar folium, in both longitudinal and transverse planes, illustrates the general organization of the cerebellar cortex. A glomerulus is a clear space where the bulbous terminal of a mossy fiber makes synaptic contact with Golgi and granule cells. (B) Bundles of parallel fibers, called beams, run transversely and excite the dendrites of Purkinje cells flanking the parallel fiber beam. (C) Synaptic organization of the basic cerebellar circuit module. Mossy and climbing fibers convey output from the cerebellum via a main excitatory loop through the deep nuclei. This loop is modulated by an inhibitory side-loop passing through the cerebellar cortex. This figure shows the excitatory (+) and inhibitory (–) connections among the cell types. Parts B & C show the geometry of the divergence and convergence of these basic connections. (Reproduced with permission from Ghez C and Thach WT. The cerebellum. In Kandel ER, Schwartz JH, and Jessell TM (eds). Principles of Neural Science, 4th ed. New York: McGraw-Hill, Inc., 2000, pp. 836–837 [Figs 41–4, 41–5, and 41–6].)

(GABA) them.[13] Pc generate two different kinds of action potential. The "simple spike," so called because of its bipolar waveform,[9,10] fires at maintained rates of 40–50/s and during movement well above and below this baseline: this exerts inhibitory restraint on the firing of the deep nuclear cells.[13] The Pc simple spike is driven by excitatory throughput from mossy fiber/granule cell/parallel fibers (Fig. 41–2), which are also tonically and phasically active. Collaterals from the mossy fibers excite the deep nuclear cells directly, which accounts for their maintained firing despite the maintained Pc inhibition.[13]

By contrast, the Pc "complex spike" is so called because of its multiphasic waveform.[9,10] It is driven by excitatory contacts on the Pc by climbing fibers from the inferior olive (Fig. 41–2). These in turn fire irregularly at close to 1/s, and increase only when the postures or movements are in error from those intended. The

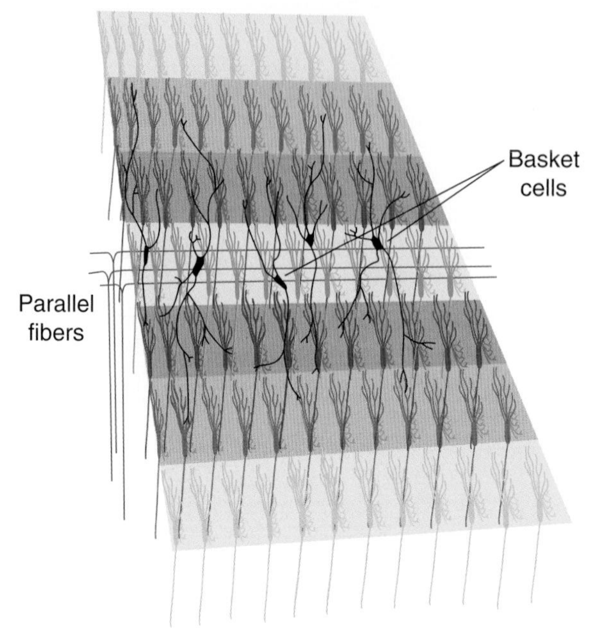

B

Parallel fibers
Basket
cell
Stellate
cell
Golgi
cell
Purkinje
cell
Climbing
fiber
Mossy
fiber
Inhibitory
cortical
side loop
Deep
cerebellar
neurons
Main
exciatory
loop
Precerebellar
nucleus cell
(spinocerebellar
pathways, brainstem
reticular nuclei,
pontine nuclei, etc.)
Inferior olivary
nucleus cell
Descending
motor
systems

C

Figure 41-2. (*continued*)

error-driven increase acts to lower the strength of the parallel fiber contact onto the Pc. Over trial-by-trial repetition, the climbing fiber action progressively changes the parallel fiber drive on the Pc, which serves to correct the nuclear cell output to generate postures and movements closer to those intended.

ACTIVITY IN INDIVIDUAL DEEP CEREBELLAR NUCLEI CORRELATES WITH (AND LESIONS IMPAIR) BEHAVIOR

The fastigial nuclei control all musculature involved in stance and gait (Fig. 41–3). They receive input from the vermal cortex, vestibular complex, lateral reticular nucleus, and (indirectly) spinocerebellar pathways. Single-unit recordings in the fastigius and vermal cortex of decerebrate cats have shown neural discharge that is correlated with both walking and scratching movements.[14,15]

Ablations of the fastigial nuclei (Fig. 41–3) in cat and monkey dramatically impair movements requiring control of equilibrium, such as unsupported sitting, stance, and gait.[15–17] Longitudinal splitting of the cerebellar cortex in humans along the midline also produces very significant and long lasting disturbances of equilibrium.[18] These data suggest that the fastigial nuclei may be preferentially involved in the postures and movements of stance and gait.

Interpositus neurons fire when the holding position of a limb is perturbed. In doing so, these neurons appear to control antagonist muscles that check the reflex movement of the limb to its prior hold position.[10,19] Interpositus neurons also modulate their activity in relation to sensory feedback, including that from tremor accompanying movement.[10,19,20] This finding is consistent with the idea that the interpositus is involved in controlling the antagonist muscle to dampen the tremor[20] (Fig. 41–3). Other evidence suggests that the interpositus is important in determining whether the pattern of activity in muscles acting at a joint represents reciprocal activation or co-contraction.[21,22] During behaviors that involve co-contraction, interpositus cells fire as if activating both agonist and antagonist muscles, and Pc are silent. In behaviors where agonists and antagonists are reciprocally active, both interpositus cells and Purkinje cells fire in similar patterns. One interpretation of these results is that alternating firing in Pc creates (through inhibition) a reciprocal pattern of activity the interpositus cells, which in turn produces the alternation between agonist and antagonist muscles.

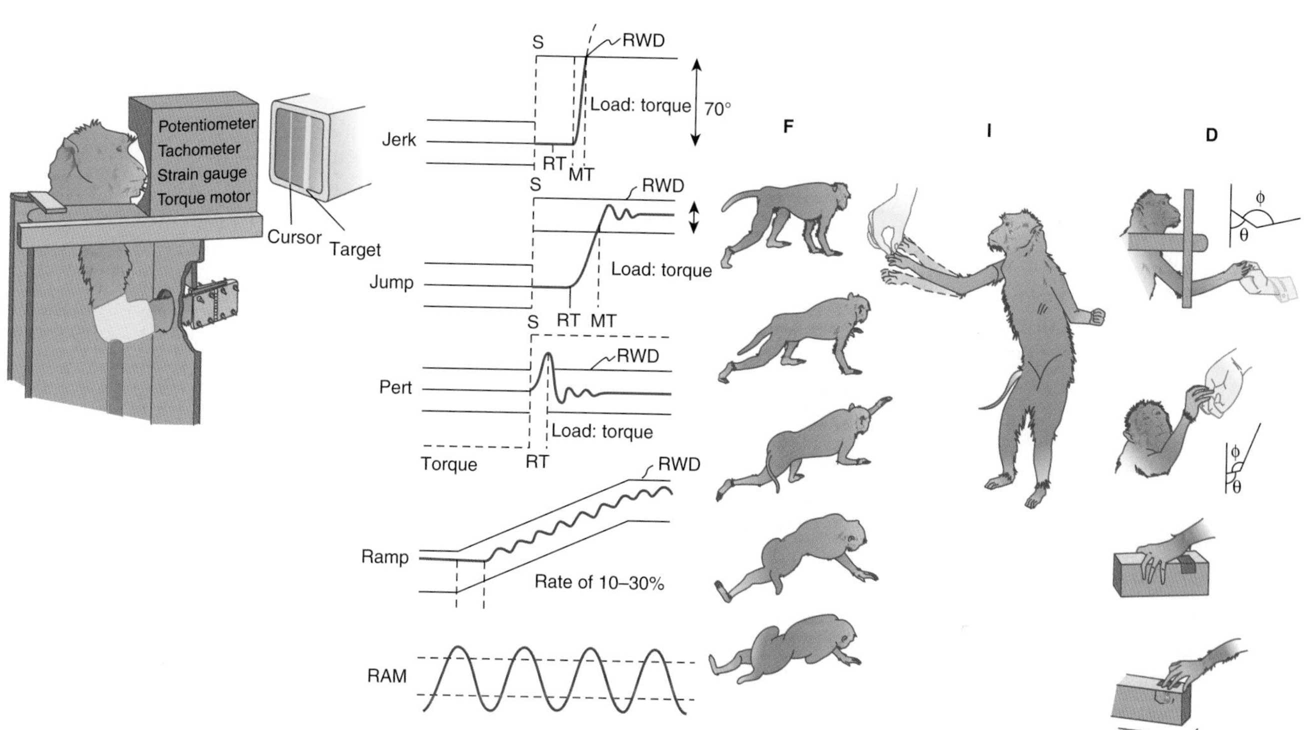

Figure 41–3. Cerebellar inactivation impairs compound movements more than simple movements. (*Left*) While seated in a chair, monkeys were trained to follow a visual target by making movements isolated to the wrist. Then portions of the cerebellum were transiently inactivated by injections of lidocaine. The performance of the simple wrist movements, except for tremor on slow ramp movements, was scarcely affected by the inactivation. (*Right*) However, upon leaving the chair, the effect of the inactivation was very apparent on compound body movements, and varied according to the site of injection: Fastigial (F): falls to the side of the inactivation, with a wide-based stance and gait; Interposed (I): in reaching to target, delay of onset of antagonist muscle producing overshoot of target, with a terminal action tremor; Deentate (D): in reaching to target, errors in *x*, *y*, and *z* dimensions, together with finger incoordination. (Reproduced with permission from Thach WT, Goodkin HP, and Keating JG. The cerebellum and the adaptive coordination of movement. Annu Rev Neurosci 1992;15:403–442.)

Ablation of the interpositus nucleus in monkeys primarily causes tremor[23,24] (Fig. 41–3). In monkeys, interpositus inactivation disturbs gait minimally but causes a large-amplitude, 3-to 5-Hz action tremor as the animals reach for food. These studies support the idea that the interpositus in monkeys is most concerned with balancing the agonist-antagonist muscle activity of a limb as it moves. The interpositus may use the abundant afferent input it receives from the periphery to generate predictive signals that decrease alternating stretch reflexes capable of causing limb oscillation.

Neuronal activity in the dentate precedes the onset of movement and may also precede firing in the motor cortex.[12,25] Dentate cells fire preferentially at the onset of movements that are triggered by mental associations, with either visual or auditory stimuli. Activity in the dentate, interpositus, and fastigial nuclei relate more to movements involving multiple joints than to those involving single joints.

Ablation of the dentate nucleus in monkeys produces slight reaction time delays, poor endpoint control, and impaired multijointed movements far beyond any deficits found in single-jointed movements[26–28] (Fig. 41–3). The same is true in humans.[29] In multijointed movements, dentate ablation results in profoundly impaired reaching patterns with abnormally increased angulation of the shoulder and elbow and excessive overshoot of the target. Dentate inactivation in monkeys and humans causes difficulty pinching small bits of food out of a narrow well; instead, the animals use one finger as a scoop to retrieve the food.[27,29]

Damage to the cerebellar cortex causes disability similar to but less severe than that resulting from damage to the deep nuclei. Damage to the cortex and the inferior olive also prevents many kinds of motor adaptation, including the acquisition of new and novel muscle synergies.

THE CEREBELLUM PARTICIPATES IN MOTOR LEARNING

David Marr,[30] James Albus[31] and Masao Ito[13] proposed that the cerebellum plays an important role in motor learning. Experiments have since shown that climbing fiber input to Purkinje neurons modifies the response of the neurons to mossy fiber–parallel fiber inputs and does so for a prolonged period.[32] Specifically, climbing fibers can selectively induce *long-term depression* in the Pc in response to parallel fibers that are activated concurrently with the climbing fibers. Furthermore, concurrent stimulation of climbing fibers and parallel fibers depresses the Pc responses to subsequent stimulation of the same parallel fibers but not to the stimulation of other parallel fibers that had not been stimulated earlier along with climbing fibers.

What functional effects might this long-term depression have? Altering the strength of certain parallel fiber–Pc synapses would alter the discharge of deep cerebellar nuclear neurons in such a way as to shape or correct eye or limb movements. During an inaccurate movement, the climbing fibers would respond to specific movement errors and depress the synaptic strength of parallel fibers involved with those errors, namely those that had been activated with the climbing fiber. With successive movements, the parallel fiber inputs conveying the flawed central command would be increasingly suppressed, a more appropriate pattern of simple-spike activity would emerge, and eventually the climbing-fiber error signal would disappear.

THE CEREBELLUM LEARNS AND STORES INTERNAL MODELS OF POSTURE AND MOVEMENT

Since the cerebellum has an accurate internal model of the physical properties of the body, it can use that model to convert the desired final movement end point into a sequence of kinematically scaled and dynamically timed commands for muscular contraction. Recordings from neurons within the cerebellum have provided evidence compatible with the idea that the cerebellum contains models of kinematics and dynamics for both arm movements and eye movements.

Studies of the movements of patients with cerebellar disorders have implied that another mechanical property of a multisegment limb, interaction torques, is also represented by an internal model in the cerebellum (Fig. 41–4).[33] Because of the structure of the arm and the momentum it develops when moving, movement of the forearm alone causes forces that move the upper arm. If a subject wants to flex or extend the elbow without simultaneously moving the shoulder, then muscles acting at the shoulder must contract to prevent its movement. These stabilizing contractions of the shoulder joint occur almost perfectly in control subjects, but not in patients with cerebellar damage. Thus, internal models allow the cerebellum to anticipate the forces that result from the mechanical properties of a moving limb and may use its learning capabilities to customize internal models to anticipate those forces accurately.

As a result of disruption of the compensation for interaction torques, patients with cerebellar ataxia experience difficulty in controlling the inertial interactions among multiple segments of a limb. This accounts for the greater inaccuracy of multijoint versus single-joint movements. Over time and practice, patients develop a strategy of decomposing the movement into serial actions at single joints. Since they can move one joint at a time with relatively little impairment, they do so rather than attempting multijointed movements. This, we shall

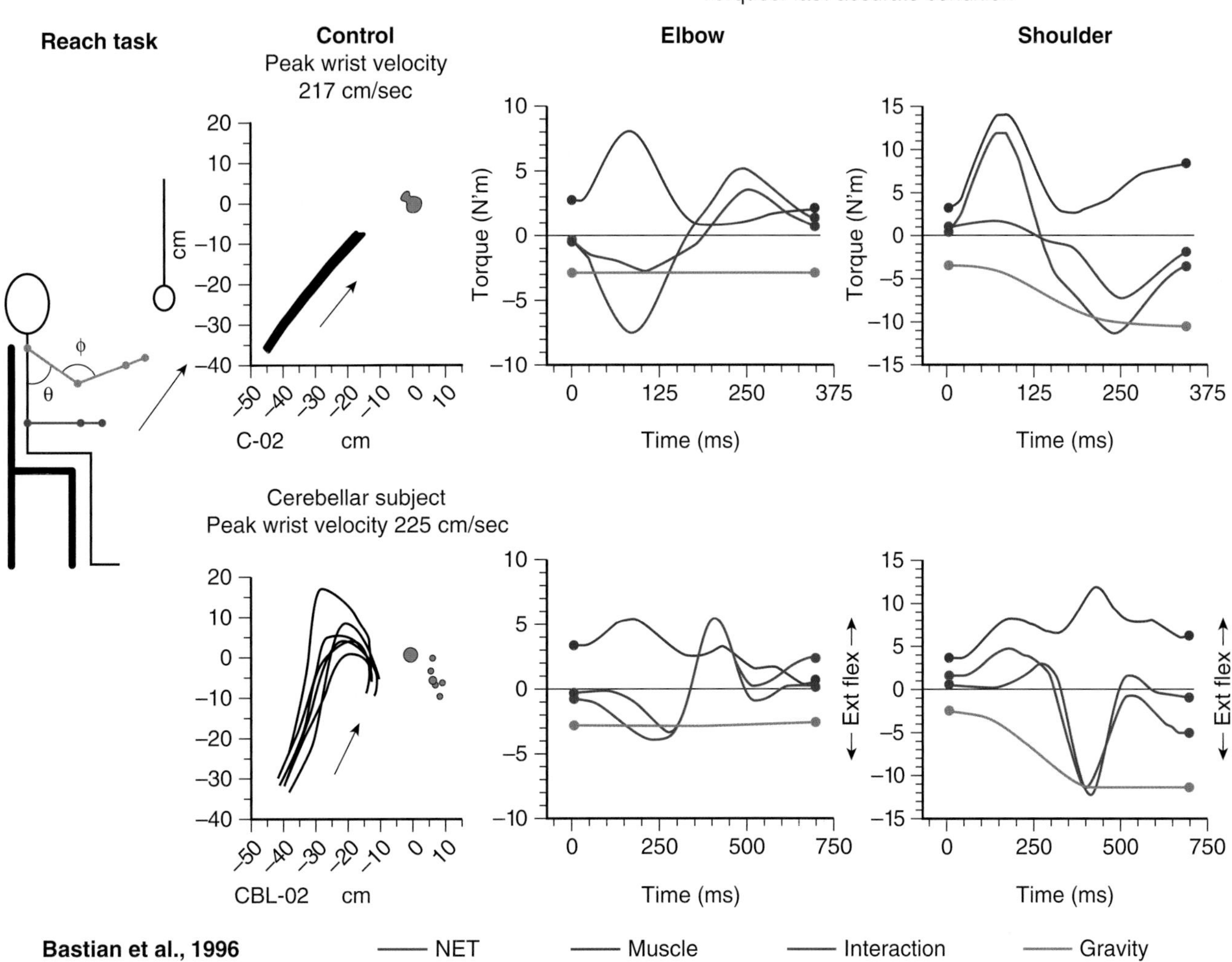

Figure 41–4. Ataxic reach: inability to compensate for interaction torques in multijoint movements. Normal human subjects (*left*) and those with lateral hemispheric cerebellar infarction (*right*) were asked to make a straight line reach to a target in space. Normal subject made the straight line reach without endpoint error; cerebellar subjects made a curved-path reach with endpoint errors in *x*, *y*, and *z* dimensions. Calculation of the interaction torques caused by the movement of one arm segment n another arm segment from estimates of the segment masses and the acceleration at connecting joints (Newtonian mechanics) suggested that the failure of the cerebellar subjects was attributable to an inability to compensate for the interaction torques. (Reproduced with permission from Bastian AJ, et al. Cerebellar ataxia: Abnormal control of interaction torques across multiple joints. J Neurophysiol 1996;76(1):492–509.)

argue later, can be the basis for rehabilitation of cerebellar movement disorders.

PARALLEL FIBERS AND PURKINJE CELL BEAMS ACT IN THE COORDINATION OF LINKED NUCLEAR CELLS

The relationship between cerebellar somatotopic maps and parallel fiber anatomy is consistent with a cerebellar role in movement coordination (Fig. 41–5). In each body representation in the deep nuclei, the rostrocaudal axis of the body is mapped onto the sagittal axis of the nucleus.[34,35] The hindlimbs are represented anteriorly, the head posteriorly, distal parts medially, and proximal parts laterally. This orientation would suggest that the myotomes, which are arranged orthogonal to the rostrocaudal axis of the body, are represented primarily in the coronal dimension of the cerebellum and thus orthogonal to the trajectory of the parallel fibers.[34,35] Because the parallel fibers are connected to the deep nuclear cells by Pc, a coronal "beam" of parallel fibers would control the nuclear cells that influence the synergistic muscles in a myotome. In this way, the parallel fiber would be

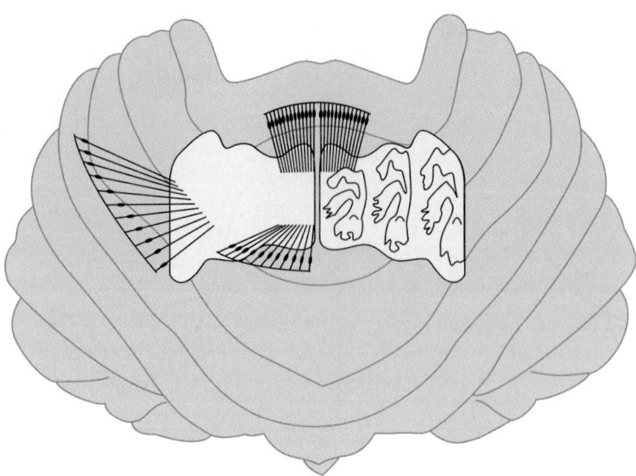

Figure 41–5. Parallel fibers are long enough to link together Purkinje cells projecting to different body parts within one nuclear body map, and multiple maps (Reproduced with permission from Thach WT, Goodkin HP, and Keating JG. The cerebellum and the adaptive coordination of movement. Annu Rev Neurosci 1992;15:403–442 [Fig. 2]). Within each of fastigial, interposed, and dentate nuclei there is a complete somatotoic representation of the body musculature. (Data from Asanuma C, Thach WT, and Jones EG. Anatomical evidence for segregated focal groupings of efferent cells and their terminal ramifications in the cerebellothalamic pathway of the monkey. Brain Res 1983 May;286(3):267–297 [Fig. 21]). The length of the parallel fibers in monkey is long enough to connect a beam of Purkinje cells projecting down onto a complete nucleus and adjacent nuclei. (Data from Mugnaini E. The length of cerebellar parallel fibers in chicken and rhesus monkey. J Comp Neurol 1983;220(1):7–15.). In rats trained to reach for an object, those Purkinje cells along a parallel fiber beam fired with simple spikes in synchrony and liked to forelimb muscles EMG during reaching. (Data from Heck DH, Thach WT, and Keating JG. On-beam synchrony in the cerebellum as the mechanism for the timing and coordination of movement. Proc Natl Acad Sci U S A 2007;104(18)(May):7658–7663.). Midline section of parallel fibers caused specific deficits suggesting that the parallel fibers coordinated the activities of the two legs. (Data from Bastian AJ, Mink JW, Kaufman BA, et al. Posterior vermal split syndrome. Ann Neurol 1998; 44:601–610.)

a single neural element spanning and coordinating the activities of multiple synergistic muscles and joints.

Anatomical studies indicate that parallel fibers in the monkey are about 6 mm long,[36] spanning a strip of cerebellar cortex that projects across the width of one or more of the deep nuclei (Fig. 41–5). Thus, the strip of Pc under the influence of a beam of parallel fibers of the same origin and length will control a strip of nuclear cells across an entire nucleus. Depending on which portion of the somatotopic map is involved, that nuclear strip may influence synergistic muscles of the eyes, head, neck, arm, trunk, or leg.

In a recent study in trained reaching rats,[37] simple spikes of pairs of Pc were recorded that, with respect to each other, were either aligned on a beam of shared parallel fibers or instead were located off beam. Firing rates of simple spikes firing in both on-beam and off-beam Pc pairs commonly showed large variation during reaching behavior. But with respect to timing, on-beam Pc pairs had simple spikes that were tightly time-locked to each other and to movement, despite the variability in rate. By contrast, off-beam Pc pairs had simple spikes that were not time-locked to each other.

What is the consequence of the on-beam synchronicity? Parallel fibers in the cerebellar cortex run roughly parallel to the myotomes of the body maps in the deep nuclei. On-beam parallel fiber activity may thus recruit Pc inhibition to modulate coordination and timing of the natural myomeric synergists mapped within the deep nuclei.

In addition, parallel fibers would be long enough to span (via Pc projections) two or more adjacent nuclei, fastigius controlling stance and gait, interpositus agonist/antagonist coordination at a single joint, and dentate eye–limb coordination in reaching and of digits in multi-digit movements.

Bastian and colleagues[20] reported how this might explain the inability to coordinate bilateral body movements in gait and balance after vermal section in humans. In five children who had surgical midline division of the posterior cerebellar vermis to remove fourth ventrical tumors (Fig.41–6 *top*), individuals could hop on one leg as well as normal controls (Fig. 41–6 *bottom*). Yet these same individuals could not do tandem heel-to-toe walking along a straight line without falling to one side or the other (Fig. 41–6 *bottom*). Fortunately, regular gait was little impaired. These observations suggested that vestibular information could be used to control one leg, but that the two legs could not be so coordinated. The division of parallel fibers crossing the midline seemed best able to explain this dissociation.

▶ IN SUMMARY

1. The cerebellum serves chiefly to coordinate movements involving many joints and muscles. Early studies of Flourens and Babinski emphasized that compound movements (those involving many joints and muscles) were severely affected by cerebellar lesions, while simple movements involving a single muscle or joint were affected little or not at all. These observations of the compound/simple dissociation have been replicated in animals. This leads to the generalization that the cerebellum serves as a "combiner" of simpler

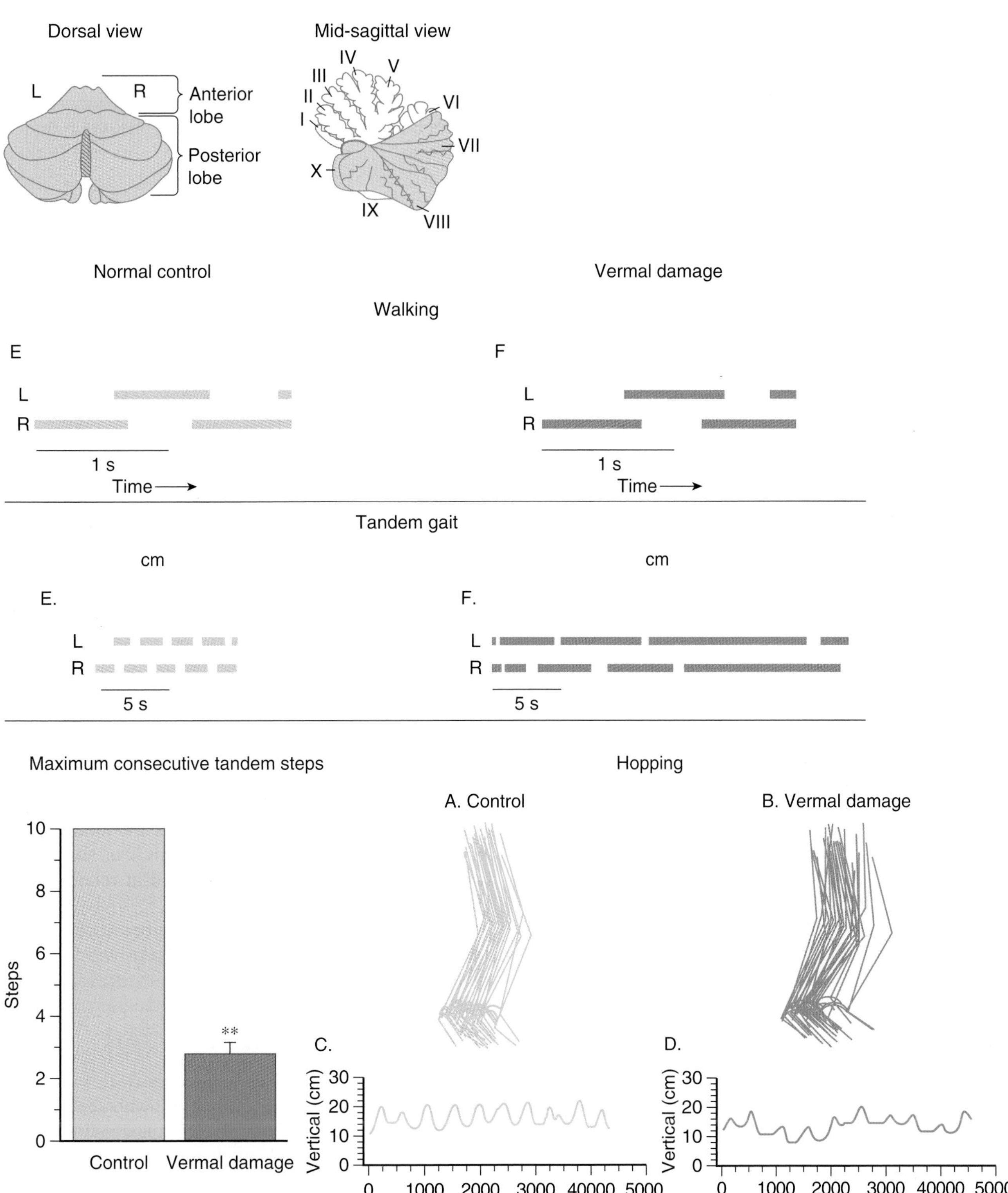

Figure 41–6. (*Top*) Five children ages 6–15 had posterior vermal splits to remove medulloblastomas from within the 4th ventricle. (Reproduced with permission from Bastian AJ, Mink JW, Kaufman BA, et al. Posterior vermal split syndrome. Ann Neurol 1998; 44:601–610 [Fig. 2].) (*Bottom*) Following surgery, the children could not perform heel-to-toe tandem gait without falling to one side. By contrast, they could hop on one leg as well as age matched control subjects. This suggested that cutting the parallel fibers in the midline prevented their linking the Purkinje cells on either side of the incision, in turn prevention the coordinated motions of the two legs together, while sparing the motions of either isolated leg. (Modified with permission from Bastian AJ, Mink JW, Kaufman BA, et al. Psoterior vermal split syndrome. Ann Neurol 1998; 44:601–610.)

movement elements controlled by other parts of the nervous system. Furthermore, the cerebellum contains learned programs for compensating for interaction torques that affect one body or limb segment when moving another segment.

2. The output of the cerebellum is from cells of the deep nuclei, which project to and excite many target cells in the nervous system, including motor and interneurons in the spinal cord, brain stem, and (via thalamus) cerebral cortex.

   (The nuclear cells are under tonic inhibitory control from Pc of the cerebellar cortex, whose firing rates are modifiable through learning to guarantee that the nuclear cell firing frequency is "just right" to optimally control cerebellar targets.)
3. The output of the cerebellum helps initiate movement: The excitatory nuclear cell output increases before that of its targets, and nuclear lesions delay or prevent firing change in the targets. Again, this is true mainly/only for compound movements.
4. The cerebellum has been shown to play a key role in motor learning by actions of the inferior olive climbing fiber ("teacher") on Purkinje and other cells in the cortex and nuclei. What is learned includes programs for the combination of muscles and body parts for use in specific contexts, and for compensation for interaction torques generated by the movement of one body part upon another. These torques are greatest when the moving body parts have large mass, and accelerate/decelerate quickly.

▶ OTHER PROPOSED MODELS OF CEREBELLAR FUNCTION

TIMER/CLOCK MODEL?

Numerous investigators have proposed that the cerebellum performs a pure timing function. Braitenberg and colleagues proposed that a wave of activity propagated along a parallel fiber could be "tapped off" by successive Pc, each tap occurring at an incremental delay after the onset of the wave.[38] This delay could be used to time movements for up to 50 ms or so. Lamarre[39] and Llinas[40] each proposed motor clock functions for the cerebellum on the basis of presumed periodic discharge of the inferior olive. This proposal was founded on the effects of the drug harmaline, which induced a whole-body, 10-Hz tremor in cats and a correlated synchronous discharge in inferior olive cells. It was also supported by studies showing a tendency for olivary neurons to fire periodically and in synchrony, and on the electronic coupling between olivary neurons, which theoretically might serve synchronize their discharge.[40] However, this interpretation is challenged by other studies showing that olivary discharge in the awake, performing monkey is not only nonperiodic but indeed random.[41,42] Ivry and colleagues[43] proposed, based on different evidence, that the cerebellum functions as a general purpose timer. Patients with lateral cerebellar injury are impaired in their ability to perceive differences in intervals between tone pairs of the order of half a second. This observation has been interpreted as indicative of a general clock not only for movement but also for perception. These timer/clock models maintain that the cerebellum (or the inferior olive) controls only the timing of muscle activity.

Arguing against these ideas is the absence of any demonstrated clocklike periodicity of cerebellar nuclear cell discharge. Instead, these cells produce a graded, tonic discharge that correlates with muscle pattern and force, limb position, and movement direction.[41,42]

▶ A CEREBELLAR ROLE IN REHABILITATION?

Patients with cerebellar disease have long been known to make compensatory behavioral adjustments to account for their incoordination. Yet, there is relatively little written about or using these adjustments to train patients in rehabilitation: the assumption is all too often that "there is nothing that can be done about it." What follow are some of these behavioral compensations that patients have developed on their own. While some of them, such as the wide-based gait, are well known, others have more rarely been appreciated. The following examples have all been documented by film in patients in chronic care programs. The suggestion here is that they be formally instituted in rehabilitation training practice.

The general philosophy is *to recognize and encourage decomposition of movement, and train the use of the simple motor elements.*

UPRIGHT STANCE AND GAIT

In standing and walking, encourage the wide base. Developing a fixed angle at both hips, with feet widely laterally placed on the floor. This forms a stable tripod that helps to prevent falling. It may also prove to be helpful in having lockable knee braces to prevent knee movement. It might also prove beneficial to have a trunk brace to restrict unwanted axial movements.

In walking, use canes to assist balance and restrict movement of trunk with emphasis on controlling movement at hip and shoulder. Use Loftstrand canes to minimize need for combined wrist/elbow activities that are required for simpler canes.

In walking, keep head and neck extended (rather than looking down at floor/feet) to enlist brain stem postural antigravity reflexes (A number of workers have begun to comment on this—John Milton, Thomas L. Clouse.

Use walkers and, ultimately, wheel chairs, progressing from arm operated to motorized ones.

SITTING, RISING FROM SITTING

In sitting upright in bed, abduct arms at the shoulder and place hands on the bed, developing a "tripod" for the trunk as in the wide-based stance and gait.

In rising from sitting, in standing, in walking, hold on with hands and arms to fixed objects—table tops, car doors, stair rails, walls.

ARM MOVEMENTS

In drinking from a glass, place elbow on table and move only at the elbow to avoid use of combined elbow-shoulder movement.

FINGER MOVEMENTS

Substitute single digit movements for combined movements (e.g., "winkling" of forefinger, replacing attempted thumb–forefinger "precision pinching").

GO SLOW!

Encourage *slowing* of movements to minimize interaction torques.

▶ A CEREBELLAR ROLE IN SHIFTING CONTROL FROM ONE CEREBRAL CORTICAL HEMISPHERE TO THE OPPOSITE

A series of patients sustained infarct of the left cerebral cortical frontal speech area with immediate onset of aphasia. After time and speech training, they recovered the ability to speak. fMRI study showed that on speaking, symmetrically opposite portions of the opposite right cerebral hemisphere were active. Further, the regions of the cerebellum now active in speech had shifted to the left cerebellar hemisphere. This suggests that (1) the primary property of the cerebellar hemispheres is not speech (right) or spatial operations (left), but rather (2) their cooperation/training of the opposite cerebral hemisphere cortex, whatever activities it is engaged in.[44]

An ongoing series of studies is exploring this potential role in neurorehabilitation of gait after hemiplegia due to cerebral hemispheric cortical infarcts or hemispherectomy for seizure control. Subjects repeatedly walk on a split treadbelt. The belt on the defective side can be made to move faster to bring gait in the impaired leg up to match that on the normal side. This training appears to carry over to "over ground" gait for a period of time. Further studies will determine whether additional intensive training can induce a permanent learning effect [Bastian, in progress].

REFERENCES

1. Holmes G. The cerebellum of man. The Hughlings Jackson memorial lecture. Brain 1939;62:1–30.
2. Dow RS and Moruzzi G. The Physiology and Pathology of the Cerebellum. 1958, Minneapolis: Univ. of Minnesota Press.
3. Gilman S, Bloedel JR, and Lechtenberg R. Disorders of the Cerebellum. Philadelphia, PA: FA Davis Co., 1981.
4. Gilman S. The mechanism of cerebellar hypotonia. An experimental study in the monkey. Brain 1969;92(3): 621–638.
5. Gilman S and Newman SW. Manter and Gatz's Essentials of Clinical Neuroanatomy and Neurophysiology. 8th ed. Philadelphia, PA: FA Davis Co., 1992, p. 179
6. Flourens P. Recherches Experimentales sur les Proprietes et les Fonctions du Systeme Nerveux, dans les Animaux Vertebres. Paris: Crevot, 1824.
7. Babinski J. De l'asynergie cerebelleuse. Rev Neurol (Paris) 1899;7:806–816.
8. Babinski J. Asynergie et inertie cerebelleuses. Rev Neurol (Paris) 1906;14:685–686.
9. Thach WT. Discharge of Purkinje and cerebellar nuclear neurons during rapidly alternating arm movements in the monkey. J Neurophysiol 1968;31(5):785–797.
10. Thach WT. Discharge of cerebellar neurons related to two maintained postures and two prompt movements. II. Purkinje cell output and input. J Neurophysiol, 1970;33(4):537–547.
11. Thach WT. Discharge of cerebellar neurons related to two maintained postures and two prompt movements. I. Nuclear cell output. J Neurophysiol 1970;33(4):527–536.
12. Thach WT, Correlation of neural discharge with pattern and force of muscular activity, joint position, and direction of intended next movement in motor cortex and cerebellum. J Neurophysiol 1978;41(3):654–676.
13. Ito M. Neural design of the cerebellar control system. Brain Res 1972;40:80–82.
14. Andersson G and Armstrong DM. Complex spikes in Purkinje cells in the lateral vermis (b zone) of the cat cerebellum during locomotion. J Physiol 1987;385:107–134.
15. Botterell EH and Fulton JF. Functional localizaton in the cerebellum of primates. II. Lesions of midline structures (vermis) and deep nuclei. J Comp Neurol 1938;69:47–62.
16. Dow RS. Effect of lesions in the vestibular part of the cerebellum in primates. Arch Neurol Psychiatry 1938;40: 500–520.
17. Chambers WW and Sprague JM. Functional localization in the cerebellum. II. Somatotopic organization in cortex and nuclei. AMA Arch Neurol Psychiatry 1955;74(6):653–680.
18. Bastian AJMink JW, Kaufman BA, et al. Posterior vermal split syndrome. Ann Neurol, 1998;44:601–610.

19. Soechting JF, Burton JE, and Onoda N. Relationships between sensory input, motor output and unit activity in interpositus and red nuclei during intentional movement. Brain Res 1978;152(1):65–79.
20. Elble RJ, Schieber MH, and Thach WT, Jr. Activity of muscle spindles, motor cortex and cerebellar nuclei during action tremor. Brain Res 1984;323(2):330–334.
21. Frysinger RC, Bourbonnais D, Kalaska JF, et al. Cerebellar cortical activity during antagonist cocontraction and reciprocal inhibition of forearm muscles. J Neurophysiol 1984;51(1):32–49.
22. Wetts R, Kalaska JF, and Smith AM. Cerebellar nuclear cell activity during antagonist cocontraction and reciprocal inhibition of forearm muscles. J Neurophysiol 1985;54(2):231–244.
23. Vilis T, and Hore J. Effects of changes in mechanical state of limb on cerebellar intention tremor. J Neurophysiol 1977;40(5):1214–1224.
24. Vilis T. and Hore J. Central neural mechanisms contributing to cerebellar tremor produced by limb perturbations. J Neurophysiol 1980;43(2):279–291.
25. Lamarre Y, Spidalieri G, and Chapman CE. A comparison of neuronal discharge recorded in the sensori-motor cortex, parietal cortex, and dentate nucleus of the monkey during arm movements triggered by light, sound or somesthetic stimuli. Exp Brain Res Suppl 1983;7:140–156.
26. Meyer-Lohmann J, et al. Effects of dentate cooling on precentral unit activity following torque pulse injections into elbow movements. Brain Res 1975;94(2):237–251.
27. Thach WT, Goodkin HP, and Keating JG. The cerebellum and the adaptive coordination of movement. Annu Rev Neurosci 1992;15:403–442.
28. Spidalieri G, Busby L, and Lamarre Y. Fast ballistic arm movements triggered by visual, auditory, and somesthetic stimuli in the monkey. II. Effects of unilateral dentate lesion on discharge of precentral cortical neurons and reaction time. J Neurophysiol 1983;50(6):1359–1379.
29. Goodkin HP, et al. Preserved simple and impaired compound movement after infarction in the territory of the superior cerebellar artery. Can J Neurol Sci 1993; 20(suppl 3):S93–104.
30. Marr D. A theory of cerebellar cortex. J. Physiol 1969;202:437–470.
31. Albus JS. A theory of cerebellar function. Math Biosci 1971;10:25–61.
32. Ito M, M Sakurai M, and Tongroach P. Climbing fibre induced depression of both mossy fibre responsiveness and glutamate sensitivity of cerebellar Purkinje cells. J Physiol 1982;324:113–134.
33. Bastian AJ, et al., Cerebellar ataxia: Abnormal control of interaction torques across multiple joints. J Neurophysiol 1996;76(1):492–509.
34. Asanuma C, Thach WT, and Jones EG. Anatomical evidence for segregated focal groupings of efferent cells and their terminal ramifications in the cerebellothalamic pathway of the monkey. Brain Res 1983;286(3):267–297.
35. Thach WT, et al., Cerebellar nuclei: Rapid alternating movement, motor somatotopy, and a mechanism for the control of muscle synergy. Rev Neurol (Paris) 1993;149(11): 607–628.
36. Mugnaini E. The length of cerebellar parallel fibers in chicken and rhesus monkey. J Comp Neurol 1983;220(1):7–15.
37. Heck DH, Thach WT, and Keating JG, On-beam synchrony in the cerebellum as the mechanism for the timing and coordination of movement. Proc Natl Acad Sci U S A 2007;104(18)(May):7658–7663.
38. Braitenberg V. Is the cerebellar cortex a biological clock in the millisecond range? Prog Brain Res 1967;25:334–346.
39. Lamarre Y and Mercier LA. Neurophysiological studies of harmaline-induced tremor in the cat. Can J Physiol Pharmacol 1971;49(12):1049–1058.
40. Llinas R and Yarom Y. Oscillatory properties of guinea-pig inferior olivary neurones and their pharmacological modulation: an in vitro study. J Physiol 1986;376:163–182.
41. Keating JG and Thach WT. Nonclock behavior of inferior olive neurons: interspike interval of Purkinje cell complex spike discharge in the awake behaving monkey is random. J Neurophysiol 1995;73(4):1329–1340.
42. Keating JG and Thach WT. No clock signal in the discharge of neurons in the deep cerebellar nuclei. Journal of Neurophysiology 1997;77:2232–2234.
43. Ivry RB, Keele SW, and Diener HC. Dissociation of the lateral and medial cerebellum in movement timing and movement execution. Exp Brain Res 1988; 73(1):167–180.
44. Connor LT, et al. Cerebellar activity switches hemispheres with cerebral recovery in aphasia. Neuropsychologia 2006;44(2):171–177.
45. Vesalius A. De Humani corporis fabrica libri septem (On the fabric of the human body in seven books) Muscles 1543; (Pt 2):174.
46. Ghez C and Thach WT. The Cerebellum. In Kandel ER, Schwartz JH, and Jessell TM (eds). Principles of Neural Science, 4th ed. New York: McGraw-Hill, Inc, 2000, pp.836–837 [Figs. 41–4, 41–5, and 41–6].

VI. OTHER MOVEMENT DISORDERS

CHAPTER 42

Wilson's Disease

Ronald F. Pfeiffer

In 1912, Wilson penned, as his doctoral thesis, his now-classic treatise describing the clinical and pathological features of the disease he labeled progressive hepatolenticular degeneration.[1] He was not, however, the first to describe the illness that now bears his name. Case descriptions of what likely was Wilson's disease (WD) were published by Frerichs in 1860,[2] Westphal in 1885,[3] Gowers in 1888,[4] Ormerod in 1890,[5] Homen in 1892,[6] and Strümpell in 1898,[7] but it was Wilson who accurately and in exhausting detail delineated the characteristics of this illness and distilled the information into a coherent clinical picture.

Since Wilson's description, our present-day understanding of WD has evolved and matured, with contributions from many individuals. Kayser in 1902[8] and Fleischer in 1903 and 1912[9,10] first described the rings of corneal pigmentation that are now so firmly linked with WD. Although Rumpel first described increased hepatic copper content in WD in 1913,[11] it was not until 1948, when Mandelbrote and colleagues[12] noted increased urinary excretion of copper and Cumings[13] documented copper deposits in both liver and brain, that WD was finally recognized as a disturbance of copper metabolism. Ceruloplasmin deficiency was subsequently documented independently by Scheinberg and Gitlin[14] and by Bearn and Kunkel[15] in 1952. The presence of impaired biliary excretion of copper in WD was first reported by Frommer in 1974.[16] The last six decades have been marked by dramatic advances in our ability to treat WD, and the last 15 years have witnessed the identification and characterization of the genetic abnormality responsible for WD.

▶ EPIDEMIOLOGY AND GENETICS

Although not recognized by Wilson himself—he noted it to be familial but believed that a toxin was the likely cause—WD was identified as a hereditary process by Hall in 1921.[17] It is an autosomal-recessive disease. Estimates of prevalence vary widely, but WD is by all accounts a rare disorder. A prevalence rate of 30 cases per million is often quoted,[18] but both lower and higher estimates have also been published, with more recent studies tending to show higher rates, perhaps due to improved diagnostic capability.[19] There is considerable geographic variability in prevalence rates for WD; in Europe a prevalence rate of 12–29 per million has been reported, which pales in comparison to a reported rate of 33–68 in Japan[20] A birth incidence rate of 17 per million (1 per 59,000) was reported in Ireland for the years 1950–1969;[21] others report incidence rates in the range of 1 per 30,000–40,000.[22,23] The incidence of WD in the United States has been estimated to be approximately one in 55,000 births.[23] It also has been estimated that there are approximately 6000 cases of WD in the United States and that approximately 1% of the population are carriers.[22]

In 1985, Frydman and colleagues proposed chromosome 13 as the location of the mutation responsible for WD.[24] This was subsequently confirmed in 1993, when several groups of investigators specifically localized, identified, and characterized the gene, now labeled the ATP7B (or WND) gene, which maps to 13q14.3 and covers a region of approximately 80 kilobase (kb) and contains 21 exons that encode a transcript of approximately 7.5 kb.[25–29] The protein encoded by the gene, also known as ATP7B (or WNDP), has been identified as a copper-transporting ATPase that binds six copper molecules[30,31] and is expressed primarily, but not exclusively, in liver and kidney. Two specific functions have been proposed for ATP7B within the liver. Under basal or steady-state conditions the protein is found primarily in the trans-Golgi network in hepatocytes, where it transports copper across organelle membranes so that the copper can be incorporated into apoceruloplasmin, forming ceruloplasmin.[32] Under high copper conditions, however, ATP7B is redistributed to cytoplasmic vesicles where it transports excess copper across the hepatocyte apical membrane into the bile canaliculus for subsequent biliary excretion.[33,34] In WD, mutation at the ATP7B locus results in defective ATP7B protein that is not capable of performing these functions, with consequent reduced amounts of ceruloplasmin in the serum and gradually increasing amounts of copper within the liver.

ATP7B is also expressed in stomach and small intestine.[35] Its function in the intestine is uncertain, but some investigators have proposed that it plays a role in maintaining copper homeostasis within enterocytes, most likely either by sequestering copper within the enterocytes or by facilitating apical excretion of copper, thus modulating intestinal copper uptake.

WD is an autosomal-recessive disorder in which the affected individual must receive a defective copy of the gene from each parent. It has become abundantly clear, however, that no single mutation of the ATP7B gene is responsible for all cases of WD. In fact, approximately 380 different mutations have now been documented in WD patients[36] and this number will almost certainly continue to grow. While missense mutations are most frequent, deletions, insertions, nonsense, and splice-site mutations all occur.[37] Most individuals with WD are actually compound heterozygotes, having inherited different mutations from each parent. In those in the United States and in individuals of northern European origin, the most frequent mutation appears to be the H1069Q mutation in exon 14 in which glutamine is substituted for histidine, but this mutation accounts for only 28–45% of the identified mutations in these groups.[22,38,39] It is this mutational heterogeneity that has made the development of commercially viable genetic testing for WD impractical thus far, although with the current pace of technical advances this certainly soon may change.

It has been speculated that the genotypic variability in WD may also play a role in the phenotypic variability so characteristic of WD, but studies have not clearly borne this out. It appears that additional factors must also be operative, since even individuals with the same mutation may vary widely in age of symptom onset and clinical presentation.[40] Even monozygotic twins with WD may display markedly different clinical manifestations of the disorder.[41]

▶ PATHOPHYSIOLOGY

As a vital component of enzyme systems such as cytochrome *c* oxidase, dopamine beta-hydroxylase, superoxide dismutase and tyrosinase, copper is an essential element for cellular functioning.[42] Dietary copper intake is typically in the range of 2–5 mg per day, with quite efficient (55–75%) intestinal absorption by enterocytes that is not regulated; instead, normal copper balance is maintained by regulation of excretion, which predominantly takes place via the hepatobiliary route.[43,44] On its own, free copper is an extremely toxic substance that can produce irreversible cellular damage and death. To protect against such injury, elegant systems have evolved that bind the copper molecule so that it can be safely absorbed, proper amounts can be transported to required sites, and excess copper can be eliminated from the body. When these delivery systems malfunction, cellular damage and death can result, either from too much or too little copper.

The mechanism by which copper produces cellular and neuronal damage and death is presumed to be via oxidative and nitrosative stress.[45] A copper-induced rise in levels of tumor necrosis factor-alpha (TNF-α), interferon-gamma (IFN-γ), and interleukin-6 (IL-6) has also been reported in patients with WD, suggesting the presence of cytokine-mediated inflammation as another factor in the pathogenesis of WD.[46]

First isolated in 1948, ceruloplasmin is an α2-glycoprotein that binds and transports 6 copper molecules.[47] It also has ferroxidase activity and may play a role in iron metabolism.[42,48] There are actually multiple forms of ceruloplasmin, with molecular weights varying from 115,000 to 200,000.[49] Although ceruloplasmin is characteristically decreased in WD, this is not absolute and WD is not, in its essence, a disease of ceruloplasmin deficiency. In fact, 5–15% of individuals with WD may have normal or only slightly reduced ceruloplasmin, whereas 10–20% of heterozygotes who are clinically asymptomatic may have reduced ceruloplasmin.[50] Ceruloplasmin deficiency in WD is due to reduced transport of copper for incorporation into apoceruloplasmin to form ceruloplasmin because of the reduced or defective ATP7B. The ceruloplasmin gene itself is on chromosome 3,[51] and is normal in WD.

Ceruloplasmin deficiency is not unique to WD. It is also characteristic of Menkes' disease. Hereditary ceruloplasmin deficiency, now labeled aceruloplasminemia, has also been described and is characterized by only modest hepatic copper accumulation, but dramatic iron deposition in liver, pancreas, and brain.[52,53] Transient ceruloplasmin deficiency may occur in a variety of conditions, including protein-losing enteropathy, nephrotic syndrome, sprue, as well as other situations in which both protein and calorie intake are deficient.[50] Ceruloplasmin deficiency also can be found in patients with chronic liver disease of any cause, including hepatitis C infection.[54]

The primary route of elimination of copper is the gastrointestinal tract.[55] Copper is also excreted in the urine, but this is normally only a secondary route. It has been firmly established that impairment of gastrointestinal elimination of copper is the fundamental basis of copper accumulation in WD. Copper is routinely secreted in saliva, gastric juice, and bile, but the copper from salivary and gastric sources is reabsorbed more distally in the gut, leaving biliary excretion as the primary source of copper elimination.[56,57] As noted earlier, the fundamental abnormality that characterizes WD is impaired biliary excretion of copper because of the genetically determined deficiency or defective function of ATP7B. This defect in biliary excretion of copper results in slow, but steady accumulation of copper in the body. Initially, the copper is stored in the liver, but eventually the storage capacity of the liver is exceeded and unbound copper spills out of the liver and finds its way to other organs and tissues, where it also begins to accumulate. As the excess copper escapes from the liver, urinary copper excretion markedly increases but is not able to compensate fully for the defect in biliary excretion. This results in a positive copper balance, with consequent relentless deposition of copper in other tissues.

▶ CLINICAL FEATURES

Although the fundamental pathogenetic defect in WD has its source in the hepatobiliary system, the consequences of the defect play themselves out in multiple organs and systems. This multisystem involvement lends itself to an extremely diverse clinical picture that, at times, presents a formidable diagnostic challenge for even the most astute clinician.

To aid in the diagnosis and assessment of individuals with WD, a number of scoring systems and scales have been devised. A scoring system was devised and published by a group of experts following the Eighth International Meeting on Wilson Disease and Menkes disease.[58] Aggarwal and colleagues have recently proposed and tested a global assessment scale intended for use in routine clinical practice to allow more objective assessment of patients with WD.[59] The Unified Wilson's Disease Rating Scale (UWDRS) has also been developed and tested.[60,61]

HEPATIC MANIFESTATIONS

Hepatic symptoms or signs of hepatic dysfunction are the most frequent mode of clinical presentation of WD, representing the initial feature in approximately 40–50% of cases (Table 42–1).[22,62] This percentage is even higher in Asian populations.[63] The average age of onset for individuals with WD who present with hepatic symptoms is 11.4 years.[64] It is rare for hepatic symptoms to appear before age 6, although elevation of liver enzymes has been noted in asymptomatic WD children as young as two years;[19] hepatic presentation beyond age 40 is unusual, but has been reported by numerous investigators.[19] In one center's experience, 17% of patients were over age 40 at the time of diagnosis.[65] One report describes a woman who, despite the absence of treatment, did not develop liver function abnormalities until age 74.[66]

▶ **TABLE 42–1. HEPATIC MANIFESTATIONS OF WD**

Asymptomatic spleen and liver enlargement
Acute transient hepatitis
Chronic hepatitis
Acute fulminant hepatitis
Progressive cirrhosis

Hepatic dysfunction in WD can follow one of several routes in its evolution. There may simply be asymptomatic enlargement of both liver and spleen. Liver function tests, however, may be elevated and spider angiomata may appear.

Acute transient hepatitis is a second, more common, mode of presentation. This occurs in 25% of individuals and is typically characterized by jaundice, anorexia, and easy fatigability with a reduced sense of energy. This may be all too easily passed off as a viral-induced hepatitis or infectious mononucleosis, especially when family history is silent. However, the concomitant presence of a hemolytic anemia should serve as an important portent of the presence of WD.[22] Other abnormalities that may also be clues to a diagnosis of WD in this setting include elevated unconjugated (indirect) bilirubin and reduced uric acid.

A picture indistinguishable from autoimmune hepatitis (chronic active hepatitis) occurs in 10–30% of individuals with WD.[67,68] One diagnostically treacherous aspect of this presentation of WD is the potential for the serum ceruloplasmin, as an acute-phase reactant, to become "elevated" into the low normal range.[22,67]

Acute, fulminant hepatitis, with rapidly progressive liver failure, encephalopathy, and coagulopathy is yet another potential mode of hepatic presentation of WD. It is the initial presentation in 5% of cases.[69] It carries with it an extremely high mortality rate. Individuals presenting in this fashion typically are younger than age 30, often in their teens; two-thirds are female.[70] Although most studies would suggest that the acute liver failure is superimposed upon a background of chronic hepatic injury,[71] fulminant failure without evidence of cirrhosis has been reported.[72] The acute hepatic failure results in massive release of copper, with marked elevation of serum copper (often >200 μg/dL), in contrast to the usual reduction in serum copper evident in WD.[44] A severe Coombs-negative hemolytic anemia, presumably as a result of intravascular hemolysis precipitated by the sudden release of hepatic copper into the bloodstream, is often present.[73] The sudden release of copper may also produce renal toxicity, with renal tubular dysfunction and consequent glycosuria, hypophosphatemia, and hypouricemia.[69] In contrast to fulminant hepatic failure in the setting of viral hepatitis, alkaline phosphatase and even aminotransferase levels are often disproportionately low, while bilirubin may be disproportionately elevated because of the hemolysis.[22,74,75] It can be very difficult to diagnose WD in a patient with fulminant hepatic failure. It may be impossible to perform liver biopsy because of coagulopathy, and 24-hour urinary copper levels, in addition to taking too long to collect, may be unreliable because of the development of hepatorenal syndrome.[76] Ceruloplasmin levels also become unreliable in the setting of fulminant hepatic failure.[71] Korman and colleagues have suggested that the combination of an alkaline phosphatase:total bilirubin (AP:TB) ratio of less than 4 and an aspartate aminotransferase:alanine aminotransferase (AST:ALT) ratio of greater than 2.2 in the setting of fulminant hepatic failure is highly accurate in predicting a diagnosis of WD, especially if hemoglobin concentration is also reduced.[71]

The most frequent hepatic manifestation of WD is the development of progressive cirrhosis. Individuals typically develop slowly progressive hepatic failure with splenomegaly (with or without hepatomegaly), ascites, esophageal varices, and encephalopathy. There are no specific identifying characteristics of the cirrhosis.

Because of the absence of any pathognomonic clinical characteristics of hepatic dysfunction due to WD, any individual under age 50 with unexplained liver disease, whether viral negative hepatitis, chronic hepatitis, cirrhosis or acute fulminant hepatic failure, should be screened for WD.[22]

NEUROLOGICAL MANIFESTATIONS

Left untreated, most individuals with WD will eventually develop symptoms or signs of neurological dysfunction (Table 42–2). In 40–60% of affected persons, however, neurological symptoms are actually the initially recognized clinical feature.[22,62] As might be suspected from the pathophysiology of WD, the average age at which neurological features appear is significantly later than the average age of onset of hepatic WD manifestations (18.9–20.2 years versus 11.4–15.5 years),[77,78] although neurological symptoms have been reported as early as age 6.[77] There is also a longer delay in diagnosis when the presenting symptoms are neurological rather than hepatic in nature; the difference was 44.4 versus 14.4 months in one study.[78] Although it is also infrequent, onset of neurological dysfunction after age 50 may occur[22,79] and onset of neurologic symptoms has even been described as late as age 72.[80]

▶ TABLE 42–2. NEUROLOGICAL MANIFESTATIONS OF WD

Frequently present
Tremor
Dysarthria
Cerebellar dysfunction
Dystonia
Gait abnormality
Occasionally present
Autonomic dysfunction
Headache
Seizures
Sleep disturbances
Muscle cramps
Pseudobulbar emotional lability
Typically absent
Upper motor neuron dysfunction
Weakness
Spasticity
Hyperreflexia
Babinski response
Lower motor neuron dysfunction
Hyporeflexia
Sensory loss
Sphincter dysfunction

Tremor is the most frequent neurological presenting feature in WD, occurring in approximately 50% of individuals.[81] The tremor may be resting, postural or kinetic in character. Asymmetry is the rule. The tremor may be fine or coarse, proximal or distal. A proximal component of tremor in the arms can endow the tremor with a "wing-beating" appearance. Head titubation may also be present. An unusual presentation of tremor in WD is isolated tongue tremor.[82,83] The importance of considering WD in the differential diagnosis of tremor presenting in young persons, even when the family history does not seem to be compatible with a recessive disorder, has been stressed.[84]

Dysarthria is another common feature of neurological WD, eventually developing in the vast majority of patients. In one series, it was the most frequent neurological manifestation of WD.[85] Several broad categories of dysarthria have been described, although typically the dysarthria is mixed in character.[85] Hypokinetic dysarthria resulting from extrapyramidal dysfunction, particularly dystonia, affecting the tongue, face, and pharynx, commonly occurs. Speech can be severely compromised. The dysarthria can become so severe that the patient becomes virtually mute. Drooling, another frequent feature of WD, is also a consequence of the dystonia, as is the "risus sardonicus," or fixed grimace-smile, seen in some individuals with WD. In addition to the risus sardonicus, some investigators have described a distinctive facial appearance that has been labeled the "Wilson's facies," which is characterized by a variable combination of open mouth, pseudoptosis, decreased eye contact, drooping angle of the mouth, and delayed or absent changes in facial expression that collectively produce a dull expressionless face.[59] An unusual "whispering dysphonia" has also been described in WD,[86] as has a very unusual laugh in which most of the sound is generated during inspiration.[87] Another type of dysarthria observed in WD is cerebellar in character, typified by scanning, explosive speech. It is the result of cerebellar and brain stem involvement. Dysphagia, with prolonged oral transit duration and increased oral residue, may also develop in individuals with WD.[88] Impaired pharyngeal function and esophageal dysmotility have also been described.[89,90]

Cerebellar dysfunction, which initially gave rise to the term "pseudosclerotic" as a type of WD, is seen in approximately 25% of WD patients with neurological dysfunction.[91] In addition to the scanning speech described earlier, individuals may display impaired coordination and kinetic (intention) tremor as part of the clinical picture. Deterioration of handwriting is often evident.

Dystonia, which can involve limbs and trunk in addition to the facial and pharyngeal muscles noted earlier, is seen quite frequently in WD, affecting 37% of patients in one series.[92] Cervical dystonia may be the presenting feature of the illnness.[93] Chorea is uncommon in WD; both tics and myoclonus are very unusual.

Gait abnormalities are another hallmark of WD. As with dysarthria, both extrapyramidal and cerebellar patterns of impairment have been described. An individual with WD may display a parkinsonian gait, a wide-based ataxic gait, or a combination of the two.

Seizures have been reported in up to 6% of patients with WD, especially in younger individuals.[94] The combination of seizures and psychiatric disturbances may indicate the presence of frontal white matter lesions.[95] Pseudobulbar emotional lability,[96] hypersomnia,[97] altered REM (rapid eye movement) sleep function,[98] and even priapism[99] have been reported in WD. Muscle cramps can be a source of discomfort for some individuals. Headache can be the presenting neurological symptom, according to some investigators, in approximately 10% of patients with WD.[18] Although often not mentioned in reviews of WD clinical features, autonomic dysfunction, presumably due to central mechanisms, has been reported to be present in 26–30% of persons with WD.[100,101]

Neither upper motor neuron signs (weakness, spasticity, hyperreflexia, Babinski responses) nor lower motor neuron signs (hyporeflexia) are typically seen in WD. Sensory loss and sphincter dysfunction are also unusual.

Historically, neurological WD has been separated into two types, the classic (dystonic) and the pseudosclerotic (Westphal) forms, with the former characterized primarily by extrapyramidal dysfunction and the latter by cerebellar dysfunction. A more recent classification scheme has included pseudoparkinsonian, pseudosclerotic, and dyskinetic categories. However, these attempts at classification are of limited practical value, since considerable variability and overlap exist.

PSYCHIATRIC MANIFESTATIONS

The psychiatric features of WD are often underappreciated and under diagnosed. Most reports indicate that psychiatric symptoms are the presenting clinical feature in approximately 20% of individuals with WD. However, some investigators have reported that psychiatric symptoms were evident at the time of initial presentation in 65% of individuals with WD, and that these symptoms were sufficiently severe to warrant psychiatric intervention in almost 50% before the diagnosis of WD was ever made.[102] Delay in diagnosis is common when psychiatric features are the presenting manifestation of WD, and such delays adversely affect treatment outcome.[103]

Most individuals with WD will experience psychiatric symptomatology at some point during the course of their illness (Table 42–3). Not surprisingly, psychiatric manifestations of WD are most frequently present in individuals who also display neurological dysfunction.

Therefore, WD should be considered and excluded in any young person, at least up to age 50, who develops otherwise unexplained psychiatric dysfunction, especially when signs of associated neurological impairment are also evident.[104] Brewer has also observed that it is important to consider the possibility of WD in young persons suspected of drug abuse, since the symptoms can be very similar.[22,104]

As with the neurological picture of WD, there is no archetypal psychiatric WD presentation. Subtle changes in personality and behavior may develop, including emotional lability, irritability, impulsiveness, childishness, reduced anger threshold, aggressiveness, recklessness, and disinhibition.[105,106] In a study of 50 patients with WD, excessive talkativeness, aggressive behavior, loss of interest in surroundings, and abusiveness were labeled as key psychiatric symptoms.[107] Bipolar affective disorder was diagnosed in nine of the 50 individuals. Deterioration in school or work performance may be an early clue of developing symptomatic WD.[22,106] Disturbances in mood, especially depression, are reported in 27% of patients[108] and may be unrecognized in many more. In one alarming study, almost 16% of patients had a history of suicide attempts.[108] Mania may occur and be the initial manifestation of the disorder.[109] WD may also present as an isolated obsessive–compulsive disorder.[110] Circadian rhythm abnormalities, with disturbances in temperature, pulse and blood pressure, have been noted in WD patients with psychiatric symptoms, suggesting hypothalamic dysfunction.[111]

▶ TABLE 42–3. PSYCHIATRIC MANIFESTATIONS OF WD

- Frequent
  - Personality changes
  - Emotional lability
  - Irritability
  - Impulsiveness
  - Childishness
  - Reduced anger threshold
  - Aggressiveness
  - Recklessness
  - Disinhibition
- Mood disturbances
  - Depression
  - Mania
- Infrequent
  - Psychosis
  - Dementia

Although clear-cut dementia is uncommon in WD, it may develop in patients with advanced WD, where structural central nervous system (CNS) damage has occurred. Patients with neurological symptoms of WD do, however, demonstrate a range of cognitive impairments that can involve frontal executive ability, visuospatial processing, and some aspects of memory.[112] Formal neuropsychological testing may demonstrate a spectrum of abnormalities.[113–116] It has been suggested that cognitive impairment in WD is a result of subclinical hepatic encephalopathy,[117] but this assessment is controversial.[106] The appearance of an individual with WD, who may display dysarthria, drooling, impaired coordination, and bradykinesia, can also be mistakenly perceived as indicative of cognitive impairment when, in fact, intellect is intact.

Psychosis, although unusual in WD, may occur and be characterized by paranoid thinking, delusional thoughts, hallucinations, and even catatonia.[118–120] These psychiatric features often respond poorly to conventional psychiatric medical management. Antisocial or criminal behavior has also been reported in individuals with WD.[121] Sexual preoccupation and disinhibition may develop in WD,[18,102] as may anorexia nervosa.[122]

Psychiatric symptoms often improve with appropriate treatment of WD, but the improvement may be delayed for as long as 6–18 months. Permanent psychiatric impairment may persist, despite adequate treatment, especially if diagnosis and appropriate treatment have been delayed. Re-emergence of psychiatric symptoms may also occur if treatment for WD is discontinued.[123] Development of severe psychosis in tandem with recovery of motor function following initiation of copper chelation treatment has been described in individuals who were severely impaired and mute prior to treatment and has been labeled emergent psychosis.[59] The presumption is that prior to treatment the psychosis was masked by severe motor disability and mutism. The psychosis resolves with continued decoppering therapy.

OPHTHALMOLOGIC MANIFESTATIONS

As noted earlier, Kayser's initial description of the pigmented corneal rings that now bear his name was published in 1902, fully 10 years before Wilson's clinical compilation. Kayser's patient was believed at the time to be suffering from multiple sclerosis.[8] Fleischer described similar ocular changes in 1903, and in 1912 connected the corneal pigmented rings with the neurological picture of "pseudosclerosis."[9,10]

Kayser–Fleischer rings (KFRs) are formed by the deposition of copper in Descemet's membrane (See Table 42–4). The excess copper is actually deposited throughout the cornea, but it is only in Descemet's membrane that sulfur-copper complexes are formed, producing the visible copper deposits.[124,125] They are almost always bilateral, but unilateral KFRs have been described.[126] Vision is neither obstructed nor impaired by the KFRs. Their color is quite variable and typically ranges from gold to brown to green. Ruby red, bright green, and ultramarine blue coloration are also described.[127] Because of their usual color composition, fully developed KFRs are often quite readily seen in blue eyes, but can be very difficult to discern when the iris is brown. The visible KFR pigment appears first in the periphery of the cornea at the limbus and then spreads centrally. In some individuals, a clear area between the pigment and the corneoscleral junction may be present.[128] The superior aspect of the cornea is involved initially, followed by the inferior aspect and then, finally, the medial and lateral regions of the cornea fill in.

Because of this pattern of evolution, it is important always to lift the eyelid when examining for KFRs, so that the entire cornea is exposed and inspected, lest an incomplete KFR be overlooked.[129] Furthermore, in many individuals, especially those with brown eyes or in whom the KFRs are not mature, it may be impossible to see the KFRs under routine ophthalmological examination. This mandates that slit-lamp examination by a neuro-ophthalmologist or experienced ophthalmologist be the routine, rather than the exception, in the evaluation of the patient with neurological or psychiatric features suspected of WD. (See Table 42–4.)

Corneal pigment deposition can occur in conditions other than WD. Copper-containing corneal rings indistinguishable from KFRs on slit-lamp examination have been

▶ TABLE 42–4. OPHTHALMOLOGICAL, MUSCULOSKELETAL, AND OTHER SYSTEMIC MANIFESTATIONS OF WD

Ophthalmological features
- Kayser–Fleischer rings
- Sunflower cataracts

Musculoskeletal features
- Osteoporosis
- Joint involvement
- Vertebral column abnormalities

Hematologic features
- Hemolytic anemia
- Thrombocytopenia

Renal features
- Nephrocalcinosis
- Hypercalciuria
- Hyperphosphaturia
- Aminoaciduria
- Proteinuria

Dermatological features
- Hyperpigmentation
- Azure lunulae

described in a variety of hepatic conditions, including primary biliary cirrhosis,[128,130] autoimmune (chronic active) hepatitis,[131] possible partial biliary atresia,[131] cirrhosis, and chronic cholestatic jaundice.[132] Estrogen-based oral contraceptives can elevate serum copper levels and have been reported to produce corneal pigment deposition within Descemet's membrane.[133] Intraocular copper-containing foreign bodies, or "grinders," can stain the iris and cornea (chalcosis) and mimic KFRs.[124] Copper sulfate-containing ophthalmic solutions, used to treat trachoma, can also stain the cornea.[134] In some individuals with multiple myeloma,[135,136] and in others with pulmonary carcinoma,[137] marked elevations of gamma-globulin and copper have led to corneal ring formation, but in a central rather than a peripheral pattern.

In several other situations, corneal staining unrelated to copper deposition can occur. Arcus senilis is usually easily distinguishable from KFRs by its whitish color, even though its location coincides with KFR territory. However, if an individual has superimposed carotenemia, the arcus senilis may assume a yellowish tint or cast and can be mistaken for KFRs.[138] Corneal heme staining following cataract removal may also transiently mimic KFRs.[131] Fleischer's ring, seen in keratoconus as a result of iron deposition in basal epithelial cells, develops as a greenish or brownish ring in the peripheral cornea and can be mistaken for KFR.[127]

KFRs are virtually always present in patients with WD who have developed neurological or psychiatric dysfunction, but they may not yet be apparent in persons with only hepatic symptoms or in presymptomatic individuals. In one large cohort of patients, KFR were present in 100% of patients with neurological dysfunction but in only 86% of those with hepatic presentation and 59% of presymptomatic individuals.[139] Other investigators contend that KFR are present at the time of diagnosis in only 44–62% of all patients presenting with hepatic dysfunction and that they are usually absent in children presenting with liver disease.[44] There are case reports documenting the absence of KFRs in WD patients with neurological symptoms, but this must be an exceedingly rare occurrence.[79]

Another ocular manifestation of WD is the sunflower cataract, which was first described by Siemerling and Oloff in 1922.[140] The sunflower cataract is much less common than KFRs, occurring in only 17% of untreated individuals.[124] It consists of copper deposits in the lens that have a green, gold, brown, or grey coloration and a sunburst or sunflower-like appearance, with a central powder-like disc and radiating petal-like spokes.[124,141] The sunflower cataract typically does not interfere with vision and in most instances can only be seen during slit-lamp examination.

Other ophthalmologic abnormalities may also be seen in WD. Eye movement abnormalities have been described by a number of investigators; over 90% of patients demonstrated abnormalities of ocular motility in one study[142,143] Impairment of voluntary control of saccades and disturbed smooth pursuit eye movements, with preservation of reflexive saccades, has been noted.[144] White retinal spot formation,[145] night blindness,[146] rapidly progressive visual loss due to optic neuropathy,[147] difficulty with gaze fixation,[148] eyelid-opening apraxia,[149] and oculogyric crisis[150] have all been described in WD, but whether they are rare features of WD or simply coincidental findings is uncertain.

MUSCULOSKELETAL MANIFESTATIONS

Joint and bone involvement is an under-recognized component of WD. (See Table 42–4) It has been reported with especially high frequency in Asian populations,[63] and the term "osteomuscular type" has been employed to describe such individuals with skeletal involvement and additional muscle weakness and wasting.[63,151] This higher frequency of musculoskeletal manifestations has been noted in Chinese,[152,153] Japanese,[154] and Indian[151] populations.

Osteoporosis, characterized by radiographic evidence of decreased bone density, may develop in up to 88% of persons with WD.[155,156] Osteomalacia, rickets, and localized bone demineralization all may occur.[157] These bone changes may lead to frequent, sometimes spontaneous, fractures. In a study of 31 children with newly diagnosed WD, osteopenia was present in 22.6% and osteoporosis in 67.7%.[158]

Joint involvement, especially at the knees, may lead to joint hypermobility or, alternatively, to joint stiffness and pain suggesting premature osteoarthritis.[155,156,159,160] Periarticular and intra-articular calcifications can also develop.[157] Joint pain can be the presenting symptom of WD.[156] A variety of vertebral column abnormalities have also been described in WD patients, with radiological evidence of this in 20–33%.[155,161]

The mechanism of bone and joint damage in WD is not clear. With the use of X-ray microprobe spectrometry, synovial copper, and iron deposition have been documented in WD, and it has been suggested that tissue destruction, mediated by free radical formation, may be responsible for the cartilage and synovial damage.[162]

OTHER MANIFESTATIONS

Hemolytic anemia may be the initial manifestation of WD in 10–15% of cases.[157,163,164] (See Table 42–4) The hemolysis is probably the result of free copper-induced oxidative injury to erythrocytes.[163,165,166] In the setting of transient hepatitis, the hemolytic anemia may also be transient. However, severe hemolytic anemia can develop in patients with WD who develop fulminant hepatic failure.[22,157,167] Additional complications, such as acute renal failure and pancreatitis, have also been reported in WD patients who develop severe hemolytic anemia.[168]

Brewer stresses that the concomitant occurrence of hemolysis and liver disease, especially in the setting of fulminant hepatic failure, is a very useful diagnostic clue to the presence of WD.[22] Furthermore, any young person with an otherwise-unexplained nonspherocytic, Coombs-negative hemolytic anemia should also be investigated for possible WD. Thrombocytopenia may develop in conjunction with hemolytic anemia, but isolated thrombocytopenia has also been reported.[169,170]

Renal involvement may also be part of the WD clinical spectrum. Excessive amounts of copper in the urine induce renal tubular dysfunction, which, in turn, can produce hypercalciuria and hyperphosphaturia with consequent nephrocalcinosis.[171] Hypercalciuria and nephrocalcinosis may even be the presenting features of WD.[172] Aminoaciduria and total proteinuria may also be present in WD.[77,173]

Wilson mentioned the presence of hyperpigmentation of the legs and a dark complexion in his initial description of WD.[1] Skin changes seem to develop with particular frequency in Chinese WD patients,[63] with anterior lower leg hyperpigmentation noted in 60% of patients in one series.[174] These changes can be misinterpreted as Addison's disease by the unwary. Bluish discoloration of the lunulae of the nails[42,175] and acanthosis nigricans[176] have also been reported in WD. Reduced sweat volume may also be present in untreated WD patients; it increases with either medical treatment of liver transplantation.[177]

Menstrual irregularity,[178–180] delayed puberty,[181] and gynecomastia have all been reported in WD, as have congestive heart failure, cardiac arrhythmia, glucose intolerance, and parathyroid insufficiency.[157]

▶ DIAGNOSIS

McIntyre has aptly stated, "the most important single factor in early diagnosis [of WD] is suspicion of the disease."[182] When the diagnosis is not considered, the diagnosis will not be made. WD should be considered and excluded in any "young" person (certainly up to age 50, but perhaps even to age 60) who develops unexplained neurological dysfunction, especially if the basal ganglia or cerebellum is involved. Moreover, because of its protean manifestations, similar consideration and exclusion of WD are equally important in similarly "young" individuals presenting with unexplained hepatic, psychiatric, and even other symptoms.

There currently is no single fail-safe diagnostic test for WD. The large numbers of mutations that occur in WD make genetic testing impractical as a screening tool at the present time. Moreover, either one or both causative mutations are not found in up to 20% of individuals with unequivocal WD who undergo genetic testing, probably because the responsible mutations are in the promotor region of the ATP7B gene, which is not analyzed during routine genetic analysis.[183] Thus, even negative genetic testing does not unequivocally exclude a diagnosis of WD. Future advances in technology likely will solve these barriers, but for the present, certain identification of WD can only be reached with judicious use of a combination of studies, the most important of which include serum ceruloplasmin, 24-hour urinary copper determination, slit-lamp examination for KFRs, and liver biopsy for determination of hepatic copper content (Table 42–5). Additional studies,

▶ **TABLE 42–5. DIAGNOSTIC TESTING FOR WD**

Diagnostic Test	Advantages	Disadvantages
Liver biopsy	The diagnostic gold standard Virtually always diagnostically elevated in WD	Potential morbidity May be elevated in other long-standing liver diseases
Ceruloplasmin	Readily available Abnormal in presymptomatic patients	Normal in 10–20% of WD patients Abnormal in 20% of carriers Is acute-phase reactant
24-h urinary copper	Virtually always elevated in untreated symptomatic patients	Cumbersome to collect Not always elevated in presymptomatic patients May be mildly elevated in carriers May be elevated in long-standing liver disease Chelation therapy complicates interpretation
Kayser–Fleischer rings (slit-lamp exam)	Virtually always present in patients with CNS symptoms (neurologic and psychiatric)	Requires referral to ophthalmologist Not reliably present in presymptomatic patients Not always present in hepatic WD
Free (unbound) copper	Measures potentially toxic portion of serum copper Typically elevated in symptomatic WD Useful for monitoring treatment compliance	Laboratories often unfamiliar with test Not reliably elevated in presymptomatic WD
Radiocopper incorporation	Useful when other tests show conflicting or nondiagnostic results	Somewhat complex to perform Can be abnormal in carriers
DNA analysis	Would be diagnostic in all patients	Vast number of potential mutations make it impractical

such as determination of the rate of incorporation of radiocopper into ceruloplasmin, neuroimaging studies, neurophysiological studies, serum free (nonceruloplasmin bound) copper levels, and even cerebrospinal fluid (CSF) copper levels, may be useful in some situations. However, it is not necessary to obtain each of the studies in every patient, and the testing typically necessary to diagnose the patient who presents with hepatic disease is different from that necessary in the individual with a neurological or psychiatric presentation.

It is important to perform the necessary studies in laboratories where the procedures are run frequently and the reported values are reliable. Care must be taken in collecting samples for analysis. Urine collections should always be in copper-free jugs supplied by the laboratory. Precautions must also be taken to avoid specimen contamination by the biopsy needle when performing liver biopsy.

LIVER BIOPSY

Determination of hepatic copper content via liver biopsy is the single most sensitive and accurate test for WD. Hepatic copper content will be significantly elevated in virtually all individuals with WD, even those who are clinically asymptomatic. Some investigators suggest that, because copper is not uniformly distributed in the liver, it is possible for a sampling error to give a falsely low copper level when a sufficiently sized biopsy (1–2 cm of tissue) is not obtained,[184] although Brewer believes such findings are more probably the consequence of inadequate laboratory technique.[22] Hepatic copper elevation in WD is typically quite striking, generally greater than 250 μg/g dry tissue, compared to normal values of 15–55 μg/g.

Hepatic copper elevation is not, by itself, pathognomonic for WD and can develop in obstructive liver diseases such as primary biliary cirrhosis, biliary atresia, extrahepatic biliary obstruction, primary sclerosing cholangitis, intrahepatic cholestasis of childhood, Indian childhood cirrhosis (Brewer has postulated that this entity actually occurs in WD heterozygotes exposed to excess dietary copper[22]), and autoimmune (chronic active) hepatitis.[185–189]

Deceptively low hepatic copper levels may also be found in individuals with WD if the biopsy is performed just as copper is being mobilized from the liver and released into the general circulation. In this situation, the hepatic copper content is still elevated, but levels in the range of "only" 100 μg/g may be recorded.[190] Some investigators have suggested that WD is unlikely with a hepatic copper content of less than 75 μg/g dry tissue and that levels between 75–250 μg/g are indeterminate.[19,191]

Although measurement of hepatic copper content is the most sensitive and accurate diagnostic study for WD, its invasiveness and small, but definite, risk of complication dictate that this study not be used as a universal screening procedure, but only when simpler approaches have not yielded a definitive diagnosis. This is unlikely to be necessary in persons presenting with neurological or psychiatric dysfunction, but is usually required in diagnosing those presenting with hepatic symptoms.

SLIT-LAMP EXAMINATION

Slit-lamp examination by a neuro-ophthalmologist or experienced ophthalmologist to look for KFRs is a vital part of the diagnostic evaluation for suspected WD. The presence of KFRs, although not absolutely specific for WD, is strong supportive evidence of the diagnosis in an individual with neurological or psychiatric features suggesting WD. It has been stated that the absence of KFRs in a patient with CNS symptoms or signs excludes the diagnosis of WD,[18] but exceptions to this doctrine have been reported and individuals with neurological WD but no KFRs described.[79,108,192,193] In persons with only hepatic symptoms or signs, where copper deposition may not yet have overwhelmed the storage capacity of the liver and systemic release of copper may not yet have occurred, KFRs are often absent. The same is true for presymptomatic individuals. It is worth repeating that KFRs can be difficult, and sometimes impossible, to see during routine office examination, especially if the patient has brown eyes, which makes it vital that slit-lamp examination be performed to accurately assess the presence or absence of KFRs.

CERULOPLASMIN

As a screening test for WD, assay of serum ceruloplasmin is both simple and practical, but not sufficient by itself. While it should be obtained on every individual in whom the diagnosis of WD is being considered, it is important to recognize that both false positive and false negative values may occur.

Ceruloplasmin may fall within or only slightly below the normal range in 5–15% of persons with WD.[18,22] Moreover, 10–20% of WD heterozygotes, who have only one defective copy of the WD gene and do not develop symptomatic WD or require WD treatment, may have ceruloplasmin levels that fall into the subnormal range.[18,22,44] Serum ceruloplasmin may also be reduced in a number of other conditions, as mentioned earlier. Because it is an acute-phase reactant, ceruloplasmin may increase in pregnancy, while taking birth control pills, during estrogen or steroid administration, or with infection or inflammation (including hepatitis).[22,50] It is possible, therefore, for ceruloplasmin to transiently reach normal or near-normal levels in persons with WD who also develop these conditions.[67] However, Yarze and colleagues believe that a serum ceruloplasmin level greater than 30 mg/dL virtually excludes the possibility of WD,[157] while Snow chooses a level of 40.[184]

24-HOUR URINARY COPPER EXCRETION

Urinary copper excretion rises dramatically in symptomatic WD, even though the increase is never sufficient to establish a negative copper balance. Urinary copper levels in symptomatic WD typically exceed 100 µg/day, but in presymptomatic individuals, where copper is still accumulating in the liver, urinary copper may still be in the normal range. Heterozygous carriers of WD may have modestly elevated urinary copper levels, but still less than 100 µg/day.[22] Moreover, obstructive liver disease, such as primary biliary cirrhosis, can also produce elevation of urinary copper.[189,194] Despite these caveats, a 24-hour urinary copper determination is, perhaps, the single best screening test for WD. The 24-hour nature of the test is a somewhat limiting factor in the use of the test as a screening tool, but the information obtained makes the test worth the trouble. Mak and Lam have drawn attention to a number of potential sources of contamination in collecting urine for copper determination: rinsing collection bottles with tap water may falsely elevate copper if the tap water has a high copper content, copper-free funnels should be used for pouring urine into containers, urine collection bags for pediatric patients may not be copper-free, and urine collected through a Foley catheter is not suitable for copper measurement.[19] Brewer routinely obtains two separate 24-hour urinary copper determinations and maintains that the 24-hour urinary copper will always be elevated in individuals with symptomatic WD; he believes that reports to the contrary[65,195] reflect laboratory error.[22]

Some investigators advocate the penicillamine challenge test (penicillamine-stimulated urinary copper excretion) as a useful non-invasive test in the diagnosis of WD,[196] although others qualify this by maintaining that the test is valuable in individuals with active liver disease but unreliable in asymptomatic siblings of WD patients.[197]

SERUM COPPER

Routine serum copper levels, which measure total serum copper, are frequently obtained as a screening test for WD, but are actually of little real value. Copper bound to ceruloplasmin normally represents approximately 90% of total serum copper.[22] Even though this percentage is lower in WD, total serum copper is usually reduced in WD simply as a reflection of reduced ceruloplasmin, and thus provides no additional useful diagnostic information.[22,157,198] The exception to this is fulminant hepatic failure, where serum copper levels may be markedly elevated because of sudden release of copper from tissue stores.[44]

FREE (NONCERULOPLASMIN-BOUND) COPPER

Determination of free (nonceruloplasmin-bound) serum copper directly measures the unbound (actually loosely albumin-complexed) copper in the blood.[157] It is this component that is free to be deposited in tissue and, thus, is potentially toxic. This copper fraction is typically elevated in symptomatic WD and may be used as another screening test for WD.[199] It's greater value, however, may be in monitoring response to and compliance with therapy. The serum free (nonceruloplasmin-bound) copper level is often calculated, rather than directly measured. Brewer notes that it can be calculated by determining total serum copper and ceruloplasmin on the same blood sample. The number for the ceruloplasmin level (reported in µg/dL) is multiplied by three and subtracted from the total serum copper level (reported in µg/dL), producing the calculated serum free copper level, which is 10–15 µg/dL in normal individuals.[22] It is higher than 25 µg/dL in most untreated WD patients.[44] Cut-off levels may vary and are not necessarily transferable between laboratories, however, so it is important to be familiar with the normal level for the laboratory one is using.[200] A method for direct measurement of free copper concentrations in serum or plasma by means of inductively coupled mass spectrometry has recently been reported.[201] Some investigators, however, hold the opinion that serum free copper levels, regardless of the way they are determined, are not helpful and may actually foment confusion.[19]

RADIOCOPPER INCORPORATION

Measurement of the incorporation of radioactive copper (^{64}Cu) into ceruloplasmin may also be of value in selected situations in the diagnostic evaluation of suspected WD, but is not used as a screening test. Difficulty obtaining the radioactive isotope also limits its availability.[44] In the normal individual there is an initial rise in ^{64}Cu after its oral or intravenous administration as it enters the blood and is complexed with albumin and amino acids. Serum ^{64}Cu levels then drop as the copper is cleared by the liver, only to show a secondary rise, peaking at 48 hours, as the ^{64}Cu is incorporated into newly synthesized ceruloplasmin by the liver and released into the circulation. This secondary rise in ^{64}Cu does not occur in WD because of defective ATP7B function, as described earlier. This defect will be evident even in individuals with normal or near-normal ceruloplasmin. Thus, this study can be useful in identifying such "covert" WD patients,[202] although some overlap between persons with WD and heterozygous carriers can exist.[22]

CSF COPPER

CSF copper levels have been measured in WD and found to be elevated in persons with neurological symptoms.[203] Levels also may decline in concert with symptomatic neurological improvement, leading some to suggest that CSF copper levels may be the most accurate reflection of the brain copper load.[204] In one study, the average treatment time necessary to normalize CSF copper content (<20 μg/L) was 47 months.[205] However, this method of copper monitoring is not performed on a routine clinical basis, and such use would require extensive additional validation.

NEUROIMAGING STUDIES

Neuroimaging studies frequently demonstrate abnormalities in WD. The changes are not specific for WD, but characteristic patterns of abnormality have been identified. As might be expected, magnetic resonance imaging (MRI) is a more sensitive indicator of brain involvement in WD than is computed tomography (CT). Some reports, in fact, have documented MRI abnormalities in 100% of individuals with WD who have neurological dysfunction.[206,207] The most consistent abnormalities are found in the basal ganglia; thalamus and brain stem are also frequently affected.[208,209] Increased signal intensity on T_2-weighted images is the characteristic abnormality; the increased signal intensity sometimes surrounds an area of decreased signal intensity.[209] It has been suggested that either edema or demyelination may account for the increased signal intensity, whereas either iron or copper deposition (both are paramagnetic substances) may produce the area of reduced signal intensity.[209,210] Certain abnormalities, such as the "face of the giant panda" midbrain sign[211,212] and the "bright claustrum" sign,[213] have been suggested to be characteristic of WD, but are not consistently present. Other disease processes, such as Leigh disease, hypoxic-ischemic encephalopathy, methyl alcohol poisoning, Japanese B encephalitis, and selective extrapontine myelinolysis, can show MRI changes similar to those seen in WD.[214] Thus clinical correlation is vitally important in assessing neuroimaging abnormalities. Abnormalities on diffusion MRI[215] and proton MR spectroscopy[216] have been described in WD. Although an earlier study did not find the latter procedure to be useful in either diagnosis or follow-up of WD patients,[210] more recently another group of investigators advocated the accuracy of the technique in monitoring treatment efficacy.[217]

Positron emission tomography (PET) scanning, both with ^{18}F-deoxyglucose[218,219] and ^{18}F-dopa,[220] typically demonstrates abnormalities in persons with WD, but PET still is not routinely available and, therefore, not part of the standard evaluation of the patient with suspected WD. Evoked potentials of various types may be abnormal in many patients with WD, often early in the course of the disease,[221] but are nonspecific and of no definitive diagnostic value.[222] Pilot studies with transcranial sonography suggest that this procedure may be useful in identifying copper accumulation in the basal ganglia preclinically, but more extensive evaluation is needed before this can be routinely employed.[223]

▶ TESTING GUIDELINES

In persons with WD presenting with hepatic dysfunction, KFRs are not consistently present, but 24-hour urinary copper content is usually elevated and serum ceruloplasmin often reduced. Liver biopsy is generally used to confirm the diagnosis by measurement of hepatic copper content and to assess the degree of hepatic injury. Individuals with longstanding hepatic failure or obstruction, regardless of cause, can demonstrate hepatic copper content that is elevated into the WD range. In these individuals, radiocopper assay may be considered in confirming or refuting the diagnosis of WD. Of course, genetic testing, if available, provides the most accurate diagnostic assessment.

In individuals with suspected WD presenting with neurological or psychiatric dysfunction, the presence of KFRs on slit-lamp examination, coupled with appropriately elevated 24-hour urinary copper and reduced serum ceruloplasmin, virtually confirms the diagnosis and obviates the need for liver biopsy. There may be instances, such as when KFRs are present and 24-hour urinary copper elevated but ceruloplasmin is not markedly reduced, that liver biopsy is still necessary.

▶ TREATMENT

Treatment strategies in WD center on restoring and maintaining appropriate copper balance within body tissues. With the exception of liver transplantation, treatment of WD is palliative rather than curative; the underlying defect that produces WD is not corrected, and treatment must be continued for the individual's lifetime. Four approaches to WD treatment have been employed, as discussed later.

DIETARY THERAPY

Limitation of dietary copper intake would seem, on the surface, to be a prudent and sensible maneuver in treating WD. In practice, however, it is difficult to achieve and has not been demonstrated to confer significant benefit. Brewer suggests that only shellfish and liver, both of which are especially high in copper content, be eliminated from the diet of WD patients.[22] Others would add nuts, chocolate and mushrooms to this list.[44]

In contrast to the general ineffectiveness of dietary therapy in WD, there have been anecdotal descriptions in which a strict lactovegetarian diet seemed to control WD adequately without other therapy,[224] presumably because the bioavailability of dietary copper was sufficiently reduced by the dietary fiber and phytate in these individuals. For most individuals, however, such a restrictive diet is not feasible.

Copper content in the primary drinking sources (home, work, school) of an individual with WD should be measured, and if the level is above 0.1 ppm alternative water sources, such as bottled water, should be used.[22] Brewer advises that such elevations are likely to be found for approximately 10% of WD patients.[22] It should also be remembered that domestic water softeners increase the copper content of water.[157] Copper content in any vitamin/mineral supplements that the WD patient might be taking should also be scrutinized.

INHIBITION OF INTESTINAL COPPER ABSORPTION POTASSIUM

Potassium iodide or potassium sulfide has been advocated in the past as a means of decreasing dietary copper absorption by interacting with copper to form insoluble copper iodide or copper sulfide. However, this approach is of no proven practical value and is not typically used in the treatment of WD.

ZINC

Zinc, administered as acetate, sulfate, or gluconate, provides another mechanism to limit gastrointestinal copper absorption in WD. The effect of zinc is mediated through the cysteine-rich 61-amino acid protein, metallothionein, which is present in many body tissues including brain, liver, and intestinal cells.[225,226] The presumed primary role of metallothionein in the body is as a zinc-binding ligand that is important for zinc homeostasis and transport.[226] Metallothionein has a high affinity for zinc, but an even higher affinity for copper.[227] When given on an empty stomach, supplemental oral zinc administration induces metallothionein formation in the intestinal enterocytes. The increased metallothionein then binds zinc and limits zinc absorption,[228] but it also binds dietary copper.[229] The bound copper, like the bound zinc, is then trapped and stored within the intestinal mucosal cells until the cells are eventually sloughed and excreted in the feces.[228,230] Reabsorption of copper that has been secreted into the gastrointestinal tract via saliva and gastric juices is also blocked by this mechanism. The net result of these actions is the induction of a small, but real, negative copper balance.

The role of zinc administration in the treatment of WD has become more clearly defined in recent years.[231] It is generally well tolerated, and this scant toxicity makes zinc very appealing as primary therapy of WD in the presymptomatic individual.[230–232] Its place in the treatment of the symptomatic patient has also been clarified. The effect of zinc administration on copper absorption does not become evident for 1–2 weeks because the induction of metallothionein is a rather slow process. Moreover, the negative copper balance induced by zinc is relatively small. In the eyes of most investigators these characteristics make zinc monotherapy unsuitable as initial therapy in the individual with WD who is already experiencing neurological symptoms,[22,231,233] although not all agree and zinc monotherapy has actually been used successfully in this clinical situation.[234,235] With the accumulation of extensive favorable experience, there is now consensus support for the use of zinc as "maintenance" therapy following (or in conjunction with) initial treatment with other more potent decoppering agents in neurologically symptomatic individuals.[19,22,44,235] Zinc therapy has also been reported to be safe and effective as maintenance management in both children and pregnant women.[236,237] It should be noted, however, that some investigators still view the use of zinc as monotherapy in WD as controversial.[238]

A dosage regimen of 50 mg of elemental zinc three times daily is generally employed. Dosage designation can be confusing, however. Zinc sulfate tablets, which are readily available without prescription in the US, are listed as containing 220 mg of zinc sulfate salt, but this translates to 50 mg of elemental zinc. Zinc acetate and zinc gluconate are labeled by their elemental zinc content.

Although zinc is almost always well tolerated, adverse effects may occur. Gastric irritation, typically with the morning dose, is more frequent with zinc sulfate than with zinc acetate.[230] For patients who are experiencing gastric discomfort with zinc administration, concomitant consumption of a small amount of a protein-containing snack (Jell-O, luncheon meat) often obviates the problem without significantly compromising efficacy.[22] Sideroblastic anemia resulting from impaired iron utilization has been reported with zinc therapy.[239] Zinc can lower high-density lipoprotein (HDL) cholesterol in both men and women by about 10%.[240,241] Serum amylase and lipase may increase early in the course of zinc therapy, later returning to normal.[242] The same phenomenon may be noted with alkaline phosphatase.[242] Whether neurological deterioration can develop as a direct result of initiating zinc therapy, as can occur with penicillamine, is disputed.[243–245] However, both neurological and hepatic deterioration have occurred in symptomatic individuals[246–248] and progression from asymptomatic to symptomatic has also been reported during zinc monotherapy.[249]

TETRATHIOMOLYBDATE

Ammonium tetrathiomolybdate (TM), although first tested in the treatment of WD in 1984,[243] has only in recent years received sustained attention[22,250] as potential WD therapy, and still remains an experimental agent that is not available for general use. Nevertheless, available evidence is sufficiently encouraging that inclusion of TM, despite its experimental status, seems warranted in a review such as this.

TM has a distinct, dual mechanism of action that distinguishes it from other available treatment modalities. It is able to reduce the copper load in WD by working at two distinct sites.[22,251] TM, like zinc, is able to limit gastrointestinal absorption of copper, but it does so by an entirely different mechanism of action. In the gut lumen, TM forms a tripartite complex with copper and albumin; the complexed copper cannot be absorbed by the intestinal mucosal cells and is excreted in the feces.[22,251] Both food-derived and endogenously secreted copper are complexed by TM. Unlike zinc, the negative copper balance produced by TM is present immediately because metallothionein induction is not necessary.

Inhibition of copper absorption, however, is not the only weapon that TM possesses in opposing copper toxicity. When TM is given without food, it is readily absorbed into the bloodstream. Once absorbed, it forms the same tripartite complex with albumin and unbound (free) copper in the blood, which renders the copper unavailable for cellular uptake and, therefore, nontoxic.[22,251] Other investigators, working with an animal model of WD, have reported that TM chelates copper within the liver, potentially binding up to six copper ions by forming copper-molybdenum multimetallic clusters.[252,253] Thus, TM can reduce the copper load in the WD patient systemically, in addition to its action in the gut lumen.

Unlike other available medications for WD, TM has not thus far been evaluated for chronic, or maintenance, therapy, but solely as an induction agent that is employed for an 8-week course of treatment and then discontinued and replaced with another agent, such as zinc, for chronic treatment. It is administered in a rather complex dosage regimen that is designed to maximize its effectiveness both in the gut and in the bloodstream. Six daily doses of 20 mg each are employed: three at mealtimes to reduce copper absorption via the gut and three between mealtimes to enhance TM absorption and maximize its action in the bloodstream.[22]

When administered as the initial therapy in the fashion described above to individuals with neurologically symptomatic WD, prompt and significant reduction in unbound (free) copper has been documented in open-label studies.[22,251,254,255] In Brewer's experience, neurological deterioration has occurred in less than 4% (2/56) of patients to whom TM has been administered.[22] Although generally tolerated quite well, several potential complications have been recognized. Bone marrow depression, with resultant anemia and occasional leukopenia, has occurred and is presumed to be a consequence of copper depletion in the marrow; it resolves with drug discontinuation.[22] Mild transaminase elevations have also been noted.[22] In rats, TM has also been shown to damage epiphyses in growing bone,[256] leading Walshe and Yealland to suggest that TM not be used for more than short courses in children or adolescents with unfused epiphyses.[257]

COPPER-CHELATION THERAPY

British Anti-Lewisite (BAL)

Dimercaprol, or British anti-Lewisite (BAL), was the initial copper-chelating agent used in the treatment of WD, but has now been virtually abandoned because of the necessity to administer it parenterally and because of its proclivity to produce a plethora of adverse effects such as headache, nausea, dizziness, and pain at the injection site.

Penicillamine

Penicillamine (dimethylcysteine) is a metabolic by-product of penicillin that avidly chelates copper; the resulting complexed copper is then excreted in the urine. Although it has generally been accepted that penicillamine produces its primary effect by copper chelation and subsequent cupriuresis, additional actions, including induction of metallothionein, have been proposed.[157] Following its introduction by Walshe in 1956 as a treatment for WD,[258] the consistent efficacy of penicillamine in inducing a negative copper balance and reducing the body's copper load was quickly recognized and penicillamine became the mainstay of WD treatment.

Improvement in function may begin within 2 weeks of initiating penicillamine therapy, but more typically, it is delayed for 2–3 months.[259] With continued therapy, gradual improvement may continue for up to 1–2 years.[230] Improvement in virtually all facets of clinical dysfunction may occur. From a neurological standpoint, tremor and cerebellar signs seem to improve more readily than dystonia, whereas the fixed smile and dysarthria may show no improvement at all. KFRs recede gradually in a sequence inverse to their appearance.[129] This languid resolution of KFR typically unfolds over 8–12 months.[59] Sunflower cataracts also clear, often more rapidly than KFRs.[124,129] Psychiatric symptoms improve with penicillamine therapy, although not as fully or as consistently as neurological symptoms and signs.[53,106] The same is true of psychometric testing.[260] Neuroimaging abnormalities, both on CT[261] and MRI,[206,207,262] may improve on penicillamine.

Penicillamine should always be given on an empty stomach. The bioavailability of penicillamine is reduced by approximately 50% if it is taken with food, although the absorption rate is not affected.[263] The traditionally recommended initial dose is 1–2 g daily, divided into four doses, but lower doses are recommended by some. Concomitant administration of pyridoxine has also been recommended by some because penicillamine is a pyridoxine antagonist;[157,264] however, others believe that penicillamine-induced pyridoxine deficiency only occurs in special circumstances, such as during pregnancy, during a growth spurt, or with dietary pyridoxine deficiency.[257,265]

A troublesome aspect of penicillamine is its propensity to produce initial deterioration in neurological function as treatment is initiated. The frequency with which this occurs is the subject of some dispute.[243–245] Walshe and Yealland[257] noted it in 22% (30 of 137) of patients that they treated, while Brewer and colleagues[22,266] reported it in 52% (13 of 25) in a retrospective survey. More ominously, Brewer adds that 50% of those in whom neurological deterioration occurred on initiation of penicillamine therapy did not fully recover to their baseline level of functioning.[22,266] Lethal status dystonicus has recently been reported following initiation of penicillamine treatment.[267] Emergence of neurological dysfunction in previously neurologically asymptomatic individuals has also been described after starting penicillamine.[268,269] The reason for this deterioration is not absolutely certain. Mobilization of copper from the liver with subsequent redistribution to the brain has been suggested,[266] but studies of CSF copper levels during this deterioration do not support this hypothesis.[204]

This potential for neurological deterioration has led some investigators to propose more gentle initiation of penicillamine therapy, with lower doses, and others to advocate induction of therapy with zinc or TM instead of penicillamine. Brewer and colleagues have been most vocal in their opposition to the use of penicillamine in the treatment of WD, and strongly advocate that it not be used at all, with the possible exception of the patient with fulminant hepatic failure awaiting liver transplantation, since safer alternatives are available.[22,244] Walshe, on the other hand, believes that a place for penicillamine still exists.[243] Thus, the controversy continues.[238,245]

A variety of other problems may also attend penicillamine therapy. Acute sensitivity reactions develop in 20–30% of individuals on penicillamine in conventional doses.[270,271] Consisting of skin rash, fever, eosinophilia, thrombocytopenia, leukopenia, and lymphadenopathy, these reactions typically develop within 2 weeks of initiation of treatment and should prompt discontinuation of the penicillamine. Even in the face of a severe reaction, however, it is not always necessary to abandon penicillamine therapy permanently. Therapy may be reinstituted at a reduced dose following resolution of the symptoms, initially with steroid co-administration.[272] However, with the current availability of alternative medications, such as trientine, such measures are usually not necessary and resumption of penicillamine is not recommended.[44] Up to 30% of patients are ultimately unable to tolerate penicillamine.[44,230] Agranulocytosis induced by penicillamine can be fatal.[273]

With chronic penicillamine administration a variety of other adverse effects may occur. Nephrotic syndrome,[274] Goodpasture's syndrome,[275] a lupus-like syndrome,[276] a myasthenia-like syndrome,[277] acute polyarthritis,[155] thrombocytopenia,[18] and retinal hemorrhages[278] have all been reported. Subclinical hypothyroidism has been described in children with WD receiving penicillamine.[279] Loss of the sense of taste may also occur with penicillamine therapy; a favorable response of this dysgeusia to zinc administration has been demonstrated.[280,281] Serum IgA deficiency has been noted with penicillamine.[282] Adverse reactions to penicillamine may still develop after prolonged therapy. There is a report of lupus developing after 30 years of therapy.[257]

Dermatologic problems may also develop with chronic penicillamine treatment. Penicillamine dermatopathy is characterized by brownish skin discoloration, which develops as a consequence of recurrent subcutaneous bleeding during incidental trauma.[283] The bleeding is attributed to penicillamine-induced inhibition of collagen and elastin cross linking.[284] Penicillamine can also impair wound healing,[285] which has led to the recommendation that penicillamine dosage should be reduced to 250–500 mg daily during perioperative periods.[18] Elastosis perforans serpiginosa,[286,287] pemphigus,[288] and aphthous stomatitis[289] are other reported penicillamine-induced dermatologic processes.

Trientine

Triethylene tetramine dihydrochloride, or trientine, is a copper-chelating agent with a mechanism of action similar to that of penicillamine.[290–293] However, the two compounds may act on different pools of copper in that trientine, in contrast to penicillamine, appears to compete for copper bound to albumin and does not enter the liver.[294] Trientine appears to be somewhat less potent than penicillamine and, thus, does not induce as vigorous decoppering, which may make it less likely to provoke the initial neurological deterioration that penicillamine can invoke, and thus be safer to use.

As with penicillamine, trientine should be taken on an empty stomach; a typical daily dose is 750–2000 mg, divided into three doses.[157] Once daily trientine administration has been effectively employed by some patients as a means to improve medication compliance, but such a treatment regimen should probably only be considered in special circumstances.[295] Experience with trientine has been less extensive than with penicillamine, but trientine appears to be a less toxic compound. Both lupus nephritis[292] and sideroblastic anemia[296] have been reported with trientine. Trientine will also chelate and form a toxic complex with iron, so concomitant administration of iron and trientine should be avoided.[44]

In the past, trientine was primarily used as an alternative copper-chelation therapy when penicillamine was not tolerated. With increasing recognition of the potential for initial neurological deterioration with the use of penicillamine, however, trientine has been increasingly advocated as a first line of treatment in the WD patient with neurological symptoms,[22,233,297] with subsequent switching to zinc for maintenance therapy.

LIVER TRANSPLANTATION

The most dreaded complication of WD is the development of fulminant hepatic failure. When treatment of Wilsonian fulminant hepatic failure is confined to medical management, the mortality rate is virtually 100%.[298–300] Because of this ghastly statistic, orthotopic liver transplantation (OLT) has been used with increasing frequency in this desperate situation. Chronic, severe hepatic insufficiency unresponsive to medical treatment measures is also seen as an appropriate indication for OLT in WD.[298]

A serious impediment to the employment of OLT in the setting of liver failure is the limited availability of donor organs, and it is not uncommon for patients to succumb, especially in the setting of fulminant hepatic failure, before a donor organ becomes available. Living-related liver transplantation, in which the donor is a living relative of the affected patient and donates part of his or her liver, has been successfully employed in WD in an effort to combat this limited liver availability.[301,302]

A form of modified dialysis in which albumin is utilized as a dialysate, the molecular adsorbents recirculating system (MARS), has been successfully employed in the setting of fulminant hepatic failure in WD patients as a bridge to buy time while awaiting an available liver for OLT.[303–305] Repeated utilization of MARS can significantly reduce serum copper levels and improve hepatic encephalopathy. Other temporizing approaches have also been devised for use while awaiting liver availability. Single-pass albumin dialysis[303,306] and plasmapheresis[307,308] also have been reported to be successful. Even a single session of plasma exchange may be beneficial when multiple sessions are not possible.[309] Extracorporeal perfusion through porcine liver cells has also been employed for the same purpose.[310]

Schilsky and colleagues have reviewed the experience with OLT in the treatment of WD at 15 transplant centers in the US and three in Europe.[298] Data on 55 patients were reviewed. The survival rate at 1 year was 79%. Similar survival rates have been noted by other investigators.[299,311] More recently, a survival rate of 100% with a median follow-up time of 10 years has been reported in 13 patients transplanted at a single center.[312] In addition to correction of hepatic dysfunction, improvement has been observed in the neurological, psychiatric, and ophthalmological features of WD following OLT.[298] However, the appearance of neurological symptoms shortly following OLT also has been reported and attributed to acute CNS injury due to massive release of copper from the damaged liver just prior to and during its removal.[313] Because the transplanted liver is free of the genetic defect responsible for WD, copper metabolism normalizes after OLT and continued chelation or other WD therapy is generally not necessary.[22,298,299] Although OLT may thus be viewed as curative therapy, it should be remembered that, if the transplant is received from a living related donor, such as a parent, the transplanted liver will carry the features of a heterozygote and, thus, may not have completely normal liver function.[314] Moreover, transplanted individuals still retain the genetic abnormality in other body tissues and will pass on the trait to all children.

Because of the success of OLT in treating WD patients with hepatic failure, the question as to whether patients with stable hepatic function but severe neurological dysfunction not responding to medical therapy should also be considered for OLT has been raised. There have been case reports of OLT performed in this situation,[315,316] but most investigators view such a treatment approach as experimental and not as the current standard of therapy. Brewer makes the point that improvement in neurological function following OLT is the result of normalized copper excretion with reduced brain copper load, which is also accomplished by medical management, and advocates that OLT be reserved for treatment of hepatic, not neurological, indications.[22]

Other surgical treatment approaches to WD have also been reported. Unilateral stereotactic thalamotomy has been employed successfully to ameliorate severe bilateral postural-kinetic tremor in one patient with WD.[317]

A possible glimpse into the future may have been provided by recent reports of the success of hepatocyte transplantation with subsequent hepatic repopulation in the Long-Evans rat model of WD.[318] Adenovirus-mediated gene transfer therapy has also been transiently effective in the same rat model.[319]

▶ TREATMENT GUIDELINES

In the individual with WD who is still asymptomatic (presymptomatic), most investigators recommend that therapy be initiated and maintained with zinc alone.

In the individual who has hepatic, but not neurological or psychiatric, symptoms, introduction of both a chelating agent and zinc may be ideal. Penicillamine has been the standard chelating agent in this situation in the past, but trientine is receiving increased attention because of the perception that it is less likely than penicillamine to induce neurological deterioration upon initiation of treatment.

It is in the individual who has developed neurological dysfunction that the most controversy regarding treatment choice has been evident. Available evidence suggests that TM may be the ideal agent for initiation of treatment in this situation, but, until formal approval from regulatory agencies is granted, its availability will remain limited. Thus, for most clinicians the choice for initial therapy will be between trientine and penicillamine. Both have their advocates, but a shift toward the use of trientine, because of its perceived lesser potential for inducing neurological deterioration, seems apparent in the literature. Zinc is recommended by some investigators for initiation of therapy in neurologically symptomatic individuals, but most reserve its use for maintenance therapy after initial decoppering.

For the individual with either fulminant hepatic failure or severe chronic liver failure, OLT may be the only viable treatment option.

Adequate monitoring of patients following initiation of treatment is an extremely important and often neglected aspect of WD management. Assuring patient compliance in taking prescribed medication is vital for successful outcome. Even with close, dedicated follow-up of patients and extensive educational measures, intermittent compliance problems become evident in 30% of WD patients, and severe compliance problems are noted in approximately 10%. Compliance with zinc therapy can be assessed by measurement of 24-hour urinary zinc and copper levels. A 24-hour urinary zinc level of less than 2 mg (normal is 0.1–0.4 mg) indicates inadequate compliance.[22] Monitoring compliance with trientine or penicillamine therapy is a bit more difficult, but a spike in a previously gradually decreasing 24-hour urinary copper level may indicate inadequate compliance.[22] In patients with WD on chronic, stable penicillamine therapy, the 24-hour urinary copper level should be in the range of 200–500 μg/day; levels below 200 μg/day may indicate either noncompliance or overtreatment.[44] The serum nonceruloplasmin (free) copper can also be useful as a monitoring tool; elevation above 15 μg/dL suggests inadequate compliance.[22,44]

It should also be remembered that prolonged treatment, both with zinc and with chelating agents, can actually induce copper deficiency in patients with WD. Anemia, sometimes with associated leukopenia, may be the initial sign of copper deficiency.[22] In patients on zinc maintenance therapy, a 24-hour urinary copper level below 35 μg is suggestive of copper deficiency due to overtreatment.[22] For individuals on trientine or penicillamine, a serum nonceruloplasmin (free) copper level below 5 μg/dL suggests overtreatment.[22,44]

A guideline for the diagnosis and treatment of WD, approved by the American Association for the Study of Liver Diseases (AASLD), has recently been published and provides an excellent in-depth review with 23 specific diagnostic and treatment recommendations.[44]

▶ SUMMARY

In the near-century since Wilson's seminal description, our understanding of and ability to treat WD effectively has dramatically advanced. Nevertheless, because of its protean clinical features, WD remains a tremendous diagnostic and therapeutic challenge to the clinician. The palliative nature of most WD therapy dictates constant vigilance on the part of the treating physician to ensure ongoing patient compliance and to watch closely for treatment complications. The reward, however, of prompt diagnosis and attentive therapy can be an asymptomatic and healthy individual faced with an otherwise fatal disease.

REFERENCES

1. Wilson SAK. Progressive lenticular degeneration: A familial nervous disease associated with cirrhosis of the liver. Brain 1912;34:295–507.
2. Frerichs FT. A Clinical Treatise on Diseases of the Liver. London: The New Sydenham Society, 1860.
3. Westphal C. Über eine dem Bilde der cerebrospinalen grauen Degeneration ähnliche Erkrankung des centralen Nervensystems ohne anatomischen Befund, nebst einigen Bermerkungen über paradoxe Contraction. Arch Psychiatr Nervenkrank 1883;14:87–134.
4. Gowers W. A Manual of Diseases of the Nervous System. London: J & A Churchill, 1988.
5. Ormerod JA. Cirrhosis of the liver in a boy, with obscure and fatal nervous symptoms. St Bart Hosp Rep 1890;XXVI:57.
6. Homen EA. Eine Eigenthümliche bei drei Geschwistern auftretende typische Krankheit unter der Form einer progressiven Dementia, in Verbindung mit ausgedehnten Gefässveränderungen (wohl lues hereditaria tarda). Arch Psychiatr 1892;XXIV:191–228.
7. Strümpell A. über die Westphal'sche Pseudosklerose und über diffuse Hirnsklerose, inbesondere bei Kindern. Dtsch Z Nervenheilk 1898;12:115–149.
8. Kayser B. Über einen Fall von angeborener grünlicher Verfärbung der Kornea. Klin Monatsbl Augenheilkd 1902;40:22–25.
9. Fleischer B. Zwei weiterer Falle von grünlicher Verfärbung der Kornea. Klin Monatsbl Augenheilkd 1903;41:489–491.
10. Fleischer B. Über eine der "Pseudosklerose" nahestehende, bisher unbekannte Krankheit (gekennzeichnet durch tremor, psychische storungen, braunliche Pigmentierung bestimmter gewebe, inbesondere auch der Hornhautperipherie, Lebercirrhose). Dtsch Z Nervenheilkd 1912;44:179–201.

11. Rumpel A. Über das Wesen und die Bedeutung der Leberveränderungen und der Pigmentierunen bei den damit verbundenen Fällen von Pseudosklerose, zugleich ein Beitrag zur Lehre von der Pseudosklerose (Westphal-Strümpell). Dtsch Z Nervenheilkd 1913;49:54–73.
12. Mandelbrote BM, Stanier MW, Thompson RHS, et al. Studies on copper metabolism in demyelinating diseases of the central nervous system. Brain 1948;71:212–228.
13. Cumings JN. The copper and iron content of brain and liver in the normal and in hepato-lenticular degeneration. Brain 1948;71:410–415.
14. Scheinberg IH and Gitlin D. Deficiency of ceruloplasmin in patients with hepatolenticular degeneration (Wilson's disease). Science 1952;116:484–485.
15. Bearn AG and Kunkel HG. Biochemical abnormalities in Wilson's disease. J Clin Invest 1952;31:616.
16. Frommer DJ. Defective biliary excretion of copper in Wilson's disease. Gut 1974;15:125–129.
17. Hall HC. La Dégénérescence Hépato-lenticulaire: Maladie de Wilson-Pseudosclérose. Paris: Paul Masson, 1921.
18. Scheinberg IH and Sternlieb I: Wilson's Disease. Philadelphia: WB Saunders, 1984.
19. Mak CM and Lam C-W: Diagnosis of Wilson's disease: a comprehensive review. Crit Rev Clin Lab Sci 2008; 45:263–290.
20. Meenakshi-Sundaram S, Mahadevan A, Taly AB, et al. Wilson's disease: A clinico-neuropathological autopsy study. J Clin Neurosci 2008;15:409–417.
21. Reilly M, Daly L, and Hutchinson M. An epidemiological study of Wilson's disease in the Republic of Ireland. J Neurol Neurosurg Psychiatry 1993;56:298–300.
22. Brewer GJ. Wilson's Disease: A Clinician's Guide to Recognition, Diagnosis, and Management. Boston: Kluwer, 2001.
23. Olivarez L, Caggana M, Pass KA, et al. Estimate of the frequency of Wilson's disease in the US Caucasian population: A mutation analysis approach. Ann Hum Genet 2001;65:459–463.
24. Frydman M, Bonné-Tamir B, Farrer LA, et al. Assignment of the gene for Wilson's disease to chromosome 13. Proc Natl Acad Sci U S A 1985;82:1819–1821.
25. Bull PC, Thomas GR, Rommens JM, et al. The Wilson disease gene is a putative copper transporting P-type ATPase similar to the Menkes gene. Nat Genet 1993;5:327–337.
26. Petrukhin K, Fischer SG, Piratsu M, et al. Mapping, cloning and genetic characterization of the region containing the Wilson disease gene. Nat Genet 1993;5:338–343.
27. Yamaguchi Y, Heiny ME, and Gitlin JD. Isolation and characterization of a human liver cDNA as a candidate gene for Wilson disease. Biochem Biophys Res Commun 1993;197:271–277.
28. Petrukhin K, Lutsenko S, Chernov I, et al. Characterization of the Wilson's disease gene encoding a P-type copper transporting ATPase: Genomic organization, alternative splicing, and structure/function predictions. Hum Mol Genet 1994;3:1647–1656.
29. Terada K, Schilsky M, Miura N, et al. ATP7B (WND) protein. Int J Biochem Cell Biol 1998;30:1063–1067.
30. Lutsenko S, Petrukhin K, Cooper MJ, et al. N-Terminal domains of human copper-transporting adenosine triphosphatases (the Wilson's and Menkes disease proteins) bind copper selectively in vivo and in vitro with stoichiometry of one copper per metal-binding repeat. J Biol Chem 1997;272:18939–18944.
31. DiDonato M, Narindrasorasak S, Forbes JR, et al. Expression, purification, and metal binding properties of the N-terminal domain from the Wilson disease putative copper-transporting ATPase (ATP7B). J Biol Chem 1997;272:33279–33282.
32. Hung IH, Suzuki M, Yamaguchi Y, et al. Biochemical characterization of the Wilson disease protein and functional expression in the yeast Saccharomyces cerevisiae. J Biol Chem 1997;272:21461–21466.
33. La Fontaine S, Theophilos MB, Firth SD, et al. Effect of the toxic milk mutation (tx) on the function and intracellular localization of Wnd, the murine homologue of the Wilson copper ATPase. Hum Mol Genet 2001;10:361–370.
34. Forbes JR and Cox DW. Copper-dependent trafficking of Wilson disease mutant ATP7B proteins. Hum Mol Genet 2000;9:1927–1935.
35. Weiss KH, Wurz J, Gotthardt D, et al. Localization of the Wilson disease protein in murine intestine. J Anat 2008;213:232–240.
36. Wilson AM, Schlade-Bartusiak K, Tison JL, et al. A minigene approach for analysis of ATP7B splice variants in patients with Wilson disease. Biochimie 2009 [epub ahead of print].
37. Loudianos G, Lovicu M, Dessi V, et al. Abnormal mRNA splicing resulting from consensus sequence splicing mutations of ATP7B. Hum Mutat 2002;20:260–266.
38. Tanzi RE, Petrukhin K, Chernov I, et al. The Wilson disease gene is a copper transporting ATPase with homology to the Menkes disease gene. Nat Genet 1993;5:44–50.
39. Thomas GR, Forbes JR, Roberts EA, et al. The Wilson disease gene: Spectrum of mutations and their consequences. Nat Genet 1999;9:210–217.
40. Shah AB, Chernov I, Zhang HT, et al. Identification and analysis of mutations in the Wilson disease gene (ATP7B): Population frequencies, genotype-phenotype correlation, and functional analyses. Am J Hum Genet 1997;61:317–328.
41. Czlonkowska A, Gromadzka G, and Chabik G. Monozygotic female twins discordant for phenotype of Wilson's disease. Mov Disord 2009;24:1066–1069.
42. Peña MMO, Lee J, and Thiele DJ. A delicate balance: Homeostatic control of copper uptake and distribution. J Nutr 1999;129:1251–1260.
43. Roberts EA and Sarkar B. Liver as a key organ in the supply, storage, and excretion of copper. Am J Clin Nutr 2008;88(suppl):851S–854S.
44. Roberts EA and Schilsky ML. Diagnosis and treatment of Wilson disease: An update. Hepatology 2008;47:2089–2111.
45. Reddy PV, Rao KV, and Norenberg MD. The mitochondrial permeability transition, and oxidative and nitrosative stress in the mechanism of copper toxicity in cultured neurons and astrocytes. Lab Invest 2008;88:816–830.
46. Goyal MK, Sinha S, Patil SA, et al. Do cytokines have any role in Wilson's disease? Clin Exp Immunol 2008;154:74–79.

47. Holmberg CG and Laurell CB. Investigations in serum copper. II. Isolation of the copper containing protein and a description of some of its properties. Acta Chem Scand 1948;2:550–556.
48. Shiono Y, Wakusawa S, Hayashi H, et al. Iron accumulation in the liver of male patients with Wilson's disease. Am J Gastroenterol 2001;96:3147–3151.
49. Sato M, Schilsky ML, Stockert RJ, et al. Detection of multiple forms of human ceruloplasmin: A novel Mr 2,000,000 form. J Biol Chem 1990;265:2533–2537.
50. Gibbs K and Walshe JM. A study of the ceruloplasmin concentrations found in 75 patients with Wilson's disease, their kinships and various control groups. Q J Med 1979;48:447–463.
51. Yang F, Naylor SL, Lum JB, et al. Characterization, mapping, and expression of the human ceruloplasmin gene. Proc Natl Acad Sci U S A 1986;83:3257–3261.
52. Morita H, Ikeda S, Yamamoto K, et al. Hereditary ceruloplasmin deficiency with hemosiderosis: A clinicopathological study of a Japanese family. Ann Neurol 1995;37:646–656.
53. Hellman NE and Gitlin JD. Ceruloplasmin metabolism and function. Annu Rev Nutr 2002;22:439–458.
54. Jones RJ, Lewis SJ, Smith JM, et al. Undetectable serum ceruloplasmin in a woman with chronic hepatitis C infection. J Hepatol 2000;32:703–704.
55. van Berge Henegouwen GP, Tangedahl TN, Hofman AF, et al. Biliary secretion of copper in healthy man. Gastroenterology 1977;72:1228–1231.
56. O'Reilly S, Weber PM, Oswald H, et al. Abnormalities of the physiology of copper in Wilson's disease. Arch Neurol 1971;25:28–32.
57. Owen CA Jr. Absorption and excretion of Cu^{64}-labeled copper by the rat. Am J Physiol 1964;207:1203–1206.
58. Ferenci P, Caca K, Loudianos G, et al. Diagnosis and phenotypic classification of Wilson disease. Liver Int 2003;23:139–142.
59. Aggarwal A, Aggarwal N, Nagral A, et al. A novel global assessment scale for Wilson's disease (GAS for WD). Mov Disord 2009;24:509–518.
60. Czlonkowska A, Tarnacka B, Möller JC, et al. Unified Wilson's Disease Rating Scale – a proposal for the neurological scoring of Wilson's disease patients. Neurol Neurochir Pol 2007;41:1–12.
61. Leinweber B, Möller JC, Scherag A, et al. Evaluation of the Unified Wilson's Disease Rating Scale (UWDRS) in German patients with treated Wilson's disease. Mov Disord 2008;23:54–62.
62. Walshe JM. Wilson's disease: The presenting symptoms. Arch Dis Child 1962;37:253–256.
63. Chu N-S and Hung T-P. Geographic variations in Wilson's disease. J Neurol Sci 1993;117:1–7.
64. Walshe JM. Wilson's disease (HLD), in Vinken PJ, Bruyn GW (eds): Handbook of Clinical Neurology. Vol 27. Amsterdam: North-Holland, 1976, pp. 379–414.
65. Gow PJ, Smallwood RA, Angus PW, et al. Diagnosis of Wilson's disease: An experience over three decades. Gut 2000;46:415–419.
66. Czlonkowska A, Rodo M, and Gromadzka G. Late onset Wilson's disease: Therapeutic implications. Mov Disord 2008;23:896–898.
67. Sternlieb I and Scheinberg IH. Chronic hepatitis as a first manifestation of Wilson's disease. Ann Intern Med 1972;76:59–64.
68. Scott J, Gollan JL, Samourian S, et al. Wilson's disease presenting as chronic active hepatitis. Gastroenterology 1978;74:645–651.
69. Lech T, Hydzik P, and Kosowski B. Significance of copper determination in late onset of Wilson's disease. Clin Toxicol (Phila) 2007;45:688–694.
70. Schilsky ML, Scheinberg IH, and Sternlieb I. Liver transplantation for Wilson's disease: Indications and outcome. Hepatology 1994;19:583–587.
71. Korman JD, Volenberg I, Balko J, et al. Screening for Wilson disease in acute liver failure: A comparison of currently available diagnostic tests. Hepatology 2008;48:1167–1174.
72. Enomoto K, Ishibashi H, Irie K, et al. Fulminant hepatic failure without evidence of cirrhosis in a case of Wilson's disease. Jpn J Med 1989;28:80–84.
73. Roche-Sicot J and Benhamou J-P. Acute intravascular hemolysis and acute liver failure associated as a first manifestation of Wilson's disease. Ann Intern Med 1977;86:301–303.
74. Hoshino T, Kumasaka K, Kawano K, et al. Low serum alkaline phosphatase activity associated with severe Wilson's disease. Is the breakdown of alkaline phosphatase molecules caused by reactive oxygen species? Clin Chim Acta 1995;238:91–100.
75. Kenngott S and Bilzer M. Inverse correlation of serum bilirubin and alkaline phosphatase in fulminant Wilson's disease. J Hepatol 1998;29:683.
76. Markiewicz-Kijewska M, Szymczak M, Ismali H, et al. Liver transplantation for fulminant Wilson's disease in children. Ann Transplant 2008;13:28–31.
77. Strickland GT and Leu ML. Wilson's disease: Clinical and laboratory manifestations in 40 patients. Medicine 1975;54:113–137.
78. Merle U, Schaefer M, Ferenci P, et al. Clinical presentation, diagnosis, and long-term outcome of Wilson's disease: a cohort study. Gut 2007;56:115–120.
79. Ross E, Jacobson IM, Dienstag JL, et al. Late onset Wilson's disease with neurologic involvement in the absence of Kayser-Fleischer rings. Ann Neurol 1985;17:411–413.
80. Ala A, Borjigin J, Rochwarger A, et al. Wilson disease in septuagenarian siblings: raising the bar for diagnosis. Hepatology 2005;41:668–670.
81. Walshe JM. Wilson's disease. In Vinken PJ, Bruyn GW, Klawans HL (eds). Handbook of Clinical Neurology. Vol 49. New York: Elsevier, 1986, pp. 223–238.
82. Topaloglu H and Renda Y. Tongue dyskinesia in Wilson disease. Brain Dev 1992;14:128.
83. Topaloglu H, Gucuyener K, Orkun C, et al. Tremor of tongue and dysarthria as the sole manifestation of Wilson disease. Clin Neurol Neurosurg 1990;92:295–296.
84. Nicholl DJ, Ferenci P, Polli C, et al. Wilson's disease presenting in a family with an apparent dominant history of tremor. J Neurol Neurosurg Psychiatry 2001;70:514–516.
85. Machado A, Chien HF, Deguti MM, et al. Neurological manifestations in Wilson's disease: Report of 119 cases. Mov Disord 2006;21:2192–2196.
86. Parker N. Hereditary whispering dysphonia. J Neurol Neurosurg Psychiatry 1985;48:218–224.

87. Cartwright GE. Diagnosis of treatable Wilson's disease. N Engl J Med 1978;298:1347–1350.
88. da Silva-Júnior FP, Carrasco AEAB, da Silva Mendes AM, et al. Swallowing dysfunction in Wilson's disease: A scintigraphic study. Neurogastroenterol Motil 2008;20:285–290.
89. Gulyas AE and Salazar-Grueso EF. Pharyngeal dysmotility in a patient with Wilson's disease. Dysphagia 1988;2:230–234.
90. Haggstrom G and Hirschowitz BI. Disordered esophageal motility in Wilson's disease. J Clin Gastroenterol 1980;2:273–275.
91. Walshe JM and Yealland M. Wilson's disease: The problem of delayed diagnosis. J Neurol Neurosurg Psychiatry 1992;55:692–696.
92. Svetel M, Kozic D, Stefanova E, et al. Dystonia in Wilson's disease. Mov Disord 2001;16:719–723.
93. Basir A, Bougteba A, and Kissani N. Torticollis révélant une maladie de Wilson. Arch Pediatr 2009;16:402–404.
94. Dening TR, Berrios GE, and Walshe JM. Wilson disease and epilepsy. Brain 1988;111:1139–1155.
95. Huang C-C and Chu N-S. Psychosis and epileptic seizures in Wilson's disease with predominantly white matter lesions in the frontal lobe. Parkinsonism Relat Disord 1995;1:53–58.
96. Mingazzini G. Über das Zwangsweinen und-lachen. Klin Wochenschr (Wien) 1928;41:998–1002.
97. Firneisz G, Szalay F, Halasz P, et al. Hypersomnia in Wilson's disease: an unusual symptom in an unusual case. Acta Neurol Scand 2000;101:286–288.
98. Portala K, Westermark K, Ekselius L, et al. Sleep in patients with treated Wilson's disease. A questionnaire study. Nord J Psychiatry 2002;56:291–297.
99. Nair KR and Pillai PG. Trunkal myoclonus with spontaneous priapism and seminal ejaculation in Wilson's disease. J Neurol Neurosurg Psychiatry 1990;53:174.
100. Bhattacharya K, Velickovic M, Schilsky M, et al. Autonomic cardiovascular reflexes in Wilson's disease. Clin Auton Res 2002;12:190–192.
101. Meenakshi-Sundaram S, Taly AB, Kamath V, et al. Autonomic dysfunction in Wilson's disease: A clinical and electrophysiological study. Clin Auton Res 2002;12:185–189.
102. Akil M, Schwartz JA, Dutchak D, et al. The psychiatric presentations of Wilson's disease. J Neuropsychiatry Clin Neurosci 1991;3:377–382.
103. Srinivas K, Sinha S, Taly AB, et al. Dominant psychiatric manifestations in Wilson's disease: A diagnostic and therapeutic challenge! J Neurol Sci 2008;266:104–108.
104. Brewer GJ. Recognition, diagnosis, and management of Wilson's disease. Proc Soc Exp Biol Med 2000;223:39–46.
105. Walshe JM. Missed Wilson's disease. Lancet 1975;ii:405–406.
106. Akil M and Brewer GJ. Psychiatric and behavioral abnormalities in Wilson's disease. Adv Neurol 1995;65:171–178.
107. Shanmugiah A, Sinha S, Taly AB, et al. Psychiatric manifestations in Wilson's disease: a cross-sectional analysis. J Neuropsychiatry Clin Neurosci 2008;20:81–85.
108. Oder W, Grimm G, Kollegger H, et al. Neurological and neuropsychiatric spectrum of Wilson's disease: A prospective study of 45 cases. J Neurol 1991;238:281–287.
109. Machado AC, Deguti MM, Caixeta L, et al. Mania as the first manifestation of Wilson's disease. Bipolar Disord 2008;10:447–450.
110. Kumawat BL, Sharma CM, Tripathi G, et al. Wilson's disease presenting as isolated obsessive-compulsive disorder. Indian J Med Sci 2007;61:607–610.
111. Matarazzo EB. Psychiatric features and disturbance of circadian rhythm of temperature, pulse, and blood pressure in Wilson's disease. J Neuropsychiatry Clin Neurosci 2002;14:335–339.
112. Seniow J, Bak T, Gajda J, et al. Cognitive functioning in neurologically symptomatic and asymptomatic forms of Wilson's disease. Mov Disord 2002;17:1077–1083.
113. Portala K, Westermark K, von Knorring L, et al. Psychopathology in treated Wilson's disease determined by means of CPRS expert and self-ratings. Acta Psychiatr Scand 2000;101:104–109.
114. Portala K, Levander S, Westermark K, et al. Pattern of neuropsychological deficits in patients with treated Wilson's disease. Eur Arch Psychiatry Clin Neurosci 2001;251:262–268.
115. Portala K, Westermark K, Ekselius L, et al. Personality traits in treated Wilson's disease determined by means of the Karolinska Scales of Personality (KSP). Eur Psychiatry 2001;16:362–371.
116. Rathbun JK. Neuropsychological aspects of Wilson's disease. Int J Neurosci 1996;85:221–229.
117. Tarter RE, Switala J, Carra J, et al. Neuropsychological impairment associated with hepatolenticular degeneration (Wilson's disease) in the absence of overt encephalopathy. Int J Neurosci 1987;37:67–71.
118. Scheinberg IH, Sternlieb I, and Richman J. Psychiatric manifestations in patients with Wilson's disease. In Bergsma D, Scheinberg IH, Sternlieb I (eds). Wilson's Disease: Birth Defects, Original Article Series. Vol 4. New York: The National Foundation—March of Dimes, 1968, pp. 85–87.
119. Dening TR. Psychiatric aspects of Wilson's disease. Br J Psychiatry 1985;147:677–682.
120. Davis EJ and Borde M. Wilson's disease and catatonia. Br J Psychiatry 1993;162:256–259.
121. Kaul A and McMahon D. Wilson's disease and offending behavior: A case report. Med Sci Law 1993;33:353–358.
122. Gwirtsman HE, Prager J, and Henkin R. Case report of anorexia nervosa associated with Wilson's disease. Int J Eat Disord 1993;13:241–244.
123. Spyridi S, Diakogiannis I, Michaelides M, et al. Delusional disorder and alcohol abuse in a patient with Wilson's disease. Gen Hosp Psychiatry 2008;30:585–586.
124. Wiebers DO, Hollenhorst RW, and Goldstein NP. The ophthalmologic manifestations of Wilson's disease. Mayo Clin Proc 1977;52:409–416.
125. Johnson RD and Campbell RJ: Wilson's disease: Electron microscopic, X-ray energy spectroscopic and atomic absorption spectroscopic studies of corneal copper deposition and distribution. Lab Invest 1982;46:546–569.
126. Innes JR, Strachan IM, and Triger DR. Unilateral Kayser-Fleischer ring. Br J Ophthalmol 1979;70:469–470.
127. Suvarna JC. Kayser-Fleischer ring. J Postgrad Med 2008;54:238–240.
128. Tauber J and Steinert RF. Pseudo-Kayser-Fleischer ring of the cornea associated with non-Wilsonian liver disease: A case report and literature review. Cornea 1993;12:74–77.
129. Sussman W and Scheinberg IH. Disappearance of Kayser-Fleischer rings. Effects of penicillamine. Arch Ophthalmol 1969;82:738–741.

130. Fleming CR, Dickson ER, Wahner HW, et al. Pigmented corneal rings in non-Wilsonian liver disease. Ann Intern Med 1977;86:285–288.
131. Frommer D, Morris J, Sherlock S, et al. Kayser-Fleischer-like rings in patients without Wilson's disease. Gastroenterology 1977;72:1331–1335.
132. Kaplinsky C, Sternlieb I, Javitt N, et al. Familial cholestatic cirrhosis associated with Kayser-Fleischer rings. Pediatrics 1980;65:782–788.
133. Garmizo G and Frauens BJ. Corneal copper deposition secondary to oral contraceptives. Optom Vis Sci 2008;85:E802-E807.
134. Stephenson S. Cases illustrating an unusual form of corneal opacity due to the long-continued application of copper sulphate to the palpebral conjunctiva. Trans Ophthalmol Soc UK 1902;23:25–27.
135. Goodman SI, Rodgerson DO, and Kaufman J. Hypercupremia in a patient with multiple myeloma. J Lab Clin Med 1967;70:57–62.
136. Lewis RA, Falls HF, and Troyer DO. Ocular manifestations of hypercupremia associated with multiple myeloma. Arch Ophthalmol 1995;93:1050–1053.
137. Martin NF, Kincaid MC, Stark WJ, et al. Ocular copper deposition associated with pulmonary carcinoma, IgG monoclonal gammopathy and hypercupremia: A clinicopathologic correlation. Ophthalmology 1983;90:110–116.
138. Giorgio AJ, Cartwright GE, and Wintrobe MM. Pseudo-Kayser-Fleischer rings. Arch Intern Med 1964;113:817–818.
139. Taly AB, Meenakshi-Sundaram S, Sinha S, et al. Wilson disease: description of 282 patients evaluated over 3 decades. Medicine (Baltimore) 2007;86:112–121.
140. Siemerling E and Oloff H. Pseudosklerose (Westphal-Strümpell) mit Cornealring (Kayser-Fleischer) und doppelseitiger Scheinkatarakt, die nur bei seitlicher Beleuchtnung sichtbar ist und die der nach Verletzung durch Kupfersplitter entstehenden Katarakt ähnlich ist. Klin Wochenschr 1922;1:1087–1089.
141. Cairns JE, Williams HP, and Walshe JM. "Sunflower cataract" in Wilson's disease. Br Med J 1969;3:95–96.
142. Goldberg MF and von Noorden GK. Ophthalmologic findings in Wilson's hepatolenticular degeneration: With emphasis on ocular motility. Arch Ophthalmol 1966;75:162–170.
143. Ingster-Moati I, Quoc EB, Pless M, et al. Ocular motility and Wilson's disease: a study on 34 patients. J Neurol Neurosurg Psychiatry 2007;78:1199–1201.
144. Leśniak M, Czlonkowska A, and Seniów J. Abnormal antisaccades and smooth pursuit eye movements in patients with Wilson's disease. Mov Disord 2008;14:2067–2073.
145. Pillat A. Changes in the eyegrounds in Wilson's disease (pseudosclerosis). Am J Ophthalmol 1933;16:1–6.
146. Walsh FB and Hoyt WF. Clinical Neuroophthalmology, 3rd ed. Vol 2. Baltimore: Williams & Wilkins, 1969, p. 1140.
147. Gow PJ, Peacock SE, and Chapman RW. Wilson's disease presenting with rapidly progressive visual loss: another neurologic manifestation of Wilson's disease? J Gastroenterol Hepatol 2001;16:699–701.
148. Lennox G and Jones R. Gaze distractibility in Wilson's disease. Ann Neurol 1989;25:415–417.
149. Keane JR. Lid-opening apraxia in Wilson's disease. J Clin Neuroophthalmol 1988;8:31–33.
150. Lee MS, Kim YD, and Lyoo CH. Oculogyric crisis as an initial manifestation of Wilson's disease. Neurology 1999;52:1714–1715.
151. Dastur DK, Manghani DK, and Wadia NH. Wilson's disease in India. I. Geographic, genetic, and clinical aspects in 16 families. Neurology 1968;18:21–31.
152. Tu JB. A genetic, biochemical and clinical study of Wilson's disease among Chinese in Taiwan. Acta Paediatr Sin 1963;4:81–84.
153. Xu XH, Yang BX, and Feng YK. Wilson's disease (hepatolenticular degeneration): Clinical analysis of 80 cases. Chin Med J 1981;94:673–678.
154. Saito T. Presenting symptoms and natural history of Wilson's disease. Eur J Pediatr 1987;146:261–265.
155. Golding DN and Walshe JM. Arthropathy of Wilson's disease: Study of clinical and radiological features in 32 patients. Ann Rheum Dis 1977;36:99–111.
156. Canelas HM, Carvalho N, Scaff M, et al. Osteoarthropathy of hepatolenticular degeneration. Acta Neurol Scand 1978;57:481–487.
157. Yarze JC, Martin P, Munoz SJ, et al. Wilson's disease: Current status. Am J Med 1992;92:643–654.
158. Selimoglu MA, Ertekin V, Doneray H, et al. Bone mineral density of children with Wilson disease: Efficacy of penicillamine and zinc therapy. J Clin Gastroenterol 2008;42:194–198.
159. Feller E and Schumacher HR: Osteoarticular changes in Wilson's disease. Arthritis Rheum 1972;15:259–266.
160. Balint G, Szebenyi B: Hereditary disorders mimicking and/or causing premature osteoarthritis. Baillieres Best Pract Res Clin Rheumatol 2000;14:219–250.
161. Mindelzun R, Elkin M, Scheinberg IH, et al. Skeletal changes in Wilson's disease: A radiological study. Radiology 1970;94:127–132.
162. Kramer U, Weinberger A, Yarom R, et al. Synovial copper deposition as a possible explanation of arthropathy in Wilson's disease. Bull Hosp Jt Dis 1993;52:46–49.
163. McIntyre N, Clink HM, Levi AJ, et al. Hemolytic anemia in Wilson's disease. N Engl J Med 1967;276:439–444.
164. Sternlieb I. Wilson's disease: Indications for liver transplants. Hepatology 1984;4:15S–17S.
165. Meyer RJ and Zalusky R. The mechanisms of hemolysis in Wilson's disease: Study of a case and review of the literature. Mt Sinai J Med 1977;44:530–538.
166. Forman SJ, Kumar KS, Redeker AG, et al. Hemolytic anemia in Wilson disease: Clinical findings and biochemical mechanisms. Am J Hematol 1980;9:269–275.
167. Lee JJ, Kim HJ, Chung IJ, et al. Acute hemolytic crisis with fulminant hepatic failure as the first manifestation of Wilson's disease: A case report. J Korean Med Sci 1998;13:548–550.
168. Druml W, Laggner AN, Lenz K, et al. Pancreatitis in acute hemolysis. Ann Hematol 1991;63:39–41.
169. Prella M, Baccala R, Horisberger JD, et al. Haemolytic onset of Wilson disease in a patient with homozygous truncation of ATP7B at Arg1319. Br J Haematol 2001;114:230–232.
170. Donfrid M, Jankovic G, Strahinja R, et al. Idiopathic thrombocytopenia associated with Wilson's disease. Hepatogastroenterology 1998;45:1774–1776.
171. Wiebers DO, Wilson DM, McLeod RA, et al. Renal stones in Wilson's disease. Am J Med 1979;67:249–254.

172. Hoppe B, Neuhaus T, Superti-Furga A, et al. Hypercalciuria and nephrocalcinosis, a feature of Wilson's disease. Nephron 1993;65:460–462.
173. Sozeri E, Feist D, Ruder H, et al. Proteinuria and other renal functions in Wilson's disease. Pediatr Nephrol 1997;11:307–311.
174. Leu ML, Strickland GT, Wang CC, et al. Skin pigmentation in Wilson's disease. J Am Med Assoc 1970;211:1542–1543.
175. Bearn AG and McKusick VA. Azure lunulae: An unusual change in the fingernails in two patients with hepatolenticular degeneration (Wilson's disease). J Am Med Assoc 1958;166:904–906.
176. Ezzo JA, Rowley JF, and Finnegin JV. Hepatolenticular degeneration associated with acanthosis nigricans. Arch Intern Med 1957;100:827–832.
177. Schaefer M, Schellenberg M, Merle U, et al. Wilson protein expression, copper excretion and sweat production in sweat glands of Wilson disease patients and controls. BMC Gastroenterol 2008;8:29.
178. Scheinberg IH and Sternlieb I. Wilson's disease. Annu Rev Med 1965;16:119–134.
179. Lau JY, Lai CL, Wu PC, et al. Wilson's disease: 35 years' experience. Q J Med 1990;75:597–605.
180. Erkan T, Aktuglu C, Gulcan EM, et al. Wilson disease manifested primarily as amenorrhea and accompanying thrombocytopenia. J Adolesc Health 2002;31:378–380.
181. Sternlieb I and Scheinberg IH. Wilson's disease. In Wright R, Alberti KGM, Karran S, et al. (eds). Liver and Biliary Disease. London: Bailliere Tindall, 1985, pp. 949–961.
182. McIntyre N. Neurological Wilson's disease. Q J Med 1993;86:349–350.
183. Houwen RHJ. Copper: Two sides of the same coin. Neth J Med 2008;66:325–326.
184. Snow B. Laboratory diagnosis and monitoring of Wilson's disease. In Neurological Aspects of Wilson's Disease, American Academy of Neurology Course 411. 1995, pp. 25–30.
185. Smallwood RA, Williams HA, and Rosenauer VM. Liver copper levels in liver disease: Studies using neutron activation analysis. Lancet 1968;ii:1310–1313.
186. Benson GD. Hepatic copper accumulation in primary biliary cirrhosis. Yale J Biol Med 1979;52:83–88.
187. Evans J, Newman S, and Sherlock S. Liver copper levels in intrahepatic cholestasis of childhood. Gastroenterology 1978;75:875–878.
188. Tanner MS, Portmann B, Mowat AP, et al. Increased hepatic copper concentration in Indian childhood cirrhosis. Lancet 1979;i:1203–1205.
189. LaRusso NF, Summerskill WH, and McCall JT. Abnormalities of chemical tests for copper metabolism in chronic active liver disease: Differentiation from Wilson's disease. Gastroenterology 1976;70:653–655.
190. Sternlieb I, Giblin DR, and Scheinberg IH. Wilson's disease. In Marsden CD, Fahn S (eds). Movement Disorders. Vol 2. London: Butterworth, 1987, pp 288–302.
191. Ferenci P, Steindl-Munda P, Vogel W, et al. Diagnostic value of quantitative hepatic copper determination in patients with Wilson's disease. Clin Gastroenterol Hepatol 2005;3:811–818.
192. Willeit J and Kiechl SG. Wilson's disease with neurologic impairment but no Kayser-Fleischer rings. Lancet 1991;337:1426.
193. Vidaud D, Assouline B, Lecoz P, et al. Misdiagnosis revealed by genetic linkage analysis in a family with Wilson disease. Neurology 1996;46:1485–1486.
194. Frommer DJ. Urinary copper excretion and hepatic copper concentrations in liver disease. Digestion 1981;21:169–178.
195. Steindl P, Ferenci P, Dienes HP, et al. Wilson's disease in patients presenting with liver disease: A diagnostic challenge. Gastroenterology 1997;113:212–218.
196. Foruny JR, Boixeda D, López-Sanroman A, et al. Usefulness of penicillamine-stimulated urinary copper excretion in the diagnosis of adult Wilson's disease. Scand J Gastroenterol 2008;43:597–603.
197. Müller T, Koppikar S, Taylor RM, et al. Re-evaluation of the penicillamine challenge test in the diagnosis of Wilson's disease in children. J Hepatol 2007;47:270–276.
198. Cumings JN. Trace metals in the brain and in Wilson's disease. J Clin Pathol 1968;21:1–7.
199. Stremmel W, Meyerrose K-W, Niederau C, et al. Wilson disease: Clinical presentation, treatment, and survival. Ann Intern Med 1991;115:720–726.
200. Twomey PJ, Viljoen A, Reynolds TM, et al. Non-ceruloplasmin-bound copper in routine clinical practice in different laboratories. J Trace Elem Med Biol 2008;22:50–53.
201. McMillin GA, Travis JJ, and Hunt JW. Direct measurement of free copper in serum or plasma ultrafiltrate. Am J Clin Pathol 2009;131:160–165.
202. Sternlieb I and Scheinberg IH. The role of radiocopper in the diagnosis of Wilson's disease. Gastroenterology 1979;77:138–142.
203. Weisner B, Hartard C, and Dieu C. CSF copper concentration: A new parameter for diagnosis and monitoring therapy of Wilson's disease with cerebral manifestation. J Neurol Sci 1987;79: 229–237.
204. Hartard C, Weisner B, Dieu C, et al. Wilson's disease with cerebral manifestation: Monitoring therapy by CSF copper concentration. J Neurol 1993;241:101–107.
205. Stuerenburg HJ. CSF copper concentrations, blood-brain barrier function, and coeruloplasmin synthesis during the treatment of Wilson's disease. J Neural Transm 2000;107:321–329.
206. Thuomas KA, Aquilonius SM, Bergstrom K, et al. Magnetic resonance imaging of the brain in Wilson's disease. Neuroradiology 1993;35:134–141.
207. Roh JK, Lee TG, Wie BA, et al. Initial and follow-up brain MRI findings and correlation with the clinical course in Wilson's disease. Neurology 1994;44:1064–1068.
208. Selwa LM, Vanderzant CW, Brunberg JA, et al. Correlation of evoked potential and MRI findings in Wilson's disease. Neurology 1993;43:2059–2064.
209. Magalhaes ACA, Caramelli P, Menezes JR, et al. Wilson's disease: MRI with clinical correlation. Neuroradiology 1994;36:97–100.
210. Alanen A, Komu M, Penttinen M, et al. Magnetic resonance imaging and proton MR spectroscopy in Wilson disease. Br J Radiol 1999;72:749–756.
211. Hitoshi S, Iwata M, and Yoshikawa K. Midbrain pathology of Wilson's disease: MRI analysis of three cases. J Neurol Neurosurg Psychiatry 1991;54:624–626.
212. Liebeskind DS, Wong S, and Hamilton RH. Faces of the giant panda and her cub: MRI correlates of Wilson's disease. J Neurol Neurosurg Psychiatry 2003;74:682.

213. Sener RN. The claustrum on MRI: Normal anatomy, and the bright claustrum as a new sign in Wilson's disease. Pediatr Radiol 1993;23:594–596.
214. Das SK and Ray K. Wilson's disease: an update. Nat Clin Pract Neurol 2006;2:482–493.
215. Sener RN. Diffusion MRI findings in Wilson's disease. Comput Med Imaging Graph 2003;27:17–21.
216. Jayasundar R, Sahani AK, Gaikwad S, et al. Proton MR spectroscopy of basal ganglia in Wilson's disease: Case report and review of literature. Magn Reson Imaging 2002;20:131–135.
217. Tarnacka B, Szeszkowski W, Golebiowski M, et al. MR spectroscopy in monitoring the treatment of Wilson's disease patients. Mov Disord 2008;23:1560–1566.
218. Hawkins RA, Mazziotta JC, and Phelps ME. Wilson's disease studied with FDG and positron emission tomography. Neurology 1987;37:1707–1711.
219. Hefter H, Kuwert T, Herzog H, et al. Relationship between striatal glucose consumption and copper excretion in patients with Wilson's disease treated with D-penicillamine. J Neurol 1993;241:49–53.
220. Snow BJ, Bhatt MH, Martin WRW, et al. The nigrostriatal dopaminergic pathway in Wilson's disease studied with positron emission tomography. J Neurol Neurosurg Psychiatry 1991;54:12–17.
221. Topcu M, Topcuoglu MA, Kose G, et al. Evoked potentials in children with Wilson's disease. Brain Dev 2002;24:276–280.
222. Grimm G, Madl C, Katzenschlager R, et al. Detailed evaluation of evoked potentials in Wilson's disease. Electroencephalogr Clin Neurophysiol 1992;82:119–124.
223. Bartova P, Skoloudik D, Bar M, et al. Transcranial sonography in movement disorders. Biomed Pap Med Fac Univ Palacky Olomouc Czech Repub 2008;152:251–258.
224. Brewer GJ, Yuzbasiyan-Gurkan V, Dick R, et al. Does a vegetarian diet control Wilson's disease? J Am Coll Nutr 1993;12:527–530.
225. Ebadi M, Paliwal VK, Takahashi T, et al. Zinc metallothionein in mammalian brain. UCLA Symp Mol Cell Biol 1989;98:257–267.
226. Ebadi M. Metallothionein and other zinc-binding proteins in brain. Methods Enzymol 1991;205:363–387.
227. Day FA, Panemangelore M, and Brady FO. In vivo and ex vivo effects of copper on rat liver metallothionein. Proc Soc Exp Biol Med 1981;168:306–310.
228. Brewer GJ, Hill GM, Prasad AS, et al. Oral zinc therapy for Wilson's disease. Ann Intern Med 1983;99:314–320.
229. Hall AC, Young BW, and Bremner I. Intestinal metallothionein and the mutual antagonism between copper and zinc in the rat. J Inorg Biochem 1979;11:57–66.
230. Brewer GJ and Yuzbasiyan-Gurkan V. Wilson's disease. In Klawans HK, Goetz CG, Tanner CM (eds). Textbook of Clinical Neuropharmacology and Therapeutics. New York: Raven Press, 1992, pp. 191–205.
231. Brewer GJ. Zinc acetate for the treatment of Wilson's disease. Expert Opin Pharmacother 2001;2:1473–1477.
232. Brewer GJ, Yuzbasiyan-Gurkan V, Lee DY, et al. Treatment of Wilson's disease with zinc. VI. Initial treatment studies. J Lab Clin Med 1989;114:633–638.
233. Schilsky ML. Treatment of Wilson's disease: What are the relative roles of penicillamine, trientine, and zinc supplementation? Curr Gastroenterol Rep 2001;3:54–59.
234. Rossaro L, Sturniolo GC, Giacon G, et al. Zinc therapy in Wilson's disease: Observations in five patients. Am J Gastroenterol 1990;85:665–668.
235. Hoogenraad T. Wilson's Disease. London: WB Saunders, 1996.
236. Brewer GJ, Dick RD, Johnson VD, et al. Treatment of Wilson's disease with zinc XVI: Treatment during the pediatric years. J Lab Clin Med 2001;137:191–198.
237. Brewer GJ, Johnson VD, Dick RD, et al. Treatment of Wilson's disease with zinc XVII: Treatment during pregnancy. Hepatology 2000;31:364–370.
238. Subramanian I, Vanek ZF, and Bronstein JM. Diagnosis and treatment of Wilson's disease. Curr Neurol Neurosci Rep 2002;2:317–323.
239. Simon SR, Branda RF, Tindle BH, et al. Copper deficiency and sideroblastic anemia associated with zinc ingestion. Am J Hematol 1988;28:181–183.
240. Brewer GJ, Yuzbasiyan-Gurkan V, and Lee D-Y. Molecular genetics and zinc-copper interactions in human Wilson's disease and canine copper toxicosis. In Prasad AS (ed). Essential and Toxic Trace Elements in Human Health and Disease: An Update. New York: Wiley-Liss, 1992, pp. 129–145.
241. Hooper PL, Visconti L, Garry PJ, et al. Zinc lowers high-density lipoprotein-cholesterol levels. J Am Med Assoc 1980;244:1960–1961.
242. Yuzbasiyan-Gurkan V, Brewer GJ, Abrams GD, et al. Treatment of Wilson's disease with zinc: V. Changes in serum levels of lipase, amylase and alkaline phosphatase in Wilson's disease patients. J Lab Clin Med 1989;114:520–526.
243. Walshe JM. Penicillamine: The treatment of first choice for patients with Wilson's disease. Mov Disord 1999;14:545–550.
244. Brewer GJ. Penicillamine should not be used as initial therapy in Wilson's disease. Mov Disord 1999;14:551–554.
245. LeWitt PA. Penicillamine as a controversial treatment for Wilson's disease. Mov Disord 1999;14:555–556.
246. Lang CJG, Rabas-Kolminsky P, Engelhardt A, et al. Fatal deterioration of Wilson's disease after institution of oral zinc therapy. Arch Neurol 1993;50:1007–1008.
247. Walshe JM and Munro NAR. Zinc induced deterioration in Wilson's disease aborted by treatment with penicillamine, dimercaprol, and a novel zero copper diet. Arch Neurol 1995;52:10–11.
248. Castilla-Higuero L, Romero-Gomez M, Suarez E, et al. Acute hepatitis after starting zinc therapy in a patient with presymptomatic Wilson's disease. Hepatology 2000;32:877.
249. Mishra D, Kalra V, and Seth R. Failure of prophylactic zinc in Wilson's disease. Indian Pediatr 2008;45:151–153.
250. Brewer GJ. The use of copper-lowering therapy with tetrathiomolybdate in medicine. Expert Opin Investig Drugs 2009;18:89–97.
251. Brewer GJ, Dick RD, Johnson V, et al. Treatment of Wilson's disease with ammonium tetrathiomolybdate. I. Initial therapy in 17 neurologically affected patients. Arch Neurol 1994;51:545–554.
252. George GN, Pickering IJ, Harris HH, et al. Tetrathiomolybdate causes formation of hepatic copper-molybdenum clusters in an animal model of Wilson's disease. J Am Chem Soc 2003;125:1704–1705.

253. Zhang L, Lichtmannegger J, Summer KH, et al. Tracing copper-thiomolybdate complexes in a prospective treatment for Wilson's disease. Biochemistry 2009;48:891–897.
254. Brewer GJ, Dick RD, Yuzbasiyan-Gurkan V, et al. Initial therapy of patients with Wilson's disease with tetrathiomolybdate. Arch Neurol 1991;48:42–47.
255. Brewer GJ, Johnson V, Dick RD, et al. Treatment of Wilson disease with ammonium tetrathiomolybdate. II. Initial therapy in 33 neurologically affected patients and follow-up with zinc therapy. Arch Neurol 1996;53:1017–1025.
256. Spence JA, Suttle NF, Wenham G, et al. A sequential study of the skeletal abnormalities, which develop in rats given a small dietary supplement of ammonium tetrathiomolybdate. J Comp Pathol 1980;90:139–153.
257. Walshe JM and Yealland M. Chelation treatment of neurological Wilson's disease. Q J Med 1993;86:197–204.
258. Walshe JM. Penicillamine: A new oral therapy for Wilson's disease. Am J Med 1956;21:487–495.
259. Deiss A. Treatment of Wilson's disease. Ann Intern Med 1983;99:398–399.
260. Goldstein NP, Ewert JC, Randall RV, et al. Psychiatric aspects of Wilson's disease (hepatolenticular degeneration): Results of psychometric tests during long-term therapy. Am J Psychiatry 1968;124:1555–1561.
261. Williams FJB and Walshe JM. Wilson's disease. An analysis of the cranial computerized tomographic appearances found in patients and the changes in response to treatment with chelating agents. Brain 1981;104:735–752.
262. Nazer H, Brismar J, Al-Kawi MZ, et al. Magnetic resonance imaging of the brain in Wilson's disease. Neuroradiology 1993;35:130–133.
263. Schuna A, Osman MA, Patel RB, et al. Influence of food on the bioavailability of penicillamine. J Rheumatol 1983;10:95–97.
264. Marsden CD. Wilson's disease. Q J Med 1987;248:959–966.
265. Gibbs KR and Walshe JM. Interruption of the tryptophan-nicotinic acid pathway by penicillamine-induced pyridoxine deficiency in patients with Wilson's disease and in experimental animals. Ann N Y Acad Sci 1969;111:158–169.
266. Brewer GJ, Terry CA, Aisen AM, et al. Worsening of neurological syndrome in patients with Wilson's disease with initial penicillamine therapy. Arch Neurol 1987;44:490–493.
267. Svetel M, Sternic N, Pejovic S, et al. Penicillamine-induced lethal status dystonicus in a patient with Wilson's disease. Mov Disord 2001;16:568–569.
268. Glass JD, Reich SG, and DeLong MR. Wilson's disease: Development of neurological disease after beginning penicillamine therapy. Arch Neurol 1990;47:595–596.
269. Brewer GJ, Turkay A, and Yuzbasiyan-Gurkan V. Development of neurologic symptoms in a patient with asymptomatic Wilson's disease. Arch Neurol 1994;51:304–305.
270. Sternlieb I and Scheinberg IH. Penicillamine therapy in hepatolenticular degeneration. J Am Med Assoc 1964;189:748–754.
271. Haggstrom GC, Hirschowitz BI, and Flint A. Long-term penicillamine therapy for Wilson's disease. South Med J 1980;73:530–531.
272. Chan C-Y and Baker AL. Penicillamine hypersensitivity: Successful desensitization of a patient with severe hepatic Wilson's disease. Am J Gastroenterol 1994;89:442–443.
273. Corcos JM, Soler-Bechera J, Mayer K, et al. Neutrophilic agranulocytosis during administration of penicillamine. J Am Med Assoc 1964;189:265–268.
274. Hirschman SZ and Isselbacher KJ. The nephrotic syndrome as a complication of penicillamine therapy of hepatolenticular degeneration (Wilson's disease). Ann Intern Med 1965;62:1297–1300.
275. Sternlieb I, Bennett B, and Scheinberg IH. D-Penicillamine induced Goodpasture's syndrome in Wilson's disease. Ann Intern Med 1975;82:673–675.
276. Walshe JM. Penicillamine and the SLE syndrome. J Rheumatol 1981;8(suppl 7):155–160.
277. Czlonkowska A. Myasthenia syndrome during penicillamine treatment. Br Med J 1975;2:726–727.
278. Bigger JF. Retinal hemorrhages during penicillamine therapy of cystinuria. Am J Ophthalmol 1968;66:954–955.
279. Hanukoglu A, Curiel B, Berkowitz D, et al. Hypothyroidism and dyshormonogenesis induced by D-penicillamine in children with Wilson's disease and healthy infants born to a mother with Wilson's disease. J Pediatr 2008;153:864–866.
280. Shoulson I, Goldblatt D, Plassche W, et al. Some therapeutic observations in Wilson's disease. Adv Neurol 1983;37:239–246.
281. Henkin RI, Keiser HR, Jaffe IA, et al. Decreased taste sensitivity after D-penicillamine reversed by copper administration. Lancet 1967;ii:1268–1271.
282. Proesman W, Jaeken J, and Eckels R. D-Penicillamine induced IgA deficiency in Wilson's disease. Lancet 1976;ii:804–805.
283. Sternlieb I, Fisher M, and Scheinberg IH. Penicillamine-induced skin lesions. J Rheumatol 1981;8(suppl 7):149–154.
284. Nimni ME. Mechanism of inhibition of collagen cross-linking by penicillamine. Proc R Soc Med 1977;70(suppl 3):65–72.
285. Morris JJ, Seifter E, Rettura G, et al. Effect of penicillamine upon wound healing. J Surg Res 1969;9:143–149.
286. Kirsch N and Hukill PB. Elastosis perforans serpiginosa by penicillamine. Electron microscopic observations. Arch Dermatol 1977;113:630–635.
287. Pass F, Goldfischer S, Sternlieb I, et al. Elastosis perforans serpiginosa after penicillamine therapy for Wilson's disease. Arch Dermatol 1973;108:713–715.
288. Eisenberg E, Ballow M, Wolfe SH, et al. Pemphigus-like mucosal lesions: A side effect of penicillamine therapy. Oral Surg Oral Med Oral Pathol 1981;51:409–414.
289. Bennett RA and Harbilas E. Wilson's disease with aseptic meningitis and penicillamine-related cheilosis. Arch Intern Med 1967;120:374–376.
290. Walshe JM. The management of penicillamine nephropathy in Wilson's disease: A new chelating agent. Lancet 1969;ii:1401–1402.
291. Walshe JM. Assessment of the treatment of Wilson's disease with triethylene tetramine 2HCl (Trien 2HCl). In Sarker B (ed). Biological Aspects of Metal Related Diseases. New York: Raven Press, 1983, pp. 243–261.
292. Walshe JM. Treatment of Wilson's disease with trientine (triethylene tetramine) dihydrochloride. Lancet 1982;i:643–647.
293. Walshe JM. Copper chelation in patients with Wilson's disease: A comparison of penicillamine and triethylene tetramine hydrochloride. Q J Med 1973;42:441–452.

294. Sarkar B, Sass-Kortsak A, Clarke R, et al. A comparative study of in vitro and in vivo interaction of D-penicillamine and triethylenetetramine with copper. Proc R Soc Med 1977;70(suppl 3):13–18.
295. Fox AN and Schilsky M. Once daily trientine for maintenance therapy of Wilson disease. Am J Gastroenterol 2008;103:494–495.
296. Condamine L, Hermine O, Alvin P, et al. Acquired sideroblastic anaemia during treatment of Wilson's disease with triethylene tetramine dihydrochloride. Br J Hematol 1993;83:166–168.
297. Brewer GJ. Wilson's disease. Curr Treat Options Neurol 2000;2:193–204.
298. Schilsky ML, Scheinberg IH, and Sternlieb I. Liver transplantation for Wilson's disease: Indications and outcome. Hepatology 1994;19:583–587.
299. Rela M, Heaton ND, Vougas V, et al. Orthotopic liver transplantation for hepatic complications of Wilson's disease. Br J Surg 1993;80:909–911.
300. Shafer DF and Shaw BW Jr. Fulminant hepatic failure and orthotopic liver transplantation. Semin Liver Dis 1989;9:189–194.
301. Cheng F, Li GO, Zhang F, et al. Outcomes of living-related liver transplantation for Wilson's disease: a single-center experience in China. Transplantation 2009;87:751–757.
302. Yoshitoshi EY, Takada Y, Oike F, et al. Long-term outcomes for 32 cases of Wilson's disease after living-donor liver transplantation. Transplantation 2009;87: 261–267.
303. Sen S, Felldin M, Steiner C, et al. Albumin dialysis and molecular adsorbents recirculating system (MARS) for acute Wilson's disease. Liver Transpl 2002;8:962–967.
304. Kreymann B, Seige M, Schweigart U, et al. Albumin dialysis: Effective removal of copper in a patient with fulminant Wilson disease and successful bridging to liver transplantation: A new possibility for the elimination of protein-bound toxins. J Hepatol 1999;31:1080–1085.
305. Chiu A, Tsoi NS, and Fan ST. Use of the molecular adsorbents recirculating system as a treatment for acute decompensated Wilson disease. Liver Transpl 2008;14:1512–1516.
306. Collins KL, Roberts EA, Adeli K, et al. Single pass albumin dialysis (SPAD) in fulminant Wilsonian liver failure: A case report. Pediatr Nephrol 2008;23:1013–1016.
307. Kiss JE, Berman D, and Van Thiel D. Effective removal of copper by plasma exchange in fulminant Wilson's disease. Transfusion 1998;38:327–331.
308. Jhang JS, Schilsky ML, Lefkowitch JH, et al. Therapeutic plasmapheresis as a bridge to liver transplantation in fulminant Wilson disease. J Clin Apher 2007;22:10–14.
309. Hursitoglu M, Kara O, Cikrikcioglu MA, et al. Clinical improvement of a patient with severe Wilson's disease after a single session of therapeutic plasma exchange. J Clin Apher 2009;24:25–27.
310. Mazariegos GV, Kramer DJ, Lopez RC, et al. Safety observations in phase I clinical evaluation of the Excorp Medical Bioartificial Liver Support System after the first four patients. ASAIO J 2001;47:471–475.
311. Chen CL and Kuo YC. Metabolic effects of liver transplantation in Wilson's disease. Transplant Proc 1993;25:2944–2947.
312. Pabón V, Dumortier J, Gincul R, et al. Long-term results of liver transplantation for Wilson's disease. Gastroenterol Clin Biol 2008;32:378–381.
313. Litwin T, Gromadzka G, and Czlonkowska A. Neurological presentation of Wilson's disease in a patient after liver transplantation. Mov Disord 2008;23:743–746.
314. Komatsu H, Fujisawa T, Inui A, et al. Hepatic copper concentration in children undergoing living related liver transplantation due to Wilsonian fulminant hepatic failure. Clin Transplant 2002;16:227–232.
315. Mason AL, Marsh W, and Alpers DH. Intractable neurological Wilson's disease treated with orthotopic liver transplantation. Dig Dis Sci 1993;38:1746–1750.
316. Stracciari A, Tempestini A, Borghi A, et al. Effect of liver transplantation on neurological manifestations in Wilson disease. Ar ch Neurol 2000;57:384–386.
317. Pal PK, Sinha S, Pillai S, et al. Successful treatment of tremor in Wilson's disease by thalamotomy: a case report. Mov Disord 2007;22:2287–2290.
318. Malhi H, Irani AN, Volenberg I, et al. Early cell transplantation in LEC rats modeling Wilson's disease eliminates hepatic copper with reversal of liver disease. Gastroenterology 2002;122:438–447.
319. Ha-Hao D, Merle U, Hofmann C, et al. Chances and shortcomings of adenovirus-mediated ATP7B gene transfer in Wilson disease: Proof of principle demonstrated in a pilot study with LEC rats. Z Gastroenterol 2002;40:209–216.

CHAPTER 43

Stiff-Person Syndrome

Oscar S. Gershanik

The stiff-person syndrome (SPS) is a rare neurologic disorder of uncertain cause, characterized by severe and incapacitating axial and proximal limb rigidity due to continuous motor unit activity. Rigidity is often enhanced by anxiety, sudden movements, or external stimuli causing intermittent painful muscle spasms, often leading to skeletal deformity. Variants of this disorder include focal involvement of one limb ("stiff-limb syndrome"), or additional neurological symptoms suggestive of involvement of subcortical gray matter ("progressive encephalomyelitis with rigidity and myoclonus") (PEWR) and occasionally secondary to malignant disease (paraneoplastic SPS). Antineuronal antibodies often associated with other autoimmune diseases are characteristic features of this disorder. The disease follows a progressive, unremitting course, resulting in pronounced disability, if left untreated.

Since the publication of the previous edition of this book, several advances have been made in the understanding of the immunobiology and pathogenesis of SPS and PEWR; a better delineation of the clinical features and boundaries of these disorders; as well as establishing clear guidelines for its treatment. Newer therapeutic options have also been added.

▶ HISTORICAL BACKGROUND

This unusual syndrome was first described by Moersch and Woltman in 1956.[1] The authors coined the term "stiff-man syndrome" in reporting 14 patients with clinical features of progressive fluctuating muscular rigidity and spasms. Their first case, a 49-year-old man, initially complained of a feeling of tightness of the neck musculature of variable occurrence. Over a period of 4 years, this disorder progressively affected the muscles of the shoulder, back, abdomen, and thighs, causing the muscles to appear stiff and "board-like." Continuous muscle contraction causing pronounced stiffness of the axial and limb muscles forced the patient to walk in a peculiar way that was both slow and awkward. Voluntary movement or passive displacement of the limbs triggered prolonged and painful muscle spasms. If severe enough, the spasms caused postural instability and falls. In the words of the authors, the patient would fall like a "wooden man." The additional 13 patients in the original report were similar in all respects.

The clinical features of this previously unreported condition were described in detail in Moersch and Woltman's paper. No other signs of central or peripheral nervous system involvement were present in their 14 patients. The only additional clinical abnormality found in 4 of the 14 original patients was diabetes mellitus. Five of their 14 patients underwent electromyographic (EMG) studies, revealing motor unit activity resembling "that which accompanies contraction of voluntary muscle." In their 1967 review on the subject, Gordon and colleagues[2] summarized the EMG findings reported in the literature until then as "one of persistent tonic contraction reflected in constant firing even at rest." No attempt at relaxation could alter the continuous motor unit discharges according to these authors. Their observations provided the electrophysiological substrate of muscle stiffness in these patients.

Since the publication of Moersch and Woltman's description of the syndrome, more than 100 cases have been reported from different regions of the world.

The first successful attempt at treatment of this condition was that of Howard in 1963[3] with the use of diazepam to reduce stiffness and spasms.

A major breakthrough in the understanding of the pathogenesis of SPS came through the work of Solimena and colleagues in 1988,[4] who reported the presence of antibodies against glutamic acid decarboxylase (anti-GAD), an enzyme involved in the synthesis of γ-aminobutyric acid (GABA) in a patient with SPS, diabetes mellitus, and evidence of additional immunological involvement. Since then, SPS has been postulated as an immunological disorder.

Gordon and colleagues[2] and later Lorish and colleagues[5] defined the clinical criteria necessary for the diagnosis of SPS. These criteria have been widely accepted and are currently used for the identification of cases of SPS. A significant number of patients fall outside these criteria, and are considered atypical SPS. In their recent review of cases seen at the National Hospital in

London, Barker and colleagues[6] assigned cases into three distinct categories: SPS, PEWR, and stiff-limb syndrome (a focal form of the disorder). Brown and Marsden,[7] in a follow-up, reviewed the clinical, immunological, and pathophysiological features of their own, and published cases presenting with features suggestive of SPS; they proposed a new classification, separating the classic form (stiff-man or stiff-person, SPS) from a distinct group designated the "stiff-man plus" syndrome, which includes both the clinically atypical presentations and the paraneoplastic forms of this disorder.

Numerous attempts at therapeutic intervention followed Howard's observation of clinical improvement with diazepam in patients with SPS. Benzodiazepines and baclofen have been recognized as the drugs of choice,[8] although reports of improvement with other drugs, such as sodium valproate, tizanidine, steroids, gabapentin, tiagabine, vigabatrin, rituximab, levetiracetam, propofol, immunoglobulin, and plasmapheresis, have been published in recent years.[6,9–11]

▶ CLINICAL ASPECTS

The disease is sporadic, affecting individuals of both sexes in variable proportion. In their analysis of 34 "valid" cases, Gordon and colleagues[2] found a 2:1 male–female preponderance. This ratio, however, is not maintained in subsequent cases in the more recent literature; interestingly, in the recently published series from the National Institute of Neurological Disorders and Stroke (NINDS), up to 70% of the patients were female.[5,12,13] Although the age at onset varies considerably, the majority of those afflicted are adults ranging from 29 to 59 years of age. Both older and younger cases have been occasionally reported (extreme range 7–71 years).[14–16] Although families with "congenital" SPS have been described, doubts have been raised concerning their identity with sporadic SPS of later onset.[8,17,18] Mean age at onset in the original Mayo Clinic series was 45.5 ± 9.3 years.[5] In the series of Dalakas and colleagues, the average age at symptom onset was 41.2 years. Time to diagnosis, however, was delayed from 1 year to 18 years.[12]

Symptoms usually start slowly and insidiously; patients often complaining of episodic aching and tightness of the axial musculature (neck, paraspinal, and abdominal muscles). Muscle tightness, stiffness, and rigidity become constant within several weeks or months. Involvement is usually symmetrical, spreading on to include proximal muscle groups in all four limbs,[5,8] although gross asymmetry is seen in 10% of cases according to Meinck.[9] Interestingly, this figure goes up to almost 70% in the series reported by Dalakas and colleagues,[10] taking into account all degrees of asymmetry. Sparing of distal muscles of the limbs and facial musculature is usually the rule in these patients; however, the hands or feet may be involved in up to 25% of cases,[9] and involvement of the cranial musculature has been reported occasionally (e.g., difficulty swallowing, dysphagia, changes in facial expression, pursing of the lips, etc.).[2] Stiffness due to involvement of antagonistic muscles causes significant restriction of voluntary movements. Patients are almost unable to bend over and find walking extremely difficult. They adopt a typical hyperlordotic lumbar posture, causing folding of the skin in that region; the neck is held in a somewhat extended position, and there is marked limitation of back and hip movement. Of importance is the fact that lumbar hyperlordosis persists even when lying down on their back. This peculiar pattern of stiffness "has prompted patients and physicians to use such descriptions as 'stiff as a board' and 'he walks like a wooden man' or 'looks like a tin soldier…" as it was colorfully reported by Lorish and colleagues[5] in their 1989 update on SPS. The rigidity or stiffness may fluctuate in intensity from hour to hour or from day to day, usually disappearing during sleep. Activities of daily living become severely impaired in these patients, as they find it extremely difficult to dress by themselves, leaning forward to tie their shoelaces or put on their socks. When severe rigidity of the cervical spine is present, patients must discontinue driving, as they are limited in their capacity to rotate their head to look back or to the side.[5]

An additional incapacitating symptom is the occurrence of intermittent severe spasms in affected muscles.[1,2,5,19] Spasms are precipitated by a wide range of triggering factors. A sudden noise, an unexpected movement, a simple touch, or just being gently nudged may often be the cause of severe spasmodic contraction of the affected muscles. Passive stretching of the muscles will also cause spasms. Emotional stimuli, as well as stress or fatigue may prompt a paroxysm. Spasms are short-lasting (minutes) and gradually disappear if the triggering stimulus is removed. Muscle spasms are often associated with pain. Painful sensation has been variably reported in the literature, either as an acute, sharp or excruciating pain, or more often as a dull, cramping feeling of fatigue.[1,2,5] Spasms may occur in rapid succession ("spasmodic storm") and the clinical picture may then resemble tetanus.[9] Patients experiencing a bout of spasms present a distressful picture, as they "appear to be in a shock-like state associated with sweating, tachycardia and restlessness."[2] An increase in blood pressure has been documented during these crises.[16] Spasms are a compounding factor of motor disability in these patients as they frequently are the cause of sudden falls. Anecdotal reports abound in the literature: patients complaining of spasmodic fits triggered by the ringing of the phone, being awaken in the middle of the night by a soft nudge by a spouse, being ejected from a chair while attempting to sit down.[5] The magnitude and intensity of the spasms is quite variable. In a few reported cases, they became severe enough to cause fracture of long bones.[2]

In a recent analysis of clinical and laboratory findings in SPS patients, Meinck and colleagues[20] extended the repertoire of symptoms in this disorder, adding three new and distinct clinical features to those previously described. Five of their 8 patients reported an "aura"-like feeling preceding spontaneous spasmodic attacks. In the majority of their cases, spasmodic jerks adopted a stereotyped motor pattern, consisting of brief opisthotonos, stiffening of the slightly abducted legs, and inversion of the plantar-flexed feet. In addition, their patients reported a feeling of paroxysmal fear invading them whenever they crossed an open space unaided. Moreover, even the thought of doing it would precipitate it. More than 50% of patients report a characteristic fear of open spaces, which is frequently associated with spasms.[9] The presence of anxiety and task-specific phobias is a frequent manifestation, which at times are so severe that they can dominate the clinical picture and lead to an erroneous diagnosis of a psychiatric disorder. The phobias, however, stem from a realistic fear of falling caused by the neurologic disability rather than from a primary psychogenic disorder.[21] Interestingly, the presence of excessive startle, space phobia, and spasms induced by emotional upset probably are the reasons behind almost 70% of initial misdiagnoses in SPS patients and a frequent label of hysteria that is attached to them.[9]

The illness follows a variable course, with a duration ranging from 6 to 28 years, measured from the onset of symptoms to either death or last follow-up visit.[5] In the majority of cases, the disease slowly and steadily progresses over time. There are, however, some cases for which stabilization is achieved through medication. Lorish and colleagues[5] reported on the follow-up of 13 patients seen at the Mayo Clinic during the period 1955–1985. These patients had a disease duration ranging from 1 to 28 years. All 13 cases were under treatment with variable doses of diazepam and the great majority remained independently mobile in spite of the long duration of the disease in some of them. The rate of progression of the disease and the final outcome will depend in part on several factors: (1) whether the clinical presentation was typical and corresponded to classical SPS; (2) or belonged to the type of disorders grouped under the "stiff-man plus" rubric according to Brown and Marsden;[6] and (3) the conditions usually associated with these disorders (e.g., diabetes, malignancy, etc.). Unexpected sudden death has been reported in SPS cases.[22] Two patients carrying a diagnosis of SPS experienced sudden death, apparently secondary to autonomic instability. Of these two cases, however, 1 had atypical clinical signs and inflammatory changes in the basal ganglia, brain stem and spinal cord, more suggestive of encephalomyelitis.[23,24] It has been reported that approximately 10% of SPS patients may experience sudden death due in most cases to autonomic dysfunction.[25] Severe autonomic symptomatology may be precipitated in SPS patients by the occurrence of repeated spasms in close succession or by sudden withdrawal of medication. This contingency should always be entertained when making changes in medication in SPS patients.

PHYSICAL EXAMINATION

Neurologic examination is usually noncontributory except for those findings related to muscle rigidity. Palpatory examination of the affected muscles will reveal a "tight, rock-hard, board-like quality." Postural changes have been described in detail in the preceding paragraphs. Gait is slow and cautious to avoid precipitation of spasms and falls. Cognitive function, cranial nerves, muscle strength, sensory function, and coordination are all normal; deep-tendon reflexes have often been found to be increased, without further evidence of pyramidal tract involvement. Some investigators have reported mild atrophy and weakness in the advanced stages of the disease. Studies of respiratory function may reveal in some cases a restrictive pattern due to involvement of the thoracic musculature.[1,2,5,8]

In the NINDS series,[12] the authors made an attempt to define the clinical presentation and physical findings of SPS patients on the basis of strict and homogeneous criteria. To that effect, they studied 20 patients with SPS selected by the presence of anti-GAD antibody positivity in high titers. The neurologic signs in these 20 patients are summarized in Table 43–1. In their conclusions, these authors remarked that, although a hallmark diagnostic sign remains, the presence of hyperlordosis and axial rigidity and co-contractures, the presence of asymmetric involvement with predominant stiffness in one leg was very common in their patients. Moreover, all of their patients with initial asymmetric presentation progressed to generalized symptomatology. Another important finding was the presence of stiffness in the facial muscles in almost 70% of the patients, which could erroneously lead to the diagnosis of an akinetic-rigid syndrome in these cases.

The finding of central nervous system (CNS) involvement (myoclonus, brain stem signs, long tract signs, lower motor neuron signs, cognitive changes, autonomic failure/sphincter involvement) or rigidity not confined to the trunk but also involving the distal limbs, often exclusively, would be suggestive of the "stiff-man plus" syndrome (PEWR and related conditions).[7] Although exclusive involvement of one limb ("stiff-limb syndrome") is considered by some to be a separate entity from SPS, the findings of Dalakas and colleagues[12] would challenge this concept to some extent.

▶ **TABLE 43–1. NEUROLOGIC SIGNS IN 20 PATIENTS WITH STIFF-PERSON SYNDROME**

Type	*n* (%)
Increased tone	
Paraspinal muscles	20 (100)
Face	13 (65)
Asymmetry with one leg predominant	15 (70)
Asymmetry with one arm predominant	7 (41)
Only in one leg (stiff-limb)	3 (17)
Prominent stiffness in the cervical paraspinal region	1 (6)
Mild proximal muscle weakness with coexisting signs of myopathy	1 (6)
Functional impairment resulting in:	
Stiff gait	20 (100)
Hyperlordosis	14 (65)
Need for cane	12 (65)
Need for walker	7 (35)
Inability to work	12 (65)
Shortness of breath	10 (50)
Task-specific phobias	10 (50)

Data from Dalakas MC, Fujii M, Li M, et al. The clinical spectrum of anti-GAD antibody-positive patients with stiff-person syndrome. Neurology 2000;55:1531–1535.

LABORATORY

Routine laboratory examinations are usually within normal limits, except in those cases in whom insulin-dependent diabetes mellitus (IDDM), thyroid disorders, malignancy, or other associated conditions are present (see associated conditions later).[1,2,5,8,13] Creatinuria is a rare finding in these patients and is most probably linked to disuse atrophy.[2] Immunological determinations reveal the presence of antibodies directed against GABAergic neurons, more specifically to GAD in a large proportion of SPS patients (60–90% according to different authors;[4,6,9–13,26,27] auto-antibodies directed against other cellular systems are also frequently found in these patients.[6,9,12,13,26] Oligoclonal IgG banding, both in serum and cerebrospinal fluid (CSF), had been reported as an occasional finding by several authors.[4,13,26,28–30] In a recent study including 18 patients, Dalakas and colleagues[31] found oligoclonal IgG bands in 67% of the cases, and an increased anti-GAD-65-specific IgG index in 85%; GABA was found to be lower in SPS patients than in controls. Similar findings regarding oligoclonal banding had been reported by Barker.[6] The presence of GAD - in the CSF is indicative of de novo intrathecal antibody production,[9] which is important in the diagnosis of SPS. Elevated CSF IgG has been reported in isolated cases.[32] The presence of significant CSF abnormalities is, on the contrary, the rule in encephalomyelitis and related conditions ("stiff-man plus" syndrome) (see differential diagnosis later).[7,23,24] Certain human lymphocyte antigen (HLA) phenotypes appear to be more frequent than others in cases of SPS.[11,33–35] All of the aforementioned point in the direction of an immunological disorder as the underlying cause of SPS (see pathophysiology later).

ELECTROMYOGRAPHY (EMG)

The presence of continuous motor unit activity at rest and its persistence despite attempts at relaxation is a constant finding in SPS patients. There are no abnormalities in the morphology of motor units; peripheral nerve motor and sensory conduction velocities are normal, and no signs of denervation, such as fasciculations, fibrillations, and positive sharp waves, can be found. No evidence of grouping of rhythmic discharges or atypical high-frequency bursts are usually found. EMG recordings show this pattern of continuous motor unit activity to be more prominent in paraspinal muscles (thoracolumbar, and rectus abdominis), and proximal arm and leg muscles. Involvement of both agonist and antagonist muscle groups is common. Peripheral stimulation (gentle touching or stroking of the skin) of the muscles explored is followed by marked enhancement of motor unit activity, either continuous or intermittent (spasms) (Fig. 43–1). A stereotyped motor response to electrical stimulation of peripheral nerves is usually obtained when recording in the trunk muscles of all patients with SPS. This response is termed spasmodic reflex myoclonus or reflex-induced spasms.[36] Reflex-induced spasms have a short-onset latency (below 80 ms), are highly reproducible, and are composed of one or more hypersynchronous bursts of EMG activity. EMG bursting is interrupted by short pauses followed by slowly ceasing activity.[9]

The abnormal EMG activity is absent during sleep. Peripheral nerve or spinal nerve root block, spinal anesthesia and general anesthesia, or intravenous injection of diazepam can also abolish this pattern of motor unit activity.[2,5,8,37]

MUSCLE BIOPSY

Histologic study of muscle is usually noncontributory. Most studies performed have reported normal findings in muscle biopsy specimens. In some cases, nonspecific findings, such as minimal atrophy, slight fibrosis, occasional degeneration and regeneration of muscle fibers with associated sprouting of nerve terminals, edema, perivascular infiltration, and proliferation of connective tissue, have been described.[2] The majority of authors are in agreement in the interpretation of these findings as secondary to prolonged ischemia linked to intense muscular contraction.[2] However, in two cases that came to autopsy and were recently published,[38,39] microscopic examination of skeletal muscle showed signs of neurogenic atrophy.

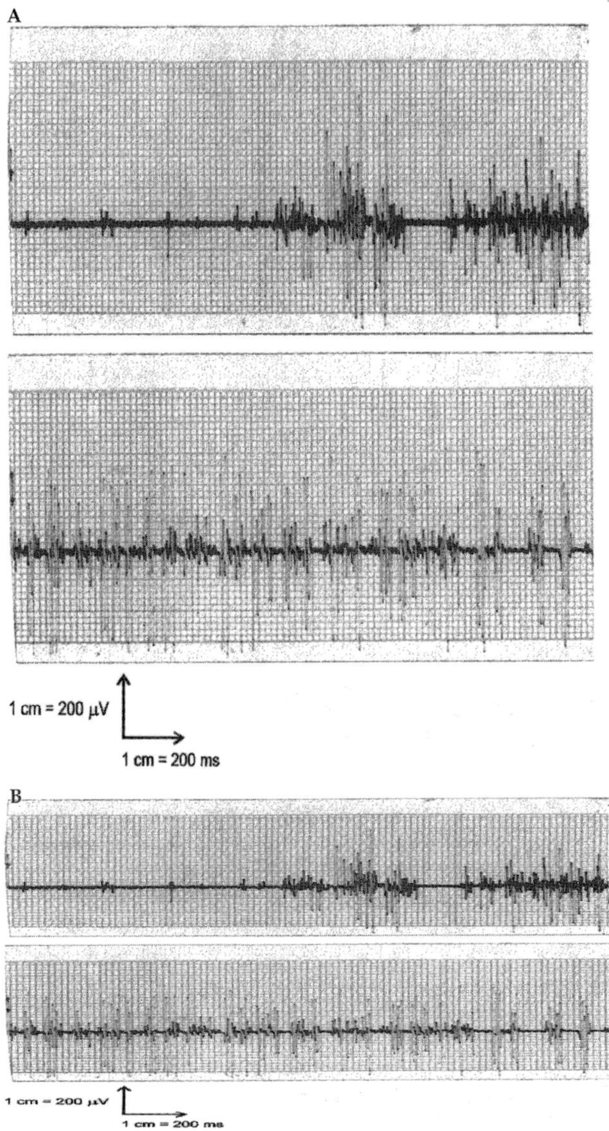

Figure 43–1. (A) Simultaneous EMG recording of antagonist muscles of the upper extremity (biceps and triceps brachialis), showing bursts of motor unit discharges at rest. (B) EMG recording of biceps brachialis, showing intermittent bursts of motor unit discharges after a mechanical stimulus (light tapping).

IMAGING STUDIES

Plain X-ray films of the spine may reveal signs of spondylosis and ossification of spinal ligaments.[1] Although these findings have been reported in SPS patients, they probably represent common, nonspecific phenomena, equally present in the general population.[2] Cortical atrophy on computed tomography and white matter lesions on magnetic resonance imaging (MRI) have been reported in isolated cases of SPS, although its relevance to this condition has not been discussed.[8,27,32] It is indeed possible that the abovementioned abnormalities would correspond to underlying encephalomyelitis. PEWR is often misdiagnosed as SPS (see differential diagnosis below). In cases with typical clinical presentation, positive for GAD autoantibodies, and typical neurophysiological findings, imaging studies might be dispensed with.[9]

▶ ASSOCIATED CONDITIONS AND CLINICAL VARIANTS

A number of medical conditions are commonly associated with SPS and are useful in validating its diagnosis as well as providing clues concerning the pathogenesis of this disorder.

In Blum and Jankovic's review of reported cases until 1991,[13] of 84 patients fulfilling Gordon's criteria for SPS, 18% had definite clinical evidence of one or more organ-specific autoimmune diseases. These included pernicious anemia, vitiligo, myasthenia gravis, hypothyroidism, hyperthyroidism, and Hashimoto's thyroiditis. Dalakas and colleagues[12] in their initial review of 20 cases of SPS with anti-GAD positivity found that 8/20 had IDDM, 8/20 thyroid disease, 3/20 pernicious anemia, and 1/20 celiac disease. Moreover, family history in these patients was positive for IDDM in seven, thyroid disease in four, and one each had family history of systemic lupus erythematosus, rheumatoid arthritis, myasthenia gravis, and vitiligo. A higher percentage of associated immune diseases (>50%) was reported by Meinck.[9] In Dalakas' expanded series,[10] including 40 patients under follow-up, diabetes, thyroiditis, and pernicious anemia were the most common associated conditions, with diabetes occurring in up to 35% of the patients. Moreover, the co-existence of another autoimmune disorder or autoantibodies, especially type 1 diabetes and antithyroglobulin or antiparietal cell antibodies, should raise the clinical suspicion of SPS in a patient presenting with rigidity and spasms. In addition, strong immunogenetic association with the DRb1 locus (0301, 0101 alleles) and DQb1 locus (0201, 0203, and 0205 alleles) has been found in these patients.[10]

Of special importance is the relationship of SPS and IDDM, not only because of the frequent association of these two conditions, but because the reason of its simultaneous occurrence may also bear upon the pathogenesis of SPS.[13] Four of the original 14 patients reported in Moersch and Woltman's paper,[1] and 8 out of 13 patients in Lorish and colleagues' update on SPS published in 1989[5] had diabetes. The type of diabetes was not mentioned in these two reports. It is currently accepted that diabetes is present in one-third to two-thirds of patients with SPS. Blum and Jankovic's review of the literature[13] found that in 8% of the published cases IDDM was present, while 13 additional patients had diabetes but without further characterization of its type. According to these authors, the frequency of IDDM in SPS patients is therefore more than 30 times that of the general population (0.25%). In recent years, this association has been further confirmed and found to be more frequent than previously reported; 40% of the patients reported by Dalakas and colleagues[12] had IDDM, while in Meinck's series[9] the figure reached 41%. These findings are of relevance in the light of the current hypothesis on the pathogenesis of IDDM. It is presently accepted that an abnormal immune response directed against pancreatic islet cells is triggered by an exogenous agent, possibly a virus, causing the development of IDDM in genetically predisposed individuals.[13] A similar mechanism may be involved in the pathogenesis of SPS (see pathophysiology later).

Epilepsy, ataxia, nocturnal myoclonus, eye movement abnormalities and vertigo have also been reported in association with SPS.[10,40–45] These symptoms can be observed from the outset, or they may appear later on in the course of the disease.[10] In their 1978 publication, Martinelli and colleagues[40] calculated, from a review of the literature, that the prevalence of epilepsy in SPS cases was close to 10%, which is exactly the figure reported recently by Dalakas and colleagues[12] in their own patients. They concluded that this figure was much higher than the prevalence of epilepsy in the general population, supporting the concept that this association was not by chance. However, this assertion has been contested by others, justifying the higher prevalence of epilepsy in SPS patients as a withdrawal phenomenon in individuals under diazepam therapy for extended periods.[46] Ataxia was also present in up to 10% of the cases in Dalakas' series.[10,41] The SPS cerebellar variant has a specific clinical phenotype. These patients present with severe stiffness and spasms; prominent cerebellar or truncal ataxia; dysarthria; very ataxic gait with prominent stiffness in the legs and trunk; and abnormal eye movements (see later). In the patients reported by Rakocevic, imaging studies were normal, high titers of anti-GAD antibodies were detected, and the serum IgG bound to cerebellar interneurons in vitro.[41]

Besides nocturnal myoclonus, other types of myoclonic jerks have been reported in cases diagnosed as SPS. Leigh and colleagues[45] published the clinical and electrophysiological findings in a 38-year-old patient with reflex myoclonus and muscle rigidity. The authors coined the term "jerking stiff-man syndrome" in view of the prominent jerking with similar characteristics to reticular reflex myoclonus, present in their patient. Although the patient had many of the clinical features necessary for the diagnosis of SPS, the presence of clinical and radiological signs of brain stem and cerebellar involvement would be more in favor of either encephalomyelitis or an atypical form of sporadic cerebellar system degeneration. An additional case reported by Alberca and colleagues[47] shares many of the clinical features described in the previous patient, although no evidence of structural involvement of the CNS was found. This concept has been more recently elaborated by Brown and Marsden,[7] who propose that the "jerking stiff-man syndrome" should be included as one of the variants of the "stiff-man plus syndrome" with prominent brain stem involvement, as opposed to the "stiff-limb syndrome" in which the spinal cord is primarily involved.

The "stiff-limb syndrome," presenting with only focal involvement has been described as a clinical variant of SPS. However, some cases, which at onset presented with stiffness restricted to one limb, went on to develop a more generalized involvement with the features of typical SPS.[6,10]

Abnormalities of eye movements including gaze-holding nystagmus (downbeat), limited abduction, vertical and horizontal ocular misalignment, deficient smooth pursuit and impaired saccade initiation (longer latencies) have been reported in SPS patients. In addition in patients with SPS and cerebellar signs a rare saccade velocity profile consisting of multicomponent saccades was observed, which has been attributed to impairment of GABAergic neurotransmission[42,43] Another isolated finding has been the occurrence of progressively delayed saccade latency together with supranuclear ophtalmoparesis in a patient fullfilling criteria for SPS but with additional features reminiscent of PSP.[48] Vertigo as an accompanying manifestation of SPS has been reported in a single case, in which it was noted that pharmacological treatment not only significantly improved rigidity and stiffness, but it also helped in resolving the vertiginous sensations.[44]

▶ DIAGNOSIS

Gordon and colleagues[2] were the first to establish a set of criteria for the diagnosis of SPS. They were based on the analysis of the original 14 cases of Moersch and Woltman and subsequent reports from the world literature. Their criteria included clinical and neurophysiologic findings, as well as a number of supportive tests. Clinical criteria were subdivided into six "key features" as follows:

1. *Prodromes* ("episodic aching and tightness of the axial musculature").
2. *Progression* ("...symmetrical, continuous stiffness characterized by tight, stony-hard, board-like muscles spreads to involve most of the limb, trunk and neck musculature").
3. *Painful spasms and precipitating factors* ("superimposed upon this persistent rigidity of muscles, sudden stimuli often precipitate paroxysms of

muscle spasm of such intensity as to lead, although not invariably, to excruciating pain").

4. *Sleep* ("In this state rigidity is abolished,...").
5. *Neurologic findings* ("Normal motor and sensory examinations are the rule, except for the difficulty in active movement and the board-hard muscles referred to under 'Progression"').
6. *Intellect* ("Invariably intellect has been found intact,...").

According to Gordon and colleagues' criteria, the EMG "defines the peculiar state of voluntary muscle in stiff-man syndrome as one of persistent tonic contraction reflected in constant firing even 'at rest'." Additional supportive tests included: (1) response to myoneural blocking agents, (2) effect of chemical block of peripheral motor fibers, and (3) response to general anesthesia. Furthermore, the beneficial effect of diazepam upon muscle stiffness was included as a final supportive criteria.

Thompson,[8] and, later on, Dalakas,[49] modified and expanded the criteria for diagnosis proposed by Gordon and colleagues[2] and Lorish and colleagues[5] (Table 43–2). The basic criteria for the diagnosis, however, can be summarized as follows: (1) muscular rigidity in the limbs and axial (trunk) muscles, prominent in the abdominal and thoracolumbar paraspinals; (2) continuous co-contraction of agonist and antagonist muscles, confirmed clinically and electrophysiologically; (3) episodic spasms precipitated by unexpected noises, tactile stimuli, or emotional upset; (4) absence of any other neurologic disease that could explain stiffness and rigidity; and (5) positive antiglutamic acid decarboxylase (GAD)65 (or amphiphysin) antibodies assessed by immunocytochemistry, Western blot, or radioimmunoassay.[10]

▶ **TABLE 43–2. CRITERIA FOR THE DIAGNOSIS OF THE STIFF-PERSON SYNDROME**

Clinical
Gradual and insidious onset of aching and tightness (rigidity) of limb and axial muscles
Slow progression; stiffness spreads from axial muscles to limbs (legs > arms) (according to Dalakas, a significant proportion may start with asymmetrical involvement of one limb and progressive generalization)
Continuous co-contraction of agonist and antagonist muscles with inability to relax, as confirmed clinically and electrophysiologically
Persistent contraction of thoracolumbar, paraspinal, and abdominal muscles
Abnormal hyperlordotic posture of lumbar spine
Board-like rigidity of abdominal muscles
Rigidity abolished by sleep
Stimulus-sensitive painful muscle spasms (precipitants: unexpected noises, tactile stimuli, or emotional upset)
No other abnormal neurological signs
Intellect normal
Cranial muscles rarely (if ever) involved (disputed by Dalakas)
Neurophysiological
Continuous motor unit activity
EMG activity abolished by sleep, peripheral nerve block, spinal or general anesthesia
Normal peripheral nerve conduction; normal motor unit morphology
Other observations that may be helpful but are of uncertain diagnostic specificity
Autoantibodies directed against GABAergic neurons, in particular to GAD
Association with autoimmune endocrine disease

Data from Thompson PD. Stiff people. In Marsden CD, Fahn S (eds). Movement Disorders 3. Oxford: Butterworth-Heinemann, 1994, pp. 373–405; with modifications according to Dalakas MC. The stiff-person syndrome: An autoimmune disorder affecting neurotransmission of gamma-aminobutyric acid. Ann Intern Med 1999;131:522–530.

▶ DIFFERENTIAL DIAGNOSIS

Any patient presenting with muscle stiffness, rigidity, and cramps or muscle spasms may at one time be considered as a possible case of SPS. Moreover, there are several conditions with clinical features resembling SPS but with demonstrable CNS pathology that have been reported in the literature as atypical cases of this disorder. The list of conditions is long and includes disorders of muscle contraction of both central and peripheral origin (Table 43–3). Dealing with each of these disorders exceeds the scope of this chapter (for a review see Refs. 8 and 37).

Strict adherence to the criteria carefully delineated by Gordon and colleagues,[2] Lorish and colleagues,[5] and more recently Thompson[8] and Dalakas,[10,49] will help in identifying cases of SPS, differentiating them from the conditions listed in Table 43–3.

Some of the disorders included in Table 43–3 deserve special consideration because of the difficulties they may present in the differential diagnosis with SPS.

PEWR is a rare, usually paraneoplastic, disorder featuring, in addition to the cardinal symptoms of SPS, evidence of brain stem, and spinal cord involvement.[23,24,50] The latter may manifest by cranial nerve signs, segmental and long tract spinal cord symptomatology. Myoclonus and opsoclonus have also been reported in this disorder. Imaging studies may reveal cortical, brain stem, and cerebellar atrophy and sometimes hyperintense signals in the white matter on MRI examination. Abnormal findings in the CSF are frequent (lymphocytic pleocytosis, elevated protein levels, increased immunoglobulins, and oligoclonal IgG bands). In a single case, diagnosed as having PEWR on the basis of a few atypical features

TABLE 43-3. DIFFERENTIAL DIAGNOSIS OF STIFF-PERSON SYNDROME

	Peripheral	
Central	Nerve	Muscle
Encephalitis (including brain stem, spinal cord ["progressive encephalomyelitis with rigidity"])	Myokimia, neuromyotonia, and pseudomyotonia Idiopathic	Myotonic syndromes (channelopathies)
		Myotonic dystrophy
		Myotonia congenital
Dystonia	Isaacs syndrome (continuous muscle fiber activity)	Paramyotonia
Idiopathic		
Symptomatic		
	Associated with neuropathy	Myopathies
	Hereditary	Metabolic
	Inflammatory	Inflammatory
Akinetic-rigid syndromes	Toxic	Endocrine
Parkinson's disease	Radiation	Congenital
Multiple-system atrophy	Paraneoplastic	
Progressive supranuclear palsy		Contracture
Drug-induced parkinsonism	Schwartz–Jampel syndrome	Arthritis
Toxic parkinsonism (MPTP, carbon monoxide, manganese)	Tetanus	Ankylosing spondylitis
		Volkmann's ischemic contracture
Neuroleptic malignant syndrome		
	Cramps	
Myelopathies (multiple sclerosis, infectious, trauma, ischemia, hemorrhage, spondylosis)		
Spinal cord tumor		
Spinal cord AVM		
Toxins (tetanus, strychnine, etc.)		
Motor neuron disease (primary lateral sclerosis, amyotrophic lateral clerosis)		
Psychiatric illness (phobic neurosis, hysteria, malingering)		

Abbreviations: MPTP, 1-methyl-4-phenyl-1,2,3,6-tetrahydropyridine; AVM, arteriovenous malformation.

(pattern of distribution of rigidity, loss of tendon jerks, nuclear and supranuclear gaze palsies, and reticular reflex myoclonus), GAD autoantibodies were detected.[51] However, no confirmation of an inflammatory process within the CNS was available. Results of biopsy or postmortem examination in PEWR cases show an inflammatory process, with perivascular lymphocytic infiltration, gliosis, and severe neuronal loss, involving mainly the lower brain stem and spinal cord (encephalomyelitis). In some cases there is a more widespread involvement, including brain cortical regions (hippocampus), and subcortical gray nuclei (basal ganglia). The most striking pathological changes are usually restricted to the central gray zones of the spinal cord containing inhibitory interneurons. The disease follows a relentless course ending in death in a few months or years. This condition has been reported either as an isolated illness or more frequently associated with malignancy (oat-cell carcinoma of the lung, Hodgkin's disease).[6,52,53]

The question of SPS as a paraneoplastic autoimmune disorder in isolated cases has been raised in several publications. In three women with breast cancer, presenting with clinical features fulfilling the criteria necessary for the diagnosis of SPS, and in whom none of the conditions frequently associated with SPS (IDDM and other immunological disorders) and no GAD autoantibodies were detected, an extensive immunological screening detected the presence of a humoral autoimmune response against a neuronal protein of 128 kDa.[54] This antigen was found to be concentrated at synapses and its distribution outside the nervous system was highly restricted. Similar to GAD, the 128-kDa antigen is localized in the cytoplasmic compartment and is not a membrane surface protein. In a follow-up study, this 128-kDa antigen has been identified as the synaptic vesicle-associated protein amphiphysin.[55] Both GAD and amphiphysin are concentrated in nerve terminals, associated to the cytoplasmic surface of synaptic vesicles. In a recently reported case of a patient who developed SPS, including disabling shoulder subluxation and wrist ankylosis, in association with breast cancer, immunologic investigations disclosed autoimmunity directed against not only amphiphysin but also GAD positivity. The patient improved after surgery and corticosteroid treatment and was reported to be stable for nearly 4 years on only antiestrogens. The triad of SPS, breast cancer, and autoantibodies against amphiphysin identifies a rather specific autoimmune paraneoplastic syndrome of the CNS in the view of these authors.[56] The presence of anti-amphiphysin antibodies is not specific to SPS as they have been detected in patients with various paraneoplastic neurological syndromes and tumors (e.g., sensory neuronopathy, encephalomyelitis, and breast cancer; limbic encephalitis, and small-cell lung cancer; encephalomyelitis and ovarian carcinoma; Lambert-Eaton myasthenic syndrome, and small-cell lung cancer), and in association with other autoantibodies.[57] In addition to amphiphysin, Butler and colleagues[58] recently reported a patient with clinical features of SPS and mediastinal cancer in whom high-titer autoantibodies directed against gephyrin were detected. Gephyrin is a cytosolic protein selectively concentrated at the postsynaptic membrane of inhibitory synapses, associated with $GABA_A$ and glycine receptors. Indeed, an antibody to glycine receptors was recently identified in patients with PEWR a form of SPS that has been identified as a probable paraneoplastic syndrome.[59]

These findings suggest a possible link between the mechanism of autoimmunity in SPS and some paraneoplastic cases. It is also worth underlying that 40% of SPS cases lack autoantibodies directed against GAD and not all patients suffer from IDDM as an associated condition.

Therefore, it is possible that SPS be in fact a heterogeneous disorder in which different pathogenetic mechanisms, including a paraneoplastic immune response with or without inflammatory changes (PEWR), play a role.[51,52,60] As previously mentioned, Brown and Marsden,[7] in an analysis of their own and previously published cases, tried to sort out cases with typical presentation (axial stiffness, GAD positivity, and high incidence of IDDM) from those with atypical symptomatology, signs of CNS involvement, poor response to medication, and worse prognosis. To that effect they grouped together these atypical cases under the label of "stiff-man plus syndrome" or, more correctly, "stiff-person plus syndrome."

The first of the "plus" cases in the view of these authors corresponds to PEWR, running a subacute course and being pathologically characterized by subcortical demyelination (encephalomyelitis). Clinical features include widespread rigidity, painful myoclonus and spasms, and long tract and brain stem signs. Survival is short (less than 3 years), and its relentless progression and histological features are suggestive of a paraneoplastic etiology, which has been confirmed in occasional cases.

In contrast to PEWR, the remaining "plus" cases are chronic and, unlike the former, have a relative absence of long tract signs in the presence of significant rigidity. In cases where there is predominant brain stem involvement, the clinical picture is dominated by the presence of reflex myoclonus involving all four limbs ("jerking stiff-person syndrome"). The paroxysmal nature of the jerks may be so severe as to compromise respiration and lead to a fatal outcome. If properly treated (assisted ventilation, antimyoclonic agents) these patients may have a long survival (10 years or more), which makes a paraneoplastic etiology unlikely, at least in a large proportion of cases. In others, there are no signs of brain stem dysfunction and myoclonus is absent. The rigidity and painful spasms in these cases is restricted to the limbs, especially distally ("stiff-limb syndrome"), suggesting spinal involvement.[61] These cases have been found to have a particular pattern of EMG activity with an unusual segmented appearance due to an abnormally synchronous discharge of motor units, in contrast to the normal-looking interference pattern found in SPS. Only in 15% of these cases is there anti-GAD positivity, which has led some to consider these cases to be a "focal" form of SPS. However, in one reported case that came to autopsy, the pathological findings were consistent with an inflammatory process restricted to the spinal cord. This condition runs a protracted course, often measured in decades, and although many have a variety of autoantibodies, the autoimmune profile in these patients is quite different from that usually observed in typical cases of SPS. Similar cases have been reported to be associated to breast or small-cell lung carcinoma and have antibodies against the presynaptic vesicle-associated protein amphiphysin.[57]

▶ PATHOPHYSIOLOGY AND PATHOGENESIS

PATHOLOGY

Postmortem examination of the CNS including the spinal cord, in patients with SPS has not yielded evidence of any significant abnormality in the majority of autopsied cases.[1,2,5,8,14] One exception is a case reported by Nakamura and colleagues,[62] showing involvement of the anterior columns of the spinal cord; an additional case was published by Warich-Kirches and colleagues,[39] who found a decrease of GABAergic cells in the cerebellar cortex, and a size reduction of Renshaw cells in the spinal cord. More recently, a case reported by Ishizawa and colleagues[38] showed reduction in the density of anterior horn neurons with somal areas up to 1500 μm^2 (corresponding to the smaller α-motor neurons and γ-motor neurons) and relative sparing of the larger (>1500 μm^2) α-motor neurons. Interestingly, GAD-like immunoreactivity in the spinal gray matter and density of GAD-containing Purkinje cells were not significantly reduced, in contrast to the observations of Warich-Kirches and colleagues[39] No consistent macroscopic or microscopic changes have been found in the few remaining cases that underwent autopsy. The lack of pathological correlates to the marked derangement of motor unit activity and muscle contraction appears to indicate that SPS is a functional rather than a structural disorder.

PHYSIOLOGY

All evidence suggests a central origin for the spasms, rigidity, and continuous motor unit activity. This is substantiated by their disappearance with sleep, peripheral nerve block, general anesthesia, and systemic administration of diazepam.[1,2,5] Several hypotheses have been proposed to explain this enhancement of spinal motor neuron activity, including increased primary excitability of α-motor neurons, a disorder of presynaptic inhibition of Ia terminals in the spinal cord, increased fusimotor activity, defective Renshaw cell function, and abnormalities in the suprasegmental descending pathways controlling spinal interneuronal systems. Several authors have addressed these hypotheses using different investigative techniques.

Monosynaptic stretch reflexes and F-waves are normal in SPS patients.[63] In addition, assessment of the ratio of the maximal H-reflex to M-wave size in the soleus muscle has failed to reveal any abnormality, excluding a primary enhancement of α-motor neuron excitability.[63]

Evaluation of the recovery curve of the soleus H-reflex after a conditioning stimulus in patients with SPS yielded normal results, thus ruling out the Ia afferent system as the source of abnormal inputs to the motor neurons of the spinal cord.[40,64]

Although there is no conclusive evidence for or against the presence of increased γ-motor neuron (fusimotor) activity, most authors consider it unlikely in view of the normal tendon reflexes and particular pattern of distribution of muscle rigidity.[2,63]

Involvement of the recurrent inhibitory loop mediated by Renshaw cells has also been ruled out as the silent period following a supramaximal peripheral nerve stimulus was found to be normal in SPS patients.[63–66]

Evidence in favor of a disorder of presynaptic inhibition of Ia terminals in the spinal cord is based on the lack of depression in amplitude of the soleus H-reflex conditioned by tonic vibration applied to the Achilles tendon in SPS cases.[64] In a recent study, however, vibration-induced inhibition of H-reflexes was diminished in eight of nine patients tested, but the presynaptic period of reciprocal inhibition was found to be normal. Both neural circuits underlying these responses are presumed to involve presynaptic inhibition and GABAergic interneurons. In the same group of patients, occasional abnormalities were found in the first period of reciprocal inhibition and nonreciprocal (Ib) inhibition, which presumably involve glycinergic circuits. Recurrent inhibition was normal. The authors speculate that differences between the two presumptive GABAergic circuits may indicate that not all populations of GABAergic neurons are uniformly affected in SPS. On the other hand, the involvement of presumptive glycinergic circuits in some patients could point to impairment of non-GABAergic neurons, unrecognized involvement of GABAergic neurons in these inhibitory circuits, or, more likely, alterations of supraspinal systems that exert descending control over spinal circuits.[67] The finding of hyperexcitability of the motor cortex (decreased inhibition and markedly increased facilitation) in SPS patients, using transcranial magnetic stimulation, lends further support to this hypothesis.[68]

Another consistent abnormal finding in SPS patients is the presence of a widespread enhancement of exteroceptive reflexes, probably due to the proposed disorder of descending pathways controlling segmental interneuronal systems.[63,69] The responses to exteroceptive stimuli have been found to be grossly exaggerated, with abnormally short transmission times and the presence of abnormal excitatory reflex phases in face, arm, and leg muscles. Both somatosensory and acoustic stimuli are the most effective in evoking an abnormal reflex response. The presence of an abnormally exaggerated blink reflex has also been noted in SPS cases.[63] A more prominent and persistent response of the acoustic startle reflex has been found in SPS patients in comparison to controls.[70] Most nonnociceptive reflexes have been found to behave abnormally, showing a low stimulation threshold, lacking habituation phenomena, and exhibiting co-contraction, suggesting nonspecific disturbances of the polysynaptic system.[40,63]

BIOCHEMISTRY AND PHARMACOLOGY

The existence of a disorder involving suprasegmental influences on inhibitory interneuronal systems at the spinal cord level is supported by a number of biochemical and pharmacological studies.

An increase in the severity of spasms induced by catecholamine precursors (e.g., L-dopa) or serotonin reuptake inhibitors (e.g., clorimipramine) has been reported.[15,63,69,71] On the contrary, opposite effects were observed with the use of drugs reducing aminergic activity within the CNS (e.g., clonidine and tizanidine),[63] or drugs that probably act by enhancing GABAergic transmission (e.g., diazepam and baclofen).[72] In addition, diazepam may also act indirectly through inhibition of catecholaminergic transmission.[15,63] These findings suggest an imbalance between noradrenergic and GABAergic neurotransmitter systems descending from the brain stem to the spinal cord.[15,63] The detection of reduced levels of GABA in the CSF of SPS patients would lend further support to this hypothesis.[13]

Neither physostigmine, a cholinergic drug, glycine, a putative inhibitory neurotransmitter at the spinal cord level, nor milacemide, a glycine precursor, produce any modification in the clinical status of SPS patients.[3,72,73] These observations lend little support to theories proposing a defective synaptic transmission either at the cholinergic synapse of recurrent axons of α-motor neurons, involving Renshaw cells or at the proposed glycinergic synapse between axons of spinal cord interneurons and cell bodies of α-motor neurons.

The hypothesis of an imbalance between a descending excitatory catecholamine neuronal system and a GABAergic counterpart with net inhibitory effects on α-motor neurons was further bolstered by findings of increased 3-methoxy-4-hydroxyphenylglycol (MHPG) excretion in a patient with SPS.[74] MHPG is the major metabolite of brain norepinephrine. Pharmacologic manipulations in this patient showed a direct correlation between clinical status and levels of MHPG in the urine, suggesting the presence of an overactive catecholamine system as one of the underlying mechanisms of rigidity and spasms.[15,63,74] However, a subsequent report failed to confirm these findings.[65] Nevertheless, the possibility that disturbances in the inhibitory descending GABAergic systems are indeed responsible for the development of rigidity and spasms is underscored by recent findings confirming the capacity of anti-GAD autoantibodies of inhibiting enzyme activity ("in vitro"), leading to reduced GABA synthesis.[75]

Although, on the basis of the therapeutic response to drugs and additional experimental evidence, most authors agree on the possibility of such an imbalance, there is as yet no firm "in vivo" evidence to substantiate this.

IMMUNOLOGY

Young, in 1966,[76] was the first to advance the hypothesis of an autoimmune mechanism in the pathogenesis of SPS, based on the findings of pernicious anemia and possibly Hashimoto's thyroiditis in a patient with this disorder. The coexistence of diseases of autoimmune origin in patients with SPS is a consistent finding, suggesting a possibly common pathogenetic mechanism. As mentioned earlier, in Blum and Jankovic's review of 84 published cases, including two of their own, 18% had clinical evidence of one or more autoimmune diseases.[13]

A compelling argument in favor of the autoimmune origin of SPS came through the work of Solimena and colleagues.[4] These authors detected the presence of autoantibodies against several nonneuronal tissues in the serum of a patient with SPS, epilepsy and IDDM, carrying an autoimmunity predisposing HLA phenotype. These included complement-fixing islet-cell antibodies, gastric parietal-cell antibodies and thyroglobulin and thyroid microsomal antibodies. In addition, both the serum and the CSF of the patient contained antibodies to mammalian CNS antigens. Antibodies were detected through immunocytochemistry and Western blot analysis. The cellular and subcellular distribution of immunoreactivity was identical to that of GAD, an enzyme involved in the synthesis of GABA. GAD is concentrated in GABAergic nerve terminals and, outside the CNS, in pancreatic beta cells. Cross-immunoreactivity was found in this patient. An important additional evidence in support of the hypothesis of an autoimmune process directed against the CNS was the finding of elevated levels of IgG with an oligoclonal pattern in the CSF of the patient.

In a subsequent publication, Solimena and colleagues[26] reported on the results of a systematic immunological study of patients with SPS. They studied the serum of 32 patients with an established diagnosis of SPS; in 24 of the cases, the CSF was also available. Control serum samples of 218 individuals were used, including 16 healthy subjects, 111 patients with varied neurological disorders, 74 with IDDM, 20 with other organ-specific autoimmune disorders and 3 with systemic autoimmune disease. The techniques used in the study included immunocytochemical assays to detect autoantibodies against GABAergic neurons, standard laboratory procedures to detect different organ-specific auto-antibodies (islet-cell, gastric parietal-cell, thyroglobulin, and thyroid microsomal-fraction antibodies), immunoblotting, immunoprecipitation, isoelectric focusing and silver staining of serum and CSF to detect oligoclonal IgG bands. Sixty percent of the sera of SPS patients tested were positive for autoantibodies against GABAergic neurons, while 50% of the CSF samples were also positive. Twenty-seven percent of the CSF samples tested revealed the presence of oligoclonal IgG bands, including two patients negative for GABAergic neuron autoantibodies. In all patients that tested positive for GABAergic neuron antibodies there was cross-immunoreactivity directed against pancreatic beta cells. Other organ-specific autoantibodies that were positive in the same patient group included gastric parietal-cell antibodies (15/19), thyroid microsomal-fraction antibodies (9/19) and thyroglobulin antibodies (4/15). In the control population, only four patients (1.8%) tested positive for GABAergic neuron autoantibodies. A Western blot assay was performed to investigate whether GAD was the autoantigen responsible for the positive immunoreactivity against brain and pancreas. A band comigrating with GAD was detected in the large majority of serum and CSF samples that were positive for autoantibodies against GABAergic neurons, confirming GAD as the antigen responsible for the autoimmune response.

More recent studies have attempted to better characterize the immunological response in both SPS and IDDM. GAD, the major autoantigen in both disorders, is present in two isoforms, GAD-65 and GAD-67; the isoforms have different molecular weights and are the products of two different genes.[77] The majority of SPS patients carry autoantibodies that react with the smaller isoform and specifically identify a dominant autoreactive target region (epitope) in the antigen.[78] The pattern of reactivity is somewhat different in IDDM, suggesting differences in epitope recognition in these two disorders.[79] These findings may indicate that, during the development of these diseases, the autoantigen is presented to the immune system through separate pathogenetic mechanisms.[80] The specificity of the immune response in SPS was further elaborated by Dalakas and colleagues[31] in a study of 18 patients with positive immunoreactivity to GABAergic neurons. Serum and CSF reactivity to purified GAD antigen was examined by Western blots, and the anti-GAD-65 antibody titers were quantified by ELISA and compared with 70 disease controls (11 patients with IDDM and 49 with other autoimmune disorders). In the serum of all patients with SPS, there were significantly high anti-GAD-65 antibody titers (7.5–214 μg/mL), whereas in IDDM patients and in those carrying other autoimmune disorders the antibody titers were much lower. Moreover, only patients with SPS had detectable CSF anti-GAD-65 antibodies. Using immunoblotting techniques, both the serum and the CSF of SPS recognized a 65-kDa protein in brain homogenates corresponding to GAD-65, which was further confirmed with the monoclonal antibody against GAD-65. Epitope recognition of recombinant GAD-65 was specific for serum and CSF of SPS patients, while none of the patients with IDDM or other autoimmune disorders immunoreacted with purified GAD-65.

Moreover, there is other evidence indicating differences in the immune response between SPS and IDDM patients at both the cellular and the humoral level. Blood T-cells of SPS patients recognize different immunodominant epitopes of GAD-65 compared with T-cells from IDDM patients. Although IgG1 is dominant in both conditions, SPS patients, however, are more likely to have isotypes other than IgG1, in particular, IgG4 or IgE isotypes, which are not present in IDDM patients.[81]

Depending on the method of detection used, autoantibodies against the larger GAD-67 isoform and to an 80-kDa antigen can also be identified in SPS cases.[77,82] In a recent report, Johnstone and Nussey[30] detected the presence of autoantibodies reacting against the large isoform of human GAD (GAD-67) using recombinant techniques, providing direct evidence for a clonally restricted response to GAD in SPS patients. These findings confirm previous observations suggesting immunological heterogeneity in SPS.[83] They also underline the need to perform different immunological techniques to identify the specific antigen involved in the production of anti-GABAergic autoantibodies in SPS cases.

High anti-GAD antibody titers are considered to be specific markers for SPS, however, they can be seen occasionally in patients with other neuro logic manifestations without SPS, such as myoclonus, epilepsy, cerebellar ataxia, and thymoma associated neuromyotonia.[84–88] GAD antibodies have also been seen in some patients with neurologic complications of thymoma and, rarely, in lung and breast carcinomas, suggesting that these antibodies may also be associated with paraneoplastic disorders.[89] In Batten's disease, the juvenile form of neuronal ceroid lipofuscinosis, an autosomal recessive disorder due to deletions in the *CLN3* gene is also associated with high anti-GAD antibody titers.[90] Furthermore, *cln3* knockout mice, the animal model of Batten's disease, also develop anti-GAD antibodies.[10] The broad variation in symptomatology observed between typical SPS or combined with cerebellar involvement, and disorders presenting with cerebellar dysfunction alone, myoclonus, or epilepsy, all having anti-GAD antibodies, could be explained by differences in recognition of GAD epitopes.[41]

The possibility of a genetically determined susceptibility to the development of SPS has been discussed by different authors. Several studies have reported on the detection of specific HLA haplotypes frequently linked to this disorder. The original patient of Solimena and colleagues[4] with autoantibodies to GAD was found to have the B44 and DR-3/4 antigens as major haplotypes. In the same year, Williams and colleagues[33] found that four of their five SPS patients, all suffering from autoimmune endocrinopathies, also typed to the B44 antigen, which is in linkage disequilibrium with DR4. HLA DR3 and DR4 are the alleles most commonly associated with IDDM in whites. Subsequently, Blum and Jankovic[13] speculated on the possibility that the specific organization of HLA-determined immunoregulatory molecules apparently involved in the development of IDDM possibly constitute the pathogenetic mechanism of autoimmunity to GABAergic cells in the CNS. The demonstration of HLA phenotypes common to both IDDM and SPS would lend further support to this hypothesis. In a more recent study on the genetics of susceptibility and resistance to IDDM in SPS, Pugliese and colleagues[34] found that, as in IDDM, SPS was associated with the allele DQB1*0201. In addition, the presence or absence of the related allele DQB1*0602 would in turn confer either a protective or a predisposing factor for the development of IDDM in SPS patients.[35] Although there is an overlap of the DQB1 allele between SPS and IDDM patients, the former are by themselves more frequently associated with the DRB1*0301 allele.[12] These findings are, according to the authors, further evidence of the importance of the HLA genetic background in the development of SPS and related autoimmune disorders.

ETIOLOGY AND PATHOGENESIS

Although as yet there is no definitive answer concerning the etiology and pathogenesis of SPS, all the available evidence, already discussed in previous paragraphs, suggests an autoimmune mechanism as responsible for its development. Moreover, this autoimmune mechanism woulds somehow interfere with inhibitory neurotransmitter pathways in the brain and spinal cord as suggested by the physiological findings. As GABA is the most important inhibitory neurotransmitter in the brain, the obvious conclusion is that GABAergic pathways should be involved. A hypothesis that is supported by the presence of high-titer antibodies against GAD (the rate-limiting enzyme for the synthesis of GABA) in more than 85% of patients[26,91] and the reduction of GABA in the motor cortex as measured through magnetic resonance spectroscopy.[92] There is also evidence of dysfunction of GABAergic pathways, found on positron emission tomography (PET) scans of SPS patients.[93]

One possibility would envision that an unknown noxious stimulus could trigger a cascade of events leading to the exposure of intracellular GAD to the immune system causing the production of autoantibodies against this enzyme and GABA-containing neurons. However, GAD65, like the two other autoantigens identified in paraneoplastic SPS (amphiphysin and gephyrin),[57,58] are cytosolic, and the mechanism by which these antibodies could gain access to GABAergic interneurons to recognize cytosolic antigens remains unknown. If this were the case, there could be a selective impairment of GABAergic transmission in suprasegmental systems influencing the inhibitory activity of spinal interneurons. The resulting imbalance between excitatory and inhibitory influences at the segmental level would be the cause of the enhancement of spinal motor neuron activity.

However, although the possibility that the anti-GAD antibodies may be pathogenic is also supported by the observation that anti-GAD–specific IgG from SPS patients inhibits GAD activity and GABA synthesis in vitro,[94] the degree of inhibition, despite being dose dependent, is unrelated to GAD titers.[95] In addition, no correlation between the cerebrospinal fluid GAD-specific IgG index and disease severity or duration, even within individual patients, has been found.[96] Moreover, GAD-specific T cells are inconsistently present in only a small number of SPS patients,[10] and anti-GAD65 antibodies do not transfer the disease from mothers to infants.[97] In addition, there is a significant number of patients with typical SPS symptomatology that test negative for anti-GAD antibodies. All these evidences and observations put together cast doubt on the causative role of anti-GAD antibodies in disease pathogenesis. Indeed, other autoantigens have been recently proposed as being responsible for SPS pathogenesis.[10] A study by Raju and colleagues[98] has recently demonstrated the presence of a newly discovered autoantigen, GABA receptor associated protein (GABARAP). This protein is responsible for the stability and surface expression of the $GABA_A$ receptors.[99] Antibodies against this protein have been found in 70% of SPS patients compared to controls.[98] Moreover, it has been shown that GABARAP IgG is capable of inhibiting the expression of $GABA_A$ receptors in vitro, suggesting that antibodies against this autoantigen may play a role in the pathogenesis of SPS.[98] Likewise, GABARAP IgG of patients with SPS but not of controls has been found to inhibit significantly the surface expression of $GABA_A$ receptors. This is highly suggestive that in SPS, circulating anti-GABARAP antibodies may be the ones responsible of the impaiment of GABAergic transmission.[98]

Despite all the advances that have been made in the understanding of the immunobiology of SPS, the pathogenesis of this disorder still remains elusive.[100,101]

▶ TREATMENT

Benzodiazepines have become the cornerstone of treatment of SPS, ever since Howard[3] first reported dramatic improvement of muscle spasms with diazepam in three patients with this disorder. The rationale behind Howard's approach was that, since diazepam blocked strychnine convulsions in mice and spinal reflexes in cats, he speculated that this drug would suppress the constant discharges originated in the motor neurons of the spinal cord believed to be the cause of rigidity and stiffness in individuals affected with this syndrome. His patients were treated with up to 60 mg/day of diazepam in four divided doses achieving significant functional improvement. Moreover, with the use of this drug, in addition to symptomatic benefit there were modifications in the EMG at rest. Unfortunately, the dose of diazepam usually needed to produce functional improvement is often associated with untoward side-effects, mainly profound sedation.[5,8] The dose range of diazepam presently used is between 10 and 100 mg daily in most cases. With this treatment regimen, patients tend to stabilize, and maintain some degree of functional capacity.[5] However, most patients experience their symptoms on a continued basis and some cases continue to deteriorate. Other benzodiazepines such as clonazepam have also been used in doses of 4–6 mg/day (1 mg of clonazepam is equivalent to 4–5 mg of diazepam) with apparent benefit in a few selected cases.[102] The second drug of choice according to several authors is baclofen in doses up to 100 mg/day to achieve maximum benefit.[65,72,103] A relative absence or unavailability of GABA, a putative inhibitory neurotransmitter at the level of the γ-motor neuron system in the spinal cord, had been proposed by Gordon[2] as the underlying mechanism for rigidity in SPS. The beneficial effects of baclofen would derive from its properties as a GABA analog ($GABA_B$ receptor agonist).[72,104] As with diazepam, the main side-effect observed with this drug is sedation. The administration of intrathecal baclofen through an infusion pump has been recently proposed.[104] The rationale behind this approach is to provide sufficiently high concentrations of the drug to the spinal cord receptors without the systemic side-effects usually seen with oral administration. Only a few patients have been treated with this method of drug delivery, and the results so far have been variable.[105] In a more recent double-blind, placebo-controlled trial of intrathecal baclofen, this approach resulted in significant improvement in reflex EMG activity compared with placebo that did not correlate with clinical improvement.[106] Special attention should be paid to the adequate operation of the drug-delivery system, as pump malfunctioning has been responsible for severe autonomic complications, delirium, and spasmodic storms.[107,108]

The standard treatment regimen in clinical practice today is a combination of diazepam and baclofen in lower doses than those used when each drug is given alone.[8] Furthermore, the best strategy is to titrate gradually the dosage of both to minimize the sedative effects of these drugs. The best results are obtained in the control of spontaneous and stimulus-sensitive muscle spasms, while axial rigidity, abnormal posturing, and limitations of mobility respond less well. Valproic acid has also been advocated, and anecdotal reports of marked benefit in some cases can be found in the literature.[109] As an anticonvulsant, valproic acid is thought to augment GABAergic transmission and perhaps its beneficial effect could be attributed to its ability to compensate a deficiency of GABA at the spinal cord level. Newly introduced anticonvulsants (gabapentin, tiagabine, vigabatrin, levetiracetam) with proposed mechanism of action at the GABA level have been tried successfully in selected cases.[9,110–112] Vigabatrin, is a structural analogue of GABA, which acts by irreversible inhibition of GABA-transaminase (the enzyme responsible for the breakdown of GABA); Tiagabine, is an inhibitor of GABA catabolism; Gabapentin, is a GABA analogue; and Levetiracetam, is a GABAergic inhibitor.[10]

Several other drugs, including tizanidine, carbamazepine, sodium dantrolene, phenytoin, phenobarbital, cyclobenzaprine, mephenesin, L-dopa, 5-hydroxytryptophan, glycine, biperiden, dipropylacetate, γ-hydroxybutyric acid, milacemide, have also been tried with inconsistent or detrimental results.[13,15,63,73,113]

Plasmapheresis became an obvious choice, after reports on the presence of antibodies reacting against GAD both in serum and CSF of patients with SPS and additional evidence of immunological involvement. The few cases undergoing this treatment obtained variable results. Two patients reported in separate papers had an excellent response to plasmapheresis; improvement was observed at variable times during the course of treatment in these two cases.[114,115] In one of them, clinical response was evident immediately after the second exchange, while subjective improvement lagged behind. Return to almost normal was reported by the patient almost 2 weeks after the end of plasmapheresis. Parallel to the reduction of rigidity and spasms there were signs of improvement in EMG studies and the areas of evoked exteroceptive reflex responses were dramatically reduced. In one of the cases, antibody levels remained unchanged, while, in the other, GAD-like immunoreactivity fell from 1:1280 to 1:80 during plasmapheresis. In contrast, in the two additional cases reported by Harding and colleagues,[29] results were disappointing, although the immunological markers in these patients were similar to the previous ones. In patients without anti-GAD positivity, plasma exchange has produced disappointing results according to a recent report.[116] Double filtration plasma exchange followed by immunoadsorption has been reported to be effective in another anti-GAD-negative SPS patient.[117] Plasmapheresis remains a promising therapeutic strategy, although controlled studies on the efficacy of this intervention have not been yet conducted.

The benefits of steroid treatment and immunosuppressive drugs have been reported on an anecdotal basis.[29,118,119] Most patients appear to require a daily dose of 30–60 mg of prednisone to achieve noticeable improvement; however, reappearance of symptoms develops whenever the steroid dosage is tapered.[119] The use of high-dose long-term steroids in the treatment of a chronic disorder, frequently associated with IDDM, does not seem convenient. Other immunosupressants like azathioprine, methotrexate, and mycophenolate have been tried with minimal benefit.[10] More recently there have been anecdotal reports with the use of Rituximab, a B cell-depleting monoclonal antibody, including its use in a case of PEWR.[120] A recently completed controlled trial yielded inconclusive results in patients with SPS.[121]

Several recent publications have reported on the beneficial effects of intravenous immunoglobulin (IVIg) in the treatment of SPS.[121–123] A total of 15 out of 17 cases showed significant subjective and functional improvement following treatment with IVIg, although this improvement has been reported to be sustained in only three cases in the reports cited earlier. However, Dalakas and colleagues[124] have tested IVIg, given at 2g/kg divided into tow daily doses in a placebo-controlled trial. They reported that treatment with IVIG significantly reduced the mean number of stiff areas three months after therapy. These authors conclude that IVIG is the preferred treatment among the immunotherapeutic options.[10]

These results lend additional support to the hypothesis of an immune origin of SPS. As with other immune disorders, IVIg therapy could be effective through either neutralization of autoantibodies or downregulation of antibody production.

Anecdotal reports on the benefits of botulinum toxin A in a patients with SPS were published a few years ago.[125,126] Significant reduction of rigidity at the paraspinal and thigh muscles, improvement of ambulation, and cessation of pain were obtained with the use of this medication.Benefits of up to four months have been reported.[126] However, the efficacy and indications of botulinum toxin A in patients with SPS have not yet been systematically explored.[10]

In summary, present-day strategies for the treatment of SPS can be divided into two separate categories. The first category includes drugs known to interact with the pharmacological mechanisms underlying the production of muscle rigidity (diazepam, baclofen, valproic acid, clonidine, tizanidine, etc.) and the benefit derived from their use is purely symptomatic. On the other hand, the use of plasmapheresis, steroids, and other immunomodulating agents (immunosuppressive drugs, IVIg) would be an attempt to modify or control the immunologic factors potentially involved in the pathogenesis of SPS. For a more extensive review on therapeutic options see Dalakas 2009.[10]

REFERENCES

1. Moersch FP and Woltman HW. Progressive fluctuating muscular rigidity and spasm ("stiff-man" syndrome): Report of a case and some observations in 13 other cases. Mayo Clin Proc 1956;31:421–427.
2. Gordon EE, Januszko DM, and Kaufman L. A critical survey of stiff-man syndrome. Am J Med 1967;42:582–599.
3. Howard FM. A new and effective drug in the treatment of stiff-man syndrome: Preliminary report. Mayo Clin Proc 1963;38:203–212.
4. Solimena M, Folli F, Denis-Donini S, et al. Autoantibodies to glutamic acid decarboxylase in a patient with stiff-man syndrome, epilepsy, and type I diabetes mellitus. N Engl J Med 1988;318:1012–1020.
5. Lorish TR, Thorsteinsson G, and Howard FM. Stiff-man syndrome updated. Mayo Clin Proc 1989;64:629–636.
6. Barker RA, Revesz T, Thom M, et al. Review of 23 patients affected by the stiff man syndrome: Clinical subdivision into stiff trunk (man) syndrome, stiff limb syndrome, and progressive encephalomyelitis with rigidity. J Neurol Neurosurg Psychiatry 1998;65:633–640.
7. Brown P and Marsden CD. The stiff man and stiff man plus syndromes. J Neurol 1999;246:648–652.
8. Thompson PD. Stiff people. In Marsden CD, Fahn S (eds). Movement Disorders 3. Oxford: Butterworth-Heinemann, 1994, pp. 373–405.
9. Meinck HM. Stiff man syndrome. CNS Drugs 2001;15: 515–526.
10. Dalakas MC. Stiff person syndrome: Advances in pathogenesis and therapeutic interventions. Curr Treat Options Neurol 2009;11(2):102–110.
11. Hattan E, Angle MR, and Chalk C. Unexpected benefit of propofol in Stiff-Person Syndrome. Neurology 2008;70:1641–1642.
12. Dalakas MC, Fujii M, Li M, et al. The clinical spectrum of anti-GAD antibody-positive patients with stiff-person syndrome. Neurology 2000;55:1531–1535.
13. Blum P and Jankovic J. Stiff-person syndrome: An autoimmune disease. Mov Disord 1991;6:12–20.
14. Trethowan WH, Allsop JL, and Turner B. The stiff-man syndrome. Arch Neurol 1960;3:114–122.
15. Isaacs H. Stiff-man syndrome in a black girl. J Neurol Neurosurg Psychiatry 1979;42:988–994.
16. Kugelmass N. Stiff-man syndrome in a child. N Y State J Med 1961;61:2483–2487.
17. Klein R, Haddow JE, and De Luca C. Familial congenital disorder resembling the stiff-man syndrome. Am J Dis Child 1972;124:730–731.
18. Sander JE, Layzer RB, and Goldsobel AB. Congenital stiff-man syndrome. Ann Neurol 1979;8:195–197.
19. Spay AJ and Chen R. Rigidity and spasms from autoimmune encephalomyelopathies: Stiff-person syndrome. MuscleNerve 2006;34:677–690.
20. Meinck HM, Ricker K, Hulser PJ, et al. Stiff man syndrome: Clinical and laboratory findings in eight patients. J Neurol 1994;241:157–166.
21. Ameli R, Snow J, Rakocevic G, et al. A neuropsychological assessment of phobias in patients with stiff person syndrome. Neurology 2005;64:1961–1963.
22. Schwartzman MJ, Mitsumoto H, Chou SM, et al. Sudden death in stiff-man syndrome with autonomic instability. Ann Neurol 1989;26:166.
23. Kasperek S and Zebrowski S. Stiff-man syndrome and encephalomyelitis. Arch Neurol 1971;24:22–31.
24. Whiteley AM, Swash M, and Urich H. Progressive encephalomyelitis with rigidity. Brain 1976;99:27–42.
25. Meinck HM and Thompson PD. Stiff man syndrome and related conditions. Mov Disord 2002 Sep;17(5):853–866.
26. Solimena M, Folli F, Morello F, et al. Autoantibodies to GABAergic neurones and pancreatic beta cells in stiff-man syndrome. N Engl J Med 1990;322:1555–1560.
27. Baekkeskov S, Aanstoot H-J, Christgau S, et al. Identification of the 64K autoantigen in insulin dependent diabetes mellitus as the GABA-synthesizing enzyme glutamic acid decarboxylase. Nature 1990;347:151–156.
28. Meinck HM and Ricker K. Long-standing "stiff-man" syndrome: A particular form of disseminated inflammatory CNS disease? J Neurol Neurosurg Psychiatry 1987;50:1556–1557.
29. Harding AE, Thompson PD, Kocen RS, et al. Plasma exchange and immunosuppression in the stiff-man syndrome. Lancet 1989;ii:915.
30. Johnstone AP and Nussey SS. Direct evidence for limited clonality of antibodies to glutamic acid decarboxylase (GAD) in stiff-man syndrome using baculovirus expressed GAD. J Neurol Neurosurg Psychiatry 1994;57:659.
31. Dalakas MC, Li M, Fujii M, et al. Stiff person syndrome: Quantification, specificity, and intrathecal synthesis of GAD65 antibodies. Neurology 2001;57:780–784.
32. Maida E, Reisner T, Summer K, et al. Stiff-man syndrome with abnormalities in CSF and computerized tomography findings. Arch Neurol 1980;37:182–183.
33. Williams AC, Nutt JG, and Hare T. Autoimmunity in stiff-man syndrome. Lancet 1988;ii:22.
34. Pugliese A, Gianani R, Eisenbarth GS, et al. Genetics of susceptibility and resistance to insulin-dependent diabetes in stiff-man syndrome. Lancet 1994;344:1027–1028.
35. Pugliese A, Solimena M, Awdeh ZL, et al. Association of HLADQB1*0201 with stiff-man syndrome. J Clin Endocrinol Metab 1993;77:1550–1553.

36. Meinck HM, Ricker K, Hulser PJ, et al. Stiff man syndrome: Neurophysiological findings in eight patients. J Neurol 1995;242:134–142.
37. Auger RG. AAEM minimonograph 44: Diseases associated with excess motor unit activity. Muscle Nerve 1994;17:1250–1263.
38. Ishizawa K, Komori T, Okayama K, et al. Large motor neuron involvement in stiff-man syndrome: A qualitative and quantitative study. Acta Neuropathol (Berl) 1999;97:63–70.
39. Warich-Kirches M, Von Bossanyi P, Treuheit T, et al. Stiff-man syndrome: Possible autoimmune etiology targeted against GABA-ergic cells. Clin Neuropathol 1997;16:214–219.
40. Martinelli P, Pazzaglia P, Montagna P, et al. Stiff-man syndrome associated with nocturnal myoclonus and epilepsy. J Neurol Neurosurg Psychiatry 1978;41:458–462.
41. Rakocevic G, Raju R, Semino-Mora C, et al. Stiff person syndrome with cerebellar disease and high-titer anti-GAD antibodies. Neurology 2006;67:1068–1070.
42. Economides JR and Horton JC. Eye movement abnormalities in stiff person syndrome. Neurology 2005;65: 1462–1464.
43. Zivotofsky AZ, Siman-Tov T, Gadoth N, et al. A rare saccade velocity profile in stiff-person syndrome with cerebellar degeneration. Brain Res 2006;1093:135–140.
44. Teggi R, Piccioni LO, Martino G, et al. Stiff-person syndrome with acute recurrent peripheral vertigo: possible evidence of gamma aminobutyric acid as a neurotransmitter in the vestibular periphery. J Laryngol Otol 2008;122(6):636–638.
45. Leigh PN, Rothwell JC, Traub M, et al. A patient with reflex myoclonus and muscle rigidity: "Jerking stiff-man syndrome". J Neurol Neurosurg Psychiatry 1980;43:1125–1131.
46. Meinck HM: Exteroceptive reflexes abnormalities in stiff-man syndrome. J Neurol Neurosurg Psychiatry 1985;48:92–93.
47. Alberca R, Romero M, and Chaparro J. Jerking stiff-man syndrome. J Neurol Neurosurg Psychiatry 1982;45: 1159–1160.
48. Oskarsson B, Pelak V, Quan D, et al. Stiff-eyes in Stiff-person Syndrome. Neurology 2008;71;378–380.
49. Dalakas MC. The stiff-person syndrome: An autoimmune disorder affecting neurotransmission of gamma-aminobutyric acid. Ann Intern Med 1999;131:522–530.
50. McCombe PA, Chalk JB, Searle JW, et al. Progressive encephalomyelitis with rigidity: A case report with magnetic resonance imaging findings. J Neurol Neurosurg Psychiatry 1989;52:1429–1431.
51. Burn DJ, Ball J, Lees AJ, et al. A case of progressive encephalomyelitis with rigidity and positive antiglutamic acid dehydrogenase antibodies. J Neurol Neurosurg Psychiatry 1991;54:449–451.
52. Bateman DE, Weller RO, and Kennedy P. Stiff-man syndrome. J Neurol Neurosurg Psychiatry 1990;53:695–696.
53. Ferari P, Fedeico M, Grimaldi LME, et al. Stiff man syndrome in a patient with Hodgkin's disease: An unusual paraneoplastic syndrome. Haematologica 1990;75:570–572.
54. Folli F, Solimena M, Cofiell R, et al. Autoantibodies to a 128-kd synaptic protein in three women with the stiff-man syndrome and breast cancer. N Engl J Med 1993;328: 546–551.
55. De Camilli P, Thomas A, Cofiell R, et al. The synaptic vesicle-associated protein amphiphysin is the 128-kD autoantigen of stiff-man syndrome with breast cancer. J Exp Med 1993;178:2219–2223.
56. Rosin L, DeCamilli P, Butler M, et al. Stiff-man syndrome in a woman with breast cancer: An uncommon central nervous system paraneoplastic syndrome. Neurology 1998;50:94–98.
57. Antoine JC, Absi L, Honnorat J, et al. Antiamphiphysin antibodies are associated with various paraneoplastic neurological syndromes and tumors. Arch Neurol 1999;56:172–177.
58. Butler MH, Hayashi A, Ohkoshi N, et al. Autoimmunity to gephyrin in stiff-man syndrome. Neuron 2000;26: 307–312.
59. Hutchinson M, Waters P, McHugh J, et al. Progressive encephalomyelitis, rigidity, and myoclonus: a novel glycine receptor antibody. Neurology 2008;71:1291–1292.
60. Piccolo G and Cosi V. Stiff-man syndrome, dysimmune disorder and cancer. Ann Neurol 1989;25:105.
61. Brown P, Rothwell JC, and Marsden CD. The stiff leg syndrome. J Neurol Neurosurg Psychiatry 1997;62:31–37.
62. Nakamura N, Fujiya S, Yahara O, et al. Stiff-man syndrome with spinal cord lesion. Clin Neuropathol 1986;5:40–46.
63. Meinck HM, Ricker K, and Conrad B. The stiff-man syndrome: New pathophysiological aspects from abnormal exteroceptive reflexes and the response to clomipramine, clonidine and tizanidine. J Neurol Neurosurg Psychiatry 1984;47:280–287.
64. Rossi B, Massetani R, Guidi M, et al. Electrophysiological findings in a case of stiff-man syndrome. Electromyogr Clin Neurophysiol 1988;28:137–140.
65. Mamoli B, Heiss WD, Maida E, et al. Electrophysiological studies on the stiff-man syndrome. J Neurol 1977;217: 111–121.
66. Boiardi A, Crenna P, Negri S, et al. Neurological and pharmacological evaluation of a case of stiff-man syndrome. J Neurol 1980;223:127–133.
67. Floeter MK, Valls-Sole J, Toro C, et al. Physiologic studies of spinal inhibitory circuits in patients with stiff-person syndrome. Neurology 1998;51:85–93.
68. Sandbrink F, Syed NA, Fujii MD, et al. Motor cortex excitability in stiff-person syndrome. Brain 2000;123: 2231–2239.
69. Meinck HM and Conrad B. Neuropharmacological investigations in the stiff-man syndrome. J Neurol 1986;233: 340–347.
70. Matsumoto JY, Caviness JN, and McEvoy KM. The acoustic startle reflex in stiff-man syndrome. Neurology 1994;44:1952–1955.
71. Guilleminault C, Sigwald J, and Castaigne P. Sleep studies and therapeutic trial with L-dopa in a case of stiff-man syndrome. Eur Neurol 1973;10:89–96.
72. Miller F and Korsvik H. Baclofen in the treatment of stiff-man syndrome. Ann Neurol 1981;9:511–512.
73. Brown P, Thompson PD, Rothwell JC, et al. A therapeutic trial of milacemide in myoclonus and the stiff person syndrome. Mov Disord 1991;6:73–75.

74. Schmidt RT, Stahl SM, and Spehlmann R. A pharmacologic study of the stiff-man syndrome. Neurology 1975;25: 622–626.
75. Dinkel K, Meinck HM, Jury KM, et al. Inhibition of gamma-aminobutyric acid synthesis by glutamic acid decarboxylase autoantibodies in stiff-man syndrome. Ann Neurol 1998;44:194–201.
76. Young W. The stiff-man syndrome. Br J Clin Pract 1966;20:507–510.
77. Butler MH, Solimena M, Dirkx R Jr, et al. Identification of a dominant epitope of glutamic acid decarboxylase (GAD-65) recognized by autoantibodies in stiff-man syndrome. J Exp Med 1993;178:2097–2106.
78. Li L, Hagopian WA, Brashear HR, et al. Identification of auto-antibody epitopes of glutamic acid decarboxylase in stiff-man syndrome patients. J Immunol 1994;152:930–934.
79. Kim J, Namchuk M, Bugawan T, et al. Higher autoantibody levels and recognition of a linear NH2-terminal epitope in the autoantigen GAD65, distinguish stiff-man syndrome from insulin-dependent diabetes mellitus. J Exp Med 1994;180:595–606.
80. Bjork E, Velloso LA, Kampe O, et al. GAD autoantibodies in IDDM, stiff-man syndrome, and autoimmune polyendocrine syndrome type I recognize different epitopes. Diabetes 1994;43:161–165.
81. Lohmann T, Hawa M, Leslie RD, et al. Immune reactivity to glutamic acid decarboxylase 65 in stiffman syndrome and type 1 diabetes mellitus. Lancet 2000;356:31–35.
82. Darnell RB, Victor J, Rubin M, et al. A novel antineuronal antibody in stiff-man syndrome. Neurology 1993;43: 114–120.
83. Gorin F, Baldwin B, Tait R, et al. Stiff-man syndrome: A disorder with autoantigenic heterogeneity. Ann Neurol 1990;28:711–714.
84. Peltola J, Kulmala P, Isojarvi J, et al. Autoantibodies to glutamic acid decarboxylase in patients with therapy resistant epilepsy. Neurology 2000;55:46–50.
85. Honnorat J, Saiz A, Giometto B, et al. Cerebellar ataxia with anti-glutamic acid decarboxylase antibodies: Study of 14 patients. Arch Neurol 2001;58:225–230.
86. Dalakas MC. The role of IVIg in the treatment of patients with stiff person syndrome and other neurological diseases associated with anti-GAD antibodies. J Neurol 2005;252 (suppl 1):I19–I25.
87. Antozzi C, Frassoni C, Vincent A, et al. Sequential antibodies to potassium channels and glutamic acid decarboxylase in neuromyotonia. Neurology 2005;64:1290–1293.
88. Vulliemoz S, Vanini G, Truffert A, et al. Epilepsy and cerebellar ataxia associated with anti-glutamic acid decarboxylase antibodies. J Neurol Neurosurg Psychiatry 2007;78:187–189.
89. Vernino S and Lennon VA. Autoantibody profi les and neurological correlations of thymoma. Clin Cancer Res 2004;10:7270–7275.
90. Pearce DA, Atkinson M, and Tagle DA. Glutamic acid decarboxylase autoimmunity in Batten disease and other disorders. Neurology 2004;63:2001–2005.
91. Murinson BB, Butler M, Marfurt K, et al. Markedly elevated GAD antibodies in SPS: effects of age and illness duration. Neurology 2004;63:2146–2148.
92. Levy LM, Levy-Reis I, Fujii M, et al. Brain gamma-aminobutyric acid changes in stiff-person syndrome. Arch Neurol 2005;62:970–974.
93. Perani D, Garibotto V, Moresco RM, et al. PET evidence of central GABAergic changes in stiff-person syndrome. Mov Disord 2007;22:1030–1033.
94. Dinkel K, Meinck HM, Jury KM, et al. Inhibition of gamma-aminobutyric acid synthesis by glutamic acid decarboxylase autoantibodies in stiff-man syndrome. Ann Neurol 1998;44:194–201.
95. Raju R, Foote J, Banga JP, et al. Analysis of GAD65 autoantibodies in stiff-person syndrome patients. J Immunol 2005;175:7755–7762.
96. Rakocevic G, Raju R, and Dalakas MC. Anti-glutamic acid decarboxylase antibodies in the serum and cerebrospinal fluid of patients with stiff-person syndrome: Correlation with clinical severity. Arch Neurol 2004;61:902–904.
97. Burns TM, Phillips LH 2nd, and Jones HR. Stiff person syndrome does not always occur with maternal passive transfer of GAD65 antibodies. Neurology 2005;64: 399–400.
98. Raju R, Rakocevic G, Chen Z, et al. Autoimmunity to GABAA-receptor-associated protein in stiff-person syndrome. Brain 2006;129(pt 12):3270–3276.
99. Leil TA, Chen ZW, Chang CS, et al. GABAA receptor associated protein traffics GABAA receptors to the plasma membrane in neurons. J Neurosci 2004;24:11429–11438.
100. Raju, Raghavan and Hampe, Christiane S. Immunobiology of Stiff-Person Syndrome. Int Rev Immunol 2008;27:1, 79–92.
101. Vincent A. Stiff, twitchy or wobbly: Are GAD antibodies pathogenic? [editorial]. Brain 2008;131:2536–2537.
102. Westblom U. Stiff-man syndrome and clonazepam. JAMA 1977;237:1930.
103. Whelan JL. Baclofen in the treatment of the "stiff-man" syndrome. Arch Neurol 1980;37:600–601.
104. Penn RD and Mangieri EA. Stiff-man syndrome treated with intrathecal baclofen. Neurology 1993;43:2412.
105. Ford B and Fahn S. Intrathecal baclofen. Neurology 1994;44:1367–1368.
106. Silbert PL, Matsumoto JY, McManis PG, et al. Intrathecal baclofen therapy in stiff-man syndrome: A double-blind, placebo-controlled trial. Neurology 1995;45:1893–1897.
107. Meinck HM, Tronnier V, Rieke K, et al. Intrathecal baclofen treatment for stiff-man syndrome: Pump failure may be fatal. Neurology 1994;44:2209–2210.
108. Stayer C, Tronnier V, Dressnandt J, et al. Intrathecal baclofen therapy for stiff-man syndrome and progressive encephalomyelopathy with rigidity and myoclonus. Neurology 1997;49:1591–1597.
109. Spehlmann R, Norcross K, Rasmus SC, et al. Improvement of stiff-man syndrome and sodium valproate. Neurology 1981;31:1162–1163.
110. Sharoqi IA. Improvement of stiff-man syndrome with vigabatrin. Neurology 1998;50:833–834.
111. Murinson BB and Rizzo M. Improvement of stiff-person syndrome with tiagabine. Neurology 2001;57:366.
112. Ruegg SJ, Steck AJ, and Fuhr P. Levetiracetam improves paroxysmal symptoms in a patient with stiff-person syndrome. Neurology 2004;62:338.

113. Gordon MF, Diaz Olivo R, Hunt AL, et al. Therapeutic trial of milacemide in patients with myoclonus and other intractable movement disorders. Mov Disord 1993;8:484–488.
114. Brashear HR and Phillips LH. Autoantibodies to GABAergic neurones and response to plasmapheresis in stiff-man syndrome. Neurology 1991;41:1588–1592.
115. Vicari AM, Folli F, Pozza G, et al. Plasmapheresis in the treatment of stiff-man syndrome. N Engl J Med 1989;320:1499.
116. Shariatmadar S and Noto TA. Plasma exchange in stiff-man syndrome. Ther Apher 2001;5:64–67.
117. Hayashi A, Nakamagoe K, Ohkoshi N, et al. Double filtration plasma exchange and immunoadsorption therapy in a case of stiff-man syndrome with negative anti-GAD antibody. J Med 1999;30:321–327.
118. George TM, Burke JM, Sobotak PA, et al. Resolution of stiff-man syndrome with cortisol replacement in a patient with deficiencies of ACTH, growth hormone, and prolactin. N Engl J Med 1984;310:1511–1513.
119. Piccolo G, Cosi V, Zandrini C, et al. Steroid-responsive and dependent stiff-man syndrome: A clinical and electrophysiological study of two cases. Ital J Neurol Sci 1988;9:559–566.
120. Baker MR, Das M, Isaacs J, et al. Treatment of stiff person syndrome with rituximab. J Neurol Neurosurg Psychiatry 2005;76:999–1001.
121. Amato AA, Cornman EW, and Kissel JT. Treatment of stiff-man syndrome with intravenous immunoglobulin. Neurology 1994;44:1652–1654.
122. Karlson EW, Sudarsky L, Ruderman E, et al. Treatment of stiff-man syndrome with intravenous immune globulin. Arthritis Rheum 1994;37:915–918.
123. Gerschlager W and Brown P. Effect of treatment with intravenous immunoglobulin on quality of life in patients with stiff-person syndrome. Mov Dis 2002;17:590–593.
124. Dalakas MC, Fujii M, Li M, et al. High-dose intravenous immunoglobulin for stiff-person syndrome. N Engl J Med 2001;345:1870–1876.
125. Davis D and Jabbari B. Significant improvement of stiff-person syndrome after paraspinal injection of botulinum toxin A. Mov Disord 1993;8:371–373.
126. Liguori R, Cordivari C, Lugaresi E, et al. Botulinum toxin A improves muscle spasms and rigidity in stiff-person syndrome. Mov Disord 1997;12:1060–1063.

UNCITED REFERENCE

127. Saidha S, Elamin M, Mullins G, et al. Treatment of progressive encephalomyelitis with rigidity and myoclonic jerks with rituximab: a case report. Eur J Neurol 2008;15:e33.

CHAPTER 44

Gait Disorders

Lewis Sudarsky

Gait is an important motor function, which is unconscious and automatic. It is also a distinctive attribute; we can recognize people by their walk.[1] Disorders of gait are common, and may be the presenting feature of neurologic disease. Reliable estimates of prevalence are difficult to obtain, as there are no standard diagnostic criteria. In a study from Durham, North Carolina, 15% of volunteers over 60 were found to exhibit some abnormality of gait on neurologic examination.[2] In the East Boston Neighborhood Health Study, a degree of shuffling or difficulty with turns was noted in 15% of the population aged 67–74, 29% of those aged 75–84, and 49% of the population aged 85 and above.[3] Gait disorders are particularly important in the elderly because they compromise independence and contribute to the risk of falls and injury.[4,5] Our job as a neurologist is not finished until the gait has been examined.

▶ ANATOMY AND PHYSIOLOGY OF GAIT

Humans and other bipeds have two principal gaits: walking and running. Walking is our preferred mode. The biomechanical events of the gait cycle are illustrated with respect to time in Fig. 44–1. The stance phase begins as the right-heel strikes the floor, where it remains for 60% of the gait cycle. The stance phase for the two legs overlap, such that 20% of the gait cycle is spent with both feet planted on the ground, while the center of mass continues its forward progression. Surface electromyographic (EMG) recorded from the leg muscles reveals an orderly, phasic pattern of activation: flexor muscles during the swing phase, extensor muscles during stance. There are two tasks that the nervous system must attend to initiate and maintain walking. (1) The brain and spinal cord generate a series of stepping movements; locomotor centers specify the timing, advance position, and instructions for loading and unloading of the limbs. (2) At the same time, balance must be managed to maintain the upright posture and a stable progression.

NEURAL NETWORKS THAT SUPPORT LOCOMOTION

In quadrupedal animals, locomotion is produced by the activity of a spinal pattern generator. Cats and dogs with high spinal transection achieve a crude pattern of walking on the treadmill, provided their balance is supported. This "fictive locomotion" can be stimulated with L-dopa or clonidine, and occurs independent of sensory feedback.[6] In the spinal cord, central pattern generators for stepping are linked by the propriospinal tract. It is difficult to produce sustained spinal locomotion in primates,[7] although efforts have been made to harness spinal stepping in the rehabilitation of spinal injury patients.[8]

Primate bipedal locomotion depends on higher command and control centers in the brain stem and cerebellum.[9] Physiologists describe four areas where postural change and stepping can be evoked by electrical stimulation in animals: a subthalamic and a mesencephalic locomotor region, and a dorsal and ventral tegmental field in the caudal pons. The fastigial nucleus in the cerebellum can also induce expression of locomotor programs from the brain stem and spinal cord.[10,11] Eidelberg and colleagues evoked a form of "controlled locomotion," more natural than spinal stepping, by stimulation of the mesencephalic locomotor region (MLR) in primates. The animals swing their arms as they walk, and display a range of associated movements. With increasing stimulation, they pick up the pace of their walking, and ultimately shift into a running gait.[7] The MLR is an area near the nucleus cuneifomis, just below the superior cerebellar peduncle. The physiologically defined MLR is of particular interest as it overlaps the pedunculopontine nucleus (PPN).

There is a great deal of interest in the PPN as a locomotor center.[12] It sits at the convergence of important motor pathways. Afferents to the PPN come from the basal ganglia output (globus pallidus internal segment, substantia nigra pars reticulata) and motor cortex. The PPN projects to the brain stem reticular nuclei and spinal cord. In the cat, stimulation of the PPN produces stepping, and inhibition slows walking.[13] A complex pattern of activity is recorded from cells in the PPN during locomotor activity.[12] The dorsal midbrain (home of the

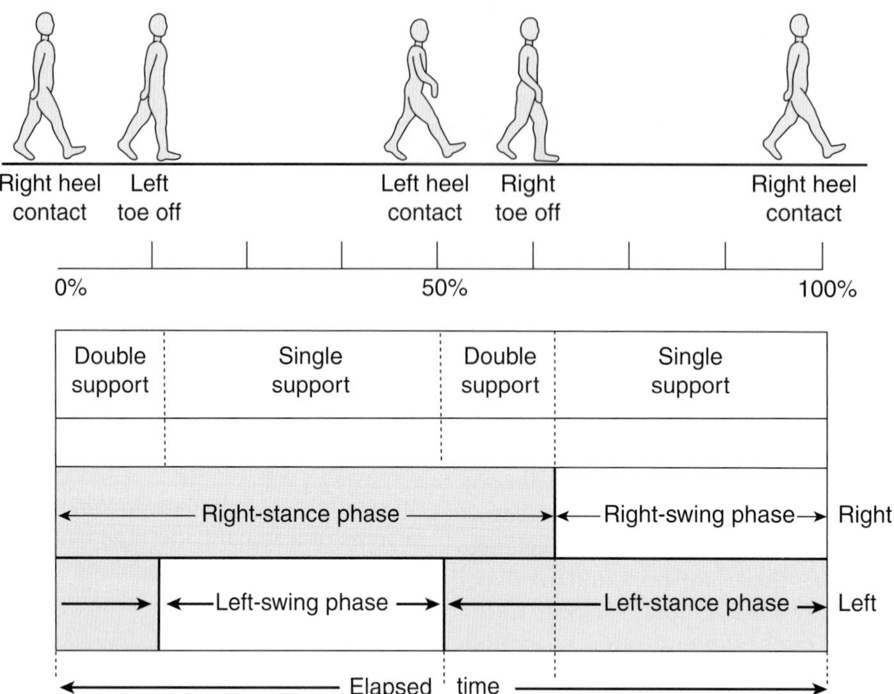

Figure 44–1. Events of the gait cycle are depicted with respect to time. From the point of right-heel strike, the right foot is in contact with the floor 60% of the time. This is the stance phase for the right leg. Roughly 20%of the gait cycle is spent in double limb support, during which forward motion of the center of mass continues. (Reproduced with permission from Ropper AH and Samuels MA. Adams & Victor's Principles of Neurology, 9th ed. McGraw-Hill, Inc., 2009. Fig. 7–1.)

PPN) is among the areas activated by walking in single-photon emission computed tomography (SPECT) imaging studies of human subjects.[14]

Locomotor commands from the brain stem are passed along phylogenetically older, descending pathways in the spinal cord, including the reticulospinal and vestibulospinal tracts. Through a series of lesion experiments, Lawrence and Kuypers demonstrated that the ventromedial spinal pathways (reticulospinal, vestibulospinal) are necessary for the recovery of postural control and locomotion in primates.[15] Eidelberg observed that primates with partial spinal transection can recover the capacity for locomotion, provided that one ventral quadrant of the spinal cord is preserved.[7]

CEREBRAL CONTROL OF WALKING

A clinician approaching the literature on gait physiology faces a paradox: an apparently natural locomotion can be expressed by a nervous system reduced to its fundamental elements (the brain stem, cerebellum, and spinal cord). Yet many of the gait disorders we struggle with in the clinic result from pathology in the forebrain (the basal ganglia, motor cortex, and frontal subcortical circuits). How does the cerebral control of locomotion operate and what does it contribute? Armstrong,[16] Garcia Rill,[17] and Mori[18] have reviewed this complex topic, and several elements stand out. The forebrain provides a *goal and purpose* for walking. It specifies when to start, when to stop, where to change direction, and it animates the performance. Cerebral control provides an element of *skill and finesse*. Cats with pyramidotomy recover an ability to walk on flat ground, but fail to walk on a narrow beam or across a ladder. Cerebral control is also involved in *context-dependent adaptation*, and *avoidance of obstacles*. Recording from awake behaving cats, Drew observed early and substantial changes in the discharge patterns of corticospinal tract neurons, which occur as the animals respond to obstacles placed in their path.[19]

MANAGEMENT OF DYNAMIC BALANCE

A hierarchy of postural responses maintains balance in the upright posture during quiet stance and during locomotion. Standing balance requires that the center of mass be maintained over the base of support, an area defined by the foot-floor contact. Unconscious postural adjustments are necessary to maintain this relationship. Long latency responses can be recorded from the trunk and leg muscles 110 ms after a perturbation in the support surface.[20–22] These responses provide a defense against slipping and tripping falls. While the physiology has been studied, the anatomic substrate for human postural control is not well defined. The vestibular nuclei and midline cerebellum are presumed to coordinate the motor response, and imbalance is evident if these systems are compromised.

Walking at a steady velocity along a flat surface poses little challenge, as the dynamics are inherently stable. The trajectory of the center of mass runs slightly ahead of the foot-floor contact, which helps maintain a propulsive force.[23] Walking on uneven ground in a poorly illuminated area requires a greater degree of sensory-motor integration. Postural defense reactions (rescue response) and anticipatory postural responses are called as needed.

While step generation does not depend on sensory feedback, sensory information is critical for balance. Romberg observed the particular importance of dorsal column afferents from the lower limbs in maintenance of standing balance.[24] Sensory information from the vestibular system, the visual system, plantar touch, and musculoarticular proprioception are all utilized in dynamic balance during locomotion. There are some indications that muscle spindle afferents and cervical mechanoreceptors also play a role, particularly during more complex motor tasks.[25,26]

▶ CLASSIFICATION OF GAIT DISORDERS

Because of the multiplicity of neural systems that support postural control and locomotion, many problems can arise. Consequently, gait disorders encountered in clinical practice are heterogeneous and sometimes multifactorial. Neurologic disorders overlap with arthritic and antalgic gaits. Failing gaits may appear fundamentally similar even when they are mechanistically different. The disorder of gait we observe in the clinic is the product of a physiological abnormality and the compensatory response. Some of the salient features such as widened stance and increased double support time are nonspecific, and represent biomechanical adaptations to improve stability and efficiency. The classification and diagnosis of gait disorders based on observational gait analysis is thus a difficult challenge.

Neurologic disorders of gait can be classified based on (1) common clinical syndromes, (2) underlying physiologic mechanisms, or (3) etiologic factors. Each classification has its proponents and its limitations. Nutt has proposed a classification of gait disorders into eight groups based on clinical characteristics: cautious, weak, stiff, ataxic, veering, freezing, marche á petit pas, and bizarre.[27,28] The advantage of this syndrome-based approach is that it lends itself to observational analysis, and is easily understood and applied. It tends to cluster together cases that share similar physiologic mechanisms, although many complex cases are not easily handled.

A physiologic, systems-based approach was outlined by Nutt and colleagues in 1993.[29] The lowest level gait disorders include those due to arthritis, neuromuscular disease, and sensory loss. Middle level gait disorders include hemiplegic gait, cerebellar gait, and the extrapyramidal syndromes. The highest-level gait disorders are the major focus of this review, and are subdivided further into five categories: cautious gait, subcortical disequilibrium, frontal disequilibrium, isolated gait ignition failure (i.e., pure freezing gait), and frontal gait. The major difficulty with this approach is that the criteria for the five highest-level gait disorders are somewhat arbitrary and are not always uniformly applied. The categories do not correlate well with etiologic diagnosis, and may change in the same patient over time. A patient with progressive supranuclear palsy, for example, might begin with a subcortical disequilibrium or freezing gait, and progress to a frontal gait with progression of the disease.

Classification of gait disorders based on etiology is practical.[30] Etiologic diagnosis is the first step in therapeutic intervention. Neurologic evaluation of 50 patients aged over 65 with an undiagnosed neurologic disorder of gait was successful at identifying the principal etiologic factor in 85%of cases. Treatable disorders were identified in 25 percent.[31] The categories of disease encountered are summarized in Table 44–1. Sometimes an etiology is not known and cannot be established, or the disorder is multifactorial. This system is not easily applied to older patients with higher-level gait disorders, and patients with more advanced disability. Efforts have been made to incorporate the strengths of each system into a single framework, or to develop a hybrid system.[32]

Classification is useful as it facilitates communication among clinicians, and it helps focus clinical investigation. Literature from the late 19th and early 20th centuries can be more easily approached when older terms such as Bruns' ataxia, trepidant abasia, senile gait, and gait apraxia are placed in a contemporary perspective. There is an evolving literature dealing with problem areas such as frontal gait disorder and freezing gait. Still none of these classifications is totally satisfactory, and they should not be considered the last word.

▶ COMMON PATTERNS OF GAIT DISORDER

THE CAUTIOUS GAIT

In their landmark paper on higher-level gait disorders, Nutt and colleagues introduced the concept of the "cautious gait."[29] The pattern of reduced stride, widened base, shorter swing phase with preservation of rhythmic stepping is, in essence, an adaptation to perceived

TABLE 44–1. CLASSIFICATION OF GAIT DISORDER IN 120 PATIENTS, ACCORDING TO ETIOLOGIC CAUSE

	1980–1982	1990–1994	Total	Percent
Myelopathy	8	12	20	16.7
Parkinsonism	5	9	14	11.7
Hydrocephalus	2	6	8	6.7
Multiple infarcts	8	10	18	15.0
Cerebellar degeneration	4	4	8	6.7
Sensory deficits	9	13	22	18.3
Toxic/metabolic	3	0	3	2.5
Psychogenic	1	3	4	3.3
Other	3	3	6	5.0
Unknown cause	7	10	17	14.2
Total	50	70	120	100

The initial 50 patients are from Sudarsky L and Ronthal M. Gait disorders among elderly patients: A survey study of 50 patients. Arch Neurol 1983;40:740–743. (From Masdeu J, Sudarsky L, Wolfson L (eds). Gait Disorders of Aging: Falls and Therapeutic Strategies. Lippincott-Raven, 1997, pp. 147–157 with permission from Lippincott Williams & Wilkins [http://lww.com].)

imbalance. Older people commonly adopt this guarded or cautious pattern of locomotion to achieve better stability.[33] While this pattern of gait is nonspecific, there may be underlying neurologic deficits that pose a postural threat. As noted by Nutt and colleagues, "Early in the course of such disorders, the cautious gait may dominate, but with progression of the condition, the characteristic gait disorder will emerge." The cautious gait was the most frequently observed higher-level gait disorder, occurring in 16 of 43 patients in Nutt's series.

Despite a narrow intent, the designation cautious gait is often appropriated to include a variety of psychogenic gait disorders dominated by anxiety and fear of falling. Consider the older patient with apprehension and recent falls, who locomotes with the arms abducted, clutching at walls and furniture, as if walking on a slippery surface.[34] A better description for this phenomenon is inappropriately cautious or phobic gait. It is particularly amenable to rehabilitation therapies.

STIFF-LEGGED GAIT

A variety of stiff-legged gaits are observed among patients with cerebral palsy, demyelinating disease, and spinal disorders. The common denominator in these conditions is an element of spasticity, but there are several distinct patterns of abnormal locomotion, and "spastic gait" is not a unitary disorder.[35] There may be inappropriate flexion at the hip or knee. Some patients have adductor spasm, with circumduction and scissoring. Equinovarus is another common pattern. The shoes often reflect uneven wear, and with progression, there may be a bouncy toe-walking. Intervention with botulinum toxin, nerve block, or surgery will be successful only if the intervention is appropriately targeted.[36] It is not clear how much benefit oral spasticity medications provide for stiff-legged gait. There are no good randomized clinical trials, though patients report subjective benefits. Intrathecal baclofen has been used for treatment failures, particularly among the cerebral diplegia population.

A different stiff-legged gait is observed in patients with autoimmune stiff-person syndrome (see Chapter 44). The disorder is characterized by antiglutamic acid decarboxylase (GAD) antibodies, and a deficiency of γ-aminobutyric acid (GABA)–mediated synaptic inhibition at a brain and spinal level.[37] There is spasm with hyperlordosis of the lumbar spine, and the patient walks as if the limbs and trunk were fused in a solid block. This "Frankenstein gait" improves with treatments that release muscle overactivity in the disorder, including high-dose benzodiazepines, intrathecal baclofen, and immunotherapy. There have been several reports of success with intravenous immunoglobulin (IVIg) in stiff-person syndrome.[38,39]

FREEZING GAIT

Freezing of gait is a remarkable and distinctive phenomenon, first described in patients with Parkinson's disease (PD) (see Chapter 14). Good descriptions appear in the writings of Charcot from the 19th century and Martin in the mid-20th.[40,41] Freezing of gait has been described as "an episodic inability to generate effective stepping, in the absence of any known cause other than parkinsonism or a high level gait disorder."[42] Patients feel their feet "glued to the floor." They experience a transient arrest of movement when walking, often during gait initiation or when turning to change direction. There may be a series of quick, ineffective stepping movements with side-to-side shifting of weight, but no forward engagement ("the slipping clutch phenomenon"). Locomotor movements can be normal or near normal once the patient is in motion, but freezing may return as the patient attempts to navigate the door threshold. There is variability, in that the same doorway may be a problem on one occasion, but not the next. One characteristic of gait freezing is its relation to context: it can be triggered by spatial constraint or by distraction, and can be overcome with the aid of visual or auditory cueing.

Freezing of gait is common in PD; the frequency increases with disease duration and motor disability.[43] Freezing of gait was reported in 7% of patients in the first 2 years, in 26% at 5 years, and 39% at 10 years.[44,45] It is more common with advanced disease and is correlated with dysarthria and postural instability. There has been a re-examination of the phenomenon in the past few years, as it was appreciated to be distinct from bradykinesia and is not always correlated with the development of motor fluctuations.[46] In patients with motor fluctuations, gait freezing is most often observed during off-time. "Off-period" gait freezing may respond to an upward adjustment or redistribution of antiparkinsonian medication, but "on-period" gait freezing is more difficult to treat.

Pharmacotherapy specifically targeting freezing of gait in PD has proved difficult (see Chapter 16). In randomized clinical trials comparing levodopa with a dopamine agonist, agonist patients show more freezing of gait.[46] Randomized clinical trials with selegiline and rasagiline suggest less freeing of gait with an MAO-B inhibitor, but in none of these studies was gait freezing a primary end point.[47,48] Amantadine, L-threo-3,4-dihydroxyphenylserine (DOPS), and methylphenidate have all been advocated, but an evidence-based review by Giladi does not support efficacy.[49–52] Experience is variable with surgical procedures like pallidotomy and deep brain stimulation, which improve spatiotemporal characteristics of gait, but do not consistently help freezing.[53,54] Pahapill and Lozano speculate about the role of cell loss in the pedunculopontine nucleus in the gait freezing of PD.[12] Consequently the PPN has emerged as a therapeutic target for deep brain stimulation. In a pilot study, six patients with PD who had persistent gait difficulty after STN-DBS had additional electrodes implanted in the PPN with benefit.[55] In general, the phenomenon responds best to rehabilitation-based interventions. Cueing to lengthen stride seems to be the most productive strategy.[56–58]

Gait freezing is also seen in various forms of atypical PD, such as progressive supranuclear palsy, multiple-system atrophy, corticobasal degeneration, and dementia with Lewy bodies (see Chapters 19 and 21–23). In each of these disorders, gait freezing is more common than in PD, and is often an early sign. In a retrospective review of records informed by neuropathology in patients with atypical PD by Muller and colleagues, freezing of gait was noted in 25% of those with PSP at initial visit, 53% at the final visit.[59] Prevalence of the phenomenon was similarly high in MSA. Gait freezing in these disorders is correlated with postural instability, dysarthria, and palilalia (freezing of speech).

A syndrome of pure akinesia unresponsive to levodopa was described in 1970 by Narabayashi, the principal manifestations being gait freezing, micrographia, and festinating speech. Some patients with pure akinesia have been found to exhibit the neuropathology of progressive supranuclear palsy at postmortem.[60] A similar disorder was reported in 1993 by Achiron and colleagues in 18 patients with gait freezing as the primary presentation, and salient features of their disorder at 2–3 years.[61,62] Factor and colleagues reported on the natural history of 30 patients with primary progressive freezing gait.[63] Long-term follow-up has confirmed that features of another neurodegenerative disorder ultimately emerge in such patients, suggesting that primary progressive freezing gait is not a distinct morbid entity.[64]

FRONTAL GAIT (MARCHE À PETIT PAS)

Marche à petit pas was described by von Malaise in 1910, in a group of patients with shuffling gait and multiple lacunar infarctions.[29] The frontal gait is a combination of impaired stepping (shuffling, freezing gait) and some degree of disequilibrium. The major cause of this phenomenon is cerebrovascular disease, particularly small-vessel disease involving the basal ganglia and periventricular white matter. In this context, the frontal gait is sometimes described as vascular parkinsonism or lower body parkinsonism,[65] although it is not primarily a dopamine-deficiency disorder. Meyer and Barron[66] and Denny-Brown[67] described the "slipping clutch" difficulty (initial hesitation or freezing) in such patients and termed this ineffectiveness of locomotion gait apraxia, although it is really a higher-level motor control disorder as opposed to an apraxia. Walking depends on the successful integration of stepping with postural control, and these patients cannot achieve this objective consistently. The anatomic basis for the phenomenon is presumed to involve the disconnection of the cortical motor areas from the basal ganglia and brain stem locomotor centers. White matter lesions within this network produce a gait disorder in patients with hypertensive cerebrovascular disease and patients with hydrocephalus.

Thompson and Marsden characterized the gait disorder and postural control in 12 patients with subcortical arteriosclerotic encephalopathy (Binswanger's disease), based on observational analysis of the patients' chair rise and gait. Start and turn hesitation were salient features; festination was not observed. Postural instability was a salient feature, and falls were frequent; several patients in the study were not independently ambulatory[68] Elble and colleagues studied the physiology of gait initiation in five patients with vascular disease (lower body parkinsonism). The basic architecture of the first step was preserved in these patients, though steps were irregular and sometimes aborted. Postural shifts necessary to initiate forward movement were not effectively generated (see Chapter 25).[69] Yanagisawa and colleagues captured episodes of gait freezing in patients with PD and vascular parkinsonism using surface EMG and analysis of ground reaction forces. An increase in step frequency was observed before freezing. Co-contraction was observed in antagonist muscles in the legs, which interferes with phasic activation of locomotor movements and restrains forward motion.[70] Co-contraction has also been described in studies of patients with normal-pressure hydrocephalus.[71] Ebersbach and colleagues reported variability in the timing and size of stepping in patients with subcortical arteriosclerotic encephalopathy. They noted compensations for imbalance and some ataxic features, in addition to short steps and freezing.[72]

The major avenue of treatment for the frontal gait disorder of cerebrovascular small-vessel disease is physical therapy. Morris and colleagues trained patients with gait freezing using a paradigm of balance training, attentional cues, and stride lengthening.[73] As with freezing in PD, medications that promote the bioavailability of monoamine neurotransmitters are often tried (L-dopa, selegiline, L-threo-3,4-dihydroxyphenylserine), and some patients benefit.[74] Amantadine has also helped reduce unsteadiness and increase stride length in some patients.[75]

DYSTONIC GAIT

Dystonia may be focal or generalized (see Chapters 29, 30, and 32). Whatever the cause, dystonia can produce unusual and sometimes bizarre disorders of gait. The two principal gaits (walking and running) may be differentially affected. For many patients, dystonia may disappear when walking backwards. In patients with generalized dystonia, there may be torsion of the trunk, and the twisted posture of the lower body may make walking difficult altogether.

The most common focal disorder is dystonic inversion at the ankle, sometimes associated with extension of the great toe. Dystonic toe flexion also occurs, as do more complex proximal lower limb dystonias. Focal dystonia is generally amenable to botulinum toxin injection, provided the active muscles can be successfully identified and targeted. Dynamic EMG or kinematic gait studies can sometimes be of help.[36] Dystonic flexion of the thoracolumbar spine (camptocormia) has been identified in patients with PD. It is activated as the patient stands to walk, and remits when lying supine, which helps distinguish the disorder from contracture.[76] Many patients with PD and related disorders have kyphoscoliosis caused by tone abnormalities from their extrapyramidal disease.

CEREBELLAR GAIT

Holmes characterized the gait ataxia in studies of patients with penetrating head injury.[77] Cerebellar disease produces imbalance (disequilibrium) and a distinct locomotor disorder (see Chapter 42). The gait is often slow and halting, with a widened base of support. Stepping is irregular, which results in a lurching quality as the upper body segments struggle to maintain alignment. The patient may stumble or veer off to the side. Truncal instability is more pronounced when attempting to walk on a narrow base, or tandem, heel-to-toe. Patients also exhibit imbalance when they turn or change direction. Control of gait and balance is localized within the cerebellum to the midline structures, including the efferent pathways of the interposed and fastigial nucleus.[78]

Kinematic studies in cerebellar patients confirm the features described above. The essential physiologic abnormality is irregular stepping: increased variability of timing, direction, and amplitude.[72] Palliyath and colleagues noted a reduced velocity and stride length in 10 patients with cerebellar degeneration.[79] While the gait was not wide based in this study, other centers have demonstrated an increased base of support in cerebellar patients.[80] Analysis of moments about the knee and ankle joints revealed poor intralimb coordination, indicating a decomposition of multijoint movement. Other characteristic features included reduced dorsiflexion of the ankle at the onset of the swing phase, which might predispose to tripping.[79] Studies by Horak and Diener show that postural responses in cerebellar patients have a normal latency, but are hypermetric in force, contributing to truncal titubation. Patients often fall in a direction opposite to the force by which they were perturbed.[81]

Patients with alcoholic cerebellar degeneration, which affects primarily the midline vermis, often have a gait ataxia out of proportion to findings in the oculomotor system and limbs. Many patients with neurodegenerative ataxia have a form of hereditary cerebellar degeneration. There has been great progress over the last 10 years in understanding the hereditary ataxias, many of which can be identified through DNA diagnostic testing. The cost of genetic testing in ataxia patients is roughly comparable to the cost of one or two magnetic resonance imaging (MRI) scans, and the information is very helpful for prognosis and genetic counseling.

Pharmacotherapy of ataxia has not been a dramatic success to date. The neurodegenerative ataxias differ in how they prune the cerebellar circuit anatomy, and it is not apparent which neurotransmitter to replace. Bus-

▶ **TABLE 44–2 CLINICAL DISTINCTION OF ATAXIC AND UNSTEADY GAITS**

	Cerebellar Ataxia	Sensory Ataxia	Frontal Gait
Stance	Wide based	Looks down	Wide based
Velocity	Variable	Slow	Very slow
Stride	Irregular, lurching	High-stepping	Short, shuffling
Romberg	±	Unsteady, falls	±
Heel–shin	Abnormal	±	Normal
Initiation	Normal	Normal	Hesitant
Turns	Veers away	±	Hesitant, fragmented
Postural instability	+	+++	++++, poor postural synergies
Falls	Uncommon	Frequent	Frequent

pirone and tandospirone have been explored, as these drugs stimulate 5-HT_{1A} receptors in the cerebellar cortex.[82,83] Individual patients may benefit, but randomized clinical trials do not show efficacy. Therapeutic trials may be more informative when they are based on homogeneous, genetically defined subgroups of ataxia patients.

SENSORY ATAXIA

Locomotor ataxia was described in the 19th century in patients with tabetic neurosyphilis. There is excess motion of the center of mass and lateral path deviation, but patients tend to have a regular stride. Most patients are visually dependent in their walking, and do poorly in the dark. Features that distinguish sensory ataxia from cerebellar are summarized in Table 44–2. While there is a healthy redundancy of sensory information about the position of the body in space during locomotion, humans are particularly dependent on proprioception. Patients with peripheral neuropathy affecting large fibers are at a substantially increased risk for falls.[84] Causes of a predominantly ataxic neuropathy in clinical practice include cobalamin deficiency, vincristine and cisplatin toxicity, paraproteinemia, and subacute sensory neuropathy, which may be autoimmune or paraneoplastic.[85]

Several studies have examined the impact of proprioceptive deficits on postural control and gait. Horak demonstrated increased body sway during stance, and displacement of the center of mass while walking in patients with diabetic neuropathy. To compensate for excess motion of the center of mass, patients alter lateral step placement. Somatosensory information derived from fingertip contact with a stable object (haptic information) can help with balance compensation.[86] Lajoie and colleagues reported kinematic studies in a patient with advanced sensory neuropathy, who had absent proprioception in the limbs by clinical measures. The focus of the discussion was on the compensatory strategies that enable locomotion to proceed in the absence of somatosensory feedback. This patient walked with a widened base of support and reduced stride, biomechanical adaptations to improve stability. A forward tilt was observed, with flexion of the neck such that the patient could monitor the performance visually. EMG demonstrated co-activation of the vastus lateralis and medial hamstring during weight acceptance, effectively bracing the leg during the stance phase. Although the gait appeared more mechanical, this strategy effectively reduces the number of degrees of freedom and simplifies the task of postural control.[87]

Vestibular deficits can also impair control of the head and center of mass during locomotion.[86] Fife and Baloh found bilateral vestibular deficits in 7 of 26 patients aged over 75 with disequilibrium of uncertain cause.[88] This syndrome is most often associated with a cautious gait and a feeling of unsteadiness, as opposed to a gross sensory ataxia.[89]

PSYCHOGENIC GAIT DISORDERS

Functional disorders of gait are well described in the medical literature, dating back to the 19th century (see Chapter 49). A variety of psychogenic gait disorders were observed among combatants in the World War I, when astasia–abasia was the most common conversion disorder.[90] Psychogenic disorders of gait occur at all ages, although extra caution should be used in making this diagnosis in the elderly.[91] Older people often exhibit a combination of imbalance and an exaggerated compensatory response, particularly if there is apprehension and fear of falling.

Lempert and colleagues characterized the recognition features that help identify psychogenic disorders of gait, from a review of video in 37 cases.[92] The abnormalities are often distinctive, and psychiatric history is sometimes revealing. Extreme slow motion may occur, as if the patient were walking through a viscous substance. Uneconomical postures with wastage of muscular effort (astasia–abasia) is another classic example. Dramatic fluctuations may occur over minutes, which is unusual for patients with neurologic disease. Observation and distraction may activate and/or suppress the findings. A video atlas, published by Hayes and colleagues, elaborates on these criteria and notes some diagnostic pitfalls.[91] Prognosis is often good for those patients in whom the history is recent and the decompensation of walking is acute. Dramatic cures are often possible in this setting.[93] When psychogenic disorders of gait persist for 6 months or more and become part of an established pattern of dependence and disability, it is often difficult to restore function.[94,95]

▶ METHODS FOR INVESTIGATION OF GAIT DISORDERS

LABORATORY GAIT ANALYSIS

In the 19th century, Eadweard Muybridge worked with a series of still cameras and a timing device to produce detailed kinematic studies of human walking. Laboratory gait analysis matured with the technology available in the late 20th century (see Chapter 2). Data captured by video camera are reconstructed on the computer to track trunk and limb movement in three dimensions. Some clinical gait laboratories and most research laboratories also provide information on ground reaction forces and surface EMG.

The principal strength of this technique is its ability to monitor the success of a specific therapeutic intervention. Kinematic studies document the efficacy of intrathecal baclofen for stiff-legged gait, and L-dopa, and surgery for PD.[96,54] Gait analysis is also used to target therapeutic interventions such as botox and orthopedic surgery in patients with cerebral palsy and stiff-legged gait.[97,98] Clinical investigation has been done using kinematic data to help understand the pathophysiology of gait disorders.[99,100] Laboratory gait analysis is not always helpful with diagnostic problem cases and bizarre gaits that defy classification on clinical grounds. There is not yet enough sophisticated pattern recognition built into the software.

OBSERVATIONAL GAIT ANALYSIS

Observational gait analysis provides a less costly alternative to laboratory gait analysis.[101] With a stopwatch and a tape measure, the principal parameters of the gait can be recorded, including cadence, velocity, and stride. Videotape (or digital) replay provides an opportunity to slow down the performance, achieve objectivity, and look for subtle diagnostic clues. A timed test of walking is used as part of the CAPSIT protocol for measuring the success of surgical interventions in PD.[102] Foot-switches can be affixed to the sole of the shoe, allowing an analysis of cadence and stride variability. Increased variability of stepping has been observed, particularly among those PD patients with a history of gait freezing.[103]

WALKING AND COGNITIVE FUNCTION (DUAL TASK WALKING)

While locomotor movements are produced by brain stem and spinal centers, walking is often abnormal in patients with dementia and cognitive impairment. Recent studies have focused on the attentional demands and cerebral control of gait, and abnormalities in performance when cognitive function is impaired or attention divided.[104] Ble and colleagues timed 900 older subjects walking through an obstacle course. Abnormalities in executive function were correlated with reduced gait speed in response to this more challenging locomotor task.[105] In an elegantly simple study often cited, Lundin-Olsson and colleagues found that older adults who "stopped walking when talking" were at increased risk of falls.[106]

One approach to investigate this phenomenon is to measure changes in gait performance (velocity, stride, stride variability) when a cognitive task (digit span, serial 7's, verbal fluency) is introduced. While the methods have not been standardized, a literature has emerged on dual task walking.[104] In studies with healthy adults, walking speed is diminished to a degree when a second, cognitive task is introduced. Slowing is more pronounced in older adults, but there is no increase in the variability of stepping.[104,107] When patients with Alzheimer's disease or PD are studied in a similar fashion, there is a significant interference effect, with loss of automaticity, stride time variability as well as reduced walking speed.[108–110] Bloem has observed that patients with PD fail to prioritize their attentional resources when walking, and use a maladaptive "posture second" strategy.[111] This failure to place the feet first is apparent is studies of elderly at known risk for falls.[112]

IMAGING

Imaging tests play an important role in the diagnostic evaluation of gait disorders, particularly higher-level gait disorders. MRI is often obtained in patients with gait problems to screen for vascular disease, demyelination, posterior fossa malformation, cerebellar degeneration, and hydrocephalus. The presence of white matter disease in the periventricular region or centrum semiovale on MRI has been correlated with gait and balance problems in numerous studies.[89,113] A modest amount of white matter change on MRI is not unusual in older patients, and careful clinical correlation is required.

Functional imaging techniques such as functional MRI, positron emission tomography (PET), and SPECT may be able to identify parts of the neural network active during integrative control of gait and balance. One disadvantage of fMRI is that it is not presently possible to study the patient during locomotion. With radiotracer studies, the image can be collected after an activation task. In PET studies, the anterior lobe of the cerebellum displays increased regional cerebral blood flow during quiet stance.[114] Fukuyama and colleagues used SPECT imaging with ^{99}Tc-HMPAO to identify a number of structures active in normal subjects during locomotion, including supplementary motor area, primary sensorimotor cortex, striatum, and cerebellar vermis.[115] In a group of 10 PD patients studied with this technique, there was underactivation of the medial frontal area.[14] Matsui and colleagues used SPECT imaging to study regional cerebral blood flow in 24 patients with PD and freezing of gait, for comparison with 31 patients with PD who did not exhibit gait freezing. A decrease in rCBF in orbitofrontal cortex (Brodmann's area 11) was noted in the group with freezing of gait.[116] Reductions of rCBF in this area have also been recorded in patients with fear of falling, a fear which is sometimes expressed by patients with freezing of gait.[117]

GAIT, BALANCE, AND WHITE MATTER DISEASE

Even absent a history of stroke, white matter abnormalities on MRI have been correlated with functional decline in gait and balance in the elderly.[118,119] Patchy areas of white matter hyperintensity are common the periventricular and subcortical regions on the T2 and flair images from MRI in older people. White matter abnormality is also apparent on computed tomography, and is sometimes referred to as leukoaraiosis. When there is no history of infection, demyelinating disease, subcortical stroke, and so on, these lesions are generally attributed to small-vessel change, and have been correlated with ischemic gliosis at post mortem. Brooks and colleagues used MR spectroscopy to distinguish symptomatic from incidental white matter lesions, and found abnormal spectra in those patients with white matter change and abnormal gait.[120]

In a prospective study, Baloh and colleagues followed 59 healthy subjects over 75 with serial gait and balance examinations, and found a correlation between volume of white matter hyperintensity (WMH) and yearly decline in performance on the Tinetti gait and balance score.[121] Silbert and colleagues followed a cohort of 104 cognitively intact elderly with volumetric analysis of serial MRIs, and found that burden of WMH in the periventricular region was correlated with a decline over time in gait velocity and stride.[122] In a large prospective, multicenter study of 639 elderly (the LADIS study), white matter abnormality was graded mild, moderate, and severe. Correlations were established with decline in a short physical performance battery (similar to the Tinetti scale), gait velocity, and single limb stance.[123] Tests of this nature have been found to be robust predictors for risk of falls in the elderly.[124]

REFERENCES

1. http://www.sciencedaily.com/releases/2008/06/080609141241.htm.
2. Newman G, Dovermuehle RH, and Busse EW. Alterations in neurologic status with age. J Am Geriatr Soc 1960;8:915–917.
3. Odenheimer G, Funkenstein HH, Beckett L, et al. Comparison of neurologic changes in successfully aging persons vs the total aging population. Arch Neurol 1994;51:573–580.
4. Tinetti ME, Speechley M, and Ginter SF. Risk factors for falls among elderly persons living in the community. N Engl J Med 1988;137:342–354.
5. Rubenstein L and Josephson KR. Interventions to reduce the multifactorial risks for falling. In Masdeu J, Sudarsky L, Wolfson L (eds). Gait Disorders of Aging: Falls and Therapeutic Strategies. Philadelphia: Lippincott-Raven, 1997, pp. 13–36.
6. Grillner S and Wallen P. Central pattern generators for locomotion, with special reference to vertebrates. Annu Rev Neurosci 1985;8:233–261.
7. Eidelberg E, Walden JG, and Nguyen LH. Locomotor control in Macaque monkeys. Brain 1981;104:647–663.
8. Dietz V, Colombo DM, Jensen DM, et al. Locomotor capacity of spinal cord in paraplegic patients. Ann Neurol 1995;37:574–582.
9. Orlovsky GN. The effect of different descending systems on flexor and extensor activity during locomotion. Brain Res 1972;40:359–371.
10. Mori S, Matsui T, Mori F, et al. Instigation and control of tread-mill locomotion in high decerebrate cats by stimulation of the hook bundle of Russell in the cerebellum. Can J Physiol Pharmacol 2000;78:945–957.
11. Mori S, Matsuyama K, Mori F, et al. Supraspinal sites that induce locomotion in the vertebrate central nervous system. Adv Neurol 2001;87:25–40.
12. Pahapill PA and Lozano AM. The pedunculopontine nucleus and Parkinson's disease. Brain 2000;123:1767–1783.
13. Garcia-Rill E. The pedunculopontine nucleus. Prog Neurobiol 1991;36:363–389.
14. Hanakawa T, Katsumi Y, Fukuyama H, et al. Mechanisms underlying gait disturbance in Parkinson's disease: A single-photon emission computed tomography study. Brain 1999;122:1271–1282.
15. Lawrence DG and Kuypers HGJM. The functional organization of the motor system in the monkey: II. The effects of lesions of the descending brain stem pathways. Brain 1968;91:15–36.
16. Armstrong DM. The supraspinal control of mammalian locomotion. J Physiol 1988;405:1–37.
17. Garcia-Rill E. The basal ganglia and the locomotor regions. Brain Res Rev 1986;11:47–63.
18. Mori S. Neurophysiology of locomotion: Recent advances in the study of locomotion. In Masdeu J, Sudarsky L, Wolfson L (eds). Gait Disorders of Aging: Falls and Therapeutic Strategies. Philadelphia: Lippincott-Raven, 1997, pp. 55–78.
19. Drew T. Discharge patterns of pyramidal tract neurons in motor cortex during a locomotion task requiring a precise control of limb trajectory. Soc Neurosci Abstr 1987;72:17.

20. Horak FB and Nashner LM. Central programming of postural movements: Adaptation to altered support surface configurations. J Neurophysiol 1986;55:1369–1381.
21. Nashner LM. Balance adjustments of humans perturbed while walking. J Neurophysiol 1980;44:650–664.
22. Allum JHJ. Vestibulospinal and proprioceptive reflex assessment of balance control. In Bronstein AD, Brandt T, Woollacott M (eds). Clinical Disorders of Balance Posture and Gait. London: Arnold, 1996, pp. 114–130.
23. Winter DA. The Biomechanics and Motor Control of Human Gait. 2nd ed. Waterloo: University of Waterloo Press, 1991.
24. Romberg MH[trans by Sieveking EH]. Manual of the Nervous System of Man. Vol 2, . London: Sydenham Society, 1853.
25. Roll JP, Vedel JP, and Roll R. Eye, head, and skeletal muscle spindle feedback in the elaboration of body references. Prog Brain Res 1989;80:113–123.
26. Pozzo T, Berthoz A, and Lefort L. Head stabilization during various locomotor tasks in humans. I. Normal subjects. Exp Brain Res 1990;82:97–106.
27. Nutt JG. Gait and balance disorders, a syndrome approach. In Jankovic J, Tolosa E (eds). Parkinson's Disease and Movement Disorders, 3rd ed. Baltimore: Williams & Wilkins, 1998, pp. 697–699.
28. Nutt JG. Classification of gait and balance disorders. Adv Neurol 2001;87:135–141.
29. Nutt JG, Marsden CD, and Thompson PD. Human walking and higher-level gait disorders, particularly in the elderly. Neurology 1993;43:268–279.
30. Sudarsky L. Gait disorders: Prevalence, morbidity, and etiology. Adv Neurol 2001;87:111–117.
31. Sudarsky L and Ronthal M. Gait disorders among elderly patients: A survey study of 50 patients. Arch Neurol 1983;40:740–743.
32. Jankovic J, Nutt JG, and Sudarsky LR. Classification, diagnosis, and etiology of gait disorders. Adv Neurol 2001;87:119–134.
33. Murray MP, Kory RC, and Clarkson BH. Walking patterns in healthy old men. J Gerontol 1969;24:169–178.
34. Murphy J and Isaacs B. The post-fall syndrome: A study of 36 elderly patients. Gerontology 1982;82:265–270.
35. Mayer NH, Esquenazi A, and Keenan MA. Patterns of upper motoneuron dysfunction in the lower limb. Adv Neurol 1999;87:311–320.
36. O'Brien CF. Chemodenervation with botulinum toxin for spasticity and dystonia: The effects on gait. Adv Neurol 1999;87:265–270.
37. Levy LM, Dalakas MC, and Floeter MK. The stiff-person syndrome: An autoimmune disorder affecting neurotransmission of GABA. Ann Intern Med 1999;131:522–530.
38. Karlson EW, Sudarsky L, Ruderman E, et al. Treatment of stiff-man syndrome with intravenous immune globulin. Arthritis Rheum 1994;37:915–918.
39. Souza-Lima CFL, Ferraz HB, Braz CA, et al. Marked improvement in a stiff-limb patient treated with intravenous immunoglobulin. Mov Disord 2000;15:358–359.
40. Charcot JM [trans by G Sigerson]. Clinical Lectures on Disease of the Nervous System. Vol 1. London: New Sydenham Society, 1877, pp. 145–146.
41. Martin JP. The basal ganglia and posture. Philadelphia, Lippincott, 1967.
42. Giladi N and Nieuwboer A. Understanding and treating freezing of gait in Parkinsonism. Mov Disord 2008;23:s423–s425.
43. Giladi N, McDermott MP, Fahn S, et al. Freezing of gait in PD. Neurology 2001;56:1712–1721.
44. Giladi N, Treves TA, Simon ES, et al. Freezing of gait in patients with advanced Parkinson's disease. J Neural Transm 2001;108:53–61.
45. Lamberti P, Armenise S, Castaldo V et al. Freezing gait in Parkinson's disease, Eur Neurol 1997;38:297–301.
46. Parkinson Study Group. Pramipexole vs levodopa as initial treatment for Parkinson disease. JAMA 2000;248:1931–1938.
47. Shoulson I, Oakes D, Fahn S et al. Impact of sustained deprenyl (selegiline) in levodopa-treated Parkinson's disease: A randomized placebo-controlled extension of the deprenyl and tocopherol anti-oxydative therapy of Parkinsonism trial. Ann Neurol 2002;51:604–612.
48. Giladi N, Rascol O, Brooks E, et al. Rasagiline treatment can improve freezing of gait in advanced Parkinson's disease: A prospective randomized, double blind placebo and entacapone controlled study. Mov Disord 2004;19:s191
49. Uitti RJ, Rajput AH, Ahlskog JE, et al. Amantadine treatment is an independent predictor of improved survival in Parkinson's disease. Neurology 1996;46:1551–1556.
50. Quinn N, Perlmutter J, and Marsden CD. Acute administration of DL-threo DOPS does not affect the freezing phenomenon in parkinsonian patients. Neurology 1984;34:149.
51. Devos D, Krystkowiak P, Clement F, et al. Improvement of gait by chronic, high doses of methylphenidate in patients with advanced Parkinson's disease. J Neurol Neurosurg Psychiatry 2007;78:470–475.
52. Giladi N. Medical treatment of freezing of gait, Mov Disord 2008;23:s482–s488.
53. Allert N, Volkmann J, Dotse S, et al. Effects of bilateral pallidal or subthalamic stimulation on gait in advanced Parkinson's disease. Mov Disord 2001;16:1076–1085.
54. Stolze H, Klebe S, Poepping M, et al. Effects of bilateral subthalamic nucleus stimulation on parkinsonian gait. Neurology 2001;57:144–146.
55. Stefani A, Lozano AM, Peppe A, et al. Bilateral deep brain stimulation of the pedunculopontine and subthalamic nuclei in severe Parkinson's disease. Brain 2007;130:1596–1607.
56. Morris ME, Iansek R, Matyas TA, et al. The pathogenesis of gait hypokinesia in Parkinson's disease. Brain 1994;117:1169–1181.
57. Rubenstein TC, Giladi N, and Hausdorff JM. The power of cueing to circumvent dopamine deficits: A review of physical therapy treatment of gait disturbances in Parkinson's disease. Mov Disord 2002;17:1148–1160.
58. Niewboer A. Cueing for freezing of gait in patients with Parkinson's disease, a rehabilitation perspective. Mov Disord 2008;23:s475–s481.
59. Muller J, Seppi K, Stefanova N, et al. Freezing of gait in postmortem-confirmed atypical parkinsonism. Mov Disord 2002;17:1041–1045.

60. Riley DE, Fogt N, and Leigh RJ. The syndrome of "pure akinesia" and its relationship to progressive supranuclear palsy. Neurology 1994;44:1025–1029.
61. Achiron A, Ziv I, Goren M, et al. Primary progressive freezing gait. Mov Disord 1993;8:293–297.
62. Atchison PR, Thompson PD, Frackowiak RSJ, et al. The syndrome of gait ignition failure. Mov Disord 1993;8:285–292.
63. Factor SA, Jennings DL, Molho ES, et al. The natural history of the syndrome of primary progressive freezing gait. Arch Neurol 2002;59:1778–1183.
64. Factor SA, Higgins DS, and Qian J. Primary progressive freezing gait: A syndrome with many causes, Neurology 2006;66:411–414.
65. Fitzgerald PM and Jankovic J. Lower body parkinsonism: Evidence for a vascular etiology. Mov Disord 1989;4:249–260.
66. Meyer JS and Barron DW. Apraxia of gait: A clinicophysiologic study. Brain 1960;83:261–284.
67. Denny-Brown D. The nature of apraxia. J Nerv Ment Disord 1958;126:9–32.
68. Thompson PD and Marsden CD. Gait disorder of subcortical arteriosclerotic encephalopathy: Binswanger's disease. Mov Disord 1987;2:1–8.
69. Elble RJ, Cousins R, Leffler K, et al. Gait initiation by patients with lower-half parkinsonism. Brain 1996;119:1705–1716.
70. Yanagisawa N, Hayashi R, and Mitoma H. Pathophysiology of frozen gait in parkinsonism. Adv Neurol 2001;87:199–207.
71. Sudarsky L and Simon S. Gait disorder in late-life hydrocephalus. Arch Neurol 1987;44:263–267.
72. Ebersbach G, Sojer M, Valldeoriola F, et al. Comparative analysis of gait in Parkinson's disease, cerebellar ataxia, and subcortical arteriosclerotic encephalopathy. Brain 1999;122:1349–1355.
73. Iansek R, Ismail NH, Bruce M, et al. Frontal gait apraxia: Pathophysiologic mechanisms and rehabilitation. Adv Neurol 2001;87:363–374.
74. Narabayashi H, Kondo T, Yokochi F, et al Clinical effects of L-threo-3,4-dihydroxyphenylserine in cases of parkinsonism and pure akinesia. Adv Neurol 1987;45:593–602.
75. Baezner H, Oster M, Henning O, et al. Amantadine increases gait steadiness in frontal gait disorder of subcortical vascular encephalopathy: A double-blind randomized placebo-controlled trial based on quantitative gait analysis. Cerebrovasc Dis 2001;11:235–244.
76. Nieves AF, Miyasaki JM, and Lang AE. Acute onset dystonic camptocormia caused by lenticular lesions. Mov Disord 2001;16:177–180.
77. Holmes G. Clinical symptoms of cerebellar disease and their interpretation, the Croonian lectures. Lancet 1922;ii:59–65.
78. Lechtenberg R and Gilman S. Localization of function in the cerebellum. Neurology 1978;28:376.
79. Palliyath S, Hallett M, Thomas SL, et al. Gait in patients with cerebellar ataxia. *Mov Disord* 1998;13:958–964.
80. Cueman-Hudson C and Krebs DE. Frontal plane dynamic stability and coordination in subjects with cerebellar degeneration. Exp Brain Res 2000;132:103–113.
81. Horak FC and Diener HC. Cerebellar control of postural scaling and central set in stance. J Neurophysiol 1994;72:479–493.
82. Trouillas P and Fuxe K: Serotonin, the Cerebellum and Ataxia. New York: Raven Press, 1993.
83. Lou J, Goldfarb L, McShane L, et al. Use of buspirone for treatment of cerebellar ataxia. Arch Neurol 1995;52:982–988.
84. Richardson JK, Ching C, and Hurvitz EA. The relationship between electromyographically documented peripheral neuropathy and falls. J Am Geriatr Soc 1992;40:1008–1012.
85. Sabin TD. Peripheral neuropathy: Disorders of proprioception. In Masdeu J, Sudarsky L, and Wolfson L (eds). Gait Disorders of Aging: Falls and Therapeutic Strategies. Lippincott-Raven, 1997, pp. 273–282.
86. Horak F. Postural ataxia related to somatosensory loss. Adv Neurol 2001;87:111–117.
87. Lajoie Y, Teasdale N, Cole JD, et al. Gait of a deafferented subject without large myelinated sensory fibers below the neck. Neurology 1996;47:109–115.
88. Fife TD and Baloh RW. Disequilibrium of unknown cause in older people. Ann Neurol 1993;34:694–702.
89. Kerber KA, Enrietto JA, Jacobson BA, et al. Disequilibrium in older people. Neurology 1998;51:574–580.
90. Lhermitte JJ and Toussy G [trans by Christophersen W]. The Psychoneuroses of War. London: University of London Press, 1918.
91. Hayes MW, Graham S, Heldorf P, et al. A video review of the diagnosis of psychogenic gait: Appendix and commentary. Mov Disord 1999;14:914–921.
92. Lempert T, Brandt T, Dieterich M, et al. How to identify psychogenic disorders of stance and gait. J Neurol 1991;238:140–146.
93. Keane JR. Hysterical gait disorders: 60 cases. Neurology 1989;39:586–589.
94. Bhatia K. Psychogenic gait disorders. Adv Neurol 2001;87:251–254.
95. Sudarsky L. Psychogenic gait disorders, Semin Neurol 2006;26:351–356.
96. Dimanico U, Coletti Moja M, Knafitz M, et al. Role of gait analysis in decision making in long-term spasticity treatment by baclofen pump in de-ambulatory patients. Mov Disord 2002;17(suppl 5):336.
97. Mayer NH, Esquenazi A, and Keenan MA. Patterns of upper motoneuron dysfunction in the lower limb. Adv Neurol 2001;87:311–320.
98. Wissel J, Muller J, Baldauf A, et al. Gait analysis to assess the effects of botulinum toxin A treatment in cerebral palsy. Eur J Neurol 1999;6(suppl 4):63–68.
99. Stolze H, Kuhtz-Buschbeck JP, Drucke H, et al. Gait analysis in idiopathic normal pressure hydrocephalus: Which parameters respond to the CSF tap test. Clin Neurophysiol 2000;111:1678–1686.
100. Stolze H, Kuhtz-Buschbeck JP, Drucke H, et al. Comparative analysis of the gait disorder of normal pressure hydrocephalus and Parkinson's disease. J Neurol Neurosurg Psychiatry 2001;70:289–297.
101. Ebersbach G and Poewe W. Simple assessments of mobility: Methodology and clinical application of kinetic gait analysis. Adv Neurol 2001;87:101–110.

102. Defer GL, Widner H, Marie RM, et al. Core assessment program for surgical interventional therapies in Parkinson's disease. Mov Disord 1999;14:572–574.
103. Hausdorff JM, Schaafsma JM, Balash J, et al. Impaired regulation of stride variability in Parkinson's disease subjects with freezing of gait. Exp Brain Res 2003;149:187–194.
104. Yogev-Seligmann G, Hausdorff JM, and Giladi N. The role of executive function and attention in gait. Mov Disord 2007;23:329–342.
105. Ble A, Volpato S, Zuliani G, et al. Executive function correlates with walking speed in older persons. J Am Geriatr Soc 2005;53:410–415.
106. Lundin-Olsson L, Nyberg L, and Gustafson Y. "Stops walking when talking" as a predictor of falls in elderly people. Lancet 1997;349:617.
107. Springer S, Giladi N, Peretz C, et al. Dual-tasking effects on gait variability: The role of aging, falls, and executive function. Mov Disord 2006;21:950–957.
108. Baddeley AD, Baddeley HA, Bucks RS, et al. Attentional control in Alzheimer's disease, Brain 2001;124:1492–1508.
109. Camicioli R, Oken BS, Sexton G, et al. Verbal fluency task affects gait in Parkinson's disease with motor freezing, J Geriatr Psych Neurol 1998;11:181–185.
110. Hausdorff JM, Balash J, and Giladi N. Effects of cognitive challenge on gait variability in patients with Parkinson's disease, J Geriatr Psychiatry Neurology 2003;16:53–58.
111. Bloem BR, Valkenburg VV, Slabbekoorn M, et al. The multiple tasks test: Strategies in Parkinson's disease. Exp Brain Res 2001;137:478–486.
112. Chapman GJ and Hollands MA. Evidence that older adult fallers prioritise the planning of future stepping actions over the accurate execution of ongoing steps during complex locomotor tasks. Gait Posture 2007;26:59–67.
113. Tell GS, Lefkowitz DS, Diehr P, et al. Relationship between balance and abnormalities in cerebral magnetic resonance imaging in older adults. Arch Neurol 1998;55:73–79.
114. Ouchi Y, Okada H, Yoshikawa E, et al. Brain activation during maintenance of standing postures in humans. Brain 1999;122:329–338.
115. Fukuyama H, Ouchi Y, Matsuzaki S, et al. Brain functional activity during gait in normal subjects: A SPECT study. Neurosci Lett 1997;228:183–186.
116. Matsui H, Udaka F, Miyoshi T, et al. Three dimensional stereotactic surface projection study of freezing of gait and brain perfusion image in Parkinson's disease. Mov Disord 2005;20:1272–1277.
117. Kent JM, Coplan JD, Mawlawi O, et al. Prediction of panic response to a respiratory stimulant by reduced orbitofrontal cerebral blood flow in panic disorder. Am J Psychiatry 2005;162:1379–1381.
118. Guttmann CR, Benson R, Warfield SK, et al. White matter abnormalities in mobility-impaired older persons. Neurology 2000;54:1277–1283.
119. Starr JM, Leaper SA, Murray AD, et al. Brain white matter lesions detected by magnetic resonance imaging are associated with balance and gait speed. J Neurol Neurosurg Psychiatry 2003;74:94–98.
120. Brooks WM, Wesley MH, Kodituwakku PW, et al. 1H-MRS differentiates white matter hyperintensities in subcortical arteriosclerotic encephalopathy from those in normal elderly. Stroke 1997;28:1940–1943.
121. Baloh RW, Ying SH, and Jacobson KM.A longitudinal study of gait and balance dysfunction in normal older people. Arch Neurol 2003;60:835–839.
122. Silbert LC, Nelson C, Howieson DB, et al. Impact of white matter hyperintensity volume progression on rate of cognitive and motor decline. Neurology 2008;71:108–113.
123. Baezner H, Blahak C, Poggessi A, et al. Association of gait and balance disorders with age-related white matter changes. Neurology 2008;70:935–942.
124. Thurman DJ, Stevens JA, and Rao JK. Practice parameter: Assessing patients in a neurology practice for risk of falls (an evidence-based review). Neurology 2008;70:473-479.
125. Inman VT, Ralston H, and Todd F. Human Walking. Baltimore: Williams & Wilkins, 1981.
126. Sudarsky L. Clinical approach to gait disorders. In Masdeu J, Sudarsky L, Wolfson L (eds). Gait Disorders of Aging: Falls and Therapeutic Strategies. Lippincott-Raven, 1997, pp. 147–157.

VII. SPECIAL CONSIDERATIONS

CHAPTER 45

Movement Disorders in Childhood

Erika Augustine, Jonathan Mink, and Leon S. Dure

Movement disorders in the pediatric age group appear phenomenologically the same as those in adults. Therefore, when considering the topic of pediatric movement disorders, a classification scheme based on the specific kinds of abnormality, whether they are tics, chorea, myoclonus, and so on, has great utility in this patient population. However, when evaluating a child with a movement disorder, it is important to consider the inherent dynamism related to growth and development, and the contribution of this state to the presentation and evolution of various diseases. While children may manifest the gamut of dyskinetic conditions, whether bradykinetic or hyperkinetic, it must not be presumed that children are miniature adults, nor should it be expected that the course of a disorder will exactly parallel that seen in adults. Having introduced this element of uncertainty, which is familiar to all child neurologists, it is still worthwhile to try to formulate a cogent overview of childhood movement disorders. Indeed, several other chapters in this book deal with conditions that are primarily diseases of childhood (Tourette's syndrome [see Chapter 39], idiopathic torsion dystonia [see Chapter 28]), and the reader is directed to these for comprehensive reviews. This chapter, however, considers the various movement disorders that may present in childhood, with special emphasis on the more common presentations.

▶ EPIDEMIOLOGY

Although centers specializing in movement disorders are not uncommon, clinics with a special emphasis on childhood conditions relating to movement are relatively rare. Thus, there are few reports in the literature that address the question of what the most common disorders might be in childhood. An exception has been the review of Fernandez-Alvarez and Aicardi, who in a large series of children with movement disorders, reported an occurrence of tics (39%), dystonia (24%), tremor (19%), chorea (5%), myoclonus (3%), akinetic-rigid syndromes (2%), and mixed disorders (8%) of a total of 684 patients, excluding those with cerebral palsy (Figure 45–1).[1] These figures may not be representative of the general population, given that the source is a tertiary referral center, but no other broadly based data are currently available. It is striking, however, how these percentages differ from an adult movement disorder population, in which essential tremor and akinetic-rigid syndromes such as Parkinson's disease (PD) would certainly be more predominant.

Probably the most well-studied movement disorder to date in terms of epidemiology in childhood is that of tics. Large-scale studies of school-age children have estimated the prevalence at between 10% and 20%.[2,3] Studies of Tourette's syndrome (TS) have varied over the years in their estimations of prevalence, but recent reports indicate it to be as high as 3–4% in school-age children, with a much higher percentage in special needs populations.[4–9] Although this may seem quite high, it is interesting to note that some of these estimates are of patients who met clinical criteria for TS, but may never have received a diagnosis due to lack of impairment or disability. In any event, it would appear that tics would probably be the most frequently encountered childhood

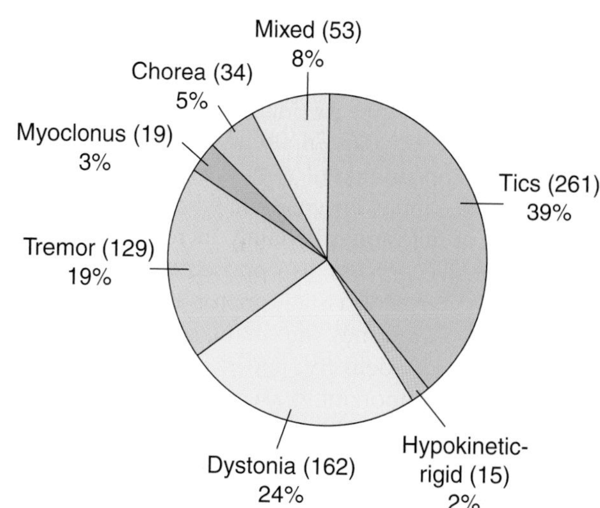

Figure 45–1. Distribution of movement disorders in 673 children seen in a tertiary referral center. (Adapted from Fernandez-Alvarez E and Aicardi J. Movement Disorders in Children. London: MacKeith Press, 2001. Used with permission.)

movement disorder, although characterization as a disease is not always true.

Among other disorders of movement, dystonia is a condition that may be seen in a number of contexts. The majority of epidemiologic studies of dystonia, however, primarily capture adult-onset focal or segmental dystonias, and do not report the incidence or prevalence of childhood-onset primary dystonia.[10] Moreover, dystonia in childhood may be seen in association with a variety of conditions, making ascertainment quite difficult. For example, dyskinetic cerebral palsy is thought to represent a subgroup of children who manifest a form of secondary dystonia. However, reports of the actual incidence of this form of movement disorder are quite disparate,[11–14] making any generalizations regarding frequency problematic.

The next most commonly encountered childhood movement disorder, tremor, has seldom been reported specifically in childhood.[15–18] This is despite the fact that essential tremor (ET) and tremor associated with other conditions are not uncommonly encountered in the clinical setting. Similarly, no data exist for chorea, myoclonus, or akinetic-rigid syndromes. Clearly, one area of potential research for the future will be to better examine and define the epidemiology of these disorders.

▶ APPROACH TO THE CHILD WITH A MOVEMENT DISORDER

As is true for most neurologic problems, when evaluating a child for a disorder of movement, the history is of paramount importance. Unlike the evaluation of an adult, however, the complaint under scrutiny must be taken in the context of the child's stage of development.[19] For example, newborns and young infants may be described as manifesting myoclonus, which at that age and in many cases is a benign and transient finding.[20,21] This is also true for infants who may manifest chorea or dystonia.[22] Careful attention must be paid to the tempo of appearance of a movement disorder, the timing, and the course. Progression, worsening of symptoms or loss of milestones certainly increases the likelihood of an active process, as opposed to the relatively unchanging features of a static motor encephalopathy. Family history is at times important, as are details regarding pregnancy, delivery, and developmental progress. Finally, it is important to ascertain any disability or impairment associated with the disorder, as well as any neurobehavioral correlates.

The examination of a child with a movement disorder can be quite challenging, and will often test the patience of the clinician. Indeed, sometimes the only way that a movement disorder can be witnessed by the clinician is for the family to provide a videotape demonstrating the child's movements. This is especially true for tics and stereotypies, which are often suppressible or state-dependent, and there are published recommendations on obtaining a home video assessment.[23] However, for many conditions, the movements are quite evident in the clinical setting. In all cases, a thorough neurologic examination is warranted, with the caveat that some parts of the examination are quite unreliable in many children (e.g., sensory testing, complex motor tasks, and some testing of higher cognitive function). Assessment of organomegaly, birthmarks, and detailed ophthalmologic examinations may be required in some cases.

Undoubtedly, the most important part of the assessment is to designate accurately the type of movement disorder. Definitions of tics, chorea, myoclonus, and such are given elsewhere in this volume, but, despite the wealth of descriptive detail regarding the various disorders, practical determination of the type of movement can be very difficult. Tics are often characterized by premonitory urges, suppressibility, and a sense of relief upon performance. However, none of these features may be reported by young children who may exhibit frequent tics yet can be oblivious to their presence. Hypertonic states such as spasticity, dystonia, and rigidity can be confusing for the less-experienced clinician, and, when occurring in the same patient, can engender disagreements even among those with significant expertise. Finally, disorders that may be difficult to differentiate upon observation, but are neurophysiologically distinct, such as rhythmic myoclonus and tremor, do not easily lend themselves to evaluation in the young child. Despite these difficulties, accurate characterization of movement disorders is usually possible, and serves as an adequate starting point to ultimate diagnosis and management. The subsequent discussion will be organized according to these standard categories of movement classification.

▶ TICS

Probably the most common movement disorder of childhood, it must be stressed that not all tics are even worthy of the designation as a pathologic entity, and could even be considered a component of normal development. Tics may be either motor or phonic, are involuntary, and may involve any part of the body.[24] One feature of tics that may distinguish them from other movement disorders is that they may be produced upon request, are stereotyped, and can often be imitated by the examiner or a family member. Common motor manifestations include head shaking, eye blinking, facial grimacing, shoulder shrugging, mouth opening, and abdominal contractions. Phonic tics can be either simple sounds, such as sniffing or throat clearing, or take the form of more complex noises or utterances. Tics often occur in bouts, which in themselves may be the consequence of suppression. Children tend to become aware of premonitory urges at an average age of 10 years, although the ability to suppress tics may come first.[25,26] This is important when considering referral for non-pharmacologic therapies or behavioral therapeutic approaches, which may require awareness of premonitory sensory phenomena.

As stated previously, tics have been observed in as many as 20% of school-aged children, but the exact frequency is not known. When tics are diagnosed by primary care physicians, the recommended practice is to provide some education and reassurance to families, since it is felt that, in the majority of these children, the tics will resolve spontaneously and not recur.[27] It is for this reason that the evaluating physician must take into account the developmental context of the patient in question. A young child with a recent onset of tics does not necessarily need a comprehensive set of investigations, since there is probably some likelihood that the tics will resolve. The formal diagnosis for this entity would be most closely approximated by a transient tic disorder (*DSM-IV-TR* 307.21, Table 45–1),[28] with the exception that most children are not adversely affected by their tics, nor do they suffer significant impairment. For a more comprehensive discussion of chronic tic disorders, the reader is referred to Chapter 40. Historical features of importance in the characterization of tics in childhood include the duration and repertoire of tics. Families often will relate that children with tic disorders have exhibited behavior in the past that would certainly be consistent with prior tics, even though the behavior contemporaneous to the evaluation may be thought of as the "first" episode of tics. Before the diagnosis, parents are usually unaware that sniffing, throat clearing, and blinking could be due to processes other than inflammatory conditions. Finally, a family history of tics, habits, or repetitive behaviors certainly points very strongly to a diagnosis within the spectrum of chronic tic disorders.

When considering TS in childhood, even when tics are not especially problematic, episodic rage or explosive outbursts can be quite disruptive within the home and in social situations or at school. Rage attacks occur in approximately 35% of children in comparison to 8% of adults. Patients demonstrate episodes of unpredictable, uncontrolled irritability, rage, or aggression, far out of proportion to the provoking event. Spells are typically less than an hour in duration, followed by significant remorse. Some series suggest that this specific behavior may co-segregate with other TS comorbidities such as attention deficit hyperactivity disorder ADHD, or obsessive compulsive disorder (OCD), but not necessarily tic severity.[29]

One issue relating to tic disorders in childhood that bears further discussion is that of "tourettism." This term is used to describe patients who may meet criteria for TS (Table 45–2) or another chronic tic disorder, but within the context of some other disorder affecting the nervous system.[30–37] Tics that fluctuate over time both in location and intensity may be seen in the context of mental retardation, pervasive developmental disorders, stroke, encephalitis, trauma and have been attributed to neuroleptic and anticonvulsant use.[38,39] Although tempting to consider this association as somehow contributing to the pathophysiology of TS, it must be kept in mind that tics and TS are relatively common, and a coincidental comorbidity is not unlikely. The answer to this question will await the development of a biological marker for TS.

▶ TABLE 45-1: DIAGNOSTIC CRITERIA – TRANSIENT TIC DISORDER (DATA FROM[28])

1. Presence of at least one motor and/or phonic tic.
2. Tics are present daily or almost daily for greater than 4 weeks but less than 12 months.
3. Onset before age 18 years.
4. The involuntary movements are not a direct result of medication administration or a general medical condition.
5. Absence of a prior diagnosis of a chronic tic disorder or Tourette Syndrome.

▶ TABLE 45-2: DIAGNOSTIC CRITERIA – TOURETTE SYNDROME (DATA FROM[28])

A. Multiple motor and at least one phonic tic have been present at some time.
B. Tics are present daily or almost daily for greater than 12 months without a tic-free interval of greater than 3 months.
C. Onset before age 18 years.
D. The involuntary movements are not a direct result of medication administration or a general medical condition.

▶ STEREOTYPIES

A clear definition of stereotypies can be somewhat difficult to elaborate, especially since elements of stereotypies are very similar to tics. It is perhaps more illustrative to describe them. These are stereotyped, rhythmic, purposeless movements that most often involve the arms, head, and face, sometimes with a vocalization. Arm-flapping, rocking, and head-banging are common examples. Stereotypies usually begin during infancy, occur multiple times per day, and may evolve in their appearance over time. This is not the same as with tics, where there is a clear migration of tic behaviors from, for example, the eyes, to the mouth, to the head. By contrast, stereotypies tend to remain relatively constant in terms of the body parts involved, and, although they may vary in terms of intensity or frequency, the movements made by a child at 2 years will have a fundamental similarity to those the child makes at 5 years. Furthermore, stereotypies are typically rhythmic, whereas tics are usually discrete. A strong association with state is another feature, usually being most prominent with excitement, stress, fatigue, anxiety, or boredom.

Most literature regarding stereotypies in children deals with repetitive behaviors in the setting of some form of sensory deprivation or developmental disability.[40–44] Stereotypies are seen commonly in children with autism, mental retardation, and visual impairment (blindisms). Hand stereotypies are a hallmark of Rett syndrome, where near continuous washing, wringing, or clapping movements may be seen.[45–47] Stereotypies in most children are symmetric, while some patients with Rett syndrome perform independent stereotypies with each hand simultaneously. Stereotypies in Rett syndrome can be quite complex early on, decreasing in prominence as hypokinesia and rigidity evolve. The etiology of these behaviors is unknown, and it has been implied that the movements are a form of self-stimulation, but this is nothing more than an inference.

Although the literature has dwelt on these behaviors in the disabled, stereotypies also occur commonly in children with seemingly normal development.[48] However, recent data suggests that stereotypies in this group are chronic, and these children may have increased risk of neurobehavioral comorbidities such as ADHD.[49,50]

At times, a home video is often the only way that a clinician will have to determine the nature of the activity, owing to situation and state sensitivity of stereotypies. Historically, it can be helpful to determine how easy or difficult it is to redirect a child who is engaged in stereotypic behavior, as well as to identify specific times and places in which they manifest.

In terms of an evaluation, the history and observation should be sufficient to make the diagnosis. Occasionally, if the events are suspicious, an electrencephalography (EEG) could be indicated to investigate the possibility of epilepsy. However, it must be kept in mind that, given the state sensitivity, a routine office EEG may be insufficient to capture a clinical event.

There is no proven therapy for stereotypies in the otherwise neurologically normal child, and it can be argued that one is seldom required. However, in some cases, stereotypies have been felt to negatively impact on self-esteem and peer relationships. In these situations, habit reversal therapy may be of benefit.[51]

▶ TREMOR

CLINICAL CHARACTERISTICS

The clinical phenotype of tremor in childhood is much the same as that in adults. Oscillatory movements about a joint or joints that may occur at rest or with action have a similar appearance in all ages, although rest tremor in children is quite uncommon because of the relative paucity of akinetic-rigid syndromes. Kinetic or postural tremors due to cerebellar disease, rubral lesions, or peripheral processes are rare in pediatrics, in parallel to the incidence of the underlying diseases that occur in this age group. Despite a dearth of research in this area, ET is probably the most common type seen in childhood, discussed in detail in Chapter 26.[1] Tremor as a manifestation of a conversion reaction is also seen.

In newborn infants, jitteriness is a rhythmic tremor of the chin and limbs that may be seen in up to 44% of healthy children during the first few hours of life, most frequently occurring in alert, startled, or crying states.[52,53] Although occasionally an accompaniment of central nervous system or systemic pathology such as hypoxic-ischemic encephalopathy, intracerebral hemorrhage, drug withdrawal, sepsis, or metabolic disturbance, in normal full-term babies, jitteriness decreases significantly in the first few weeks of life, and resolves in the vast majority of patients within the first year of life.[53,54]

In a child with kinetic or postural tremor, it is important to determine if indeed the condition is monosymptomatic, with no other medical or neurologic history that could point towards a primary process that would cause tremor as part of another disorder. Family history of tremor may be helpful, but actual examination of the biological parents is often warranted. Assessment of exacerbating factors such as exercise or anxiety can help focus the diagnosis. Besides the routine neurologic examination, some specific techniques are necessary. Examination of tremor at rest, with the extremities held in a stable posture, or while reaching for an object, are maneuvers that, with encouragement, most children can perform. In the reluctant child, observation as a tower of blocks is constructed, or the careful placement of an object by the child into the examiner's hand, can be informative. Children who are able to use a pen, pencil, or even a crayon can be encouraged to draw an Archimedes spiral, although in younger children a rather large drawing may be necessary. In cases where tremor is suspected to be the manifestation of a conversion disorder, examination for changes in frequency or amplitude of tremor by using a weight in the affected limb is useful.[55]

ESSENTIAL TREMOR (ET)

The most common type of tremor in adults is ET, and, in large retrospective studies of familial tremor, age of onset in childhood is certainly reported.[17,18,56] A case series of childhood ET in 19 patients found a mean age of 12.7 years at the time of diagnosis. Although detailed neurophysiologic testing was not performed, the clinical course and examination of these patients suggests that childhood ET is very similar to the adult variety. However, head tremor is relatively uncommon, and in contrast to the female predominance seen in adulthood, childhood ET is observed predominantly in males (68–74%).[16,57–59] Family history of tremor has been strongly associated with younger age of onset, with positive family history of ET in 91% of patients with tremor onset before age 20.[58] What is unknown, however, is if the long-term prognosis of ET differs if onset is in childhood. In adults, tremor severity has been reported to be independently associated with both age and duration of illness.[60] It would be tempting to speculate that earlier-onset ET may lead to greater disability in adulthood, but the lack of continuing prospective follow-up in childhood ET makes counseling difficult.

There are no published series of treatment strategies in childhood ET. However, pharmacologic agents such as β-adrenergic blockers, primidone, and topiramate have proven useful, as they have in adults.[58,61–63] Care should be taken, though, to assess treatment goals, as younger children seldom require more than education and perhaps modifications in school regarding handwriting. On the other hand, adolescents will often request a treatment trial to avoid exhibiting tremor in public.

There are two entities described in children that have been characterized as ET variants. These conditions are geniospasm (hereditary chin trembling),[64,65] and shuddering attacks.[66,67] Both of these conditions may present as early as infancy, and, in the case of geniospasm, most cases reported are within families, in an autosomal-dominant inheritance pattern. Geniospasm is a trembling of the chin that may be asymmetric, paroxysmal, and state-dependent, appearing more prominent with emotional stress, concentration, or extreme temperature change. It is seldom disabling and usually does not require attention, as most episodes are seconds to minutes in duration. For the rare patient who experiences nocturnal tongue biting or social embarrassment due effects on speech or eating, botulinum toxin to the mentalis muscle may be considered.[68] Geniospasm gradually decreases in intensity throughout adulthood, particularly in women.[65] In the case of shuddering attacks, children present with a history of paroxysms of fine shaking of the whole body, as if they are experiencing a chill, typically in seated or standing positions. Events are seconds in length and are not associated with a change in consciousness. Shuddering attacks are quite difficult to diagnose by history alone, and it is rare that a child will manifest an attack during a clinic visit, even though they may occur daily. Often, these patients undergo video EEG monitoring to rule out epilepsy, but a home videotape of the events should suffice to make the diagnosis. Although episodes can be very frequent, like geniospasm, shuddering attacks do not require any therapy. Moreover, they tend to disappear with time.

OTHER TREMORS

Another tremor that is seldom described, but is seen with some frequency, is in the context of an underlying neurologic or developmental disorder. Tremor may accompany static encephalopathies such as cerebral palsy, and has been described in apraxic children.[69] Since these and other conditions are commonly seen by child neurologists, it is possible that they represent the occurrence of two diseases in the same child, similar to the situation described above regarding tourettism. However, until larger series are assembled for study, this issue remains unresolved.

Palatal tremor, or palatal myoclonus, is further detailed in Chapter 38, however, it should be noted that essential palatal tremor involving the tensor veli palatini occurs primarily in children as compared with symptomatic palatal tremor of the levator veli palatini in adulthood. The essential type can sometimes be distinguished from symptomatic palatal tremor by the presence of ear clicks, tendency to diminish or extinguish during sleep, and absence of facial or extremity musculature involvement. Neuroimaging is normal. Onset of symptoms is most commonly between 6 and 9 years of age, with gradual resolution over a period of years.[70]

In terms of tremors that are specific to childhood, spasmus nutans and the bobblehead doll syndrome must be considered. Spasmus nutans presents most commonly within the first year of life, and is described as the constellation of head tremor, high-frequency pendular nystagmus, and inconsistently with torticollis.[71] The tremor is slow (2–4 Hz), and is typically in a "no-no" direction. Nystagmus may be monocular or asymmetric and can be associated with strabismus and torticollis. These symptoms have also been described with optic nerve tumors, therefore imaging is warranted.[72] Head shaking associated with congenital nystagmus and retinal dystrophies may mimick spasmus nutans, thus ophthalmology evaluation, possibly including electroretinography should be considered.[73] However, barring an abnormality of cranial imaging or vision, spasmus nutans almost always resolves spontaneously, with good visual acuity, without intervention, although subclinical nystagmus may persist through late childhood.[74] On the other hand, the bobblehead doll syndrome is an episodic 2–3Hz head tremor in a "yes-yes" direction, associated with communicating hydrocephalus due to lesions near the third ventricle, including tumors, aqueductal stenosis, or arachnoid cysts.[75,76] When confronted with a child with this type of up-and-down tremor, the clinician should look for other signs of hydrocephalus or increased intracranial pressure. As opposed to spasmus nutans, this syndrome will not resolve without alleviation of the hydrocephalus.

Finally, tremor is a known side-effect of anticonvulsant drugs, lithium, and adrenergic agents, among others.[77,78] These drugs in particular are used with some frequency in children. A syndrome of transient tremor has also been reported in infants who have received supplemental vitamin B_{12} for megaloblastic anemia.[79,80]

▶ DYSTONIA

CLINICAL FEATURES

Defined as a condition in which there is an abnormality of posture that may be static or dynamic, dystonia in childhood is most frequently thought of as being synonymous with idiopathic torsion dystonia (ITD). This disorder is explored in Chapter 29, and probably represents the most commonly diagnosed primary dystonia in childhood. The emphasis on "diagnosed" relates to the growing realization that dystonia is felt to be underrecognized and may be part of the clinical phenotype of a number of childhood disorders. Family and population-based studies have tended to focus on the typical adult forms of dystonia, such as blepharospasm, writer's cramp, and torticollis, which are certainly more common than ITD.[10] However, taking elements of the definition of dystonia (postural abnormalities, fluctuation of tone, a twisting quality), clinicians who take care of children with neurologic disorders can often detect this abnormality of movement.

As an example of the potential prevalence of dystonia in childhood, it is informative to consider the entity of static motor encephalopathy, or cerebral palsy (CP). There are several subtypes of CP based on the distribution and character of the clinical findings. These include diplegic, triplegic, and quadriplegic, each of which is typically associated with spasticity, hypotonic, ataxic, dyskinetic, and mixed. Of these subtypes, dyskinetic CP has the appearance of what is typically referred to as a hyperkinetic movement disorder and is often described as "choreic," "athetoid," or "choreoathetoid."[11–13,81,82] Population-based studies of the epidemiology of CP usually include any and all of these types as part of the analysis. The overall incidence of CP varies from study to study, but 1–2/1000 live births is a reasonable range. What is interesting, however, is the steadily increasing appreciation for mixed forms of CP (approaching 25% of cases), with the common feature of "dyskinesia." These dyskinetic patients often manifest some component of dystonia, although formal definitions of dystonia in this context are not necessarily well formulated. Attempts are being made to return to first principles and develop consensus guidelines for the characterization of these dyskinetic movements.[83] Should these movements be clearly accepted as dystonic, then incidence and prevalence rates of dystonia will clearly need to be reevaluated.

When evaluating a child with dystonia, historical information relating to onset, course, distribution, and family history are necessary. Moreover, the clinician needs to remain cognizant of the fact that dystonia may be a finding in other disorders, particularly CP. A list of other conditions in which childhood dystonia may be present is described in Table 45–3. Examination of children for dystonia can be quite difficult, owing not so much to a lack of cooperation as much as to the fluctuating nature of the movement. Sometimes, the only way to appreciate subtle dystonias in childhood is to observe the child while playing or ambulating.

DYSTONIC CONDITIONS IN CHILDHOOD

The differential diagnosis and steps in evaluation are discussed in Chapters 29 and 32, but there is one entity that deserves some emphasis, if only because it is often unrecognized. Dystonia has been reported to develop in patients with a history of CP, sometimes years after what has been considered a stable clinical state.[84,85] Why this occurs is not known, although it is believed that maturational processes may result in an "evolving" motor disturbance in children and does not necessarily indicate the development of a new disease.

Another group of disorders that have been recently described as causing a dystonic phenotype are those of neurotransmitter synthesis or breakdown, particularly monoamine metabolism.[86–88] Deficiencies of tyrosine-hydroxylase and aromatic acid decarboxylase have been described in infancy, and are characterized by abnormalities in cerebrospinal fluid neurotransmitter metabolites and documentation of enzyme hypoactivity. The incidence of these disorders is not known, but the index of suspicion should be high in infants with progressive encephalopathy and dystonia. Therapeutic trials of L-dopa can be quite helpful in these children, but not all, indicating that there may be other enzymatic or metabolic disturbances leading to this phenotype.

DOPA-RESPONSIVE DYSTONIA (DRD)

One of the more satisfying dystonias to diagnose and treat in childhood is that of dopa-responsive dystonia (DRD) (see Chapter 28). In most cases, DRD is due to a mutation affecting GTP cyclohydrolase 1 (GCH_1), an enzyme necessary for tetrahydrobiopterin synthesis, which is in turn a cofactor for dopamine and serotonin production. DRD is characterized by onset of dystonia with diurnal fluctuation in the first decade of life, often presenting with focal lower extremity dystonia. Bradykinesia and postural tremor are sometimes

▶ TABLE 45–3. **DISORDERS ASSOCIATED WITH DYSTONIA IN CHILDHOOD**

Primary
Genetic
Idiopathic torsion dystonia (DYT_1)
Dopa-responsive dystonia (GCH_1)
Myoclonus dystonia (SCGE)
Rapid-onset dystonia parkinsonism
X-linked dystonia deafness syndrome
Deafness-dystonia-optic neuropathy syndrome
Paroxysmal
- Paroxysmal kinesigenic dyskinesia
- Paroxysmal nonkinesigenic dyskinesia
- Paroxysmal exercise-induced dyskinesia
- Transient idiopathic dystonia of infancy
- Benign paroxysmal torticollis of infancy
- Benign paroxysmal upgaze of infancy
- Alternating hemiplegia of childhood

Neurodegenerative disorders
- Juvenile Parkinson's disease
- Juvenile Huntington's disease
- Pantothenate kinase-associated neurodegeneration
- Rett syndrome
- Ataxia-telangiectasia
- Neuronal ceroid lipofuscinosis
- DRPLA
- Machado Joseph
- Neuroaxonal dystrophy
- Pelizaeus Merzbacher
- Intranuclear neuronal inclusion disease

Benign hereditary chorea
Neurodegeneration with brain iron accumulation
Neuroacanthocytosis

Secondary
Metabolic
Neurotransmitter disorders
- Tyrosine hydroxylase deficiency
- Aromatic L-amino acid decarboxylase deficiency.
- Succinic semialdehyde dehydrogenase deficiency.
- Sepiapterin reductase deficiency

Organic acidurias
- Glutaric aciduria
- Methylmalonic academia
- Propionic academia
- Maple syrup urine disease
- 4-hydroxybutyric aciduria

Neimann–Pick type C
Juvenile metachromatic leukodystrophy
Lesch–Nyhan syndrome
Wilson's disease
Biotinidase deficiency
Gangliosidosis (juvenile GM_1 and GM_2)
Mitochondrial encephalomyelopathies
- Leigh
- Kearns–Sayre syndrome
- MELAS

Secondary (cont.)
Metabolic (cont.)
Glucose transporter 1 deficiency ($GLUT_1$)
Galactosemia
Hartnup's disease
Infantile Gaucher
Krabbe's disease
Mucopolysaccharoidoses
Pyruvate dehydrogenase deficiency
Sulfite oxidase deficiency
Glutaryl-CoA dehydrogenase deficiency
3-Hydroxyisobutyric aciduria
6-Pyruvoyl-tetrahydrobiopterin synthase deficiency

Static/Structural
Posterior fossa tumors
Basal ganglia infarction
Hypoxic-ischemic encephalopathy, anoxic brain injury
Pontocerebellar hypoplasia
Holoprosencephaly

Systemic/Immune-Mediated/Parainfectious
Multiple sclerosis
Acute disseminated encephalomyelitis
Recessive hereditary methemoglobinemia
Celiac disease
HIV, *Mycoplasma pneumoniae*
Neurocysticercosis
Tuberculous meningitis

Vascular
Moyamoya
Arteriovenous malformations
Spinal epidural hematoma

Drugs/Toxins
Anticonvulsants
Neuroleptics
Metaclopramide, cisapride
Cetirizine
Carbon monoxide

Other
Hypomyelination with atrophy of the basal ganglia and cerebellum
Trauma
ARX
Reflex-sympathetic dystrophy
Neurofibromatosis type 1
Alagille's syndrome

associated features.[88–93] It has been reported in children mistakenly labeled as having CP, presenting with hypertonicity, abnormal gait, and developmental delay. In these cases, a family history of first-degree relatives with "cerebral palsy" and evidence of dystonia make DRD a possibility, and a trial of levodopa–carbidopa is indicated. As opposed to most dystonias of childhood, DRD is exquisitely sensitive to treatment, with sometimes sensational reduction in symptoms. These treatment responses are apparently still present after as long as 20 years of therapy.[94,95]

The significance of the relationship between CP and dystonia has a clear therapeutic implication. Due to the desire to detect cases of DRD, it is generally recommended that all children with dystonia be given a therapeutic trial of L-dopa. Likewise, it is clear that the usual therapeutic interventions for CP may be neither beneficial nor indicated in children with significant dystonia. In some children, surgical or pharmacologic therapies directed at lessening spasticity may have a deleterious effect on children who are primarily dystonic. In conclusion, it is of paramount importance to recognize dystonia, keeping in mind that, unlike in adults, dystonia may be only one part of the neurologic process.

TRANSIENT DYSTONIAS

Another type of presumably primary dystonia of childhood is that collection of entities with the common feature of transience. These include transient idiopathic dystonia of infancy, benign paroxysmal torticollis of infancy, and benign paroxysmal upgaze.[96] Transient idiopathic dystonia of infancy presents in the first year of life, resolving within some months.[22] Often unilateral, it has more of a focal or segmental distribution. The dystonia may fluctuate and can be difficult to elicit in a clinical setting, but a home videotape will demonstrate dystonic posturing in the child that may or may not interfere with acquisition of developmental milestones. Little is known about this disorder from either an etiologic or pathologic perspective, because these children "outgrow" the dystonia, with complete resolution. A similar presentation and course has also been reported to occur in the setting of fever.[97]

Paroxysmal torticollis is usually thought of as an entity of little impact, hence the descriptor of "benign" paroxysmal torticollis of infants (BPT). Children have episodes of torticollis that may alternate sides or involve retrocollis, sometimes associated with significant discomfort, vomiting, diaphoresis, ataxia, and irritability. Furthermore, episodes can last days to weeks, causing significant morbidity, suggesting that denoting this condition as "benign" may be inappropriate. Between spells there is no neurologic abnormality; neuroimaging and electrophysiologic studies are normal. Considered a migraine equivalent, benign paroxysmal torticollis has been described in families with familial hemiplegic migraine and mutations of the CACNA1A gene. In some, episodes are triggered upon waking or in association with specific events such as teething or illness. Symptoms begin in the first months of life and gradually resolve by 3–5 years of age, however patients may later develop other migraine spectrum phenomena, including cyclic vomiting, episodic abdominal pain, benign paroxysmal vertigo, or migraine headache. There have been no comprehensive studies of treatment, although agents such as acetazolamide and calcium-channel blockers have been used.[98–100]

In benign paroxysmal upgaze or paroxysmal tonic upgaze of infancy patients experience recurrent episodes of sustained conjugate upward deviation of the eyes, lasting 10 to 30 seconds, at times occurring in clusters with ataxia. With attempts at downward gaze, downbeat nystagmus occurs; horizontal eye movements are normal. Symptoms worsen with fatigue and are alleviated by sleep. The neurologic examination, electrophysiologic and imaging studies are generally normal. Symptoms develop in the first year of life with spontaneous resolution observed within 1–2 years without neurologic sequelae. Treatment with levodopa is rarely indicated.[101]

Paroxysmal dyskinesias, a group of disorders with childhood-onset, including paroxysmal kinesigenic dyskinesia, paroxysmal nonkinesigenic dyskinesia, and paroxysmal exercise-induced dyskinesia, characterized by intermittent episodes of dystonia, choreoathetosis, or ballismus are discussed in Chapter 37. There is often prolonged delay in diagnosis or referral to a neurologist due to lack of awareness of this subset of disorders with initial consideration of psychogenic or conversion disorders.

Of particular note for the general pediatric neurologist is infantile convulsions and childhood paroxysmal choreoathetosis (ICCA), where children first present with afebrile seizures in infancy or early childhood only later in childhood or adolescence develop of episodes of chorea. Seizure onset is between 3 and 12 months of age with a favorable course as seen in benign infantile convulsions. The choreoathetotic events are brief, lasting less than 1 minute, occurring several times daily, mainly triggered by sudden movement, exertion, emotional stress but spontaneously at times as well. ICCA has been linked to a pericentromeric region of chromosome 16, although a specific gene has not been identified.[102,103] This disorder should be high on the differential diagnosis for developmentally normal children who present for evaluation of chorea with a history of epilepsy in infancy.

Alternating hemiplegia of childhood (AHC) consists of a triad of abnormal eye movements, dystonia, and episodes of hemiplegia, although these features are not necessarily simultaneous. Furthermore, despite the name, initial presentation is not usually with hemiplegia. In a series of 44 patients with AHC, first symptoms were abnormal eye movements in 65%, dystonia in 60%, and hemiplegia in 32%. The initial phase of the disorder begins in the early months of life and lasts approximately 1 year. Patients display mild developmental delay with intermittent episodes of nystagmus or sustained eye deviation. Episodic dystonia or hemiplegia does occur, although these are not prominent symptoms during this phase. Symptoms worsen in the second phase of illness with new development of or worsening of prior episodic of hemiplegia. As seen in other paroxysmal movement disorders, spells are often triggered by emotional stress, fatigue, excitement, or sudden change in environmental temperature. Hemiplegia may alternate sides, including during a single attack. During periods of transition of hemiplegia from one side to the other, quadriplegia with respiratory compromise may occur, and some patients experience quadriplegia from the very start of an episode. Hemiplegic attacks last minutes to days, and attacks of multiple weeks have been reported with associated autonomic phenomena. In the 1- to 5-year duration of the second phase, developmental regression with loss of milestones occurs along with evolution of spastic hemiplegia, quadriplegia, or hypotonia. Between distinct attacks, chorea and clonic seizures may develop in this period. In the final stage, fits become less frequent and less severe over time, with resolution of hemiplegic attacks generally by 7 years of age. However 91% of patients are left with developmental delay and permanent chorea, spasticity, or hypotonia. Younger age of onset has been correlated with poorer neurodevelopmental outcome. Flunarizine is effective in shortening the duration of episodes in a majority of patients, but may not impact developmental outcome.[104] Association with family history of migraine and similarity of certain features to familial hemiplegic migraine has raised question of AHC representing a migraine variant. Most cases are sporadic, but mutations in ATP1A2 in families have been reported.[105,106] In benign familial nocturnal alternating hemiplegia of childhood (BNAHC), recurrent episodes of hemiplegia occur out of sleep, typically less than 30 minutes in duration. In contrast to AHC, these children have an older age of onset, and do not experience episodes of abnormal eye movements, nor progressive cognitive or motor impairment. Spells do not respond to flunarizine.[107]

Infantile masturbation has been described as a transient or paroxysmal behavior that may appear dystonic, and some of these children have been evaluated for epileptic tonic spasms.[108,109] Dystonic posturing of the trunk and/or head has been seen in the setting of hiatal hernia or gastroesophageal reflux, the Sandifer's syndrome.[110–113]

▶ CHOREA

CLINICAL FEATURES

Chorea is defined as a hyperkinetic movement disorder that is rapid, nonrhythmic, unpredictable in amplitude with some dependence on state, and can be variable in terms of location. As is true in the case of tics, chorea is quite a common finding in early childhood, and "chorea minima," or a piano-playing movement seen with the arms outstretched, is present in many children in a general pediatrics setting.[114] Pathologic chorea, though, most often is described in the setting of rheumatic fever, or Sydenham's chorea (SC) (see Chapter 36). In fact, other choreas being so unusual in childhood, a previously normal child who presents with chorea is considered to have SC until proven otherwise.

Examination of the child with chorea can be among the more difficult challenges facing a neurologist, because children are quite frequently reluctant to cooperate. Children with chorea often will not participate for a sufficient time in holding their hands outstretched, and it is sometimes easier to detect that a child with chorea will often sit on his/her hands in order to limit their movements. Likewise, motor impersistence seems to predominate, and maneuvers employed by the examiner to demonstrate this feature will prove more rewarding.

Chorea may be an accompaniment to the static motor encephalopathy that is a consequence of kernicterus, and this has been called choreoathetotic CP. However, the term "choreoathetosis" lends no further precision to the type of movements being described and is essentially a vague means of conveying a dyskinesia that actually has elements of dystonia, athetosis, and chorea. The same is true for the word "choreiform," which has been used to describe adventitious movements in the context of the pediatric autoimmune neuropsychiatric disorder associated with streptococcus (PANDAS).[115] This illustrates the difficulty in recognition of chorea; however, since chorea can actually be thought of as the intrusion of fragments of movement into purposeful activity. Using this as a defining quality, then choreiform is less than informative.

SYDENHAM'S CHOREA (SC)

SC is one of the major criteria defining postinfectious rheumatic fever, occurring in approximately one-third of patients.[116–118] Usually presenting on the order of weeks to months after a group A β-hemolytic streptococcus infection, SC is classically defined by the triad of chorea, emotional lability, and hypotonia. The abnormal movements present as a hemichorea in 20–42% of patients.[118] The behavioral manifestations have been demonstrated to be quite striking, and at times are the main indication for therapy.[119–122] Patients with SC may be less likely to develop other features of rheumatic fever, such as carditis and arthritis; when present, these systemic manifestations tend to be of lesser severity. Although there is no significant gender difference in the occurrence of rheumatic fever, large series have shown a higher incidence of SC in girls. In most cases, SC resolves spontaneously over time, although there are reports of chronic and apparently permanent chorea associated with rheumatic fever.[123,124] Recrudescence of the chorea has been reported with reactivation of rheumatic fever and pregnancy (chorea gravidarum).[125]

The pathogenesis of SC is in all likelihood related to molecular mimicry and streptococcal antigens. Antibodies from the serum of patients with SC cross-react with human basal ganglia tissue.[126–130] Imaging studies in some patients with SC indicate the presence of an inflammatory process within caudate and putamen.[131] It is presumed that this immune process disrupts basal ganglia function in such a way as to produce choreic movements.

Although neuroleptic agents are quite effective in the treatment of SC, these agents are not often necessary for the chorea itself, as children are seldom debilitated significantly by the movements. On the other hand, the behavioral manifestations may be of such severity that neuroleptics make an excellent therapeutic intervention. Benzodiazepines, carbamazepine, and valproic acid have also been reported as useful for the movement disorder.[132,133] The role of immunosuppression has been examined, and there may be a role for steroids, intravenous gamma-globulin, and even plasmapheresis.[134] However, the possible side-effects of such therapies must be weighed carefully against the actual impairment.

BENIGN HEREDITARY CHOREA

Benign hereditary chorea (BHC) is a relatively rare condition, unless the practitioner happens to live in some proximity to a family with the disorder. Most often autosomal-dominant, this is one occasion in which family history is of the utmost importance. Care must be taken to delineate the clinical features of the condition, as another autosomal-dominant chorea, Huntington's disease (HD) (see Chapter 33), presents quite differently in childhood (see later). Nevertheless, because of lack of information or education about benign hereditary chorea, patients may believe that they are at risk for HD. The typical history is one of delayed motor development, with complaints consistent with a nonprogressive chorea with onset in infancy or early childhood. Children may be reported to be clumsy, hyperactive, and slow to master fine motor skills. Examination reveals diffusely distributed chorea. Manifestations within a single family may be quite varied in terms of severity and symptomatology, including dystonia, myoclonus, tremor, or dysarthria. Patients have normal or slightly diminished intelligence without reports of dementia. A mutation of a thyroid transcription factor gene (TITF-1) on chromosome 14 has been established in both an Alabama and a Dutch pedigree,[135,136] while excluded in other families. Congenital hypothyroidism, neonatal respiratory distress, or recurrent pulmonary infections in infancy are common associated findings with this mutation, leading to a suggested Brain-Thyroid-Lung syndrome name for this specific phenotype.

OTHER CHOREAS

Other choreas in childhood that may be encountered are seldom seen in the context of an otherwise normal child. Table 45–4 lists a number of potential etiologies for chorea (see also Chapter 36). A secondary chorea which often has a poor outcome is that of "postpump" chorea, described in children who have undergone open-heart surgery with hypothermia.[137–139] Usually presenting within the first postoperative week, this disorder is characterized by chorea affecting the entire body, often so severe as to appear ballistic. Gaze abnormalities have been described as well. Factors associated with postpump chorea include surgery occurring in children past infancy and prolonged bypass times. The cause is not known, but microembolic phenomena have been suggested. Treatment is often unsuccessful, and long-term follow-up of patients indicates significant morbidity.[140,141]

Drug-induced choreas have been reported in childhood secondary to a variety of medications, including digoxin,[142] valproate,[143] and pemoline.[144] Chorea has also been described as part of the syndromes of moyamoya,[145] antiphospholipid antibodies,[146] and hypoparathyroidism.[147]

▶ MYOCLONUS

Myoclonus, sudden involuntary muscle contraction, must be differentiated from epileptic myoclonus, particularly in children, in whom seizure disorders are more frequent when compared to adults. As with other types of disorders of movement, it is important to establish whether myoclonus is isolated or part of a broader neurologic syndrome (Table 45–5) (see Chapters 37 and 38).

OPSOCLONUS-MYOCLONUS ATAXIA SYNDROME (OMS)

OMS is an immune-mediated paraneoplastic disorder observed in 2–3% young of children with neuroblastoma, although it may occur in other malignant, infectious, or para-infectious states, presenting with the same constellation of signs and symptoms. Neuroblastoma, the most common extracranial solid tumor of childhood, presents at a mean age of 2 years; although the tumor is often

▶ **TABLE 45-4. DISORDERS IN CHILDHOOD ASSOCIATED WITH CHOREA**

Primary	Secondary (cont.)
Genetic	***Systemic/Immune mediated***
Benign hereditary chorea	Behçet's disease
Paroxysmal kinesigenic choreoathetosis	Systemic lupus erythematosus
Infantile convulsions and choreoathetosis	Antiphospholipid antibodies/antibody syndrome
Huntington chorea	***Infectious/Parainfectious***
Familial inverted choreoathetosis	Rheumatic fever (Sydenham's chorea)
Alternating hemiplegia of childhood	Bacterial meningitisç
Friedreich's ataxia	Viral encephalitis
Ataxia telangiectasia	Endocarditis
Secondary	HIV
Metabolic/Neurodegenerative	Neurocysticercosis
Glutaric aciduria type 1	***Drugs/Toxins***
Gangliosidosis (GM_1, GM_2)	Methylphenidate
Biopterin dependent hyperphenylalanemia	Anticonvulsants (phenytoin, valproate, lamotrigine)
Mucopolysaccharidosis type II	Neuroleptics
Neuronal ceroid lipofuscinosis	Trimethoprim-sulfamethoxazole
Galactosemia	Oral contraceptives
Lesch–Nyhan	Digoxin
PKU	Levodopa, dopamine agonists
Wilson disease	Lithium
3-Methylglutaconic aciduria	Pemoline
Propionic academia	Carbon monoxide
Neuroacanthocytosis	Methyl alcohol
Rett syndrome	Manganese
Pantothenate kinase deficiency	Toluene
Dentatorubral–pallidoluysian atrophy	***Vascular***
Machado Joseph	Cyanotic heart disease
Leigh's syndrome	Moyamoya
Static/Structural	Polycythemia
Hypoxic ischemic encephalopathy	Transient cerebral ischemia
Kernicterus	Postanoxic
Holoprosencephaly	Cavernous angioma
Olivoontocerebellar atrophy	***Other***
Infantile bilateral striatal necrosis	Trauma
	Postpump chorea
	Poststatus epilepticus

occult at the time of presentation with symptoms of OMS. As the name indicates, patients with OMS present with acute or subacute onset of opsoclonus (conjugate, chaotic, multidirectional, involuntary eye movements precipitated by saccades), polymyoclonus, and cerebellar ataxia. In the initial phases of illness, prominent irritability, sleep disturbance, and night terrors are common.[148] Tumor removal is often insufficient to induce OMS remission, and prolonged courses of immunosuppressant therapy are required. Children with OMS and neuroblastoma are more likely to demonstrate favorable tumor histology, absence of *N-myc* amplification, and improved survival when compared to neuroblastoma patients without OMS. Unfortunately, long-term sequelae of OMS include cognitive impairment, behavioral dysfunction, dysphoric mood, dysarthria, delays in speech, language, and motor development, as well as problems of attention in a majority of patients, up to 69%, even when involuntary movements and ataxia improve.[149–155] Clinical courses with multiple relapses have been associated with poorer developmental outcome.[156] In addition to a multiphasic course early on, patients may relapse

▶ TABLE 45-5. CHILDHOOD DISORDERS ASSOCIATED WITH MYOCLONUS

Primary	Secondary (cont.)
Genetic	***Static/Structural***
Essential myoclonus	Central pontine myelinolysis
Benign myoclonus of early infancy	Pontocerebellar hypoplasia
Benign neonatal sleep myoclonus	***Systemic/Parainfectious/Autoimmune***
Myoclonus-dystonia	Opsoclonus-myoclonus ataxia syndrome
Essential palatal myoclonus	Viral encephalitis
Febrile myoclonus	Subacute sclerosing panencephalitis
Hyperekplexia	Systemic lupus erythematosus
Secondary	Acute disseminated encephalomyelitis
Epileptic myoclonus	Hashimoto's encephalopathy
Metabolic/Neurodegenerative	Vitamin E deficiency
Niemann–Pick type C	Ramsay–Hunt syndrome
Wilson's disease	***Drugs/Toxins***
Sialidosis type I	Heavy metal poisoning, Manganese
Neuronal ceroid lipofuscinoses	Anticonvulsants
Friedreich's ataxia	Selective serotonin reuptake inhibitors
Gaucher's disease	Midazolam
PKAN	Propofol
Cerebral lipidoses	***Vascular***
Biotin deficiency	Posthypoxic
Nonketotic hyperglycinemia	***Other***
Rett syndrome	Reflex sympathetic dystrophy
Mitochondrial disorders	Trauma
Dentatorubral–pallidoluysian atrophy	

with cerebellar ataxia decades after the initial diagnosis of OMS, often in the setting of infectious illness.[157] Despite normal imaging early on, cerebellar atrophy may be seen upon late follow-up.[154] OMS also occurs as paraneoplastic phenomenon in adults, further described in Chapter ___, and has been reported in an adolescent with ovarian teratoma,[158] in association with celiac disease,[159] Lyme disease,[160] enterovirus,[161] and group A strep infection.[162,163]

Isolated opsoclonus without myoclonus has also been reported as an initial sign of neonatal HSV encephalitis.[164] Benign opsoclonus has been described in both premature and term infants without other associated neurologic phenomena. Due to the aforementioned associations, further workup is warranted, but in these patients, opsoclonus generally resolves between 1 and 6 months of age.[165]

OTHER MYOCLONIC CONDITIONS IN CHILDHOOD

Benign neonatal sleep myoclonus (BNSM) is a benign disorder of infancy characterized by rhythmic myoclonic jerks during the drowsy and sleeping states only, lasting seconds to minutes.[166] As the spells can be quite prolonged, and are recurrent, the movements are commonly mistaken for seizure, including status epilepticus.[167,168] Myoclonus starts within the first few days of life, with outliers of up to 28 days. In a series of 38 cases of BNSM, spells ceased on average by the age of 2 months, but lasted up to 10 months in some. Synchronous bilateral myoclonic jerks of the distal limbs during sleep were observed with sparing of the face, although focal myoclonus can occur. Neurodevelopmental outcome was normal at the time of follow-up for 30, with mild abnormalities of tone in eight at the time of follow up.[166] Prompt cessation of myoclonus upon awakening in the setting of a normal electroencephalogram and normal development is diagnostic. Maneuvers such as rocking or loud repetitive auditory stimuli may help to provoke events, again helping to distinguish this from other disorders.[169] BNSM is typically a sporadic disorder, although familial cases have been described.[170] This is an important entity to recognize to avoid unnecessary treatment with anticonvulsants and to provide parent reassurance concerning the benign natural history and positive prognosis.

In contrast to the poor developmental outcome seen in West's syndrome (infantile spasms), patients with benign myoclonus of early infancy (BMEI) display spells of identical clinical appearance but have an excellent prognosis. Clusters of tonic head/trunk flexion or head drops start in the first year of life in infants with normal neurological development. Imaging and electrophysiologic studies are normal, including ictal and interictal EEGs. Events resolve without intervention by 2 years of age, regardless of treatment, and increased risk for later development of seizures is not demonstrated.[171]

HYPEREKPLEXIA

Hyperekplexia is a rare disorder with onset in the neonatal period characterized by pathologic exaggerated startle response to auditory and tactile stimuli due to mutations in the glycine receptor α_1 ($GLRA_1$) or β-subunit (GLRB), with autosomal-dominant or recessive inheritance, although sporadic cases do occur. Two forms of this disorder have been described. In the major form, excessive startle reaction is followed by generalized stiffening or tonic spasms. In the neonatal period, patients also demonstrate generalized muscular rigidity, hypokinesia, and nocturnal myoclonus that diminishes over time. Generalized tonic spasms may result in falls in ambulatory patients; however, in infants, potentially life-threatening apneic spells may occur, which can be aborted by forced flexion of the neck and lower extremities towards the trunk. Apneic episodes typically resolve by 2 years of age, although patients are at increased risk for sudden infant death syndrome during this interval. Tapping the bridge of the nose or blowing air onto the nose can elicit a tonic spell or an exaggerated head retraction reflex, which are slow to habituate. In the minor form, excessive startle is present without associated hypertonicity or spasms. In both forms, symptoms improve over time with normal long-term neurodevelopmental outcome.[172] Treatment with benzodiazepines is indicated for severe cases, particularly patients with apneic spells. Hyperekplexia-like states have been described without typical $GLRA_1$ mutations, in association with refractory status epilepticus, spastic paraparesis, and in secondary states of intracranial hemorrhage, molybdenum cofactor deficiency, brainstem infarction, and posterior fossa malformations.

▶ AKINETIC-RIGID SYNDROMES

Hypokinetic or parkinsonian symptoms are rare in childhood. Primary causes of such a syndrome would include such entities as juvenile HD,[173–175] the juvenile form of neuronal ceroid lipofuscinosis (JNCL, Batten's disease),[176] inherited forms of PD with juvenile-onset,[177,178] neurotransmitter disorders, and some cases of DRD.[89,90] Each of these disorders is relatively uncommon, thus emphasizing the exceptional circumstance of a child presenting with such features as a primary complaint. The hallmark features of parkinsonism, tremor at rest, bradykinesia, and postural instability are seldom seen in isolation in the pediatric age group. Each of the entities mentioned above will usually manifest other movement disorders, with the hypokinetic features being a part of a larger phenotype. For example, in juvenile HD, myoclonus, seizures, dystonia, and a rapidly progressive dementia are often more striking than the parkinsonism. Similarly, JNCL and DRD are accompanied by blindness and dementia in the former, and dystonia in the latter.

Juvenile HD (clinical onset before age 20 years), accounts for approximately 10% of all HD patients, with onset in the first decade occurring in less than 2% (childhood-onset HD). Given the rarity of childhood-onset HD, it is not uncommon for a delay in diagnosis of years, particularly in patients with very early onset of disease who may to present with cognitive or behavioral decline easily mistaken for ADHD, or speech/language delay. Furthermore, imaging studies may be normal early in the disease course. Oropharyngeal dysfunction often develops prior to the onset of extrapyramidal signs.[179–182]

Secondary causes of parkinsonism are quite varied in scope,[183] but would of course include a variety of drug exposures. Neuroleptic use and acute or subacute parkinsonian symptoms are well described in adults and children, and a history of ingestion makes this a relatively simple diagnosis to make.[184–186] Interestingly, in children overmedicated with stimulants for the treatment of ADHD, hypomimia, and bradykinesia can be seen, although a rest tremor has not been described. Other drugs reported to be associated with emergent parkinsonism include sodium valproate[187] and certain chemotherapeutic agents.[188] Hydrocephalus is another problem of childhood that unusually manifests as a parkinsonian phenotype.[189] Occasionally, the pseudodementia seen with untreated or refractory depression can certainly be associated with a masklike face, although again, this is quite rare. Finally, parkinsonism continues to be seen rarely after encephalitis, but nowhere near to the extent of that described in the influenza epidemics of the early 1900s.[190–194]

▶ OTHER MOVEMENT DISORDERS

RESTLESS LEGS SYNDROME

Restless legs syndrome (RLS), a common sensorimotor disorder of adulthood, with prevalence of up to 15% reported,[195] is likely underdiagnosed in the pediatric population (see Chapter 46). This may be in part due to lack of knowledge of the occurrence of this disorder in childhood, but also due to lack of specificity of the complaints, and decreased ability of children to clearly express the symptoms in question. In a review of 133 adults with RLS, 38% reported onset before the age of 20 years, with onset before age 10 year in 13%.[196]

TABLE 45–6. DIAGNOSTIC CRITERIA FOR ADULT AND CHILDHOOD RLS

Essential Criteria for Adults

1. Desire to move the limbs, particularly the legs usually associated with paresthesias/dysesthesias.
2. Motor restlessness.
3. Symptoms are worse or exclusively present at rest with partial and temporary relief by activity.
4. Symptoms are worse in evening/night.

Diagnostic Criteria of Definite RLS in Childhood

1. The child fulfills all four essential adult criteria for RLS.
2. The child provides a description in his own words of leg discomfort.

or

1. The child fulfills all four essential adult criteria for RLS.
2. The child meets two of three following supportive criteria:
   a) sleep disturbance for age,
   b) family history of RLS (parents or siblings), and
   c) polysomnography demonstrates periodic limb movement index ≥5/hr of sleep

Note: Use standard adult criteria after age 12 years. (Data adapted from 2003 NIH Workshop diagnostic criteria for RLS in children.)

Through a large-scale survey using 2003 NIH criteria for diagnosis of RLS in children (Table 45–6), pediatric prevalence was estimated at 2%.[197] In another series (23 children with definite RLS), the mean age of symptom onset was 5.1 years, with an average age at diagnosis of 9.1 years. All patients reported leg symptoms, with all extremities affected in 17%.[195]

Often attributed to growing pains or ADHD by primary providers, there may in fact be some overlap or comorbidity of these conditions. Growing pains are a common disorder of childhood, occurring in approximately 30%, however up to 80% of children with RLS report a history of growing pains. Family history can provide an important clue, as an estimated 70% of children with RLS have at least one affected parent.[195,197–199]

A study of sleep habits of 872 children from a general pediatric clinic population found a significant association between parent reported symptoms of conduct problems and patients at high risk for periodic limb movement disorder. Twenty-four percent of children with RLS had high scores on a conduct problem index as compared with 12% of controls.[200] It is possible that a small proportion of children with disorders of conduct may benefit from sleep evaluation, at least by detailed history. Within the same group, patients with historical evidence of periodic limb movements in sleep (PLMS) had increased levels of hyperactivity and inattention as compared to controls. Similarly, 18% of children with RLS displayed elevated inattention and hyperactivity scores compared with 11% of controls.[201] The converse also holds true. In a series of 14 patients with ADHD, 64% of ADHD demonstrated more than five periodic limb movements in sleep per hour.[202] Several hypotheses have been proposed, including iron deficiency, given low ferritin frequently found in RLS patients and iron's role as a cofactor in the dopamine synthesis pathway.[203,204]

Given the distressing nature of RLS symptoms, associated sleep disturbance, and above-mentioned potential comorbidities, symptoms of RLS should be carefully evaluated in at-risk groups. As with adults, data suggests that children also demonstrate positive symptomatic response to dopaminergic therapy.[205]

PEDIATRIC AUTOIMMUNE NEUROPSYCHIATRIC DISORDERS ASSOCIATED WITH STREPTOCOCCAL INFECTION (PANDAS)

As referenced earlier, the neuropsychiatric features of Sydenham's chorea have been well described. Exploration of a postinfectious autoimmune mechanism led to broader theories that other neuropsychiatric disorders of childhood without chorea could share a similar underlying pathophysiology of molecular mimicry. PANDAS is a proposed group of immune-mediated neurobehavioral disorders that may include signs and symptoms of obsessions, compulsions, anxiety, affective disorders, hyperactivity, impulsivity, tics, and/or chorea following group A β-hemolytic streptococcal (GABHS) infection as measured by positive throat culture or positive antistreptococcal antibodies (Table 45–7). Following the initial inciting infection, there are recurrent exacerbations in temporal relation to new streptococcal infections over time, corresponding with a rise and fall in antistreptococcal serum antibodies, although exacerbations are also be seen in the setting of other infectious illnesses.

Although antineuronal antibodies have been demonstrated in PANDAS, it remains unclear if there are clear correlations between GABHS infection, the presence of these antibodies, and clinical symptoms. The first large series

TABLE 45–7. PANDAS CRITERIA

1. Presence of OCD or a tic disorder.
2. Onset between 3 years of age and the beginning of puberty.
3. Abrupt onset of symptoms or a course characterized by dramatic exacerbations of symptoms.
4. The onset or the exacerbations of symptoms is temporally related to infection with GABHS.
5. Abnormal results of neurologic examination (hyperactivity, choreiform movements, and/or tics) during an exacerbation.

of patients were described in detail 1998, yet PANDAS remains a controversial entity over a decade later, in part due to lack of specificity of the spectrum of symptoms, overlap in the age of onset with that of Tourette syndrome, waxing and waning nature of other tic and OCD disorders independent of infection, as well as the commonality and frequency of streptococcal infections in childhood making specific temporal association difficult.[206a–209]

▶ CONCLUSION

As previously stated, movement disorders in childhood have significant phenomenologic similarities to those in adults. Although in the aggregate rarer than in adults, there are still a fairly large number of children, particularly those with other neurologic vulnerabilities, who may manifest a movement disorder at some time during their lives. What this chapter has endeavored to provide the reader is not an exhaustive list of those disorders that "can" be associated with dystonia, chorea, and such, since most of the clinical conditions causing movement pathology in adults have been described in children. The goal of this discussion is to emphasize conditions that are either unique to or have their typical onset in childhood, to better familiarize the readers with what they may encounter in clinical practice.

When considering a number of these disorders, it is apparent from the limited information that is available how incomplete is our understanding, and by extension how limited are the treatment options. What is clear, though, is the need for accurate classification of childhood movement disorders into well-defined categories. This task will not be without effort, since so many children seem to manifest mixed types of disorders. However, once there is consensus regarding phenotypic characterizations, the process of defining both pathophysiology and rational treatment strategies may begin.

REFERENCES

1. Fernandez-Alvarez E and Aicardi J. Movement Disorders in Children. London: MacKeith Press, 2001.
2. Scahill L, Tanner C, and Dure L. The epidemiology of tics and Tourette syndrome in children and adolescents. Adv Neurol 2001;85:261–271.
3. Costello EJ, Angold A, Burns BJ, et al. The Great Smoky Mountains Study of Youth. Goals, design, methods, and the prevalence of DSM-III-R disorders. Arch Gen Psychiatry 1996;53:1129–1136.
4. Apter A, Pauls DL, Bleich A, et al. A population-based epidemiological study of Tourette syndrome among adolescents in Israel. Adv Neurol 1992;58:61–65.
5. Eapen V, Robertson MM, Zeitlin H, et al. Gilles de la Tourette's syndrome in special education schools: A United Kingdom study. J Neurol 1997;244:378–382.
6. Kurlan R, McDermott MP, Deeley C, et al. Prevalence of tics in schoolchildren and association with placement in special education. Neurology 2001;57:1383–1388.
7. Mason A, Banerjee S, Eapen V, et al. The prevalence of Tourette syndrome in a mainstream school population. Dev Med Child Neurol 1998;40:292–296.
8. Tanner CM, and Goldman SM. Epidemiology of Tourette syndrome. Neurol Clin 1997;15:395–402.
9. Kurlan R, Como PG, Miller B, et al. The behavioral spectrum of tic disorders: A community-based study. Neurology 2002;59:414–420.
10. Epidemiological Study of Dystonia in Europe (ESDE) Collaborative Group: A prevalence study of primary dystonia in eight European countries. J Neurol 2000;247:787–792.
11. Surveillance of Cerebral Palsy in Europe. Surveillance of cerebral palsy in Europe: A collaboration of cerebral palsy surveys and registers. Dev Med Child Neurol 2000;42:816–824.
12. Albright L. Spasticity and movement disorders in cerebral palsy. J Child Neurol 1996;11(suppl 1):S1–S4.
13. Pharoah P, Platt M, and Cooke T. The changing epidemiology of cerebral palsy. Arch Dis Child 1996;75: F169–F173.
14. Pharoah PO, Cooke T, Johnson MA, et al. Epidemiology of cerebral palsy in England and Scotland, 1984–9. Arch Dis Child Fetal Neonatal Ed 1998;79:F21–F25.
15. Paulson GW. Benign essential tremor in childhood: Symptoms, pathogenesis, treatment. Clin Pediatr 1976;15: 67–70.
16. Louis ED, Dure LSI, and Pullman S. Essential tremor in childhood: A series of nineteen cases. Mov Disord 2001;16:921–923.
17. Findley LJ and Koller WC. Essential tremor: A review. Neurology 1987;37:1194–1197.
18. Bain PG, Findley LJ, Thompson PD, et al. A study of hereditary essential tremor. Brain 1994;117(pt 4):805–824.
19. Pranzatelli MR. An approach to movement disorders of childhood. Pediatr Ann 1993;22:13–17.
20. Lombroso CT and Fejerman N. Benign myoclonus of early infancy. Ann Neurol 1977;1:138–143.
21. Resnick TJ, Moshe SL, Perotta L, et al. Benign neonatal sleep myoclonus. Relationship to sleep states. Arch Neurol 1986;43:266–268.
22. Rothfield K, Behr J, McBride M, et al. Developmental chorea and dystonia of infancy. Neurology 1987;37:99.
23. Goetz CG, Leurgans S, and Chmura TA. Home alone: methods to maximize tic expression for objective videotape assessments in Gilles de la Tourette syndrome. Mov Disord 2001;16:693–697.
24. Leckman JF. Tourette's syndrome. Lancet 2002;360: 1577–1586.
25. Leckman JF, Walker DE, and Cohen DJ. Premonitory urges in Tourette's syndrome. Am J Psychiatry 1993;150:98–102.
26. Banaschewski T, Woerner W, and Rothenberger A. Premonitory sensory phenomena and suppressibility of tics in Tourette syndrome: Developmental aspects in children and adolescents. Dev Med Child Neurol 45:700–703, 2003.
27. Brett EM. Some syndromes of involuntary movements. In EM Brett (ed). Paediatric Neurology, 3rd ed. New York: Churchill Livingstone, 1997, pp. 275–290.

28. American Psychiatric Association. Diagnostic and Statistical Manual of Mental Disorders, Fourth Edition. Washington, DC: American Psychiatric Association, 1994.
29. Budman CL, Bruun RD, Park KS, et al. Explosive outbursts in children with Tourette's disorder. J Am Acad Child Adolesc Psychiatry 2000;39:1270–1276.
30. Angelini L, Sgro V, Erba A, et al. Tourettism as clinical presentation of Huntington's disease with onset in childhood. Ital J Neurol Sci 1998;19:383–385.
31. Barabas G: Tourettism. Pediatr Ann 1988;17:422–423.
32. Bharucha KJ and Sethi KD. Tardive tourettism after exposure to neuroleptic therapy. Mov Disord 1995;10:791–793.
33. Collacott RA and Ismail IA. Tourettism in a patient with Down's syndrome. J Ment Defic Research 1988;32(pt 2):163–166.
34. Jankovic J and Ashizawa T. Tourettism associated with Huntington's disease. Mov Disord 1995;10:103–105.
35. Kwak CH and Jankovic J. Tourettism and dystonia after subcortical stroke. Mov Disord 2002;17:821–825.
36. Saiki S, Hirose G, Sakai K, et al. Chorea-acanthocytosis associated with Tourettism. Mov Disord 2004;19:833–836.
37. Dale RC, Church AJ, and Heyman I. Striatal encephalitis after varicella zoster infection complicated by Tourettism. Mov Disord 2003;18:1554–1556.
38. Alkin T, Onur E, and Ozerdem A. Co-occurence of blepharospasm, tourettism and obsessive-compulsive symptoms during lamotrigine treatment. Prog Neuropsychopharmacol Biol Psychiatry 2007;31:1339–1340.
39. Lombroso CT. Lamotrigine-induced tourettism. Neurology 1999;52:1191–1194.
40. Aichner F, Gerstenbrand F, and Poewe W. Primitive motor patterns and stereotyped movements. A comparison of findings in early childhood and in the apallic syndrome. Int J Neurol 1982;17:21–29.
41. MacLean WE Jr, Ellis DN, Galbreath HN, et al. Rhythmic motor behavior of preambulatory motor impaired, Down syndrome and nondisabled children: A comparative analysis. J Abnorm Child Psychol 1991;19:319–330.
42. Rojahn J. Self-injurious and stereotypic behavior of noninstitutionalized mentally retarded people: prevalence and classification. Am J Ment Defic 1986;91:268–276; published erratum appears in Am J Ment Defic 1987;91:619.
43. Brown R, Hobson RP, Lee A, et al. Are there "autistic-like" features in congenitally blind children? J Child Psychol Psychiatry 1997;38:693–703.
44. FitzGerald PM, Jankovic J, and Percy AK. Rett syndrome and associated movement disorders. Mov Disord 1990;5:195–202.
45. Nomura Y, Segawa M, and Hasegawa M. Rett syndrome: Clinical studies and pathophysiological consideration. Brain Dev 1984;6:475–486.
46. Nomura Y and Segawa M. Characteristics of motor disturbances of the Rett syndrome. Brain Dev 1990;12:27–30.
47. Temudo T, Ramos E, Dias K, et al. Movement Disorders in Rett Syndrome: An Analysis of 60 Patients with Detected MECP2 mutation and correlation with mutation type. Mov Disord 2008;23:1384–1390.
48. Tan A, Salgado M, and Fahn S. The characterization and outcome of stereotypic movements in nonautistic children. Mov Disord 1997;12:47–52.
49. Harris KM, Mahone M, and Singer HS. Nonautistic motor stereotypies: Clinical features and longitudinal follow-up. Pediatric Neurology 2008;38:267–272.
50. Mahone EM, Bridges D, Prahme C, et al. Repetitive Arm and hand movements (complex motor stereotypies) in children. J Pediat 2004;145:391–395.
51. Miller JM, Singer HS, Bridges DD, et al. Behavioral therapy for treatment of stereotypic movements in nonautistic children. J Child Neurol 2006;21:119–125.
52. Kramer U, Nevo Y, and Harel S. Jittery babies: A short-term follow-up. Brain Dev 1994;16:112–114.
53. Parker S, Zuckerman B, Bauchner H, et al. Jitteriness in full-term neonates: Prevalence and correlates. Pediatrics 1990;85:17–23.
54. Shuper A, Zalzberg J, Weitz R, et al. Jitteriness beyond the neonatal period: A benign pattern of movement in infancy. J Child Neurol 1991;6:243–245.
55. Deuschl G, Koster B, Lucking CH, et al. Diagnostic and pathophysiological aspects of psychogenic tremors. Mov Disord 1998;13:294–302.
56. Jankovic J, Beach J, Pandolfo M, et al. Familial essential tremor in 4 kindreds. Prospects for genetic mapping. Arch Neurol 1997;54:289–294.
57. Tan EK, Lum SY, and Prakash KM. Clinical features of childhood onset essential tremor. Eur J Neurol 2006;13:1302–1305.
58. Louis ED and Ottman R. Study of possible factors associated with age of onset in essential tremor. Mov Disord 2006;21:1980–1986.
59. Louis ED, Fernandez-Alvarez E, Dure LS, et al. Association between male gender and pediatric essential tremor. Mov Disord 2005;20:904–906.
60. Louis ED, Jurewicz EC, and Watner D. Community-based data on associations of disease duration and age with severity of essential tremor: implications for disease pathophysiology. Mov Disord 2003;18:90–93.
61. Danek A. Geniospasm: Hereditary chin trembling. Mov Disord 1993;8:335–338.
62. Soland VL, Bhatia KP, Sheean GL, et al. Hereditary geniospasm: Two new families. Mov Disord 1996;11:744–746.
63. Holmes GL and Russman BS. Shuddering attacks. Evaluation using electroencephalographic frequency modulation radiotelemetry and videotape monitoring. Am J Dis Child 1986;140:72–73.
64. Vanasse M, Bedard P, and Andermann F. Shuddering attacks in children: An early clinical manifestation of essential tremor. Neurology 1976;26:1027–1030.
65. Goraya JS, Virdi V, and Parmar V. Recurrent nocturnal tongue biting in a child with hereditary chin trembling. J Child Neurol 2006;21:985–987.
66. Ondo W and Jankovic J. Essential tremor. CNS Drugs 1996;6:178–191.
67. Galvez-Jimenez N. Topiramate and essential tremor. Ann Neurol 2000;47:837–838.
68. Connor GS. A double-blind placebo-controlled trial of topiramate treatment for essential tremor. Neurology 2002;59:132–134.
69. Gubbay SS, Ellis E, Walton JN, et al. Clumsy children. A study of apraxic and agnosic defects in 21 children. Brain 1965;88:295–312.

70. Campistol-Plana J, Majumdar A, and Fernandez-Alvarez E. Palatal tremor in childhood: Clinical and therapeutic considerations. Dev Med Child Neurol 2006;48:982–984.
71. Antony JH, Ouvrier RA, and Wise G. Spasmus nutans: A mistaken identity. Arch Neurol 1980;37:373–375.
72. Farmer J and Hoyt CS. Monocular nystagmus in infancy and early childhood. Am J Ophthalmol 1984;98:504–509.
73. Smith DE, Fitzgerald K, Stass-Isern M, et al. Electroretinography is necessary for Spasmus Nutans Diagnosis. Pediatric Neurology 2000;23:33–36.
74. Gottlob I, Wizov S, and Reinecke S. Spasmus Nutans. A long-term follow-up. Invest Opthalmol Vis Sci 1995;36:2768–2771.
75. Benton JW, Nellhaus G, and Huttenlocher PR. The bobblehead syndrome. Report of a unique truncal tremor associated with third ventricular cyst and hydrocephalus in children. Neurology 1966;16:725–729.
76. Mussell HG, Dure LS, Percy AK, et al. Bobble-head doll syndrome: Report of a case and review of the literature. Mov Disord 1997;12:810–814.
77. Zesiewicz TA and Hauser RA. Phenomenology and treatment of tremor disorders. Neurol Clin 2001;19:651–680.
78. Deuschl G. Differential diagnosis of tremor. J Neural Transm Suppl 1999;56:211–220.
79. Emery ES, Homans AC, and Colletti RB. Vitamin B12 deficiency: A cause of abnormal movements in infants. Pediatrics 1997;99:255–256.
80. Ozer EA, Turker M, Bakiler AR, et al. Involuntary movements in infantile cobalamin deficiency appearing after treatment. Pediatr Neurol 2001;25:81–83.
81. Morris JG, Grattan-Smith P, Jankelowitz SK, et al. Athetosis II: The syndrome of mild athetoid cerebral palsy. Mov Disord 2002;17:1281–1287.
82. Russman BS. Cerebral palsy. Curr Treat Options Neurol 2000;2:97–108.
83. Sanger TD, Delgado MR, Gaebler-Spira D, et al. Classification and definition of disorders causing hypertonia in childhood. Pediatrics 2003;111:e89–97.
84. Scott BL and Jankovic J. Delayed-onset progressive movement disorders after static brain lesions. Neurology 1996;46:68–74.
85. Saint Hilaire MH, Burke RE, Bressman SB, et al. Delayed-onset dystonia due to perinatal or early childhood asphyxia. Neurology 1991;41:216–222.
86. Hyland K, Surtees RA, Rodeck C, et al. Aromatic L-amino acid decarboxylase deficiency: Clinical features, diagnosis, and treatment of a new inborn error of neurotransmitter amine synthesis. Neurology 1992;42:1980–1988.
87. Rondot P and Wevers RA. Dystonie dopa-sensible forme recessive mutation du gene de la tyrosine-hydroxylase. Bull Acad Natl Med 1999;183:639–646, discussion 646–647.
88. Furukawa Y, Graf WD, Wong H, et al. Dopa-responsive dystonia simulating spastic paraplegia due to tyrosine hydroxylase (TH) gene mutations. Neurology 2001;56:260–263.
89. Hwang WJ, Calne DB, Tsui JK, et al. The long-term response to levodopa in dopa-responsive dystonia. Parkinsonism Relat Disord 2001;8:1–5.
90. Rajput AH. Levodopa prolongs life expectancy and is non-toxic to substantia nigra. Parkinsonism Relat Disord 2001;8:95–100.
91. Fernandez Alvarez E. Transient movement disorders in children. J Neurol 1998;245:1–5.
92. Nagatsu T and Ichinose H. GTP cyclohydrolase I gene, dystonia, juvenile parkinsonism, and Parkinson's disease. J Neural Transm Suppl 1997;49:203–209.
93. Nygaard TG, Trugman JM, de YJ, et al. Dopa-responsive dystonia: The spectrum of clinical manifestations in a large North American family. Neurology 1990;40: 66–69.
94. Steinberger D, Korinthenberg R, Topka H, et al. Dopa-responsive dystonia: Mutation analysis of GCH1 and analysis of therapeutic doses of L-dopa. German Dystonia Study Group. Neurology 2000;55:1735–1737.
95. Nygaard TG, Wilhelmsen KC, Risch NJ, et al. Linkage mapping of dopa-responsive dystonia (DRD) to chromosome 14q. Nat Genet 1993;5:386–390.
96. Muller U, Steinberger D, and Topka H. Mutations of GCH1 in dopa-responsive dystonia. J Neural Transm 2002;109:321–328.
97. Dooley JM, Furey S, Gordon KE, et al. Fever-induced dystonia. Pediatr Neurol 2003;28:149–150.
98. Drigo P, Carli G, and Laverda AM. Benign paroxysmal torticollis of infancy. Brain Dev 2000;22:169–172.
99. Al-Twaijri WA and Shevell MI. Pediatric migraine equivalents: occurrence and clinical features in practice. Pediatr Neurol 2002;26:365–368.
100. Giffin NJ, Benton S, and Goadsby PJ. Benign paroxysmal torticollis of infancy: Four new cases and linkage to CACNA1A mutation. Dev Med Child Neurol 2002;44:490–493.
101. Verrotti A, Trotta D, Blasetti A, et al. Paroxysmal Tonic Upgaze of childhood: Effect of age-of-onset on prognosis. Acta Paediatrica 2001;90:1343–1355.
102. Thiriaux A, de St Martin A, Vercueil L, et al. Co-occurrence of infantile epileptic seizures can childhood paroxysmal choreoathetosis in one family: Clinical, EEG, and SPECT characterization of episodic events. Mov Disord 2002;17:98–104.
103. Szepetowski P, Rochette J, Berquin P, et al. Familial infantile convulsions and paroxysmal choreoathetosis: A new neurological syndrome linked to the pericentromeric region of human chromosome 16. Am J Hum Genet 1997;61:889–898.
104. Mikati MA, Kramer U, Zupanc ML, et al. Alternating hemiplegia of childhood: Clinical manifestations and long-term outcome. Pediatric Neurology 2000;23:134–141.
105. Bassi MT, Bresolin N, Tonelli A, et al. A novel mutation in the ATP1A2 gene causes alternating hemiplegia of childhood. J Med Genet 2004;41:621–628.
106. Swoboda KJ, Kanavakis E, Xaidara A, et al. Alternating hemiplegia of childhood or familial hemiplegic migraine?: A novel ATP1A2 mutation. Ann Neurol 2004;55:884–887.
107. Chaves-Vischer V, Picard F, Andermann E, et al. Benign nocturnal alternating hemiplegia of childhood: Six patients and long-term follow-up. Neurology 2001;57:1491–1493.
108. Deda G, Caksen H, Suskan E, et al. Masturbation mimicking seizure in an infant. Indian J Pediatr 2001;68:779–781.
109. Wulff CH, Ostergaard JR, and Storm K. Epileptic fits or infantile masturbation? Seizure 1992;1:199–201.

110. O'Donnell JJ and Howard RO. Torticollis associated with hiatus hernia (Sandifer's syndrome). Am J Ophthalmol 1971;71:1134–1137.
111. Kotagal P, Costa M, Wyllie E, et al. Paroxysmal non-epileptic events in children and adolescents. Pediatrics 2002;110:e46.
112. Golden GS. Nonepileptic paroxysmal events in childhood. Pediatr Clin North Am 1992;39:715–725.
113. Dias E, Ramachandra C, D'Cruz AJ, et al. An unusual presentation of gastro-oesophageal reflux: Sandifer's syndrome. Trop Doct 1992;22:131.
114. Swaiman KF. Movement disorders. In KF Swaiman (ed). Pediatric Neurology Principles and Practice, Vol 1, 1st edn. St. Louis: Mosby, 1989, pp. 205–218.
115. Swedo SE, Leonard HL, Garvey M, et al. Pediatric autoimmune neuropsychiatric disorders associated with streptococcal infections: Clinical description of the first 50 cases. Am J Psychiatry 1998;155:264–271; published erratum appears in Am J Psychiatry 1998;155:578.
116. Jummani R and Okun M. Sydenham chorea. Arch Neurol 2001;58:311–313.
117. Marques-Dias MJ, Mercadante MT, Tucker D, et al. Sydenham's chorea. Psychiatr Clin North Am 1997;20:809–820.
118. Walker AR, Tani LY, Thompson JA, et al. Rheumatic chorea: Relationship to systemic manifestations and response to corticosteroids. J Pediatr 2007;151:679–683.
119. Freeman JM, Aron AM, Collard JE, et al. The emotional correlates of Sydenham's chorea. Pediatrics 1965;35:42–49.
120. Swedo SE. Sydenham's chorea: A model for childhood autoimmune neuropsychiatric disorders. JAMA 1994;272:1788–1791.
121. Bird MT, Palkes H, Prensky AL. A follow-up study of Sydenham's chorea. Neurology 1976;26:601–606.
122. Swedo SE, Rapoport JL, Cheslow DL, et al. High prevalence of obsessive-compulsive symptoms in patients with Sydenham's chorea. Am J Psychiatry 1989;146:246–249.
123. Berrios X, Quesney F, Morales A, et al. Are all recurrences of "pure" Sydenham chorea true recurrences of acute rheumatic fever? J Pediatr 1985;107:867–872.
124. Cardoso F, Vargas AP, Oliveira LD, et al. Persistent Sydenham's chorea. Mov Disord 1999;14:805–807.
125. Nausieda PA, Bieliauskas LA, Bacon LD, et al. Chronic dopaminergic sensitivity after Sydenham's chorea. Neurology 1983;33:750–754.
126. Husby G, van de Rijn I, Zabriskie J, et al. Antibodies reacting with cytoplasm of subthalamic and caudate nuclei neurons in chorea and acute rheumatic fever. J Exp Med 1976;144:1094–1110.
127. Singer HS, Loiselle CR, Lee O, et al. Anti-basal ganglia antibody abnormalities in Sydenham chorea. J Neuroimmunol 2003;136:154–161.
128. Church AJ, Cardoso F, Dale RC, et al. Anti-basal ganglia antibodies in acute and persistent Sydenham's chorea. Neurology 2002;59:227–231.
129. Church AJ, Dale RC, Cardoso F, et al. CSF and serum immune parameters in Sydenham's chorea: Evidence of an autoimmune syndrome? J Neuroimmunol 2003;136:149–153.
130. Morshed SA, Parveen S, Leckman JF, et al. Antibodies against neural, nuclear, cytoskeletal, and streptococcal epitopes in children and adults with Tourette's syndrome, Sydenham's chorea, and autoimmune disorders. Biol Psychiatry 2001;50:566–577.
131. Castillo M, Kwock L, and Arbelaez A. Sydenham's chorea: MRI and proton spectroscopy. Neuroradiology 1999;41:943–945.
132. Genel F, Arslanoglu S, Uran N, et al. Sydenham's chorea: clinical findings and comparison of the efficacies of sodium valproate and carbamazepine regimens. Brain Dev 2002;24:73–76.
133. Harel L, Zecharia A, Straussberg R, et al. Successful treatment of rheumatic chorea with carbamazepine. Pediatr Neurol 2000;23:147–151.
134. Garvey MA and Swedo SE. Sydenham's chorea. Clinical and therapeutic update. Adv Exp Med Biol 1997;418:115–120.
135. Breedveld GJ, van Dongen JW, Danesino C, et al. Mutations in TITF-1 are associated with benign hereditary chorea. Hum Mol Genet 2002;11:971–979.
136. Breedveld GJ, Percy AK, MacDonald ME, et al. Clinical and genetic heterogeneity in benign hereditary chorea. Neurology 2002;59:579–584.
137. Ferry PC. Neurologic sequelae of open-heart surgery in children. An "irritating question." Am J Dis Child 1990;144:369–373.
138. Robinson RO, Samuels M, and Pohl KR. Choreic syndrome after cardiac surgery. Arch Dis Child 1988;63:1466–1469.
139. Curless RG, Katz DA, Perryman RA, et al. Choreoathetosis after surgery for congenital heart disease. J Pediatr 1994;124:737–739.
140. Wong PC, Barlow CF, Hickey PR, et al. Factors associated with choreoathetosis after cardiopulmonary bypass in children with congenital heart disease. Circulation 1992;86:II118–126.
141. Medlock MD, Cruse RS, Winek SJ, et al. A 10-year experience with postpump chorea. Ann Neurol 1993;34:820–826.
142. Sekul EA, Kaminer S, Sethi KD. Digoxin-induced chorea in a child. Mov Disord 1999;14:877–879.
143. Lancman ME, Asconape JJ, and Penry JK. Choreiform movements associated with the use of valproate. Arch Neurol 1994;51:702–704.
144. Nausieda PA, Koller WC, Weiner WJ, et al. Pemoline-induced chorea. Neurology 1981;31:356–360.
145. Watanabe K, Negoro T, Maehara M, et al. Moyamoya disease presenting with chorea. *Pediatr Neurol* 1990;6:40–42.
146. Okun MS, Jummani RR, and Carney PR. Antiphospholipid-associated recurrent chorea and ballism in a child with cerebral palsy. Pediatr Neurol 2000;23:62–63.
147. Christiansen NJ and Hansen PF. Choreiform movements in hypoparathyroidism. N Engl J Med 1972;287:569–570.
148. Pranzatelli MR, Tate ED, Dukar WS, et al. Sleep disturbance and rage attacks in opsoclonus-myoclonus syndrome: Response to trazodone. J Pediatr 2005;147:32–378.
149. Klein A, Schmitt B, and Boltshauser E. Long-term outcome of ten children with opsoclonus-myoclonus syndrome. Eur J Pediatr 2007;166:359–363.
150. Hammer MS, Larsen MB, and Stack CV. Outcome of children with opsoclonus-myoclonus regardless of etiology. Pediatric Neurology 1995;13:21–24.
151. Turkel SB, Brumm VL, Mitchell WG, et al. Mood and behavioral dysfunction with opsoclonus-myoclonus ataxia. J Neuropsychiatry Clin Neurosci 2006;18:239–241.

152. Rudnick E, Khakoo Y, Antunes NL, et al. Opsoclonus-myoclonus-ataxia syndrome in neuroblastoma: Clinical outcome and antineuronal antibodies – A report from the Children's Cancer Group Study. Med Pediatr Oncol 2001;36:612–622.
153. Mitchell WG, Davalos-Gaonzalez Y, Brumm VL, et al. Opsoclonus-ataxia caused bychildhood neuroblastoma: Developmental and neurologic sequelae. Pediatrics 2002;109:86–98.
154. Hayward K, Jeremy RJ, Jenkins S, et al. Long-term neurobehavioral outcomes in children with neuroblastoma and opsoclonus-myoclonus-ataxia syndrome: Relationship to MRI findings and anti-neuronal antibodies. J Pediatr 2001;139:552–559.
155. Russo C, Cohn SL, Petruzzi MJ, et al. Long-term neurologic outcome in children with opsoclonus-myoclonus associated with neuroblatoma: A report from the pediatric oncology group. Med Pediatr Oncol 1997;29:284–288.
156. Mitchell WG, Brumm VL, Azen CG, et al. Longitudinal neurodevelopmental evaluation of children with opsoclonus-ataxia. Pediatrics 2005;116:901–907.
157. Pranzatelli MR, Tate ED, Kinsbourne M, et al. Forty-one-year follow-up of childhood –onset opsoclonus-myoclonus-ataxia: Cerebellar atrophy, multiphasic relapses, and response to IVIG. Mov Disord 2002;17:1387–1390.
158. Fitzpatrick AS, Gray OM, McConville J, et al. Opsoclonus-myoclonus syndrome associated with benign ovarian teratoma. Neurology 2008;70:1292–1293.
159. Deconinck N, Scaillon M, Segers V, et al. Opsoclonus-myoclonus associated with celiac disease. Pediatric Neurology 2006;34:312–314.
160. Vukelic D, Bozinovic D, Mororvic M, et al. Opsoclonus-myoclonus syndrome in a child with neuroborreliosis. J Infect 2000;40:189–191.
161. Tabarki B, Palmer P, Lebon P, et al. Spontaneous recovery of opsoclonus-myoclonus syndrome caused by enterovirus infection. J Neurol Neurosurg Psychiatry 1998;64:406–422.
162. Jones CE, Smyth DPL, Faust SN. Opsoclonus-myoclonus syndrome associated with group a streptococcal infection. J Pediatr Infect Dis J 2007;26:358–359.
163. Candler PM, Dale RC, Griffin S, et al. Post-streptococcal opsoclonus-myoclonus syndrome associated with anti-neuroleukin antibodies. J Neurol Neurosurg Psychiatry 2006;77:507–512.
164. Krolczyk S, Pacheco E, Valencia P, et al. Opsoclonus: an early sign of neonatal herpes encephalitis. J Child Neurol 2003;18:356–358.
165. Morad Y, Benyamini OG, and Avni I. Benign opsoclonus in preterm infants. Pediatric Neurology 2004;31:275–278.
166. Paro-Panjan D, and Neubauer D. Benign neonatal sleep myoclonus: Experience from the study of 38 infants. Eur J Paediatr Neurol 2008;12:14–18.
167. Egger J, Grossmann G, and Auchterionie GG. Benign sleep myoclonus in infancy mistaken for epilepsy. Br Med J 2003;326:975–976.
168. Turanli G, Senbil N, Altunbasak S, et al. Benign neonatal sleep myoclonus mimicking status epilepticus. J Child Neurol 2004;19:62–63.
169. Alfonso I, Papazian O, Aicardi J, et al. A simple maneuver to provoke benign neonatal sleep myoclonus. Pediatrics 1995;96:1161–1163.
170. Cohen R, Shuper A, and Straussberg R. Familial benign neonatal sleep myoclonus. Pediatr Neurol 2007;36: 334–337.
171. Maydell BV, Berenson F, Rothner AD, et al. Benign myoclonus of early infancy: An imitator of West's syndrome. J Child Neurol 2001;16:109–112.
172. Shahar E and Raviv R. Sporadic major hyperekplexia in neonates and infants: Clinical manifestations and outcome. Pediatr Neurol 2004;31:30–34.
173. Bird MT and Paulson GW. The rigid form of Huntington's chorea. Neurology 1971;21:271–276.
174. Byers RK, Gilles FH, and Fung C. Huntington's disease in children. Neurology 1973;23:561–569.
175. Jervis GA. Huntington's chorea in childhood. Arch Neurol 1963;9:244–257.
176. Rasmussen A, Macias R, Yescas P, et al. Huntington disease in children: Genotype-phenotype correlation. Neuropediatrics 2000;31:190–194.
177. Aberg LE, Rinne JO, Rajantie I, et al. A favorable response to antiparkinsonian treatment in juvenile neuronal ceroid lipofuscinosis. Neurology 2001;56:1236–1239.
178. Golbe LI. Young-onset Parkinson's disease: A clinical review. Neurology 1991;41:168–173.
179. Muthane UB, Swamy HS, Satishchandra P, et al. Early onset Parkinson's disease: Are juvenile- and young-onset different? Mov Disord 1994;9:539–544.
180. Waugh JL, Miller VS, Chudnow RS, et al. Juvenile Huntington disease exacerbated by methylphenidate: Case report. J Child Neurol 2008;23:807–809.
181. Gonzalez-Alegre P and Afifi AK. Clinical characteristics of childhood-onset (juvenile) Huntington disease: report of 12 patients and review of the literature. J Child Neurol 2006;21:223–229.
182. Yoon G, Kramer J, Zanko A, et al. Speech and language delay are early manifestations of juvenile-onset Huntington disease. Neurology 2006;67:1265–1267.
183. Pranzatelli MR, Mott SH, Pavlakis SG, et al. Clinical spectrum of secondary parkinsonism in childhood: A reversible disorder. Pediatr Neurol 1994;10:131–140.
184. Bateman DN, Darling WM, Boys R, et al. Extrapyramidal reactions to metoclopramide and prochlorperazine. Q J Med 1989;71:307–311.
185. Richardson MA, Haugland G, and Craig TJ. Neuroleptic use, parkinsonian symptoms, tardive dyskinesia, and associated factors in child and adolescent psychiatric patients. Am J Psychiatry 1991;148:1322–1328.
186. Roberts MD. Risperdal and parkinsonian tremor. J Am Acad Child Adolesc Psychiatry 1999;38:230.
187. Alvarez-Gomez MJ, Vaamonde J, Narbona J, et al. Parkinsonian syndrome in childhood after sodium valproate administration. Clin Neuropharmacol 1993;16:451–455.
188. Boranic M and Raci F. A Parkinson-like syndrome as side effect of chemotherapy with vincristine and adriamycin in a child with acute leukaemia. Biomedicine 1979;31:124–125.
189. Curran T and Lang AE. Parkinsonian syndromes associated with hydrocephalus: Case reports, a review of the literature, and pathophysiological hypotheses. Mov Disord 1994;9:508–520.
190. Hsieh JC, Lue KH, and Lee YL. Parkinson-like syndrome as the major presenting symptom of Epstein-Barr virus encephalitis. Arch Dis Child 2002;87:358.

191. Mellon AF, Appleton RE, Gardner-Medwin D, et al. Encephalitis lethargica-like illness in a five-year-old. Dev Med Child Neurol 1991;33:158–161.
192. Misra UK and Kalita J. Prognosis of Japanese encephalitis patients with dystonia compared to those with parkinsonian features only. Postgrad Med J 2002;78:238–241.
193. Murgod UA, Muthane UB, Ravi V, et al. Persistent movement disorders following Japanese encephalitis. Neurology 2001;57:2313–2315.
194. Ravenholt RT and Foege WH. 1918 influenza, encephalitis lethargica, parkinsonism. Lancet 1982;ii:860–864.
195. Muhle H, Neumann A, Lohmann-Hedrich K, et al. Childhood-onset restless legs syndrome: Clinical and genetic features of 22 families. Mov Disord 2008;23:1113–1121.
196. Montplaisir J, Boucher S, Poirier G, et al. Clinical, polysomnographic, and genetic characteristics of restless legs syndrome: A study of 133 patients diagnosed with new standard criteria. Mov Disord 1997;12:61–65.
197. Picchietti D, Allen RP, Walters AS, et al. Restless legs syndrome: Prevalence and impact in children and adolescents – the Peds REST study. Pediatrics 2007;120:253–266.
198. Evans AM and Scutter SD. Prevalence of "growing pains" in young children. J Pediatr 2004;145:255–258.
199. Kotagal S and Silber MH. Childhood-onset restless legs syndrome. Ann Neurol 2004;56:803–807.
200. Chervin RD, Dillon JE, Archbold KH, et al. Conduct problems and symptoms of sleep disorders in children. J Am Acad Child Adolesc Psychiatry 2003;42:201–208.
201. Chervin, RD, Archbold KH, Dillon JE, et al. Associations between symptoms of inattention, hyperactivity, restless legs, and periodic limb movements. *Sleep* 2002;25: 213–218.
202. Picchietti DL, Underwood DJ, Farris WA, et al. Further studies on periodic limb movement disorder and restless legs syndrome in children with attention-deficit hyperactivity disorder. Mov Disord 1999;14:1000–1007.
203. Cortese S, Lecendreux M, Bernardina BD, et al. Attention-deficit/hyperactivity disorder, Tourette's syndrome, and restless legs syndrome: the iron hypothesis. Med Hypotheses 2008;70:1128–1132.
204. Oner P, Dirik EB, Taner Y, et al. Association between low serum ferritin and restless legs syndrome in patients with attention deficit hyperactivity disorder. Tohoku J Exp Med 2007;213:269–276.
205. Walters AS, Mandelbaum DE, Lewin DS, et al. Dopaminergic therapy in children with restless legs/periodic limb movements in sleep and ADHD. Dopaminergic Therapy Study Group. Pediatr Neurol 2000;22:182–186.
206. Swedo SE, Leonard HL, Garvey M, et al. Pediatric autoimmune neuropsychiatric disorders associated with streptococcal infections: clinical description of the first 50 cases. Am J Psychiatry 1998;155:264271.
207. Singer HS, Hong JJ, Yoon DY, et al. Serum autoantibodies do not differentiate PANDAS and Tourette syndrome from controls. Neurology 2005;65:1701–1707.
208. Dale RC, Heyman I, Giovannoni G, et al. Incidence of anti-brain antibodies in children with obsessive-compulsive disorder. Br J Psychiatry 2005;187:314–319.
209. Singer HS, Loiselle CR, Lee O, et al. Anti-basal ganglia antibodies in PANDAS. Mov Disord 2004;19:406–415.

CHAPTER 46

Restless Legs Syndrome and Periodic Leg Movements of Sleep

David B. Rye and Lynn Marie Trotti

Restless legs syndrome (RLS) is characterized by a compelling, often insatiable, need to move the legs, accompanied by unpleasant sensations located mainly in the ankles and calves. Because symptoms are brought on by inactivity, distress intrudes upon everyday activities such as air travel, car rides, attending school, meetings, or the theatre, and sleep. The first comprehensive description of RLS in 1945 by Ekbom noted its key features: (1) a prevalence of at least 5%; (2) a diurnal preference for the evening and night; (3) a subpopulation with pain; (4) a proclivity to affect pregnant women; (5) heritability; and (6) a favorable response to iron supplementation. A second advance came with recognition that periodic limb movements in sleep (PLMs) are present in the anterior tibialis muscles of the legs in 85–95% of RLS subjects. Coincident with PLMs are elevations of heart rate and blood pressure, and peripheral vasoconstriction that are increasingly viewed as causal to cardio- and cerebrovascular morbidity. A third major advance has come with demonstration that pharmacologic agents acting at D_2 and D_3 dopamine receptors relieve both the sensory (RLS) *and* motor (PLMs) symptoms. A fourth advance has been demonstration of brain iron reductions in a subpopulation of RLS cases. The fifth seminal advance has been the identification of five genetic loci in four genes that account for a majority of the population attributable risk of RLS.

▶ EPIDEMIOLOGY AND NATURAL HISTORY

RLS is conventionally defined by a symptom complex that includes (1) an intense urge to move the legs that is often uncomfortable or painful; (2) a worsening at rest; (3) relief with movement; and (4) a circadian preference to emerge in the evening and at night.[1] Variability in symptom expressivity is the rule rather than exception.[2–5] Symptoms begin as mild and infrequent and slowly progress, thereby delaying most diagnoses until the fourth to sixth decades of life. RLS prevalence in populations of European descent ranges from 3–15%.[6–12] "Clinically significant" RLS, that is, symptoms that are deemed frequent or severe enough to require treatment, is less common, occurring in about 1.6% to 2.8% of these populations.[7,8,13]

Symptoms of RLS *and* PLMs exhibit a genuine circadian pattern,[14–18] and are influenced by age, sex, pregnancy, genetic factors, and common medical conditions. RLS affects 2% of school-aged children,[19–20] 3% of 30 year-olds, and 20% aged 80 and older.[10] Women are affected more often than men are in a roughly 2:1 ratio, and exhibit greater night-to-night variability in PLMs.[21] Nearly one-in-three pregnant women experience RLS in their third trimester[22–23] and the risk of RLS increases linearly with the number of live births (OR = 3.57 for >3 births).[24] Familial aggregation of RLS is well documented,[25] and the proportion of phenotypic variation attributable to genes, that is, heritability, is 54–83%.[26–29] Prevalence in non-European ethnic groups are notably low: 0.1% in Singapore,[30] 0.9% in South Korea,[31] 2.0% in Ecuador,[32] 3.2% in Turkey,[33] and 3.3% in Japan;[34] implicating genetic, environmental, or sociocultural factors in expressivity or reporting. The frequency that RLS is encountered in many common medical conditions—ostensibly 'secondary' RLS—exceeds that which would be expected by chance and includes: iron deficiency,[28] frequent blood donation,[35] end-stage renal disease,[36] rheumatologic disorders,[37] diabetes,[38] pulmonary hypertension,[39] chronic obstructive pulmonary disease,[40–41] liver disease,[42] Crohn's[43] and celiac disease,[44–45] gastric surgery,[46] and irritable bowel syndrome.[47] Neurologic conditions associated with RLS include migraine, [48–49] Parkinson's disease,[50–54] myelopathy,[55] Charcot-Marie-Tooth type 2,[56] spinocerebellar ataxias types 1, 2, and 3,[57–60] and multiple sclerosis.[60] In summary, the expressivity of RLS is influenced by a substantial genetic component, and further impacted by circadian, medical, environmental, and additional

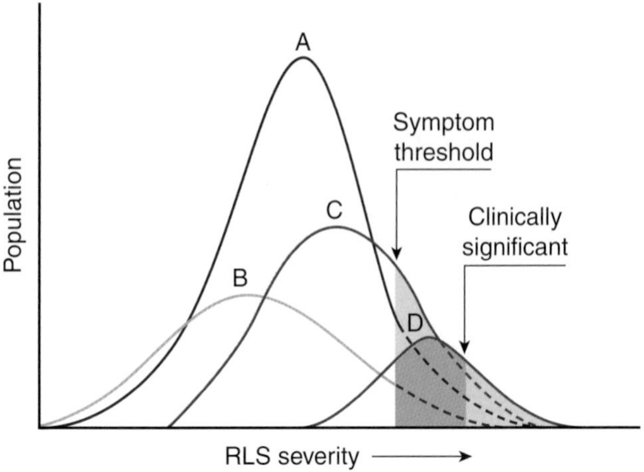

Figure 46–1. Expressivity of RLS symptoms is influenced by genetic and environmental/medical factors. Curve A is representative of an adult population of Northern-European descent. The area under the curve to the right of the arrow designated "Symptom threshold" defines the proportion of the population affected by RLS symptoms. The area under the curve to the right of the arrow marked "Clinically significant" represents the proportion in whom symptoms are frequent or intense enough to necessitate treatment. The remaining curves depict populations in whom expressivity varies from this baseline population. Curve B is representative of adolescent Northern Europeans or adult populations of Asian descent, whose diatheses to RLS are substantially lower due to age-related or genetic factors, respectively. Curve C represents the nearly 50% of Northern Europeans who are homozygous for the susceptibility variant in the *BTBD9* gene, and thus, a correspondingly greater proportion who surpass the RLS symptom and clinically significant thresholds. Curve D is illustrative of the small population of patients with end-stage renal disease requiring dialysis and in whom RLS is nearly ubiquitous. (From Trotti LM, Bhadriraju S, and Rye DB. An update on the pathophysiology and genetics of restless legs syndrome. Curr Neurol Neurosci Rep 2008;8(4):281–287. Reprinted, with permission, from Current Medicine Group LLC.)

genetic factors through mechanisms that remain poorly defined (Fig. 46–1).

DIFFERENTIATING RLS SYMPTOMS

The four RLS diagnostic criteria are considered sufficient for a diagnosis in adults, but several features formally codified as 'supportive' are often useful in confirming a diagnosis in ambiguous cases. These features include periodic limb movements of sleep (PLMs) (see later), a favorable response to dopaminergic therapy, and a family history. Empiric trials of dopamine agonists are often used in practice and may improve diagnostic accuracy by excluding conditions that mimic RLS.[61–62] In addition, a history of intolerance to, or symptom exacerbation with, a variety of over-the-counter and prescribed medications often proves a useful diagnostic clue. Exacerbation of both the signs (e.g., PLMs)[63–64] and symptoms[65–66] of RLS have also been noted with selective serotonin, and particularly, norepinephrine reuptake inhibitors. Symptom worsening with nonspecific antihistamines (e.g., diphenhydramine), sympathomimetics (e.g., ephedrine and pseudoephedrine), and antidopaminergics (e.g., metaclopramide and prochlorperazine) are common but have not been comprehensively catalogued as to the frequency of their occurrence. Antagonism with normal dopamine signaling also likely underlies the clinical experience and anecdotal reports of symptom worsening with typical and atypical antipsychotics. Reports of dramatic worsening of RLS/PLMs following regional anesthesia or during spinal anesthesia are likely due to the use of sympathomimetic amines in these clinical scenarios.[67–71]

Self-administered questionnaires of about RLS symptoms (based on consensus criteria) exhibit sensitivities and specificities of approximately 0.75. False positives are often due to the presence of conditions that "mimic" RLS.[72–74] With careful attention to diagnostic and supportive criteria and the medication history both past and present, one is usually able to distinguish RLS from mimics. For instance, in myelopathy and radiculopathy, there may be discomfort in the legs provoked by sitting or lying down, but there is no urge to move nor response to dopaminergics.[75] Neuropathy can cause uncomfortable leg sensations with a nocturnal predominance, albeit less pronounced than in RLS, but typically without an associated urge to move or improvement with movement.[75] Additionally, while neuropathy is most often symmetric and predominantly affects the feet, RLS often exhibits asymmetry and typically spares the feet. The urge to move of RLS is similar to that seen in neuroleptic-induced akathisia, but akathisia is typically described as an inner, "psychic" restlessness that does not preferentially affect the legs, does not have a circadian pattern of symptom expression, and is not associated with uncomfortable sensory symptoms accompanying the urge to move.[76] Nocturnal leg cramps have a circadian pattern and preferentially affect the legs, but are not associated with an urge to move and do not improve with movement.[76] The syndrome of painful legs and moving toes (PLMT) bears a remarkable resemblance to RLS as emphasized in original descriptions by Marsden and coworkers.[77–78] Anecdotal reports that PLMT exhibits familiality,[79] can be exacerbated by neuroleptics,[80] persists into sleep,[81] and is associated with some of the same pathologies known to exacerbate RLS/PLMs (e.g., brain pathology, radiculopathy, sympathetic nervous system overactivity, and spinal cord compression),[81] lends credence to our personal belief that PLMT and RLS/PLMs are part of the same phenotypic spectrum.

DIFFERENTIATING THE SIGNS OF RLS: PERIODIC LEG MOVEMENTS AND OTHER STEREOTYPIES

The diagnostic criteria for RLS are a human construct, necessarily informed by physician experience, clinical expediency, and regulatory agencies, but are an imperfect reflection of the underlying biology of the disorder. PLMs, on the other hand, are a genetically mediated, objective, biologic phenomenon and remain an important tool in our understanding of RLS. Nearly all patients with RLS also experience periodic leg movements while awake (PLMw) or asleep (PLMs). These movements originally coined "nocturnal myoclonus" by Symonds are involuntary, highly stereotyped, and regularly occurring. They are evident at a rate of >5/hour from anterior tibialis surface electrodes (employed in routine polysomnography [PSG]) in 80% of RLS subjects, increasing to 88% on two consecutive recording nights.[82] PLMs detected by ambulatory accelerometry on a single leg are manifest at a rate of >5/hour on at least one of five nights in 91% of subjects who seek treatment for RLS.[21] Enhanced sensitivity with additional recording nights emphasizes that the night-to-night variability in PLMs is significant, and may be particularly so in younger and less severely affected subjects, and women.

Videographically, PLMs emulate a flexor-withdrawal response, which belies their origin in hyperexcitable spinal and associated supraspinal circuits.[83–84] Sudden extension of the big toe (i.e., extensor hallicus longus) occurs in concert with dorsiflexion of the ankle, and occasionally with flexion of the knee and hip. Surface electromyographic recordings from the extensor hallicus longus reveal periodic movements in a greater proportion of RLS subjects and enhance sensitivity (~95%), but are not routinely performed. PLMs are characterized by bursts of electromyographic activity of 0.5- to 10-second duration, 5–90 seconds apart, but with inter-movement intervals concentrating around 22 seconds.[85–86] Four consecutive movements whose amplitude is at least an 8 μV increase in voltage above baseline are required for a movement to be scored. A PLMs index (PLMsI; PLMs per hour) >5/hour is generally considered pathologic. PLMs are conventionally taught to be nonspecific, occurring in other conditions such as narcolepsy, REM-sleep behavior disorder, in subjects treated with antidepressant medications, and in seemingly asymptomatic elderly. Quantification of PLMw (>15/hour) occurring during bouts of wakefulness following sleep onset exhibits good specificity (~90%) for diagnosing RLS.[87] A combination of PLMsI of >5/hour with self-reported symptoms as a criteria for RLS improves diagnostic certainty substantially (positive predictive value of >95%).[88] The PLMsI also exhibits reasonable ability to discriminate RLS from insomnia at a threshold of 10/hour.[82] Correlations of PLMsI with the International RLS Study Group Rating Scale are not robust (Pearson's correlations r = 0.22–0.46),[89–91] but nonetheless PLMs are quite sensitive, as are subjective measures, to medication effects.[91] In summary, assessment of PLMs, and particularly PLMw, are useful as a supportive diagnostic tool as well as an objective means of assessing treatment response in RLS.

While PLMs are not specific for RLS, they have attracted considerable attention as they are linked to the biology of RLS, are likely to portend some of the disorder's morbidity and mortality, and are typically sensitive to treatments that also bring relief from the distressing sensory components of RLS. PLMs are thought to reflect disinhibition of spinal cord somatomotor and autonomic pathways that originate from brain networks responsive to dopamine and opiate receptor agonists (see later).[84] PLMs are one component of a repetitive, sleep-related phenomenon that also includes cardiovascular and cerebrocortical arousals occurring at regular intervals of approximately 20–30 seconds. Elevations in heart rate[92–94] and robust systolic and diastolic blood pressure upsurges[95–96] temporally coincide with PLMs in RLS and exceed those observed with volitional leg movements (e.g., the exercise pressor reflex), and random, nonperiodic movements in sleep. These cardiovascular responses are of the same magnitude as the sympathetically mediated elevations in blood pressure that accompany the hyperventilatory phase of sleep apnea,[97–99] and that have been implicated in the development of cardiovascular disease[100] and stroke.[101]

Prevalences for PLMs range from 5 to 11% for rates ≥5/hour,[102] to 4.3% for African Americans and 9.3% for European Americans meeting a threshold of 15 PLMs/hour on a single night of polysomnography.[103] There are no population-based or longitudinal data that tell us what proportion of individuals with PLMs fulfill, or eventually develop, a portion, or all of the diagnostic criteria for RLS. Asymptomatic PLMs are often a precursor to RLS,[5,104–106] are more common in RLS families,[2,5,107–108] and are more prevalent and abundant in ethnic groups that have the highest frequencies of RLS/PLMs risk alleles (e.g., North Americans of European versus African descent).[103,109] The *BTBD9* gene variant conferring risk for RLS, in fact, is a more powerful predictor of PLMs in individuals who experience symptoms atypical of RLS, or none at all, than those with RLS.[72] Sympathetically mediated elevations in heart rate[110] and repetitive peripheral vasoconstriction that coincide with PLMs in the absence of RLS symptoms[111] mimic those observed in RLS, and PLMs are more predictive of cardiovascular medication burden than is sleep disordered breathing in the Bay Area Sleep Cohort.[112] Thus, PLMs, irrespective of the absence or presence of RLS symptoms, share common pathophysiologies and cardiovascular consequences.

Polysomnography is expensive and incapable of capturing between night variability in RLS symptoms, PLMw, and PLMs, so that actigraphic monitoring has seen increased use in the study and assessment of RLS. Such devices, which detect and store the occurrence of movements, can also be used to detect PLMw and PLMs. Miniaturized accelerometers placed on the big toe, ankle, or foot capture movement that manifests as limb acceleration, as opposed to EMG activity. Actigraphy is less expensive than PSG and has the advantage that it can be conducted in the home environment over many nights. More recent versions such as the PAM–RL triaxial accelerometer (Respironics; Murrysville, PA), which samples and stores movement activity at 10 Hz, have proven useful for diagnostic purposes and in large clinical trials. This small (65 gm), wristwatch-sized accelerometer is affixed via a hook-and-loop strap to the subject's most affected ankle for 5 consecutive nights and from it one can derive a PLMsI. The PAM-RL device provides an accurate "naturalistic" assessment of polysomnographically derived PLMsI (Pearson's correlation $r = 0.87$, $p < 0.0001$),[113] discriminates between PLMs and random nocturnal motor activity,[114] and is sensitive to treatment effects. [115–116] Actigraphy has further practical advantages to PSG including reliability and durability,[72] and engages the patient in their assessment and care. All this being said, actigraphy cannot differentiate between PLMw and PLMs. In employing such devices, it is therefore important to use them in conjunction with a sleep–wake diary to identify reliably the rest portion of the rest–activity cycle, and to be fairly confident that detected movements are impacting sleep.

The presence, character, and potential diagnostic utility of voluntary and involuntary movements manifest by RLS subjects during the waking state has not been comprehensively assessed. It has been our clinical experience that many patients exhibit stereotypies in their feet and legs that involve volitional, repetitive foot tapping, flexion, and extension at the knee, and abduction and adduction at the hip. One gets the sense that these movements reflect a compelling necessity to move or an underlying comorbid anxiety that often crescendos in an abrupt arising from the examination chair and pacing. Less frequently (~3–5% in our tertiary referral center), these movements are unequivocally nonvolitional and pathologic and have the appearance of a dyskinesia,[117] fanning or clawing of the toes as described in PLMT, brief myoclonic jerks in isolated muscles of the feet, or an unambiguous spontaneous flexor-withdrawal sequence best interpreted as a PLMw. One recent attempt to capture this diversity videographically and to differentiate it as distinct to RLS/PLMs has appeared.[118] Other than representing unusual and dramatic phenotypic variants of RLS, the clinical significance of these movements remains unclear. Our clinical experience suggests that these myoclonic-like, nonvolitional movements occur more commonly in the setting of augmentation[1] and may be a manifestation of opioid withdrawal in individuals in whom opiates have been prescribed for symptomatic relief of RLS/PLMs or pain.[119–121] We have encountered myoclonic phenomena in several young, unmedicated RLS patients in whom they precipitated falls while walking or negatively impacted coordination in skilled motor behaviors. It is of interest that Ekbom in his seminal description of RLS made note of a similar discoordination in his patients, as well as of leg weakness and fatiguability. Application of modern technologies to analysis of gait indeed suggests the presence of abnormal electromyographic activation patterns during wake in RLS subjects that is fortunately subclinical.[122]

▶ HEALTH-RELATED SIGNIFICANCE OF RLS

Quality of life is poor in RLS patients and is lower than that experienced by type 2 diabetics.[123] Sensory symptoms often manifest as childhood growing pains[20,124] and are painful in 35–55% of adults.[125–126] Treatments are symptomatic, not curative, and since RLS is a chronic, progressive disorder, a diagnosis portends life-long pharmacotherapy.[127] Even with improved treatment options, 10–20% of subjects experience life altering exacerbation of symptoms with chronic dopaminergic therapy (i.e., augmentation).[128] Impulse control disorders (e.g., compulsive spending, pathologic gambling, punding, and hypersexuality) have also been reported to develop in from 3–9% of RLS subjects treated with dopamine agonists.[129] If these quality of life issues were not substantial enough, newer epidemiologic data suggests that the economic costs associated with RLS are substantial. Additionally, we now know that RLS reliably produces sleep disruption and is associated with dramatically increased cross-sectional rates of mood, anxiety, and panic disorders.[31,130–132] Cardiovascular disease (CVD) is twice as common in those describing RLS symptoms in the large Sleep Heart Health Study cohort after controlling for other risk factors and the association is stronger in those experiencing more frequent or debilitating symptoms.[133] Additional data show that PLMs in excess of 30/hour in RLS patients predicts a doubling of the risk of prevalent hypertension after controlling for known contributors to hypertension.[134] At a systems level, dramatic, repetitive, nocturnal elevations of blood pressure time-locked to PLMs deriving from spinal sympathetic hyperactivity (vide supra), is the most parsimonious explanation for the association between RLS and CVD, and PLMs-related mortality in end-stage kidney disease.[36,135–137] Although the causal basis for these associations is not yet firmly established, the magnitude of the impact of RLS/PLMs upon public health is becoming increasingly clear.

▶ GENETICS OF RLS

The picture of how variants in the sequence of the human genome confer risk of RLS and PLMs is emerging. The proportion of phenotypic variation in RLS attributable to genes (i.e., heritability) ranges from 54 to 83%.[26–27, 29] Linkage studies have identified several regions of interest,[138–140] but only RLS1 on chromosome 12 is evident in families of diverse origin (e.g., in French-Canadian, Icelandic, and German families) with a specific gene being implicated—that is, neuronal nitric oxide synthase (NOS1).[133] Three recent genome-wide-association studies have yielded five significant associations to specific regions in four genes. We have reported genome-wide significant association of a SNP (rs3923809) in an intron of the *BTBD9* gene on chromosome 6 in both Icelandic and American subjects with an increased risk of RLS and PLMs of 70% to 80%. Because this at-risk variant is common, being present in two-thirds of those of northern European ancestry, it accounts for at least 50% of the population-attributable risk for RLS/PLMs. This association is notable for being "driven" by PLMs; that is, the SNP confers greatest risk (OR = 2.3) for PLMs in a group of asymptomatic RLS family members and subjects with atypical RLS sensory symptoms. Additional associations were reported simultaneously in Germans and French-Canadians with clinically diagnosed RLS (PLMs status unknown) to the *Meis1* gene on chromosome 2p14 and intergenic regions of the *MAP2K5* and *LBXCOR1* genes on chromosome 15q23. The credibility of these findings is undeniable. The associations are robust, have been replicated in five different populations of European descent, and the effect sizes are comparable across study populations populations.[72,141–142] Yet to be published studies confirm that variants in *Meis1* confer the greatest risk to the individual carrying them, and that these are also intimately linked to PLMs. A fourth and fifth signal, both with nominal risk for clinically diagnosed RLS in an intron of *PTPRD* (chr 9p23–24) have also been reported.[143] Together, these five genetic variants implicating four unique genes account for nearly 80% of the population attributable risk for RLS.

These findings explain much that we have learned from epidemiologic surveys of RLS and provide a solid footing upon which to build a model of the molecular pathophysiology of RLS/PLMs. Their biologic plausibility derives from (1) a dose-dependent relationship of the *BTBD9* variant to decrements in iron stores; and (2) a dose-dependent relationship of the *BTBD9 and Meis1* risk variants to PLMs. As each copy of the *BTBD9* at-risk variant predicts a 13% lower average serum ferritin, iron deficiency commonly encountered in RLS appears attributable to, or a factor influencing, expressivity of this at-risk variant. The notable differences in worldwide RLS prevalences mimic the disparate frequencies of the at-risk alleles in various ethnic groups[144] (http://www.hapmap.org). Finally, the phenomenon of anticipation manifest in many RLS families likely reflects the commonality of the at-risk variants in otherwise asymptomatic or presymptomatic individuals, as opposed to expanded triplet repeats previously excluded as contributors to RLS.[145–146]

▶ PATHOPHYSIOLOGY OF RLS/PLMS

MOLECULAR GENETIC INSIGHTS

Echoing a theme that is emerging from genome-wide association studies (GWAS) of common diseases, the variants conferring susceptibility to RLS/PLMs do not provide a comprehensive accounting for how and why symptoms emerge. The at-risk SNPs in each instance are common, present within noncoding, intronic, or intergenic regions, and implicate genes that are widely expressed in the central nervous system and other organs. Exceedingly little is known about the normal function of *BTBD9*, which is named for its BTB domain (i.e., "broad complex, tramtrack, and bric a brac"), and whose *Drosophila* ortholog *(CG1826)* is widely expressed, and most robustly during embryonic and larval stages.[147] Though much is known of the functionally versatile BTB-domain-containing protein family, the function of *BTBD9* is unknown. This protein harbors three highly conserved peptide domains, in order from amino to carboxy terminus: a BTB domain, a BACK domain, and several Kelch repeats. The BTB domain is a phylogenetically conserved protein-protein interaction motif that participates in a wide range of cellular functions, including transcriptional regulation, cytoskeleton dynamics, ion channel assembly and gating, and targeting proteins for ubiquitination.[148–149] The BACK (for BTB And C-terminal Kelch) domain is highly conserved across metazoan genomes, and may facilitate substrate orientation during ubiquitin ligation.[150–151] Kelch repeats interact with actin and play a role in cytoskeletal/microfilament orientation.[152] *Meis1* (Myeloid Ecotropic viral Integration Site 1), in contrast, is a well studied homeobox gene whose *Drosophila* homologue is critical to distal limb formation and the patterning of motor neuron connectivity.[153–154] The Xenopus homolog of *Meis1* specifies neural crest cell fate,[155] and *Meis1* is also essential to leukemogenesis and normal hematopoiesis,[156] and vascular patterning/endothelial cell development in both mice[157] and zebrafish.[158] *Meis1* has also been hypothesized to regulate the expression of Substance P in the central amygdala, a brain region universally recognized as a common final output pathway that coordinates mood and autonomic nervous system activity.[159] The *MAP2K5* gene, one of the mitogen-activated protein kinases, is implicated in muscle differentiation[160] and dopamine neuroprotection.[161] The *LBXCOR1* gene is another homeobox gene that, acting as a corepressor of Lbx1,[162] determines a GABAergic cell fate in dorsal spinal cord interneurons that are critical to gating sensory perception of pain and temperature.[163] Finally, *PTPRD* (protein tyrosine phosphatase receptor type delta) functions in the guidance and termination of mammalian motor neuron axons,[164] and its expression is dampened in a dose-dependent fashion by **estradiol**.[165]

FUNCTIONAL ANATOMY

The pathophysiologic substrates underlying RLS and PLMs are presumed to be similar as they frequently coexist, respond to, and are aggravated by the same medications and share some electrophysiologic characteristics and susceptibility genes in common. The neural networks implicated in their expression are many and diverse and include both the peripheral and central nervous systems. The characteristics of both the sensory disturbances and wake- and sleep-related movements in RLS favor a final common pathway that resides in the spinal cord. As a site of convergence for peripheral sensory afferents and descending tracts that modulate sensorimotor and autonomic excitability, the spinal cord provides a utilitarian substrate that (1) accounts for much of what has been gleaned from clinical experience and electrophysiogic investigations of RLS/PLMs; and (2) justifies the logic in a neurologic exam that begins from the periphery and ascends to the cranium in individuals being evaluated for RLS/PLMs.

The sensory component of RLS suggests involvement of the peripheral nervous system, especially the small caliber A-delta and C-fibers that carry pain signals and that mediate somatosympathetic reflexes. While associations between diffuse, small-fiber axonopathies and RLS have been described,[3,166] they are most evident in some hereditary neuropathies,[56,167] or are limited to selective, small case-series in which the neuropathy was "subclinical" and evident only by electrophysiologic[168] or microscopic[169] examination of the peripheral nerves. Conventional electromyograms (EMGs) and nerve conduction velocities (NCVs), somatosensory evoked potentials (SEPs), and sympathetic skin responses are generally normal in idiopathic RLS[170–174] and PLMs in isolation,[175–176] and EMG-NCVs are also normal for RLS encountered in the setting of iron-deficiency.[177] The prevalence of RLS in patients with acquired neuropathies is no greater than that encountered in population controls, except in individuals with family histories for RLS.[167] Thus, a patient's genetic predisposition is an important determinant of whether RLS will occur in an acquired neuropathy. Anecdotal reports and our personal clinical experiences that RLS can acutely worsen when a diffuse neuropathy develops, or preferentially lateralize to the leg or foot after damage to a spinal root or peripheral nerve, injury or surgery to a soft or bony tissue, or a thrombosed vein, emphasizes that the peripheral nervous system does indeed modulate RLS expressivity. The mechanisms acting in the periphery that precipitate the sensory RLS experience and the neural substrates that convey them are unknown. They are likely to involve ectopic or ephaptic excitation in damaged peripheral nerves and abnormal impulse generation in their sensory and/or sympathetic components. Pharmacologics effective for neuropathic pain such as gabapentin and its derivatives might derive their efficacy for RLS, particularly painful forms of RLS, from actions upon peripheral nerves.[178] Sympathetic mechanisms in the periphery are likely also important mediators, given the complete relief from painful RLS (i.e., asthenia crurum dolorosa) experienced by three of four patients of Ekbom after lumbar sympathetic ganglia blockade,[179] but have been inadequately studied.

In contrast to the modest amount of evidence that RLS symptoms do not take origin from a primary dysfunction of the peripheral nervous system, there is an abundance of data pointing to a generalized disinhibition of spinal sensorimotor and autonomic circuits. Evidence derives from both electrophysiologic examinations and functional imaging of patients with idiopathic RLS or PLMs in the absence of a sensory complaints, as well as accountings of the effects of stimulation, structural lesions, or diseases of the central nervous system upon both the sensory symptoms and motor signs (i.e., PLMs) of RLS. The picture that emerges is one of global hyperexcitability in widespread premotor circuits that includes both extra-pyramidal and pyramidal pathways that ultimately converge upon the spinal sensorimotor apparatus. No single descending inhibitory pathway has yet been identified whose dysfunction is either necessary or sufficient to produce RLS or PLMs. That said, converging lines of evidence point to monoaminergic pathways (i.e., noradrenergic, serotonergic, and dopaminergic) that innervate multiple spinal cord segments in their descent,[180] as important modulators of ascending sensory impulses such as those occurring in RLS via postsynaptic actions on dorsal horn neurons or presynaptic actions on the terminal axons of dorsal root afferents.[84,181–184] Among these, a dopaminergic diencephalospinal pathway originating from the posterior hypothalamic A11 cell group is particularly relevant given the efficacy of D_2-like dopamine receptor agonists in alleviating RLS/PLMs[84] (Fig. 46–2). Electrical[181] and pharmacologic[185] manipulations targeting the A11 cell group are antinociceptive and suppress neuropathic hypersensitivity, respectively. Lesioning of the A11 cell group in animals yields a phenotype reminiscent of RLS/PLMs[186–189] that

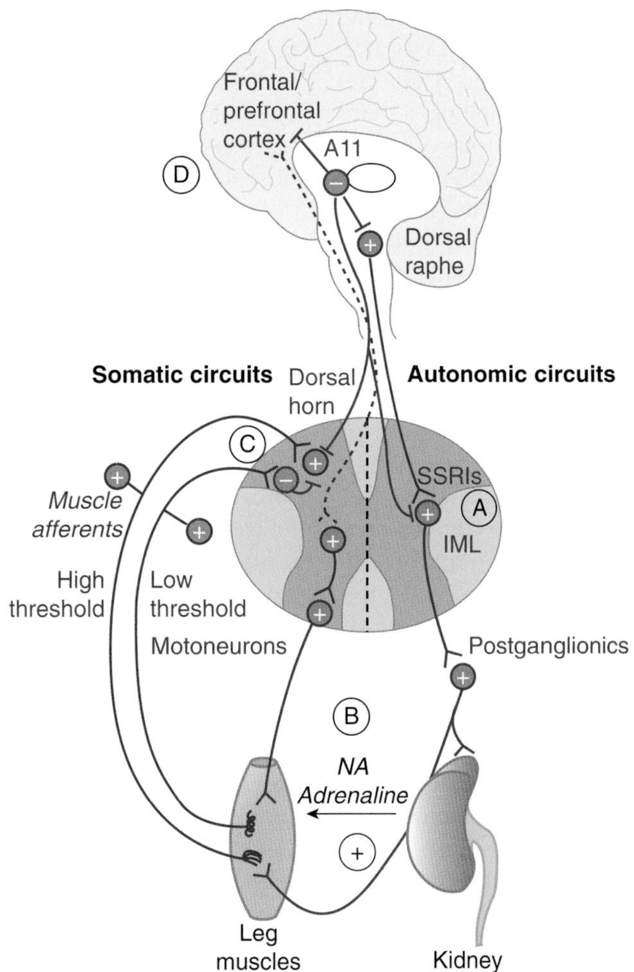

Figure 46–2. Schematic of supraspinal monoaminergic pathway modulation of RLS and PLMs related spinal networks. The diencephalopsinal dopaminergic pathway predominantly inhibits somatosensory (*left*) and sympathetic autonomic circuits (*right*) via dense innervation of the dorsal horn and intermediolateral cell column (IML), respectively. Hypothetical consequences of compromise to these circuits, or the D_2 and D_3 receptors that subserve them, are presented as a sequential series numbered 1 through 4. (A) Interference with normal inhibitory actions shifts the balance of supraspinal control of sympathetic preganglionics in the IML towards excitation. (B) Heightened sympathetic drive increases neurally mediated noradrenaline release (and adrenal gland mediated release of adrenaline) that, in turn, contributes to aberrant activation of high-threshold muscle afferents. (C) Loss of inhibitory dopaminergic 'tone' in lamina I, a region responsible for relaying deep afferent inputs to the brain, prevents normal dampening of the sensations originating from high-threshold muscle afferents. (D) Perception of these sensations (i.e., a focal akathisia), higher-order sensory processing, and the affective and cognitive consequences of RLS may be mediated by collateral innervation of the frontal and prefrontal cortices known to derive from A11 neurons. The attractiveness of this heuristic model derives further from its ability to account for the transient, movement related improvement in RLS symptoms, and potential aggravation by serotonin reuptake inhibitors. A consequence of movement is segmental activation of non-pain-encoding muscle proprioceptors known to inhibit high-threshold muscle afferent pathways by 'gate-control' mechanisms. While serotonin is known to gate sensory input at spinal dorsal horn sites, it also has robust excitatory actions in the IML—a competing influence that would favor expression of RLS symptoms. (From Clemens, S, Rye D, and Hochman S. Restless legs syndrome: Revisiting the dopamine hypothesis from the spinal cord perspective. Neurology 2006;67(1):125–130. Reprinted, with permission, from Lippincott, Williams and Wilkins, Baltimore, MD.)

includes hyperlocomotion, a disrupted diurnal pattern of locomotion, and partial reversal with dopamine agonists. Dietary iron deficiency augments the hyperlocomotion[187] and spinal D_2 and D_3 receptor reductions[188] that follow A11 lesions, and alters gene expression in the spinal dorsal horn and accentuates behavioral responsivity to both acute and chronic pain.[190] The absence of gross histopathologic changes in the A11 cell group[191] (as is also the case for other brain regions surveyed by conventional neuropathologic examinations), does not take away from these experimental findings. They are entirely consistent with RLS patients exhibiting a static mechanical hyperalgesia that derives from centrally mediated sensitization to A-delta fiber, high-threshold mechanoreceptor input (a hallmark sign of the hyperalgesic type of neuropathic pain).[192] In a similar vein, the cutaneous silent period (CSP), which is a spinal reflex mediated by A-delta fibers, is prolonged in RLS.[193] A parsimonious explanation for documented normalization of mechanical hyperalgesia [192] and duration of the CSP[193] by dopamine agonist therapy, are actions on the diencephalospinal dopamine network.[84] The contribution of reductions in dopaminergic tone to pain hypersensitivity might involve alternate supraspinal circuits such as the basal ganglia, insular and anterior cingulate cortices, and thalamus,[194–195] as well as functional polymorphisms in dopamine metabolic pathway genes.[196] The spinal cord is probably the most reliable site from which a wide array of pathologies can elicit RLS or PLMs lacking RLS sensory symptoms.[55,197–201] Irrespective of the disease process, rostrocaudal level, or extent and pattern of involvement of spinal grey and white matter, the RLS and PLMs that emerge appear indistinguishable from "idiopathic" RLS/PLMs, inclusive of their reversibility with dopamine agonists.[55] Given the heterogeneous nature of these spinal insults, the universality of treatment response points to intact spinal networks distal to the lesion—as opposed to proximal—as the critical site(s) mediating dopaminergic efficacy in RLS/PLMs.

The additional contribution of disparate supraspinal pathways and widespread disinhibition to the expression of RLS/PLMs is supported by many additional observations. Co-activation of axial, upper limb,[172] and bulbar (personal observations) muscles with PLMs, albeit uncommon, unequivocally implicates supraspinal networks in the pathophysiology of RLS. While the basal ganglia and their associated thalamocortical pathways are implicated by a plethora of correlative studies, there is little in the way of concrete data that establishes cause and effect. Lesioning of the internal globus pallidus to treat medically refractory Parkinson's disease (PD) improved bilateral RLS sensory symptoms, and preferentially benefited the contralateral leg, in a single patient.[202] Bilateral subthalamic nucleus stimulation produces inconsistent effects upon RLS in patients with coincident PD, with both detrimental[203] or beneficial[204] effects reported in small proportions of patients undergoing such surgeries, whereas deep brain stimulation of the ventralis intermedius nucleus of the thalamus does not benefit RLS in patients with coexistent essential tremor.[205] RLS with PLMs, and PLMs in isolation are common in the setting of strokes[206] and multiple sclerosis,[201,207] and are more frequently encountered with pathology located subcortically, and especially, infratentorially.

Neural hyperexcitability reflective of generalized disinhibition in RLS/PLMs has been documented in the motor cortex (notable in being reversible with dopamine agonists),[208–209] the brainstem,[175,210–211] and spinal sensorimotor circuits.[83,212–213] Cinematography demonstrates that PLMs involve flexion of the hip and knee, dorsiflexion of the ankle, and extension of the great toe that resemble the spinal defense reflex mechanism designed to withdraw the limb from painful stimuli (i.e., a Babinski response). This is a primitive, pathologic reflex that belies heightened excitability in neural elements comprising the flexor-reflex arc studied extensively by Sherrington. In RLS patients, the threshold to elicit this flexor-reflex is reduced in a state-dependent manner (i.e., during sleep), and it is exaggerated as manifest in spread of the response to muscles beyond the segmental reflex arc.[83,212] This likely reflects disruption of pre- and postsynaptic inhibitory mechanisms acting within the spinal cord, a pattern also present in PLMs occurring in the absence of sensory symptoms of RLS.[213] While we have discussed multiple brain circuits that may affect disinhibition of spinal cord sensorimotor and autonomic networks, it is undeniable that wherever their origin, they are exquisitively responsive to D_2-like dopamine, and opiate receptor agonists. The efficacy of dopamine agonists in symptomatic RLS/PLMs that emerges below the level of spinal cord injury,[55,214] the normal role of spinal D_3 dopamine receptors in dampening of the flexor-reflex[215] and sympathetic tone,[84] and the complete resolution of medically refractory RLS realized with intrathecal opiate delivery, [216–218] all reinforce the central role that the spinal cord networks play in the pathophysiology of RLS/PLMs.

Pain being closely related to pruritus (viz., itch) offers additional insights into the pathophysiologic basis of the sensory RLS experience. Face validity for comparisons between pruritus and RLS derives from shared urgencies to act to relieve the unpleasant sensations that attend both conditions. Construct validity derives from observations that spinothalamic neurons are integral to the transmission of itch and pain, *and* the sensory component of RLS,[55] and that movement inhibits both spinothalamic, itch-related neural activity in a state dependent manner,[219] and the obligatory urges of RLS. The interactions of itch and pain—and by inference, RLS—at the spinal level are complex,[220] yet increasingly direct attention to distinct neural and molecular substrates that could be exploited in the future as novel targets for relief from RLS.[221–222] The central representation of the sensorial/affectional aspects of pain, itch, and RLS also exhibit many similarities as revealed by a number of functional imaging modalities. Pain,[194] itch,[223] urges to move,[224] and sensory RLS[225–226] all activate the thalamus and anterior cingulate cortex which are components of a wider distributed brain network that subserves perception of unpleasant sensations and their cognitive and emotive qualities.[194] This network exhibits tremendous plasticity evident in reorganization of peripheral, spinal, and central substrates that impact wake–sleep state dependent perception and gating of sensory impulses. These considerations are relevant to RLS because it is generally a chronic and progressive condition with attendant affective comorbidites that often go untreated. Significance derives not only from the potential to advance discovery of novel treatment targets, but also because plasticity confounds attempts to distinguish the neuropharmacologic substrates underlying RLS sui generis from those possibly more reflective of disease chronicity or treatment.

In summary, because they are influenced by multiple genes and heterogenous molecular networks, RLS and PLMs are best viewed as complex traits. Both are influenced not by a single brain circuit that goes awry, but rather by any one of a multitude of peripheral and central nervous system pathways that converge upon the spinal cord. On the backdrop of a strong genetic diathesis, the expression of RLS/PLMs is favored. What remain to be discovered are how and where the implicated genes interact with the functional anatomy of RLS/PLMs, and whether these interactions identify unique pathways that can be exploited to predict, prevent, and better treat these disorders.

IRON AND DOPAMINE ALTERATIONS AND ADDITIONAL NEUROPHARMACOLOGIC CONSIDERATIONS

Theories about the pathophysiologic basis of RLS/PLMs have historically been dominated by discussions of iron deficiency as an environmental contributor to 'secondary' RLS, and the efficacy of dopaminomimetics in relieving both the sensory symptoms *and* motor signs of RLS.[227] An intimate interplay between systemic and brain iron and central dopaminergic tone is supported by clinical investigations, several neuroimaging modalities, analyses of autopsy tissue and cerebrospinal fluid, and experimental models of dietary iron deficiency.[28,227–229] Careful perusal of these data, together with clinical experience and newer experimental findings, much of it presented above, challenge the monolithic construct of brain iron deficiency, and a hypodopaminergic state, or a global brain 'dopaminergic abnormality', as inextricably bound to the causality of all RLS/PLMs. Simply put, there is scant evidence that either iron deficiency or a disorder of dopamine signaling is sufficient or necessary to cause RLS/PLMs in the general population of subjects who comprise idiopathic or 'primary' RLS/PLMs.

The incidence of RLS increases in normal and pathologic conditions in which iron deficiency is common and includes pregnancy, gastrointestinal conditions that interfere with iron absorption, and end-stage renal disease (ESRD). The degree of iron deficiency revealed by reductions in serum ferritin in idiopathic RLS correlates with sensory symptom severity.[230] Symptoms improve with oral repletion in confirmed iron deficiency,[230–232] and with intravenous iron repletion in ESRD-related iron deficiency.[233] One older uncontrolled study even suggested that irrespective of peripheral iron status, intravenous iron brought complete and prolonged symptom relief in 21 of 22 RLS subjects.[234] It was therefore reasoned that (1) iron deficiency is the mechanism underlying idiopathic RLS/PLMs; and (2) that this deficiency is restricted largely to the confines of the brain (and, therefore, not necessarily revealed by assessments of serum iron parameters). These are seductive hypotheses because diurnal variation in serum iron exhibits a robust amplitude with the peak to trough difference approaching 30–40% of the circardian mean[235–236]—the evening nadir coinciding with the peak time for RLS symptoms. Brain iron in animals is also influenced by diurnal cycle, sex, and systemic iron status, albeit, in complex ways,[237] and dietary iron deficiency impairs recycling and signaling of synaptic dopamine (see later).[238–240] A causal effect between iron deficiency and the sleep phenotype of RLS/PLMs is suggested by a single animal study,[241] but is difficult to establish because of a lack of consensus criteria for what constitutes validity in an animal model,[28] and because the transient fluxes in iron that attend blood donation may aggravate sleep in a non-specific manner (viz., RLS is not universally encountered).[242] Nonetheless, brain markers of iron metabolism have been interpreted to "consistently show evidence of iron insufficiency" in idiopathic RLS/PLMs and include studies of cerebrospinal fluid (CSF),[243–244] post-mortem brain tissue,[245–246] and magnetic resonance brain images.[247–249] A wide range or skewed distribution of values for some of the dependent variables of interest, an inability to control for their known or suspected diurnal fluctuations in the brain, small sample sizes (10–16 for CSF, 8 for autopsy tissue, and 5–40 for magnetic imaging), potential confounds such as age, sex, and disease and treatment duration, and selection bias, warrant pause before generalization of these findings to the RLS/PLMs population at large. Reductions in brain iron might be unique only to a subgroup of patients with early life disease onset and selectively affect the substantia nigra through mechanisms that remain obscure.[248] Transcranial B-mode sonography (TCS) has reasonable power to discriminate presumptive depletion of iron from the substantia nigra (SN) in idiopathic RLS,[250–251] particularly familial cases,[252] from healthy controls (positive predictive value of approximately 0.90). While ventral midbrain hypoechogenicity has been interpreted as reflective of decrements in cellular iron in the SN, this is not well established given that the same investigators noted *hyper*echogenecity in the adjacent, iron-rich red nucleus in the same RLS subjects,[252] and widespread abnormalities of cerebral white matter have been reported in RLS by diffusion tensor imaging.[253] Nigral hypoechogenecity also appears to be common in peripheral polyneuropathies, both a potential mimic and modifier of RLS—not only complicating interpretation of the biologic meaning of hyper- and hypoechogenicity, but also taking away from the diagnostic utility of TCS.[254]

The view that brain iron deficiency is a unifying mechanism causal to idiopathic and many "secondary" cases of RLS/PLMs does not translate smoothly to the bedside. First, clinical experience with iron deficient states and epidemiologic considerations are unambiguous that systemic iron deficiency is neither sufficient nor necessary to produce RLS/PLMs. A small cross-sectional study in a hematology clinic, for example, diagnosed RLS in only 40% of subjects documented to be iron deficient.[177] While RLS can emerge or worsen in nearly one-third of pregnant women, the correlations to iron parameters bear little to no relation to symptoms that otherwise resolve quickly after delivery despite the attendant loss of blood, and presumably iron.[23,255–257] Similarly, although RLS has been noted in frequent blood donors,[35] a systematic study failed to find a relationship of RLS symptoms to donation of three or less units of blood in 2000 donors in England.[258–259] Neither was an association between RLS and iron deficiency found in the only large, rigorous, population-based study of RLS that probed carefully for iron deficiency using sensitive metrics (e.g., soluble transferrin receptor).[260] Second, one open-label study,[261] and two randomized, double-blind, placebo-controlled studies[262–263] of intravenous iron for RLS have failed to conclusively demonstrate reliable efficacy. In a study of 1 gm of iron-dextran in 10 RLS subjects, there were 4 non-responders and there were few, if any, complete responders as assessed for PLMs (44 ± 27% reduction in PLMs).[261] This was despite posttreatment confirmation of iron accumulation in the prefrontal cortex and a trend for the substantia nigra for *both* nonresponders and responders. One placebo-controlled study of RLS subjects with normal systemic iron status demonstrated no benefit in an interim analysis and was therefore halted prematurely.[262] In a second study of intravenous iron sucrose in RLS with mild-to-moderate evidence of systemic iron deficiency, some positive symptom benefit was demonstrable, but not at all time points or in all subjects.[263] Much of the inconsistency between the iron deficiency hypothesis of RLS and these realities likely reflects a selection bias for more severely affected or refractory individuals who are more likely to present to specialized centers. Pathologically low mobilizable stores of iron as revealed by serum ferritin, in fact, are more frequently encountered in these settings than they are in the general population: 25% in 113 RLS subjects in one retrospective study,[264] and 14.6% and 44.4% with values of $\leq$15 ng/mL and $\leq$40 ng/mL, respectively, in our database of 437 RLS subjects. An additional counterweight to the hypothesis that iron deficiency is universal to RLS/PLMs, is the fact that the RLS susceptibility allele in the *BTBD9* gene predicts 13% lower ferritin per copy and accounts for only 50% of the population attributable risk.[72] Rather than a molecular network involving iron metabolism that is common to all individuals with idiopathic RLS/PLMs, this finding alone argues that it is potentially unique to the 65% of Europeans who carry this genetic variant.

In summary, when all the data is considered and given its appropriate weight, systemic or brain iron deficiency emerges as recognizable and reversible state that appears to modulate expression of RLS in a proportion of, but in no way approaching all, individuals with idiopathic RLS who are of northern European descent. The relationship of iron to PLMs, particularly their treatment, is much less clear. A reliable marker or algorithm for diagnosing RLS based on assessment of an iron metric derived from the brain or blood,[265] inclusive of testing for genetic at-risk variants, has not found its way to the clinic. Thus, despite the high prevalence of iron deficiency amongst subjects seeking treatment, there is still little data to go on to guide one's selection of patients who are deserving of treatment with iron, and which mode of delivery and formulation of iron should be used.

Given the efficacy of levodopa and dopamine agonists in relieving RLS/PLMs, and the basal ganglia being a principal arbiter of hypo- and hyperkinetic movement disorders, the original hypothesis of RLS/PLMs pathophysiogy focused around a hypodopaminergic state in nigrostriatal circuits. This hypothesis has endured because of several compelling correlates that include (1) the natural nadir in dopamine's synthesis, release, and signaling coinciding with the peak time for RLS/PLMs symptoms;[266] (2) iron being a cofactor for the rate-limiting enzyme in dopamine's synthesis (i.e., tyrosine hydroxylase; TH);[267–268] and (3) dietary iron deficiency impairing the recycling and signaling of synaptic dopamine in the basal ganglia.[238–240] Evidence of a hypodopaminergic state in the basal ganglia occurring independently, or because of, iron deficiency has not been forthcoming despite substantial and repeated efforts. Imaging modalities including SPECT and PET have failed to demonstrate significant or consistent alterations in pre- and post-synaptic markers that subserve dopamine signaling in the basal ganglia.[87,269–273] A deficiency of dopamine or disorder of alternate monoamines manifesting in lumbar CSF is also absent,[274–277] although finer discriminative analysis of metabolites suggests excess, as opposed to insufficient, quantities of dopamine.[278] Taken together with observations that lesions or stimulation of the basal ganglia have inconsistent effects upon RLS that occurs in the setting of PD (see earlier), evidence for diurnal fluctations in the efficiency of dopamine signaling in tuberoinfundibular pathways,[16] and the face and construct validities to alternate constructs that emphasize dopaminergic diencephalospinal pathways (see earlier), there is very little compelling reason to continue to envisage that the pathophysiologic basis of RLS/PLMs resides in hypo-functioning of dopamine related signaling pathways in the basal ganglia.

The diversity of dopaminergic pathways that govern wake–sleep states, the dose and receptor dependent characteristics of dopaminergic drugs, as well as the robust plasticity of the proteins involved in the synthesis, recycling, and signaling of dopamine, are significant challenges that need to be carefully accounted for as the field continues to endeavor to explain the efficacy of dopaminomimetics in idiopathic RLS/PLMs.[266] We have already touched upon the potential importance of pathways outside the confines of the basal ganglia as being involved in modulating RLS/PLMs. It is as important to recognize that pharmacologic agents targeted at dopaminergic signaling exhibit a biphasic dose-response relationship with many physiologic and behavioral readouts such as locomotion, pain sensitivity, blood pressure, prolactin secretion, oxytocin release, and heart rate.[279] It is therefore not unreasonable to presume that the same biologic substrates governing such biphasic relationships are also relevant to RLS/PLMs. Dose-dependency is in part accounted for by autoreceptor mediated presynaptic inhibition being a primary mechanism by which dopamine neuron excitability is governed.[266] Because D_2-like ($D_{2,3,4}$) receptors are the principal autoreceptors, and exhibit 10-fold higher affinities for dopamine, they appear best poised to mediate the benefits observed with the low doses of dopaminomimetics employed in RLS/PLMs. Particular interest in the D_3 receptor derives from the efficacy of the newer relatively, D_3 preferring agonists in treating RLS/PLMs, its exhibiting the lowest K_d for endogenous dopamine, and the fact that mice lacking a functional D_3 receptor exhibit electrophysiogic features at the spinal level[84,215] and behavioral attributes[189,280] that are consistent with what is observed in RLS/PLMs. Thus, peculiarities and heterogeneity intrinsic to dopamine pathways and receptors, render equal plausibility to two competing, but not necessarily mutually exclusive hypotheses. One that posits insufficient signaling at higher affinity G_i-coupled D_2-like receptors that are otherwise strategically positioned at supraspinal and spinal levels to suppress sensorimotor reponsiveness, and a second that emphasizes that higher levels recruit additional, lower-affinity G_s-coupled D_1-like and post-synaptic receptors that might facilitate sensorimotor processing. In this regard, it is interesting to note that dietary models of iron deficiency have consistently demonstrated an excess in extracellular striatal dopamine due to disordered pre-synaptic mechanisms governing dopamine's release (e.g., reductions in the dopamine-transporter and D_2-like receptors) as opposed to its synthesis.[238–240] Human RLS striatal autopsied tissue, and animals and cell lines depleted of iron, exhibit complementary reductions in D_2 receptors and particularly, elevations in active, phosphorylated tyrosine hydroxylase (THp) that have been interpreted as seminal evidence for an altered dopaminergic profile in RLS (albeit, one of hyper- versus hypodopaminergic functioning), and justification for continued investigation of dopamine signaling abnormalities in the basal ganglia as the bridge between iron deficiency and RLS/PLMs.[246] The claims hinge on analysis of brain tissue from only eight women with chronic RLS under varied treatment conditions are correlative as opposed to causal and did not comprehensively interrogate the status of other monoamines or brain regions relevant to expression of RLS/PLMs. The magnitude of natural physiologic variations in nearly all proteins that participate in dopamine signaling is also well within the ranges of those observed in this handful of RLS brains and cast further doubt on the saliency these results. Tyrosine hydroxylase and tetrahydrobiopterin (both necessary for dopamine synthesis), THp,[281] levodopa kinetics, the dopamine transporter, and dopamine receptor density and affinity are each influenced by diurnal and circadian factors, sex, and sleep deprivation in species as diverse as fruit flies[282] and humans[16] (reviewed in Ref. 266). Additional plasticity and complexity is evident in the membrane trafficking of many of the synaptic proteins that govern dopaminergic signaling.[283–286] Therefore, the precise mechanisms by which deficiencies in iron produce RLS/PLMs, and whether this occurs primarily, if not exclusively, by way of dopamine signaling abnormalities in nigrostriatal circuits, remain unknown. Distinguishing the contributions of individual dopamine neurons and dopaminoceptive structures to RLS/PLMs requires additional and substantial, anatomical, physiologic, and clinicopharmacologic data. A lot of heavy lifting remains before dopaminergic circuitry can be properly incorporated into a comprehensive heuristic model of RLS and PLMs.

The emerging view of RLS/PLMs is therefore one of complex traits, whose expression is not exclusively predicated upon any single nutrient or neurotransmitter. Undeniably, iron and dopaminergic tone are important determinants of trait expressivity in *some* patients, possibly a unique, more severely affected, medically refractory subpopulation of RLS sufferers who seek relief and volunteer for studies at tertiary referral centers. A final common pathway governing the expression of RLS/PLMs remains the holy grail of researchers in the field. Reliable animal or drosophila models and valid metrics that allow repeated, preferably noninvasive, assessments are necessary tools critical to unraveling the mysteries inherent to variable symptom expressivity.

▶ ASSESSMENT AND TREATMENT

The factors that impact diagnostic precision in RLS have been discussed in detail earlier. We now turn to aspects of the assessment that impact management and treatment of the patient. Realization of symptom relief from RLS demands a thorough clinical evaluation to rule out coexisting conditions that enhance RLS expressivity. There is an absence of evidence-based medicine as to the positive or negative effects of lifestyle and diet on RLS/PLMs. That said, sleep restriction, tobacco, alcohol, and caffeine have all been implicated in worsening of RLS[287] and should be avoided as recommended by consensus of expert opinion.[288] It has been our clinical experience that foods rich in vasoactive biogenic amines (e.g., tyramine and phenylethylamines) such as aged cheeses, red wine, chocolate, and fermented foods tend to exacerbate RLS. Medications known or suspected to worsen RLS should be discontinued when feasible. These include the nonspecific antihistamines (e.g., diphenhydramine and meclizine), dopamine antagonists, antidepressants, neuroleptics, and lithium.[66,287,289–290] Of the selective serotonin (SSRI) norepinephrine (SNRI) and mixed reuptake inhibitors, mirtazapine appears to have the highest rate of new or worsened RLS (occurring in 28% of treated patients, versus 9% of patients treated with any SSRI or SNRI).[66] If treatment of comorbid depression is necessary, we prefer agents with the least evidence for norepinephrine reuptake blockade, and often prescribe bupropion because it and its metabolite are relatively selective for the dopamine transporter, and by itself has been anecdotally noted to improve RLS symptoms.[291–292] Proton pump inhibitors (PPI) also have the potential to aggravate RLS by interfering with iron absorption secondary to increased duodenal pH.[293] We have encountered this phenomenon within weeks of a PPI being prescribed, suggesting that the curve describing the relationship of systemic iron availability to RLS symptom severity might be quite steep in some individuals.

Another common exogenous factor influencing RLS expressivity is iron deficiency, and this should be routinely assessed for at the initial evaluation and at yearly follow-up. Because a substantial number (~two-thirds of our clinic population) of iron-deficient RLS patients do not exhibit coexisting anemia (i.e., they have preanemic iron deficiency), and ferritin being an acute-phase reactant prone to false elevations, a complete serum iron panel (iron, total iron binding capacity, percent transferrin saturation, and ferritin) is preferred. We are particularly vigilant in assessing serum iron parameters in subjects with comorbid gastrointestinal pathologies (e.g., gastric stapling or bypass and celiac disease) in whom iron deficiency is common and appears contributory to RLS.[44–47] We also regularly assess for vitamin B_{12} and folate as their malabsorption can also occur in these conditions, and theoretically interfere with dopamine synthesis since each is required for the biosynthesis of tetrahydrobiopterin (a cofactor for tyrosine hydroxylase).[294] One small open-label study of oral folate to treat RLS in the setting of documented deficiencies of folate demonstrated good results.[295] In the larger population of idiopathic, primary RLS, folate and vitamin B_{12} deficiencies are no more common than observed in controls.[230,296]

The RLS Foundation treatment algorithm recommends iron repletion when ferritin is below 20 ng/mL and consideration of iron repletion on a case-by-case basis when the ferritin is between 20 and 50 ng/mL.[288] Although this is an expert guideline, data to support iron supplementation are still mixed, as already discussed. A randomized, controlled trial of oral iron sulfate in RLS patients not stratified by iron status did not reflect a benefit on sleep or RLS symptoms.[297] The subset of patients whose RLS improved were those who exhibited significant increases in iron parameters. A more recent randomized, controlled trial of oral iron in RLS patients with low-normal ferritin did show a significant reduction in RLS severity.[232] The use of intravenous (IV) iron formulations is less clear as we have already discussed, with benefits reasonably well established only in patients with end-stage renal disease.[233] Although a ferritin of ≤50 ng/mL does not appear to interfere with response to dopaminergic therapy for RLS,[298] very low ferritins of ≤20 ng/mL do increase the risk of treatment complications, specifically, augmentation.[299] If reduced availability of iron is suspected or confirmed, the first step is to educate the patient on factors that can interfere with absorption of dietary or supplemental sources of iron. Dietary iron comes in two sources: heme- and nonheme iron. The former is derived from animal sources and in red greater than white meat, and is efficiently absorbed due to its solubility. Nonheme iron, derived from vegetables and grains, is less efficiently absorbed in the presence of phytates, oxalates, and phenols, metallic elements (e.g., magnesium, manganese, zinc, calcium, and copper) with which it competes for absorption, and in alkalinized environments where it has a proclivity to form insoluble complexes. Thus, dietary or supplemental iron should preferably be ingested on an empty stomach absent excessive additional nutritional supplements, antacids, or beverages containing tannic acid (e.g., teas, coffees, and many red wines). Ascorbic acid (i.e., vitamin C) containing supplements or foods/juices significantly enhance absorption of nonheme iron when taken on an empty stomach. A number of formulations of both nonheme and heme iron are available when oral supplementation is desired. In oral form, there are several different salts and formulations, including ferrous sulfate, ferrous gluconate, and ferrous fumarate. Dosing that provides 100–200 mg of elemental iron per day is preferred over conventional, daily multivitamins and prenatal vitamins that contain 27–65 mg of iron. Many preparations cause gastrointestinal side effects such as constipation, diarrhea, nausea, and abdominal pain. These side effects can be minimized by reducing the amount of elemental iron absorbed, either by taking the iron with food, lowering the dose of iron, or using a preparation with a relatively low amount of elemental iron such as ferrous gluconate.[300] The time to repletion of iron with a goal of ferritin >50 ng/mL and a transferrin saturation >20% is dependent on many factors and therefore highly variable. We typically institute treatment for 6–8 weeks before adjusting recommendations on the basis of a reassessment of serum iron parameters. Several intravenous formulations of iron are also available. Of these, iron dextran has the highest rate of serious anaphylaxis (0.6–0.7%) and other adverse events, present in up to 50% of patients.[301] Iron sucrose and ferric gluconate have lower rates of serious anaphylaxis (0.002% and 0.04%, respectively) and adverse events (36% and 35%),[301] although their use outside of chronic renal failure constitutes off-label use and the single negative study of iron sucrose in RLS raises questions about its efficacy relative to iron dextran. We reserve use only for those patients with documented severe iron deficiency (e.g., ferritin <10 ng/mL, transferrin saturations <15%, and/or iron <25 ug/dL [females]/45ug/dL [males]) *and* refractoriness to pharmacologic interventions, *and* in whom the risks associated with RLS related sleep restriction to <3–4 hours/night are greater than those posed by a course of intravenous iron treatments.

When pharmacologic treatment for RLS is needed, the first line of treatment is dopaminergic agents. It is important to bear in mind that many clinical trials establishing efficacy of dopaminomimetics excluded individuals with suspected iron deficiency because this was a suspected "cause" of secondary RLS/PLMs (e.g., ferritin <15–20 ng/mL) and were largely derived from patient populations that are two-thirds women, and therefore might not be generalizable to every clinician's practice. The only two medications presently approved by the United States Food & Drug Administration (FDA) for treatment of RLS are the dopamine agonists ropinirole and pramipexole. Dopamine agonists alleviate RLS symptoms in 70–90% of patients in randomized trials.[302] Placebo effects in RLS are notable,[303] consistent with evolving views that they are more common in disorders such as RLS where "top-down" mechanisms are implicated in disease pathophysiology.[304] Pramipexole is a non-ergot-derived dopamine D_3- and D_2-receptor agonist that has been proven efficacious for both RLS and PLMs.[305–309] The mean effective daily dose ranges from 0.25 to 1 mg,[310] although little added benefit is evident at doses exceeding 0.5 mg in most patients. The authors' clinical experience, particularly in older men, suggests that higher total doses (0.5–1.5 mg) given in a divided manner may be needed for complete symptom relief. Pramipexole is exclusively excreted by the kidneys, and dosing guidelines therefore suggest a more cautious, slower dosing titration in the setting of impaired creatinine clearances and ESRD. Ropinirole is another non-ergot-derived dopamine agonist that also acts preferentially on D_3 and D_2 receptor subtypes, and is effective for RLS and PLMs.[311–315] The mean effective daily dose of ropinirole is approximately 2 mg.[310] Ropinirole is metabolized through the CYP1A2 isoenzyme of the cytochrome P450 system, and has important drug interactions with inhibitors and inducers (including nicotine) of this system. Because of this, warfarin levels can be increased by concomitant use of ropinirole, making pramipexole a potentially safer choice in patients on warfarin. Since plasma concentrations for both pramipexole and ropinirole peak nearly 2 hours after ingestion, it is critical to dose these medications several hours before symptom onset. We often split dosing at the evening meal and again at bedtime rather than dosing on an as-needed basis to enhance compliance and achieve efficacy that persists throughout the entire rest and sleep periods. A direct comparison of these two agents has not been conducted, although one industry-sponsored meta-analysis suggests a slight superiority for pramipexole, as assessed by improvement in the International RLS Study Group's rating scale, and a more favorable side effect profile.[316] Extended release formulations of both pramipexole and ropinirole exist and are approved for use in PD, however, there are no published controlled trial data for RLS. Cabergoline is an ergot-derived dopamine agonist that is a particularly effective RLS treatment given its very long elimination half-life,[317–320] but because ergot-derived dopamine agonists carry some risk for valvular heart disease, albeit minor,[321] cabergoline is not considered a first line therapy for RLS.

Transdermal delivery of dopamine agonists has also been investigated for the treatment of RLS. Continuous administration via transdermal application potentially could lead to fewer side effects by maintaining more stable plasma levels[322] and benefit patients with daytime symptoms.[323] Pilot and open-label data support the use of rotigotine[323–324] and lisuride[322] for RLS. Rotigotine is available in parts of Europe, although it was recently removed from the market in the United States due to crystallization of medication within the patch substrate. Lisuride is an ergot-derived dopamine agonist, but long-term safety (especially regarding the potential for development of fibrotic disease) is not known.[310] The adverse effects associated with dopamine agonists include nausea, somnolence, headache, dizziness, rhinitis, and peripheral edema.

Dopamine can also be supplied directly in the form of levodopa for the treatment of RLS. Although levodopa is effective for RLS, it appears to be more reliably associated with the development of augmentation than the dopamine agonists, which can limit its usefulness.[325] However, for patients with sporadic symptoms who need a "rescue" medication but not a daily prophylactic medication, levodopa (100 to 200 mg) is a good choice because of its rapid onset of action. Side effects of levodopa are similar to those of the dopamine agonists and include hypotension, hallucinations, sleepiness, and gastrointestinal discomfort.

▶ **TABLE 46–1. PHARMACOLOGIC TREATMENTS FOR RLS**

First Line	
Dopamine agonists	
Pramipexole	0.25–0.75 mg
Ropinirole	0.25–4 mg
Second Line[a]	
Gabapentin	800–3000 mg
Levodopa	100–200 mg
Third Line[a]	
Oxycodone	5–30 mg
Carbamazepine	200–400 mg
Valproic acid	600 mg
Clonidine	0.1–0.5 mg
Transdermal rotigotine	0.5–4 mg
Cabergoline	0.5–2 mg
Investigational[a]	
Methadone	10–40 mg
Tramadol	50–200 mg
Clonazepam	0.25–1 mg
Zolpidem	2.5–10 mg
Amantadine	100–300 mg
Transdermal lisuride	3–6 mg q.o.d.

[a]Use of these medications constitutes "off-label" use in the United States.

Several other classes of medications have been used for the treatment of RLS (Table 46–1). The Movement Disorders Society (MDS) recently appointed a task force to review the evidence for RLS treatments. Based on this systematic review, the MDS task force classified gabapentin as effective for RLS (in addition to dopaminergic agents).[310] The mean effective daily dose of gabapentin was 1855 mg/day, divided into two daily doses.[178] Patients with painful RLS benefited more than patients without pain did. Open-label investigation of pregabalin, a related compound, has shown preliminary support for its benefit in RLS.[326] A larger, placebo controlled trial has extended this experience in demonstrating clinical and polysomnographic improvements with pregabalin.[327] A gabapentin prodrug (currently designated XP13512/GSK 1838262) is under development for use in RLS, with data from two randomized, controlled trials suggesting that a single daily dose can significantly improve RLS signs and symptoms with a positive benefit upon sleep.[328,329]

The MDS task force identified several other medications as "likely efficacious" in RLS based on the level of evidence supporting their use. These included oxycodone, carbamazepine, valproic acid, and clonidine.[310] Given concerns about long-term use of opioid treatment, Walters and colleagues reviewed their experience with 36 patients who had attempted opioid monotherapy for RLS.[330] Of these, 20 patients remained on monotherapy for an average of almost 6 years. Of the one-third of patients who did not remain on monotherapy, eight had discontinued due to side effects, seven had an incomplete response, and only one patient developed signs of tolerance and addiction. Of note, when 7 of the 20 patients who remained on monotherapy were studied with polysomnography, 2 had developed new sleep apnea and a third showed exacerbation of previously diagnosed apnea.[330] These results suggest that opioids may have long-term effectiveness for some patients with RLS, but that side effects and sleep-disordered breathing may interfere with treatment in a subgroup. Clonidine was shown to be effective for RLS, but not PLMs, in a single small, controlled trial.[331] Other medications considered investigational by the MDS task force include methadone, tramadol, clonazepam, zolpidem, and amantadine.[310]

Several nonpharmacologic or nonprescription interventions are also under investigation for use in RLS. A small randomized, controlled trial comparing pneumatic compression devices to sham devices, both used for at least 1 hour a day before typical symptom onset, showed significant benefits in RLS severity.[332] In patients with coexisting superficial venous insufficiency and RLS, treatment with endovascular laser ablation significantly reduced RLS symptoms compared to a no-treatment placebo group.[333] Several groups have investigated the use of acupuncture for RLS, but presently there is insufficient evidence to support or refute its use.[334] Botulinum toxin injection has been attempted as treatment for RLS, with promising early results from a case series[335] that has not been corroborated by a single, small but blinded and controlled clinical trial.[336] Magnesium and folate supplementation do not have sufficient evidence to support their use except as experimental therapy.[310] Exercise (aerobic and lower body conditioning) may reduce RLS symptoms,[337] but is still considered investigational.[310] Transcutaneous, neuromuscular stimulation of the legs for 30 minutes before sleep significantly reduces PLMs in the absence of RLS with a trend for improvement in sleep continuity.[338]

TREATMENT COMPLICATIONS

Augmentation is a troubling clinical phenomenon, unique to RLS, that follows a period of effective pharmacologic intervention and then tolerance, and manifests as worsening of RLS symptoms. Augmentation needs to be distinguished from symptom rebound, which is the emergence of symptoms at a time consistent with the half-life of the drug. Rebound is encountered more frequently with dopaminergic agents with shorter half-lives and typically manifests late in the sleep period or early in the morning. It occurs in at least one-quarter of patients treated with levodopa,[339] yet it is rarely a clinically relevant problem. Management includes switching to an agent with a longer half-life, or split dosing with the latter dose taken immediately at bedtime. In the instance of augmentation, symptoms typically become more frequent and severe than in the pretreatment condition. Increased severity manifests as either the occurrence of symptoms by at least 4 hours earlier in the day or at least two of the following: spread of symptoms to previously unaffected body parts such as the arms; more rapid symptom onset on becoming inactive; increase in symptom intensity; shorter duration of treatment effect; or the appearance of PLMw.[340] The most specific feature of augmentation, appears to be the emergence of RLS symptoms earlier in the day, while the most sensitive symptom is an increase in symptom intensity.[325] Augmentation can range from a minor problem to a severe clinical complication. Augmentation occurs predominantly with dopaminergic medications but has also been reported to occur with tramadol.[341] Estimates of augmentation rates are limited by the short duration of most RLS clinical trials (weeks to months) in comparison with the length of time augmentation takes to develop (months to years) and by a lack of systematic methods to evaluate augmentation[310] before the recent publication of an augmentation rating scale.[342] Data suggest that levodopa has a rate of augmentation as high as 60–73%[128,342] while rates for pramipexole are lower (8–56%); reliable rates for ropinirole have not published.[128] It is the authors' clinical experience that augmentation rates with ropinirole are as least as high as those reported for pramipexole. Risk for augmentation is higher amongst individuals free of neuropathy who have previously experienced augmentation with alternate dopaminergics, a family history of RLS,[343] and those with serum ferritins <20 ng/mL.[299] The latter being modifiable, we routinely reassess serum iron parameters when tolerance or augmentation are encountered, and prescribe oral iron supplements to replete ferritins to >50 ng/mL. Mild cases of augmentation may be treated by moving the medication dosage earlier in the day,[128] or by split dosing. For more severe cases, the patient should be transitioned to a different medication, typically gabapentin or an opiate.[128] In our and others'[344] experience, methadone (10–40 mg) in divided doses is an effective alternative in severe, refractory RLS, and particularly in severe cases of augmentation. Changing from one dopamine agonist to another in cases of augmentation is controversial[128] but can be beneficial.[288] To avoid the development of tolerance and augmentation, a strategy of rotation amongst agents from various drug classes (e.g., dopaminergics, opiates, gabapentin, and even benzodiazepines) has been advocated.[345]

There have been recent reports of compulsive behaviors associated with the treatment of RLS with dopaminergic agents.[346–347] One questionnaire-based study found that 6% of RLS patients experienced increased urges to gamble and increased time spent gambling after starting dopaminergic medications and 4% noted increased sexual desire.[348] In patients with either RLS or PD taking dopamine agonists, younger age and higher doses of dopamine agonists were risk factors for the development of increased gambling, spending, or sexual activity.[349] A preliminary controlled trial suggests that impulse control disorders (e.g., compulsive spending, pathologic gambling, punding, and hypersexuality) develop in from 3–9% of RLS subjects treated with dopamine agonist therapy.[350] Patients should be alerted to this potentially serious complication, although prospective, longitudinal studies with validated measures of impulse control are needed to clarify any cause–effect relationship. Recent functional imaging in RLS patients suggests that this potential propensity to impulse control disorders may reside in dopaminergic activation of ventral striatal reward circuits.[351]

TREATMENT IN SPECIAL CLINICAL SITUATIONS

Patients with ESRD have a high prevalence of RLS, ranging from 6.6 to 62% of dialysis patients, with similar prevalence in patients receiving peritoneal dialysis and hemodialysis.[352] Dialysis itself does not relieve the symptoms of RLS, but renal transplantation frequently does.[353–354] As with idiopathic RLS, dopaminergic medications are considered first line therapy for patients with ESRD.[352] Pramipexole and levodopa are both effective in this population.[352,355] Nondopaminergic therapies used in primary RLS have also been studied and shown to be beneficial in uremic patients, including clonazepam, gabapentin, and clonidine.[352] Since gabapentin is renally excreted, it is critical to limit its dosing to the postdialysis period and not nightly.

RLS in pregnancy presents a particular challenge because medications typically used in the treatment of RLS are not considered safe in pregnancy. RLS medications that are FDA class C (for which animal data demonstrate harm but no human data exist, or for which neither animal nor human data exist) include ropinirole, pramipexole, levodopa, clonidine, and gabapentin. Medications that are pregnancy class D (having evidence of fetal risk in human studies) include carbamazepine and some benzodiazepines. Additionally, infants born to mothers taking benzodiazepines or opioids near the end of pregnancy are at risk for withdrawal symptoms.[356] Thus, nonpharmacologic therapies should be used when possible. Iron deficiency should be corrected when present in pregnancy and some authors propose the use of magnesium for the treatment of RLS based on cases of RLS improving when pregnant women are given intravenous magnesium for tocolysis.[357] Contributions of iron, vitamin B_{12}, or folate deficiencies to pregnancy related RLS are unclear, yet, attention to serum folate status might be most relevant. Lower serum folates as opposed to ferritin or vitamin B_{12} have been associated with RLS in the 3rd trimester,[255] and addition of folate to multivitamin and iron supplementation demonstrated superiority in alleviating pregnancy related RLS.[358] Similarly, while no differences in serologic measures of ferritin, vitamin B_{12} or folate were noted in another study of pregnant women with RLS, RLS was less frequently observed in those taking prenatal vitamins.[256]

REFERENCES

1. Allen R, Hening W, Montplaisir J, et al. Restless legs syndrome: Diagnostic criteria, special considerations, and epidemiology: A report from the RLS diagnosis and epidemiology workshop at the national instititutes of health. Sleep Med 2003;4:101–119.
2. Lazzarini A, Walters AS, Hickey K, et al. Studies of penetrance and anticipation in five autosomal-dominant restless legs syndrome pedigrees. Mov Disord 1999;14(1):111–116.
3. Ondo W and Jankovic J. Restless legs syndrome: Clinicoetiologic correlates. Neurology 1996;47:1435–1441.
4. Trenkwalder C, Collado-Seidel V, Gasser T, et al. Clinical symptoms and possible anticipation in a large kindred of familial restless legs syndrome. Mov Disord 1996;11: 389–394.
5. Walters A, Picchietti D, Hening W, et al. Variable expressivity in familial restless legs syndrome. Arch Neurol 1990;47:1219–1220.
6. Hening W, Walters A, Allen R, et al. Impact, diagnosis and treatment of restless legs syndrome (rls) in a primary care population: The rest (rls epidemiology, symptoms, and treatment) primary care study. Sleep Med 2004;5:237–246.
7. Allen RP, Walters AS, Montplaisir J, et al. Restless legs syndrome prevalence and impact: Rest general population study. Arch Intern Med 2005;165(11):1286–1292.
8. Happe S, Vennemann M, Evers S, et al. Treatment wish of individuals with known and unknown restless legs syndrome in the community. J Neurol 2008;255:1365–1371.
9. Lavigne G and Montplaisir J: Restless legs syndrome and sleep bruxism: Prevalence and association among canadians. Sleep 1994;17:739–743.
10. Phillips B, Young T, Finn L, et al. Epidemiology of restless legs symptoms in adults. Arch Int Med 2000;160: 2137–2141.
11. Ulfberg J, Bjorvatn B, Leissner L, et al. Comorbidity in restless legs syndrome among a sample of swedish adults. Sleep Med 2007;8:768–772.
12. Ulfberg J, Nystrom B, Carter N, et al. Prevalence of restless legs syndrome among men aged 18 to 64 years: An association with somatic disease and neuropsychiatric symptoms. Mov Disord 2001;16:1159–1163.
13. O'Keeffe ST, Egan D, Myers A, et al. The frequency and impact of restless legs syndrome in primary care. Ir Med J 2007;100(7):539–542.
14. Michaud M, Dumont M, Selmaoui B, et al. Circadian rhythm of restless legs syndrome: Relationship with biological markers. Ann Neurol 2004;55:372–380.
15. Trenkwalder C, Hening WA, Walters AS, et al. Circadian rhythm of periodic limb movements and sensory symptoms of restless legs syndrome [in process citation]. Mov Disord 1999;14(1):102–110.
16. Garcia-Borreguero D, Larrosa O, Granizo J, et al. Circadian variation in neuroendocrine response to l-dopa in patients with restless legs syndrome. Sleep 2004;27:669–673.
17. Duffy J, Lowe A, Winkelman J, et al. Peak circadian occurrence of plms during the biological nighttime. Sleep 2005;Abst Suppl:A275.
18. Baier P and Trenkwalder C. Circadian variation in restless legs syndrome. Sleep Med 2007;8(6):645–650.
19. Picchietti D, Allen R, Walters A, et al. Restless legs syndrome: Prevalence and impact in children and adolescents-the peds rest study. Sleep (in press).
20. Picchietti D and Stevens H. Early manifestations of restless legs syndrome in childhood and adolescence. Sleep Med 2007;22:297–300.
21. Trotti LM Bliwise D, Greer SA, et al. Correlates of plms variability over multiple nights and impact upon rls diagnosis. Sleep Med 2009;10(6):668–671.
22. Lamberg L: Sleeping poorly while pregnant may not be "Normal". JAMA 2006;295(12):1357–1361.
23. Manconi M, Govoni V, De Vito A, et al. Restless legs syndrome and pregnancy. Neurology 2004;63:1065–1069.
24. Berger K, Luedemann J, Trenkwalder C, et al. Sex and the risk of restless legs syndrome in the general population. Arch Int Med 2004;164:196–202.
25. Kemlink D, Polo O, Montagna P, et al. Family-based association study of the restless legs syndrome loci 2 and 3 in a european population. Mov Disord 2007;22(2):207–212.
26. Desai A, Cherkas L, Spector T, et al. Genetic influences in self-reported symptoms of obstructive sleep apnoea and restless legs syndrome: A twin study. Twin Res 2004;7:589–595.
27. Ondo WG, Vuong KD, and Wang Q. Restless legs syndrome in monozygotic twins. Neurology 2000;55(9): 1404–1406.
28. Earley C, Allen R, Beard J, et al. Insight into the pathophysiology of restless legs syndrome. J Neurosci Res 200062(5):623–628.
29. Chen S, Ondo W, Rao S, et al. Genomewide linkage scan identifies a novel susceptibility locus for restless legs syndrome on chromosome 9p. Am J Hum Genet 2004;74:876–885.
30. Tan E, Seah A, See S, et al. Restless legs syndrome in an asian population: A study in singapore. Mov Disord 2001;16:577–579.
31. Cho SJ, Hong JP, Hahm BJ, et al. Restless legs syndrome in a community sample of korean adults: Prevalence, impact on quality of life, and association with dsm-iv psychiatric disorders. Sleep 2009;32(8):1069–1076.
32. Castillo PR, Kaplan J, Lin SC, et al. Prevalence of restless legs syndrome among native South Americans residing in coastal and mountainous areas. Mayo Clin Proc 2006;81(10):1345–1347.
33. Sevim S, Dogu O, Camdeviren H, et al. Unexpectedly low prevalence and unusual characteristics of rls in mersin, turkey. Neurology 2003;61(11):1562–1569.
34. Inoue Y, Ishizuka T, and Arai H. Surveillance on epidemiology and treatment of restless legs syndrome in japan. J New Rem Clim 2000;49:244–254.
35. Silber M and Richardson J. Multiple blood donations associated with iron deficiency in patients with restless legs syndrome. Mayo Clin Proc 2003;78:52–54.

36. Winkelman JW, Chertow GM, and Lazarus JM. Restless legs syndrome in end-stage renal disease. Am J Kidney Dis 1996;28(3):372–378.
37. Hening WA and Caivano CK. Restless legs syndrome: A common disorder in patients with rheumatologic conditions. Semin Arthritis Rheu 2008;38(1):55–62.
38. Merlino G, Fratticci L, Valente M, et al. Association of restless legs syndrome in type 2 diabetes: A case-control study. Sleep 2007;30(7):866–871.
39. Minai OA, Malik N, Foldvary N, et al. Prevalence and characteristics of restless legs syndrome in patients with pulmonary hypertension. J Heart Lung Transplant 2008;27(3):335–340.
40. Kaplan Y, Inonu H, Yilmaz A, et al. Restless legs syndrome in patients with chronic obstructive pulmonary disease. Can J Neurol Sci 2008;35(3):352–357.
41. Lo Coco D, Mattaliano A, Lo Coco A, et al. Increased frequency of restless legs syndrome in chronic obstructive pulmonary disease patients. Sleep Med 2009;10(5): 572–576.
42. Franco RA, Ashwathnarayan R, Deshpandee A, et al. The high prevalence of restless legs syndrome symptoms in liver disease in an academic-based hepatology practice. J Clin Sleep Med 2008;4(1):45–49.
43. Weinstock LB, Bosworth BP, Scherl EJ, et al. Crohn's disease is associated with restless legs syndrome. Inflamm Bowel Dis 2009.
44. Manchanda S, Davies CR, and Picchietti D. Celiac disease as a possible cause for low serum ferritin in patients with restless legs syndrome. Sleep Med 2009;10(7):763–765.
45. Weinstock LB, Walters AS, Mullin GE, et al. Celiac disease is associated with restless legs syndrome. Dig Dis Sci 2009.
46. Banerji NK and Hurwitz LJ. Restless legs syndrome, with particular reference to its occurrence after gastric surgery. Br Med J 1970;4(5738):774–775.
47. Weinstock LB, Fern SE, and Duntley SP. Restless legs syndrome in patients with irritable bowel syndrome: Response to small intestinal bacterial overgrowth therapy. Dig is Sci. 2008;53(5):1252–1256.
48. Cologno D, Cicarelli G, Petretta V, et al. High prevalence of dopaminergic premonitory symptoms in migraine patients with restless legs syndrome: A pathogenetic link? Neurol Sci 2008;29(suppl 1):S166–S168.
49. Rhode AM, Hosing VG, Happe S, et al. Comorbidity of migraine and restless legs syndrome-a case-control study. Cephalalgia 2007;27(11):1255–1260.
50. Poewe W, and Hogl B: Akathisia, restless legs, and periodic limb movements in sleep in Parkinson's disease Neurology 2004;63(suppl 3):S12–S16.
51. Nomura T, Inoue Y, Miyake M, et al. Prevalence and clinical characteristics of restless legs syndrome in japanese patients with parkinson's disease. Mov Disord 2006;21(3):380–384.
52. Gomez-Esteban, JC, Zarranz JJ, Tijero B, et al. Restless legs syndrome in parkinson's disease. Mov Disord 2007;22(13):1912–1916.
53. Calzetti S, Negrotti A, Bonavina G, et al. Absence of comorbidity of parkinson disease and restless legs syndrome: A case-control study in patients attending a movement disorders clinic. Neurol Sci 2009;30:119–122.
54. Lee J, Shin H, Kim K, et al. Factors contributing to the development of restless legs syndrome in patients with parkinson disease. Mov Disord 2009;24(4):579–582.
55. Trotti LM, and Rye DB. Functional anatomy and treatment of rls/plms emerging after spinal cord lesions. Sleep 2007;30:A306.
56. Gemignani F, Marbini A, Di Giovanni G, et al. Charcot-marie-tooth disease type 2 with restless legs syndrome. Neurology 1999;52(5):1064–1066.
57. Abele M, Burk K, Laccone F, et al. Restless legs syndrome in spinocerebellar ataxia types 1, 2, and 3. J Neurol 2001;248(4):311–314.
58. Schöls L, Haan J, Riess O, et al. Sleep disturbance in spinocerebellar ataxias. Is the sca3 mutation a cause of restless leg syndrome? J Neurol 1998;51:1603–1607.
59. Tuin I, Voss U, Kang JS, et al. Stages of sleep pathology in spinocerebellar ataxia type 2 (sca2). Neurology 2006;67(11):1966–1972.
60. Manconi M, Fabbrini M, Bonanni E, et al. High prevalence of restless legs syndrome in multiple sclerosis. Eur J Neurol 2007;14(5):534–539.
61. Benes H, von Eye A, and Kohnen R. Empirical evaluation of the accuracy of diagnostic criteria for restless legs syndrome. Sleep Med 2008;10(5):524–530.
62. Stiasny-Kolster K, Kohnen R, Moller JC, et al. Validation of the "L-dopa test" For diagnosis of restless legs syndrome. Mov Disord 2006;21(9):1333–1339.
63. Salin-Pascual R, Galicia-Polo L, and Drucker-Colin R: Sleep changes after 4 consecutive days of venlafaxine administration in normal volunteers. J Clin Psychiatry 1997;58(8):348–350.
64. Yang C, White DP, and Winkelman JW. Antidepressants and periodic leg movements of sleep. Biol Psychiatry 2005;58(6):510–514.
65. Page RL, 2nd, Ruscin JM, Bainbridge JL, et al. Restless legs syndrome induced by escitalopram: Case report and review of the literature. Pharmacotherapy 2008;28(2): 271–280.
66. Rottach KG, Schaner BM, Kirch MH, et al. Restless legs syndrome as side effect of second generation antidepressants. J Psychiatr Res 2008;43(1):70–75.
67. Fox EJ, Villanueva R, and Schutta HS. Myoclonus following spinal anesthesia. Neurology 1979;29(3):379–380.
68. Lee MS, Lyoo CH, Kim WC, et al. Periodic bursts of rhythmic dyskinesia associated with spinal anesthesia. Mov Disord 1997;12(5):816–817.
69. Nadkarni AV and Tondare AS. Localized clonic convulsions after spinal anesthesia with lidocaine and epinephrine. Anesth Analg 1982;61(11):945–947.
70. Watanabe S, Sakai K, Ono Y, et al. Alternating periodic leg movement induced by spinal anesthesia in an elderly male. Anesth Analg 1987;66(10):1031–1032.
71. Hogl B, Frauscher B, Seppi K, et al. Transient restless legs syndrome after spinal anesthesia: A prospective study. Neurology 2002;59(11):1705–1707.
72. Stefansson H, Rye DB, Hicks A, et al. A genetic risk factor for periodic limb movements in sleep.[see comment]. New Eng J Med 2007;357(7):639–647.
73. Hening WA. Subjective and objective criteria in the diagnosis of the restless legs syndrome. Sleep Med 2004;5(3):285–292.

74. Hening W, Allen R, Washburn M, et al. The four diagnostic criteria for restless legs syndrome are unable to exclude confounding conditions ("Mimics"). Sleep Med 2009;10(9):976–981.
75. Benes H, Walters AS, Allen RP, et al. Definition of restless legs syndrome, how to diagnose it, and how to differentiate it from rls mimics. Mov Disord 2007;22(suppl 18):S401–S408.
76. Chaudhuri KR, Rye DB, and Muzerengi S. Differential diagnosis of RLS. In Chaudhuri KR, Ferini-Strambi L, and Rye DB (eds). Restless Legs Syndrome. Oxford: Oxford University Press, 2008, pp. 35–43.
77. Spillane JD, Nathan PW, Kelly RE, et al. Painful legs and moving toes. Brain 1971;94(3):541–556.
78. Dressler D, Thompson PD, Gledhill RF, et al. The syndrome of painful legs and moving toes. Mov Disord 1994;9(1):13–21.
79. Dziewas R, Kuhlenbaumer G, Okegwo A, et al. Painless legs and moving toes in a mother and her daughter. Mov Disord 2003;18(6):718–722.
80. Sandyk R. Neuroleptic-induced "Painful legs and moving toes" Syndrome: Successful treatment with clonazepam and baclofen. Ital J Neurol Sci 1990;11(6):573–576.
81. Alvarez MV, Driver-Dunckley EE, Caviness JN, et al. Case series of painful legs and moving toes: Clinical and electrophysiologic observations. Mov Disord 2008;23(14): 2062–2066.
82. Montplaisir J, Boucher S, Poirier G, et al. Clinical, polysomnographic, and genetic characteristics of restless legs syndrome: A study of 133 patients diagnosed with new standard criteria. Mov Disord 1997;12:61–65.
83. Bara-Jimenez W, Aksu M, Graham B, et al. Periodic limb movements in sleep—state dependent excitability of the spinal flexor reflex. Neurology 2000;54:1609–1615.
84. Clemens S, Rye D, and Hochman S. Restless legs syndrome: Revisiting the dopamine hypothesis from the spinal cord perspective. Neurology 2006;67(1):125–130.
85. Ferri, R, Zucconi M, Manconi M, et al. New approaches to the study of periodic leg movements during sleep in restless legs syndrome. Sleep 2006;29(6):759–769.
86. Pennestri MH, Whittom S, Adam B, et al. Plms and plmw in healthy subjects as a function of age: Prevalence and interval distribution. Sleep 2006;29(9):1183–1187.
87. Michaud M, Soucy J, Chabli A, et al. Spect imaging of striatal pre- and postsynaptic dopaminergic status in restless legs syndrome with periodic leg movements in sleep. J Neurol 2002;249:164–170.
88. Rye D, Bliwise D, Iranzo A, et al. A novel 2-step diagnostic approach for rls disease classification. Sleep 2004;27 (suppl S):306–307.
89. Aksu M, Demirci S, and Bara-Jimenez W: Correlation between putative indicators of primary restless legs syndrome severity. Sleep Med 2007;8(1):84–89.
90. Garcia-Borreguero D, Larrosa O, de la Llave Y, et al. Correlation between rating scales and sleep laboratory measurements in restless legs syndrome. Sleep Med 2004;5(6):561–565.
91. Hornyak M, Feige B, Voderholzer U, et al. Polysomnography findings in patients with restless legs syndrome and in healthy controls: A comparative observational study. Sleep 2007;30(7):861–865.
92. Ferri R, Zucconi M, Rundo F, et al. Heart rate and spectral eeg changes accompanying periodic and nonperiodic leg movements during sleep. Clin Neurophysiol 2007;118(2):438–448.
93. Sforza E, Pichot V, Cervena K, et al. Cardiac variability and heart-rate increment as a marker of sleep fragmentation in patients with a sleep disorder: A preliminary study. Sleep 2007;30(1):43–51.
94. Winkelman J. The evoked heart rate response to periodic leg movements of sleep. Sleep 1999;22:575–580.
95. Pennestri MH, Montplaisir J, Colombo R, et al. Nocturnal blood pressure changes in patients with restless legs syndrome. Neurology 2007;68(15):1213–1218.
96. Siddiqui F, Strus J, Ming X, et al. Rise of blood pressure with periodic limb movements in sleep and wakefulness. Clin Neurophysiol 2007;118(9):1923–1930.
97. Morgan BJ, Dempsey JA, Pegelow DF, et al. Blood pressure perturbations caused by subclinical sleep-disordered breathing. Sleep 1998;21(7):737–746.
98. Roman MJ, Pickering TG, Schwartz JE, et al. Relation of blood pressure variability to carotid atherosclerosis and carotid artery and left ventricular hypertrophy. Arterioscler Thromb Vasc Biol 2001;21(9):1507–1511.
99. Zakopoulos NA, Tsivgoulis G, Barlas G, et al. Time rate of blood pressure variation is associated with increased common carotid artery intima-media thickness. Hypertension. 2005;45(4):505–512.
100. Frattola A, Parati G, Cuspidi C, et al. Prognostic value of 24-hour blood pressure variability. J Hypertens 1993;11(10):1133–1137.
101. Pringle E, Phillips C, Thijs L, et al. Systolic blood pressure variability as a risk factor for stroke and cardiovascular mortality in the elderly hypertensive population. J Hypertens 2003;21(12):2251–2257.
102. Bixler E, Kales A, Vela-Bueno A, et al. Nocturnal myoclonus and nocturnal myoclonic activity in the normal population. Res Commun Chem Pathol Pharmacol. 1982;36(1):129–140.
103. Scofield H, Roth T, and Drake C. Periodic limb movements during sleep: Population prevalence, clinical correlates, and racial differences. Sleep 2008;31(9):1221–1227.
104. Allen R and Earley C. Augmentation of the restless legs syndrome with carbidopa/levodopa. Sleep 1996;19: 205–213.
105. Picchietti MA and Picchietti DL. Restless legs syndrome and periodic limb movement disorder in children and adolescents. Semin Pediatr Neurol 2008;15(2):91–99.
106. Santamaria J, Iranzo A, and Tolosa E. Development of restless legs syndrome after dopaminergic treatment in a patient with periodic leg movements in sleep. Sleep Med. 2003;4:153–155.
107. Birinyi PV, Allen RP, Hening W, et al. Undiagnosed individuals with first-degree relatives with restless legs syndrome have increased periodic limb movements. Sleep Med 2006;7(6):480–485.
108. Bonati M, Ferini-Strambi L, Aridon P, et al. Autosomal dominant restless legs syndrome maps on chromosome 14q. Brain 2003;126:1485–1492.
109. O'Brien, LM, Holbrook CR, Faye Jones V, et al. Ethnic difference in periodic limb movements in children.[see comment]. Sleep Med 2007;8(3):240–246.

110. Guggisberg AG, Hess CW, and Mathis J. The significance of the sympathetic nervous system in the pathophysiology of periodic leg movements in sleep. Sleep 2007;30(6): 755–766.
111. Ware J, Blumoff R, and Pittard J. Peripheral vasoconstriction in patients with sleep related periodic leg movements. Sleep 1988;11:182–186.
112. Bliwise, D. Sleep and aging. In (ed) Understanding Sleep: The Evaluation and Treatment of Sleep Disorders Washington, DC, 1997.
113. Sforza, E, Johannes M, and Claudio B. The pam-rl ambulatory device for detection of periodic leg movements: A validation study.[see comment]. Sleep Med 2005;6(5):407–413.
114. Tuisku K, Holi M, Wahlbeck K, et al. Quantitative rest activity in ambulatory monitoring as a physiological marker of restless legs syndrome: A controlled study. Mov Disord 2003;18:442–448.
115. Tuisku K, Holi M, Wahlbeck K, et al. Actometry in measuring the symptom severity of restless legs syndrome. Eur J Neurol 2005;12:385–387.
116. Rye D, Allen R, Carson S, et al. Ropinirole decreases bedtime periodic leg movements in patients with rls: Results of a 12-week us study. Sleep 2005;28 (Suppl S):A270.
117. Hening W, Walters A, Kavey N, et al. Dyskinesias while awake and periodic movements in sleep in restless legs syndrome: Treatment with opiods. Neurology 1986;36:1363–1366.
118. Hogl B, Zucconi M, and Provini F. RLS, PLM, and their differential diagnosis: A video guide. Mov Disord 2007;22(suppl 18):S414–S419.
119. Han PK, Arnold R, Bond G, et al. Myoclonus secondary to withdrawal from transdermal fentanyl: Case report and literature review. J Pain Symptom Manage 2002;23(1):66–72.
120. Lauterbach EC. Hiccup and apparent myoclonus after hydrocodone: Review of the opiate-related hiccup and myoclonus literature. Clin Neuropharmacol 1999;22(2):87–92.
121. Mercadante S. Pathophysiology and treatment of opioid-related myoclonus in cancer patients. Pain. 74(1):5-9,1998.
122. Paci D, Lanuzza B, Cosentino FI, et al. Subclinical abnormal emg activation of the gastrocnemii during gait analysis in restless legs syndrome: A preliminary report in 13 patients. Sleep Med 2009;10(3):312–316.
123. Kushida C, Martin M, Nikam P, et al. Burden of restless legs syndrome on health-related quality of life. Quality Life Res 2007;16(4):617–624.
124. Walters AS. Is there a subpopulation of children with growing pains who really have restless legs syndrome? A review of the literature. Sleep Med 2002;3(2):93–98.
125. Bassetti CL, Mauerhofer D, Gugger M, et al. Restless legs syndrome: A clinical study of 55 patients. European Neurol 2001;45(2):67–74.
126. Holmes R, Tluk S, Metta V, et al. Nature and variants of idiopathic restless legs syndrome: Observations from 152 patients referred to secondary care in the uk. J Neural Transm 2007;114(7):929–934.
127. Earley C. Restless legs syndrome. NEJM 2003;348: 2103–2109.
128. Garcia-Borreguero, D, Allen RP, Benes H, et al. Augmentation as a treatment complication of restless legs syndrome: Concept and management. Mov Disord 2007;22 Suppl 18:S476–S484.
129. Cornelius J, Tippmann-Piekert M, Slocumb N, et al. Impulse control disorders with use of dopaminergic agents in restless legs syndrome: A case-control study. Sleep 2010;33(1):81–87.
130. Kushida CA. Clinical presentation, diagnosis, and quality of life issues in restless legs syndrome. Am J Med 2007;120(1 suppl 1):S4–S12.
131. Lee HB, Hening WA, Allen RP, et al. Restless legs syndrome is associated with dsm-iv major depressive disorder and panic disorder in the community. J Neuropsychiatry Clin Neurosci 2008;20(1):101–105.
132. Winkelmann J, Prager M, Lieb R, et al. "Anxietas tibiarum". Depression and anxiety disorders in patients with restless legs syndrome. J Neurol 2005;252(1):67–71.
133. Winkelmann J, Lichtner P, Schormair B, et al. Variants in the neuronal nitric oxide synthase (nnos, nos1) gene are associated with restless legs syndrome. Mov Disord 2008;23(3):350–358.
134. Billars L, Hicks A, Bliwise D, et al. Hypertension risk and plms in restless legs syndrome. Sleep 2007;30: A297–A298.
135. Benz RL, Pressman MR, Hovick ET, et al. Potential novel predictors of mortality in end-stage renal disease patients with sleep disorders.[see comment]. Am J Kidney Dis 2000;35(6):1052–1060.
136. Molnar MZ, Szentkiralyi A, Lindner A, et al. Restless legs syndrome and mortality in kidney transplant recipients. Am J Kidney Dis 2007;50(5):813–820.
137. Unruh ML, Levey AS, D'Ambrosio C, et al. Restless legs symptoms among incident dialysis patients: Association with lower quality of life and shorter survival. Am J Kidney Dis 2004;43(5):900–909.
138. Kemlink D, Plazzi G, Vetrugno R, et al. Suggestive evidence for linkage for restless legs syndrome on chromosome 19p13. Neurogenetics 2008;9(2):75–82.
139. Winkelmann J, Polo O, Provini F, et al. Genetics of restless legs syndrome (RLS): State-of-the-art and future directions. Mov Disord 2007;22(suppl 18):S449–S458.
140. Lohmann-Hedrich K, Neumann A, Kleensang A, et al. Evidence for linkage of restless legs syndrome to chromosome 9p: Are there two distinct loci? Neurology 2008;70(9):686–694.
141. Winkelmann J, Schormair B, Lichtner P, et al. Genome-wide association study of restless legs syndrome identifies common variants in three genomic regions.[see comment]. Nature Genet 2007;39(8):1000–1006.
142. Vilarino-Guell C, Farrer MJ, and Lin SC. A genetic risk factor for periodic limb movements in sleep. N Engl J Med 2008;358(4):425–427.
143. Schormair B, Kemlink D, Roeske D, et al. Ptprd (protein tyrosine phosphatase receptor type delta) is associated with restless legs syndrome. Nature Genet 2008;40(8): 946–948.
144. Mignot, E: A step forward for restless legs syndrome. [comment]. Nature Genet 2007;39(8):938–939.
145. Desautels A, Turecki G, Montplaisir J, et al. Analysis of cag repeat expansions in restless legs syndrome. Sleep 2003;26(8):1055–1057.
146. Konieczny M, Bauer P, Tomiuk J, et al. Cag repeats in restless legs syndrome. Am J Med Genet. Part B, Neuropsychiatr Genet 2006;141(2):173–176.

147. Arbeitman MN, Furlong EE, Imam F, et al. Gene expression during the life cycle of drosophila melanogaster. [erratum appears in science 2002 nov 8;298(5596):1172]. Science 2002;297(5590):2270–2275.
148. Bilic I and Ellmeier W. The role of btb domain-containing zinc finger proteins in t cell development and function. Immunol Lett 2007;108(1):1–9.
149. Perez-Torrado R, Yamada D, and Defossez P: Born to bind: The btb protein-protein interaction domain. Bioessays Rev 2006;28:1194–1202.
150. Stogios P, Downs G, Jauhal J, et al. Sequence and structural analysis of btb domain proteins. Genome Biol 2005;6:R82.
151. Stogios P and Privé G. The back domain in btb-kelch proteins. Trends Biochem Sci 2004;29:634–637.
152. Adams J, Kelso R, and Cooley L. The kelch repeat superfamily of proteins: Propellers of cell function. Trends Cell Biol 2000;10:17–24.
153. Casares F and Mann RS. Control of antennal versus leg development in drosophila. Nature 1998;392(6677):723–726.
154. Kurant E, Pai CY, Sharf R, et al. Dorsotonals/homothorax, the drosophila homologue of meis1, interacts with extradenticle in patterning of the embryonic PNS. Development. 1998;125(6):1037–1048.
155. Maeda R, Mood K, Jones TL, et al. Xmeis1, a protooncogene involved in specifying neural crest cell fate in xenopus embryos. Oncogene 2001;20(11):1329–1342.
156. Argiropoulos B, Yung E, and Humphries RK: Unraveling the crucial roles of meis1 in leukemogenesis and normal hematopoiesis.[comment]. Genes Dev 2007;21(22):2845–2849.
157. Azcoitia V, Aracil M, Martinez AC, et al. The homeodomain protein meis1 is essential for definitive hematopoiesis and vascular patterning in the mouse embryo. Dev Biol 2005;280(2):307–320.
158. Minehata K, Kawahara A, and Suzuki T. Meis1 regulates the development of endothelial cells in zebrafish. Biochem Biophys Res Comm 2008;374(4):647–652.
159. Davidson S, Miller KA, Dowell A, et al. A remote and highly conserved enhancer supports amygdala specific expression of the gene encoding the anxiogenic neuropeptide substance-p. Molecular Psychiatry 2006;11(4):323.
160. Dinev D, Jordan BW, Neufeld B, et al. Extracellular signal regulated kinase 5 (erk5) is required for the differentiation of muscle cells. EMBO Reports 2001;2(9):829–834.
161. Cavanaugh JE, Jaumotte JD, Lakoski JM, et al. Neuroprotective role of erk1/2 and erk5 in a dopaminergic cell line under basal conditions and in response to oxidative stress. J Neurosci Res 2006;84(6):1367–1375.
162. Mizuhara E, Nakatani T, Minaki Y, et al. Corl1, a novel neuronal lineage-specific transcriptional corepressor for the homeodomain transcription factor lbx1. J Biol Chem 2005;280(5):3645–3655.
163. Cheng L, Samad OA, Xu Y, et al. Lbx1 and tlx3 are opposing switches in determining gabaergic versus glutamatergic transmitter phenotypes.[erratum appears in Nat Neurosci 2005 Dec;8(12):1791]. Nat Neurosci 2005;8(11):1510–1515.
164. Uetani N, Chagnon MJ, Kennedy TE, et al. Mammalian motoneuron axon targeting requires receptor protein tyrosine phosphatases sigma and delta. J Neurosci 2006;26(22):5872–5880.
165. Naciff JM, Overmann GJ, Torontali SM, et al. Gene expression profile induced by 17 alpha-ethynyl estradiol in the prepubertal female reproductive system of the rat. Toxicol Sci 2003;72(2):314–330.
166. Rutkove S, Matheson J, and Logigian E: Restless legs syndrome in patients with polyneuropathy. Muscle Nerve 1996;19(5):670–672.
167. Hattan E, Chalk C, and Postuma R. Is there a higher risk of restless legs syndrome in peripheral neuropathy? Neurology 2009;72(11):955–960.
168. Iannaccone S, Zucconi M, Marchettini P, et al. Evidence of peripheral axonal neuropathy in primary restless legs syndrome. Mov Disord 1995;10(1):2–9.
169. Polydefkis M, Allen R, Hauer P, et al. Subclinical sensory neuropathy in late-onset restless legs syndrome. Neurology 2000;55(8):1115–1121.
170. Montplaisir J, Godbout R, Boghen D, et al. Familial restless legs with periodic movements in sleep: Electrophysiologic, biochemical, and pharmacologic study. Neurology1985;35:130–134.
171. Bliwise D, Ingham R, Date E, et al. Nerve conduction and creatinine clearance in aged subjects with periodic movements in sleep. J Gerontol Med Sci 1989;44:M164–M167.
172. Provini F, Vetrugno R, Meletti S, et al. Motor pattern of periodic limb movements during sleep. Neurology 2001;57(2):300–304.
173. Ferreri F, and Rossini P: Neurophysiological investigations in restless legs syndrome and other disorders of movement during sleep. Sleep Med 2004;5:397–399.
174. Tyvaert L, Laureau E, Hurtevent J, et al. A-delta and c-fibres function in primary restless legs syndrome. Neurophysiol Clin 2009;39(6):267–274.
175. Wechsler L, Stakes J, Shahani B, et al. Periodic leg movements of sleep (nocturnal myoclonus): An electrophysiological study. Ann Neurol 1986;19:168–173.
176. Smith R, Gouin P, Minkley P, et al. Periodic limb movement disorder is associated with normal motor conduction latencies when studied by central magnetic stimulation—successful use of a new technique. Sleep 1992;15(4):312–318.
177. Akyol A, Kiylioglu N, Kadikoylu G, et al. Iron deficiency anemia and restless legs syndrome: Is there an electrophysiological abnormality? Clin Neurol Neurosurg 2003;106:23–27.
178. Garcia-Borreguero D, Larrosa O, de la Llave Y, et al. Treatment of restless legs syndrome with gabapentin: A double-blind, cross-over study. Neurology 2002;59:1573–1579.
179. Ekbom K. Restless legs. Acta Med Scand Suppl 1945;158:1–123.
180. Pedersen L, Nielsen A, and Blackburn-Munro G: Antinociception is selectively enhanced by parallel inhibition of multiple subtypes of monoamine transporters in rat models of persistent and neuropathic pain. Psychopharmacology(Berl) 2005;182(4):551–561.
181. Fleetwood-Walker S, Hope P, and Mitchell R. Antinociceptive actions of descending dopaminergic tracts on cat and rat dorsal horn somatosensory neurones. J. Physiol (Lond) 1988;399:335–348.

182. Garraway S and Hochman S. Modulatory actions of serotonin, norepinephrine, dopamine, and acetylcholine in spinal cord deep dorsal horn neurons. J. Neurophysiol 2001;86:2183–2194.
183. Millan MJ and Colpaert FC. Alpha2 receptors mediate the antinociceptive action of 8-oh-dpat in the hot-plate test in mice. Brain Res 1991;539;342–346.
184. Yoshimura M and Furue H. Mechanisms for the antinociceptive actions of the descending noradrenergic and serotonergic systems in the spinal cord. J Pharmacol Sci2006;101(2):107–117.
185. Wei H, Viisanen H, and Pertovaara A. Descending modulation of neuropathic hypersensitivity by dopamine d2 receptors in or adjacent to the hypothalamic a11 cell group. Pharmacol Res 2009;59(5):355–363.
186. Ondo WG, He Y, Rajasekaran S, et al. Clinical correlates of 6-hydroxydopamine injections into a11 dopaminergic neurons in rats: A possible model for restless legs syndrome. Mov Disord 2000;15(1):154–158.
187. Qu S, Le W, Zhang X, et al. Locomotion is increased in a11-lesioned mice with iron deprivation: A possible animal model for restless legs syndrome. J Neuropathol Exp Neurol 2007;66(5):383–388.
188. Zhao H, Zhu W, Pan T, et al. Spinal cord dopamine receptor expression and function in mice with 6-ohda lesion of the a11 nucleus and dietary iron deprivation. J Neurosci Res 2007;85(5):1065–1076.
190. Dowling P, Klinker F, Amaya F, et al. Iron-deficiency sensitizes mice to acute pain stimuli and formalin-induced nociception. J Nutr 2009;139(11):2087–2092.
191. Earley C, Allen R, Connor J, et al. The dopaminergic neurons of the a11 system in rls autopsy brains appear normal. Sleep Med 2009;10(10):1155–1157.
192. Stiasny-Kolster K, Magerl W, Oertel W, et al. Static mechanical hyperalgesia without dynamic tactile allodynia in patients with restless legs syndrome. Brain 2004;127: 773–782.
193. Han JK, Oh K, Kim BJ, et al. Cutaneous silent period in patients with restless leg syndrome. Clin Neurophysiol 2007;118(8):1705–1710.
194. Rye D and Freeman A. Pain and its' interaction with thalamocortical excitability states. In Lavigne G, Choinière M, Sessle B, et al (eds). Sleep and Pain. Seattle: IASP Press 2007, pp. 77–97.
195. Wood PB. Role of central dopamine in pain and analgesia. Expert Rev Neurother 2008;8(5):781–797.
196. Treister R, Pud D, Ebstein RP, et al. Associations between polymorphisms in dopamine neurotransmitter pathway genes and pain response in healthy humans. Pain 2009;147(1–3):187–193.
197. Yokota T, Hirose K, Tanabe H, et al. Sleep-related periodic leg movements (nocturnal myoclonus) due to spinal cord lesion. J.Neurol.Sci 1991;104:13–18.
198. Dickel M, Renfrow S, Moore P, et al. Rapid eye movement sleep periodic leg movements in patients with spinal cord injury. Sleep 1994;17(8):733–738.
199. Lee M, Choi Y, and Lee S: Sleep-related periodic leg movements associated with spinal cord lesions. Mov Disord 1996;11(6):719–722.
200. de Mello M, Lauro F, Silva A, et al. Incidence of periodic leg movements and of the restless legs syndrome during sleep following acute physical activity in spinal cord injury subjects. Spinal Cord 1996;34(5):294–296.
201. Manconi M, Rocca M, Ferini-Strambi L, et al. Restless legs syndrome is a common finding in multiple sclerosis and correlates with cervical cord damage. Mult Scler 2008;14(1):86–93.
202. Rye D and DeLong M. Amelioration of sensory limb discomfort of restless legs syndrome by pallidotomy. Ann Neurol 1999;46(5):800–801.
203. Kedia S, Moro E, Tagliati M, et al. Emergence of restless legs syndrome during subthalamic stimulation for parkinson disease. Neurology 2004;63(12):2410–2412.
204. Driver-Dunckley E, Evidente VG, Adler CH, et al. Restless legs syndrome in parkinson's disease patients may improve with subthalamic stimulation. Mov Disord 2006;21(8):1287–1289.
205. Ondo W. Vim deep brain stimulation does not improve pre-existing restless legs syndrome in patients with essential tremor. Parkinsonism Relat Disord 2006;12(2): 113–114.
206. Lee SJ, Kim JS, Song IU, et al. Poststroke restless legs syndrome and lesion location: Anatomical considerations. Mov Disord 2008.
207. Ferini-Strambi L, Filippi M, Martinelli V, et al. Nocturnal sleep study in multiple sclerosis: Correlations with clinical and brain magnetic resonance imaging findings. J. Neurological Sciences 1994;125:194–197.
208. Scalise A, Cadore IP, and Gigli GL: Motor cortex excitability in restless legs syndrome. Sleep Med 2004;5(4):393–396.
209. Nardone R, Ausserer H, Bratti A, et al. Cabergoline reverses cortical hyperexcitability in patients with restless legs syndrome. Acta Neurol Scand 2006;114(4):244–249.
210. Wechsler L, Stakes J, Shahani B, et al. Nocturnal myoclonus, restless legs syndrome, and abnormal electrophysiological findings. Ann Neurol1987; 21:515.
211. Briellmann R, Rosler K, and Hess C. Blink reflex excitability is abnormal in patients with periodic leg movements in sleep. Mov Disord 1996;11(6):710–714.
212. Aksu M and Bara-Jimenez W. State dependent excitability changes of spinal flexor reflex in patients with restless legs syndrome secondary to chronic renal failure. Sleep Med 2002;3(5):427–430.
213. Rijsman R, Stam C, and de Weerd A: Abnormal h-reflexes in periodic limb movement disorder; impact on understanding the pathophysiology of the disorder. Clin Neurophysiol 2005;116:204–210.
214. de Mello MT, Poyares DL, and Tufik S: Treatment of periodic leg movements with a dopaminergic agonist in subjects with total spinal cord lesions. Spinal Cord 1999;37(9):634–637.
215. Clemens S, and Hochman S: Conversion of the modulatory actions of dopamine on spinal reflexes from depression to facilitation in d3 receptor knock-out mice. J. Neurosci 2004;24:11337–11345.
216. Jakobsson B, and Ruuth K: Successful treatment of restless legs syndrome with an implanted pump for intrathecal drug delivery. Acta Anaesthesiologica Scandinavica 2002;46(1):114–117.
217. Lindvall P, Ruuth K, Jakobsson B, et al. Intrathecal morphine as a treatment for refractory restless legs syndrome. Neurosurgery 2008;63(6):E1209; author reply E1209.

218. Ross DA, Narus MS, and Nutt JG. Control of medically refractory restless legs syndrome with intrathecal morphine: Case report. Neurosurgery 2008;62(1):E263; discussion E263.
219. Davidson S, Zhang X, Khasabov S, et al. Relief of itch by scratching: State-dependent inhibition of primate spinothalamic tract neurons. Nature Neuroscience 2009;12:544–5462009.
220. Ikoma A, Steinhoff M, Ständer S, et al. The neurobiology of itch. Nat Rev Neurosci 2006;7(7):535–547.
221. Sun Y, Zhao Z, Meng X, et al. Cellular basis of itch sensation. Science. 2009;325(5947):1531–1534.
222. Handwerker H and Schmelz M. Itch without pain—: A labeled line for itch sensation? Nat Rev Neurol 2009;5: 640–641.
223. Hseih J, Hagermark O, Stahle-Backdahl M, et al. Urge to scratch represented in the human cerebral cortex during itch. J Neurophysiol 1994;72(6):3004–3008.
224. Lerner A, Bagic A, Hanakawa T, et al. Involvement of insula and cingulate cortices in control and suppression of natural urges. Cereb Cortex 2009;19(1):218–223.
225. Bucher S, Seelos K, Oertel W, et al. Cerebral generators involved in the pathogenesis of the restless legs syndrome. Ann Neurol 1997;41(5):639–645.
226. San Pedro EC, Mountz JM, Mountz JD, et al. Familial painful restless legs syndrome correlates with pain dependent variation of blood flow to the caudate, thalamus, and anterior cingulate gyrus. J Rheumatol 1998;25(11):2270–2275.
227. Allen R. Dopamine and iron in the pathophysiology of restless legs syndrome (rls). Sleep Med 2004;5(4):385–391.
228. Allen R, and Earley C. The role of iron in restless legs syndrome. Mov Disord 2007;22(Suppl 18):S440–S448.
229. Connor J. Pathophysiology of restless legs syndrome: Evidence for iron involvement. Curr Neurol Neurosci Rep 2008;8(2):162–166.
230. O'Keeffe S, Gavin K, and Lavan J. Iron status and restless legs syndrome in the elderly. Age Ageing 199423:200–203.
231. Ekbom K. Restless legs syndrome. Neurology 1960;10: 868–875.
232. Wang J, O'Reilly B, Venkataraman R, et al. Efficacy of oral iron in patients with restless legs syndrome and a low-normal ferritin: A randomized, double-blind, placebo-controlled study. Sleep Med 2009.
233. Sloand J, Shelly M, Feigin A, et al. A double-blind, placebo-controlled trial of intravenous iron dextran therapy in patients with esrd and restless legs syndrome. Am J Kidney Dis 2004;43:663–670.
234. Nordlander N. Therapy in restless legs. Acta Med Scand 1953;145:453–457.
235. Tarquini B. Iron metabolism: Clinical chronobiological aspects. Chronobiologia 1978;5:315–336.
236. Nicolau G, Haus E, Lakatua D, et al. Chronobiology of serum iron concentration in subjects of different ages at different geographic locations. Rev Roum Med Endocrinol 1987;25(2):63–82.
237. Unger EL, Earley CJ, and Beard JL. Diurnal cycle influences peripheral and brain iron levels in mice. J Appl Physiol 2009;106(1):187–193.
238. Nelson C, Erikson K, Pinero D, et al. In vivo dopamine metabolism is altered in iron-deficient anemic rats. J Nutr 1997;127:2282–2288.
239. Bianco LE, Wiesinger J, Earley CJ, et al. Iron deficiency alters dopamine uptake and response to l-dopa injection in sprague-dawley rats. J Neurochem 2008;106(1): 205–215.
240. Bianco L, Unger E, Earley C, et al. Iron deficiency alters the day-night variation in monoamine levels in mice. Chronobiol. Int 2009;26(3):447–463.
241. Dean Jr T, Allen R, O'Donnell C, et al. The effects of dietary iron deprivation on murin circadian sleep architecture. Sleep Med 2006;7(8):634–640.
242. Kryger M, Shepertycky M, Foerster J, et al. Sleep disorders in repeat blood donors. Sleep 2003;26:625–626.
243. Earley CJ, Connor JR, Beard JL, et al. Abnormalities in csf concentrations of ferritin and transferrin in restless legs syndrome. Neurology 2000;54(8):1698–1700.
244. Mizuno S, Mihara T, Miyaoka T, et al. Csf iron, ferritin and transferrin levels in restless legs syndrome. J Sleep Res 2005;14(1):43–47.
245. Connor J, Boyer P, Menzies S, et al. Neuropathological examination suggests impaired brain iron acquisition in restless legs syndrome. Neurology 2003;61:304–309.
246. Connor JR, Wang XS, Allen RP, et al. Altered dopaminergic profile in the putamen and substantia nigra in restless leg syndrome. Brain 2009;132(pt 9):2403–2412.
247. Allen R, Barker P, Wehrl F, et al. Mri measurement of brain iron in patients with restless legs syndrome. Neurology 2001;56:263–265.
248. Earley C, Barker P, Horska A, et al. Mri-determined regional brain iron concentrations in early- and late-onset restless legs syndrome. Sleep Med 2006;7(5):458–461.
249. Godau J, Klose U, Di Santo A, et al. Multiregional brain iron deficiency in restless legs syndrome. Mov Disord 2008;23(8):1184–1187.
250. Schmidauer C, Sojer M, Seppi K, et al. Transcranial ultrasound shows nigral hypoechogenicity in restless legs syndrome. Ann Neurol 2005;58(4):630–634.
251. Godau J, Schweitzer K, Liepelt I, et al. Substantia nigra hypoechogenicity: Definition and findings in restless legs syndrome. Mov Disord 2007;22(2):187–192.
252. Godau J, Wevers AK, Gaenslen A, et al. Sonographic abnormalities of brainstem structures in restless legs syndrome. Sleep Med 2008;9(7):782–789.
253. Unrath A, Muller HP, Ludolph AC, et al. Cerebral white matter alterations in idiopathic restless legs syndrome, as measured by diffusion tensor imaging. Mov Disord. 2008;23(9):1250–1255.
254. Godau J, Manz A, Wevers A, et al. Sonographic substantia nigra hypoechogenicity in polyneuropathy and restless legs syndrome. Mov Disord 2009;24(1):133–137.
255. Lee K, Zaffke M, and Baratte-Beebe K. Restless legs syndrome and sleep disturbance during pregnancy: The role of folate and iron. J Women Health Gend Based Med 2001;10(4):335–341.
256. Tunc T, Karadag Y, Dogulu F, et al. Predisposing factors of restless legs syndrome in pregnancy. Mov Disord 2007;22(5):627–631.
257. Dzaja, A, Wehrle R, Lancel M, et al. Elevated estradiol plasma levels in womeb with restless legs during pregnancy. Sleep. 32(2):169–174,2009.
258. Burchell BJ, Allen RP, Miller JK, et al. Rls and blood donation. Sleep Med 2009;10(8):844–849.

259. Becker PM. Bleed less than 3: Rls and blood donation. Sleep Med. 10(8):820–821,2009.
260. Berger K, von Eckardstein A, Trenkwalder C, et al. Iron metabolism and the risk of restless legs syndrome in an elderly general population—the memo study. J Neurol 2002;249:1195–1199.
261. Earley C, Heckler D, and Allen R. The treatment of restless legs syndrome with intravenous iron dextran. Sleep Med 2004;5:231–235.
262. Earley CJ, Horska A, Mohamed MA, et al. A randomized, double-blind, placebo-controlled trial of intravenous iron sucrose in restless legs syndrome. Sleep Med 2009;10(2):206–211.
263. Grote L, Leissner L, Hedner J, et al. A randomized, double-blind, placebo controlled, multi-center study of intravenous iron sucrose and placebo in the treatment of restless legs syndrome. Mov Disord 2009;24(10):1445–1452.
264. Aul EA, Davis BJ, and Rodnitzky RL. The importance of formal serum iron studies in the assessment of restless legs syndrome. Neurology 1998;51(3):912.
265. Earley C, Ponnuru P, Wang X, et al. Altered iron metabolism in lymphocytes from subjects with restless legs syndrome. Sleep 2008;31(6):847–852.
266. Freeman A, and Rye D. Dopamine in behavioral state control. In Sinton C, Perumal P, and Monti J (eds). The Neurochemistry of Sleep and Wakefulness. Cambridge, Cambridge University Press, 2008, pp. 179–223.
267. Ramsey A, Hillas P, and Fitzpatrick P. Characterization of the active site iron in tyrosine hydroxylase. Redox states of the iron. J Biol Chem 1996;271:24395–24400.
268. Nagatsu I. Tyrosine hydroxylase: Human isoforms, structure and regulation in physiology and pathology. Essays Biochem 1995;30:15–35.
269. Trenkwalder C, Walters AS, Hening WA, et al. Positron emission tomographic studies in restless legs syndrome. Mov Disord 1999;14(1):141–145.
270. Turjanski N, Lees A, and Brooks D. Striatal dopaminergic function in restless legs syndrome. Neurology 1999;52:932–937.
271. Ruottinen HM, Partinen M, Hublin C, et al. An fdopa pet study in patients with periodic limb movement disorder and restless legs syndrome. Neurology 2000;54(2):502–504.
272. Tribl GG, Asenbaum S, Klosch G, et al. Normal ipt and ibzm spect in drug naive and levodopa-treated idiopathic restless legs syndrome. Neurology 2002;59(4):649–650.
273. Cervenka S, Palhagen SE, Comley RA, et al. Support for dopaminergic hypoactivity in restless legs syndrome: A pet study on d2-receptor binding. Brain 2006;129(pt 8): 2017–2028.
274. Earley C, Hyland K, and Allen R. Csf dopamine, serotonin, and biopterin metabolites in patients with restless legs syndrome. Mov Disord 2001;16:144–149.
275. Stiasny-Kolster, K Moller J, Zschocke J, et al. Normal dopaminergic and serotonergic metabolites in cerebrospinal fluid and blood of restless legs syndrome patients. Mov Disord 2004;19:192–196.
276. Earley CJ, Hyland K, and Allen RP. Circadian changes in csf dopaminergic measures in restless legs syndrome. Sleep Med 2006;7(3):263–268.
277. Poceta J, Parsons L, Engelland S, et al. Circadian rhythm of csf monoamines and hypocretin-1 in restless legs syndrome and parkinson's disease. Sleep Med 2009;10(1):129–133.
278. Allen RP, Connor JR, Hyland K, et al. Abnormally increased csf 3-ortho-methyldopa (3-omd) in untreated restless legs syndrome (RLS) patients indicates more severe disease and possibly abnormally increased dopamine synthesis. Sleep Med 2008;10(1):123–108.
279. Calabrese, EJ: Dopamine: Biphasic dose responses. Crit Rev Toxicol 2001;31(4–5):563–583.
281. McClung C, Sidiropoulou K, Vitaterna M, et al. Regulation of dopaminergic transmission and cocaine reward by the clock gene. Proc Natl Acad Sci U S A 2005;102:9377–9381.
282. Andretic, R, and Hirsh J: Circadian modulation of dopamine receptor responsiveness in drosophila melanogaster. Proc Natl Acad Sci U S A 2000;97(4):1873–1878.
283. Mortensen O, and Amara S: Dynamic regulation of the dopamine transporter. Eur J Pharmacol 2003;479(1–3): 159–170.
284. Robertson S, Matthies H, and Galli A: A closer look at amphetamine-induced reverse transport and trafficking of the dopamine and norepinephrine transporters. Mol Neurobiol 2009;39(2):73–80.
285. He Y, Yu L, and Jin G: Differential distribution and trafficking properties of dopamine d1 and d5 receptors in nerve cells. Brain Res Bull 2009;25(2):43–53.
286. Eriksen J, Rasmussen S, Rasmussen R, et al. Visualization of dopamine transporter trafficking in live neurons by use of fluorescent cocaine analogs. J Neurosci 2009;29(21):6794–6808.
287. Hening WA: Current guidelines and standards of practice for restless legs syndrome. Am J Med 2007;120(1 Suppl 1): S22–S27.
288. Silber, M, Ehrenberg B, Allen R, et al. An algorithm for the management of restless legs syndrome. Mayo Clin Proc 2004;79:916–922.
289. Hornyak M, Feige B, Riemann D, et al. Periodic leg movements in sleep and periodic limb movement disorder: Prevalence, clinical significance and treatment. Sleep Med Rev 2006;10(3):169–177.
290. Urbano MR, and Ware JC: Restless legs syndrome caused by quetiapine successfully treated with ropinirole in 2 patients with bipolar disorder. J Clin Pharmacol 2008;28(6):704–705.
291. Kim S, Shin I, Kim J, et al. Bupropion may improve restless legs syndrome: A report of three cases. Clin Neuropharmacol 2005;28(6):298–301.
292. Lee J, Erdos J, Wilkoosz M, et al. Bupropion as a possible treatment option for restless legs syndrome. Ann Pharmacotherap 2009;43(2):370–374.
293. Smith HS, Dhingra R, Ryckewaert L, et al. Proton pump inhibitors and pain. Pain Physician 2009;12(6):1013–1023.
294. Numata Y, Kato T, Nagatsu T, et al. Effects of stereochemical structures of tetrahydrobiopterin on tyrosine hydroxylase. Bichim Biophys Acta 1977;480(1):104–112.
295. Botez M, Fontaine F, Botez T, et al. Folate-responsive neurological and mental disorders: Report of 16 cases. Neuropyschological correlates of computerized transaxial tomography and radionuclide cisternography in folic acid deficiencies. Eur Neurol. 1977;16(1–6):230–246.
296. Bachmann C, Guth N, Helmshmied K, et al. Homocysteine in restless legs syndrome. Sleep Med 2008;9(4):388–392.

297. Davis BJ, Rajput A, Rajput ML, et al. A randomized, double-blind placebo-controlled trial of iron in restless legs syndrome. Eur Neurol 2000;43(2):70–75.
298. Morgan JC, Ames M, and Sethi KD: Response to ropinirole in restless legs syndrome is independent of baseline serum ferritin. J Neurol Neurosurg Psychiatry 2008;79(8):964–965.
299. Trenkwalder C, Hogl B, Benes H, et al. Augmentation in restless legs syndrome is associated with low ferritin. Sleep Med 2008;9(5):572–574.
300. Umbreit J. Iron deficiency: A concise review. Am J Hematol 2005;78(3):225–231.
301. Silverstein SB, and Rodgers GM. Parenteral iron therapy options. Am J Hematol 2004;76(1):74–78.
302. Happe S, and Trenkwalder C: Role of dopamine receptor agonists in the treatment of restless legs syndrome. CNS Drugs 2004;18(1):27–36.
303. Fulda S, and Wetter TC: Where dopamine meets opioids: A meta-analysis of the placebo effect in restless legs syndrome treatment studies. Brain 2008;131(pt 4):902–917.
304. Diederich NJ, and Goetz CG: The placebo treatments in neurosciences: New insights from clinical and neuroimaging studies. Neurology 2008;71(9):677–684.
305. Montplaisir J, Nicolas A, Denesle R, et al. Restless legs syndrome improved by pramipexole: A double-blind randomized study. Neurology 1999;52:938–943.
306. Montplaisir J, Denesle R, and Petit D: Pramipexole in the treatment of restless legs syndrome: A follow-up study. Eur J Neurol 2000;Suppl 1:27–31.
307. Winkelman JW, Sethi KD, Kushida CA, et al. Efficacy and safety of pramipexole in restless legs syndrome. Neurology 2006;67(6):1034–1039.
308. Ferini-Strambi L, Aarskog D, Partinen M, et al. Effect of pramipexole on rls symptoms and sleep: A randomized, double-blind, placebo-controlled trial. Sleep Med 2008;9:874–881.
309. Partinen M, Hirvonen K, Jama L, et al. Efficacy and safety of pramipexole in idiopathic restless legs syndrome: A polysomnographic dose-finding study--the prelude study. Sleep Med 2006;7(5):407–417.
310. Trenkwalder C, Hening WA, Montagna P, et al. Treatment of restless legs syndrome: An evidence-based review and implications for clinical practice. Mov Disord 2008.
311. Adler CH, Hauser RA, Sethi K, et al. Ropinirole for restless legs syndrome: A placebo-controlled crossover trial. Neurology 2004;62(8):1405–1407.
312. Walters AS, Ondo WG, Dreykluft T, et al. Ropinirole is effective in the treatment of restless legs syndrome. Treat rls 2: A 12-week, double-blind, randomized, parallel-group, placebo-controlled study. Mov Disord 2004;19(12):1414–1423.
313. Allen R, Becker PM, Bogan R, et al. Ropinirole decreases periodic leg movements and improves sleep parameters in patients with restless legs syndrome. Sleep 2004;27(5):907–914.
314. Bliwise DL, Freeman A, Ingram CD, et al. Randomized, double-blind, placebo-controlled, short-term trial of ropinirole in restless legs syndrome. Sleep Med 2005;6(2):141–147.
315. Bogan RK, Fry JM, Schmidt MH, et al. Ropinirole in the treatment of patients with restless legs syndrome: A us-based randomized, double-blind, placebo-controlled clinical trial. Mayo Clin Proc 2006;81(1):17–27.
316. Quilici S, Abrams K, Nicolas A, et al. Meta-analysis of the efficacy and tolerability of pramipexole versus ropinirole in the treatment of restless legs syndrome. Sleep Med. 2008;9(7):715–726.
317. Stiasny-Kolster K, Benes H, Peglau I, et al. Effective cabergoline treatment in idiopathic restless legs syndrome (rls): A randomized, double-blind, placebo-controlled, multicenter dose-finding study followed by an open long-term extension. Neurology. 2004;63(12):2272–2279.
318. Benes H, Heinrich CR, Ueberall MA, et al. Long-term safety and efficacy of cabergoline for the treatment of idiopathic restless legs syndrome: Results from an open-label 6-month clinical trial. Sleep 2004;27(4):674–682.
319. Oertel WH, Benes H, Bodenschatz R, et al. Efficacy of cabergoline in restless legs syndrome: A placebo-controlled study with polysomnography (cator). Neurology. 2006;67(6):1040–1046.
320. Trenkwalder C, Benes H, Grote L, et al. Cabergoline compared to levodopa in the treatment of patients with severe restless legs syndrome: Results from a multi-center, randomized, active controlled trial. Mov Disord 2007;22(5):696–703.
321. Zanettini R, Antonini A, Gatto G, et al. Valvular heart disease and the use of dopamine agonists for parkinson's disease. N Engl J Med 2007;356(1):39–46.
322. Benes H. Transdermal lisuride: Short-term efficacy and tolerability study in patients with severe restless legs syndrome. Sleep Med 2006;7(1):31–35.
323. Stiasny-Kolster K, Kohnen R, Schollmayer E, et al. Patch application of the dopamine agonist rotigotine to patients with moderate to advanced stages of restless legs syndrome: A double-blind, placebo-controlled pilot study. Mov Disord 2004;19(12):1432–1438.
324. Oertel WH, Benes H, Garcia-Borreguero D, et al. One year open-label safety and efficacy trial with rotigotine transdermal patch in moderate to severe idiopathic restless legs syndrome. Sleep Med 2008;9:865–873.
325. Paulus W, and Trenkwalder C. Less is more: Pathophysiology of dopaminergic-therapy-related augmentation in restless legs syndrome. Lancet Neurol 2006;5(10):878–886.
326. Sommer M, Bachmann CG, Liebetanz KM, et al. Pregabalin in restless legs syndrome with and without neuropathic pain. Acta Neurol Scand 2007;115(5):347–350.
327. Garcia-Borreguero D, Larrosa O, Alvares J, et al. Effective treatment of idiopathic restless legs syndrome with pregabalin: A twelve-week, double-blind, placebo-controlled study with clinical and polysomnographic assessment. Sleep 200932(Abstract Suppl):A294.
328. Kushida C, Walters A, Becker PM, et al. A randomized, double-blind, placebo-controlled, crossover study of xp1351/gsk183262 in the treatment of patients with primary restless legs syndrome. Sleep 2009;32(2):159–168.
329. Kushida CA, Becker PM, Ellenbogen AL, et al. Randomized, double-blind, placebo-controlled study of xp13512/gsk1838262 in patients with RLS. Neurology 2009;72(5):439–446.
330. Walters AS, Winkelmann J, Trenkwalder C, et al. Long-term follow-up on restless legs syndrome patients treated with opioids. Mov Disord 2001;16(6):1105–1109.

331. Wagner ML, Walters AS, Coleman RG, et al. Randomized, double-blind, placebo-controlled study of clonidine in restless legs syndrome. Sleep 1996;19(1):52–58.
332. Lettieri CJ, and Eliasson AH. Pneumatic compression devices are an effective therapy for restless legs syndrome: A prospective, randomized, double-blinded, sham-controlled trial. Chest 2009;135(1):74–80.
333. Hayes CA, Kingsley JR, Hamby KR, et al. The effect of endovenous laser ablation on restless legs syndrome. Phlebology 2008;23(3):112–117.
334. Cui Y, Wang Y, and Liu Z. Acupuncture for restless legs syndrome. Cochrane Database Sys Rev 2008;4:CD006457.
335. Rotenberg JS, Canard K, and Difazio M: Successful treatment of recalcitrant restless legs syndrome with botulinum toxin type-a. J Clin Sleep Med 2006;2(3):275–278.
336. Nahab FB, Peckham EL, and Hallett M. Double-blind, placebo-controlled, pilot trial of botulinum toxin a in restless legs syndrome. Neurology 2008;71(12): 950–951.
337. Aukerman MM, Aukerman D, Bayard M, et al. Exercise and restless legs syndrome: A randomized controlled trial. J Am Board Fam Med 2006;19(5):487–493.
338. Kovacevic-Ristanovic R, Cartwright RD, and Lloyd S. Nonpharmacologic treatment of periodic leg movements in sleep. Arch Phys Med Rehabil 1991;72(6):385–389.
339. Guilleminault C, Cetel M, and Philip P: Dopaminergic treatment of restless legs and rebound phenomenon. Neurology 1993;43(2):445.
340. Garcia-Borreguero D, Allen RP, Kohnen R, et al. Diagnostic standards for dopaminergic augmentation of restless legs syndrome: Report from a world association of sleep medicine-international restless legs syndrome study group consensus conference at the max planck institute. Sleep Med 2007;8(5):520–530.
341. Earley CJ, and Allen RP. Restless legs syndrome augmentation associated with tramadol. Sleep Med 2006;7(7): 592–593.
342. Garcia-Borreguero D, Kohnen R, Hogl B, et al. Validation of the augmentation severity rating scale (asrs). Sleep Med 2007;8:455–463.
343. Ondo W, Romanyshyn J, Vuong K, et al. Long-term treatment of restless legs syndrome with dopamine agonists. Arch Neurol 2004;61:1393–1397.
344. Ondo WG. Methadone for refractory restless legs syndrome. Mov Disord 2005;20(3):345–348.
345. Kurlan R, Richard I, and Deeley C. Medication tolerance and augmentation in restless legs syndrome: The need for drug class rotation. J Gen Intern Med 2006;21(12): C1–C4.
346. Quickfall J, and Suchowersky O. Pathological gambling associated with dopamine agonist use in restless legs syndrome. Parkinsonism Relat Disord 2007;13(8):535–536.
347. Tippmann-Peikert M, Park JG, Boeve BF, et al. Pathologic gambling in patients with restless legs syndrome treated with dopaminergic agonists. Neurology 2007;68(4):301–303.
348. Driver-Dunckley ED, Noble BN, Hentz JG, et al. Gambling and increased sexual desire with dopaminergic medications in restless legs syndrome. Clin Neuropharmacol. 2007;30(5):249–255.
349. Ondo WG, and Lai D: Predictors of impulsivity and reward seeking behavior with dopamine agonists. Parkinsonism Relat Disord 2008;14(1):28–32.
350. Cornelius JR, Tippmann-Peikert M, Slocumb NL, et al. Impulse control disorders with the use of dopaminergic agents in restless legs syndrome: A case-control study. Sleep 2010;33(1):81–87.
351. Abler B, Hahlbrock R, Unrath A, et al. At-risk for pathological gambling: Imaging neural reward processing under chronic dopamine agonists. Brain 2009;132(pt 9): 2396–2402.
352. Kavanagh D, Siddiqui S, and Geddes CC: Restless legs syndrome in patients on dialysis. Am J Kidney Dis 2004;43(5):763–771.
353. Winkelmann J, Stautner A, Samtleben W, et al. Long-term course of restless legs syndrome in dialysis patients after kidney transplantation. Movement Disorders. 2002;17(5):1072–1076.
354. Molnar MZ, Novak M, Ambrus C, et al. Restless legs syndrome in patients after renal transplantation. Am J Kidney Dis 2005;45(2):388–396.
355. Miranda M, Kagi M, Fabres L, et al. Pramipexole for the treatment of uremic restless legs in patients undergoing hemodialysis. Neurology 2004;62(5):831–832.
356. Chesson AL, Jr., Wise M, Davila D, et al. Practice parameters for the treatment of restless legs syndrome and periodic limb movement disorder. An american academy of sleep medicine report. Standards of practice committee of the american academy of sleep medicine. Sleep 1999;22(7):961–968.
357. Bartell S, and Zallek S: Intravenous magnesium sulfate may relieve restless legs syndrome in pregnancy. J Clin Sleep Med 2006;2(2):187–188.
358. Botez M, and Lambert B: Folate deficiency and restless legs syndrome in pregnancy. New Eng J Med 1977;297(12):670.
359. Trotti LM, Bhadriraju S, and Rye DB: An update on the pathophysiology and genetics of restless legs syndrome. Curr Neurol Neurosci Rep 2008;8(4):281–287.

CHAPTER 47

Movement Disorders Specific to Sleep and Sleep in Waking Movement Disorders

Donald L. Bliwise, Lynn Marie Trotti, and David B. Rye

In this chapter, we will review movement disorders in sleep. The disorders reviewed below encompass an extraordinarily wide range of movements and behaviors. For ease of presentation, we have divided this review into movement disorders known to be specific to sleep versus those movement disorders characteristic of wakefulness that may be modulated by sleep. Additionally, we will focus on practical guidelines for treatment that are, in part, driven by anatomic and physiological considerations of movement in sleep, using Parkinson's disease (PD) as the prototypical disorder. The similarity of the sleep-related manifestations of many of these disorders and their assumed common underlying pathophysiology lead to treatment considerations that are parallel, despite heterogeneity of waking clinical disease. It is our belief that the various states of sleep may represent an exquisitely sensitive window on the functional anatomy and pharmacology of the basal ganglia and related structures, which may enhance our knowledge of the mechanisms underlying these conditions.

Much of our knowledge of sleep and movement disorders derives from studies on small groups of patients, including many individual patient reports. There are sparingly few comprehensive studies that (1) evaluate the natural history of disordered sleep in various movement disorders; (2) control adequately for all variables that may confound clinical presentation, including aging, dementia, and affective state; and (3) evaluate response to treatment in a placebo-controlled fashion. This is not surprising, given the existence of multiple interacting variables that hinder identification of homogeneous patient populations. Moreover, complex combinations of pathology in brain regions such as the basal forebrain, raphe nuclei, locus ceruleus, and pedunculopontine nucleus occur in many movement disorders and would be expected to contribute appreciably to the manifestations of most of the conditions discussed below.

▶ NORMAL MOVEMENT IN SLEEP

To define abnormal quantities or qualities of nocturnal movement, it is first necessary to establish the parameters of what constitutes normal movement during sleep. In some cases (e.g., paroxysmal nocturnal dystonia (PND) or rapid eye movement sleep behavior disorder (RBD)), the pattern and amplitude of movement is clearly abnormal. Conversely, in other cases, either by virtue of the widespread prevalence of a condition (e.g., periodic leg movements in sleep (PLMS)) or its transient expression during development (e.g., somnambulism), defining the limits of normality may be problematic. Undoubtedly, some of the complexity stems from the varying sensitivities of the techniques used to detect movements; that is, can they be documented videographically or do they require more sophisticated detection methods, such as accelerometers (e.g., actigraphy), surface, or even needle electromyography (EMG)? Muscle activity recorded from surface electrodes, as is used in most polysomnographic studies, for example, may reveal some information regarding individual motor units when those units are located closer to the skin surface, but in other situations involving higher threshold force or when the muscle group of interest is further from skin, such surface (EMGs may be insufficient.[1] Additionally, determining whether movement in sleep is focal or is a manifestation of a more complex pattern of movement adds another dimension of complexity. Polysomnographic studies often rely on surface EMG recordings of only several muscle groups (mentalis, anterior tibialis), which may show somewhat different patterns of activation relative to other muscles. Using actigraphic measures, for example, van Hilten and colleagues[2] have shown that the upper limbs consistently reflect more movement during sleep relative to body trunk.

Although most skeletal muscles show reduced tonic activity during sleep,[3,4] it has long been known that the body of the sleeper is far from still throughout the night.

Seminal studies from the first part of this century by Kleitman and colleagues[4] and Johnson and colleagues,[5] using primitive techniques, confirmed that the average sleeper exhibits from 40 to 50 movements during a night of sleep. Later work, using video time-lapse photography, confirmed these findings[6]. Gardner and Grossman[7] maintain that gross body movements represent the end points of afferent stimulation as the sleeper adjusts position to maintain comfort. For example, a hard bed surface has been associated with a greater number of body movements relative to a more comfortable bed.[8] Generally, however, the characteristic number of such gross body movements during sleep has been demonstrated to be a relatively stable individual trait[9] that predicts change in sleep state,[10] decreases during post-sleep deprivation recovery sleep,[11] and is often preceded by autonomic activation.[12]

In contrast to these, gross body movements are brief twitches of distal limb muscles also known to occur during sleep. These were originally described in humans by De Lisi[13] and have been associated with both sleep onset ("hypnic jerks" or "sleep starts")[14] and REM sleep, as recorded in the finger,[15] in the leg,[16] and in the mimetic muscles.[17,18] Hypnic jerks are classified as an apparently normal variant that is "essentially universal" during sleep onset by the International Classification of Sleep Disorders.[19] Middle ear muscle activity has been investigated extensively during sleep and has been shown to relate at above chance levels with motor activity in the face, neck, and extremities.[20,21] Brief isolated twitches in rapid eye movement (REM) sleep have also been described in normal animals, including the cat[22] and baboon.[23] In humans, they have been likened to fasciculations and are without pathological significance.[24] Fasciculations in patients with lower motor neuron disease appear unaffected by sleep.[25]

Although limb jerks and twitches can be seen in normal sleepers, an increasingly large body of evidence suggests that waking movement disorders in general and neurodegenerative disorders centered on the basal ganglia may be characterized by excessive amounts of such activity within sleep.[26,27] Parkinsonian patients undergoing long-term L-dopa therapy are known to demonstrate myoclonic-like limb activity.[28] Such activation of motor systems during sleep in disorders of the basal ganglia may be distinguished from the normal activity during sleep described above because of its duration, frequency, and/or widespread distribution across muscle groups. A more complete description of these movements, as well as potential mechanisms underlying their occurrence, is explored in greater detail below.

▶ MOVEMENT DISORDERS SPECIFIC TO SLEEP

In recent years, the development of the multidisciplinary field of sleep disorders has led clinicians and researchers to examine movement patterns during sleep. In this section, we briefly review several of the movement disorders confined to or exacerbated by sleep. The enormous range and rich panoply of movements observed in otherwise neurologically normal individuals challenge the assumption that human sleep is a period of virtual quiescence.

IDIOPATHIC RAPID EYE MOVEMENT SLEEP BEHAVIOR DISORDER (RBD)

Description

In the mid-1980s, Schenck and colleagues described patients (predominantly older males in their 50s and 60s) with purposeful nocturnal motor activity, often violent in nature, that resembled dream enactment.[29] This condition, now termed idiopathic RBD, is "...characterized by the intermittent loss of REM sleep EMG atonia and by the appearance of elaborate motor activity associated with dream mentation."[30] The behaviors are nonstereotyped, emotionally laden, and semipurposeful. Frequently these are accompanied by vocalization and are violent in nature, appearing to correlate with defensive dream content. Some behaviors have been described as potentially lethal,[31] although occasionally more pleasant behaviors (e.g., laughing, singing, clapping) have been noted.[32] These behaviors are differentiated from other parasomnias by their nonstereotypy, coincidence with dream recall, restriction to REM sleep, and nonepileptiform nature. Differentiating RBD from panic attacks or nocturnal terrors by history alone can be problematic given variability in dream recall. Panic attacks and terrors, however, arise from stage 2 at the transition to stage 3 and from stage 3/4 sleep, respectively.[33] Nocturnal motor behavior with lack of dream recall, abrupt arousal accompanied by diffuse autonomic symptoms, and amnesia for the event suggest the diagnosis of panic attacks. Nocturnal terrors also manifest with extreme autonomic activation and retrograde amnesia; however, motor behaviors are usually more pronounced and marked by confusion and violence on attempted arousal.[33] An important discrimination when discussing RBD is whether the term is being used diagnostically or descriptively. As originally described by Schenck and colleagues, patients with the diagnosis of idiopathic RBD were neurologically normal and did not have signs or symptoms of PD. However, it is now understood that many patients with parkinsonism also show dream enactment behaviors, often accompanied by dream recall, and this constellation is often referred to as "RBD." In the remainder of this section, we will specifically discuss idiopathic RBD and its clinical and prognostic correlates. Later in this chapter (see the section "Sleep in parkinsonism"), we will describe dream enactment behavior (i.e., "RBD") and its possible significance in the broader context of this particular movement disorder.

Clinical Correlates of RBD

Perhaps the most striking feature of idiopathic RBD is that it appears to represent a prodrome for the development of parkinsonism, which has been documented in at least four separate case series and one well-documented case report.[34] The original quasi-prospective series reported by Schenck and colleagues[35] noted an incidence of parkinsonism of 38% at 12.7 years after initiation of dream enactment symptoms, with this figure increasing to 65% 7 years subsequent to that.[36] In the largely retrospective Mayo series, 52% of patients with PD with current RBD type symptoms developed their symptoms a median of 3 years *before* PD diagnosis, whereas 57% of the total patients presenting with RBD carried a concurrent diagnosis of prevalent neurologic disease.[37] A follow-up of the idiopathic RBD cases at Mayo suggested an incidence of 65% over a mean follow-up interval of 11.2 years.[38] Iranzo and colleagues[39] reported that 45% of idiopathic RBD patients studied for a mean interval of 11.5 years after onset of symptoms developed Lewy body disease (e.g., PD, multiple-system atrophy (MSA), or dementia with Lewy bodies (DLB)). In the most recently published case series, Postuma and colleagues[40] reported 5-year, 10-year, and 12-year risks for such synucleinopathies of 19.5%, 38.0%, and 55.0%, respectively, subsequent to initiation of dream enactment behaviors. Although based largely on about 100 patients each, these case series provide highly suggestive evidence that idiopathic RBD represents a prodrome for parkinsonism. In fact, the strength of these relationships is so strong that some authors have questioned whether so-called idiopathic RBD can really be termed "idiopathic."[41]

Such provocative findings, all based on neurology clinic or sleep clinic populations, otherwise beg the question as to the prevalence and significance of dream enactment behaviors in more representative populations, which has been estimated to be as high as 2.1% across a broad age range (15–100 years) with male predominance and association with psychiatric disorders.[42] The association with psychopathology and/or medications has been confirmed in a tertiary clinic and VA populations as well.[43,44] Specifically in an older, Chinese population the prevalence has been estimated at 0.8%.[45] A few cases in the latter study were confirmed polysomnographically, but studies of apparent RBD in the general population have been based exclusively on self-report, and no population-based studies have examined incident Lewy body disease in such unselected populations. A recent analysis of questionnaire responses from college students suggests that to some extent frequency of response can be increased by how questions are worded[46]; when specific examples are provided, higher rates of endorsement are noted.

Because idiopathic RBD may represent a harbinger for the development of broadly defined Lewy body diseases, considerable effort has been directed to examining the relationships between such symptoms and other early indicators of incipient synucleinopathy, such as impaired olfaction. Braak[47] has reported early (stage 1 and 2) neuronal loss in both the olfactory bulb and anterior olfactory nucleus in parkinsonism. Not surprisingly, olfactory impairment co-occurs in conjunction with idiopathic RBD,[48,49] often at levels seen in fully developed PD[40,50,51] and is also more likely in narcoleptic patients who have RBD than those who do not.[52] Identification of several particular odors (e.g., paint thinner, gasoline) showed particularly strong discrimination from controls.[53]

In addition to olfaction, focus on RBD as a *forme fruste* of Lewy body disease comes from studies of the autonomic nervous system (ANS). Deposition of alpha-synuclein within cardiac and gut plexuses, known to be an early sign of parkinsonism,[54,55] has been confirmed in postmortem studies, and biopsies from 16 patients undergoing abdominopelvic surgeries demonstrated a strong association between positive immunochemistry for alpha-synuclein and histories of dream enactment behavior.[56] Functionally, such alterations manifest as altered R-R intervals indicative of impairment to both the sympathetic and parasympathetic branches of the ANS,[57] and reductions in presynaptic markers in nerves innervations the heart in idiopathic RBD, of similar magnitude to that seen in PD and DLB.[58,59] The latter finding has been replicated[60,61] in several cases and was also shown to discriminate idiopathic RBD versus apparent dream enactment associated with sleep apnea.[62] Postuma and colleagues[48] noted that impaired color vision, self-reported autonomic symptoms involving urinary, erectile and bowel dysfunction, and slow motor speed (e.g., timed up and go test) all occurred significantly more frequently or with greater magnitude of impairment in idiopathic RBD relative to controls. The impairment of color vision was interpreted as consistent with retinal alpha-synuclein deposition, often seen in Lewy body disease.[63]

Functional brain neuroimaging studies in patients with idiopathic RBD have demonstrated some abnormalities, though the effects are not always consistent. Striatal dopamine transporter is downregulated in idiopathic RBD as shown by both single photon emission computed tomography (SPECT)[64,65] and PET[66] relative to control subjects but still somewhat higher than in PD. MSA patients with RBD were shown to show decreased striatal, but not thalamic, monoaminergic binding on SPECT.[67] Differences in SPECT were somewhat less pronounced when comparing narcoleptic patients with and without dream enactment behaviors.[49] Whole-brain perfusion is increased bilaterally in the pons and putamen in idiopathic RBD, with some evidence of decreased cortical perfusion in frontal and temporoparietal regions,[68] findings that have been interpreted as reflecting a potential compensatory network for midbrain dopaminergic depletion. By contrast, otherwise healthy older adults with some report of dream enactment (but not polysomnographically confirmed RBD) demonstrated lower glucose utilization in parietal, temporal, and posterior cingulate cortex.[69] A study examining brain stem and midbrain metabolism in idiopathic RBD using magnetic resonance spectroscopy was unable to document differences in metabolism relative to controls.[70] These imaging studies are complemented by reports demonstrating neuropsychological impairments across the domains of visuospatial function,[71,72] verbal memory,[73,74] attention,[73,75] executive function[73,74,76] or more broadly defined mild cognitive impairment,[77] in idiopathic RBD.

Diagnosis of idiopathic RBD can be made through the clinical history, and may involve patients' recollection for aggressive dream content, often involving excessive physical activity and interactions with animals (but, curiously, not sexuality),[78] as well as history supplemented by questionnaires administered to the spouse or bed partner, in those cases where one may be available. Regarding the latter, several different approaches have been undertaken, and although no single scale has achieved universal acceptance, versions employed by the Mayo,[79] Ann Arbor,[80] and Marburg[81] groups are the best validated. An artificial intelligence-based phone interview,[82] which apparently relies on similar content to these published scales, has generated some epidemiologic estimates of prevalence (see above) but cannot be easily incorporated into clinical practice.

For reasons that remain unclear, there is a strong male predominance (at least 4:1) for RBD, although attempts to link such behaviors to free testosterone levels have shown no clear associations in either idiopathic RBD[83] or PD[84] and the male predominance may even be higher in idiopathic RBD, than either PD or MSA.[83]

As a complement to caregiver reports, videotapes, either made at home or collected during overnight polysomnography in the laboratory, constitute important objective corroborating evidence of RBD. Although dream enactment behaviors may show both inter- and intranight variability, Zhang and colleagues[85] reported that one night of video-polysomnographic monitoring was usually sufficient to screen for behavioral enactment. Bliwise and Rye[86] reported that even if behavioral episodes were not apparent, the elevation of phasic muscle activity during sleep (particularly REM, but also to some degree in nonrapid eye movement (NREM) as well) could clearly differentiate idiopathic RBD from controls. Definitive diagnosis may necessitate that video NPSG be accompanied by an expanded electroencephalography (EEG) montage to rule out nocturnal frontal lobe seizures. Manni and colleagues[87,88] reported on the comorbidity epilepsy variants and RBD, suggesting that as many of 12.5% of patients over age 60 with known seizure disorders may also demonstrate RBD.

In RBD, phasic muscle activity occurs at higher than expected rates in both REM and NREM sleep.[86,89] The polysomnogram (PSG) in the prototypical RBD patient also demonstrates periodic movements in NREM sleep,[90] which are more often unilateral, have a longer inter movement interval, and are also more likely to occur in REM relative to restless leg syndrome (RLS) patients.[91] Elevated amounts of visually scored stages 3 and 4 NREM sleep have been noted in idiopathic RBD,[92] a finding also reflected in increased spectral power in the delta band in sleep.[93] However, these findings, particularly in view of the slowing of the waking[74] and REM[94] EEG, are probably best interpreted as evidence of diffuse slowing, rather than a normal sleep EEG variant. During REM, behavioral events have been reported to occur more often during phasic eye movement activity, rather than periods of tonic REM.[95,96] Phasic EMG activity has been reported to become worse over time in idiopathic RBD,[97] although it appears stable over the short-term (i.e., night-to-night) in some studies,[85] but not others.[98] Some of this variability may be methodological in origin; novel digitized approaches to quantification of phasic EMG during sleep are under development,[98–100] though to date no consensus has been achieved on the best approach.

Finally, it should be emphasized that dream enactment behaviors are neither sensitive nor specific as a diagnostic indicator for idiopathic PD and have been associated with many other neurodegenerative conditions. Those commonly reported include DLB,[34,101–103] Alzheimer's disease (AD),[104] MSA,[105] pure autonomic failure,[106] and pontine lesions.[107,108] Disorders less frequently associated with dream enactment include olivopontocerebellar degeneration (OPCD),[109] corticobasal ganglionic degeneration,[110] spinocerebellar ataxia (SCA) type 3 (Machado–Joseph disease),[111–113] and tauopathies, such as progressive supranuclear palsy (PSP),[114] (although conflicting data exist for this association[115]) as well as atypical Guadeloupean Parkinsonism,[116] also thought to be a tauopathy. Nocturnal motor dyscontrol including RBD is frequently encountered in narcolepsy–cataplexy[117–119] and in many neurologic conditions that affect the brain stem.[109,120–123] Idiopathic RBD also has been associated with encephalitis of various forms.[124,125] Obstructive sleep apnea can mimic idiopathic RBD, with behavioral awakenings from both REM and NREM sleep, showing such apparent similarities.[126] Additionally, numerous pharmacological agents in humans have been associated with some loss of REM atonia, including tricyclic antidepressants, monoamine oxidase inhibitors, monoamine reuptake inhibitors, selective serotonin reuptake inhibitors, and alcohol.[127–133] Ingestion of chocolate may exacerbate RBD.[134]

Pathophysiology of RBD

Pathophysiological understanding of the substrates of RBD takes origin in a feline disease model that predates clinical recognition of the condition. The dorsolateral pons inclusive of the subceruleal region has been the focus of much attention since bilateral lesions here in cats release elaborate behavior suggestive of dream enactment[135,136]. The absence of REM atonia in cats correlates best with degree of loss of glutamatergic versus cholinergic neurons in the subceruleal region.[137] The subceruleal region is extremely heterogeneous anatomically, neurochemically, and physiologically, with significant interspecies variability, making it difficult to confidently discern the substrates responsible for RBD with precision. Recent experimental findings in rats point to the importance of mutually inhibitory gamma-aminobutyric acid (GABA)ergic circuits intrinsic to this region (e.g., the ventrolateral periaqueductal gray and sublaterodorsal tegmental nucleus) in coordinating REM-atonia with the desynchronized EEG and other hallmarks of REM sleep.[138,139]

It is tempting to implicate neurons intrinsic to the dorsolateral mesopontine tegmentum as the ultimate mediators of RBD as a subgroup of these exhibit REM sleep-specific increases in discharge. Descending pathways from the tegmentum to ventromedial medullary regions are known to be essential in maintaining REM atonia. When these pathways are interrupted, REM sleep-specific motor behaviors can be seen in humans.[109,121–123] The most parsimonious explanation for RBD therefore posits that it derives from loss of REM sleep-specific glutamatergic drive from the dorsolateral tegmentum to atonia generating premotor, glycinergic elements in the ventromedial medulla. As RBD predates or accompanies diseases that have in common waking features of parkinsonism, it has been suggested that the pathophysiological basis of RBD may lie in loss of noradrenergic subceruleal or cholinergic pedunculopontine tegmental nucleus (PPN) region neurons that are frequently involved by the primary pathology of many neurodegenerative conditions. This hypothesis, however, is inconsistent with experimental work. Loss of noradrenergic function, for example, might be expected to promote atonia but appears to eliminate it,[140] and loss of cholinergic PPN neurons also produces a contrary result with enhancement, rather than loss of phasic motor elements of REM sleep.[137] Postmortem human studies cast some doubt on either PPN or LDT having a specific role in RBD, however, because neuronal loss in both the PPN and the LDT was unrelated to antemortem findings of RBD in patients with DLB or MSA.[141]

Alternatively, a more complex circuit may be involved in producing enhanced phasic and tonic REM sleep-specific motor activity and a continuum to dream enactment behaviors. This could reflect increased excitatory drive to motor circuits from supratentorial brain regions (e.g., the basal ganglia and ventral forebrain) that modulate emotive behaviors and exhibit multisynaptic connections with the ventromedial medulla by way of the dorsolateral mesopontine tegmentum. This is supported by several observations, including (1) cats with RBD exhibit significant increases in open field, exploratory activity in wake[142]; (2) drugs that enhance prolocomotor monoaminergic neurotransmission can release or exacerbate RBD[131–133] (personal observations); and (3) there is a paradoxically heightened REM sleep-specific, serotonergic neural activity in cats exhibiting RBD features.[143]

As the particular behavior released in REM sleep in cats depends on the site and size of lesions[134,144] in a brain region exhibiting a wide array of forebrain afferents,[145] there are potentially numerous other structures in the hypothalamus, amygdala, or basal ganglia that might modify RBD. Of these structures that link themselves with lower motor centers via the dorsolateral pons, clinical and experimental evidence argues that the basal ganglia nuclei may be most relevant to the pathophysiology of "idiopathic" RBD. Each of the neurodegenerative conditions in which RBD is commonly observed, for example, share in common loss of nigrostriatal dopamine pathways, and imaging studies in "idiopathic" RBD demonstrate loss of dopamine transporter activity in nigrostriatal axons but no detectable alterations of D_2 receptor density.[65,66] Rats[146] and nonhuman primates[147] depleted of striatal dopamine lack overt behavioral manifestations suggestive of RBD, but do exhibit heightened phasic and tonic somatomotor activity in REM sleep that predominates in limb versus axial musculature (personal observations). Enhancement of phasic motor phenomena of REM sleep ultimately derives from transient hyperpolarization of subpopulations of glutamatergic and cholinergic PPN region neurons that exhibit low-threshold calcium spikes, as might be expected given pathologically elevated phasic bursting of GABAergic basal ganglia output nuclei in PD.[148,149] Enhancement of tonic EMG activity in REM sleep, on the other hand, may reflect excessive inhibition of alternate subpopulations of glutamatergic and cholinergic neurons whose REM sleep-specific activation is otherwise necessary for engaging REM atonia premotor elements in the ventromedial medulla. Thus, removal of excessive, inhibitory pallidal influences on the upper brain stem by pallidotomy might account for reversal of REM sleep elevations in somatomotor activity observed in some PD patients[150] (personal observations). Pharmacologic dampening of pathologic pallidal firing with low doses of L-dopa/carbidopa may similarly account for the reported benefits of this agent in treating RBD.[121,151] Reversal of RBD by surgical and pharmacologic interventions is by no means universal, and is increasingly viewed as the exception rather than the rule. Bilateral subthalamic nucleus stimulation, for example, appears ineffective in reversing RBD,[152,153] while treatment with L-dopa/carbidopa may enhance rather than suppress REM sleep-specific EMG activity early in the course of PD.[154] These mixed experiences likely reflect the heterogeneous nature of parkinsonian pathologies, the complicated effects of dopamine on behavioral state-related muscle activity (see below), and our relative lack of knowledge concerning the full spectrum of parkinsonian-related neuropathological alterations. The novel suggestion that disease burden in idiopathic PD progresses rostrally from the medulla[155] is particularly germane to the clinicopathophysiology of parkinsonian-related RBD. Early involvement of REM atonia regions in the ventromedial medulla, for example, might account for the fact that RBD can presage overt waking manifestations of PD by years, and the ineffectiveness of surgical interventions in universally reversing RBD.

Treatment of RBD

Treatment of RBD needs to be highly individualized and includes avoidance of suspected aggravators such as caffeine, nicotine, alcohol, sleep deprivation, antidepressants with significant blockade of serotonin or norepinephrine reuptake, and traditional antidopaminergics. There have been no randomized, controlled trials of RBD treatment. Clonazepam (typically 0.5–2.0 mg qhs) is the mainstay of treatment, with partial or complete response documented in up to 90% of patients in several large case series.[92,121,156,157] Long-term use of clonazepam for RBD does not appear to be associated with a significant risk of tolerance,[158] but side effects such as excessive daytime sleepiness, confusion, and cognitive impairment may be seen in up to 58% of patients, resulting in medication discontinuation in up to one third.[159] Three smaller series suggest efficacy of melatonin (response rates 71–83%, dosages of 3–12 mg), with side effects including morning sleepiness and morning headache in 36%.[160–162] Donepezil[163,164] and zopiclone[159] have also been shown to be effective in smaller series, and data are mixed for pramipexole, showing benefit in some,[165,166] but not all,[167] series. Because RBD may result in serious injury to patients and bed partners, management should also employ measures to insure safe sleeping arrangements, including: removal of objects from nightstands, placement of pillows on the bedside floor, alternative sleeping arrangements for the bed partner, and using beds with padded bedrails.

SLEEP-RELATED RHYTHMIC MOVEMENT DISORDER

Rhythmic movement disorder (RMD) consists of repetitive, rhythmic, and stereotyped movements such as head banging, head rolling, or body rocking. Body rocking often occurs with the sleeper on his knees in bed with anteroposterior thrusting of the entire body into the pillow. Other variants may exist as well, as in a case of repetitive, nocturnal tongue biting in a 2-year-old child that was not associated with epileptiform activity in waking or sleep.[168] Movements occur during drowsiness and at sleep onset,[169] but can persist during NREM or REM sleep.[170,171] In some patients, movements occur exclusively during NREM or REM sleep.[169,172] While the RMD occurring during REM sleep typically occurs in the setting of normal REM sleep, cases of RMD occurring during episodes of idiopathic RBD have been reported.[173] The typical frequency of RMD movements is 0.5–2 Hz, and movements occur in bouts lasting from a few seconds up to 114 minutes.[169] RMD is most commonly seen in infants, for whom a prevalence of 60% at age 9 months has been reported.[174] RMD is much less frequent in older children and adults, but when present typically dates back to early childhood.[169] Spontaneous presentations in adults have been noted; one report implied that head banging may have resulted from closed-head injury.[175] A male:female ratio of 5:1 in older children and adults has been reported.[169] Psychopathology, especially ADHD, has been found in 21–60% of children and adults with RMD.[169,176]

There is no clear consensus on treatment, but it seems warranted in severe cases with self-injurious behavior. A minority of adult cases are triggered by respiratory arousals from sleep apnea, and treatment with continuous positive airway pressure (CPAP) may be beneficial in this group.[169] The judicious use of clonazepam at bedtime is supported by case reports.[177,178] In milder cases, behavioral modification that involves audio masking with a metronome may be of benefit. Over practicing of rhythmic behavior in a rocking chair or more vigorous rhythmic exercises before retiring may be of additional benefit, and self-hypnosis has also been reported to be successful.[179] A small series of children were treated successfully with a 3-week regimen of sleep restriction combined with a single week of chloral hydrate administration.[180]

BRUXISM

Bruxism is defined as tooth grinding or tooth clenching during sleep that is associated with tooth wear, temporomandibular joint or jaw pain, or masseter muscle hypertrophy. Bruxism is reported by 8% of the adult population[181] and declines with age. Patients with bruxism are more likely to have anxious personality traits, be single, have at least a college level of education, and use tobacco daily.[182] In adults with sleep apnea, bruxism is associated with tension headaches.[183] In children, bruxism is associated with tension headaches in some,[184] but not all.[185] Subjects who self-report bruxism are more likely to also report difficulties with sleep initiation and sleep maintenance than those who do not report bruxism,[186] although small PSG comparisons of bruxers versus nonbruxers have not shown differences in sleep latency and have shown only nonsignificant trends toward more time awake after sleep onset and less total sleep duration. The majority of events (88%) occur during light NREM sleep.[187] Of note, 75–85% of bruxing events co-occur with more generalized body movements, typically in the anterior tibialis.[188] Current literature supports the view that bruxism represents a terminal event in a sequence of repetitive brain and autonomic activations termed "micro-arousal during sleep."[187,189,190] Patients with bruxism have higher levels of urinary catecholamines[191] and increased cardiac sympathetic activity as measured by analysis of heart rate variability.[192,193]

Alcohol has been reported to increase bruxism.[194] Moreover, as for most other nocturnal movements, sleep bruxism has been associated with the use of agents that lead to excess amounts of prolocomotor monoamines, including serotonin reuptake inhibitors.[195,196] Antagonism[197] or enhancement[198–200] of dopaminergic neurotransmission has also been anecdotally noted to predispose to sleep bruxism. Mandibular advancement devices and clonidine have both been shown to be effective treatments, although are associated with side effects.[201] Occlusal splints tend to be better tolerated and are thus recommended by some authors,[202] but meta-analyses do not provide clear evidence of their benefit.[202,203] Modest, but significant, reductions in sleep bruxism have also been reported with L-dopa,[204] pergolide,[205] clonazepam,[206] and the beta-adrenergic receptor blocker propranolol,[207,208] but these findings await confirmation with larger, double-blind studies before formal recommendation and widespread clinical use. Muscle relaxation, biofeedback, and psychotherapy may be of some benefit, but their effectiveness has not been well defined.[209]

NIGHT TERRORS (PAVOR NOCTURNUS)

Night terrors are characterized by dramatic awakenings accompanied by extraordinarily loud vocalizations, screaming, and a heightened affective state. Tachycardia, tachypnea, sweating, and enlarged pupils have been described.[210] Retrograde amnesia usually exists, although the sleeper may have a vague recollection of frightening experiences. Events typically occur during arousals from stage 3 sleep.[211] This condition is usually seen in children rather than in adults, and may represent a transiently normal developmental event. Psychopathology and coexisting sleep disorders that increase arousals (such as sleep apnea)[212] are implicated in adults. Individual cases of night terrors arising in an adult with a thalamic lesion[213] and a teen with a brain stem lesion[214] have been described, but the anatomy of this phenomenon is not known. Night terrors frequently respond to benzodiazepines[158,215] and have also been shown to respond to paroxetine[216] and L-5-hydroxytryptophan.[217] In our clinical experience, trazodone (25–150 mg), carbamazepine (200–300 mg), or valproate (125–500 mg) at bedtime may also be of some benefit.

SLEEPTALKING (SOMNILOQUY)

This phenomenon has been investigated extensively by Arkin,[218] who reported that episodes may arise from both NREM and REM sleep and have varying levels of complexity and semantic structure. There was little relationship with psychopathology.[208] MacNeilage[219] reported that episodes of sleeptalking were preceded by an average of 10 sec of muscle activity, as recorded in the genioglossus and other orobuccal muscles. Additionally, individuals who characteristically talked in their sleep showed a greater abundance of such muscle activity, even during periods without vocalization.[209] Adults who talk in their sleep typically report a history of sleep talking during childhood, and genetic influences explain over 50% of the phenotypic variance in child twin pairs.[220] Sleeptalking is more common in children with sleep-disordered breathing than those without,[221] and can also occur during night terrors. In adults, vocalizations during sleep are common during episodes of RBD. Treatment of sleeptalking is targeted toward other associated parasomnias or sleep disorders, if present. Isolated sleeptalking is of unknown significance and has no known specific treatment.

SLEEPWALKING (SOMNAMBULISM)

Classic sleepwalking (somnambulism) was described polysomnographically in the 1960s,[222] reportedly appearing to occur largely in stage 4 sleep and not uncommonly in children. More recent reports have confirmed these findings.[223] Because the condition derives out of slow-wave sleep (SWS) and often involves incomplete awakening, some have considered the condition as a disorder of arousal.[224] Adult sleepwalkers have been shown to have higher amounts of stages 3 and 4 sleep and have more spontaneously occurring disruptions of these stages as well.[225] It is distinguished from complex partial seizures by a normal EEG during both waking and sleep. Somnambulism should be differentiated from the phenomenon of sundowning in geriatric patients.[226] A sleepwalker remains amnestic during and after the event and, unlike the complex, purposeful movements of RBD, the sleeper's movements are awkward and gangly. Somnambulism is common in children, with a prevalence as high as 39–48% in 4 to 6-year-olds noted in some epidemiological studies.[227] It is thought to be of little psychopathological consequence in childhood, although adults who sleepwalk have been reported to have schizoid tendencies.[228] Childhood trauma or post-traumatic stress disorder are risk factors. A study of twins has suggested genetic contributions in 36–80% of adult sleepwalking (for women and men, respectively).[229] The HLA subtype DQB1*05 is associated with sleepwalking in Caucasians.[230]

At all ages, the sleepwalker should be considered potentially dangerous to self and others. Review of medications should be performed as there are anecdotal reports of somnambulism associated with buproprion,[231] quetiapine,[232] metoprolol,[233] and zolpidem.[234] Sleep deprivation should be avoided as it can precipitate episodes of sleepwalking events in patients with a predisposition to sleepwalking.[235] Symptomatic treatment with clonazepam is often effective.[158] Sleepwalking may respond to psychotherapy[236] and/or hypnosis.[223,237]

NOCTURNAL EATING

Two distinct syndromes of nocturnal eating have been described. Nocturnal eating syndrome (NES) is a condition where patients eat a significant fraction of total daily calories after their last meal (i.e., dinner) and during awakenings in the night. They are fully awake and eat similar foods to those eaten in the daytime, except tend to choose foods higher in carbohydrates. NES is thought to represent a problem with circadian timing of food intake.[238]

In contrast, sleep-related eating disorder (SRED) consists of episodes of eating after arousals from sleep that typically occur during a dissociated state.[239,240] Patients are usually amnestic for the experiences or have a sensation that the eating is happening without their control, although full consciousness is reported in some.[238,241] Unlike in NES, patients with SRED often eat foods during their nocturnal arousals that they do not eat during the daytime.[242] SRED can result in the consumption of unpalatable or unsafe foods (such as raw bacon)[243] or in injury from dangerous preparation of food.[242] SRED is associated with sleepwalking, PLMS, RLS, and OSA.[238,242] SRED has also been associated with the use of triazolam, zolpidem, tricyclic antidepressants, anticholinergics, lithium, olazapine, and risperdal.[238,242,244–246]

The first step in treating SRED, as in other disorders of arousal, is to treat any associated periodic limb movements or sleep apnea.[238] Offending medications should be discontinued. If further treatment is needed, topirimate[247] or dopaminergics (L-dopa/carbidopa,[248] pramipexole[249]) or buproprion[238] appear promising, although clinical trial data is limited to support their use. Favorable responses to serotonin reuptake inhibitors, representing a smaller subset of patients, have also been reported[242].

PAROXYSMAL NOCTURNAL DYSTONIA (PND)

Originally considered to be a movement disorder specific to sleep lacking an EEG correlate, it now appears that PND is caused by partial seizures of frontal lobe origin.[250,251] Patients experience spells that arise abruptly from NREM sleep and consist of uni- or bilateral dystonic posturing, and choreoathetoid or ballistic movements lasting 10–60 sec. On some occasions, vocalizations occur.[252] Often these behaviors appear grossly "unusual" and may not suggest seizures to the inexperienced clinician despite their stereotypic quality and tendency to cluster. They may be only occasional, or recur 30–40 times nightly. A 10–40-sec modal interval between attacks appears causally related to waxing and waning in thalamocortical arousability as manifest in the cyclic alternating pattern of normal NREM sleep.[253,254] In some patients, semipurposeful arm activity or even sexual automatisms may be seen. Thus, NPD patients share some features with RBD; however, the episodes in NPD clearly evolve from NREM (typically stage 4) sleep. Typical patients exhibit normal interictal EEG activity during both sleep and wakefulness.[255] Less often, spike wave complexes, prominent in frontal regions, may be observed during a behavioral episode.[256] Diagnosis is therefore often made through the clinical history and home videotapes because localization of a frontal epileptic focus is difficult, particularly with the limited EEG montages employed by routine PSG. A definitive diagnosis of PND (e.g., versus psychogenic seizures) may necessitate video PSG with an expanded EEG montage, or even inpatient or outpatient video EEG monitoring. Treatment includes the use of carbamazepine (200–400 mg qhs) that seems to produce more effective results than other anticonvulsants. Treatment failures should alert one to the possibility of a primary sleep disorder, since for PND, as with any seizure disorder, sleep disruption or deprivation can increase seizure frequency.

GENERAL CONSIDERATIONS ON THE TREATMENT OF OTHER MOVEMENT DISORDERS SPECIFIC TO SLEEP

Historical or PSG identification of the specific form of nocturnal movement disorder will dictate the course of treatment. Once the proper diagnosis is established, the majority are treatable by either behavioral or pharmacological means. Because their etiologies are likely to be diverse, however, the proposed treatments are legion and usually lack validated objective results. The physician should first attempt to rule out any associated condition and/or medication that may account for nocturnal movements or parasomnic behaviors. Methylphenidate, for example, may worsen bruxism,[198] whereas cardiac antiarrhythmic agents and some antidepressants may exacerbate night terrors.[257,258] Before pharmacological interventions, the physician should always counsel the patient and family on proper sleep hygiene, including (1) avoidance of sleep deprivation; (2) maintenance of a strict sleep-wake schedule; and (3) avoidance of nicotine, alcohol, and caffeinated beverages because of their tendencies to fragment sleep.

Sleeptalking, sleepwalking, night terrors, and SRED comprise a group of parasomnias that frequently coexist.[259] One of the most important aspects of the treatment of these disorders is ruling out coexistent depression or other psychopathology, particularly in the elderly patient.

A wide variety of stimuli, such as PLMS, apnea, and gastroesophageal reflux, may also present with complaints of parasomnic behavior, presumably secondary to their precipitating nocturnal arousals. PSG, therefore, is frequently indicated to consider these etiologies that demand distinct treatment strategies. Nocturnal seizures less commonly present with complaints simulating one of these parasomnias or head banging/body rocking. Video monitoring and PSG with EEG montages that are more elaborate than those typically used in routine studies are, therefore, only occasionally required for proper diagnosis.

▶ SLEEP IN WAKING MOVEMENT DISORDERS

SLEEP IN PARKINSONISM

Nocturnal Sleep

Disorders of sleep in patients with PD have long been recognized; however, their pathophysiological basis remains ill-defined, and universal treatment strategies have not been established. Reasons for these deficiencies are many, and they include the pathological heterogeneity of PD and coincident factors such as medication use, aging, dementia, and mood disturbances, each of which independently affect sleep parameters. The sleep of PD patients is profoundly disturbed, even relative to other neurodegenerative conditions. One survey placed the prevalence of nocturnal sleep disturbance in PD at 98%.[260] PSG studies of PD patients, extending back into the 1960s, consistently demonstrate poor sleep efficiency, decrease in stages 3 and 4 sleep, and marked sleep fragmentation.[261–266] These changes are related to disease duration.[267] The sleep state-specific EEG also changes in PD, with sleep spindles being reduced during SWS[264,268,269] and alpha activity intruding into REM sleep.[261] Reported changes in REM sleep are variable across studies and appear highly dependent on dose and length of dopaminomimetic treatment, disease duration, and individual patient differences.[262–264,267,270–273] Given the REM sleep-suppressant effects of L-dopa,[274] many have hypothesized that REM sleep rebound underlies hallucinations experienced by many PD patients.[275–281] The recent demonstration of REM sleep intrusions into daytime naps in hallucinating and nonhallucinating patients provides electrophysiologic evidence supporting these conclusions.[282–285]

Disordered sleep in the form of excessive nocturnal movement in PD was first noted in Parkinson's 19th century *Essay on the Shaking Palsy*, and these findings have subsequently been confirmed and extended. A detailed account of previous studies and the development of this line of investigation is presented in earlier editions of this book.[286] Despite the widely held belief that involuntary movements associated with disease of the extrapyramidal motor system disappear during sleep, motor dyscontrol in sleep in the form of tremor (Figs. 47–1 and 47–2), aperiodic (Fig. 47–3) and periodic leg movements (Fig. 47–4), increased phasic and tonic EMG activity in REM sleep (Fig. 47–3), and frank RBD predate or accompany neurodegenerative disease involving nuclei of the basal ganglia.

In summary insofar as nighttime sleep is concerned:

1. Sleep can be punctuated by parkinsonian tremor (Figs. 47–1 and 47–2), although tremor may be preceded by microawakenings, and, during REM, isolated muscle contractions are common (Fig. 47–3).
2. NREM and REM sleep are characterized by large numbers of isolated and periodic limb movements (Fig. 47–4).
3. Stages 3 and 4 of NREM sleep are least likely to manifest movements.
4. Nocturnal movements are common in both upper and lower extremities.
5. Nocturnal movements are common in both flexor and extensor muscles.
6. Nocturnal movements are generally best controlled when waking motor symptomatology is best treated, although movement may persist even in the presence of antiparkinsonian medication.
7. As mentioned earlier in this chapter, RBD can accompany and even precede waking signs of PD, as well as other degenerative conditions affecting the basal ganglia and/or brain stem.

The prevalence of nocturnal motor dyscontrol in PD is difficult to establish because most published data derive from PSG studies carried out at referral centers, thereby selecting for patients with disturbed sleep. PLMs lacking subjective RLS complaints are common in PD, occurring at a greater prevalence than in conditions lacking severe nigrostriatal dopamine neuron loss, such as aging, AD,[287] and MSA.[288] Historical accounts from patients and their bed partners estimate that RBD in idiopathic PD is also relatively common, possibly reaching 15%,[289,290] although as documented polysomnographically, the prevalence of REM sleep without atonia (RWA) could approach 60% in PD patients unselected for symptomatic dream enactment behavior.[289] The degree to which nocturnal movements contribute to sleep fragmentation, and whether these are disease-specific or treatment-related phenomena, remain controversial issues that are still to be resolved. The intrinsic pathology in PD itself is likely to be the major contributor because early and/or untreated PD patients exhibit disturbed sleep that includes excessive nocturnal movement.[262–264,291] Moreover, rats[146] and nonhuman primates[147] depleted of striatal dopamine bilaterally exhibit excessive nocturnal movement, and sleep in the parkinsonian patient deteriorates with disease progression.[269,271,292] The fact that nocturnal movements are generally best controlled when waking motor

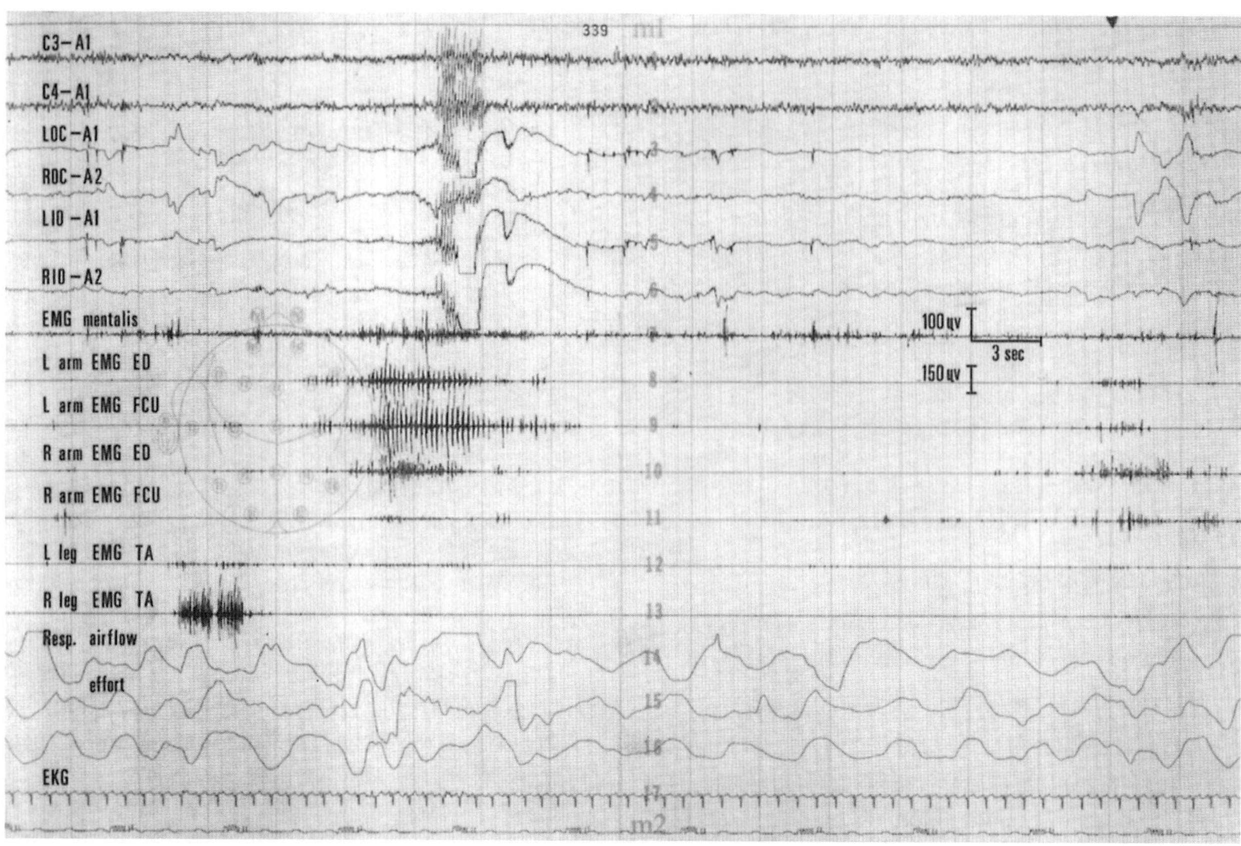

Figure 47–1. PSG recording of an episode of tremor intruding on an epoch of REM sleep in a patient with PD. Also note the increased level of tonic activity in the chin EMG (EMG mentalis). Abbreviations: R, right; L, left; ED, extensor digitorum; FCU, flexor carpi ulnaris; TA, tibialis anterior.

symptomatology is best treated medically, argues further that their pathophysiological bases are firmly rooted in nigrostriatal dopaminergic neuron loss. Clinical improvements of PD seen with surgical interventions that restore balance in basal ganglia neurotransmission also improve sleep architecture.[145,152,153] A systematic analysis of this phenomenon is warranted given potential differential effects that pallidotomy[145] and bilateral subthalamic nucleus stimulation[152,283–285,293–296] have on PLM, RBD, and overall sleep duration and quality, though not necessarily on reported daytime sleepiness.[294,295] The precise substrates accounting for the detrimental effects of nigrostriatal dopamine loss on nocturnal movement are ill-defined. It is tempting to speculate that dopamine modulates brain stem circuits effecting PLM and REM sleep atonia. This does not occur via direct dopaminergic innervation of the brain stem, but rather by indirect, multisynaptic routes linking the basal ganglia output nuclei with pontomedullary reticulospinal pathways via the dorsolateral pons, including the subceruleal region (see Fig. 47–6). Accentuated blink reflexes[297–299] and acoustic stimulation of spinal reflexes,[300] argue for the presence of heightened excitability in brain stem circuits. Similar reflex pathway abnormalities in patients with PLM, but not suffering from PD, suggest that PLM in PD are modulated by the same neuropharmacologic substrates. Interestingly, recent use of deep brain stimulation specifically within the pedunculopontine nucleus resulted in increased REM sleep but without obvious introduction of symptomatic RBD in patients with advanced PD.[301]

Other neuromodulatory systems are frequently involved by the neuropathology of PD, and may potentially account for alterations in sleep architecture. Neuronal degeneration in PD, for example, has been described in the serotonergic dorsal and median raphe, noradrenergic locus ceruleus, and cholinergic PPN neurons.[302–305] Cell loss has been estimated at between 30% and 90%, and is proposed to underlie many of the functional waking deficits observed in PD, particularly akinesia, depression, and dementia.[305,306] Decrements in spinal norepinephrine and serotonin and their metabolites suggest additional degeneration of descending cerulospinal and raphespinal pathways, but quantitative estimates of death in the cells of origin are not available.[307] The significance of these alternate pathologies to the etiology of nocturnal movement disorders of PD is unknown. The majority of experimental findings argue against a significant role for serotonergic, noradrenergic or cholinergic pathologies

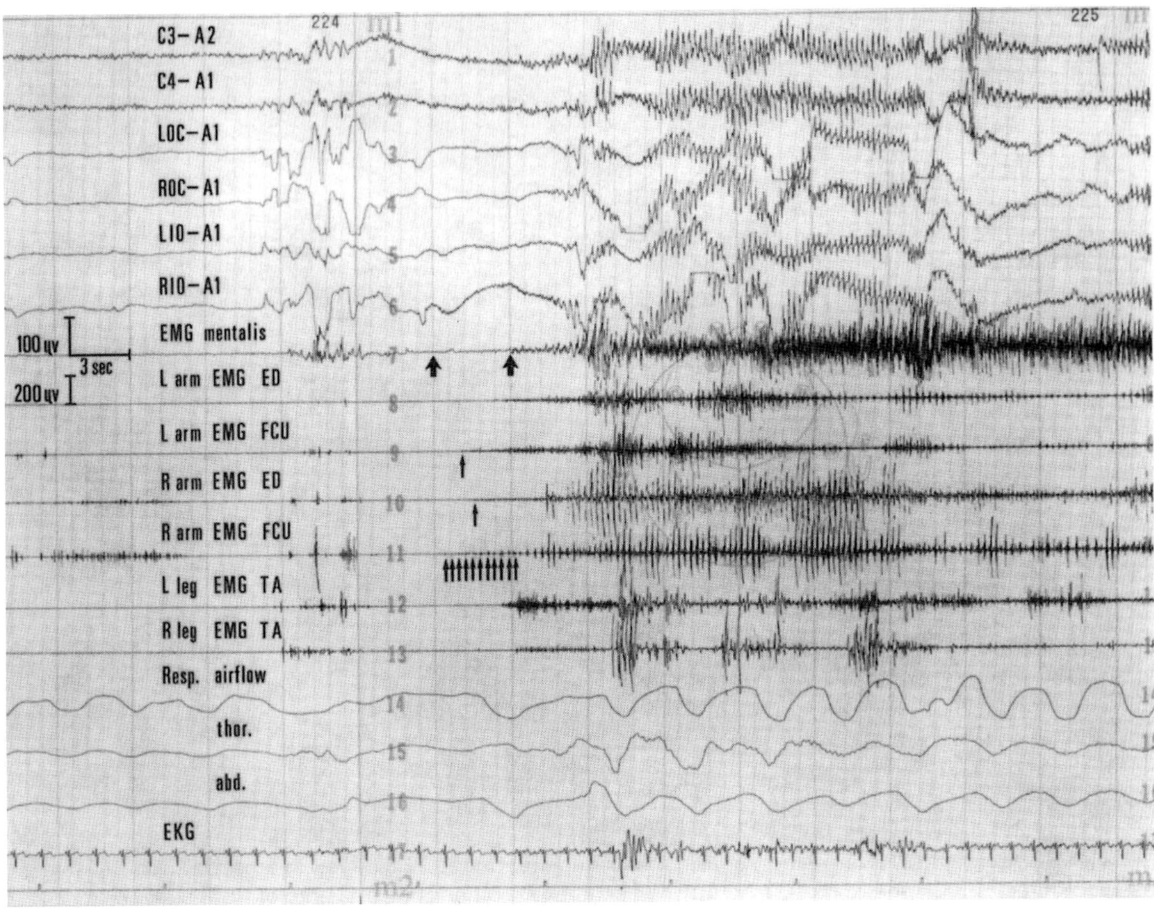

Figure 47–2. PSG recording of an episode of tremor intruding on REM sleep with subsequent arousal in a patient with PD. Multiple small arrows denote tremor that begins in the right flexor carpi ulnaris (FCU), coincident with the development of tonic activity in the right extensor digitorum (ED) and left flexor carpi ulnaris (small arrows). During this 3-sec epoch there is no change in chin muscle activity, as detected by the mentalis EMG (two broad arrows) or in the cortical EEG. Arousal from REM sleep, therefore, clearly occurs after these EMG changes. Abbreviations are as designated in Fig. 47–1.

in the nocturnal motor disturbances of PD. Loss of central and spinal monoamines, for example, might be expected to protect against, rather than increase, the incidence of PLM in NREM sleep given the prolocomotor effects of systemic serotonin and nornepinephrine during sleep.[308] With respect to REM sleep, lack of serotonergic and adrenergic innervation of the cholinergic PPN would diminish rather than enhance RBD-related phasic EMG events by removing sources of transient hyperpolarization necessary for a burst firing mode. Loss of cholinergic PPN neurons themselves would also favor less, rather than more, phasic EMG activity in REM sleep.[137] Extranigral, nondopaminergic pathology in sporadic PD is increasingly recognized to involve medullary and pontine regions containing multiple neuron types with presumed influences on wake/sleep-related somatomotor activity.[309] The proposition that this pathology predates the extensive loss of midbrain dopaminergic neurons traditionally thought to underly PD[47,310] may account for the near ubiquitous occurrence of sleep-related movements in PD, and the experience that disturbed sleep, particularly RBD, can presage the development of the waking manifestations of parkinsonism.

The daytime consequences of sleep fragmentation have not been systematically investigated, although patients and their spouses frequently volunteer that activities of daily living are improved when sleep is undisturbed.[311] Sleep and levels of arousal have generally accepted benefits on mobility in parkinsonism and remain an area of active investigation.[281,311–315] An expected consequence of disturbed sleep in PD might be excessive daytime somnolence (EDS), but the results of questionnaire-based surveys paint a conflicting picture,[316,317] and recent quantitative assessments argue that short, fragmented sleep is less, rather than more, likely to be associated with EDS.[283,285] Our own and others' experiences with PD patients suggests a wide range of daytime sleep latencies between and within subjects that

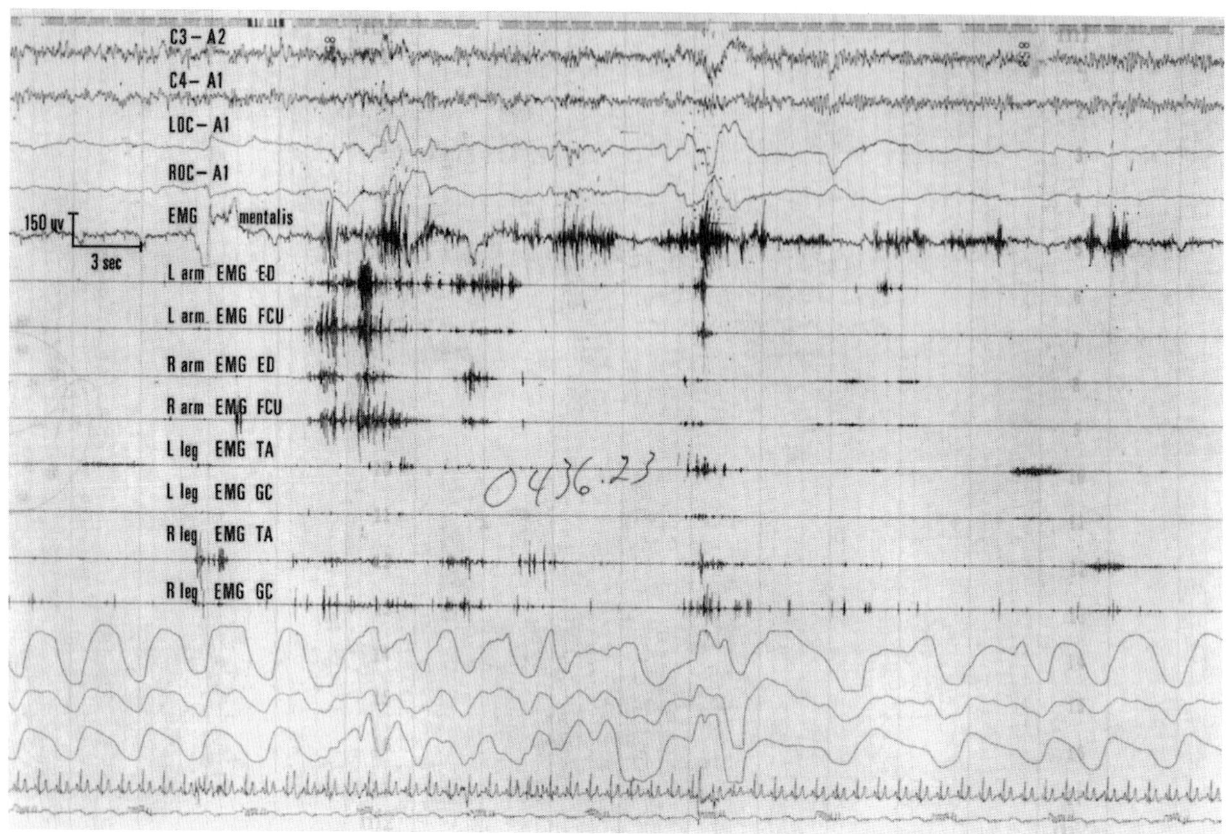

Figure 47–3. PSG recording of intermittent, phasic muscle activity during REM sleep in a patient with PD. It is not unusual to detect similar phasic muscle activity coincident with other phasic events of REM sleep (e.g., eye movements) in normals. Note, however, the occurrence of heightened phasic and tonic muscle activity in the chin (EMG mentalis) that occurs independent of eye movements in the parkinsonian patient. REM sleep appears to persist despite these EMG changes. Abbreviations as for Fig. 47–1; GC, gastrocnemius.

reflects principally the pathology in brain regions critical for maintaining arousal (see below), and also a complex interplay between medications, the "on-off" phenomenon (Fig. 47–5), disease-related sleep fragmentation, and disruption secondary to PLM or sleep apnea.

Daytime Sleepiness

Sleepiness in PD is common, very real, yet underrecognized. As captured by Oliver Sacks' familiar memoir *Awakenings*, the sleepiness of the parkinsonian patient transcends the metaphor. It is undeniably verifiable, and likely as much a consequence of the disease as its treatment. Treatment of PD with psychostimulants in the pre-L-dopa era, in fact, may owe its partial benefit to alleviation of sleepiness.[318–321] Intrinsic sleepiness therefore represents an important target in disease management, as much as a fear of pharmacologic intervention, and nonmotor daytime symptoms, including sleepiness and fatigue, are increasingly recognized as essential components influencing quality of life in PD.[322,323] There are also population-based data that suggest that sleepiness in middle-aged men or sleep durations longer than 9 hours in women can portend later development of PD.[324,325] It is important to recognize that not all patients or clinicians recognize sleepiness as a symptom of PD and instead may describe their symptoms under the rubric of fatigue;[326,327] some data suggest that this descriptor may be more closely related to depression.[328] Some attempts have been made to differentiate these conditions psychometrically,[326,328] although the existence of objective, polysomnographic procedures such as the multiple sleep latency test (MSLT)[282,283,285,292,329–331] or maintenance of wakefulness test (MWT)[331,332] allow for more valid measurements of state instability and provide better documentation of such phenomena.

Dopamine cell death in PD profoundly alters not only nocturnal movement but also thalamocortical arousal state. This manifests as daytime sleepiness, and intrusion of REM sleep into daytime naps (sleep-onset REM sleep (SOREM)).[282,283,333] The initial report of dose-related "sleep attacks" with pramipexole and ropinirole was interpreted as a novel, idiosyncratic response specific

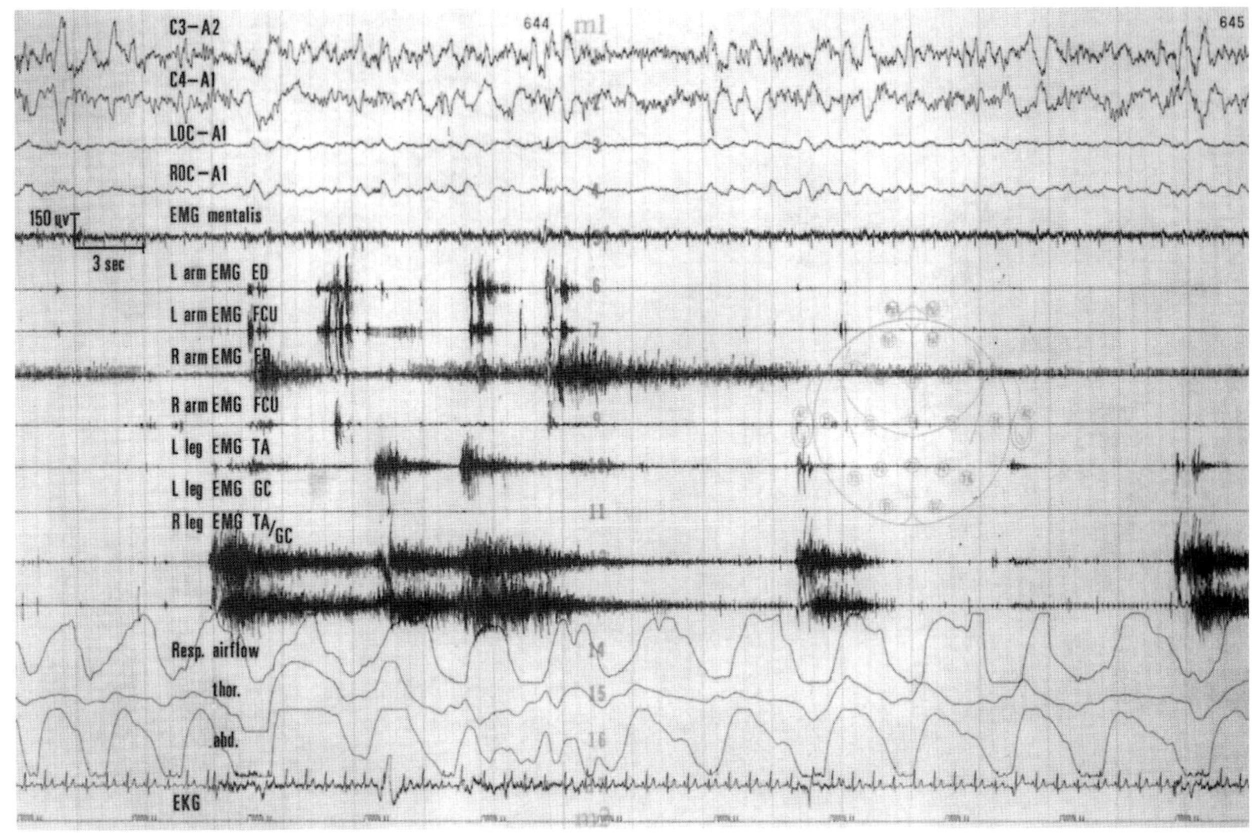

Figure 47–4. PSG recording of periodic leg movements during stage 2 NREM sleep in a PD patient. Note the periodic cocontraction of the right tibialis anterior (TA) and gastrocnemius (GC) indicative of PLMs. In the parkinsonian patient, this is more likely to occur coincident with, as well as independent of, activity in several other upper- and lower-extremity muscle groups. Arousal from sleep clearly does not accompany these EMG changes.

to the new nonergot D_2/D_3 receptor agonists.[334] Clinical experience and more comprehensive assessments agree that sleepiness has long been under-recognized in PD, but that it is a phenomenon not restricted to a specific class of dopaminomimetics.[335–338]

In community-based samples of PD patients, the rate of self-reported sleepiness ranges from 6% to 29% as compared to 1–2% in healthy, elderly controls.[339–342] Depending on the criterion and self-reported measurement instrument used, estimates as high as 43% have been reported.[343,344] Longitudinal studies have demonstrated that the rate increases by about 6% per year.[345] Higher rates are generally noted in clinic-based samples,[338,346–348] even up to 76% of patients in one clinic.[349]

A wide variety of questionnaires have been used to attempt to assess sleepiness in PD patients. These include the Epworth Sleepiness Scale (ESS),[283,285,338,339,342,346,350–357] a 15-item visual analog scale, the Parkinson's Disease Sleep Scale (PDSS),[358–360] the Scales for Outcomes in PD-Sleep Scale (SCOPA-S),[343,359,361] and the more general Non-motor Symptoms Questionnaire for Parkinson's Disease (NMSQuest).[322,323] Although marginally adequate psychometric properties have been derived for most of these scales, the widespread use of the ESS for both PD and non-PD patients experiencing subjective sleepiness probably favors use of this scale for the assessment of self-reported sleepiness per se. Detailed analyses of the hierarchical item structure of the ESS in PD patients revealed a two-factor solution comparable with analyses of the ESS made in patients having daytime sleepiness from other disorders.[362]

Employing a standardized measure of physiological sleep tendency across five daytime nap opportunities, we and others have objectively documented "pathological" sleepiness in 30–50% of patients, and a narcolepsy-like phenotype in a similar number[282,283,285,329–332] (Fig. 47–5). Sleepiness bears little relationship to the primary motor manifestations of disease (e.g., disability scale, medication burden), or sleep architecture measures (e.g., total sleep time, and stage). These findings argue that parkinsonism itself accounts for impairments in the expression of wake and REM sleep, an important concept that finds further support from animal models of parkinsonism. Remarkably, contrary to what one would expect based on the demands of sleep homeostatic mechanisms, poor nocturnal sleep is generally associated with greater, rather than lesser, degrees of daytime alertness. The dissociation of arousal state from the motor manifestations

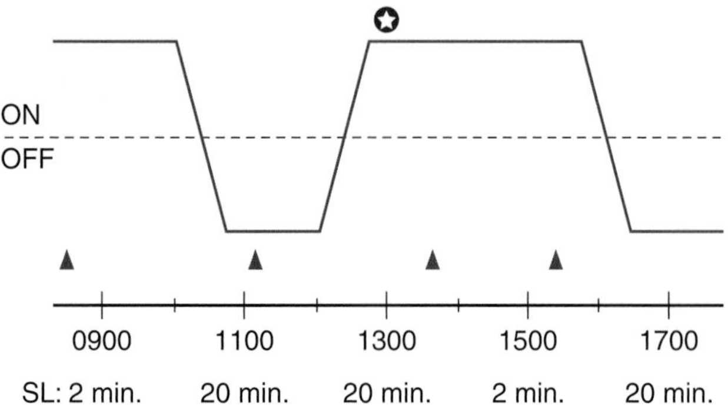

Figure 47–5. Multiple sleep latencies (SL) in a patient with PD demonstrate extreme variability across time of day and are likely to reflect complex inter-relationships among circadian factors, medications, and "on-off" status. Note SL of 2 minutes at 9 am (0900) and 3 pm (1500) while the patient was "on," versus no sleep (i.e., SL of 20 minutes) during "off"-periods or peak-dose dyskinesias (star). Arrowheads indicate times of dosing of one-half tablet of controlled-release carbidopa/L-dopa 50/200 (Sinemet-CR).

of disease and homeostatic sleep drives (viz., sleep propensity should be inversely rather directly related to the quality and quantity of prior nights' sleep) in PD has several implications. First, it emphasizes that dopamine pathway integrity is critical for maintaining homeostatic sleep mechanisms. Second, it points to the pathophysiological basis of impaired thalamocortical arousal state residing outside of the sensorimotor subcircuit of nigrostriatal pathways traditionally thought to underlie parkinsonian motor disabilities. A threshold of 60–90% dopamine loss in the sensorimotor putamen is necessary for the emergence of waking clinical manifestations,[363] and then proceeds in an orderly fashion through associative (i.e., caudate), and eventually limbic (i.e., nucleus accumbens) striatal subcircuits. Thus, it is loss of dopamine in these latter circuits, most characteristic of advanced disease, that is, a potential factor in the expression of sleepiness and SOREM in PD.

The objective findings in a small number of newly diagnosed, unmedicated or young PD patients[283,291] emphasize that the parkinsonian state itself is a major factor in the expression of sleepiness and SOREM. For example, one study reported that the likelihood of EDS may increase over 8 years within patients even when dopamine agonists were not used,[364] although this has been disputed in many descriptive[331,338,342,344,346,349,351,355] and some interventional[365,366] studies that indicate an independent role for medications in these effects. The point is best made in animal models of disease that control for potentially confounding variables such as age, comorbid conditions, and medications. Rats spend less of their subjective day awake following destruction of nigrostriatal pathways with bilateral, intrastriatal infusions of the dopamine toxin 6-hydroxydopamine.[146] Similarly, daytime sleepiness and SOREM have been reported in a single nonhuman primate following systemic delivery of the dopamine neurotoxin 1-methyl,4-phenyl-1,2,3,6-tetrahydropyridine (MPTP),[147] and this has been confirmed in two additional animals (personal observations). The cellular and subcellular substrates underlying these disease-related effects remain ill-defined. These phenomena may reflect loss of dopamine's effects on neural excitability in any one of a number of brain regions necessary for maintaining normal states of thalamocortical excitability. One plausible substrate given the narcolepsy-like phenotype seen in nearly half of "sleepy" PD patients is hypocretin-containing neurons in the lateral hypothalamus known to degenerate in primary narcolepsy/cataplexy.[367] Other plausible neural substrates that deserve future investigation include targets of ventral tegmental area (VTA) dopamine neurons, including the prefrontal cortex, the cholinergic magnocellular basal forebrain, and midline thalamic nuclei. This hypothesis is supported by the results of several studies, including one which demonstrated that D_2 receptor antagonists microinjected into the VTA block the sedation seen with systemic administration of dopamine agonists,[368] and another which demonstrated that infusions of amphetamine directly into ventral forebrain targets of the VTA neurons both initiated and maintained alert wakefulness.[369] Alternatively, sleepiness and SOREM may reflect extranigral pathology[305] (e.g., in nuclei comprising the traditional ascending reticular activating system such as the dorsal raphe, locus ceruleus, and PPN). Dysregulation of the PPN region, an area known to promote thalamocortical arousal and REM sleep, may also be an important factor secondary to its position as a principal brain stem target of pathological basal ganglia outflow[145] (see Fig. 47–6).

Recently, attention has focused on dysfunction of the orexin/hypocretin system, a potent regulatory neuropeptide diffusely projecting to many monoaminergic, histaminergic and dopaminergic cell groups, as the primary neuronal substrate for sleepiness in the PD patient. Interest in hypocretin was prompted by low or undetectable levels of this peptide in the brain and cerebrospinal fluid (CSF) of patients with the prototypical disorder of inability to maintain daytime alertness, narcolepsy.[370,371] Postmortem data have demonstrated loss of hypocretin cell bodies throughout the hypothalamus in PD,[372] although CSF derived from living PD patients was noted to be normal in several studies of PD,[371,373,374] but not all.[375] The neuropathologic findings were confirmed by Fronczek and colleagues,[376] who also showed that postmortem CSF hypocretin levels were similarly decreased in those same patients. CSF hypocretin levels were reported as normal in MSA, DLB, PSP and corticobasal degeneration (CBD),[377–380] though in PSP, more severely affected patients were noted to have the lowest levels.[379]

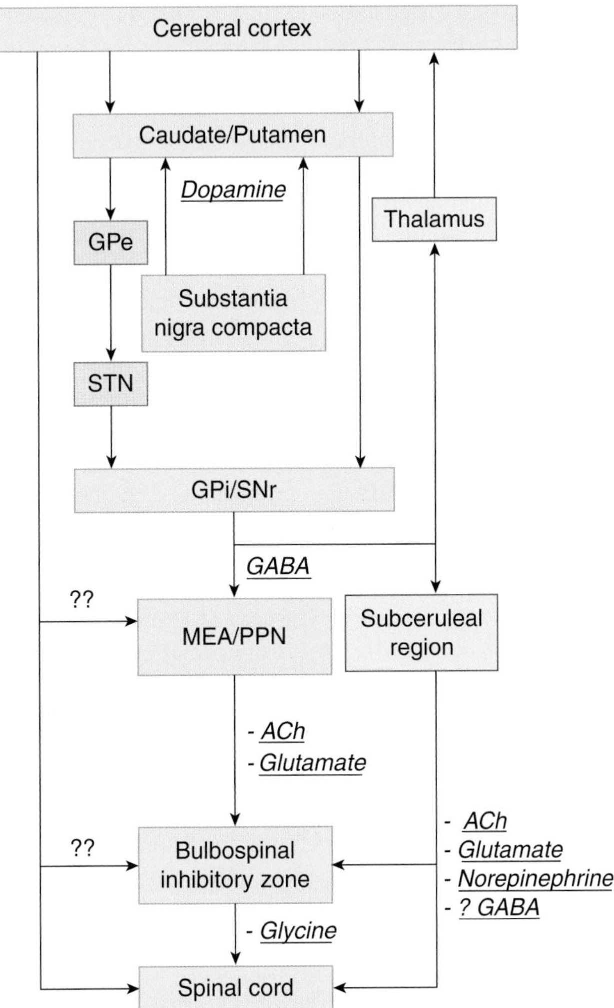

Figure 47–6. Schematic representation of established pathways linking dopamine-sensitive basal ganglia circuits with premotor elements in the brain stem and, in turn, to spinal motor circuits. The dorsolateral mesopontine tegmentum including the midbrain extrapyramidal area (MEA), adjacent pedunculopontine tegmental nucleus (PPN), and subceruleal region are key elements that can relay GABAergic influences from the internal segment of the globus pallidus (GPi) and substantia nigra pars reticulata (SNr) to the ventromedial medulla (i.e., the bulbospinal inhibitory zone of Magoun and Rhines). Descending pathways from these structures employ glutamate and/or acetylcholine and are ultimately responsible for REM sleep-specific tonic and phasic increases in ventromedial medullary neuronal activity. Because this increased neural activity is necessary to maintain atonia, any alterations in glutamatergic, cholinergic, or glycinergic influences on, or exiting from, the ventromedial medulla will impact on EMG activity in REM sleep. These alterations may take the form of neuronal loss in the BIZ or MEA/PPN region that accompanies many neurodegenerative conditions, or alternatively, of abnormal modulation of these neurons by pathological influences originating in one of their many afferent sources (e.g., amygdala, hypothalamus, basal ganglia). As the pathophysiologic basis of many movement disorders specific to sleep are envisioned to lie in the basal ganglia, these brain stem pathways may also represent the substrates mediating many additional motor disturbances in sleep. Abbreviations: ACH, acetylcholine; GPe, external segment of the globus pallidus; STN, subthalamic nucleus.

Reduced density of hypocretin neurons was noted in the posterior hypothalamus in MSA, though CSF was not analyzed in that study.[381] More recently, interest has focused on a different neuroregulatory peptide, cocaine and amphetamine regulated transcript (CART) with stimulant properties,[382] which has been reported to be decreased in the CSF of DLB patients.[383]

Separate from the neurobiological substrates governing PD, other factors may influence expression of sleepiness and SOREM. Advanced disease or disease duration have been contributing factors noted in several studies.[283,337,345,346,348] Other potential risk factors include older age of onset,[364] benzodiazepine use,[283] male sex in some[346,364] (but not all[349]) studies, comorbid dementia or psychosis,[345] and autonomic failure (e.g., orthostatic hypotension).[347] A wrist actigraphic study reported that hallucinating PD patients showed a reduced amplitude of their sleep/wake rhythm over 5 days, consistent with greater daytime sleepiness relative to nonhallucinating patients.[384] Many of these clinical features are also shared by patients exhibiting DLB,[385] suggesting that sleepiness may be a phenotypic characteristic of this subtype of parkinsonism. This is supported by a longitudinal study that found that nearly two-thirds of PD patients with sleepiness went on to develop dementia.[345] Additionally, AD patients demonstrating parkinsonian signs have been reported to nap more frequently than AD patients without such signs,[386] although AD patients generally appear to be less sleepy than PD or DLB patients, as based on caregiver reports of the ESS.[387] Neuroimaging studies using SPECT have suggested that PD patients who are the most sleepy showed cortical hypoperfusion in selected left cortical regions and right caudate with hyperperfusion in right thalamus and brain stem,[354] however, whether these patients had bilateral clinical signs is unknown. A study examining unilaterally presenting PD noted that patients with left-side onset reported greater daytime sleepiness, consistent with right hemisphere-mediated neural networks affecting levels of waking arousal and activtation.[388] On the other hand, using SPECT, Happe and colleagues[389] reported that lower binding of dopamine transporter on both ipsilateral and contralateral side of maximal involvement in striatum, putamen and caudate were highly correlated with greater sleepiness on the ESS.

Some evidence suggests that genetics may also play a role in the daytime sleepiness of selected PD patients. For example, Frauscher and colleagues[390] reported that patients carrying both alleles of a single nucleotide substitution in a functional polymorphism of the catechol-O-methyltranferase receptor (suggesting decreased dopamine transport) were more likely to be sleepy during the day. An attempted replication by the same group, however, was unable to repeat the result,[391] although noting receptor polymorphisms on the D_2 receptor differentiated PD patients with and without sudden onset of sleep.[392] Another group was unable to confirm the this association but reported significant allelic variation in the DRD4 region.[393] A parallel, but independent, hypocretin-related polymorphism was also reported to play a role.[394] As with many genetic association studies, replication across populations will be essential to document relevance of such findings to the sleepiness of the PD patient.

Despite the fact that sleepiness may be intrinsic to the disease process per se, a number of reports in PD link sleepiness to sudden onset of sleep or "sleep attacks" and dopaminomimetic use.[334,395–400] The apparent prevalence of daytime sleepiness in PD notwithstanding, the prevalence of such events appears, at least in studies that have measured both, to be less in some studies.[339,342] To a certain extent, the emphasis on the lexicon of "sleep attacks" may essentially be a surrogate marker for what can be more objectively quantified as more severe levels of sleepiness.[329] One study even noted that the frequency of "sleep attacks" was similar in PD patients and controls, despite having very different distributions of sleepiness, as measured by the ESS,[356] further arguing that defining sudden onset of sleep phenomenologically is difficult in PD patients. Some authors have contended that the inability of some PD patients to self-perceive their own levels of sleepiness amounts to anosognosia for such state instability.[401] At least one survey of over 6,000 PD patients noted that nearly 50% acknowledged sleep attacks but that nearly 5% of this population claimed that they never experienced any daytime sleepiness whatsoever,[344] and a small laboratory study contended that PD patients with and without sudden onset of sleep could not be differentiated on the basis of MSLT, with means of both groups falling within the normal range.[402] The latter group, however, reported somewhat different results in a later study in which two similar groups of patients were monitored with continuous daytime polysomnography, revealing a greater number of spontaneous microsleep episodes in patients with a history of "sleep attacks."[403] Other studies using MSLT are consistent with the spontaneous sleep results.[282]

Regardless of whether called sleepiness or "sleep attacks," such phenomena in PD can be associated with dopaminomimetics in dose-related manner. They are not clearly related to specific class of agent (e.g., L-dopa versus ergot- and nonergot-derived D_2/D_3 receptor-like agonists),[331,337,338,346,349,351,355,400] although some have contended that nonergot agonists may present the greater risk.[344] One study reported that L-dopa induced greater subjectively assessed sleepiness in MSA relative to PD.[404] These reports are based on self-reports and only a few have documented or investigated the nature of such medication effects systematically using MSLT or MWT.[405,406] While sleepiness observed with dopaminomimetic use in PD is now well recognized, it remains unresolved how often this use contributes and how much of a contributing factor it is. L-Dopa,[365] ropinirole,[366] and pramipexole,[407] for example, can exacerbate sleepiness even in drug-naïve controls. It has been suggested that obstructive sleep apnea and PLMs coexisting with PD may also contribute to sleepiness and SOREM,[285,351] although studies attempting to confirm such associations with sleep apnea largely have been negative.[282,408] Yet, this is controversial since sleepiness in nonparkinsonian patients is not completely explained by the severity of obstructive sleep apnea and PLMs. A final important determinant of sleepiness in PD is premorbid sleepiness level, which is increasingly recognized to be a heritable trait in the general population. One survey of sudden-onset sleep in a large number of movement disorder clinics, in fact, found that 20% of PD patients reporting sudden onset of sleep while driving experienced similar events prior to the diagnosis of PD being made.[338] In summary, the pathophysiological bases underlying the spectrum of PD-related changes in sleep-wake tendencies are complex and unique to the individual patient. Until more data are forthcoming, the most prudent clinical and experimental approaches should proceed from the assumption that the parkinsonian condition represents an underlying diathesis to sleepiness and SOREM expression that can be exaggerated by numerous coexistent factors, including use of dopamine agonists and L-dopa, sedative-hypnotic and potentially other medications, primary sleep disorders, and potentially comorbid conditions such as dementia and depression.

Daytime somnolence experienced by idiopathic PD patients is thus potentially as severe and disabling as that manifest by narcoleptics. Proper treatment can dramatically enhance quality of life and prevent the significant morbidity and mortality that attends pathological sleepiness. Physicians treating PD should therefore educate patients and their families on the potential detrimental effects of this disease and its treatment not only on motor symptoms but also on the ability to maintain an active, awake state. Patients should be informed about the potential dangers of driving. Administration of the ESS,[409] possibly completed by the caregiver or significant other, and queries about unintended sleep episodes, particularly while driving, should be routine. Anywhere from 11% to 22% of PD patients experience sleepiness while driving, and this risk tends to correlate with higher ESS scores.[338,346,410] The frequency of sudden-onset sleep while driving is reported to be about 3.8%,[338] with the majority of these preceded by drowsiness or warning signs (about 85%). If significant or unpredictable sleepiness is suspected, driving should be temporarily restricted until the sleepiness resolves.

Treatments for Daytime Sleepiness and Disturbed Nocturnal Sleep

General Considerations

Clinicians treating patients with PD and other neurodegenerative diseases of the basal ganglia should always carefully inquire about sleep quality, since disturbed nocturnal sleep and impaired daytime alertness can presage the development of further more troublesome sleep disorders.[278] When sleep disturbances in patients with PD do occur, their management is highly individualized. In general, appropriate management of waking motor symptoms generally reduces nocturnal movement and improves sleep efficiency.[411] Although amelioration of waking motor symptoms is always the desired outcome, the fact that anywhere from 74% to 98% of medicated PD patients complain of sleep disturbances[260,278] suggests that suboptimal management may well be the rule rather than the exception. Because a typical pattern of disordered sleep has not been clearly delineated and etiology is generally unknown, no clear-cut algorithms exist for approaching the treatment of PD patients with disordered sleep. Specific treatments need to be customized to complaints only after an adequate sleep history and review of PSG findings, as discussed in detail below, have been completed. History should not rely on subjective reports of sleep alone, since reliability of personal assessments is well known to be poor secondary to sleep state misperception. Information from a caregiver and preferably a bed partner is a *sine qua non* to guide treatment decisions, as is historical information on the timing of medications and nocturnal symptoms, as well as the relationship of symptoms to any changes in medication. Whenever historical evidence exists for nocturnal motor behavior, abnormal respiratory patterns, or EDS, PSG, including either MSLT or MWT, should be performed. Before pharmacological interventions, the physician should always counsel the patient and family on proper sleep hygiene, which includes, but is not restricted to, avoidance of alcoholic beverages, nicotine, and caffeine.

Daytime Sleepiness

The first step in effecting resolution of parkinsonian-related sleepiness demands a careful review of medications and defining any temporal relationship between dosing and symptoms, as dosage reduction or discontinuation of dopaminomimetics, particularly agonists, or long-lasting benzodiazepines might reverse sleepiness. Nightly benzodiazepine use intended to improve daytime alertness by lengthening total sleep time and preventing nocturnal arousals seems particularly unwarranted given the strong inverse correlation of parkinsonian sleepiness with the quantity or quality of prior nights' sleep. If medication adjustments are ineffectual, the diagnostic "yield" for routine PSG and mean sleep latency evaluation of PD patients could be considerable (15% prevalence of PLMs, 20% prevalence of obstructive sleep apnea, 40% prevalence of "secondary" narcolepsy). Treatment strategies may then need to be targeted at alleviating PLMs and obstructive sleep apnea, if present. If sleepiness persists, treatments that until now have focused primarily on minimizing waking motor disability should include agents specifically designed to promote daytime alertness. Prescribing wake-promoting agents such as bupropion,[412] traditional psychostimulants,[319,320] and modafinil are justified on identification of a narcolepsy-like phenotype or mean sleep latencies of <8 minutes. While the initial open-label experiences with modafinil in PD patients with drug-related drowsiness are encouraging, a double-blind, randomized, placebo-controlled study is needed to corroborate and extend the results.[413–416] Although optimistic insofar as some subjective fatigue outcomes are concerned, more recent trials have been disappointing for primary end points of daytime sleepiness such as ESS or MSLT.[417–420] The use of selegiline in treating the EDS in PD is also deserving of investigation, given its metabolization to amphetamine derivatives,[421] tendency to improve memory and learning of word associations in PD patients,[422,423] increased theta EEG frequency bands over delta activity,[424] and utility in treating the EDS accompanying other disorders such as narcolepsy.[425–427] A medication dosed nocturnally that is approved for treating narcolepsy with cataplexy, sodium oxybate, was shown in an open-label trial to increase subjective alertness and decrease daytime fatigue in PD, both effects attributed to an increase in SWS seen with this drug.[428]

Selection of the most appropriate drug and its dosing for maximizing wakefulness in PD will require future clinical trials. As the problem of PD-related sleepiness has only recently been recognized, there are no comprehensive studies on how it might be best reversed. Pharmacologic treatment is employed only for those patients in whom identification and treatment of other causes of daytime sleepiness has proved ineffectual (Table 47–1). In the nonhuman MPTP primate model of PD, sleepiness and SOREM have been reversed with the dopamine precursor L-dopa, the dopamine reuptake blocker bupropion,[429] but not the $D_{2\text{-like}}$ receptor agonist pergolide.[147] L-Dopa and bupropion require presynaptic integrity to enhance synaptic availability of dopamine by promoting its synthesis, or by blockade of dopamine transporter, respectively. Thus, the abilities of these agents to reverse sleepiness and SOREM likely reflect actions on surviving mesocorticolimbic dopamine circuits that are less vulnerable to MPTP and affected only later in the course of idiopathic PD. Enhancement of synaptic dopamine availability in mesocorticolimbic circuits, in fact, may underlie the success of amphetamines in the treatment of PD described nearly 30 years ago,[319,320] providing beneficial alerting effects in truly "sleepy" patients.

TABLE 47–1. TREATMENT OF SLEEPINESS IN PD

Medication adjustments
Reduce over-the-counter sleeping aids with antihistaminergic activity
Minimize benzodiazepine use
Minimize "sedating" antidepressant use
Dopaminomimetic dose adjustment if dosing temporally associated with sleepiness
Treat-documented sleep or other disturbance
Continuous positive airway pressure for sleep apnea
Nighttime dosing of dopaminomimetics, opiates, or gabapentin for periodic leg movements of sleep
Consider treatment of orthostatic hypotension
Treat "residual" daytime sleepiness
Hygiene measures
Scheduled naps
More frequent, smaller meals
Pharmacologic measures
Bupropion (75–150 mg two or three times per day)
Modafinil (100–200 mg each morning and noon)
Dextroamphetamine sulfate (5–30 mg each morning and noon), combination of sustained-release and regular tablets
Sodium oxybate (3.0–4.5 g qhs and again 4 hours later)

Sleep-onset Insomnia

Sleep-onset insomnia appears to be no greater a problem in the PD patient than in the general aged population, based on questionnaire data.[260,280,316,317] In most instances, sleep-onset problems can be related to anxiety or to agitated depression, which should then be the focus of treatment. Additional contributors to sleep-onset insomnia in subpopulations of PD patients include RLS and akathisia, which are discussed in more detail below.

When treatment with L-dopa is instituted, some patients may experience sleep-onset insomnia that typically resolves with time.[430] Sleep-onset insomnia, at the outset of L-dopa therapy, is best treated by administering medications earlier and waiting patiently. When insomnia is severe enough to produce a significant and persistent phase delay in sleep onset, the use of fairly rapidly absorbed and/or short-acting benzodiazepines, such as temazepam (15–30 mg), alprazolam (0.125–0.25 mg), estazolam (1–2 mg) or triazolam (0.125–0.25 mg), seems warranted. In our own experience, we have been most satisfied with triazolam, with the comment that it should be used with caution in elderly and demented patients. Our own repeated attempts to treat advanced patients with zolpidem (5–10 mg), a very rapidly absorbed and short-acting benzodiazepine-like medication, as well as other sedative-hypnotics (chloral hydrate, pentobarbital), have met with limited success.

Sleep-Maintenance Insomnia

Sleep-maintenance insomnia (i.e., sleep fragmentation) is the most common nocturnal complaint in PD patients. When examined subjectively with sleep diaries over 2 weeks, PD patients barely average 6 hours of sleep per night[431] (which probably translates to even less than 6 hours with polysomnographic measurements), though several longitudinal studies using more general questionnaires over periods of 6 to 8 years suggest that symptoms of poor sleep tend to wax and wane over disease course.[432,433] Studies that have directly compared MSA and PD patients have shown even greater sleep continuity problems in the former.[434] It is of primary importance to first rule out, by history, other comorbid conditions that might present as a complaint of sleep-maintenance insomnia. For example, poor sleep characterized by early morning awakenings can signal the appearance of depression, the use of alcohol as a sedative, or the natural effect of aging in phase advancing the wake-sleep cycle. Having ruled out these possibilities, the clinician should recognize that the complaint of sleep fragmentation in PD manifests in PSG as a continuum from unexplained spontaneous awakenings to awakenings associated with quite specific nocturnal motor disturbances. Each of the latter conditions can be associated with either under- or overtreatment of the daytime symptoms of PD, or represent side effects of adjunct medications and, therefore, require very different treatment strategies.

Clinical experience dictates that, early in the course of treatment with L-dopa, daytime administration improves motor symptoms and may not disrupt sleep. Frequent awakenings, for the most part unassociated with movements, are treated with sedating antidepressants, such as trazodone, nefazodone, nortriptyline, amitriptyline, or clomipramine. Some caution should be exercised in prescribing antidepressants because they may precipitate confusion/hallucinosis,[430] worsen PD,[435] or worsen PLMs (see above). Because the latter two side effects appear related to serotonergic mechanisms, the antidepressants listed above are presented in order of preference, based on their increasing potencies in blocking serotonin reuptake.[436]

As PD progresses and/or L-dopa use becomes long term, patients may experience "off" phenomena during the night. These patients, usually advanced in their disease, typically relate a history of marked interdose motor fluctuations during the day. Not only dyskinesia but also immobility with subsequent inability to turn over, or to rise to use the bathroom, may be troubling for the patient at night.[260] In this instance, historical documentation frequently uncovers the presence of nocturnal movements, severe akinesia, and/or prolonged awakenings that occur later in the night. This situation should be carefully distinguished, preferably by PSG, from nocturnal movements early in the night, which are more suggestive for nocturnal myoclonus secondary to overtreatment or PLMs. Treatment for PD patients with distinct nocturnal motor disabilities such as tremor, dyskinesias, akinesia, and prolonged awakenings should begin with dosing L-dopa closer to bedtime, particularly in sustained-release form, because this is felt to diminish sleep fragmentation by nocturnal movements.[437,438] Alternatively, selegiline and bromocriptine have been shown to improve sleep in patients with PD, even when L-dopa has minimal effect.[273,430] High evening doses, however, might increase sleep latency and disrupt sleep in the first half of the night, despite improving sleep continuity in the second half of the night.[263,264] When PSG-documented nocturnal movements persist, we complement treatment with benzodiazepines, which are known to attenuate phasic sleep events and small and large body movements.[439] We prefer the use of triazolam (0.125–0.25 mg qhs) in nondemented patients because of its documented benefit for elderly patients with PLMs, sleep fragmentation, and daytime sleepiness.[440] A double-blind, placebo-controlled trial suggested that very high dosages of melatonin (50 mg) resulted in actigraphically defined improvements in total sleep time of about 10 minutes, as well as improving subjective alertness,[441] but a much smaller double-blind trial employing 3 mg and using polysomnographic measurements was unable to show any significant effects.[442] There are no published trials in PD with ramelteon, a prescription medication with selective affinity for the melatonin type 1 and 2 receptors. As mentioned above, an open label trial identified sodium oxybate as a potential agent to enhance SWS in PD.[428]

Frequently encountered in our practice has been the worsening of nocturnal myoclonus and PLMs with antidepressants, particularly norepinephrine and serotonin reuptake inhibitors, which is an infrequently recognized side effect but is commonly accepted among sleep clinicians (see above).[443,444] This phenomenon is consistent with reports of benefits from methysergide, a serotonin antagonist, in alleviating the nocturnal myoclonus of PD (see below).[16,28,279] Treatment options include discontinuation of antidepressant medication or its substitution with an antidepressant, whose potency in blocking serotonin reuptake is less. We have also observed worsening of PLMs in PD secondary to the inadvertent prescription of metaclopromide for the gastrointestinal symptoms of PD, which presumably reflects its dopamine antagonist action.

Fragmentary Nocturnal Myoclonus

The chronic administration of L-dopa can lead to the development of fragmentary nocturnal myoclonus during SWS.[28,279] Historical data that may suggest the presence of nocturnal myoclonus include the complaint of troubling daytime dyskinesias related to L-dopa dosing,[28] or that of exaggerated axial myoclonus at sleep onset that may precipitate abrupt arousals from sleep. This phenomenon is thought to reflect L-dopa-induced upregulation of serotonergic neurotransmission because it is alleviated by methysergide (2 mg), a serotonergic antagonist, and by discontinuing L-dopa but not by altering anticholinergic medications.[28] Treatment options include a reduction in nighttime dosing of dopamine agonists, addition of a benzodiazepine such as temazepam, clonazepam, or triazolam, and possibly a trial with methysergide (2 mg) shortly before bedtime.

Periodic Leg Movements of Sleep (PLMS)

PLMs are an entity distinct from fragmentary nocturnal myoclonus, although their presence early in NREM sleep disrupts sleep in a similar manner. They can be differentiated clinically from myoclonus because they are more often unilateral and prolonged, spaced at very regular intervals, and characterized by a flexor withdrawal-type movement typically restricted to the lower extremities. Although a careful history from a spouse or bed partner may, therefore, distinguish between these two entities, PSG is sometimes required and warranted since treatment modalities are distinct. Although PLMs exhibit high prevalence rates in the general population over the age of,[445–448] they are more prevalent in PD patients.[287,449] By history, PD patients with RBD appear more likely to show these as well.[450] Because the neurophysiological abnormalities delineated in patients with PLMs but not suffering from PD[445,451] approximate those seen in PD patients,[300,452] a common pathophysiology is suggested. Although comparably high levels of PLMS were seen in idiopathic RBD and PD patients, multiple system atrophy patients had even higher levels[453] and MSA patients have also been noted to have higher rates of isolated phasic EMG acivity as well.[99,453] In treating PD patients with coexistent PLMs, we follow the strategies outlined above for PLMs in the nonparkinsonian population. Given the decreased capacity of the pathologically effected substantia nigra to synthesize dopamine from L-dopa, trials with low doses of dopamine agonists seem particularly warranted. When dopaminomimetics are unsatisfactory, aggravate insomnia, produce troubling nocturnal myoclonus, or result in "rebound" leg movements in the early morning, we will substitute gabapentin (300–1800 mg in divided doses), oxycodone (5–15 mg), or propoxyphene (65–100 mg) at bedtime for the dopaminomimetics. We reserve the use of benzodiazepines for patients who are refractory to these approaches to avoid problems associated with the development of tolerance and possible worsening of coexistent depression.

Restless Legs Syndrome (RLS)

Several investigators have failed to note the coincidence of RLS in patients with PD.[430,454] However, in our experience and that of others,[346] the two frequently coexist. One case control study reported a higher prevalence of RLS in PD than in age, sex and race-matched controls, although even within the PD patients the prevalence was relatively low (3%).[455] Suspected RLS in a PD patient should be very carefully differentiated from akathisia, which is also encountered in PD patients. An anecdotal report of alleviation of RLS in PD with pallidotomy is consistent with suggestions that the basal ganglia and their connections are intimately involved in the expression of RLS.[456]

Akathisia

Nocturnal akathisia is a reported problem in a small subgroup of PD patients and should be carefully differentiated from RLS. Akathisia is not associated with prominent paresthesias, and symptoms are not typically relieved by movements or pacing, unlike those of RLS. Moreover, there is no PSG-documented hallmark that has yet been defined in the PD patient experiencing akathisia. Akathisia is frequently described by the PD patient as a vague sensation of an "inner restlessness." Moreover, akathisia is thought to be precipitated by L-dopa,[457,458] which would be expected to suppress the symptoms of RLS. While one report suggests that akathisia more commonly occurs in PD patients with bradykinesia and "stiffness,"[457] another notes that it is unrelated to motor or mental state or time of day.[458] Successful treatments include alterations in the timing or dosage of L-dopa[457] and bedtime dosing of clozapine, which has the added benefit of reducing nighttime tremor.[458] Successful treatment of akathisia has also been reported, using fluoxetine alone or together with amitriptyline, in 1 depressed PD patient.[459]

REM Sleep Behavior Disorder (RBD) (See also Preceding Section on Idiopathic RBD, Treatments)

As mentioned previously, the recognition that RBD predates and is associated with neurodegenerative diseases that share waking manifestations of parkinsonism has captured considerable attention. This clinical entity is more frequently encountered in the male PD patient, as is the case with "idiopathic" RBD.[92] In MSA, the male/female ratio is closer to 1:1, and RBD may be even more common than in PD.[434] An interesting feature of RBD in PD is the coordinated quality and speed of purposeful movements that occur during sleep, in contrast to the somewhat more discontinuous and bradykinetic portrait of movement seen in the waking state.[460] Histories consistent with RBD can be obtained from nearly one in six patients with idiopathic PD.[289,290] PSG analysis reveals "subclinical" evidence of RBD in nearly 60% of PD patients,[289] and this muscle activity (when quantified as a phasic electromyographic metric, PEM) distinguishes parkinsonian subjects from age-matched controls.[289,461] The yield for elucidating a history of RBD seems particularly high in those suffering from L-dopa or dopamine agonist-induced hallucinations.[281,462–465] In MSA, history of RBD may occur in as many as 90% of patients.[466]

PD patients with and without RBD can be differentiated by a number of clinical disease features. In some studies,[467,468] but not all,[450] such patients are less likely to be tremor-predominant. Although evidence is clearly mixed, some data suggest that RBD in PD may be associated with current or future psychotic signs, such as hallucinations,[281,284,462,463,469,470] though conflicting data exist.[432,471–474] One study noted later development of hallucinations in PD patients with RBD only if executive dysfunction existed at the time of initial study.[475] Dream enactment behaviors are more likely to occur in PD cases with dementia,[476] and even nondemented PD patients with RBD are more likely to show more subtle cognitive impairments,[76,477] particularly in the domains of verbal memory, executive function, and visuospatial processing when compared to nondemented PD patients without RBD. Although the presence of RBD in PD may vary over periods of nearly a decade,[465] several investigators have suggested that its presence at one time is almost predictive of a documented synucleinopathy.[101,478] This has been confirmed in a recent neuropathologic investigation of RBD plus dementia or parkinsonism.[479] The clinicopathologic associations are so strong that the consensus criteria now include RBD as a core clinical feature strongly suggestive of a diagnosis of DLB.[480] Waking EEG slowing in nondemented PD patients with RBD history has been reported,[481] although neuroimaging approaches attempting to differentiate such patients using magnetic resonance spectroscopy[482] were not revealing. Conversely, SPECT studies have suggested a decreased gradient of presynaptic striatal dopamine transporter from normals, to idiopathic RBD patients to PD patients with clinically manifest RBD.[64]

As was the case for idiopathic RBD, the presence of dream enactment behaviors in PD patients is associated with orthostatic hypotension,[473] and other autonomic signs such as constipation[474] but associations with impaired olfaction are not as strong.[473] In MSA, associations between RBD and impaired cardiac sympathetic ganglionic function are less apparent than in PD.[59]

The treatment of choice for RBD is clonazepam (0.5–2.0 mg qhs), which is effective in 75–90% of cases. Dopaminomimetics and/or antidepressants, which exhibit some ability to block dopamine reuptake (e.g., buproprion and sertraline), may theoretically prove to be useful alternative or adjunct medications in the PD patient with RBD (see also section above on treatments for idiopathic RBD).

Other Parasomnias

Parasomnia is a term that includes a variety of complex sleep-related behavioral phenomena in addition to RBD. In PD patients, these include sleeptalking, sleepwalking (i.e., somnambulism), altered dream content, nocturnal hallucinations, nocturnal terrors, and panic disorder. Difficulties in differentiating between parasomnias on the basis of history and the lack of specific PSG features in PD have precluded accurate delineation of their pathophysiology and treatment. Because many of these parasomnias have been reported as prodromes to the development of full-blown RBD,[483,484] they may describe a continuum reflecting a common pathophysiology. The sleep of patients experiencing nocturnal terrors, however, lacks any distinct alterations in sleep architecture,[430] whereas that of patients with nocturnal hallucinations is markedly fragmented and approximates that seen in RBD.[281] Although panic disorder could theoretically manifest nocturnally in PD, it is rarely encountered and typically occurs during the "off" phase in depressed PD patients taking L-dopa but not direct agonists.[485] Most studies attribute parasomnias in PD to the long-term effects of L-dopa treatment.[276–278,430,454] Pathological differences between individual PD patients are as likely to contribute to parasomnias because nocturnal hallucinations[281] and nocturnal wandering/disruptive behavior[486] in PD can be unrelated to medication type or dose. A greater prevalence of parasomnia-type behaviors in the subpopulation of PD patients with dementia further supports this contention.[454] There is little information on the treatment of patients with nocturnal terrors or panic attacks, particularly those with coexistent PD. Instruction on proper sleep hygiene, and sedating antidepressants, alone or together with an anxiolytic such as alprazolam, are the mainstays of treatment. The parasomnia condition most familiar to the clinician treating PD patients is that of nocturnal hallucinations/delirium, where preexisting sleep complaints are more common,[278] sleep deprivation markedly aggravates the severity of symptoms,[487] and sleep efficiency, total REM sleep time, and percentage are significantly reduced.[281] Other than reducing the dosage of dopaminomimetics, the mainstays of treatment include clozapine (6.25–50 mg qhs),[488,489] risperidone (0.5–2.0 mg qhs),[490,491] or quetiapine (12.5–150 mg ghs). Quetiapine appears to exhibit less tendency for motor worsening.[492–494] The nature of the beneficial effects of atypical neuroleptics in the PD population has been attributed to antagonism of 5-HT_{2A} receptors and may reflect their tendency to enhance sedation, improve sleep continuity, reduce gross body movements, and enhance REM sleep.[495–498] Sedating antidepressants such as amitriptyline or trazodone may be of additional added benefit.

Sleep Apnea

Central or obstructive sleep apnea, hypoventilation, and irregular patterns of respiration likely contribute to sleep fragmentation in a small subpopulation of PD patients; however, few detailed studies have been reported.[499,500] With the possible exception of MSA, nocturnal respiratory disturbances probably are no more likely to occur in PD or other movement disorders, despite their high prevalence in the normal adult population.[283,288,454,501] A recent study reports a lower apparent prevalence than in age, sex, and body mass index-matched controls.[408] Increased tone or dyskinesias in the upper airway muscles, caused by either the disease itself or medications,[502] can predispose the PD patient to obstructive apneas. Dyscoordination of respiratory muscle activity and abnormalities in respiratory drive have also been observed that might contribute to nocturnal respiratory disturbances.[503–505] The severity of respiratory abnormalities is greater in patients with coincident autonomic dysfunction,[449,500] possibly accounting for the fact that EDS is more regularly present in patients with MSA-P and MSA-C.

In both MSA-P and MSA-C, obstructive and central sleep apnea, respirations with variable amplitude, and arrhythmic respiration are commonly observed.[506–509] Gilman and colleagues[510] noted that decreased cholinergic binding within the thalamus was positively associated with severity of sleep apnea in MSA patients, a finding interpreted as suggesting decreased cholinergic activity deriving from mesopontine structures more intimately involved in respiratory control. MSA patients may have particularly severe sleep apnea when vocal cord abductor paralysis is present.[511,512] A relatively high prevalence of snoring was noted to be approximately equal in both MSA-C and MSA-P subtypes.[513] Nocturnal stridor, indicating elevated expiratory resistance, often accompanies the widespread snoring (most typically representing increased respiratory resistance) seen in such patients, although the respiratory disturbance index may not be grossly elevated.[514] A neuropathologic study indicated neuronal loss in the medullary arcuate nucleus in MSA,[515] a finding consistent with decreased central chemoresponsiveness and central type sleep apnea.

Although in PD it is generally felt that respiratory disturbances correlate with the severity of rigidity and tremor, they do not typically improve with administration of L-dopa.[454] Treatment of the sleep-related respiratory disturbances in PD is, therefore, similar to that when these problems are encountered in the normal adult population. For obstructive and central sleep apnea, treatment with CPAP offers the best chance of success and can be used effectively by most patients. In MSA, two case series, one reporting modest[516] and the other relatively high[517] adherence to CPAP have been published. In patients who cannot tolerate CPAP, we first explore the use of bilevel PAP before adding adjunct medications such as sedative antidepressants or the extremely short-acting sedative/hypnotic zolpidem (5–10 mg qhs). One anecdotal report notes successful treatment of central sleep apnea in OPCD using trazadone (50 mg qhs).[518] The clinician should always recognize that the risk of sudden nocturnal death remains high in MSA patients[519] and may even be exacerbated by tracheostomy.[520]

PROGRESSIVE SUPRANUCLEAR PALSY (PSP)

The sleep of patients with PSP has been reported to show a near absence of REM sleep by some[114,521] but not all authors.[522] Decreased sleep efficiency and increased sleep latency are seen in PSP patients compared with PD patients.[522] The severity of reduced sleep efficiency and increased sleep fragmentation has been correlated with extent of dementia,[114] although body movement in these patients appears to be no more severe than in age-matched controls.

Despite RBD being more common in synucleinopathies than tauopathies,[523] RWA/RBD also occurs in PSP. While overt, disruptive or injurious dream enactment was not reported by the bedpartners of 10 PSP patients,[524] some degree of dream enactment was endorsed by 20% of PSP patients or their caregivers.[525] Eighty-five percent of PSP patients had some degree of RWA by PSG,[522] although the amount was significantly less than that seen in age-matched PD patients. PSG-documented RBD was less common than RWA, occurring in 35% of the PSP patients.[522]

PLM indices are significantly higher in PSP patients than PD patients.[522] Eleven of twenty PSP patients were found to have previously undiagnosed sleep-disordered breathing (defined as an AHI > 5) in one series.[522] Despite overall poorer PSG-determined sleep quality in the PSP group, there were no differences between the PSP and PD groups on self-evaluation of sleep on the PDSS, and spontaneous reports of poor sleep quality in PSP are rare.[522]

Hypocretin-1 levels in CSF are significantly lower in patients with PSP than those with PD and inversely correlated with PSP disease duration.[526]

CORTICOBASAL DEGENERATION (CBD)

Subjective reports of poor sleep are present in 33.3–100% of CBD patients, with lower rates based on the Neuropsychiatric Inventory (NPI) and higher on Pittsburgh Sleep Quality Index (PSQI) scores > 5.[527,528] Sleep efficiency and REM sleep percentage are reduced.[528,529] SWS amounts are variable, with absent, severely reduced, normal, or increased (up to nearly 40%) amounts of SWS being reported.[528,529]

Systematic, questionnaire-based studies of patients with CBD have shown a prevalence of dream enactment of 5–7%.[524,525] RBD or RWA has been reported in isolated case reports or small case series of CBD.[110,529,530] A PSG study of five patients meeting diagnostic criteria for "probable CBD," however, found no RBD or RWA in any of the patients.[528]

RLS was seen in two of five CBD patients.[528] PLMS were present in three of these five patients, only one of whom had coexisting RLS. In one reported case of PLMS in a CBD patient, PLMS were unilateral and contralateral to the more severely affected hemisphere.[531] Sleep-disordered breathing was seen in two of five patients (severe central and obstructive apnea in one and upper airway resistance syndrome in the other).[528]

Hypocretin-1 levels in CSF are significantly lower in CBD than in PD, with a mean level of 246 pg/mL.

A pathologically low level (defined as a level less than 110 pg/mL) was seen in one of 7 CBD patients.[526]

HUNTINGTON'S DISEASE (HD)

Dyskinesias have been reported to occur in sleep in Huntington's disease (HD),[532] with lowest frequency during SWS (stages 3 and 4). REM sleep, by contrast, appeared to be a time of relative activation of the chorea. Fish and colleagues[533] reported that HD patients showed a larger number of movements across the entire sleep period relative to PD patients, although they contended that such apparent sleep-related movements were preceded by several seconds of EEG arousal before the movement itself.

PSG studies of HD have demonstrated disturbance of sleep architecture, including reduced sleep efficiency. Prolonged sleep latency and reduced SWS have been shown by some[534] but not other[535] investigators. Early studies claimed an absence of REM sleep in HD,[536] but this has not been confirmed by others,[534,537] although reduced amounts of REM and prolonged REM latency can be seen.[535] In one report, REM percentage decreased with disease severity from premanifest disease through moderately severe disease.[535] Increased density of sleep spindle (12–14 Hz) activity has been noted in the stage 2 sleep of HD patients.[371,373]

Insomnia, largely of sleep maintenance, was reported by 64% of HD patients.[535] Thirty-six percent of patients had PSG-documented sleep onset prior to 9 pm, a marker for advanced sleep phase, but this was not more common in HD patients with insomnia than those without.[535] Daytime sleepiness, as measured by an ESS score >10, is not different between HD patients and controls, although 16% of HD patients demonstrated an abnormally short mean sleep latency of less than 8 minutes on MSLT.[535] Three of 25 HD patients exhibited PSG-documented RBD and an additional one patient had evidence for RWA.[535] A single kindred with comorbid HD and RLS has been reported,[538] but other investigators have found that HD patients have significantly more PLMs than controls without an increased frequency of RLS.[535]

Despite reports of hypocretin neuronal loss in HD patients, two or more sleep onset REM periods are not seen during MSLT[535] and CSF levels of hypocretin are normal.[539]

OTHER FORMS OF CHOREA

In Morvan's chorea, severe insomnia is prominent and PSG recordings show loss of typical sleep architecture, with both day and night recordings showing stage 1 sleep interrupted by short bouts of REM sleep without atonia. Sleep spindles and deep sleep are severely reduced. These features are similar to those seen in familial fatal insomnia.[540]

WILSON'S DISEASE (WD)

Portala and colleagues[541] investigated subjective sleep complaints in a group of 24 treated WD patients compared to a population-based control group. WD patients had longer sleep latencies and more nocturnal awakenings. The WD patients estimated their sleep need as higher than did controls, and were more likely to endorse daytime fatigue, unrefreshing sleep, and taking daytime naps. Sleep paralysis was reported by 20.8% of WD patients in the presleep period and 25% on awakening, significantly more than was reported by controls. These sleep symptoms were present in treated patients, although there is a single case of a patient presenting with hypersomnia that resolved with treatment of HD.[542]

DYSTONIA

There is a general consensus that the elevated muscle tone seen in many conditions characterized by dystonia decreases in sleep.[532,543,544] Several studies have demonstrated that the movements associated with blepharospasm and hemifacial spasm decrease in amplitude and frequency through sleep stages, with the lowest values seen in REM sleep.[545,546] REM atonia is generally unchanged in both primary and secondary dystonia.[547]

Impaired sleep quality (as measured subjectively by patients through the PSQI) is seen in hemifacial spasm and cervical dystonia,[548] with excessive daytime sleepiness seen in some,[549] but not all[548] studies of cervical dystonia. Fish and colleagues[533] contend that, in both primary and secondary torsion dystonia, sleep-related movements emerge only after brief awakenings. However, other investigators have noted that muscle tension in the affected sternocleidomastoid in spasmodic torticollis can appear as a specific sleep-related event.[292,550] Emser and colleagues[292] even suggested a temporal linkage of such EMG activity with vertex sharp waves during stage 1 sleep. Mano and colleagues[532] also concluded that the long-lasting EMG discharges corresponding to the waking clinical dystonic condition can "...appear in any sleep stage with the same EMG characteristics as in wakefulness."

Segawa and colleagues[544] and others[551] have described diurnal variation in dopa-responsive dystonia, with symptoms greatly improved during and immediately subsequent to sleep.

HEMIBALLISMUS

A small number of cases detailing sleep in hemiballismus have been reported. Movements are decreased in NREM sleep but continue to be detectable.[532]

TOURETTE'S SYNDROME (TS)

Clinical data indicate that sleep disturbance is present in 62% (69/112) of TS patients, with tics during sleep reported in about one-third of these patients, and somnambulism and bruxism reported in a lower percentage of these.[552] Sandyk and Bamford[553] have suggested that decreases in tic frequency during sleep may be a useful indicator of improvement on waking clinical state in these patients.

Early PSG studies of TS patients did not report on movement during sleep,[554] but did note normalization of sleep architecture after haloperidol administration. Some studies have reported reduced REM sleep percentages or SWS in these patients,[554] but these results may reflect the fact that the subjects in these studies were not drug-naïve.[555] Among 34 patients studied by PSG, motor activity was reported to be present in 23,[552] although quantified PSG data were not presented. Numerous other studies have confirmed the persistence of PSG-defined movement during sleep in TS.[556–558] Movements were reported to decrease from wakefulness to sleep, although they reoccurred during the sleep period. As was the case for several movement disorders studied by Fish and colleagues,[533] these authors contend that most of the sleep-related movements in TS, although technically occurring during the "sleep period," actually represent events that are preceded by brief microawakenings or by lightening of sleep stages to stage 1. Movements were rare, according to these authors, during stages 2, 3, 4, or REM. Several more recent studies, however, have noted an increased prevalence of PLMs in TS, which, by definition, occur from sleep and are not preceded by microarousals.[559,560]

Glaze and colleagues[555] noted "unusual" behavior episodes in TS that originated from stage 4 sleep and consisted of high-amplitude delta activity accompanied by disorientation, confusion, or combativeness. Unlike typical episodes of night terrors or somnambulism, there was no evidence of elevated heart rate or breathing rate during these episodes.

Lesperance and colleagues[561] demonstrated a higher than expected frequency of RLS in TS patients (10%) and their parents (23%), with inheritance of RLS linked to maternal, but not paternal, RLS.

TIC DISORDER

Children with tic disorder have decreased sleep efficiency, prolonged sleep latency, increased REM sleep, increased microarousals in REM sleep, and increased numbers of short motor-related arousals compared to children without tic disorder.[562]

PALATAL MYOCLONUS

Chokroverty and Barron[563] first noted persistence of palatal myoclonus in sleep in patients with brain stem infarcts. Later, Kayed and colleagues[564] reported several cases of palatal myoclonus that clearly persisted in sleep in patients without infarcts. Although rates of movement typically declined from high rates during wakefulness (120–200/min) to rates as low as 80/min, the data of Kayed and colleagues conclusively indicated continued presence of palatal myoclonus during EEG-defined sleep. Of particular interest was that, in REM sleep, the amplitude of the movements showed considerable clustering with 2–4 high-amplitude movements alternating with lower-amplitude movements. This did not appear to be related to bursting of eye movements. Yokota and colleagues[565] reported that palatal myoclonus was exacerbated in REM sleep.

ESSENTIAL TREMOR

RLS has been found in 33% of patients with essential tremor,[566] with family history of RLS (present in 57.6% of this group) being the only significant predictor of RLS. Conversely, patients with RLS have an increased frequency of low amplitude, nonpathologic tremor,[566] but not overt ET.[566,567]

PRION DISEASE

In Creutzfeldt–Jakob disease, generalized paroxysmal spike activity precludes normal identification of NREM sleep stages and REM sleep is typically difficult to discern.[568] Diffuse myoclonus is seen in all limbs and is apparent throughout sleep and wakefulness.

In fatal familial insomnia, early symptoms include insomnia and daytime sleepiness.[569] Sleep spindles and SWS are progressively lost during the course of the disease.[540] The disease progresses to a pattern of alternating wake, stage 1, and brief REM periods occurring both day and night.[540] Some patients ultimately lapse into a persistent vegetative state.[569] Normal circadian oscillations, as measured by hormonal and autonomic measures, are eventually completely lost.[540] Dream enactment behavior is common.[569]

A study of two sisters with Gerstmann–Straussler–Scheinker (GSS) disease revealed normal or near-normal amounts of REM and SWS but decreased sleep efficiency, thought to be a nonspecific marker of neurodegenerative disease.[570] Unlike in FFI, the two patients with GSS had preserved circadian core body temperature rhythms.[570]

STIFF-PERSON SYNDROME

Case reports and small case series have established that the continuous muscle activity and rigidity seen in stiff-person syndrome are abolished during sleep,[571,572] although muscle contractions persist into drowsiness and can interfere with sleep onset.[573] Muscle contractions may reappear repeatedly during awakenings from sleep.[574]

SPINOCEREBELLAR ATAXIA (SCA)

Sleep has been studied in two groups of SCA2 patients with medium size SCA2 expansions (38-44 or 49 CAG repeats).[575,576] Subjective sleep quality was almost universally reported as good[575] and dream enactment was denied.[575,576] Despite this, sleep was not normal, with decreased sleep efficiency and increased wake after sleep onset in most patients.[575] REM sleep was absent in the most severely affected patients, and some degree of RWA was seen in almost all patients with REM sleep.[575,576] Based on their series, Tuin and colleagues propose that sleep alterations in SCA2 progress with disease severity, from nonspecific increased wakefulness without clear REM abnormalities in the mildly affected, to RWA in those of medium disease severity, to absent REM sleep in the most severely affected. SWS percentages were also increased in the most severely affected patients[575] PLMS were seen in 10–80% of patients with SCA2[575,576] and RLS was present in 27% (compared to 10% of controls).[577]

EDS has been found in some,[578] but not all[579,580] studies of SCA3. Insomnia, RLS, RBD, snoring, and apnea are all reported by SCA3 patients more than by controls.[577,579,580] On PSG, SCA3 patients have decreased sleep efficiency, total sleep time, and REM percentage.[112] PLMS were seen in 100% of nine SCA3 patients and RBD in five of nine.[112]

Scores on the PSQI (a measure of sleep quality) and ESS are higher in patients with SCA6 than in controls,[581] and PLMS > 15/hr were found in 80% of SCA6 patients in one series (with corresponding RLS in only 40%).[582]

RLS is more common in SCA1 than in controls, occuring in 23%.[577]

SUMMARY

The nature and prevalence of disturbed sleep across the spectrum of waking movement disorders is complex, and the pathophysiology is poorly defined. It is not, therefore, surprising that scientifically validated objective results documenting specific treatments of disturbed sleep in each waking movement disorder rarely exist. Nonetheless, it has been our impression that effective treatment of the core symptoms of the underlying waking movement disorder will often result in a corresponding improvement in any associated sleep disturbances. When sleep complaints persist after the successful treatment of the core waking motor disturbance, a re-evaluation of the patient for a possible underlying sleep disorder should be performed, including PSG.

▶ ACKNOWLEDGMENTS

The authors would like to extend their greatest appreciation to Drs. Dainis Irbe, Bhupesh Dihenia, Lisa Johnston, and Paul Gurecki for their assistance in performing and scoring polysomnographic records from a variety of movement disorder patients, as well as Dr. Robert Turner for his critical help in recording sleep/wake-specific neuronal discharge in the primate globus pallidus. Supported in part by US Public Health Service grants NS-36697 (DBR), NS-40221 (DBR), NS-43374 (DBR), and the Restless Legs Syndrome Foundation (DBR), NS-050595 (DLB), NS-35345 (DLB) and AG-10643 (DLB), and KL2 RR025009 (LMT).

REFERENCES

1. Fujimoto T, Nishizono H. Muscle contractile properties by surface electrodes compared with those by needle electrodes. Electroencephalogr Clin Neurophysiol 1993;89:247–251.
2. van Hilten J, Kabel J, Middelkoop H, et al. Assessment of response fluctuations in parkinson's disease by ambulatory wrist activity monitoring. Acta Neurol Scand 1993;87:171–177.
3. Jacobson A, Kales A, Lehmann D, et al. Muscle tonus in human subjects during sleep and dreaming. Exp Neurol 1964;10:418–424.
4. Kleitman N, Cooperman N, Mullin F. Studies on the physiology of sleep ix. Motility and body temperature during sleep. Am J Physiol 1933;105:574–584.
5. Johnson H, Swan T, Weigand G. In what positions do healthy people sleep? JAMA 1930;94:2058–2062.
6. Hobson J, Spagna T, Malenka R. Ethology of sleep studied with time-lapse photography: Postural immobility and sleep-cycle phase in humans. Science 1978;204: 251–253.
7. Gardner J, R, Grossman W. Normal motor patterns in sleep in man. In Advances in Sleep Research. New York: Spectrum Publications, Inc., 1975, 67–107.
8. Suckling E, Koenig E, Hoffman B, et al. The physiological effects of sleeping on hard or soft beds. Hum Biol 1957;29:274–288.
9. Moses J, Lubin A, Naitoh P, et al. Methodology: Reliability of sleep measures. Psychophysiology 1972;9:78–82.
10. Muzet A, Naitoh P, Townsend R, et al. Body movements during sleep as a predictor of stage change. Psychon Sci 1972;29(1):7–10.
11. Naitoh P, Muzet A, Johnson L, et al. Body movements during sleep after sleep loss. Psychophysiology 1973;10(4): 363–368.
12. Townsend R, Johnson L, Naitoh P. Heart rate preceding motility in sleep. Psychophysiology 1975;12:217–219.
13. De Lisi L. Su di un fenomeno motorio constate del sonno normale: Le mioclonie ipniche fisiologiche. Riv Pat Nerv Ment 1932;39:481–496.
14. Oswald I. Sudden bodily jerks on falling asleep. Brain 1959;82:92–103.

15. Stoyva J Finger electromyographic activity during sleep: Its relation to dreaming in deaf and normal subjects. J Abnorm Psychol 1965;70(5):343–349.
16. Askenasy J, Yahr M, Davidovitch S. Isolated phasic discharges in anterior tibial muscle: A stable feature of paradoxical sleep. J Clin Neurophysiol 1988;5(2):175–181.
17. Chokroverty S. Phasic tongue movements in human rapid-eye-movement sleep. Neurology 30:665–668.
18. Bliwise D, Coleman R, Bergmann B, et al. Facial muscle tonus during rem and nrem sleep. Psychophysiology 1974;11:447–508.
19. Sateia MJ. The International Classification of Sleep Disorders. Westchester, IL: American Academy of Sleep Medicine, 2005.
20. Slegel D, Benson K, VP Zarcone J, et al. Middle-ear muscle activity (mema) and its association with motor activity in the extremities and head in sleep. Sleep 1991;14(5): 454–459.
21. Pessah M, Roffwarg H. Spontaneous middle ear muscle activity in man: A rapid eye movement sleep phenomenon. Science 178(62):773–776.
22. Gassel MM, Marchiafava PL, Pompeiano O. Phasic changes in muscular activity during desynchronized sleep in unrestrained cats. Arch Ital Biol 1964;102:449–470.
23. Cepeda C, Naquet R. Physiological sleep myoclonus in baboons. Electroencephalogr Clin Neurophysiol 1985;60: 158–162.
24. Montagna P, Liguori R, Zucconi M, et al. Physiological hypnic myoclonus. Electroencephalogr Clin Neurophysiol 1988;70:172–175.
25. Montagna P, Liguiori R, Zucconi M, et al. Fasciculations during wakefulness and sleep. Acta Neurol Scand 1987;76:152–154.
26. van Hilten B, Hoff J, Middelkoop H, et al. Sleep disruption in parkinson's disease. Assessment by continuous activity monitoring. Arch Neurol 1994;51:922–928.
27. Laihinen A, Alihanka J, Raitasuo S, et al. Sleep movements and associated autonomic nervous activities in patients with parkinson's disease. Acta Neurol Scand 1987;76:64–68.
28. Klawans H, Goetz C, Bergen D. Levodopa-induced myoclonus. Arch Neurol 1975;32:331–334.
29. Schenck C, Bundlie S, Ettinger M, et al. Chronic behavioral disorders of human rem sleep: A new category of parasomnia. Sleep 1986;9:293–308.
30. ICSD-International Classification of of Sleep Disorders: Diagnostic and Coding Manual. Diagnostic Classification Steering Commitee, Thorpy MH, Chairman, Rochester, Minnesota: American Sleep Disorders Association, 1990.
31. Schenck C, Lee S, Bornemann M, et al. Potentially lethal behaviors associated with rapid eye movement sleep behavior disorder: Review of the literature and forensic implications. J Forensic Sci 2009;54(6):1475–1484.
32. Oudiette D, De Cock V, Lavault S, et al. Nonviolent elaborate behaviors may also occur in rem sleep behavior disorder. Neurology 2009;72:551–557.
33. Uhde T. The anxiety disorders. In Kryger M, Roth T, Dement W (eds) Principles and practice of sleep medicine. Philadelphia: WB Saunders Company, 1994, 871–898.
34. Turner R, Chervin R, Frey K, et al. Probable diffuse lewy body disease presenting as rem sleep behavior disorder. Neurology 1997;49:523–527.
35. Schenck C, Bundlie S, Mahowald M. Delayed emergence of a parkinsonian disorder in 38% of 29 older men initially diagnosed with idiopathic rapid eye movement sleep behavior disorder. Neurology 1996;46:388–393.
36. Schenck C, Bundlie S, Mahowald M. Rem behavior disorder (rbd): Delayed emergence of parkinsonism or dementia in 65% of older men initially diagnosed with idiopathic rbd, and an analysis of the minimum and maximum tonic and/or phasic electromyographic abnormalities found during rem sleep. Sleep 2003;26 (suppl):A316.
37. Olson EJ, Boeve BF, Silber MH. Rapid eye movement sleep behaviour disorder: Demographic, clinical and laboratory findings in 93 cases. Brain 2000;123(Pt 2): 331–339.
38. Tippmann-Peikert M, Olson E, Boeve B, et al. Idiopathic rem sleep behavior disorder: A follow-up of 39 patients. Sleep 2006;29(abstract suppl):A272.
39. Iranzo A, Molinuevo J, Santamaria J, et al. Rapid-eye-movement sleep behaviour disorder as an early marker for a neurodegenerative disorder: A descriptive study. Lancet Neurol 2006;5(7):572–577.
40. Postuma, R, Gagnon J, Vendette M, et al. Quantifying the risk of neurodegenerative disease in idiopathic rem sleep behavior disorder. Neurology 2009;72:1296–1300.
41. Mahowald M. Does "idiopathic" Rem sleep behavior disorder exist? Sleep 2006;29(7):874–875.
42. Ohayon M, Caulet M, Priest R. Violent behavior during sleep. J Clin Psychiatry 1997;58(8):369–376.
43. Husain A, Miller P, Carwile S. Rem sleep behavior disorder: Potential relationship to post-traumatic stress disorder. J Clin Neurophysiol 2001;18(2):148–157.
44. Teman P, Tippmann-Peikert M, Silber M, et al. Idiopathic rapid-eye-movement sleep disorder: Associations with antidepressants, psychiatric diagnoses, and other factors, in relation to age of onset. Sleep Med 2009;10:60–65.
45. Chiu H, Wing Y, Lam L, et al. Sleep-related injury in the elderly--an epidemiological study in hong kong. Sleep 2000;23(4):513–517.
46. Nielsen T, Svob C, Kuiken D. Dream-enacting behaviors in a normal population. Sleep 2009;32(12):1629–1636.
47. Braak H, Tredici K, Rub U, et al. Staging of brain pathology related to sproadic parkinson's disease. Neurobiol Aging 2003;24:197–211.
48. Postuma R, Lang A, Massicotte-Marquez J, et al. Potential early markers of parkinson disease in idiopathic rem sleep behavior disorder. Neurology 2006;66:845–851.
49. Stiansky-Kolster K, Doerr Y, Moller J. Combination of 'idiopathic' rem sleep behaviour disorder and olfactory dysfunction as possible indicator for alpha-synucleinopathy demonstrated by dopamine transporter fp-cit-spect. Brain 2005;128:126–137.
50. Postuma R, Gagnon J, Vendette M, et al. Idiopathic rem sleep behavior disorder in the transition to degenerative disease. Mov Disord 2009;24(15):2225–2232.
51. Miyamoto T, Miyamoto M, Iwanami M, et al. Odor identification test as an indicator of idiopathic rem sleep behavior disorder. Mov Disord 2009;24(2):268–273.
52. Stiansky-Kolster K, Clever S, Moller J, et al. Olfactory dysfunction in patients with narcolepsy with and without rem sleep behaviour disorder. Brain 2007;130: 442–449.

53. Fantini M, Postuma R, Montplaisir J. Olfactory deficit in idiopathic rapid eye movements sleep behavior disorder. Brain Research Bulletin 2006;70:386–390.
54. Amino T, Orimo S, Itoh Y, et al. Profound cardiac sympathetic denervation occurs in parkinson disease. Brain Pathology 2005;15(1):29–34.
55. Wakabayashi K, Takahashi H. Neuropathology of autonomic nervous system in parkinson's disease. European Neurology 1997;38(suppl 2):2–7.
56. Minguez-Castellanos A, Chamorro C, Escamilla-Sevilla F, et al. Do alpha synuclein aggregates in autonomic plexuses predate lewy body disorders? Neurology 2007;68: 2012–2018.
57. Lanfranchi P, Fradette L, Gagnon J, et al. Cardiac autonomic regulation during sleep in idiopathic rem sleep behavior disorder. Sleep 2007;30(8):1019–1025.
58. Miyamoto T, Miyamoto M, Inoue Y, et al. Reduced cardiac ^{123}I-MIBG scintigraphy in idiopathic rem sleep behavior disorder. Neurology 2006;67(12):2236–2238.
59. Miyamoto T, Miyamoto M, Suzuki K, et al. I-mibg cardiac scintigraphy provides clues to the underlying neurodegenerative disorder in idiopathic rem sleep behavior disorder. Sleep 2008;31(5):717–723.
60. Koyama S, Tachibana N, Masaoka Y, et al. Decreased myocardial ^{123}I-MIBG uptake and impaired facial expression recognition in a patient with rem sleep behavior disorder. Mov Disord 2007;22:746–747.
61. Oguri T, Tachibana N, Mitake S, et al. Decrease in myocardial ^{123}I-MIBG radioactivity in rem sleep behavior disorder: Two patients with different clinical progression. Sleep Med 2008;9(583–585.
62. Miyamoto T, Miyamoto M, Suzuki K, et al. Comparison of severity of obstructive sleep apnea and degree of accumulation of cardiac 123-i-mibg radioactivity as a diagnostic marker for idiopathic rem sleep behavior disorder. Sleep Med 2009;10:577–580.
63. Devos D, Tir M, Maurage C, et al. Erg and anatomical abnormalities suggesting retinopathy in dementia with lewy bodies. Neurology 2005;65(7):1107–1110.
64. Eisensehr, I, Linke R, Tatsch K, et al. Increased muscle activity during rapid eye movement sleep correlates with decrease of striatal presynaptic dopamine transporters. Ipt and ibzm spect imaging in subclinical and clinically manifest idiopathic rem sleep behavior disorder, parkinson's disease, and controls. Sleep 2003;26(5): 507–512.
65. Eisensehr I, Linke R, Noachtar S, et al. Reduced striatal dopamine transporters in idiopathic rapid eye movement behaviour disorder. Comparison with parkinson's disease and controls. Brain 2000;123(6):1155–1160.
66. Albin R, Koeppe R, Chervin R, et al. Decreased striatal dopaminergic innervation in rem sleep behavior disorder. Neurology 2000;55:1410–1412.
67. Gilman S, Koeppe RA, Chervin RD, et al. Rem sleep behavior disorder is related to striatal monoaminergic deficit in msa. Neurology 2003;61(1):29–34.
68. Mazza S, Soucy J, Gravel P, et al. Assessing whole brain perfusion changes in patients with rem sleep behavior disorder. Neurology 2006;67:1618–1622.
69. Caselli R, Chen K, Bandy D, et al. A preliminary fluorodeoxyglucose positron emission tomography study in healthy adults reporting dream-enactment behavior. Sleep 2006;29(7):927–933.
70. Iranzo A, Santamaria J, Pujol J, et al. Brainstem proton magnetic resonance spectroscopy in idiopathic rem sleep behavior disorder. Sleep 2002;25:867–870.
71. Ferini-Strambi L, Di Gioia M, Castronovo V, et al. Neuropsychological assessment in idiopathic rem sleep behavior disorder (rbd): Does the idiopathic form of rbd really exist? Neurology 2004;62:41–45.
72. Iranzo A, Molinuevo JL, Santamaria J, et al. Rapid-eye-movement sleep behaviour disorder as an early marker for a neurodegenerative disorder: A descriptive study. Lancet Neurol 2006;5(7):572—577.
73. Terzaghi M, Sinforiani E, Zucchella C, et al. Cognitive performance in rem sleep behaviour disorder: A possible early marker of neurodegenerative disease? Sleep Med 2008;9(4):343–351.
74. Massicotte-Marquez J, Decary A, Gagnon J, et al. Executive dysfunction and memory impairment in idiopathic rem sleep behavior disorder. Neurology 2008;70: 1250–1257.
75. Massicotte-Marquez J, Decary A, Gagnon JF, et al. Executive dysfunction and memory impairment in idiopathic rem sleep behavior disorder. Neurology 2008;70(15): 1250–1257.
76. Gagnon J, Vendette M, Postuma R, et al. Mild cognitive impairment in rapid eye movement sleep behavior disorder and parkinson's disease. Ann Neurol 2009;66: 39–47.
77. Gagnon JF, Vendette M, Postuma RB, et al. Mild cognitive impairment in rapid eye movement sleep behavior disorder and parkinson's disease. Ann Neurol 2009;66(1):39–47.
78. Fantini M, Corona A, Clerici S, et al. Aggressive dream content without daytime aggressiveness in rem sleep behaviour disorder. Neurology 2005;65:1010–1015.
79. Boeve BF, Molano JR, Ferman T, et al. Validation of the Mayo Sleep Questionnaire to screen for REM Sleep Behavior Disorder in an aging and dementia cohort. Sleep Med;2011 in press.
80. Consens F, Chervin R, Koeppe R, et al. Validation of a polysomnographic score for rem sleep behavior disorder. Sleep 2005;28(8):993–997.
81. Stiansky-Kolster K, Mayer G, Schafer S, et al. The rem sleep behavior disorder screening questionnaire- a new diagnostic instrument. Mov Disord 2007;22(16):2386–2393.
82. Ohayon MM, Caulet M, Priest RG. Violent behavior during sleep. J Clin Psychiatry 1997;58(8):369–376; quiz 377.
83. Iranzo A, Santamaria J, Vilaseca I, et al. Absence of alterations in serum sex hormone levels in idiopathic rem sleep behavior disorder. Sleep 2007;30(6):803–806.
84. Chou K, Moro-de-Casillas M, Amick M, et al. Testosterone not associated with violent dreams or rem sleep behavior disorder in men with parkinson's. Mov Disord 2007;22:411–414.
85. Zhang J, Lam P, Ho C, et al. Diagnosis of rem sleep behavior disorder by video-polysomnographic study: Is one night enough? Sleep 2008;31(8):1179–1185.
86. Bliwise D, Rye D. Elevated pem (phasic electromyographic metric) rates identify rapid eye movement behavior disorder patients on nights without behavioral abnormalities. Sleep 2008;31(6):853–857.

87. Manni R, Terzaghi M, Zambrelli E. Rem sleep behavior disorder and epileptic phenomena: Clinical aspects of the comorbidity. Epilepsia 2006;47(uppl 5):78–81.
88. Manni R, Terzaghi M, Zambrelli E. Rem sleep behaviour disorder in elderly subjects with epilepsy: Frequency and clinical aspects of the comorbidity. Epilepsy Res 2007;77(2–3):128–133.
89. Lapierre O, Montplaisir J. Polysomnographic features of rem sleep behavior disorder: Development of a scoring method. Neurology 1992;42:1371–1374.
90. Fantini M, Michaud M, Gosselin N, et al. Periodic leg movements in rem sleep behavior disorder and related autonomic and eeg activation. Neurology 2002;59: 1889–1894.
91. Manconi M, Ferri R, Zucconi M, et al. Time structure analysis of leg movements during sleep in rem sleep behavior disorder. Sleep 2007;30(12):1779–1785.
92. Olson E, Boeve B, Silber M. Rapid eye movement sleep behaviour disorder: Demographic, clinical and laboratory findings in 93 cases. Brain 2000;123:331–339.
93. Massicotte-Marquez J, Carrier J, Decary A, et al. Slow-wave sleep and delta power in rapid eye movement sleep behavior disorder. Ann Neurol 2005;57:277–282.
94. Fantini M, Gagnon J, Petit D. Slowing of electroencephalogram in rapid eye movement sleep behavior disorder. Ann Neurol 2003;53:774–780.
95. Frauscher B, Gschliesser V, Brandauer E, et al. The relation between abnormal behaviors and rem sleep microstructure in patients with rem sleep behavior disorder. Sleep Med 2009;10:174–181.
96. Manni R, Terzaghi M, Glorioso M. Motor-behavioral episodes in rem sleep behavior disorder and phasic events during rem sleep. Sleep 2009;32(2):241–245.
97. Iranzo A, Ratti P, Casanova-Molla J, et al. Excessive muscle activity increases over time in idiopathic rem sleep behavior disorder. Sleep 2009;32(9):1149–1153.
98. Burns J, Consens F, Little R, et al. Emg variance during polysomnography as an assessment for rem sleep behavior disorder. Sleep 2007;30(12):1771–1778.
99. Ferri R, Manconi M, Plazzi G, et al. A quantitative statistical analysis of the submentalis muscle emg amplitude during sleep in normal controls and patients with rem sleep behavior disorder. J Sleep Res 2008;17(1): 89–100.
100. Mayer G, Kesper K, Ploch T, et al. Quantification of tonic and phasic muscle activity in rem sleep behavior disorder. J Clin Neurophysiol 2008;25(1):48–55.
101. Boeve B, Silber M, Ferman T, et al. Rem sleep behavior disorder and degenerative dementia – An association likely reflecting lewy body disease. Neurology 1998;51: 363–370.
102. Turner R. Idiopathic rapid eye movement sleep behavior disorder is a harbinger of dementia with lewy bodies. J Geriatr Psychiatry Neurol 2002;(15):195–199.
103. Boeve B, Silber M, Ferman T, et al. Association of rem sleep behavior disorder and neurodegenerative disease may reflect an underlying synucleinopathy. Mov Disord 2001;16:622–630.
104. Gagnon JF, Petit D, Fantini ML, et al. Rem sleep behavior disorder and rem sleep without atonia in probable alzheimer disease. Sleep 2006;29(10):1321–1325.
105. Tison F, Wenning G, Quinn N, et al. Rem sleep behaviour disorder as the presenting symptom of multiple system atrophy. J Neurol Neurosurg Psychiatr 1995;58:379–385.
106. Kashihara K, Ohno M, Kawada S, et al. Frequent nocturnal vocalization in pure autonomic failure. J Int Med Res 2008;36(3):489–495.
107. Xi Z, Luning W. Rem sleep behavior disorder in a patient with pontine stroke. Sleep Med 2009;10(1):143–146.
108. Mathis J, Hess C, Bassetti C. Isolated mediotegmental lesion causing narcolepsy and rapid eye movement sleep behaviour disorder: A case evidencing a common pathway in narcolepsy and rapid eye movement sleep behaviour disorder. J Neurol Neurosurg Psychiatr 2007;78(4):427–429.
109. Shimizu T, Inami Y, Sugita Y, et al. Rem sleep without muscle atonia (stage 1-rem) and its relation to delirious behavior during sleep in patients with degenerative diseases involving the brain stem. Jap J Psychiatr Neurol 1990;44(4):681–692.
110. Kimura K, Tachibana N, Aso T, et al. Subclinical rem sleep behavior disorder in a patient with corticobasal degeneration. Sleep 1997;20(10):891–894.
111. Syed B, Rye D, Singh G. Rem sleep behavior disorder and sca-3 (machado-joseph disease). Neurology 2003;14:148.
112. Iranzo A, Munoz E, Santamaria J, et al. Rem sleep behavior disorder and vocal cord paralysis in machado-joseph disease. Mov Disord 2003;18(10):1179–1183.
113. Friedman J. Presumed rapid eye movement behavior disorder in machado-joseph disease (spinocerebellar ataxia type 3). Mov Disord 2002;17:1350–1353.
114. Aldrich M, Foster N, White R, et al. Sleep abnormalities in progressive supranuclear palsy. Ann Neurol 1989;25: 577–581.
115. Arnulf I, Merino-Andreu M, Bloch F, et al. Rem sleep behavior disorder and rem sleep without atonia in patients with progressive supranuclear palsy. Sleep 2005;28(3):349–354.
116. de Cock V, Lannuzel A, Verhaeghe S, et al. Rem sleep behavior disorder in patients with guadeloupean parkinsonism, a tauopathy. Sleep 2007;30(8):1026–1032.
117. Dauvilliers Y, Rompre S, Gagnon J, et al. Rem sleep characteristics in narcolepsy and rem sleep behavior disorder. Sleep 2007;30(7):844–849.
118. Schenck C, Mahowald M. Motor dyscontrol in narcolepsy: Rapid-eye-movement (rem) sleep without atonia and rem sleep behavior disorder. Ann Neurol 1992;32:3–10.
119. Nightingale S, Orgill J, Ebrahim I, et al. The association between narcolepsy and rem behavior disorder (rbd). Sleep Med 2005;6(3):253–258.
120. Limousin N, Dehais C, Gout O, et al. A brainstem inflammatory lesion causing rem sleep behavior disorder and sleepwalking (parasomnia overlap disorder). Sleep Med 2009;10(9):1059–1062.
121. Mahowald M, Schenck C. Rem sleep parasomnias. In Kryger M, Roth T, Dement W (eds). Principles and Practice of Sleep Medicine. St. Louis: WB Saunders Company, 2000, pp. 724–743.
122. Culebras A, Moore J. Magnetic resonance findings in rem sleep behavior disorder. Neurology 1989;39:1519–1523.
123. Kimura K, Tachibana N, Kohyama J, et al. A discrete pontine ischemic lesion coud cause rem-sleep behavior disorder. Neurology 2000;55:894–895.

124. Compta Y, Iranzo A, Santamaria J, et al. Rem sleep behavior disorder and narcoleptic features in anti-ma2-associated encephalitis. Sleep 2007;30(6):767–769.
125. Iranzo A, Graus F, Clover L, et al. Rapid eye movement sleep behavior disorder and potassium channel antibody-associated limbic encephalitis. Ann Neurol 2006;59:178–182.
126. Iranzo A, Santamaria J. Severe obstructive sleep apnea/hypopnea mimicking rem sleep behavior disorder. Sleep 2005;28(2):203–206.
127. Gross M, Goodenough D, Tobin M, et al. Sleep disturbances and hallucinations in the acute alcoholic psychoses. J Nerv Ment Dis 1966;142:493–514.
128. Winkelman JW, James L. Serotonergic antidepressants are associated with rem sleep without atonia. Sleep 2004;27(2):317–321.
129. Yeh Y, Chen C, Feng H, et al. New onset somnambulism associated with different dosage of mirtazapine: A case report. Clin Neuropharmacol 2009;32(4):232–233.
130. Greenberg R, Pearlman C. Delirium tremens and dreaming. Am J Psychiatry 1967;124:37–46.
131. Guilleminault C, Raynal D, Takahaski S, et al. Evaluation of short-term and long-term treatment of the narcolepsy syndrome with clomipramine hydrochloride. Acta Neurol Scand 1976;54:71–87.
132. Akindele M, Evans J, Oswald I. Mono-amine oxidase inhibitors, sleep and mood. Electroencephalogr Clin Neurophysiol 1970;29:47–56.
133. Schenck C, Mahowald M, Kim S, et al. Prominent eye movements during nrem sleep and rem sleep behavior disorder associated with fluoxetine treatment of depression and obsessive-compulsive disorder. Sleep 1992;15:226–235.
134. Vorona R, Ware J. Exacerbation of rem sleep behavior disorder by chocolate ingestion: A case report. Sleep Med 2002;3(4):365–367.
135. Hendricks JC, Morrison AR, Mann GL. Different behaviors during paradoxical sleep without atonia depend on pontine lesion site. Brain Res 1982;239:81–105.
136. Morrison, A. Paradoxical sleep without atonia. Arch Italian Biol 1988;126:275–289.
137. Shouse M, Siegel J. Pontine regulation of rem sleep components in cats: Integrity of the pedunculopontine tegmentum (ppt) is important for phasic events but unnecessary for atonia during rem sleep. Brain Res 1992;571:50–63.
138. Fuller PM, Saper CB, Lu J. The pontine rem switch: Past and present. J Physiol 2007;584(Pt 3):735–741.
139. Lu J, Sherman D, Devor M, et al. A putative flip-flop switch for control of rem sleep. Nature 2006;441(7093):589–594.
140. Morrison AR, Mann GL, Hendricks JC. The relationship of excessive exploratory behavior in wakefulness to paradoxical sleep without atonia. Sleep 1981;4(3):247–257.
141. Trulson ME, Jacobs BL, Morrison AR. Raphe unit activity across the sleep-waking cycle in normal cats and in pontine lesioned cats displaying rem sleep without atonia. Brain Res 1981;226:75–91.
142. Wu MF, Gulyani SA, Yau E, et al. Locus coeruleus neurons: Cessation of activity during cataplexy. Neuroscience 1999;91(4):1389–1399.
143. Schmeichel A, Buchhalter L, Low P, et al. Mesopontine cholinergic neuron involvement in lewy body dementia and multiple system atrophy. Neurology 2008;70(5):368–373.
144. Morrison A. The pathophysiology of rem-sleep behavior disorder. Sleep 1998;21(5):446.
145. Rye D. Contributions of the pedunculopontine region to normal and altered rem sleep. Sleep 1997;20(9):757–788.
146. Decker M, Keating G, Freeman A, et al. Parkinsonian-like sleep-wake architecture in rats with bilateral striatal 6-ohda lesions. Soc Neurosci Abstr 2000;26:1514.
147. Daley J, Turner R, Bliwise D, et al. Nocturnal sleep and daytime alertness in the mptp-treated primate. Sleep 1999;22(suppl):S218–S219.
148. Vitek J, Kaneoke Y, Turner R, et al. Neuronal activity in the internal (gpi) and external (gpe) segments of the globus pallidus (gp) of parkinsonian patients is similar to that in the mptp-treated primate model of parkinsonism. Soc Neurosci Abstr 1993;19:1584.
149. Magnin M, Morel A, Jeanmonod D. Single-unit analysis of the pallidum, thalamus and subthalamic nucleus in parkinsonian patients. Neuroscience 2000;96(3):549–564.
150. Rye D, Dempsay J, Dihenia B, et al. Rem-sleep dyscontrol in parkinson's disease: Case report of effects of elective pallidotomy. Sleep Res 1997;26:591.
151. Tan A, Salgado M, Fahn S. Rapid eye movement sleep behavior disorder preceding parkinson's disease with therapeutic response to levodopa. Mov Disord 1996;11(2):214–216.
152. Arnulf I, Bejjani B, Garma L, et al. Improvement of sleep architecture in pd with subthalamic nucleus stimulation. Neurology 2000;55:1732–1734.
153. Iranzo A, Valldeoriola F, Santamaria J, et al. Sleep symptoms and polysomnographic architecture in advanced parkinson's disease after chronic bilateral subthalamic stimulation. J Neurol Neurosurg Psychiatry 2002;72:661–664.
154. Garcia-Borreguero D, Caminero A, de la Llave Y, et al. Decreased phasic emg activity during rem-sleep in treatment-naive parkinson's disease: Effects of treatment with l-dopa and progression of illness. Mov Disord 2002;17:934-941.
155. Braak H, Rub U, Gai W, et al. Idiopathic parkinson's disease: Possible routes by which vulnerable neuronal types may be subject to neuroinvasion by an unknown pathogen. J Neural Transm 2003;110:517–536.
156. Wing YK, Lam SP, Li SX, et al. Rem sleep behaviour disorder in hong kong chinese: Clinical outcome and gender comparison. J Neurol Neurosurg Psychiatry 2008;79(12):1415-1416.
157. Sforza E, Krieger J, Petiau C. Rem sleep behavior disorder: Clinical and physiopathological findings. Sleep Med Rev 1997;1(1):57–69.
158. Schenck CH, Mahowald MW. Long-term, nightly benzodiazepine treatment of injurious parasomnias and other disorders of disrupted nocturnal sleep in 170 adults. Am J Med 1996;100(3):333–337.
159. Anderson KN, Shneerson JM. Drug treatment of rem sleep behavior disorder: The use of drug therapies other than clonazepam. J Clin Sleep Med 2009;5(3):235–239.
160. Kunz D, Bes F. Melatonin as a therapy in rem sleep behavior disorder patients: An open- labeled pilot study on the possible influence of melatonin on rem-sleep regulation. Mov Disord 1999;14(3):507–511.
161. Boeve BF, Silber MH, Ferman TJ. Melatonin for treatment of rem sleep behavior disorder in neurologic disorders: Results in 14 patients. Sleep Med 2003;4(4):281–284.

162. Takeuchi N, Uchimura N, Hashimuze Y, et al. Melatonin therapy for rem sleep behavior disorder. Psychiatry Clin Neurosci 2001;55:267–270.
163. Ringman J, Simmons J. Treatment of rem sleep behavior disorder with donepezil: A report of three cases. Neurology 2000;55:870–871.
164. Massironi G, Galluzzi S, Frisoni GB. Drug treatment of rem sleep behavior disorders in dementia with lewy bodies. Int Psychogeriatr 2003;15(4):377–383.
165. Fantini ML, Gagnon JF, Filipini D, et al. The effects of pramipexole in rem sleep behavior disorder. Neurology 2003;61(10):1418–1420.
166. Schmidt MH, Koshal VB, Schmidt HS. Use of pramipexole in rem sleep behavior disorder: Results from a case series. Sleep Med 2006;7(5):418–423.
167. Kumru H, Iranzo A, Carrasco E, et al. Lack of effects of pramipexole on rem sleep behavior disorder in parkinson disease. Sleep 2008;31(10):1418–1421.
168. Tuxhorn I, Hoppe M. Parasomnia with rhythmic movements manifesting as nocturnal tongue biting. Neuropediatrics 1993;24:167–168.
169. Mayer G, W-FJ, Kurella B. Sleep related rhythmic movement disorder revisited. J Sleep Res 2007;16:110–116.
170. Regestein Q, Hartmann E, Reich P. A head movement disorder occurring in dreaming sleep. J Nerv Ment Disease 1977;16:432–435.
171. Gagnon P, Koninck JD. Repetitive head movements during rem sleep. Biol Psychiatry 1985;20:176–178.
172. Anderson KN, Smith IE, Shneerson JM. Rhythmic movement disorder (head banging) in an adult during rapid eye movement sleep. Mov Disord 2006;21(6):866–879.
173. Manni R, Terzaghi M. Rhythmic movements in idiopathic rem sleep behavior disorder. Mov Disord 2007;22(12):1797–1800.
174. Klackenberg G. Rhythmic movements in infancy and early childhood. Acta Pediatr Scand 1971;224(suppl):74.
175. Drake J, ME: Jactatio nocturna after head injury. Neurology 1986;36:867–867.
176. Stepanova I, Nersimalova S, Hanusova J. Rhythmic movement disorder in sleep persisting into childhood and adulthood. Sleep 2005;28(7):851–857.
177. Merlino G, Serafini A, Dolso P, Canesin Ret al. Association of body rolling, leg rolling, and rhythmic feet movements in a young adult: A video-polysomnographic study performed before and after one night of clonazepam. Mov Disord 2008;23(4):602–607.
178. Chisholm T, Morehouse RL. Adult headbanging: Sleep studies and treatment. Sleep 1996;19(4):343–346.
179. Rosenberg C. Elimination of a rhythmic movement disorder with hypnosis – A case report. Sleep 1995;18(7):608–609.
180. Etzioni T, Katz N, Hering E, Ravid S, et al. Controlled sleep restriction for rhythmic movement disorder. J Pediatr 2005;147:393–395.
181. Lavigne GJ, Khoury S, Abe S, Yamaguchi T, et al. Bruxism physiology and pathology: An overview for clinicians. J Oral Rehabil 2008;35(7):476–494.
182. Johansson A, Unell L, Carlsson G, et al. Associations between social and general health factors and symptoms related to temporomandibular disorders and bruxism in a population of 50-year-old subjects. Acta Odontol Scand 2004;62(4):231–237.
183. Bailey DR. Tension headache and bruxism in the sleep disordered patient. Cranio 1990;8(2):174–182.
184. Vendrame M, Kaleyias J, Valencia I, Legido A, et al. Polysomnographic findings in children with headaches. Pediatr Neurol 2008;39(1):6–11.
185. Nagamatsu-Sakaguchi C, Minakuchi H, Clark GT, Kuboki T. Relationship between the frequency of sleep bruxism and the prevalence of signs and symptoms of temporomandibular disorders in an adolescent population. Int J Prosthodont 2008;21(4):292–298.
186. Ahlberg K, Jahkola A, Savolainen A, et al. Associations of reported bruxism with insomnia and insufficient sleep symptoms among media personnel with or without irregular shift work. Head Face Med 2008;4:4.
187. Macaluso G, Pavesi G, De Laat A. Sleep bruxism is a disorder related to periodic arousals during sleep. J Dent Res 1998;77:565–573.
188. Sjöholm T, Polo O, Alihanka J. Sleep movements in teethgrinders. J Craniomandib Disord Facial Oral Pain 1992;6:184–191.
189. Lavigne G, Kato T, Kolta A, et al. Neurobiological mechanisms involved in sleep bruxism. Crit Rev Oral Biol Med 2003;14:30–46.
190. Kato T, Rompre P, Montplaisir J, et al. Sleep bruxism: An oromotor activity secondary to microarousal. J Dent Res 2001;80:1940–1944.
191. Seraidarian P, Seraidarian PI, das Neves Cavalcanti B, et al. Urinary levels of catecholamines among individuals with and without sleep bruxism. Sleep Breath 2009;13:85–88.
192. Huynh N, Kato T, Rompre PH, et al. Sleep bruxism is associated to micro-arousals and an increase in cardiac sympathetic activity. J Sleep Res 2006;15(3):339–346.
193. Marthol H, Reich S, Jacke J, et al. Enhanced sympathetic cardiac modulation in bruxism patients. Clin Auton Res 2006;16(4):276–280.
194. Hartmann E. Alcohol and bruxism. N Engl J Med 1979;301:334.
195. Ellison J, Stanziani P. Ssri-associated nocturnal bruxism in four patients. J Clin Psychiatry 1993;54:432–434.
196. Por C, Watson L, Doucette D, et al. Sertraline-associated bruxism. Can J Clin Pharmacol 1996;3:123–125.
197. Kamen S. Tardive dyskinesia, a significant syndrome for geriatric dentistry. Oral Surg Oral Med Oral Path 1975;39:52.
198. Mendhekar DN, Andrade C. Bruxism arising during monotherapy with methylphenidate. J Child Adolescent Psychopharmacol 2008;18(5):537–538.
199. Pohto P. Experimental aggression and bruxism in rats. Acta Odontol Scand 1979;37:117–126.
200. Magee K. Bruxism related to levodopa therapy. JAMA 1970;214:147.
201. Huynh NT, Rompre PH, Montplaisir JY, et al. Comparison of various treatments for sleep bruxism using determinants of number needed to treat and effect size. Int J Prosthodont 2006;19(5):435–441.
202. Huynh N, Manzini C, Rompre PH, et al. Weighing the potential effectiveness of various treatments for sleep bruxism. J Can Dent Assoc 2007;73(8):727–730.
203. Macedo CR, Silva AB, Machado MA, et al. Occlusal splints for treating sleep bruxism (tooth grinding). Cochrane Database Syst Rev 2007;4:CD005514.

204. Lobbezoo F, Lavigen G, Tanguay R, et al. The effect of the catecholamine precursor l-dopa on sleep bruxism: A controlled clinical trial. Mov Disord 1997;12:73–78.
205. Van der Zaag J, Lobbezoo F, Van der Avoort PG, et al. Effects of pergolide on severe sleep bruxism in a patient experiencing oral implant failure. J Oral Rehabil 2007;34(5):317–322.
206. Saletu A, Parapatics S, Saletu B, et al. On the pharmacotherapy of sleep bruxism: Placebo-controlled polysomnographic and psychometric studies with clonazepam. Neuropsychobiology 2005;51(4):214–225.
207. Sjoholm T, Lehtinen I, Piha S. The effect of propranolol on sleep bruxism: Hypothetical considerations based on a case study. Clin Autonom Res 1996;6:37–40.
208. Amir I, Hermesh H, Gavish A. Bruxism secondary to antipsychotic drug exposure: A positive response to propranolol. Clin Neuropharmacol 1997;20:86–89.
209. Hartmann E Bruxism. In Kryer M, Roth T, Dement W (eds). Principles of Practice of Sleep Medicine. Philadelphia: WB Saunders Company, 1994, pp. 598–601.
210. Rogozea R, Florea-Ciocoiu V. Orienting reaction in patients with night terrors. Biol Psychiatry 1985;20: 894–905.
211. Kales J, Kales A, Soldatos C, et al. Night terrors. Arch Gen Psychiatry 1980;37:1413–1417.
212. Espa F, Dauvilliers Y, Ondze B, et al. Arousal reactions in sleepwalking and night terrors in adults: The role of respiratory events. Sleep 2002;25(8):871–875.
213. Di Gennaro G, Autret A, Mascia A, et al. Night terrors associated with thalamic lesion. Clin Neurophysiol 2004;115(11):2489–2492.
214. Mendez MF. Pavor nocturnus from a brainstem glioma. J Neurol Neurosurg Psychiatry 55(9):860.
215. Popoviciu L, Corfariu O. Efficacy and safety of midazolam in the treatment of night terrors in children. Br J Clin Pharmacol 1983;16 Suppl 1:97S–102S.
216. Wilson SJ, Lillywhite AR, Potokar JP, et al. Adult night terrors and paroxetine. Lancet 1997;350(9072):185.
217. Bruni O, Ferri R, Miano S, et al. L -5-hydroxytryptophan treatment of sleep terrors in children. Eur J Pediatr 2004;163(7):402–7.
218. Arkin A. Sleep-Talking:Psychology and Psychophysiology Hillsdale, NJ:Lawrence Erlbaum, 1981.
219. MacNeilage L. Activity of the speech apparatus during sleep and its relation to dream reports. Unpublished doctoral disseration, Columbia University, 1971.
220. Hublin C, Kaprio J, Partinen M, et al. Sleeptalking in twins: Epidemiology and psychiatric comorbidity. Behav Genet 1998;28(4):289–298.
221. Goodwin JL, Kaemingk KL, Fregosi RF, et al. Parasomnias and sleep disordered breathing in caucasian and hispanic children - the tucson children's assessment of sleep apnea study. BMC Med 2004;2:14.
222. Jacobson A, Kales A. Somnambulism: All-night eeg and related studies. In Baltimore Maryland (ed). Sleep and altered states of consciousness. The Williams & Wilkins Company, 1967, pp. 424–455.
223. Kavey N, Whyte J, SR Resor J, et al. Somnambulism in adults. Neurology 1990;40:749–752.
224. Broughton R. Sleep disorders: Disorders of arousal? Science 1968;159:1070.
225. Blatt I, Peled R, Gadoth N, et al. The value of sleep recording in evaluating somnambulism in young adults. Electroencephalogr Clin Neurophysiol 1991;78:407–412.
226. Bliwise D. What is sundowning? J Am Geriatr Soc 1994;42:1009–1011.
227. Cirignotta F, Zucconi M, Mondini S, et al. Enuresis, sleepwalking, and nightmares: An epidemiological survey in the republic of san marino. In Guilleminault C, Lugaresi E (eds). Sleep/wake disorders: Natural history, epidemiology, and long-term evolution. New York: Raven Press, 1983, pp. 237–241.
228. Kales A, Soldatos C, Caldwell A, et al. Somnambulism. Arch Gen Psychiatry 1980;37:1406–1410.
229. Hublin C, Kaprio J, Partinen M, et al. Prevalence and genetics of sleepwalking: A population-based twin study. Neurology 1997;48(1):177–181.
230. Lecendreux M, Bassetti C, Dauvilliers Y, et al. Hla and genetic susceptibility to sleepwalking. Mol Psychiatry 2003;8(1):114–117.
231. Khazaal Y, Krenz S, Zullino DF. Bupropion-induced somnambulism. Addict Biol 2003;8(3):359–362.
232. Hafeez ZH, Kalinowski CM. Two cases of somnambulism induced by quetiapine. Prim Care Companion J Clin Psychiatry 2007;9(4):313.
233. Hensel J, Pillmann F. Late-life somnambulism after therapy with metoprolol. Clin Neuropharmacol 2008;31(4): 248–250.
234. Yang W, Dollear M, Muthukrishnan SR. One rare side effect of zolpidem--sleepwalking: A case report. Arch Phys Med Rehabil 2005;86(6):1265–1266.
235. Zadra A, Pilon M, Montplaisir J. Polysomnographic diagnosis of sleepwalking: Effects of sleep deprivation. Ann Neurol 2008;63(4):513–519.
236. Fisher C, Kahn E, Edwards A, et al. A psychophysiological study of nightmares and night terrors. Psychoanal Contemp Sci 1974;3:317–398.
237. Reid W. Treatment of somnambulism in military trainees. Am J Psychiatry 1975;29:101–105.
238. Howell MJ, Schenck CH, Crow SJ. A review of nighttime eating disorders. Sleep Med Rev 2009;13:34–35.
239. Schenck C, Hurwitz T, Bundlie S, et al. Sleep-related eating disorders: Polysomnographic correlates of a heterogeneous syndrome distinct from daytime eating disorders. Sleep 1991;14:419–431.
240. Spaggiari M, Granella F, Parrino L, et al. Nocturnal eating syndrome in adults. Sleep 1994;17(4):339–344.
241. Winkelman JW. Clinical and polysomnographic features of sleep-related eating disorder. J Clin Psychiatry 1998;59(1):14–19.
242. Schenck CH, Mahowald MW. Review of nocturnal sleep-related eating disorders. Int J Eat Disord 1994;15(4): 343–356.
243. Whyte J KN. Somnambulistic eating: A report of three cases. Int J Eat Disord 1990;9(5):577–581.
244. Lu, ML, Shen WW. Sleep-related eating disorder induced by risperidone. J Clin Psychiatry 2004;65(2):273–274.
245. Najjar M. Zolpidem and amnestic sleep related eating disorder. J Clin Sleep Med 2007;3(6):637–638.
246. Paquet V, Strul J, Servais L, et al. Sleep-related eating disorder induced by olanzapine. J Clin Psychiatry 2002;63(7):597.

247. Winkelman JW. Efficacy and tolerability of open-label topiramate in the treatment of sleep-related eating disorder: A retrospective case series. J Clin Psychiatry 2006;67(11):1729–1734.
248. Schenck C, Hurwitz T, O'Connor K, et al. Additional categories of sleep-related eating disorders and the current status of treatment. Sleep 1993;16(5):457–466.
249. Provini F, Albani F, Vetrugno R, et al. A pilot double-blind placebo-controlled trial of low-dose pramipexole in sleep-related eating disorder. Eur J Neurol 2005;12(6): 432–436.
250. Provini F, Plazzi G, Lugaresi E. From nocturnal paroxysmal dystonia to nocturnal frontal lobe epilepsy. Clin Neurophysiol 2000;111 (suppl 2):S2–S8.
251. Provini F, Plazzi G, Tinuper P, et al. Nocturnal frontal lobe epilepsy. A clinical and polygraphic overview of 100 consecutive cases. Brain 1999;122:1017–1031.
252. Sforza E, Montagna P, Rinaldi R, et al. Paroxysmal periodic motor attacks during sleep: Clinical and polygraphic features. Electroencephalogr Clin Neurophysiol 1993;86:161–166.
253. Terzano M, Parrino L, Spaggiari M. The cyclic alternating pattern sequences in the dynamic organization of sleep. Electroencephalogr Clin Neurophysiol 1988;69: 437–447.
254. Terzano M, Monge-Strauss M, Mikol F, et al. Cyclic alternating pattern as a provocative factor in nocturnal paroxysmal dystonia. Epilepsia 1997;38:1015–1025.
255. Lugaresi E, Cirignotta F. Hypnogenic paroxysmal dystonia: Epileptic seizure or a new syndrome? Sleep1981;4(2): 129–138.
256. Tinuper P, Cerullo A, Cirignotta F, et al. Nocturnal paroxysmal dystonia with short-lasting attacks: Three cases with evidence for an epileptic frontal lobe origin of seizures. Epilepsia 1990;31:549–556.
257. Huapaya L: Somnambulsim and bedtime medication. Am J Psychiatry 1976;133:1207.
258. Huapaya L: Seven cases of somnambulsim induced by drugs. Am J Psychiatry 1979;36:985.
259. Keefauver SP, Guilleminault C. Parasomnias. Sleep terrors and sleewalking. In Kryger M, Roth T, Dement W. Principles and Practice of Sleep Medicine. Philadelphia, WB Saunders Company, 1994, pp. 567–573.
260. Lees A, Blackburn N, Campbell V. The nightime problems of parkinson's disease. Clin Neuropharmacol 1988;11: 512–519.
261. Mouret J. Differences in sleep in patients with parkinson's disease. Electroencephalogr Clin Neurophysiol 1975;38: 653–657.
262. Kales A, Ansel R, Markham C, et al. Sleep in patients with parkinson's disease and normal subjects prior to and following levodopa administration. Clin Pharmacol Ther 1971;12:397–406.
263. Bergonzi P, Chiurulla C, Cianchetti C, et al. Clinical pharmacology as an approach to the study of biochemical sleep mechanisms: The action of l-dopa. Confin Neurol 1974;36:5–22.
264. Bergonzi P, Chiurulla C, Gambi D, et al. L-dopa plus dopa-decarboxylase inhibitor. Sleep organization in parkinson's syndrome before and after treatment. Acta Neurol Belg 1975;75(1):5–10.
265. Wilson W, Nashold B, Green R. Studies of the cortical and subcortical electrical activity during sleep of patients with dyskinesias. Third Symp Park Dis 1969;160–164.
266. Traczynska-Kubin D, Atef E, Petre-Quadens O. Le sommeil dans la maladie de parkinson. Acta Neurol Belg 1969;69:727–733.
267. Diederich N, Vaillant M, Mancuso G, et al. Progressive sleep 'destructuring' in parkinson's disease. A polysomnographic study in 46 patients. Sleep Med 2005;6:313–318.
268. Puca F, Bricolo A Rurella G. Effect of l-dopa or amantadine therapy on sleep spindles in parkinsonism. Electroencephalogr Clin Neurophysiol 1973;35:327–330.
269. Friedman A: Sleep pattern in parkinson's disease. Acta Med Pol 1980;21:193–199.
270. Rabey J, Vardi J, Glaubman H, et al. Eeg sleep: Study in parkinsonian patients under bromocryptine treatment. Eur Neurol 1978;17:345–350.
271. Schneider E, Ziegler B, Maxion H, et al. Sleep in parkinsonior patients under levodopa. Results of a long-term follow-up study. In 3rd Europeon Congress Sleep Research Montpellier. Basel, Switzerland, Karger, 1976, pp.447–450
272. Lavie P, Bental E, Goshen H, et al. Rem ocular activity in parkinsonian patients chronically treated with levodopa. J Neural Transm 1980;47:61–67.
273. Lavie P, Wajsbort J, Youdim M. Deprenyl does not cause insomnia in parkinsonian patients. Commun Psychopharmacol 1980;4:303–307.
274. Gillin J, Post R, Wyatt R, et al. Rem inhibitory effect of l-dopa infusion during human sleep. Electroencephalogr Clin Neurophysiol 1973;35:181–186.
275. Lesser R, Fahn S, Sniker S, et al. Analysis of the clinical problems in parkinsonism and the complications of long-term levodopa therapy. Neurol 1979;29:1253–1260.
276. Moskovitz C, H Moses I, Klawans H. Levodopa-induced psychosis: A kindling phenomenon. Am J Psychiatry 1978;135(6):669–675.
277. Sharf B, Moskovitz C, Lupton M, et al. Dream phenomena induced by chronic levodopa therapy. J Neural Transm 1978;43:143–151.
278. Nausieda P, Weiner W, Kaplan L. Sleep disruption in the course of chronic levodopa therapy: An early feature of the levodopa psychosis. Clin Neuropharmacol 1982;5: 183–194.
279. Nausieda P, Tanner C, Klawans H. Serotonergically active agents in levodopa-induced psychiatric toxicity reactions. In Fahn S, Calne D, Shoulson I (eds). Advances in Neurology. New York: Raven Press, 1983, pp. 23–32.
280. Nausieda P, Glantz R, Weber S, et al. Psychiatric complications of levodopa therapy of parkinson' disease. In Hassler R, Christ J (eds). Advances in Neurology. New York: Raven Press, 1984, pp. 271–277.
281. Comella C, Tanner C, Ristanovic R. Polysomnographic sleep measures in parkinson's disease patients with treatment-induced hallucinations. Ann Neurol 1993;34:710–714.
282. Monaca C, Duhamel A, Jacquesson J, et al. Vigilance troubles in parkinson's disease: A subjective and objective polysomnographic study. Sleep Med 2006;7:448–453.
283. Rye DB, Bliwise DL, Dihenia B, et al. Fast track: Daytime sleepiness in parkinson's disease. J Sleep Res 2000;9(1): 63–69.

284. Arnulf I, Bonnet A, Damier P, et al. Hallucinations, rem sleep, and parkinson's disease: A medical hypothesis. Neurology 2000;55(2):281–288.
285. Arnulf I, Konofal E, Merino-Andreu M, et al. Parkinson's disease and sleepiness: An integral part of pd. Neurology 2002;58:1019–1024.
286. Rye D, Bliwise D. Movement disorders specific to sleep and the nocturnal manifestations of waking movement disorders. In Watts R, keller W (eds). Movement disorders:Neurologic principles and practice. New York: McGraw-Hill, Inc., 1997, pp. 687–713.
287. Bliwise D, Rye D, Dihenia B, et al. Periodic leg movements in elderely patients with parkinsonism. Sleep 1998;21(suppl):196.
288. Wetter T, Collado-Seidel V, Pollmacher T, et al. Sleep and periodic leg movement patterns in drug-free patients with parkinson's disease and multiple system atrophy. Sleep 2000;23(3):361–367.
289. Gagnon J, Bedard M-A, Fantini M, et al. Rem sleep behavior disorder and rem sleep without atonia in parkinson's disease. Neurology 2002;59:585–589.
290. Comella C, Nardine T, Diedrich N, et al. Sleep-related violence, injury, and rem sleep behavior disorder in parkinson's disease. Neurology 1998;51:526–529.
291. Rye D, Johnston L, Watts R, et al. Juvenile parkinson's disease with rem behavior disorder, sleepiness and daytime rem-onsets. Neurology 1999;53:1868–1870.
292. Emser W, Hoffmann K, Stolz T, et al. Sleep disorders in diseases of the basal ganglia. In Karger, Basel Switzerland (eds). Interdisciplinary Topics in Gerontology. 1987, pp. 144–157.
293. Cicolin A, Lopiano L, Zibetti M, et al. Effects of deep brain stimulation of the subthalamic nucleus on sleep architecture in parkinsonian patients. Sleep Med 2004;5(2):207–210.
294. Hjort N, Ostergaard K, Dupont E. Improvement of sleep quality in patients with advanced parkinson's disease treated with deep brain stimulation of the subthalamic nucleus. Mov Disord 2004;19(2):196–199.
295. Lyons K, Pahwa R. Effects of bilateral subthalamic nucleus stimulation on sleep, daytime sleepiness, and early morning dystonia in patients with parkinson disease. J Neurosurg 2006;104:502–505.
296. Monaca C, Ozsancak C, Jacquesson J, et al. Effects of bilateral subthalamic stimulation on sleep in parkinson's disease. J Neurol 2004;251(2):214–218.
297. Nakashima K, Shimoyama R, Yokoyama Y, et al. Auditory effects on the electrically elicited blink reflex in patients with parkinson's disease. Electroenceph Clin Neurophysiol 1993;89:108–112.
298. Penders C, Delwaide P. Blink reflex studies in patients with parkinsonism before and during therapy. J Neurol Neurosurg Psychiatry 1971;34:674–678.
299. Kimura J. Disorder of interneurons in parkinsonism. The orbicularis oculi reflex to paired stimuli. Brain 1973;96: 87–96.
300. Delwaide P, Pepin J, Noordhout Md. The audiospinal reaction in parkinsonian patients reflects functional changes in reticular nuclei. Ann Neurol 1993;33:63–69.
301. Lim A, Moro E, Lozano A, et al. Selective enhancement of rapid eye movement sleep by deep brain stimulation of the human pons. Ann Neurol 2009;66(1):110–114.
302. Jellinger K. The pedunculopontine nucleus in parkinson's disease, progressive supranuclear palsy and alzheimer's disease. J Neurol Neurosurg Psychiatry 1988;51:540–543.
303. Hirsch E, Graybiel A, Duyckaerts C, et al. Neuronal loss in parkinson's disease and in progressive supranucleur palsy. Proc Natl Acad Sci USA 1987;84:5976–5980.
304. Gai W, Halliday G, Blumbergs P, et al. Substance p-containing neurons in the mesopontine tegmentum are severely affected in parkinson's disease. Brain 1991;114: 2253–2267.
305. Jellinger K. Pathology of parkinson's disease. Changes other than the nigrostriatal pathway. Mol Chem Neuropathol 1991;14:153–197.
306. Paulus W, Jellinger K. The neuropathologic basis of different clinical subgroups of parkinson's disease. J Neuropathol Exp Neurol 1991;50(6):743–755.
307. Scatton B, Dennis T, L'Heureux R, et al. Degeneration of noradrenergic and serotonergic but not dopaminergic neurones in the lumbar spinal cord of parkinsonian patients. Brain Research 1986;380:181–185.
308. Rye D. Modulation of normal and pathologic motoneuron activity during sleep. In Chokroverty S, Hening W, Walters A (eds). Sleep and movement disorders. Philadelphia: Butterworth-Heinemann, 2003, pp. 94–119.
309. Braak H, Rub U, Sandmann-Keil D, et al. Parkinson's disease: Affection of brain stem nuclei controlling premotor and motor neurons of the somatomotor system. Acta Neuropathol (Berl) 2000;99:489–495.
310. Braak H, Tredici K, Bratzke H, et al. Staging of the intracerebral inclusion body pathology associated with idiopathic parkinson's disease (preclinical and clinical stages). J Neurol 2002;249(suppl 3):III/1–IIII/5.
311. Marsden, C, Parkes J, Quinn N. Fluctuations of disability in parkinson's disease - clinical aspects. In C Marsden, S Fahn (eds). Movement Disorders. London: Butterworth Scientific, 1982, pp. 96–122.
312. Comella C, Bohmer J, Stebbins G. The frequency and factors associated with sleep benefit in parkinson's disease. Sleep Res 1995;24:386.
313. Schwab R, Zieper I. Effects of mood, motivation, stress and alertness on the performance in parkinson's disease. Psychiatr Neurol Basel 1965;150:345–357.
314. Hogl BE, Gomez-Arevalo G, Garcia S, et al. A clinical, pharmacologic, and polysomnographic study of sleep benefit in parkinson's disease. Neurology 1998;50(5): 1332–1339.
315. Ploski H, Levita E, Riklan M. Impairment of voluntary movement in parkinson's disease in relation to activation level, autonomic malfunction, and personality rigidity. Psychosomatic Med 1966;28:70–77.
316. Factor S, McAlarney T, Sanchez-Ramos J, et al. Sleep disorders and sleep effect in parkinson's disease. Mov Disord 1990;5(4):280–285.
317. van Hilten J, Weggeman M, Velde Evd, et al. Sleep, excessive daytime sleepiness and fatigue in parkinson's disease. J Neural Transm [P-D Sect] 1993;5:235–244.
318. Nakano K, Hasegawa Y, Tokushige A, et al. Topographical projections from the thalamus, subthalamic nucleus and pedunculopontine tegmental nucleus to the striatum in the japanese monkey, macaca fuscata. Brain Res 1990;537:54–68.

319. Miller E, Nieburg H. Amphetamines. Valuable adjunct in treatment of parkinsonism. N Y State J Med 1973;73: 2657–2661.
320. Parkes JD, Tarsy D, Marsden CD, et al. Amphetamines in the treatment of parkinson's disease. J Neurol Neurosurg Psychiatry 1975;38(3):232–237.
321. Cantello R, Aguggia M, Gilli M, et al. Major depression in parkinson's disease and the mood response to intravenous methylphenidate: Possible role of the "Hedoni" Dopamine synapse. J Neurol Neurosurg Psychiatry 1989;52:724–731.
322. Chaudhuri K, Martinez-Martin P, Brown R, et al. The metric properties of a novel non-motor symptoms scale for parkinson's disease: Results from an international pilot study. Mov Disord 2007;22(13):1901–1911.
323. Chaudhuri K, Martinez-Martin P, Schapira A, et al. International multicenter pilot study of the first comprehensive self-completed nonmotor symptoms questionnaire for parkinson's disease: The nmsquest study. Mov Disord 2006;21(7):916–923.
324. Abbott R, Ross G, White L, et al. Excessive daytime sleepiness and subsequent development of parkinson disease. Neurology 2005;65:1442–1446.
325. Chen H, Schernhammer E, Schwarzschild M, et al. A prospective study of night shift work, sleep duration, and risk of parkinson's disease. Am J Epidemiol 2006;163(8): 726–730.
326. Friedman J, Brown R, Comella C, et al. Fatigue in parkinson's disease: A review. Mov Disord 2007;22(3):297–308.
327. Hagell P, Hoglund A, Reimer J, et al. Measuring fatigue in parkinson's disease: A psychometric study of two brief generic fatigue questionnaires. J Pain Symptom Management 2006;32(5):420–432.
328. Havlikova E, Van Dijk J, Rosenberger J, et al. Fatigue in parkinson's disease is not related to excessive sleepiness or quality of sleep. J Neurol Sci 2008;270:107–113.
329. Roth T, Rye D, Borchert L, et al. Assessment of sleepiness and unintended sleep in parkinson's disease patients taking dopamine agonists. Sleep Med 2003;4(4):275–280.
330. Shpirer I, Miniovitz A, Klein C, et al. Excessive daytime sleepiness in patients with parkinson's disease: A polysomnography study. Mov Disord 2003;21(9):1432–1438.
331. Razmy A, Lang A, Shapiro C. Predictors of impaired daytime sleep and wakefulness in patients with parkinson disease treated with older (ergot) vs newer (nonergot) dopamine agonists. Arch Neurol 2004;61:97–102.
332. Stevens S, Comella C, Stepanski E. Daytime sleepiness and alertness in patients with parkinson disease. Sleep 2004;27(5):967–972.
333. Rye DB Jankovic J. Emerging views of dopamine in modulating sleep/wake state from an unlikely source:Pd. Neurology 2002;58(3):341–346.
334. Frucht S, Rogers J, Greene P, et al. Falling asleep at the wheel: Motor vehicle mishaps in persons taking pramipexole and ropinirole. Neurology 1999;52(9):1908–1910.
335. Hening W, Allen R, Earley C, et al. The treatment of restless legs syndrome and periodic limb movement disorder: An american academy of sleep medicine review. Sleep 1999;22:970–999.
336. Sanjiv CC, Schulzer M, Mak E, et al. Daytime somnolence in patients with parkinson's disease. Parkinsonism Relat Disord 2001;7:283–286.
337. O'Suilleabhain PE, Dewey RB. Contributions of dopaminergic drugs and disease severity to daytime sleepiness in parkinson disease. Arch Neurol 2002;59:986–989.
338. Hobson DE, Lang AE, Martin WRW, et al. Excessive daytime sleepiness and sudden-onset sleep in parkinson disease. JAMA 2002;287(4):455–463.
339. Ghorayeb I, Loundou A, Auquier P, et al. A nationwide survey of excessive daytime sleepiness in parkinson's disease in france. Mov Disord 2007;22(11):1567–1572.
340. Tandberg E, Larsen J, Karlsen K. Excessive daytime sleepiness and sleep benefit in parkinson's disease: A community based study. Mov Disord 1999;14:922–927.
341. Tan EK, Lum SY, Fook-Chong SMC, et al. Evaluation of somnolence in parkinson's disease: Comparison with age and sex matched controls. Neurology 2002;58(3): 465–468.
342. Paus S, Brecht H, Koster J, et al. Sleep attacks, daytime sleepiness, and dopamine agonists in parkinson's disease. Mov Disord 2003;18(6):659–667.
343. Verbaan D, Marinus J, Visser M, et al. Patient-reported autonomic symptoms in parkinson disease. Neurology 2007;69(4):333–341.
344. Korner Y, Meindorfner C, Moller J, et al. Predictors of sudden onset of sleep in parkinson's disease. Mov Disord 2004;19(11):1298–1305.
345. Gjerstad MD, Aarsland D, Larsen JP. Development of daytime somnolence over time in parkinson's disease. Neurology 2002;58:1544–1546.
346. Ondo WG, Vuong KV, Khan H, et al. Daytime sleepiness and other sleep disorders in parkinson's disease. Neurology 2001;57:1392–1396.
347. Montastruc J-L, Brefel-Courbon C, Senard J-M, et al. Sleep attacks and antiparkinsonian drugs: A pilot prospective pharmacoepidemiologic study. Clin Neuropharmacol 2001;24:181–183.
348. Kumar S, Bhatia M, Behari M. Sleep disorders in parkinson's disease. Mov Disord 2002;17(775–781.
349. Brodsky M, Godbold J, Roth T, et al. Sleepiness in parkinson's disease: A controlled study. Mov Disord 2003;18(6):668–672.
350. Johns MW. A new method for measuring daytime sleepiness: The epworth sleepiness scale. Sleep 1991;14(6): 540–545.
351. Hogl B, Seppi K, Brandauer E, et al. Increased daytime sleepiness in parkinson's disease: A questionnaire survey. Mov Disord 2003;18(3):319–323.
352. Brodsky M, Godbold J, Roth T, et al. Sleepiness in parkinson's disease: A controlled study. Mov Disord 2003;18:668–672.
353. Razmy A, Lang A, Shapiro C. Predictors of impaired daytime sleep and wakefulness in patients with parkinsons disease treated with older (ergot) vs newer (nonergot) dopamine agonists. Arch Neurol 2004;61:97–102.
354. Matsui H, Nishinaka K, Oda M, et al. Excessive daytime sleepiness in parkinson disease: A spect study. Sleep 2006;29(7):917–920.
355. Suzuki K, Miyamoto T, Miyamoto M, et al. Excessive daytime sleepiness and sleep episodes in japanese patients with parkinson's disease. J Neurol Sci 2008;271:47–52.
356. Ferreira J, Desboeuf K, Galitzky M, et al. Sleep disruption, daytime somnolence and 'sleep attacks' in parkinson's

diseases: A clinical survey in pd patients and age-matched healthy volunteers. Eur J Neurol 2006;13:209–214.

357. Fabbrini G, Barbanti P, Aurilia C, et al. Excessive daytime sleepiness in de novo and treated parkinson's disease. Mov Disord 2002;17:1026–1030.

358. Chaudhuri K, Pal S, DiMarco A, et al. The parkinson's disease sleep scale: A new instrument for assessing sleep and nocturnal disability in parkinson's disease. J Neurol Neurosurg Psychiatry 2002;73(6):629–635.

359. Martinez-Martin P, Visser M, Rodriguez-Blazquez C, et al. Scopa-sleep and pdss: Two scales for assessment of sleep disorder in parkinson's disease. Mov Disord 2008;23(12): 1681–1688.

360. Tse W, Liu Y, Barthlen G, et al. Clinical usefulness of the parkinson's disease sleep scale. Parkinsonism Relat Disord 2005;11:317–321.

361. Marinus J, Visser M, van Hilten J, et al. Assessment of sleep and sleepiness in parkinson disease. Sleep 2003;26(8): 1049–1054.

362. Hagell P, Broman J. Measurement properties and hierarchical item structure of the epworth sleepiness scale in parkinson's disease. J Sleep Research 2007;16:102–109.

363. Agid Y. Parkinson's disease: Pathophysiology. Lancet 1991;337:1321–1324.

364. Gjerstad M, Alves G, Wentzel-Larsen T, et al. Excessive daytime sleepiness in parkinson disease: Is it the drugs or the disease? Neurology 2006;67:853–858.

365. Andreau N, Chale J, Senard J, et al. L-dopa induced sedation: A double-blind cross-over controlled study versus triazolam and placebo in healthy volunteers. Clin Neuropharmacol 1999;22:15–23.

366. Ferreira JJ, Galitzky M, Thalamas C, et al. Effect of ropinirole on sleep onset: A randomized placebo controlled study in healthy volunteers. Neurology 2002;58(3):460–462.

367. Silber MH, Rye DB. Solving the mysteries of narcolepsy. Neurology 2001;56:1616–1618.

368. Bagetta G, Sarro GD, Priolo E, et al. Ventral tegmental area: Site through which dopamine d_2-receptor agonists evoke behavioral and electrocortical sleep in rats. Br J Pharmacol 1988;95(860–866.

369. Berridge C, O'Neil J, Wifler K. Amphetamine acts within the medial basal forebrain to initiate and maintain alert waking. Neuroscience 1999;93:885–896.

370. Thannickal T, Moore R, Nienhuis R, et al. Reduced number of hypocretin neurons in human narcolepsy. Neuron 2000;27(3):469–474.

371. Mignot E, Lammers G, Ripley B, et al. The role of cerebrospinal fluid hypocretin measurement in the diagnosis of narcolepsy and other hypersomnias. Arch Neurol 2002;59(10):1553–1562.

372. Thannickal T, Lai Y, Siegel J. Hypocretin (orexin) cell loss in parkinson's disease. Brain 2007;130:1586–1595.

373. Baumann C, Ferini-Strambi L, Waldvogel D, et al. Parkinsonism with excessive daytime sleepiness: A narcolepsy-like disorder? J Neurol 2005;252:139–145.

374. Ripley B, Overeem S, Fujiki N, et al. Csf hypocretin/orexin levels in narcolepsy and other neurological conditions. Neurology 2001;57(12):2253–2258.

375. Drouot X, Moutereau S, Nguyen J, et al. Low levels of ventricular csf orexin/hypocretin in advanced pd. Neurology 2003;61(4):540–543.

376. Fronczek R, Overeem S, Lee S, et al. Hypocretin (orexin) loss in parkinson's disease. Brain 2007;130:1577–1585.

377. Martinez-Rodriguez J, Seppi K, Cardozo A, et al. Cerebrospinal fluid hypocretin-1 levels in multiple system atrophy. Mov Disord 2007;22(12):1822–1824.

378. Abdo W, Bloem B, Kremer H, et al. Csf hypocretin-1 levels are normal in multiple-system atrophy. Parkinsonism Relat Disord 2008;14(4):342–344.

379. Yasui K, Inoue Y, Kanbayashi T, et al. Csf orexin levels of parkinson's disease, dementia with lewy bodies, progressive supranuclear palsy and corticobasal degeneration. J Neurol Sci 2006;250:120–123.

380. Baumann C, Dauvilliers Y, Mignot E, et al. Normal dsf hypocretin-1 (orexin a) levels in dementia with lewy bodies associated with excessive daytime sleepiness. Eur Neurol 2004;52:73–76.

381. Benarroch E, Schmeichel A, Sandroni P, et al. Involvement of hypocretin neurons in multiple system atrophy. Acta Neuropathologica 2007;113(1):75–80.

382. Keating G, Kuhar M, Bliwise D, et al. Wake promoting effect of cocaine and amphetamine-regulated transcript (cart). Neuropeptides 2010;44:241–246.

383. Schultz K, Wiehager S, Nilsson K, et al. Reduced csf cart in dementia with lewy bodies. Neurosci Lett 2009;453: 104–106.

384. Whitehead D, Davies A, Playfer J, et al. Circadian rest-activity rhythm is altered in parkinson's disease patients with hallucinations. Mov Disord 2008;23(8):1137–1145.

385. Mega M, Masterman D, Benson F, et al. Dementia with lewy bodies: Reliability and validity of clinical and pathologic criteria. Neurology 1996;47:1403–1409.

386. Park M, Comella C, Leurgans S, et al. Association of daytime napping and parkinsonian signs in alzheimer's disease. Sleep Med 2006;7:614–618.

387. Boddy F, Rowan E, Lett D, et al. Subjectively reported sleep quality and excessive daytime somnolence in parkinson's disease with and without dementia, dementia with lewy bodies and alzheimer's disease. Int J Geriatr Psychiatry 2007;22(6):529–535.

388. Stavitsky K, McNamara P, Durso R, et al. Hallucinations, dreaming and frequent dozing in parkinson's disease: Impact of right-hemisphere neural networks. Cogn Behavior Neurol 2008;21(3):143–149.

389. Happe S, Baier P, Halmschmied K, et al. Association of daytime sleepiness with nigrostriatal dopaminergic degeneration in early parkinson's disease. J Neurol 2007;254:1037–1043.

390. Frauscher B, Hogl B, Maret S, et al. Association of daytime sleepiness with comt polymorphism in patients with parkinson disease: A pilot study. Sleep 2004;27(4): 733–736.

391. Rissling I, Frauscher B, Kronenberg F, et al. Daytime sleepiness and the comt val^{158}met polymorphism in patients with parkinson disease. Sleep 2006;29(1):108–111.

392. Rissling I, Geller F, Bandmann O, et al. Dopamine receptor gene polymorphisms in parkinson's disease patients reporting "sleep attacks". Mov Disord 2004;19(11):1279–1284.

393. Paus S, Seeger G, Brecht H, et al. Association study of dopamine d2, d3, d4 receptor and serotonin transporter gene polymorphisms with sleep attacks in parkinson's disease. Mov Disord 2004;19(6):705–707.

394. Rissling I, Korner Y, Geller F, et al. Preprohypocretin polymorphisms in parkinson disease patients reporting "sleep attacks". Sleep 2005;28(7):871–875.
395. Fabbrini G, Barbanti P, Aurilia C, et al. Excessive daytime sleepiness in de novo treated parkinson's disease. Mov Disord 2002;17(5):1026–1030.
396. Frucht S, Rogers J, Greene P, et al. Falling asleep at the wheel: Motor vehicle mishaps in people taking pramipexole and ropinirole - letters to the editor. Neurology 2000;54: 274–277.
397. Olanow CW, Schapira AHV, Roth T. Waking up to sleep episodes in parkinson's disease. Mov Disord 2000;15: 212–215.
398. Ryan M, Slevin J, Wells A. Non-ergot dopamine agonist-induced sleep attacks. Pharmacotherapy 2000;20:724–726.
399. Hauser RA, Gauger L, Anderson WM, et al. Pramipexole-induced somnolence and episodes of daytime sleep. Mov Disord 2000;15(4):658–663.
400. Ferreira J, Galitzky M, Montastruc J, et al. Sleep attacks and parkinson's disease treatment. Lancet 2000;355(9212): 1333–1334.
401. Merino-Andreu M, Arnulf I, Konofal E, et al. Unawareness of naps in parkinson's disease and in disorders with excessive daytime sleepiness. Neurology 2003;60:1553–1554.
402. Moller J, Rethfeldt M, Korner Y, et al. Daytime sleep latency in medication-matched parkinsonian patients with and without sudden onset of sleep. Mov Disord 2005;20(12):1620–1622.
403. Moller J, Unger M, Stiasny-Kolster K, et al. Continuous sleep eeg monitoring in pd patients with and without sleep attacks. Parkinsonism Relat Disord 2009;15:238–241.
404. Seppi K, Hogl B, Diem A, et al. Levodopa-induced sleepiness in the parkinson variant of multiple system atrophy. Mov Disord 2006;21(8):1281–1283.
405. Tracik F, Ebersbach G. Sudden daytime sleep onset in parkinson's disease: Polysomnographic recordings. Mov Disord 2001;16:500–506.
406. Ulivelli M, Rossi S, Lombard C, et al. Polysomnographic characterization of pergolide-induced "Sleep attacks" In an idiopathic pd patient. Neurology 2002;58(3):462–465.
407. Micallef J, Rey M, Eusebio A, et al. Antiparkinsonian drug-induced sleepiness: A double-blind placebo-controlled study of l-dopa, bromocriptine and pramipexole in healthy subjects. Br J Clin Pharmacol 2009;67(3):333–340.
408. Cochen De Cock V, Abouda M, Leu S, et al. Is obstructive sleep apnea a problem in parkinson's disease? Sleep Med 2010;11:247–252.
409. Johns M A new method for measuring daytime sleepiness: The epworth sleepiness scale. Sleep 1991;14(6):540–545.
410. Moller JC, Stiasny K, Hargutt V, et al. Evaluation of sleep and driving performance in six patients with parkinson's disease reporting sudden onset of sleep under dopaminergic medication: A pilot study. Mov Disord 2002;17:474–481.
411. Askenasy J, Yahr M. Reversal of sleep disturbance in parkinson's disease by antiparkinsonian therapy: A preliminary study. Neurology 1985;35:527–532.
412. Goetz C, Tanner C, Klawans H. Bupropion for parkinson's disease. Neurology 1984;34:1092–1094.
413. Hauser RA, Wahba MN, Zesiewicz TA, et al. Modafinil treatment of pramipexole-associated somnolence. Mov Disord 2000;15:1269–1271.
414. Rabinstein A, Shulman LM, Weiner WJ. Modafinil for the treatment of excessive daytime sleepiness in parkinson's disease: A case report. Park Rel Disord 2001;7:287–288.
415. Nieves AV, Lang AE. Treatment off excessive daytime sleepiness in patients with parkinson's disease with modafinil. Clin Neuropharmacol 2002;25:111–114.
416. Hogl B, Saletu M, Brandauer E, et al. Modafinil for the treatment of daytime sleepiness in parkinson's disease: Double-blind, randomized, cross-over, placebo-controlled polygraph trial. Sleep 2002;25:905–909.
417. Adler C, Caviness J, Hentz J, et al. Randomized trial of modafinil for treating subjective daytime sleepiness in patients with parkinson's disease. Mov Disord 2003;18(3): 287–293.
418. Ondo W, Fayle R, Atassi F, et al. Modafinil for daytime somnolence in parkinson's disease: Double blind, placebo controlled parallel trial. J Neurol Neurosurg Psychiatry 2005;76(12):1636–1639.
419. Tyne H, Taylor J, Baker GA, Steiger M. Modafinil for parkinson's disease fatigue. J Neurol 2010;257:252–256.
420. Lou J, Dimitrova D, Park B, et al. Using modafinil to treat fatigue in parkinson disease: A double-blind, placebo-controlled pilot study. Clin Neuropharmacol 2009;32(6):305–310.
421. Reynolds G, Elsworth J, Blau K, et al. Deprenyl is metabolized to methamphetamine and amphetamine in man. Br J Clin Pharmacol 1978;6:542–544.
422. Hietanen M. Selegiline and cognitive function in parkinson's disease. Acta Neurol Scand 1991;84:407–410.
423. Portin R, Rinne U. The effect of deprenyl (selegiline) on cognition and emotion in parkinsonian patients undergoing long-term levodopa treatment. Acta Neurol Scand 1983;Suppl 95:135–144.
424. Nickel B, Borbe H, Szelenyi I. Effect of selegiline and desmethyl-selegiline on cortical electric activity in rats. J Neural Transm [Suppl] 1990;32:139–144.
425. Hublin C, Partinen M, Heinonen E, et al. Selegiline in the treatment of narcolepsy. Neurology 1994;44:2095–2101.
426. Reinish L, MacFarlane J, Sandor P, et al. Rem changes in narcolepsy with selegiline. Sleep 1995;18(5):362–367.
427. Mayer G, Meier K, Hephata K. Selegeline hydrochloride treatment in narcolepsy. A double-blind placebo-controlled study. Clin Neuropharmacol 1995;18(4):306–319.
428. Ondo W, Perkinson T, Swick T, et al. Sodium oxybate for excessive daytime sleepiness in parkinson disease. Arch Neurol 2008;65(10):1337–1340.
429. Cooper B, Wang C, Cox R, et al. Evidence that the acute behavioral and electrophysiological effects of bupropion (wellbutrin) are mediated by a noradrenergic mechanism. Neuropsychopharmacology 1994;11:133–141.
430. Nausieda P. Sleep in parkinson disease. In Thorpy N (ed). Handbook of Sleep Disorders. New York: Marcel Dekker, 1990, pp. 719–733.
431. Happe S, Klosch G, Lorenzo J, et al. Perception of sleep: Subjective versus objective sleep parameters in patients with parkinson's disease in comparison with healthy elderly controls. Sleep perception in parkinson's disease and controls. J Neurol 2005;252:936–943.
432. Goetz C, Wuu J, Curgian L, et al. Hallucinations and sleep disorders in pd: Six-year prospective longitudinal study. Neurology 2005;64:81–86.

433. Gjerstad M, Wentzel-Larsen T, Aarsland D, et al. Insomnia in parkinson's disease: Frequency and progression over time. J Neurol Neurosurg Psychiatry 2007;78:476–779.
434. Ghorayeb I, Yekhlef F, Chrysostome V, et al. Sleep disorders and their determinants in multiple system atrophy. J Neurol Neurosurg Psychiatry 2002;72(6):798–800.
435. Steur E. Increase of parkinson disability after fluoxetine medication. Neurol 1993;43:211–213.
436. Richelson E. Pharmacology of antidepressants-characteristics of the ideal drug. Mayo Clin Proc 1994;69:1069–1081.
437. Lees A. A sustained release formulation of l-dopa (madopar hbs) in the treatment of nocturnal and early morning disabilities in parkinson's disease. Eur Neurol 1987;27(suppl 1):126–134.
438. Kerchove MVd, Jacquy J, Gonce M, et al. Sustained-release levodopa in parkinsonian patients with nocturnal disabilities. Acta Neurol Belg 1993;93:32–39.
439. Gaillard J. Benzodiazepines and gaba-ergic transmission. In Kryger M, Roth T, Dement W (eds). Principles and Practice of Sleep Medicine. Philadelphia: WB Saunders Company, 1994, pp. 349–354.
440. Bonnet M, Arand D. The use of triazolam in older patients with periodic leg movements, fragmented sleep, and daytime sleepiness. J Gerontol 1990;45(4):M139–144.
441. Dowling G, Mastick J, Colling E, et al. Melatonin for sleep disturbance in parkinson's disease. Sleep Med 2005;6(5):459–66.
442. Medeiros C, Carvalhedo de Bruin P, Lopes L, et al. Effect of exogenous melatonin on sleep and motor dysfunction in parkinson's disease. A randomized, double blind, placebo-controlled study. J Neurol 2007;2007(254):4.
443. Morgan JL, Brown TM, Wallace ER 4th. Monoamine oxidase inhibitors and sleep movements. Am J Psychiatry 1994;151(5): 782–783.
444. Ware J, Brown F, PJ Moorad J, et al. Nocturnal myoclonus and tricyclic antidepressants. Sleep Res 1984;13:72.
445. Wechsler L, Stakes J, Shahani B, et al. Periodic leg movements of sleep (nocturnal myoclonus): An electrophysiological study. Ann Neurol 1986;19:168–173.
446. Wechsler L, Stakes J, Shahani B, et al. Nocturnal myoclonus, restless legs syndrome, and abnormal electrophysiological findings. Ann Neurol 1987;21:515.
447. Ancoli-Israel S, Kripke D, Klauber M, et al. Periodic limb movements in sleep in community dwelling elderly. Sleep 1991;14:496–500.
448. Roehrs T, Zorick F, Sicklesteel J, et al. Age-related sleep-wake disorders at a sleep disorder center. J Am Geriatr Soc 1983;31:364–370.
449. Wetter TC, Collado-Seidel V, Pollmacher T, et al. Sleep and periodic leg movement patterns in drug-free patients with parkinson's disease and multiple system atrophy. Sleep 2000;23(3):361–367.
450. Scaglione C, Vignatelli L, Plazzi G, et al. Rem sleep behaviour disorder in parkinson's disease: A questionnaire-based study. Neurol Sci 2005;25:316–321.
451. Smith R. Confirmation of babinski-like response in periodic movements in sleep (nocturnal myoclonus). Biol Psychiatry 1987;22:1271–1273.
452. Delwaide P, Pepin J, Noordhout AMd. Short-latency autogenic inhibition in patients with parkinsonian ridigity. Ann Neurol 1991;30:83–89.
453. Iranzo A, Santamaria J, Rye D, et al. Characteristics of idiopathic rem sleep behavior disorder and that associated with msa and pd. Neurology 2005;65(2):247–52.
454. Aldrich M. Parkinsonism. In MH Kryger T Ruth, WC Dement (eds). Principles and Practice of Sleep Medicine. Philadelphia: WB Saunders Company, 1994, pp. 783–789.
455. Loo H-V, Tan E-K. Case-control study of restless leg syndrome and quality of sleep in parkinson's disease. J Neurol Sci 2008;266:145–49.
456. Rye D, DeLong M. Amelioration of sensory limb discomfort of restless legs syndrome by pallidotomy. Ann Neurol 1999;46(5):800–801.
457. Lang A, Johnson K. Akathisia in idiopathic parkinson's disease. Neurology 1987;37(477–481.
458. Linazasoro G, Masso JM, Suarez J. Nocturnal akathisia in parkinson's disease: Treatment with clozapine. Mov Disord 1993;8(2):171–174.
459. Fischer P, Naske R. Akathisia-like motor restlessness in major depression responding to serotonin-reuptake inhibition. J Clin Psychopharmacol 1992;12(4):295–296.
460. de Cock V, Vidailhet M, Leu S, et al. Restoration of normal motor control in parkinson's disease during rem sleep. Brain 2007;130:450–456.
461. Bliwise D, He L, Ansari F, et al. Quantification of electromyographic activity during sleep: A phasic electromyographic metric. J Clin Neurophysiol 2006;23(1):59–67.
462. Onofrj M, Thomas A, D'Andreamatteo G, et al. Incidence of rbd and hallucination in patients affected by parkinson's disease: 8-year follow-up. Neurol Sci 23 suppl 2:S91–94.
463. Pacchetti C, Manni R, Zangaglia R, et al. Relationship between hallucinations, delusions, and rapid eye movement sleep behavior disorder in parkinson's disease. Mov Disord 2005;20(11):1439–1448.
464. Ozekmekci S, Apaydin H, Kilic E. Clinical features of 35 patients with parkinson's disease displaying rem behavior disorder. Clin Neurol Neurosurg 2005;107(4): 306–309.
465. Gjerstad M, Boeve B, Wentzel-Larsen T, et al. Occurrence and clinical correlates of rem sleep behaviour disorder in patients with parkinson's disease over time. J Neurol Neurosurg Psychiatry 2008;79:387–391.
466. Plazzi G, Corsini R, Provini F, et al. Rem sleep behavior disorders in multiple system atrophy. Neurology 1997;48(4):1094–1097.
467. Postuma RB, Gagnon JF, Vendette M, et al. Manifestations of parkinson disease differ in association with rem sleep behavior disorder. Mov Disord 2008;23(12):1665–1672.
468. Kumru H, Santamaria J, Tolosa E, et al. Relation between subtype of parkinson's disease and rem sleep behavior disorder. Sleep Med 2007;8(7–8):779–783.
469. Manni R, Pacchetti C, Terzaghi M, et al. Hallucinations and sleep-wake cycle in pd: A 24-hour continuous polysomnographic study. Neurology 2002;59(12):1979–1981.
470. Nomura T, Inoue Y, Mitani H, et al. Visual hallucinations as rem sleep behavior disorders in patients with parkinson's disease. Mov Disord 2003;18(7):812–817.
471. Sinforiani E, Zangaglia R, Manni R, et al. Rem sleep behavior disorder, hallucinations, and cognitive impairment in parkinson's disease. Mov Disord 2006;21(4): 462–466.

472. Meral H, Aydemir T, Ozer F, et al. Relationship between visual hallucinations and rem sleep behavior disorder in patients with parkinson's disease. Clin Neurol Neurosurg 2007;109:862–867.
473. Postuma RB, Gagnon JF, Vendette M, et al. Rem sleep behaviour disorder in parkinson's disease is associated with specific motor features. J Neurol Neurosurg Psychiatry 2008;79(10):1117–1121.
474. Yoritaka A, Ohizumi H, Tanaka S, et al. Parkinson's disease with and without rem sleep behaviour disorder: Are there any clinical differences? Eur Neurol 2009;61(3): 164–170.
475. Sinforiani E, Pacchetti C, Zangaglia R, et al. Rem behavior disorder, hallucinations and cognitive impairment in parkinson's disease: A two-year follow up. Mov Disord 2008;23(10):1441–1445.
476. Marion M, Qurashi M, Marshall G, et al. Is rem sleep behaviour disorder (rbd) a risk factor of dementia in idiopathic parkinson's disease? J Neurol 2008;255(2):192–226.
477. Vendette M, Gagnon JF, Decary A, et al. Rem sleep behavior disorder predicts cognitive impairment in parkinson disease without dementia. Neurology 2007;69(19):1843–1849.
478. Turner R, D'Amato C, Chervin R, et al. The pathology of rem-sleep behavior disorder with comorbid lewy body dementia. Neurology 2000;55:1730–1732.
479. Boeve B, Silber M, Pirisi J, et al. Synucleinopathy pathology and rem sleep behavior disorder plus dementia or parkinsonism. Neurology 2003;61:40–45.
480. McKeith IG, Ballard CG, Perry RH, et al. Prospective validation of consensus criteria for the diagnosis of dementia with lewy bodies [in process citation]. Neurology 2000;54(5):1050–1058.
481. Gagnon J, Fantini M, Bedard M, et al. Association between waking eeg slowing and rem sleep behavior disorder in pd without dementia. Neurology 2004;62(3):401–406.
482. Hanoglu L, Ozer F, Meral H, et al. Brainstem ^{1}H-MR spectroscopy in patients with parkinson's disease with rem sleep behavior disorder and ipd patients without dream enactment behavior. Clin Neurol Neurosurg 2006;108(2):129–134.
483. Mahowald M, Schenck C. Rem sleep behavior disorder. In Kryger M, Roth T, Dement W (eds). Principles and Practices of Sleep Medicine. Philadelphia: WB Saunders Company, 1994, pp. 574–588.
484. Schenck C, Boyd J, Mahowald M. A parasomnia overlap disorder involving sleepwalking, sleep terrors, and rem sleep behavior disorder in 33 polysomnographically confirmed cases. Sleep 1997;20(11):972–981.
485. Vazquez A, Jimenez-Jimenez F, Garcia-Ruiz P, et al. "Panik attacks" In parkinson's disease. A long-term complication of levodopatherapy. Acta Neurol Scand 1993;87:14–18.
486. Bliwise D, Watts R, Watts N, et al. Disruptive nocturnal behavior in parkinson's disease and alzheimer's disease. J Geriatr Psychiatry Neurol 1995;8:107–110.
487. Lauterbach E. Sleep benefit and sleep deprivation in subgroups of depressed patients with parkinson's disease. Am J Psychiatry 1994;151(5):782–783.
488. Friedman J, Lannon M. Clozapine in the treatment of psychosis in parkinson's disease. Neurology 1989;39: 1219–1221.
489. Wolters E, Hurwitz T, Mak E, et al. Clozapine in the treament of parkinsonian patients with dopaminomimetic psychosis. Neurology 1990;40:832–834.
490. Meco G, Alessandria A, Bonifati V, et al. Risperidone for hallucinations in levodopa-treated parkinson's disease patients. Lancet 1994;343(8909):1370–1371.
491. Tavares J, AR. Risperidone in parkinson's disease. J Neurol Neurosurg Psychaitry 1995;58(4):521.
492. Morgante L, Epifanio A, Spina E, et al. Quetiapine versus clozapine: A preliminary report of comparative effects on dopaminergic psychosis in patients with parkinson's disease. Neurol Sci 2002;23(suppl 2)(S89–90.
493. Fernandez H, Trieschmann M, Burke M, et al. Quetiapine for psychosis in parkinson's disease versus dementia with lewy bodies. J Clin Pyschiatry 2002;63:513–515.
494. Menza M, Palermo B, Mark M. Quetiapine as an alternative to clozapine in the treatment of dopamimetic psychosis in patients with parkinson's disease. Ann Clin Psychiatry 1999;11:141–144.
495. Touyz S, Beumont P, Saayman G, et al. A psychophysiological investigation of the short-term effects of clozapine upon sleep parameters of normal young adults. Biological Psychiatry 1977;12(6):801–822.
496. Touyz S, Saayman G, Zabow T. A psychophysiological investigation of the long-term effects of clozapine upon sleep patterns of normal young adults. Psychopharmacology 1978;56:69–73.
497. Blum A. Triad of hyperthermia, increased rem sleep, and cataplexy during clozapine treatment? J Clin Psychiatry 1990;51(6):259–260.
498. Blum A, Girke W. Marked increase in rem sleep produced by a new antipsychotic compound. Clin Electroencephalogr 1973;4(2):80–84.
499. Hardie R, Efthimiou J, Stern G. Respiration and sleep in parkinson's disease (letter). J Neurol Neurosurg Psychiatry 1986;49:1326.
500. Apps M, Sheaff P, Ingram D, et al. Respiration and sleep in parkinson's disease. J Neurol Neurosurg Psychiatry 1985;48:1240–1245.
501. Bliwise D, Watts R, Watts N, et al. Nocturnal behavior disruption in parkinson's disease and alzheimer's disease (abstract). Sleep Res 1994;23:352.
502. Vincken W, Gauthier S, Dollfuss R, et al. Involvment of upper-airway muscles in extrapyramidal disorders. N Engl J Med 1984;311:438–442.
503. Hovestadt A, Bogaard J, Meerwaldt J, et al. Pulmonary function in parkinson's disease. J Neurol Neurosurg Psychiatry 1989;52:329–333.
504. Feinsilver S, Friedman J, Rosen J. Respiration and sleep in parkinson's disease. J Neurol Neurosurg Psychiatry 1986;49:964.
505. Rosen J, Feinsilver S, Friedman J. Increased co_2 responsiveness in parkinson's disease: Evidence for a role of dopamine in respiratory control. Am Rev Respir Dis 1985;131:A297.
506. Guilleminault C, Briskin J, Greenfield M, et al. The impact of autonomic nervous system dysfunction on breathing during sleep. Sleep 1981;4(3):263–278.
507. McNicholas W, Rutherford R, Grossman R, et al. Abnormal respiratory pattern generation during sleep in pa-

tients with autonomic dysfunction. Am Rev Respir Dis 1983;128:429–433.
508. Bergonzi P, Gigli G, Laudisio A, et al. Sleep and human cerebellar pathology. Int J Neurosci 1981;15:159–163.
509. Chokroverty S, Sachdeo R, Masdeu J. Autonomic dysfunction and sleep apnea in olivopontocerebellar degeneration. Arch Neurol 1984;41:926–931.
510. Gilman S, Chervin R, Koeppe R, et al. Obstructive sleep apnea is related to a thalamic cholinergic deficit in msa. Neurology 2003;61(1):35–39.
511. Sadaoka T, Kakitsuba N, Fujiwara Y, et al. Sleep-related breathing disorders in patients with multiple system atrophy and vocal fold palsy. Sleep 1996;19(6):479–484.
512. Shimohata T, Shinoda H, Nakayama H, et al. Daytime hypoxemia, sleep-disordered breathing, and laryngopharyngeal findings in multiple system atrophy. Arch Neurol 2007;64(6):856–861.
513. Schmidt C, Herting B, Prieur S, et al. Autonomic dysfunction in different subtypes of multiple system atrophy. Mov Disord 2008;23(12):1766–1772.
514. Vetrugno R, Provini F, Cortelli P, et al. Sleep disorders in multiple system atrophy: A correlative video-polysomnographic study. Sleep Med 2004;5(1):21–30.
515. Benarroch E, Schmeichel A, Low P, et al. Depletion of putative chemosensitive respiratory neurons in the ventral medullary surface in multiple system atrophy. Brain 2007;130(Pt 2):469–475.
516. Ghorayeb I, Yekhlef F, Bioulac B, et al. Continuous positive airway pressure for sleep-related breathing disorders in multiple system atrophy: Long-term acceptance. Sleep Med 2005;6(4):359–362.
517. Iranzo A, Santamaria J, Tolosa E, et al. Long-term effect of cpap in the treatment of nocturnal stridor in multiple system atrophy. Neurology 2004;63(5):930–932.
518. Salazar-Grueso E, Rosenberg R, Roos R. Sleep apnea in olivopontocerebellar degeneration: Treatment with trazodone. Ann Neurol 1988;23:399–401.
519. Shimohata T, Ozawa T, Nakayama H, et al. Frequency of nocturnal sudden death in patients with multiple system atrophy. J Neurol 2008;255(10):1483–1485.
520. Jin K, Okabe S, Chida K, et al. Tracheostomy can fatally exacerbate sleep-disordered breathing in multiple system atrophy. Neurology 2007;68(19):1618–1621.
521. Gross R, Spehlmann R, Daniels J. Sleep disturbances in progressive supranuclear palsy. Electroencephalogr Clin Neurophysiol 1978;45:16–25.
522. Sixel-Doring F, Schweitzer M, Mollenhauer B, et al. Polysomnographic findings, video-based sleep analysis and sleep perception in progressive supranuclear palsy. Sleep Med 2009;10:407–415.
523. Boeve BF, Silber MH, Ferman TJ, et al. Association of rem sleep behavior disorder and neurodegenerative disease may reflect an underlying synucleinopathy. Mov Disord 2001;16(4):622–630.
524. Cooper AD, Josephs KA. Photophobia, visual hallucinations, and rem sleep behavior disorder in progressive supranuclear palsy and corticobasal degeneration: A prospective study. Parkinsonism Relat Disord 2009;15:59–61.
525. Diederich NJ, Leurgans S, Fan W, et al. Visual hallucinations and symptoms of rem sleep behavior disorder in parkinsonian tauopathies. Int J Geriatr Psychiatry 2008;23(6):598–603.
526. Yasui K, Inoue Y, Kanbayashi T, et al. Csf orexin levels of parkinson's disease, dementia with lewy bodies, progressive supranuclear palsy and corticobasal degeneration. J Neurol Sci 2006;250(1–2):120–3.
527. Borroni B, Turla M, Bertasi V, et al. Cognitive and behavioral assessment in the early stages of neurodegenerative extrapyramidal syndromes. Arch Gerontol Geriatr 2008;47(1):53–61.
528. Roche S, Jacquesson JM, Destee A, et al. Sleep and vigilance in corticobasal degeneration: A descriptive study. Neurophysiol Clin 2007;37(4):261–4.
529. Wetter TC, Brunner H, Collado-Seidel V, et al. Sleep and periodic limb movements in corticobasal degeneration. Sleep Med 2002;3(1):33–6.
530. Gatto EM, Uribe Roca MC, Martinez O, et al. Rapid eye movement (rem) sleep without atonia in two patients with corticobasal degeneration (cbd). Parkinsonism Relat Disord 2007;13(2):130–132.
531. Iriarte J, Alegre M, Arbizu J, et al. Unilateral periodic limb movements during sleep in corticobasal degeneration. Mov Disord 2001;16(6):1180–1183.
532. Mano T, Shiozawa Z, Sobue I. Extrapyramidal involuntary movements during sleep. In Broughton R (ed). Neurosciences. Amsterdam: Elsevier Biomedical Press, 1982, pp. 431–442.
533. Fish D, Sawyers D, Allen P, et al. The effect of sleep on the dyskinetic movements of parkinson's disease, gilles de la tourette syndrome, huntington's disease, and torsion dystonia. Arch Neurol 1991;48:210–214.
534. Wiegand M, Moller A, Lauer C-J, et al. Nocturnal sleep in huntington's disease. J Neurol 238:203–208.
535. Arnulf I, Nielsen J, Lohmann E, et al. Rapid eye movement sleep disturbances in huntington disease. Arch Neurol 2008;65(4):482–488.
536. Starr A. A disorder of rapid eye movements in huntington's chorea. Brain 1967;90(3):545–564.
537. Emser W, Brenner M, Stober T, et al. Changes in nocturnal sleep in huntington's and parkinson's disease. J Neurol 1988;235:177–179.
538. Evers S, Stogbauer F. Genetic association of huntington's disease and restless legs syndrome? A family report. Mov Disord 2003;18(2):225–227.
539. Meier A, Mollenhauer B, Cohrs S, et al. Normal hypocretin-1 (orexin-a) levels in the cerebrospinal fluid of patients with huntington's disease. Brain Res 2005;1063(2):201–203.
540. Provini F, Lombardi C, Lugaresi E. Insomnia in neurological diseases. Semin Neurol 2005;25(1):81–89.
541. Portala K, Westermark K, Ekselius L, et al. Sleep in patients with treated wilson's disease. A questionnaire study. Nord J Psychiatry 2002;56(4):291–297.
542. Firneisz G, Szalay F, Halasz P, et al. Hypersomnia in wilson's disease: An unusual symptom in an unusual case. Acta Neurol Scand 2000;101(4):286–288.
543. Jankel W, Allen R, Niedermeyer E, et al. Polysomnographic findings in dystonia musculorum deformans. Sleep 6(3):281–285.
544. Segawa M, Hosaka A, Miyagawa F, et al. Hereditary progressive dystonia with marked diurnal fluctuation. In El-

dridge R, Fahn S (eds). Advances in Neurology. New York: Raven Press, 1976, pp. 215–233.
545. Montagna P, Imbriaco A, Zucconi M, et al. Hemifacial spasm in sleep. Neurology 1986;36(270–273.
546. Silvestri R, Domenico PD, Rosa AD, et al. The effect of nocturnal physiological sleep on various movement disorders. Mov Disord 1990;5(1):8–14.
547. Fish D, Sawyers D, Smith S, et al. Motor inhibition from the brainstem is normal in torsion dystonia during rem sleep. J Neurol Neurosurg Psychiatry 1991;54(2): 140–144.
548. Avanzino L, Martino D, Marchese R, et al. Quality of sleep in primary focal dystonia: A case-control study. Eur J Neurol 2010;17:576–581.
549. Trotti LM, Esper CD, Feustel PJ, et al. Excessive daytime sleepiness in cervical dystonia. Parkinsonism Relat Disord 2009;15(10):784–786.
550. Forgach L, Eisen A, Fleetham J, et al. Studies on dystonic torticollis during sleep. Neurology 1986;36(suppl 1):120.
551. Sunohara N, Mano Y, Ando K, et al. Idiopathic dystonia - parkinsonism with marked diurnal fluctuation of symptoms. Ann Neurol 1985;17:39–45.
552. Jankovic J, Rohaidy H. Motor, behavioral and pharmacologic findings in tourette's syndrome. Can J Neurol Sci 1987;14:541–546.
553. Sandyk R, Bamford C. Sleep disorders in tourette's syndrome. Interm J Neurosci 1987;37:59–65.
554. Mendelson W, Caine E, Goyer P, et al. Sleep in gilles de la tourette syndrome. Biol Psychiatry 1980;15(2):339–343.
555. Glaze D, Frost J, Jankovic J. Sleep in gilles de la tourette's syndrome: Disorder of arousal. Neurology 1983;33: 586–592.
556. Silvestri R, Domenico PD, Gugliotta M, et al. Gilles de la tourette's syndrome: Arousal and sleep polygraphic findings. A case report. Acta Neurol (Napoli) 1987;9(4):263–272.
557. Hashimoto T, Endo S, Fukuda K, et al. Increased body movements during sleep in gilles de la tourette syndrome. Brain Dev 1981;3:31–35.
558. Drake ME Jr, Hietter SA, Bogner JE, Andrews JM et al. Cassette eeg sleep recordings in gilles de la tourette syndrome. Clin Electroencephalogr 1992;23(3):142–146.
559. Voderholzer U, Muller N, Haag C, et al. Periodic limb movements during sleep are a frequent finding in patients with gilles de la tourette's syndrome. J Neurol 1997;244(8):521–526.
560. Cohrs S, Rasch T, Altmeyer S, et al. Decreased sleep quality and increased sleep related movements in patients with tourette's syndrome. J Neurol Neurosurg Psychiatry 2001;70:192–197.
561. Lesperance P, Djerroud N, Diaz Anzaldua A, et al. Restless legs in tourette syndrome. Mov Disord 2004;19(9): 1084–1087.
562. Kirov R, Kinkelbur J, Banaschewski T, et al. Sleep patterns in children with attention-deficit/hyperactivity disorder, tic disorder, and comorbidity. J Child Psychol Psychiatry 2007;48(6):561–570.
563. Chokroverty S, Barron K. Palatal myoclonus and rhythmic ocular movements: A polygraphic study. Neurology 1969;19:975–982.
564. Kayed K, Sjaastad O, Magnussen I, et al. Palatal myoclonus during sleep. Sleep 1983;6(2):130–136.
565. Yokota T, Atsumi Y, Uchiyama M, et al. Electroencephalographic activity related to palatal myoclonus in rem sleep. J Neurol 1990;237:290–294.
566. Ondo WG, Lai D. Association between restless legs syndrome and essential tremor. Mov Disord 2006;21(4): 515–518.
567. Walters AS, LeBrocq C, Passi V, et al. A preliminary look at the percentage of patients with restless legs syndrome who also have parkinson disease, essential tremor or tourette syndrome in a single practice. J Sleep Res 2003;12(4):343–345.
568. Calleja J, Carpizo R, Berciano J, et al. Serial waking-sleep eegs and evolution of somatosensory potentials in creutzfeldt-jakob disease. Electroencephalogr Clin Neurophysiol 1985;60:504–508.
569. Montagna P, Gambetti P, Cortelli P, et al. Familial and sporadic fatal insomnia. Lancet Neurol 2003;2(3): 167–176.
570. Provini F, Vetrugno R, Pierangeli G, et al. Sleep and temperature rhythms in two sisters with p102l gerstmann-straussler-scheinker (gss) disease. Sleep Med 2009;10: 374–377.
571. Mamoli B, Heiss WD, Maida E, et al. Electrophysiological studies on the "Stiff-man" Syndrome. J Neurol 1977;217(2):111–121.
572. Piovano C, Piattelli M, Spina T, et al. The stiff-person syndrome. Case report. Minerva Anestesiol 2002;68(11): 861–865.
573. Armon C, McEvoy KM, Westmoreland BF, et al. Clinical neurophysiologic studies in stiff-man syndrome: Use of simultaneous video-electroencephalographic-surface electromyographic recording. Mayo Clin Proc 1990;65(7): 960–967.
574. Martinelli P, Pazzaglia P, Montagna P, et al. Stiff-man syndrome associated with nocturnal myoclonus and epilepsy. J Neurol Neurosurg Psychiatry 1978;41(5):458–462.
575. Tuin I, Voss U, Kang JS, et al. Stages of sleep pathology in spinocerebellar ataxia type 2 (sca2). Neurology 2006;67(11):1966–1972.
576. Boesch SM, Frauscher B, Brandauer E, et al. Disturbance of rapid eye movement sleep in spinocerebellar ataxia type 2. Mov Disord 2006;21(10):1751–1754.
577. Abele M, Burk K, Laccone F, et al. Restless legs syndrome in spinocerebellar ataxia types 1, 2, and 3. J Neurol 2001;248(4):311–314.
578. Friedman JH, Amick MM. Fatigue and daytime somnolence in machado joseph disease (spinocerebellar ataxia type 3). Mov Disord 2008;23(9):1323–1324.
579. D'Abreu A, Franca Jr M, Conz L, et al. Sleep symptoms and their clinical correlates in machado-joseph disease. Acta Neurol Scand 2009;119:277–280.
580. Friedman JH, Fernandez HH, Sudarsky LR. Rem behavior disorder and excessive daytime somnolence in machado-joseph disease (sca-3). Mov Disord 2003;18(12): 1520–1522.
581. Howell MJ, Mahowald MW, Gomez CM. Evaluation of sleep and daytime somnolence in spinocerebellar ataxia type 6 (sca6). Neurology 2006;66(9):1430–1431.
582. Boesch SM, Frauscher B, Brandauer E, et al. Restless legs syndrome and motor activity during sleep in spinocerebellar ataxia type 6. Sleep Med 2006;7(6):529–532.

CHAPTER 48

Psychogenic Movement Disorders

Daniel S. Sa, Néstor Gálvez-Jiménez, and Anthony E. Lang

In 1922, Sir Henry Head wrote: "...Hysteria is sometimes said to imitate organic affections; but this is a highly misleading statement. The mimicry can only deceive an observer ignorant of the signs of hysteria or content with perfunctory examination."[1] Although in many cases of psychogenic movement disorders (PMDs) the nature of the problem is quite obvious from the first patient encounter, in the majority the diagnosis requires careful analysis of the history and the phenomenology of the abnormal movements and occasionally prolonged periods of observation and assessment. In general, abnormal movements and postures due to primary psychiatric disease are among the most difficult diagnostic problems in neurology even for the most experienced neurologist.

More recently, legal problems have increased the burden on such diagnoses. With the increasing risk of being sued by a mistake either way, either subjecting a patient to potentially dangerous diagnostic procedures and treatment options or denying potentially effective treatment options, the responsibility for accurate diagnosis has increased tremendously. Disputes involving work-related injuries and resulting compensation have become a major legal issue in most countries, and the increasing frequency of psychogenic or factitious disorders in these circumstances have taken the diagnosis of a PMD to a greater dimension while we are still looking for good biological markers to aid us in the diagnosis of organic forms of movement disorders. A recent survey of Movement Disorder Society members has shown that the majority (51%) of treating physicians still go through extensive, and expensive testing even when patients present with definitive evidence of a PMD (A. Espay, personal communication).

In this chapter, we will review the varied manifestations of PMDs and provide guidelines for the diagnosis and approach to therapy of these patients.

▶ HISTORY

In the 1880s, Charcot was fascinated by "hysteria" directing much attention to its definition, analysis, treatment, and research.[2] In one of his Tuesday lessons at the Salpêtrière, he presented a young woman who developed a contracture and deformity of her right foot 5 days following a fall. In his teachings, such a contracture should have been corrected as soon as it appeared. In this particular case, he decided to watch the progression of the disorder over 4 days without interfering. He taught that in such cases the treatment involved inducing a second attack to make the "fixed" contracture completely disappear. He used "hysterogenic points" to provoke such a transient attack as a form of therapy in the treatment of static hysteric signs. From the patient description, it appears that Charcot was dealing with a case of what we would now term "psychogenic dystonia."

According to Charcot, posttraumatic contractures were more frequently seen in hysterics. Charcot proposed that hysteria was not restricted to women but was also common in males, especially working-men,[3] children,[4] and effeminate men.[5] Freud[3] also reported Charcot's observations that many conditions previously ascribed to alcoholic or lead poisonings were, in fact, hysterical.

Contrary to what is frequently believed, however, in his original classification of diseases, Charcot included hysteria under "nevroses," diseases or states well-characterized clinically but lacking an identifiable lesion.[6] He believed that similar to seizures, also classified under "névroses", there was a specific neuroanatomic basis to hysteria, but such changes were transient[7] Charcot's approach to hysteria was criticized by many (among others, Paul Broca,[8] Sigmund Freud,[9] and later Gowers[10]), especially in regard to the therapeutic use of suggestion and hypnosis.[11] Freud in his writings on hypnosis and suggestion said that "...if the supporters of the suggestion theory are right, all the observations made at the Salpêtrière are worthless" because there were many who believed (especially in Germany) that the power of suggestion was due to "...a combination of credulity on the part of the observers and of simulation on the part of the subjects of the experiments."[9] Charcot had the patients repeat their crises in front of physicians and medical students.[4] Furthermore, Charcot's experiments on hypnosis were performed by his chiefs of clinic, interns, and other assistants but they were never personally checked with the result that inadequacies and failures of this form of therapy were not known to him.[4] Because the majority of his hysterics were housed together with the epileptics ("...the old wards of the chronic patients"[9]), it was well known that many of the postures or attacks demonstrated by hysterics were nothing more than colorful imitations of real epileptic seizures further reinforced by public demonstrations in his Tuesday clinics in front of not only his pupils but also society people, actors, writers, magistrates, and journalists.[4] Since then, the clinical manifestations and pathophysiological mechanisms underlying hysteria have been a matter of controversy. Late in his life, Charcot made passing remarks that hysteria could be "for the most part a mental illness," marking a significant change in his long-held beliefs.[7] Gowers[12] wrote "there are few organic diseases of the brain that the great mimetic neurosis may not simulate. Palsy and spasm, coma ...almost every symptom of positive disease find its counterpart in the repertoire of ...the nervous system." He insisted that "...given symptoms of hysteria, we must never infer that this is the primary disease until we have searched for, and excluded, the symptoms of organic disease."[12] He described "psychogenic laryngeal spasms" and "psychogenic pharyngeal spasms" in his writings on epilepsy and hysteria[10] and used hypnosis to determine if these spasms could be altered during sleep attempting to distinguish attacks due to hysteria from those due to real organic disease (although we now recognize that true organic dystonia can disappear during sleep or with hypnosis). Gowers believed that hysteria could occur in both sexes[13] observing that "...hysteroid attacks are not very rare in lads and young men including transient paralysis, or contractures, of a limb, precisely similar to those met with in the female sex."[10]

In his address to the London Hospital Medical Society, Sir Henry Head[1] described a variety of PMDs. He described hysterical tremor as a positive repetitive movement of a high "voluntary" type, varying in rapidity, and ceasing with distraction: "...a soldier with a severe tremor of the right hand and arm was able to play the banjo perfectly and I used this musical aptitude for affecting his cure." He also described abnormal focal postures in a limb or a single joint, "...any attempt to break down a spasm of this kind, to open the closed hand, or to straighten the flexed knee, meets with intense resistance" and in describing what he felt was "psychogenic torticollis" he stated that "... resistance may be experience not only in pushing the head towards the normal shoulder, but also in moving it farther in the direction of the affected side."[1] In the same address, he referred to "psychogenic ataxia," which differs fundamentally from "ataxy of organic origin."[1] On attempting to touch the nose with the index finger, there was past-pointing "...to the same side of the head," but if the head was pushed in the direction of the past-pointed finger as to make contact with it, the affected limb would deviate even further away from the head.

In general, many of the observations of these earlier writers have been corroborated with time as experience with specific PMDs has accumulated. However, older and even more modern medical literature contains many examples of organic movement disorders mistakenly attributed to primary psychological factors. Tourette's syndrome is possibly the best example of a condition once thought to have a psychological origin that is now accepted to be due to a disorder of the central nervous system (CNS). The same applies to the wide range of idiopathic dystonias, all of which at one time or another have been considered psychogenic. Reasons for this include the unusual nature of the movements, their appearance only on certain actions but not others using the same muscles, their relief by certain peculiar "sensory tricks," the common worsening of the movements in response to mental or social stress, and until very recently the failure to find any underlying anatomical, physiological, or biochemical abnormalities. These factors "supported" the common belief that such patients had an underlying psychiatric disturbance, which then encouraged the development of psychopathological hypotheses to explain the significance of the abnormal movements. Examples of these included the "turning away" from responsibilities or avoidance of conflict in the patient with dystonic head turning or the phallic symbolism of a pen extruding ink causing writer's cramp. However, several studies of patients with focal dystonias such as torticollis[14] and writer's cramp[15,16] have failed to demonstrate evidence for abnormal premorbid personalities or an association with underlying causative psychopathology. Where abnormalities are found (e.g., depression, poor body image, and self-esteem), it is possible that they are a result of the dystonia rather than the cause. The broader modern recognition of the spectrum organic movement disorders, in part, led by David Marsden and Stanley Fahn, initially increased the reluctance to consider a psychogenic etiology. However, further clinical observations, again particularly by Dr. Fahn, began to recognize the occurrence of psychogenic counterparts for most forms of movement disorders and the term "psychogenic" has largely replaced "hysteria," given the negative connotations of the latter.

The historical pendulum has swung back and forth over the past century. Most of the neurologists trained under the National Hospital, Queen Square, during the twentieth century were taught to avoid the term hysteria, and a much criticized study by Slater and Glithero reported finding an underlying organic diagnosis in 49 of 85 patients diagnosed with hysteria. It is important to note that, even accepting most of their conclusions as valid, still 57% of their patients had no organic diagnoses.[17] Subsequent follow-up studies[18] have shown that misdiagnosis of organic disorders as due to "hysteria" or a "conversion disorder" following detailed neurological assessment and modern imaging occurs in no more than 5–10% of patients.[19]

▶ PSYCHIATRIC DEFINITIONS

It would be helpful to begin our review of PMDs with a brief discussion of the current terminology recommended by the American Psychiatric Association's *Diagnostic and Statistical Manual of Mental Disorders, Fourth Edition* (DSM IV)[20] related to psychiatric disturbances that can be seen in such patients. The new version, the DSM V, is expected to be released by May 2012.

Somatoform disorders have as a feature the occurrence of symptoms suggesting a systemic medical condition, but these symptoms do not fit or cannot be fully explained by the presence of a known medical disorder, the exposure to a substance or drug, or by another psychiatric condition. These symptoms must cause significant distress or impairment in social, occupational, or other areas of functioning. Somatoform disorders include somatization disorders, factitious disorders, malingering, and conversion disorders. **Somatization disorders** (Table 48–1) were formerly referred to as hysteria or Briquet's syndrome. Somatization disorders begin before age 30 and consist of recurrent and multiple clinically significant somatic complaints that result in medical intervention or social or occupational impairment. The differential diagnosis of these disorders must include major depressive, anxiety, and adjustment disorders.

Somatization disorders must be differentiated from **factitious disorders** including Münchausen's syndrome (Table 48–2) and **malingering** (Table 48–3) where the symptoms are intentionally produced or feigned. The difference between these two is that in the former there is a motivation to assume a sick role to obtain medical evaluation and treatment, whereas in the latter there are external incentives such as financial gain or compensation, avoidance of duty, evasion of criminal prosecution, or obtaining drugs.

Conversion disorders (Table 48–4) are characterized by the presence of symptoms or signs affecting voluntary motor or sensory function suggesting a neurological deficit ("pseudoneurological") associated with psychological conflicts or other stressors resulting in significant alterations in social or occupational functioning. These symptoms are not intentionally produced or feigned as in factitious disorders or malingering. Some patients with a **histrionic personality disorder** add to the clinical presentation a pattern of excessive emotionality and attention-seeking behavior (Table 48–5). Histrionic personality disorder occurs more frequently in women.[20,21]

Only recently have studies begun to assess the pathogenesis of the neurological dysfunction accompanying conversion disorders. For example, a recent imaging study in patients with hysterical unilateral sensorimotor loss demonstrated decreased regional cerebral blood flow in the contralateral thalamus and basal ganglia that resolved after recovery. Lower activation of the caudate predicted a poorer outcome. The authors proposed the presence of a "functional disorder in striatothalamocortical circuits controlling sensorimotor function and voluntary motor behavior." Although similar studies in patients with PMDs will be exceedingly interesting, as discussed later in this chapter, it will be critical to control for the presence, nature, and duration of abnormal movements.

▶ TABLE 48–1. DIAGNOSTIC CRITERIA FOR SOMATIZATION DISORDER (DSM IV)

1. History of many physical complaints beginning before age 30 years occurring over a period of many years, resulting in medical treatment or significant impairment in social, occupational, or other areas of functioning.
2. The following criteria must have been met, with the symptoms occurring any time during the course of the disturbance:
   (A) four pain symptoms in at least four different sites
   (B) two gastrointestinal symptoms other than pain
   (C) one sexual symptom other than pain
   (D) one pseudoneurological symptom suggesting a neurological condition not limited to pain.

Adapted with permission from American Psychiatric Association: Diagnostic and statistical mamnual of mental disorders, 4th edition (DSM IV). Washington, American Psychiatric Association, 1994.

▶ TABLE 48–2. DIAGNOSTIC CRITERIA FOR FACTITIOUS DISORDER (DSM IV)

1. Intentional production or feigning of physical or psychological symptoms or signs (Münchausen syndrome).
2. The motivation for the behavior is to assume the sick role.
3. External incentives for the behavior are absent (economic gain, avoidance of legal responsibilities, or improving physical well-being).

Adapted with permission from American Psychiatric Association: Diagnostic and statistical mamnual of mental disorders, 4th edition (DSM IV). Washington, American Psychiatric Association, 1994.

▶ TABLE 48–3. FEATURES SUGGESTIVE OF MALINGERING (MODIFIED FROM DSM IV)

1. The essential feature is the intentional production of false or grossly exaggerated physical or psychological symptoms, motivated by external incentives (i.e., avoiding work, obtaining financial compensation).
2. Malingering may represent adaptive behavior.
3. Malingering should be suspected if there is a medicolegal issue, that is, the person has been referred by his/her attorney.
4. Marked discrepancy between the person's claimed stress and disability and the objective findings.
5. Lack of cooperation during the diagnostic evaluation and in complying with the prescribed treatment.
6. Presence of antisocial personality disorder.

Adapted with permission from American Psychiatric Association: Diagnostic and statistical mamnual of mental disorders, 4th edition (DSM IV). Washington, American Psychiatric Association, 1994.

TABLE 48-4. DIAGNOSTIC CRITERIA FOR CONVERSION DISORDER (DSM IV)

1. One or more symptoms or deficits affecting voluntary motor or sensory functions that suggest a neurological or other general medical condition.
2. Psychological factors judged to be associated with the symptom or deficit because the onset of symptoms is preceded by conflicts or other stressors.
3. The symptom is not intentionally produced or feigned.
4. The symptom cannot be explained by a general medical condition after a thorough medical and laboratory evaluation, or as a direct effect of a substance, or culturally sanctioned behavior or experience.
5. The symptom causes significant distress or impairment in social, occupational, or other important areas of functioning or warrants medical evaluation.
6. The symptom is not limited to pain or sexual dysfunction, does not occur exclusively during the course of somatization disorder, and is not better accounted for by another mental disorder.

With permission from American Psychiatric Association: Diagnostic and statistical mamnual of mental disorders, 4th edition (DSM IV). Washington, American Psychiatric Association, 1994.

EPIDEMIOLOGY

Accurate epidemiological data is limited, but psychogenic disorders are relatively common. The Mannheim Cohort project has estimated that up to 25% of the population at some time or the other would fulfill criteria for psychogenic disorders.[23] Snyder and Strain, in a hospital-based study, found that somatoform disorders were responsible for 2.6% of the main discharge diagnoses in a group of 1801 patients.[24]

TABLE 48-5. CRITERIA FOR HISTRIONIC PERSONALITY DISORDER (DSM IV)

1. Constantly seeks or demands reassurance, approval, or praise.
2. Is inappropriately sexually seductive in appearance or behavior.
3. Overly concerned with physical attractiveness.
4. Expresses emotion with inappropriate exaggeration, for example, embraces casual acquaintances with excessive ardor, sobbing on minor sentimental occasions, or has temper tantrums.
5. Is uncomfortable in situations in which he or she is not the center of attention.
6. Displays rapidly shifting and shallow expression of emotions.
7. Is self-centered, actions being directed toward obtaining immediate satisfaction; has no tolerance for the frustration of delayed gratification.
8. Has a style of speech that is exceedingly impressionistic and lacking in detail.

Data from American Psychiatric Association: Diagnostic and statistical mamnual of mental disorders, 4th edition (DSM IV). Washington, American Psychiatric Association, 1994.

In patients with neurological signs and symptoms, psychogenic disorders are also relatively frequent, being estimated to account for 1–9% of all diagnoses.[25,26,27]

It has been reported that at Charcot's Tuesday clinic, 7% (244 patients out of 3168) of the total population seen during one academic year were diagnosed as having hysteria.[4,5,28] This figure is probably influenced by ascertainment bias because Charcot's interest in hysteria was well known at that time. The extent of Charcot's overdiagnosis or false positive labeling of patients as hysterical is also uncertain.

Among the psychogenic neurological disorders that can be seen, movement disorders are not uncommon. In a group of 842 consecutive patients evaluated on a specialty clinic, 28 (3.3%) were ultimately diagnosed as having a PMD.[29] Phenomenologically, the most common movement disorders were tremor, dystonia, myoclonus, and parkinsonism in that order. A recent update on those numbers yielded nearly identical figures, with 135 of 3826 (3.5%).[19] In a recent review of a large general neurology clinic in one of our institutions, PMDs represented approximately 1% of the 19,755 total neurology cases evaluated during the calendar year 2008 (N.G.-J., personal observations). When considering only those new patients presenting with a disorder of movement evaluated during the same time period at the same center, PMD represented 2.2% of the total movement disorders patient assessed. This number is in keeping with those reported from other specialty clinics (see above).

A report from the movement disorders unit at New-York-Presbyterian/Columbia University Medical Center in 1988 (CPMC),[30] which housed a dystonia research center, described experience with 131 patients diagnosed as having PMDs. Many patients had more than one movement disorder subtype. Eighty-two (53%) had psychogenic dystonia, 21 (13%) psychogenic tremor, 14 (9%) psychogenic gait disturbances, 11 (7%) psychogenic myoclonus, 4 (2%) blepharospasm and facial movements, 3 (1.9%) parkinsonism, and 2 (1.3%) tics and stiff person syndrome was seen in one case (0.6%). Nine percent of their cases (14) were categorized as having paroxysmal dyskinesias/shaking and undifferentiated movements. Better defined movements or postures (e.g., dystonia) occurring in a paroxysmal fashion are a relatively common manifestation of a PMD.

The Toronto Western Hospital Movement Disorders Clinic diagnosed a total of 279 patients with a PMD between 1990 and 2004. The most common predominant movement abnormality recorded was tremor in 91 patients (32.6%), followed by dystonia in 89 (31.9%), myoclonus in 51(18.3%), gait disorders in 16 (5.7%), and parkinsonism in 14 (5%). The remaining cases included paroxysmal movements, chorea, tics, dysphonia, and "spasms"[31] Interestingly, in contrast to other disorders, there is a small preponderance of males (9:8) in patients with parkinsonism.[29,32,33]

In a recent review of the Movement Disorders Program of the Cleveland Clinic Florida (CCFla) database, in a 10-year span between 1998 and 2008, 162 cases of PMDs were evaluated. The most common movement diagnosis was tremor (38%), followed by dystonia in 36% and myoclonus in 12%. Combinations of movement disorders were also common, and movements resembling hemifacial spasm were seen in 5 cases (see below) accounting for 0.2% of all hemifacial spasm cases seen over a 7-year span. Two of these had associated psychogenic blepharospasm.

In the Movement Disorders Clinic of The Marshfield Clinic Neurology Department, between July 2006 and December 2008, a total of 92 patients with a new diagnosis of PMD were seen. Of these, tremor was the main abnormal movement in 33 (35.8%), dystonia in 22 (24%), myoclonus in 22 (24%), parkinsonism in 4 (4.3%), and a gait disorder in 11 (11.9%). Women predominated in this series as in most, accounting for 62 patients (67.3%) (Sa D, unpublished data).

Table 48–6 combines the data of multiple institutions, although the data collection and presentation varied from reporting the predominant movement to reporting all observed movements. The combination of these experiences encompassing a total of 959 patients seen at various centers suggests that psychogenic tremor is the most common PMD (34.7%)—followed by psychogenic dystonia (33.8%), psychogenic myoclonus (13%), gait disorders (6.7%), and parkinsonism (3.3%).

However, all these results must be considered cautiously since referral bias is a likely consideration for all of such established referral centers. Another important confounding factor that cannot be overlooked is the possibility of an associated organic movement disorder along with the PMD. As in the case of pseudoseizures in known epileptic patients, patients with PMDs have been reported to have a concomitant organic disorder.[29,33–36] In the recent series of Factor and colleagues, 25% of their patients with PMDs had a concomitant organic problem. Other series, including the collected data at the Marshfield Clinic Movement Disorders Center, shows a significantly smaller proportion with a concomitant organic problem (7.6%) (Sa D, unpublished data).

The pediatric population is not free from PMDs. Schwingenshuh and colleagues recently reported 15 pediatric patients with a diagnosis of PMD. The mean onset age was 12.3 years; only 13% had onset before age 10. Dystonia (47%), tremor (40%), and gait disorders (13%) were the most common movement disorders.[37] Ferrara and Jankovic published a series of 54 pediatric patients with PMD, accounting for 3.1% of their pediatric movement disorder population. Tremor, dystonia, and myoclonus were the most commonly reported movements.[38]

In one series of 405 patients with conversion disorders requiring admission to hospital, Lempert and colleagues found that the most common underlying psychiatric disorder was depression (38%), followed by "anxiety and compulsion" (13%) and hysterical personality disorders (9%).[27] The nature of the primary

TABLE 48-6. COMBINED DATA ON PSYCHOGENIC MOVEMENT DISORDER SEEN AT SEVERAL MOVEMENT DISORDERS CENTERS*

Abnormal Movement	Toronto Western Hospital†	NewYork-Presbyterian/ Columbia University Medical Center‡	Cleveland Clinic Florida§	Marshfield Clinic‖	Baylor College of Medicine¶	Total
	(%)	(%)	(%)	(%)	(%)	(%)
Dystonia	89(31.9)	82(54)	43(26.5)	22 (24)	89(39)	325(33.8)
Tremor	91(32.6)	21(14)	61(37.6)	33 (35.8)	127(55.7)	333(34.7)
Myoclonus	51(18.3)	11(7)	8((4.9)	22 (24)	30(13.2)	122(12.7)
Gait disorder	16(5.7)	14(9)	17(10.5)	11 (11.9)	7(3.1)	65(6.7)
Parkinsonism	14(5)	3(2)	5(3.0)	4 (4.3)	6(2.6)	32(3.3)
Tics	3(1.1)	2(1)	9(5.5)	–	15 (6.6)	29(3.0)
Other	15(5.4)	19(13)	19(11.7)	–	–	53(5.5)
Total	279	152	162	92	274	959

*Data collection varied from listing predominant movement as in †, §, and ‖ to all movements observed.[3]
†Baik JS, Lang AE. Gait abnormalities in psychogenic movement disorders. Movement Disord 2007;22(3):395–399.
‡Williams DT, Ford B, Fahn S. Phenomenology and psychopathology related to psychogenic movement disorders. Adv Neurol 1995;65:231–258.
§Galvez-Jimenez N. Unpublished data (Cleveland Clinic Florida (CCFla) 1998–2008).
‖Sa D. Unpublished data. Collected July 2006–December 2008.
¶Thomas M, Jankovic J. Psychogenic movement disorder: Diagnosis and management. CNS Drug 2008;18:437–452.

psychiatric abnormality did not predict the type of presenting neurological symptoms, although paroxysmal vertigo was seen more often in patients with anxiety and compulsion. In Marsden's experience, depression was present in 18% of the 34 "hysterical" patients admitted to hospital over a 5-year period, whereas 20% had Briquet's syndrome and 6% had anxiety.[26] Feinstein and colleagues (from our unit in Toronto), interviewing 42 patients with a diagnosis of documented or clinically established PMD (most often fulfilling criteria for a conversion disorder), found a variety of additional psychiatric disorders, including anxiety disorders in 16 (38.1%), major depression in 8 (19.1%), and a combination of the two in 5 (11.9%). Other lifetime psychiatric diagnoses included adjustment disorder in 9.5% (4), schizoaffective disorders in 2.4% (1), bipolar disorder in 2.4% (1), and alcohol or sedative abuse in 2.4% (1) each. This study was conducted an average of 3.2 years after the initial assessment, and therefore these disorders could also represent consequences of long-standing disability.[39]

Ford and colleagues[40] from the movement disorders unit at CPMC found that the majority of patients with PMDs had no underlying organic neurological disorder. However, "...there are individuals who manifest psychogenic symptomatology that represents an exaggeration or elaboration of a neurological condition."[40] In this series of 24 patients with PMDs, the profile of a typical patient consisted of a young person (mean age 36 years, range 11–60), most often female (79%), of average or above average intelligence (96% combined), with a mean duration of symptoms of 5 years (range <1 month to 23 years) unable to work and on disability (70% of patients). The principal psychiatric diagnoses were conversion disorder (75%), followed by somatization (12.5%), factitious disorder (8%), and malingering (4%). Dysthymia, as a secondary psychiatric diagnosis, was present in 67% of patients. The rest included a variety of different psychiatric conditions such as major depression, adjustment disorder, organic mood or organic delusional disorders, obsessive-compulsive disorder, panic attacks, bipolar disorder, and others.

Therefore, it appears that the three most common psychiatric disturbances seen in patients presenting with psychogenic neurological disorders are depression, hysterical (somatization) personality disorders, and anxiety disorders.

▶ CLUES TO THE DIAGNOSIS

There are a number of important historical and clinical features that can give a clue to the psychogenic nature of a movement disorder (Table 48–7).[30,41,42] Many of these are generally applicable to all patients and others relate to a specific type of abnormal movement (e.g., tremor and dystonia). These clues may be evident on taking the patient's history, on clinical examination, or on assessment of response to therapeutic interventions. The general clues are listed in Table 48–7, while the more specific clues are considered in the sections dealing with specific disorders.

▶ TABLE 48–7. GENERAL CLUES SUGGESTING THAT A MOVEMENT DISORDER MAY BE PSYCHOGENIC[30,41,42]

(A) *Historical*
1. Abrupt onset
2. Static course
3. Spontaneous remissions (inconsistency over time)
4. Obvious psychiatric disturbance
5. Multiple somatizations
6. Employed in a health-related profession
7. Pending litigation or compensation
8. Presence of secondary gain
9. Young female

(B) *Clinical*
1. Inconsistent character of the movement (amplitude, frequency, distribution, selective disability)
2. Paroxysmal movement disorder
3. Movements increase with attention or decrease with distraction
4. Ability to trigger or relieve the abnormal movements with unusual or nonphysiological interventions (e.g., trigger points on the body, tuning fork)
5. False weakness
6. False sensory complaints
7. Self-inflicted injuries
8. Deliberate slowness of movements
9. Functional disability out of proportion to exam findings
10. Movement abnormality that is bizarre, multiple or difficult to classify

(C) *Therapeutic responses*
1. Unresponsive to appropriate medications
2. Response to placebos
3. Remission with psychotherapy

Most organic movement disorders have a relatively slow course; therefore, abrupt onset and rapid progression are suggestive of a PMD. Paroxysmal movements (i.e., attacks) are also strongly suggestive of a PMD, as well as spontaneous remissions, no progression, relationship to minor injury, and involvement in litigation. On the examination, selective disabilities, when a patient is unexpectedly able to do some tasks that would have been considered exceedingly difficult, if not impossible, on the basis of his alleged dysfunction and bizarre, mixed movement disorders should also suggest this possibility. Inconsistencies on the exam are also important, including variability, distractibility, entrainability, and changes in pattern induced by suggestion or placebo. Additional atypical findings that can direct the attention to a PMD include "give-way" weakness, nonanatomical sensory disturbances, and extreme slowness or difficulty performing examination tasks along with excessive grimacing or sighing.

It should be noted, however, that taken individually, most of these "clues" are no more than that; more substantive evidence is generally required before a diagnosis of a psychogenic disorder can be confirmed. All of the mentioned clues can be seen in organic disorders. Abrupt onset and rapid progression can occur in rapid-onset dystonia parkinsonism, Wilson's disease, and some postlesional movement disorders. The same is true for paroxysmal movements, which can be due to a variety of relatively uncommon paroxysmal dyskinesias. Organic movement disorders, especially dystonia and tremor, can be task-specific. Although uncommon, spontaneous remissions may also occur in a number of organic disorders including idiopathic dystonias (especially cervical dystonia) and Tourette's syndrome.

Other supportive evidence can be derived from the existence of multiple undiagnosed somatic complaints and known psychiatric disorders; however, it must be borne in mind that psychiatric patients frequently have an organic movement disorder due to their medication side effects or unrelated reasons. It is also important to remember the potential for an initial presentation with psychiatric alterations to be followed only later by abnormal movement disorders in a variety of diseases including Wilson's disease, Huntington's disease, dentatorubropallidoluysian atrophy (DRPLA), Tourette's syndrome, and neuroacanthocythosis.

Obviously, surreptitious observation of a symptom-free period remains the most useful evidence for this diagnosis. Attempts to induce such periods utilizing placebo or suggestion can be extremely helpful, although it is known that patients with organic movement disorders can overcome the disability voluntarily, and therefore this could happen during suggestion; placebo responses in organic movement disorders have been documented in the past.[43] The use of placebos in these circumstances is somewhat controversial, and will be discussed in detail in the diagnosis section.

Throughout these assessments, as mentioned earlier, it is important to remember that patients with organic neurological disorders can have hysterical or psychogenic dysfunction as well. Weir Mitchell is quoted by Gowers[10] as saying "...the symptoms of many organic diseases of the nervous system are pictures painted on an hysterical background." Gowers[10] in his writings on epilepsy and hysteria said "...hysteria, it must be remembered, is common not only as an isolated, but also as a conjoined, morbid state and that hysteria can be the consequence of organic disease. Striking symptoms of hysteria are often seen, for instance, in cases of tumors of the brain." The clinician should be cautious in attributing all symptoms to "hysteria" alone because up to 30% of patients thought to have a psychogenic disorder are eventually found to have a disease that could account for their symptoms.[42] Just as pseudoseizures often occur on a background of true epilepsy, PMDs may occur in patients with underlying organic movement disorders. For example, Ranawaya and colleagues reported six such cases.[36] The new movement disorders were considered psychogenic because of the historical, clinical, and behavioral features and the responses to placebo and suggestion. Importantly, the PMD was typically the source of greater concern and disability than the preexisting organic condition. In Fahn and Williams'[30] series of psychogenic dystonia one patient developed "psychogenic worsening" of organic idiopathic familial dystonia due to his inability to compete with other students and teasing by his friends. Recently, psychogenic dystonia has been described in a nonmanifesting carrier of the DYT1 gene, the mother and caregiver of a child who was extremely disabled by DYT1 dystonia.[44]

"Pseudo-tics" have been reported in patients with Tourette's syndrome.[34] However, as mentioned previously, it is important to note that in patients who have been completely and adequately assessed and an underlying organic disorder has been excluded, it is rare for subsequent evaluation to uncover such an illness must many months or years later.[18] This is important to note since failure to deal properly with a PMD and repeated investigations looking for an alternative explanation for the symptoms can be very detrimental to the long-term prognosis of these patients.

▶ PSYCHOGENIC HYPERKINETIC MOVEMENT DISORDERS

PSYCHOGENIC DYSTONIA

Dystonia refers to a syndrome dominated by sustained muscle contractions, frequently causing twisting and repetitive movements resulting in abnormal or dystonic postures.[45] Dystonias can be classified as primary or idiopathic where no cause can be found after exhaustive neurological evaluation and secondary or symptomatic where a cause is evident. Dystonia can also be classified according to age of onset (childhood, adolescence, and adult) or by distribution (focal, segmental, multifocal, generalized, or hemidystonia).

Earlier we mentioned that certain symptoms and signs may occur in organic movement disorders that can encourage the misdiagnosis of a psychogenic cause. This error probably occurs more often in the case of dystonia, especially the idiopathic dystonias, than for other hyperkinesias. In fact, it is probably more common that an organic dystonia is misdiagnosed as psychogenic than the other way around, and this is certainly due, in part, to a lack of a biological marker (with increasing exceptions

TABLE 48–8. CLINICAL FEATURES OF ORGANIC DYSTONIAS THAT SOMETIMES ENCOURAGE A MISDIAGNOSIS OF A PSYCHOGENIC DISORDER[156,157]

1. The movements in dystonic syndromes can be quite varied including prolonged spasms, sinuous writhing, brief myoclonic jerks, slow rhythmical movements, and faster tremors.
2. Dystonia can remit in up to 20% of patients, especially in those with cervical dystonia (spasmodic torticollis).
3. Patients with idiopathic torsion dystonia (ITD) have no other neurological deficits and normal ancillary investigations.
4. Dystonia can be task specific (i.e., writer's cramp) or may be purely action induced (e.g., foot dystonia when walking forward but not backward or oromandibular dystonia only when attempting to speak or alternatively only on eating).
5. Occasional patients experience dystonia at rest with improvement in action ("paradoxical dystonia").
6. Dystonia can be relieved by "sensory tricks" (geste antagoniste). The best known of these occurs in patients with cervical dystonia where light touch or pressure very often will correct the abnormal head position. Many other examples are seen in a variety of dystonias.
7. Organic dystonia can be relieved by relaxation and hypnosis and is typically worsened by emotional stress.
8. Dystonia can be paroxysmal (e.g., paroxysmal kinesigenic choreoathetosis, paroxysmal non-kinesigenic choreoathetosis) or can show diurnal variation, as seen most prominently in dopa-responsive dystonia.

related to recognized gene mutations).[46] In his original description in 1908, Schwalbe considered dystonia as a psychogenic disorder.[47] Although a full discussion of dystonia and dystonic syndromes[41,48] is beyond the scope of this chapter, Table 48–8 outlines some of the features of dystonia that encourage this confusion by those unfamiliar with the disorder.

There are certain other clinical features of organic dystonias that can be extremely useful in raising the consideration of a psychogenic diagnosis. Idiopathic dystonia rarely begins in the lower limb in adult life. When this is a manifestation of a secondary dystonia, other neurological features (e.g., parkinsonism) or laboratory abnormalities (e.g., CT or MRI) regularly accompany the dystonia. The onset of organic dystonia is almost always gradual or slow. A notable but rare exception to these two rules is an autosomal dominant disorder known as "rapid-onset dystonia-parkinsonism."[49] Idiopathic dystonia typically begins with action-induced movements (see Table 48–8) and only after a prolonged period (sometimes never) progresses to dystonia at rest. Secondary dystonia may present with rest dystonia; however, this is typically accompanied by other neurological dysfunction or abnormalities on investigation. Despite the extremely disfiguring postures, pain, other than muscle ache, is surprisingly uncommon in patients with dystonia. An important exception here is cervical dystonia, where pain can be the principal source of disability. Unusual sensory tricks markedly relieving the dystonic movements and postures are a common feature of organic (particularly idiopathic) dystonia, and their presence should strongly suggest this diagnosis. However, recently we have reported a young woman with definite psychogenic dystonia who used a variety of similar tricks to suppress her abnormal movements.[50] Finally, although primary sporadic forms of paroxysmal nonkinesigenic dystonia do occur, psychogenic dystonia is a more common cause of this presentation. In a review of 25 patients with nonkinesigenic paroxysmal dystonia, 7 were found to have a definable symptomatic CNS cause, 7 were diagnosed as having primary sporadic paroxysmal dystonia, and 11 (44%) had PMD.[51] Response to medication is sometimes an important factor in the diagnosis of specific forms of dystonia, most notably dopa-responsive dystonia (DRD). However, as we have occasionally seen (including patients with a referral diagnosis of DRD on the basis of a marked response to L-dopa), placebo response to an active medication may result in the diagnosis of inorganic dystonia when in fact the problem is psychogenic.

It is also important to recognize that psychological and psychiatric disorders are not uncommon in patients with movement disorders, and this frequently is simply a consequence of the disability caused by it. In dystonia, this disability is not only physical but also secondary to the social embarrassment related to the abnormal postures, and additional stressors related to delays in diagnosis and misdiagnosis including labeling an organic disorder as psychogenic. It should also be noted that a number of neuropsychiatric dysfunctions can be secondary to basal ganglia abnormalities, and even some forms of hereditary dystonia such as myoclonus dystonia are associated with psychiatric disturbances. In these circumstances, a psychiatric diagnosis should be considered a comorbidity rather than an etiologic factor.[52]

Before the seminal paper of Fahn and Williams,[30] very few cases of true psychogenic dystonia had appeared in the literature. A critical review of most reports claiming a psychogenic origin in individual cases suggests that an organic source was in fact more likely. Indeed, because many patients with idiopathic torsion dystonia (ITD) had been misdiagnosed as hysterical and received years of unnecessary psychotherapy, it was generally emphasized by authorities in the field that psychogenic dystonia did not exist.[30] However, rare well-documented cases of psychogenic dystonia were occasionally reported.[46] Possibly the best known of these was a case of Münchausen syndrome simulating ITD reported by Batshaw and colleagues.[53] This woman's symptoms began at age 29 with dystonia in the right foot accompanied by left-sided torticollis. Her symptoms progressed to generalized dystonia over a 7-year period despite aggressive medical therapy. The organic basis of her symptoms was questioned and a diagnosis of psychogenic dystonia was considered. Because of the bizarre and relentless progression of her disease despite aggressive psychotherapy, she underwent many consultations at centers with expertise in movement disorders, and many psychiatric evaluations and admissions to in-patient psychiatric units all without benefit. She subsequently underwent bilateral thalamotomies in hopes of improving her limb dystonia. The thalamotomies were "complicated" by the onset of dysarthria progressing to aphonia 2 months after surgery. She had episodes of periodic breathing and acute opisthotonic posturing lasting up to 6 hours. During one of these episodes, she had a "seizure" and had a respiratory arrest after intravenous diazepam requiring subsequent tracheostomy. Trismus developed and she had to be fed by nasogastric and later gastrotomy tube-feedings. She lost 13.6 kg despite these procedures. It was not until nursing home placement became a consideration that 1 day the patient awoke with normal speech, volume, and articulation. She was transferred to a psychiatric unit where she appeared delusional, hallucinating and with features of a histrionic personality disorder. During behavioral modification therapy, she sat up, began to use her arms normally, and walked. Her psychotic symptoms disappeared and medications were discontinued. By the time of discharge, all symptoms of dystonia had resolved except for a 20-degree contracture of the right achilles tendon that had resulted from the volitional maintenance of an equino posture. Later, the patient admitted to have feigned all of her symptoms. It was also learned that she had previously feigned a number of disorders to gain sympathy and attention from her family and friends. This history had not been evident earlier because the patient had kept her family apart from her physicians. During subsequent psychiatric evaluations, it was found that she was bisexual with difficulty maintaining long-term relationships and had difficulty communicating her needs. She had been abandoned by her father early in her life and had been diagnosed with a number of other medical disorders including lymphoma and multiple sclerosis for which she claimed to have received therapy.

In 1988, Fahn and Williams[30] clearly defined the features of psychogenic dystonia reviewing 39 patients, 21 of who fulfilled their criteria for documented or clinically established psychogenic dystonia. The mean age of onset in these 21 patients was 26 years (ages ranging from 8 to 56 years). All patients but two were female (10.5:1). The duration of symptoms before a correct diagnosis of psychogenic dystonia varied between less than 1 month and 15 years. The most common clue suggesting psychogenic dystonia was the incongruity or inconsistency of the dystonic movements that were present in 85% (18). Other clues included false weakness (14), onset of dystonia at rest (11), pain (9), multiple somatizations (8), bizarre nature of the movements (7), sudden weakness (6), nonanatomic sensory changes (5), "seizures" (5), excessive slowness of movements (5), tenderness to light touch (4), and startle-induced "elaborate" movements (2). All patients except two had more than one such clue to the diagnosis. Fahn and Williams emphasized the presence of pain or tenderness in 62% (13/21), onset at rest in 11 out of the 15 patients who had continual instead of paroxysmal psychogenic dystonia, and onset in a lower limb, mostly the foot in 66% (14). In this series, before the authors' diagnosis of psychogenic dystonia all but two patients had a diagnosis of an organic movement disorder (12) or a combination of psychogenic and organic dystonia (7). None had been diagnosed as pure psychogenic dystonia.

In 1995, Lang[54] reported a 10-year experience with 18 patients diagnosed as having clinically definite psychogenic dystonia excluding cases with isolated paroxysmal movements. The clinical characteristics of the dystonia were inconsistent or incongruous with established forms of organic dystonia. The female to male ratio was 2.6:1. The mean age of onset was 35 years (range 17–59). The onset of dystonia was abrupt in half of the cases and progressed rapidly to fixed dystonic postures in 6. In 4 patients, the dystonia progressed over a period of weeks up to 5 years. A known precipitant for the dystonic symptoms was evident in 14 cases, trauma being the most common (a motor vehicle accident in 5 and a local injury in 6 including hand surgery, a fall, a poorly described work injury, and a fractured patella with later surgery). The dystonia began in a leg in 7 and the upper extremity was initially affected in 4. Four had generalized dystonia from the onset and three had dystonia of the neck and shoulder. The dystonia was present at rest from the onset in 12, and 7 of these had persistent unchanging dystonia without spontaneous or action-induced changes in posturing. Five had periods in which they were free of dystonia; 11 had dystonia at least part of the time brought out or aggravated by action with only 1 experiencing dystonia exclusively at these times (i.e., pure action-induced dystonia). Ten patients had paroxysmal symptoms superimposed on the persistent dystonia. The final distribution of dystonia at time of diagnosis was segmental in 28% (5), focal in 22% (4), generalized in 44% (8), and 1 (6%) had hemidystonia. Pain was present in 88% (16) of patients and was a prominent

▶ **TABLE 48–9. CLINICAL FEATURES OF PSYCHOGENIC DYSTONIA**

	Fahn and Williams[30]	Lang[54]	Totals/means
Number of patients	21	18	39
Mean age of onset	23 years	35 years	29 y
Female/male ratio	9.5:12	6:14	5:1
Duration between onset and diagnosis	<1 months–15 years	2 months–30 years	<1 months–30 years
Onset-at-rest dystonia	11/14 (78%)	12/18 (66%)	23/39 (59%)
Pain/tenderness	13/21 (62%)	16/18 (88%)	29/39 (74%)
Distribution of dystonia at onset			
Upper limb	0	4(22%)	4(10%)
Neck/shoulder	4 (19%)	3 (17%)	7 (18%)
Trunk	1 (5%)	0	1 (2%)
Lower limb	14 (67%)	7 (39%)	21 (54%)
Hemidystonia	2 (9%)	0	2 (5%)
Generalized	0	4 (22%)	4 (10%)
Final distribution			
Focal	6 (28%)	4 (22%)	10 (26%)
Segmental	5 (24%)	5 (28%)	10 (26%)
Hemidystonia	0	1 (6%)	1 (3%)
Generalized	10 (48%)	8 (44%)	18 (46%)
Other psychogenic neurological findings			
Give-way weakness/paralysis	20/21 (95%)	11/18 (61%)	31/39 (79%)
Excessive slowness	5/21 (24%)	5/18 (28%)	10/39 (26%)
Marked resistance to passive movements	0	3(17%)	3/39 (7.6%)
Nonanatomic sensory changes	5/21 (24%)	8/18 (44%)	13/39 (33%)
Multiple somatizations	8/21 (38%)	8/18 (14%)	16/39 (41%)

feature in 14 of the 18 patients. One of these had well-established reflex sympathetic dystrophy (RSD). Ten patients had accompanying other PMDs including three with multiple forms (5 tremor, 2 myoclonus, and 6 miscellaneous). Other psychogenic neurological features included give-way weakness 61% (11/18), excessive slowness in 28% (5/18), marked resistance to passive movements in 17% (3), and nonanatomic neurological changes in 44% (8/18). The primary psychiatric diagnosis most often was a conversion disorder, or somatoform disorder and none had known factitious or malingering disorders.

Table 48–9 summarizes and combines the data from these two large series. As can be seen, psychogenic dystonia affects mostly young women, with abrupt "onset-at-rest" dystonia involving the lower limb, most often a foot, accompanied by excessive pain and tenderness with nonanatomic sensory dysfunction, give-way weakness or paralysis, excessive slowness of movement and multiple somatizations. The dystonia will most often become generalized, followed in frequency by segmental or focal distribution. Rarely symptoms will begin as hemidystonia or progress to hemidystonia.

DYSTONIA ± REFLEX SYMPATHETIC DYSTROPHY FOLLOWING PERIPHERAL INJURY

Although the criteria discussed above are largely accepted, the relationship of dystonia with RSD, or complex regional pain syndrome (CRPS) as it has more recently been renamed, is much more controversial, and target of multiple publications and debates over the past 20 years. Similar to the nature of CRPS itself, particularly type I, the pathogenesis of the frequent accompanying movement disorders has been hotly debated.

There have been a number of reports describing a variety of movement disorders, most notably dystonia, following peripheral injury. When dystonia predominates, it may occur in isolation but more often occurs in association with other movement disorders (particularly tremor and myoclonus), severe pain ("causalgia"), and sometimes full-blown RSD. A variety of case series of patients with typical idiopathic dystonia have mentioned the potential role of preceding local trauma in anywhere from 5%[55,56] to 16.4%.[57] However, Fletcher and colleagues failed to show an association between idiopathic dystonia

▶ **TABLE 48–10. DIFFERENCES BETWEEN "CAUSALGIA-DYSTONIA" AND PRIMARY TORSION DYSTONIA***

Causalgia Dystonia	Idiopathic Dystonia
Clear preponderance of women	No preponderance of women
No family history	Positive family history (not uncommon)
Painful (causalgia)	Usually painless
Vasomotor, sudomotor, and trophic changes	Such changes not seen
Fixed spasm	Mobile spasms
Contractures common and early	Contractures (uncommon and late)
No geste antagoniste	Geste frequent
No improvement in sleep	Sleep often improves
Poor response to botulinum toxin and other therapy	Often responds to botulinum toxin and others
Onset in leg in adult	Adult leg onset very rare
Rapid spread → slow progression	

*Adapted with permission from Bhatia KP, Bhatt MH, Marsden CD. The causalgia-dystonia syndrome. Brain 1993;116:843–851.

and a history of previous injury.[58] Importantly, if one reviews the descriptions of movement disorders following peripheral trauma, it is clear that the majority of patients have a clinical syndrome quite distinct from "classical" movement disorder syndromes such as ITD. Bhatia and colleagues[59] outlined a number of clinical characteristics that distinguished "causalgia-dystonia" from primary torsion dystonia (Table 48–10). Importantly, many of the clinical characteristics of this form of dystonia are similar to those seen in patients with well-defined psychogenic dystonia (see above). This, then, represents one of the most problematic and controversial areas in movement disorders.

There is an extensive early literature on the role of trauma in a large number of neurological diseases.[60] With respect to modern movement disorder literature, Marsden and colleagues described five female patients developing dystonic posturing variably combined with tremor and myoclonus associated with RSD.[61] This syndrome followed minor injury to the limb in three of the five patients. Schott in 1986 described a series of 10 patients with 6 demonstrating features of dystonia.[62] In 1988, Jankovic and Van der Linden described 23 patients with movement disorders following peripheral injury.[63] Ten of the 23 had RSD. Fifteen had dystonia as the primary movement disorder with four demonstrating additional tremor. In contrast to other studies of such patients, the authors felt that the movement disorders seen in their cases were "clinically similar to those typically seen in patients with ITD or ET." Also in contrast to other studies, they found that fully 65% had evidence of "predisposing factors" such as a family history of a movement disorder or previous neuroleptic use. Although the authors felt that their patients represented examples of organic disorders, they admitted that "psychiatric disease may have contributed." In 1990, Schwartzman and Kerrigan described 43 of 200 RSD patients who demonstrated a movement disorder.[64] All 43 had dystonia, 10 of whom showed only "subtle features." Thirty-one of the 43 also had tremor. The features of dystonia were similar to those outlined in Table 48–7. In addition to the dystonia, all patients demonstrated "spasms" as well as difficulty initiating movement. Most demonstrated increased tone and reflexes. As in other reports, minor injuries were causative in most cases. No predisposing factors were mentioned in this report. Sympathetic blocks were said to improve the symptoms temporarily in 90% of patients. In 1993, Bhatia and colleagues coined the term "causalgia-dystonia syndrome" describing 18 patients who developed fixed dystonic postures, usually after minor injury.[65] In contrast to Schwartzman and Kerrigan's report, they found that sympathetic blockade, sympathectomies, and a variety of medications were entirely unhelpful. These authors admitted the potential for psychogenic factors to have played an important role in the development of this problem recognizing that the absence of overt psychopathology is not uncommon in isolated conversion reactions, contrary to the opinion of Schwartzman and Kerrigan.[66] More recently, Van Hilten and colleagues have reported a series of papers describing dystonia accompanying RSD.[67–69] Once again, many features, particularly the rapid onset, unusual progression (sometimes to generalized involvement), posturing at rest from the outset, and marked resistance to passive movement (indeed, increased resistance similar to that described by Head as quoted in the History section of this chapter), might suggest the alternative diagnosis of psychogenic dystonia. These authors described a marked response to intrathecal infusion of baclofen.[68] Although this was a placebo-controlled study, we would argue that a placebo response is still a possible explanation for this benefit.

The movement disorders accompanying RSD (which recently has had its name changed to CRPS, types I (clinical syndrome not limited to a peripheral nerve distribution) and type II (after documented damage to a particular nerve)) have been the subject of an important study by Verdugo and Ochoa. In their group of 53 patients with an involuntary movement and CRPS, 74.2% had dystonia or some abnormal muscle spasm. The striking finding was that no patients with CRPS type II had an abnormal movement. All of their patients with movement disorders (100% with CRPS type I) had other signs of a psychogenic component, including "give-way" weakness, erratic fluctuations, distractibility, response to placebo and psychotherapy, and nonanatomic sensory disturbances. Another important feature was a clear relationship to a minimal precipitating event, work related in 81% of the cases.[70]

We have observed similar findings studying a group of patients with peripheral trauma-induced cervical "dystonia" {Sa, 2003 16452 /id}. In this group of 13 patients who developed muscle spasms with abnormal posturing of neck and shoulder soon after local injury, several characteristics were identified: (1) precipitants were always trivial with no serious injury detected, usually work related and frequently involving the neck/shoulder area; (2) abnormal movements developed quickly, with a fixed posture consisting of shoulder elevation and head tilt being present no later than 2 weeks after the inciting event; (3) pain was a prominent feature; (4) litigation or compensation was involved in the majority of patients; (5) psychological interview utilizing the Minnesota Multiphasic Personality Inventory was suggestive of conversion disorders; Sodium amytal interview resulted in improvement in pain and posture in most patients; (6) other findings suggestive of a psychogenic disorder were frequent, including "give-way" weakness, nonanatomic sensory loss; distractibility, improvement with sham botulinum toxin injections, symmetrical neck tan and surreptitious observation of a symptom-free period. We applied the term "post-traumatic painful torticollis" to avoid confusion between this group (where we believe there are important underlying psychological factors, and the pathogenesis is quite distinct from other forms of dystonia), and patients with more typical cervical dystonia preceded or not by peripheral injury.

Range of motion was affected in all of our patients. This finding raises concerns over "established" long-standing disability related to traumatic injuries; one recent study implicated impaired range of motion as a prognostic factor in whiplash injuries {Kasch, 2001 12284 /id}. Even more important was the fact that despite the clinical impression of the presence of muscle hypertrophy, this was excluded during amytal interview or general anesthesia in all but one patient.

In a large study, involving 103 patients with fixed dystonia, association with a minor peripheral trauma preceding the development of "dystonia" was found in 63% of the patients.[71] Here, dystonia largely affected the limbs (90%), with only 6% affecting neck or shoulder region. Similar to our study, however, besides the trauma association pain was prominent in 41%. More importantly, 37% fulfilled criteria for PMD, 29% for a somatization disorder and 24% for both. Dissociative and affective disorders were significantly more common than in a control group, and as expected, medical and surgical treatments were largely unsuccessful, whereas a small proportion of patients who had multidisciplinary treatment including psychotherapy experienced some degree of remission.

Adding to the controversy in CRPS, a recent report by Munts attempted to characterize clinical and physiologic aspects of myoclonus in such patients.[72] However, it was subsequently argued that the electrophysiological characteristics reported were strongly suggestive of a psychogenic etiology.[73]

Various forms of evidence have been presented to support a causative role of peripheral trauma in dystonia, suggesting a variety of pathophysiologic explanations mostly related to an aberrant response of the CNS to such traumatic injury.[62,74–80] Compounding the problem further, the criteria proposed for the diagnosis of peripheral trauma-induced dystonia, early medical visits, injury anatomically related to the site of dystonia, and the development of an abnormal (dystonic) posture within a year of the trauma,[80] are common features of psychogenic dystonia. Given the frequent nature of traumatic injuries, it might be expected that we would encounter such patients extremely frequently in specialized clinics, which is not the case. Samii and colleagues found a history of local injury within a year in 12% of their group of 114 consecutive patients with cervical dystonia, and recall bias was an important possible contribution to this figure. Furthermore, Jankovic and colleagues, from their highly specialized database of 3500 patients, found only 18 patients who could have a trauma-related dystonia, not limited to the neck.[63] In fact, that group of patients did not show any major clinical difference from idiopathic dystonia patients except for the temporal relationship to injury, pain, poor response to conventional treatment and persistence of dystonic posturing at rest (all features strikingly similar to those found in psychogenic dystonia and in our patients with posttraumatic cervical posturing).

A genetic predisposition has been postulated to explain the relative rarity of the syndrome, when compared to the common occurrence of peripheral injury. Van Hilten and colleagues reported an association between dystonia complicating RSD and HLA-DR13.[69] Dryness of the eyes and mouth and bladder and bowel disturbances were also common in these patients. However, in a later paper, they did not mention this finding (or some of the other accompanying symptoms)[67] and so it is unclear whether it was borne out in studying larger numbers of patients. Bressman and colleagues and Gasser and colleagues failed to find a correlation between the DYT1 founder mutation and dystonia in a group of patients with dystonia following peripheral trauma and repetitive stress, respectively.[81,82]

Based on the explanation of an aberrant CNS response to a peripheral injury, one might expect that the more severe the nerve damage, the more likely aberrant responses, and therefore abnormal movements would develop. However, Verdugo and Ochoa failed to identify involuntary movements in CRPS type II (evidence of nerve damage),[70] and Bhatia and colleagues found no overt nerve damage in their group of 18 patients with similar symptoms.[65]

The controversy surrounding this syndrome is not limited to the movement disorders aspect. Similar controversy flourishes in the field of CRPS where some authors have argued that patients who lack clear evidence of nerve injury constitute a "pseudoneuropathy of psychogenic origin."[83] We would argue that an unquestioning acceptance of all cases of dystonia following injury as organic "peripheral trauma-induced dystonia" explaining them with a variety of peripheral and secondary suprasegmental pathophysiological mechanisms of unproven relevance legitimizes and intellectualizes the problem without sufficient justification. With respect to the acceptance of the diagnosis of RSD without nerve injury, Ochoa states "It is dangerous to diagnose RSD because that term carries the illusion of pathophysiology and the illusion of efficacious treatment. These unfortunate patients are the pariahs of our incompetent health system. While they do carry a genuine health disorder, they have been cursed by diagnostic adjudication of a disease of medical understanding."[83] We would argue that a similar statement could be made of many patients who have been diagnosed as having "post-traumatic dystonia."

▶ PSYCHOGENIC TREMOR

Tremor is defined as an involuntary, rhythmic, sinusoidal movement due, in part, to regular rhythmical contractions of reciprocally innervated muscles.[45,84] In the series presented in Table 48–6, it accounted for 35% of a total of 959 PMDs.

There is a long history of writing on this subject. Charcot described proximal tremors (involving the shoulder or hip), as almost unique to hysterical disorders referring to them (unfortunately) as "rhythmical chorea." Another variant was "hammering chorea," where the patient alternately flexed and extended the elbow as though using a hammer. We now recognized that both of these forms of tremor, although uncommon, may also be seen in organic neurological disease (e.g., the wing-beating tremor sometimes seen in Wilson's disease). Of the two, a rhythmic hammering movement is more characteristic of psychogenic tremor.

Gowers[12,10] described the presence of hysterical tremor in patients with hysterical paralysis. He stated that "...when the paralysis is incomplete, movement is slow, and is attended by characteristic irregular, coarser tremor than simple tremor." This is accompanied by interference of voluntary movements by the "...undue contractions in the opponents of the muscles that should effect the movement."

Kinnier Wilson[85] referring to hysterical tremors said that "... they present no separate or contrasting features when set alongside those of so-called 'organic' type." He disagreed with Gowers who firmly believed that hysterical tremor could be differentiated from organic tremor based on its variability, the influence of physical and emotional stimuli, and dependence on the attention paid to it because "...numerous organic tremors can be affected by a whole series of factors, exhibit marked fluctuations and fluidity, are highly irregular, shift their incidence and are aggravated when the subject is under observation." He considered both hysterical and organic tremors, "escape phenomena of infracortical level" therefore, part of an individual's "physiologic" repertoire. This would explain why "...hysterical subjects exhibiting such movements do not complain of fatigue, or at least appear to be less conscious of it than does a normal subject who executes them intentionally." In the person who intentionally produces a tremor, fatigue sets in easily because the "artifactual" tremor forms no part of their habitual function.

Fahn reported two cases of psychogenic tremor[86] and subsequently Koller and colleagues[87] described 24 patients with clinically established or documented psychogenic tremor. In this latter series, the female to male ratio was 1.7:1. The mean age was 43.4 years with a range of 15–78 years. The onset of tremor was abrupt in 87.5% of cases and the duration of tremor ranged from 1 month to 10 years. The majority of patients showed no change in their tremors over time (45%), while 25% experienced improvement to complete resolution, 4% worsened, and a 16% had a fluctuating course. Ninety-one percent of the patients had other features suggestive of a functional disorder such as nonphysiologic weakness, atypical gait disturbances, and nonanatomical sensory changes. The psychiatric diagnosis in order of frequency was a conversion reaction, depression, an anxiety disorder, and malingering. The tremors were characterized by resting, postural, and kinetic components. The postural component was the most prominent followed by resting and action tremors (i.e., resting<postural>action). Twelve percent of patients had an associated head tremor. With distraction all patients showed a reduction in the amplitude of tremor as well as variability in tremor frequency.

Our subsequent experience with psychogenic tremor continues to support these earlier observations.[88] The general historical and clinical features of PMDs all apply. Possibly more than in most forms of PMDs, the abrupt onset and the early (sometimes immediate) attainment of maximal severity are very useful clues since these features are rarely if ever seen in organic tremors. As with other PMDs, abrupt onset often follows a known precipitant (e.g., minor trauma). Psychogenic tremors are often present equally at rest, with postural maintenance and during action, whereas organic tremors uncommonly persist in all states and when they do the tremor tends to increase in amplitude from one to another (i.e., rest < posture < intention). We would agree with Wilson's criticism of overemphasis on tremor variability given the pronounced variation seen in organic tremors. However, complete suppression with distraction is not seen in organic tremors. More often the opposite is seen, the tremor increases with patient concentration on mental or physical tasks. Suppression with distraction is an especially useful sign when the movement disorder is continuous or constant as are most examples of psychogenic tremor. Another extremely useful clinical sign is the entrainment of the tremor to a new frequency or pattern. When the patient is asked to beat out a slow rhythmical or complex irregular pattern with the uninvolved limb (or the opposite limb to that being observed in cases of bilateral psychogenic tremor), the tremor will often change frequency or character to match the imposed contralateral movement. Rarely organic mirror movements might be confused with this phenomenon, although these would not normally suppress the underlying tremor. Alternatively, the tremor continues unabated but the requested movement is performed poorly and incompletely. This is often seen when asking the patient to make a full, smooth, side-to-side movement with the tongue. Occasionally, forcefully restraining a tremulous limb will result in a tremor developing in a previously unaffected limb. Psychogenic tremor may affect a single limb or multiple limbs and axial structures. The arms are most often involved, followed by the head and then the legs. Interestingly, although arms are commonly affected and fingers are rarely involved,[89] it seems to depend on a clonus mechanism, and therefore be mediated by reflex mechanisms.[90] Psychogenic tremor may be continuous or intermittent; in the upper limbs it is often continuous but it rarely if ever has this course in the legs, typically occurring intermittently or paroxysmally, often precipitated by attention, movement, or some other activity. Thomas and Jankovic reported a group of 127 consecutive patients with a diagnosis of psychogenic tremor, where the most common characteristics included abrupt onset in 100 (78.7%), distractibility in 92 (72.4%), variable amplitude and frequency in 79 (62.2%), and a multitude of other observations including intermittent occurrence, inconsistency, variable direction, and irregular pattern.[91] Entrainment did not differ in the two groups; however, the method used for such evaluation (i.e., wrist extension and flexion for 10 sec in the unaffected arm) may not be an adequate test for this feature since we have found it necessary to use a variety of frequencies or more complex patterns in many patients.

The combination of general clues to psychogenicity with the specific features listed above permits the experienced clinician sufficient diagnostic certainty to categorize most typical cases as "clinically established" psychogenic tremor. In long-standing, well-established cases, it is remarkable how persistent and seemingly invariable the tremor is and, like Wilson, one cannot help remarking on the lack of an expected fatiguing component. However careful, sometimes prolonged or repeated assessments will demonstrate clinical inconsistencies or incongruities with organic tremors. These criteria must be reliably demonstrated and convincingly evident before accepting a psychogenic diagnosis.

In common form of psychogenic tremor involves the palate and is readily mistaken for what has been termed "essential palatal tremor." Recognizing this problem, Zadikoff and colleagues propose the term "isolated palatal tremor" to include a heterogeneous group of patients, some with a presumed organic disorder, others with tics, learned movements, and indeed a psychogenic disorder supported by clear distractibility and entrainability.[92] Such patients have also been reported to demonstrate sensory tricks akin to the geste antagoniste seen in organic dystonias.[93] Electrophysiological studies may be helpful in both diagnosing and understanding psychogenic tremor, and this will be further discussed below under the section "establishing a diagnosis/investigations."

▶ PSYCHOGENIC MYOCLONUS

Myoclonus is defined as brief, shock-like muscle contractions (positive myoclonus) or sudden lapses in tone (negative myoclonus) as exemplified by asterixis. Psychogenic myoclonus represents approximately 13% of all psychogenic movements disorders seen (Table 48–6).

The only reported series of psychogenic myoclonus is that of Monday and Jankovic,[94] who described 18 patients seen over a 10-year period. The female to male ratio was 2.6:1 with a mean age of 42.5 years (range 22–75 years). None had a family history of myoclonus. Eighty-three percent of patients (15/18) had a precipitating event, and the abnormal involuntary movement began suddenly in 61% of patients (11) with gradual onset over several days in 38%. Eighty-three percent of patients (15) experienced exacerbations of the myoclonus with stress, and 77% (14) had definite worsening of the myoclonus during periods of anxiety. The most common distribution of the myoclonus was segmental in 10 (55%), followed by generalized in 39% and focal in 5% of patients. The myoclonus was present at rest in all and exacerbated by movement in 77% (14). Light and noise worsened myoclonus in one and four patients, respectively.

Other neurological findings included tremor (postural 3, kinetic 2, and resting 1), focal (posttraumatic) dystonia in one, and gait abnormalities in six. In most, these neurological findings were believed to be also of psychogenic origin. Neurological evaluation showed no abnormalities except for these movement disorders. All patients had normal electroencephalography and other neurological investigations were unrevealing.

Overt psychiatric disturbances were present in 55% of patients before the onset of myoclonus and 61% had a demonstrable psychiatric pathology by psychiatric interview or neuropsychological testing. The most common diagnoses were depression in four, anxiety disorder and panic attacks in two, and personality disorders in two. Eighty-eight percent of the patients had a variety of different predisposing factors. Six had trauma before the onset of myoclonus: three had "on-the-job" related injuries, one slipped in a shopping mall and two patients were involved in motor vehicle accidents. Only one had a worker's compensation suit.

Follow-up was available in 12/18 patients (67%). Fifty-eight percent reported improvement in the myoclonus over time, while 25% thought that the myoclonus was much worse after evaluation. The authors emphasized that spontaneous resolution of the myoclonus can be regarded as a strong indication of psychogenicity, provided that reversible causes of myoclonus are ruled out such as infections, metabolic encephalopathies, or neurodegenerative disorders and there is no family history of myoclonus. Reduction in myoclonus with distraction was found to be a very helpful finding in establishing the diagnosis. However, because psychogenic myoclonus is often intermittent or discontinuous, this sign is probably less useful than in cases of more persistent psychogenic movements (e.g., psychogenic tremor).

Electrophysiological testing may be very helpful in problematic cases, and this is discussed in further detail in the section dealing with establishing a diagnosis/investigations.

Brief mention should be made of three related disorders first described approximately 100 years ago in different populations. Latah, Jumping Frenchmen of Maine and Myriachit all variably demonstrate excessive startle, echolalia, echopraxia, and automatic obedience.[95] Considerable debate exists about the true origins of these disorders. Careful clinical and modern electrophysiological assessments of these uncommon conditions are lacking. Some authors believe that they are organically mediated neuropsychiatric disorders akin to Tourette's syndrome.[96] In fact, Gilles de la Tourette himself thought of these disorders as part of the "syndrome of tic convulsive."[97,98] Others argue that they represent forms of "culturally mediated behaviour"[95,96,98,99] and as such might be considered types of "psychogenic movement disorders" in the broadest sense (Kinnier Wilson called them "collective psychoneurosis"[85]). Having reviewed videotapes of Latah patients from Indonesia[100] and cases from Louisiana with a disorder related to Jumping Frenchmen of Maine ("Ragin' Cajuns")[101,102] the authors favor the latter opinion. However, further study of these unusual conditions is clearly required.

▶ PSYCHOGENIC CHOREA/BALLISM

As mentioned in the section on psychogenic tremors, earlier medical writings used the term chorea to described bizarre movement disorders that would not be consistent with the current definition of chorea. Terms such as "rhythmical chorea," "hammering chorea," and "dancing chorea" were popularized by Charcot for very spectacular movements seen in hysterical patients. True chorea, defined as random fleeting movements that flow from one part of the body to another in an unpredictable fashion, is exceedingly rare in PMD patients. We have seen only one patient who could be considered as having psychogenic chorea. Importantly, unlike most cases of organic chorea, his movements were purely paroxysmal. There was a very clear psychiatric history and the patient lacked other features of organic paroxysmal dyskinesias. Given the rare occurrence of psychogenic chorea, we would recommend caution in making this diagnosis even by clinicians with considerable experience in the field of movement disorders.

▶ PSYCHOGENIC TICS

Little has been written about psychogenic tics. Psychogenic tics accounted for only 3% of PMDs in the series reviewed in Table 48–6. The disparate frequencies probably relate to the definitions utilized

Recently, Kurlan and colleagues[34] reported a young woman with long-standing Tourette's syndrome and obsessive–compulsive disorder (OCD) who developed complex movements such as slumping in a chair or to the floor or bed along with tonic–clonic like movements suggestive of pseudoseizures. No alteration of consciousness or incontinence was noted. These episodes were referred to by the patient as "bad spells" and her physicians believed they represented poorly controlled tics. However, multiple adjustments of her antitic medications failed to improve the movements. After careful analysis, it became clear that these "bad spells" were psychogenic in nature. The patient received psychotherapy and was found to fulfill criteria for a borderline personality disorder. There were clear secondary "gains" such as the need for financial support from her parents and avoidance of social, educational, and domestic responsibilities.

What is not clear from the description of this case is whether the patient had any premonitory feelings or symptoms of an urge to perform her usual tics or the newly developed movements, and if in trying to control the movements she had a buildup of tension with a subsequent worsening. The absence of this urge may have helped differentiate these "tics" from true tics. In our experience, a very high proportion of tic patients experience a subjective urge to perform the tics (at one time or another). The performance of the tic is commonly appreciated as a partially volitional capitulation to this urge.[103] In some of our tic patients who have had other concomitant movement disorders (e.g., dystonia, tardive dyskinesia), a similar subjective feeling has never been present and the patient has always been able to distinguish between their tics and these other movements. In addition, none of our PMDs patients have admitted to the "voluntary" performance of the movement (see below for a possible exception), and we are aware of only one patient in the literature with psychogenic tremor associated with posttraumatic stress disorder[104] who admitted to the purposeful performance of the movement. Thus, patients' responses to this line of questioning may be very helpful in defining bizarre or unusual movements as forms of tics or psychogenic movements.

Although Kurlan and colleagues[34] chose to term the movements "psychogenic tics" based on the diagnostic confusion that had existed in their patient, it could be argued that the movements would be better classified as "pseudo-seizures" or a mixed form of bizarre psychogenic movements given their paroxysmal nature and the complexity of the movements that did not conform to those usually seen in the Tourette's syndrome. We believe that this broader, arguably inappropriate, use of the term tic in similar cases accounts for the varied frequencies from the movement disorders clinic's summarized in Table 48–6.

In contrast, we have seen a 52-year-old man who, over a 2-week period after sustaining a minor injury to his lower back, developed paroxysmal episodes of flexion of shoulders and extension with twisting of the neck. These movements were associated with an inner urge and a preceding feeling of tightness in the neck that forced him to contract the shoulders and neck. The urges gradually disappeared but the movements continued to occur spontaneously in paroxysms with periods of remission. At this time the movements were described as "having a mind of their own" (in contrast to the purposeful or volitional performance of the same movements earlier in the course of his symptoms). There was a pronounced reduction in the frequency and severity of the movements after the patient's disability support was approved. He had been exposed to phentermine hydrochloride for appetite suppression but had only taken it intermittently for a total of 90 days over a 12-month period and had stopped taking the medication 2 months before the trauma and onset of the movements. He had no family history of neurological or psychiatric disorders and denied any tic-like symptomatology or obsessive compulsive behavior at any time earlier in life. During the examination he demonstrated intermittent, abrupt, brief contraction of the trapezius muscle with "pulling" of the shoulders backwards, followed by extension of the neck and contraction of the platysma muscle. At times he had alternating contraction of the sternocleidomastoid muscles giving a brief rotatory component to the neck movement. During the examination he sometimes stated that he needed to move his neck because of a "build-up" feeling in his neck. As with most cases of both tics and PMDs, distraction completely suppressed the movements. In contrast to tics, but like many psychogenic movements, the neck movements "entrained" with synkinetic and alternating finger-counting movements of his hands.

Although this may be an unusual case of trauma-induced adult-onset tics with the additional theoretic predisposition from prior stimulant use, some of the clinical features outlined above encourage a diagnosis of psychogenic tics. Without further support one could only classify such a case as "probable" or "possible."

▶ PSYCHOGENIC HEMIFACIAL SPASM AND OTHER FACIAL DYSKINESIAS

Scant information is available on the frequency and clinical features of psychogenic hemifacial spasm or other facial dyskinesias. In Tan and Jankovic's report, the diagnosis of psychogenic hemifacial spasm was made in 2.4% of 210 consecutive patients suffering from hemifacial spasm who were evaluated at their center during an unspecified period of time.[105] All patients were women with a median age at diagnosis of 34.6 years, and a mean duration of illness of 1.1 years. Except for the one patient who had other associated PMDs, all other patients had isolated psychogenic hemifacial spasm without the accompaniment of other movements. This is in contrast to the experience of Galvez-Jimenez and Hargreave,[106] who over a 7-year period reported an incidence of psychogenic hemifacial spasm of 0.3% of all movement disorder cases and 6% of all hemifacial spasm patients seen during that same period of time. Four were women and one male, with an average age at diagnosis of 39.6 years, and all had more striking PMDs such as psychogenic gait in two (robotic in one, astasia–abasia in one), psychogenic parkinsonism in one, psychogenic tremor in two, and psychogenic dystonia and alternating psychogenic hemifacial spasm in one. The initial reason for consultation in these patients was the other psychogenic movements; the presence of the psychogenic hemifacial spasm became evident during the examination. The onset was abrupt in four and progressive in one. All routine ancillary testing and imaging studies were normal. Clues to the diagnosis included the abrupt onset in most, multiple somatizations in four, and secondary gains in three patients. Clinically, the character of the movement was variable in all, with exacerbations and reduction with attention or distraction in all. Abrupt resolution of the movement was noted in two after psychiatric care and response to placebo in one. This experience suggests that psychogenic hemifacial spasm is uncommon but that it is also probably underreported as more dramatic psychogenic movements may distract the examiner when cataloging the presence of movements in a given patient.

▶ PSYCHOGENIC PARKINSONISM

Walters and colleagues[32] described a case of psychogenic parkinsonism in a 64-year-old man with onset of symptoms in his lower limbs, later accompanied by stuttering, halting speech, and tremor over a 3-year period. His gait was slow and shuffling but atypical for parkinsonism. The patient would slide one foot "glued" to the floor a long distance and then would slide the other foot in the same manner to a point "equally" distant from the first foot. Finger tapping, alternating movements, and foot tapping were slowed. His speech was also very uncharacteristic of Parkinson's disease. Tremor in his hands was equally prominent at rest, with postural maintenance and on action. The rest of the neurological examination was normal. The patient's symptoms did not respond to L-dopa therapy but resolved spontaneously 1 year after discontinuing levodopa.

More recently, one of us reported 14 cases of psychogenic parkinsonism seen at three University Movement Disorders Centers.[33] Thirteen had pure psychogenic parkinsonism and one had psychogenic parkinsonism superimposed on milder features of true parkinsonism. There was a 1:1 male to female ratio. The average age of the patients was 47 years with a range of 21–63 years. The mean duration of symptoms before diagnosis was 5 years with a range between 4 months and 13 years. In 71% (10), the symptoms of parkinsonism began suddenly after a minor work-related injury or motor vehicle accident except in one case who had sustained a serious head injury 9 years earlier complicated by a subdural hematoma. Parkinsonian symptoms were bilateral in 57% of the patients and unilateral in the remainder, typically involving the dominant side. Reduced facial expression, probably related to depression in most, was present in 6 of the 14 patients. Tremor was present in 85%. An isolated postural and action tremor was seen in only one case. More often, the tremor had characteristic features of a psychogenic tremor, as outlined earlier. It was typically present at rest and persisted in postures and with action, lacking the characteristic dampening of true parkinsonian rest tremor that occurs on adopting a new posture or with movement. In all cases, the tremor dampened or disappeared with distraction. This is the opposite of what is usually seen in patients with true resting tremor of Parkinson's disease where the performance of mental exercises typically accentuates or brings out the tremor. The entrainment of the tremor to the frequency of other repetitive movements performed in another limb (typical of psychogenic tremor) contrasts with what may be seen with true parkinsonian tremor where it is the tremor that entrains the rate and rhythm of an attempted repetitive task (e.g., finger tapping). "Bradykinesia" was seen in all cases, but the marked degree of slowness seen in most was atypical for true parkinsonian bradykinesia. Movements were often performed painstakingly slowly. However, the fatigue with decremental amplitude and arrest in ongoing movement so common in organic bradykinesia were lacking. Rigidity was present in 42% of cases. This often had features of voluntary resistance or difficulty relaxing. Several patients complained of associated pain in the limb that contributed to this increased resistance to passive movements. The increased tone usually diminished during the performance of synkinetic movements of an opposite limb in contrast to the normal accentuation of true parkinsonian rigidity (i.e., "activated rigidity"). No true cogwheeling was appreciated. Abnormal gait and postural instability were present in 85% of patients. Arm swing was diminished or absent on the affected side. However, the arm might have been held stiffly extended and adducted at the side (even while running) or flexed across the chest rather than in the typical flexed posture with reduced swing characteristic of true Parkinson's disease. The gait also demonstrated a variety of other bizarre or atypical features including a component of antalgia when pain was associated. Minimal force applied to the pull-test often resulted in very exaggerated or extreme responses; however, no patient fell. The nature of this response often confirmed the psychogenicity of other features. For example, the distraction might have suppressed tremor. In one patient whose dominant arm was slow and stiff and held tightly at the side while walking and running, both arms flailed upward equally rapidly in her extreme response to minimal posterior trunk displacements.

The 15 patients reported with psychogenic parkinsonism demonstrated a combination of features (i.e., tremor, rigidity, bradykinesia, postural disturbances, and gait instability) that justify their classification as a form of parkinsonism. However, all of these features were somewhat atypical for Parkinson's disease and other akinetic-rigid syndromes. As with all PMDs, the recognition of the clinical incongruities with known disease required considerable experience in the assessment and management of the "organic" counterparts (i.e., parkinsonian disorders). Other important clues to the psychogenicity of the movement disorder (see Table 48–7) were present in all patients. Abrupt onset, inconsistencies in the character of the movements, alterations of the movements with attention, or distraction and associated false neurological signs were characteristically present in all patients in different combinations. Disability from psychogenic parkinsonism was often considerable. Patients were either on full disability pensions or had been forced to take early retirement. Despite the recognition of a psychogenic cause in all 15 (documented in nine, one with additional mild organic parkinsonism and clinically established in 6) outcome varied considerably. In some, the symptoms and signs resolved completely, either spontaneously or with psychiatric therapy and in others, symptoms and resulting disability persisted unabated.

In very difficult or questionable cases of psychogenic parkinsonism, PET or single photon emission computed tomography (SPECT) scanning of the presynaptic dopamine system or PET using FDG may provide useful supportive diagnostic information.[107] Some series have included a majority of patients with what was felt to be a combination of psychogenic parkinsonism plus Parkinson's disease, the latter supported by abnormalities on an imaging study.[108] However, it is not clear that these patients should have been classified as having psychogenic parkinsonism rather than simply the more common "psychogenic overlay" that not infrequently complicates organic neurological disease.

▶ PSYCHOGENIC GAIT DISORDERS

In 1860, Jaccoud described "ataxia from want of automatic coordination," reporting a patient with normal use of his legs but inability to stand or walk properly.[109] Mills and Gowers recognized gait abnormalities as a manifestation of hysteria in the late nineteenth century.[12,110,]

The French school headed by Charcot also devoted some time to these disorders[111] (Table 48–11). In Woolsey's experience, the nature of the gait disturbance seen in hysteria related to the type of motor disability the patient imagined himself/herself to have.[28] For example, in the most common hysterical gait disorder observed by Woolsey a supposed paretic limb was dragged behind with the foot rotated outward contacting the floor on the medial aspect of the heel and the base of the great toe. Alternatively, if the patient believed himself to be unsteady or "ataxic" the gait would zig-zag from side to side with frequent lurches from one support to another "...making it in the nick of time to the next," but without falls or injuries.

In a review videotape, the most useful features to distinguish a psychogenic gait from organic causes included exaggerated effort or fatigue, excessive slowness, fluctuations, convulsive shaking, uneconomic postures such as camptocormia (discussed in more detail later) and a bizarre gait.[109] Morris and colleagues, in a recent review, added knee buckling and appearance of pain suggested by grimaces or antalgic features as signs suggestive of a psychogenic gait disorder.[112]

Psychogenic gait disorders accounted for 6.7% of all PMDs reported in Table 48–6. At the Los Angeles County/University of Southern California Medical Center, of all patients admitted to a neurological service with "functional neurological disorders" over a 10-year period, 26% (60/228) of patients had hysterical gait disorders. Hysterical gait disorders accounted for 1.5% (68/4470) of neurological admissions to the Munich University Clinic, over a 3-year period.[113] At the TWH, out of 279 patients with PMDs seen over a 14-year period, 16 (5.7%) had a pure psychogenic gait disorder, but an additional 102 (36.6%) had another dominant movement disorder (documented or established) along with gait abnormalities fulfilling criteria for a psychogenic gait disorder. Thus, although a pure psychogenic gait disorder was uncommon in this population, 42.3% of patients with a PMD demonstrated some form of psychogenic gait abnormality. In that series, the gait abnormalities consisted of slowing (18.6%), dystonic (17.8%), bizarre/unclassifiable (11.9%), astasia–abasia (11.9%), and buckling of the knee (7.6%). Taking into account only the patients with a pure gait abnormality, buckling of the knee followed by asatasia–abasia was the most common subtype, although overall numbers were small. Typical characteristics of the psychogenic gait abnormality included abrupt onset, inconsistencies and incongruencies, multiple simultaneous symptoms, and a previous history of minor injury.[31] Keane[111] reported his experience with 60 patients with hysterical gait disorders seen over a 10-year period. There were 37 women and 23 males (1.6:1) with a mean age of 36.3 (19–80 years). He found that 43% (26/60) of patients had associated hysterical eye findings including 13 with visual field cuts, 6 with decreased visual acuity, 4 with eye movement limitation, and 3 with monocular diplopia (this high incidence of eye movement abnormalities may relate to referral bias given the author's interest in neuro-ophthalmology). Other "false" neurologic signs were present in 71% (43/60) of patients; motor

▶ TABLE 48–11. FRENCH-SCHOOL CLASSIFICATION OF HYSTERICAL GAIT DISORDERS AT THE TURN OF THE CENTURY[111]

Charcott and Tourette	Roussy and Lhermitte
Astasia–abasia	Astasia–abasia
Paralytic	Pseudotabetic
Ataxic	Pseudopolyneuritic
Choreiform	Tightrope walker
Trepidant	Robot
Habit limping	
Choreic	
Knock-kneed	
As on a sticky surface	
As through water	

From Keane JR.[111] with permission.

abnormalities were the most common (hemiparesis in 12, quadriparesis in 7, paraparesis in 4, and triparesis in 1). Other findings included voice abnormalities, tremor, contractures, and abnormal finger-to-nose testing where three patients had either finger-to-eye or finger-to-cheek alterations. The most common gait abnormalities (some patients had more than one type of gait disturbance) included ataxia (38%), hemiparesis (20%), paraparesis (16%), and trembling gait (14%). Other unusual seen patterns included dystonic, myoclonic, stiff-legged, and slapping gaits and one case of camptocormia (from the Greek for bent tree trunk). Camptocormia as a feature of "hysteria" has been emphasized previously, for example, by Eames,[114] whose patient developed an hysterical gait after head trauma resulting in her walking around the hospital bent over with her palms down almost touching the floor. The term was first applied to a presumed hysterical gait in soldiers returning from the Balkan War and World Wars I and II. It is important to recognize that camptocormia may also occur in organic dystonia or parkinsonian disorders, and we have seen 2 cases with unilateral basal ganglia infarcts in which the onset of camptocormia was abrupt.[115]

Other associated features in Keane's series[111], which were present in 23 of 60 patients, included a scissoring gait, a knee giving-way with quick recovery, posturing of an "arm-above-head" while walking (however, we have patients with organic axial dystonia who hold the arm above the head as a trick to allow them to walk with a more upright posture), and ataxic (tandem) gaits that blended into trembling although "tremblers" usually had additional arm or truncal tremors while lying on bed. Six patients in the ataxic group had a history of intentional overdose with phenytoin that had been prescribed for pseudoseizures.

In another series of psychogenic gait disturbances,[113] 37 patients seen at the Munich University Clinic over 9 years (1980–1989) were video-analyzed (22 prospectively and 15 retrospectively) for the purposes of establishing diagnostic criteria and to determine if a diagnosis of psychogenic gait disturbance was possible on phenomenological grounds alone. In this series, the most salient features seen included (1) hesitation (16.2%), (2) excessive slowness of movements (35%), (3) fluctuations in the gait impairment with "uneconomic" postures and wasting of muscle energy (51%), (4) a "walking on ice" gait pattern (30%), and (5) a "psychogenic Romberg" test (32%). The authors concluded that if one or more of these six features were present, a diagnosis of a psychogenic gait disturbance could be made on phenomenological grounds alone with over 90% certainty (97% of patients had one or more of these six characteristics).

Other features included sudden knee buckling in 27%; however, over 80% of patients did not fall despite this feature. Eleven percent of patients had astasia and vertical shaking tremor was present in 8% of cases. A suffering or strained facial expression was seen in 19 patients, associated in all with moaning, mannered posturing of hands, and grasping of the leg along with hyperventilation.

These 37 patients had a total of 116 associated hysterical findings. The most common abnormalities included other motor disturbances in 53 (45%) that often added to the gait disorder. These included hemiparesis (23%), quadriparesis (13%), scissoring (9%), knee giveway with recovery (9%), assuming a tandem gait (9%), dragging a leg (7.5%), paraparesis (7.5%), and flailing of the arms (5%). Other associated hysterical findings included eye movement abnormalities (22%), bizarre tremors (12%), pseudoataxia (8%), and voice abnormalities (7%).

In Keanes' experience, the most common initial diagnostic error was in not insisting that the patient attempt to walk.[111] Wilson's disease and Huntington's disease were the most frequent neurological disorders, where a misdiagnosis of a hysterical gait was made. In his experience, a few minutes of observation are sufficient to determine that the pattern of gait disturbance is psychogenic in origin, provided that spontaneous gait, tandem, heel, and toe walking are examined. This is in keeping with Lempert and colleagues'[113] finding that the diagnosis of an hysterical gait disorder can reliably be made on phenomenological grounds if unusual postures and gait patterns, striking slowness of locomotion, momentary fluctuations, and a psychogenic Romberg test are seen. Other clues helpful in diagnosis are incongruities in the neurological examination (e.g., normal reflexes in a chronically paralyzed leg), give-way weakness, and elimination of symptoms with suggestion or placebo. We agree with Lempert and colleagues'[113] word of caution that the presence of muscle atrophy or joint contractures do not necessarily argue against a psychogenic disorder; they can represent secondary changes due to lack of use or prolonged maintenance of a tonic posture.

▶ ESTABLISHING A DIAGNOSIS/ INVESTIGATIONS

As discussed extensively so far, a diagnosis of PMD should be carefully established since an incorrect classification either way will subject the patient to additional psychological stress, increased costs of further diagnostic tests, and possibly even denial of a potentially helpful treatment or untoward side effects of a wrongly prescribed drug.

Clinical diagnoses, even in experienced hands, are extremely difficult and filled with pitfalls. It should be established by an experienced neurologist, or preferably by a movement disorders specialist since one of the most useful and important features is how the movement compares to the organic equivalent, and therefore extensive experience in the field is required. The differential diagnosis of PMDs encompasses the entire field of movement disorders; therefore, the neurologist should be alert to these diagnostic possibilities in any patient who fulfills some of the characteristics mentioned above. Although it is important to keep an open mind to the possibility of an incorrect diagnosis, a protracted course, pronounced disability, or resistance to therapy should never be used as criteria against a diagnosis of a PMD when all other historical and clinical criteria are satisfied.

Admission to hospital can prove beneficial in some cases, providing continuous observation, and sometimes video-monitoring can provide additional evidence. It can also provide ancillary tests to exclude organic diseases and convince the patient that a reasonable effort to exclude them was undertaken.[30,47] However, once the diagnosis is established, additional investigations should be avoided as it could convey the feeling of diagnostic uncertainty to the patient.

Imaging of the nigrostriatal dopamine system, for example, with fluorodopa positron emission tomography (FDOPA-PET) and betaCIT or ^{123}I-isoflupane SPECT, can be quite helpful in the diagnosis of parkinsonian disorders. It is abnormal even in very early Parkinson's disease[116] as well as in most other neurodegenerative forms of parkinsonism[117,118] but is expected to be normal in patients with pure psychogenic parkinsonism.[108,119] Electrophysiological studies can be of particular help in the diagnosis of psychogenic tremors and myoclonus. In the particular case of tremors, electrophysiological tests can evaluate the consistency of frequency and whether distractability is present. Increased amplitude with weighting of a limb and the "co-activation sign," whereby the tremor only persists while there is ongoing muscle contraction and immediately abates when this subsides, are two important features.[89] Entrainment, which can be used on a clinical basis, acquires a more definitive and measurable aspect when assessed with electrophysiological techniques. Coherence analysis is also helpful in this differentiation.[120] Deuschl and colleagues have also proposed, based on electrophysiological studies, that psychogenic tremor seems to depend on either a clonus mechanism, presumably mediated by reflex pathways, or a voluntary mechanism.[120] These two types would be expected to differ in clinical and electrophysiological characteristics.

Electrophysiological measurements can also be quite helpful in the diagnosis of psychogenic myoclonus. The characteristics of organic myoclonus are well known, and can be used to contrast the findings in patients suspected of a psychogenic origin.[121]

The temporal pattern of muscle activation in various forms of pathologic myoclonus is stereotypic and depends on the location of the generator or origin of the myoclonus (e.g., cortex, brainstem, and spinal cord). Myoclonic jerks originating in the cortex (EMG burst of 10–50 ms[122]) and brainstem (EMG burst >100 ms[122]) induced by sensory input (i.e., reflex myoclonus) usually have a short latency (~60–70 ms[123]) between stimulus and resulting jerk that is typically just long enough for the sensory input to reach the site of origin and for a return volley to travel down rapidly conducting descending pathways (e.g., the corticospinal tract) to the anterior horn cells and thence to the muscle. Less commonly, electrophysiological testing demonstrates evidence of much slower, presumably polysynaptic, propagation of the response, as in propriospinal myoclonus, although it has recently been shown that the electrophysiological characteristics of propriospinal myoclonus can be mimicked purposefully and have been seen in a case of psychogenic axial jerks.[124]. Electrophysiological studies using EMG surface electrodes in patients with psychogenic myoclonus may show variable and inconsistent muscle activation patterns, and more importantly the stimulus-induced responses tend to habituate as seen in the normal startle response.[125] More useful is the timing of responses (in stimulus-sensitive forms) where the latency from stimulus to jerk is much longer than that seen in pathological forms of myoclonus, and typically falls within the range of voluntary reaction time (~100–120 ms, P. Ashby, personal communication). Terada and colleagues[126] reported an assessment of the readiness potential or Bereitschaftspotential (BP) in patients with psychogenic myoclonus. The BP is a negative shift in the EEG that occurs 1.5 sec before a voluntary movement takes place.[127] Terada and colleagues hypothesized that an involuntary movement (such as that seen in pathological forms of myoclonus) would lack a preceding BP. They found that BPs preceded the jerks in patients with psychogenic myoclonus and concluded that this feature was consistent with the movements being generated through voluntary mechanisms. Although BPs can rarely be associated with involuntary movements due to neuroacanthocytosis[128] and mirror movements[129,130] and are typically absent before triggered as opposed to spontaneous (internally driven) movements, the presence of a BP can be a extremely useful in identifying a spontaneous movement as psychogenic. As mentioned earlier, the electrophysiological characteristics of myoclonus accompanying CRPS reported by Munts and colleagues[72] included many of the features of psychogenic myoclonus as outlined above.[73] Unfortunately, the investigators did not include an evaluation of the BP in their patients.

This same type of electrophysiological assessment is very helpful in cases where sound is the inducing stimulus (i.e., psychogenic startle). The normal startle response might be considered a form of physiological myoclonus that occurs in an exaggerated fashion in a familial disorder known as hyperekplexia or startle disease. Electrophysiological study[131–133] of a startle response demonstrates progression of muscle contraction first involving closure of the eyes (onset latency of 30–40 msec), followed by facial grimacing and forward flexion of the head (55–85 msec), flexion of the elbows (85–100 msec), abduction of the shoulders, pronation of the forearms, and clenching of the fists. Onset latency of the muscle activity in hamstrings and quadriceps is about 100–125 msec and for the tibialis anterior 130–140 msec. Some patients only manifest closure of the eyes. The rostrocaudal progression of the muscle contraction follows a similar pattern to that seen in reticular reflex myoclonus or reflex myoclonus of brainstem origin.[125] The normal physiological behavior of the startle response includes sensitization (resulting in increased amplitude and/or shorter latency of a response) that is masked by the habituation resulting from several repetitive stimuli. In startle disease, patients have an exaggerated response and lack of habituation. Many patients with psychogenic myoclonus demonstrate an exaggerated response to startle. Typically, this startle response habituates over several trials as expected in normal physiological startle. Simple visual analysis of the muscle contractions may show moment-to-moment variability (i.e., inconsistency) in the latency from stimulus to response and in the pattern of muscle activation and these inconsistencies can be confirmed by multichannel EMG assessment.

A variety of electrophysiological findings have been described in organic dystonic syndromes, but it is unclear how useful they are in differentiating organic from psychogenic dystonia. Tijssen and colleagues proposed that a short-term synchronization between sternocleidomastoid and splenius capitis, along with a lack of phase differences in organic cervical dystonia, could help in this differentiation.[134]

In a 2001 review, Brown and Thompson[135] pointed out findings that potentially could be useful in the evaluation of organic versus psychogenic dystonia. Diminished reciprocal inhibition at intermediate and long latencies, as well as the absence of broad-peak synchronization of co-contracting antagonist muscles could be useful in supporting the diagnosis of organic dystonia.[134] Espay and colleagues found increased cortical excitability in psychogenic dystonia, suggesting that changes such as decreased short- and long-interval intracortical inhibition and decreased intracortical facilitation might be a consequence of the dystonic posture as opposed to a pathophysiological mechanism associated with dystonia.[136]

In the case of ataxias, it has been suggested that kinematic differences between centripetal and centrifugal phases of movements in the vertical plane might be useful to diagnose a psychogenic condition.[137]

Utilization of placebo or suggestion is a more controversial subject. Suggestion is a relatively benign approach: the reinforcement that there is no serious underlying degenerative disease coupled sometimes with directed physiotherapy training and biofeedback techniques can be extremely helpful.

The use of placebos can be hazardous. First, there are ethical and legal concerns about the use of nonactive drugs, negating the patient's autonomy. Second, it can endanger the physician–patient relationship, with the latter feeling deceived and therefore abandoning treatment.[138] This is particularly the case since most authorities do not inform the patient in advance of the possible "inactive" nature of the therapy because this clearly reduces the likelihood of a response. Patients are generally told that they are going to receive a drug that has the potential to markedly improve or ameliorate their symptoms. Sometimes, patients are told they will receive a drug that can worsen the symptoms (useful when the movements are exclusively paroxysmal) followed by another ("an antidote") that will have the opposite effect. Usually these challenges are given intravenously. An alternative (which we have not used) is a small alcohol swab or gauze patch soaked in a very mild chemical irritant that causes a slight tingling or burning sensation on the skin. One of the major concerns or criticisms of the use of placebo is that the patient may respond to being told (or especially if they learn "by accident" in some other way) of the nature of the placebo test with the conviction that they have been tricked by the medical profession.[139] The resulting resentment is very counterproductive to the therapeutic relationship necessary for ongoing management of these patients. However, when the nature and results of placebo testing are shared with the patient in a supportive milieu as part of the overall treatment program, this can be an extremely effective tool with both diagnostic and therapeutic effects.

Little has been written on the use of placebos in PMDs possibly because there is no "gold standard" for the confirmation of diagnosis with that to compare the results of this testing as in the case of EEG and epilepsy. Lancman and colleagues[140] have reported that in patients with psychogenic seizures an "induction test" had a sensitivity of 77.4% and a specificity of 100% with a positive predictive value of 100%. The negative predictive value was 48.7%. They used a "patch" placed on the skin, and the patients were told that the medication would be absorbed into the circulation and reach the brain in 30 sec. They were also told not to control the seizures and that removal of the patch would stop the resulting seizure if one developed. Similar approaches[141,142] usually using intravenous injections of saline are considered safe and effective,[140] although Walczack and colleagues[143] found that in a minority of patients, placebo injections produced atypical events or epileptic seizures that could lead to an incorrect diagnosis. There is also the potential for both severe psychogenic "reactions" on the challenge and false-positive responses in suggestible patients with organic disease. Placebo effects are widely recognized in a variety of diseases, including movement disorders.[43] However, the use of a placebo enables a direct observation and can establish a diagnosis and even a therapeutic approach. One must remember that as soon as the diagnosis of a PMD can be established with a reasonable degree of certainty, it is possible to both withdraw and avoid therapies with potential harmful side effects. As previously mentioned, patients have been subjected to hazardous treatments, including neurosurgical procedures due to incorrect diagnoses.

In general, we reserve the use of placebo saline injections for patients in whom there remains diagnostic uncertainty after a full clinical assessment. This would include patients with a history of paroxysmal events that could not be triggered by simpler means such as the application of a tuning fork to the forehead or sternum combined with the suggestion that vibration often triggers such attacks in other patients. The use of pressure points in a somewhat similar fashion is effective in some patients. Attacks are sometimes precipitated by asking the patient to look up quickly. In others, applying pressure to the top of the head when the head is held steady for evaluation of eye movements is an effective precipitant. Any of these same maneuvers (e.g., tuning fork, "trigger pressure points") can also be used with suggestion to induce transient remissions of persistent symptoms and if the improvement is profound and inconsistent with an organic disorder, such a response can provide strong evidence for a psychogenic etiology. The results of these triggering or relieving maneuvers, including placebo challenges, should be incorporated in the presentation of the diagnosis to the patient.

As with placebo challenges, little has been written on the use of sodium amytal testing in patients with PMDs. It is critical to remember that barbiturates or other sedatives may have a nonspecific but pronounced ameliorative effect on a variety of organic movement disorders. Alternatively, PMDs, especially when long standing, may change little in response to this agent. In our case series of posttraumatic cervical spasms, the amytal interview resolved the associated sensory abnormality seen in those patients, helping to establish a PMD diagnosis. Recently, symptom persistence during sodium amytal infusion test[144] has been reported useful in differentiating organic spasmodic dysphonia from psychogenic vocal cord dystonia, where improvement in speech symptoms was commonly evident. Family history, neurological and psychiatric evaluations, electrical stimulation of the superior laryngeal nerve, and standard speech testing did not help in distinguishing these two conditions. Schneider and Bhatia have discussed the therapeutic use of a videotape obtained during an amytal/benzodiazepine interview to provide feedback to enhance patient recovery.[145]

When the diagnosis is confirmed by other means, amytal testing may provide useful insights into the psychodynamic factors causing the problem. However, caution must be exercised not to overinterpret information volunteered during this testing, especially if the diagnosis of a PMD is not supported or established by other evidence.

In our experience, the most difficult diagnostic problems arise in two situations: (1) when there is a clear evidence of a PMD but an underlying organic component cannot be excluded and (2) when the movement disorder is an unchanging tonic ("dystonic") contraction of muscles usually precipitated by a seemingly inconsequential injury. In most examples of the former, it is the psychogenic movements that are the predominant complaint and the chief source of disability and concern.[36] We suggest dealing with these cases in a similar manner to other psychogenic movements disorders, keeping in mind the potential contribution (sometimes progressively so) of the underlying organic condition. This point was recently emphasized by Mai,[146] who stated that "... the diagnosis of conversion disorders and neurological disorders are not mutually exclusive; they may occur in the same patient either concurrently or consecutively and are particularly common in chronic relapsing diseases such as multiple sclerosis and epilepsy." In the second situation, the nature of tonic muscle contraction ("dystonia" or "spasm") occurring after injury represents a major source of controversy in the field of movement disorders as discussed previously.

Psychiatric consultation should be obtained for assistance with primary diagnosis and therapy. However, as stated previously, the diagnosis of a PMD is made on the basis of positive criteria by the neurologist independent of the psychiatric assessment. It should never be a diagnosis of exclusion largely supported by the presence of concurrent psychiatric illness. However, once the diagnosis is made, further establishing a psychiatric diagnosis is of paramount importance to the management of patients with PMDs. In difficult uncertain diagnoses, a positive response to psychotherapy lends further support to the PMD diagnosis. However, it is important to reiterate that patients with organic movement disorders may have additional coincident or secondary psychopathology.

It should also be noted that in many patients with PMDs, the underlying psychopathology is not overt even after an extended psychiatric assessment. It is not uncommon for such patients to have received "psychiatric clearance" with the final opinion expressed that there is no underlying psychiatric problem, and therefore an organic cause of the movement disorder must be present. This is comparable to a time when psychiatrists found evidence for psychopathology in patients with organic dystonia and blamed these "disturbances" for the movement disorder, whereas we would now either disregard this evidence or recognize it as a consequence rather than as a cause of the motor dysfunction. The diagnosis of a PMD is made by a neurologist with experience in the field of movement disorders and should not be made or refuted by a psychiatrist, especially one inexperienced with movement disorders. As Ford and colleagues[40] pointed out, there are three basic errors in dealing with such patients that can lead to devastating consequences: (1) the patient may be misdiagnosed as having a psychogenic disorder when in fact it is organic, (2) a truly psychogenic disorder can be misdiagnosed as organic, and (3) the clinician fails to provide the appropriate care and therapy for these patients.

▶ CATEGORIES OF DIAGNOSTIC CERTAINTY

The level of diagnostic certainty that the physician has for a psychogenic cause of a movement disorder varies greatly, depending on the clinical features of the movement disorder and the accompanying symptoms and signs. The four degrees of certainty for the diagnosis of psychogenic dystonia were developed by Fahn and Williams over 20 years ago[30] are now commonly applied to all forms of PMDs. These degrees of certainty are divided into documented, clinically established, probable, and possible PMDs.

In **documented** PMDs, the movements must be persistently relieved by psychotherapy, suggestion, and administration of placebos, or the patient is witnessed as being free of symptoms when left alone unobserved. **Clinically established** PMDs are inconsistent over time or are incongruent with the classical definitions of movement disorders. For example, in the case of dystonia, the patient cannot move the limb on request and resist passive movements but can easily groom him- or herself in daily life. Along with these incongruities, the patient must show additional features that suggest psychogenicity such as other neurological signs that are definitely psychogenic (e.g., false weakness or false sensory findings or self-inflicted injuries, multiple somatizations, and an obvious psychiatric condition). Caution needs to be exercised in the case of self-inflicted injuries since these can occasionally be symptoms of an organic movement disorder such as Tourette's syndrome or neuroacanthocytosis. These first two categories were subsequently combined under "clinically definite."[147] **Probable** PMDs apply to those patients who fall into the following categories: (1) The movement disorder is inconsistent or incongruent with classical definitions, but there are no other features suggesting psychogenicity, (2) The movement disorder is consistent and congruent with organic disease, but accompanying neurological signs are definitely psychogenic such as false weakness or sensory findings (3) The movement disorder is consistent with a classical condition, but multiple somatizations are present. In the case of the second and third categories, it is important to consider the diagnostic alternative of an organic movement disorder accompanied by coincidental or associated psychiatric disturbances (see below). Finally, the diagnosis of a PMD is **possible** when an obvious emotional disturbance is present in a patient with a movement disorder that is otherwise consistent with a known organic disease.

However, there are problems with this classification scheme, and it is probably time to consider revising it (Table 48–12). Many patients falling into the last two categories (probable and possible) have organic movement disorders with additional psychiatric disturbances (i.e., with "functional overlay"), while other patients with unequivocal PMDs (e.g., completely distractible or fully entrainable tremor) who lack other psychogenic features (e.g., false neurological signs and multiple somatizations) can only be classified as "Probable." This scheme also does not take into account the possibility of confirming that the movement disorder is psychogenic with additional electrophysiological testing. For these reasons, a new simplified classification scheme has been proposed for both research and clinical use applying the following categories[148]: (1) *documented* (as in the original); (2a) *clinically definite + other features* (as in the original); (2b) *clinically definite minus other features* (unequivocal clinical features incompatible with organic disease and no other features suggesting underlying neurological or psychiatric problems) (1 + 2a + 2b could be combined as "clinically definite") and (3) *laboratory supported definite* (primarily in the case of psychogenic tremor and psychogenic myoclonus). When the movement disorder demonstrates clinical features (or electrophysiology) that are strongly suggestive but not diagnostic of a psychogenic cause the category of "Possible" could be used, and where the movements are consistent and congruous with an organic movement disorder combined with "false" neurological signs or psychiatric features such as multiple somatizations a classification of a PMD would not be applied (Table 48–12).

▶ APPROACH TO THERAPY OF PSYCHOGENIC MOVEMENTS DISORDERS

When a diagnosis is firmly established, empathy and understanding on the part of the physician are of paramount importance. The diagnosis should be presented carefully avoiding conveyance of uncertainty. We agree with Ford and colleagues[40] that the use of a neurobiological explanation for the patient's symptoms helps in establishing trust, acceptance, and understanding of their diagnosis and will help in the recovery of the symptoms. The nature of the movement disorder should be confirmed (i.e., the patient is told he/she has a form of dystonia, tremor, myoclonus, etc.), but that the problem

TABLE 48-12. DIAGNOSTIC CLASSIFICATION OF PSYCHOGENIC MOVEMENT DISORDERS

Traditional Classification of Degrees of Certainty in Diagnosis*	Proposed Revision of Classification of Degrees of Certainty in Diagnosis†
1. Documented: Remittance with suggestion, physiotherapy, psychotherapy, and placebos "while unobserved"	1. Documented (as in original)
2. Clinically established: Inconsistent over time/incongruent with clinical condition + other manifestations: other "false" signs, multiple somatizations, obvious psychiatric disturbance	2a. Clinically established + other features (as in original) 2b. Clinically established − other features Unequivocal clinical features incompatible with organic disease with no features, suggesting another underlying or logical or psychiatric problem
1 + 2 = Clinically definite	1 + 2a + 2b = Clinically definite
3. Probable: Inconsistent/incongruent − no other features Consistent/congruent −/+ "false" neurological signs Consistent/congruent + multiple somatizations	3. Laboratory supported definite: Electrophysiological evidence proving a psychogenic movement disorder (primarily in cases of psychogenic tremor and psychogenic myoclonus)
4. Possible: Consistent/congruent + obvious emotional disturbance	

*From Fahn S, Williams PJ. Psychogenic dystonia. Adv Neurol 1988;50:431–455.
†From Gupta A, Lang AE. Psychogenic movement disorders. Curr Opin Neurol 2009;(in press).

is not due to severe or permanent structural brain disease. This should be done in a nonjudgmental fashion reassuring the patient that it is not believed that they are "crazy" or that they purposefully feigning or causing the movements to occur and acknowledging that this problem can result in considerable disability.

It is of paramount importance that a referral to psychiatry is accompanied by clear and unequivocal documentation and discussion about the diagnosis. This should avoid the extremely detrimental pronouncement by a psychiatrist that "there is nothing psychologically wrong" with the patient, which creates further doubt in the patient's mind, generating additional consultation and opinions, further testing increasing the patient's uncertainty and fruitless spending. Depending on the circumstances, one may have to introduce the need for psychiatric consultation by stating that it is strictly for the purposes of evaluating and assisting the patient in their strategies of coping with the disability caused by the abnormal movements. This approach is often necessary in patients with long-standing symptoms who have had multiple investigations, have been given a diagnosis of an organic movement disorder, and have undergone extensive therapeutic trials. In others, it may be possible to introduce the concept of a psychological cause even before obtaining the psychiatric consultation.

The patient should be reassured and counselled to the effect that there is a strong possibility of improvement. Further management approaches depend largely on the nature and severity of the underlying psychopathology. Treatment is largely empirical as there are no published controlled trials in PMDs. It frequently requires the variable combinations of physiotherapy, biofeedback, and other motor retraining paradigms, psychotherapy, suggestion, psychopharmacology,[149] and obviously aggressive treatment of any underlying psychiatric disorders identified. Hypnosis might be considered, however, this had no additional benefit on treatment outcome of conversion disorders of the motor type in a recent study of 45 patients.[150]

Placebo treatments have been widely used and reported in noncontrolled fashion. Although there are clear advantages of using such approach instead of potentially habit-forming pharmacological agents, it also poses multiple ethical and legal problems that go beyond the scope of this chapter, and cannot be generally recommended.

Some patients with acute short-lived symptoms may only require reassurance, support, and active follow-up. Further discussion of the management of the causative psychiatric disorders is beyond the scope of this text.

PROGNOSIS

Despite the reassurance given to patients suffering from PMDs, it should be emphasized that the prognosis must be guarded. Some patients will remain refractory to all treatment. However, a systematic approach involving a team composed of a neurologist, psychiatrist, nurses, physiotherapists, and others may be rewarded with striking successes even in long-lasting, extremely disabled cases. Despite the suggestion that settlement resolves the problem in patients involved in legal or compensation issues, the natural intuitive thinking that abnormal movements of psychogenic origin will eventually settle and previous uncontrolled findings that 25% of these patients improve spontaneously, it now seems that quite a high proportion of patients will have long-standing or persistent disability.[39,47]

The poor prognosis and profound negative impact of PMDs were emphasized in a recent study that compared 66 patients with PMDs to 704 with Parkinson's disease, and the PMD had significantly increased psychiatric comorbidity, more severe mental health disturbances, and more importantly, similar disability and quality of life indicators despite overall shorter disease duration and younger age.[151] Feinstein and colleagues interviewed 42 patients out of a group of 88 subjects seen in our unit in Toronto with either documented or clinically established PMD[39] At the time of the study interview, on average 3.2 years after the initial assessment, all but 4 patients still had the abnormal movement (90.5%). Of these four patients, two had replaced the abnormal movement by a different somatoform disorder. Although there was no formal assessment at baseline, the psychiatric status showed a significant array of disorders; only two patients did not have a psychiatric diagnosis at follow-up (4.8%). Diagnosis at the time of interview included anxiety disorders in 16 patients (38.1%), major depression in eight (19.1%), and a combination of the two in five (11.9%). A schizoaffective disorder was diagnosed in one patient (2.4%).

Twenty three of our previously diagnosed PMD patients (most of them participating in the study of Feinstein described above) agreed to a follow-up detailed neurological examination (J. Fine, A. Nieves, and A. Lang unpublished observations). In this subset, all patients were still manifesting PMD at the time of follow-up, with a mean duration of symptoms of 8.6±8.5 years. Activities of daily living such as eating, dressing, and hygiene were reported impaired in 19 of the examined patients (82.6%). Of the patients whose symptoms had improved or stabilized, 66.6% experienced this change within the first year of illness. This overall poor prognosis for recovery and substantial disability has been reported by other groups, for example, studying psychogenic tremor.[89]

Not all studies, however, support a necessarily bleak outcome. Although McKeon and colleagues found a 65% disability rate on patient-reported disability scales in their psychogenic tremor patients, Jankovic and colleagues reported a better prognosis with a 60% improvement rate.[152,153] Differences in data ascertainment that could potentially explain such marked differences in outcomes include the facts that Jankovic and colleagues included any degree of improvement, their study lacked a prospective follow-up design and electrophysiological assessments, as the study of McKeon did. Furthermore, symptom duration was shorter in the Jankovic study, a fact that has been suggested to relate to better prognosis.

The outcome of PMDs depends greatly on the underlying psychiatric basis. One study evaluating conversion disorders showed that patients with a conversion disorder admitted to hospital who were young (<40 years) and, similar to the case in pseudoepileptic disorders, had a recent onset of symptoms (usually a few days before admission to hospital) generally had a good prognosis.[154] The strongest predictive factor was found to be the condition of the patient on discharge. If the symptoms improved while in hospital, a good outcome was observed in up to 96% of patients. In this study, only two patients mistakenly diagnosed as having a conversion disorder were later found to develop an organic neurological disease (left middle cerebral artery territory infarct and multiple sclerosis, respectively). The authors concluded that neurological disease will emerge only rarely in patients with conversion disorders, and although neuroimaging is helpful in difficult cases, it can also be a source of confusion by "...showing harmless anatomical variants." They found that apraxia, focal dystonia, and the combination of organic deficits with a conversion disorder are areas of most frequent diagnostic error and confusion. Finally, it was emphasized that recovery of a conversion disorder is rare if improvement does not occur during the initial hospital evaluation.

Thus, in summary, PMDs seem to carry a poor prognosis, both for psychiatric and motor function. Patients who fare better seem to be the ones whose symptoms improve and stabilize within the first year, suggesting that long-standing disease when first assessed carries a particularly poor prognosis. Other studies have suggested that additional features that may predict a good outcome in psychogenic neurological syndromes include a clear emotional trigger or precipitant, and lack of long-standing psychopathology.[154]

As expected, factitious disorders and malingering respond poorly. When litigation or compensation issues are pending, it is important to resolve them as quickly as possible. However, response to this approach is often disappointing or unpredictable. Malingerers may either keep up the act to justify the settlement or will have a striking improvement once a settlement has been reached. In our experience, although somatoform disorders less commonly improve in response to a financial settlement, spontaneous or therapeutically induced remissions are much less likely to occur while economic issues remain unresolved.

The experience of Williams and his colleagues[155] contrasts with the rather negative impressions outlined above. They found that age, gender, intelligence, chronicity of illness, and PMD symptomatology had no influence on outcome. In PMD patients with either a conversion or somatoform disorder, the response to treatment was considered "successful" in all (except in three patients with either malingering or a factitious disorder), and they concluded that "...patients with many years of established psychogenic symptomatology were able to make full recoveries."[155] However, their treatment often entailed intensive, extended hospitalization (that is now rather impractical or even impossible in the era of managed care) and long-term follow-up documenting sustained improvement, once the patient left the intensive therapeutic milieu, was generally not available. This highlights an urgent need for accurate outcome data documenting long-term prognosis in patients managed with a variety of treatment approaches. As emphasized previously, PMDs are common and frequently result in pronounced disability with consequent impact on both the individual and society. Future research must be directed at advancing our understanding of the pathogenesis of these disorders and improving their management.

REFERENCES

1. Head H. The diagnosis of hysteria. Brit Med J 1922;1: 827–829.
2. Charcot J-M. Hystero-epilepsy: A young woman with a convulsive attack in the auditorium. In Goetz CG (ed). Charcot The Clinician. The Tuesday Lessons. New York: Raven Press, 1987, pp. 102–122.
3. Freud S. Charcot. In Sutherland JD (ed). Collected Papers—Volume 1. London: The Hogarth Press, 1957, 9–23.
4. Guillain G. J.M. Charcot, 1825-1893, His Life—His Work. New York: Paul B. Hoeber, Inc., 1959.
5. Havens LL. Charcot and hysteria. J Nerv Ment Dis 1966;141:505–516.
6. Goetz C. Neuroscience across the centuries. London: Smith-Gordon, 1989.
7. Goetz C. Charcot and psychogenic movement disorders. In Hallet M, Fahn S, Jankovic J, et al. (eds). Psychogenic Movement Disorders Neurology and Neuropsychiatry. Philadelphia: Lippincott Williams & Wilkins, 2006, pp. 3–13.
8. Schiller F. Paul Broca—Founder of French Anthropology, Explorer of the Brain. New York: Oxford University Press, 1992.
9. Freud S. Hypnotism and suggestion (1888). In Strachey J (ed). Collected Papers. London, England: Hogarth Press, 1957, pp. 11–24.
10. Gowers WR. Epilepsy and Other Chronic Convulsive Diseases: Their Causes, Symptoms & Treatment. New York: Dover Publications, Inc., 1964.
11. Lecrubier Y. Images in psychiatry—Jean-Martin Charcot, 1825-1893. Am J Psychiatry 1995;151:1:121.
12. Gowers WR. A Manual of Diseases of the Nervous System. Philadelphia: Blakiston, 1888.
13. Walshe SF. Diagnosis of hysteria. Brit Med J 1965;2:1451–1454.
14. Cockburn JJ. Spasmodic torticollis: A psychogenic condition? J Psychosomat Res 1971;15:471–477.
15. Harrington RC, Wieck A, Marks IM, et al. Writer's cramp: Not associated with anxiety. Mov Disord 1988;3:195–200.
16. Grafman J, Cohen LG, Hallett M. Is focal hand dystonia associated with psychopathology? Mov Disord 1991;6: 29–35.
17. Slater E. Diagnosis of "hysteria". Brit Med J 1965;1: 1395–1399.
18. Crimlisk HL, Bhatia K, Cope H, et al. Slater revisited: 6 year follow up study of patients with medically unexplained motor symptoms. BMJ 1998;316(7131):582–586.
19. Lang AE. General overview of psychogenic movement disorders: Epidemiology, diagnosis, and prognosis. In Hallett M, Fahn S, Jankovic J, et al. (eds). Psychogenic Movement Disorders—Neurology and Neuropsychiatry. Lippincott Williams & Wilkins, 2006, pp. 35–41.
20. American Psychiatric Association: Diagnostic and Statistical Manual of Mental Disorders, 4th edn, (DSM IV). Washington: American Psychiatric Association, 1994.
21. Thompson DJ, Goldberg D. Hysterical personality disorder. Br J Psychiatry 1987;150:241–245.
22. Vuilleumier P, Chicherio C, Assal F, et al. Functional neuroanatomical correlates of hysterical sensorimotor loss. Brain 2001;124(6):1077–1090.
23. Schepank H, Hilpert H, Honmann H, et al. The Mannheim Cohort Project—Prevalence of psychogenic diseases in cities. Z Psychosom Med Psychoanal 1984;30(1):43–61.
24. Snyder S, Strain JJ. Somatoform disorders in the general hospital inpatient setting. Gen Hosp Psychiatry 1989;11(4):288–293.
25. Franz M, Schellberg D, Reister G, et al. Incidence and follow-up characteristics of neurologically relevant psycogenic symptoms. Nervenarzt 1993;64(6):369–376.
26. Marsden CD. Hysteria—A neurologist's view. Psychol Med 1986;16(2):277–288.
27. Lempert T, Dieterich M, Huppert D, et al. Psychogenic disorders in neurology: frequency and clinical spectrum. Acta Neurol Scand 1990;82:335–340.
28. Woolsey RM. Hysteria: 1875 to 1975. Dis Nerv Syst 1976;37:379–386.
29. Factor SA, Podskalny GD, Molho ES. Psychogenic movement disorders: Frequency, clinical profile, and characteristics. J Neurol Neurosurg Psychiatry 1995;59(4):406–412.
30. Fahn S, Williams PJ. Psychogenic dystonia. Adv Neurol 1988;50:431–455.
31. Baik JS, Lang AE. Gait abnormalities in psychogenic movement disorders. Movement Disord 2007;22(3):395–399.
32. Walters AS, Boudwin J, Wright D, et al. Three hysterical movement disorders. Psychol Reports 1988;62:979–985.
33. Lang AE, Koller WC, Fahn S. Psychogenic Parkinsonism. Arch Neurol 1995;52:802–810.
34. Kurlan R, Deeley C, Comon PG. Psychogenic movement disorder (pseudo-tics) in a patient with Tourette's syndrome. J Neuropsychiatry Clin Neurosci 1992;4:347–348.
35. Kanner AM, Parra J, Frey M, et al. Psychiatric and neurologic predictors of psychogenic pseudoseizure outcome. Neurology 1999;53:933–938.
36. Ranawaya R, Riley D, Lang AE. Psychogenic dyskinesias in patients with organic movement disorders. Mov Disord 1990;5:127–133.
37. Schwingenschuh P, PontSunyer C, Surtees R, et al. Pychogenic Movement Disorders in Children: A Report of

15 Cases and a Review of the Literature. Movement Disord 2008;23(13):1882–1888.

38. Ferrara J, Jankovic J. Psychogenic movement disorders in children. Movement Disord 2008;23(13):1875–1881.
39. Feinstein A, Stergiopoulos V, Fine J, et al. Psychiatric outcome in patients with a psychogenic movement disorder: A prospective study. Neuropsychiatry Neuropsychol Behav Neurol 2001;14(3):169–176.
40. Ford B, Williams DT, Fahn S. Treatment of Psychogenic Movement Disorders. In Kurlan R (ed). Treatment of Movement Disorders. J.B. Lippincott Company, 1995, pp. 475–485.
41. Barclay CL, Lang AE. Other Secondary Dystonias. In Tsui J, Calne DB (eds). Handbook of Dystonia. New York: Marcel Dekker, 1995, pp. 267–305.
42. Koller W. Movement Disorders: Which Ones are Real? Malingering and Conversion Reactions. American Academy of Neurology Annual Meeting, Washington, D.C., 1994, #222-3-225-25.
43. Goetz CG, Leurgans S, Raman R, et al. Objective changes in motor function during placebo treatment in PD. Neurology 2000;54(3):710–714.
44. Bentivoglio AR, Loi M, Valente EM, et al. Phenotypic variability of DYT1-PTD: Does the clinical spectrum include psychogenic dystonia? Mov Disord 2002;17(5):1058–1063.
45. Weiner WJ, Lang AE. Movement Disorders—A Comprehensive Survey. New York: Futura Publishing, 1989.
46. Lesser RP, Fahn S. Dystonia: A disorder often misdiagnosed as a conversion reaction. Am J Psychiat 1978;153:349–352.
47. Marsden CD. Psychogenic problems associated with dystonia. Adv Neurol 1995;65:319–326.
48. Weiner WJ, Lang AE. Idiopathic torsion dystonia. In Weiner WJ, Lang AE (eds). Movement Disorders: A Comprehensive Survey. Mount Kisco, NY: Future Publishing, 1989, pp. 1–725.
49. Dobyns WB, Ozelius LJ, Kramer PL, et al. Rapid-onset dystonia-parkinsonism. Neurology 1993;43:2596–2602.
50. Munhoz RP, Lang AE. *Gestes antagonistes* in psychogenic dystonia. Mov Disord 2004;19(3):331–332.
51. Bressman SB, Fahn S, Burke RE. Paroxysmal non-kinesigenic dystonia. In Fahn S, Marden CD, Calne DB (eds). Advances in Neurology. New York: Raven Press, 1988, Vol. 50, pp. 403–413.
52. Saint-Cyr JA, Taylor AE, Nicholson K. Behavior and the basal ganglia. Adv Neurol 1995;65:1–28.
53. Batshaw ML, Wachtel RC, Deckel AW, et al. Munchausen's syndrome simulating torsion dystonia. N Engl J Med 1985;312:1437–1439.
54. Lang AE. Psychogenic dystonia: A review of 18 cases. Can J Neurol Sci 1995;22:136–143.
55. Sheehy MP, Marsden CD. Writer's Cramp—A focal dystonia. Brain 1982;461:480.
56. Sheehy MP, Marsden CD. Trauma and pain in spasmodic torticollis. Lancet 1980;1:777–778.
57. Fletcher NA, Harding AE, Marsden CD. The relationship between trauma and idiopathic torsion dystonia. J Neurol Neurosurg Psychiatry 1991;54:713–717.
58. Fletcher NA, Harding AE, Marsden CD. A case-control study of idiopathic torsion dystonia. Mov Disord 1991;6:304–309.
59. Eidelberg D, Takikawa S, Wilhelmsen K, et al. Positron emission tomographic findings in Filipino X-linked dystonia-parkinsonism. Ann Neurol 1993;34:185–191.
60. Koller WC, Wong GF, Lang A. Posttraumatic movement disorders: A review. Mov Disord 1989;4:20–36.
61. Marsden CD, Obeso JA, Traub MM, et al. Muscle spasms associated with Sudeck's atrophy after injury. BMJ 1984;288:173–176.
62. Schott GD. The relationship of peripheral trauma and pain to dystonia. J Neurol Neurosurg Psychiatry 1985;48: 698–701.
63. Jankovic J, Van Der Linden C. Dystonia and tremor induced by peripheral trauma:predisposing factors. J Neurol Neurosurg Psychiatry 1988;51:1512–1519.
64. Schwartzman RJ, Kerrigan J. The movement disorder of reflex sympathetic dystrophy. Neurology 1990;40:57–61.
65. Bhatia KP, Bhatt MH, Marsden CD. The causalgia-dystonia syndrome. Brain 1993;116:843–851.
66. Schwartzman RJ. Movement disorder of RSD—Letter. Neurology 1990;40:1477–1478.
67. Van Hilten JJ, Van de Beek WJT, Vein AA, et al. Clinical aspects of multifocal or generalized tonic dystonia in reflex sympathetic dystrophy. Neurology 2001;56(12):1762–1765.
68. Van Hilten BJ, Van de Beek WJT, Hoff JI, et al. Intrathecal baclofen for the treatment of dystonia in patients with reflex sympathetic dystrophy. N Engl J Med 2000;343(9):625–630.
69. Van Hilten JJ, Van de Beek WJT, Roep BO. Multifocal or generalized tonic dystonia of complex regional pain syndrome: A distinct clinical entity associated with HLA-DR13. Ann Neurol 2000;48(1):113–116.
70. Verdugo RJ, Ochoa JL. Abnormal movements in complex regional pain syndrome: Assessment of their nature. Muscle Nerve 2000;23(2):198–205.
71. Schrag A, Trimble M, Quinn N, et al. The syndrome of fixed dystonia: an evaluation of 103 patients. Brain 2004;127(10):2360–2372.
72. Munts AG, Van Rootselaar AF, Van Der Meer JN, et al. Clinical and neurophysiological characterization of myoclonus in complex regional pain syndrome. Mov Disord 2008;23(4):581–587.
73. Lang AE, Angel M, Bhatia K, et al. Myoclonus in Complex Regional Pain Syndrome. Movement Disord 2009;24(2):314–316.
74. Tarsy D. Comparison of acute- and delayed-onset posttraumatic cervical dystonia. Mov Disord 1998;13(3):481–485.
75. Truong DD, Dubinsky R, Hermanowicz N, et al. Posttraumatic torticollis. Arch Neurol 1991;48(2):221–223.
76. Goldman S, Ahlskog JE. Posttraumatic cervical dystonia. Mayo Clin Proc 1993;68(5):443–448.
77. Samii A, Pal PK, Schulzer M, et al. Post-traumatic cervical dystonia: A distinct entity? Can J Neurol Sci 2000;27(1):55–59.
78. Wright RA, Ahlskog JE. Focal shoulder-elevation dystonia. Mov Disord 2000;15(4):709–713.
79. Höllinger P, Burgunder JM. Posttraumatic focal dystonia of the shoulder. Eur Neurol 2000;44(3):153–155.
80. Jankovic J. Post-traumatic movement disorders: Central and peripheral mechanisms. Neurology 1994;44: 2006–2014.

81. Bressman SB, De Leon D, Raymond D, et al. Secondary dystonia and the *DYT1* gene. Neurology 1997;48(6): 1571–1577.
82. Gasser T, Bove CM, Ozelius LJ, et al. Haplotype analysis at the DYT1 locus in Ashkenazi Jewish patients with occupational hand dystonia. Mov Disord 1996;11(2):163–166.
83. Ochoa J. Reflex Sympathetic Dystrophy—Fact or Fiction. Malingering and Conversion Reactions. American Academy of Neurology Annual Meeting, Washington, D.C., 1994, #222-41-222-56.
84. Elble RJ, Koller WC. The Definition and Classification of Tremor. Baltimore: The Johns Hopkins University Press, 1990, pp. 1–9.
85. Wilson SAK. The approach to the study of hysteria. J Neurol Psychopath 1931;11:193–206.
86. Fahn S. Atypical tremors, rare tremors and unclassified tremors. In Findley LJ, Capildeo R (eds). Movement Disorders. London: The MacMillan Press Ltd., 1984, pp. 431–443.
87. Koller W, Lang AE, Vetere-Overfield B, et al. Psychogenic tremors. Neurology 1989;39:1094–1099.
88. Kim YJ, Pakiam AS, Lang AE. Historical and clinical features of psychogenic tremor: a review of 70 cases. Can J Neurol Sci 1999;26(3):190–195.
89. Deuschl G, Köster B, Lücking CH, et al. Diagnostic and pathophysiological aspects of psychogenic tremors. Mov Disord 1998;13(2):294–302.
90. Deuschl G, Raethjen J, Lindemann M, et al. The pathophysiology of tremor. Muscle Nerve 2001;24(6):716–735.
91. Thomas M, Jankovic J. Psychogenic movement disorder: Diagnosis and management. CNS Drug 2008;18:437–452.
92. Zadikoff C, Lang AE, Klein C. The 'essentials' of essential palatal tremor: a reappraisal of the nosology. Brain 2006;129(4):832–840.
93. Silverdale MA, Schneider SA, Bhatia KP, et al. The spectrum of orolingual tremor—A proposed classification system. Movement Disord 2008;23(2):159–167.
94. Monday K, Jankovic J. Psychogenic myoclonus. Neurology 1993;43:349–352.
95. Chapel JL. Latah, myriachit, and jumpers revisited. New York State J Med 1970.
96. Andermann F, Andermann E. Excessive startle syndromes: Startle disease, jumping and startle epilepsy. Adv Neurol 1986;43:321–338.
97. Stevens H. "Jumping Frenchmen of Maine". Arch Neurol 1965;12:311–314.
98. Kunkle EC. The "jumpers" of Maine: A reappraisal. Arch Intern Med 1967;119:355–358.
99. Saint-Hilaire MH, Saint-Hilaire JM, Granger L. Jumping Frenchmen of Maine. Neurology 1986;36:1269–1271.
100. Tanner CM, Chamberland J. Latah in Jakarta, Indonesia. Mov Disord 2001;16:526–529.
101. Saint-Hilaire M-H, Saint-Hilaire J.M. Jumping Frenchmen of Maine. Mov Disord 2001;16:530.
102. McFarling DA. The "Ragin' Cajuns" of Louisiana. Mov Disord 2002;16:531–532.
103. Lang AE. Patient perception of tics and other movement disorders. Neurology 1991;41:223–228.
104. Walters AS, Hening WA. Noise-induced psychogenic tremor associated with post-traumatic stress disorder. Mov Disord 1992;7:333–338.
105. Tan EK, Jankovic J. Psychogenic hemifacial spasm. J Neuropsychiatry Clin Neurosci 2001;13(3):380–384.
106. Galvez-Jimenez N, Hargreaves MJ. Psychogenic hemifacial spasm (Psych-HFS); incidence and clinical features. Psychogenic Movement Disorders, AAN 2006;Abstracts:332–334.
107. Morgan JC, Sethi K. Psychogenic parkinsonism. In Hallet M, Fahn S, Jankovic J, et al. (eds). Psychogenic Movement Disorders, Neurology and Neuropsychiatry. Philadelphia: Lippincott Williams & Wilkins, 2006, pp. 62–68.
108. Benaderette S, Fregonara PZ, Apartis E, et al. Psychogenic parkinsonism: A combination of clinical, electrophysiological, and [123I]-FP-CIT SPECT scan explorations improves diagnostic accuracy. Mov Disord 2006;21(3):310–317.
109. Hayes MW, Graham S, Heldorf P, et al. A video review of the diagnosis of psychogenic gait. Mov Disord 1999;14:914–921.
110. Mills CK. Hysteria. In Pepper W, Starr L, (eds). A System of Practical Medicine. Philadelphia: Lea Brothers, 1886, pp. 205–287.
111. Keane JR. Hysterical gait disorders: 60 cases. Neurology 1989;39:586–589.
112. Morris JG, De Moore GM, Heberstein M. Psychogenic gait. In Hallet M, Fahn S, Jankovic J, et al. (eds). Psychogenic Movement Disorders Neurology and Neuropsychiatry. Philadelphia: Lippincott Williams & Wilkins, 2006, pp. 69–75.
113. Lempert T, Brandt T, Dieterich M, et al. How to identify psychogenic disorders of stance and gait. J Neurol 1991;238:140–146.
114. Eames P. Hysteria following brain injury. J Neurol Neurosurg Psychiatry 1992;55:1046–1053.
115. Nieves AV, Miyasaki JM, Lang AE. Acute Onset Dystonic Camptocormia Caused by Lenticular Lesions. Mov Disord 2001;16:177–180.
116. Jennings DL, Seibyl JP, Oakes D, et al. (^{123}I) β-CIT and single-photon emission computed tomographic imaging vs clinical evaluation in Parkinsonian syndrome - Unmasking an early diagnosis. Arch Neurol 2004;61(8):1224–1229.
117. Felicio AC, Shih MC, Godeiro-Junior C, et al. Molecular imaging studies in Parkinson disease: reducing diagnostic uncertainty. Neurologist 2009;15(1):6–16.
118. Scherfler C, Schwarz J, Antonini A, et al. Role of DAT-SPECT in the diagnostic work up of Parkinsonism. Movement Disord 2007;22(9):1229–1238.
119. Gaig C, Marti MJ, Tolosa E, et al. 123I-Ioflupane SPECT in the diagnosis of suspected psychogenic Parkinsonism. Mov Disord 2006;21(11):1994–1998.
120. Deuschl G, Raethjen J, Kopper F, et al. The diagnosis and physiology of psychogenic tremor. In Hallet M, Fahn S, Jankovic J, et al. (eds). Psychogenic Movement Disorders Neurology and Neuropsychiatry. Philadelphia: Lippincott Williams &Wilkins, 2006, pp. 265–273.
121. Brown P. Clinical neurophysiology of myoclonus. In Hallet M, Fahn S, Jankovic J, et al. (eds). Psychogenic Movement Disorders Neurology and Neuropsychiatry. Philadelphia: Lippincott Williams & Wilkins, 2006, pp. 131–143.
122. Obeso JA, Artieda J, Martinez-Lage JM. The physiology of myoclonus in man. In Quinn NP, Jenner PG (eds).

Disorders of Movement. Clinical, Pharmacological and Physiological Aspects. London: Academic Press, 1989, pp. 437–444.
123. Hallett M, Chadwick D, Marsden CD. Cortical reflex myoclonus. Neurology 1979;29:1107–1125.
124. Kang SY, Sohn YH. Electromyography patterns of propriospinal myoclonus can be mimicked voluntarily. Mov Disord 2006;21(8):1241–1244.
125. Thompson PD, Colebatch JG, Brown P, et al. Voluntary Stimulus-Sensitive Jerks and Jumps Mimicking Myoclonus or Pathological Startle Syndromes. Mov Disord 1992;7:257–262.
126. Terada K, Ikeda A, Van Ness PC, et al. Presence of Bereitschaftspotential preceding psychogenic myoclonus: clinical application of jerk-locked back averaging. J Neurol Neurosurg Psychiatry 1995;58:745–747.
127. Rothwell J. Cerebral Cortex. Control of Human Voluntary Movement. London: Chapman & Hall, 1994, pp. 293–386.
128. Shibasaki H, Sakai T, Nishimura H, et al. Involuntary movements in chorea-acanthocytosis: A comparison with Huntington's chorea. Ann Neurol 1982;12:311–314.
129. Shibasaki H, Nagae K. Mirror movement: application of movement-related cortical potentials. Ann Neurol 1984;15:299–302.
130. Cohen LG, Meer J, Tarkka I, et al. Congenital mirror movements: abnormal organization of motor pathways in two patients. Brain 1991;114:381–403.
131. Hallett MD. The Pathophysiology of Tics, Startle Reactions, and Other Complex Involuntary Movements. Motor Control. Seattle: American Academy of Neurology, 1995, pp. 77–92.
132. Matsumoto J, Hallett M. Startle syndromes. In Marsden CD, Fahn S (eds). Movement Disorders 3. Butterworth Heinemann, 1994, pp. 418–433.
133. Matsumoto J, Fuhr P, Nigro M, et al. Physiological abnormalities in hereditary hyperekplexia. Ann Neurol 1992;32:41–50.
134. Tijssen MA, Marsden JF, Brown P. Frequency analysis of EMG activity in patients with idiopathic torticollis. Brain 2000;123:677–686.
135. Brown P, Thompson PD. Electrophysiological aids to the diagnosis of psychogenic jerks, spasms, and tremor. Mov Disord 2001;16(4):595–599.
136. Espay AJ, Morgante F, Purzner J, et al. Cortical and spinal abnormalities in psychogenic dystonia. Ann Neurol 2006;59(5):825–834.
137. Manto MU. Discrepancy between dysmetric centrifugal movements and normometric centripetal movements in psychogenic ataxia. Eur Neurol 2001;45:261–265.
138. Markus AC. The ethics of placebo prescribing. Mt Sinai J Med 2000;67(2):140–143.
139. Bok S. The ethics of giving placebos. Sci Am 1974;231:17–23.
140. Lancman ME, Asconape JJ, Craven WJ, et al. Predictive value of induction of psychogenic seizures by suggestion. Ann Neurol 1994;35:359–361.
141. Levy RS, Jankovic J. Placebo-induced conversion reaction: A neurobehavioural and EEG study of hysterical aphasia, seizure, and coma. J Abnorm Psychol 1983;92:243–249.
142. Friedman WE, Rothner AD, Luders H, et al. Psychogenic seizures in children and adolescents. Outcome after diagnosis by ictal video and electroencephalographic recording. Pediatrics 1990;85:480–484.
143. Walczak TS, Williams DT, Berten W. Utility and reliability of placebo infusion in the evaluation of patients with seizures. Neurology 1994;44:394–399.
144. Ludlow CL, Martinez P, Braun AR, et al. Differential diagnosis between psychogenic and neurogenic dysphonias. Neurology 1995;45:A393.
145. Schneider SA, Bhatia KP. Sodium amytal and benzodiazepine interview and its possible application in psychogenic movement disorders. In Hallet M, Fahn S, Jankovic J, (eds). Psychogenic Parkinsonism Neurology and Neuropsychiatry. Philadelphia: Neurology Reference Series, 2006, pp. 249–255.
146. Mai FM. "Hysteria" in clinical neurology. Can J Neurol Sci 1995;22:101–110.
147. Williams DT, Ford B, Fahn S. Phenomenology and psychopathology related to psychogenic movement disorders. Adv Neurol 1995;65:231–258.
148. Gupta A, Lang AE. Psychogenic movement disorders. Curr Opin Neurol. 2009;(In Press)
149. Voon V, Lang AE. Antidepressant treatment outcomes of psychogenic movement disorder. J Clin Psychiatry 2005;66(12):1529–1534.
150. Moene FC, Spinhoven P, Hoogduin KA, et al. A randomised controlled clinical trial on the additional effect of hypnosis in a comprehensive treatment programme for in-patients with conversion disorder of the motor type. Psychother Psychosom 2002;71(2):66–76.
151. Anderson KE, GruberBaldini AL, Vaughan CG, et al. Impact of psychogenic movement disorders versus Parkinson's on disability, quality of life, and psychopathology. Movement Disord 2007;22(15):2204–2209.
152. McKeon A, Ahlskog JE, Bower JH, et al. Psychogenic tremor: long term prognosis in patients with electrophysiologically-confirmed disease. Mov Disord 2009;24(1):72–76.
153. Jankovic J, Vuong KD, Thomas M. Psychogenic tremor: long-term outcome. CNS Spectr 2006;11(7):501–508.
154. Couprie W, Wijdicks EFM, Rooijmans HGM, et al. Outcome in conversion disorder: a follow up study. J Neurol Neurosurg Psychiatry 1995;58:750–752.
155. Williams DT, Ford B, Fahn S. Phenomenology and psychopathology related to psychogenic movement disorders. In Weiner WJ, Lang AE (eds). Behavioural Neurology in Movement Disorders. New York: Raven Press, 1994, pp. 231–257.
156. Herz E. Dystonia II. Clinical classification. Arch Neurol Psychiat (Chicago) 1944;51:319–355.
157. Marsden CD, Harrison MJG. Idiopathic torsion dystonia (Dystonia Musculorum Deformans). A review of forty-two patients. Brain 1974;97:793–810.

CHAPTER 49

Systemic Illnesses that Cause Movement Disorders

Amy Colcher and Howard I. Hurtig

Movement disorders often complicate systemic illnesses. They occur in conjunction with metabolic encephalopathy, infection, neoplasms, and disorders of the endocrine, immune, and hematological systems. Movement disorders associated with systemic illness run the gamut from an exaggerated physiological tremor to hemiballismus, and also include the akinetic-rigid syndromes. In some cases, the movement disorder is what causes the patient to consult a physician. The underlying disorder may or may not be known at the time the movement disorder becomes obvious. In some cases, the pathophysiology of the systemic disorder causing the movement disorder is known. In some cases, there is a structural lesion in the brain responsible for the neurological problem. In other cases, there is no clear explanation for the movement disorder in the context of the systemic disease.

▶ ENDOCRINE DISORDERS

HYPERTHYROIDISM

Endocrine abnormalities are commonly recognized causes of hyperkinetic movement disorders. Hyperthyroidism is associated with an exaggerated physiological tremor. Up to 97% of patients with hyperthyroidism will exhibit a tremor,[1] the oscillatory frequency of which is the same as a physiological tremor, but the amplitude is greater. The hands are predominantly affected, although the feet, tongue, and eyelids can be affected as well. The pathophysiology is thought to be mediated by changes in peripheral β-adrenergic receptor tone. This theory is supported by the fact that β-blockers, including propranolol, will dampen the tremor. It is unclear whether there is a central generator for tremor. Positron emission tomography (PET) studies of patients with essential tremor reveal abnormal bilateral cerebellar, red nuclear, and thalamic activation.[2] When thyrotoxicosis is the etiology of the tremor, the tremor is reversible by returning thyroid function to normal.

Chorea is a rare complication of hyperthyroidism, occurring in less than 2% of patients with thyrotoxicosis.[1] The pathophysiology is not well understood, but the chorea is reversible with treatment of the hyperthyroidism.[1,3–5] Baba and colleagues described a young woman with unilateral chorea and thyrotoxicosis with normal computed tomography (CT), magnetic resonance imaging (MRI), and single-photon emission CT (SPECT) scans.[3] Autopsy studies of patients with hyperthyroid chorea reveal no pathological lesion within the basal ganglia.[1,6] Measurements of dopamine metabolites in the cerebrospinal fluid (CSF) of patients with and without hyperthyroidism reveal lower levels of homovanillic acid (HVA) in patients with hyperthyroidism than in normals.[6] Decreased HVA levels suggest an alteration in dopamine metabolism in hyperthyroid individuals.[6] Thyroid abnormalities may alter the sensitivity of dopaminergic receptors.[1,6] An alteration in basal ganglia metabolism or function, such as heightened sensitivity of dopamine receptors in the basal ganglia of hyperthyroid individuals, is one postulated mechanism for the chorea.[6] It is possible that there may need to be preexisting damage to the basal ganglia to predispose a hyperthyroid individual to develop chorea. Fischbeck and Layzer described a patient who had an anoxic event prior to the development of hyperthyroidism and later developed chorea.[7] The initial insult may have made the basal ganglia more susceptible to the altered receptor sensitivity induced by the change in thyroid function.[6] The chorea of hyperthyroidism is responsive to dopamine receptor-blocking agents such as haloperidol.

HYPOTHYROIDISM

Myxedema is associated with cerebellar dysfunction in a percentage of patients,[1] most of whom complain of unsteadiness,[8] difficulty walking, and incoordination. Examination of patients with these complaints reveals a truncal ataxia, although appendicular ataxia is also seen. Rare patients will exhibit dysarthria. A 3-Hz body oscillation has been described.[8] Dysfunction of the cerebellum or cerebellar connections is a postulated mechanism for the ataxia seen with myxedema. Autopsy of patients with myxedema and alcoholism reveal degeneration of the cerebellar cortex and glycogen-containing inclusions within cerebellar cortical neurons.[1] It is not clear that the pathology is related purely to the thyroid disorder. The ataxia improves as the patient becomes euthyroid.

DIABETES

Both hyper- and hypoglycemia have been reported as uncommon causes of choreoathetosis.[9,10] SPECT studies on a patient with hemichorea/hemiballism secondary to hyperglycemia reveal increased blood flow in the contralateral striatum and thalamus.[11] Haan's description of an 80-year-old woman who had paroxysmal choreoathetosis when her blood glucose was both high and low raises interesting questions about pathogenesis. A possible theory is that a prolonged blood glucose level resets the osmoreceptors in the brain, and any rapid change from that level is poorly tolerated.[12] Hyperglycemia without ketosis is a recognized cause of chorea. The chorea associated with blood glucose abnormalities may resolve with correction of the blood glucose, or it may be slow, taking months to resolve,[13] or it may be permanent.[14] The patients described with chorea associated with abnormal blood glucose have, for the most part, been elderly. A multifactorial etiology may play a role here in that some preexisting structural damage such as lacunar infarction or hemorrhage may be necessary to make the striatum more susceptible to the effects of hyperglycemia,[15] or an ischemic episode in small arterioles occurring at the time of the hyperglycemia may contribute.

HYPOPARATHYROIDISM

Hypoparathyroidism results in hypocalcemia, hypophosphatemia, and hypomagnesemia. Metabolic derangements, primarily hypocalcemia, are responsible for the frequently encountered neurological complications such as tetany, neuromuscular irritability, and seizures. Pseudohypoparathyroidism is a hereditary parathyroid resistance syndrome caused by a defect in the parathyroid hormone (PTH) receptor. Pseudohypoparathyroidism produces the same metabolic abnormalities in association with pathognomonic phenotypic changes such as short metacarpal bones, short stature, round face, mental retardation, dental abnormalities, and obesity. Inheritance is X-linked or autosomal-dominant. Most patients have a defect of the PTH receptor-adenylate cyclase system.[16] Calcifications of the basal ganglia are seen in the majority of patients with primary hypoparathyroidism.[17] Calcification, described as early as 1855, is not limited to the basal ganglia. It can be present in the cerebral hemispheres and in the dentate nucleus of the cerebellum.[16] Basal ganglia calcification does not correlate with the presence of movement disorders.[18] Chorea is a described complication of both hypoparathyroidism[19] and pseudohypoparathyroidism.[18]

Paroxysmal dystonias are seen in some metabolic disorders, including hypoparathyroidism and hyperthyroidism. Hypoparathyroidism with basal ganglia calcification has been associated with paroxysmal dystonic choreoathetosis.[20] This has been described infrequently, but seems to represent basal ganglia dysfunction secondary to disordered calcium metabolism.[21] The movement disorder responds to treatment of the underlying disorder with calciferol. The structural alterations in the basal ganglia from the calcification do not seem to be responsible for the dystonic syndrome, as the calcifications do not resolve with treatment of the hypoparathyroidism.

Parkinsonism can occur in the setting of hypoparathyroidism[22] and pseudohypoparathyroidism (4–12% of patients) with or without basal ganglia calcifications.[23] It has been reported to occur at ages ranging from 20 to 73 years. The pathogenesis of parkinsonism in these patients initially was presumed to result in some way from calcification in the basal ganglia, although cases without basal ganglia calcification have been reported. Evans and Donley hypothesize that parkinsonism may be related to a defect of G protein,[23] intermediaries in neurotransmission as well as hormonal neuromodulation. An alteration in G protein function could impair neurotransmission in the striatum and produce parkinsonism. Untreated hypoparathyroidism often results in basal ganglia calcification, but it is rare that it is associated with parkinsonism. When the two occur together it is usually in the setting of symptomatic hypocalcemia. In this setting, the parkinsonism is slowly progressive, as in idiopathic Parkinson's disease (PD), and is responsive to L-dopa therapy. Cases have been described without symptomatic hypocalcemia in which the parkinsonism was responsive to vitamin D, calcium, and magnesium replacement.[22]

▶ METABOLIC/NUTRITIONAL DISORDERS

TETRAHYDROBIOPTERIN DEFICIENCY

Tetrahydrobiopterin (BH_4) is a cofactor necessary for the enzymatic synthesis of biogenic amines. Deficiency states lead to defective production of serotonin and catecholamines in addition to hyperphenylalaninemia. Symptoms occur in infancy and include developmental delay, seizures, hypotonia, and dystonia. Three patients have been reported with tremor and orofacial dyskinesias as presenting symptoms. In the case described by Factor and colleagues an episodic high-amplitude coarse flapping tremor initially appeared at 3 months of age and recurred twice before 6 months.[24] Each episode lasted several hours and improved with sedation. The tremor was present both at rest and with action. The child was also found to be hypotonic. Treatment with L-dopa led to cessation of the movements. Improvement was seen within 24 hours, and further development was normal when followed up at 18 months. The significant improvement with L-dopa implies that the pathogenesis of movement disorders associated with BH_4 deficiency relates to insufficient dopamine synthesis.

MALABSORPTION SYNDROMES

Any disease that causes fat malabsorption or steatorrhea has the potential to cause tocopherol (vitamin E) deficiency. Deficiency of tocopherol must be present for years before neurological sequelae are evident. The associated syndrome of spinocerebellar ataxia and peripheral neuropathy may resemble B_{12} deficiency. Patients are dysarthric with oculomotor abnormalities, ataxia, and position and vibratory sense loss. Pathologically there is a loss of myelinated nerve fibers in the posterior columns and central nervous system (CNS). Ataxia has been reported in patients with cystic fibrosis, chronic cholestasis, after small bowel resection, blind loop syndromes, and intestinal lymphangiectasia in addition to other malabsorption syndromes.[25]

HEPATIC FAILURE

Hepatic failure is a well-known cause of tremor, asterixis, and other involuntary movements. Asterixis is seen in the setting of an underlying encephalopathy and can be associated with metabolic derangements secondary to failure of various organ systems. It is encountered in hepatic encephalopathy, uremia, hypercarbia, alcohol withdrawal, cardiac failure, sepsis, and sometimes as a result of the treatment used for these disorders, such as hemodialysis.[26] The mechanism of pathogenesis is unknown. Asterixis can be caused by a variety of focal lesions in the thalamus (especially the ventrolateral portion), midbrain, parietal cortex, and medial frontal cortex,[26] but in cases of encephalopathy no structural lesion is evident on imaging studies. In most cases, electroencephalography reveals diffuse rather than focal brain disturbance.[27] MRI scans can show increased signal on T_1-weighted images of the caudate. Generalized myoclonus, ataxia, and chorea can be seen in the setting of hepatic or renal failure.[27]

KWASHIORKOR

Kwashiorkor is a nutritional deficiency of protein and calories, which can produce movement disorders. Kwashiorkor can produce a combination of myoclonus, rigidity, and bradykinesia.[28] Tremors are also apparent in children when they are treated for malnutrition.[28,29]

ALCOHOLISM

A tremor can be prominent among alcoholics when they are not actively drinking or are withdrawing from alcohol. The alcoholic tremor is postural, usually mild, and it causes little if any functional limitation. It is often of a higher frequency than essential tremor, the majority of patients having a tremor frequency of less than 7 Hz,[30] although patterns similar to those seen with essential tremor are described. Postural tremor with a frequency of 6–11-Hz can be seen. The tremor of chronic alcoholism has two components. There is a 4–7-Hz peak and a 9.4–9.6-Hz peak. Increasing the speed of movement of the arm decreases the low-frequency peak without changing the high-frequency peak. Increasing effort increases the amplitude of the low-frequency peak.[31] The tremor of chronic alcoholism is usually asymmetric and can persist for years during complete abstinence. Treatment with β-blockers is usually effective.

A second type of tremor that is seen in alcoholics is a 3-Hz tremor of the legs. The tremor is slow and rhythmic, involves flexion and extension of the muscles of the hip girdle, and can affect the gait. It does not disappear with cessation of alcohol consumption.[32]

Transient parkinsonism has been described in intoxicated patients or within days of the last drink.[33,34] Symptoms include bradykinesia, shuffling gait, stooped posture, cogwheel rigidity, and resting tremor. The condition is self-limited and usually resolves within a few weeks.[32] Alcohol causes decreased dopamine release, and this may explain the parkinsonism.[35]

Alcoholic cerebellar degeneration is a well-known complication of alcohol abuse. It is postulated to be nutritional in origin. PET scans of ataxic patients reveal hypometabolism in the superior vermis.[36] MRI reveals atrophy of the cerebellar vermis, and, when severe, the cerebellar hemispheres. Pathologically, there is degeneration of the anterior superior aspect of the cerebellar vermis, and, when severe, atrophy of the cerebellar hemispheres. There is a striking loss of Purkinje cells as well as other neural cells.

KERNICTERUS

Prolonged untreated hyperbilirubinemia in the perinatal period damages nuclei of the basal ganglia, especially the globus pallidus and subthalamic nucleus. The cerebellum and the auditory and vestibular pathways are also involved. Children may show signs of damage early with high-tone hearing loss, dysarthria, and athetosis. Usually symptomatic children will have delayed motor development and show signs of dystonia, choreoathetosis, tremor, and rigidity by the time they are 10 years old.[37] Other

▶ **TABLE 49–1. METABOLIC DISORDERS OF CHILDHOOD THAT CAUSE DYSTONIA**

Hexosaminidase A and B deficiency
GM1 and GM2 gangliosidosis
Phenylketonuria
Triose phosphate isomerase deficiency
Tetrahydrobiopterin deficiency
Metachromatic leukodystrophy
Glutaric acidemia
Methylmalonic acidemia
Wilson's disease
Homocystinuria
Pyruvate decarboxylase deficiency
D-Glyceric acidemia
Lesch–Nyhan's syndrome
Ceroid lipofuscinosis
Hartnup's disease

children may be asymptomatic, and dystonia can occur up to 20 years after the initial insult.[38] In children who die early in the course of the disease, pathological findings reveal yellow staining of the subthalamic nucleus, Ammon's horn, globus pallidus, dentate nucleus, and olives. In children who live longer these areas reveal cell loss, demyelination, and gliosis.[37]

HOMOCYSTINURIA

Many metabolic disorders of childhood have dystonia as a prominent symptom. These will not all be discussed here but are listed in Table 49–1.

Homocystinuria is not commonly associated with dystonia, but the combination has been described. A deficiency of cystathione synthetase leads to a buildup of homocysteine and methionine. Patients generally are mentally retarded, have lens dislocations, seizures, bony abnormalities, and are predisposed to strokes. In a report of two sisters, symptoms began at ages 3 and 4, with dysarthria in one and foot inversion in the other.[39] Dystonia progressed over the next few years until it was generalized and both girls severely disabled. MRI studies revealed bilateral low-intensity lesions in the basal ganglia on T_2 imaging. Other patients with dystonia had later onset of dystonic symptoms, starting in the teenage years.[38] Other patients described had typical features of homocystinuria, which the two sisters did not. As homocystinuria is associated with thromboembolic events, it is possible that the dystonia is secondary to basal ganglia infarcts.[38] Others postulate that a neurochemical derangement (i.e., a defect in sulfur amino acid metabolism) is responsible.[39]

▶ HEMATOLOGICAL DISORDERS

POLYCYTHEMIA

Polycythemia vera usually has its onset in middle age. There is an increase in all myeloid elements, although the increase in hemoglobin concentration is the primary hematological manifestation of this disease. Neurological symptoms are primarily related to increased blood volume and viscosity. These include headache, dizziness, visual changes, and syncope.[40] Chorea occurs in less than 1% of patients with polycythemia vera and is more common in females than males.[6] It is usually bilaterally symmetrical and can be short-lived, lasting only weeks, or persistent. Two thirds of patients who have chorea in the setting of polycythemia do not know that they have polycythemia when the chorea is initially evaluated, although the associated symptoms of a ruddy complexion and splenomegaly are often seen.

The pathophysiology of polycythemic chorea is unclear. Some patients have a history of rheumatic fever in childhood, which may in some way predispose them to the development of chorea later on. Hyperviscosity due to the polycythemia can lead to small infarctions or hemorrhage in the basal ganglia, especially the caudate and putamen. Neuropathological specimens support this, although demyelination in the interior globus pallidus has also been reported.[3] Treatment of the polycythemia is not always correlated with amelioration of the chorea. A presynaptic catechol-depleting drug such as reserpine or tetrabenazine is the treatment of choice, although dopamine receptor-blocking agents (neuroleptics) may be required in resistant cases.

MASTOCYTOSIS

Mastocytosis is a hematological disorder in which mast cells proliferate and deposit themselves in various tissues in the body. Most often their distribution is limited to cutaneous structures. CNS dysfunction has been reported with systemic mastocytosis, but usually takes the form of headache, seizures, and encephalopathy. One case of chorea has been described in association with this disorder in a 13-year-old girl.[41] The chorea resolved spontaneously within 5 days and did not recur. According to one theory of pathogenesis, mast cells release various substances (histamine, prostaglandins, and other peptide mediators), which induce alterations in the basal ganglia neurotransmission. This may be responsible for the chorea.

▶ INFECTION

SYDENHAM'S CHOREA

Sydenham's chorea (SC), a sequela of infection with group A streptococcus, is the most celebrated example of a movement disorder resulting from an infection. Chorea occurs 1–6 months after the initial febrile illness, which most often presents with pharyngitis. The onset is usually insidious, progressing over weeks to months. Women are more often affected than men. The movements are usually bilateral, but can be unilateral, and the face is usually involved. Dysarthria and hypotonia are frequently seen. Behavioral changes include psychosis, irritability, confusion, and obsessive–compulsive disorder (OCD).[42] These symptoms usually begin several days to weeks before the onset of the chorea. The behavioral as well as the motoric symptoms can wax and wane during the course of the syndrome.[42] Antineuronal antibodies are present in the majority of children affected. The initial bout of chorea is self-limiting, but recurrences are well documented, independent of the natural history of rheumatic fever, which is, for the most part, a monophasic illness. Recurrences usually occur within 2 years of the initial chorea.[43] SC is known to recur during pregnancy in women who have had rheumatic fever as a child[43] and in patients who later take medications such as oral contraceptives and phenytoin.[43]

Few PET studies have been done on patients with SC. Weindl and colleagues, using two patients, found increased striatal regional cerebral glucose consumption in both patients.[44] This study was done without age-matched controls.

Circulating antibodies to brain and cardiolipin have been described in association with SC. Streptococcal proteins can induce antibodies that will cross-react with human brain.[45] Others have reported finding IgG antibodies that cross-react with nuclear protein of caudate and subthalamus.[46] This may begin to explain the pathophysiology of SC. Figueroa and colleagues found that 80% of patients with acute rheumatic fever had anticardiolipin antibodies during an acute attack.[47] There was no difference in the percentage of patients with antibodies when comparing those with SC (76%) and those without chorea (83%). All patients with cardiac valvular abnormalities had antibodies.

The neuropathology in patients with SC is not specific. There are reports of a broad spectrum of abnormalities, including hemorrhage, inflammation, and vasculopathy.[6]

SC is self-limited in most cases. Therefore, treatment with dopamine blockers, which may have permanent tardive sequelae, should be avoided unless the chorea is incapacitating. Presynaptic dopamine-depleting agents (reserpine and tetrabenazine) can be used. There is no treatment that has been proven to shorten the course of the chorea.

Poststreptococcal autoimmune movement disorders have also been described. The most controversial of these is pediatric autoimmune neuropsychiatric disorders associated with streptococcal infection (PANDAS).[48] Symptoms of PANDAS closely resemble Tourette's syndrome (see Chapter 40). Children develop complex motor and vocal tics associated with behavioral abnormalities, weeks to months after a streptococcal infection. Behavioral abnormalities include OCD, ritualistic behaviors, attention deficit hyperactivity disorders (ADHD), oppositional behavior, nightmares, sleep disturbance. The onset of symptoms is acute, and the symptoms follow a relapsing remitting course. More recently, a case of paroxysmal dystonic choreoathetosis has been described in a poststreptococcal setting.[49] Symptoms in this case were the acute onset of dystonic posturing, choreoathetosis, visual hallucinations, and behavioral disturbance. Episodes lasted from 10 minutes to 4 hours. Symptoms continued with variable severity for 6 months. MRI of the brain was normal. Antibodies to basal ganglia structures were detected.

LYME DISEASE

Lyme disease, which in the last decade has become the great imitator, can produce chorea along with a myriad of other neurological abnormalities.[50] The disease is transmitted through the bite of the deer tick *Ixodes dammini*. The causative organism is a spirochete, *Borrelia burgdorferi*. The initial manifestation is usually an expanding red rash (erythema chronicum migrans). As the rash expands, the center clears, creating the appearance of a target. The rash occurs most commonly 1–3 weeks after the tick bite. At the time of the rash, constitutional symptoms, headache, fever, arthralgias, and myalgias may occur. Secondary Lyme disease causes myocarditis, cranial neuritis, and myositis. Stage 3 or chronic Lyme disease occurs months after the initial onset and may persist for years. Clinical findings associated with this stage are arthritis, myositis, peripheral neuropathies, chronic meningitis, and acrodermatitis chronica atrophicans. Cranial nerve palsies are common, including facial diplegia. Patients with meningitis will have positive CSF antibody to *B. burgdorferi*.[51] Serological testing for Lyme disease (ELISA and indirect fluorescent antibody staining) should be positive in most cases of disseminated Lyme infection.[52] False-positive tests do occur in patients with other infections (syphilis), autoimmune disorders (systemic lupus erythematosus, SLE), and some malignancies.[51] A Western blot analysis should be done to confirm the diagnosis before therapy is initiated. MRI findings in patients with focal CNS findings reveal white matter changes representing leukoencephalitis, which can improve with antibiotic therapy.[53] Movement disorders have been reported in the setting of Lyme disease.[50] Chorea and synkinesis are associated with encephalitis.[53] Cerebellar ataxia also has been described.[53] These symptoms usually improve with treatment of the underlying infection and/or with steroids.

HIV-1

A tremor at rest resembling a parkinsonian tremor is seen in the HIV-1-associated cognitive motor complex.

The resting tremor and slowness of movement parallel the slowness in thought processing associated with HIV-1 dementia. Pathological studies reveal white matter pallor, reactive gliosis, and microglial nodules. The caudate, putamen, and pons are involved early, and cortical structures later.[54] Parkinsonism is seen as part of the HIV-cognitive-motor complex. Patients manifest psychomotor slowing, bradykinesia, bradyphrenia, stooped posture, shuffling gait, and postural instability clinically similar to that seen in PD.[55] It appears from primate models that there is early dopaminergic cell loss in HIV-infected patients.[56] Highly active antiretroviral therapy may improve symptoms.[57,58] Imaging should be performed on patients presenting with parkinsonism as structural lesions need to be excluded. Cerebral toxoplasmosis in combination with HIV infection is another rare cause of parkinsonism. A woman with enhancing lesions in the anterior limb of both internal capsules was found to have decreased facial expression, cogwheel rigidity, monotone speech, and drooling.[59] Toxoplasmosis was found in these lesions. Neither antitoxoplasmosis therapy nor L-dopa/carbidopa combinations improved her condition. Bradykinesia, rigidity, facial masking and grimacing, and gait instability were described in a young girl with HIV and progressive multifocal leukoencephalopathy (PML).[60] MRI lesions involved the basal ganglia and deep white matter, centrum semiovale, and corona radiata and enhanced slightly with the administration of gadolinium. Brain biopsy in this case revealed demyelination, Alzheimer type 1 astrocytes, and intranuclear eosinophilic inclusions within oligodendroglial cells. The biopsy as well as the CSF and blood were positive for JC virus by polymerase chain reaction (PCR). A patient with granulomas in the basal ganglia was also described.[61]

HIV can cause movement disorders, as can the opportunistic infections associated with it. Toxoplasmosis, the most common opportunistic infection causing neurological symptoms in HIV-positive patients, has been associated with akathisia, chorea, athetosis, and hemiballism, especially when the lesions are in the basal ganglia.[59] When ring-enhancing lesions are seen on CT or MRI, empiric antitoxoplasmosis therapy is indicated. If treatment causes resolution of the lesions on imaging studies, but the movement disorder persists, treatment with dopamine-depleting or -blocking agents may become necessary. In general, patients without HIV infection who have cerebral toxoplasmosis do not have movement disorders associated with it.[59] There may be an interaction between the two infections, making HIV-positive patients more susceptible to developing a movement disorder when they are coinfected with toxoplasmosis.

Cerebral toxoplasmosis has also been associated with dystonia. Nath and colleagues described a man with HIV and toxoplasmosis who presented with dystonic posturing of the left arm.[59] An enhancing lesion was seen on CT scan in the right globus pallidus and right thalamus. In this case, the dystonia was not improved by treatment of the toxoplasmosis.

Paroxysmal dyskinesias have been reported in association with HIV infection.[62] Both kinesogenic and nonkinesogenic chorea have been described. Associated myoclonus, tremor, and dysarthria were seen. In some patients dystonic posturing was evident. Gliosis and neuronal loss in the subcortical gray matter was found on autopsy of one patient with nonkinesogenic dyskinesia. Chorea itself can be the result of structural lesions such as PML or toxoplasmosis, bacterial encephalitis, or direct HIV infection.[63]

ENCEPHALITIS

Mycoplasma is a microorganism that accounts for a large number of cases of pneumonia each year. Uncommon complications of infection with this organism include myopathy and encephalitis. Beskind and Keim described a boy with encephalitis who presented with acute choreoathetosis, dysarthria, and fever who was found to have serological evidence of *Mycoplasma pneumoniae* infection.[64] Choreoathetosis and hemiballismus are rarely associated with encephalitis of viral etiology. This may be a direct result of the infection or a postinfectious phenomenon.[65] The movements may be difficult to control, necessitating the use of dopamine-depleting agents (reserpine).

WHIPPLE'S DISEASE

Whipple's disease (WD) is an infectious disease of the small intestine, causing malabsorption, lymphadenopathy, arthritis, and neurological symptoms. Gastrointestinal manifestations usually bring the patient to medical attention. These include diarrhea, steatorrhea, abdominal pain, and weight loss. WD and its symptoms respond to antibiotics if therapy is initiated early in the course of the illness. The pathology in the small intestine reveals periodic acid-Schiff (PAS)-positive macrophages and Gram-positive bacilli. Neurological complications of WD occur in 10% of patients,[66] including encephalopathy, myoclonus, seizures, tremor, and ophthalmoplegia. A dystonic syndrome characterized by involuntary bruxism[67] and abnormalities of extraocular movement has been designated an oculomasticatory myorhythmia (OMM).[36] Myorhythmia is a repetitive, regular 2–4-Hz involuntary movement affecting the face (lips, chin, and jaw) and neck. Myorhythmia in WD occurs in conjunction with cognitive deterioration and ophthalmoparesis.[68] Neurological symptoms occur late in the disease and generally indicate a poor prognosis. OMM can improve with antibiotic therapy. Neurological sequelae can occur even after successful treatment of the gastrointestinal symptoms with antibiotics. This may be due to poor CNS penetration of some antibiotics. Penicillin, trimethoprim–sulfamethoxazole, and streptomycin should be used. There is a high incidence of CNS relapse, so antibiotic therapy should be continued for a prolonged course of many months.[25] Patients have been reported with neurological symptoms and no gastrointestinal complaints.[69] In patients with OMM, WD should be suspected with or without gastrointestinal symptoms.

Pathological studies of patients with WD affecting the nervous system have revealed nodules and granulomas throughout the brain. Locations include the cortex, basal ganglia, cerebellum, hypothalamus. Cases of WD with myorhythmia are rare and consistent clinicopathological correlation has not been done.

Eye movement abnormalities in the form of supranuclear gaze palsies without myorhythmia have been described in patients with WD.[70] One patient described had rigidity and bradykinesia similar to that seen in progressive supranuclear palsy.[71]

HEMOLYTIC–UREMIC SYNDROME

Hemolytic–Uremic syndrome (HUS) is a postviral illness causing acute renal failure in children and adults. Hemolytic anemia, thrombocytopenic purpura, and oliguric renal failure are the major components of the illness, which mimics thrombocytopenic thrombotic purpura. CNS involvement in HUS is uncommon and can cause seizures, encephalopathy, and stroke. Pathological studies in these patients reveal multiple small infarctions secondary to the ischemic effect of small arteriolar thrombi. Dystonia has been described in association with seizures in HUS.[72]

SARCOIDOSIS

Sarcoidosis is a systemic granulomatous disease without known etiology. Granulomas form in various organ systems, resulting in a varied clinical picture. CNS involvement is rare. Most patients with neurological symptoms have evidence of sarcoidosis in other organ systems (i.e., hilar adenopathy, hypercalcemia, or anergy). As in polycythemia, neurological symptoms can be the reason the patient seeks medical attention. Sarcoid most often causes meningitis, primarily at the base of the brain, affecting cranial nerves, hypothalamus, and the pituitary.[73] Facial nerve palsies and optic neuritis are the most common cranial neuropathies. Movement disorders can take the form of chorea and hemiballismus if granulomas infiltrate the basal ganglia.[73] Myelopathy and myopathy can also occur.

Neurosarcoid can produce akinetic-rigid syndromes or parkinsonism. Schlegel and colleagues reported a case of cerebral sarcoidosis that presented with vertical gaze palsy, bradykinesia, and rest tremors.[74] The patient had had systemic sarcoidosis for 11 years before these symptoms became apparent. The parkinsonism and gaze palsy resolved with the use of corticosteroids and antiparkinson medications. Treatment of neurosarcoidosis usually requires the temporary use of corticosteroids. The response of the movement disorder to this treatment is variable.

One concept of pathogenesis is that basilar meningitis leads to obstructive hydrocephalus, which compresses the tectal region of the brainstem and nuclei in the basal ganglia causing upgaze palsy and parkinsonism, respectively. This is a rare complication of neurosarcoidosis. Other reports of sarcoidosis causing parkinsonism have noted granulomatous infiltration of the basal ganglia.[73]

▶ AUTOIMMUNE DISORDERS

AUTOIMMUNE DISEASE

Autoimmune diseases have also been reported to cause dystonic syndromes. Craniocervical dystonia (Meige's syndrome) was described in a patient with rheumatoid arthritis and Sjögren's syndrome. Other combinations of autoimmune disease and cranial dystonia have been described.[75] Patients with myasthenia gravis have been reported to have coexistent dystonic syndromes.[76] Autoimmune thyroid disease also has an unusually high association with dystonia.[77] In two cases of blepharospasm described by Jankovic and Patten, one with SLE and the other with myasthenia, both cases responded to immunosuppressive therapy.[78] The mechanism underlying blepharospasm and other dystonic disorders in the setting of autoimmune disease is unclear.

SJÖGREN'S SYNDROME

Sjögren's syndrome (SS) is an immune-mediated disorder in which salivary and lacrimal glands are destroyed, resulting in mucosal and conjunctival dryness (the sicca syndrome). Xerostomia, xerophthalmia, and conjunctivitis are the principal manifestations. Other organs can be involved, including kidney, lungs, and blood vessels. SS is often associated with other autoimmune diseases. The most common neurological manifestations are mononeuritis multiplex, peripheral neuropathy, and myositis. CNS dysfunction has been reported and can be either focal or diffuse. Some patients have anti-Ro (SS-A) antibodies that are directed against a 60-kDa peptide and may be implicated in the production of a small vessel angiitis.[79] Cerebellar degeneration has been described in association with SS. In one reported case of SS, antineuronal antibodies were found.[80] These antibodies stained cytoplasmic elements in the cerebellum and hippocampus primarily. The antibodies found in this patient were not anti-Yo or anti-Hu antibodies, although they were similarly immunoreactive. The patient described improved after immunosuppression with corticosteroids. Parkinsonism has also been described in association with SS.[81] MRI in this case showed increased signal on T_2-weighted images in the pons and basal ganglia. The parkinsonism did not respond to treatment with L-dopa, but did respond to immunosuppression with corticosteroids. Chorea has also been described at a manifestation of SS in a limited number of case reports.[82,83] Generalized chorea has been reported with sudden onset. The chorea in these patients did not respond to immunosuppression to treat the SS, but rather to dopamine-blocking medications.

SYSTEMIC LUPUS ERYTHEMATOSUS

SLE is an autoimmune disease that affects multiple organ systems, including both the CNS and the peripheral nervous system. Chorea is by far the most common movement disorder associated with SLE[5] (see Chapter 37). Involuntary movements account for 2% of all neurological symptoms in SLE and frequently precede the diagnosis of lupus. The patients who develop chorea are usually young and female. Chorea may be intermittent or persistent and is usually unilateral, although it can be generalized. The pathology is inconsistent, although widespread microinfarcts are the classic pathological hallmark of CNS SLE. There is no consistent change in the basal ganglia. PET scans do not reveal any change in striatal glucose metabolism that could be responsible for the chorea. Antiphospholipid antibodies are seen in 45–70% of patients with SLE, but they can occur without other findings of lupus in primary antiphospholipid antibody syndrome[84] (see below). The lupus anticoagulant is any phospholipid antibody that prolongs the phospholipid-dependent coagulation steps when there is not a coagulation factor deficiency. The antiphospholipid antibody reacts with the platelet membrane and leads to recurrent thrombotic events. Blepharospasm and torticollis have been described in the setting of SLE.[85] The clinicopathological correlation is not known, but vasculitis involving the brainstem and diencephalon is one postulated mechanism.[78] As in SC, another postulated mechanism is the cross-reactivity of antibodies with neurons.[85]

ANTIPHOSPHOLIPID ANTIBODY SYNDROME

Antiphospholipid antibody syndrome is a condition in which antibodies that bind to the negatively charged phospholipids in the membrane of endothelial cells somehow cause recurrent arterial and venous thrombotic and embolic events. The syndrome is clinically expressed by thrombocytopenia, spontaneous abortion, thromboembolism, and chorea.[84] In SLE, imaging studies of the brain do not reveal infarcts in the basal ganglia in patients with chorea in spite of the frequency of infarction in this patient population as a whole. In some cases, an embolic source is identified, such as a cardiac valvular vegetation, and an infarct can be demonstrated on brain imaging studies. Kirk and Harding reported a patient with antiphospholipid antibody and chorea who had an infarct in the head of the caudate.[86] Recent PET studies in patients with antiphospholipid antibody syndrome using ^{18}F-fluorodeoxyglucose revealed contralateral striatal hypermetabolism.[87] Scans were done when the patient had chorea and later when the chorea had resolved. The hypermetabolism was present regardless of the presence of chorea. Chorea can occur in association with anticardiolipin antibodies with or without the associated thromboembolic events.

GLUTEN ENTEROPATHY

Gluten ataxia is now recognized as a form of episodic ataxia.[88,89] Testing patients with genetically confirmed or familial ataxias also yields 14% serum positivity for antigliadin antibodies.[90] Only one in eight patients with gluten sensitivity will present with gastrointestinal symptomatology. A rash, dermatitis herpetiformis, or neurological symptoms, most commonly ataxia, may be the presenting complaints. The mean age of onset is 48 years. Symptoms include eye movement disturbance, slow saccades or gaze-evoked nystagmus, dysarthria, limb ataxia, and gait disorder. MRI reveals cerebellar atrophy in most patients and white matter hyperintensity in a few patients. Sensorimotor axonal neuropathy was found on EMG (electromyography) evaluation in 45% of patients. Duodenal biopsy yields the typical pathology of celiac disease in less than a quarter of patients. Antigliadin antibodies are seen in 12% of the population at large. Pathological specimens show perivascular cuffing with both CD4 and CD8 cells in the white matter of the cerebellum. There was also significant Purkinje cell loss. This does have implications for treatment.[91] Ataxia for the most part is not amenable to therapeutic intervention. Patients with antigliadin antibodies may benefit from a gluten-free diet with resultant improvement in their symptoms. Further study is needed.

▶ PREGNANCY

This heading does not imply that pregnancy is a systemic illness; rather, it is a systemic change from a woman's usual state that makes a woman susceptible to particular illnesses. Chorea gravidarum (CG) is a rare example of a movement disorder that occurs during pregnancy. The term does not specify etiology and is clinically indistinguishable from any other kind of chorea. CG occurs most frequently in young women during first pregnancies. Half of the cases will start in the first trimester and one-third in the second trimester.[92] The majority of women with CG have previously had chorea due to SC prior to pregnancy; it spontaneously remits in about a third. In the rest, the chorea will last until the child is born. In about one fifth of patients, the chorea will recur with subsequent pregnancies. SLE, which can also be worsened by pregnancy, can be responsible for CG in some cases.

▶ NEOPLASMS

Cerebellar dysfunction is seen in systemic illness, most commonly in the form of pancerebellar degeneration, one of the paraneoplastic syndromes. This syndrome can occur with any malignancy, but is most often associated with small cell lung cancer, ovarian cancer, and Hodgkin's lymphoma. The paraneoplastic cerebellar syndrome frequently precedes the diagnosis of cancer.

The ataxia in this syndrome usually has a subacute onset that may begin with dizziness, nausea, and vomiting, and progress to truncal and gait ataxia to dysarthria, diplopia, dysphagia, and limb ataxia over a few months. Frequently the neurological deficit stabilizes, but the patient may remain significantly impaired. Treatment of the underlying malignancy is rarely helpful.

Pathologically there is cerebellar atrophy with almost total loss of Purkinje cells in the cerebellum. There is thinning of the molecular layer with gliosis, and mild thinning of the granular layer. The deep cerebellar nuclei show inflammatory infiltrates and gliosis. Other areas of the CNS may be affected, including the corticospinal tracts, dorsal columns, and spinocerebellar tracts, which show varying degrees of degeneration. Patchy demyelination is seen in the brainstem, spinal cord, and dorsal root ganglia.[93]

In some patients, antibodies associated with the underlying malignancy cross-react with Purkinje cells and result in their destruction.[94,95] These antibodies bind to membrane-bound and free ribosomes within the Purkinje cell.[96] A putative protein kinase C substrate protein has been detected in some patients with paraneoplastic cerebellar degeneration.[97] Anti-Yo antibodies are present in the serum and CSF of some patients.[98] The onset of this syndrome is similar to patients without antibodies in that the syndrome is subacute, progressing over a few weeks. These patients typically have ataxia of the trunk and limbs, dysarthric speech, and nystagmus.[98] Common malignancies associated with the anti-Yo antibody are, in order of frequency, ovarian, breast, endometrial, and adenocarcinoma with unknown primary. In the majority of patients, the neurological symptoms precede the diagnosis of cancer. Neuropathological findings in these patients reveal critical atrophy of the cerebellum with reduction in the number of Purkinje cells as in antibody-negative cases.

Treatment of the underlying malignancy rarely will improve the ataxia. Plasmapheresis to remove the anti-Yo antibody does not usually improve the ataxia.[98] Corticosteroids and immunosuppression have not been beneficial. It is not clear how the anti-Yo antibody causes cerebellar disease.

Hodgkin's disease is also associated with cerebellar degeneration.[99] In most of these patients, the cerebellar syndrome begins after the diagnosis of lymphoma. The onset of the ataxia is sudden or subacute. Gait instability is the most common complaint, followed by limb ataxia and truncal ataxia. Nystagmus and dysarthria are frequently present in this syndrome, especially downbeat nystagmus. Some of these patients have anti-Purkinje cell antibodies.[99] Anti-Tr antibodies have been detected in some patients.[100] This adds support to an autoimmune mechanism as there are similar antigens in both Purkinje cells and T-lymphocytes.[99] The patients with Hodgkin's disease have had more variable responses to treatment of their malignancies. Some patients will stabilize, some recover, and some recover and then remit.

Opsoclonus–myoclonus syndrome associated with malignancies is more commonly seen in children, but has been described in adults. Opsoclonus, or rapid multidirectional saccades, is associated with ataxia and myoclonus. Associated adult malignancies include lung and breast cancer.[101] Anti-Ri antibodies are associated with breast and gynecological malignancies. Anti-Hu, anti-Yo, and anti-Ma2 antibodies have also been described. Pathology is variable, with some specimens showing normal findings and others with Purkinje cell loss and degeneration with inflammatory infiltrates in the brainstem and basilar meninges. The prognosis in adults is poor if the tumor is untreated. Patients progress to encephalopathy, coma, and death. The syndrome itself may respond to treatment with steroids or intravenous immunoglobulin (IVIG).

In children, the most frequent associate malignancy is neuroblastoma; 50% of children with opsoclonus myoclonus have neuroblastoma. Median age of onset of symptoms is 18 months. The syndrome is seen in conjunction with hypotonia, ataxia, and irritability. Treatment of the underlying malignancy is helpful as are immunosuppressive therapies including ACTH (adrenocorticotrophic hormone), steroids, and IVIG. Unfortunately, even though the opsoclonus and myoclonus may resolve, the majority of children are left with psychomotor retardation, behavioral difficulties, and sleep disturbance. Relapses of the opsoclonus–myoclonus syndrome have been reported in 68% of patients in one study.[102]

Stiff-man syndrome presents as severe rigidity affecting the axial muscles, as well as spasms triggered by sensory and emotional stimuli. The spasms can be severe and painful. Most commonly the symptoms affect the leg and lower trunk, but neck and arm symptoms have been reported. EMG studies are helpful, demonstrating continuous motor unit activity. Antibodies have been described to cytoplasmic proteins that are associated with GABA (γ-aminobutyric acid)-glycine synapses.[103] Most common are anti-amphiphysin antibodies, but anti-gephyrin antibodies have been described.[104] The most common associated malignancies are breast, lung, colon, and Hodgkin's lymphoma. The pathology in this disorder involves inhibitory interneurons in the spinal cord, vacuolar degeneration or motor neurons, and inflammatory infiltrates.[105] Treatment includes benzodiazepines, baclofen, valproate, steroids, and treatment of the underlying malignancy.

Chorea has been described associated with the anti-Hu antibody syndrome.[106] It is very rare. MRI abnormalities such as caudate atrophy or hyperintensity in the neostriatum can be seen, but in some cases the MRI is normal. In all reported cases the chorea preceded the diagnosis of the malignancy. In most cases the underlying malignancy was small cell lung cancer. Chorea in these patients varied in severity. Generalized chorea has been reported as well as oral, buccal, lingual chorea, and hemiballismus. It can be associated with dystonia, ataxia, visual loss, and encephalitis. Some cases improved with chemotherapy IVIG or dopamine blockers. Some patients with anti-Hu antibodies also had CRMP-5 neuronal antibodies, but this can be the only antibody found in some patients with chorea.[107] In this syndrome patients can present with involuntary movements. Chorea can be asymmetrical, generalized, affecting only the face with resultant dysarthria, or combined with dystonia. Basal ganglia abnormalities can be seen on MRI in some patients with increased T_2 signal in the caudate and putamen.[107] Small cell lung cancer is the most common malignancy. A subset of patients responded to chemotherapy, and a few to steroids with improvement in their chorea.

REFERENCES

1. Swanson JW, Kelly JJ Jr, McConahey WM. Neurologic aspects of thyroid dysfunction. Mayo Clin Proc. 1981 Aug; 56(8):504–512.
2. Wills AJ, Jenkins IH, Thompson PD, et al. A positron emission tomography study of cerebral activation associated with essential and writing tremor. Arch Neurol 1995;52:299.
3. Baba M, Terada A, Hishida R, et al. Persistent hemichorea associated with thyrotoxicosis. Intern Med 1992;31:1144.
4. Lucantoni C, Grottoli S, Moretti A. Chorea due to hyperthyroidism in old age. A case report. Acta Neurol (Napoli) 1994;16:129.
5. Pozzan GB, Battistella PA, Rigon F, et al. Hyperthyroid-induced chorea in an adolescent girl. Brain Dev 1992;14:126.
6. Weiner WJ. Movement Disorders: A Comprehensive Survey. Mt. Kisco, NY: Futura, 1989.
7. Fischbeck KH, Layzer RB. Paroxysmal choreoathetosis associated with thyrotoxicosis. Ann Neurol 1979; 6:453.
8. Harayama H, Ohno T, Miyatake T. Quantitative analysis of stance in ataxic myxoedema. J Neurol Neurosurg Psychiatry 1983;46:579.
9. Newman RP, Kinkel WR. Paroxysmal choreoathetosis due to hypoglycemia. Arch Neurol 1984;41:341.
10. Rector WG Jr, Herlong HF, Moses H 3rd. Nonketotic hyperglycemia appearing as choreoathetosis or ballism. Arch Intern Med 1982;142:154.
11. Nabatame H, Nakamura K, Matsuda M, et al. Hemichorea in hyperglycemia associated with increased blood flow in the contralateral striatum and thalamus. Intern Med 1994;33:472.
12. Haan J, Kremer HP, Padberg GW. Paroxysmal choreoathetosis as presenting symptom of diabetes mellitus. J Neurol Neurosurg Psychiatry 1989;52:133.
13. Linazasoro G, Urtasun M, Poza JJ, et al. Generalized chorea induced by nonketotic hyperglycemia. Mov Disord 1993;8:119.
14. Hefter H, Mayer P, Benecke R. Persistent chorea after recurrent hypoglycemia. A case report. Eur Neurol 1993;33:244.
15. Lin JJ, Chang MK. Hemiballism-hemichorea and nonketotic hyperglycaemia. J Neurol Neurosurg Psychiatry 1994;57:748.
16. O'Doherty DS CJ. Neurologic aspects of endocrine disturbances. In RI J (ed). Clinical Neurology, Vol. 4. Philadelphia, PA: J.B. Lippincott, 1990.
17. Sachs C, Sjoberg HE, Ericson K. Basal ganglia calcifications on CT: Relation to hypoparathyroidism. Neurology 1982;32:779.
18. Kaminski HJ, Ruff RL. Neurologic complications of endocrine diseases. Neurol Clin 1989;7:489.
19. Salti I, Faris A, Tannir N, et al. Rapid correction by 1-alpha-hydroxycholecalciferol of hemichorea in surgical hypoparathyroidism. J Neurol Neurosurg Psychiatry 1982;45:89.
20. Barabas G, Tucker SM. Idiopathic hypoparathyroidism and paroxysmal dystonic choreoathetosis. Ann Neurol 1988;24:585.
21. Yamamoto K, Kawazawa S. Basal ganglion calcification in paroxysmal dystonic choreoathetosis. Ann Neurol 1987;22:556.
22. Tambyah PA, Ong BK, Lee KO. Reversible parkinsonism and asymptomatic hypocalcemia with basal ganglia calcification from hypoparathyroidism 26 years after thyroid surgery. Am J Med 1993;94:444.
23. Evans BK, Donley DK. Pseudohypoparathyroidism, parkinsonism syndrome, with no basal ganglia calcification. J Neurol Neurosurg Psychiatry 1988;51:709.
24. Factor SA, Coni RJ, Cowger M, et al. Paroxysmal tremor and orofacial dyskinesia secondary to a biopterin synthesis defect. Neurology 1991;41:930.
25. Albers JW, Nostrant TT, Riggs JE. Neurologic manifestations of gastrointestinal disease. Neurol Clin 1989;7:525.
26. Young RR, Shahani BT. Asterixis: One type of negative myoclonus. Adv Neurol 1986;43:137.
27. Rothstein JD, Herlong HF. Neurologic manifestations of hepatic disease. Neurol Clin 1989;7:563.

28. Swaiman KF. Disorders of the basal ganglia. In Swaiman KF (ed). Pediatric Neurology: Principles and Practice. St. Louis, MO: CV Mosby, 1989, p. 819.
29. Thame M, Gray R, Forrester T. Parkinsonian-like tremors in the recovery phase of kwashiorkor. West Indian Med J 1994;43:102.
30. Koller WC, Busenbark K, Gray C, et al. Classification of essential tremor. Clin Neuropharmacol 1992;15:81.
31. Aisen ML, Adelstein BD, Romero J, et al. Peripheral mechanical loading and the mechanism of the tremor of chronic alcoholism. Arch Neurol 1992;49:740.
32. Neiman J, Lang AE, Fornazzari L, et al. Movement disorders in alcoholism: A review. Neurology 1990; 40:741.
33. Carlen PL, Lee MA, Jacob M, et al. Parkinsonism provoked by alcoholism. Ann Neurol 1981;9:84.
34. Shandling M, Carlen PL, Lang AE. Parkinsonism in alcohol withdrawal: A follow-up study. Mov Disord 1990;5:36.
35. Brust A. Neurologic Aspects of Substance Abuse. Stoneham, MA: Butterworth-Heinemann, 1993.
36. Gilman S, Adams K, Koeppe RA, et al. Cerebellar and frontal hypometabolism in alcoholic cerebellar degeneration studied with positron emission tomography. Ann Neurol 1990;28:775.
37. Swaiman KF JR. Developmental abnormalities of the central nervous system. In RI J (ed). Clinical Neurology. Philadelphia, PA: JB Lippincott, 1988.
38. Calne DB, Lang AE. Secondary dystonia. Adv Neurol 1988;50:9.
39. Berardelli A, Thompson PD, Zaccagnini M, et al. Two sisters with generalized dystonia associated with homocystinuria. Mov Disord 1991;6:163.
40. Massey EW, Riggs JE. Neurologic manifestations of hematologic disease. Neurol Clin 1989;7:549.
41. Iriarte LM, Mateu J, Cruz G, et al. Chorea: A new manifestation of mastocytosis. J Neurol Neurosurg Psychiatry 1988;51:1457.
42. Swedo SE, Leonard HL, Schapiro MB, et al. Sydenham's chorea: Physical and psychological symptoms of St Vitus dance. Pediatrics 1993;91:706.
43. Riley DE LA. Movement disorders. In Bradley WG DR, Fenichel GM, Marsden CD (eds). Neurology in Clinical Practice. Vol. 2. Stoneham, UK: Butterworth-Heinemann, 1991, p. 1584.
44. Weindl A, Kuwert T, Leenders KL, et al. Increased striatal glucose consumption in Sydenham's chorea. Mov Disord 1993;8:437.
45. Bronze MS, Dale JB. Epitopes of streptococcal M proteins that evoke antibodies that cross-react with human brain. J Immunol 1993;151:2820.
46. Husby G, van de Rijn I, Zabriskie JB, et al. Antibodies reacting with cytoplasm of subthalamic and caudate nuclei neurons in chorea and acute rheumatic fever. J Exp Med 1976;144:1094.
47. Figueroa F, Berrios X, Gutierrez M, et al. Anticardiolipin antibodies in acute rheumatic fever. J Rheumatol 1992;19:1175.
48. Swedo SE, Leonard HL, Garvey M, et al. Pediatric autoimmune neuropsychiatric disorders associated with streptococcal infections: Clinical description of the first 50 cases. Am J Psychiatry 1998;155:264.
49. Dale RC, Church AJ, Surtees RA, et al. Post-streptococcal autoimmune neuropsychiatric disease presenting as paroxysmal dystonic choreoathetosis. Mov Disord 2002;17:817.
50. Reik L, Steere AC, Bartenhagen NH, et al. Neurologic abnormalities of Lyme disease. Medicine (Baltimore) 1979;58:281.
51. Pachner AR. Early disseminated Lyme disease: Lyme meningitis. Am J Med 1995;98:30S.
52. Magnarelli LA. Current status of laboratory diagnosis for Lyme disease. Am J Med 1995;98:10S.
53. Garcia-Monco JC, Benach JL: Lyme neuroborreliosis. Ann Neurol 1995;37:691.
54. Kieburtz K, Schiffer RB. Neurologic manifestations of human immunodeficiency virus infections. Neurol Clin 1989;7:447.
55. Mirsattari SM, Power C, Nath A. Parkinsonism with HIV infection. Mov Disord 1998;13:684.
56. Koutsilieri E, Sopper S, Scheller C, et al. Parkinsonism in HIV dementia. J Neural Transm 2002;109:767.
57. Hersh BP, Rajendran PR, Battinelli D. Parkinsonism as the presenting manifestation of HIV infection: Improvement on HAART. Neurology 2001;56:278.
58. Sacktor NC, Skolasky RL, Lyles RH, et al. Improvement in HIV-associated motor slowing after antiretroviral therapy including protease inhibitors. J Neurovirol 2000;6:84.
59. Nath A, Hobson DE, Russell A. Movement disorders with cerebral toxoplasmosis and AIDS. Mov Disord 1993;8:107.
60. Singer C, Berger JR, Bowen BC, et al. Akinetic-rigid syndrome in a 13-year-old girl with HIV-related progressive multifocal leukoencephalopathy. Mov Disord 1993;8:113.
61. Maggi P, de Mari M, Moramarco A, et al. Parkinsonism in a patient with AIDS and cerebral opportunistic granulomatous lesions. Neurol Sci 2000;21:173.
62. Mirsattari SM, Berry ME, Holden JK, et al. Paroxysmal dyskinesias in patients with HIV infection. Neurology 1999;52:109.
63. Piccolo I, Causarano R, Sterzi R, et al. Chorea in patients with AIDS. Acta Neurol Scand 1999;100:332.
64. Beskind DL, Keim SM. Choreoathetotic movement disorder in a boy with *Mycoplasma pneumoniae* encephalitis. Ann Emerg Med 1994;23:1375.
65. Thiele EA SM, Siffert JO. Severe choreoathetosis associated with presumed encephalitis: A series of five cases. Ann Neurol 1994;36:541.
66. Weiner SR, Utsinger P. Whipple disease. Semin Arthritis Rheum 1986;15:157.
67. Tison F, Louvet-Giendaj C, Henry P, et al. Permanent bruxism as a manifestation of the oculo-facial syndrome related to systemic Whipple's disease. Mov Disord 1992;7:82.
68. Hausser-Hauw C, Roullet E, Robert R, et al. Oculo-facio-skeletal myorhythmia as a cerebral complication of systemic Whipple's disease. Mov Disord 1988;3:179.
69. Adams M, Rhyner PA, Day J, et al. Whipple's disease confined to the central nervous system. Ann Neurol 1987;21:104.
70. Lee AG. Whipple disease with supranuclear ophthalmoplegia diagnosed by polymerase chain reaction of cerebrospinal fluid. J Neuroophthalmol 2002;22:18.

71. Averbuch-Heller L, Paulson GW, Daroff RB, et al. Whipple's disease mimicking progressive supranuclear palsy: The diagnostic value of eye movement recording. J Neurol Neurosurg Psychiatry 1999;66:532.
72. Whiting S FK, McCormic AQ, Carter JEJ. Retinal and neurologic involvement in the hemolytic uremic syndrome (HUS). Neurology 1985;35:248.
73. Delaney P. Neurologic manifestations in sarcoidosis: Review of the literature, with a report of 23 cases. Ann Intern Med 1977;87:336.
74. Schlegel U, Clarenbach P, Cordt A, et al. Cerebral sarcoidosis presenting as supranuclear gaze palsy with hypokinetic rigid syndrome. Mov Disord 1989;4:274.
75. Jankovic J, Ford J. Blepharospasm and orofacial-cervical dystonia: Clinical and pharmacological findings in 100 patients. Ann Neurol 1983;13:402.
76. Jankovic J. Etiology and differential diagnosis of blepharospasm and oromandibular dystonia. Adv Neurol 1988;49:103.
77. Nutt JG CJ, DeGarmo, Hammerstad JP. Meige syndrome and thyroid dysfunction. Neurology 1984;34:222.
78. Jankovic J, Patten BM. Blepharospasm and autoimmune diseases. Mov Disord 1987;2:159.
79. Alexander EL, Ranzenbach MR, Kumar AJ, et al. Anti-Ro (SS-A) autoantibodies in central nervous system disease associated with Sjögren's syndrome (CNS-SS): Clinical, neuroimaging, and angiographic correlates. Neurology 1994;44:899.
80. Terao Y, Sakai K, Kato S, et al. Antineuronal antibody in Sjögren's syndrome masquerading as paraneoplastic cerebellar degeneration. Lancet 1994;343:790.
81. Nishimura H, Tachibana H, Makiura N, et al. Corticosteroid-responsive parkinsonism associated with primary Sjögren's syndrome. Clin Neurol Neurosurg 1994;96:327.
82. Nakazato Y, Yamanoto T, Tamura N, Shimazu K, Ishii K. Primary Sjogren's syndrome presenting with choreoathetosis. Rinsho Shinkeigaku 2002;42(10):946–948.
83. Venegas FP, Sinning M, Miranda M. Primary Sjogren's syndrome presenting as a generalized chorea. Parkinsonism Relat Disord 2005;11(3):193–194.
84. Coull BM, Levine SR, Brey RL. The role of antiphospholipid antibodies in stroke. Neurol Clin 1992;10:125.
85. Rajagopalan N, Humphrey PR, Bucknall RC. Torticollis and blepharospasm in systemic lupus erythematosus. Mov Disord 1989;4:345.
86. Kirk A, Harding SR. Cardioembolic caudate infarction as a cause of hemichorea in lupus anticoagulant syndrome. Can J Neurol Sci 1993;20:162.
87. Furie R, Ishikawa T, Dhawan V, et al. Alternating hemichorea in primary antiphospholipid syndrome: Evidence for contralateral striatal hypermetabolism. Neurology 1994;44:2197.
88. Burk K, Bosch S, Muller CA, et al. Sporadic cerebellar ataxia associated with gluten sensitivity. Brain 2001;124:1013.
89. Luostarinen LK, Collin PO, Peraaho MJ, et al. Coeliac disease in patients with cerebellar ataxia of unknown origin. Ann Med 2001;33:445.
90. Hadjivassiliou M, Grunewald R, Sharrack B, et al. Gluten ataxia in perspective: Epidemiology, genetic susceptibility and clinical characteristics. Brain 2003;126:685.
91. Bushara KO, Goebel SU, Shill H, et al. Gluten sensitivity in sporadic and hereditary cerebellar ataxia. Ann Neurol 2001;49:540.
92. Donaldson J. Neurology of Pregnancy, 2nd ed. London: WB Saunders, 1989.
93. Posner JB. Paraneoplastic syndromes. Neurol Clin 1991;9:919.
94. Furneaux HM, Rosenblum MK, Dalmau J, et al. Selective expression of Purkinje-cell antigens in tumor tissue from patients with paraneoplastic cerebellar degeneration. N Engl J Med 1990;322:1844.
95. Hetzel DJ, Stanhope CR, O'Neill BP, et al. Gynecologic cancer in patients with subacute cerebellar degeneration predicted by anti-Purkinje cell antibodies and limited in metastatic volume. Mayo Clin Proc 1990;65:1558.
96. Hida C, Tsukamoto T, Awano H, et al. Ultrastructural localization of anti-Purkinje cell antibody-binding sites in paraneoplastic cerebellar degeneration. Arch Neurol 1994;51:555.
97. Gandy SE, Grebb JA, Rosen N, et al. General assay for phosphoproteins in cerebrospinal fluid: A candidate marker for paraneoplastic cerebellar degeneration. Ann Neurol 1990;28:829.
98. Peterson K, Rosenblum MK, Kotanides H, et al. Paraneoplastic cerebellar degeneration. I. A clinical analysis of 55 anti-Yo antibody-positive patients. Neurology 1992;42:1931.
99. Hammack J, Kotanides H, Rosenblum MK, et al. Paraneoplastic cerebellar degeneration. II. Clinical and immunologic findings in 21 patients with Hodgkin's disease. Neurology 1992;42:1938.
100. Graus F, Gultekin SH, Ferrer I, et al. Localization of the neuronal antigen recognized by anti-Tr antibodies from patients with paraneoplastic cerebellar degeneration and Hodgkin's disease in the rat nervous system. Acta Neuropathol (Berl) 1998;96:1.
101. Wirtz PW, Sillevis Smitt PA, Hoff JI, et al. Anti-Ri antibody positive opsoclonus-myoclonus in a male patient with breast carcinoma. J Neurol 2002;249:1710.
102. Pranzatelli MR, Tate ED, Wheeler A, et al. Screening for autoantibodies in children with opsoclonus-myoclonus-ataxia. Pediatr Neurol 2002;27:384.
103. Bataller LDJ. Paraneoplastic neurologic syndromes. Neurol Clin North Am 2003;21:221.
104. Butler MH, Hayashi A, Ohkoshi N, et al. Autoimmunity to gephyrin in stiff-man syndrome. Neuron 2000;26:307.
105. Saiz A, Minguez A, Graus F, et al. Stiff-man syndrome with vacuolar degeneration of anterior horn motor neurons. J Neurol 1999;246:858.
106. Tremont-Lukats IW, Fuller GN, Ribalta T, Giglio P, Groves MD. Paraneoplastic chorea: Case study with autopsy confirmation. Neuro-Oncology 2002;4:192–195.
107. Vernino S, Tuite P, Adler CH, et al. Paraneoplastic chorea associate with CRMP-5 neuronal antibody and Lung carcinoma. Ann Neurol 2002;51:625–630.

INDEX

Note:Page numbers followed by *f* and *t* indicate figures and tables, respectively.

H

N